Essentials of Physical Medicine and Rehabilitation

Musculoskeletal Disorders, Pain, and Rehabilitation

Essentials of Physical Medicine and Rehabilitation

Musculoskeletal Disorders, Pain, and Rehabilitation

THIRD EDITION

Walter R. Frontera, MD, PhD
Professor and Chair (inaugural)
Department of Physical Medicine and Rehabilitation
Vanderbilt University School of Medicine
Medical Director of Rehabilitation Services
Vanderbilt University Medical Center
Nashville, Tennessee
Adjunct Professor
Department of Physiology
University of Puerto Rico School of Medicine
San Juan, Puerto Rico

Julie K. Silver, MD
Associate Professor
Department of Physical Medicine and Rehabilitation
Harvard Medical School
Boston, Massachusetts

Thomas D. Rizzo, Jr., MD
Consultant, Department of Physical Medicine and Rehabilitation
Mayo Clinic
Jacksonville, Florida
Assistant Professor, Physical Medicine and Rehabilitation
Mayo Clinic College of Medicine
Rochester, Minnesota

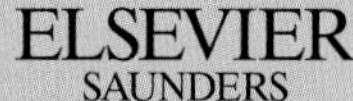

ELSEVIER
SAUNDERS

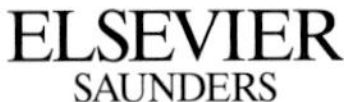

ELSEVIER
SAUNDERS

1600 John F. Kennedy Blvd.
Ste 1800
Philadelphia, PA 19103-2899

ESSENTIALS OF PHYSICAL MEDICINE AND REHABILITATION: MUSCULOSKELETAL DISORDERS, PAIN, AND REHABILITATION ISBN: 978-1-4557-7577-4

Library of Congress Cataloging-in-Publication Data

Essentials of physical medicine and rehabilitation (Frontera)
Essentials of physical medicine and rehabilitation : musculoskeletal disorders, pain, and rehabilitation/edited by] Walter R. Frontera, Julie K. Silver, Thomas D. Rizzo, Jr.—Third edition.
p. ; cm.
Includes bibliographical references and index.
ISBN 978-1-4557-7577-4 (hardcover : alk. paper)
I. Frontera, Walter R., 1955- editor of compilation. II. Silver, J. K. (Julie K.), 1965- editor of compilation. III. Rizzo, Thomas D., 1959- editor of compilation. IV. Title.
[DNLM: 1. Musculoskeletal Diseases–rehabilitation. 2. Pain–rehabilitation. 3. Pain Management. WE 140]
RM700
617′.03—dc23

2014004422

Senior Content Strategist: Don Scholz
Senior Content Development Specialist: Anne Snyder
Publishing Services Manager: Patricia Tannian
Senior Project Manager: Claire Kramer
Designer: Ellen Zanolle

Printed in China

Last digit is the print number: 9 8 7 6 5 4 3 2 1

We dedicate this book to our mentors, teachers, colleagues, and students, who have encouraged us to pursue academic careers with their enthusiasm for knowledge and learning; to our patients, who often are our greatest teachers; and to our families, who support us and provide the foundation for our pursuits.

Walter R. Frontera, MD, PhD
Julie K. Silver, MD
Thomas D. Rizzo, Jr., MD

Contributors

ANTOINNE C. ABLE, MD, MSCI
Associate Professor/Clinical, Physical Medicine and Rehabilitation, Orthopedics and Rehabilitation, Vanderbilt University Medical Center, Nashville, Tennessee
Stroke in Young Adults

SOL M. ABREU SOSA, MD, FAAPMR
Clinica de Medicina Fisica y Electrodiagnostico (CMFE), Auguada, Puerto Rico
Ulnar Collateral Ligament Sprain
Stress Fractures of the Lower Limb

FARSHAD ADIB, MD
Division of Sports Medicine, Boston Children's Hospital, Harvard Medical School, Boston, Massachusetts
Posterior Cruciate Ligament Sprain
Quadriceps Tendinopathy and Tendinitis

MEENA AGARWAL, MD, PhD, MS, Dip Urol, FRCS, FRCS(Urol)
Consultant Urological Surgeon and Senior Lecturer, University Hospital of Wales and Cardiff University, Heath Park, Cardiff, United Kingdom
Neurogenic Bladder
Neurogenic Bowel

MARYAM R. AGHALAR, DO
Cancer Rehabilitation Fellow, Rehabilitation Medicine Service, Memorial Sloan Kettering Cancer Center, New York, New York
Chemotherapy-Induced Peripheral Neuropathy

VENU AKUTHOTA, MD
Professor and Vice Chair, Physical Medicine and Rehabilitation, University of Colorado School of Medicine, Aurora, Colorado
Collateral Ligament Sprain
Iliotibial Band Syndrome
Meniscal Injuries

JOHN D. ALFONSO, MD
Assistant Professor, Department of Rehabilitation Medicine, University of Texas Health Science Center, University Hospital Wound Care Center, San Antonio, Texas
Plexopathy—Brachial
Plexopathy—Lumbosacral

JOSEPH T. ALLEVA, MD, MBA
Division Head, Division of Physical Medicine and Rehabilitation, Department of Medicine, NorthShore University HealthSystem; Clinical Assistant Professor, University of Chicago, Pritzker School of Medicine, Chicago, Illinois
Cervical Sprain or Strain
Piriformis Syndrome
Patellar Tendinopathy (Jumper's Knee)
Patellofemoral Syndrome

ERIC L. ALTSCHULER, MD, PhD
Associate Professor, Department of Physical Medicine and Rehabilitation, Rutgers New Jersey Medical School, Newark, New Jersey
Complex Regional Pain Syndrome
Central Post-Stroke Pain (Thalamic Pain Syndrome)

JOAO E.D. AMADERA, MD, PhD
School of Medicine, University of São Paulo; Director of the Spine Center, Hospital do Coração, São Paulo, Brazil
Low Back Strain or Sprain
Baker Cyst

EDUARDO AMY, MD
Assistant Professor, Physical Medicine, Rehabilitation, and Sports Medicine Department, University of Puerto Rico School of Medicine, San Juan, Puerto Rico
Anterior Cruciate Ligament Tear

ANNA BABUSHKINA, MD
Assistant in Orthopaedic Surgery, Hand Surgery, Massachusetts General Hospital, Boston, Massachusetts
Wrist Osteoarthritis

JOHN R. BACH, MD
Professor and Vice-Chairman, Department of Physical Medicine and Rehabilitation; Professor of Neurosciences, Rutgers New Jersey Medical School, Newark, New Jersey
Pulmonary Rehabilitation for Patients with Lung Disease
Pulmonary Rehabilitation (Neuromuscular)

ALLISON BAILEY, MD
Director and Founder, Integrated Health and Fitness Associates; Instructor, Harvard Medical School, Mount Auburn Hospital, Cambridge, Massachusetts
Pelvic Pain

MOON SUK BANG, MD, PhD
Department of Rehabilitation Medicine, Seoul National University College of Medicine, Seoul, South Korea
Cervical Dystonia
Phantom Limb Pain

ALPESHKUMAR BAVISHI, MD
Pulmonary Fellow, Rutgers New Jersey Medical School, Newark, New Jersey
Pulmonary Rehabilitation for Patients with Lung Disease

WILLIAM J. BECKWORTH, MD
Assistant Professor, Physical Medicine and Rehabilitation and Orthopaedic Surgery, Emory University, Atlanta, Georgia
Intercostal Neuralgia

KEITH A. BENGTSON, MD
Director of Hand Rehabilitation, Physical Medicine and Rehabilitation, Mayo Clinic, Rochester, Minnesota
Trigger Finger

ANDREW R. BERMAN, MD
Associate Professor of Clinical Medicine, Rutgers New Jersey Medical School, Newark, New Jersey
Pulmonary Rehabilitation for Patients with Lung Disease

OMAR M. BHATTI, MD
Clinical Assistant Professor, Department of Rehabilitation Medicine, University of Washington, Seattle, Washington
Hamstring Strain

PETER BIENKOWSKI, MD
Orthopaedic Surgeon, Carlton Sports Medicine Clinic, Carlton University, Ottawa, Ontario, Canada
Posterior Cruciate Ligament Sprain
Quadriceps Tendinopathy and Tendinitis

WILLIAM L. BOCKENEK, MD
Chief Medical Officer, Carolinas Rehabilitation; Chair, Department of Physical Medicine and Rehabilitation, Carolinas Medical Center, Charlotte, North Carolina
Heterotopic Ossification

KATH BOGIE, DPhil
Adjunct Assistant Professor, Department of Orthopaedics and Biomedical Engineering, School of Medicine, Case Western Reserve University; Senior Research Scientist, Advanced Platform Technology Center, Louis Stokes Cleveland Department of Veterans Affairs Medical Center, Cleveland, Ohio
Pressure Ulcers

KRISTIAN BORG, MD, PhD
Department of Rehabilitation Medicine, Karolinska Institutet, Danderyd University Hospital, Stockholm, Sweden
Myopathies

JOANNE BORG-STEIN, MD
Associate Professor of Physical Medicine and Rehabilitation, Harvard Medical School; Director, Harvard/Spaulding Sports Medicine Fellowship, Boston, Massachusetts; Medical Director, Spine Center and Chief of Physical Medicine and Rehabilitation, Newton-Wellesley Hospital, Newton, Massachusetts
Cervicogenic Vertigo
Fibromyalgia

GLENDALIZ BOSQUES, MD
Clinical Assistant Professor, Physical Medicine and Rehabilitation, University of Texas Health Science Center; Chief of Pediatric Rehabilitation Medicine, TIRR Memorial Hermann, Houston, Texas
Neural Tube Defects

JAY E. BOWEN, DO
New Jersey Sports Medicine, LLC, Cedar Knolls, New Jersey; Assistant Professor, Physical Medicine and Rehabilitation, Rutgers New Jersey Medical School, Newark, New Jersey
Rotator Cuff Tendinopathy
Rotator Cuff Tear

JEFFREY S. BRAULT, DO
Physical Medicine and Rehabilitation, Mayo Clinic, Rochester, Minnesota
Extensor Tendon Injuries
Flexor Tendon Injuries

COLONEL STEVEN E. BRAVERMAN, MD
Commander, Walter Reed Army Institute of Research, Silver Spring, Maryland
Ankylosing Spondylitis

DIANE W. BRAZA, MD
Chair, Physical Medicine and Rehabilitation, Medical College of Wisconsin, Milwaukee, Wisconsin
Upper Limb Amputations
Diabetic Foot and Peripheral Arterial Disease

DAVID T. BURKE, MD, MA
Professor and Chairman, Department of Rehabilitation Medicine, Emory University School of Medicine, Atlanta, Georgia
Median Neuropathy (Carpal Tunnel Syndrome)
Traumatic Brain Injury

MABEL CABAN, MD, MS
Physical Medicine and Rehabilitation, University of Texas Southwestern, Dallas, Texas
Lymphedema

ALISON L. CABRERA, MD
Tennessee Orthopaedic Alliance, Clarksville, Tennessee
Total Hip Replacement
Knee Chondral Injuries

JUAN A. CABRERA, MD
Assistant Professor, Department of Physical Medicine and Rehabilitation, Vanderbilt University Medical Center, Nashville, Tennessee
Total Hip Replacement

MARK CAMPBELL, MD, MSc
Assistant Professor, Department of Medicine, Division of Physical Medicine and Rehabilitation, University of Ottawa, Ottawa, Ontario, Canada
Joint Contractures

GREGORY T. CARTER, MD, MS
Medical Director, St. Luke's Rehabilitation Institute, Spokane, Washington; Clinical Professor, Physical Medicine and Rehabilitation, University of California Davis School of Medicine, Sacramento, California; Clinical Faculty, MEDEX, University of Washington School of Medicine, Seattle, Washington
Motor Neuron Disease

CHARLES CASSIDY, MD
Henry H. Banks Associate Professor and Chairman, Orthopaedics, Tufts Medical Center, Boston, Massachusetts
Elbow Arthritis
Olecranon Bursitis
Hand and Wrist Ganglia
Kienböck Disease

DAVID A. CASSIUS, MD
Physiatrist, Seattle, Washington
Costosternal Syndrome

ANDREA CHEVILLE, MD, MSCE
Associate Professor, Physical Medicine and Rehabilitation, Mayo Clinic, Rochester, Minnesota
Cancer-Related Fatigue

KELVIN CHEW, MBBCh, MSpMed
Senior Consultant, Sports Medicine Department, Changi General Hospital, Singapore
Greater Trochanteric Pain Syndrome

MARTIN K. CHILDERS, DO, PhD
Professor, Department of Rehabilitation Medicine, University of Washington, Seattle, Washington
Myofascial Pain Syndrome

SALLAYA CHINRATANALAB, MD
Assistant Professor of Medicine, Division of Rheumatology, Department of Internal Medicine, Vanderbilt University Medical Center, Nashville, Tennessee
Systemic Lupus Erythematosus

CHIEN CHOW, MD
Anesthesia Service Medical Group, San Diego, California
Elbow Arthritis

VICTOR CHUNG, MD
Clinical Associate, Otolaryngology, Head and Neck Surgery, Tufts Medical Center, Boston, Massachusetts
Hand and Wrist Ganglia

DANIEL M. CLINCHOT, MD
Vice Dean for Education, College of Medicine; Associate Professor, Physical Medicine and Rehabilitation, The Ohio State University, Columbus, Ohio
Femoral Neuropathy
Lateral Femoral Cutaneous Neuropathy

RICARDO COLBERG, MD
Primary Care Sports Medicine, American Sports Medicine Institute, Birmingham, Alabama
Hip Adductor Strain

MELISSA COLBERT, MD
Resident Physician, Physical Medicine and Rehabilitation, Harvard Medical School/Spaulding Rehabilitation Hospital, Boston, Massachusetts
Cervicogenic Vertigo
Fibromyalgia

EARL J. CRAIG, MD
Clinical Assistant Professor, Department of Physical Medicine and Rehabilitation; Clinical Assistant Professor, Department of Medicine, Indiana University School of Medicine, Indianapolis, Indiana
Femoral Neuropathy
Lateral Femoral Cutaneous Neuropathy

DI CUI, MD
Department of Rehabilitation Medicine, Emory University School of Medicine, Atlanta, Georgia
Traumatic Brain Injury

CHRISTINE CURTIS, MD
Manhattan Beach, California
Posterior Cruciate Ligament Sprain
Quadriceps Tendinopathy and Tendinitis

CHRISTIAN M. CUSTODIO, MD
Assistant Attending, Rehabilitation Medicine Service, Memorial Sloan Kettering Cancer Center; Assistant Professor, Department of Rehabilitation Medicine, Weill Cornell Medical College, New York, New York
Chemotherapy-Induced Peripheral Neuropathy

ALAN M. DAVIS, MD, PhD
Associate Professor, Physical Medicine and Rehabilitation, University of Utah School of Medicine, Salt Lake City, Utah
Cardiac Rehabilitation

GEORGE W. DEIMEL IV, MD
Department of Physical Medicine and Rehabilitation, Mayo Clinic, Rochester, Minnesota
Ankylosing Spondylitis

DAVID R. DEL TORO, MD
Professor, Physical Medicine and Rehabilitation, Medical College of Wisconsin, Milwaukee, Wisconsin
Tibial Neuropathy (Tarsal Tunnel Syndrome)

MATTHEW M. DIESSELHORST, MD
Southwest Orthopaedic Specialists, Oklahoma City, Oklahoma
Hip Labral Tears

TIMOTHY R. DILLINGHAM, MD, MS
Professor and Chairman, Physical Medicine and Rehabilitation, The University of Pennsylvania, Philadelphia, Pennsylvania
Upper Limb Amputations
Diabetic Foot and Peripheral Arterial Disease

SUSAN J. DREYER, MD
Associate Professor, Physical Medicine and Rehabilitation, Orthopaedic Surgery, Emory University, Atlanta, Georgia
Intercostal Neuralgia

NANCY DUDEK, MD, MEd
Associate Professor, Department of Medicine, Division of Physical Medicine and Rehabilitation, University of Ottawa, Ottawa, Ontario, Canada
Joint Contractures

ISRAEL DUDKIEWICZ, MD
Orthopaedic Surgeon, Consultant in Physical Medicine and Rehabilitation, Tel Aviv, Israel
Cervical Spondylotic Myelopathy
Cervical Degenerative Disease

SHEILA DUGAN, MD
Associate Professor, Physical Medicine and Rehabilitation, Rush Medical College, Chicago, Illinois
Ulnar Collateral Ligament Sprain
Stress Fractures of the Lower Limb

BLESSEN C. EAPEN, MD
Section Chief, Polytrauma Rehabilitation Center, South Texas Veterans Health Care System; Assistant Professor, Department of Rehabilitation Medicine, University of Texas Health Science Center, San Antonio, Texas
Deep Venous Thrombosis

JENNIFER L. EARLE, MD
Physical Medicine and Rehabilitation, Spaulding Rehabilitation Hospital, Harvard Medical School, Boston, Massachusetts
Lumbar Spondylolysis and Spondylolisthesis

GEROLD R. EBENBICHLER, MD
Physical Medicine and Rehabilitation, Vienna Medical University, General Hospital of Vienna, Vienna, Austria
Chronic Fatigue Syndrome

RACHEL EGYHAZI, MD
Clinical Fellow, Pain Medicine, Department of Anesthesiology, Massachusetts General Hospital, Harvard Medical School, Boston, Massachusetts
Cervical Spinal Stenosis

OMAR EL ABD, MD
Assistant Professor, Physical Medicine and Rehabilitation, Harvard Medical School, Boston, Massachusetts
Low Back Strain or Sprain

JEFFREY B. ELIASON, MD
Assistant Professor, Physical Medicine and Rehabilitation Department, Emory University; Veterans Affairs Medical Center, Atlanta, Georgia
Heterotopic Ossification

MAURY ELLENBERG, MD
Clinical Professor, Physical Medicine and Rehabilitation, Wayne State University School of Medicine, Detroit, Michigan
Lumbar Radiculopathy

MICHAEL J. ELLENBERG, MD
Rehabilitation Physicians PC, Novi, Michigan
Lumbar Radiculopathy

JESSE D. ENNIS, MD, FRCP(C)
Physical Medicine and Rehabilitation, Neurorehabilitation Unit, Victoria General Hospital, Victoria, British Columbia, Canada
Spinal Cord Injury (Thoracic)

ERIK ENSRUD, MD
Department of Neurology, Brigham and Women's Hospital, Boston, Massachusetts
Myopathies
Plexopathy—Brachial

STEPHAN M. ESSER, MD
Physical Medicine and Rehabilitation, Heekin Orthopedics, Jacksonville, Florida
Chronic Ankle Instability

AVITAL FAST, MD
Chief, Rehabilitation Medicine, Tel Aviv Sourasky Medical Center, Tel Aviv, Israel; Professor Emeritus, Albert Einstein College of Medicine, Bronx, New York
Cervical Spondylotic Myelopathy
Cervical Degenerative Disease

RICHARD FEENEY, DO
University of California Davis Medical Center, Sacramento, California
Sacroiliac Joint Dysfunction

JEFFERY B. FELDMAN, PhD
Section of Neuropsychology, Department of Neurology; Director, Center for Integrative Medicine; Associate, Translational Science Institute;
Director, Occupational Rehabilitation Programs, Wake Forest University, Winston-Salem, North Carolina
Myofascial Pain Syndrome

JONATHAN T. FINNOFF, DO
Physician, Tahoe Orthopedics and Sports Medicine, South Lake Tahoe, California; Clinical Professor, Department of Physical Medicine and Rehabilitation, University of California Davis School of Medicine, Sacramento, California
Suprascapular Neuropathy
Hip Labral Tears

LESLIE S. FOSTER, DO
Parkway Neuroscience and Spine Institute, Hagerstown, Maryland
Plantar Fasciitis

PATRICK M. FOYE, MD
Interim Chair and Associate Professor, Physical Medicine and Rehabilitation, Rutgers New Jersey Medical School, Newark, New Jersey
Hip Osteoarthritis

MICHAEL FREDERICSON, MD
Professor, Orthopedic Surgery and Physical Medicine and Rehabilitation; Director, Physical Medicine and Rehabilitation Sports Medicine, Stanford University Medical Center, Palo Alto, California
Greater Trochanteric Pain Syndrome

JOEL E. FRONTERA, MD
Assistant Professor, Department of Physical Medicine and Rehabilitation, University of Texas Medical School at Houston (UTHealth), Houston, Texas
Spasticity

WALTER R. FRONTERA, MD, PhD
Professor and Chair (inaugural), Department of Physical Medicine and Rehabilitation, Vanderbilt University School of Medicine; Medical Director of Rehabilitation Services, Vanderbilt University Medical Center, Nashville, Tennessee; Adjunct Professor, Department of Physiology, University of Puerto Rico School of Medicine, San Juan, Puerto Rico

MICHELLE GITTLER, MD
Residency Program Director, Associate Medical Director for Academic Affairs, Schwab Rehabilitation Hospital; Clinical Associate Professor of Surgery, Orthopedic Surgery, and Rehabilitation Medicine, University of Chicago, Chicago, Illinois
Lower Limb Amputations

MEL B. GLENN, MD
Director, Outpatient and Community Brain Injury Rehabilitation, Spaulding Rehabilitation Hospital; Associate Professor, Department of Physical Medicine and Rehabilitation, Harvard Medical School, Boston, Massachusetts; Medical Director, NeuroRestorative-Massachusetts, Braintree, Massachusetts; Medical Director, Community Rehab Care, Newton and Medford, Massachusetts
Postconcussion Symptoms

PETER GONZALEZ, MD
Associate Professor, Department of Physical Medicine and Rehabilitation, Eastern Virginia Medical School, Norfolk, Virginia
Iliotibial Band Syndrome

MARLÍS GONZÁLEZ-FERNÁNDEZ, MD, PhD
Assistant Professor, Physical Medicine and Rehabilitation, Johns Hopkins University School of Medicine; Medical Director Outpatient Clinics, Physical Medicine and Rehabilitation, Johns Hopkins Hospital, Baltimore, Maryland
Cerebral Palsy

THOMAS E. GROOMES, MD
Vanderbilt University Medical Center and Vanderbilt Stallworth Rehabilitation Hospital, Nashville, Tennessee
Total Knee Replacement

DAWN M. GROSSER, MD
Orthopaedic Surgeon, South Texas Bone and Joint, Corpus Christi, Texas
Ankle Arthritis
Bunion and Bunionette
Hallux Rigidus
Posterior Tibial Tendon Dysfunction

H. MICHAEL GUO, MD, PhD
Assistant Professor, Director, Neurorehabilitation Fellowship Program, Section of Physical Medicine and Rehabilitation, Department of Neurology, Wake Forest University School of Medicine, Winston Salem, North Carolina
Myofascial Pain Syndrome

NAVNEET GUPTA, MD
Johnson City, Tennessee
Knee Bursitis

HOPE S. HACKER, MD
Chief, Physical Medicine and Rehabilitation Services, Central Texas Veterans Health Care Systems, Temple, Texas
Plexopathy—Lumbosacral

LORI HALL, PT, MS, CLT-LANA
Physical Medicine and Rehabilitation Department, Parkland Health and Hospital System, Dallas, Texas
Lymphedema

ED HANADA, MD
Assistant Professor, Department of Medicine, Dalhousie University; Staff Physiatrist, Department of Medicine/Division of Physical Medicine and Rehabilitation, Capital District Health Authority, Halifax, Nova Scotia, Canada
Knee Bursitis

TONI J. HANSON, MD
Assistant Professor, Physical Medicine and Rehabilitation, Mayo Clinic, College of Medicine, Rochester, Minnesota
Thoracic Compression Fracture

AMANDA L. HARRINGTON, MD
Assistant Professor, Physical Medicine and Rehabilitation, University of Pittsburgh School of Medicine; Program Director, Spinal Cord Injury Medicine Fellowship, University of Pittsburgh Medical Center; Director of Spinal Cord Injury Services, University of Pittsburgh Medical Center Rehabilitation Institute, Pittsburgh, Pennsylvania
Heterotopic Ossification

DAVID E. HARTIGAN, MD
Department of Orthopedic Surgery, Mayo Clinic, Rochester, Minnesota
Labral Tears of the Shoulder

SETH D. HERMAN, MD
Physiatrist, Brain Injury Rehabilitation Program, Spaulding Rehabilitation Hospital; Associate Program Director, Neurological Rehabilitation Fellowship, Harvard Medical School/Spaulding Rehabilitation Hospital; Instructor, Department of Physical Medicine and Rehabilitation, Harvard Medical School, Boston, Massachusetts
Postconcussion Symptoms

JOSEPH E. HERRERA, DO
Residency Program Director, Rehabilitation Medicine; Fellowship Director, Interventional Spine and Sports Medicine Division, Department of Rehabilitation; Director of Sports Medicine, Icahn School of Medicine at Mount Sinai Department of Rehabilitation Medicine, New York, New York
Compartment Syndrome of the Leg

CHESTER H. HO, MD
Associate Professor and Head, Division of Physical Medicine and Rehabilitation, Department of Clinical Neurosciences and Hotchkiss Brain Institute, University of Calgary, Calgary, Alberta, Canada
Pressure Ulcers

ANNE Z. HOCH, DO
Professor, Department of Orthopedic Surgery, Director, Women's Sports Medicine Program and Fellowship, Medical College of Wisconsin, Milwaukee, Wisconsin
Hamstring Strain

JASON HOLM, MD
Twin Cities Orthopedics, Burnsville, Minnesota
Suprascapular Neuropathy

ALICE J. HON, MD
Department of Physical Medicine and Rehabilitation, Rutgers New Jersey Medical School, Newark, New Jersey
Central Post-Stroke Pain (Thalamic Pain Syndrome)

THOMAS H. HUDGINS, MD
Associate Division Head, Division of Physical Medicine and Rehabilitation, NorthShore University HealthSystem; Assistant Professor, Department of Orthopedics, University of Chicago, Pritzker School of Medicine, Chicago, Illinois
Cervical Sprain or Strain
Piriformis Syndrome
Patellar Tendinopathy (Jumper's Knee)
Patellofemoral Syndrome
Foot and Ankle Bursitis

KATARZYNA IBANEZ, MD
Assistant Attending Physiatrist, Department of Neurology, Rehabilitation Service, Memorial Sloan Kettering Cancer Center; Assistant Professor of Rehabilitation Medicine, Weill Cornell Medical College, New York, New York
Radiation Fibrosis Syndrome

MAHMUD M. IBRAHIM, MD
Fellow, Interventional Spine and Sports Medicine Division, Department of Rehabilitation, Icahn School of Medicine at Mount Sinai Department of Rehabilitation Medicine, New York, New York
Compartment Syndrome of the Leg

MARTA IMAMURA, MD
Affiliated Professor and Chief of Staff, Technical Session, Division of Physical Medicine and Rehabilitation, Department of Orthopaedics and Traumatology; Coordinator, Clinical Research Center at the Institute of Physical and Rehabilitation Medicine, University of São Paulo School of Medicine, São Paulo, Brazil
Costosternal Syndrome
Tietze Syndrome

SATIKO T. IMAMURA, MD
Professor, Division of Rehabilitation Medicine, Clinics Hospital, University of São Paulo School of Medicine, São Paulo, Brazil
Tietze Syndrome

ZACHARIA ISAAC, MD
Director, Interventional Physical Medicine and Rehabilitation, Harvard Medical School; Medical Director, Comprehensive Spine Care Center, Brigham and Women's Hospital, Boston, Massachusetts
Lumbar Spinal Stenosis
Sacroiliac Joint Dysfunction

RATHI L. JOSEPH, DO
Sports Medicine Fellow, Department of Sports Medicine and Family Medicine, Advocate Lutheran General Hospital, Park Ridge, Illinois
Piriformis Syndrome
Patellar Tendinopathy (Jumper's Knee)
Patellofemoral Syndrome
Foot and Ankle Bursitis

SHIVANG JOSHI, MD, MPH, BPharm
Neurologist, New England Regional Headache Center, University of Massachusetts Medical School, Worcester, Massachusetts
Headaches

NANETTE C. JOYCE, DO, MAS
Assistant Professor, Physical Medicine and Rehabilitation, University of California, Davis, Sacramento, California
Motor Neuron Disease

SE HEE JUNG, MD, PhD
Department of Rehabilitation Medicine, Seoul National University Boramae Medical Center, Seoul, South Korea
Phantom Limb Pain

JONATHAN KAY, MD
Professor of Medicine, Director of Clinical Research, Division of Rheumatology, University of Massachusetts Medical School and UMass Memorial Medical Center
Hand Rheumatoid Arthritis

AYAL M. KAYNAN, MD, FACS
Director, Minimally Invasive and Robotic Surgery; Vice-Chairman, Section of Urology, Department of Surgery, Morristown Medical Center, Morristown, New Jersey
Neurogenic Bladder

JOHN C. KEEL, MD
Department of Physical Medicine and Rehabilitation, Harvard Medical School; The Spine Center, New England Baptist Hospital, Boston, Massachusetts
Lumbar Spondylolysis and Spondylolisthesis

ROBERT KENT, DO, MHA, MPH
Pain Spine Sports Physiatry at the Kent Clinic, Orlando, Florida
Temporomandibular Joint Dysfunction
Polytrauma Rehabilitation

FLORIAN S. KEPLINGER, MD
Rehab Medical Associates of Arkansas, Sherwood, Arkansas
Knee Bursitis

STUART KIGNER, DPM
Attending Staff, Podiatry Service, Massachusetts General Hospital; Attending Staff, Podiatry Division, Brigham and Women's Hospital, Boston, Massachusetts
Metatarsalgia

TODD A. KILE, MD
Consultant, Department of Orthopedic Surgery, Mayo Clinic, Scottsdale, Arizona; Assistant Professor, Mayo Clinic College of Medicine, Rochester, Minnesota
Ankle Arthritis
Bunion and Bunionette
Hallux Rigidus
Posterior Tibial Tendon Dysfunction

JOHN C. KING, MD
Professor, Rehabilitation Medicine, University of Texas Health Science Center; Medical Director, Reeves Rehabilitation Center, University Health System, San Antonio, Texas
Peroneal Neuropathy
Plexopathy—Brachial
Plexopathy—Lumbosacral

NEIL KIRSCHBAUM, DO
Physical Medicine and Rehabilitation Residency Program, Morsani College of Medicine, University of South Florida, Tampa, Florida
Polytrauma Rehabilitation

MELISSA A. KLAUSMEYER, MD
Hand Surgery Fellow, Department of Orthopedics, Division of Hand and Upper Extremity, Harvard Medical School, Boston, Massachusetts
Wrist Rheumatoid Arthritis

JASON H. KORTTE, MS, CCC-SLP
Speech-Language Pathologist, Medstar Good Samaritan Hospital; Affiliate Faculty, Loyola University, Baltimore, Maryland
Speech and Language Disorders

BRIAN J. KRABAK, MD, MBA, FACSM
Clinical Associate Professor, Rehabilitation, Orthopedics, and Sports Medicine, University of Washington and Seattle Children's Sports Medicine, Seattle, Washington
Adhesive Capsulitis
Biceps Tendinopathy
Ankle Sprain

GAIL LATLIEF, DO
Physical Medicine and Rehabilitation Service, James A. Haley Veterans' Hospital; Assistant Professor, Department of Neurology, Division of Physical Medicine and Rehabilitation, Morsani College of Medicine, University of South Florida, Tampa, Florida
Polytrauma Rehabilitation

SAMMY M. LEE, DPM
Attending Staff, Podiatry Service, Massachusetts General Hospital, Boston, Massachusetts
Morton Neuroma

SHI-UK LEE, MD, PhD
Department of Rehabilitation Medicine, Seoul National University College of Medicine; Department of Physical Medicine and Rehabilitation, Seoul National University Boramae Medical Center, Seoul, Korea
Cervical Dystonia

TED A. LENNARD, MD
Clinical Assistant Professor, Department of Physical Medicine and Rehabilitation, University of Arkansas for Medical Sciences, Little Rock, Arkansas; Medical Director, WorkComplete CoxHealthCare Systems, Springfield Neurological and Spine Institute, Springfield, Missouri
Cervical Facet Arthropathy
Lumbar Facet Arthropathy

PAUL LENTO, MD
Associate Professor, Physical Medicine and Rehabilitation, Temple University School of Medicine, Philadelphia, Pennsylvania
Collateral Ligament Sprain
Iliotibial Band Syndrome
Meniscal Injuries

JAN LEXELL, MD, PhD
Professor of Rehabilitation Medicine, Department of Health Sciences, Lund University; Medical Director and Consultant Physician, Department of Neurology and Rehabilitation Medicine, Skåne University Hospital in Lund, Lund, Sweden
Postpoliomyelitis Syndrome

PETER A.C. LIM, MD
Clinical Professor, Physical Medicine and Rehabilitation, Baylor College of Medicine, Houston, Texas; Adjunct Associate Professor, Medicine, Duke–National University of Singapore Graduate Medical School; Senior Consultant, Rehabilitation Medicine, Singapore General Hospital, Singapore
Transverse Myelitis

CINDY LIN, MD
Attending Physician, Sports Medicine and Rehabilitation Medicine, Sports Medicine Department, Changi General Hospital, Singapore
Greater Trochanteric Pain Syndrome

KARL-AUGUST LINDGREN, MD, PhD
ORTON Rehabilitation Centre, Helsinki, Finland
Thoracic Outlet Syndrome

VASILIOS A. LIROFONIS, DPM
Attending Staff, Podiatry Service, Massachusetts General Hospital, Boston, Massachusetts
Mallet Toe

ELIZABETH LODER, MD
Chief, Division of Headache and Pain, Department of Neurology, Brigham and Women's Hospital, Boston, Massachusetts
Headaches

EDRICK LOPEZ, MD, JD
Harvard Medical School, Department of Physical Medicine and Rehabilitation, Spaulding Rehabilitation Hospital, Boston, Massachusetts
Lumbar Spinal Stenosis

GERARD A. MALANGA, MD
New Jersey Sports Medicine, LLC, Cedar Knolls, New Jersey; Clinical Professor, Physical Medicine and Rehabilitation, University of Medicine and Dentistry of New Jersey–New Jersey Medical School, Newark, New Jersey
Rotator Cuff Tendinopathy
Rotator Cuff Tear

JULIE MARTIN, PT
Lead Outpatient Physical Therapist, James A. Haley Veterans' Hospital, Tampa, Florida
Temporomandibular Joint Dysfunction

RAFAEL MASCARINAS, MD
Attending Physician, Physical Medicine and Rehabilitation Service, James A. Haley Veterans' Hospital; Assistant Professor, Department of Neurology, Division of Physical Medicine and Rehabilitation, Morsani College of Medicine, University of South Florida, Tampa, Florida
Polytrauma Rehabilitation

JILL MASSENGALE, MS, ARNP
Physical Medicine and Rehabilitation Service, James A. Haley Veterans' Hospital, Tampa, Florida
Temporomandibular Joint Dysfunction
Polytrauma Rehabilitation

KOICHIRO MATSUO, DDS, PhD
Professor, Department of Dentistry, School of Medicine, Fujita Health University, Aichi, Japan
Dysphagia

MARISSA McCARTHY, MD
Assistant Professor, Department of Neurology, Division of Physical Medicine and Rehabilitation, Morsani College of Medicine, University of South Florida; Medical Director, Traumatic Brain Injury/Polytrauma Unit, James A. Haley Veterans' Hospital, Tampa, Florida
Temporomandibular Joint Dysfunction
Polytrauma Rehabilitation

KELLY C. McINNIS, DO
Instructor, Physical Medicine and Rehabilitation, Harvard Medical School; Clinical Associate, Physical Medicine and Rehabilitation, Massachusetts General Hospital, Boston, Massachusetts
Repetitive Strain Injuries

PETER M. McINTOSH, MD
Assistant Professor, College of Medicine, Mayo Clinic, Rochester, Minnesota; Consultant, Department of Physical Medicine and Rehabilitation, Mayo Clinic, Jacksonville, Florida
Scapular Winging
Adhesive Capsulitis of the Hip

ALEC L. MELEGER, MD
Assistant Professor of Physical Medicine and Rehabilitation, Harvard Medical School, Boston, Massachusetts; Medical Director, Spaulding Outpatient Center, Medford, Massachusetts
Cervical Spinal Stenosis

BRYAN MERRITT, MD
Physical Medicine and Rehabilitation Service, James A. Haley Veterans' Hospital; Assistant Professor, Department of Neurology, Division of Physical Medicine and Rehabilitation, Morsani College of Medicine, University of South Florida, Tampa, Florida
Polytrauma Rehabilitation

LYLE J. MICHELI, MD
Program Director, Sports Medicine, Harvard University, Boston, Massachusetts
Posterior Cruciate Ligament Sprain
Quadriceps Tendinopathy and Tendinitis

WILLIAM MICHEO, MD
Professor and Chairman, Physical Medicine and Rehabilitation and Sports Medicine Department; Sports Medicine Program Director, University of Puerto Rico, San Juan, Puerto Rico
Glenohumeral Instability
Anterior Cruciate Ligament Tear

MATTHEW E. MILLER, MD
Captain, United States Army Medical Corps; Residency Associate Program Director and Staff Physiatrist, Physical Medicine and Rehabilitation, Walter Reed National Military Medical Center, Bethesda, Maryland
Plantar Fasciitis

GERARDO MIRANDA, MD
Assistant Professor, Physical Medicine and Rehabilitation and Sports Medicine, San Juan, Puerto Rico
Glenohumeral Instability

NATHAN MOHR, BA
Pre-medical Student, University of Northern Iowa, Cedar Falls, Iowa
Cervical Sprain or Strain

DANIEL P. MONTERO, MD
Mayo Clinic Florida, Jacksonville, Florida
Hammer Toe

S. JIT MOOKERJEE, DO
Physical Medicine and Rehabilitation Service, James A. Haley Veterans' Hospital; Assistant Professor, Department of Neurology, Division of Physical Medicine and Rehabilitation, Morsani College of Medicine, University of South Florida, Tampa, Florida
Polytrauma Rehabilitation

ALI MOSTOUFI, MD, FAAPMR, FAAPM
Assistant Professor, Physical Medicine and Rehabilitation, Tufts University; Medical Director, Boston Spine Center, Boston, Massachusetts
Cervical Radiculopathy
Chronic Pain Syndrome

CHAITANYA S. MUDGAL, MD, MS (Orth), MCh (Orth)
Chief and Director, Hand Fellowship Program, Orthopaedic Hand Service, Massachusetts General Hospital, Boston, Massachusetts
Wrist Osteoarthritis
Wrist Rheumatoid Arthritis

LARRY V. NAJERA III, MD
Schwab Rehabilitation Hospital, Chicago, Illinois; Pain Treatment Centers of Illinois, Orland Park, Illinois
Cervical Sprain or Strain

SHANKER NESATHURAI, MD, MPH, FRCP(C)
Professor of Medicine and Division Director of Physical Medicine and Rehabilitation, Michael G. DeGroote School of Medicine, McMaster University; Chief of Physical Medicine and Rehabilitation, Hamilton Health Sciences and St. Joseph's Healthcare, Hamilton, Ontario, Canada; Lecturer in Physical Medicine and Rehabilitation, Harvard Medical School, Spaulding Hospital, Boston, Massachusetts
Spinal Cord Injury (Thoracic)

JESS NORDIN, DO
Resident, Johns Hopkins Department of Physical Medicine and Rehabilitation, Baltimore, Maryland
Neural Tube Defects

CARINA J. O'NEILL, DO
Physical Medicine and Rehabilitation, Spaulding Rehabilitation, Braintree, Massachusetts; Clinical Instructor, Physical Medicine and Rehabilitation, Harvard Medical School, Boston, Massachusetts
de Quervain Tenosynovitis

ANDREA K. ORIGENES
Pre-medical Student, University of Illinois, Chicago, Illinois
Cervical Sprain or Strain

CEDRIC J. ORTIGUERA, MD
Consultant, Department of Orthopedics, Mayo Clinic, Jacksonville, Florida; Assistant Professor, Mayo Clinic, College of Medicine, Rochester, Minnesota
Labral Tears of the Shoulder

MICHAEL D. OSBORNE, MD
Assistant Professor, Physical Medicine and Rehabilitation, Mayo Clinic, Jacksonville, Florida
Chronic Ankle Instability
Arachnoiditis

JEFFREY B. PALMER, MD
Lawrence Cardinal Shehan Professor and Chair, Department of Physical Medicine and Rehabilitation; Professor, Physical Medicine and Rehabilitation, Otolaryngology–Head and Neck Surgery, and Functional Anatomy and Evolution; Johns Hopkins University; Physiatrist-in-Chief, Department of Physical Medicine and Rehabilitation, Johns Hopkins Hospital; Chair, Department of Physical Medicine and Rehabilitation, Medstar Good Samaritan Hospital, Baltimore, Maryland
Dysphagia
Speech and Language Disorders

PAUL F. PASQUINA, MD
United States Army Medical Corps (Colonel Ret.); Residency Director and Chair, Physical Medicine and Rehabilitation, Uniformed Services University of the Health Sciences, Walter Reed National Military Medical Center, Bethesda, Maryland
Plantar Fasciitis

ATUL T. PATEL, MD, MHSA
Kansas City Bone and Joint Clinic, Overland Park, Kansas; Medical Director of Adult Program, Rehabilitation Institute of Kansas City; Adjunct Associate Professor, Physical Therapy, University of Kansas Medical Center, Kansas City, Kansas
Trapezius Strain
Pubalgia

JOSEMARIA PATERNO, MD
Fellow, Interventional Pain, Brigham and Women's Hospital, Harvard Medical School, Boston, Massachusetts
Trigeminal Neuralgia

INDER PERKASH, MD, FRCS, FACS
Professor of Urology (emeritus), Paralyzed Veterans of America Professor of Spinal Cord Injury Medicine (emeritus), Professor of Medicine (Gastrointestinal) and Physical Medicine and Rehabilitation, Stanford University, Stanford, California
Neurogenic Bladder
Neurogenic Bowel

EDWARD M. PHILLIPS, MD
Assistant Professor of Physical Medicine and Rehabilitation; Director and Founder, Institute of Lifestyle Medicine, Joslin Diabetes Center, Harvard Medical School; Adjunct Scientist, United States Department of Agriculture, Jean Mayer Human Nutrition Research Center on Aging, Tufts University, Boston, Massachusetts
Knee Osteoarthritis
Osteoarthritis

DANIEL C. PIMENTEL, MD
Interventional Physiatrist, Director of Spine Center HCor; Assistant Professor, University of São Paolo, School of Medicine, São Paulo, Brazil
Thoracic Radiculopathy
Thoracic Sprain or Strain

THOMAS E. POBRE, MD
Director of Outpatient Services, Physical Medicine and Rehabilitation, Nassau University Medical Center, East Meadow, New York
Radial Neuropathy

REBECCA POSTHUMA, MD
Clinical Research Fellow, Female Pelvic and Reconstructive Surgery, Massachusetts General Hospital, Boston, Massachusetts
Pelvic Pain

ALISON R. PUTNAM, DO
Department of Physical Medicine and Rehabilitation, Virginia Mason Medical Center, Seattle, Washington
Iliotibial Band Syndrome

JAMES RAINVILLE, MD
Assistant Clinical Professor, Physical Medicine and Rehabilitation, Harvard Medical School; Chief, Physical Medicine and Rehabilitation, Orthopedics, New England Baptist Hospital, Boston, Massachusetts
Lumbar Spondylolysis and Spondylolisthesis

V.S. RAMACHANDRAN, MD, PhD
Professor, Department of Psychology, University of California, San Diego, California
Complex Regional Pain Syndrome

DAVID RING, MD, PhD
Associate Professor of Orthopaedic Surgery, Harvard Medical School, Chief of Hand Surgery, Massachusetts General Hospital, Boston, Massachusetts
Hand Osteoarthritis
Hand Rheumatoid Arthritis

JUSTIN RIUTTA, MD, FAAPMR
Department of Physical Medicine and Rehabilitation, William Beaumont Hospital, Royal Oak, Michigan
Post-Mastectomy Pain Syndrome
Post-Thoracotomy Pain Syndrome

ALEXANDRA RIVERA-VEGA, MD
Assistant Professor, Department of Physical Medicine and Rehabilitation at University of Arkansas for Medical Sciences, Little Rock, Arkansas
Glenohumeral Instability

THOMAS D. RIZZO, JR., MD
Consultant, Department of Physical Medicine and Rehabilitation, Mayo Clinic, Jacksonville, Florida; Assistant Professor, Physical Medicine and Rehabilitation, Mayo Clinic College of Medicine, Rochester, Minnesota
Acromioclavicular Injuries

DARREN ROSENBERG, DO
Assistant Professor, Physical Medicine and Rehabilitation, Harvard Medical School, Boston, Massachusetts
Thoracic Radiculopathy
Thoracic Sprain or Strain
Baker Cyst

SEWARD B. RUTKOVE, MD
Professor, Neurology, Harvard Medical School/Beth Israel Deaconess Medical Center, Boston, Massachusetts
Peripheral Neuropathies

SUNIL SABHARWAL, MD
Assistant Professor, Department of Physical Medicine and Rehabilitation, Harvard Medical School; Chief, Spinal Cord Injury, Veterans Affairs Boston Health Care System, Boston, Massachusetts
Spinal Cord Injury (Cervical)
Spinal Cord Injury (Lumbosacral)

FRANCISCO H. SANTIAGO, MD
Attending Physician, Physical Medicine and Rehabilitation, Bronx-Lebanon Hospital, Bronx, New York
Median Neuropathy
Ulnar Neuropathy (Wrist)

ROBERT J. SCARDINA, DPM
Chief, Podiatry Service; Residency Program Director, Podiatry Service, Massachusetts General Hospital; Instructor in Orthopaedic Surgery, Harvard Medical School, Boston, Massachusetts
Mallet Toe
Metatarsalgia
Morton Neuroma

MICHAEL K. SCHAUFELE, MD
Pain Solutions Treatment Centers, Marietta, Georgia
Lumbar Degenerative Disease

JEFFREY C. SCHNEIDER, MD
Medical Director, Trauma, Burn, and Orthopedic Program, Spaulding Rehabilitation Hospital; Assistant Professor, Physical Medicine and Rehabilitation, Harvard Medical School, Boston, Massachusetts
Burns

STEVEN SCOTT, DO
Assistant Professor, Department of Neurology, Division of Physical Medicine and Rehabilitation; Chief, Physical Medicine and Rehabilitation, University of South Florida, Tampa, Florida
Temporomandibular Joint Dysfunction
Polytrauma Rehabilitation

MICHAEL SEIN, MD
Department of Anesthesiology, University of California, San Diego, San Diego, California
Knee Osteoarthritis

FERNANDO SEPÚLVEDA, MD
Chief Resident, Physical Medicine and Rehabilitation Residency Training Program, University of Puerto Rico School of Medicine, San Juan, Puerto Rico
Anterior Cruciate Ligament Tear

JOHN SERGENT, MD
Professor of Medicine, Division of Rheumatology, Department of Internal Medicine, Vanderbilt University Medical Center, Nashville, Tennessee
Systemic Lupus Erythematosus

VIVEK M. SHAH, MD
Clinical Instructor in Orthopaedic Surgery, New England Baptist Hospital, Longwood Orthopedic Associates, Inc., Chestnut Hill, Massachusetts
Kienböck Disease

NUTAN SHARMA, MD, PhD
Associate Professor, Neurology, Harvard Medical School; Associate Neurologist, Massachusetts General Hospital; Associate Neurologist, Brigham and Women's Hospital, Boston, Massachusetts
Parkinson Disease

HUMA SHEIKH, MD
Clinical Instructor, Brigham and Women's Hospital–Neurology, Harvard Medical School, Boston, Massachusetts
Headaches

SARAH SHUBERT, MD
Falmouth Orthopaedic Center, Falmouth, Maine
Olecranon Bursitis

IMRAN J. SIDDIQUI, MD
Department of Physical Medicine and Rehabilitation, Spaulding Rehabilitation Hospital, Harvard Medical School, Boston, Massachusetts
Lumbar Spondylolysis and Spondylolisthesis

JULIE K. SILVER, MD
Associate Professor, Department of Physical Medicine and Rehabilitation, Harvard Medical School, Boston, Massachusetts
Trigger Finger

KENNETH H. SILVER, MD
Department of Physical Medicine and Rehabilitation, Johns Hopkins University School of Medicine; Medstar Good Samaritan Hospital, Baltimore, Maryland
Movement Disorders

ANEESH SINGLA, MD, MPH
Physician, National Spine and Pain Centers; Medical Director, Rockville, Maryland; Lecturer, Harvard Medical School, Boston, Massachusetts
Occipital Neuralgia
Trigeminal Neuralgia

MICHAEL SLESINSKI, DO
Instructor, Department of Physical Medicine and Rehabilitation, Michigan State University–College of Osteopathic Medicine, East Lansing, Michigan
Quadriceps Contusion

DAVID M. SLOVIK, MD
Associate Professor of Medicine, Harvard Medical School, Boston, Massachusetts; Chief, Division of Endocrinology, Newton-Wellesley Hospital, Newton, Massachusetts; Physician, Endocrine Unit, Massachusetts General Hospital, Boston, Massachusetts
Osteoporosis

KURT SPINDLER, MD
Vanderbilt Orthopaedic Institute, Nashville, Tennessee
Knee Chondral Injuries

JOSEPH STANDLEY, DO
Physical Medicine and Rehabilitation Service, James A. Haley Veterans' Hospital, Tampa, Florida
Polytrauma Rehabilitation

JOEL STEIN, MD
Simon Baruch Professor and Chair, Rehabilitation and Regenerative Medicine, Columbia University College of Physicians and Surgeons; Professor and Chief, Division of Rehabilitation Medicine, Weill Cornell Medical College; Physiatrist-in-Chief, New York–Presbyterian Hospital, New York, New York
Stroke

SONJA K. STILP, MD
Boulder, Colorado
Iliotibial Band Syndrome

TODD P. STITIK, MD
Professor, Physical Medicine and Rehabilitation; Director, Occupational/Musculoskeletal Medicine, Rutgers New Jersey Medical School, Newark, New Jersey
Hip Osteoarthritis

MICHAEL F. STRETANSKI, DO
Medical Director/Fellowship Director, Interventional Spine and Pain Rehabilitation Center, Mansfield, Ohio; Spine and Pain Services Director, Wyandot Memorial Hospital, Upper Sandusky, Ohio; Full Professor, Rehabilitation Medicine, Pain Medicine, Ohio University College of Osteopathic Medicine, Columbus, Ohio
Biceps Tendon Rupture
Shoulder Arthritis
Dupuytren Contracture
Shin Splints
Achilles Tendinopathy

MICHAEL D. STUBBLEFIELD, MD
Associate Attending Physiatrist and Chief, Rehabilitation Service, Department of Neurology, Memorial Sloan Kettering Cancer Center; Associate Professor of Rehabilitation Medicine, Weill Cornell Medical College, New York, New York
Radiation Fibrosis Syndrome

JORDAN L. TATE, MD, MPH
Physical Medicine and Rehabilitation, Emory University, Atlanta, Georgia
Lumbar Degenerative Disease

MAYA THERATTIL, MD
Assistant Professor, Clinical Rehabilitation Medicine, Albert Einstein College of Medicine, Bronx, New York
Scoliosis and Kyphosis

ANN-MARIE THOMAS, MD, PT
Assistant Professor, Physical Medicine and Rehabilitation, Harvard Medical School; Staff Physiatrist, Physical Medicine and Rehabilitation, Spaulding Rehabilitation Hospital; Clinical Associate, Physical Medicine and Rehabilitation, Massachusetts General Hospital; Associate Physiatrist in Medicine, Brigham and Women's Hospital, Boston, Massachusetts
Multiple Sclerosis

MARK A. THOMAS, MD
Associate Professor, Physical Medicine and Rehabilitation, Albert Einstein College of Medicine; Program Director, Physical Medicine and Rehabilitation, Montefiore Medical Center, Bronx, New York
Scoliosis and Kyphosis

JIAXIN TRAN, MD
Rutgers New Jersey Medical School, Newark, New Jersey
Complex Regional Pain Syndrome

GUY TRUDEL, MD, MSc, FRCPC, DABPMR
Professor of Medicine, Surgery, and Biochemistry, Faculty of Medicine, University of Ottawa, Ottawa, Ontario, Canada
Joint Contractures

TONY URBISCI, BS
Morsani College of Medicine, University of South Florida, Tampa, Florida
Temporomandibular Joint Dysfunction

SATHYA VADIVELU, DO
Fellow, Pediatric Rehabilitation Medicine, Kennedy Krieger Institute, Physical Medicine and Rehabilitation, Johns Hopkins University, Baltimore, Maryland
Cerebral Palsy

RAMON VALLARINO, JR., MD
Attending Physician, Department of Neurosciences, New York Methodist Hospital, Brooklyn, New York; Clinical Assistant Professor, Department of Physical Medicine and Rehabilitation, Albert Einstein College of Medicine of Yeshiva University, Bronx, New York
Median Neuropathy
Ulnar Neuropathy (Wrist)

MONICA VERDUZCO-GUTIERREZ, MD
Assistant Professor, Department of Physical Medicine and Rehabilitation, University of Texas Medical School at Houston (UTHealth), Houston, Texas
Spasticity

ARIANA VORA, MD
Instructor, Physical Medicine and Rehabilitation, Harvard Medical School; Staff Physiatrist, Massachusetts General Hospital; Staff Physiatrist, Spaulding Rehabilitation Hospital, Boston, Massachusetts
Coccydynia
Postherpetic Neuralgia

ADAM WALLACE, MD
Pain Management of Tulsa, Tulsa, Oklahoma
Arachnoiditis

BETH M. WEINMAN, DO
Sports Medicine Fellow, Department of Orthopedic Surgery, Medical College of Wisconsin, Milwaukee, Wisconsin
Hamstring Strain

JAY M. WEISS, MD
Medical Director, Long Island Physical Medicine and Rehabilitation, Jericho, New York
Lateral Epicondylitis
Medial Epicondylitis
Ulnar Neuropathy (Elbow)

LYN D. WEISS, MD
Chairman and Program Director, Physical Medicine and Rehabilitation, Nassau University Medical Center, East Meadow, New York
Lateral Epicondylitis
Medial Epicondylitis
Radial Neuropathy
Ulnar Neuropathy (Elbow)

DAVID WEXLER, MD, FRCS (Tr & Orth)
Orthopaedic Surgeon, Center for Joint Replacement, St. Mary's Regional Medical Center, Lewiston, Maine
Ankle Arthritis
Bunion and Bunionette
Hallux Rigidus
Posterior Tibial Tendon Dysfunction

JANE WIERBICKY, RN, BSN
National Spinal Cord Injury Association, Gloucester, Massachusetts
Spinal Cord Injury (Thoracic)

J. MICHAEL WIETING, DO, MEd, FAOCPMR, FAAPMR
Interim Dean; Associate Dean, Clinical Medicine; and Assistant Vice President, New Program Development, DeBusk College of Medicine/Division of Health Sciences; Professor of Physical Medicine and Rehabilitation; Professor of Osteopathic Manipulative Medicine, Lincoln Memorial University–DeBusk College of Osteopathic Medicine, Harrogate, Tennessee
Quadriceps Contusion

ALLEN N. WILKINS, MD
Assistant Professor of Clinical Rehabilitation and Regenerative Medicine, Weill Cornell Medical College; Associate Medical Director, Manhattan Physical Medicine and Rehabilitation, LLP, New York, New York
Knee Osteoarthritis
Osteoarthritis

FAREN H. WILLIAMS, MD, MS
Chief and Clinical Professor, Physical Medicine and Rehabilitation Division, Department of Physical Rehabilitation and Orthopedics, University of Massachusetts Medical School, Worcester, Massachusetts
Rheumatoid Arthritis

AMY X. YIN, MD
Resident Physician, Physical Medicine and Rehabilitation, Harvard Medical School/Spaulding Rehabilitation Hospital, Boston, Massachusetts
Coccydynia
Postherpetic Neuralgia
Burns
Osteoarthritis

MARK YOUNG, MD
Massachusetts General Hospital, Boston, Massachusetts
Occipital Neuralgia

MEIJUAN ZHAO, MD
Instructor, Physical Medicine and Rehabilitation, Harvard Medical School; Staff Physiatrist, Spaulding Rehabilitation Hospital, Massachusetts General Hospital, Boston, Massachusetts
Median Neuropathy (Carpal Tunnel Syndrome)

Preface

When the first edition of this work was created, we wanted to publish a book that covered a variety of medical conditions that any physiatrist, internist, family physician, orthopedist, rheumatologist, or neurologist could encounter in his or her medical practice. We particularly wanted to emphasize the clinical aspects of both musculoskeletal injuries and chronic medical conditions requiring rehabilitation from the perspective of a practitioner in an ambulatory setting. In the second edition we maintained the structure of the book and added an entirely new section on the ambulatory management of pain conditions.

This, the third edition of *Essentials of Physical Medicine and Rehabilitation,* again covers many diagnoses in a deliberately succinct and specific format. The first section contains 94 chapters on specific musculoskeletal diagnoses, conveniently organized by anatomic region. The second section describes the management of pain conditions in 23 specific conditions. The third section covers 45 common medical conditions that are typically chronic and benefit from long-term rehabilitative interventions. Although some of these conditions require hospitalization, we have tried to focus on the rehabilitation that takes place in an ambulatory setting. The content of the third edition includes new topics such as labral tears (shoulder and hip) and conditions associated with cancer and its treatment. Each chapter includes the same sections in the same order (Synonyms, ICD-9 Codes, new ICD-10 Codes, Definition, Symptoms, Physical Examination, Functional Limitations, Diagnostic Studies, Differential Diagnosis, Treatment [Initial, Rehabilitation, Procedures, and Surgery], Potential Disease Complications, Potential Treatment Complications, and References). In this edition we are including both the ICD-9 and ICD-10 codes. The new ICD-10 codes allow for greater specificity in describing a patient's diagnosis, and we hope that they will help busy clinicians in their practices.

It is our hope that physicians in all specialties and allied health care providers will find that this book complements the excellent existing rehabilitation textbooks and that it will be an efficient and useful reference tool in the office setting.

We are extremely grateful for the hard work of our colleagues who authored these chapters and who represent many different specialties and come from excellent institutions. Their generous support of our work has made this book possible.

Finally, we would like to thank our editorial team at Elsevier. Their assistance was invaluable in bringing this book to publication. Anne Snyder, our senior content development specialist, deserves special recognition for her commitment to this project.

Walter R. Frontera, MD, PhD
Julie K. Silver, MD
Thomas D. Rizzo, Jr., MD

Contents

PART 1
MUSCULOSKELETAL DISORDERS

PART 1

MUSCULOSKELETAL DISORDERS

SECTION I

Head, Neck, and Upper Back

CHAPTER 1

Cervical Spondylotic Myelopathy

Avital Fast, MD

Israel Dudkiewicz, MD

Synonyms

Cervical radiculitis
Degeneration of cervical intervertebral disc
Cervical spondylosis without myelopathy
Cervical pain

ICD-9 Codes

721.0 Cervical spondylosis without myelopathy
722.4 Degeneration of cervical intervertebral disc
723.3 Cervical pain
723.4 Cervical radiculitis

ICD-10 Codes

M47.812 Cervical spondylosis without myelopathy or radiculopathy
M48.02 Spinal stenosis in cervical region
M48.03 Spinal stenosis in cervicothoracic region
M50.30 Degeneration of cervical disc
M50.32 Degeneration of mid-cervical region
M50.33 Degeneration of cervicothoracic region
M54.2 Cervical pain
M54.12 Cervical radiculitis
M54.13 Cervicothoracic radiculitis

Definition

Cervical spondylotic myelopathy (CSM) is a frequently encountered entity in middle-aged and elderly patients. The condition affects both men and women. Progressive degeneration of the cervical spine involves the discs, facet joints, joints of Luschka, ligamenta flava, and laminae, leading to gradual encroachment on the spinal canal and spinal cord compromise. CSM has a fairly typical clinical presentation and, frequently, a progressive and disabling course.

As a consequence of aging, the spinal column goes through a cascade of degenerative changes that tend to affect selective regions of the spine. The cervical spine is affected in most adults, most frequently at the C4-C7 region [1,2]. Degeneration of the intervertebral discs triggers a cascade of biochemical and biomechanical changes, leading to decreased disc height, among other changes. As a result, abnormal load distribution in the motion segments causes cervical spondylosis (i.e., facet arthropathy) and neural foraminal narrowing. Disc degeneration also leads to the development of herniations (soft discs), disc calcification, posteriorly directed bone ridges (hard discs), hypertrophy of the facets and the uncinate joints, and ligamenta flava thickening. On occasion, more frequently in Asians but not infrequently in white individuals, the posterior longitudinal ligament and the ligamenta flava ossify [3]. These degenerative changes narrow the dimensions and change the shape of the cervical spinal canal. In normal adults, the anteroposterior diameter of the subaxial cervical spinal canal measures 17 to 18mm, whereas the spinal cord diameter in the same dimension is about 10mm. Severe CSM gradually decreases the space available for the cord and brings about cord compression in the anterior-posterior axis. Cord compression usually occurs at the discal levels [4–6].

The encroaching structures may also compress the anterior spinal artery, resulting in spinal cord ischemia that usually involves several cord segments beyond the actual compression site. Spinal cord changes in the form of demyelination, gliosis, myelomalacia, and eventually severe atrophy may develop [4,7–9]. Dynamic instability, which can be diagnosed in flexion or extension lateral x-ray views, further complicates matters. Disc degeneration leads to laxity of the supporting ligaments, bringing about anterolisthesis or retrolisthesis in flexion and extension, respectively. This may further compromise the spinal cord and intensify the presenting symptoms [2,4].

Symptoms

CSM develops gradually during a lengthy period of months to years. Not infrequently, the patient is unaware of any functional compromise, and the first person to notice that something is amiss may be a close family member. Whereas pain appears rather early in cervical radiculopathy and alerts the patient to the presence of a problem, this is usually not the case in CSM. A long history of neck discomfort and intermittent pain may frequently be obtained, but these are not prominent at the time of CSM presentation.

Most patients have a combination of upper motor neuron symptoms in the lower extremities and lower motor neuron symptoms in the upper extremities [4]. Patients frequently present with gait dysfunction resulting from a combination of factors, including ataxia due to impaired joint proprioception, hypertonicity, weakness, and muscle control deficiencies.

Studies have demonstrated that severely myelopathic patients display abnormalities of deep sensation, including vibration and joint position sense, which is attributed to compression of the posterior columns [10,11]. Paresthesias and numbness may be frequently mentioned. Compression of the pyramidal and extrapyramidal tracts can lead to spasticity, weakness, and abnormal muscle contractions. These sensory and motor deficits result in an unstable gait. Patients may complain of stiffness in the lower extremities or plain weakness manifesting as foot dragging and tripping [5]. Symptoms related to the upper extremities are mostly the result of fine motor coordination deficits. At times, the symptoms in the upper extremities are much more severe than those related to the lower extremities, attesting to central cord compromise [4]. Most patients do not have urinary symptoms. However, urinary symptoms (i.e., incontinence) may occasionally develop in patients with long-standing myelopathy [12]. As CSM develops in middle-aged and elderly patients, the urinary symptoms may be attributed to aging, comorbidities, and cord compression. Bowel incontinence is rare.

Physical Examination

Because of sensory ataxia, the patient may be observed walking with a wide-based gait. Some resort to a cane to increase the base of support and to enhance safety during ambulation. Patients with severe gait dysfunction frequently require a walker and cannot ambulate without one. Many patients lose the ability to tandem walk. The Romberg test result may become positive. Examination of the lower extremities may reveal muscle atrophy, increased muscle tone, abnormal reflexes—clonus or upgoing toes (Babinski sign), and abnormalities of position and vibration sense. Muscle fasciculations may be observed. The foot tapping test (number of sole tappings while the heel maintains contact with the floor in 10 seconds) is an easy and useful quantitative tool for lower extremity function in these patients [13].

In the upper extremities, weakness and atrophy of the small muscles of the hands may be noted. The patient may have difficulties in fine motor coordination (e.g., unbuttoning the shirt or picking a coin off the table). The patient frequently displays difficulty in performing repetitive opening and closing of the fist. In normal individuals, 20 to 30 repetitions can be performed in 10 seconds.

Weakness can occasionally be documented in more proximal muscles and may appear symmetrically. Fasciculations may appear in the wasted muscles. Hypesthesia, paresthesia, or anesthesia may be documented. On occasion, the sensory findings in the hands are in a glove distribution. As in the lower extremities, the vibration and joint position senses may be disturbed. Hyporeflexia or hyperreflexia may be found. The Hoffmann response may become positive and can be facilitated in early myelopathy by cervical extension [14]. In some patients, severe atrophy of all the hand intrinsic muscles is observed [1,5,15,16].

The neck range of motion may be limited in all directions. Many patients cannot extend the neck beyond neutral and may feel electric-like sensation radiating down the torso on neck flexion, known as the Lhermitte sign. Often, when a patient stands against the wall, the back of the head stays an inch to several inches away, and the patient is unable to push the head backward to bring it to touch the wall.

Functional Limitations

Patients with CSM have difficulties with activities of daily living. Patients may have difficulties inserting keys, picking up coins, buttoning a shirt, or manipulating small objects. Handwriting may deteriorate. Patients may drop things from the hands and occasionally can complain of numbness affecting the fingers or the palms, mimicking peripheral neuropathy [2,5,15,17,18]. They may have problems dressing and undressing. When weakness is a predominant feature, they will be unable to carry heavy objects. Unassisted ambulation may become difficult. The gait is slowed and becomes inefficient. In late stages of CSM, patients may become almost totally disabled and require assistance with most activities of daily living.

Diagnostic Studies

Plain radiographs usually reveal multilevel degenerative disc disease with cervical spondylosis. Dynamic studies (flexion and extension views) may reveal segmental instability with anterolisthesis on flexion and retrolisthesis on extension. In patients with ossification of the posterior longitudinal ligament, the ossified ligament may be detected on lateral plain films. The Torg-Pavlov ratio may help diagnose congenital spinal stenosis. This ratio can be obtained on plain films by dividing the anteroposterior diameter of the vertebral body by the anteroposterior diameter of the spinal canal at that level. The canal diameter can be measured from the posterior wall of the vertebra to the spinolaminar line [19]. A ratio of 0.8 and below is indicative of spinal stenosis (Fig. 1.1) [20].

Magnetic resonance imaging, the study of choice, provides critical information about the extent of stenosis and the condition of the compressed spinal cord. Sagittal and axial cuts clearly show the offending structures (discs, thickened ligamenta flava), and the cord shape and signal provide critical information about the extent of cord compression and the prognosis (Fig. 1.2). Increased cord signal on T2-weighted images is abnormal and points to the presence of edema, demyelination, myelomalacia, or gliosis. Decreased cord signal on T1-weighted images may also be observed. However, these cord signal changes are of limited value in predicting functional outcome. A newer magnetic resonance imaging technique, diffusion tensor imaging of the cervical cord, holds considerable promise in predicting the severity of cord injury and may help guide the clinician in deciding whether to operate because it may show cord abnormalities before the development of T2 hyperintensity on conventional sequences [21,22]. Severe cord atrophy denotes a poor prognosis even when decompressive surgery is performed.

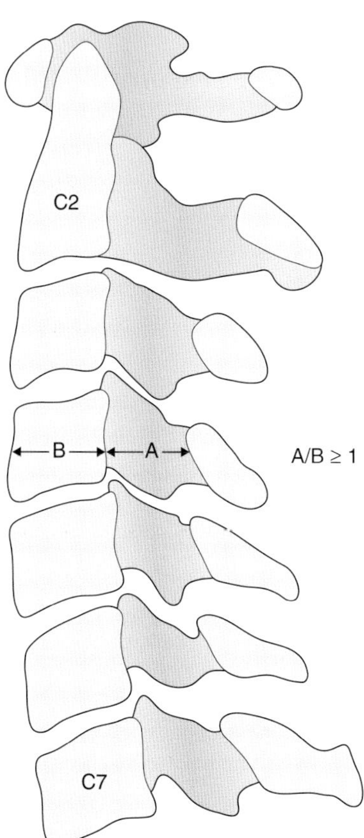

FIGURE 1.1 Schematic lateral view of the cervical spine. The canal diameter (*A*) can be measured by drawing a line between the posterior border of the vertebral body and the spinolaminar line. The vertebral diameter is reflected by line *B*. *(From Fast A, Goldsher D. Navigating the Adult Spine. New York, Demos Medical Publishing, 2007.)*

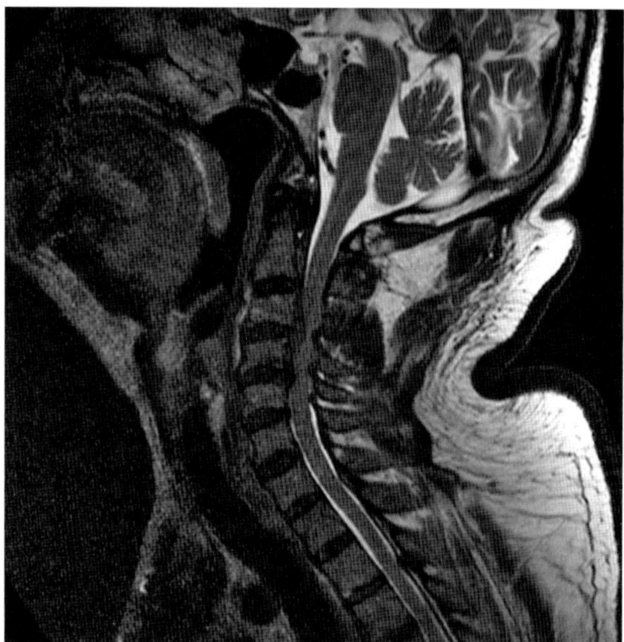

FIGURE 1.2 Sagittal T2-weighted image of the cervical spine showing degenerative disc disease involving the C4-5 and C5-6 intervertebral discs.

Computed tomographic myelography provides fine and detailed information on the amount and location of neural compression and is frequently obtained before surgery. Electrodiagnostic studies play an important role, especially in diabetic patients with peripheral neuropathy, which may confound the clinical diagnosis.

Differential Diagnosis

Amyotrophic lateral sclerosis
Multifocal motor neuropathy [23]
Multiple sclerosis
Syringomyelia
Peripheral neuropathy

Treatment

Initial

The treatment of CSM depends on the stage in which it is discovered. No conservative treatment can be expected to decompress the spinal cord. In the initial stages, education of the patient is of paramount importance. The patient is instructed to avoid cervical spinal hyperextension. As the cervical spinal canal diameter decreases and the spinal cord diameter increases during cervical hyperextension, this position may lead to further cord compression [24]. The patient is advised to drink with a straw and to avoid prolonged overhead activities.

Rehabilitation

Because the course of CSM may be unpredictable and a significant percentage of patients deteriorate in a slow stepwise course, close monitoring of the patient's neurologic condition and spine is indicated. Patients with mild CSM may be managed conservatively. A biannual detailed neurologic examination and an annual magnetic resonance imaging evaluation are indicated. Special attention should be devoted to the cord cross-sectional area and the cord signal; these are important prognostic factors and may help determine whether surgery is indicated. In the interim, patients should be instructed in *static* neck exercises. Weak muscles in the upper or lower extremities should be strengthened with progressive resistance exercise techniques. Judicial use of anti-inflammatory medications is called for, especially in elderly individuals. Soft cervical collars are frequently used (recommended by physicians or obtained by patients without the physician's recommendations) without a sound scientific basis. Assistive devices, such as a cane or walker, should be provided when ambulation safety is compromised.

Procedures

No existing procedures affect the course or symptoms of cervical myelopathy.

Surgery

Patients with moderate to severe progressive CSM (unsteady gait, limited function in the upper extremities) who have significant cord compression or cord signal changes should be referred for decompressive surgery. Two main approaches exist—anterior and posterior.

Anterior Approach

The anterior approach is usually reserved for patients with myelopathy affecting up to three spinal levels. This approach allows adequate decompression of "anterior" disease. Anterior disease refers to pathologic changes that are anterior to the spinal cord (e.g., soft disc, hard disc, vertebral body spurs, and ossified posterior longitudinal ligament). Through this approach, the offending structures can be removed without disturbing the spinal cord. The anterior approach allows adequate decompression in patients with cervical kyphotic deformity. After anterior decompression (anterior cervical decompression and fusion, corpectomies), bone grafting and instrumentation ensure stabilization and fusion. This approach is not indicated in patients whose predominant pathologic process is posterior to the cord (i.e., hypertrophied ligamentum flavum) or in patients with disease affecting more than three or four segments because this may lead to an increased rate of complications, including pseudarthrosis [6,16].

Posterior Approach

The posterior approach consists of two basic procedures, laminectomy and laminoplasty.

Cervical laminectomy can be easily performed by most spinal surgeons and is less technically demanding than anterior corpectomies are. This approach allows easy access to posterior disease, such as hypertrophied laminae and ligamenta flava. The main disadvantage of the laminectomy procedure is that it requires stripping of the paraspinal muscles and thus tends to destabilize the cervical spine. This may result in loss of the cervical lordosis or frank kyphotic deformity and instability (stepladder deformity), especially when it is performed over several spinal levels or when the facet joints have to be sacrificed.

Laminoplasty, another procedure performed through the posterior approach, has been developed in Japan and addresses some of the shortcomings of laminectomy. Unlike laminectomy, cervical laminoplasty preserves the cervical facets and the laminae. In this procedure, the laminae are hinged away (lifted by an osteotomy) from the site of main pathologic change, resulting in an increase of sagittal canal diameter [25]. Unilateral or bilateral hinges can be performed; the bilateral hinge approach allows symmetric expansion of the spinal canal. It is hoped that after posterior decompression, the spinal cord will "migrate" away from the anterior pathologic process, and thus cord decompression will be achieved [16,26]. This has been confirmed in magnetic resonance imaging studies after laminoplasty.

Regardless of the surgical approach, poor outcome and higher complication rate can be expected in elderly patients with long-standing myelopathy and spinal cord atrophy [27].

Potential Disease Complications

Left untreated, a patient with progressive myelopathy may develop severe disability. Patients may become totally dependent and nonambulatory. In some cases, neurogenic bladder may develop and further compromise the quality of life.

Potential Treatment Complications

Pseudarthrosis, restenosis, spinal instability, postoperative radiculopathy, kyphotic deformity, and axial pain are among the surgical complications [14].

References

[1] Heller J. The syndromes of degenerative cervical disease. Orthop Clin North Am 1992;23:381–94.
[2] Bernhardt M, Hynes RA, Blume HW, White III AA. Cervical spondylotic myelopathy. J Bone Joint Surg Am 1993;75:119–28.
[3] Yu YL, Leong JCY, Fang D, et al. Cervical myelopathy due to ossification of the posterior longitudinal ligament. A clinical, radiological and evoked potentials study in six Chinese patients. Brain 1988;111:769–83.
[4] Rao R. Neck pain, cervical radiculopathy, and cervical myelopathy. Pathophysiology, natural history, and clinical evaluation. J Bone Joint Surg Am 2002;84:1872–81.
[5] Law MD, Bernhardt M, White III AA. Evaluation and management of cervical spondylotic myelopathy. Instr Course Lect 1995;44:99–110.
[6] Truumees E, Herkowitz HN. Cervical spondylotic myelopathy and radiculopathy. Instr Course Lect 2000;49:339–60.
[7] Taylor AR. Vascular factors in the myelopathy associated with cervical spondylosis. Neurology 1964;14:62–8.
[8] Breig A, Turnbull I, Hassler O. Effects of mechanical stresses on the spinal cord in cervical spondylosis. J Neurosurg 1966;25:45–56.
[9] Doppman JL. The mechanism of ischemia in anteroposterior compression of the spinal cord. Invest Radiol 1975;10:543–51.
[10] Takayama H, Muratsu H, Doita M, et al. Impaired joint proprioception in patients with cervical myelopathy. Spine (Phila Pa 1976) 2004;30:83–6.
[11] Okuda T, Ochi M, Tanaka N, et al. Knee joint position sense in compressive myelopathy. Spine (Phila Pa 1976) 2006;31:459–62.
[12] Misawa T, Kamimura M, Kinoshita T, et al. Neurogenic bladder in patients with cervical compressive myelopathy. J Spinal Disord Tech 2005;18:315–20.

[13] Numasawa T, Ono A, Wada K, et al. Simple foot tapping test as a quantitative objective assessment of cervical myelopathy. Spine (Phila Pa 1976) 2012;37:108–13.
[14] Denno JJ, Meadows GR. Early diagnosis of cervical spondylotic myelopathy. A useful clinical sign. Spine (Phila Pa 1976) 1991;16:1353–5.
[15] Dillin WH, Watkins RG. Cervical myelopathy and cervical radiculopathy. Semin Spine Surg 1989;1:200–8.
[16] Edwards CC, Riew D, Anderson PA, et al. Cervical myelopathy: current diagnostic and treatment strategies. Spine J 2003;3:68–81.
[17] Ono K, Ebara S, Fiji T, et al. Myelopathy hand. New clinical signs of cervical cord damage. J Bone Joint Surg Br 1987;69:215–9.
[18] Ebara S, Yonenobu K, Fujiwara K, et al. Myelopathy hand characterized by muscle wasting. A different type of myelopathy hand in patients with cervical spondylosis. Spine (Phila Pa 1976) 1988;13:785–91.
[19] Pavlov H, Torg JS, Robie B, Jahre C. Cervical spinal stenosis: determination with vertebral body ratio method. Radiology 1987;164:171–5.
[20] Lebl DR, Hughes A, Cammisa FP, et al. Cervical spondylotic myelopathy: pathophysiology, clinical presentation, and treatment. Eur Spine J 2011;7:170–8.
[21] Kara B, Celik A, Karadereler S, et al. The role of DTI in early detection of cervical spondylotic myelopathy: a preliminary study with 3-T MRI. Neuroradiology 2011;53:609–16.
[22] Rajasekaran S, Kanna RM, Shetty AP. Diffusion tensor imaging of the spinal cord and its clinical applications. J Bone Joint Surg Br 2012;94:1024–31.
[23] Olney RK, Lewis RA, Putnam TD, Campellone Jr JV. Consensus criteria for the diagnosis of multifocal motor neuropathy. Muscle Nerve 2003;27:117–21.
[24] Lauryssen C, Riew KD, Wang JC. Severe cervical stenosis: operative treatment or continued conservative care. SpineLine 2006;January/February;1–25.
[25] Hirabayashi K, Watanabe K, Wakano K, et al. Expansive open-door laminoplasty for cervical spinal stenotic myelopathy. Spine (Phila Pa 1976) 1983;8:693–9.
[26] Aita I, Hayashi K, Wadano T, Yabuki T. Posterior movement and enlargement of the spinal cord after cervical laminoplasty. J Bone Joint Surg Br 1998;80:33–7.
[27] Fehlings M, Smith JS, Kopjar B, et al. Perioperative and delayed complications associated with surgical treatment of cervical spondylotic myelopathy based patients from the AOSpine North America Cervical Spondylotic Myelopathy study. J Neurosurg Spine 2012;16:425–32.

CHAPTER 2

Cervical Facet Arthropathy

Ted A. Lennard, MD

Synonyms

Facet joint arthritis
Apophyseal joint pain
Spondylosis
Z-joint pain
Zygapophyseal joint pain
Posterior element disorder

ICD-9 Codes

715.1 **Osteoarthrosis, localized, primary**
715.2 **Osteoarthrosis, localized, secondary**
719.4 **Pain in joint**
721.0 **Cervical spondylosis without myelopathy**
723.1 **Cervicalgia**
723.3 **Cervicobrachial syndrome**
723.9 **Unspecified musculoskeletal disorders and symptoms referable to neck**
847.0 **Neck: atlanto-occipital (joints), atlantoaxial (joints), whiplash injury**

ICD-10 Codes

M43.02 **Cervical spondylosis**
M54.2 **Cervicalgia**
S13.4 **Neck: Sprain of atlanto-axial (joints), sprain of atlanto-occipital (joints), whiplash injury**

Definition

Cervical facet joints are located in the posterior portion of the cervical spine (Fig. 2.1). These paired synovial joints allow mobility and provide stability to the head and neck. Each of these joints is innervated by the medial branch of the posterior primary ramus [1–3]. Cervical facet arthropathy refers to any acquired, degenerative, or traumatic process that affects the normal function of the facet joints in the cervical region, often resulting in a source of neck pain and cervicogenic headaches. It may be a primary source of pain (e.g., after a whiplash injury) but often is secondary to a degenerative or injured cervical disc, fracture, or ligamentous injury. Common causes of cervical facet pain include acceleration-deceleration cervical injuries (whiplash), a sudden torque motion to the head and neck with extension and rotation, and a cervical compression force. In some cases, simply looking upward may cause facet pain. The cervical facet joints may also become painful in conjunction with a cervical disc herniation, after a cervical discectomy or fusion, or after a cervical compression fracture.

Cervical facet arthrosis appears to increase with age and occurs more commonly in the upper cervical spine. In cadaveric studies, the prevalence of cervical arthrosis was greatest for the C4-C5 level, followed by the C3-C4 level [4]. The C6-C7 level was least involved. Abnormal findings within the cervical facet joints appear to be independent of race and gender [5].

Symptoms

Patients typically complain of generalized posterior neck and suboccipital pain but may present with localized tenderness over the posterolateral aspect of the neck. Pain provoked with cervical extension and axial rotation is common. These joints may refer pain anywhere from the midthoracic spine to the cranium and often in the suboccipital region [6–8]. Neurologic symptoms, such as sensory complaints and muscle weakness in the upper limbs, are not expected in patients with primary cervical facet pain. Concomitant nerve root or cord injury is more likely if these symptoms are present.

Physical Examination

The essential element of the examination is manual palpation of the spinal segments and elicitation of reproducible pain over the involved joints [9]. Localized point tenderness over the cervical paraspinal muscles is common and is precipitated by excessive cervical lordosis, causing abnormal joint forces. The fluidity of motion of the involved spinal area–cervical region may suggest extension pain with relief on flexion. Patients may present with loss of cervical motion

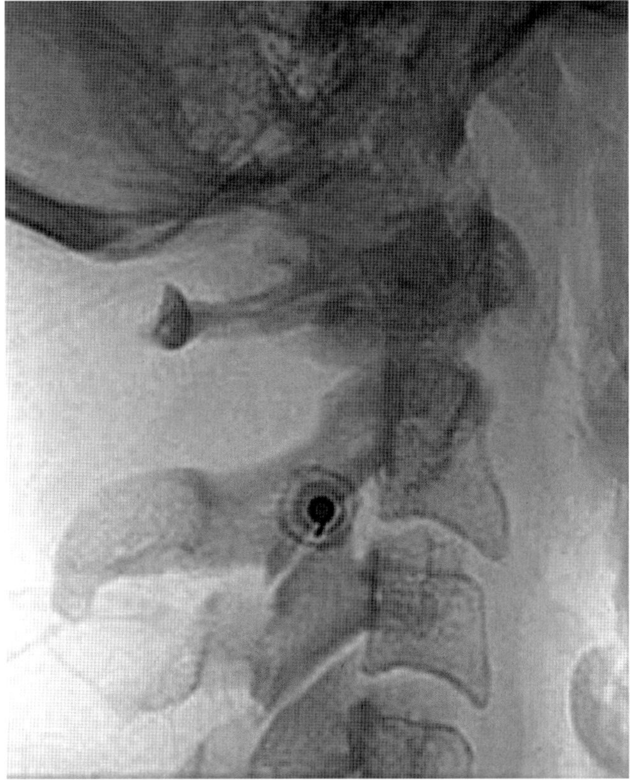

FIGURE 2.1 Lateral fluoroscopic view of the right C2-3 zygapophyseal joint with the needle tip inside the joint. *(From Dreyfuss P, Kaplan M, Dreyer SJ. Zygapophyseal joint injection techniques in the spinal axis. In Lennard TA, ed. Pain Procedures in Clinical Practice, 3rd ed. Philadelphia, Elsevier/Saunders, 2011: 373.)*

and paraspinal spasms. Unless cervical disc or nerve root disease is also present, the findings of the neurologic examination are otherwise typically normal.

Functional Limitations

Cervical extension and rotation, overhead lifting, and overhead reaching may be difficult when the cervical spine is involved. This may interfere with activities such as bathing, grooming, and driving.

Diagnostic Studies

Fluoroscopically guided intra-articular arthrography confirmed that anesthetic injections are the "gold standard" for diagnosis (Fig. 2.2) [10–13]. Abnormalities detected on radiography, computed tomography, or magnetic resonance imaging have not been shown to correlate with facet joint pain. A single-photon emission computed tomographic scan can be used in refractory cases of suspected cervical facet disorders to rule out underlying bone processes that may mimic facet pain (e.g., spondylolysis, infection, tumor) [14]. When an abnormality is detected, the scan may confirm the proposed diagnosis and determine which specific joint is affected.

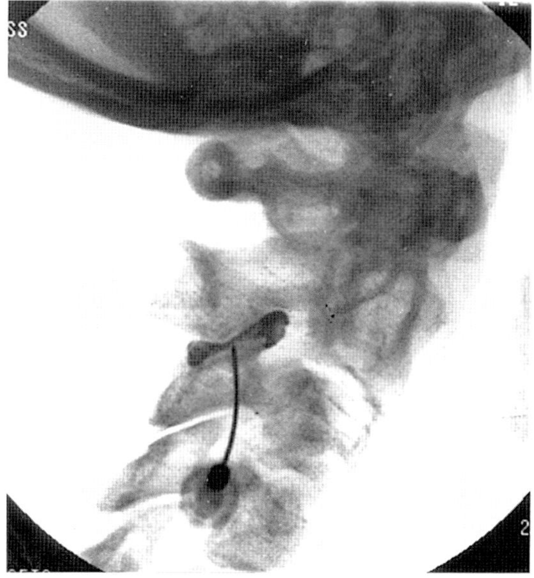

FIGURE 2.2 Lateral radiograph of a C2-3 Z-joint arthrogram by a lateral approach. *(From Dreyfuss P, Kaplan M, Dreyer SJ. Zygapophyseal join injection techniques in the spinal axis. In Lennard TA, ed. Pain Procedures in Clinical Practice, 2nd ed. Philadelphia, Hanley & Belfus, 2000:291.)*

Differential Diagnosis

Degenerative disc disease
Myofascial pain syndrome
Internal disc disruption
Disc herniation
Cervical stenosis
Nerve root compression
Spondylolysis, spondylolisthesis
Osteoid osteoma
Tumor
Infection

Treatment

Initial

Initial treatment emphasizes local pain control with ice, stretching, nonsteroidal anti-inflammatory drugs and oral analgesics, topical creams, transcutaneous electrical nerve stimulation, local periarticular corticosteroid injections, and avoidance of exacerbating activities [15]. Specialized pillows may be helpful, but rarely are cervical collars indicated.

Rehabilitation

Manual forms of therapy (e.g., myofascial release, muscle energy, soft tissue mobilization, and strain-counterstrain techniques) and low-velocity manipulations (e.g., osteopathic manipulation) are commonly used for isolated facet disorders, but their effectiveness has been questioned [16,17]. In healthy patients with no associated spinal disease (e.g., disc abnormalities, stenosis, radiculopathy, fracture), low-velocity manipulations may be used on a limited basis in cases unresponsive to routine conservative care [18–20]. Use in the cervical region should be approached with extreme caution and performed only by experienced practitioners.

Physical therapy may consist of passive modalities such as electrical stimulation, ultrasound, and traction to reduce local pain. However, these modalities have not been shown to change long-term outcomes [18–21]. Regional manual therapy with facet gapping techniques can be helpful. Advancement into a flexion-biased exercise program with regional stretching is the mainstay of rehabilitation. Cervical exercises include both static and dynamic resisted forward and lateral flexion movements. Following cervical facet injections, passive modalities, stretching, and exercises can be useful to reduce pain and to maximize functional recovery. For recurrent episodes of pain, a change in daily and work activity or in sporting technique and other biomechanical adjustments may eliminate the underlying forces at the joint level.

Procedures

Intra-articular, fluoroscopically guided, contrast-enhanced facet injections are considered critical for proper diagnosis and can be instrumental in the treatment of facet joint arthropathies [22,23]. Ultrasound guidance for facet injections is gaining in popularity [24,25]. A patient can be examined both before and after injection to determine what portion of his or her pain can be attributed to the joints injected. Typically, small amounts of anesthetic or corticosteroid are injected directly into the joint. Another step may be to perform medial branch blocks of the affected joints with small volumes (0.1 to 0.3 mL) of anesthetic. If the facet joint is found to be the putative source of pain, a denervation procedure by use of radiofrequency, cryotherapy, or chemicals (e.g., phenol) may be considered [26,27]. Acupuncture may also be considered [28].

Surgery

Surgery is rarely necessary in isolated facet joint arthropathies. Surgical spinal fusion may be performed for discogenic pain, which may affect secondary cases of facet joint arthropathies.

Potential Disease Complications

Because facet joint arthropathy is usually degenerative in nature, this disorder is often progressive, resulting in chronic, intractable spinal pain. It usually coexists with spinal disc abnormalities, further leading to chronic pain. This subsequently results in diminished spinal motion, weakness, and loss of flexibility.

Potential Treatment Complications

Treatment-related complications may be caused by medications; analgesics may cause constipation or liver dysfunction, and nonsteroidal anti-inflammatory drugs may cause gastrointestinal and renal problems. Local periarticular injections and acupuncture may cause local transient needle pain. Facet injections may cause transient local spinal pain, swelling, and possibly bruising. More serious injection complications may include infection, injury to a blood vessel or nerve, injury to the spinal cord, and allergic reaction to the medications [13]. Fortunately, major complications are rare [29]. Exacerbation of symptoms often transiently occurs after injection. Cervical injections may also precipitate headaches.

References

[1] Lee KE, Davis MB, Mejilla RM, et al. In vivo cervical facet capsule distraction: mechanical implications for whiplash and neck pain. Stapp Car Crash J 2004;48:373–95.
[2] Ebraheim NA, Patil V, Liu J, et al. Morphometric analyses of the cervical superior facets and implications for facet dislocation. Int Orthop 2008;32:97–101.
[3] Zhou HY, Chen AM, Guo FJ, et al. Sensory and sympathetic innervation of cervical facet joint in rats. Chin J Traumatol 2006;9:377–80.
[4] Lee MJ, Riew KD. The prevalence of cervical facet arthrosis: an osseous study in a cadaveric population. Spine J 2009;9:711–4.
[5] Master DL, Toy JO, Eubanks JD, Ahn NU. Cervical endplate and facet arthrosis: an anatomic study of cadaveric specimens. J Spinal Disord Tech 2012;25:379–82.
[6] Bogduk N, Marsland A. The cervical zygapophyseal joints as a source of neck pain. Spine (Phila Pa 1976) 1988;13:610–7.
[7] Dwyer A, Aprill C, Bogduk N. Cervical zygapophyseal joint pain patterns. I: a study in normal volunteers. Spine (Phila Pa 1976) 1990;15:453–7.
[8] Fukui S, Ohseto K, Shiotani M. Referred pain distribution of the cervical zygapophyseal joints and cervical dorsal rami. Pain 1996;68:79–83.
[9] King W, Lau P, Lees R, et al. The validity of manual examination in assessing patients with neck pain. Spine J 2007;7:22–6.
[10] Bogduk N. International spinal injection society guidelines for the performance of spinal injection procedures. Part I. Zygapophysial joint blocks. Clin J Pain 1997;13:285–302.
[11] Hechelhammer L, Pfirrmann CW, Zanetti M, et al. Imaging findings predicting the outcome of cervical facet joint blocks. Eur Radiol 2007;17:959–64.
[12] Kim KH, Choi SH, Kim TK, et al. Cervical facet joint injections in the neck and shoulder pain. J Korean Med Sci 2005;20:659–62.
[13] Heckmann JG, Maihofner C, Lanz S, et al. Transient tetraplegia after cervical facet joint injection for chronic neck pain administered without imaging guidance. Clin Neurol Neurosurg 2006;108:709–11.
[14] Pneumaticos SG, Chatziioannou SN, Hipp JA, et al. Low back pain: prediction of short-term outcomes of facet joint injection with bone scintigraphy. Radiology 2006;238:693–8.
[15] Mazanec D, Reddy A. Medical management of cervical spondylosis. Neurosurgery 2007;60(Suppl 1):S43–50.
[16] Bronfort G, Haas M, Evans R, et al. Effectiveness of manual therapies: the UK evidence report. Chiropr Osteopat 2010;18:3.
[17] Patel KC, Gross A, Graham N, et al. Massage for mechanical neck disorders. Cochrane Database Syst Rev 2012;9: CD004871.
[18] Bronfort G, Haas M, Evans RL, Bouter LM. Efficacy of spinal manipulation and mobilization for low back pain and neck pain: a systematic review and best evidence synthesis. Spine J 2004;4:335–56.
[19] Bronfort G, Evans R, Nelson B, et al. A randomized clinical trial of exercise and spinal manipulation for patients with chronic neck pain. Spine (Phila Pa 1976) 2001;26:788–97.
[20] Jordan A, Bendix T, Nielsen H, et al. Intensive training, physiotherapy, or manipulation for patients with chronic neck pain. A prospective, single-blinded, randomized clinical trial. Spine (Phila Pa 1976) 1998;23:311–8.
[21] Skargren EI, Oberg BE, Carlsson PG, Gade M. Cost and effectiveness analysis of chiropractic and physiotherapy treatment for low back and neck pain. Six month follow up. Spine (Phila Pa 1976) 1997;22:2167–77.
[22] Park SC, Kim KH. Effect of adding cervical facet joint injections in a multimodal treatment program for long-standing cervical myofascial pain syndrome with referral pain patterns of cervical facet joint syndromes. J Anesth 2012;5:738–45.
[23] Falco FJ, Datta S, Manchikanti L. An updated review of the diagnostic utility of cervical facet joint injections. Pain Physician 2012;15:807–38.
[24] Galiano K, Obwegeser AA, Bodner G, et al. Ultrasound guidance for facet joint injections in the lumbar spine: a computed feasibility study. Anesth Analg 2005;101:579–83.
[25] Loizides A, Obernauer J, Peer S, et al. Ultrasound-guided injections in the middle and lower cervical spine. Med Ultrason 2012;3:235–8.

[26] Manchikanti L, Damron K, Cash K. Therapeutic cervical medial branch blocks in managing chronic neck pain: a preliminary report of a randomized, double-blind, controlled trial. Pain Physician 2006;9:333–46.
[27] Boswell MV. Therapeutic cervical medial branch blocks: a changing paradigm in interventional pain management. Pain Physician 2006;9:279–81.
[28] Cherkin DC, Sherman KJ, Deyo RA, et al. A review of the evidence for the effectiveness, safety, and cost of acupuncture, massage therapy, and spinal manipulation for back pain. Ann Intern Med 2003;138:898–906.
[29] Manchikanti L, Malla Y, Wargo BW, et al. Complications of fluoroscopically directed facet joint nerve blocks: a prospective evaluation of 7,500 episodes with 43,000 nerve blocks. Pain Physician 2012;15:143–50.

CHAPTER 3

Cervical Degenerative Disease

Avital Fast, MD
Israel Dudkiewicz, MD

Synonyms

Spinal stenosis of cervical region
Intervertebral disc disorder with myelopathy
Cervical spondylosis with myelopathy

ICD-9 Codes

721.0 **Cervical spondylosis without myelopathy**
721.1 **Cervical spondylosis with myelopathy**
722.7 **Intervertebral disc disorder with myelopathy**
723.3 **Cervical pain**
722.4 **Degeneration of cervical intervertebral disc**
723.0 **Spinal stenosis of cervical region**

ICD-10 Codes

M47.12 **Cervical spondylosis with myelopathy**
M47.13 **Cervicothoracic spondylosis with myelopathy**
M48.02 **Spinal stenosis of cervical region**
M48.03 **Spinal stenosis of cervicothoracic region**
M50.00 **Intervertebral disc disorder with myelopathy, cervical region**
M50.03 **Intervertebral disc disorder with myelopathy, cervicothoracic region**
M50.30 **Degeneration of cervical disc**
M50.33 **Degeneration of cervicothoracic region**
M50.32 **Degeneration of mid-cervical region**
M54.2 **Cervical Pain**

Definition

The term *cervical degenerative disease* encompasses a wide range of pathologic changes affecting all the components of the cervical spine that may lead to axial or radicular pain.

The mechanisms underlying cervical degenerative disease are complex and multifactorial. Genetics, aging, and attrition and trauma may all play an important role. It is believed that disc degeneration results in altered, abnormal load distribution, which in turn leads to a cascade of structural changes that affect the various components of the spinal column. These structural changes may change spinal posture and stability and may compromise neural function. The pathomechanisms underlying axial and radicular pain are still not completely clear. Increased vascularization after discal herniation and the presence of inflammatory mediators such as nitric oxide, prostaglandin E_2, interleukin-6, matrix metalloproteinase, and others play an important role in the pathogenesis of pain [1].

In the seventh and eighth decades of life, most if not all individuals display diffuse degenerative changes throughout the cervical spine. Only a fraction of these individuals, however, have clinical signs and symptoms. Not uncommonly, individuals who are symptomatic early on become asymptomatic as the degenerative process evolves.

The lowest five cervical vertebrae are connected by five structural elements: the intervertebral disc, the facet joints, and the neurocentral joints (joints of Luschka) [2]. The neurocentral joints are unique to the cervical spine and do not appear anywhere else in the spinal column. These joints, located in the posterolateral aspect of the vertebral bodies, consist of bone projections that articulate with the vertebral body above them (Fig. 3.1). They provide some stability to the very mobile cervical spine and protect the exiting nerve roots from pure lateral disc herniations. Once the disc degenerates, however, these joints may hypertrophy, narrow the intervertebral foramina, and modify their shape, thus compromising the radicular nerves or the dorsal root ganglia. A similar degenerative process may involve the facet joints that are posteriorly located, and they in turn

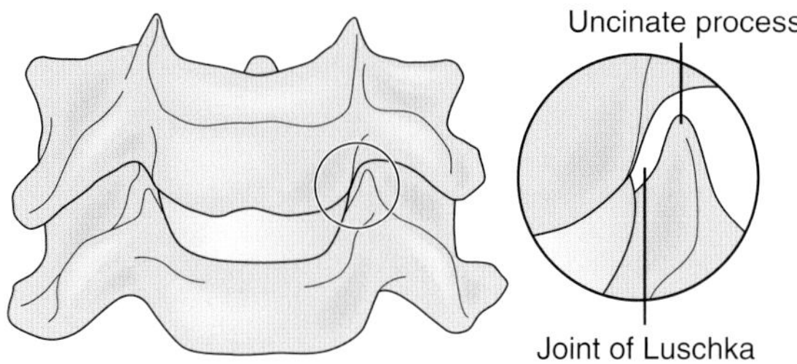

FIGURE 3.1 Schematic representation of the joint of Luschka in the coronal plane. *(From Fast A, Goldsher D. Navigating the Adult Spine. New York, Demos Medical Publishing, 2007.)*

may compress the exiting neural elements from the back. Indeed, the most common cause of cervical radiculopathy is foraminal narrowing due to facet or neurocentral joint hypertrophy [3]. The lower cervical spine, especially C4-C5, C5-C6, and to a lesser extent C6-C7, is the source of pain in most symptomatic individuals. Unlike in the lumbar spine, nucleus pulposus herniation is less frequent and is the cause of radicular pain in only 20% to 25% of cases [3,4]. As the spinal cord occupies a substantial proportion of the cervical spinal canal, posteriorly directed herniations can result in significant cord compression as well as radicular symptoms.

Symptoms

The most common symptom, one that drives most of the patients to the physician's office, is pain. In the general population, the point prevalence for neck pain ranges between 9.5% and 22%, whereas lifetime prevalence may be as high as 66%. The annual incidence is higher in men and peaks around 50 to 54 years of age [5,6].

In this respect, two large groups of patients can be recognized: patients whose main complaint is limited to axial pain and patients with radicular pain. Patients with axial pain typically complain of stiffness and pain in the cervical spine. The pain is usually more severe in the upright position and relieved only with bed rest. Cervical motion, especially hyperextension and side bending, increases the pain. In patients with pathologic changes involving the upper cervical joints or degeneration of upper cervical discs, the pain may radiate into the head, typically into the occipital region. In patients with lower cervical disease, the pain radiates into the region of the superior trapezius or the interscapular region. On occasion, patients present with atypical symptoms, such as jaw pain or chest pain–cervical angina.

Identification of the pain generator and its management are far more challenging in patients with axial pain because imaging studies frequently show multilevel pathologic changes, such as multilevel disc degeneration, facet arthropathy, and uncovertebral joint disease. It is often difficult and quite challenging to identify the exact source of pain. As the facets and the uncovertebral joints, peripheral discs, and ligaments all contain nerve endings, each one or a combination of them could be the source of pain [4].

Patients with radicular pain have symptoms commensurate with the involved nerve root. The pain usually follows a myotomal distribution and is frequently described as boring, aching, deep-seated pain. The pain is made worse by tilting the head toward the affected side or by hyperextension and side bending. Infrequently, patients find that the pain may be made more tolerable when the hand of the symptomatic side is placed over the top of the head (shoulder abduction release) [7]. The sensory symptoms (numbness, tingling, and burning sensation) usually follow the dermatomal distribution. When carpal tunnel syndrome accompanies cervical radiculopathy (double crush syndrome), the sensory changes may be in median nerve distribution. Indeed, there is a high concurrent incidence of cervical radiculopathy and carpal tunnel syndrome [8]. Sclerotomal pain, frequently overlooked or interpreted as trigger points, may be present and commonly resides in the medial or lateral scapular borders [9,10]. On occasion, patients complain of arm or hand weakness as they may drop things or find difficulty with routine activities of daily living.

Physical Examination

Because of severe axial pain, the patient may keep the head and neck immobile as cervical movements may increase the symptoms. Frequently, the only comfortable position is when the patient reclines and the neck is unloaded. Axial pain may increase with cervical extension or side bending. The Spurling test, whereby simultaneous axial loading and tilting of the head toward the symptomatic side in the upright position are performed, elicits neck and radicular pain. This test may elicit a specific dermatomal pain pattern and has high specificity and sensitivity of 95% for identifying nerve root compression [11]. Manual neck distraction may alleviate the symptoms. Tender spots are frequently found over the cervical paraspinal muscles, within the superior trapezius muscles, or in muscles supplied by the compromised root. These spots refer to areas within the muscles that, when stimulated, elicit a sensation of local pain [10]. Tender spots may be of diagnostic significance, especially when they are found unilaterally or in conjunction with other symptoms of cervical radiculopathy.

In patients with radicular pain, depending on the root involved, examination may reveal weakness in myotomal distribution, sensory changes in dermatomal distribution, and reflex changes (Table 3.1). Meticulous physical examination helps identify the compromised root: C5 root compromise will affect shoulder abductors; C6, elbow flexors; C7, elbow extensors; and C8, finger flexors. Finding of concomitant sensory and reflex changes is helpful. Dermatomal arrangement is not fixed and may vary in different patients because of aberrant rootlets or anastomoses between peripheral nerves. Frequently, dermatomes represent only a portion of the root's domain [12]. The dermatomal charts are useful, however, and play a role in the patient's diagnosis. Radicular pain frequently occurs without weakness, reflex, or apparent sensory changes. The most frequently affected roots are C5, C6, and C7 [3,6]. In the cervical region, unlike in other regions of the spine, the nerve roots exit the spine above their respective vertebrae; the C5 nerve root exits above C5 vertebra and hence may be compromised by herniation of the C4-5 intervertebral disc. The C8 nerve root exits below

Table 3.1 Salient Features of the Most Frequently Affected Roots

	Predominantly Affected Muscles	Sensory Distribution	Reflex Changes
C5	Deltoid, supraspinatus, and infraspinatus	Shoulder and lateral aspect of arm	Supinator reflex
C6	Elbow flexors: biceps brachialis, brachioradialis, and radial extensors of the wrist	Distal lateral forearm, thumb, and index fingers	Biceps reflex
C7	Triceps, wrist flexors	Dorsal aspects of forearm and middle finger	Triceps reflex
C8	Flexor digitorum superficialis and profundus	Ulnar aspects of forearm, hand, and fourth and fifth fingers	No reflex changes

the C7 vertebral body; all the subsequent nerves below that level follow the same pattern.

Looking for long tract signs is of paramount importance because their presence points toward cord compression and may modify the treatment plan. The diagnostic accuracy of the physical examination is fairly reliable and may correlate well with imaging studies [9,11,13,14].

Functional Limitations

The functional limitations associated with cervical degenerative disease depend on the extent of the degenerative changes and the neurologic involvement. Not infrequently, patients are asymptomatic, and the only functional limitation noted is loss of cervical range of motion. They tend to hold the neck in a forward stooped posture; the neck is held in forward flexion and cannot achieve extension. When these patients stand against a wall, the back of the head may be inches away from it, and they cannot straighten the cervical spine. These patients may function well but have limited range of motion in all planes and cannot look up. When weakness is present, patients may have functional deficits corresponding with their spinal level of involvement (e.g., patients with C8-T1 involvement may drop things and have difficulties with movements requiring fine motor coordination).

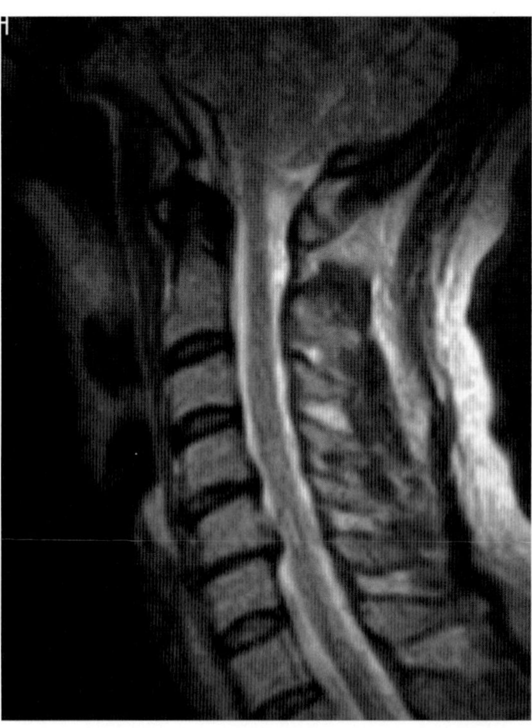

FIGURE 3.2 Sagittal T2-weighted image of the cervical spine showing spinal cord compression at the C3-C4 and C4-C5 levels. At the C3-C4 level, the cord is compressed from the front and from the back. No cerebrospinal fluid is visible in the compressed regions.

Diagnostic Studies

Radiographs (anteroposterior, lateral, oblique, and flexion and extension views) are frequently obtained but may be of limited use. The vertebral components are clearly seen in these studies but not the intervertebral discs, spinal cord, or peripheral nerves. The x-ray films clearly show degenerative changes (narrowing intervertebral discs; spurs and calcified or ossified soft tissues). Frequently, there is no good correlation between the symptoms and the extent of degenerative findings on radiographs [14]. Diffuse multilevel changes are frequently observed but are, for the most part, irrelevant to the patient's symptoms. Flexion and extension views are important as they can detect degenerative instability that is responsible for the symptoms and that may not be seen in the static views [6]. Radiographs are not helpful in the early stages of infection and tumors.

Magnetic resonance imaging is the diagnostic modality of choice because it allows visualization of the whole cervical spine without irradiation and enables the clinician to assess the neural structures (cord, roots) as well as the soft tissues (discs, ligaments). Correlation of the imaging studies with the history and clinical examination is of utmost importance because in many individuals, the magnetic resonance imaging studies reveal significant pathologic changes (herniated discs, neural foraminal stenosis) that are totally irrelevant to the patient's complaints and symptoms (Fig. 3.2). Computed tomography should be obtained after trauma because it may identify fractures that could be otherwise missed on plain radiography and even magnetic resonance imaging studies. Computed tomographic myelography is frequently obtained before surgery but should not be obtained on a routine basis. Patients with axial pain who do not respond to conservative measures can be referred for discography to identify the pain generator. Discography may be the only way to identify the disc responsible for the symptoms; however, this procedure remains controversial and should be performed only in selected patients. Electrodiagnostic studies play an important role, especially in diabetic patients or whenever peripheral neuropathies are suspected [8,15].

Differential Diagnosis [16]

Rotator cuff tendinitis
Rotator cuff tear
Peripheral neuropathies
Carpal tunnel syndrome
Spine tumors
Spinal infection
Brachial plexopathy
Thoracic outlet syndrome

Treatment

Initial

The management of patients with axial pain without radicular symptoms is much more challenging than the management of radicular pain. In the case of axial pain, it is often difficult to identify the pain generator and thus to initiate a direct therapeutic response. Anti-inflammatory drugs along with analgesics should be prescribed as a first line of treatment in the initial stages of the disease. Patients with severe radicular pain may be managed with systemic steroids, such as methylprednisolone (Dosepak), when they do not respond to other anti-inflammatory drugs. Steroids may be beneficial in relieving pain because they reduce inflammation and swelling, thereby facilitating neural nutrient and blood supply, and stabilize neural membranes, thus suppressing ectopic discharges within the affected nerve fibers. They may be administered during the course of a week to 10 days in tapering dose. For severe pain, a starting dose of 70 mg of prednisone decreasing by 10 mg daily may be recommended. Methylprednisolone is quite handy, as the daily dose is prearranged separately within the package. A substantial percentage of patients with spondylotic radicular nontraumatic pain are expected to improve significantly after fluoroscopically guided therapeutic selective nerve root injections (see later) [17,18]. Patients with severe burning pain may respond favorably to gabapentin (Neurontin) or pregabalin (Lyrica).

The patient should be instructed to try the shoulder abduction release maneuver as a therapeutic measure (i.e., put the affected hand over the head) with the hope that this might decrease the tension on the affected nerve root and bring some symptomatic relief [19].

Rehabilitation

Conclusive high-quality studies that clearly define the most efficient rehabilitation approach to patients with neck pain are still lacking [5]. The more commonly applied methods are summarized here.

Activity modifications are of paramount importance. It has been demonstrated in vivo that the neural foraminal dimensions vary with flexion and extension. It has been shown that cervical flexion increases foraminal height, width, and cross-sectional area, whereas extension has the opposite effects [20,21]. Because foraminal narrowing plays a major clinical role in patients with cervical radicular pain, patients should be advised to avoid activities in which cervical extension is involved. The patients should be instructed to drink with a straw, to avoid overhead activities, to face the sink while shampooing the hair, to adjust the monitor height, and the like. Temporary immobilization of the cervical spine may bring about some relief. This can be accomplished with a collar when the patient is mobile but should be used only temporarily. Cervical traction, provided it is administered in the supine position with the head held in slight flexion, may be of value in patients with radicular pain. Traction could be administered manually or, preferably, through a mechanized approach. The mechanized approach allows accurate traction forces to be administered. The distraction forces that are applied to the neck can, to some extent, relieve nerve compression by increasing the foraminal height and the intervertebral distance [22]. Traction application in the supine position is preferable because the weight of the head is eliminated and all the traction forces are effectively directed to the cervical spine. Despite its common use, no conclusive evidence that proves its therapeutic efficacy exists, however [23,24]. Superficial heat should be applied concomitantly with the traction as an adjunct therapy to relax the muscles before and during traction. Isometric neck exercises should be recommended as they may preserve muscle tone and strength without leading to pain. Cervical range of motion exercises are not recommended during the acute pain period.

Manual medicine (massage, mobilization, manipulation), acupuncture, and electrical stimulation are also widely used. Although these approaches are popular, studies demonstrating their efficacy are still lacking [25–32].

Procedures

Translaminar and transforaminal (selective nerve root) steroid administration may provide significant and at times long-term relief in patients with radicular pain. Properly selected, up to 60% of patients who are managed with selective nerve root injection may have good to excellent outcome [3,17]. Because there may be a significant risk with these injections (i.e., vertebral artery injury), they should be fluoroscopically guided and administered only by physicians with proper training.

Surgery

The main indications for surgery are severe or progressive neurologic deficits and persistent pain that does not respond to conservative measures.

The standard surgical treatment of cervical radiculopathy for many decades has been anterior cervical decompression and fusion. This approach prevailed because in most patients with cervical radiculopathy, the symptoms are caused by osteophytes compressing the nerves within the intervertebral foramina, and laminectomy is not effective in these cases.

The anterior approach permits excellent access to anteriorly impinging structures, such as discs and spondylotic spurs. Some surgeons add instrumentation (i.e., plate) to increase the fusion rate and the postoperative stability [13]. Adequate foraminal decompression can result in early pain relief and enhanced muscle strength. Long term, however, no significant differences in pain or function have been found between conservatively and surgically treated patients [25,33]. Dysphagia, which frequently follows the anterior approach, usually subsides several weeks postoperatively.

The negative long-term effects of fusion have only recently been appreciated. Fusion leads to stiffness and lost range of motion, and over the years, it results in next-level degeneration (i.e., accelerated discal degeneration above and below the fused vertebrae). This has led to the development of disc replacement surgery—arthroplasty. Whereas the concept of disc replacement is attractive as disc replacement maintains the intervertebral discal height while preserving spinal motion [34], the advantages of this approach and its long-term effects have not yet been established [35].

Patients with single-level soft disc herniation may be operated on from the back. In these patients, laminotomy with foraminotomy may bring about relief without fusion and its complications while maintaining cervical stability [13].

Potential Disease Complications

Chronic pain and permanent neurologic deficits may develop in some patients. These may compromise the quality of life and interfere with activities of daily living.

Potential Treatment Complications

Steroid administration carries certain risks, and these should be considered before steroid administration. Surgical complications include infection, nerve injury, pain, stiffness, pseudarthrosis, and next-level degeneration.

References

[1] Peng B, Hao J, Hou S, et al. Possible pathogenesis of painful intervertebral disc degeneration. Spine (Phila Pa 1976) 2006;31:560–6.

[2] Macnab I. Cervical spondylosis. Clin Orthop 1973;109:69–77.

[3] Carette S, Fehlings MG. Cervical radiculopathy. N Engl J Med 2005;353:392–9.

[4] Bogduk N, Windsor M, Inglis A. The innervation of the cervical intervertebral discs. Spine (Phila Pa 1976) 1988;13:2–8.

[5] Davidson RI, Dunn EJ, Metzmaker JN. The shoulder abduction test in the diagnosis of radicular pain in cervical extradural compressive monoradiculopathies. Spine (Phila Pa 1976) 1981;6:441–6.

[6] Haymaker W, Woodhall B. Peripheral nerve injuries. Principles of diagnosis. Philadelphia: WB Saunders; 1953, 47–53.

[7] Letchuman R, Gay RE, Shelerud RA, VanOstrand LA. Are tender points associated with cervical radiculopathy? Arch Phys Med Rehabil 2005;86:1333–7.

[8] Lo SF, Chou LW, Meng NH. Clinical characteristics and electrodiagnostic features in patients with carpal tunnel syndrome, double crush syndrome, and cervical radiculopathy. Rheumatol Int 2012;32:1257–63.

[9] Slipman CW, Plastaras CT, Palmitier RA, et al. Symptom provocation of fluoroscopically guided cervical nerve root stimulation. Are dynatomal maps identical to dermatomal maps? Spine (Phila Pa 1976) 1998;23:2235–42.

[10] Rao R. Neck pain, cervical radiculopathy, and cervical myelopathy. J Bone Joint Surg Am 2002;84:1872–81.

[11] Bridwell KH, Anderson PA, Boden SD, et al. Specialty update: What's new in spine surgery. J Bone Joint Surg Am 2012;94:1140–8.

[12] Wainner RS, Fritz JM, Irrgang JJ, et al. Reliability and diagnostic accuracy of the clinical examination and patient self-report measures for cervical radiculopathy. Spine (Phila Pa 1976) 2003;28:52–62.

[13] Heller JG. The syndrome of degenerative cervical disease. Orthop Clin North Am 1993;23:381–94.

[14] Truumees E, Herkowitz HN. Cervical spondylotic myelopathy and radiculopathy. Instr Course Lect 2000;49:339–60.

[15] Wainner RS, Gill H. Diagnosis and nonoperative management of cervical radiculopathy. J Orthop Sports Phys Ther 2000;30:728–44.

[16] Honet JC, Ellenberg MR. What you always wanted to know about the history and physical examination of neck pain but were afraid to ask. Phys Med Rehabil Clin N Am 2003;14:473–91.

[17] Slipman CW, Lipetz JS, Jackson HB, et al. Therapeutic selective nerve root block in the nonsurgical treatment of atraumatic cervical spondylotic radicular pain: a retrospective analysis with independent clinical review. Arch Phys Med Rehabil 2000;81:741–6.

[18] Bush K, Hillier S. Outcome of cervical radiculopathy treated with periradicular/epidural corticosteroid injections: a prospective study with independent clinical review. Eur Spine J 1996;5:319–25.

[19] Fast A, Parikh S, Marin EL. The shoulder abduction relief sign in cervical radiculopathy. Arch Phys Med Rehabil 1989;70:402–3.

[20] Hoving JL, Gross AR, Gasner D, et al. A critical appraisal of review articles on the effectiveness of conservative treatment for neck pain. Spine (Phila Pa 1976) 2001;26:196–205.

[21] Kitagawa T, Fujiwara A, Kobayashi N, et al. Morphologic changes in the cervical neural foramen due to flexion and extension. In vivo imaging study. Spine (Phila Pa 1976) 2004;29:2821–5.

[22] Craig Humphreys S, Chase J, Patwardhan A, et al. Flexion and traction effect on C5-C6 foraminal space. Arch Phys Med Rehabil 1998;79:1105–9.

[23] van der Heijden GJ, Beurskens AJ, Koes BW, et al. The efficacy of traction for back and neck pain: a systematic, blinded review of randomized clinical trial methods. Phys Ther 1995;75:93–104.

[24] Raney NH, Petersen EJ, Smith TA, et al. Development of a clinical prediction rule to identify patients with neck pain likely to benefit from cervical traction and exercise. Eur Spine J 2009;18:382–91.

[25] Wang WTJ, Olson SL, Campbell AH, et al. Effectiveness of physical therapy for patients with neck pain: an individualized approach using a clinical decision-making algorithm. Am J Phys Med Rehabil 2003;82:203–18.

[26] Klaber Moffett JA, Hughes GI, Griffiths P. An investigation of the effects of cervical traction. Part 1. Clinical effectiveness. Clin Rehabil 1990;4:205–11.

[27] Persson LCG, Carlsson CA, Carlsson JY. Long-lasting cervical radicular pain managed with surgery, physiotherapy, or a cervical collar. Spine (Phila Pa 1976) 1997;22:751–8.

[28] Taimela S, Takala EP, Asklof T, et al. Active treatment of chronic neck pain: a prospective randomized intervention. Spine (Phila Pa 1976) 2000;25:1021–7.

[29] Kjellman GV, Skargren EI, Oberg BE. A critical analysis of randomised clinical trials on neck pain and treatment efficacy: a review of the literature. Scand J Rehabil Med 1999;31:139–52.

[30] Wolff L, Levine LA. Cervical radiculopathies: conservative approaches to management. Phys Med Rehabil Clin N Am 2002;13:589–608.

[31] Weintraub MI. Complementary and alternative methods of treatment of neck pain. Phys Med Rehabil Clin N Am 2003;14:659–74.

[32] Langevin P, Roy JS, Desmeules F. Cervical radiculopathy: study protocol of a randomised clinical trial evaluating the effect of mobilisations and exercises targeting the opening of intervertebral foramen. BMC Musculoskelet Disord 2012;13:10–7.

[33] Fouyas IP, Statham PF, Sandercock AG. Cochrane review on the role of surgery in cervical spondylotic radiculomyelopathy. Spine (Phila Pa 1976) 2002;27:736–47.

[34] Phillips FM, Garfin SR. Cervical disc replacement. Spine (Phila Pa 1976) 2005;30:S27–33.

[35] Jiang H, Zhu Z, Qiu Y, et al. Cervical disc arthroplasty versus fusion for single-level symptomatic cervical disc disease: a meta-analysis of randomized controlled studies. Arch Orthop Trauma Surg 2012;132:141–51.

CHAPTER 4

Cervical Dystonia

Moon Suk Bang, MD, PhD
Shi-Uk Lee, MD, PhD

Synonyms

Spasmodic torticollis
Idiopathic torsion dystonia
Symptomatic torsion dystonia

ICD-9 Codes

333.6 Idiopathic torsion dystonia
333.7 Symptomatic torsion dystonia

ICD-10 Codes

G24.1 Idiopathic torsion dystonia
G24.2 Symptomatic torsion dystonia

Definition

Idiopathic cervical dystonia, the most common form of adult-onset focal dystonia, is twisting and turning of the neck caused by abnormal involuntary muscle contractures [1]. Cervical dystonia has also been known as spasmodic torticollis, which implies head jerking or neck spasms. However, these features are absent in 25% to 35% of patients with this condition [2]. Furthermore, the term *spasmodic torticollis* fails to emphasize the dystonic nature of the condition and the frequent association of cervical dystonia with dystonia in adjacent or remote body parts.

The incidence of cervical dystonia has been estimated at 1.07 per 100,000 person-years [3]. Women are affected 1.5 to 1.9 times more often than men are [2,4]. In 70% to 90% of cases, the disease begins between the fourth and sixth decades, with a peak incidence in the fifth decade of life [5].

The pathogenetic mechanisms are unclear, but increasing evidence suggests that cervical dystonia is influenced by genetic factors. Many patients with cervical dystonia have a family history [2]. Several gene loci, such as *DYT1*, *DYT6*, and *DYT7*, have recently been reported to be associated with cervical dystonia [6].

Cervical dystonia has also been reported to develop secondary to head, neck, and shoulder trauma [7]. The role of the sensory system is important in the pathogenesis of this condition (see section on symptoms) [8]. Impaired inhibition of sensory Ia afferent fibers, impairment of central sensory pathways, and increased spindle responsiveness secondary to overactive gamma spindle efferent fibers have been proposed as pathogenic mechanisms [9]. Other proposed mechanisms are vestibular impairment, dysfunction of the subcortical-cortical motor network, and dopaminergic dysfunction [9].

The natural course of dystonia has been reported [10], and in 68.1% of patients, dystonia remained focal. Progression of dystonia to sites other than the neck was noted in 31.9% of patients. The only risk factor for progression of dystonia to other body parts was longer duration of the disease. The rate of spontaneous remission was 20.8%. In most of the cases (87%), the remission occurred during the first 5 years after the onset of symptoms. The remission was sustained in 60% of the patients, and in 40% of the patients who had experienced remission, the disorder relapsed (nonsustained remission). The duration of the disease before remission was an important discriminating factor between sustained and nonsustained remission. The patients who experienced nonsustained remission had all done well within the first 2 years of the disorder; whereas in the patients who had sustained remission, the duration of dystonia before remission was more than 2 years.

Symptoms

Symptoms usually begin insidiously with complaints of a pulling or drawing in the neck or an involuntary twisting or jerking of the head. In most patients, the manifesting symptoms are sensory in nature (described variously as pain, pulling, or stiffness) or a degree of head rotation or deviation, with jerking and tremor of the head being distinctly less common complaints [2,4,11]. In 83% of patients, head deviation was constant rather than jerky (i.e., nonspasmodic) and demonstrated some degree of rotation (97%). Only a fraction of patients showed head jerks (35%) and neck spasms (37%), which are the cardinal features of "spasmodic" torticollis [2].

Several provocative and palliative factors are characteristic of idiopathic dystonia. Most notable is the use of a sensory trick or *geste antagoniste*. Gently touching the chin, back of the head, or top of the head relieves the symptoms. The use of sensory tricks to keep the head in the body midline position was reported by 88.9% of patients in one series [12]. The physiologic mechanism of sensory tricks remains unknown. Other effective maneuvers include leaning against a high-backed chair, placing something in the mouth, and pulling the hair. Early in the illness, these tricks are helpful in most patients, but they tend to lose effectiveness as the disease progresses. Less common palliative factors are relaxation, alcohol, and "morning benefit," when symptoms are improved for a while after waking. Cervical dystonia is commonly exacerbated by activity (e.g., walking), fatigue, or stress [13].

Pain is a major source of disability in two thirds to three quarters of patients with cervical dystonia [2,3,14,15]. Pain severity was related to the intensity of dystonia and muscle spasms [2] but not to the duration of cervical dystonia and severity of motor dysfunction [14]. Pain was commonly described as tiring, radiating, tugging, aching, and exhausting [14].

Physical Examination

Inspection of the patient's head posture is enough for the diagnosis of cervical dystonia. A wide variety of abnormal head and neck postures can occur (Fig. 4.1). Rotational torticollis is a rotation of the chin around the longitudinal axis toward the shoulder. Laterocollis is a rotation of the head in the coronal plane, moving the ear toward the shoulder. Anterocollis and retrocollis are rotations of the head in the sagittal plane; anterocollis brings the chin toward the chest, and retrocollis elevates the chin and brings the occiput toward the back. By convention, the direction of the rotation is defined by the chin, so right-turning torticollis means that the chin is turning to the right. There may also be sagittal or lateral deviation of the base of the neck from the midline [13]; 66% to 80% of patients present with a combination of these movements [2,4]. The most common component of complex deviations is rotational torticollis, followed by head tilt, retrocollis, and anterocollis. Isolated deviations (e.g., in a single plane) are seen in less than one third of patients. Notably, idiopathic cases of pure anterocollis are extremely uncommon. There is no statistically significant preponderance of right or left deviation [2,4,5,16]. The abnormal posture is present for more than 75% of the time in most patients, but findings may change in nature and directional preponderance over time [2].

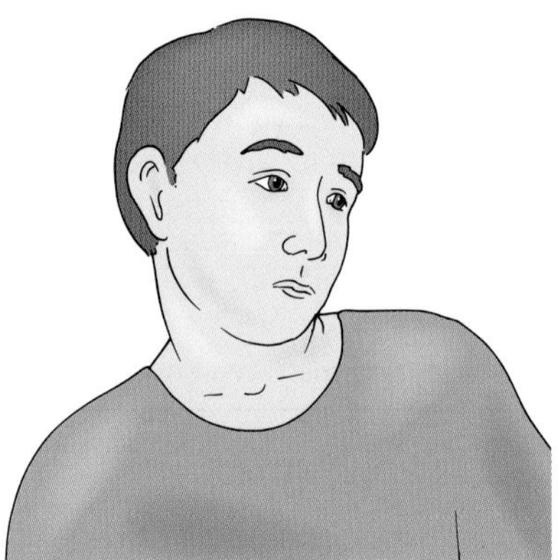

FIGURE 4.1 Drawing of a patient with left rotational torticollis and laterocollis showing prominent left rotation, left tilt, and shoulder elevation.

Many patients have signs of dystonia involving other body segments at the time of presentation. Extracervical dystonia is found in 10% to 20% of patients [2,4]; the jaw (oromandibular), eyelids (blepharospasm), arm or hand (writer's cramp), and trunk (axial) are the most frequently affected parts. A postural or kinetic hand tremor is found on physical examination in up to 25% of patients.

Although the term *spasmodic torticollis* implies head jerking or neck spasms, this feature is absent in 25.33% of patients. The adjectives *spasmodic* and *spastic* are misleading because there is no evidence that cervical dystonia is a spastic disorder or caused by dysfunction of the pyramidal tracts. Furthermore, the movements are not always spasmodic but may be sustained.

Although abnormal head position is enough for the diagnosis, physical examination in patients with cervical dystonia must be focused on detection of "pseudodystonia" secondary to structural abnormalities [17]. Normal findings in a complete neurologic examination are mandated to exclude secondary dystonia. The presence of corticospinal, sensory, cerebellar, oculomotor, or cortical signs with cervical or extracervical dystonia suggests secondary dystonia.

Functional Limitations

Functional limitations due to cervical dystonia are found in almost all patients (99% of 220 patients) [16]. The severity of disability ranges from mild (subjective feeling of discomfort in social conditions without objective consequences on social life) to severe (qualitative and quantitative modification of the occupational level with resulting impairment of social life). One report documented depression in 24% of 67 patients with idiopathic cervical dystonia [18].

At some point during the illness, 75% of patients complain of pain, and patients usually consider the pain a major source of disability [2,4,10,15]. Pain is associated with constant head turning, greater severity of head turning, and presence of spasms [2]. Disability is also caused by task-specific limitations (e.g., inability to drive) and avoidance of social interaction due to abnormal posture. Questioning of patients about disability and clarification of the contributing factors are crucial for the optimal care of patients with idiopathic cervical dystonia [19].

Diagnostic Studies

Screening biochemical studies (blood chemistry screening test, complete blood count, thyroid function) in addition to a ceruloplasmin level should be performed to rule out other medical conditions that might cause dystonic features. Because various central nervous system lesions are known to be associated with cervical dystonia, magnetic resonance imaging of the brain and cervical spine should be considered in all patients with a fixed painful neck posture [20]. If there is scoliosis, it may be evaluated with plain radiographs to document the baseline abnormality. In addition,

Wilson disease should be excluded in all patients younger than 50 years by measurement of serum ceruloplasmin and a slit-lamp examination.

Differential Diagnosis

Atlantoaxial dislocation
Cervical fracture
Degenerative disc
Osteomyelitis
Klippel-Feil syndrome
Congenital torticollis associated with absence or fibrosis of cervical muscles
Postirradiation fibrosis
Acute stiff neck
Pharyngitis
Painful lymphadenopathy, adenitis
Vestibulo-ocular dysfunction (head tilt with fourth nerve paresis or labyrinthine disease)
Posterior fossa tumor
Arnold-Chiari syndrome
Bobble-head doll syndrome (with third ventricle cyst)
Nystagmus
Sandifer syndrome
Spinal cord tumor or syrinx
Extraocular muscle palsies, strabismus
Head thrusts with oculomotor apraxia
Hemianopia
Spasmus nutans
Focal seizures

Treatment

Initial

The goals of treatment are to palliate, to improve the quality of life, and to prevent secondary complications. Reassurance is most important. Patients should be reassured that cervical dystonia is not dangerous and be reminded that cervical dystonia does not become generalized but may spread locally. However, they should also be told that treatment is symptomatic, not curative. Physicians must understand which aspects of the illness are most limiting because disability in cervical dystonia may be caused by many factors, such as pain, abnormal posture, functional limitation, social embarrassment, and depression. Detection of concomitant depression is crucial because it is a major source of disability, will limit therapeutic benefit, and is itself treatable. Secondary complications, such as radiculopathy, myelopathy, and dysphagia, must be recognized and treated. The evaluation of therapies for cervical dystonia is difficult: the abnormal postures, pain, and disability are not easy to quantitate; there are spontaneous remissions; and most studies are small and not randomized controlled trials [21]. Therefore, no universally accepted treatment protocol exists. However, the treatment of cervical dystonia has been revolutionized by chemodenervation with botulinum toxin. Medications are generally used as adjuncts to botulinum toxin. Adjunctive medications can prevent development of neutralizing antibodies because it is possible to lower dosages and frequency of botulinum toxin injections. Anticholinergics, benzodiazepines, and baclofen are the most widely used.

Other medications, such as dopamine-depleting agents (e.g., tetrabenazine) [22], are available, and many patients will require combination therapy. If therapy with botulinum toxin and oral medications fails, surgery may be required [9].

Rehabilitation

Patients with mild symptoms may be managed with physical measures or pharmacotherapy. Physical measures include the simple *geste antagoniste* (i.e., sensory tricks), biofeedback, mechanical braces, and physiotherapy. Use of the manipulative approach in the treatment of cervical dystonia is not appropriate under the assumption that the condition results from a spinal or orthopedic abnormality. In most patients, it is not possible to physically overcome the brain's disordered central processing commands to displace the head position. Therefore physiotherapists and chiropractors are advised not to use orthopedic techniques or physical force as this may result in further discomfort or injury to the patient. However, it is beneficial to assist patients to use their own resources to improve head control by strengthening and enhanced flexibility.

Physical therapy is recommended as an adjunct to botulinum toxin injection. After treatment with botulinum toxin, there is less opposition from the dystonic musculature. The goal is to facilitate the patient's increased control over head movement and posture once the antagonists are weakened. In a case report, reduction of the effective dose of botulinum toxin was also possible when physiotherapy management was added to a long-term treatment regimen [23].

Procedures

The prognosis of patients with cervical dystonia has been radically changed after the introduction of chemodenervation with botulinum toxin. Compared with all previous therapies, botulinum toxin benefits the highest percentage of patients in the shortest time, has been proved effective in many double-blind placebo-controlled and open trials [24], and has fewer side effects than other pharmacologic therapies [25]. For idiopathic cervical dystonia, serotype A is most widely used. The use of serotypes B and F is under investigation in patients who have become immunologically resistant to serotype A [26].

The identification of the sites of pain and the muscles responsible for the abnormal posture is the most important factor in botulinum toxin administration. The sternocleidomastoid, trapezius, splenius capitis, and levator scapulae are most commonly injected. An electromyographic study of 100 patients found that two or three muscles are most commonly abnormal [27]. In a recent study, ^{18}F-fluorodeoxyglucose positron emission tomography/computed tomography was suggested to be a useful modality to identify dystonic cervical muscles [28]. The most commonly found abnormal muscles in each head posture are shown in Table 4.1. There is wide variability in the number of muscles injected, the number of injections per muscle, the concentration of botulinum toxin employed, and the use of electromyography-assisted injections, among other technical details. Which technique provides optimal results remains to be determined [29]. The average optimal dose

Table 4.1 Head Postures and the Muscles Most Commonly Responsible for the Posture

Head Posture	Responsible Muscles
Rotational torticollis	Contralateral SCM Ipsilateral SC With or without contralateral SC
Laterocollis	Ipsilateral SCM, SC, TPZ
Retrocollis	Bilateral SC

SCM, sternocleidomastoid; *SC,* splenius capitis; *TPZ,* trapezius.
Modified from Deuschl G, Heinen F, Kleedorfer B, et al. Clinical and polymyographic investigation of spasmodic torticollis. J Neurol 1992;239:9-15.

for patients with cervical dystonia is varied between trials (mean Botox dose: 188 units [50 to 280 units]; mean Dysport dose: 577 units [250–1000 units]) [30]. It is important to customize the dosage and the muscles to suit the needs of the individual patients. The optimal dosing in a particular muscle has been assessed only for the sternocleidomastoid muscle by quantitative electromyography. Doses as small as 20 units of Botox reduced dystonic activity in the sternocleidomastoid muscle, whereas doses larger than 20 units offered minimal additional improvement [31]. Similarly, for Dysport, 100 units was sufficient to reduce the sternocleidomastoid muscle activity [31]; doses larger than 100 units were associated with a greater occurrence of dysphagia [32].

A benefit from botulinum toxin is generally seen within the first week but rarely may be delayed for up to 8 weeks. The benefit lasts an average of 12 weeks, and most physicians suggest that the injections be repeated every 3 to 4 months. The response to toxin is not affected by the pattern of deviation. Continued toxin injections provide progressive improvement of dystonia [29].

Patients with cervical dystonia who never benefit from botulinum toxin injection are considered primary nonresponders. This occurs in approximately 15% to 30% of patients [33]. In addition to the occurrence of primary treatment failure (patients never responding to injection), secondary failure may also occur in 10% to 15% of patients. These patients with initial improvement after treatment fail to respond to subsequent injections. Of the secondary failures, 35.7% were found to have antibodies to botulinum toxin by the mouse neutralization assay [33].

Surgery

Surgical therapy is recommended only for patients whose dystonia is prolonged, unresponsive to adequate trials of medication and botulinum toxin injections, and associated with significant pain or disability. Since the introduction of botulinum toxin, surgery is rarely required. Peripheral denervation procedures designed to denervate dystonic muscles selectively are the most widely practiced surgical procedures. Selective ramisectomy is a procedure that involves the selective section of dorsal rami of the upper cervical spinal nerves [34]. Selective denervation procedures are often combined with selective spinal accessory nerve section, anterior rhizotomy, or myotomy. Deep brain stimulation is becoming the standard of care for medically intractable, disabling dystonias. Advantages of deep brain stimulation include reversibility, adjustability, and continued access to the therapeutic target. Initial reports describing the use of deep brain stimulation in generalized dystonia have been encouraging, and experience in the use of deep brain stimulation to treat various forms of dystonia is continually growing [35].

Potential Disease Complications

Patients may develop cervical spondylosis with resulting radiculopathy or myelopathy [36]. Extracervical spread of dystonia is a progression of dystonia to a segmental pattern of dystonia. In one third of 72 patients who first had isolated cervical dystonia, the dystonia typically spread to the face, jaw, arms, or trunk [10].

Potential Treatment Complications

Side effects of botulinum toxin injections have been reported in 20% to 30% of patients per treatment cycle and approximately 50% of patients at some time during therapy. Dysphagia, neck weakness, and local pain at the injection site are the most commonly reported side effects, but dizziness, dry mouth, influenza-like syndrome, lethargy, dysphonia, and generalized weakness have been reported. The frequency of side effects varies widely, apparently on the basis of the dosage used [26].

Failure to spare ventral roots in selective ramisectomy injures the cervical and brachial plexuses and leads to the complications of diaphragmatic paralysis and dysphagia. Other sequelae of the selective denervation procedure include sensory loss in the distribution of the greater occipital nerve, paresthesias, and occasional sudden tic-like pain.

References

[1] Fahn S, Marsden CD, Calne DB. Classification and investigation of dystonia. In: Marsden CD, Fahn S, editors. Movement disorders. 2nd ed. London: Butterworth; 1987. p. 332–58.
[2] Chan J, Brin MF, Fahn S. Idiopathic cervical dystonia: clinical characteristics. Mov Disord 1991;6:119–26.
[3] Steeves TD, Day L, Dykeman J, et al. The prevalence of primary dystonia: a systemic review and meta-analysis. Mov Disord 2012;27:1789–96.
[4] Jankovic J, Leder S, Warner D, et al. Cervical dystonia: clinical findings and associated movement disorders. Neurology 1991;41:1088–91.
[5] Duane DD. Spasmodic torticollis. Adv Neurol 1988;49:135–50.
[6] Elia AE, Lalli S, Albanese A. Differential diagnosis of dystonia. Eur J Neurol 2010;17(Suppl 1):1–8.
[7] Tarsy D. Comparison of acute- and delayed-onset posttraumatic cervical dystonia. Mov Disord 1998;13:481–5.
[8] Tempel LW, Perlmutter JS. Abnormal cortical responses in patients with writer's cramp. Neurology 1993;43:2252–7.
[9] Dauer WT, Burke RE, Greene P, et al. Current concepts on the clinical features, aetiology and management of idiopathic cervical dystonia. Brain 1998;121:547–60.
[10] Jahanshahi M, Marion MH, Marsden CD. Natural history of adult-onset idiopathic torticollis. Arch Neurol 1990;47:548–52.
[11] Rivest J, Marsden CD. Trunk and head tremor as isolated manifestations of dystonia. Mov Disord 1990;5:60–5.
[12] Jahanshahi M. Factors that ameliorate or aggravate spasmodic torticollis. J Neurol Neurosurg Psychiatry 2000;68:227–9.
[13] Consky ES, Lang AE. Clinical assessments of patients with cervical dystonia. In: Jankovic J, Hallett M, editors. Therapy with botulinum toxin. New York: Marcel Dekker; 1994. p. 211–37.
[14] Kutvonen O, Dastidar P, Nurmikko T. Pain in spasmodic torticollis. Pain 1997;69:279–86.
[15] Lowenstein DH, Aminoff MJ. The clinical course of spasmodic torticollis. Neurology 1988;38:530–2.

[16] Rondot P, Marchand MP, Dellatolas G. Spasmodic torticollis: review of 220 patients. Can J Neurol Sci 1991;18:143–51.
[17] Weiner WJ, Lang AE. Idiopathic torsion dystonia. In: Weiner WJ, Lang AE, editors. Movement disorders: a comprehensive survey. New York: Futura; 1989. p. 347–418.
[18] Jahanshahi M. Psychosocial factors and depression in torticollis. J Psychosom Res 1991;35:493–507.
[19] Zetterberg L, Lindmark B, Soderlund A, et al. Self-perceived non-motor aspects of cervical dystonia and their association with disability. J Rehabil Med 2012;44:950–4.
[20] Comella CL, Thompson PD. Treatment of cervical dystonia with botulinum toxins. Eur J Neurol 2006;13(Suppl 1):S16–S20.
[21] Lal S. Pathophysiology and pharmacotherapy of spasmodic torticollis: a review. Can J Neurol Sci 1979;6:427–35.
[22] Jankovic J, Beach J. Long-term effects of tetrabenazine in hyperkinetic movement disorders. Neurology 1997;48:358–65.
[23] Ramdharry G. Case report: physiotherapy cuts the dose of botulinum toxin. Physiother Res Int 2006;11:117–22.
[24] Dressler D. Botulinum toxin for treatment of dystonia. Eur J Neurol 2010;17(Suppl 1):88–96.
[25] Brans JW, Lindeboom R, Snoek JW, et al. Botulinum toxin versus trihexyphenidyl in cervical dystonia: a prospective, randomized, double-blind controlled trial. Neurology 1996;46:1066–72.
[26] Jankovic J. Botulinum toxin therapy for cervical dystonia. Neurotox Res 2006;9:145–8.
[27] Swope D, Barbano R. Treatment recommendations and practical application of botulinum toxin treatment of cervical dystonia. Neurol Clin 2008;26(Suppl 1):54–65.
[28] Sung DH, Choi JY, Kim D, et al. Localization of dystonic muscles with ^{18}F-FDG PET/CT in idiopathic cervical dystonia. J Nucl Med 2007;48:1790–5.
[29] Jankovic J, Schwartz K, Donovan DT. Botulinum toxin treatment of cranial-cervical dystonia, spasmodic dysphonia, other focal dystonias and hemifacial spasm. J Neurol Neurosurg Psychiatry 1990;53:633–9.
[30] Costa J, Espirito-Santo C, Borges A, et al. Botulinum toxin type A therapy for cervical dystonia. Cochrane Database Syst Rev 2005;1:CD003633.
[31] Dresler D. Electromyographic evaluation of cervical dystonia for planning of botulinum toxin therapy. Eur J Neurol 2000;7:713–8.
[32] Borodic GE, Joseph M, Fay L, et al. Botulinum A toxin for the treatment of spasmodic torticollis: dysphagia and regional toxin spread. Head Neck 1990;12:392–9.
[33] Barnes MP, Best D, Kidd L, et al. The use of botulinum toxin type-B in the treatment of patients who have become unresponsive to botulinum toxin type-A—initial experiences. Eur J Neurol 2005;12:947–55.
[34] Braun V, Richter HP. Selective peripheral denervation for the treatment of spasmodic torticollis. Neurosurgery 1994;35:58–63.
[35] Tagliati M, Shils J, Sun C, et al. Deep brain stimulation for dystonia. Expert Rev Med Devices 2004;1:33–41.
[36] Waterston JA, Swash M, Watkins ES. Idiopathic dystonia and cervical spondylotic myelopathy. J Neurol Neurosurg Psychiatry 1989;52:1424–6.

CHAPTER 5

Cervical Radiculopathy

Ali Mostoufi, MD, FAAPMR, FAAPM

Synonyms

Radiculopathy, cervical region
Brachial neuritis or radiculitis

ICD-9 Code

723.4 Cervical radiculitis

ICD-10 Codes

M54.12 Cervical radiculitis
M54.13 Cervicothoracic radiculitis

Definition

Cervical radiculopathy is dysfunction of a cervical nerve root resulting in pain in the neck and arm with associated sensory, motor, and reflex abnormalities. Involvement of the ventral root of the spinal nerve results in motor weakness, and involvement of the dorsal root of the spinal nerve results in sensory deficits. Involvement of either root may result in reflex abnormality because the reflex arc comprises both (pertinent to C5, C6, and C7). In most cases, both the ventral and dorsal roots are affected, resulting in motor and sensory cervical radiculopathy.

Cervical radicular pain refers to neck pain radiating to the arm in a specific nerve root pattern, but it is not necessarily associated with loss of sensation, motor deficit, or reflex abnormality. A patient could experience radicular neck pain without abnormal physical examination findings that are characteristic of radiculopathy.

Cervical spine anatomy is complex (Fig. 5.1). There are seven cervical vertebrae (C1-C7). The C1 vertebra is ring shaped, and its lateral masses articulate with the occipital condyle of the skull. The vertebral body of C2 is marked by the cephalad extension of the dens, which is secured in place by the transverse ligament. There are six intervertebral discs (C2-C7) located anteriorly in between vertebral bodies of adjacent vertebrae. C2-C7 vertebrae articulate posterolaterally through facet joints, which are situated in the coronal plane with inferior angulations. C3-C7 vertebrae also have a unique articulation through the uncovertebral joint. There are eight pairs of cervical nerve roots. The names of the cervical nerves correspond to the vertebral body below the nerve, except C8. The C8 roots exit at the C7-T1 intervertebral foramen. The foramina are largest in the upper cervical spine and gradually narrow distally, with the C7-T1 foramen being the narrowest [1]. Cervical nerve roots exit through the inferior portion of the cervical intervertebral foramina [1]. The C1-C3 spinal nerves have dorsal innervations including suboccipital (C1), greater occipital (C2), and third occipital nerves (C3) [2]. The C1-C4 ventral primary rami form the cervical plexus, and the C5-C8 ventral primary rami contribute to the brachial plexus innervating the arm [3]. Each cervical intervertebral foramen is bordered posterolaterally by the zygapophyseal joint (facets), anteromedially by the uncovertebral joint, and inferiorly and superiorly by the pedicles of the adjacent vertebrae. Intervertebral discs are located anteriorly, and they separate vertebral bodies to lend height to the intervertebral foramina.

The most common radiculopathy is C7, followed by C6, C8, and C5 in descending order of incidence [4]. The most common reasons for cervical radiculopathy are posterolateral herniated disc (Fig. 5.2); narrowing of the neuroforamina due to facet spondylosis; hypertrophied uncinate process with neuroforaminal encroachment; and spondylolisthesis, with or without instability, narrowing adjacent neuroforamina. Less common causes include facet synovial cyst with encroachment of nerve root, extradural mass, spinal tumors, and abscess. Other medical conditions that resemble cervical radicular symptoms should be carefully ruled out as part of medical evaluation of neck and arm pain (Table 5.1). These include musculoskeletal, neurologic, and rheumatologic disorders.

Symptoms

The most common symptom of cervical radiculopathy is neck pain with associated unilateral arm pain in a specific

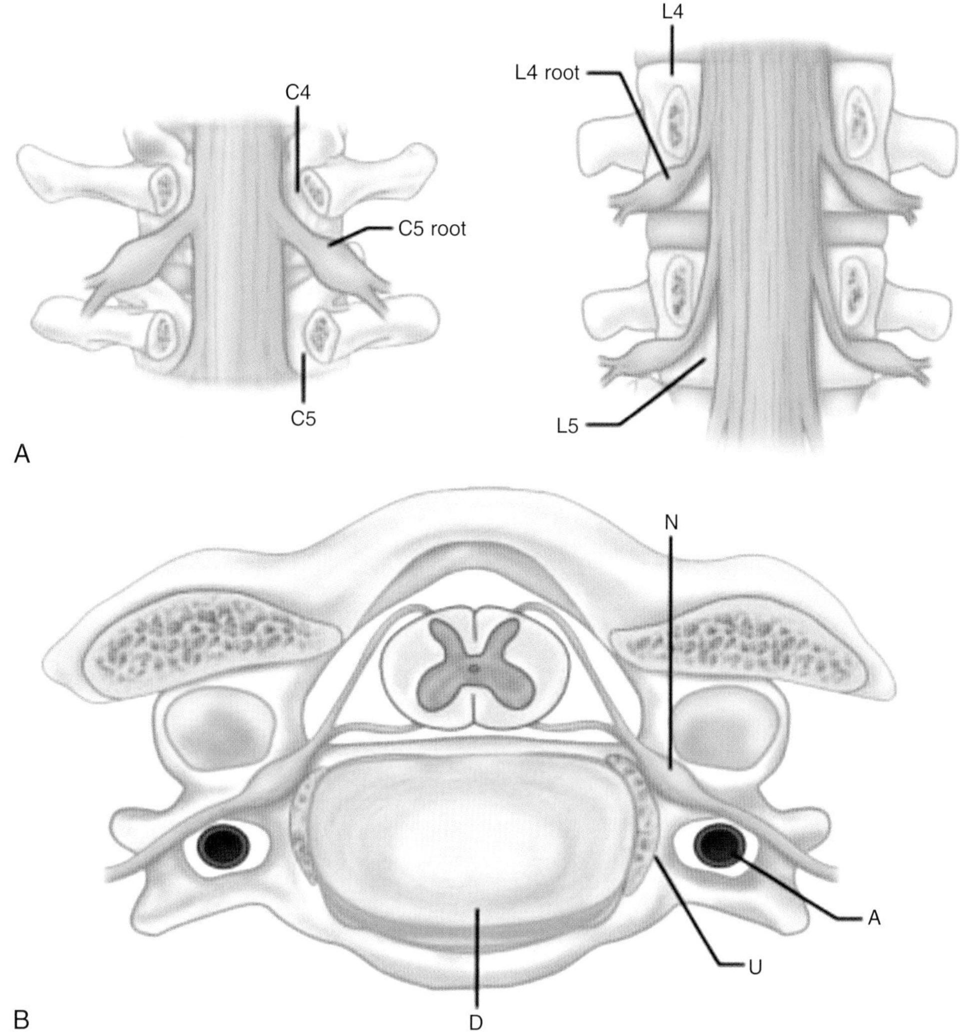

FIGURE 5.1 **A,** Comparison of points at which nerve roots emerge from cervical and lumbar spine. **B,** Cross-sectional view of cervical spine at level of disc (D). Uncinate process (U) forms ventral wall of foramen. Root (N) exits dorsal to vertebral artery (A). *(From Canale ST, Beaty JH, eds. Campbell's Operative Orthopaedics, 12th ed. St. Louis, Elsevier/Mosby, 2013.)*

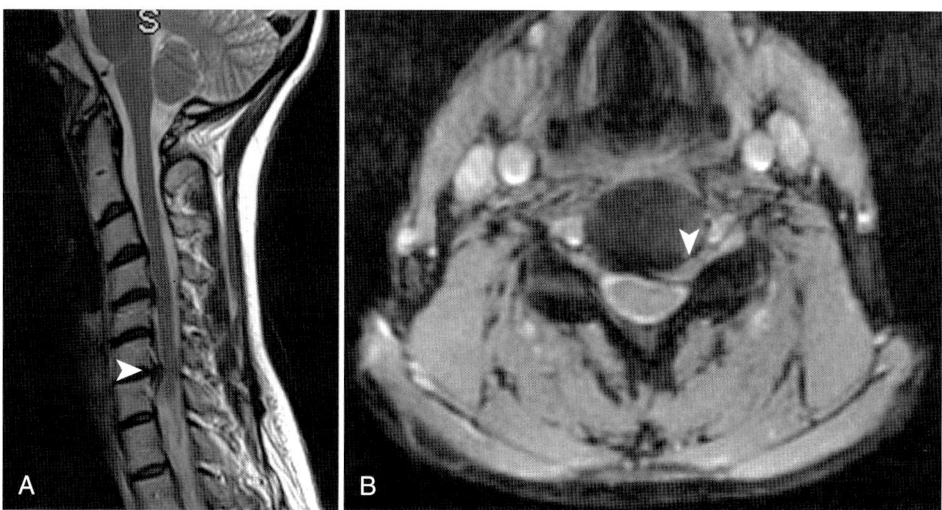

FIGURE 5.2 Sagittal (**A**) and axial (**B**) magnetic resonance images of left paracentral C6 herniated disc. Posterolateral herniated disc is the most common cause of cervical radicular pain. Traversing nerve root can be abutted, displaced, or compressed by the herniated segment, resulting in radicular pain and radiculopathy.

Table 5.1 Differential Diagnosis of Cervical Radiculopathy by System

Musculoskeletal	Tendinopathy, tenosynovitis, epicondylitis, bursitis Peripheral joint disease (shoulder, elbow, wrist, hand) Rotator cuff tear Glenoid labral defect (Bankart or SLAP lesion) Shoulder impingement syndrome Adhesive capsulitis
Neurologic	Peripheral neuropathy Peripheral entrapments Brachial plexus injury Syringomyelia Demyelinating disease Neuromuscular disease Complex regional pain syndrome
Infections	Lyme disease Herpes
Tumors	Pancoast tumor Spinal tumors (primary or metastatic)
Vascular	Thoracic outlet syndrome Aortic arch syndrome
Rheumatologic	Polymyalgia rheumatica Fibromyalgia Myofascial pain syndrome

SLAP, Superior labral tear from anterior to posterior.

nerve root pattern. Sensory complaints of numbness, tingling, burning, or electrical sensation follow a dermatomal pattern, and weakness follows the same anatomic-level myotomal pattern. Of the subjective complaints, the distribution of hand paresthesias appears to have the greatest localizing value [5]. Literature supports that suprascapular (C5-C6), interscapular (C7), and scapular (C8) pain suggests radiculopathy [6]. Symptoms can be aggravated by motion of the head toward the painful side, free hanging of the arm, lifting of heavier items, coughing, sneezing, and Valsalva maneuver. Pulling, pushing, and lifting of items are often not tolerated in the acute phase. Pain may improve when the head is tilted away from the painful side or if the affected arm is abducted over the head. Clumsiness, fine motor deficits, and mild grip weakness may precede gross weakness. Clinicians should routinely inquire about symptoms of myelopathy. Myelopathy symptoms are bilateral hand numbness or paresthesias, altered dexterity, poor balance, falls, and bowel or bladder dysfunction. These symptoms are not features of a discrete radiculopathy and should alert the clinician to rule out spinal cord compression.

Physical Examination

A complete musculoskeletal and neurologic examination is indicated in the evaluation of cervical radiculopathy. Special attention is needed to differentiate between objective findings compatible with radiculopathy and myelopathy signs. Physical examination needs to be expanded if other system involvement is suspected.

Visual Observation

Simple observation is a first step to proper diagnosis and treatment. A clinician's eyes should be trained to notice poor posture, body mechanics, spinal deformity, muscle atrophy, asymmetric gait, use of assistive devices, skin abnormalities, and nonverbal behaviors.

Gait Evaluation

Examination of gait is an important step in differentiating radicular neck pain from myelopathy. Gait should be normal in cervical radiculopathy and could be abnormal in cervical myelopathic patients.

Palpation

In patients with radiculopathy, ipsilateral tenderness and muscle spasm are common. The clinician should examine muscles for taut bands or tender points.

Range of Motion

Range of motion (ROM) of the cervical spine in all planes should be examined and deficits should be documented. Clinicians should carefully reevaluate ROM of the cervical spine to monitor progress in treatment. The normal cervical ROM is as follows: extension, 55 degrees; flexion, 45 degrees; lateral bending, 40 degrees; rotation, 75 degrees [7]. Among activities of daily living, backing up a car requires the most available range. Personal hygiene, such as hand washing, shaving, and applying makeup, necessitates a significantly greater cervical ROM relative to mobility activities of daily living, including walking and negotiating stairs [7].

Sensory Testing

Radiculopathy results in dermatomal sensory abnormality in the neck, shoulder girdle, and ipsilateral arm. On the basis of the specific dermatomal deficits, a clinician can localize the anatomic level of nerve root impingement. Light touch, pinprick, two-point discrimination, proprioception, and vibration sense should be tested in both the symptomatic and symptom-free arm. There is a degree of overlap between dermatomal innervations of the arm. To date, the International Standards for Neurological Classification of Spinal Cord Injury is the most standardized sensory testing guideline [8]. For consistent examination, the use of these guidelines is recommended to examine sensory function in the upper limb (Fig. 5.3).

Deep Tendon Reflexes

The most frequently tested reflexes in the upper limb are the biceps brachii (innervation C5/6, C5 primary), the brachioradialis (C5/6, C6 primary), and the triceps (C7 primary). Reflexes are tested bilaterally and compared. Hyporeflexia (diminished) or areflexia (complete absence) indicates involvement of the lower motor neuron, including the specific nerve root tested. Hyperreflexia (increased or brisk reflex) is an indication of central nervous system involvement. The response levels of deep tendon reflexes are graded 0 to 4+, with 2+ being normal (Table 5.2 and Fig. 5.4).

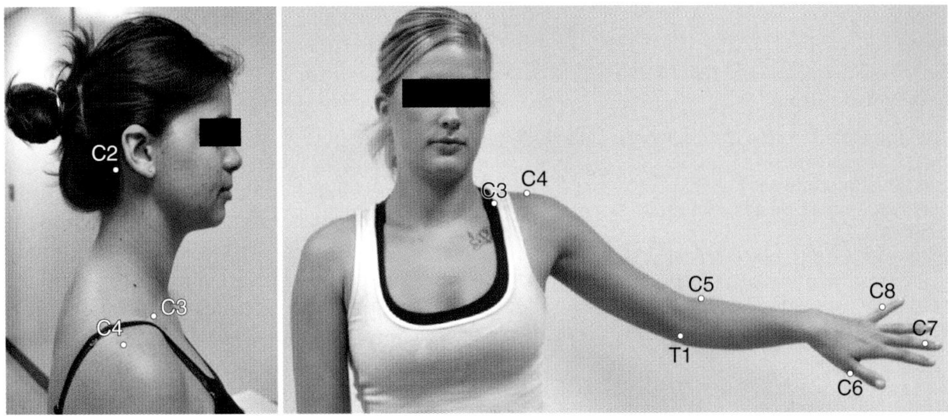

FIGURE 5.3 Key sensory points examination of the upper extremity.

Table 5.2 Muscle Group and Sensory Point Testing in Cervical Radiculopathy [8]: Upper Extremity Key Reflexes

Root	Reflex	Key Muscle Group (neck and arm)	Key Sensation Point
C2	Normal reflexes	Neck flexion	1 cm lateral to occipital protuberance
C3	Normal reflexes	Neck extension and lateral flexion	Supraclavicular fossa, mid-clavicle line
C4	Normal reflexes	Shoulder elevation	Skin over acromioclavicular joint
C5	Diminished biceps deep tendon reflex	Elbow flexor	Radial side of the antecubital fossa
C6	Diminished brachioradialis deep tendon reflex	Wrist extension	Dorsal surface, proximal phalanx of the thumb
C7	Diminished triceps deep tendon reflex	Elbow extension	Dorsal surface, proximal phalanx of the third digit
C8	Normal reflexes	Long finger flexors	Dorsal surface, proximal phalanx of the fifth digit

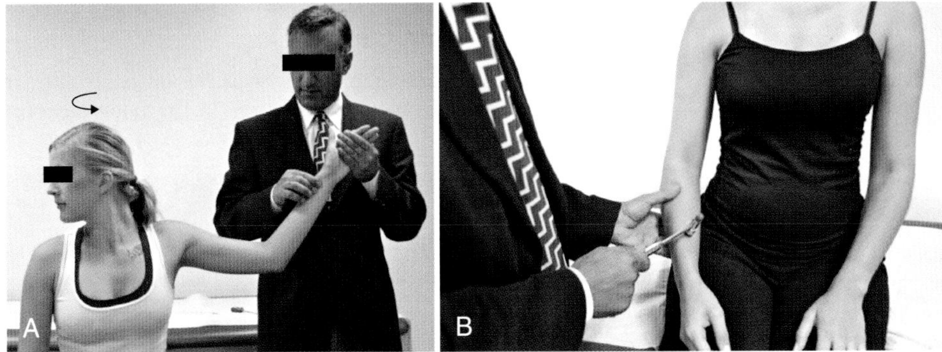

FIGURE 5.4 The Adson maneuver (**A**) tests for radial pulse obliteration and is a screening tool for thoracic outlet syndrome. The brachioradialis reflex is often diminished in C5-C6 radiculopathy (**B**).

Motor Testing

Subjective weakness in the upper limb is a common complaint in patients with radiculopathy. Patterns of weakness can help localize a lesion to a particular spinal cord level, nerve root, peripheral nerve, or muscle. Comparison of the strength of each muscle group with its contralateral counterpart allows the detection of any asymmetries. The degree of pain and the patient's effort can be limiting factors in the examination of muscle strength. Relevant to cervical radiculopathy, strength testing is often focused on muscles innervated by the C4-C8 nerve roots. The International Standards for Neurological Classification of Spinal Cord Injury has standardized and recommends testing of five key muscles in the upper limb: C5 elbow flexors, C6 wrist extensors, C7 elbow extensor, C8 long finger flexors, and T1 small finger abductor [8] (Table 5.3). Muscle strength is rated on a scale of 0/5 to 5/5. When weakness is detected in one of the key muscle groups, the clinician has to reexamine individual muscles in the arm to further localize the lesion (brachial plexus roots vs trunks vs divisions vs cord).

Joint Examination

Cervical facets can be examined by ROM testing and also by localized external pressure on them. These maneuvers may reproduce neck pain or head pain concordant with the patient's nonradicular complaint. Referred pain from facets

Table 5.3 Sample of Neck and Arm Muscles or Muscle Groups Innervated by Cervical Roots [3,33]

Root	Muscle or Muscle Group
C2	Sternocleidomastoid, rectus capitis, longus colli
C3	Trapezius, splenius capitis
C4	Trapezius, levator scapulae
C5	Elbow flexors, deltoid, biceps, supraspinatus, infraspinatus
C6	Wrist extensors, biceps, brachioradialis, supinator
C7	Elbow extensors, wrist flexors, triceps
C8	Flexor digitorum superficialis, thumb extensor and adductors, wrist ulnar deviators

to the shoulder girdle or scapular region may be confused with radicular pain of similar distribution. Careful examination of the shoulder as well as of the elbow and wrist is also important in differentiating radicular neck pain from other musculoskeletal causes of arm pain.

Special Maneuvers

The Spurling maneuver is a classic test used to identify nerve root irritation (Fig. 5.5). This test is a combination of ipsilateral tilt and forward flexion of the neck while the examiner exerts axial load. The modified Spurling test is a combination of ipsilateral rotation, extension, and axial compression of the head. Reproduction of the patient's radicular symptoms (distal to the shoulder) in either maneuver is considered a positive test result. Several studies have shown that the Spurling test has a low sensitivity (30%-40%), high specificity (80%-90%), and fair to good interexaminer reliability [9,10]. The Spurling test should be avoided if fracture or instability is suspected.

Clinicians should be familiar with the Adson and Roos tests in examining patients with neck and arm pain (see Fig. 5.4). Pain, weakness, and neurovascular deficits are associated with thoracic outlet syndrome, part of the differential diagnosis of cervical radiculopathy.

Lhermitte sign is a sudden painless electric shock–like sensation originating in the neck and spreading down the spine into the limbs when the patient's neck is flexed. This test was described in a 1924 publication by Lhermitte [11]. Although nonspecific, it is most commonly seen in multiple sclerosis as well as in myelopathy due cervical spondylosis, spinal cord tumors, epidural bleed, and postirradiation therapy.

The neck distraction sign and shoulder abduction test can also determine nerve root irritation [10]. Babinski response, Hoffmann sign, and clonus are also part of the examination of the patient with cervical radiculopathy and may suggest involvement of the central nervous system.

Functional Limitations

Pain commonly interferes with sleep, work, or social activities. With restriction in ROM, driving, overhead activity, and reading may be difficult. Desktop computer work and use of tablet computer and smartphone may result in increased pain. Loss of sensation in the fingers may negatively affect individuals who rely on tactile function for their work. Grip weakness may lead to dropping of items, and proximal muscle weakness will affect the ability to carry items or to pull and push objects. Patients with failed medical and surgical treatments often experience permanent impairment resulting in chronic disabilities.

Diagnostic Studies

Radiography

Radiography is seen as the initial imaging modality to evaluate anatomic changes in the bone structure of the cervical

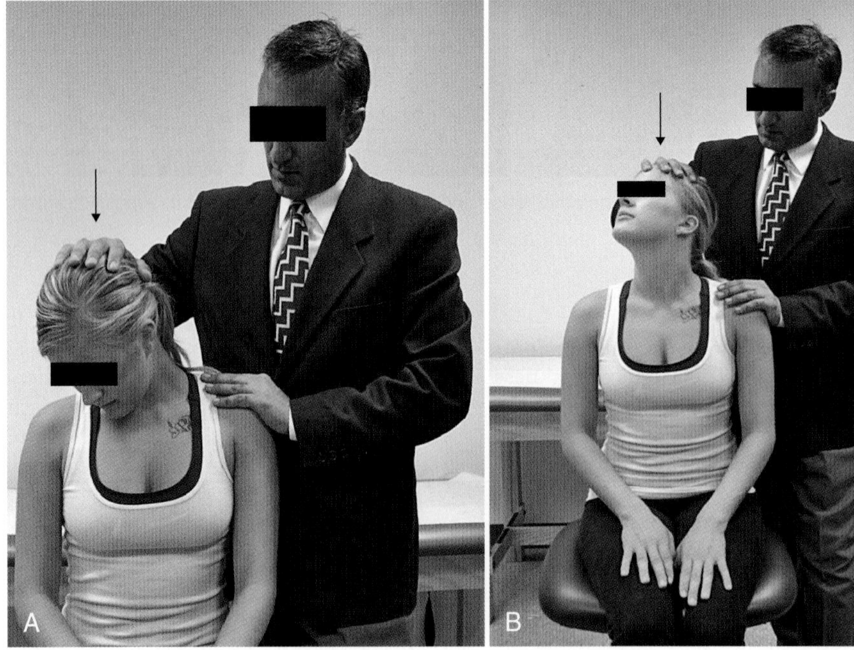

FIGURE 5.5 The Spurling maneuver (**A**) and the modified Spurling maneuver (**B**) test for cervical root irritation. A positive test result is the reproduction of pain and paresthesia in the arm.

spine. It is sensitive to evaluate fractures, misalignment, spondylolisthesis, facet arthrosis, and disc space narrowing. It can identify instability of the cervical spine by means of dynamic and open mouth views. Although it is often used in urgent care settings for patients with radicular pain, apart from showing the bone narrowing of the neuroforamina and disc space narrowing, it is of little value.

Computed Tomography

Computed tomography (CT) provides exquisite depiction of bone detail of the cervical spine. It is particularly useful in and is considered a primary imaging evaluation for acute spine trauma in adults [12]. It is an excellent modality in multitrauma workup of fractures (C1, C2, and distal cervical segments) and possible bleeding in or around the spinal canal. Because it is a cross-sectional imaging technique, it is able to identify bone narrowing of the central canal and neuroforamina and thickening of the ligamentum flavum. CT is the modality of choice in patients with implanted pacemakers and other devices that do not allow the use of magnetic resonance imaging (MRI). CT with axial and coronal reconstruction is used to identify proper fusion of the adjacent vertebrae after spinal fusion surgery. CT myelography has some indications in complex surgical revisions or postsurgical cases with persistent arm symptoms. CT is used after discography is performed to better visualize internal disc derangements, including radial tears. CT is also used in the workup of possible infection, as in spinal abscess.

Magnetic Resonance Imaging

Compared with CT, MRI is a clinically superior diagnostic test in the evaluation of patients with suspected disc herniation. It should be the diagnostic study of choice when it is available.

MRI is the "gold standard" imaging study for patients with radicular symptoms. It can clearly identify soft tissue abnormalities, including the cord, muscles, and ligaments. With axial images, clinicians can gauge the caliber of the spinal canal and the neuroforamina. With T1- and T2-weighted images, signal abnormality within the spinal cord substance (myelomalacia) and bone marrow can also be evaluated. Acuity of cervical spine fractures as well as primary or metastatic tumors of the spinal column can be assessed by this imaging modality. MRI before and after the administration of a contrast agent is necessary to define certain conditions like cancerous lesions and postsurgical scarring. In workup of a possible infection, MRI can help identify soft tissue signal abnormality, local fluid collection, osteomyelitis, discitis, and abscess formation. Interpretation of the MRI study is difficult after spinal instrumentation because of metallic artifact. In such cases, CT becomes the imaging of choice.

Bone Scan

The utility of the bone scan in spine care is limited to spondylolysis, infection, and metastatic or primary spinal tumors.

Electrodiagnosis

Nerve conduction studies and electromyography are considered an extension of the physical examination. In patients with clear cervical radicular symptoms, supportive MRI, and concordant examination findings, there is no indication for electrodiagnosis. Nerve conduction studies and electromyography can be useful if there is clinical suspicion of peripheral neuropathy or peripheral entrapment that is manifested with symptoms similar to cervical radicular pain. Electromyography can be an additional tool in those cases in which symptoms, physical examination findings, and imaging results are not concordant [13].

Myelography

Before the advent of MRI, myelography was a useful test to examine the caliber of the central canal and intervertebral foramen and possible compression on the nerve root. Its use is currently limited to complex postsurgical cases, surgical revisions, and evaluation of spinal tumors.

Diagnostic Spinal Injections

Fluoroscopically guided contrast-enhanced procedures can deliver medications to a desired target. In complex cases in which multilevel degenerative changes are seen and there is a question of which segment is contributing to the arm pain, spine surgeons may ask for a diagnostic selective nerve root injection. The degree of pain relief within the half-life of the injected anesthetic can provide valuable preoperative information to the surgeon and increase the likelihood of successful surgical treatment. The evidence for selective nerve root blocks in the preoperative evaluation of patients with normal or inconclusive imaging studies is moderate [14].

Provocative discography has been used to diagnose discogenic axial pain. For cervical discogenic pain, discography has a level II-2 support (U.S. Preventive Services Task Force classification, evidence obtained from well-designed cohort or case-control analytic studies, preferably from more than one center or research group) [15]. Complications associated with cervical discography because of the surrounding anatomy include injury to the trachea, esophagus, carotid artery, and jugular veins; nerve root or spinal cord injury; and pneumothorax [3]. The potential complication of discitis is also of concern in considering diagnostic discography [3]. Because there are no well-designed studies to support cervical discography as a diagnostic tool for discogenic neck pain, such a procedure should be considered with utmost caution.

Treatment

Initial

With conservative care, 70% to 80% of patients with cervical radicular symptoms improve [16]. Pain reduction and patient education are important initial goals. For the acute phase, one can consider the use of ice as well as passive treatment consisting of semihard cervical collar immobilization and rest from activities that aggravate the condition. Nonsteroidal anti-inflammatory drugs, muscle relaxants, and, at times, short tapering doses of an oral steroid can be the initial recommended medication treatment for most patients. Stronger pain medications are indicated on the basis of the severity of the pain. In some cases, adjunct medication like anticonvulsants, tricyclic antidepressants, or selective norepinephrine reuptake inhibitors may be used.

Timely involvement of a physical therapist appears beneficial. Manual therapy techniques in conjunction with therapeutic exercise are effective in increasing function, improving active ROM, and decreasing pain and disability [17]. The scientific literature supports the use of cervical traction for management of pain as well as improvement in function and strength in patients with cervical radiculopathy [18,19]. Acupuncture and massage can help reduce muscle tension and pain. There is moderate quality evidence that spinal manipulation is effective for the treatment of acute radiculopathy [20]. It is the responsibility of health care providers to educate patients about their condition and to suggest ways to prevent worsening and recurrence of the symptoms by activity modification, appropriate body mechanics (neutral spine), proper lifting techniques, suitable pillow and mattress use, and appropriate exercises.

Rehabilitation

In the management of cervical radicular pain, early involvement of physical and occupational therapy services is encouraged. The rehabilitation program should focus on reduction of muscle spasm, improvement in ROM, and improvement of muscle strength. Cervical stabilization, stretching (passive and active), static strengthening, and progressive resistive exercises are incorporated in the rehabilitation phase and should be transitioned to a home exercise program [21]. Thermal modalities, manual traction, and transcutaneous electrical nerve stimulation are often used by physiotherapists for temporary pain reduction during this phase. Interventional procedures and medications can reduce pain and increase the patient's compliance with rehabilitation. Within the framework of rehabilitation, the patient is educated on body mechanics, proper desk ergonomics, and use of adaptive equipment (e.g., book stand, hands-free phone or headset, and document holder).

Procedures

Interlaminar Epidural Steroid Injections

Cervical epidural steroid injection is indicated in persistent painful cervical radiculopathy despite appropriate initial medical and rehabilitation treatments. In the hands of trained physicians, when it is done with image guidance, it is a safe and effective treatment. On the basis of a systematic review of the literature, the evidence for treatment of cervical radicular pain with interlaminar epidural steroid injection is good [22,23]. There is no indication for performing these injections in a series.

Selective Nerve Root Block

Cervical selective nerve root block is a diagnostic procedure. If a patient has substantial decrease in pain with image-guided contrast-enhanced injection of anesthetics at a specific nerve root, the clinician can consider that specific nerve root to be the main cause of arm pain. Surgeons use such information to plan for surgical management of radiculopathy [24]. Selectivity of such injection is lost if there is epidural spread of the injectate. Some interventional practitioners use particulate steroids when performing a selective nerve root block to treat cervical radicular pain. Given the probability of vascular injection of steroid in this technique and potential catastrophic complications (brain and spinal cord infarction), clinicians should carefully gauge the benefit versus risk when choosing transforaminal epidural injection as a treatment for their patients [25,26]. Use of digital subtraction imaging and nonparticulate steroids is encouraged. Like all interventions, this procedure should be done by fellowship-trained physicians.

Surgery

Progressive neurologic deficit, development of myelopathy, and failed conservative care are indications for spinal surgery. Surgical intervention has been shown to provide faster improvement in pain, sensory disturbance, and muscle strength at 3 months postoperatively than conservative treatment [27]. It is not clear from the evidence that long-term outcomes are improved with the surgical treatment of cervical radiculopathy compared with nonsurgical measures [28]. It is not evident that one open surgical technique is clearly superior to others for radiculopathy [28]. Decision-making for discectomy alone or discectomy and fusion with or without foraminotomy is affected by the degree of anatomic change, previous spine surgery, existence of instability, coexisting spondylolisthesis, amount of neck pain in addition to arm pain, and preference of the surgeon. Fusion can be achieved anteriorly (anterior cervical discectomy and fusion) (Fig. 5.6) or posteriorly (posterior cervical fusion). Disc arthroplasty is a newer technique for management of cervical disc diseases; it maintains segmental height and motion. These devices have been shown to have efficacy similar to that of anterior cervical discectomy and fusion [29].

Potential Disease Complications

Possible complications of cervical radiculopathy are persistent or progressive neurologic weakness, residual neck or radicular pain, chronic pain syndrome, disability, and myelopathy (rare, usually associated with spondylosis or large central disc herniation).

Potential Treatment Complications

Medications used to treat cervical radiculopathy can result in class-specific side effects. Nonsteroidal anti-inflammatory drugs commonly have gastrointestinal and renal side effects. Muscle relaxants, selective norepinephrine reuptake inhibitors, and tricyclics can cause central nervous system suppression. Steroids result in endocrine side effects, including hyperglycemia, hypothalamus-pituitary-adrenal axis impact, and amenorrhea. Narcotics can cause nausea, constipation, respiratory suppression, mental status changes, and suppression of endogenous opioids; dependence, tolerance, and abuse may also result.

Manipulation may exacerbate symptoms. Although rare, progressive weakness, carotid dissection, and recurrence of herniation have been reported in connection with cervical spine manipulation [30].

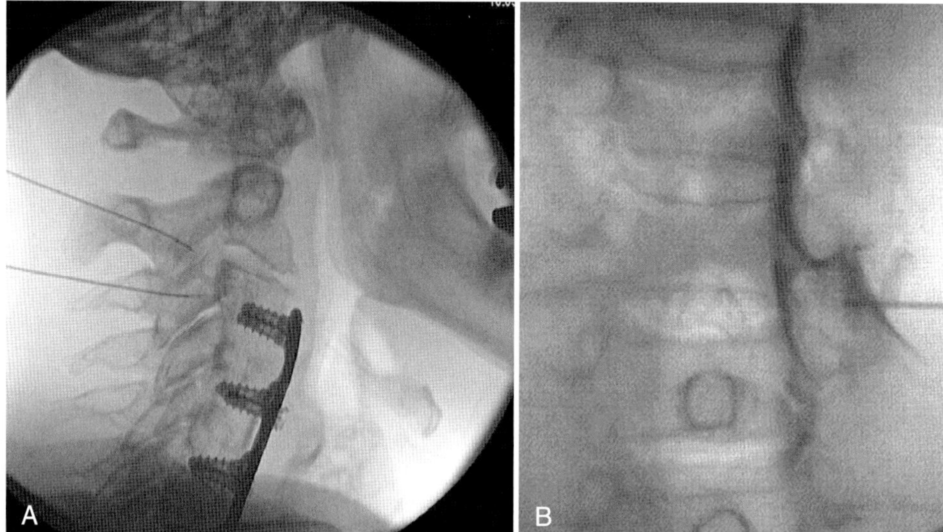

FIGURE 5.6 **A,** C3-C6 anterior cervical discectomy and fusion hardware on standard lateral fluoroscopic view (needles placed for treatment of facetogenic headache). **B,** Transforaminal needle placement in cervical spine and injection of contrast material confirm flow along the descending C6 nerve root sleeve and ipsilateral epidural gutter.

Interventional injections may result in transient increased pain, facial flushing, hyperglycemia, allergic reaction to injectate, and vasovagal reaction. Vasovagal reaction is the most common minor complication [31]. Infection, nerve injury, vascular insult, epidural hematoma, and spinal cord injury are rare but more serious complications that may occur after such invasive procedures. Experienced interventionalists can limit such complications by exercising sterile technique, performing image-guided contrast-enhanced procedures, and withholding anticoagulants and antiplatelets before elective procedures. Cervical transforaminal steroid injection carries the additional risk of vascular injection of steroid, which may lead to brain and spinal cord infarction due to the embolic phenomenon of particulate steroids [26]. Use of digital subtraction imaging and nonparticulate steroids may reduce such risk [32]. Interventional spine procedures should be performed only by fellowship-trained physicians specifically trained in such procedures.

Acknowledgment

The author would like to acknowledge Dr. Asif Jillani for his assistance with this chapter.

References

[1] Caridi J, Pumberger M, Hughes A. Cervical radiculopathy: a review. HSS J 2011;7:265–72.

[2] O'Rahilley, Müller F, Carpenter S, Swenson R. Muscles, vessels, nerves and joints of the back. Basic human anatomy: a regional study of human structure [online]. Dartmouth Medical School; 2008. Available at, www.dartmouth.edu/~humananatomy/.

[3] Gardocki RJ, Park AL. Lower back pain and disorders of intervertebral disc. In: Canale ST, Beaty JH, editors. Campbell's operative orthopaedics. 12th ed. St. Louis: Elsevier/Mosby; 2013. p. 1918.

[4] Radhakrishan K, Litchy WJ, O'Fallon WM, et al. Epidemiology of cervical radiculopathy: a population-based study from Rochester, Minnesota, 1976 through 1990. Brain 1994;117:325–35.

[5] Yoss RE, Corbin KB, MacCarty CS, et al. Recent data on significance of symptoms and signs in localization of involved root in cervical disc protrusion. Neurology 1957;7:673–83.

[6] Tanaka Y, Kokubun S, Sato T, Ozawa H. Cervical roots as origin of pain in the neck or scapular regions. Spine (Phila Pa 1976) 2006;31:E568–73.

[7] Murphey F, Simmons JCH, Brunson B. Ruptured cervical discs 1939-1972. Clin Neurosurg 1973;20:9–17.

[8] Kirshblum SC, Burns SP, Biering-Sorensen F, et al. International standards for neurological classification of spinal cord injury. J Spinal Cord Med 2011;34:535–46.

[9] Tong HC, Haig AJ, Yamakawa K. The spurling test and cervical radiculopathy. Spine (Phila Pa 1976) 2002;27:156–9.

[10] Malanga GA, Landes P, Nadler SF. Provocative tests in cervical spine examination: historical basis and scientific analyses. Pain Physician 2003;6:199–205.

[11] Lhermitte JJ, Bollak NM. Les douleurs à type décharge électrique consécutives à la flexion céphalique dans la sclérose en plaques. Un cas de la sclérose multiple. Rev Neurol 1924;2:56–7.

[12] American College of Radiology (ACR), American Society of Neuroradiology (ASNR), American Society of Spine Radiology (ASSR), and the Society for Pediatric Radiology (SPR). ACR-ASNR-ASSR-SPR practice guideline for the performance of computed tomography (CT) of the spine, revised 2011 (Resolution 34). Available at http://www.acr.org/~/media/03586F4164384C6C995E83CE68A5C835.pdf.

[13] Nardin RA, Patel MR, Gudas TF, et al. Electromyography and magnetic resonance imaging in the evaluation of radiculopathy. Muscle Nerve 1999;22:151–5.

[14] Boswell MV, Shah RV, Everett CR, et al. Interventional techniques in the management of chronic spinal pain: evidence-based practice guidelines. Pain Physician 2005;8:1–47.

[15] Manchikanti L, Dunbar EE, Wargo BW, et al. Systematic review of cervical discography as a diagnostic test for chronic spinal pain. Pain Physician 2009;12:305–21.

[16] Sampath P, Bendebba M, Davis JD, et al. Outcome in patients with cervical radiculopathy: prospective, multicenter study with independent clinical review. Spine (Phila Pa 1976) 1999;24:591–7.

[17] Boyles R, Toy P, Mellon J, Hayes M. Effectiveness of manual physical therapy in the treatment of cervical radiculopathy: a systematic review. J Man Manip Ther 2011;19:135–42.

[18] Olivero WC, Dulebohn SC. Results of halter cervical traction for the treatment of cervical radiculopathy: retrospective review of 81 patients. Neurosurg Focus 2002;12:ECP1.

[19] Joghataei MT, Arab AM, Khaksar H. The effect of cervical traction combined with conventional therapy on grip strength on patients with cervical radiculopathy (randomized controlled study). Clin Rehabil 2004;18:879–87.

[20] Leininger B, Bronfort G, Evans R, Reiter T. Spinal manipulation or mobilization for radiculopathy: a systematic review. Phys Med Rehabil Clin N Am 2011;22:105–25.

[21] Wolff MW, Levine LA. Cervical radiculopathies: conservative approaches to management. Phys Med Rehabil Clin N Am 2002;13:589–608.
[22] Benyamin RM, Singh V, Parr AT, et al. Systematic review of the effectiveness of cervical epidurals in the management of chronic neck pain. Pain Physician 2009;12:137–57.
[23] Abdi S, Datta S, Trescot AM, et al. Epidural steroids in the management of chronic spinal pain: a systematic review. Pain Physician 2007;10:185–212.
[24] Anderberg L, Annertz M, Rydholm U, et al. Selective diagnostic nerve root block for the evaluation of radicular pain in the multilevel degenerated cervical spine. Eur Spine J 2006;15:794–801.
[25] Baker R, Dreyfuss P, Mercer S, Bogduk N. Cervical transforaminal injection of corticosteroids into a radicular artery: a possible mechanism for spinal cord injury. Pain 2002;103:211–5.
[26] Malhotra G, Abbasi A, Rhee M. Complications of transforaminal cervical epidural steroid injections. Spine (Phila Pa 1976) 2009;34:731–9.
[27] Persson LC, Moritz U, Brandt L. Cervical radiculopathy: pain, muscle weakness and sensory loss in patients with cervical radiculopathy treated with surgery, physiotherapy or cervical collar. A prospective, controlled study. Eur Spine J 1997;6:256–66.
[28] Nordin M, Carragee EJ, Hogg-Johnson S, et al, Bone and Joint Decade 2000-2010 Task Force on Neck Pain and Its Associated Disorders. Treatment of neck pain: injections and surgical interventions. Spine (Phila Pa 1976) 2008;33:S101–22.
[29] Coric D, Nunley PD, Guyer RD, et al. Prospective, randomized, multicenter study of cervical arthroplasty: 269 patients from the Kineflex|C artificial disc investigational device exemption study with a minimum 2-year follow-up. J Neurosurg Spine 2011;15:348–58.
[30] Parenti G, Orlandi G, Bianchi M. Vertebral and carotid artery dissection following chiropractic cervical manipulation. Neurosurg Rev 1999;22:127–9.
[31] Pobiel RS, Schellhas KP, Eklund JA, et al. Selective cervical nerve root blockade: prospective study of immediate and longer term complications. AJNR Am J Neuroradiol 2009;30:507–11.
[32] McLean JP. The rate of detection of intravascular injection in cervical transforaminal epidural steroid injections with and without digital subtraction angiography. PM R 2009;1:636–42.
[33] Gray's Anatomy of the Human Body [online version]. Available at Bartleby.com.

CHAPTER 6

Cervical Sprain or Strain

Larry V. Najera III, MD
Joseph T. Alleva, MD, MBA
Nathan Mohr, BA
Andrea K. Origenes
Thomas H. Hudgins, MD

Synonyms

None

ICD-9 Codes

723.1 Cervicalgia
723.3 Cervical pain

ICD-10 Codes

M54.2 Cervicalgia
M60.9 Myositis, unspecified
M79.1 Myalgia
S13.4 Whiplash injury (cervical spine)
S13.9 Neck sprain, unspecified parts of the neck
S16.1 Neck strain
S23.3 Thoracic sprain
S39.012 Back strain
Add additional character for type of encounter for categories S13, S16, S23, and S39: A—initial encounter, D—subsequent encounter, S—sequela

Definition

Cervical sprain or strain typically refers to acute pain arising from injured soft tissues of the neck, including muscles, tendons, and ligaments. The most common event leading to such injuries is motor vehicle collision. The mechanism of injury is complex. During a rear-end motor vehicle collision, the initial head and neck acceleration lags behind vehicular acceleration. Eventually, head and neck acceleration reaches up to 2½ times the maximum car acceleration, which subsequently results in dramatic deceleration at end range of motion of the neck [1,2]. Whereas such injury can also result in fracture, disc, or neurologic injury, cervical strain or sprain, by definition, excludes these entities.

Although these other entities need to be excluded from the differential diagnosis, recent evidence implicates the zygapophyseal joints as a source of neck pain after whiplash injury. Specifically, in a randomized controlled trial in which the medial branches of the cervical dorsal rami were blocked with local anesthetic or treated with saline, it was shown that 60% of patients with whiplash injury had complete neck pain relief after injection of local anesthetic compared with no relief by injection of placebo [3].

Many factors have been associated with worse outcome in acceleration-deceleration injuries involving motor vehicles. Older women tend to have a worse prognosis than that of younger women and men in general. In addition, poor education and a history of prior neck pain are prognostic factors for worse pain in women. Low family income, history of prior neck pain, and lack of awareness of head position in the crash arc associated with a poor prognosis in men [4]. Additional crash-related factors associated with a worse outcome include occupancy in a truck, being a passenger, colliding with a moving object, and getting hit head-on or perpendicularly [5]. A high intensity of neck pain, a decreased onset of latency of the initial pain, and radicular symptoms are also prognostic of worse outcomes [6]. Because many of these injuries result in initiation of litigation by patients, this too is a poor prognostic indicator.

Other causes include sleeping in awkward positions, lifting or pulling heavy objects, and repetitive motions involving the head and neck.

Estimates exist that 1 million whiplash injuries each year are due to motor vehicle collisions. The annual incidence varies worldwide, but in North America and western Europe, the incidence is likely to be at least 300 per 100,000 inhabitants [6].

Symptoms

The most common presentation of patients with cervical strain or sprain is nonradiating neck pain (Fig. 6.1). Patients will also complain of neck stiffness, fatigue, and worsening of symptoms with cervical range of motion. The pain often extends into the trapezius region or interscapular region. Headache, probably the most common associated symptom, originates in the occiput region and radiates frontally. Increased irritability and sleep disturbances are common. Paresthesias, radiating arm pain, dysphagia, visual symptoms, auditory symptoms, and dizziness may be reported [7,8]. Whereas an isolated cervical sprain or strain injury should be without these symptoms, there is the possibility of concomitant neurologic or bone injury. If these symptoms are present, alternative diagnoses should be suspected. Myelopathic symptoms, such as bowel and bladder dysfunction, which suggest a different diagnosis that is more serious, must be investigated.

Physical Examination

The primary finding in a cervical sprain or strain injury is decreased or painful cervical range of motion. This may be accompanied by tenderness of the cervical paraspinal, trapezius, occiput, or anterior cervical (i.e., sternocleidomastoid) muscles (Fig. 6.2).

A thorough neurologic examination should be performed to rule out myelopathic or radicular processes. In an isolated cervical sprain injury, the neurologic examination findings should be normal.

The result of the neurocompression test, in which the patient is asked to rotate and extend the head, thereby reducing the neuroforaminal space, should be negative with cases of cervical sprain or strain.

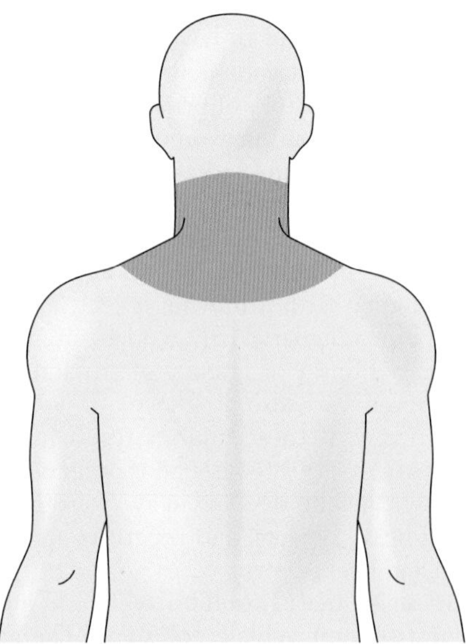

FIGURE 6.1 Typical pain distribution for a patient with an acute cervical sprain or strain injury.

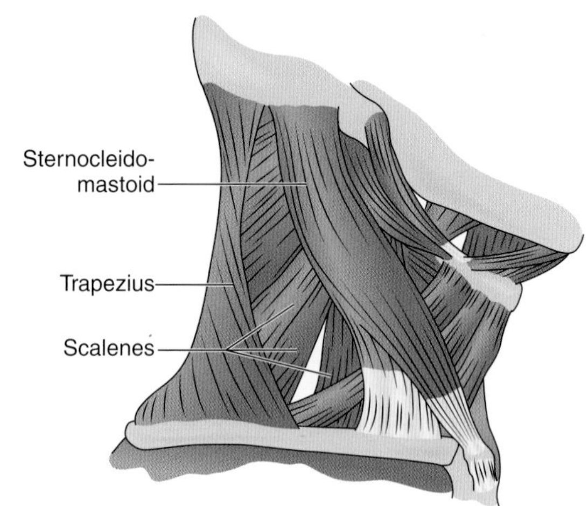

FIGURE 6.2 Muscles commonly involved in a cervical sprain or strain injury.

Functional Limitations

Restricted range of motion of the cervical spine may contribute to difficulty with daily activities, such as driving. Patients often complain of neck fatigue, heaviness, and pain with static cervical positions, such as reading and working at the computer. Sleep may be affected as well.

Diagnostic Studies

It is generally accepted that radiographs to exclude fracture should be obtained in patients involved in a traumatic event and who have altered consciousness, are intoxicated, or exhibit cervical tenderness and focal neurologic signs with decreased range of motion on physical examination [9]. Although the clinician may commonly see straightening of the cervical lordosis on the lateral cervical radiograph, this is thought to be related to spasm of the paracervical musculature and bears no other significance (Fig. 6.3).

Studies such as magnetic resonance imaging scans, computed tomographic scans, and electrodiagnostics are typically used to rule out alternative or coexisting entities.

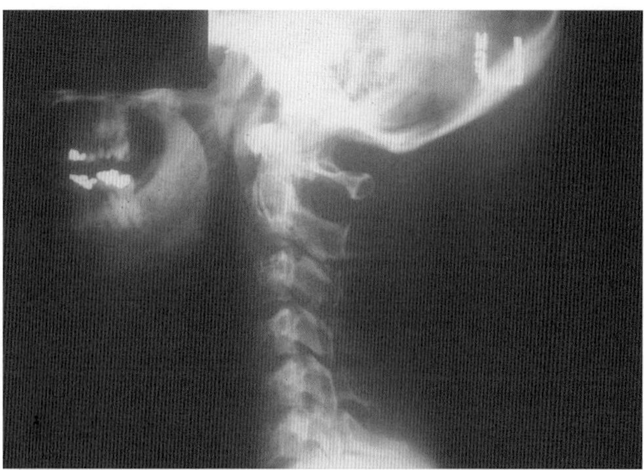

FIGURE 6.3 Cervical spine radiograph showing straightening of the spine and loss of the normal cervical lordosis.

All of these studies will have normal findings in cases of cervical sprain or strain.

Differential Diagnosis

Occult cervical fracture or dislocation
Cervical discogenic pain
Cervical herniated disc, radiculopathy
Cervical facet syndrome
Cervical spine tumor
Cervical spine infection

Treatment

Initial

Initial interventions used in patients with cervical sprain or strain have not been fully scientifically tested. Education of the patient is essential to minimize iatrogenic disability and cost of health care resources [10], and it is critical for a realistic expectation of resolution of symptoms. In most cases, symptoms will resolve within 4 to 6 weeks. In some cases, however, resolution of symptoms may be delayed up to 6 months.

It is reasonable to recommend relative rest within the first 24 hours of injury. The detriments of prolonged bed rest and the use of cervical collars have been clearly described, and these "treatments" may, in fact, promote disability [11]. The short-term use of nonsteroidal anti-inflammatory drugs, muscle relaxants, and analgesic medications on a judicious basis is accepted to promote early return to activity [12]. Muscle relaxants or low-dose tricyclic antidepressants (nortriptyline or amitriptyline, beginning with 10 to 25 mg at bedtime) are also used to help restore sleep in the patient for whom this is an issue. However, in the acute period, the addition of cyclobenzaprine to ibuprofen did not provide any added benefit in terms of improving pain scores [13].

High-dose intravenous methylprednisolone within 8 hours of the whiplash injury has been studied and was shown to be associated with decreased pain at 1 week after injury and fewer total sick days taken at 6 months. However, larger trials are needed to further evaluate the cost-benefit ratio for this treatment [14].

Rehabilitation

No rehabilitation approach has been proved unequivocally effective, although early mobilization and return to function is the key to successful rehabilitation. An early course of mobilization combined with home exercise in the acute phase of recovery is effective in minimizing disability. Cervical manipulation, massage, and mobilization on a limited basis are geared toward correction of segmental restrictions and restoration of normal range of motion. Such approaches have been shown to be more effective than passive modalities with regard to range of motion and reduction of pain [15]. Therapeutic modalities such as ultrasound and electrical stimulation can be tried for pain control but have no proven efficacy for long-term recovery. In addition, cervical traction done either manually (by a physical therapist) or with a mechanical unit (prescribed for home use) may be tried if there are no contraindications (i.e., fracture). Educational videos that make recommendations about posture, return to activity, exercise, and pain relief methods may help reduce rates of persistent symptoms at 6 months after injury [16].

Strengthening and stretching exercises for muscles with a tendency for tightness should be used in conjunction with the aforementioned techniques. Muscle imbalances must be addressed, and weak muscle groups such as the scapular stabilizers (middle-lower trapezius, serratus anterior, and levator scapulae) should be strengthened. This is typically done after muscles with a tendency for tightness (upper trapezius, sternocleidomastoid, scalenes, latissimus dorsi, and pectoralis major and minor) are stretched [17]. Cumulative data suggest that such an approach to cervical sprain injuries produces both long- and short-term benefits [9]. The overall treatment goal is to achieve an independent, customized home exercise program so that the patient can become active in his or her treatment [17]. An exercise protocol targeting shoulder and neck muscle strength and endurance was effective in decreasing chronic neck pain and disability in 180 female police officers [18].

Evaluation of the home or work environment by an occupational therapist can also be of benefit. Specifically, ergonomic alterations, such as the use of a telephone headrest and document holders, may aid in recovery.

Procedures

Trigger point injections are a reasonable adjunct to decrease pain so that patients may participate in physical therapy. A meta-analysis in 2010 stated that lidocaine injections into myofascial trigger points appear to be effective [19]. The upper trapezius, scalenes, and semispinalis capitis are the most common muscles to develop trigger points after acceleration-deceleration injuries. Other trigger points tend to arise in the splenius capitis, longus capitis, and longus colli after such injuries [20].

Botulinum toxin injections were initially thought to be effective for chronic cervical pain causing headaches [21]; however, there is more recent evidence that botulinum toxin A is not superior to saline injection for chronic mechanical neck pain [19].

Facet injections, epidural injections, and cervical traction may be instituted for conditions such as cervical radiculopathy and facet syndrome.

Surgery

Surgery is not indicated.

Potential Disease Complications

Similar to other grade I soft tissue strains, this injury will heal within 6 weeks. As such, there are no significant complications because this is not a permanent injury. There is research to suggest that the initial level of pain and degree of loss of cervical spine range of motion directly correlate with a poorer prognosis [22]. In addition, older age, lower educational achievement, part-time employment, preexisting neck or low back pain, and previous whiplash injury are associated with a significantly worse outcome. Of note, continuing litigation is associated with more severe pain [23].

Potential Treatment Complications

Analgesics and nonsteroidal anti-inflammatory drugs have well-known side effects that most commonly affect the gastric, hepatic, and renal systems. Muscle relaxants and low-dose tricyclic antidepressants can cause sedation. Overly aggressive manipulation or manipulation done when there is a concomitant unidentified injury (i.e., fracture) may result in serious injury. Injections are rarely associated with infection and allergic reactions to the medications used.

Interestingly, there is a correlation between the patient's perception of the severity of the initial injury and the expectations for recovery [24]. It is for that reason that patient education is a significant focus in the treatment of cervical strain, and therefore lack of education may have negative effects. Thus far, a meta-analysis in 2012 has not shown scientifically that education is truly beneficial [25].

References

[1] Bogduk N. The anatomy and pathophysiology of whiplash. Clin Biomech 1986;1:92–100.

[2] Stovner L. The nosologic status of the whiplash syndrome: a critical review based on methodological approach. Spine (Phila Pa 1976) 1996;21:2735–46.

[3] Lord SM, Barnsley L, Wallis BJ, Bogduk N. Chronic cervical zygapophysial joint pain after whiplash. A placebo-controlled prevalence study. Spine (Phila Pa 1976) 1996;21:1737–44.

[4] Holm LW, Carroll LJ, Cassidy JD, Ahlbom A. Factors influencing neck pain intensity in whiplash-associated disorders. Spine (Phila Pa 1976) 2006;31:E98–104.

[5] Harder S, Veilleux M, Suissa S. The effect of socio-demographic and crash-related factors on the prognosis of whiplash. J Clin Epidemiol 1998;51:377–84.

[6] Holm LW, Carroll LJ, Cassidy JD, et al. The burden and determinants of neck pain in whiplash-associated disorders after traffic collisions. Spine (Phila Pa 1976) 2008;33(Suppl):S52–9.

[7] Radanov B, Sturzenegger M. Long-term outcome after whiplash injury. A 2-year follow-up considering features of injury mechanism and somatic, radiologic, and psychosocial findings. Medicine (Baltimore) 1974;1995:281–97.

[8] Norris S, Watt I. The prognosis of neck injuries resulting from rear-end vehicle collisions. J Bone Joint Surg Br 1983;65:608–11.

[9] Spitzer W, Skovron M, Salmi LR, et al. Scientific monograph of the Quebec Task Force on whiplash-associated disorders: redefining "whiplash" and its management. Spine (Phila Pa 1976) 1995;20(Suppl): S1–5.

[10] Cote P, Soklaridis S. Does early management of whiplash-associated disorders assist or impede recovery? Spine (Phila Pa 1976) 2011; 36:S275–9.

[11] Mealy K, Brennan H, Fenelon GC. Early mobilization of acute whiplash injury. Br Med J (Clin Res Ed) 1986;292:656–7.

[12] McKinney L. Early mobilisation and outcome in acute sprains of the neck. BMJ 1989;299:1006–8.

[13] Khwaja SM, Minnerop M, Singer A. Comparison of ibuprofen, cyclobenzaprine or both in patients with acute cervical strain: a randomized controlled trial. CJEM 2010;12:39–44.

[14] Pettersson K, Toolanen G. High-dose methylprednisolone prevents extensive sick leave after whiplash injury. A prospective, randomized, double-blind study. Spine (Phila Pa 1976) 1998;23:9844–89.

[15] Rosenfeld M, Gunnarsson R, Borenstein P. Early intervention in whiplash-associated disorder. Spine (Phila Pa 1976) 2000;25:1782–7.

[16] Brison RJ, Hartling L, Dostaler S, et al. A randomized controlled trial of an educational intervention to prevent the chronic pain of whiplash associated disorders following rear-end motor vehicle collisions. Spine (Phila Pa 1976) 2005;30:1799–807.

[17] Janda V. Muscles and cervicogenic pain syndromes. In: Grant R, editor. Physical therapy of the cervical and thoracic spine. New York, Churchill Livingstone; 1998. p.153–66.

[18] Nikander R, Mälkiä E, Parkkari J, et al. Dose-response relationship of specific training to reduce chronic neck pain and disability. Med Sci Sports Exerc 2006;38:2068–74.

[19] Peloso PM, Gross A, Haines T, et al. Medicinal and injection therapies for mechanical neck disorders. Cochrane Database Syst Rev 2010;(3).

[20] Simons DG, Travell JG, Simons LS. Travell & Simons' myofascial pain and dysfunction: the trigger point manual. 2nd ed. Upper Half of Body, vol. 1. Baltimore: Williams & Wilkins; 1999, 278–307, 432–444, 445–471, 504–537.

[21] Freund JB, Schwartz M. Treatment of chronic cervical-associated headache with botulinum toxin A: a pilot study. Headache 2000;40:231–6.

[22] Sterling M, Carroll L, Kasch H, et al. Prognosis after whiplash injury. Spine (Phila Pa 1976) 2011;36:S330–4.

[23] Bannister G, Amirfeyz R, Kelley S, Gargan M. Whiplash injury. J Bone Joint Surg Br 2009;91:845–50.

[24] Ferrari R, Louw D. Correlation between expectations of recovery and injury severity perception in whiplash-associated disorders. J Zhejiang Univ Sci B 2011;12:683–6.

[25] Gross A, Forget M, St George K, et al. Patient education for neck pain. Cochrane Database Syst Rev 2012;3, CD005106.

CHAPTER 7

Cervical Spinal Stenosis

Alec L. Meleger, MD
Rachel Egyhazi, MD

Synonyms

Cervical spondylotic myelopathy
Spinal stenosis
Cervical myelopathy

ICD-9 Codes

721.0 Cervical spondylosis without myelopathy
723.0 Spinal stenosis in cervical region

ICD-10 Codes

M47.812 Cervical spondylosis without myelopathy or radiculopathy
M48.02 Spinal stenosis in cervical region
M48.03 Spinal stenosis in cervicothoracic region

Definition

Cervical spinal stenosis refers to pathologic narrowing of the spinal canal that can be either congenital or acquired. The congenital type is commonly due to short pedicles that produce an abnormally shallow central spinal canal [1]. Less frequently, congenital stenosis may be associated with developmental disorders, such as achondroplasia, Klippel-Feil syndrome, Morquio syndrome, and trisomy 21 (i.e., Down syndrome) [2,3]. The main contributing factors in development of the acquired type are the degenerative, hypertrophic, age-related changes that affect the intervertebral discs, facet joints, and uncovertebral joints as well as the ligamentum flavum (Fig. 7.1). On radiologic imaging, these degenerative changes are present in 25% to 50% of the population by the age of 50 years and in 75% to 85% by 65 years [4–6]. Some of the other factors that may contribute to pathologic narrowing of the spinal canal are degenerative spondylolisthesis, ossification of the posterior longitudinal ligament, and atlantoaxial subluxation as seen in rheumatoid arthritis; rarely, it may be secondary to such extradural pathologic processes as metastatic disease, abscess formation, and trauma [7]. Aside from age, other demographic factors do not contribute significantly to the development of cervical stenosis [8]. Whereas ossification of the posterior longitudinal ligament was once considered specific to the Japanese, it has since been well documented in Western and other Asian populations [9].

Symptomatic spinal cord compression, or cervical myelopathy, commonly occurs at the cervical levels C5-C7, given the relatively increased mobility of these segments and the subsequent development of degenerative "wear and tear." Concomitant compression of the exiting cervical nerve roots is also typically observed in cervical spondylotic disease. Symptom production can occur by constant, mechanical compression of the neural elements or be of an intermittent, dynamic nature as seen with extremes of cervical flexion and extension. Chronic compression can lead to local cord ischemia with subsequent development of cervical myelopathy [10].

Symptoms

Symptomatic presentation of cervical spinal stenosis can differ from patient to patient, depending on the pathologic process, the anatomic structures, and the cervical levels involved. Intervertebral disc degeneration and zygapophyseal joint arthritis commonly are manifested with axial neck pain. Patients with cervical foraminal stenosis may complain of radicular arm pain as well as of paresthesias, dysesthesias, numbness, and weakness of the upper extremity. On the other hand, patients with cervical central canal stenosis can present with myelopathic symptoms of the upper and lower extremities, neurogenic bladder or bowel, sexual dysfunction, and unsteady and stiff-legged gait as well as weakness, paresthesias, or numbness of the lower extremities. Lower extremity pain is not known to be a clinical symptom unless concomitant lumbar spinal disease is present.

Physical Examination

Physical examination findings of the patient with cervical stenosis should be consistent with upper or lower motor

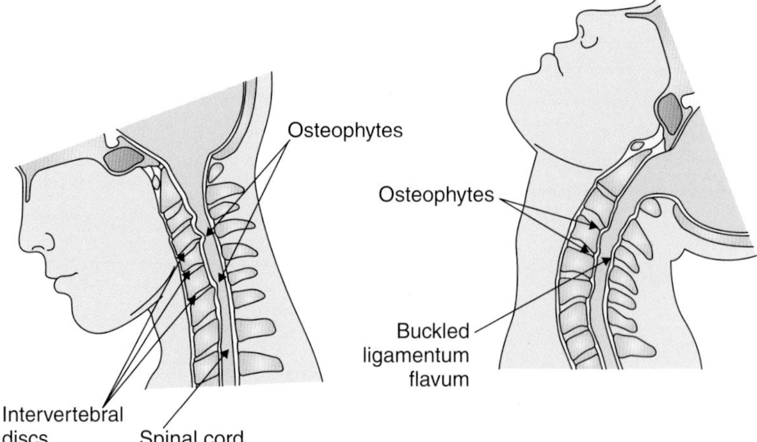

FIGURE 7.1 Cervical stenosis is a narrowing of the spinal canal that may be due to a variety of factors (e.g., congenital narrowing, osteophyte formation, and hypertrophy of the ligamentum flavum).

neuron signs, depending on the spinal level involved. Lower motor neuron findings are more commonly seen in the upper extremities; these include muscle atrophy, diminished sensation, decreased reflexes, diminished muscle tone, and weakness. Upper extremity myelopathic findings, such as hyperactive reflexes, increased tone, and present Hoffmann sign, can also be observed in cases of upper and mid cervical spinal cord involvement. A Spurling sign (radicular pain on axial loading of an extended head rotated toward the involved extremity) can also be present. A well-documented feature of cervical spondylotic myelopathy is so-called myelopathy hand, characterized by wasting of intrinsic and extrinsic hand muscles, loss of power of adduction and extension of the ulnar two or three digits, and inability to rapidly grip and release. Myelopathy hand is demonstrated by the hand grip-and-release test, which measures alternating closed-fist and full finger extension movements (normal result is 20 times in 10 seconds); the finger escape sign is tested with fingers fully extended and adducted, noting a tendency for ulnar digit spread [11].

Lower extremity examination is more consistent with upper motor neuron findings in the presence of cervical stenosis with myelopathy. Increased reflexes, Babinski sign, sustained or unsustained clonus, spasticity, weakness, decreased tactile and vibratory sensation, impaired proprioception, and neurogenic bowel or bladder can be seen. Lhermitte sign, an electric-like sensation that the patient reports going down the back when the neck is flexed (Fig. 7.2), can sometimes be elicited [12]. Refer to Chapter 1 for more detail.

Functional Limitations

The functional limitations depend on the extent of neurologic involvement. A person with mild symptoms can still be completely independent with activities of daily living, mobility, household chores, and work duties. In some cases, pain and weakness can produce various degrees of disability in self-care, such as grooming, bathing, and dressing, as well as in more physically demanding functions, especially in the community setting, such as lifting, carrying, and ambulation. Bowel and bladder incontinence as well as abnormalities of mood and sleep can further lead to social isolation and an increased level of actual and self-perceived disability.

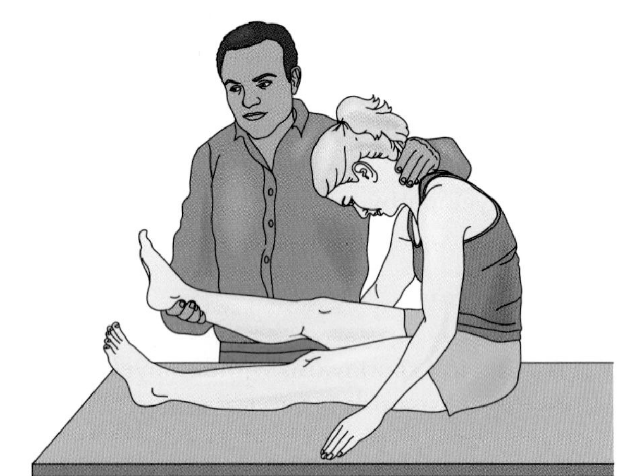

FIGURE 7.2 Lhermitte sign. The examiner flexes the patient's head and hip simultaneously.

In extreme cases, paraplegia and quadriplegia can limit nearly all functional activities.

Diagnostic Studies

Facet and uncovertebral joint arthropathy, loss of intervertebral disc space, neuroforaminal narrowing, and presence of spondylolisthesis can be evaluated with cervical spine radiographs; if dynamic instability is suspected, flexion-extension views are advised. Presence of osseous and soft tissue disease as well as the extent of nerve root and spinal cord compression can be assessed by magnetic resonance imaging (MRI) (Fig. 7.3). Cervical myelography can provide additional information on the behavior of neural elements during flexion and extension. An upright dynamic MRI study may be able to provide the same information on the behavior of neural elements with less procedural invasiveness [13] (Fig. 7.4). Somatosensory evoked potentials can confirm the presence of myelopathy, and electromyography can confirm peripheral nerve root involvement [14].

Several radiologic criteria exist to define what constitutes significant stenosis of the cervical spine. The normal anterior-posterior dimension of the spinal canal at C3 through C7 is 16 to 18 mm [15]. Neck flexion reduces canal diameter by 2 to 3 mm, whereas extension

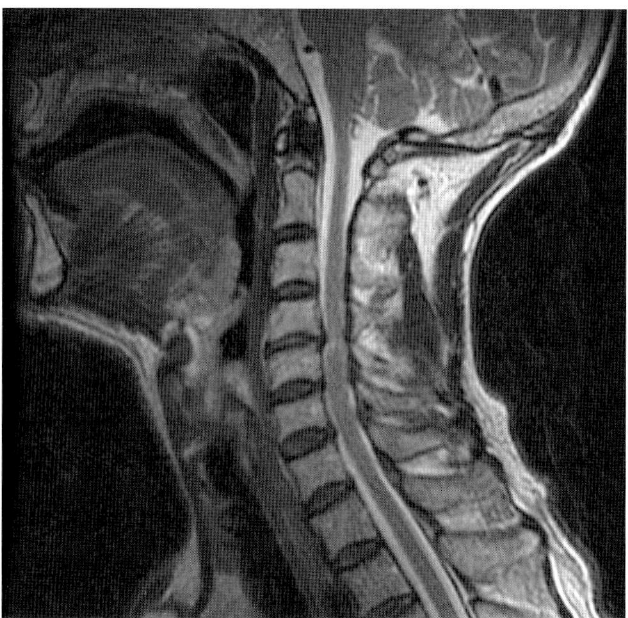

FIGURE 7.3 Severe C4-C5 cervical stenosis. Disc-osteophyte complex and hypertrophic ligamentum flavum are producing an indentation of the spinal cord. Notice an intramedullary hyperintensity signal consistent with spinal cord injury.

may decrease it up to 3.5 mm at 45 degrees because of ligamentum flavum infolding [16,17]. According to some sources, an absolute cervical spinal stenosis is present when the sagittal spinal canal diameter is less than 10 mm, and relative spinal stenosis is present when this measurement is 10 to 13 mm [18,19]. A Torg ratio of less than 0.8, which is measured by dividing the sagittal diameter of the spinal canal by the sagittal diameter of the respective vertebral body, has been used to predict the presence of significant spinal stenosis and tries to eliminate any inherent radiographic measurement errors [20]. A more widely accepted approach in evaluating the extent of stenotic pathologic changes is through the use of MRI, which permits the functional capacity of the surrounding subarachnoid space and the state of the spinal cord itself to be more definitively assessed. Several studies have demonstrated a poor correlation between Torg ratio and extent of stenosis identified on MRI [21].

Diffusion-weighted sequences, in particular a technique known as diffusion tensor imaging, allow the visualization of specific nerve tract bundles and may detect early damage to the myelin sheath. Although its utility in imaging the spinal cord is currently limited, diffusion tensor imaging has demonstrated enhanced sensitivity for detection of early cervical spondylotic myelopathy and intramedullary lesions [22,23]. The presence of intramedullary signal abnormalities warrants further investigation and a more

Differential Diagnosis

Thoracic spinal stenosis
Cervical intramedullary or extramedullary neoplasm
Cervical osteomyelitis with or without epidural abscess
Multiple sclerosis (spinal)
Transverse myelitis
Cerebrovascular accident
Syringomyelia
Spinal cord injury
Arteriovenous malformation
Tabes dorsalis
Progressive multifocal leukoencephalopathy
Tropical spastic paraparesis
Lumbar spinal stenosis
Thoracic outlet syndrome
Idiopathic brachial neuritis
Brachial plexopathy

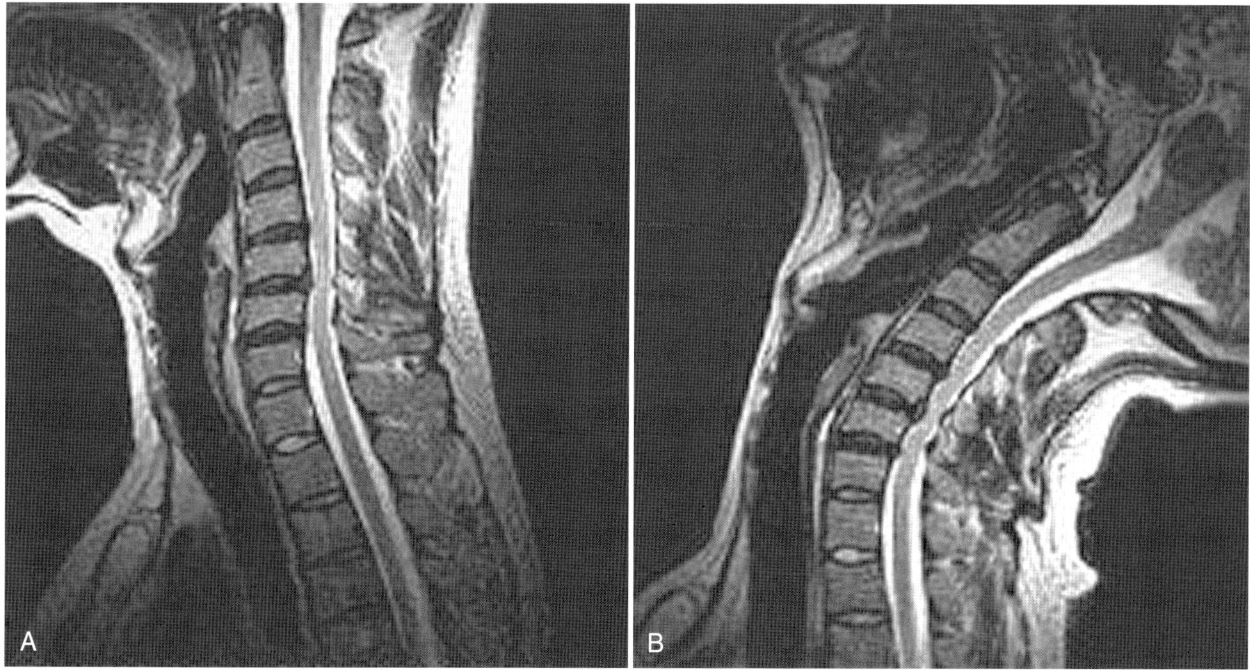

FIGURE 7.4 Sagittal magnetic resonance images of cervical spine with the patient recumbent (**A**) and standing with the neck extended (**B**).

aggressive treatment approach (see Fig. 7.3). Computed tomographic myelography continues to offer some advantages over MRI, including superior spatial resolution, ability to distinguish bone from soft tissue intrusion into the cervical foramina, and dynamic visualization of the flow of contrast material [24].

Treatment

Initial

Conservative treatment is generally undertaken in the absence of clinical evidence of cervical myelopathy. If cervical myelopathy is suspected or clearly evident, the patient must be immediately referred for an evaluation by a spine surgical specialist. When a patient is symptomatic with pain but does not have myelopathic symptoms, relative decrease in physical activity for no longer than 2 or 3 days is initially recommended. For severe cervical or radicular pain, a soft neck collar can be prescribed for a few days with subsequent self-weaning by alternating periods of collar removal [25].

Self-application of ice or heat for cervical pain and transcutaneous electrical nerve stimulation for radicular symptoms can be of benefit to some patients.

Initial analgesics of choice are acetaminophen and nonsteroidal anti-inflammatory drugs, which may show some effect in cervical as well as in radicular pain when they are taken at regular intervals. More than one family of nonsteroidals should be tried before they are deemed to be ineffective. A short course of opioids and muscle relaxants may benefit those patients with severe pain and strong contraindications to the use of acetaminophen and nonsteroidal anti-inflammatory drugs. For recalcitrant, functionally limiting radicular symptoms, a 7- to 10-day tapering course of oral steroids is recommended. Persistent radicular pain can be treated with neuropathic pain medications, such as gabapentin, pregabalin, tricyclic antidepressants, duloxetine, and others [26].

Education of the patient about the nature of cervical stenosis, its worrisome signs and symptoms (e.g., progressive difficulties with gait, urinary retention or incontinence), injury prevention, and the importance of staying active is of paramount importance. In older patients, fall prevention and fall precautions should be immediately addressed to prevent catastrophic neurologic consequences. In individuals with MRI evidence of severe cervical stenosis, certain physical activities, such as horseback or motorcycle riding, climbing ladders, and participation in contact sports, should be strongly discouraged. Patients should also be advised to avoid the extremes of repetitive cervical extension and flexion, as in swimming the breast stroke, painting a ceiling, or performing legs overhead backward stretching.

Rehabilitation

Physical and occupational therapy should focus on keeping patients as active as possible while educating them about activities that might place them at risk for further injury. Continued physical activity, such as walking and the use of a stationary bicycle, is recommended to prevent overall muscle and aerobic deconditioning. Gentle cervical traction may also be tried in the absence of severe stenosis or myelopathic findings. With passing of the acute phase, a program consisting of stretching and isometric neck exercises should be undertaken. Once the pain-free range of motion is achieved, isotonic neck strengthening is initiated [27]. Eventually, patients should be graduated to a home exercise program.

Work site evaluation and institution of certain job restrictions are recommended to prevent repetitive hyperextension or hyperflexion activities. These might include adjustment of computer monitor height, recommendation for a phone headset, and restriction of duties requiring activities above eye level. The use of bifocals should also be addressed because these require frequent head positional changes.

Depression and anxiety can lead to symptom magnification and should be addressed by a mental health care provider. Cognitive-behavioral therapy, biofeedback, self-hypnosis, and relaxation techniques must always be considered part of the comprehensive pain management treatment.

Procedures

A trial of interlaminar or transforaminal epidural steroid injections is advocated for acute or subacute radicular symptoms of severe intensity unresponsive to more conservative measures. Care should be taken to avoid the introduction of a spinal needle at the level of stenosis when an interlaminar approach is used. Transforaminal epidural steroid injections should be performed by a well-trained practitioner with the use of digital subtraction angiography and with preference toward nonparticulate steroids (e.g., dexamethasone) to avoid catastrophic complications. Patients without significant central spinal canal compromise and who continue to suffer with chronic severe radicular symptoms, unresponsive to conservative approaches, may be candidates for a spinal cord stimulator trial and implantation.

Arthritic cervical facet joints, which are innervated by medial branch nerves, can be another source of pain. Intra-articular steroid injections can provide up to several months of significant pain relief. If these fail to provide significant analgesic effect, diagnostic medial branch nerve blocks can be performed; if results are found to be positive, radiofrequency nerve ablation should follow.

Surgery

Immediate surgical intervention should be sought with symptoms of progressive weakness, bladder or bowel incontinence, unsteady gait, and upper motor neuron findings. Decompressive single-level or multilevel laminectomy, laminoplasty, discectomy, foraminotomy, and cervical fusion by use of bone graft or instrumentation are the common surgical procedures. Referral to a surgical specialist should be considered for intractable radicular symptoms [28,29].

Various classification systems have been used to grade the severity of spondylotic myelopathy and to guide the decision for surgery. The Nurick scale, used more frequently in a research setting, is based exclusively on ambulatory function [30]. The Japanese Orthopaedic Association (JOA) classification system and its modified versions evaluate additional variables, including upper extremity function and manual dexterity, sensory changes of the trunk and extremities, and bladder function [31]. Operative management is typically recommended for a JOA score of less than 13 with clinical symptoms and evidence of spinal cord compression on imaging [32].

Potential Disease Complications

If it is left untreated, progressive pressure on the exiting cervical nerve roots and the spinal cord may lead to worsening weakness, loss of sensation, dysfunction of the bladder and bowel, or tetraplegia.

The natural course of symptomatic cervical spondylotic myelopathy, when it is treated conservatively, demonstrates slow gradual decline in many patients, with periods of long quiescence or mild clinical improvement in some [33].

Potential Treatment Complications

Application of aggressive or improper physical or occupational therapy treatments can lead to further injury to the already compromised spinal cord and the exiting nerve roots. Cervical traction may promote signs and symptoms of myelopathy and radiculopathy. Atrophy of cervical musculature can occur with prolonged use of a cervical collar [34]. Aggressive cervical manual technique can cause vertebral artery dissection and severe neurologic sequelae.

Nonsteroidal anti-inflammatory medications carry well-known side effects of gastrointestinal irritation, bleeding, edema, and nephropathy. These medications are to be used cautiously or avoided in patients with a past history of peptic ulcer disease or with decreased renal function. A proton pump inhibitor or misoprostol should be considered for ulcer prophylaxis in individuals at high risk. All of the neuropathic pain medications carry significant side effects; gabapentin and pregabalin possess the best tolerance. The most common complaints are sedation, dizziness, and poor ambulatory balance. Continued use of opioids can lead to physiologic dependence, tolerance, sedation, constipation, and rarely addiction. Objective evidence of improved function and decreased level of pain is required for their continued use.

Interlaminar epidural steroid injections carry a small risk of dural puncture and subsequent development of a post–dural puncture headache. In most patients, these headaches are self-limited and respond well to bed rest, hydration, and caffeine. Improper placement of the needle tip and intravascular injection of particulate steroids with the transforaminal epidural approach can lead to spinal cord injury, stroke, and brain stem infarct. All interventions, percutaneous and surgical, carry a rare risk of spinal infection, compressive hematoma, and nerve and spinal cord injury.

References

[1] Inoue H, Ohmori K, Takatsu T, et al. Morphological analysis of the cervical spinal canal, dural tube and spinal cord in normal individuals using CT myelography. Neuroradiology 1996;38:148–51.
[2] Reeder MM. Congenital syndromes and bone dysplasias with vertebral abnormality. Gamuts in Radiology 4.0, 2003. Available at, http://gamuts.isradiology.org/data/C-1.htm, Accessed September 2012.
[3] McKay SD, Al-Omari A, Tomlinson LA, Dormans JP. Review of cervical spine anomalies in genetic syndromes. Spine (Phila Pa 1976) 2012;37:E269–77.
[4] Bohlman HH, Emery SE. The pathophysiology of cervical spondylosis and myelopathy. Spine (Phila Pa 1976) 1988;13:843–6.
[5] Adams CB, Logue V. Studies in cervical spondylotic myelopathy: I-III. Brain 1971;94:557–94.
[6] Connell MD, Wiesel SW. Natural history and pathogenesis of cervical disc disease. Orthop Clin North Am 1992;23:369–80.
[7] Ono K, Yonenobu K, Miyamoto S, Okada K. Pathology of ossification of the posterior longitudinal ligament and ligamentum flavum. Clin Orthop Relat Res 1999;359:18–26.
[8] Lee MJ, Cassinelli EH, Riew KD. Prevalence of cervical spine stenosis: anatomic study in cadavers. J Bone Joint Surg Am 2007;89:376–80.
[9] Matsunaga S, Sakou T. OPLL: disease entity, incidence, literature search, and prognosis. In: Yonenobu K, Nakamura K, Toyama Y, editors. OPLL: ossification of the posterior longitudinal ligament. 2nd ed. Springer: Tokyo; 2006. p. 11–7.
[10] Singh A, Crockard HA, Platts A, Stevens J. Clinical and radiological correlates of severity and surgery-related outcome in cervical spondylosis. J Neurosurg 2001;94(Suppl):189–98.
[11] Ono K, Ebara S, Fuji T, et al. Myelopathy hand: new clinical signs of cervical cord damage. J Bone Joint Surg Br 1987;69:215–9.
[12] Clark CR. Cervical spondylotic myelopathy: history and physical findings. Spine (Phila Pa 1976) 1988;13:847–9.
[13] Jinkins JR, Dworkin JS, Damadian RV. Upright, weight-bearing, dynamic-kinetic MRI of the spine: initial results. Eur Radiol 2005;15:1815–25.
[14] Yiannikas C, Shahani BT, Young RR. Short-latency somatosensory-evoked potentials from radial, median, ulnar, and peroneal nerve stimulation in the assessment of cervical spondylosis. Comparison with conventional electromyography. Arch Neurol 1986;43:1264–71.
[15] Cusick JF, Yoganandan N. Biomechanics of the cervical spine 4: major injuries. Clin Biomech (Bristol, Avon) 2002;17:1–20.
[16] Penning L. Functional pathology of the cervical spine. Williams & Wilkins: Baltimore; 1968.
[17] Gu R, Zhu Q, Lin Y, et al. Dynamic canal encroachment of ligamentum flavum: an in vitro study of cadaveric specimens. J Spinal Disord Tech 2006;19:187–90.
[18] Matsuura P, Waters RL, Adkins RH, et al. Comparison of computerized tomography parameters of the cervical spine in normal control subjects and spinal cord–injured patients. J Bone Joint Surg Am 1989;71:183–8.
[19] Edwards WC, LaRocca H. The developmental segmental sagittal diameter of the cervical spinal canal in patients with cervical spondylosis. Spine 1983;8:2027.
[20] Pavlov H, Torg JS, Robie B, Jahre C. Cervical spinal stenosis: determination with vertebral body ratio method. Radiology 1987;164:771–5.
[21] Cantu RC. The cervical spinal stenosis controversy. Clin Sports Med 1998;17:121–6.
[22] Rajasekaran S, Kanna RM, Shetty AP. Diffusion tensor imaging of the spinal cord and its clinical applications. J Bone Joint Surg Br 2012;94:1024–31.
[23] Song T, Chen WJ, Yang B, et al. Diffusion tensor imaging in the cervical spinal cord. Eur Spine J 2011;20:422–8.
[24] Maus TP. Imaging of the spine and nerve roots. Phys Med Rehabil Clin N Am 2002;13:487–544.
[25] Persson L, Carlsson CA, Carlsson JY. Long lasting cervical radicular pain managed with surgery, physiotherapy, or a cervical collar: a prospective, randomized study. Spine (Phila Pa 1976) 1997;22:751–8.
[26] Yildirim K, Sisecioglu M, Karatay S, et al. The effectiveness of gabapentin in patients with chronic radiculopathy. Pain Clin 2003;15:213–8.
[27] Levoska S, Keinanen-Kiukaanniemi S. Active or passive physiotherapy for occupational cervicobrachial disorders? A comparison of two treatment methods with a 1-year follow up. Arch Phys Med Rehabil 1993;74:425–30.
[28] Kavanagh RG, Butler JS, O'Byrne JM, Poynton AR. Operative techniques for cervical radiculopathy and myelopathy. Adv Orthop 2012;2012:794087.
[29] Edwards RJ, Cudlip SA, Moore AJ. Surgical treatment of cervical spondylotic myelopathy in extreme old age. Neurosurgery 1999;45:696.
[30] Nurick S. The natural history and the results of surgical treatment of the spinal cord disorder associated with cervical spondylosis. Brain 1972;95:101–8.
[31] Japanese Orthopaedic Association. Japanese Orthopaedic Association scoring system for cervical myelopathy (17-2 version and 100 version). Nippon Seikeigeka Gakkai Zasshi 1994;68:490–503 [in Japanese with English translation].
[32] Bono CM, Fisher CG. Prove it! evidence-based analysis of common spine practice. Philadelphia: Lippincott Williams & Wilkins; 2010.
[33] Matz PG, Anderson PA, Holly LT, et alJoint Section on Disorders of the Spine and Peripheral Nerves of the American Association of Neurological Surgeons and Congress of Neurological Surgeons. The natural history of cervical spondylotic myelopathy. J Neurosurg Spine 2009;11:104–11.
[34] Muzin S, Zacharia I, Walker J, et al. When should a cervical collar be used to treat neck pain? Curr Rev Musculoskelet Med 2008;1:114–9.

CHAPTER 8

Cervicogenic Vertigo

Joanne Borg-Stein, MD
Melissa Colbert, MD

Synonyms

Cervicogenic dizziness
Neck pain associated with dizziness

ICD-9 Codes

723.1	**Neck pain**
780.4	**Vertigo**
780.4	**Dizziness**

ICD-10 Codes

M54.2	**Neck pain**
R42	**Vertigo**
R42	**Dizziness**

Definition

Cervicogenic vertigo is the false sense of motion that is due to cervical musculoskeletal dysfunction. The symptoms may be secondary to post-traumatic events with resultant whiplash or postconcussive syndrome. Alternatively, cervicogenic vertigo may be part of a more generalized disorder, such as fibromyalgia or underlying cervical osteoarthritis.

Cervicogenic vertigo is thought to result from convergence of the cervical and cranial nerve inputs and their close approximation in the upper cervical spinal segments of the spinal cord [1,2]. Dizziness and vertigo, common presenting symptoms, account for 8 million primary care visits to physicians in the United States each year and represent the most common presenting complaint in patients older than 75 years [3]. In fact, 40% to 80% of patients with neck trauma experience vertigo, particularly after whiplash injury. The incidence of symptoms of dizziness and vertigo in whiplash patients has been reported as 20% to 58% [4,5].

Symptoms

Patients with cervicogenic vertigo experience a false sense of motion, often whirling or spinning. Some patients experience sensations of floating, bobbing, tilting, or drifting. Others experience nausea, visual motor sensitivity, and ear fullness [6]. The symptoms are often provoked or triggered by neck movement or sustained awkward head positioning [7–9]. Cervical pain or headache may interfere with sleep and functional activities. At times, patients with coexistent cervical radiculitis may complain of paresthesias in the upper cervical dermatomes.

Physical Examination

The essential elements of the physical examination are normal neurologic, ear, and eye examination findings for nystagmus. Abnormalities in any of these aspects of the examination indicate a need to exclude other otologic or neurologic conditions, such as Meniere disease, benign paroxysmal positional vertigo, and stroke [5,10]. A careful cervical examination should be performed, including range of motion testing and palpation of the facet joints to assess mechanical dysfunction. Myofascial trigger points should be sought in the sternocleidomastoid, cervical paraspinal, levator scapulae, upper trapezius, and suboccipital musculature. Patients with cervicogenic headache and disequilibrium have a significantly higher incidence of restricted cervical flexion or extension and painful cervical joint dysfunction and muscle tightness [11,12]. Palpation in these areas can often reproduce the symptoms experienced as cervicogenic vertigo [13].

Functional Limitations

Functional limitations may include difficulty with walking, balance, or equilibrium. As a result, patients may not feel confident with activities such as driving because cervical rotation may induce symptoms. Occupations that require balance and coordination (such as construction) are often limited. Anxiety about the occurrence of disequilibrium may contribute to secondary disability.

Diagnostic Studies

Cervicogenic dizziness is a clinical diagnosis. Testing may include cervical radiographs to rule out cervical osteoarthritis or instability. Cervical magnetic resonance imaging is indicated when cervical spondylosis is suspected, either as a cause of the condition or as an associated diagnosis. Brain magnetic resonance imaging or magnetic resonance angiography may be ordered to exclude vascular lesions or tumor (i.e., acoustic neuroma). A comprehensive neurotologic test battery and consultation are preferred if a primary otologic disorder or post-traumatic vertigo is considered [14].

Differential Diagnosis

- Meniere disease
- Benign paroxysmal positional vertigo
- Labyrinthitis
- Vestibular neuronitis
- Cardiovascular causes: arrhythmia, carotid stenosis, or postural hypotension
- Vestibular migraine
- Progressive dysequilibrium of aging
- Post-traumatic vertigo

Treatment

Initial

Initial treatment involves reassurance and education of the patient. Nonsteroidal anti-inflammatory drugs are useful to help pain control for those who have underlying cervical osteoarthritis. Muscle relaxants such as cyclobenzaprine, carisoprodol, and low-dose tricyclic antidepressants may be used at bedtime to facilitate sleep and muscle relaxation for myofascial pain. We occasionally prescribe ondansetron (4 to 8 mg every 8 hours as needed) if disequilibrium is accompanied by significant nausea.

Rehabilitation

Rehabilitation is aimed at reducing muscle spasm, increasing cervical range of motion, improving posture, and restoring function. A physical therapist with training and experience in manual therapy, myofascial and trigger point treatment, and neck and trunk stabilization techniques should evaluate and treat the patient to restore normal cervical function [15]. The use of gentle manual therapy is validated by moderate evidence, with sustained natural apophyseal glides being particularly beneficial in relief of dizziness and pain up to at least 12 weeks [16,17]. Occupational therapy can improve posture, ergonomics, and functional daily activities [18]. Vestibular rehabilitation therapy helps patients develop compensatory responses and normalizes cervical sensory input [16].

Ergonomic accessories, such as telephone earset or headset, may help the patient avoid awkward head and neck postures that contribute to symptoms. Psychological or behavioral medicine consultation and treatment can aid the patient in overcoming the fear, avoidance, and anxiety that often develop [16,19].

Procedures

Trigger point injections with local anesthetic (1% lidocaine or 0.25% bupivacaine) are often helpful to decrease cervical muscle pain (Fig. 8.1). The clinician should locate those trigger point areas that reproduce the patient's symptoms. Acupuncture with an emphasis on local treatment of muscle spasm may be an alternative to trigger point injection [20,21].

Although botulinum toxin injection may have a role in the treatment of cervicogenic headache [22,23], there are no data yet on the treatment of cervicogenic vertigo with botulinum toxin.

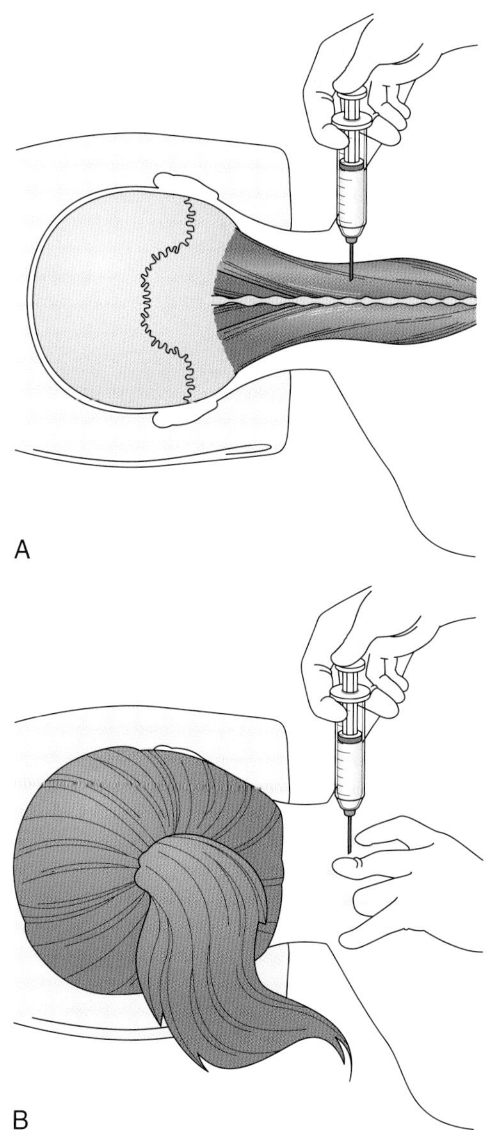

FIGURE 8.1 **A** and **B**, Trigger points in the splenius capitis muscle frequently involved in cervicogenic vertigo. *(From Simons DG, Travell JG, Simons LS. Travell & Simons' Myofascial Pain and Dysfunction: The Trigger Point Manual, 2nd ed. Upper Half of Body, vol 1. Baltimore, Williams & Wilkins, 1999:310.)*

Surgery

There is no surgery indicated for treatment of this disorder, unless there is coexistent neurologically significant cervical stenosis or disc herniation.

Potential Disease Complications

The major complications are inactivity, deconditioning, falls, fear of going outside the home, anxiety, and depression. Chronic intractable neck pain and persistent dizziness may persist in spite of treatment.

Potential Treatment Complications

Side effects from nonsteroidal anti-inflammatory drugs may include gastric, renal, hepatic, cardiovascular, and hematologic complications [24]. Muscle relaxants and tricyclics may induce fatigue, somnolence, constipation, urinary retention, and other anticholinergic side effects. Local injections may result in local pain, ecchymosis, intravascular injection, or pneumothorax if they are improperly executed.

References

[1] Norre M. Cervical vertigo. Acta Otorhinolaryngol Belg 1987; 25:495–9.
[2] Revel M, Andre-Deshays C, Mingeut M. Cervicocephalic kinesthetic sensibility in patients with cervical pain. Arch Phys Med Rehabil 1991;72:288–91.
[3] Colledge NR, Barr-Hamilton RM, Lewis SJ, et al. Evaluation of investigations to diagnose the cause of dizziness in elderly people: a community based controlled study. BMJ 1996;313:788–93.
[4] Wrisley D, Sparto P, Whitney S, Furman J. Cervicogenic dizziness: a review of diagnosis and treatment. J Orthop Sports Phys Ther 2000;30:755–66.
[5] Post RE, Dickerson LM. Dizziness: a diagnostic approach. Am Fam Physician 2010;82:361–8.
[6] Karlberg M, Magnusson M, Malmström EM, et al. Postural and symptomatic improvement after physiotherapy in patients with dizziness of suspected cervical origin. Arch Phys Med Rehabil 1996;77:874–82.
[7] Jongkees L. Cervical vertigo. Laryngoscope 1969;79:1473–84.
[8] Praffenrath V, Danekar R, Pollmann W. Cervicogenic headache—the clinical picture, radiological findings, and hypotheses on its pathophysiology. Headache 1987;25:495–9.
[9] Sjaastad O, Frediksen T, Praffenrath V. Cervicogenic headache: diagnostic criteria. Headache 1990;30:725–6.
[10] Froehling DA, Silverstein MD, Mohr DN, Beatty CW. Does this dizzy patient have a serious form of vertigo? JAMA 1994;271:385–8.
[11] Zito G, Jull G, Story I. Clinical tests of musculoskeletal dysfunction in the diagnosis of cervicogenic headache. Man Ther 2006;11:118–29.
[12] Matsui T, Ii K, Hojo S, Sano K. Cervical neuro-muscular syndrome: discovery of a new disease group caused by abnormalities in the cervical muscles. Neurol Med Chir (Tokyo) 2012;52:75–80.
[13] Simons DG, Travell JG, Simons LS. Travell & Simons' myofascial pain and dysfunction: the trigger point manual. 2nd ed Upper Half of Body. vol. 1. Baltimore: Williams & Wilkins; 1999.
[14] Ernst A, Basta D, Seidl RO, et al. Management of posttraumatic vertigo. Otolaryngol Head Neck Surg 2005;132:554–8.
[15] Reid SA, Rivett DA. Manual therapy treatment of cervicogenic dizziness: a systematic review. Man Ther 2005;10:4–13.
[16] Lystad RP, Bell G, Bonnevie-Svendsen M, Carter CV. Manual therapy with and without vestibular rehabilitation for cervicogenic dizziness: a systematic review. Chiropr Man Therap 2011;19:21.
[17] Reid SA, Rivett DA, Katekar MG, Callister R. Sustained natural apophyseal glides (SNAGs) are an effective treatment for cervicogenic dizziness. Man Ther 2008;13:357–66.
[18] Karlberg M, Persson L, Magnusson M. Impaired postural control in patients with cervico-brachial pain. Acta Otolaryngol Suppl 1995;520:440–2.
[19] Borg-Stein J, Rauch S, Krabak B. Evaluation and management of cervicogenic dizziness. Crit Rev Phys Med Rehabil 2001;13:255–64.
[20] deJong P, de Jong M, Cohen B, Jongkees LB. Ataxia and nystagmus induced by injection of local anesthetics in the neck. Ann Neurol 1997;1:240–6.
[21] Carlson J, Fahlerantz A, Augustinsson L. Muscle tenderness in tension headaches treated with acupuncture and physiotherapy. Cephalalgia 1990;10:131–41.
[22] Sycha T, Kranz G, Auff E, Schnider P. Botulinum toxin in the treatment of rare head and neck pain syndromes: a systematic review of the literature. J Neurol 2004;251(Suppl 1):I19–30.
[23] Karadaş O, Öztürk B, Ulaş UH, et al. The efficacy of botulinum toxin in patients with cervicogenic headache: a placebo-controlled clinical trial. Balkan Med J 2012;29:184–7.
[24] Trelle S, Reichenbach S, Wandel S, et al. Cardiovascular safety of non-steroidal anti-inflammatory drugs: network meta-analysis. BMJ 2011;342:c7086.

CHAPTER 9

Trapezius Strain

Atul T. Patel, MD, MHSA

Synonyms

Myofascial shoulder pain
Trapezius myositis
Myofasciitis
Tension neck ache
Nonarticular rheumatism
Fibrositis
Fibromyalgia
Repetitive stress injury

ICD-9 Codes

729.1 Myalgia and myositis, unspecified
847.0 Neck (sprain or strain); whiplash injury
847.1 Thoracic (sprain or strain)
847.9 Unspecified site of the back (sprain or strain)

ICD-10 Codes

M60.9 Myositis, unspecified
M79.1 Myalgia
S13.4 Whiplash injury (cervical spine)
S13.9 Neck sprain, unspecified parts of the neck
S16.1 Neck strain (add additional character for type of encounter)
S23.3 Thoracic sprain
S39.012 Back strain

Definition

Trapezius strain is often considered a part of the myofascial pain syndrome (MPS). This is a common diagnosis of patients who present to outpatient clinics for musculoskeletal pain disorders [1]. There is no standard definition of trapezius strain or MPS; however, MPS is described as a disorder characterized by acute and chronic nonspecific pain that affects a small number of muscles and involves single or multiple trigger points that are usually located in tight bands within the affected muscles [2]. The pain in this area must not be mistaken for cervical radicular pain that involves the shoulder girdle and the upper limb [3]. The etiology of trigger point formation is not known, but the most accepted hypothesis focuses on the existence of dysfunctional end plates leading to a perpetuated shortening of the muscle [4,5].

Trapezius strain is thought to be due to common repetitive strain or stress injury associated with carrying light loads and certain postures, such as that with working on a computer for long periods [6]. Myofascial trigger points can be the main cause of neck and upper back pain, and the trapezius muscle is the most commonly studied [7]. The condition can also result from acute causes, such as a whiplash injury.

Symptoms

Patients typically complain of a sore or aching sensation in the region of the upper trapezius muscle. Patients may also complain of posterior neck and shoulder pain. Some may have associated posterior headaches, difficulty with sleeping due to shoulder pain, and interscapular area pain. The symptoms can be constant and relieved by rest and worsened with activity. There can be increased pain with cervical movement and hence limitation in neck range of motion. The pain is regional and does not follow spinal segmental or peripheral nerve distribution. Patients may often report that the symptoms are partly relieved with the use of heat or cold modalities and focal pressure.

Physical Examination

The importance of the physical examination is to rule out other conditions that may be causing the patient's symptoms, such as a radiculopathy, peripheral nerve injury, cervical dystonia, or some other condition that may be suspected on the basis of the history. A neurologic and musculoskeletal examination focusing on the neck and upper body should be done in addition to a general examination. Other evaluations include cranial nerve function, especially checking the spinal accessory nerve; sensation to light touch and pinprick about the face, upper limbs, and torso with attention to dermatomes and cutaneous nerve distribution; muscle stretch reflexes; and strength testing. The findings on neurologic examination are typically normal in primary trapezius strain. The patient may present with a forward head posture, scapular protraction, and compensatory cervical hyperextension. Muscle palpation about the neck and shoulder girdle may reveal tender areas and trigger points, especially in the trapezius muscle. A shoulder examination should be carried out to assess for shoulder disease.

Functional Limitations

Trapezius muscle strain can limit activities requiring the arm to be outstretched in front or to the side. There can be pain with rotation of the head and hence function limitation, such as turning the head for a shoulder check when driving. Pain in certain positions may interfere with restful sleep and thus affect overall function.

Diagnostic Studies

There is no specific test that is used to diagnose trapezius strain. It is a clinical diagnosis based on the history and physical examination. Radiologic studies, electrodiagnostic testing, and laboratory testing can be helpful in ruling out other potential conditions, such as cervical radiculopathy, cervical degenerative disease, shoulder disease, or inflammatory process. Newer musculoskeletal imaging techniques show promise for future application as diagnostic tools to objectively measure the presence or absence of myofascial trigger points. Magnetic resonance elastography is a research tool that is used to measure the stiffness of biologic tissues; it has been reported to successfully identify and quantify myofascial taut bands [8]. Musculoskeletal ultrasound is another tool that is changing the approach to the diagnosis of musculoskeletal conditions, including muscle strains [9,10].

Differential Diagnosis

Cervical spondylosis
Cervical herniation
Cervical radiculopathy
Cervical facet syndrome
Peripheral nerve entrapment (e.g., suprascapular, spinal accessory)
Inflammatory disease (e.g., myositis, polymyalgia rheumatica)
Endocrine disorders (e.g., hypothyroidism)
Electrolyte abnormalities
Tumor

Treatment

Initial

Initially, the patient should be educated about the condition and its usual benign course. The importance of appropriate activity, posture, and exercise is stressed. The goal is to break the cycle of improper posture, overuse and strain, and deconditioning. This may require a short-term course of muscle relaxants, anti-inflammatory medications, analgesics, and modalities.

There is little evidence in the literature that any of the muscle relaxants provide clear benefit in patients with MPS. A Cochrane review that evaluated the efficacy of cyclobenzaprine for the treatment of MPS found that insufficient evidence supports its use because of a lack of high-quality randomized controlled trials [11]. A review article that assessed the efficacy of numerous muscle relaxants for the treatment of MPS concluded that insufficient evidence exists to support the use of tizanidine, alprazolam, or diazepam monotherapy, but evidence is supportive for the use of clonazepam in the treatment of MPS [12]. Similarly, there is insufficient evidence in favor of antidepressants (other than amitriptyline), anticonvulsants, topical analgesics, nonsteroidal anti-inflammatory medications, and other analgesics [13].

Electrical stimulation, laser therapy, and magnetic therapy did not show clear evidence to support use in the treatment of MPS. Ultrasound-based interventions appear to have a role in providing short-term and intermediate-term improvement in pain and function, especially as an adjunctive therapy [13].

Rehabilitation

The goals of therapy (occupational or physical) are to reduce pain and to improve function. Depending on the severity and chronicity of the condition, the patient may have developed secondary problems related to muscle shortening, weakness, and reduced range of motion. The initial goal of the therapy is to reduce the local muscle spasms and pain, followed by appropriate stretching and strengthening to minimize the risk of recurrent problems. Physical modalities such as heat and cold therapy combined with massage can help relieve some of the symptoms by relaxing the muscles. Stretching is initially targeted to specific portions of the trapezius muscle. The cervical extensor and scapular stabilizers are strengthened. The patient should be set up with a home program to continue with the stretching and strengthening exercises. A primary goal of rehabilitation should include evaluating and appropriately modifying tasks that exacerbate the patient's symptoms. For example, carrying heavy baskets of laundry, driving, typing on a computer keyboard, and many other daily tasks may exacerbate symptoms. If indicated, an ergonomic assessment of the patient's workstation should be carried out to help maintain an appropriate upper body posture.

Procedures

Procedures include acupuncture, dry needling, and trigger point injections. A review of dry needling therapy trials in patients with MPS shows inconclusive evidence in favor of or against the use of superficial dry needling therapy for the treatment of MPS [13]. There is insufficient evidence to conclude that trigger point injections are more effective than dry needling alone or placebo. Limited evidence exists to support the use of trigger point injections for the treatment of MPS (grade B recommendations) [13]. Botulinum toxin injections have been studied. A Cochrane review found that only one of several trials that met the selection criteria was effective in treating pain from trigger points [14–17]. The conclusion of this review was that current evidence does not support the use of botulinum toxin A for the treatment of trigger points in MPS [18]. Another review of predominantly level 1 studies found three studies in favor of botulinum toxin injections and eight against or equivalent with control intervention or placebo [13].

Surgery

Surgery is not indicated for treatment of trapezius strain.

Potential Disease Complications

If the patient's condition is left untreated, problems of reduced range of functional motion of the neck and shoulder, muscle atrophy, and secondary chronic pain may develop. These can result in personal and occupational disability.

Potential Treatment Complications

Oral medications that may be used for analgesia or muscle relaxation can have side effects or interactions with other drugs the patient may be taking. The nonsteroidal anti-inflammatory drugs may produce gastropathy, renal toxicity, hepatic toxicity, bleeding, exacerbation of asthma, and central nervous system effects. Muscle relaxants and tricyclic antidepressants may cause sedation and anticholinergic side effects, such as dry mouth, urinary retention, orthostatic hypotension, and weight gain. Botulinum toxins can cause asthenia, dysphagia, influenza-like symptoms, and muscle weakness. Trigger point injections can result in local ecchymosis and pain.

References

[1] Rickards L. The effectiveness of non-invasive treatments for active myofascial trigger point pain: a systematic review of the literature. Int J Osteopath Med 2009;12:42–3.

[2] Simons D, Travell J, Simons L. Travell and Simons' myofascial pain and dysfunction: the trigger point manual. 2nd ed. Williams & Wilkins: Baltimore, Md; 1983.

[3] Bogduk N. The anatomy and pathophysiology of neck pain. Phys Med Rehabil Clin N Am 2003;14:455–72.

[4] Gerwin RD, Dommerholt J, Shah JP. An expansion of Simons' integrated hypothesis of trigger point formation. Curr Pain Headache Rep 2004;8:468–75.

[5] Shah JP, Danoff JV, Desai MJ, et al. Biochemicals associated with pain and inflammation are elevated in sites near to and remote from active myofascial trigger points. Arch Phys Med Rehabil 2008;89:16–23.

[6] Carter JB, Banister EW. Musculoskeletal problems in VDT work: a review. Ergonomics 1994;37:1623–48.

[7] Fernandez-de-las Perias C, Alonso-Blanco C, Miangolarra JC. Myofascial trigger points in subjects presenting with mechanical neck pain: a blinded, controlled study. Man Ther 2007;12:29–33.

[8] Chen Q, Bensamoun S, Basford JR, et al. Identification and quantification of myofascial taut bands with magnetic resonance elastography. Arch Phys Med Rehabil 2007;88:1658–61.

[9] Smith J, Finnoff JT. Diagnostic and interventional musculoskeletal ultrasound. Part 1: fundamentals. PM R 2009;1:64–75.

[10] Ballyns JJ, Shah JP, Hammond J, et al. Objective sonographic measures for characterizing myofascial trigger points associated with cervical pain. J Ultrasound Med 2011;30:1331–40.

[11] Leite F, Atallah A, El Dib R, et al. Cyclobenzaprine for the treatment of myofascial pain in adults. Cochrane Database Syst Rev 2009;3, CD006830.

[12] Manfredini D, Landi N, Tognini F, et al. Muscle relaxants in the treatment of myofascial face pain. A literature review. Minerva Stomatol 2004;53:305–13.

[13] Annaswamy TM, De Luigi AJ, O'Neill BJ, et al. Emerging concepts in the treatment of myofascial pain: a review of medications, modalities, and needle-based interventions. PM R 2011;3:940–61.

[14] Graboski CL, Gray DS, Burnham RS. Botulinum toxin A versus bupivacaine trigger point injections for the treatment of myofascial pain syndrome: a randomised double blind crossover study. Pain 2005;118:170–5.

[15] Kamanli A, Kaya A, Ardicoglu O, et al. Comparison of lidocaine injection, botulinum toxin injection, and dry needling to trigger points in myofascial pain syndrome. Rheumatol Int 2005;25:604–11.

[16] Gobel H, Heinze A, Reichel G, et al. Efficacy and safety of a single botulinum type A toxin complex treatment (Dysport) for the relief of upper back myofascial pain syndrome: results from a randomized double-blind placebo-controlled multicentre study. Pain 2006;125:82–8.

[17] Qerama E, Fuglsang-Frederiksen A, Kasch H, et al. A double-blind, controlled study of botulinum toxin A in chronic myofascial pain. Neurology 2006;67:241–5.

[18] Ho KY, Tan KH. Botulinum toxin A for myofascial trigger point injection: a qualitative systematic review. Eur J Pain 2007;11:519–27.

SECTION II
Shoulder

CHAPTER 10

Acromioclavicular Injuries

Thomas D. Rizzo, Jr., MD

Synonyms

Acromioclavicular joint injuries
Acromioclavicular pain
Acromioclavicular separation
Separated shoulder
Acromioclavicular osteoarthritis
Atraumatic osteolysis of the distal clavicle

ICD-9 Codes

831.04 **Closed dislocation acromioclavicular joint**
840.0 **Acromioclavicular (joint) (ligament) sprain**

ICD-10 Codes

S43.50 **Sprain of unspecified acromiclavicular joint, ligament**
S43.51 **Sprain of right acromiclavicular joint, ligament**
S43.52 **Sprain of left acromiclavicular joint, ligament**
S43.101 **Unspecified dislocation of right acromioclavicular joint**
S43.102 **Unspecified dislocation of left acromioclavicular joint**
S43.109 **Unspecified dislocation of unspecified acromioclavicular joint**
Add seventh character for episode of care (A—initial encounter, D—subsequent encounter, S—sequela)

Definition

The acromioclavicular joint is a diarthrodial joint found between the lateral end of the clavicle and the medial side of the acromion [1]. The joint is surrounded by a fibrous capsule and stabilized by ligaments. The acromioclavicular ligaments cross the joint. Three ligaments begin at the coracoid process on the scapula and attach to the clavicle (trapezoid and conoid ligaments) or the acromion (coracoacromial ligament) (Fig. 10.1). This complex provides passive support and suspension of the scapula from the clavicle while allowing rotation of the clavicle to be transmitted to the scapula [1,2].

Injuries to the acromioclavicular complex are graded I to VI (Table 10.1). Injuries to the acromioclavicular joint were originally classified as grades 1, 2, and 3 by Tossy [3]. This classification was extended to include more complicated injuries, and grades 4, 5, and 6 were described. The extended grading system uses roman numerals [4].

The coracoacromial (lateral) ligament is not disrupted in injuries to the acromioclavicular joint. Therefore the fibrous connection persists between structures of the scapula emanating anteriorly and posteriorly [5]. In rare instances, there is an intra-articular fracture of the distal clavicle in addition to the ligamentous injuries [6].

There are few demographic data on differences of the disorder based on gender. Problems with the acromioclavicular joint can be associated with trauma and with overhead and throwing activities. Higher grade injuries are more likely to be due to trauma, such as auto accidents, falls, or sports injuries [7]. Concomitant injuries can vary on the basis of age; 86% of individuals older than 50 years have rotator cuff tears [8].

Most patients with grade I or grade II injuries respond to conservative measures and become asymptomatic within 3 weeks [9].

Symptoms

Patients often provide a history of trauma to the shoulder or in the vicinity of the acromioclavicular joint. Participants in

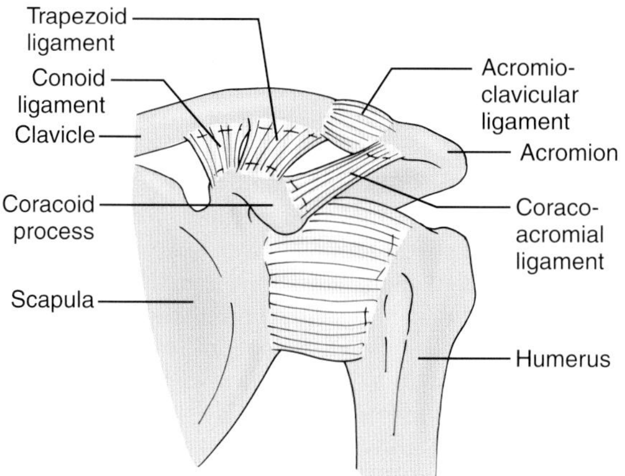

FIGURE 10.1 Normal anatomy of the ligaments associated with the acromioclavicular joint.

contact or collision sports (e.g., football, downhill skiing) are particularly susceptible. Patients seek care because of pain in the anterior and superior aspect of the shoulder [2]. This radiates into the base of the neck and the trapezius or deltoid muscles or down the arm in a radicular pattern [2,5,10].

Patients may describe pain brought on by activities of daily living that bring the arm across the chest (e.g., reaching into a jacket pocket) or behind the back (e.g., tucking in a shirt). Pain can also occur with shoulder flexion (reaching overhead) or with adduction of the arm across the chest. Patients may not have pain at rest and may be able to complete many activities without discomfort.

Physical Examination

Appropriate examination for suspected acromioclavicular injuries includes an examination of the neck and shoulder joint and girdle to eliminate the possibility of a radiculopathy or referred pain. Patients should have normal neck and neurologic examination findings. The presence of neurologic or vascular injury suggests that a greater degree of trauma has been sustained [5].

On inspection, there may be a raised area at the acromioclavicular joint. This is caused by depression of the scapula relative to the clavicle or swelling of the joint itself. This area is commonly tender to touch. On active range of motion, the patient may complain of pain or wince near the extreme of shoulder flexion.

Shoulder range of motion is typically within normal limits. Supporting the arm at the elbow and gently directing the arm superiorly may decrease the pain and allow more complete assessment of the patient's shoulder range of motion. The pain may become worse as the shoulder is further flexed, whether it is done actively or passively. This is in distinction to impingement syndromes, which often hurt at a particular point in the arc of motion but are painless as the motion proceeds. Pain is typically absent with static manual muscle testing of the rotator cuff. Rotator cuff injuries will be painful with activation of the muscles of the rotator cuff. These problems are best identified with the shoulder in a neutral position (i.e., elbow next to the body) because the rotator cuff muscles are in a lengthened position and are easily made symptomatic.

Special tests to identify acromioclavicular joint disease attempt to compress the joint. The most common test is the cross-body adduction test (Fig. 10.2). The shoulder is abducted to 90 degrees and the elbow is flexed to the same degree. The clinician then brings the arm across the patient's body until the elbow approaches the midline (or the patient reports pain) [2].

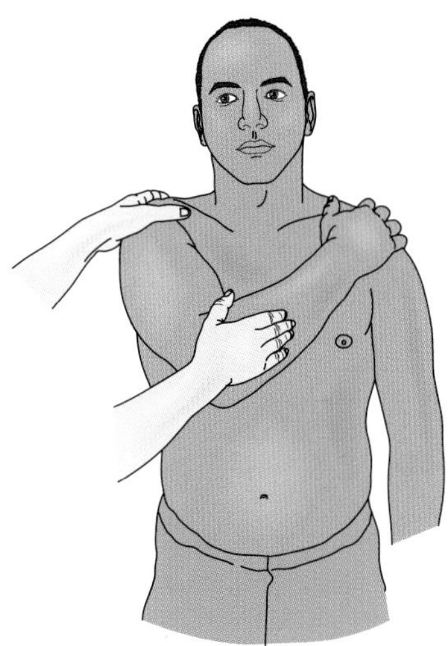

FIGURE 10.2 Cross-body adduction test for a sprain of the acromioclavicular joint.

Table 10.1 Grades of Acromioclavicular Joint Injuries and Treatments

Grade of Injury	AC Ligament	CC Ligament	Clavicle Displacement	Treatment
I	Sprain	Intact	Mild superior displacement	Conservative
II	Torn	Sprain	Definite superior displacement	Conservative
III	Torn	Torn	25%-100% increase in CC space	Conservative or surgical
IV	Torn	Torn	Posterior displacement	Surgical
V	Torn	Torn	100%-300% increase in CC space	Surgical
VI	Torn	Torn	Subacromial or subcoracoid location	Surgical

AC, acromioclavicular; *CC*, coracoclavicular.

Other tests help differentiate between impingement syndrome and acromioclavicular joint pain. If the shoulder is passively flexed while it is internally rotated, the greater tuberosity can pinch (impinge) the supraspinatus tendon and subacromial bursa. The same test performed with the shoulder externally rotated will compress the acromioclavicular joint without impinging the subacromial space [11]. In the active compression test, the shoulder is flexed to 90 degrees and then adducted to 10 degrees (Fig. 10.3). The patient first maximally internally rotates the arm and then tries to flex the shoulder against the clinician's resistance. This puts pressure on the acromioclavicular joint and may reproduce pain if disease is present. The test is repeated with the shoulder in full external rotation. This will put stress on the biceps tendon and its labral attachment while excluding the acromioclavicular joint [12].

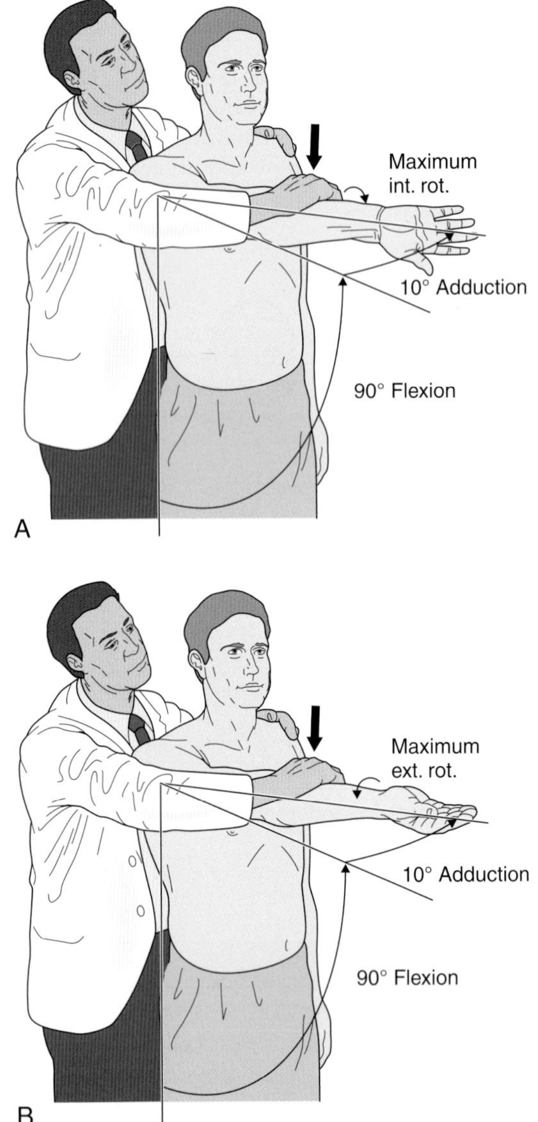

FIGURE 10.3 The active compression test. **A,** The arm is forward flexed and internally rotated maximally. Downward force is applied, and pain indicates acromioclavicular joint disease. **B,** The test is repeated with the arm externally rotated. Pain indicates disease of the biceps tendon and its labral attachment. *(From O'Brien SJ, Pagnani MJ, Fealy S, et al. The active compression test: a new and effective test for diagnosing labral tears and acromioclavicular joint abnormality. Am J Sports Med 1998;26:610-613.)*

In the acromioclavicular resisted extension test, the shoulder is abducted to 90 degrees and adducted across the body to 90 degrees (Fig. 10.4). The examiner resists active shoulder extension. A positive test result reproduces pain in the acromioclavicular joint. A combination of these tests will improve the diagnostic accuracy over isolated tests [13].

The Paxinos sign, along with bone scan, has a high degree of diagnostic accuracy in acromioclavicular joint disease [14]. The examiner stands behind the patient and, using the hand contralateral to the affected shoulder, stabilizes the clavicle and pushes the acromion into the clavicle with the thumb. The test response is considered positive if pain occurs or increases in the region of the acromioclavicular joint; the test response is considered negative if there is no change in the pain level (Fig. 10.5).

Functional Limitations

Reaching up, reaching across the body, and carrying heavy weights are limited because of pain. Patients may have no pain at rest and little or no pain with many activities. Patients may complain of difficulty with putting on a shirt, combing the hair, and carrying a briefcase or grocery bag. Most recreational activities, especially those that incorporate throwing, will be limited as well. Sleep may be affected because of pain, especially when rolling over on the affected side.

Diagnostic Studies

Because this is often a traumatic injury, radiographs are important in most cases and should be obtained to rule out fracture as well as to assess the severity of the injury (Fig. 10.6). Views should include an anteroposterior view, a lateral Y view, and an axillary view. It is important to let the radiologist know that injury to the acromioclavicular joint, not just the shoulder, is in question. Stress or weighted views are usually not helpful and cause undue pain without improving the accuracy of diagnosis [2,15]. Overpenetration of films may make the interpretation of the acromioclavicular joint and distal clavicle difficult [5].

A 15-degree cephalad anteroposterior view helps diagnose sprains by decreasing x-ray penetration and showing separation between the acromion and clavicle, whereas the 40-degree cephalic tilt anteroposterior view should be used for suspected fractures of the clavicle. If the fracture is medial to the coracoclavicular ligaments, both anterior and posterior 45-degree views should be obtained [5]. Typically, the decision to obtain these views is made by a radiologist.

Certainly, if there are concerns about a fracture or arthrosis and the x-ray images do not provide confirmation, further evaluation with a bone scan [2,5] or magnetic resonance imaging (MRI) may be indicated [16]. MRI evaluation of symptomatic acromioclavicular joints revealed that 80% had active bone edema in the distal clavicle or acromion or on both sides, but no asymptomatic patients had this finding [17]. MRI will detect the extent of acromioclavicular arthrosis more frequently than conventional radiology [18]. MRI does not appear to add any further information to the clinical assessment [19].

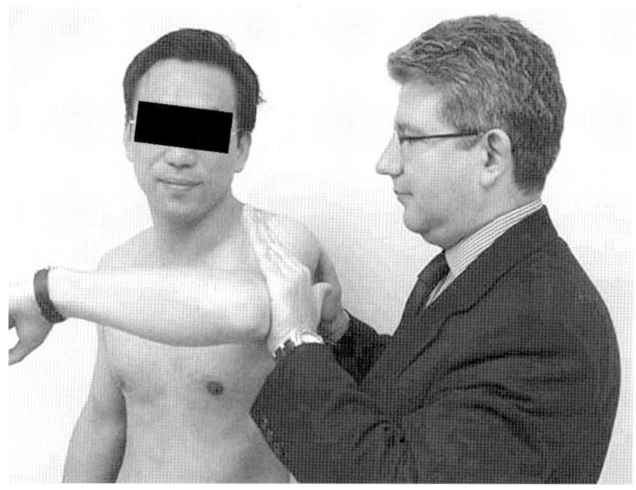

FIGURE 10.4 In the acromioclavicular resisted extension test, the examiner resists active shoulder extension. A positive test result reproduces pain in the acromioclavicular joint. *(From Chronopoulos E, Kim TK, Park HB, et al. Diagnostic value of physical tests for isolated chronic acromioclavicular lesions. Am J Sports Med 2004;32:655-661.)*

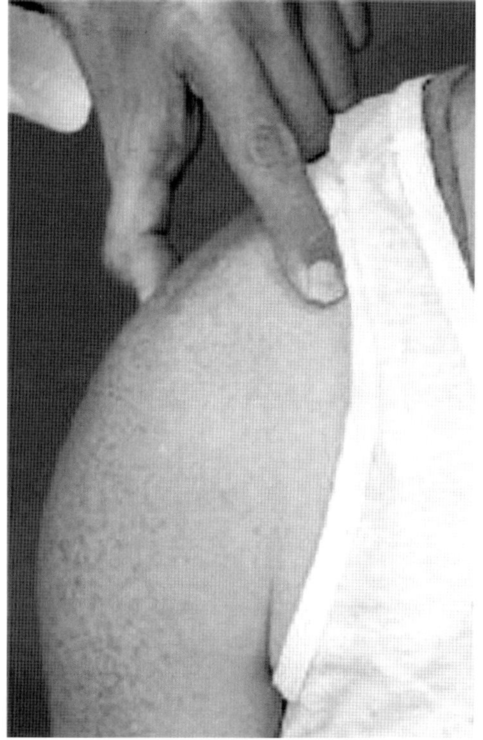

FIGURE 10.5 To elicit the Paxinos sign, stand behind the patient and use the hand contralateral to the affected shoulder. *(From Walton J, Mahajan S, Paxinos A, et al. Diagnostic values of tests for acromioclavicular joint pain. J Bone Joint Surg Am 2004;86:807-812.)*

Ultrasonography is a reproducible method of evaluating the joint space and joint capsule, but the measurements may vary from those obtained by MRI [20]. The findings on ultrasound evaluation correlate well with the diagnosis obtained by clinical examination and radiography [21].

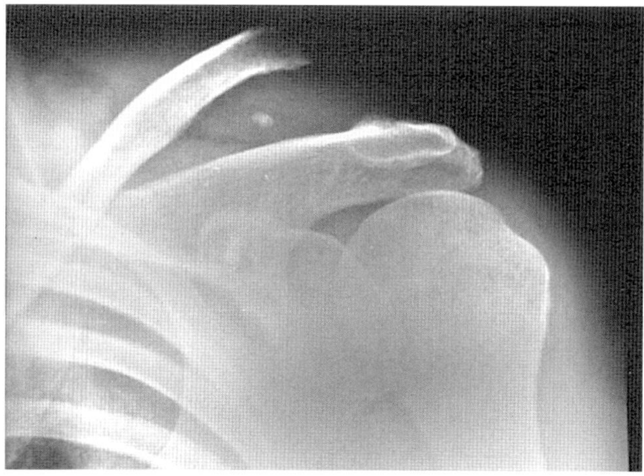

FIGURE 10.6 Grade III acromioclavicular joint dislocation. There is marked superior displacement of the distal clavicle relative to the acromion and coracoid processes. *(From Katz DS, Math KR, Groskin SA. Radiology Secrets. Philadelphia, Hanley & Belfus, 1998.)*

Differential Diagnosis

Adhesive capsulitis
Arthritis (e.g., rheumatoid, crystal induced, and septic)
Calcific tendinitis
Cervical radiculopathy
Distal osteolysis of the clavicle
Fractures of the acromion or distal clavicle
Ganglia and cysts in the acromioclavicular joint
Gout
Infection
Os acromiale syndrome
Rotator cuff tears
Shoulder impingement syndrome
Tendinitis of the long head of the biceps
Tears of the glenohumeral labrum
Tumors
Referred pain may come from cardiac, pulmonary, and gastrointestinal disease

Treatment

Initial

Initial treatment depends on the degree of injury and the patient's activity and goals.

Type I and type II injuries are exclusively treated nonoperatively, whereas type IV, type V, and type VI injuries require surgery. Treatment of type III injuries is controversial (see Table 10.1).

The initial phase of treatment for all injuries not going to surgery (i.e., type I, type II, and some type III) includes rest, ice, and possibly a sling or brace for 1 to 6 weeks (2 to 3 weeks average). Over-the-counter or prescription nonnarcotic analgesics are usually sufficient. Nonsteroidal anti-inflammatory drugs can be used for pain and inflammation. Injections into the joint can also be done in the initial phase of treatment for immediate pain control and to help confirm the diagnosis. Injections have been done acutely with immediate return to activity in low-grade injuries.

Rest should be relative, that is, the patient should avoid aggravating activities but should not be immobilized if at all possible.

Ice massage can be done over the painful area for 5 to 10 minutes every 2 hours, as needed. An ice pack can be used for 20 minutes at a time and also can be repeated every 2 hours. The usual precautions for the use of cold modalities should be followed.

Type I and type II sprains can be treated with a sling to help support the arm and shoulder. This should be used symptomatically and discontinued for painless activities and when the patient's pain is under control.

Type III injuries have been treated operatively and nonoperatively (Fig. 10.7). In the majority of published studies and reference texts, orthopedists favor nonoperative treatment as a rule, even in throwing athletes [5,15,22–24]. One study suggested greater long-term satisfaction in patients who had surgery but showed no difference in range of motion or strength [25]. Most patients have no long-term difficulty with nonoperative management. There are also reports of high complication rates with surgery [5,24]. Surgery may be considered in symptomatic individuals with type III injuries and in those who do not respond to conservative measures.

One approach for type III injuries is to treat conservatively with relative rest, support, modalities, medications for symptoms, and gradual return to activity during 6 to 12 weeks. If there is a significant limitation in function, including avocational or sport activities, or if the patient is not progressing as expected, further evaluation is warranted [5]. Unlike with musculotendinous injuries, delayed surgery does not lead to poorer outcomes.

Rehabilitation

Physical or occupational therapy can be ordered to assist with education of the patient, pain control, and, in later stages, gradual range of motion and strengthening exercises. Modalities to control pain can include, in addition to ice, ultrasound and phonophoresis with 10% lidocaine. Alternatively, interferential current can be used. As pain is controlled, motion can be obtained in a pain-free range. Codman and pendulum exercises can progress to active or active-assisted range of motion to restore shoulder flexion and abduction, both individually and in combination. In the initial phase of a rehabilitation program, it is reasonable to avoid painful positions or movements. These include extremes of flexion—even when they are done passively—and adduction across the chest. When the shoulder is pain free and has full range of motion, rehabilitation can progress to gradual strengthening and return to activity. A typical shoulder strengthening rehabilitation program can be used. Light dumbbell exercises with 1 to 5 pounds to strengthen the internal and external rotators or resistance bands can be used initially. This program can be advanced to isolate the shoulder abductors and to incorporate internal and external rotator strengthening at different degrees of shoulder abduction. Further progression depends on the patient's goals and requires incorporation of the scapular stabilizers and training in coordinated movements.

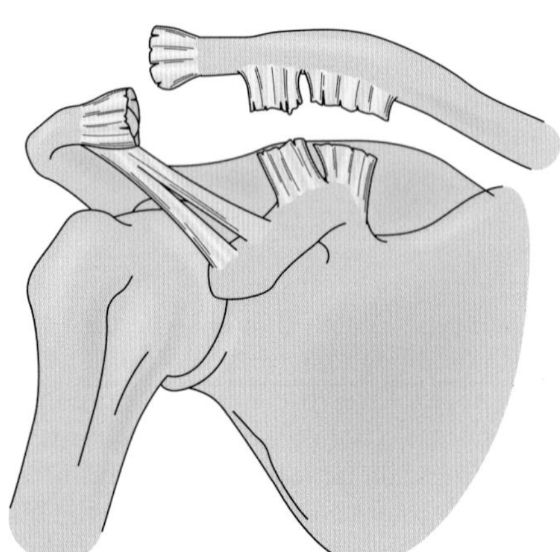

FIGURE 10.7 Grade III acromioclavicular joint sprain. *(From Mellion MB. Office Sports Medicine, 2nd ed. Philadelphia, Hanley & Belfus, 1996.)*

Postoperative rehabilitation varies by the type of injury (type III–type VI), acute versus chronic repair, surgical technique employed, and surgeon. Typically, there is a period of immobilization or support with a sling (1-6 weeks). Passive, active-assisted, or active range of motion exercises may be allowed during this time. In some instances, daily activities will be allowed, but strengthening and heavy lifting are not.

Strengthening exercises may begin as soon as 2 weeks or as many as 3 months postoperatively, depending on the repair. Return to sports may take 8 weeks and be as long as 6 months. Given the variety of recommendations, good communication with the orthopedic surgeon is essential [7,26–28].

Procedures

Patients with acromioclavicular joint pain due to type I or mild type II injuries can receive injections and return to play or work during the same day or competitive event with little risk of injury as long as they have full functional range of motion and symmetric strength. For diagnostic purposes, a local anesthetic injection may confirm the diagnosis of a type I sprain if the patient has complete pain relief immediately after the injection. Intra-articular injection of a combination of a local anesthetic and a corticosteroid may give immediate and longer acting relief. Injections into the joint can be done for higher grade injuries as well as to give quick symptomatic relief. However, this is not a substitute for relative rest in more seriously injured joints (type II and higher), and 1 week of avoiding provocative maneuvers after the injection is advised [2]. The blind or palpation approach to acromioclavicular joint injection is done with the patient sitting or supine with the shoulder propped under a pillow. The acromioclavicular joint is injected under sterile conditions with use of a 25-gauge, 1½-inch disposable needle and a local anesthetic or anesthetic and corticosteroid combination (Fig. 10.8). Typically, a 1- to 3-mL aliquot of solution is injected (e.g., 1 mL of 1% lidocaine mixed with 1 mL of betamethasone). Keep in mind that the acromioclavicular joint is small and close to the surface.

Ultrasound guidance of the acromioclavicular joint injection can improve the accuracy of the injection [29,30]. Injection by the palpation method is truly in the joint 40% to 60% of the time [29,31]. Use of ultrasound [29,30] or an image intensifier [31] ensures 100% accurate needle placement.

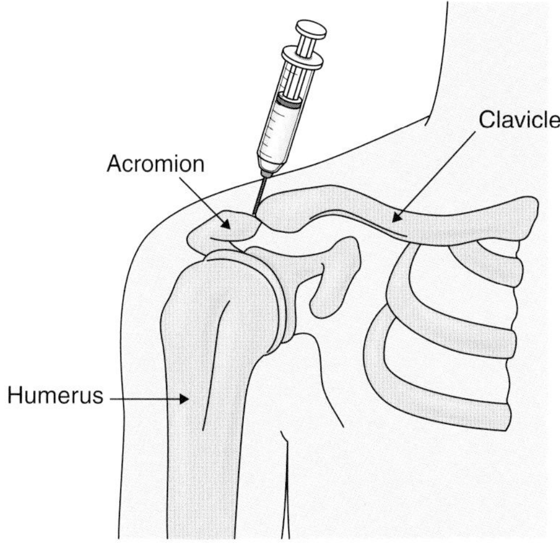

FIGURE 10.8 Internal anatomic site for injection of the acromioclavicular joint. *(From Lennard TA. Pain Procedures in Clinical Practice, 2nd ed. Philadelphia, Hanley & Belfus, 2000.)*

It is not clear that use of ultrasound improves outcome [30]. The ultrasound-guided approach is somewhat different (Fig. 10.9) as a lateral to medial approach is advocated [29].

Postinjection care should include local icing for 10 to 15 minutes and instructions to the patient to avoid aggravating activities for at least 1 week.

Surgery

Type IV, type V, and type VI injuries are forms of dislocation of the acromioclavicular joint. These need to be reduced surgically with some form of reconstruction attempted. Early referral is indicated to minimize pain and dysfunction. Because the scapula is no longer suspended from the clavicle, the deltoid and trapezius muscles will become involved in an attempt to hold the scapula in place. These muscles may have been injured directly and therefore are ill-suited to take on the role of suspending the arm. The result is more significant pain and a greater chance for prolonged disability.

If the patient has sustained a fracture, surgery may be necessary, and referral to an orthopedist is appropriate. The severity of the injury depends on whether the fracture is medial to the coracoclavicular ligaments or involves the acromioclavicular joint itself. Fractures medial to the ligaments can result in displacement of the clavicle, and the patient therefore runs the risk of delayed union or nonunion. The displacement can look like a type II or type III sprain. Careful examination of the location and degree of pain should suggest an injury to the clavicle. Regardless, radiographs are indicated to assess the possibility of fracture.

Fractures into the joint are likely to lead to arthrosis in the future. These patients may not need surgery initially—that will be decided by the patient and the orthopedist—but may require a protracted conservative course of symptomatic treatment.

Resection of the distal clavicle, tacking of the acromion to the clavicle, re-creation of the ligaments, and screw fixation of the acromioclavicular joint or of the clavicle to the coracoid process have been used to stabilize the joint. The goal of any surgical procedure is to try to re-create a stable, pain-free joint [5].

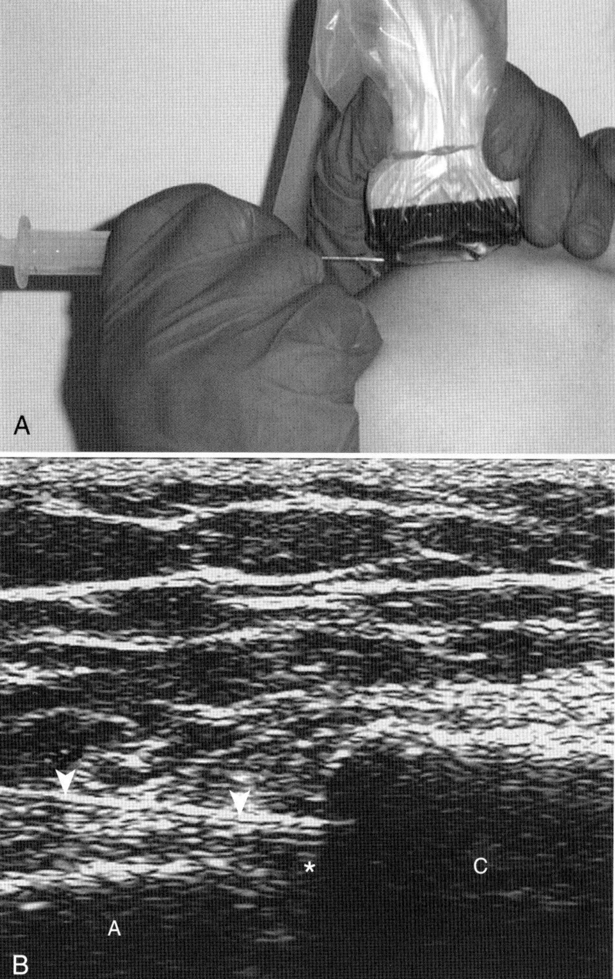

FIGURE 10.9 **A,** Needle approach and ultrasound transducer position for ultrasound-guided acromioclavicular joint injections. **B,** Ultrasound image of the acromioclavicular joint *(asterisk)* and needle *(arrowheads)* in long-axis (in-plane) view. *Left,* lateral; *top,* superficial, *A,* acromion, *C,* clavicle. (Merlin 1101 US system, B-K Medical Systems, Wilmington, Mass.) *(From Peck E, Lai J, Pawlina W, Smith J. Accuracy of ultrasound-guided versus palpation-guided acromioclavicular joint injections: a cadaveric study. PM R 2010;2:817-821.)*

Postoperative outcome of surgical repair of type V injuries was excellent in 11 of 12 patients after 2 years [7]. Twenty-one years after surgical treatment of type III injuries, 92% of patients had satisfactory results and no pain and would have the procedure again [32].

Potential Disease Complications

Patients may be left with a "bump" due to the depression of the acromion relative to the clavicle. This should be expected and is unavoidable without surgery. Acromioclavicular joint pain due to chronic instability is the most common complication [5,33]. Degenerative arthritis can occur because of the injury or instability. This can be treated symptomatically with modalities and injections. One in five patients with a grade I or grade II injury will have restriction in range of motion, but less than 10% will have symptoms that restrict daily or athletic activity [34].

If the pain persists, surgery should be considered. In one study, more than 25% of patients with grade I or grade II injuries required surgery 2 years after the injury [10].

Concomitant disorders of the glenohumeral joint complex can develop along with acromioclavicular arthrosis. These include rotator cuff tears, glenoid labrum tears, glenohumeral arthrosis, and biceps tendon disease [9].

Potential Treatment Complications

Analgesics and nonsteroidal anti-inflammatory drugs have well-known side effects that most commonly affect the gastric, hepatic, and renal systems. Cyclooxygenase 2 inhibitors may have fewer gastric side effects, but cardiovascular risks should be considered. Injection of the joint with too long a needle may result in injection into the subacromial space. This can cause diagnostic confusion, if not outright injury [2]. Injections can also be associated with infection in rare cases.

Direct complications of surgery can include infection, pain, wound or skin breakdown, and hypertrophic scar [5,23,35]. After surgery, there can be a recurrence of the deformity [23,25], hardware failure or migration [6,23,32,35], or limitation of movement. Pain may persist as a result of insufficient resection, weakness, or joint instability [2]. Acromioclavicular arthrosis may develop after surgery, although this may not adversely affect the patient's function [7,32].

Recalcification after acromioclavicular joint resection can be a cause of pain and may require revision of the distal clavicle resection [35]. Likewise, distal osteolysis of the clavicle can occur, requiring revision surgery [36]. Coracoclavicular ligament ossification may develop, although this is not typically painful [32].

References

[1] Stecco A, Sgambati E, Brizzi E, et al. Morphometric analysis of the acromioclavicular joint. Ital J Anat Embryol 1997;102:195–200.

[2] Shaffer BS. Painful conditions of the acromioclavicular joint. J Am Acad Orthop Surg 1999;7:176–88.

[3] Tossy JD, Mead NC, Sigmond HM. Acromioclavicular separations: useful and practical classification for treatment. Clin Orthop Relat Res 1963;28:111–9.

[4] Rockwood CA, Williams GR, Young DC. Acromioclavicular injuries. 3rd ed. Rockwood CA, Green DP, Bucholz RW, editors. Rockwood and Green's Fractures in Adults, vol. 1. Philadelphia: JB Lippincott; 1991. p. 1181–239.

[5] Turnbull JR. Acromioclavicular joint disorders. Med Sci Sports Exerc 1998;30:S26–32.

[6] Berg EE. An intra-articular fracture dislocation of the acromioclavicular joint. Am J Orthop 1998;7:555–9.

[7] Kim SH, Lee YH, Shin SH, et al. Outcome of conjoined tendon and coracoacromial ligament transfer for the treatment of chronic type V acromioclavicular joint separation injury. Injury 2012;43:213–8.

[8] Brown JN, Roberts SN, Hayes MG, Sales AD. Shoulder pathology associated with symptomatic acromioclavicular joint degeneration. J Shoulder Elbow Surg 2000;9:173–6.

[9] Mouhsine E, Garofalo R, Crevoisier X, Farron A. Grade I and II acromioclavicular dislocations: results of conservative treatment. J Shoulder Elbow Surg 2003;12:599–602.

[10] Gerber C, Galantay RV, Hersche O. The pattern of pain produced by irritation of the acromioclavicular joint and subacromial space. J Shoulder Elbow Surg 1998;7:352–5.

[11] Buchberger DJ. Introduction of a new physical examination procedure for the differentiation of acromioclavicular joint lesions and subacromial impingement. J Manipulative Physiol Ther 1999;22:316–21.

[12] O'Brien SJ, Pagnani MJ, Fealy S, et al. The active compression test: a new and effective test for diagnosing labral tears and acromioclavicular joint abnormality. Am J Sports Med 1998;26:610–3.

[13] Chronopoulos E, Kim TK, Park HB, et al. Diagnostic value of physical tests for isolated chronic acromioclavicular lesions. Am J Sports Med 2004;32:655–61.

[14] Walton J, Mahajan S, Paxinos A, et al. Diagnostic values of tests for acromioclavicular joint pain. J Bone Joint Surg Am 2004;86:807–12.

[15] Lemos M. Evaluation and treatment of the injured acromioclavicular joint in athletes. Am J Sports Med 1998;26:137–44.

[16] Yu JS, Dardani M, Fischer RA. MR observations of posttraumatic osteolysis of the distal clavicle after traumatic separation of the acromioclavicular joint. J Comput Assist Tomogr 2000;24:159–64.

[17] Shubin Stein BE, Ahmad CS, Pfaff CH, et al. A comparison of magnetic resonance imaging findings of the acromioclavicular joint in symptomatic versus asymptomatic patients. J Shoulder Elbow Surg 2006;15:56–9.

[18] de Abreu MR, Chung CB, Wesselly M, et al. Acromioclavicular joint osteoarthritis: comparison of findings derived from MR imaging and conventional radiography. Clin Imaging 2005;29:273–7.

[19] Jordan LK, Kenter K, Griffiths HL. Relationship between MRI and clinical findings in the acromioclavicular joint. Skeletal Radiol 2002;31:516–21.

[20] Heers G, Gotz J, Schachner H, et al. Ultrasound evaluation of the acromioclavicular joint. A comparison with magnetic resonance imaging. Sportverletz Sportschaden 2005;19:177–81 [in German].

[21] Iovane A, Midiri M, Galia M, et al. Acute traumatic acromioclavicular joint lesions: role of ultrasound versus conventional radiography. Radiol Med (Torino) 2004;107:367–75.

[22] McFarland EG, Blivin SJ, Doehring CB, et al. Treatment of grade III acromioclavicular separations in professional throwing athletes: results of a survey. Am J Orthop 1997;26:771–4.

[23] Phillips AM, Smart C, Groom AF. Acromioclavicular dislocation. Conservative or surgical therapy. Clin Orthop Relat Res 1998;353:10–7.

[24] Spencer Jr EE. Treatment of grade III acromioclavicular joint injuries: a systematic review. Clin Orthop Relat Res 2007;455:38–44.

[25] Press J, Zuckerman JD, Gallagher M, Cuomo F. Treatment of grade III acromioclavicular separations. Bull Hosp Joint Dis 1997;56:77–83.

[26] Leidel BA, Braunstein V, Kirchhoff C, et al. Consistency of long-term outcome of acute Rockwood grade III acromioclavicular joint separations after K-wire transfixation. J Trauma 2009;66:1666–71.

[27] Albers WE. Old unreduced dislocations. In: Canale ST, Beaty JH, editors. Campbell's Operative orthopaedics. 12th ed. St. Louis: Elsevier/Mosby; 2013.

[28] Mascioli AA. Acute dislocations. In: Canale ST, Beaty JH, editors. Campbell's Operative orthopaedics. 12th ed. St. Louis: Elsevier/Mosby; 2013.

[29] Peck E, Lai J, Pawlina W, Smith J. Accuracy of ultrasound-guided versus palpation-guided acromioclavicular joint injections: a cadaveric study. PM R 2010;2:817–21.

[30] Sabeti-Aschraf M, Ochsnera A, Schueller-Weidekammb C, et al. The infiltration of the AC joint performed by one specialist: ultrasound versus palpation a prospective randomized pilot study. Eur J Radiol 2010;75:e37–40.

[31] Pichler W, Weinberg AM, Grechenig S, et al. Intra-articular injection of the acromioclavicular joint. J Bone Joint Surg Br 2009;91:1638–40.

[32] Lizaur A, Sanz-Reig J, Gonzalez-Parreño S. Long-term results of the surgical treatment of type III acromioclavicular dislocations. J Bone Joint Surg Br 2011;93:1088–92.

[33] Clarke HD, McCann PD. Acromioclavicular injuries. Orthop Clin North Am 2000;31:177–87.

[34] Shaw MB, McInerney JJ, Dias JJ, Evans PA. Acromioclavicular joint sprains: the post-injury recovery interval. Injury 2003;34:438–42.

[35] Rudzki JR, Matava MJ, Paletta Jr GA. Complications of treatment of acromioclavicular and sternoclavicular joint injuries. Clin Sports Med 2003;22:387–405.

[36] Geaney LE, Miller MD, Ticker JB, et al. Management of the failed AC joint reconstruction: causation and treatment. Sports Med Arthrosc Rev 2010;18:167–72.

CHAPTER 11

Adhesive Capsulitis

Brian J. Krabak, MD, MBA, FACSM

Synonyms

Frozen shoulder
Periarthritis of the shoulder
Stiff and painful shoulder
Periarticular adhesions
Humeroscapular fibrositis

ICD-9 Code

726.0 Adhesive capsulitis of shoulder

ICD-10 Codes

M75.00 Adhesive capsulitis of shoulder, unspecified
M75.01 Adhesive capsulitis of right shoulder
M75.02 Adhesive capsulitis of left shoulder

Definition

Primary adhesive capsulitis of the shoulder is an idiopathic, progressive, painful but self-limited restriction of active and passive range of motion [1–3]. The onset is insidious and progresses through several stages, usually during the course of 1 to 2 years. These stages include the painful phase, the freezing or adhesive phase, and the thawing or resolution phase. Adhesive capsulitis occurs in approximately 2% to 5% of the general population and accounts for approximately 6% of office visits to shoulder specialists (orthopedists and physiatrists) on a yearly basis [2]. The condition preferentially affects women after the age of 50 years, involves the nondominant shoulder, and develops in the opposite shoulder in 20% to 30% of cases. The primary etiology is unknown, but it is associated with numerous secondary causes, including immobilization, diabetes, hypothyroidism, autoimmune disease, and treatment of breast cancer (Table 11.1).

The pathologic process related to adhesive capsulitis involves structures both intrinsic to the glenohumeral joint and surrounding it (Fig. 11.1). Although it is not clear, one theory is that stimulation of synovitis leads to fibrosis due to the activation of various cytokines, including growth factors such as transforming growth factor-β [4]. The pathologic findings of adhesive capsulitis ultimately depend on its stage when it is assessed [1,2]. The painful phase is characterized by synovitis that progresses to capsular thickening (particularly in the anterior and inferior portions of the capsule) with an associated reduction in synovial fluid. As the adhesive phase continues, fibrosis of the capsule is more pronounced, and thickening of the rotator cuff tendons is common. As this phase continues, the glenohumeral joint space becomes contracted and often obliterated. Pathologic change is more consistent with chronic inflammation with resolution of joint space loss during the final stage.

Symptoms

Symptoms will depend on the stage of adhesive capsulitis. In stage 1, the patients experience the gradual onset of progressive pain that is worse during the night and exacerbated by overhead activities. They will gradually report a loss of motion with symptoms lasting less than 3 months. In stage 2, there is a progressive increase in pain that is associated with a reduction in the range of motion and decreased use of the affected shoulder [1,2]. The stage can last 9 to 15 months. Stage 3, the "thawing stage," is characterized by a gradual decrease in pain and increase in the pain-free range of motion. Some individuals will return to normal, but not all (Table 11.2).

Physical Examination

The findings noted on physical examination reflect the stage of adhesive capsulitis development. During the painful and adhesive stages of adhesive capsulitis, there is a measurable reduction in *both* passive and active shoulder range of motion. Motion is painful, particularly at the extremes of external rotation and abduction [1,2,5]. This pattern of motion loss is consistent with a capsular pattern of passive range of motion loss, which demonstrates a greater limitation in external rotation and abduction followed by an increasing loss of flexion. These signs are similar to those found in osteoarthritis of the glenohumeral joint, in which there is a similar loss of motion with shoulder pain. However, this presentation is in contrast to findings seen in rotator cuff tears, in which active range of motion is restricted but passive range of motion may approximate normal values. A reduced glenohumeral glide is often noted with adhesive capsulitis, especially with

Table 11.1 Diseases and Conditions Associated with Secondary Adhesive Capsulitis

Immobilization	Pulmonary tuberculosis	Scleroderma
Diabetes mellitus	Chronic lung disease	Post mastectomy
Thyroid disease	Myocardial infarction	Cervical radiculitis
Rheumatoid arthritis	Cerebrovascular accidents	Peripheral nerve injury
Trauma	Rotator cuff disease	Lung cancer
		Breast cancer

Modified from Siegel LB, Cohen NJ, Gall EP. Adhesive capsulitis: a sticky issue. Am Fam Physician 1999;59:1843-1852.

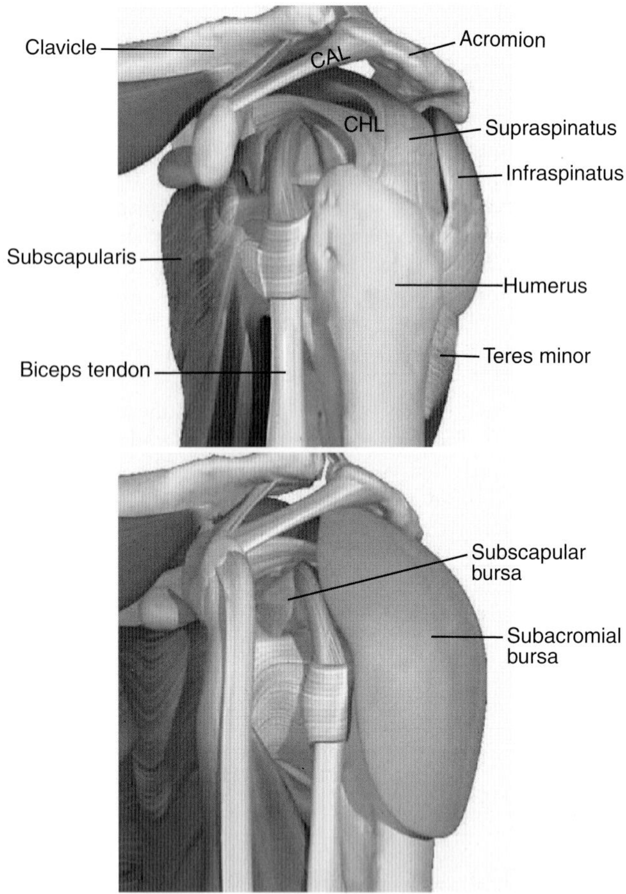

FIGURE 11.1 Relevant anatomy of the glenohumeral joint. Note the rotator cuff tendon insertion sites, biceps tendon, subacromial bursa, and coracoacromial ligament (CAL); the subcoracoid triangle is formed by the coracoid process, coracohumeral ligament (CHL), and joint capsule. *(From Stubblefield MD, Custodio CM. Upper extremity pain disorders in breast cancer. Arch Phys Med Rehabil 2006;87[Suppl 1]:S96-S99.)*

inferior translation. The relationship of glenohumeral joint movements independent of scapulothoracic motion should also be noted. Last, the shoulder is often painful to palpation around the rotator cuff tendons distally. As symptoms start to improve and the patient enters the resolution stage, there is a reversal of the loss of motion, with internal rotation being the last to improve.

Table 11.2 The Three Stages of Adhesive Capsulitis

Painful Stage

Pain with movement
Generalized ache that is difficult to pinpoint
Muscle spasm
Increasing pain at night and at rest

Adhesive Stage

Less pain
Increasing stiffness and restriction of movement
Decreasing pain at night and at rest
Discomfort felt at extreme ranges of movement

Resolution Stage

Decreased pain
Marked restriction with slow, gradual increase in range of motion
Recovery is spontaneous but frequently incomplete

Modified from Siegel LB, Cohen NJ, Gall EP. Adhesive capsulitis: a sticky issue. Am Fam Physician 1999;59:1843-1852.

Neurologic evaluation findings are usually normal in adhesive capsulitis, although manual muscle testing may detect weakness secondary to pain or disuse. However, concomitant rotator cuff involvement is common and could explain true weakness if it is noted on physical examination. The combination of myotomal weakness, altered dermatomal sensation, reflex asymmetry, and positive findings with cervical spine provocative testing is more suggestive of a neurologic cause of shoulder pain [5].

Functional Limitations

Patients often experience sleep disruption as a result of pain or inability to sleep on the affected side. Inability to perform activities of daily living (e.g., fastening a bra in the back, putting on a belt, reaching for a wallet in the back pocket, reaching for a seat belt, combing the hair) is common. Work activities may be limited, particularly those that involve overhead activities (e.g., filing above waist level, stocking shelves, lifting boards or other items). Recreational activities (e.g., difficulty serving or throwing a ball, inability to do the crawl stroke in swimming) are also affected.

Diagnostic Studies

Because adhesive capsulitis is associated with other comorbidities and a population of patients in whom neoplastic processes are common, routine blood work and radiographs should be obtained to rule out secondary causes [6–9]. Radiographs in patients with adhesive capsulitis are generally normal. In advanced stages, joint space narrowing may be noted on arthrograms as there is a reduced volume of injectable contrast material into the joint (Fig. 11.2). Magnetic resonance imaging may also prove to be a useful diagnostic tool; studies have confirmed findings seen at arthroscopy, including thickening of the coracohumeral ligament and obliteration of the subcoracoid space (Fig. 11.3) [6–8]. Ultrasonography allows a dynamic view of the shoulder region with a sensitivity of 91%, a specificity of 100%, and an accuracy of 92% for detection of adhesive capsulitis [9].

Differential Diagnosis

Labral disease
Rotator cuff disease
Subacromial bursitis
Osteoarthritis
Acromioclavicular joint disease
Calcific tendinosis
Synovitis
Fractures
Bicipital tendinosis
Cervical radiculopathy (C5, C6)
Peripheral nerve entrapment (suprascapular)
Complex regional pain syndrome
Brachial plexopathies, thoracic outlet syndrome
Neoplastic conditions
Rheumatic conditions

Treatment

Initial

The treatment goals depend on the stage of adhesive capsulitis, but the general goals are to decrease pain and inflammation while increasing the shoulder range of motion in all planes [1–3]. Initially, pain and inflammation should be managed with ice, medications, and activity modifications. Reducing inflammation and pain through the use of nonsteroidal anti-inflammatory drugs is generally advocated, although it has not been clearly shown to have an impact on the resolution of pain [2]. A short trial of oral steroids has been shown to more rapidly decrease pain compared with placebo, but the benefits are not sustained during long-term follow-up [2,10]. Similarly, intra-articular injection of corticosteroids (with or without lidocaine) has been shown to be helpful during the early stages of adhesive capsulitis compared with placebo, but it does not change long-term outcomes [2].

Rehabilitation

Despite the lack of significant well-conducted clinical trials, the standard of treatment mainly involves physical therapy and home exercises to restore range of motion for the treatment of adhesive capsulitis [1,2,10–12]. The clinician will gauge the need for physical therapy versus a home exercise program and rate of progression of therapy as adhesive capsulitis can take months to years to resolve. Factors affecting the setting and pace of rehabilitation include the severity of the patient's symptoms, physical examination findings, ability to perform the exercises appropriately, and compliance with a home exercise program. Initially, pendulum exercises, overhead stretches, and crossed adduction of the affected arm should be taught to patients while they are in the physician's office once adhesive capsulitis is suspected to prevent further loss of function (Fig. 11.4). Some physicians

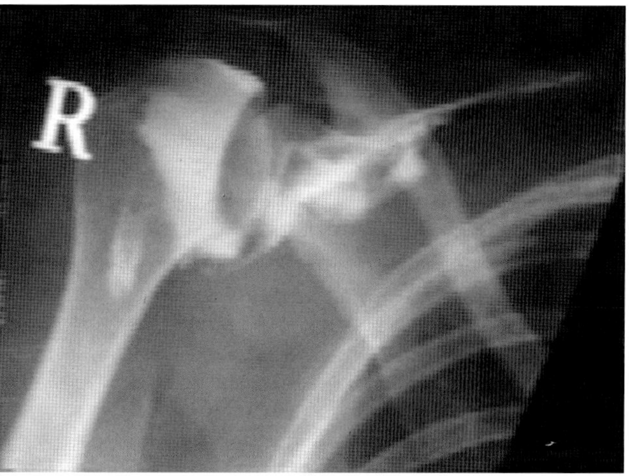

FIGURE 11.2 Arthrogram of shoulder with advanced adhesive capsulitis with a contracted joint space. Note the absence of the axillary recess and the reduced amount of contrast material injected. *(From Smith LL, Burnet SP, McNeil JD. Musculoskeletal manifestations of diabetes mellitus. Br J Sports Med 2003;37:30-35.)*

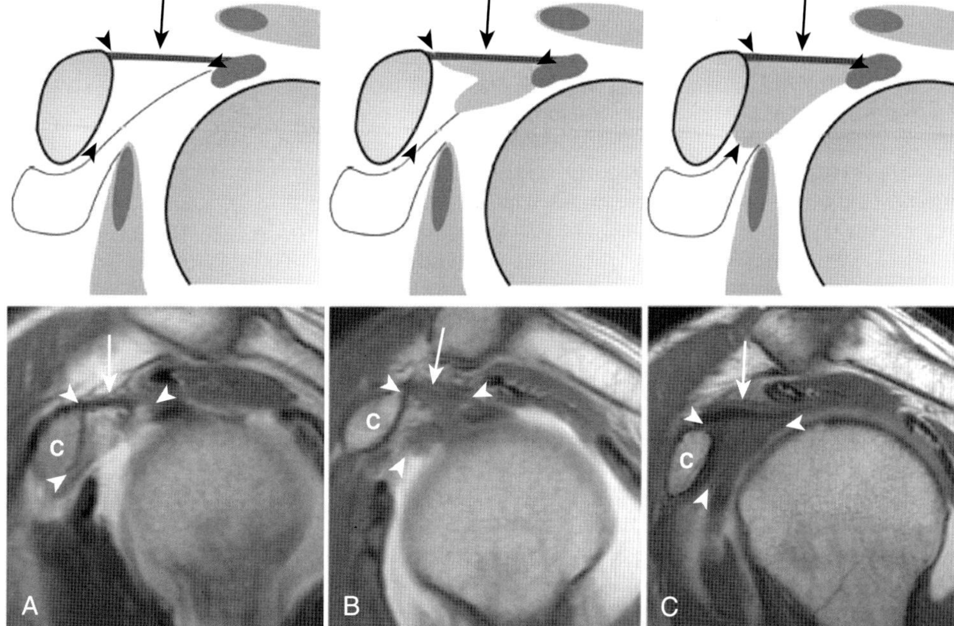

FIGURE 11.3 Note thickening of the coracohumeral ligament *(arrows)* and obliteration of the subcoracoid space *(arrowheads)* on T1-weighted magnetic resonance imaging. *C*, coracoid space. **A**, Normal shoulder. **B**, Partial obliteration of subcoracoid space. **C**, Complete obliteration of subcoracoid space. *(From Mengiardi B, Pfirrmann CW, Gerber C, et al. Frozen shoulder: MR arthrographic findings. Radiology 2004;233:486-492.)*

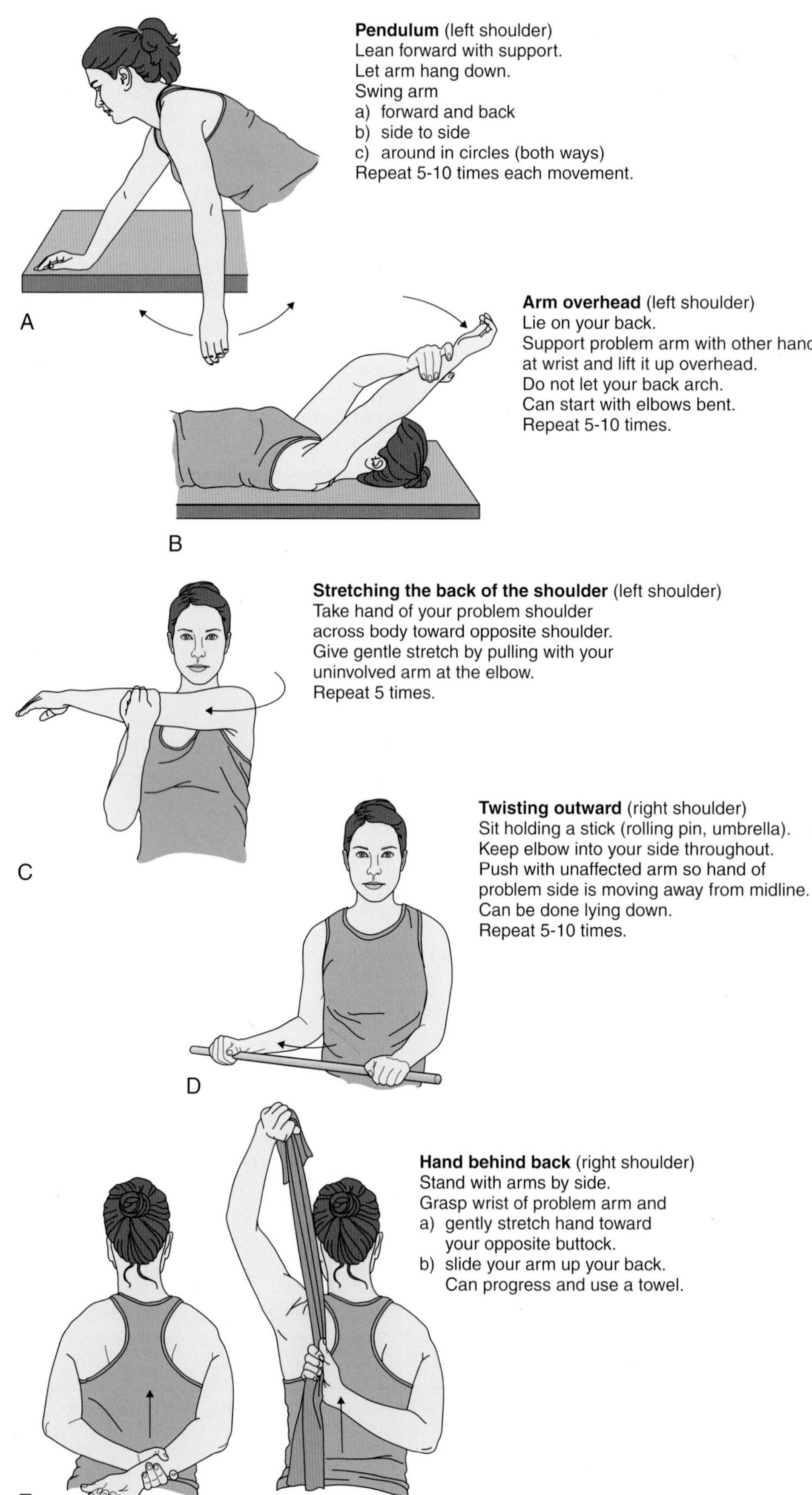

FIGURE 11.4 Pendulum and University of Washington (Jackins) exercises for improving range of motion. These exercises should be implemented early. Explanations of the procedures are provided. **A,** Pendulum exercises. **B,** Overhead stretch. **C,** Cross-body reach. **D,** External rotation. **E,** Internal rotation with adduction. *(From Yeovil Elbow and Shoulder Service. Available at www.yess.uk.com/patient_information.)*

will manage the patient through a home exercise program with periodic follow-up visits to review the patient's progress. Others will implement physical therapy early to manage pain, to improve the pain-free range of motion, and to prevent further contraction of the joint capsule. As the patient progresses with physical therapy, a more detailed home exercise program should be implemented on the basis of the patient's understanding of and compliance with the exercises. If the patient shows continued progress with less pain and improved range of motion, exercises should be graduated to strengthening of rotator cuff muscles and periscapular stabilizers. The physician should be cognizant of the cost of prolonged physical therapy and encourage the patient to maintain compliance with a home exercise program. Once symptoms resolve, patients should be encouraged to continue the home exercise program to maintain range of motion and to prevent recurrence of adhesive capsulitis.

Procedures

In the treatment of adhesive capsulitis, procedures are often performed in conjunction with physical therapy sessions and primarily involve pain-alleviating modalities. These procedures may include intra-articular joint injection, suprascapular nerve blocks, and joint capsule hydrodilation [2,13–15]. As noted before, intra-articular injections can be used to break pain cycles. Several small studies using suprascapular nerve blocks have also reported them to be helpful in breaking pain cycles associated with adhesive capsulitis [13]. Hydrodilation involves glenohumeral injections with saline or lidocaine to lyse adhesions and to distend the capsule. Unfortunately, more studies are needed to fully understand its efficacy [1,14,15].

Surgery

The decision to perform surgery is based on failure of conservative management or an unacceptable quality of life. Manipulation under anesthesia followed by immediate physical therapy focusing on improvement of range of motion of the glenohumeral joint can be helpful for refractory cases. Studies suggest that it results in short-term and long-term improvement in pain and mobility [1,15,16]. However, larger studies are needed to better understand the full impact on recovery. Finally, arthroscopic lysis of adhesions may be an effective option if all else has failed [17,18].

Potential Disease Complications

Most of the complications associated with adhesive capsulitis are related to pain and range of motion loss. Pain is usually transient but can persist for months as the condition runs its clinical course. The loss of range of motion that is seen in adhesive capsulitis is usually regained, but it has been reported that as many as 15% of patients develop permanent loss of full range of motion. This range of motion loss is often not associated with functional deficits [1–3].

Potential Treatment Complications

Treatment complications from conservative management are rare but can include side effects associated with nonsteroidal anti-inflammatory drugs and analgesic medications; these include gastrointestinal bleeds, gastritis, toxic hepatitis, and renal failure [19]. Caution should be used in the treatment of patients with congestive heart failure and hypertension because of fluid retention associated with the use of nonsteroidal anti-inflammatory drugs. Patients undergoing physical therapy could experience significant pain from too aggressive therapeutic exercises or manipulation. In patients undergoing suprascapular nerve blocks, care must be taken to prevent intraneural and intravascular injections. There has been one reported case of a patient suffering a pneumothorax during a suprascapular nerve block when a spinal needle was used [20]. A common surgical complication that can occur is a humeral fracture during manipulations under anesthesia.

References

[1] Robinson CM, Seah KT, Chee YH, et al. Frozen shoulder. J Bone Joint Surg Br 2012;94:1–9.
[2] Neviaser AS, Hannafin JA. Adhesive capsulitis: a review of current treatment. Am J Sports Med 2010;38:2346–56.
[3] Dias R, Cutts S, Massoud S. Frozen shoulder. BMJ 2005;331:1453–6.
[4] Lho YM, Ha E, Cho CH, et al. Inflammatory cytokines are overexpressed in the subacromial bursa of frozen shoulder. J Shoulder Elbow Surg 2013;22:666–72.
[5] McGee DJ. Orthopedic physical assessment. 4th ed. Philadelphia: WB Saunders; 2002, 296–308.
[6] Ahn KS, Kang CH, Oh YW, Jeong WK. Correlation between magnetic resonance imaging and clinical impairment in patients with adhesive capsulitis. Skeletal Radiol 2012;41:1301–8.
[7] Lee MH, Ahn JM, Muhle C, et al. Adhesive capsulitis of the shoulder: diagnosis using magnetic resonance arthrography, with arthroscopic findings as the standard. J Comput Assist Tomogr 2003;27:901–6.
[8] Connell D, Padmanabhan R, Buchbinder R. Adhesive capsulitis: role of MR imaging in differential diagnosis. Eur Radiol 2002;12:2100–6.
[9] Vuillemin V, Guerini H, Morvan G. Musculoskeletal interventional ultrasonography: the upper limb. Diagn Interv Imaging 2012;93:665–73.
[10] Buchbinder R, Green S, Youd JM, Johnston RV. Oral steroids for adhesive capsulitis. Cochrane Database Syst Rev 2006;4, CD006189.
[11] Hanchard NC, Goodchild L, Thompson J, et al. Evidence-based clinical guidelines for the diagnosis, assessment and physiotherapy management of contracted (frozen) shoulder: quick reference summary. Physiotherapy 2012;98:117–20.
[12] Maund E, Craig D, Suekarran S, et al. Management of frozen shoulder: a systematic review and cost-effectiveness analysis. Health Technol Assess 2012;16:1–264.
[13] Karatas GK, Meray J. Suprascapular nerve block for pain relief in adhesive capsulitis: comparison of 2 different techniques. Arch Phys Med Rehabil 2002;83:593–7.
[14] Buchbinder R, Green S, Youd JM, et al. Arthrographic distension for adhesive capsulitis (frozen shoulder). Cochrane Database Syst Rev 2008;1, CD007005.
[15] Buchbinder R, Green S. Effect of arthrographic shoulder joint distention with saline and corticosteroid for adhesive capsulitis. Br J Sports Med 2004;38:384–5.
[16] Kivimaki J, Pohjolainen T. Manipulation under anesthesia for frozen shoulder with and without steroid injection. Arch Phys Med Rehabil 2001;82:1188–90.
[17] Le Lievre HM, Murrell GA. Long-term outcomes after arthroscopic capsular release for idiopathic adhesive capsulitis. J Bone Joint Surg Am 2012;94:1208–16.
[18] Diwan D, Murrell G. An evaluation of the effects of the extent of capsular release and of postoperative therapy on the temporal outcomes of adhesive capsulitis. Arthroscopy 2005;21:1105–13.
[19] Laine L. Gastrointestinal effects of NSAIDs and coxibs. J Pain Symptom Manage 2003;25(Suppl):S32–40.
[20] Marhofer P, Greher M, Kapral S. Ultrasound guidance in regional anaesthesia. Br J Anaesth 2005;94:7–17.

CHAPTER 12

Biceps Tendinopathy

Brian J. Krabak, MD, MBA, FACSM

Synonyms

Biceps tendinosis
Bicipital tendinitis

ICD-9 Codes

726.11 Calcifying tendinitis of shoulder
726.12 Bicipital tenosynovitis

ICD-10 Codes

M75.30 Calcifying tendinitis of shoulder, unspecified
M75.31 Calcifying tendinitis of right shoulder
M75.32 Calcifying tendinitis of left shoulder
M75.20 Bicipital tenosynovitis, unspecified shoulder
M75.21 Bicipital tenosynovitis of right shoulder
M75.22 Bicipital tenosynovitis of left shoulder

Definition

First documented in 1932, the term *biceps tendinitis* was used to describe inflammation, pain, or tenderness in the region of the biceps tendon [1]. More recently, *tendinitis* has been replaced by the term *tendinopathy* to reflect the nature of injury secondary to inflammation of the tendon sheath (–itis) versus degeneration of the tendon (–osis) [2,3]. Both represent overuse injuries to the biceps tendon, which helps prevent superior translation of the humeral head during shoulder abduction and is intimately associated with the labrum [4]. The biceps tendon works in concert with the rest of the shoulder muscles to maintain mobility and function. Injury to or compromise of a single muscle of the dynamic shoulder stabilizers can adversely affect other muscles and impair function of the entire joint.

Primary biceps tendinitis describes isolated inflammation of the tendon as it runs in the intertubercular groove; it typically occurs in the younger athletic populations [4]. The precipitating forces in primary biceps tendinitis are multifactorial, including acute repetitive overuse and secondary impingement due to scapular dyskinesis, unilateral instability, and multidirectional shoulder instability [5]. A flat medial wall or shallow bicipital groove can predispose to subluxation of the long head tendon, increasing risk for inflammation [6]. On the other hand, bicipital tendinosis is typically seen in the older population (i.e., athletes older than 35 years or nonathletes older than65 years) and more commonly than primary biceps tendinitis [1,5]. Studies have found that up to 95% of patients with bicipital tendinosis have associated rotator cuff disease [7].

Symptoms

Biceps tendinopathy usually is manifested with complaints of anterior shoulder pain that is worse with activities involving elbow flexion [2]. Pain usually localizes to the bicipital groove with occasional radiation to the arm or deltoid region. Often, pain will also occur with prolonged rest and immobility, particularly at night. The throwing athlete often describes pain during the follow-through of a throwing motion and may feel a "snap" if the tendon subluxes in the groove [4]. Attention should be given to onset, duration, and character of the pain. Some individuals present with only complaints of fatigue with shoulder movement. A history of prior trauma, athletic and occupational endeavors, and systemic diseases should be considered in evaluating the shoulder. Patients with accompanying "impingement syndrome" often complain of a "pinching" sensation with overhead activities and a "toothache" sensation in the lateral proximal arm. The pain can be difficult to separate from impingement or rotator cuff syndrome [5].

Physical Examination

The physical examination begins with adequate inspection of the shoulder and neck region. Attention is given to prior scars, structural deformities, posture, and muscle bulk. Determination of the exact location of pain can be helpful for diagnosis. Biceps tendinopathy commonly presents with palpable tenderness over the bicipital groove (Fig. 12.1). Side-to-side comparisons should be made because the tendon is typically slightly tender to direct palpation. Tenderness over the lateral aspect of the shoulder suggests bursitis, tendinopathy, or strain of the deltoid muscle. Caution should be used as the accuracy for palpation of the biceps tendon was 5.3%

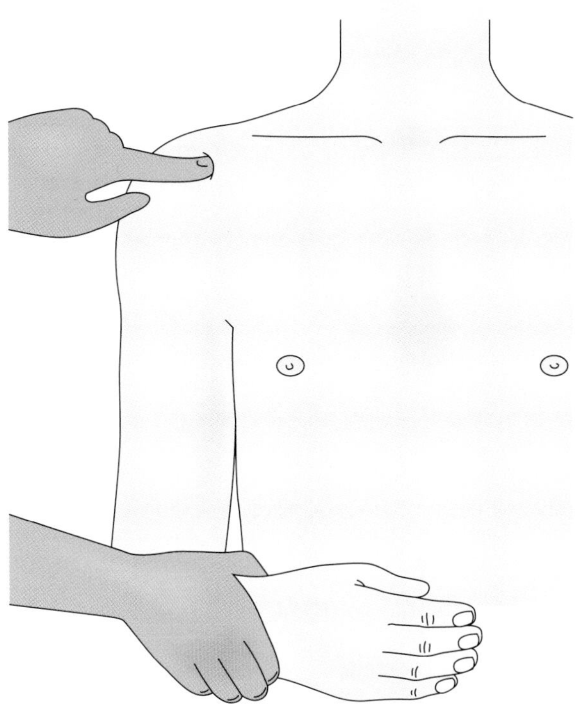

FIGURE 12.1 Palpation of the bicipital groove.

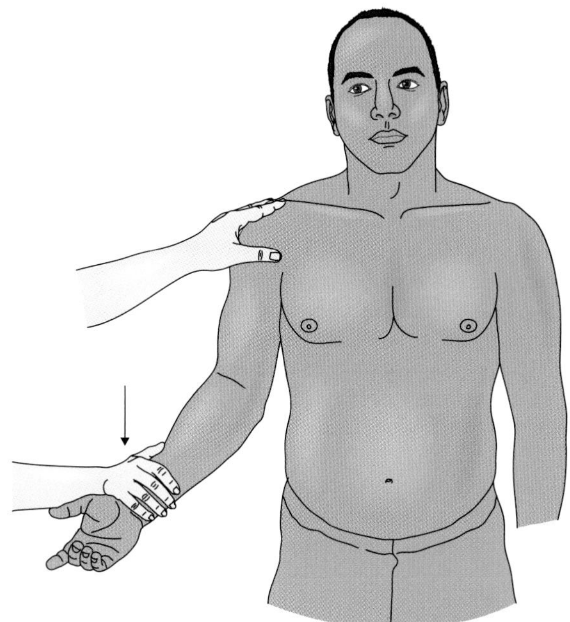

FIGURE 12.2 Demonstration of the Speed test for bicipital tendinitis. The examiner provides resistance to forward flexion of the shoulder with the elbow in extension and supination of the forearm. Pain is elicited in the intertubercular groove in a positive test result.

in residents and fellows [8]. Motion limitation is not seen in isolated tendinopathies but is often seen in concomitant degenerative joint diseases, impingement syndromes, tendon tears, and adhesive capsulitis. Shoulder range of motion may be limited if the rotator cuff is involved. The findings on neurologic examination should be normal, including sensation and deep tendon reflexes. On occasion, strength is limited by pain or disuse. Assessment of the kinetic chain, including scapular stability and spine stabilization, is important.

Special tests of the shoulder should be performed routinely. The Speed and Yergason tests (Figs. 12.2 and 12.3) are often used to help evaluate for bicipital tendinopathy. Unfortunately, a recent meta-analysis suggests that these tests are not sensitive (Speed test, 50%-63%;Yergason test, 14%-32%) or specific (Speed test, 60%-85%; Yergason test, 70%-89%) for diagnosis of biceps tendinopathy [9]. Impingement tests and supraspinatus tests will help assess for any concurrent rotator cuff tendinopathy. Other maneuvers to assess for instability (anterior apprehension, anterior-posterior load and shift), labral disease (O'Brien test), and acromioclavicular joint arthritis (scarf test) should be performed.

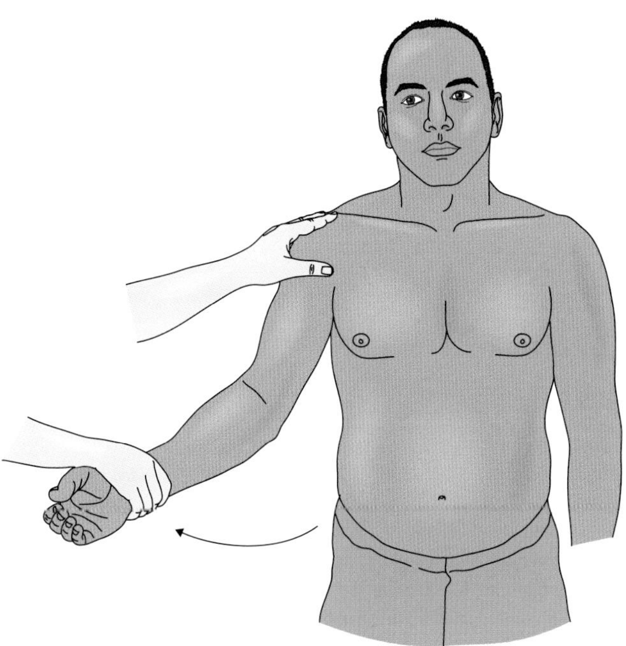

FIGURE 12.3 Demonstration of the Yergason test. The examiner provides resistance against supination of the forearm with the elbow flexed at 90 degrees. The test result is considered positive when pain is produced or intensified in the intertubercular groove.

Functional Limitations

Biceps tendinitis may cause patients to limit their activities at home and at work. Limitations may include difficulty with lifting and carrying groceries, garbage bags, and briefcases. Athletics that involve the affected arm, such as swimming, tennis, and throwing sports, may be curtailed. Pain may impair sleep.

Diagnostic Studies

Biceps tendinopathy is generally diagnosed on a clinical basis, but imaging studies are helpful to exclude other pathologic processes. Plain radiographs are usually normal [1]. They can, however, show calcifications in the tendon and degenerative disease of the joint that may predispose to tendinitis. The Fisk view is used in evaluating bicipital tendinopathy to assess the size of the intertubercular groove. This may help determine whether there is a relative risk for development of recurrent subluxation of the tendon, which is seen in individuals with short and narrow margins of the intertubercular groove [10].

Ultrasonography can be extremely helpful and a cost-effective way to evaluate the biceps and rotator cuff tendons. Ultrasound can detect increased fluid in the biceps tendon sheath and evidence of tendinosis. In addition, ultrasound allows dynamic evaluation of the shoulder region to better assess biceps tendon subluxation. Recent research suggests that ultrasound of the shoulder is more accurate in confirming a normal biceps tendon or full-thickness tear but less accurate in the diagnosis of partial-thickness tears [11].

Magnetic resonance imaging can detect partial-thickness tendon tears, examine muscle substance, evaluate soft tissue abnormalities and labral disease (magnetic resonance arthrography), and assess for masses. In biceps tendinitis, increased signal intensity is seen on T2-weighted images [12]. However, this finding is also seen with partial tears of the tendon. Tendinosis is manifested with increased tendon thickness and intermediate signal in the surrounding sheath. Arthroscopy is a useful procedure for the evaluation of intra-articular disease but does not play a role in isolated tendinitis.

Differential Diagnosis

Rotator cuff tendinitis and tears
Multidirectional instability
Biceps brachii rupture
Acromioclavicular joint sprain
Glenohumeral or acromioclavicular degenerative joint disease
Rheumatoid arthritis
Crystalline arthropathy
Adhesive capsulitis
Cervical spondylosis
Cervical radiculopathy
Brachial plexopathy
Peripheral entrapment neuropathy
Referral from visceral organs
Diaphragmatic referred pain

Treatment

Initial

The treatment of biceps tendinopathies involves activity modification, anti-inflammatory measures, and heat and cold modalities [2,4]. Overhead activities and lifting are to be avoided initially. Workstation assessment and modification can be helpful for laborers. Evaluation of athletic technique and training adaptations are important in athletes. Nonsteroidal anti-inflammatory drugs can assist with decreasing the pain and inflammation in treating tendinitis but do not play a role in tendinosis. Medications to increase blood flow to the tendon (i.e., nitro patches) may facilitate recovery. Ice is helpful after exercise for minimizing pain [3,4]. Moist heat can be useful before activity. Other modalities, such as iontophoresis and electrical stimulation, have been used, but there are no clinical trials supporting their efficacy.

Rehabilitation

Rehabilitation for biceps tendinopathy is similar to that for rotator cuff tendinopathy (see Chapter 16). Moreover, because biceps tendinitis rarely occurs in isolation, it is important to rehabilitate the patient by accounting for all of the shoulder disease that is present (e.g., instability, impingement) [1,2]. Shoulder stretching helps maintain or improve range of motion and is emphasized in all important shoulder movements of abduction, adduction, and internal and external rotation. Posterior capsule stretching is also important, particularly when impingement syndrome is also present. Once full, pain-free active range of motion is achieved, progressive resistance exercises are used to strengthen the dynamic shoulder and spine stabilizers, progressing from static to dynamic exercise as tolerated [4]. Eccentric strengthening exercises may be beneficial for biceps tendinopathy, but more research is needed. Overhead and shoulder abduction activities should be avoided early in treatment because they can exacerbate symptoms. Scapular and spine stabilization exercises should be introduced once biceps strength improves. The exercise program should progress to sport-specific functional activities, when appropriate. Athletes may return to play, gradually, when pain is minimal or absent [4].

Procedures

Steroid injections are a potentially useful adjunct for biceps tendinitis (Fig. 12.4) but should probably be avoided in cases

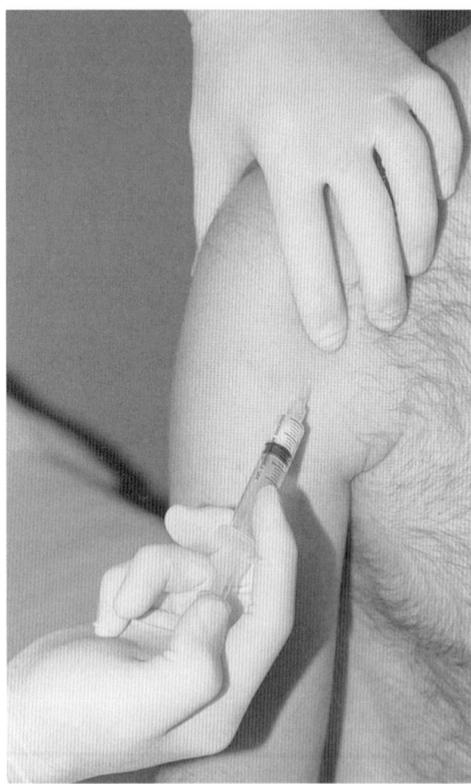

FIGURE 12.4 Injection technique for the long head of the biceps brachii (ideally performed under ultrasound guidance). Under sterile conditions with use of a 25-gauge, 1½-inch disposable needle and a local anesthetic-corticosteroid combination, the area surrounding the biceps tendon is injected. It is important to bathe the tendon sheath in the preparation rather than to inject the tendon itself. Typically, a 1- to 3-mL aliquot of the mixture is used (e.g., 1 mL of 1% lidocaine mixed with 1 mL of betamethasone). *(From Lennard TA. Pain Procedures in Clinical Practice, 2nd ed. Philadelphia, Hanley & Belfus, 2000.)*

of tendinosis. The goal of an injection would be to diminish pain and inflammation while facilitating the rehabilitation treatment program. Injections must be used judiciously to avoid weakening of the tendon substance. Ideally, injections should be performed under ultrasound guidance to improve accuracy and to avoid complications from injecting the tendon [13]. Immediate postinjection care includes icing for 5 to 10 minutes, and the patient may continue to apply ice at home for 15 to 20 minutes, two or three times daily, for several days. The patient should be instructed to avoid heavy lifting or vigorous exercise for 48 to 72 hours after injection. Injection of biologics (autologous blood and platelet-rich plasma) is potentially promising but needs further research to better define its utility [14]. Depending on the concurrent shoulder disease, other injections may also be useful (e.g., subacromial) [15].

Surgery

Surgery is generally not indicated for isolated biceps tendinitis. However, biceps tenodesis in conjunction with acromioplasty in chronic, refractory cases and in those cases associated with rotator cuff impingement has been found to have good results [16]. Tenotomy of the long head of the biceps for chronic tendinitis remains controversial, and long-term results are unknown [16,17].

Potential Disease Complications

Progressive biceps tendinitis and pain can lead to diminished activity, rotator cuff disease, and adhesive capsulitis. Compensatory problems with other tendons can develop because of their interdependence for proper shoulder movement. The development of myofascial pain of the surrounding shoulder girdle muscles is another common complication in shoulder tendinopathy.

Potential Treatment Complications

The exercise program should be properly supervised initially to prevent aggravation of tendinitis of other muscle groups. Analgesics and nonsteroidal anti-inflammatory drugs have well-known side effects that most commonly affect the gastric, hepatic, and renal systems. Repeated steroid injections in or near tendons could result in tendon rupture and should be performed under ultrasound guidance, whenever possible.

References

[1] Patton WC, McCluskey GM. Overuse injuries in the upper extremity. Clin Sports Med 2011;20:439–51.

[2] Churgay CA. Diagnosis and treatment of biceps tendinitis and tendinosis. Am Fam Physician 2009;80:470–6.

[3] Longo UG, Loppini M, Marineo G, et al. Tendinopathy of the tendon of the long head of the biceps. Sports Med Arthrosc 2011;19:321–32.

[4] Ryu JH, Pedowitz RA. Rehabilitation of biceps tendon disorders in athletes. Clin Sports Med 2010;29:229–46, vii–viii.

[5] Snyder GM, Mair SD, Lattermann C. Tendinopathy of the long head of the biceps. Med Sport Sc 2012;57:76–89.

[6] Pfahler M, Branner S, Refior HJ. The role of the bicipital groove in tendopathy of the long biceps tendon. J Shoulder Elbow Surg 1999;8:419–24.

[7] Harwood MI, Smith CT. Superior labrum, anterior-posterior lesions and biceps injuries: diagnostic and treatment considerations. Prim Care Clin Office Pract 2004;31:831–55.

[8] Gazzillo GP, Finnoff JT, Hall MM, et al. Accuracy of palpating the long head of the biceps tendon: an ultrasonographic study. PM R 2011;3:1035–40.

[9] Hegedus EJ, Goode AP, Cook CE, et al. Which physical examination tests provide clinicians with the most value when examining the shoulder? Update of a systematic review with meta-analysis of individual tests. Br J Sports Med 2012;46:964–78.

[10] Schaeffeler C, Waldt S, Holzapfel K, et al. Lesions of the biceps pulley: diagnostic accuracy of MR arthrography of the shoulder and evaluation of previously described and new diagnostic signs. Radiology 2012;264:504–13.

[11] Skendzel JG, Jacobson JA, Carpenter JE, Miller BS. Long head of biceps brachii tendon evaluation: accuracy of preoperative ultrasound. AJR Am J Roentgenol 2011;197:942–8.

[12] Tirman PF, Smith ED, Stoller DW, Fritz RC. Shoulder imaging in athletes. Semin Musculoskelet Radiol 2004;8:29–40.

[13] Hashiuchi T, Sakurai G, Morimoto M, et al. Accuracy of the biceps tendon sheath injection: ultrasound-guided or unguided injection? A randomized controlled trial. J Shoulder Elbow Surg 2011;20:1069–73.

[14] Ibrahim VM, Groah SL, Libin A, Ljungberg IH. Use of platelet rich plasma for the treatment of bicipital tendinopathy in spinal cord injury: a pilot study. Top Spinal Cord Inj Rehabil 2012;18:77–8.

[15] Elser F, Braun S, Dewing CB, et al. Anatomy, function, injuries, and treatment of the long head of the biceps brachii tendon. Arthroscopy 2011;27:581–92.

[16] Kelly AM, Drakos MC, Fealy S, et al. Arthroscopic release of the long head of the biceps tendon: functional outcome and clinical results. Am J Sports Med 2005;33:208–13.

[17] Slenker NR, Lawson K, Ciccotti MG, et al. Biceps tenotomy versus tenodesis: clinical outcomes. Arthroscopy 2012;28:576–82.

CHAPTER 13

Biceps Tendon Rupture

Michael F. Stretanski, DO

Synonyms

Biceps brachii rupture
Biceps tear
Bicipital strain

ICD-9 Codes

727.62 **Rupture of tendon of biceps (long head), nontraumatic**
840.8 **Sprain or strain of other specified site of shoulder and upper arm**

ICD-10 Codes

M66.821 **Rupture of tendon of biceps (upper arm), nontraumatic, right**
M66.822 **Rupture of tendon of biceps (upper arm), nontraumatic, left**
M66.829 **Rupture of tendon of bicep (upper arm), nontraumatic, unspecified**

Definition

Biceps tendon rupture is either complete or partial disruption of the tendon of the biceps brachii muscle that can occur proximally or distally. The more common proximal ruptures are frequently seen in older individuals who have had chronic tendinosis of the long head of the biceps tendon associated with concomitant rotator cuff disease and degenerative joint disease of the shoulder [1] (Fig. 13.1). The incidence is 1.2 per 100,000 patients, with a majority on the dominant side of men who smoke and are in the fourth decade of life [2]. Most cases involve the long head of the biceps brachii and are manifested as a partial or complete avulsion from the superior rim of the anterior glenoid labrum [3]. Rupture of the proximal biceps tendon represents 90% to 97% of all biceps ruptures; it almost exclusively involves the long head [4] and is 7.5 times more likely in smokers [2].

Recent cadaveric study suggests that the relative avascularity of the long head of the biceps tendon may be a risk factor, as seen in many other tendon ruptures. Supplied through its osteotendinous and musculotendinous junctions and rarely branches from the anterior circumflex humeral artery traveling in a mesotenon, the long head of the biceps tendon has a hypovascular region in the border of two adjacent vascular territories. This region of limited arterial supply, 1.2 to 3 cm from the tendon origin, extends midway through the glenohumeral joint to the proximal intertubercular groove [5]. The distal biceps rupture is relatively uncommon and typically occurs in middle-aged men, although acute traumatic ruptures may occur in younger individuals or in anyone engaged in predisposing activities, such as forceful explosive contraction of the biceps. Patients with a distal biceps tendon rupture carry a risk of at least 8% for a rupture on the contralateral side [6]. This often develops suddenly with stressing of the flexor mechanism of the elbow. Distal biceps rupture usually occurs as a single traumatic event, such as with heavy lifting; it is often an avulsion of the tendon from the radial tuberosity, but it can also occur as a midsubstance tendon rupture [7].

Symptoms

Proximal ruptures are often asymptomatic and are commonly discovered with awareness of distal migration of the biceps brachii muscle mass, or they may occur suddenly by a seemingly trivial event. Often, individuals will note an acute "popping" sensation. The patient often takes one finger and points directly to the bicipital groove when describing the pain. Edema and ecchymosis may be seen with tendon rupture but also with other regional pathologic processes. The proximal ruptures are typically less painful but can be preceded by chronic shoulder discomfort [8]. An acute distal rupture is often associated with pain at the antecubital fossa that is typically aggravated by resisted elbow flexion. The pain is usually sharp initially but improves with time and is often described as a dull ache [9]. Swelling, distal ecchymosis, and proximal migration of the biceps brachii muscle mass accompany this injury with a magnitude dependent on the degree of injury. Younger, healthy patients may often present with a cosmetic rather than a functional complaint.

Physical Examination

Visual inspection of the biceps brachii, including comparison with the unaffected limb, is usually the first and most

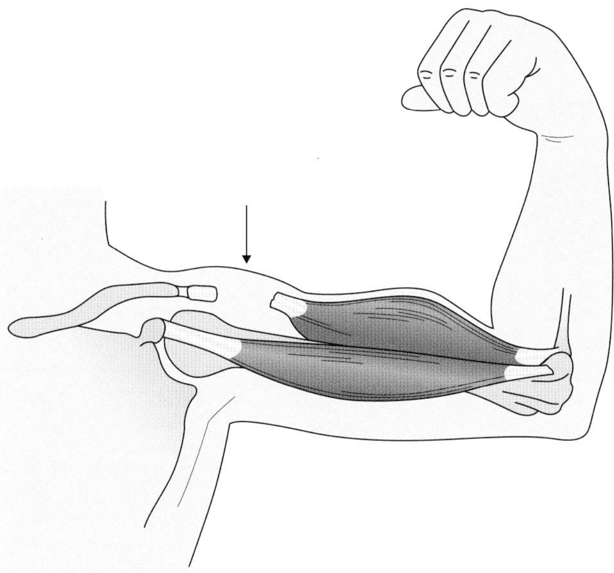

FIGURE 13.1 Proximal biceps tendon rupture.

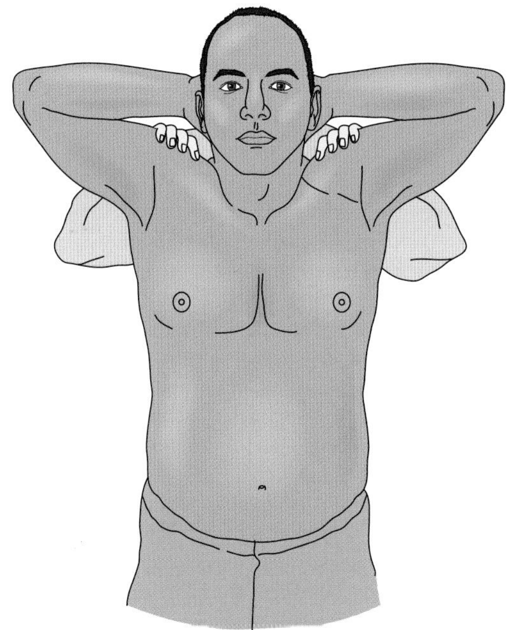

FIGURE 13.2 The Ludington test is performed by having the patient clasp both hands onto or behind the head, allowing the interlocking fingers to support the arms. This action permits maximum relaxation of the biceps tendon in its resting position. The patient then alternately contracts and relaxes the biceps while the clinician palpates the tendon and muscle. In a complete tear, contraction is not felt on the affected side.

critical element in the physical examination of this condition. Advances in portability, training, and technology have led to a larger trend among physicians in various specialties to integrate diagnostic musculoskeletal ultrasound into the early phases of routine clinical assessment [10].

The Ludington test [11] is a recommended position in which to observe differences in the contour and shape of the biceps (Fig. 13.2). Diagnosis of complete ruptures is relatively easy; patients often come in aware of the biceps muscle retraction. Partial ruptures exist along a spectrum and can be more difficult to diagnose. The clinician should also assess for the presence of ecchymosis or swelling as a sign of acute injury. Palpation for point tenderness will often reveal pain at the rupture site. An effort should also be made to determine whether the rupture is complete by palpation and observation of the tendon. Thorough assessment of the shoulder and elbow should be made for range of motion and laxity. The Yergason [12] and Speed [13] tests (see Chapter 12), which are used in the assessment of bicipital tendinitis, are also recommended. Posterior dislocation of the long head of the biceps tendon has been reported [14] and may share some common physical examination findings but not muscle retraction.

In patients with inconsistent physical examination findings and questionable secondary gains, the American Shoulder and Elbow Surgeons subjective shoulder scale [15], a standardized scale of shoulder function with patient and physician components, has demonstrated acceptable psychometric performance for outcomes assessment in patients with shoulder instability, rotator cuff disease, and glenohumeral arthritis [16]. It is important to examine the entire shoulder and to keep in mind that it is a complex, inherently unstable, well-innervated joint that tends to function, and fail, as a unit; therefore, additional lesions that are the true pain generator may be evident. One study [17] looking at shoulder magnetic resonance findings showed no statistical relationship between the level of disability and either biceps tendon rupture or biceps tendinopathy; rather, disability was linked to supraspinatus tendon lesions and bursitis.

A thorough neurologic and vascular examination is performed, and findings should be normal in the absence of concomitant problems. Caution should be used with strength testing or end-range motion to avoid worsening of an incomplete tear.

Functional Limitations

The functional limitations are generally relatively minimal with proximal biceps rupture [18], and the patient's concern is often centered around cosmetic considerations. More significant weakness of elbow flexion and supination is noted after a distal tendon disruption. Pain can be acutely limiting after both situations but is typically more of a problem in distal rupture. The primary role of the biceps brachii is supination of the forearm. Elbow flexion is functional by the action of the brachialis and brachioradialis. A degree of residual weakness with supination and elbow flexion, particularly after distal tendon rupture, can cause functional impairment for individuals who perform heavy physical labor [19]. Fatigue with repetitive work is also a common complaint with nonsurgically treated distal tendon ruptures [20]. The long head of the biceps is thought to play a role in anterior stability of the shoulder [21,22]; this is an issue for people who perform overhead activities (such as lifting, filing, and painting), powerlifting (in which the final 10% of strength is crucial), and nonsports activities in which the appearance of symmetry is important (such as modeling or bodybuilding).

Diagnostic Studies

The diagnosis of biceps brachii rupture is often made on a clinical basis alone. Magnetic resonance imaging is helpful in confirming the diagnosis and assessing the extent of the injury, but it should be performed in the FABS (flexed elbow, abducted shoulder, forearm supinated) position to obtain a true longitudinal view [23]; it is particularly useful in partial ruptures. Magnetic resonance imaging studies can also assess concomitant rotator cuff disease. Diagnostic ultrasound, which has grown in applicability and portability, may have a role in demonstrating not only proximal but also distal biceps tendon bifurcation [24]. Diagnostic ultrasound may be more cost-effective as an initial screening tool when no surgical injuries are suspected. Imaging of the entire insertion site as well as of elbow structures should be performed in distal ruptures [25]. Plain radiographs sometimes show hypertrophic bone formation related to chronic degenerative tendon abnormalities as a predisposition to rupture. Radiographs are also obtained in acute traumatic cases to rule out fractures and to identify developmental variants. Electrodiagnostic medicine consultation for possible peripheral nerve damage should be considered in cases with evidence of lower motor neuron findings or where the distribution of weakness is not fully accounted for by pain. Attention should be paid to median neuropathy at the elbow and, although it is technically difficult, to lateral antebrachial cutaneous nerve studies.

Differential Diagnosis

Musculocutaneous neuropathy
Rotator cuff disease
Brachial plexopathy
Pectoralis major muscle rupture
Tumor
Hematoma
Dislocated biceps tendon
Cervical radiculopathy
Parsonage-Turner syndrome
Isolated subscapularis tendon disease

Treatment

Initial

For most patients, treatment of proximal biceps tears is conservative. Gentle range of motion exercises for prevention of contractures of the elbow and shoulder (adhesive capsulitis) can be started almost immediately. The function of the long head of the biceps tendon and its role in glenohumeral kinematics presently remain only partially understood because of the difficulty of cadaveric and in vivo biomechanical studies. Most treatment and rehabilitation efforts remain evidence based [26]. Surgery is rarely necessary because there is little loss of function with this tear, and the cosmetic deformity is generally acceptable without surgical repair. Young athletes or heavy laborers may be the exception; they typically need the lost strength that occurs with loss of the continuity of the biceps tendon [27]. Distal tears are more commonly referred to surgery acutely. However, initial treatment of partial distal ruptures consists of splint immobilization in flexion, which should be continued for 3 weeks. This is followed by a gradual return to normal activities. Analgesics, nonsteroidal anti-inflammatory drugs, topical agents (menthol-based or other custom compounded), therapeutic ultrasound, and ice may assist with the swelling and discomfort and facilitate rehabilitation efforts in both proximal and distal ruptures.

Rehabilitation

Nonsurgical treatment includes gentle range of motion exercises of the elbow and shoulder for contracture prevention. Modalities such as iontophoresis and therapeutic ultrasound can be used for pain control and prevention of contraction. Electrical stimulation is largely contraindicated in a partial tear (because of the concern of converting it to a complete tear) and not indicated in a complete tear. Gentle strengthening can typically be done after the acute phase in complete tears that are not going to be repaired because there is little chance of further injury. Partial ruptures can scar and remain in continuity [2].

Postoperative rehabilitation for distal biceps rupture repairs consists of immobilization of the elbow in 90 degrees of flexion for 7 to 10 days, followed by the use of a hinged flexion-assist splint with a 30-degree extension block for 8 weeks after surgery. Gentle range of motion and progressive resistance exercises are started initially; unlimited activity is not typically allowed until 5 months postoperatively [28].

Procedures

No procedures are performed in the direct treatment of biceps tendon rupture. Musculocutaneous nerve, upper trunk brachial plexus, and maybe even stellate ganglion blocks may have a role either perioperatively or palliatively in selected cases. Suprascapular nerve block or subacromial infiltration of local anesthetic may have a role in facilitation of rehabilitation therapies, including maintenance of range of motion and prevention of a secondary adhesive capsulitis. The author often coordinates such local anesthetic infiltrations just before physical or occupational therapy appointments. Caution should be exercised during passive stretching, and even then only by therapists who are familiar with suppression of protective mechanisms, to avoid further soft tissue damage at what may be atypical and asymmetric end-range motion. There may be a role for steroid injection in professional or elite athletes during critical phases of their season. In such cases, the subacromial approach is preferred with avoidance of direct needle entry into the biceps tendon. Pulsed radiofrequency of the suprascapular nerve may also have a longer term role in palliation of pain and has the advantage of not requiring steroid injection.

Surgery

Prompt assessment is necessary for complete distal biceps ruptures under consideration for surgical repair because muscle shortening will occur over time. The same is true for proximal ruptures in very active individuals who require maximal upper body strength for their vocation or sport. Optimal surgical outcomes are obtained if treatment occurs within the first 4 weeks after injury. Partial distal ruptures are generally observed nonoperatively until a complete rupture occurs. Several techniques, including the two-incision, buttonhole, and Boyd-Anderson approaches, are used. More recently, a sonographically guided, mini-open technique involving one incision giving access to three peripectoral anatomic zones has been described [29]. The goal of surgical treatment is to restore strength of supination and flexion. For distal repairs, this is typically performed by a two-incision technique involving reinsertion of the biceps tendon to the radial tuberosity [30]. A single-incision technique with use of suture anchors in the bicipital tuberosity has shown excellent long-term functional results by the Disabilities of the Arm, Shoulder, and Hand (DASH) questionnaire [31].

Potential Disease Complications

Complications from isolated biceps rupture are relatively rare. Partial tears can become complete tears. Attention should be given to potential contracture formation. Median nerve compression has been reported presumably to be related to an enlarged synovial bursa associated with a partial distal biceps tendon rupture [32]. Isolated antebrachial cutaneous neuropathy, due to traction from the biceps tendon displacing the nerve laterally with alleviation of symptoms after proximal biceps tenodesis, has been reported [33]. Compartment syndrome has also been reported in proximal biceps rupture in a patient receiving systemic anticoagulation [34]. The risk-benefit ratio of discontinuing drugs known to have an association with tendon rupture should be ascertained.

Potential Treatment Complications

Analgesics and nonsteroidal anti-inflammatory drugs have well-known side effects that most commonly affect the gastric, hepatic, and renal systems. Advancement of the extent of the rupture can occur with overly aggressive strengthening measures and passive stretching. The potential for serious surgical complications is most significant with distal rupture because of the important neurovascular structures in that region, including the median and radial nerves and brachial artery and vein [26]. The complication rate increases with the length of time after rupture that surgery is performed. Proximal radial-ulnar synostosis and heterotopic ossification have also been reported as rare postsurgical complications [21], as has humeral fracture after subpectoral biceps tenodesis [35]. Stiffness and contractures are possible with or without surgical intervention.

References

[1] Neer CS. Impingement lesions. Clin Orthop 1983;173:70–7.

[2] Safran MR, Graham SM. Distal biceps tendon ruptures: incidence, demographics and the effect of smoking. Clin Orthop Relat Res 2002;404:275–83.

[3] Gilcreest EL. The common syndrome of rupture, dislocation and elongation of the long head of the biceps brachii: an analysis of one hundred cases. Surg Gynecol Obstet 1934;58:322.

[4] Elser F, Braun S, Dewing CB, et al. Anatomy, function, injuries, and treatment of the long head of the biceps brachii tendon. Arthroscopy 2011;27:581–92.

[5] Cheng NM, Pan WR, Vally F, et al. The arterial supply of the long head of biceps tendon: anatomical study with implications for tendon rupture. Clin Anat 2010;23:683–92.

[6] Green JB, Skaife TL, Leslie BM. Bilateral distal biceps tendon ruptures. J Hand Surg Am 2012;37:120–3.

[7] Le Huec JC, Moinard M, Liquois F, Zipoli B. Distal rupture of the tendon of biceps brachii: evaluation by MRI and the results of repair. J Bone Joint Surg Br 1996;78:767–70.

[8] Waugh RI, Hathcock TA, Elliott JL. Ruptures of muscles and tendons: with particular reference of rupture (or elongation of the long tendon) of biceps brachii with report of fifty cases. Surgery 1949;25:370–92.

[9] Bourne MH, Morrey BF. Partial rupture of the distal biceps tendon. Clin Orthop Relat Res 1991;271:143–8.

[10] Patil P, Dasgupta B. Role of diagnostic ultrasound in the assessment of musculoskeletal diseases. Ther Adv Musculoskel Dis 2012;4:341–55.

[11] Ludington NA. Rupture of the long head of the biceps flexor cubiti muscle. Ann Surg 1923;77:358–63.

[12] Yergason RM. Rupture of biceps. J Bone Joint Surg 1931;13:160.

[13] Gilcreest EL, Albi P. Unusual lesions of muscles and tendons of the shoulder girdle and upper arm. Surg Gynecol Obstet 1939;68:903–17.

[14] Bauer T, Vuillemin A, Hardy P, Rousselin B. Posterior dislocation of the long head of the biceps tendon: a case report. J Shoulder Elbow Surg 2005;14:557–8.

[15] Richards RR, An KN, Bigliani LU, et al. A standardized method for the assessment of shoulder function. J Shoulder Elbow Surg 1994;3:347–52.

[16] Kocher MS, Horan MP, Briggs KK, et al. Reliability, validity and responsiveness of the American Shoulder and Elbow Surgeons subjective shoulder scale in patients with shoulder instability, rotator cuff disease and glenohumeral arthritis. J Bone Joint Surg Am 2005;87:2006–11.

[17] Krief OP, Huguet D. Shoulder pain and disability: comparison with MR findings. AJR Am J Roentgenol 2006;186:1234–9.

[18] Phillips BB, Canale ST, Sisk TD, et al. Ruptures of the proximal biceps tendon in middle-aged patients. Orthop Rev 1993;22:349–53.

[19] Pearl ML, Bessos K, Wong K. Strength deficits related to distal biceps tendon rupture and repair: a case report. Am J Sports Med 1998;26:295–6.

[20] Davison BL, Engber WD, Tigert LJ. Long term evaluation of repaired distal biceps brachii tendon ruptures. Clin Orthop Relat Res 1996;333:188–91.

[21] Rodosky MW, Harner CD, Fu FH. The role of the long head of the biceps muscle and superior glenoid labrum in anterior stability of the shoulder. Am J Sports Med 1994;22:121–30.

[22] Warner JJ, McMahon PJ. The role of the long head of the biceps brachii in superior stability of the glenohumeral joint. J Bone Joint Surg Am 1995;77:366–72.

[23] Erickson SJ, Fitzgerald SW, Quinn SF, et al. Long bicipital tendon of the shoulder: normal anatomy and pathologic findings on MR imaging. AJR Am J Roentgenol 1992;158:1091–6.

[24] Tagliafico A, Michaud J, Capaccio E, et al. Ultrasound demonstration of distal biceps tendon bifurcation: normal and abnormal findings. Eur Radiol 2010;20:202–8.

[25] Chew ML, Giuffrè BM. Disorders of the distal biceps brachii tendon. Radiographics 2005;25:1227–37.

[26] Elser F, Braun S, Dewing CB, et al. Anatomy, function, injuries, and treatment of the long head of the biceps brachii tendon. Arthroscopy 2011;27:581–92.

[27] Hawkins RJ, Kennedy JC. Impingement syndrome in athletes. Am J Sports Med 1980;8:151–8.

[28] Ramsey ML. Distal biceps tendon injuries: diagnosis and management. J Am Acad Orthop Surg 1999;7:199–207.

[29] Bhatia DN, DasGupta B. Surgical correction of the "Popeye biceps" deformity: dual-window approach for combined subpectoral and deltopectoral access and proximal biceps tenodesis. J Hand Surg Am 2012;37:1917–24.

[30] Boyd HD, Anderson LD. A method for reinsertion of the distal biceps brachii tendon. J Bone Joint Surg Am 1961;43:1041–3.

[31] McKee MD, Hirji R, Schemitsch EH, et al. Patient-oriented functional outcome after repair of distal biceps tendon ruptures using a single-incision technique. J Shoulder Elbow Surg 2005;14:302–6.

[32] Foxworthy M, Kinninmonth AW. Median nerve compression in the proximal forearm as a complication of partial rupture of the distal biceps brachii tendon. J Hand Surg Br 1992;17:515–7.

[33] Brogan DM, Bishop AT, Spinner RJ, Shin AY. Shin lateral antebrachial cutaneous neuropathy following the long head of the biceps rupture. J Hand Surg Am 2012;37:673–6.

[34] Richards AM, Moss AL. Biceps rupture in a patient on long-term anticoagulation leading to compartment syndrome and nerve palsies. J Hand Surg Br 1997;22:411–2.

[35] Sears BW, Spencer EE, Getz CL. Humeral fracture following subpectoral biceps tenodesis in 2 active, healthy patients. J Shoulder Elbow Surg 2011;20:e7–e11.

CHAPTER 14

Glenohumeral Instability

William Micheo, MD
Alexandra Rivera-Vega, MD
Gerardo Miranda, MD

Synonyms

Dislocation
Subluxation
Recurrent dislocation
Multidirectional instability

ICD-9 Codes

718.81 Instability of shoulder joint
831.00 Closed dislocation of shoulder, unspecified

ICD-10 Codes

S43.004 Unspecified dislocation of right shoulder joint
S43.005 Unspecified dislocation of left shoulder joint
S43.006 Unspecified dislocation of unspecified shoulder joint
S43.014 Anterior dislocation of right humerus
S43.015 Anterior dislocation of left humerus
S43.016 Anterior dislocation of unspecified humerus
S43.024 Posterior dislocation of right humerus
S43.025 Posterior dislocation of left humerus
S43.026 Posterior dislocation of unspecified humerus
S43.034 Inferior dislocation of right humerus
S43.035 Inferior dislocation of left humerus
S43.036 Inferior dislocation of unspecified humerus
Add seventh character for episode of care (A—initial encounter, D—subsequent encounter, S—sequela)

Definitions

Shoulder instability represents a spectrum of disorders ranging from shoulder subluxation, in which the humeral head partially slips out of the glenoid fossa, to shoulder dislocation, which is a complete displacement of the humeral head out of the glenoid. It is classified as anterior, posterior, or multidirectional and on the basis of its frequency, etiology, direction, and degree. Instability can result from macrotrauma, such as shoulder dislocation, or repetitive microtrauma associated with overhead activity, and it can occur without trauma in individuals with generalized ligamentous laxity [1–4].

The glenohumeral joint has a high degree of mobility at the expense of stability. Static and dynamic restraints combine to maintain the shoulder in place with overhead activity. Muscle action, particularly of the rotator cuff and scapular stabilizers, is important in maintaining joint congruity in midranges of motion. Static stabilizers, such as the glenohumeral ligaments, the joint capsule, and the glenoid labrum, are important for stability in the extremes of motion [2].

Traumatic damage to the shoulder capsule, the glenohumeral ligaments, and the inferior labrum is a result of acute dislocation. Repeated capsular stretch, rotator cuff, and superior labral injuries are associated with overuse injury resulting in anterior instability in athletes who participate in overhead sports; a loose patulous capsule is the primary pathologic change with multidirectional instability, and patients may present with bilateral symptoms [4–6]. Shoulder instability affects, in particular, young individuals, females, and athletes, but it may also affect sedentary individuals, with an incidence of 1.7% in the general population [1,7,8].

Traumatic instability often occurs when the individual usually falls on an outstretched, externally rotated, and abducted arm with a resulting anterior dislocation. A blow to the posterior aspect of the externally rotated and abducted arm can also result in anterior dislocation. Posterior dislocation usually results from a fall on the forward flexed and adducted arm or by a direct blow in the posterior direction when the arm is above the shoulder [5].

Recurrent shoulder instability after a traumatic dislocation is common, particularly when the initial event happens at a young age. In these individuals, it may occur repeatedly in association with overhead activity, and it may even happen at night, while changing position in bed, in those with severe instability. The patients may initially require visits to the emergency department or reduction of recurrent dislocation by a team physician; but as the condition becomes more chronic, some may be able to reduce their own dislocations [9,10].

Patients with neurologic problems such as stroke, brachial plexus injury, and severe myopathies may develop shoulder girdle muscle weakness, scapular dysfunction, and resultant shoulder instability.

Symptoms

With atraumatic instability or subluxation, it may be difficult to identify an initial precipitating event. Usually, symptoms result from repetitive activity that places great demands on the dynamic and static stabilizers of the glenohumeral joint, leading to increased translation of the humeral head in overhead sports and occupational activities. Pain is the initial symptom, usually associated with impingement of the rotator cuff under the coracoacromial arch. Patients may also report that the shoulder slips out of the joint or that the arm goes "dead," and they may report weakness associated with overhead activity [1–3,9–11].

Patients with neurologic injury present with pain with motion and shoulder subluxation as well as scapular and shoulder girdle muscle weakness. In the case of a patient with acute shoulder injury, factors to identify include the patient's age, dexterity or dominant side, sports and position, activity level, mechanism of injury, and any associated symptoms such as neurologic or functional deficits. In cases of acute dislocation, the age at first dislocation is a prognostic indicator in view of a recurrence of 75% to 100%, especially in skeletally immature individuals [11].

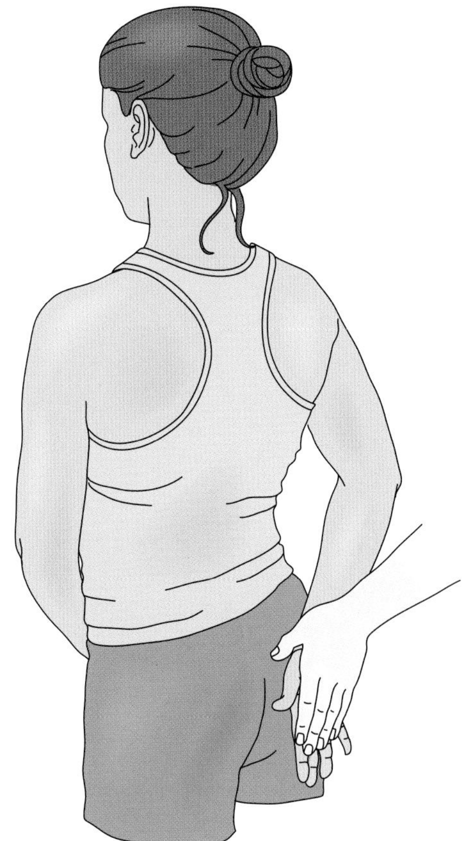

FIGURE 14.1 In the lift-off test of the subscapularis, the patient places the arm on the lower back area and attempts to forcefully internally rotate against the examiner's hand. It is important to document first that the patient has enough passive motion to allow the shoulder to be internally rotated away from the lower back area.

Physical Examination

The shoulder is inspected for deformity, atrophy of surrounding muscles, asymmetry, and scapular winging. Individuals are observed from the anterior, lateral, and posterior positions with the shoulder in neutral position on the side of the body as well as with flexion and abduction motion. Palpation of soft tissue and bone is systematically addressed and includes the four joints that compose the shoulder complex (sternoclavicular, acromioclavicular, glenohumeral, and scapulothoracic), rotator cuff, biceps tendon, and subacromial region.

Passive and active range of motion is evaluated. Differences between passive and active motion may be secondary to pain, weakness, or neurologic damage. Repeated throwing may lead to an increase in measured external rotation accompanied by a reduction in internal rotation; tennis players may present with an isolated glenohumeral internal rotation deficit [12]. These changes may be secondary to posterior capsule tightness, humeral torsion, and glenohumeral laxity that may lead to internal impingement [12].

Manual strength testing is performed to identify weakness of specific muscles of the rotator cuff and the scapular stabilizers. The supraspinatus muscle can be tested in the scapular plane with internal rotation or external rotation of the shoulder, and the external rotators are tested with the arm at the side of the body. The subscapularis muscle can be tested by the lift-off test, in which the palm of the hand is lifted away from the lower back (Fig. 14.1). The scapular stabilizers, such as the serratus anterior and the rhomboid muscles, can be tested in isolation or by doing wall pushups. Sensory examination of the shoulder girdle is performed to rule out nerve injuries.

Testing the shoulder in the position of 90 degrees of forward flexion with internal rotation (Hawkins maneuver) or in extreme forward flexion (until 180 degrees) with the forearm pronated (Neer maneuver) can assess for rotator cuff impingement and may reproduce symptoms of pain [10] (Fig. 14.2). Glenohumeral translation testing for ligamentous laxity or symptomatic instability should be documented. Apprehension testing can be performed with the patient sitting, standing, or in the supine position. The shoulder is stressed anteriorly in the position of 90 degrees of abduction and external rotation to reproduce the feeling that the shoulder is coming out of the joint (apprehension test). A relocation maneuver that reduces the symptoms of instability also aids in the diagnosis but appears to be less specific than apprehension

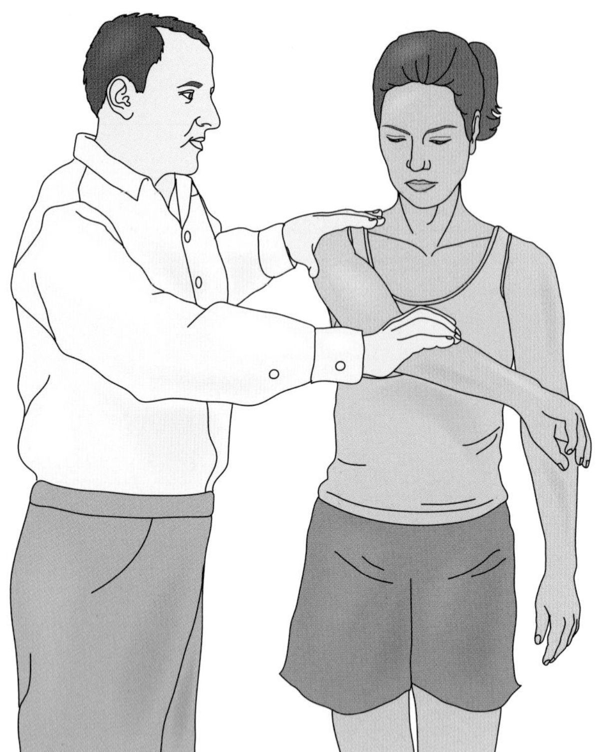

FIGURE 14.2 Impingement test for impingement against the coracoacromial arch.

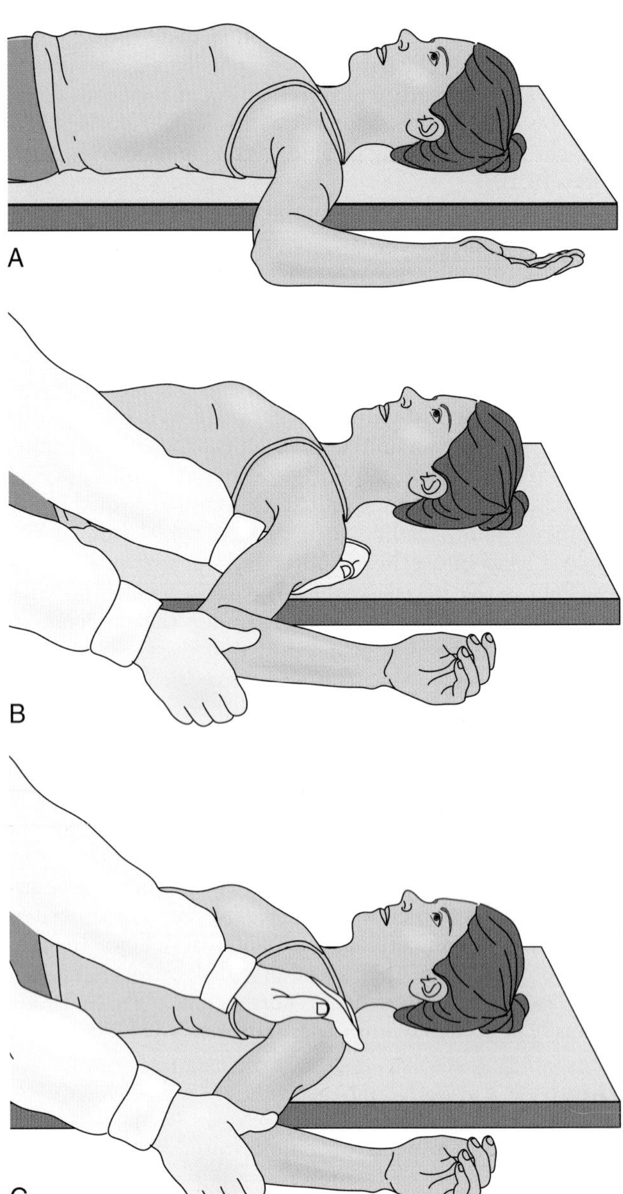

FIGURE 14.3 **A,** Apprehension relocation test in supine position with arm in 90 degrees of abduction and maximal external rotation. **B,** Reduction of symptoms of apprehension with posteriorly directed force on proximal humerus. **C,** Increased symptoms of apprehension or pain with anterior force applied on proximal humerus.

testing [11] (Fig. 14.3). The causation of posterior shoulder pain (rather than symptoms of instability) with apprehension testing may be associated with internal impingement of the rotator cuff and posterior superior labrum [13–19] (Fig. 14.4).

Other tests for shoulder laxity include the load and shift maneuver with the arm at the side to document humeral head translation in anterior and posterior directions and the sulcus sign to document inferior humeral head laxity. Labral injuries can be evaluated with a combination of tests including the active compression test described by O'Brien and colleagues in which a downward force is applied to the forward flexed, adducted, and internally rotated shoulder to reproduce pain associated with superior labral tears or acromioclavicular joint disease. In the crank test, pain and clicking are reproduced when the shoulder is abducted to 160 degrees and an axial load is placed on the humerus and the arm is internally and externally rotated. Another test is the biceps loading test, in which the patient is asked to supinate the forearm, abduct the shoulder to 90 degrees, flex the elbow to 90 degrees, and externally rotate the arm until apprehensive and the examiner provides resistance against elbow flexion. Pain would suggest a proximal biceps tendinopathy or a labral tear [13–19].

Functional Limitations

Impairment includes reduced motion, muscle weakness, and pain that interfere with activities of daily living, such as reaching into cupboards and brushing hair. Athletes, particularly those participating in throwing sports, may experience a decrease in the velocity of their pitches, and tennis players may lose control of their serve. Occupational limitations may include inability to reach or to lift weight above the level of the head or pain with rotation of the arm in a production line. Recurrent instability often leads to avoidance of activities that require abduction and external rotation because of reproduction of symptoms.

Diagnostic Studies

The standard radiographs that are obtained to evaluate the patient with shoulder symptoms include anteroposterior

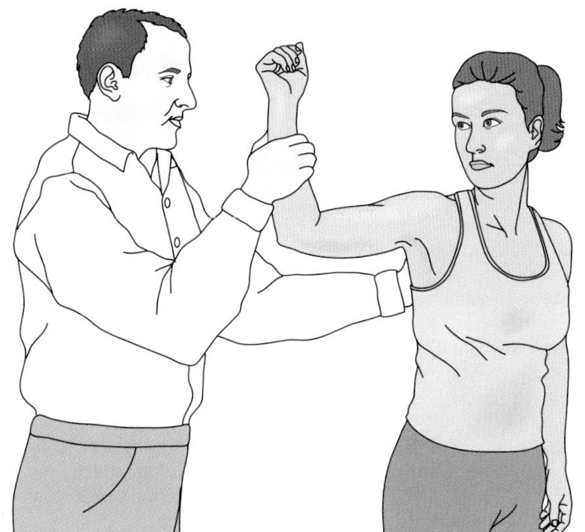

FIGURE 14.4 Internal impingement test. The arm is abducted to approximately 90 degrees and progressively externally rotated to reproduce pain in the posterior aspect of the shoulder.

views in external and internal rotation, outlet view, axillary lateral view, and Stryker notch view. These allow an assessment of the greater tuberosity and the shape of the acromion and reveal irregularity of the glenoid or posterior humeral head as well as dysplasia, hypoplasia, or bone loss that can contribute to instability [3,20].

Special tests that can also be ordered include arthrography, computed tomographic arthrography, magnetic resonance imaging, and magnetic resonance arthrography. These should be ordered to look for rotator cuff or labral abnormalities in the patient who has not responded to treatment. Magnetic resonance arthrography allows better evaluation of rotator cuff, glenoid labrum, and glenohumeral ligaments [3,21]. Gadolinium contrast enhancement and modification of the position of the arm for the test appear to increase the sensitivity of magnetic resonance imaging in identifying the specific location of capsular or labral pathologic changes associated with recurrent instability and dislocation [3,21]. Musculoskeletal sonography has grown in popularity in the last decade, and its use in shoulder disease has been well documented. Evaluation of shoulder instability is limited to visualization of the posterior labrum and the rotator cuff tendons and evaluation for paralabral cysts that may suggest labral injury [22]. Diagnostic arthroscopy can be used in some cases but is generally not necessary.

Differential Diagnosis

Glenohumeral joint instability
- Post-traumatic
- Atraumatic
- Multidirectional

Rotator cuff tendinitis or tendinosis
Rotator cuff tear or insufficiency
Glenoid labral tear
Suprascapular neuropathy

Treatment

Initial

Acute management of glenohumeral instability is nonoperative in the majority of cases. This includes relative rest, ice, and analgesic or anti-inflammatory medication. Goals at this stage are pain reduction, protection from further injury, and initiation of an early rehabilitation program.

If the injury was observed (as often occurs in athletes) and no neurologic or vascular damage is evident on clinical examination, reduction may be attempted with traction in forward flexion and slight abduction, followed by gentle internal rotation. If this fails, the patient should be transported away from the playing area; reduction may be attempted by placing the patient prone, sedating the individual, and allowing the injured arm to hang from the bed with a 5- to 10-pound weight attached to the wrist. If fracture or posterior dislocation is suspected, the patient should undergo radiologic evaluation before a reduction is attempted. After the reduction, radiologic studies should be repeated [1,3,23–25].

When acute shoulder dislocations are treated nonoperatively, they are usually managed with 1 to 4 weeks of immobilization in a sling, in which the arm is positioned in internal rotation, followed by an exercise program and gradual return to activity. Several studies have suggested that placement of the arm in a position of external rotation may be more appropriate because of better realignment of anatomic structures and reduction position [23–26]. However, this issue still merits further study because there is a lack of randomized controlled studies demonstrating a significant reduction in recurrent dislocation rates or a difference in return to activity levels in comparing the positions of immobilization after reduction or the duration of the postreduction immobilization period [25].

Rehabilitation

The rehabilitation of glenohumeral instability should begin as soon as the injury occurs. The goals of nonsurgical management are reduction of pain, restoration of full functional motion, correction of muscle strength deficits, achievement of muscle balance, and return to full activity free of symptoms. The rehabilitation program consists of acute, recovery, and functional phases [2–4,17–19] (Table 14.1).

Acute Phase (1 to 2 weeks)

This phase should focus on treatment of tissue injury and clinical signs and symptoms. The goal in this stage is to allow tissue healing while reducing pain and inflammation. Reestablishment of nonpainful active range of motion, prevention of shoulder girdle muscle atrophy, reduction of scapular dysfunction, and maintenance of general fitness are addressed.

Recovery Phase (2 to 6 weeks)

This phase focuses on obtaining normal passive and active glenohumeral range of motion, restoring posterior capsule flexibility, improving scapular and rotator cuff muscle strength, and achieving normal core muscle strength and balance. Flexibility training should include the sleeper stretch; strength training includes exercises for the lower

Table 14.1 Glenohumeral Instability Rehabilitation

	Acute Phase	Recovery Phase	Functional Phase
Therapeutic intervention	Active rest Cryotherapy Electrical stimulation Protected motion Isometric and closed chain exercise to shoulder and scapular muscles General conditioning Nonsteroidal anti-inflammatory drugs	Modalities: superficial heat, ultrasound, electrical stimulation Range of motion exercises, flexibility exercises for posterior capsule Scapular control: closed chain exercises, proprioceptive neuromuscular facilitation patterns Dynamic upper extremity strengthening exercise: isolated rotator cuff exercises Sports-specific exercises: surgical tubing, multiplanar joint exercises, core and lower extremity Gradual return to training	Power and endurance in upper extremities: diagonal and multiplanar motions with tubing, light weights, medicine balls, plyometrics Increased multiple-plane neuromuscular control Maintenance: general flexibility training, strengthening, power and endurance exercise program Sports-specific progression
Criteria for advancement	Pain reduction Recovery of pain-free motion Symptom-free progression of muscle strengthening exercises	Full nonpainful motion Normal scapular stabilizers and rotator cuff strength Correction of posterior capsule inflexibility Symptom-free progression in a sports-specific program	Normal clinical examination Normal shoulder mechanics Normal kinematic chain integration Completed sports-specific program Normal throwing motion

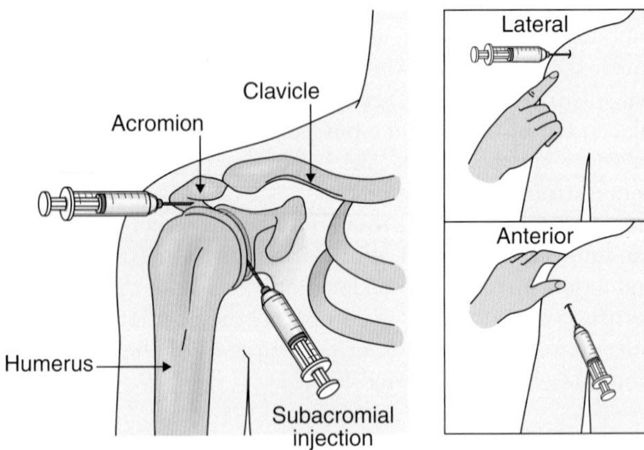

FIGURE 14.5 Approximate surface anatomy *(insets)* and internal anatomic sites for injection of the glenohumeral joint laterally and anteriorly. See also Figure 14.6. *(From Lennard TA. Physiatric Procedures. Philadelphia, Hanley & Belfus, 1995.)*

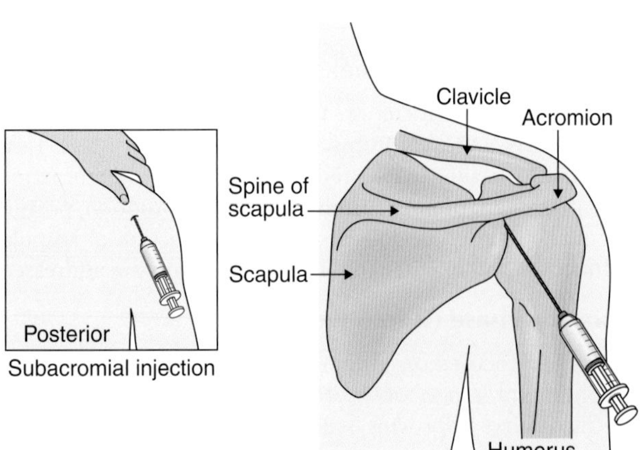

FIGURE 14.6 Posterior injection of the glenohumeral joint. *(From Lennard TA. Physiatric Procedures. Philadelphia, Hanley & Belfus, 1995.)*

trapezius and serratus anterior muscle. This phase can be started as soon as pain is controlled and the patient can participate in an exercise program without exacerbation of symptoms. Young individuals with symptomatic instability need to progress slowly to the position of shoulder abduction and external rotation. Athletes can progress rapidly through the program and emphasize exercises in functional ranges of motion. Older patients with goals of returning to activities of daily living may require slower progression, particularly if they have significant pain, muscle inhibition, and weakness. Biomechanical and functional deficits including abnormalities in the throwing motion should also be addressed.

Functional Phase (6 weeks to 6 months)

This phase focuses on increasing power and endurance of the upper extremities while improving neuromuscular control because a normal sensorimotor system is key in returning to optimal shoulder function [24]. Rehabilitation at this stage works on the entire kinematic chain to address specific functional deficits.

After the completion of rehabilitation, a continued exercise program with goals of preventing recurrent injury should be instituted for individuals who participate in sports, recreational activities, or work-related tasks in which high demands on the shoulder joint are expected. A training program that combines flexibility and strengthening exercises with neuromuscular as well as proprioceptive training should be ongoing. Patients with multidirectional instability need to work specifically on strengthening of the scapular stabilizers and balancing the force couples between the rotator cuff and the deltoid muscle.

Procedures

If the individual persists with some symptoms of pain secondary to rotator cuff irritation despite an appropriate rehabilitation program, a subacromial injection could be considered (Figs. 14.5 and 14.6). The patient at that time should be reevaluated for identification of residual functional and biomechanical deficits that need to be addressed in combination with the injection. Under sterile conditions, with use of a 23- to 25-gauge, 1½-inch disposable needle, inject an anesthetic-corticosteroid preparation by an anterior, posterior, or lateral approach with or without sonographic guidance, based on availability and clinician expertise. Typically, 3 to 8 mL is injected (e.g., 4 mL of 1% lidocaine and 2 mL of 40 mg/mL triamcinolone). Alternatively, the lidocaine may be injected first, followed by the corticosteroid. Postinjection care includes local ice for 5 to 10 minutes. The patient is instructed to ice the shoulder for 15 to 20 minutes three or four times daily for the next few days and to avoid aggressive overhead activities for the following week. Other procedures, such as prolotherapy, platelet-rich plasma injections, and ultrasound-guided infiltrations, are becoming more popular, especially in athletes for other musculoskeletal injuries, but the results of use for shoulder instability are still unknown [27].

Surgery

Because of high rates of recurrent instability after conservative treatment in the active athletic population and, in particular, throwers, early surgical intervention is gaining acceptance [28]. Open repair of Bankart lesions has been the standard surgical intervention after traumatic instability, and it is still reported by some authors as the preferred method because of predictable results in regard to recurrence of dislocation and return to activity [28]. Early arthroscopic repair of the inferior labral defect associated with acute shoulder dislocation is becoming widespread because of an apparent reduction in postoperative morbidity that may allow the athlete an early return to function [29–31].

In the individual with recurrent instability, surgical treatment may need to address abnormalities in the shoulder capsule, glenoid labrum, and rotator cuff. Arthroscopic interventions result in comparable outcomes when they are measured against open surgery, but no "gold standard" method has been established [3]. Surgical interventions include capsular procedures, such as the capsular shift, and labral as well as rotator cuff procedures, such as débridement and repair [32,33]. In many instances, these procedures need to be combined for optimal results in the patient, followed by an accelerated rehabilitation program with guidelines similar to those for the patient treated nonoperatively [34]. Rehabilitation protocols are similar for open and arthroscopic techniques. The shoulder is immobilized with an abduction pillow for 4 to 6 weeks, with therapy initiated if stiffness develops. After immobilization, strengthening exercises (similar to nonsurgical protocols) are recommended. If the rehabilitation protocol is successfully completed, the patient is allowed to return to full activity 4 to 6 months after surgery [3,34,35].

Potential Disease Complications

Complications include recurrent instability with overhead activity, pain in the shoulder region, nerve damage, and weakness of the rotator cuff and scapular muscles. These tend to occur more commonly in patients with multidirectional atraumatic instability. Loss of function may include inability to lift overhead and loss of throwing velocity and accuracy. Recurrent episodes of instability in the older individual may also be related to the development of rotator cuff tears [36].

Potential Treatment Complications

Analgesics and nonsteroidal anti-inflammatory drugs have well-known side effects that most commonly affect the gastric, hepatic, cardiovascular, and renal systems. Complications of treatment include loss of motion, failure of surgical repair with recurrent instability, and inability to return to previous level of function. Failure of conservative treatment may be associated with incomplete rehabilitation or poor technique. Recurrent dislocation after surgical treatment can be related to not addressing all the sites of pathologic change at the time of the operation [35].

References

[1] Dumont GD, Russell RD, Robertson WJ. Anterior shoulder instability: a review of pathoanatomy, diagnosis and treatment. Curr Rev Musculoskelet Med 2011;4:200–7.
[2] Buckhart S, Morgan C, Kibler B. The disabled throwing shoulder: spectrum of pathology part III: the SICK scapula, scapular dyskinesis, the kinetic chain, and rehabilitation. Arthroscopy 2003;19:641–61.
[3] Gamradt S, Warren R. Glenohumeral instabilities. In: Delee J, Drez D, Miller M, editors. Orthopaedic sports medicine: principles and practice. 3rd ed. Philadelphia: Saunders Elsevier; 2011. p. 909–31.
[4] Eckenrode B, Kelley M, Kelly J. Anatomic and biomechanical fundamentals of the thrower shoulder. Sports Med Arthrosc Rev 2012;20:2–10.
[5] Takase K, Yamamoto K. Intraarticular lesions in traumatic anterior shoulder instability. Acta Orthop 2005;76:854–7.
[6] Cordasco FA. Understanding multidirectional instability of the shoulder. J Athl Train 2000;35:278–85.
[7] Loud KJ, Micheli LJ. Common athletic injuries in adolescent girls. Curr Opin Pediatr 2001;13:317–22.
[8] Wasserlauf BL, Paletta Jr GA. Shoulder disorders in the skeletally immature throwing athlete. Orthop Clin North Am 2003;34:427–37.
[9] Satterwhite YE. Evaluation and management of recurrent anterior shoulder instability. J Athl Train 2000;35:273–7.
[10] Laurencin CT, O'Brien SJ. Anterior shoulder instability: anatomy, pathophysiology, and conservative management. In: Andrews JR, Zarims B, Wilk K, editors. Injuries in baseball. Philadelphia: Lippincott-Raven; 1998. p. 189–97.
[11] Good CR, MacGillivray JD. Traumatic shoulder dislocation in the adolescent athlete: advances in surgical treatment. Curr Opin Pediatr 2005;17:25–9.
[12] Myers JB, Laudner KG, Pasquale MR, et al. Glenohumeral range of motion deficits and posterior shoulder tightness in throwers with pathologic internal impingement. Am J Sports Med 2006;34:385–91.
[13] Bowen JE, Malanga GA, Tutankhamen P, et al. Physical examination of the shoulder. In: Malanga GA, Nadler SF, editors. Musculoskeletal physical examination: an evidence-based approach. Philadelphia: Elsevier; 2006. p. 59–118.
[14] Pappas GP, Blemker SS, Beaulieu CF, et al. In vivo anatomy of the Neer and Hawkins sign positions for shoulder impingement. J Shoulder Elbow Surg 2006;15:40–9.
[15] Farber AJ, Castillo R, Clough M, et al. Clinical assessment of three common tests for traumatic anterior shoulder instability. J Bone Joint Surg Am 2006;88:1467–74.
[16] Clarnette RC, Miniaci A. Clinical exam of the shoulder. Med Sci Sports Exerc 1998;30(Suppl):1–6.
[17] Meister K. Injuries to the shoulder in the throwing athlete. Part one: biomechanics/pathophysiology/classification of injury. Am J Sports Med 2000;28:265–75.
[18] O'Brien SJ, Pagnani MJ, Fealy S, et al. The active compression test: a new and effective test for diagnosing labral tear and acromioclavicular joint abnormality. Am J Sports Med 1998;26:610–3.
[19] Meister K. Injuries to the shoulder in the throwing athlete. Part two: evaluation/treatment. Am J Sports Med 2000;28:587–601.

[20] Moosikasuwan JB, Miller TT, Dines DM. Imaging of the painful shoulder in throwing athletes. Clin Sports Med 2006;25:433–43.
[21] Song HT, Huh YM, Kim S, et al. Antero-inferior labral lesions of recurrent shoulder dislocation evaluated by MR arthrography in an adduction internal rotation (ADIR) position. J Magn Reson Imaging 2006;23:29–35.
[22] Jacobson J. Fundamentals of musculoskeletal ultrasound. Philadelphia: WB Saunders; 2007.
[23] De Baere T, Delloye C. First-time traumatic anterior dislocation of the shoulder in young adults: the position of the arm during immobilization revisited. Acta Orthop Belg 2005;71:516–20.
[24] Funk L, Smith M. Best evidence report. How to immobilize after shoulder dislocation? Emerg Med J 2005;22:814–5.
[25] Handoll HH, Hanchard NC, Goodchild L, Feary J. Conservative management following closed reduction of traumatic anterior dislocation of the shoulder. Cochrane Database Syst Rev 2006;1, CD004962.
[26] Paterson WH, Throckmorton TW, Koester M, et al. Position and duration of immobilization after primary anterior shoulder dislocation: a systematic review and meta-analysis of the literature. J Bone Joint Surg Am 2010;92:2924–33.
[27] Borg-Stein J, Zaremski JL, Hanford MA. New concepts in the assessment and treatment of regional musculoskeletal pain and sports injury. PM R 2009;1:744–54.
[28] Nelson BJ, Arciero RA. Arthroscopic management of glenohumeral instability. Am J Sports Med 2000;28:602–14.
[29] Mohtadi NG, Bitar IJ, Sasyniuk TM, et al. Arthroscopic versus open repair for traumatic anterior shoulder instability: a meta-analysis. Arthroscopy 2005;21:652–8.
[30] Carreira DS, Mazzocca AD, Oryhon J, et al. A prospective outcome evaluation of arthroscopic Bankart repairs: minimum 2 years follow-up. Am J Sports Med 2006;34:771–7.
[31] Fabbriciani C, Milano G, Demontis A, et al. Arthroscopic versus open treatment of Bankart lesions of the shoulder: a prospective randomised study. Arthroscopy 2004;20:456–62.
[32] Ticker JB, Warner JJP. Selective capsular shift technique for anterior and anterior-inferior glenohumeral instability. Clin Sports Med 2000;19:1–17.
[33] Marquard B, Potzl W, Witt KA, et al. A modified capsular shift for atraumatic anterior-inferior shoulder instability. Am J Sports Med 2005;33:1011–5.
[34] Kim SH, Ha KI, Jung MW, et al. Accelerated rehabilitation after arthroscopic Bankart repair for selected cases: a prospective randomized clinical trial. Arthroscopy 2003;19:722–31.
[35] Tauber M, Resch H, Forstner R, et al. Reasons for failure after surgical repair of anterior shoulder instability. J Shoulder Elbow Surg 2004;13:279–85.
[36] Porcellini G, Paladini P, Campi F, et al. Shoulder instability and related rotator cuff tears: arthroscopic findings and treatment in patients aged 40 to 60 years. Arthroscopy 2006;22:270–6.

CHAPTER 15

Labral Tears of the Shoulder

David E. Hartigan, MD
Cedric J. Ortiguera, MD

Synonyms

SLAP tears (superior labral anterior-posterior)
Soft tissue Bankart lesion
Reverse soft tissue Bankart lesion

ICD-9 Codes

SLAP
840.7 Lesion superior glenoid labrum
840.8 Tear superior glenoid labrum
Bankart
718.20 Pathological dislocation
718.31 Subluxation shoulder anterior recurrent, subluxation shoulder posterior recurrent
905.6 Late effect of dislocation
905.7 Late effect of sprain and strain without mention of tendon injury

ICD-10 Codes

S43.431 SLAP lesion of right shoulder
S43.432 SLAP lesion of left shoulder
S43.439 SLAP lesion of unspecified shoulder
Add seventh character for episode of care (A—initial encounter, D—subsequent encounter, S—sequela encounter)
M75.80 Other shoulder lesions, unspecified shoulder
M75.81 Other shoulder lesions, right shoulder
M75.82 Other shoulder lesions, left shoulder

Definition

The glenoid labrum is a densely fibrous tissue that is located along the periphery of the glenoid bone [1] (Fig. 15.1). As the outer labrum transitions from the periphery to its articulation with the glenoid, the histology changes from fibrous to a small fibrocartilaginous zone at the junction with the glenoid [2]. The labrum increases the height and width of the glenoid while also giving extra depth to the joint. This provides increased stability while still allowing great range of motion [3]. The labrum also serves as an attachment point for the long head of the biceps tendon, the glenohumeral ligaments, and the long head of the triceps tendon, forming a periarticular system of fibers that gives the shoulder joint much needed stability [4]. The vascular supply to the labrum is from the posterior humeral circumflex artery, the circumflex scapular branch of the subscapular artery, and the suprascapular artery. These arteries come from the periphery of the labrum, making the articular margins of the labrum avascular [2]. It has also been shown that the superior labrum has less vascular supply than the inferior labrum. The long head of the biceps has a variable attachment to the labrum and glenoid. Approximately 40% to 60% of the biceps tendon originates from the supraglenoid tubercle, and the remaining fibers insert into the labrum [1]. The biceps insertion into the labrum is variable but most commonly is in a more posterior position.

Tears can occur in all regions of the labrum. The most studied injury to the labrum is the superior labral anterior-posterior (SLAP) tear. Anterior dislocations of the shoulder can be associated with a disruption of the anteroinferior labrum and anterior band of the inferior glenohumeral ligament, also known as a Bankart lesion. Posterior shoulder instability may result in injury to the posterior band of the inferior glenohumeral ligament as well as the posterior labrum, or a reverse Bankart lesion. Tears can extend to involve multiple regions of the labrum and have other associated injuries. The SLAP tear and Bankart lesion are the most common and for that reason are the focus of this discussion.

The most common mechanisms for SLAP tears are forced traction on the shoulder and direct compression. Direct compression can occur in the acute traumatic setting or in the chronic setting typical in the overhead throwing athlete. Overhead throwers are predisposed to SLAP

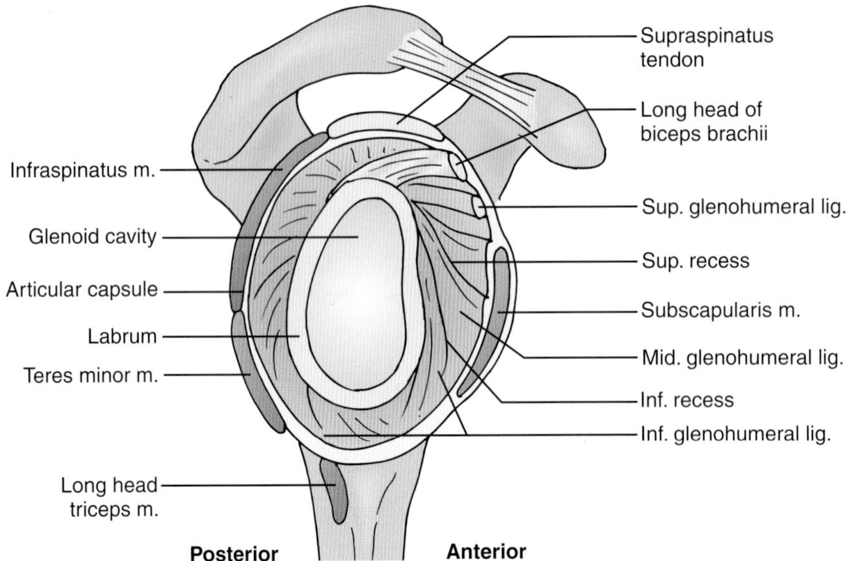

FIGURE 15.1 Normal anatomy of the shoulder.

tears secondary to their adaptive anatomy. They tend to have posterior capsular contractures, loose anterior capsular structures, and a retroverted humeral head, all increasing the amount of external rotation in the shoulder. As a result of these anatomic changes, the arm goes into an extreme externally rotated position while the biceps kinks at its insertion and assumes a more vertical and posterior position. This applies a torsional force to the biceps-labral complex superiorly, resulting in a peel back mechanism on the superior labrum [5,6]. Alternatively, as throwers externally rotate in the cocking phase, the rotator cuff may impinge on the posterior-superior glenoid, causing an "internal impingement" and tearing of the labrum [7].

Snyder [8] classified SLAP tears into four types, which was further modified by Morgan and Maffet. Most physicians think that the four-class system (Fig. 15.2) is sufficient and that the additional classifications could be placed within these basic types, so it is the preferred classification.

Bankart lesions are created by episodes of anterior instability. As the humeral head moves out anteriorly and inferiorly, anterior damage can occur to the anterior-inferior labrum, glenohumeral ligaments, joint capsule, rotator cuff, and possibly neurovascular structures. It has been shown that the Bankart lesion is created about 85% to 97% of the time in anterior dislocations [9,10]. This pathologic change is thought to be an important reason for recurrent instability.

In addition to the labrum's increasing the depth and diameter of the glenoid, the labrum and capsule also create a negative pressure that provides stability through the glenohumeral articulation. If the labrum or capsule is injured, such as in the Bankart lesion, this suction is lost, and this decreases the stability of the shoulder. Several factors may predispose patients to recurrent instability. These include fracture on the glenoid or humeral head, hyperlaxity syndromes, male gender, younger age at initial dislocation, participation in contact or overhead throwing sport, and positive correlation between number of dislocations and risk of future dislocation. Dislocations later in life increase the risk of rotator cuff injury, with tears occurring in nearly 30% of patients older than 40 years and in up to 80% of patients older than 60 years.

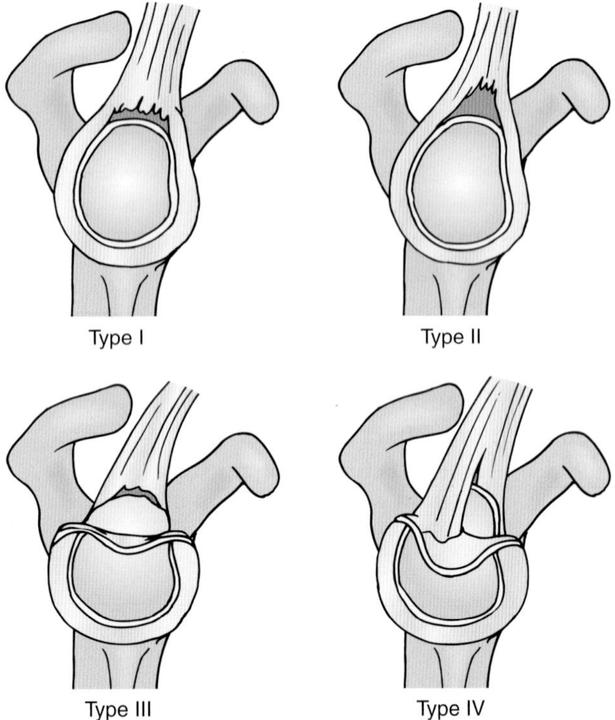

FIGURE 15.2 SLAP tear classification. Type I: degenerative tear of the undersurface of the superior labrum with the biceps anchor intact. Type II: tear of the superior labrum as well as of the biceps anchor. Type III: bucket-handle tear of the superior labrum with biceps anchor intact. Type IV: bucket-handle tear of the superior labrum with extension into biceps tendon.

Symptoms

SLAP Tear

A patient with a SLAP tear will most commonly present with symptoms of deep-seated pain, which can be sharp or dull [11]. It is usually located deep within the center of the shoulder and can be made worse with overhead activities, pushing heavy objects, lifting, or reaching behind the back. Patients may have mechanical symptoms, such as catching, popping, or grinding with rotation of the shoulder. Many patients with a SLAP tear will also have other shoulder disease, making clinical diagnosis challenging [11].

It is essential to obtain a thorough history for trauma to evaluate for traction or compression type injuries, dislocations, and sports (e.g., baseball, football, waterskiing, tennis) they play that may predispose them to this injury. Overhead throwing athletes may suffer decreased velocity and usually complain of pain in the late cocking and early acceleration phase of throwing. They may have weakness due to pain or secondary to a paralabral cyst compressing the suprascapular nerve. Compression on the nerve at the spinoglenoid notch can cause weakness in external rotation as well as deep posterior shoulder pain.

Bankart Lesion

Symptoms of anterior instability are usually obvious as the patient states that there has been a dislocation and continues to complain of pain and instability in that shoulder. Sometimes there is not a history of overt dislocation, but instead the patient has multiple episodes of instability without a complete dislocation. The patient will complain of pain and feeling of impending dislocation with the arm in abduction and external rotation. Important historical variables include the patient's age at first dislocation, need for formal reduction, number of recurrent instability episodes, voluntary instability, and anticipated future sports activities.

The most comfortable position for these patients is usually with the arm in adduction and internal rotation. They avoid abduction and external rotation because this is the position that led to the dislocation and it also stresses the injured labrum, inferior glenohumeral ligament, and subscapularis tendon.

Physical Examination

SLAP Tear

Several clinical tests are designed to assist the clinician in making the SLAP tear diagnosis [12–15]. These tests are trying to do one of two things: to pinch the torn labrum between the humeral head and the glenoid, causing pain or mechanical symptoms, or to place traction on the biceps tendon (Table 15.1). The tests have had variable ranges of sensitivity and specificity between studies, and thus no single test is considered diagnostic. The most commonly performed test is the O'Brien active compression test. This has been shown to be very sensitive but has extremely poor specificity. Accurate diagnosis requires a careful history to correlate with the examination findings.

In many cases, concomitant disease may cloud the physical examination findings [11]. On inspection of the shoulder, there may be atrophy of the supraspinatus and infraspinatus muscles. The supraspinatus atrophy is difficult to observe because of the overlying trapezius muscle. The atrophy can occur because of a paralabral cyst that compresses the suprascapular nerve, or it could be secondary to an associated rotator cuff tear. Palpation of the biceps tendon may demonstrate tenderness within the bicipital groove. The range of motion of the shoulder should be preserved, although throwing athletes may have increased external rotation and loss of internal rotation with a resulting glenohumeral internal rotation deficit [5,6].

Bankart Lesion

Evaluation for anterior instability may include a number of tests (Table 15.2). After reduction of a dislocation, a thorough neurovascular examination should be performed to rule out major vessel or brachial plexus injury. In a typical Bankart lesion with anterior instability, patients will often experience apprehension when the arm is brought

Table 15.1 Common Tests for Diagnosis of SLAP Tears

Test	Instruction	Indication of Positive Test Result
Active compression (O'Brien) test	Arm is forward flexed to 90 degrees, adducted across the body Patient resists downward force on arm in pronated and supinated position of the forearm	Pain is increased in pronated position
Crank test	Arm is abducted >100 degrees in the scapular plane; elbow is flexed to 90 degrees Axial force is applied through the humerus onto the glenohumeral joint and the shoulder is rotated (internal and external rotation)	Pain, catching, clicking
Pain provocative test	Patient abducts shoulder to 90 degrees, flexes elbow to 90 degrees, and pronates and supinates the hand	Pain is worse or present only in pronation
Biceps load test	Patient is supine; shoulder is abducted to 90 degrees; elbow is flexed to 90 degrees The shoulder is externally rotated to a point at which the patient feels pain, apprehension, or maximum external rotation; the patient then performs resisted flexion of the elbow	Worsening of pain when resisted elbow flexion is performed
Compression-rotation test	Patient is supine; shoulder is abducted to 90 degrees; elbow is flexed to 90 degrees Axial load is placed on the glenohumeral joint and the humerus is rotated	Pain, catching, clicking, snapping
Anterior slide test	Patient is sitting and places hands on the hips with thumbs facing posterior The examiner places a finger over the anterior shoulder and the other hand pushes up on the humerus superior and anterior; patient is asked to resist	Pain or click

Table 15.2 Common Tests for Diagnosis of Anterior Instability

Test	Instruction	Indication of Positive Test Result
Load and shift	Supine position Arm at 0, 45, 90 degrees of abduction Anterior directed force on the humerus	Increasing translation at higher degrees of abduction indicates that the inferior glenohumeral ligament is compromised. Grade 1: increased translation compared with contralateral Grade 2: humeral head translates to the glenoid rim Grade 3: translates over the glenoid rim
Apprehension test (crank)	Supine position Arm brought into 90 degrees of abduction and increasing external rotation	Pain, feeling of impending dislocation, or muscle guarding
Relocation (Jobe) test	Apprehension position with posteriorly directed force on the humeral head	Decreased apprehension or pain
Surprise test	Relocation test with sudden release of posteriorly directed force	Sense of instability or apprehension with release of force

into abduction and external rotation. Strength should be assessed, looking for axillary or radial nerve palsies as well as rotator cuff disease in the older patient. In a patient older than 40 years who cannot lift the arm after a dislocation, rotator cuff tear is far more common than an axillary nerve palsy [16,17]. The surprise test has been shown to be the most accurate test, with a positive predictive value of 98% and a negative predictive value of 78% [18].

Functional Limitations

SLAP Tear

Patients may have difficulty carrying or pushing heavy objects, working overhead, and throwing [1]. This pathologic process can often be asymptomatic at rest and symptomatic only with more vigorous activity. SLAP tears often are manifested with a multitude of other shoulder diseases, so limitations may vary according to what else is present in the shoulder along with the SLAP tear [11].

Bankart Lesion

Avoidance of the abducted and externally rotated position is required to limit recurrent instability. This may limit many athletic activities, particularly in contact sports and in throwers.

Diagnostic Studies

SLAP Tear

The initial imaging study for any shoulder pain is plain radiography, including anterior-posterior, scapular anterior-posterior, axillary, and outlet views. There are no typical findings for SLAP tears on radiography, but it is necessary to rule out other sources of pain.

Magnetic resonance imaging (MRI) should be the next test obtained for patients with a high clinical likelihood of labral disease. There is controversy as to whether high-resolution non–contrast-enhanced MRI or magnetic resonance arthrography is the "gold standard" for diagnosis of SLAP lesions [19,20]. With the high rate of concomitant shoulder injuries, MRI is helpful in showing both intra-articular and extra-articular pathologic changes within the soft tissues. Positioning of the arm in external rotation or abduction and external rotation can improve the ability to accurately diagnose these lesions [21,22]. Computed tomographic arthrography may also be used if MRI is contraindicated, but it is less sensitive to other soft tissue disease. Ultrasound may be useful to visualize concomitant disease, such as tears of the rotator cuff and paralabral cyst, but it has poor visualization of the labrum.

Arthroscopy has been the gold standard for diagnosis of labral disease. Many times the diagnosis is made during arthroscopy after other modalities have failed to make a conclusive diagnosis.

Bankart Lesion

Plain radiography should be performed to rule out dislocation in the acute setting. With more chronic instability, additional views could be considered. The West Point view can assist with visualization of the glenoid in an attempt to see bone disruptions of the glenoid rim; a Stryker notch view may better visualize an associated Hill-Sachs lesion of the humeral head.

In patients with soft tissue Bankart lesions, the radiographs may be unrevealing. MRI would be the next imaging study conducted (Fig. 15.3). In the acute setting,

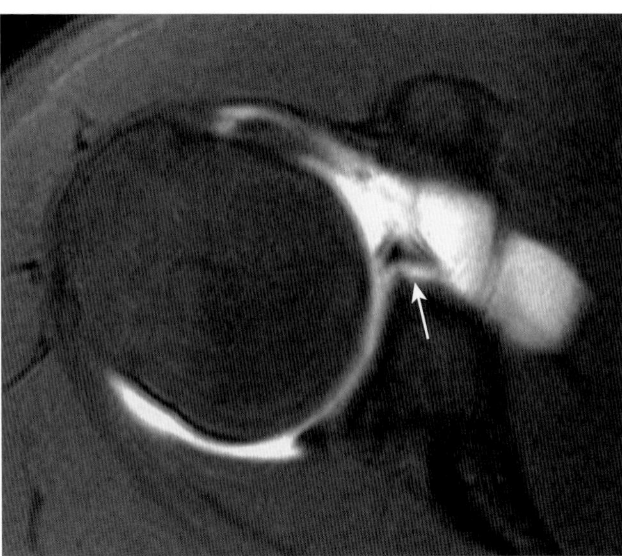

FIGURE 15.3 Axial magnetic resonance image of a Bankart lesion.

non–contrast-enhanced MRI is reasonable as the hemarthrosis from the dislocation aids in visualization of the labral process. In the chronic setting, magnetic resonance arthrography can improve labral imaging.

Differential Diagnosis

Impingement syndrome
Rotator cuff disease
Acromioclavicular joint disease
Cervical disc injury
Cervical radiculopathy
Brachial plexus injury
Refractory bicipital tendinitis
Multidirectional instability
Bony Bankart lesion
Humeral avulsion of the glenohumeral ligament
Malingering

Treatment

Initial

SLAP Tear

Overhead throwing athletes with more than 35 degrees of glenohumeral internal rotation deficit have a 60% chance of shoulder injury that requires them to miss games [5]. Regular posterior-inferior capsular stretching exercises significantly decrease the rate of shoulder injuries in overhead throwing athletes [5,6] and are now a part of preventive care for baseball players.

Initial treatment of a SLAP tear is symptomatic. Nonsteroidal anti-inflammatory medications, cryotherapy, and activity modification are the mainstays of treatment until the acute inflammation and pain subside. A short period of sling immobilization for comfort should be followed by early institution of range of motion exercises.

Bankart Lesion

The Bankart lesion is a result of anterior shoulder instability or dislocation. If the shoulder is dislocated, the initial step in treatment is to reduce the shoulder. Postreduction radiographs should be obtained and neurovascular status checked. Sling immobilization should be instituted for a short period. Recommendations for the duration of immobilization vary from days to weeks. The position of immobilization is controversial as immobilization in external rotation has been shown by some to lower the recurrence rate of instability, but it must be instituted immediately after the instability episode [23,24]. The most common recommendation is for standard sling immobilization for a period of 1 to 3 weeks.

Rehabilitation

SLAP Tear

When a SLAP tear is suspected, the recommended physical therapy focuses on strengthening the rotator cuff, capsular stretching, range of motion of the glenohumeral joint, and scapular stabilization exercises. A study by Edwards showed good results with nonoperative treatment of SLAP tears [25]; 51% of the patients in the study ended up having surgery, but the remainder reported significant pain relief, 100% returned to sports, and 70% returned to preinjury level. Patients in this study were treated with nonsteroidal anti-inflammatory drugs, scapular strengthening, and posterior capsular stretching. The results are comparable to surgical outcomes, so conservative management should be the first-line treatment.

Postoperative rehabilitation after arthroscopic labral repair involves a 4- to 6-week period of sling immobilization followed by a progressive range of motion and strengthening program. For overhead athletes, a throwing program can begin at 4 months with full return at approximately 7 to 12 months.

Bankart Lesion

After a period of sling immobilization in the acute setting, the patient is progressed through simple passive, active-assisted, and then active range of motion. Once the patient is comfortable with these exercises, the focus shifts to progressive resistance training of the rotator cuff, deltoid, and scapular stabilizers. This should continue until strength and motion are equal bilaterally. The goal is to strengthen the dynamic stabilizers of the glenohumeral joint. Activity modification should be a part of rehabilitation in some patients as well. Avoidance of the activity that led to the dislocation is often reasonable in the older patient but challenging for the young athlete who would like to return to sport. In the young athlete with first-time dislocation, surgical management is becoming more common as nonoperative treatment is not nearly as successful as in the older patient population (older than 30 years). Other nonsurgical options in addition to physical therapy that can be considered in the patient with anterior instability and a Bankart lesion are bracing and taping. Whereas these modalities are directed at preventing the position of abduction and external rotation or preventing humeral subluxation, neither has been shown to decrease the rate of instability.

Procedures

Patients with labral tears can undergo an intra-articular injection with corticosteroid and local anesthetic to help with pain and inflammation. Intra-articular injection should be done in conjunction with the physical therapy as described. This can be done under fluoroscopic or ultrasound guidance or by anatomic landmarks.

Aspiration of paralabral cysts causing compression on the suprascapular nerve can be performed with image guidance. This has been shown to provide relief in 60% of patients, although it is usually temporary. Failure to address the primary pathologic process of the labral tear may allow recurrence of the cyst.

Surgery

SLAP Tear

Surgery is indicated once the patient and physician have decided that nonoperative measures have not been adequate. It is generally recommended that patients have a trial of conservative therapy, usually involving at least a 3-month period of physical therapy and medications, before proceeding to the operating room. The following surgical procedures are based on the type of injury:

Type I: Gentle débridement of labrum back to stable tissue.

Type II: Arthroscopic labral repair with suture anchors.

Type III: Arthroscopic débridement of the bucket-handle fragment with repair of any unstable portions of the labral rim.

Type IV: Treatment of the biceps disease with débridement, tenotomy, or tenodesis combined with labral repair or débridement.

Patients older than 40 years have had less successful results of superior labral repairs compared with younger patients because pain may continue to be generated by the biceps-labral complex. In this age group, the trend for surgical treatment has been to perform biceps tenodesis with labral débridement.

Treatment of a SLAP tear with associated paralabral cyst involves arthroscopic labral repair with or without cyst decompression. Studies show acceptable outcomes with both approaches.

Bankart Lesion

Labral repair with plication of the attenuated capsule is successful in restoring stability (Fig. 15.4). Modern arthroscopic techniques allow suture anchor fixation of the labrum and capsular plication and have shown success rates comparable to those of traditional open surgery.

Outcomes

SLAP Tear

As discussed in the section on rehabilitation, the literature on nonoperative treatment of SLAP tears is sparse. Edwards and colleagues showed that about 51% of patients treated nonoperatively went on to have an operation. Of those who continued with nonoperative treatment, all returned to sports and about 70% to preinjury level [25].

With simple débridement, the patient usually is provided with good pain relief in the short term. About 80% of patients have good relief for the first year or so, but at 2 years or more, this number decreases to near 60% [26,27]. Type II SLAP tears are the most commonly encountered, so they are the most studied. Many studies report that 90% return to sport and approximately 70% to 80% return to preinjury level.

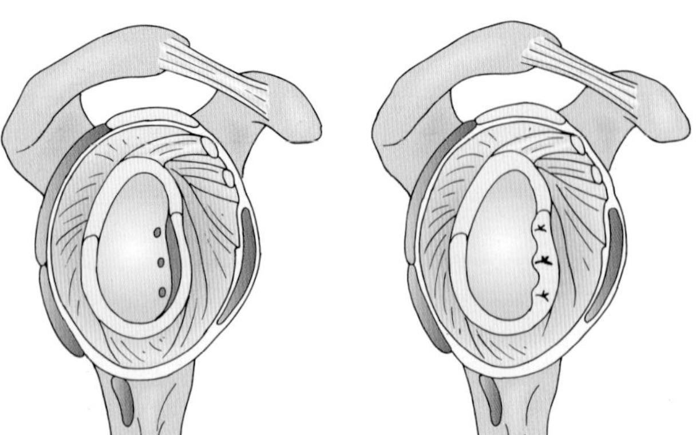

FIGURE 15.4 Suture anchor repair of Bankart lesion.

Bankart Lesion

Success of nonoperative management is dependent on multiple factors, particularly the age of the patient at first dislocation, athletic activities, associated disease, number of dislocations, and gender. In first-time dislocators older than 30 years, the chance of recurrence is approximately 27%, whereas the patient younger than 30 years has between a 40% and 90% chance of redislocation [28]. Men typically have a higher rate of recurrence than women, as do athletes involved in throwing or contact sports. An associated pathologic process, such as a bony Bankart lesion, large Hill-Sachs lesion, or rotator cuff tear or avulsion, is also predictive of failure of nonoperative treatment.

With open or arthroscopic surgical stabilization, the risk of recurrence compared with conservative treatment is about one fifth that of the nonoperative group [29].

Potential Disease Complications

SLAP tears result in a decrease in overall shoulder stability as the glenoid labrum is disrupted. This is usually well tolerated but can lead to episodes of instability and further damage of the labrum, biceps, capsule, and surrounding ligamentous structures. No data exist to suggest that nonoperative management of SLAP tears leads to significant degenerative changes.

Bankart lesions are caused by shoulder instability, and the pathologic change that they create increases the chance for further instability. This will create greater attenuation and damage to the tissues around and within the shoulder capsule, which can then cause fracture of the glenoid or the humeral head, possible neurovascular compromise, and increased risk of future glenohumeral arthritis.

Potential Treatment Complications

The risk of taking long-term nonsteroidal anti-inflammatory medication includes damage of the gastric and renal systems. Cyclooxygenase 2 inhibitors avoid some of the gastric complications, but there is a concern for cardiovascular complications, and past medical history should be taken into account. Injection of the glenohumeral joint has a small chance of causing septic arthritis.

Nonoperative management of SLAP tears has little risk as conservative management has not been shown to place the shoulder at risk for future deterioration. In the setting of a Bankart tear with anterior instability, recurrent instability episodes do risk further labral, capsular, articular cartilage, and rotator cuff damage. In the younger patient at risk for recurrent instability, this may prompt earlier surgical treatment.

Potential surgical complications specific to labral repairs include postoperative stiffness, recurrent tearing and instability, and post-traumatic arthritis.

References

[1] Keener JD, Brophy RH. Superior labral tears of the shoulder: pathogenesis, evaluation, and treatment. J Am Acad Orthop Surg 2009;17:627–37.

[2] Cooper DE, Arnoczky SP, O'Brien SJ. Anatomy, histology, and vascularity of the glenoid labrum: an anatomical study. J Bone Joint Surg Am 1992;74:46–52.

[3] Howell SM, Galinat BJ. The glenoid-labral socket: a constrained articular surface. Clin Orthop Relat Res 1989;243:122–5.

[4] Huber WP, Putz RV. Periarticular fiber system of the shoulder joint. Arthroscopy 1997;13:680–91.

[5] Burkhart SS, Morgan CD, Kibler WB. Current concepts: the disabled throwing shoulder: spectrum of pathology part I: pathoanatomy and biomechanics. Arthroscopy 2003;19:404–20.

[6] Burkhart SS, Morgan CD, Kibler WB. Current concepts: the disabled throwing shoulder: spectrum of pathology part II: evaluation and treatment of SLAP lesions in throwers. Arthroscopy 2003;19:531–9.

[7] Jobe CM. Posterior superior glenoid impingement: expanded spectrum. Arthroscopy 1995;11:530–6.

[8] Snyder SJ, Karzel RP, DelPizzo W. SLAP lesions of the shoulder. Arthroscopy 1990;6:274–9.

[9] Rowe CR, Patel D, Southmayd WW. The Bankart procedure: a long term end-result study. J Bone Joint Surg Am 1978;10:1–16.

[10] Ownes BD, Dickens JF, Kilcoyne KG, Rue JP. The management of mid-season traumatic anterior shoulder instability in athletes. J Am Acad Orthop Surg 2012;20:518–26.

[11] Kim TK, Queale WS, Cosgarea AJ, McFarland EG. Clinical features of the different types of SLAP lesions. An analysis of one hundred and thirty-nine cases. J Bone Joint Surg Am 2003;85:66–71.

[12] Tennent TD, Beach WR, Meyers JF. A review of the special tests associated with shoulder examination. Part II: laxity, instability, and superior labral anterior and posterior (SLAP) lesions. Am J Sports Med 2003;31:301–7.

[13] Berg EE, Ciullo JB. A clinical test for superior glenoid labral or SLAP lesions. Clin J Sport Med 1998;8:121–3.

[14] Kibler WB. Specificity and sensitivity of the anterior slide test in throwing athletes with superior glenoid labral tears. Arthroscopy 1995;11:296–300.

[15] Guanche CA, Jones DC. Clinical testing for tears of the glenoid labrum. Arthroscopy 2003;19:517–23.

[16] Owens BD, Dickens JF, Kilcoyne KG, et al. The management of mid-season traumatic anterior shoulder instability in athletes. J Am Acad Orthop Surg 2012;20:518–26.

[17] Neviaser RJ, Neviaser TJ, Neviaser JS. Anterior dislocation of the shoulder and rotator cuff rupture. Clin Orthop Relat Res 1993;291:103–6.

[18] Lo IK, Nonweiler B, Woolfrey M, et al. An evaluation of the apprehension, relocation, and surprise test for anterior shoulder instability. Am J Sports Med 2004;32:301–7.

[19] Major NM, Browne J, Domzalski T, et al. Evaluation of the glenoid labrum with 3-T MRI: is intraarticular contrast necessary? AJR Am J Roentgenol 2011;196:1139–44.

[20] Phillips JC, Cook C, Beaty S, et al. Validity of noncontrast magnetic resonance imaging in diagnosing superior labrum anterior-posterior tears. J Shoulder Elbow Surg 2013;22:3–8.

[21] Jung JY, Ha DH, Lee SM, et al. Displaceability of SLAP lesion on shoulder MR arthrography with external rotation position. Skeletal Radiol 2011;40:1047–55.

[22] Borrero CG, Casagranda BU, Towers JD, Bradley JP. Magnetic resonance appearance of posterosuperior labral peel back during humeral abduction and external rotation. Skeletal Radiol 2010;39:19–26.

[23] Itoi E, Sashi R, Minagawa H, et al. Position of immobilization after dislocation of the glenohumeral joint: a study with use of MRI. J Bone Joint Surg Am 2001;83:661–7.

[24] Itoi E, Hatakeyama Y, Sato T. Immobilization in external rotation after shoulder dislocation reduces the risk of recurrence: a randomized controlled trial. J Bone Joint Surg Am 2007;89:1224–2131.

[25] Edwards SL, Lee JA, Bell JE, et al. Nonoperative treatment of superior labrum anterior posterior tears. Improvements in pain, function, and quality of life. Am J Sports Med 2010;38:1456–61.

[26] Altcheck DW, Warren RF, Wickiewicz TL, et al. Arthroscopic labral debridement: a 3 year follow up study. Am J Sports Med 1992;20:702–6.

[27] Cordasco FA, Steinmann S, Flatow EL, Bigliani LU. Arthroscopic treatment of glenoid labral tears. Am J Sports Med 1993;21:425–30.

[28] Wheeler JH, Ryan JB, Arciero RA, Molinari RN. Arthroscopic versus nonoperative treatment of acute shoulder dislocations in young athletes. Arthroscopy 1989;5:213–7.

[29] Hovelius L, Olgsson A, Sandstrom B. Nonoperative treatment of primary anterior shoulder dislocation in patients 40 years of age and younger: a prospective twenty-five-year follow up. J Bone Joint Surg Am 2008;90:945–52.

CHAPTER 16

Rotator Cuff Tendinopathy

Jay E. Bowen, DO
Gerard A. Malanga, MD

Synonyms

Impingement syndrome
Rotator cuff tendinosis

ICD-9 Code

726.10 Rotator cuff syndrome

ICD-10 Codes

M75.100 Unspecified rotator cuff tear or rupture of unspecified shoulder, not specified as traumatic
M75.101 Unspecified rotator cuff tear or rupture of right shoulder, not specified as traumatic
M75.102 Unspecified rotator cuff tear or rupture of left shoulder, not specified as traumatic
M75.80 Other shoulder lesions, unspecified shoulder
M75.81 Other shoulder lesions, right shoulder
M75.82 Other shoulder lesions, left shoulder

Definition

Rotator cuff tendinopathy is a common phenomenon affecting both athletes and nonathletes. The muscles that compose the rotator cuff—supraspinatus, infraspinatus, subscapularis, and teres minor—may become inflamed or impinged by the acromion, coracoacromial ligament, acromioclavicular joint, and coracoid process [1]. Fibroblastic hyperplasia (tendinosis) may play a role as well. The supraspinatus tendon is the most commonly involved.

Rotator cuff tendinopathy may result from a variety of factors. The tendon or its musculotendinous junction can be "squeezed" along its course from a relatively narrowed space [2]. Tendinosis can be a result of degeneration from the aging process or from underlying subtle instability of the humeral head [3,4].

In chronic rotator cuff tendinopathy, the muscles of the rotator cuff and surrounding scapulothoracic stabilizers may become weak by disuse. Under these conditions, the muscles can fatigue early, resulting in altered biomechanics. The humeral head moves excessively off the center of the glenoid, usually superiorly [5-8]. From this abnormal motion, impingement of the rotator cuff occurs, causing inflammation of the tendon. This is what many refer to as impingement syndrome; it particularly occurs during forward flexion when the anterior portion of the acromion impinges on the supraspinatus tendon.

With the passage of time, modifications of the acromion occur, resulting in osteophyte formation or "hooking" of the acromion (Fig. 16.1) [1,9]. With repeated superior migration and acromial changes, degeneration of the musculotendinous junction can lead to tearing of the rotator cuff (see Chapter 17). With prolonged shoulder pain, adhesive capsulitis can develop from the lack of active motion (see Chapter 11).

Symptoms

Patients normally present with pain in the posterolateral shoulder region and, often, deltoid muscle pain, which is referred from the shoulder. The pain is described as dull and achy and often occurs at night. Complaints occur with activities above the shoulder level, usually when the arm is abducted more than 90 degrees. Pain is also noted in movements involving eccentric contractions, when sleeping on the affected side, and during overhead activities such as swimming and painting [10-14].

Physical Examination

The shoulder examination is approached systematically in every patient. It includes inspection, palpation, range of motion, muscle strength testing, and performance of special tests of the shoulder as clinically indicated.

The examination begins with observation of the patient during the history portion of the evaluation. The shoulder

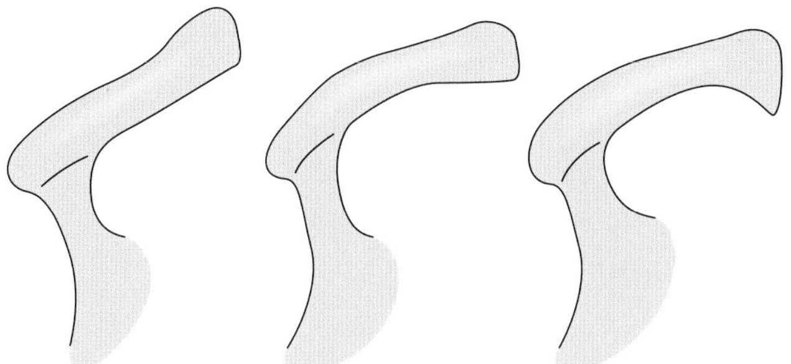

FIGURE 16.1 Types of acromial shape (lateral view).

should be carefully inspected from the anterior, lateral, and posterior positions. Because shoulder pain is usually unilateral, comparison with the contralateral shoulder is often useful. Atrophy of the supraspinatus and infraspinatus muscles can be seen in massive rotator cuff tears as well as in entrapments of the suprascapular nerve. Scapular winging is rare in rotator cuff injuries; however, abnormalities of scapulothoracic motion are often present and should be addressed as part of the treatment plan.

Tenderness is often localized to the greater tuberosity, subacromial bursa, or long head of the biceps.

Total active and passive range of motion in all planes and scapulohumeral rhythm should be evaluated. Maximal total elevation occurs in the plane of the scapula, which lies approximately 30 degrees forward of the coronal plane. Patients with rotator cuff tears tend to have altered scapulothoracic motion during active shoulder elevation. Decreased active elevation with normal passive range of motion is usually seen in rotator cuff tears secondary to pain and weakness. When both active and passive range of motion is similarly decreased, this usually suggests the onset of adhesive capsulitis. Glenohumeral internal rotation is assessed most accurately by abduction of the shoulder to 90 degrees and manual fixation of the scapula. From this point, the elbow is flexed to 90 degrees and the humerus is internally rotated. The impingement syndrome associated with rotator cuff injuries tends to cause pain with elevation between 60 and 120 degrees (painful arc), when the rotator cuff tendons are compressed against the anterior acromion and coracoacromial ligament [5,6,15].

Muscle strength testing should be done isolating the relevant individual muscles. The anterior cuff (subscapularis) can be assessed by the lift-off test (see Chapter 14, Fig. 14.1), which is performed with the arm internally rotated behind the back. Lifting of the hand away from the back against resistance tests the strength of the subscapularis muscle. The posterior cuff (infraspinatus and teres minor) can be tested with the arm at the side and the elbow flexed to 90 degrees. Significant weakness in external rotation will be seen in large tears of the rotator cuff. The supraspinatus muscle is specifically tested by abduction of the patient's arm to 90 degrees, horizontal adduction to 20 to 30 degrees, and internal rotation of the arm to the thumbs down position. Testing of the scapula rotators, the trapezius, and the serratus anterior is also important. The serratus anterior can be tested by having the patient lean against a wall; winging of the scapula as the patient pushes against the wall indicates weakness [15,16].

Drop Arm Test

The clinician abducts the patient's shoulder to 90 degrees and then asks the patient to slowly lower the arm to the side in the same arc of movement. The test result is positive if the patient is unable to return the arm to the side slowly or has severe pain when attempting to do so. A positive result indicates a tear of the rotator cuff [17].

Impingement Sign

The shoulder is forcibly forward flexed with the humerus internally rotated, causing a jamming of the greater tuberosity against the anterior inferior surface of the acromion. Pain with this maneuver reflects a positive test result and indicates an overuse injury to the supraspinatus muscle and possibly to the biceps tendon (see Chapter 14, Fig. 14.2) [18].

Apprehension Test

The arm is abducted 90 degrees and then fully externally rotated while an anteriorly directed force is placed on the posterior humeral head from behind. The patient will become apprehensive and resist further motion if chronic anterior instability is present (see Chapter 14, Fig. 14.4) [1].

Relocation Test

Perform the apprehension test with the patient supine and the shoulder at the edge of the table (Fig. 16.2). A posteriorly directed force on the proximal humerus will cause resolution of the patient's symptoms of apprehension, which is another indicator of anterior instability (see Chapter 14, Fig. 14.3) [1].

Functional Limitations

Patients with rotator cuff tendinopathy complain of limitations in the performance of overhead activities, such as throwing a baseball and painting a ceiling, particularly above 90 degrees of abduction [19-21]. Pain may also occur with internal and external rotation and may affect daily self-care activities. Women typically have difficulty hooking the bra in back. Work activities, such as filing, hammering overhead, and lifting, can be affected [22,23]. The patient can be awoken by pain in the shoulder, which impairs sleep [12].

Diagnostic Studies

In the event of trauma to the shoulder and complaints consistent with rotator cuff tendinopathy, the clinician should obtain radiographs to avoid missing an occult fracture. The anteroposterior view with internal and external rotation is sufficient for screening. If dislocation is suspected, further views should be obtained, including West Point axillary, true anteroposterior, and Y views.

Magnetic resonance imaging is the study of choice when a patient is not progressing with conservative management or to rule out an alternative pathologic process (e.g., rotator cuff tear). In tendinopathy, magnetic resonance imaging will demonstrate an increased T2-weighted signal within the substance of the tendon [22]. Diagnostic arthroscopy is used in some cases but is generally not necessary.

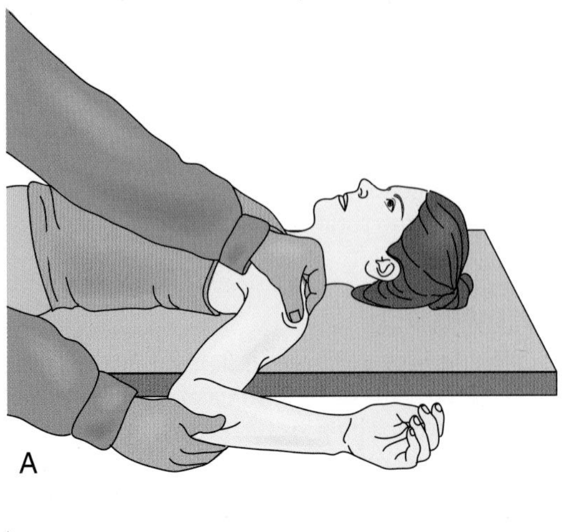

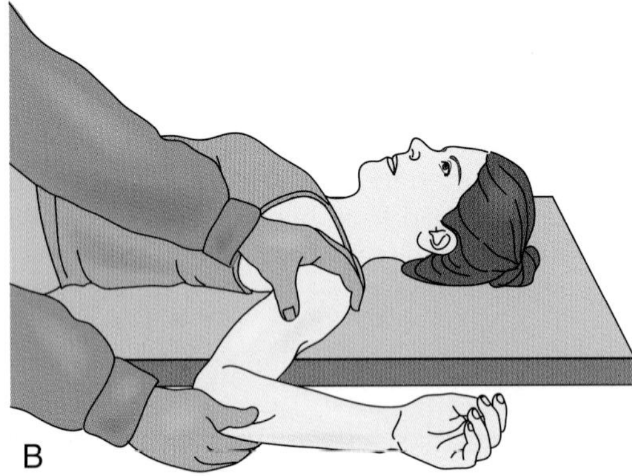

FIGURE 16.2 Relocation test. **A,** In certain shoulders, pain limits abduction and maximum external rotation. **B,** By the application of pressure on the anterior shoulder, the discomfort is eliminated and greater external rotation is noted.

Electrodiagnostic studies can be ordered to exclude alternative diagnoses as well (e.g., cervical radiculopathy) [15,24].

Subacromial anesthetic injections (see Chapter 14, Figs. 14.5 and 14.6) have been discussed as diagnostic tools to assist in the confirmation of rotator cuff tendinopathy. This procedure is not as important for diagnosis of tendinopathy as it is for ruling out a tear. If the patient cannot provide good effort to abduction during the physical examination, the clinician can inject the anesthetic into the subacromial space. After the injection, if there is significant reduction in the pain level and the patient can provide adequate and nearly maximal abduction, tendinopathy is more likely than a rotator cuff tear [10,13,14].

Differential Diagnosis

Rotator cuff tear
Glenolabral tear
Muscle strain
Subacromial bursitis
Bicipital tendinopathy
Myofascial pain
Fracture
Acromioclavicular sprain
Tumor
Myofascial or vascular thoracic outlet syndrome
Cervical radiculopathy
Traumatic or atraumatic brachial plexus disease (e.g., Parsonage-Turner [acute brachial neuritis])
Suprascapular neuropathy
Thoracic outlet syndrome

Treatment

Initial

There are five basic phases of treatment (Table 16.1). These phases may overlap and can be progressed as rapidly as tolerated, but each should be performed to speed recovery and to prevent reinjury.

Initially, pain control and inflammation reduction are required to allow progression of healing and the initiation of an active rehabilitation program. This can be accomplished with a combination of relative rest from aggravating activities, icing (20 minutes three or four times a day), and electrical stimulation. Acetaminophen may help with pain control. Nonsteroidal anti-inflammatory drugs are avoided because of their negative effect on tendon healing. Having the patient sleep with a pillow between the trunk and arm will decrease the tension on the supraspinatus tendon and prevent compromise of blood flow in its watershed region.

Rehabilitation

Physical therapy may also help with pain management. Initially, gentle, passive, prolonged stretch may be needed. The use of ultrasound should be closely monitored to avoid heating of an inflamed tendon, which will worsen the situation. Postoperative rehabilitation will progress in a similar fashion once initial healing has occurred and at the discretion of the surgeon.

Restoration of Shoulder Range of Motion

After the pain has been managed, restoration of shoulder motion can be initiated. The focus of treatment in this early stage is on improvement of range, flexibility of the posterior capsule, postural biomechanics, and restoration of normal scapular motion. Codman pendulum exercises, wall walking, stick or towel exercises, and a physical therapy program are useful in attaining full pain-free range of motion. It is important to address any posterior capsular tightness because it can cause anterior and superior humeral head migration, resulting in impingement. A tight posterior capsule and the imbalance it causes force the humeral head anteriorly, producing shearing of the anterior labrum and

Table 16.1 Treatment Phases for Rotator Cuff Tendinopathy

Pain control and reduction of inflammation
Restoration of normal shoulder motion, both scapulothoracic and glenohumeral
Normalization of strength and dynamic muscle control
Proprioception and dynamic joint stabilization
Sport- or task-specific training

causing additional injury [25]. Stretching of the posterior capsule is a difficult task. The horizontal adduction that is usually performed tends to stretch the scapular stabilizers, not the posterior capsule. However, stretching of the posterior capsule is possible if care is taken to fix and to stabilize the scapula, preventing stretching of the scapulothoracic stabilizers.

Postural biomechanics are important because with poor posture (e.g., excessive thoracic kyphosis and protracted shoulders), there is increased acromial space narrowing, resulting in greater risk for rotator cuff impingement [26,27]. Restoration of normal scapular motion is also essential because the scapula is the platform on which the glenohumeral joint rotates [28,29]. Thus, an unstable scapula can secondarily cause glenohumeral joint instability and resultant impingement. Scapular stabilization includes exercises such as wall pushups and biofeedback (visual and tactile) [30].

Strengthening

The third phase of treatment is muscle strengthening, which should be performed in a pain-free range of motion. Strengthening should begin with the scapulothoracic stabilizers and the use of shoulder shrugs, rowing, and pushups, which will isolate these muscles and help return smooth motion, allowing normal rhythm between the scapula and the glenohumeral joint. This will also provide a firm base of support on which the arm can move. Attention is then turned to strengthening of the rotator cuff muscles. Positioning of the arm at 45 and 90 degrees of abduction for exercises prevents the "wringing out" phenomenon that hyperadduction can cause by stressing the tenuous blood supply to the tendon of the exercising muscle. The thumbs down position with the arm in more than 90 degrees of abduction and internal rotation should also be avoided to minimize subacromial impingement. After the scapular stabilizers and rotator cuff muscles are rehabilitated, the prime movers are addressed to prevent further injury and to facilitate return to prior function.

There are many ways to strengthen muscles. The rehabilitation program should start with static exercises and co-contractions, progress to concentric exercises, and be completed with eccentric exercises. A therapy prescription should include the number of repetitions, the number of sets, and the intensity at which the specific exercise should be performed. When strength is restored, a maintenance program should be continued for fitness and prevention of reinjury. Local muscle endurance should also be trained.

Proprioception

The fourth phase is proprioceptive training. This is important to retrain the neurologic control of the strengthened muscles, providing improved dynamic interaction and coupled execution of tasks for harmonious movement of the shoulder and arm [31,32]. Tasks should begin with closed kinetic chain exercises (e.g., exercises done with the hand in contact with a fixed object like a wall) to provide joint stabilizing forces [33,34]. As the muscles are reeducated, exercises can progress to open chain activities, such as dumbbell exercises, that may be used in specific sports or tasks. In addition, proprioceptive neuromuscular facilitation is designed to stimulate muscle-tendon stretch receptors for reeducation [35].

Task or Sport Specific

The last phase of rehabilitation is to return to task- or sport-specific activities [36,37]. This is an advanced form of training for the muscles to relearn prior activities. This is important and should be supervised so the task is performed correctly and the possibility of reinjury or injury in another part of the kinetic chain from improper technique is eliminated [38]. The rehabilitation begins at a cognitive level but must be repeated so that it transitions to unconscious motor programming [11].

Procedures

A subacromial injection of anesthetic can be beneficial in differentiating a rotator cuff tear from tendinopathy. Patients with pain that limits the validity of their strength testing may be able to provide almost full resistance to abduction and external rotation after the injection, suggesting rotator cuff tendinopathy. On the other hand, if there is continued weakness, one must consider a rotator cuff tear.

Many clinicians include a corticosteroid with the anesthetic to avoid the need for a second injection. This procedure can be both diagnostic and therapeutic. If one makes the diagnosis of rotator cuff tendinopathy, the corticosteroid injection will decrease the inflammation and allow accelerated rehabilitation. Moreover, a percutaneous tenotomy can be performed under ultrasound guidance. The needle is localized and placed in and out of the tendon to create small perforations within the damaged tendon. This stimulates the healing response through the inflammatory cascade, enhancing tendon repair.

Refer to the injection procedure in Chapter 14.

Surgery

Surgery should be considered if the patient fails to improve with a progressive nonoperative therapy program of 3 to 6 months. Surgical procedures may include subacromial decompression arthroscopically or, less commonly, open. At that time, the surgeon may débride the tendon and explore for other pathologic changes [14,39,40].

Potential Disease Complications

The greatest risk in not treating rotator cuff tendinopathy is rupture or tear of a tendon or the development of a labral tear. As previously discussed, with prolonged impairment in motion and strength and subtle instability, hooking of the acromion can develop. Adhesive capsulitis may develop with chronic pain and decreased shoulder movement as well [18,41-44].

Potential Treatment Complications

There are minimal possible complications from nonoperative treatment of rotator cuff tendinopathy. Because nonsteroidal anti-inflammatory drugs are used frequently, one must remain vigilant to their potential side effects (e.g., gastritis, ulcers, renal impairment, bronchospasm). Injections may cause rupture of the diseased tendon.

References

[1] Hawkins RJ. Basic science and clinical application in the athlete's shoulder. Clin Sports Med 1991;10:955–71.

[2] Lohr JF, Uhthoff HK. The microvascular pattern of the supraspinatus tendon. Clin Orthop Relat Res 1990;254:35–8.

[3] Rathburn JB, Macnab I. The microvascular pattern of the rotator cuff of the shoulder. J Bone Joint Surg Br 1970;52:540.

[4] Swiontkowski M, Iannotti JP, Esterhai JL, et al. Intraoperative assessment of rotator cuff vascularity using laser Doppler flowmetry. Presented at the 56th annual meeting of the American Academy of Orthopaedic Surgeons; Las Vegas, Nev, Feb 10, 1989.

[5] Harryman DT, Sidles JA, Clark JM, et al. Translation of the humeral head on the glenoid with passive glenohumeral motion. J Bone Joint Surg Am 1990;72:1334–43.

[6] Poppen NK, Walker PS. Normal and abnormal motion of the shoulder. J Bone Joint Surg Am 1976;58:195–201.

[7] Smith L, Weiss E, Lehmkuh L. Brunnstrom's clinical kinesiology. 5th ed. Philadelphia: FA Davis; 1996.

[8] Steindler A. Kinesiology of human body under normal and pathological conditions. Springfield, Ill: Charles C Thomas; 1995.

[9] Wang JC, Shapiro MS. Changes in acromial morphology with age. J Shoulder Elbow Surg 1997;6:55–9.

[10] Cailliet R. Shoulder pain. 3rd ed. Philadelphia: FA Davis; 1991, 42–46.

[11] Malanga GA, Bowen JE, Nadler SF, Lee A. Nonoperative management of shoulder injuries. J Back Musculoskelet Rehabil 1999;12:179–89.

[12] Nicholas JA, Hershman EB. The upper extremity in sports medicine. St. Louis: Mosby; 1990.

[13] Reid DC. Sports injury assessment and rehabilitation. New York: Churchill Livingstone; 1992.

[14] Rockwood CA, Matsen FA. The shoulder. Philadelphia: WB Saunders; 1990.

[15] Malanga GA, Jenp Y, Growney E, An K. EMG analysis of shoulder positioning in testing and strengthening the supraspinatus. Med Sci Sports Exerc 1996;28:661–4.

[16] DeLateur BI. Exercise for strength and endurance. In: Basmajian JV, editor. Therapeutic exercise. 4th ed. Baltimore: Williams & Wilkins; 1984.

[17] Gross J, Fetto J, Rosen E. Musculoskeletal examination. Cambridge, Mass: Blackwell Science; 1996.

[18] Neer CS. Anterior acromioplasty for the chronic impingement syndrome in the shoulder: a preliminary report. J Bone Joint Surg Am 1972;54:41–50.

[19] Kibler WB. Role of the scapula in the overhead throwing motion. Contemp Orthop 1991;22:525–32.

[20] Kibler WB, Chandler TJ. Functional scapular instability in throwing athletes. Presented at the 15th annual meeting of the American Orthopaedic Society for Sports Medicine; Traverse City, Mich, June 19–22, 1989.

[21] Plancher KD, Litchfield R, Hawkins RJ. Rehabilitation of the shoulder in tennis players. Clin Sports Med 1995;14:116–8.

[22] Dines DM, Levinson M. The conservative management of the unstable shoulder including rehabilitation. Clin Sports Med 1995;14:799–813.

[23] Steinbeck J, Liljenqvist U, Jerosch J. The anatomy of the glenohumeral ligamentous complex and its contribution to anterior shoulder stability. J Shoulder Elbow Surg 1998;7:122–6.

[24] Basmajian J. Muscles alive: their functions revealed by electromyography. 5th ed. Philadelphia: Williams & Wilkins; 1985.

[25] Howell SM, Galinat BJ. The glenoid-labral socket—a constrained articular surface. Clin Orthop 1989;243:122–5.

[26] Inman VT, Saunders JB, Abbott LC. Observations of the function of the shoulder. J Bone Joint Surg 1944;26:1–30.

[27] Saha AK. Dynamic stability of the glenohumeral joint. Acta Orthop Scand 1971;42:491.

[28] Andrews JR. Diagnosis and treatment of chronic painful shoulder: review of nonsurgical interventions. Arthoscopy 2005;21:333–47.

[29] Rees JD, Wilson AM, Wolman RL. Current concepts in the management of tendon disorders. Rheumatology (Oxford) 2006;45:508–21.

[30] Wuelker N, Korell M, Thren K. Dynamic glenohumeral joint stability. J Shoulder Elbow Surg 1998;7:43–52.

[31] Borsa PA, Lephart SM, Kocher MS, Lephart SP. Functional assessment and rehabilitation of shoulder proprioception for the glenohumeral instability. J Sports Rehab 1994;3:84–104.

[32] Blasier RB, Carpenter JE, Huston LJ. Shoulder proprioception: effect of joint laxity, joint position, and direction of motion. Orthop Rev 1994;23:45–50.

[33] Janda DH, Loubert P. A preventive program focusing on the glenohumeral joint. Clin Sports Med 1991;10:955–71.

[34] Jenp Y, Malanga GA, Growney E, An K. Activation of the rotator cuff in generating isometric shoulder rotation torque. Am J Sports Med 1996;24:477–85.

[35] Kabat H. Proprioception facilitation in therapeutic exercise. In: Kendall HD, editor. Therapeutic exercises. Baltimore: Waverly Press; 1965. p. 327–43.

[36] Yoneda B, Welsh R. Conservative treatment of shoulder dislocation in young males. J Bone Joint Surg Br 1982;64:254–5.

[37] Burkhead Jr WZ, Rockwood Jr CA. Treatment of instability of the shoulder with an exercise program. J Bone Joint Surg Am 1992;74:890–6.

[38] Cordasco FA, Wolfe IN, Wootten ME, Bigliani LU. An electromyographic analysis of the shoulder during a medicine ball rehabilitation program. Am J Sports Med 1996;24:386–92.

[39] Brems JJ. Management of atraumatic instability: techniques and results. Instructional Course Lecture 179. In: American Academy of Orthopaedic Surgeons annual meeting; Atlanta, Ga; Feb 26, 1996.

[40] Simonet WT, Cofield RH. Prognosis in anterior shoulder dislocation. Am J Sports Med 1984;12:19–24.

[41] Biglianni LU, Morrison D, April EW. The morphology of the acromion and its relationship to rotator cuff tears. Orthop Trans 1986;10:228.

[42] Codman EA. The shoulder: rupture of the supraspinatus tendon and other lesions in or about the subacromial bursa. Boston: Thomas Todd; 1934.

[43] Flatow E, Soslowsky L, Ticker J, et al. Excursion of the rotator cuff under the acromion: patterns of subacromial contact. Am J Sports Med 1994;22:779–87.

[44] Ozaki J, Fujimoto S, Nakagawa Y, et al. Tears of the rotator cuff of the shoulder associated with pathologic changes in the acromion: a study in cadavers. J Bone Joint Surg Br 1988;70:1224–30.

CHAPTER 17

Rotator Cuff Tear

Jay E. Bowen, DO
Gerard A. Malanga, MD

Synonyms

Shoulder tear
Torn shoulder

ICD-9 Codes

726.10 Rotator cuff syndrome
727.61 Nontraumatic complete rupture of rotator cuff
840.4 Rotator cuff sprain

ICD-10 Codes

M75.100 Unspecified rotator cuff tear or rupture of unspecified shoulder, nontraumatic
M75.101 Unspecified rotator cuff tear or rupture of right shoulder, nontraumatic
M75.102 Unspecified rotator cuff tear or rupture of left shoulder, nontraumatic
S43.421 Sprain of right rotator cuff
S43.422 Sprain of left rotator cuff
S43.429 Sprain of unspecified rotator cuff

Definition

The rotator cuff has three main functions in the shoulder. It compresses the humeral head into the fossa, increases joint contact pressure, and centers the humeral head on the glenoid. Three types of tears can occur to the rotator cuff. A full-thickness tear can be massive and cause immediate functional impairments. Another type of tear, a partial-thickness tear, can be broken down into a tear on the superior surface into the subacromial space or a tear on the inferior surface on the articular side. As a result of a rotator cuff tear, the humeral head will be displaced superiorly during abduction because of the unopposed action of the deltoid. These tears can be either traumatic or degenerative [1–7] (Figs. 17.1 to 17.3).

Traumatic tears occur in the younger population of athletes and laborers, whereas degenerative tears occur in older individuals. One reason that rotator cuff tears are more common in men is because there are more male heavy laborers. The incidence of degenerative tears is increased in both sexes for individuals older than 35 years and for those with chronic impingement syndrome, repetitive microtrauma, tendon degeneration, and hypovascularity [4,6,8].

Symptoms

Symptoms are similar to those of rotator cuff tendinitis. Pain is referred to the lateral triceps and sometimes more globally in the shoulder. There is often coexisting inflammation, and the pain quality is dull and achy. Weakness occurs because of the pain, which is caused by the impaired motion or the tear itself. Persons have difficulty with overhead activities. Patients may report pain at night in a side-lying position.

Physical Examination

Examination is essentially the same as for rotator cuff tendinitis. The most common physical findings of a tear are supraspinatus weakness, external rotator weakness, and impingement. The arm drop test may demonstrate greater weakness than expected from an inflamed, intact tendon, although one can be easily fooled. As with rotator cuff tendinitis, an anesthetic injection into the subacromial space may help discern tear. Even though the pain may be improved or resolved from the injection, resisted abduction will be just as weak because the torn tendon cannot withstand the stress [9].

Remember to examine the cervical spine to avoid missing underlying pathologic changes. A rotator cuff tear develops in some individuals as a result of a radiculopathy or other nerve impairment. The dysfunction of the shoulder from a radiculopathy or suprascapular neuropathy results in weakness of the rotator cuff or the scapular stabilizers. This dysrhythmia causes impingement of the tendons with other structures and eventually leads to fraying and tearing [10–12].

Functional Limitations

The greatest limitation that patients complain of is performing overhead activities [2,7,13–15].

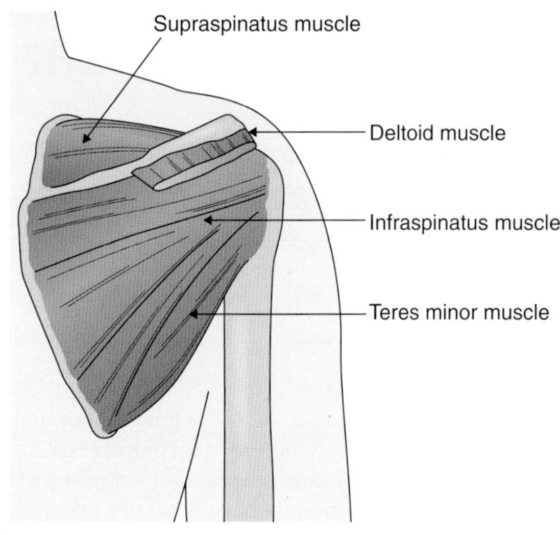

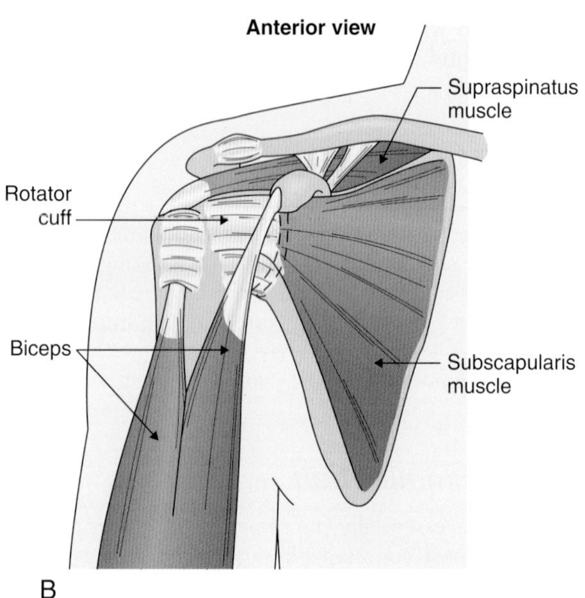

FIGURE 17.1 Muscles of the rotator cuff, posterior (**A**) and anterior (**B**) views. *(From Snider RK. Essentials of Musculoskeletal Care. Rosemont, Ill, American Academy of Orthopaedic Surgeons, 1997.)*

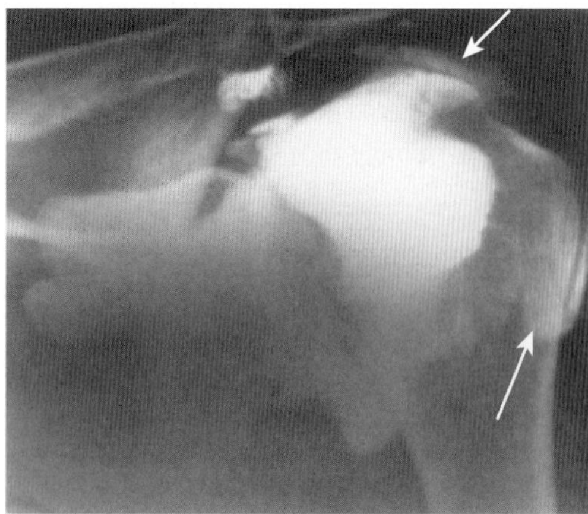

FIGURE 17.2 Rotator cuff tear with extension of contrast material into the subacromial *(short arrow)* and subdeltoid *(long arrow)* bursae. *(From West SG. Rheumatology Secrets. Philadelphia, Hanley & Belfus, 1997:373.)*

Patients with rotator cuff tendinitis complain of difficulty with overhead activities (e.g., throwing a baseball, painting a ceiling), greatest above 90 degrees of abduction, secondary to pain or weakness. Internal and external rotation may be compromised and may affect daily self-care activities. Women typically have difficulty hooking the bra in back. Work activities, such as filing, hammering overhead, and lifting, will be affected. The patient can be awakened by pain in the shoulder, which impairs his or her sleep.

Diagnostic Studies

The diagnosis of a rotator cuff tear depends mostly on the history and physical examination. However, imaging studies may be used to confirm the clinician's diagnosis and to eliminate other possible pathologic processes.

Radiographs are often obtained to rule out any osseous problem. A tear can be inferred if there is evidence of humeral head upward migration or sclerotic changes at the greater tuberosity where the tendons insert. Radiographs

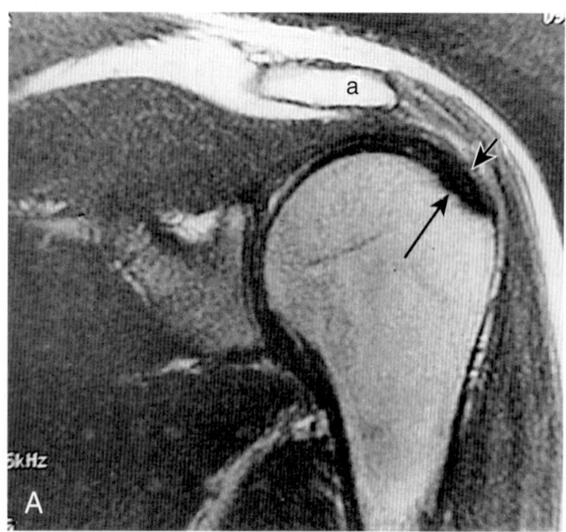

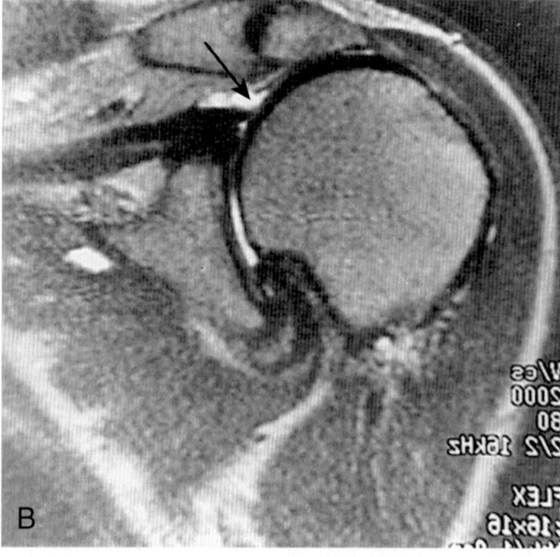

FIGURE 17.3 **A,** Normal shoulder magnetic resonance image. The supraspinatus tendon is uniformly low signal and continuous *(arrows)*. The space between the humeral head and the acromion *(a)* is maintained. **B,** Chronic rotator cuff tear. The supraspinatus tendon is completely torn and retracted to the level of the glenohumeral joint *(arrow),* where it is surrounded by fluid. Note the high-riding humeral head, close to the acromion. This is due to the atrophy of the cuff muscles associated with chronic tendon tears.

are helpful with active 90-degree abduction showing a decreased acromiohumeral distance secondary to absence of the supraspinatus and unopposed action of the deltoid.

Magnetic resonance imaging (MRI) of the shoulder is the "gold standard." [16] Computed tomographic scans show osseous structures better but are less effective at demonstrating a soft tissue injury. By evaluation of the amount of retraction, the clinician is also better able to predict the course of recovery.

As in the evaluation of a person with rotator cuff tendinitis, an anesthetic injection can be performed to differentiate a tear from tendinitis.

Shoulder arthrography is performed less often since the advent of MRI. Arthrography involves injection of contrast material into the glenohumeral joint followed by plain radiography. Dye should remain contained in the joint space. If it extravasates, this signifies a tear. Partial-thickness rotator cuff tears can be missed, especially tears on the superior surface. Some centers have been combining gadolinium dye injections with MRI. This is used mostly to identify a labral tear, not a rotator cuff tear.

Ultrasound imaging can also be used in the diagnosis of full-thickness rotator cuff tears [17]. Ultrasonography is becoming more popular in the United States, and it can be a very helpful study when it is performed in centers with clinicians who have experience in musculoskeletal ultrasound imaging. It is now believed that ultrasonography is as accurate as MRI in the diagnosis of supraspinatus tendon tears. Full-thickness tears appear hypoechoic or anechoic where fluid has replaced the area of torn tendon. Manual compression will be able to displace the fluid. In an area of torn tendon without fluid, compression will show the "sagging peribursal fat" sign.*

Diagnostic arthroscopy is done in some instances but is not generally necessary.

Differential Diagnosis

- Non-neurologic
  - Rotator cuff tendinitis
  - Glenolabral tear
  - Acromioclavicular sprain
  - Occult fracture
  - Osteoarthritis
  - Rheumatoid arthritis
  - Adhesive capsulitis
  - Myofascial pain syndrome
  - Myofascial thoracic outlet syndrome
- Neurologic
  - Cervical radiculopathy
  - Brachial plexopathy
  - Suprascapular neuropathy
  - Neurogenic (true) thoracic outlet syndrome

Treatment

Initial

Initial treatment of a rotator cuff tear is similar to that of rotator cuff tendinitis (see Chapter 16). However, if the symptoms do not respond to a rehabilitation program, the clinician should consider surgical consultation earlier in the course of injury.

*References 4,6,8,9,12,13,18,19.

Rehabilitation

Because of the interrelationship of instability and impingement previously discussed, there is a great deal of overlap in the rehabilitation of these shoulder problems. Treatment must be individualized and based on the restoration of optimal *function,* not merely surgical correction of anatomic changes. Supervised physical therapy is the mainstay of treatment and is successful in most patients.

The basic phases of rehabilitation include the following [12]: pain control and reduction of inflammation; restoration of normal shoulder motion, both scapulothoracic and glenohumeral; normalization of strength and dynamic joint stabilization; proprioception and dynamic joint stabilization; and sport-specific training. The rehabilitation phases may overlap and can be progressed as rapidly as tolerated, but all should be performed to speed recovery and to prevent reinjury.

Pain Control and Reduction of Inflammation

Initially, pain control and inflammation reduction are required to allow progression of healing and the initiation of an active rehabilitation program. These can be accomplished with a combination of relative rest, icing (20 minutes, three or four times a day), electrical stimulation, and acetaminophen or a nonsteroidal anti-inflammatory drug. The next section's rehabilitation program can be added as tolerated by the patient. Having the patient sleep with a pillow between the trunk and the arm will decrease the tension on the supraspinatus tendon and prevent compromise of blood flow in its watershed region.

Restoration of Shoulder Range of Motion

As with all musculoskeletal disorders, the entire body must be taken into consideration. Abnormalities in the kinetic chain can also affect the shoulder. If there are restrictions or limitations in range of motion or strength, the forces will be transmitted to other portions of the kinetic chain, resulting in an overload of those tissues and possibly injury.

After the pain has been managed, restoration of motion can be initiated. The use of Codman pendulum exercises, wall walking, stick or towel exercises, or a physical therapy program is beneficial in attaining full pain-free range. It is important to address any posterior capsular tightness because this can cause anterior and superior humeral head migration, resulting in impingement. A tight posterior capsule and the imbalance it causes force the humeral head anteriorly, producing shearing of the anterior labrum and causing an additional injury. Stretching of the posterior capsule is a difficult task. The horizontal adduction that is usually performed tends to stretch the scapular stabilizers rather than the posterior capsule. If care is taken to fix and to stabilize the scapula and therefore to prevent the stretching of the scapulothoracic stabilizers, stretching of the posterior capsule can be achieved. The focus of treatment in this early stage should be on improving range and flexibility of the posterior capsule, improving postural biomechanics, and restoring normal scapular motion.

Initially, ultrasound to the posterior capsule followed by gentle, passive prolonged stretch may be needed. The use of ultrasound should be closely monitored to prevent heating of an inflamed tendon, which will worsen the injury.

Postural biomechanics are important because with poor posture (e.g., excessive thoracic kyphosis and protracted shoulders), there is increased outlet narrowing, resulting in greater risk for rotator cuff impingement. Restoration of normal scapular motion is also essential because the scapula is the platform on which the glenohumeral joint rotates [20,21]. Thus, an unstable scapula can secondarily cause glenohumeral joint instability and resultant impingement. Scapular stabilization includes exercises such as wall pushups and biofeedback (visual and tactile).

Strengthening

The third phase of treatment is strengthening, and it should be performed in a pain-free range. Strengthening should begin with the scapulothoracic stabilizers and the use of shoulder shrugs, rowing, and pushups, which will isolate these muscles and help return smooth motion, allowing normal rhythm between the scapula and the glenohumeral joint. This will also provide a firm base of support on which the arm can move. Attention should then be turned toward strengthening of the rotator cuff muscles. Positioning of the arm at 45 and 90 degrees of abduction for exercises prevents the "wringing out" phenomenon that hyperadduction can cause by stressing the tenuous blood supply to the tendon of the exercising muscle. The thumbs down position with the arm in greater than 90 degrees of abduction and internal rotation should also be avoided to minimize subacromial impingement. After the scapular stabilizers and rotator cuff muscles are rehabilitated, the prime movers should be addressed to prevent further injury and to facilitate return to prior function.

There are many ways by which to strengthen muscles. The rehabilitation program should start with static contractions and co-contractions, progress to concentric exercises, and be completed with eccentric exercises and endurance training. The BodyBlade (www.BodyBlade.com) can be used for co-contraction in multiple planes and positions for rhythmic stabilization. There are many techniques to strengthen muscles, including static and dynamic exercises. A therapy prescription should include the number of repetitions, the number of sets of repetitions, and the intensity at which the specific exercise should be performed. When strength is restored, a maintenance program should be continued for fitness and prevention of reinjury.

Proprioception

The fourth phase is proprioceptive training. This is important to retrain the neurologic control of the strengthened muscles in providing improved dynamic interaction and coupled execution of tasks for harmonious movement of the shoulder and arm. Tasks should begin with closed kinetic chain exercises to provide joint stabilizing forces. As the muscles are reeducated, exercises can progress to open chain activities that may be used in specific sports or tasks. Exercises such as those using the BodyBlade or plyometrics will also address proprioception. In addition, proprioceptive neuromuscular facilitation is designed to stimulate muscle-tendon stretch receptors for reeducation. Kabat [22] has described shoulder proprioceptive neuromuscular facilitation techniques in detail.

Task or Sport Specific

The last phase of rehabilitation is to return to task- or sport-specific activities. This is an advanced form of training for the muscles to relearn prior activities. This is important and should be supervised so that the task performed is correct and the possibility of reinjury or injury in another part of the kinetic chain from improper technique is eliminated. The rehabilitation begins at a cognitive level but must be practiced so that it ultimately becomes part of unconscious motor programming.

Procedures

Subacromial injections of anesthetic and corticosteroid may be both diagnostic and therapeutic (see Chapter 16).

Surgery

If the patient's condition has not progressed with a conservative rehabilitation after 2 to 3 months, a surgical consultation should be considered. If the patient is unable to perform all the activities he or she demands (vocationally and avocationally) after 6 months of treatment and independent exercise performance, a surgical consultation should be obtained. If the patient is a high-level athlete or worker, earlier consultation may be appropriate. The population of younger patients is more amenable to surgical intervention [6,8].

If surgery is contemplated, repair, débridement, decompression, or a combination of these may be considered. A concomitant injury should be considered, such as a labral tear. The detail of these surgical procedures is beyond the scope of this text.

Potential Disease Complications

Partial rotator cuff tears can progress to full-thickness tears, especially if untreated. Rehabilitation attempts to restore biomechanics close to normal to prevent excessive wear on the tendon, which can cause further degeneration. Chronic untreated rotator cuff tears can lead to shoulder arthropathy [6,11].

Potential Treatment Complications

Analgesics and nonsteroidal anti-inflammatory drugs have well-known side effects that most commonly affect the gastric, hepatic, and renal systems. There are minimal disadvantages to coordinating a rehabilitation program that may improve the patient's symptoms to a level at which the patient is satisfied and functional. However, an overly aggressive program can progress a partial tear to a complete tear. With surgery, in general, the potential problems include bleeding, infection, worsening of the complaints, and nerve injury.

References

[1] Biglianni LU, Morrison D, April EW. The morphology of the acromion and its relationship to rotator cuff tears. Orthop Trans 1986;10:228.
[2] Codman EA. The shoulder: rupture of the supraspinatus tendon and other lesions in or about the subacromial Bursa. Boston: Thomas Todd; 1934.
[3] Flatow E, Soslowsky L, Ticker J, et al. Excursion of the rotator cuff under the acromion: patterns of subacromial contact. Am J Sports Med 1994;22:779–87.

[4] Hawkins RJ. Basic science and clinical application in the athlete's shoulder. Clin Sports Med 1991;10:693–971.
[5] Neer CS. Anterior acromioplasty for the chronic impingement syndrome in the shoulder. A preliminary report. J Bone Joint Surg Am 1972;54:41–50.
[6] Rockwood CA, Matsen FA. The shoulder. Philadelphia: WB Saunders; 2004, 795–871.
[7] Ozaki J, Fujimoto S, Nakagawa Y, et al. Tears of the rotator cuff of the shoulder associated with pathologic changes in the acromion: a study in cadavers. J Bone Joint Surg Am 1988;70:1224–30.
[8] Reid DC. Sports injury assessment and rehabilitation. New York: Churchill Livingstone; 1992.
[9] Gross J, Fetto J, Rosen E. Musculoskeletal examination. Boston: Blackwell Science; 1996.
[10] Basmajian J. Muscles alive: their functions revealed by electromyography. 5th ed. Williams & Wilkins: Baltimore; 1985.
[11] Kibler WB. Role of the scapula in the overhead throwing motion. Contemp Orthop 1991;22:525–32.
[12] Malanga GA, Bowen JE, Nadler SF, Lee A. Nonoperative management of shoulder injuries. J Back Musculoskelet Rehabil 1999;12:179–89.
[13] Dines DM, Levinson M. The conservative management of the unstable shoulder including rehabilitation. Clin Sports Med 1995;14:799–813.
[14] Harryman DT, Sidles JA, Clark JM, et al. Translation of the humeral head on the glenoid with passive glenohumeral motion. J Bone Joint Surg Am 1990;72:1334–43.
[15] Steinbeck J, Liljenqvist U, Jerosch J. The anatomy of the glenohumeral ligamentous complex and its contribution to anterior shoulder stability. J Shoulder Elbow Surg 1998;7:122–6.
[16] Chaipat L, Palmer WE. Shoulder magnetic resonance imaging. Clin Sports Med 2006;25:371–86.
[17] Moosikasuwan JB, Miller TT, Burke BJ. Rotator cuff tears: clinical, radiographic, and US findings. Radiographics 2005;25:1591–607.
[18] Cailliet R. Shoulder pain. 3rd ed. Philadelphia: FA Davis; 1991, 42–46.
[19] Nicholas JA, Hershman EB. The upper extremity in sports medicine. 2nd ed. St. Louis: Mosby; 1996, 209–222.
[20] Kibler WB, Chandler TJ. Functional scapular instability in throwing athletes. Presented at the 15th annual meeting of the American Orthopaedic Society for Sports Medicine; Traverse City, Mich, June 19-22, 1989.
[21] Nuber GW, Jobe FW, Perry J, et al. Fine wire electromyography analysis of the shoulder during swimming. Am J Sports Med 1985;13:216–22.
[22] Kabat H. Proprioception facilitation in therapeutic exercise. In: Kendall HD, editor. Therapeutic exercises. Baltimore: Waverly Press; 1965. p. 327–43.

CHAPTER 18

Scapular Winging

Peter M. McIntosh, MD

Synonyms

Scapulothoracic winging
Long thoracic nerve palsy
Spinal accessory nerve palsy
Scapula alata
Alar scapula
Rucksack palsy

ICD-9 Codes

352.4	**Spinal accessory nerve disorder**
353.3	**Neuropathy long thoracic**
353.5	**Neuralgic amyotrophy**
354.9	**Mononeuritis of upper limb, unspecified**
723.4	**Cervical radiculopathy NOS**
724.4	**Long thoracic nerve entrapment**
728.87	**Muscle weakness NOS**

ICD-10 Codes

G54.3	**Neuropathy thoracic root**
G54.5	**Neuralgic amyotrophy**
G56.9	**Mononeuritis of unspecified upper limb**
G56.91	**Mononeuritis of right upper limb**
G56.92	**Mononeuritis of left upper limb**
G58.9	**Nerve entrapment, unspecified**
M54.12	**Cervical radiculopathy**
M54.13	**Cervicothoracic radiculopathy**
M62.81	**Muscle weakness, generalized**

Definition

Scapular winging refers to prominence of the vertebral (medial) border of the scapula [1]. The inferomedial border can also be rotated or displaced away from the chest wall. This well-defined medical sign was first described by Velpeau [2] in 1837. It is associated with a wide array of medical conditions or injuries that typically result in dysfunction of the scapular stabilizers and rotators and, ultimately, glenohumeral and scapulothoracic biomechanics.

Fiddian and King [1] classified scapular winging as either static or dynamic after examination of 25 patients with 23 different causes of scapular winging. Static winging is attributable to a fixed deformity in the shoulder girdle, spine, or ribs; it is characteristically present with the patient's arms at the sides. Dynamic winging is ascribed to a neuromuscular disorder; it is produced by active or resisted movement and is usually absent at rest. Scapular winging has also been classified anatomically according to whether the etiology of the lesion is related to nerve, muscle, bone, or joint disease (Table 18.1).

The scapula is a triangular bone that is completely surrounded by muscles and attaches to the clavicle by the coracoclavicular ligaments and acromioclavicular joint capsule. Motion of the scapula along the chest wall occurs through the action of the muscle groups that originate or insert on the scapula and proximal humerus. These muscles include the rhomboids (major and minor), trapezius, serratus anterior, levator scapulae, and pectoralis minor. The rotator cuff and deltoid muscles are involved with glenohumeral motion. Innervation of these muscle groups includes all the roots of the brachial plexus and several peripheral nerves. Scapular winging may be caused by brachial plexus injuries but most often is related to a peripheral nerve injury (see Table 18.1).

Injury to the long thoracic and spinal accessory nerves with weakness of the serratus anterior and trapezius muscles, respectively, is most commonly associated with scapular winging. The serratus anterior muscle originates on the outer surface and superior border of the upper eight or nine ribs and inserts on the costal surface of the medial border of the scapula. It abducts the scapula and rotates it so the glenoid cavity faces cranially and holds the medial border of the scapula against the thorax.

The serratus anterior muscle is innervated by the pure motor long thoracic nerve, which arises from the ventral rami of the fifth, sixth, and seventh cervical roots. The nerve passes through the scalenus medius muscle, beneath the brachial plexus and the clavicle, and over the first rib. It then runs superficially along the lateral aspect of the chest wall to supply all the digitations of the serratus anterior muscles [26]. Because of its long and superficial course, the long thoracic nerve is susceptible to both traumatic and nontraumatic injuries (Fig. 18.1).

The trapezius muscle consists of upper, middle, and lower fibers. The upper fibers originate from the external occipital protuberance, superior nuchal line, nuchal ligament, and spinous process of the seventh cervical vertebra and insert on the lateral clavicle and acromion. The middle fibers arise from the spinous process of the first

Table 18.1 Etiology of Scapular Winging

Characteristic	Nerve	Muscle	Bone	Joint
Site of lesion	LTN [3] SAN [4] DSN C5-C7 nerve root lesion Brachial plexus lesion [5]	SA T R	Scapula Clavicle Spine Ribs	GHJ ACJ
Traumatic	Acute, repetitive, or chronic compression of LTN, SAN, DSN Trauma or traction injury to LTN, nerve roots, brachial plexus [6] Whiplash injury [7]	Direct muscle injury to SA, T, R [4,8] Avulsion of SA, T, R RTC disease Sports-related injury [8–10]	Nonunion Malunion Fractures of scapula [11,12], clavicle, acromion	Glenoid fracture ACJ dislocation Shoulder instability
Congenital, hereditary	Cerebral palsy	Congenital contracture of infraspinatus muscle Agenesis of SA, T, R Duchenne muscular dystrophy FSHD [13] Fibrous bands (deltoid)	Scoliosis Craniocleidodysostosis Ollier disease Sprengel deformity	Arthrogryposis multiplex congenita Congenital posterior shoulder dislocation
Degenerative, inflammatory	SLE [14] Neuritis Amyotrophic brachial neuralgia [5] Guillain-Barré syndrome [15]	Toxin exposure Infection Myositis		Abduction-internal rotation contracture from AVN of humeral head Arthropathy
Iatrogenic	Epidural or general anesthesia Radical neck dissection [16] Lymph node biopsy First rib resection [17] Radical mastectomy Posterolateral thoracotomy incision Axillary node dissection Anterior spinal surgery [18]	Postinjection fibrosis (deltoid) Division of SA		
Miscellaneous	Vaginal delivery [19] Cervical syringomyelia [20]	Chiropractic manipulation Electrocution [21]	Scapulothoracic bursa Enchondroma Subscapular osteochondroma [22–24] Exostoses of rib or scapula [25]	Voluntary posterior shoulder subluxation

ACJ, acromioclavicular joint; *AVN,* avascular necrosis; *DSN,* dorsal scapular nerve; *FSHD,* facioscapulohumeral muscular dystrophy; *GHJ,* glenohumeral joint; *LTN,* long thoracic nerve; *R,* rhomboid muscles; *RTC,* rotator cuff muscles; *SA,* serratus anterior muscle; *SAN,* spinal accessory nerve; *SLE,* systemic lupus erythematosus; *T,* trapezius muscle.
From Fiddian NJ, King RJ. The winged scapula. Clin Orthop Relat Res 1984;185:228-236.

through fifth thoracic vertebrae and insert on the superior lip of the scapular spine. The lower fibers originate from the spinous process of the sixth through twelfth thoracic vertebrae and insert on the apex of the scapular spine. They are innervated by the pure motor spinal accessory nerve (cranial nerve XI) and afferent fibers from the second through fourth cervical spinal nerves. The root fibers unite to form a common trunk that ascends to enter the intracranial cavity through the foramen magnum. It exits with the vagus nerve through the jugular foramen, pierces the sternocleidomastoid muscle, and descends obliquely across the floor of the posterior triangle of the neck to the trapezius muscle [26]. In the posterior triangle, the nerve lies superficially, covered only by fascia and skin, and is susceptible to injury. Cadaver studies have shown considerable variations in the course and distribution of the spinal accessory nerve in the posterior triangle and in the nerve's relationship to the borders of the sternocleidomastoid and trapezius muscles [27]. The trapezius muscle adducts the scapula (middle fibers), rotates the glenoid cavity upward (upper and lower fibers), and elevates and depresses the scapula. Overall, the trapezius muscles maintain efficient shoulder function by both supporting the shoulder and stabilizing the scapulae (Fig. 18.2).

A rare cause of scapular winging is dorsal scapular nerve palsy. The dorsal scapular nerve is a pure motor nerve from the fifth cervical spinal nerve that supplies the rhomboid and levator scapulae muscles. It arises above the upper trunk of the brachial plexus and passes through the middle scalene muscle on its way to the levator scapulae and rhomboids. The rhomboids (major and minor) adduct and elevate the scapula and rotate it so the glenoid cavity faces caudally [26].

The levator scapulae muscles originate on the transverse process of the first four cervical vertebrae and insert on the medial borders of the scapulae between the superior angle and the root of the spine. They elevate the scapulae and assist in rotation of the glenoid cavity caudally. They are

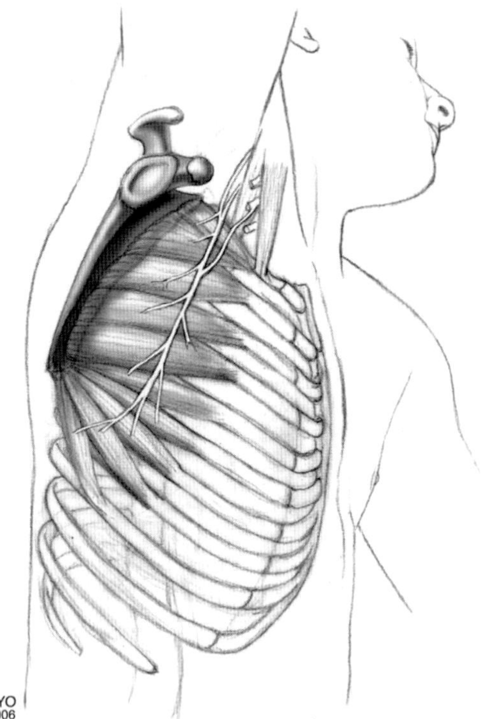

FIGURE 18.1 Anterolateral view of the right upper chest and shoulder showing the course of the long thoracic nerve and innervation of the serratus anterior muscles. Note the superficial location of the long thoracic nerve. *(From the Mayo Foundation for Medical Education and Research. © Mayo Foundation, 2007.)*

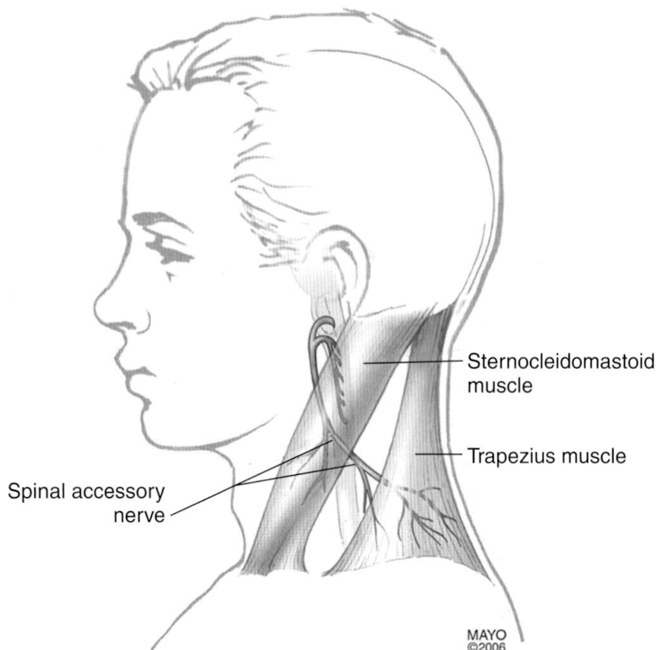

FIGURE 18.2 Lateral view of the neck showing the course of the spinal accessory nerve and innervation of the trapezius muscle. *(From the Mayo Foundation for Medical Education and Research. © Mayo Foundation, 2007.)*

innervated by the dorsal scapular nerve (emanating from the fifth cervical spinal nerve) and the cervical plexus (emanating from the third and fourth cervical spinal nerves) (Fig. 18.3).

Symptoms

A patient's presenting symptoms depend on the type and chronicity of the injury. Most patients, however, complain of upper back or shoulder pain, muscle fatigue, and weakness with use of the shoulder. The diagnosis of scapular winging is made clinically. A pain profile should be obtained, including onset and duration of pain, location, severity, and quality as well as exacerbating and relieving factors, not only to provide baseline information but also to help develop a differential diagnosis. The patient should also be questioned about hand dominance because the dominant shoulder is usually more muscular but sits lower than the nondominant shoulder. Knowledge of the patient's age, occupation and hobbies, and current and previous level of functioning may also contribute to the diagnosis and treatment plan. The mechanism of injury in patients with traumatic palsy is important, as are associated findings including muscle spasm, paresthesia, and muscle wasting or weakness [28,29]. The scapular winging of long thoracic neuropathy and serratus anterior muscle weakness must be distinguished from that of a spinal accessory neuropathy and trapezius muscle weakness as well as dorsal scapular neuropathy and rhomboid weakness. Serratus anterior muscle dysfunction is the most common cause of scapular winging. Typically, patients complain of a dull aching pain in the shoulder and periscapular region. The periscapular pain may be related to spasm from unopposed contraction of the other scapular stabilizers in the presence of serratus anterior muscle weakness. There may be "clicking" or "popping" noise emanating from the periscapular area when the patient moves, which is made worse with

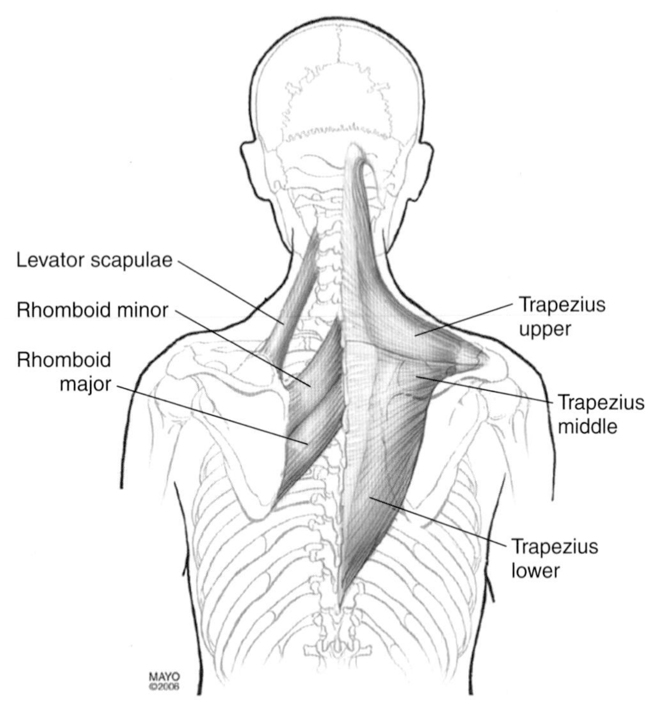

FIGURE 18.3 View of upper back showing origins and insertions of rhomboid, levator scapulae, and trapezius muscles. *(From the Mayo Foundation for Medical Education and Research. © Mayo Foundation, 2007.)*

stressful upper extremity activities [28]. Because the serratus anterior muscle rotates the scapula forward as the arm is abducted or forward flexed above the shoulder level, these movements are affected. Shoulder fatigue and weakness are related to loss of scapular rotation and stabilization.

A cosmetic deformity may occur in the upper back as a result of the winged scapula. It may be apparent at rest but usually is more obvious on raising of the arm. Patients may find it difficult to sit for prolonged periods with the back resting against a hard surface, such as driving for long periods.

With trapezius muscle weakness, the affected shoulder is depressed, and the inferior scapular border rotates laterally, which makes prolonged use of the arm painful and tiresome. Patients often complain of a dull ache around the shoulder girdle and difficulty with overhead activities and heavy lifting, especially with shoulder abduction greater than 90 degrees [29].

Physical Examination

The patient should be suitably undressed so that the examiner can observe, both front and back, the normal bone and soft tissue contours of both shoulders and scapulae for symmetry and their relationship to the thorax. The patient's overall posture is assessed, as are the presence of muscle spasm and trapezius or rhomboid muscle atrophy. Scapulothoracic motion is examined with both passive and active range of motion activities of the shoulder. The different patterns of scapulothoracic movement can assist in the differential diagnosis of scapular winging and are illustrated in Figures 18.4 to 18.6 [30].

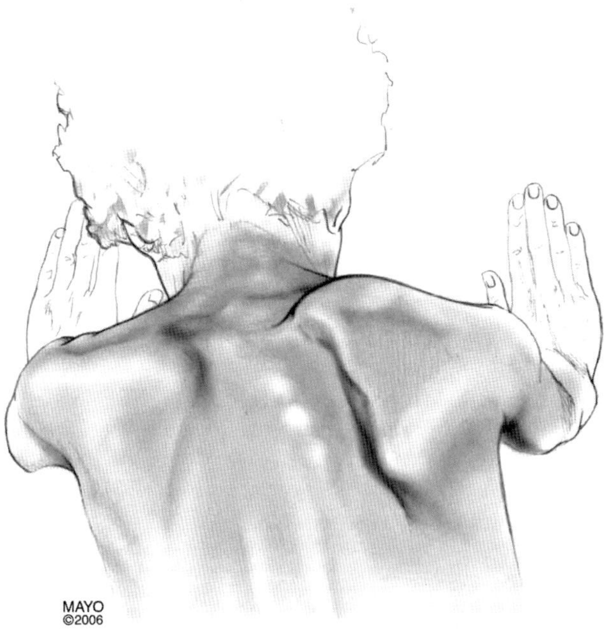

FIGURE 18.4 Winging of the right scapula with forward flexion of the extended arms due to injury of the long thoracic nerve with serratus anterior weakness. Note the upward displacement of the scapula with prominence of the vertebral border and medial displacement of the inferior angle. *(From the Mayo Foundation for Medical Education and Research. © Mayo Foundation, 2007.)*

With long thoracic neuropathy and serratus anterior muscle weakness, the cardinal sign is winging of the scapula, in which the vertebral border of the scapula moves away from the posterior chest wall and the inferior angle is rotated toward midline. This scapular winging may be visible with the patient standing normally, but if the weakness is mild, it may

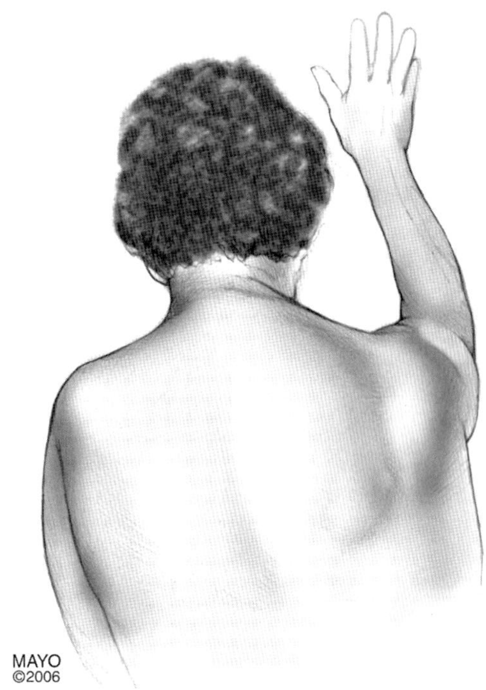

FIGURE 18.5 Right spinal accessory nerve palsy with trapezius weakness. The neckline is asymmetric, the shoulder droops, and there is lateral displacement of the superior angle of scapula with the glenoid labrum rotated downward. *(From the Mayo Foundation for Medical Education and Research. © Mayo Foundation, 2007.)*

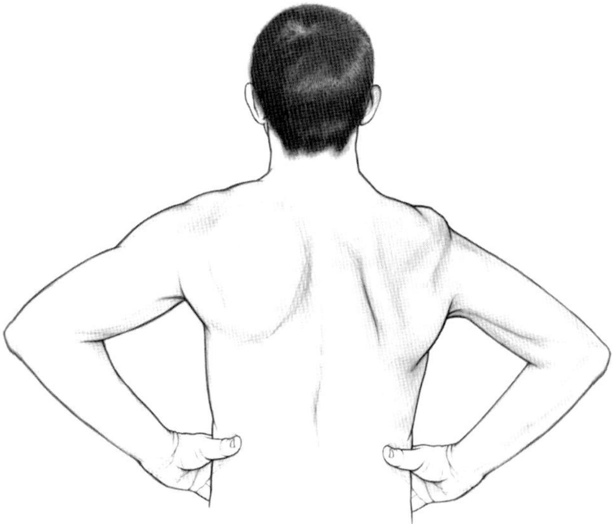

FIGURE 18.6 Dorsal scapular nerve palsy with rhomboid weakness. There is lateral displacement of the inferior angle of the right scapula that is accentuated when the patient pushes his elbows backward against resistance. Note atrophy of the rhomboid and infraspinatus muscles. *(From the Mayo Foundation for Medical Education and Research. © Mayo Foundation, 2007)*

be visible only when the patient extends the arm and pushes against a wall in a pushup position (Fig. 18.4) [3,28,31].

Spinal accessory neuropathy and trapezius muscle weakness are usually accompanied by an asymmetric neckline with noticeable shoulder droop when the patient's arms are unsupported at the sides. On the affected side, deepening of the supraclavicular fossa is evident and shoulder shrug is difficult. With shoulder elevation, the scapula is displaced laterally, rotating downward and outward. There is usually difficulty with shoulder abduction above 90 degrees, more so than with forward flexion. Weakness with attempted shoulder elevation against resistance is characteristic. Normal muscle testing can elicit weakness in the trapezius muscle (Fig. 18.5) [29,32].

With weakness of the rhomboids, winging of the scapula is usually minimal. There is lateral displacement of the inferior angle of the scapula that is best accentuated when the patient pushes the elbow backward against resistance or slowly lowers the arms from a forward elevated position. Atrophy of the rhomboids may be present. The scapula is displaced downward and laterally (Fig. 18.6) [32].

A complete neurologic and musculoskeletal examination, with manual muscle strength testing and sensory and reflex testing, should be completed to rule out underlying neuromuscular disease processes. In addition, thorough examination of the neck and shoulder with provocative maneuvers should be completed to rule out additional musculoskeletal sources of scapular winging.

Functional Limitations

Functional limitations depend not only on the cause of the scapular winging but also on the severity of weakness and pain. Difficulty with activities of daily living may be evident as a result of pain, weakness, and altered scapulothoracic and glenohumeral motion. Especially affected are activities that require arm elevation above the level of the shoulder (e.g., brushing hair or teeth or shaving). Recreational and vocational activities such as golf, tennis, and volleyball that entail working or reaching overhead may be affected. Chronic shoulder pain and dysfunction can lead to depression and anxiety, irritability, concentration difficulties, lack of sleep, and chronic fatigue. Overuse of the shoulder and scapular stabilizer muscles can lead to myofascial pain syndromes.

Diagnostic Studies

Plain radiography of the shoulder, cervical spine, chest, and scapulae is recommended as part of the initial evaluation for scapular winging, especially if the cause is not obvious. Plain radiography can help rule out other causes of scapular winging, such as subscapular osteochondroma, avulsion fracture of the scapula, or other primary shoulder and cervical spine disease. With radiographs of the scapula, oblique views are recommended because osteochondroma may be hidden on anteroposterior views [33].

Computed tomography and magnetic resonance imaging are usually not necessary unless the coexistence of other disease processes is suspected. The patient's presentation and examination findings are pivotal in deciding whether advanced imaging is necessary.

Electrodiagnostic studies, namely, electromyography and nerve conduction studies, are valuable tools clinically to aid in the evaluation of scapular winging. They can assist in localizing injury and disease of peripheral nerves or muscles related to scapular function. These studies can help evaluate patients with abnormal scapulothoracic motion but in whom it cannot be clearly established clinically whether the weakness lies in a particular muscle or in the actions of other muscles acting on the scapula.

Serial electromyographic and nerve conduction studies have been used to follow recovery in patients with isolated long thoracic or spinal accessory nerve palsies and to help in decisions of whether to undertake nerve exploration or muscle transfer [28,29]. However, caution has been advised in the use of needle electromyographic findings to predict the prognosis and to guide the timing of surgical repair [34]. Long thoracic and spinal accessory neuropathies may be associated with a good prognosis, irrespective of needle electromyographic findings.

Differential Diagnosis [42]

Rotator cuff disease
Shoulder impingement syndromes
Glenohumeral instability (especially posterior instability)
Acromioclavicular joint disease
Shoulder arthritis
Adhesive capsulitis
Bicipital tendinitis
Cervical radiculopathy (especially C5-C7)
Suprascapular nerve entrapment
Myofascial pain syndromes
Scoliosis (associated rib deformities can cause asymptomatic scapular winging on convex side of curve)
Sprengel deformity (congenital deformity of shoulder with high-riding and downward-rotated scapula, often confused with scapular winging)
Fracture or malunion of clavicle and acromion
Tumors of shoulder girdle, lung, or spine

Treatment

In most patients, scapular winging is a result of neurapraxic injuries. Fortunately, these types of injuries usually resolve spontaneously within 6 to 9 months after traumatic injury and within 2 years after nontraumatic injuries. In one study [34], traumatic long thoracic and spinal accessory nerve injuries were associated with a poor prognosis compared with nontraumatic neuropathies. Once the diagnosis is made, conservative treatment should be initiated. Some clinicians have recommended a trial of conservative treatment for at least 12 to 24 months to allow adequate time for nerve recovery [28,29].

Initial

Pain control may be achieved early with use of an analgesic or an anti-inflammatory medication. Activity modification is recommended. The patient should avoid precipitating activities and strenuous use of the involved extremity. Physical modalities, such as ice massage, superficial moist heat, and ultrasound, can be applied to help with pain control. Ice massage may additionally help control swelling and relieve associated muscle spasm [32].

Immobilization should be a part of the initial management to prevent overstretching of the weakened muscle [35]. This can be accomplished with the use of a sling to rest the arm until the patient can recover brace-free shoulder flexion or have reduced pain. In one study, this could be anywhere from 1 to 7 months [36].

Long-term use of scapular winging shoulder braces to maintain the position of the scapula against the thorax is controversial. Various shoulder braces and orthotics have been used with mixed results. Some authors [8,31] recommend against use of shoulder braces because they are cumbersome, poorly tolerated, and ineffective. Others have advocated their use to protect against muscle overstretching and scapulothoracic overuse [32,35]. One author reported successful treatment of a brachial plexus injury and winged scapula with use of Kinesio tape and exercise to facilitate the rotator cuff groups and scapular stabilizers [36].

Rehabilitation

Specific treatment varies, depending on the etiology of the scapular winging. In general, range of motion exercises should be initiated early to prevent contractures or adhesive capsulitis, especially if the affected extremity is immobilized.

A stretching and strengthening exercise program can be undertaken after pain control is achieved [32]. Stretching the scapular stabilizers and shoulder capsules without overstretching the weakened muscle as well as cross-body adduction to stretch the rhomboids is important and should be supervised by a physical therapist. The scapular stabilizer, cervical muscles, and rotator cuff muscle should be strengthened, especially the affected muscle groups. This can be accomplished by passive scapular retraction, such as scapular squeeze. Isometric strengthening exercises can include scapular protraction and retraction, shoulder packing, and shoulder shrugs to strengthen the pectoralis, serratus anterior, rhomboids, upper trapezius, and levator scapulae. Advanced exercises can include specific rotator cuff strengthening as well as shoulder circles with a ball against a wall, stabilizing ball pushups, resistance band pull-aparts and pull-downs, and chest presses both standing and lying down. Neuromuscular electrical stimulation may be used to prevent muscle atrophy. Functional glenohumeral and scapulothoracic muscle patterns must be relearned. Progression to an independent structured home exercise program is recommended, but the patient should first be able to perform the exercises appropriately under supervision of a physical therapist.

Procedures

Localized injections are not routinely administered for isolated scapular winging. Injection therapy may be indicated for other coexisting shoulder disease to help with pain control.

Surgery

Conservative treatment has been recommended for a prolonged period (12 to 24 months) to allow adequate time for recovery before surgical options are considered. [28,29,37] Surgery should be considered for patients who do not recover in this time. In patients with penetrating trauma in which the nerve may have been injured, spontaneous recovery is less likely, and early nerve exploration with neurolysis, direct nerve repair, or nerve grafting may be indicated.

Surgery may also be indicated if scapular winging appears to have been caused by a surgically treatable lesion (e.g., a subscapular osteochondroma) and the patient is symptomatic or has a cosmetic disfigurement [22,38]. In general, surgical options are many but can be divided into two categories: static stabilization procedures and dynamic muscle transfers.

Static stabilization procedures involve scapulothoracic fusion and scapulothoracic arthrodesis in which the scapula is fused to the thorax. These procedures may be effective in cases of generalized weakness (e.g., facioscapulohumeral muscular dystrophy) when the patient has disabling pain and functional loss and no transferable muscles. [32,37,39,40] They can relieve shoulder fatigue and pain and allow functional abduction and flexion of the upper extremity [13,39]. Static stabilization procedures have fallen out of favor for scapular winging related to isolated muscle weakness because the results deteriorate over time with recurrence of winging. The usual incidence of complications associated with some of these procedures is high [32,39]. Dynamic muscle transfers have shown better results for correction of scapular winging and restoration of function. Several different muscles have been used in various muscle transfer techniques to provide dynamic control of the scapula and to improve scapulothoracic and glenohumeral motion. Transfer of the sternal head of the pectoralis major muscle to the inferior angle of the scapula with fascia lata autograft reinforcement is the preferred method of treatment for scapular winging related to long thoracic nerve injury. [32,37,41] The surgical procedure of choice for scapular winging related to chronic trapezius muscle dysfunction involves the lateral transfer of the insertions of the levator scapulae and the rhomboid major and minor muscles. This procedure enables the muscles to support the shoulder girdle and to stabilize the scapula [29,32,37].

Potential Disease Complications

Disease complications are usually related to scapulothoracic dysfunction as a result of scapular winging. This can contribute to glenohumeral instability and subsequent shoulder range of motion and functional deficits as well as chronic periscapular, upper back, and shoulder pain. Secondary impingement syndromes can result from the muscle dysfunction. Adhesive capsulitis can occur from loss of shoulder mobility and function. Cosmetic deformity is a common result of scapular winging, especially if there is a combined serratus anterior and trapezius muscle weakness.

Potential Treatment Complications

Pharmacotherapy can lead to treatment complications. Nonsteroidal anti-inflammatory drugs have well-documented adverse effects that most commonly involve the gastrointestinal system. Analgesics may have adverse effects that predominantly involve the hepatorenal system. These complications can be minimized by having a working knowledge of the patient's ongoing medical problems, current medications, and potential drug interactions.

Local injections may cause allergic reactions, infection at the injection site, and, rarely, sepsis. Tendon rupture is a potential complication if inadvertent injection into a tendon occurs.

Surgical complications are numerous and include a large, cosmetically unpleasant incision over the shoulder and upper back, postoperative musculoskeletal deformities (e.g., scoliosis), infection, pulmonary complications (e.g., pneumothorax and hemothorax), hardware failure, pseudarthrosis, recurrent winging, and persistent pain.

References

[1] Fiddian NJ, King RJ. The winged scapula. Clin Orthop Relat Res 1984;185:228–36.

[2] Velpeau AALM. Luxations de l'epaule. Arch Gen Med 1837;14:269–305.

[3] Oakes MJ, Sherwood DL. An isolated long thoracic nerve injury in a Navy Airman. Mil Med 2004;169:713–5.

[4] Aksoy IA, Schrader SL, Ali MS, et al. Spinal accessory neuropathy associated with deep tissue massage: a case report. J Athl Train 2009;44:519–26.

[5] Parsonage MJ, Turner JW. Neuralgic amyotrophy: the shoulder-girdle syndrome. Lancet 1948;251:973–8.

[6] Lee SG, Kim JH, Lee SY, et al. Winged scapula caused by rhomboideus and trapezius muscles rupture associated with repetitive minor trauma: a case report. J Korean Med Sci 2006;21:581–4.

[7] Bodack MP, Tunkel RS, Marini SG, et al. Spinal accessory nerve palsy as a cause of pain after whiplash injury: case report. J Pain Symptom Manage 1998;15:321–8.

[8] Schultz JS, Leonard JA Jr. Long thoracic neuropathy from athletic activity. Arch Phys Med Rehabil 1992;73:87–90.

[9] Packer GJ, McLatchie GR, Bowden W. Scapula winging in a sports injury clinic. Br J Sports Med 1993;27:90–1.

[10] Sherman SC, O'Connor M. An unusual cause of shoulder pain: winged scapula. J Emerg Med 2005;28:329–31.

[11] Marsha M, Middleton A, Rangan A. An unusual cause of scapular winging following trauma in an army personnel. J Shoulder Elbow Surg 2010;19:24–7.

[12] Bowen TR, Miller F. Greenstick fracture of the scapula: a cause of scapular winging. J Orthop Trauma 2006;20:147–9.

[13] Rhee YG, Ha JH. Long-term results of scapulothoracic arthrodesis of facioscapulohumeral muscular dystrophy. J Shoulder Elbow Surg 2006;15:445–50.

[14] Delmonte S, Massone C, Parodi A, et al. Acquired winged scapula in a patient with systemic lupus erythematosus. Clin Exp Rheumatol 1998;16:82–3.

[15] Sivan M, Hasan A. Images in emergency medicine: winged scapula as the presenting symptom of Guillain-Barré syndrome. Emerg Med J 2009;26:790.

[16] Witt RL, Gillis T, Pratt R Jr. Spinal accessory nerve monitoring with clinical outcome measures. Ear Nose Throat J 2006;85:540–4.

[17] Wood VE, Frykman GK. Winging of the scapula as a complication of first rib resection: a report of six cases. Clin Orthop Relat Res 1980;149:160–3.

[18] Ameri E, Behtash H, Omidi-Kashani F. Isolated long thoracic nerve paralysis—a rare complication of anterior spinal surgery: a case report. J Med Case Rep 2009;3:7366.

[19] Debeer P, Devlieger R, Brys P, et al. Scapular winging after vaginal delivery. BJOG 2004;111:758–9.

[20] Niedermaier N, Meinck HM, Hartmann M. Cervical syringomyelia at the C7-C8 level presenting with bilateral scapular winging. J Neurol Neurosurg Psychiatry 2000;68:394–5.

[21] Marmor L, Bechtol CO. Paralysis of the serratus anterior due to electric shock relieved by transplantation of the pectoralis major muscle: a case report. J Bone Joint Surg Am 1963;45:156–60.

[22] Frost NL, Parada SA, Manoso MW, et al. Scapula osteochondromas treated with surgical excision. Orthopedics 2010;33:804.

[23] Ermis MN, Aykut US. Snapping scapular syndrome caused by subscapular osteochondroma. Erlem Hastalik Cerrahisi 2012;23:40–3.

[24] Scott DA, Alexander JR. Relapsing and remitting scapular winging in a pediatric patient. Am J Phys Med Rehabil 2010;89:505–8.

[25] Parsons TA. The snapping scapula and subscapular exostoses. J Bone Joint Surg Br 1973;55:345–9.

[26] Hollinshead WH. Anatomy for surgeons. Hagerstown, Md, Harper & Row; 1982, 259–340.

[27] Symes A, Ellis H. Variations in the surface anatomy of the spinal accessory nerve in the posterior triangle. Surg Radiol Anat 2005;27:404–8.

[28] Wiater JM, Flatow EL. Long thoracic nerve injury. Clin Orthop Relat Res 1999;368:17–27.

[29] Wiater JM, Bigliani LU. Spinal accessory nerve injury. Clin Orthop Relat Res 1999;368:5–16.

[30] Tsivgoulis G, Vadikolias K, Courcoutsakis N, et al. Teaching neuroimages: differential diagnosis of scapular winging. Neurology 2012;78:e109.

[31] Warner JJ, Navarro RA. Serratus anterior dysfunction: recognition and treatment. Clin Orthop Relat Res 1998;349:139–48.

[32] Meninger AK, Figuerres BF, Goldberg BA. Scapular winging: an update. J Am Acad Orthop Surg 2011;19:453–62.

[33] Banerjee A. X-rays as a diagnostic aid in winged scapula. Arch Emerg Med 1993;10:261–3.

[34] Friedenberg SM, Zimprich T, Harper CM. The natural history of long thoracic and spinal accessory neuropathies. Muscle Nerve 2002;25:535–9.

[35] Marin R. Scapula winger's brace: a case series on the management of long thoracic nerve palsy. Arch Phys Med Rehabil 1998;79:1226–30.

[36] Walsh SF. Treatment of a brachial plexus injury using kinesiotape and exercise. Physiother Theory Pract 2010;26:490–6.

[37] Galano GJ, Bigliani MD, Ahmad CS, Levine WN. Surgical treatment of winged scapula. Clin Orthop Relat Res 2008;466:652–60.

[38] Ziaee MA, Abolghasemian M, Majd ME. Scapulothoracic arthrodesis for winged scapula due to facioscapulohumeral dystrophy (a new technique). Am J Orthop 2006;35:311–5.

[39] Sewell MD, Higgs DS, Al-Hadithy N, et al. The outcome of scapulothoracic fusion for painful winging of the scapula in dystrophic and non-dystrophic conditions. J Bone Joint Surg Br 2012;94:1253–9.

[40] Jeon IH, Neumann L, Wallace WA. Scapulothoracic fusion for painful winging of the scapula in nondystrophic patients. J Shoulder Elbow Surg 2005;14:400–6.

[41] Streit JJ, Lenarz CJ, Shishani Y, et al. Pectoralis major tendon transfer for the treatment of scapular winging due to long thoracic nerve palsy. J Shoulder Elbow Surg 2012;21:685–90.

[42] Belville RG, Seupaul RA. Winged scapula in the emergency department: a case report and review. J Emerg Med 2005;29:279–82.

CHAPTER 19

Shoulder Arthritis

Michael F. Stretanski, DO

Synonyms

Glenohumeral arthritis
Osteoarthritis
Arthritic frozen shoulder

ICD-9 Codes

715.11 Primary osteoarthritis, shoulder
715.21 Secondary osteoarthritis, shoulder (rotator cuff arthropathy)
716.11 Traumatic arthropathy, shoulder
716.91 Arthropathy, unspecified, shoulder

ICD-10 Codes

M19.011 Primary osteoarthritis, right shoulder
M19.012 Primary osteoarthritis, left shoulder
M19.019 Primary osteoarthritis, unspecified shoulder
M19.211 Secondary osteoarthritis, right shoulder
M19.212 Secondary osteoarthritis, left shoulder
M19.219 Secondary osteoarthritis, unspecified shoulder
M12.511 Traumatic arthropathy, right shoulder
M12.512 Traumatic arthropathy, left shoulder
M12.519 Traumatic arthropathy, unspecified shoulder
M12.811 Other specified arthropathies, not elsewhere classified, right shoulder
M12.812 Other specified arthropathies, not elsewhere classified, left shoulder
M12.819 Other specified arthropathies, not elsewhere classified, unspecified shoulder

Definition

Osteoarthritis of the glenohumeral joint occurs when there is loss of articular cartilage that results in narrowing of the joint space (Fig. 19.1). Synovitis and osteocartilaginous loose bodies are commonly associated with glenohumeral arthritis. Pathologic distortion of the articular surfaces of the humeral head and glenoid can be due to increasing age, overuse, heredity, alcoholism, trauma, Gaucher disease (lipid storage disease), or metabolic disease of bone.

In looking at glenohumeral arthritic conditions, one must consider osteonecrosis both as an etiologic entity and as a related endpoint to the disease. Most of the information about osteonecrosis of the humeral head is extrapolated from the research findings of the disorder of the hip. The major difference between osteonecrosis of the hip and osteonecrosis of the humeral head is that the shoulder bears less weight than the hip. Risk factors are corticosteroid use, radiation therapy, and sickle cell anemia, but its presence in a medically uncomplicated adolescent competitive swimmer [1] does seem to suggest that it may be more common than previously thought.

Shoulder osteoarthritis is most commonly seen beyond the fifth decade and is more common in men. Long-standing complete rotator cuff tears, multidirectional instability from any cause, lymphoma [2] (chronic lymphocytic lymphoma or immunocytoma), or prior capsulorrhaphy for anterior instability [3] can predispose to glenohumeral arthritis.

Acute septic arthritis should not be heedlessly ruled out in the face of severe osteoarthritis [4]. The medical history should include any history of fracture, dislocation, rotator cuff tear, repetitive motion, metabolic disorder, immunosuppression, chronic glucocorticoid administration, and prior shoulder surgery

Symptoms

Symptoms include shoulder pain intensified by activity and partially relieved with rest. Pain is usually noted with all shoulder movements. Major restriction of shoulder motion and disuse weakness or pain inhibitory weakness are common and potentially progressive. Resultant adhesive capsulitis may be the primary clinical presentation. Pain is typically restricted to the area of the shoulder and may be felt around the deltoid region but not typically into the forearm. Pain is

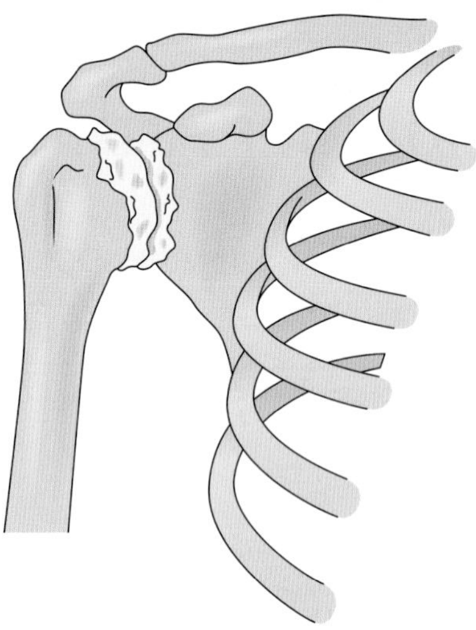

FIGURE 19.1 Osteoarthritis of the shoulder.

generally characterized as dull and aching but may become sharp at the extremes of range of motion; it is typically worse in the supine position and in attempting to sleep on the arthritic side. Pain may interfere with sleep and may be worse in the morning. Neurologic symptoms, such as numbness and paresthesias, should be absent.

Physical Examination

Restriction of shoulder range of motion is a major clinical component, especially loss of external rotation and abduction. Both active and passive range of motion is affected in shoulder arthritis, compared with only active motion in rotator cuff tears (passive range is normal in rotator cuff injuries unless adhesive capsulitis is present). Pain increases when the extremes of the restricted motion are reached, and crepitus is common with movement. Tenderness may be present over the anterior rotator cuff and over the posterior joint line.

Several well-described tests for examination of the shoulder are commonly used in clinical practice (e.g., Neer, Hawkins-Kennedy, Yergason, painful arc, and compression-rotation test). Pooled sensitivity and specificity range from 53% to 95%, yet meta-analysis has demonstrated that use of any single shoulder examination test to make a diagnosis cannot be unequivocally recommended. Combinations of tests provide better accuracy, but marginally so. These findings seem to provide support for stressing a comprehensive clinical examination [5].

If acromioclavicular joint osteoarthritis is an accompanying problem, the acromioclavicular joint may be tender. There may be wasting of the muscles surrounding the shoulder because of disuse atrophy. Sensation and deep tendon reflexes should be normal. In patients with inconsistent physical examination findings and questionable secondary gain issues, the American Shoulder and Elbow Surgeons subjective shoulder scale has demonstrated acceptable psychometric performance for outcomes assessment in patients with shoulder instability, rotator cuff disease, and glenohumeral arthritis [6]. Additional scoring systems, such as the Hospital for Special Surgery score and the validated Western Ontario Osteoarthritis of the Shoulder Index, may be of clinical or research utility [7].

Functional Limitations

Any activities that require upper extremity strength, endurance, and flexibility can be affected. Most commonly, activities that require reaching overhead in external rotation are limited. These include activities of daily living (such as brushing hair or teeth, donning or doffing upper torso clothes) and activities such as throwing or reaching for items overhead. If pain is severe and constant, sleep may be interrupted, sleep-wake cycle disruption may occur, and situational reactive depression is not uncommon, especially with a shoulder pain syndrome that has exceeded 3 months [8].

Diagnostic Studies

Routine shoulder radiographs with four views (anteroposterior internal and external rotation, axillary, and scapular Y) are generally sufficient for evaluating loss of articular cartilage and glenohumeral joint space narrowing (Fig. 19.2). Varying degrees of flattening of the humeral head, marginal osteophytes, calcific tendinitis, subchondral cysts in the humeral head and glenoid, sclerotic bone, bone erosion, and humeral head migration may be seen. Specifically, if there is a chronic rotator cuff tear that is contributing to the destruction of the articular cartilage, the humeral head will be seen pressing against the undersurface of the acromion. Associated acromioclavicular joint arthritis can be seen on the anteroposterior view.

Conventional magnetic resonance imaging is the "gold standard" to assess soft tissues for rotator cuff tear; but when more sensitive evaluation of the labrum, capsule, articular cartilage, and glenohumeral ligaments is required or when a partial-thickness rotator cuff tear is suspected, magnetic resonance arthrography with intra-articular administration of contrast material may be required to visualize these subtle findings [9]. Paralabral cysts (extraneural ganglia), which can result with posterior labrocapsular complex tears and cause suprascapular nerve compression, may be visualized on magnetic resonance imaging [10].

Computed tomography may have a unique role in finding posterior humeral head subluxation relative to the glenoid in the absence of posterior glenoid erosion [11]. A rise in popularity of diagnostic ultrasonography in musculoskeletal medicine is undeniable. The modality may play a role in the diagnosis of full-thickness rotator cuff tear in experienced hands, but significant inter-rater reliability has been

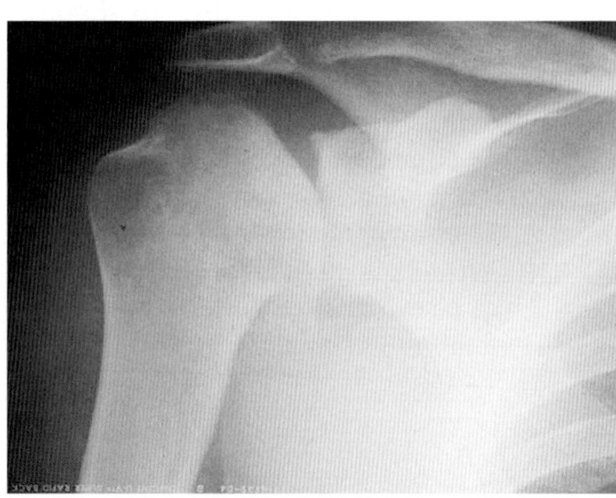

FIGURE 19.2 Radiograph typical of glenohumeral osteoarthritis.

called into question [12,13], and diagnostic ultrasonography would play a minimal role in the diagnosis of glenohumeral arthritic conditions.

Electrodiagnostic medicine consultation will help rule out idiopathic brachial plexopathy (Parsonage-Turner syndrome), cervical radiculopathy, and isolated suprascapular, dorsal scapular, or axillary neuropathy. The sensory irritative component of spinal or peripheral nerve irritation will usually yield a normal result, but H reflexes to median nerve stimulation at the level of the elbow may be suggestive of C5-C6 radiculitis, whereas findings on needle electromyography would be normal.

Complete blood counts, coagulation profile, erythrocyte sedimentation rate, and blood cultures may be in order. In addition, the author encourages that any woman with shoulder pain recalcitrant to seemingly appropriate treatment be considered for mammography.

Differential Diagnosis

Rotator cuff disease
Synovitis
Cervical osteoarthritis
Shoulder instability
Rheumatoid arthritis
Cervical radiculopathy
Labral degeneration and tear
Pseudogout
Charcot joint
Biceps tendon abnormalities
Infection
Fracture of the humerus
Adhesive capsulitis
Parsonage-Turner syndrome
Neoplasms
Leukemic arthritis
Avascular necrosis

Treatment

Initial

Shoulder arthritis is a chronic condition, but acute exacerbations in pain can be managed conservatively. Nonsteroidal anti-inflammatory drugs or analgesic medications can help with pain and enable rehabilitation. Capsaicin cream, lidocaine patches, ice, or moist heat may be used topically as needed. Gentle stretching exercises help maintain the range of motion and prevent secondary adhesive capsulitis and sequelae of immobility.

Rehabilitation

The shoulder is a complicated structure composed of several joints with both static and dynamic stabilizers that tend to function, and fail, as a unit. A well-designed rehabilitation program must take this into account and treat glenohumeral arthritic conditions within this context. The rehabilitative efforts are dedicated to the restoration of strength, endurance, and flexibility of the shoulder musculature. Supervised physical or occupational therapy should focus on the upper thoracic, neck, and scapular muscle groups but address the entire upper extremity kinetic chain, including the rotator cuff, arm, forearm, wrist, and hand. Patients benefit from aquatic therapy and can easily be taught exercises and then transitioned to an independent pool exercise program that they can continue long term. In cases of severe rheumatoid arthritis, joint-sparing static exercises may prevent atrophy and maintain strength of dynamic stabilizers of the shoulder without placing undue stress on the remaining articular surfaces. Joint-sparing exercises such as isometric contraction within normal range of motion will strengthen shoulder stabilizers, minimize joint damage, and decrease induction of the inflammatory cascade that often drives arthritic patients to seek health care. The consensus [14] on glenohumeral involvement in rheumatoid arthritis is that narrowing of the joint space is a turning point indicating a risk of rapid joint destruction, and surgical interventions should be considered before musculoskeletal sequelae are too severe to enable adequate recovery. Postoperative care, although it depends on the operative intervention, should focus on maintenance of functional range of motion and prevention of adhesive capsulitis but be balanced with avoidance of dislocation or damage to the repaired labrum. Range of motion after total shoulder arthroplasty will be considerably less than in the shoulder not operated on. Suprascapular nerve block may have a role in helping the patient tolerate postoperative therapies.

The success of flexibility exercises will be determined by the extent of mechanical bone blockade, which in turn is determined by the magnitude of glenohumeral incongruous distortion, presence of loose bodies, and osteophyte formation. Pain control can be assisted with modalities such as ultrasound and iontophoresis. Electrical stimulation may have a limited role in posterior shoulder strengthening in patients with poor posture and "rounded shoulders" on examination, but it should not take the place of volitional contraction and not be used routinely across arthritic joints. In caring for arthroplasty patients, the Neer protocol for postoperative total shoulder arthroplasty rehabilitation is widely used and based on tradition and the basic science of soft tissue and bone healing [15].

Procedures

If therapies fail or are impossible because of pain, the patient has several options. Periarticular injections may offer some help to control pain of associated problems, such as subacromial bursitis and rotator cuff tendinopathy. Wide variations exist in local anesthetic doses and techniques. On the other hand, steroid doses do not vary as widely with methylprednisolone acetate and triamcinolone acetonide, the most commonly used agents [16]. Intra-articular glenohumeral joint injections may also afford some pain relief, particularly in the early stages. The accuracy of intra-articular injections not fluoroscopically guided is less than perfect at 80%; the anterior approach is slightly more accurate than the posterior approach at 50% [17]. However, injections have not been shown to alter the underlying arthritis pathoanatomy (Fig. 19.3). Great care should be taken in anticoagulated patients. Viscosupplementation (hylan G-F 20) is not approved by the Food and Drug Administration for the glenohumeral joint, but the author has empirically seen it play a role in comprehensive care of mild osteoarthritis.

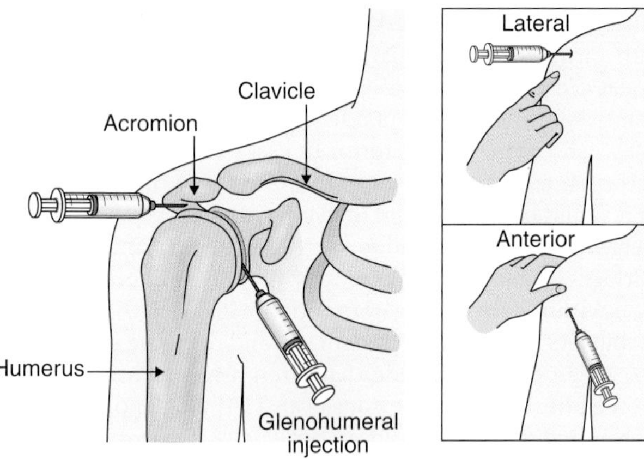

FIGURE 19.3 Approximate surface anatomy *(insets)* and internal anatomic sites for injection of the glenohumeral joint laterally and anteriorly. *(From Lennard TA. Physiatric Procedures in Clinical Practice. Philadelphia, Hanley & Belfus, 1995.)*

The initial setup can be identical for either intra-articular glenohumeral or subacromial injection. With the patient seated with the arm either in the lap or hanging down by the side, the internal rotation and gravity pull of the arm will open the space, leading to the glenohumeral joint or subacromial space. Several approaches have been described. Most commonly for a subacromial injection, the skin entry point is 1 cm inferior to the acromion, and the needle is tracked anteriorly at a lateral to medial 45-degree angle in the axial plane and slightly superior (under the acromion). The injectate should flow with minimal resistance into this potential space. If resistance is encountered, the needle should be repositioned to avoid intratendinous injection, which can increase the risk of tendon rupture. For glenohumeral injection, a more inferior and medial approach is used (Fig. 19.4).

Postinjection care includes awareness of the local anesthetic effects and avoidance of impingement or maneuvers at end range of motion. Patients are cautioned to avoid aggressive activities for the first few days after the injection. If the adhesive capsulitis component is specifically being treated, a suprascapular nerve block with 5 to 10 mL of 0.25% bupivacaine (Marcaine) with or without epinephrine can be performed immediately before therapy, with an appropriately trained therapist aware of the safe handling of such an anesthetized joint. The author typically employs a combined suprascapular and subacromial approach in these cases and coordinates follow-up appointments with occupational therapy. This should be done only with properly trained therapists who are aware of the postinjection proprioceptive loss.

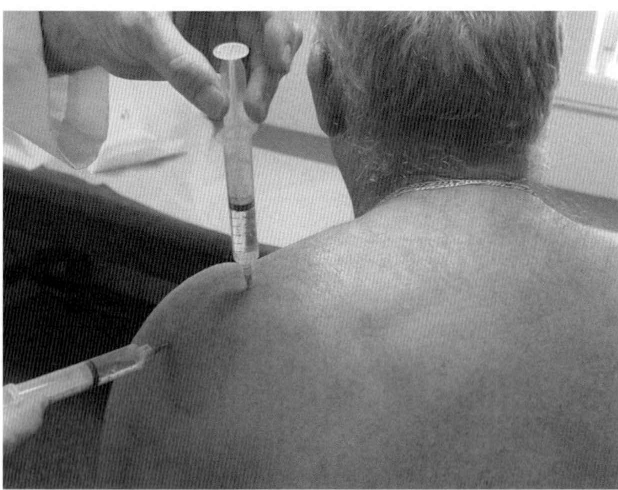

FIGURE 19.4 Combined subacromial and suprascapular injection. The site is marked for intra-articular glenohumeral injection.

Surgery

If unacceptable symptoms persist despite conservative treatment, the patient may decide to reduce his or her activity level to minimize pain or proceed with one of a number of surgical interventions. It is important to inform the patient that regardless of the treatment approach, with osteoarthritis, a return to normal shoulder function, by either rehabilitation or surgery, is not possible. However, pain control and some increased function are usually achievable.

Surgical options include débridement of the glenohumeral joint by open or arthroscopic techniques and hemiarthroplasty or total shoulder arthroplasty. If reasonable congruity between the humeral head and glenoid is present, good improvement in pain control and some functional improvement can be anticipated with débridement, even in the presence of severe chondromalacia. The glenoid may be amenable to arthroscopic resurfacing with a meniscal allograft [18]. Other biologic surfaces include anterior capsule, fascia lata autograft, Achilles tendon allograft, and cartilage-preserving arthroscopic spongioplasty [19]. However, inconsistent results and high complication rates are seen, and a trend toward arthroplasty is occurring. Other arthroscopic techniques are successful, provided osteophytes and loose bodies are removed (Fig. 19.5) [20]. Hemiarthroplasty may be indicated in the absence of advanced glenohumeral disease if the glenoid can at least be converted to a smooth concentric surface [21]. Shoulder hemiarthroplasty volumes and rates increased at annual rates of 6% to 13% from 1993 to 2007, with a revision increase from 4.5% to 7%, and procedures are predicted to increase by 192% to 322% by 2015 [22]. Hemiarthroplasty has also been suggested as the procedure of choice in moderate to severe glenohumeral arthritis and irreparable rotator cuff tears [23]; it may have other indications in avascular

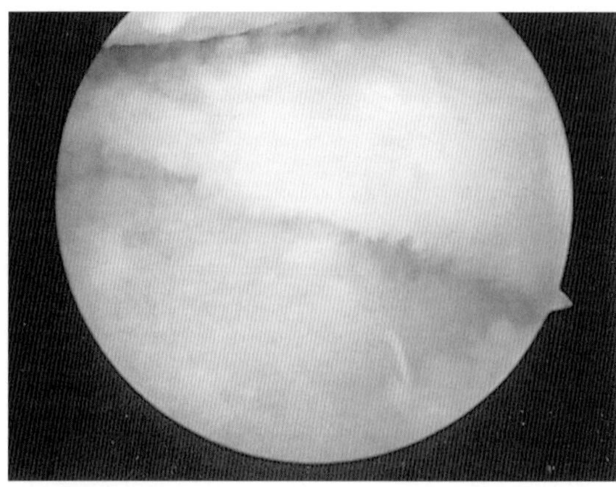

FIGURE 19.5 Arthroscopic surgical view of osteoarthritis.

necrosis, glenohumeral chondrolysis, tumor, or complete deltoid denervation with subluxation and secondary osteoarthritis [24].

If major incongruity is present between the humeral head and glenoid, total shoulder arthroplasty may be indicated [25]. There is some suggestion of better long-term outcomes when biceps tenodesis is performed concomitantly with shoulder arthroplasty [26]. Although it may seem counterintuitive, proprioception actually improves after total shoulder arthroplasty over prearthroplasty measurements [27]. This is important from the standpoint of activities of daily life in osteoarthritic patients. Most shoulders, however, can be aided arthroscopically with appropriate technique, which often necessitates a second posterior portal and a highly experienced shoulder arthroscopist [20]. Although a greater risk of more advanced glenohumeral arthritis is associated with arthroscopic procedures that result in limited external rotation [28], arthrodesis may be required for irreversible and non-reconstructible massive rotator cuff tears, tumor, and deltoid muscle denervation as well as for detachment of the deltoid from its origin or to stabilize the glenohumeral joint after many failed attempts at shoulder reconstruction [29]. Arthrodesis for failed prosthetic arthroplasty or tumor resection presents additional challenges and additional risk of the aforementioned complications. A newer procedure, thermal capsulorrhaphy, has come in and out of favor; it is usually used more in high-functioning athletes for isolated posterior instability without labral detachment rather than in isolated glenohumeral osteoarthritis [30].

Potential Disease Complications

Disease complications include chronic intractable pain and loss of shoulder range of motion. These result in diminished functional ability to use the arm, disuse weakness, difficulty with sleep, inability to perform work and recreational activities, and reactive depression. Isolated nerve injury or brachial plexopathy may result.

Potential Treatment Complications

Analgesics and nonsteroidal anti-inflammatory drugs have well-known side effects that most commonly affect the gastric, hepatic, and renal systems. Infection, hemarthrosis, and allergic reaction to the medications are rare side effects of injections. In particular, there may be an association between subdeltoid septic bursitis and concomitant systemic isotretinoin (Accutane) [31]. Fluid retention or transient hyperglycemia may be seen with a single exogenous glucocorticoid injection. Arthroscopic complications are not common, but the usual possibilities, including neurovascular issues, have been reported. Arthrodesis complications include nonunion, malposition, pain associated with prominent hardware, and periarticular fractures. Arthrodesis after cancer reconstruction has a higher risk of complication [29].

References

[1] Zuo J, Sano H, Yamamoto N, et al. Humeral head osteonecrosis in an adolescent amateur swimming athlete: a case report. Sports Med Arthrosc Rehabil Ther Tech 2012;4:39.

[2] Braune C, Rittmeister M, Engels K, Kerschbaumer F. Non-Hodgkin lymphoma (immunocytoma) of low malignancy and arthritis of the glenohumeral joint. Z Orthop Ihre Grenzgeb 2002;140:199–202 [in German].

[3] Green A, Norris TR. Shoulder arthroplasty for advanced glenohumeral arthritis after anterior instability repair. J Shoulder Elbow Surg 2001;10:539–45.

[4] Martínez Oviedo A, Gracia Sánchez P, Pueo E, Chopo JM. Septic arthritis as an initial manifestation of bacterial endocarditis caused by *Staphylococcus aureus*. An Med Interna 2006;23:184–6.

[5] Hegedus EJ, Goode AP, Cook CE, et al. Which physical examination tests provide clinicians with the most value when examining the shoulder? Update of a systematic review with meta-analysis of individual tests. Br J Sports Med 2012;46:964–78.

[6] Kocher MS, Horan MP, Briggs KK, et al. Reliability, validity and responsiveness of the American Shoulder and Elbow Surgeons subjective shoulder scale in patients with shoulder instability, rotator cuff disease and glenohumeral arthritis. J Bone Joint Surg Am 2005;87:2006–11.

[7] Wright RW, Baumgarten KM. Shoulder outcomes measures. J Am Acad Orthop Surg 2010;18:436–44.

[8] Cho CH, Jung SW, Park JY, et al. Is shoulder pain for three months or longer correlated with depression, anxiety, and sleep disturbance? J Shoulder Elbow Surg 2013;22:222–8.

[9] Chaipat L, Palmer WE. Shoulder magnetic resonance imaging. Clin Sports Med 2006;25:371–86.

[10] Spinner RJ, Amrami KK, Kliot M, et al. Suprascapular intraneural ganglia and glenohumeral joint connections. J Neurosurg 2006;104:551–7.

[11] Walch G, Ascani C, Boulahia A, et al. Static posterior subluxation of the humeral head: an unrecognized entity responsible for glenohumeral osteoarthritis in the young adult. J Shoulder Elbow Surg 2002;11:309–14.

[12] Naredo E, Miller I, Moragues C, et al. Interobserver reliability in musculoskeletal ultrasonography: results from a "Teach the Teachers" rheumatologist course. Ann Rheum Dis 2006;65:14–9.

[13] O'Connor PJ, Rankine J, Gibbon WW, et al. Interobserver variation in sonography of the painful shoulder. J Clin Ultrasound 2005;33:53–6.

[14] Thomas T, Nol E, Goupille P, et al. The rheumatoid shoulder: current consensus on diagnosis and treatment. Joint Bone Spine 2006;73:139–43.

[15] Wilcox RB, Arslanian LE, Millett P. Rehabilitation following total shoulder arthroplasty. J Orthop Sports Phys Ther 2005;35:821–36.

[16] Skedros JG, Hunt KJ, Pitts TC. Variations in corticosteroid/anesthetic injections for painful shoulder conditions: comparisons among orthopaedic surgeons, rheumatologists, and physical medicine and primary-care physicians. BMC Musculoskelet Disord 2007;8:63.

[17] Sethi PM, El Attrache N. Accuracy of intra-articular injection of the glenohumeral joint: a cadaveric study. Orthopedics 2006;29:149–52.

[18] Lee BK, Vaishnav S, Rick Hatch 3rd GF, Itamura JM. Biologic resurfacing of the glenoid with meniscal allograft: long-term results with minimum 2-year follow-up. J Shoulder Elbow Surg 2013;22:253–60.

[19] Heid A, Dickschas J, Schoeffl V. Cortisone-induced humerus head necrosis in acute myeloid leukemia: cartilage-preserving arthroscopic spongioplasty. Unfallchirurg 2013;116:180–4 [in German].

[20] Nirschl RP. Arthroscopy in the treatment of glenohumeral osteoarthritis. Presented to the Brazilian Congress of Upper Extremity Surgeons; Belo Horizonte, Brazil, Sept 29, 2000.

[21] Wirth MA, Tapscott RS, Southworth C, Rockwood CA. Treatment of glenohumeral arthritis with a hemiarthroplasty: a minimum of five-year follow-up outcome study. J Bone Joint Surg Am 2006;88:964–73.

[22] Day JS, Lau E, Ong KL, et al. Prevalence and projections of total shoulder and elbow arthroplasty in the United States to 2015. J Shoulder Elbow Surg 2010;19:1115–20.

[23] Laudicina L, D'Ambrosia R. Management of irreparable rotator cuff tears and glenohumeral arthritis. Orthopaedics 2005;28:382–8.

[24] Gartsman GM, Edwards TB. Shoulder arthroplasty. Philadelphia: WB Saunders; 2008.

[25] Schenk T, Iannotti JP. Prosthetic arthroplasty for glenohumeral arthritis with an intact or repairable rotator cuff: indications, techniques, and results. In: Iannotti J, Williams G, editors. Disorders of the shoulder: diagnosis and management. Philadelphia: Lippincott Williams & Wilkins; 1999.

[26] Fama G, Edwards TB, Boulahia A, et al. The role of concomitant biceps tenodesis in shoulder arthroplasty for primary osteoarthritis: results of a multicentric study. Orthopedics 2004;27:401–5.
[27] Cuoma F, Birdzell MG, Zuckerman JD. The effect of degenerative arthritis and prosthetic arthroplasty on shoulder proprioception. J Shoulder Elbow Surg 2005;14:345–8.
[28] Brophy RH, Marx RG. Osteoarthritis following shoulder instability. Clin Sports Med 2005;24:47–56.
[29] Safran O, Iannotti JP. Arthrodesis of the shoulder. J Am Acad Orthop Surg 2006;14:145–53.
[30] Bisson LJ. Thermal capsulorrhaphy for isolated posterior instability of the glenohumeral joint without labral detachment. Am J Sports Med 2005;33:1898–904.
[31] Drezner JA, Sennett BJ. Subacromial/subdeltoid septic bursitis associated with isotretinoin therapy and corticosteroid injection. J Am Board Fam Pract 2004;17:299–302.

CHAPTER 20

Suprascapular Neuropathy

Jason Holm, MD

Jonathan T. Finnoff, DO

Synonyms

Infraspinatus syndrome
Volleyball shoulder
Neurogenic shoulder pain
Suprascapular nerve rotator cuff compression syndrome

ICD-9 Codes

354.8 Other mononeuritis of upper limb
354.9 Mononeuritis of upper limb, unspecified

ICD-10 Codes

G56.80 Other mononeuritis of unspecified upper limb
G56.81 Other mononeuritis of right upper limb
G56.82 Other mononeuritis of left upper limb
G56.90 Unspecified mononeuritis of unspecified upper limb
G56.91 Unspecified mononeuritis of right upper limb
G56.92 Unspecified mononeuritis of left upper limb

Definition

Suprascapular neuropathy is a demyelinating or axonal injury to the suprascapular nerve. Once considered a diagnosis of exclusion, suprascapular neuropathy is now becoming a well-recognized condition stemming from traction or compression of the nerve at some point along its course. Epidemiologic data are limited, but the prevalence of suprascapular neuropathy is reportedly between 12% and 33% in overhead athletes and between 8% and 100% in patients with massive rotator cuff tears [1].

To understand the pathophysiologic mechanism, it is imperative to have a good knowledge of the anatomy (Fig. 20.1). The suprascapular nerve arises from the upper trunk of the brachial plexus and receives contributions mainly from the fifth and sixth cervical nerve roots, with variable contribution from the fourth cervical nerve root. It courses posterolaterally, deep to the trapezius and clavicle, on its way to the suprascapular notch. Here, it passes beneath the transverse scapular ligament to enter the supraspinous fossa. Within the supraspinous fossa, the suprascapular nerve sends two motor branches to the supraspinatus muscle and receives sensory branches from multiple surrounding structures, including the posterior aspect of the glenohumeral joint, the acromioclavicular joint, and the subacromial bursa. The nerve then courses inferolaterally around the lateral aspect of the scapular spine. This region is referred to as the spinoglenoid notch and is a common area of suprascapular nerve compression. Finally, the nerve enters the infraspinous fossa, where its terminal motor branches innervate the infraspinatus muscle.

The indirect course of the nerve as well as its passage through two notches makes it particularly vulnerable to injury. Static forms of compression or traction can stem from anatomic variations, particularly at the suprascapular notch, where the transverse scapular ligament can hypertrophy or ossify. At the spinoglenoid notch, compression is most frequently due to a space-occupying paralabral cyst that develops as a result of a labral tear [1].

Dynamic forms of suprascapular neuropathy are often seen in overhead athletes because of tightening of the spinoglenoid ligament during the overhead motion [2]. This leads to the so-called infraspinatus syndrome because only the infraspinatus is affected. Large rotator cuff tears can also cause a suprascapular neuropathy because the medially retracted muscle belly places a traction force on the nerve [3,4].

Less commonly, suprascapular neuropathy may result from shoulder girdle trauma or from iatrogenic injury as a complication of surgery. Three-dimensional mapping of operatively treated scapular fractures has shown extension of the fracture to the spinoglenoid notch in 22% of patients [5].

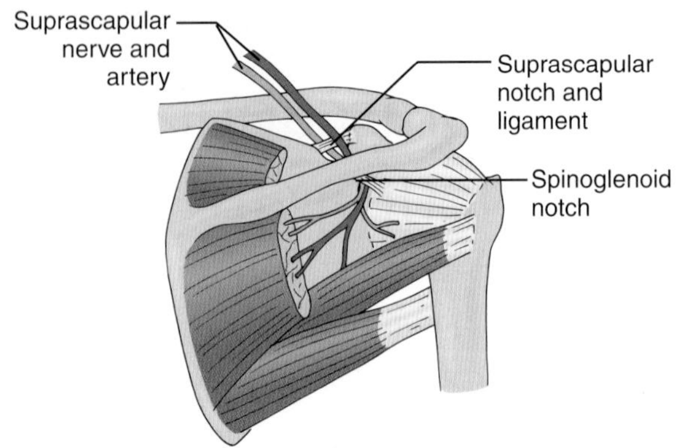

FIGURE 20.1 Posterior view of the scapula demonstrating the course of the suprascapular nerve through the suprascapular and spinoglenoid notches.

Symptoms

A range of symptoms may be associated with suprascapular neuropathy. Patients' complaints are often similar to those of patients with other pathologic processes about the shoulder, including pain, weakness, and functional impairment. Some patients, however, may present only after recognizing painless atrophy. Suprascapular neuropathy is therefore difficult to diagnose on the basis of history alone. The pain, when it is present, can be poorly localized but is often located along the posterolateral shoulder and described as a deep, dull ache. This pain pattern coincides with the diffuse sensory contribution of the suprascapular nerve, as it carries sensory afferents from up to 70% of the shoulder [6]. For nontraumatic injuries, the onset is typically insidious and night pain is variable. Although it is less common, trauma can cause suprascapular neuropathy, and in this case, symptom onset is rapid.

For athletes, overhead sport-specific motions can intensify typical pain symptoms, and a decline in throwing velocity or hitting speed may be seen. Weakness is often described as a sense of fatigue during these activities.

Physical Examination

A complete physical examination of the shoulder is critical to identify a suprascapular nerve lesion and its underlying cause. Inspection may demonstrate atrophy in the supraspinatus or infraspinatus fossa. Atrophy of the supraspinatus may be difficult to visualize, given the bulk of the overlying trapezius. Isolated atrophy of the infraspinatus suggests compression of the nerve at the spinoglenoid notch. Palpation may elicit tenderness along the course of the nerve, particularly at the level of the suprascapular notch, within the supraspinous fossa or at the spinoglenoid notch. The tenderness may be enhanced with horizontal shoulder adduction, which tightens the spinoglenoid ligament. Strength testing may demonstrate weakness in abduction or external rotation. Weakness may be subtle because of compensatory muscle action. Other special tests should be performed to evaluate for labral disease, given its association with spinoglenoid notch cysts that can compress the suprascapular nerve. The examiner should also perform a thorough upper extremity neurovascular examination and evaluate the contralateral shoulder and cervical spine.

Functional Limitations

Functional limitations will vary significantly, depending on the patient's activity level. As previously mentioned, overhead athletes may see a decrease in their pitching or throwing velocity or overhead swing speed. Strength deficits are particularly prevalent in volleyball players, up to 68% of whom have external rotation strength deficits in their hitting arm [7]. Weakness may be subtle and have limited effect on performance because of compensatory muscle action. In those patients with a proximal neuropathy affecting both the supraspinatus and infraspinatus, functional declines, especially with overhead activities, are more apparent.

Diagnostic Studies

A thorough history and physical examination can heighten suspicion for a suprascapular neuropathy and lead to the initiation of further testing. Whereas standard shoulder radiographs are most often unremarkable, a Stryker notch view can be helpful as it allows visualization of anatomic variations at the suprascapular notch. If bone variations are suspected, three-dimensional computed tomography is helpful to further delineate the anatomy and to plan interventions. Magnetic resonance imaging allows evaluation of the suprascapular nerve along its course, demonstrating points of tethering or compression. Rotator cuff edema or atrophy may be appreciated, giving a sense of the severity or chronicity of the nerve compression. Magnetic resonance arthrography is the diagnostic test of choice for labral disease and also will identify an associated spinoglenoid notch cyst. Ultrasonography can also identify rotator cuff disease and paralabral cysts.

Electrodiagnostic studies are the "gold standard" test for confirming the diagnosis of suprascapular neuropathy and grading the injury severity. A demyelinating injury is suggested by a prolonged distal motor latency with stimulation at Erb point and recording over the supraspinatus or infraspinatus. The presence of fibrillation potentials, positive sharp waves, increased motor unit amplitude or duration and polyphasia, and decreased recruitment pattern on needle electromyography suggest the presence of an axonal injury [8].

A diagnostic suprascapular nerve block can also assist with diagnosis of this disorder. The nerve block should be performed with ultrasound or fluoroscopic guidance to ensure accuracy. Temporary resolution of the patient's symptoms in response to a suprascapular nerve block confirms the diagnosis of suprascapular neuropathy.

Differential Diagnosis

Rotator cuff tendinopathy or tear
Cervical radiculopathy
Cervical disc degeneration
Brachial plexopathy
Subacromial impingement
Labral disease
Parsonage-Turner syndrome

Treatment

Initial

An appropriate workup to accurately determine the cause and location of the suprascapular nerve injury is imperative as treatment strategies will vary according to the precise location and cause of the pathologic process. In the absence of an identified space-occupying lesion, such as a paralabral cyst, the first line of treatment is nonoperative. Patients should be instructed to avoid repetitive overhead activities or other exacerbating arm positions. Nonsteroidal anti-inflammatory drugs or acetaminophen can be used for pain relief. As with most shoulder-related disease, physical therapy plays an important role in nonoperative management.

Rehabilitation

Physical therapy has been demonstrated to be particularly effective when injury to the nerve is the result of a dynamic process, such as in overhead athletes. Ferretti and coworkers successfully treated 35 of 38 (92%) competitive volleyball players with isolated atrophy of the infraspinatus, and although the atrophy remained unchanged at long-term follow-up, the patients were asymptomatic [9]. Early rehabilitation should focus on flexibility of the scapular protractors and elevators, such as the pectoralis minor and superior belly of the trapezius. Strengthening should include the scapular stabilizers, with particular attention to the rhomboideus major and minor, inferior and middle bellies of the trapezius, and serratus anterior. The rotator cuff should also be strengthened, with a focus on the external rotators. Proprioceptive exercises improve shoulder stability and neuromuscular control. The exercise program should initially avoid positions of abduction and external rotation and gradually progress to exercises that enter this range of motion as the patient's symptoms resolve. The final phase of rehabilitation should incorporate sports-specific training in preparation for return to sports. On completion of the final phase of supervised rehabilitation, the patient should be transitioned to a home exercise program to maintain the therapeutic gains.

Procedures

Procedures for management of suprascapular neuropathy typically serve a diagnostic purpose or provide temporary palliation. Suprascapular nerve blocks, as previously mentioned, can help localize the pain source. The suprascapular nerve can be blocked at the suprascapular notch or spinoglenoid notch. Because of the deep location and sensitive nature of the suprascapular nerve, image guidance (e.g., fluoroscopy or ultrasound) should be used in performing a suprascapular nerve block.

If a patient has a paralabral cyst causing suprascapular nerve compression in the spinoglenoid notch, an ultrasound-guided spinoglenoid notch cyst aspiration can be performed. However, this procedure frequently provides only temporary relief as the underlying pathologic change leading to the cyst (i.e., glenoid labral tear) is not addressed by this procedure [10]. Patients with chronic shoulder pain refractory to other treatments may respond to radiofrequency ablation of the suprascapular nerve.

Surgery

In the setting of failed nonoperative management, surgical intervention has been shown to provide effective pain relief and restoration of function in most patients [11]. Optimal surgical timing and approach are ongoing areas of debate. The goal of surgery is direct or indirect decompression of the nerve. For isolated suprascapular neuropathy, direct decompression can be achieved through open or arthroscopic means. The nerve is released at the suprascapular or spinoglenoid notch, depending on the cause. Some authors have advocated for routine release of both the transverse scapular ligament and spinoglenoid ligament to optimize the likelihood of a full neurologic recovery [12,13]. When underlying disease, such as a paralabral cyst or rotator cuff tear, is present, debate exists as to whether indirect decompression through addressing the primary pathologic process is sufficient to alleviate the neuropathy or whether concomitant direct nerve decompression is also necessary [1,12,13]. Further research is required to answer this question.

Potential Disease Complications

Ongoing compression of the suprascapular nerve could lead to permanent muscle weakness and progressive shoulder dysfunction that is usually not reversible when atrophy is significant. Given the role of the supraspinatus and infraspinatus in stabilizing the humeral head within the glenoid, one could speculate that rotator cuff arthropathy would be the end-result of long-term suprascapular neuropathy. It has been suggested that earlier surgical decompression may improve the likelihood for restoration of full muscle strength and normalization of shoulder function [11].

Potential Treatment Complications

Patients who are treated with mild oral analgesics such as acetaminophen and nonsteroidal anti-inflammatory drugs are at risk for complications associated with these medications, such as liver or renal toxicity and peptic ulcer disease. Suprascapular nerve blocks can result in direct trauma to the suprascapular nerve. The complex anatomy of the suprascapular nerve places it at risk for injury during any surgical approach. Injuries can include nerve traction and nerve laceration. Ongoing pain, continued muscle atrophy, or recurrence can occur despite attempts at treatment.

References

[1] Freehill MT, Shi LL, Tompson JD, et al. Suprascapular neuropathy: diagnosis and management. Phys Sportsmed 2012;40:72–83.
[2] Plancher KD, Luke TA, Peterson RK, et al. Posterior shoulder pain: a dynamic study of the spinoglenoid ligament and treatment with arthroscopic release of the scapular tunnel. Arthroscopy 2007;23:991–8.
[3] Albritton MJ, Graham RD, Richards RS, et al. An anatomic study of the effects on the suprascapular nerve due to retraction of the supraspinatus muscle after a rotator cuff tear. J Shoulder Elbow Surg 2003;12:497–500.
[4] Massimini DF, Singh A, Wells JH, et al. Suprascapular nerve anatomy during shoulder motion: a cadaveric proof of concept study with implications for neurogenic shoulder pain. J Shoulder Elbow Surg 2013;22:463–70.
[5] Armitage BM, Wijdicks CA, Tarkin IS, et al. Mapping of scapular fractures with three-dimensional computed tomography. J Bone Joint Surg Am 2009;91:2222–8.

[6] Brown DE, James DC, Roy S, et al. Pain relief by suprascapular nerve block in glenohumeral arthritis. Scand J Rheumatol 1988;17:411–5.
[7] Lajtai G, Wieser K, Ofner M, et al. Electromyography and nerve conduction velocity for the evaluation of the infraspinatus muscle and the suprascapular nerve in professional beach volleyball players. Am J Sports Med 2012;40:2303–8.
[8] Buschbacher RM, Weir SK, Bentley JG, et al. Normal motor nerve conduction studies using surface electrode recording from the supraspinatus, infraspinatus, deltoid, and biceps. PM R 2009;1:101–6.
[9] Ferretti A, De Carli A, Fontana M. Injury of the suprascapular nerve at the spinoglenoid notch: the natural history of infraspinatus atrophy in volleyball players. Am J Sports Med 1998;26:759–63.
[10] Bathia N, Malanga G. Ultrasound-guided aspiration and corticosteroid injection in the management of a paralabral ganglion cyst. PM R 2009;1:1041–4.
[11] Shah AA, Butler RB, Sung SY, et al. Clinical outcomes of suprascapular nerve decompression. J Shoulder Elbow Surg 2011;20:975–82.
[12] Sandow MJ, Hie J. Suprascapular nerve rotator cuff compression syndrome in volleyball players. J Shoulder Elbow Surg 1998;7:516–21.
[13] Moen TC, Babatunde OM, Hsu SH, et al. Suprascapular neuropathy: what does the literature show? J Shoulder Elbow Surg 2012;21:835–46.

SECTION III
Elbow and Forearm

CHAPTER 21

Elbow Arthritis

Charles Cassidy, MD
Chien Chow, MD

Synonyms

Rheumatoid elbow
Primary degenerative arthritis
Osteoarthritis of the elbow

ICD-9 Codes

714.12	**Rheumatoid arthritis of the elbow**
715.12.1	**Osteoarthritis, primary, of the elbow**
715.22	**Osteoarthritis, secondary, of the elbow**
716.12	**Traumatic arthritis of the elbow**

ICD-10 Codes

M06.821	**Rheumatoid arthritis, right elbow**
M06.822	**Rheumatoid arthritis, left elbow**
M06.829	**Rheumatoid arthritis, unspecified elbow**
M19.021	**Primary osteoarthritis, right elbow**
M19.022	**Primary osteoarthritis, left elbow**
M19.029	**Primary osteoarthritis, unspecified elbow**
M19.221	**Secondary osteoarthritis, right elbow**
M19.222	**Secondary osteoarthritis, left elbow**
M19.229	**Secondary osteoarthritis, unspecified elbow**
M12.521	**Traumatic arthropathy, right elbow**
M12.522	**Traumatic arthropathy, left elbow**
M12.529	**Traumatic arthropathy, unspecified elbow**

Definition

In the simplest of terms, arthritis of the elbow reflects a loss of articular cartilage in the ulnotrochlear and radiocapitellar articulations. Destruction of the articulating surfaces and bone loss or, alternatively, excess bone formation in the form of osteophytes can be present. Joint contractures are common. Joint instability can result from inflammatory or traumatic injury to the bone architecture, capsule, and ligaments. The spectrum of disease ranges from intermittent pain or loss of motion with minimal changes detectable on radiographs to the more advanced stages of arthritis with a limited, painful arc of motion and radiographic demonstration of osteophyte formation, cysts, and loss of joint space. Ultimately, these destructive processes may result in complete ankylosis or total instability of the elbow.

The major causes of elbow arthritis are the inflammatory arthropathies, of which rheumatoid arthritis is the predominant disease. Arthritis of the elbow eventually develops in approximately 20% to 50% of patients with rheumatoid arthritis [1]. Involvement of the elbow in juvenile rheumatoid arthritis is not uncommon. Other inflammatory conditions affecting the elbow joint are systemic lupus erythematosus, the seronegative spondyloarthropathies (ankylosing spondylitis, psoriatic arthritis, Reiter syndrome, and enteropathic arthritis), and crystalline arthritis (gout and pseudogout). Post-traumatic arthritis may result from intra-articular fractures of the elbow. Osteonecrosis of the capitellum or trochlea, leading to arthritis, has also been described [2,3]. Primary osteoarthritis of the elbow is a rare condition, responsible for less than 5% of elbow arthritis [4]. Interestingly, the incidence is significantly higher in the Alaskan Eskimo and Japanese populations [5]. Primary elbow arthritis usually affects the dominant arm of men in their 50s. Repetitive, strenuous arm use appears to be a risk factor; primary elbow arthritis has been reported in heavy laborers, weightlifters, and throwing athletes. Synovial chondromatosis is another rare cause of elbow arthritis [3].

Symptoms

The symptoms of elbow arthritis reflect, in part, the underlying etiology and severity of the disease process. Regardless of the etiology, however, the inability to fully straighten (extend) the elbow is a nearly universal complaint of patients with elbow arthritis. Associated symptoms of cubital tunnel syndrome (ulnar neuropathy at the elbow) include numbness in the ring and small fingers, loss of hand dexterity, and aching pain along the ulnar aspect of the forearm. Cubital tunnel syndrome is neither uncommon nor unexpected, given the proximity of the ulnar nerve to the elbow joint (see Chapter 27).

Patients with early rheumatoid involvement complain of a swollen, painful joint with morning stiffness. Progressive loss of motion or instability is seen in later stages. Compression of the posterior interosseous nerve by rheumatoid synovitis can occasionally produce the inability to extend the fingers.

Patients with crystalline arthritis of the elbow may complain of severe pain, swelling, and limited motion; an expedient evaluation is warranted to rule out a septic elbow in such cases.

Post-traumatic or idiopathic arthritis of the elbow, in contrast, usually is manifested with painful loss of motion without the significant effusions, warmth, or constant pain associated with an inflamed synovium. These patients usually complain of pain at the extremes of motion secondary to osteophyte impingement, and they typically have more trouble extending the elbow than flexing it. Pain throughout the arc of motion implies advanced arthritis. The final stages of arthritis, irrespective of cause, can include complaints of severe pain and decreased motion that hinder activities of daily living as well as the cosmetic deformity of the flexed elbow posture.

Physical Examination

Physical examination findings vary according to the cause and stage of the elbow arthritis. A flexion contracture is almost always present. The range of motion should be monitored at the initial examination and at subsequent follow-up examinations.

Normal adult elbow range of motion in extension-flexion is from 0 degrees to about 150 degrees; pronation averages 75 degrees, and supination averages 85 degrees. A functional range of motion is considered to be 30 to 130 degrees, with 50 degrees of both pronation and supination [6].

All other joints should be assessed as well. Strength should be normal but may be impaired in long-standing elbow arthritis because of disuse or, in more acute cases, pain. Weakness may also be noted in the presence of associated neuropathies. In the absence of associated neuropathies, deep tendon reflexes and sensation should be normal.

Associated ulnar nerve irritation can produce a sensitive nerve with the presence of Tinel sign over the cubital tunnel, diminished sensation in the small finger and ulnar half of the ring finger, and weakness of the intrinsic muscles (see Chapter 27). Numbness provoked by acute flexion of the elbow for 30 to 60 seconds is a positive elbow flexion test result.

Effusions, synovial thickenings, and erythema are commonly noted in the inflammatory arthropathies during acute flares. Loss of motion in flexion and extension as well as in pronation and supination can be present because the synovitis affects all articulating surfaces in the elbow. Pain, limited motion, and crepitus worsen as the disease progresses. On occasion, rheumatoid destruction of the elbow will produce instability, which may be perceived by the patient as weakness or mechanical symptoms. Examination of such elbows will demonstrate laxity to varus and valgus stress; posterior instability may also be seen.

In contrast, progressive primary or post-traumatic arthritis of the elbow results in stiffness. The loss of extension is usually worse than the loss of flexion. Pain is present with forced extension or flexion. Crepitus may be palpable throughout the arc of flexion-extension or with forearm rotation.

Functional Limitations

The elbow functions to position the hand in space. Significant loss of extension can hinder an individual's ability to interact with the environment, making activities that require nearly full extension, like carrying groceries or briefcases, painful. Significant loss of flexion can interfere with activities of daily living such as eating, shaving, and washing. A normal shoulder can compensate well for a lack of pronation, whereas a normal shoulder, wrist, and cervical spine can compensate, albeit awkwardly, for a lack of full elbow flexion. There is no simple solution for a significant lack of elbow extension; the body must be moved closer to the desired object. Compensatory mechanisms are often impaired in patients with rheumatoid arthritis, magnifying the impact of the elbow arthritis on function.

Diagnostic Studies

Anteroposterior, lateral, and oblique radiographic views of the elbow are usually sufficient for diagnosis of elbow arthritis. The radiographs should be inspected for joint space narrowing, osteophyte and cyst formation, and bone destruction. For the rheumatoid patient, the Mayo Clinic radiographic classification of rheumatoid involvement is useful (Table 21.1) [7]. Dramatic loss of bone is evident as the disease progresses (Fig. 21.1). This pattern of destruction is not seen, however, in the post-traumatic or idiopathic patient. Radiographic features in these patients include spurs or osteophytes on the coronoid and olecranon, loose bodies, and narrowing of the coronoid and olecranon fossae (Fig. 21.2).

Magnetic resonance arthrography or computed tomographic arthrography may help localize suspected loose bodies. Magnetic resonance imaging is most valuable for confirmation of suspected osteonecrosis.

Table 21.1 Radiographic Classification of Rheumatoid Arthritis [7]

I	Synovitis with a normal-appearing joint
II	Loss of joint space but maintenance of the subchondral architecture
IIIa	Alteration of the subchondral architecture
IIIb	Alteration of the architecture with deformity
IV	Gross deformity

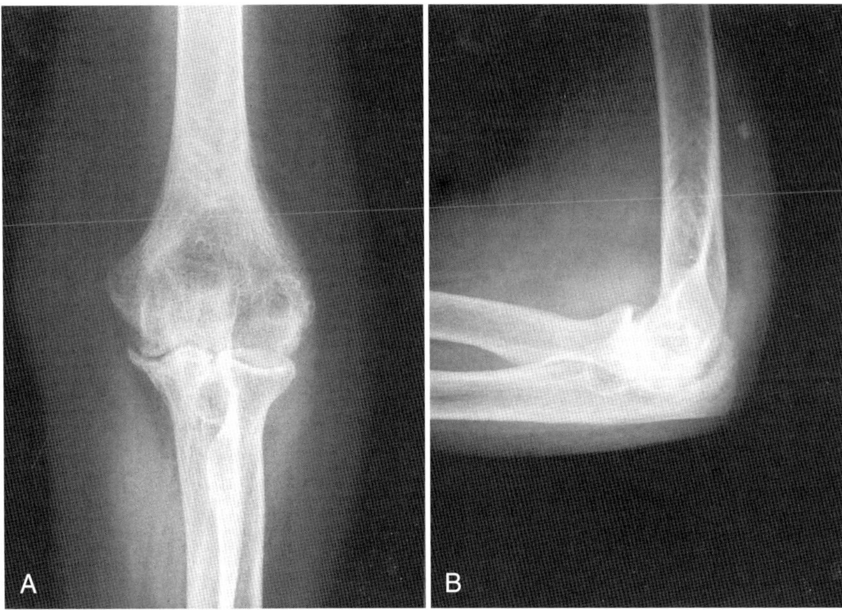

FIGURE 21.1 Rheumatoid arthritis. Anteroposterior (**A**) and lateral (**B**) elbow radiographs of a 40-year-old woman with long-standing elbow pain. Osteopenia and symmetric joint space narrowing are present. The lateral radiograph demonstrates early bone loss in the ulna. This is categorized as stage IIIa.

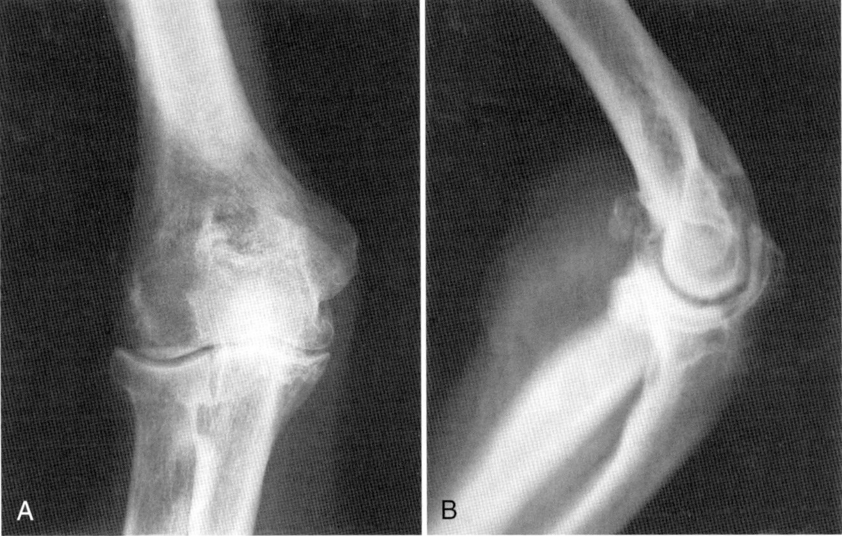

FIGURE 21.2 Primary degenerative elbow arthritis. Anteroposterior (**A**) and lateral (**B**) elbow radiographs of a 52-year-old man with dominant right elbow pain at the extremes of motion. **A,** Joint space narrowing and obliteration of the coronoid fossa. **B,** Coronoid and olecranon spurs and a large anterior loose body are evident.

The diagnosis of rheumatoid arthritis will have already been made in the majority of patients who present with rheumatoid elbow involvement. When isolated inflammatory arthritis of the elbow is suspected, appropriate serologic studies may include analysis of rheumatoid factor, antinuclear antibody, HLA-B27, and erythrocyte sedimentation rate. Elbow aspiration may be needed to rule out a crystalline or infectious cause in patients who present with a warm, stiff, swollen, and painful joint with no history of trauma or inflammatory arthritis.

Differential Diagnosis

Medial or lateral epicondylitis
Median nerve compression
Elbow instability
Radial tunnel syndrome
Septic arthritis
Cervical radiculopathy
Acute fracture
Elbow contracture
Cubital tunnel syndrome

Treatment

Initial

Treatment of elbow arthritis depends on the diagnosis, degree of involvement, functional limitations, and pain. When the elbow is one of a number of joints actively involved with inflammatory arthritis, the obvious treatment is systemic. Disease-modifying agents have had a dramatic effect in relieving symptoms and retarding the progression of arthritis for many of these patients. For systemic disease, a rheumatology consultation can be beneficial.

The initial local treatment of an acutely inflamed elbow joint includes rest. A simple sling places the elbow in a relatively comfortable position. The patient should be encouraged to remove the sling for gentle range of motion exercises of the elbow and shoulder several times daily. Icing of the elbow for 15 minutes several times a day for the first few days may be beneficial.

Nonoperative treatment of primary osteoarthritis of the elbow primarily consists of rest, activity modification, and nonsteroidal anti-inflammatory drugs. Oral analgesics may help with pain control. Topical treatments such as capsaicin can be tried as well.

Patients who have associated cubital tunnel symptoms are instructed to avoid direct pressure over the elbow and to avoid prolonged elbow flexion. A static night splint that maintains the elbow in about 30 degrees of flexion may help alleviate cubital tunnel symptoms (see Chapter 27).

Rehabilitation

Once the acute inflammation has subsided, physical or occupational therapy may be instituted to regain elbow motion and strength and to educate the patient in activity modification and pain control measures.

Therapy should focus on improving range of motion and strength throughout the upper body with a goal of improving function regardless of the degree of elbow arthritis. Adaptive equipment, such as reachers, can be recommended. Ergonomic workstation equipment may also be useful (e.g., voice-activated computer software, forearm rests).

Modalities such as ultrasound and iontophoresis may help with pain control.

Nighttime static, static-progressive, or dynamic extension splinting may be indicated to relieve significant elbow contractures. Braces may be effective in the setting of instability. The goal of therapy is *functional* rather than full elbow motion.

In primary osteoarthritis of the elbow, corrective splinting is not indicated because bone impingement is usually present. Similarly, therapy may actually aggravate the symptoms and should be ordered judiciously.

Rehabilitation is critical to the success of surgical procedures around the elbow. The rheumatoid patient commonly has multiple joint problems that must not be neglected during treatment of the elbow. The shoulder is at particular risk for stiffness. A good operation, a motivated patient, and a knowledgeable and skillful therapist are necessary to optimize postoperative results. Postoperative rehabilitation depends on the procedure and the surgeon's preference. However, in general, physical or occupational therapy should be recommended to restore range of motion and strength.

Procedures

For recalcitrant symptoms, intra-articular steroid injections are effective in relieving the pain associated with synovitis (Fig. 21.3).

The elbow joint is best accessed through the "soft spot," the center of the triangle formed by the lateral epicondyle, the tip of the olecranon, and the radial head. The patient is placed with the elbow between 50 and 90 degrees of flexion. For the posterolateral approach, the lateral epicondyle and the posterior olecranon are palpated. Under sterile conditions, with use of a 25-gauge, 1½-inch needle, 3 to 4 mL of an anesthetic-corticosteroid mixture (e.g., 1 mL of 80 mg/mL methylprednisolone and 3 mL of 1% lidocaine) is injected. The needle is directed proximally toward the head of the radius and medially into the elbow joint. No resistance should be noted as the needle enters the joint. If an effusion is present, aspiration may be done before the anesthetic-corticosteroid mixture is injected.

For the posterior approach, the olecranon fossa is palpated just proximal to the tip of the olecranon. The needle is then inserted above the superior aspect of and lateral to the olecranon. Again, it should enter the joint without resistance.

Postinjection care may include icing of the elbow for 10 to 20 minutes after the injection and then two or three times daily thereafter. The patient should be informed that the pain may worsen for the first 24 to 36 hours and that the medication may take 1 week to work.

In general, repeated injections are not recommended. Although the intra-articular steroids are effective in treating synovitis, they also temporarily inhibit chondrocyte synthesis, an effect that could potentially accelerate arthritis.

Surgery

Patients who have failed to respond to treatment after 3 to 6 months of adequate medical therapy are potential candidates for surgery. Refractory pain is the best indication for surgery. In assessment of the surgical candidate with primary elbow arthritis, it is important to listen carefully to the patient's complaints. Many patients are dissatisfied with the simple fact that they cannot fully straighten the elbow. Such patients will not be fully satisfied with surgery.

Intermittent locking or catching, suggestive of a loose body, is often best treated with arthroscopy. Pain at the extremes of motion is consistent with olecranon and coronoid osteophyte impingement. An ulnohumeral arthroplasty, or surgical débridement of the elbow joint, may be recommended. Traditionally, open surgical techniques have been performed to remove impinging osteophytes. More recent arthroscopic advances have permitted this débridement to be performed in a less invasive manner, with potentially less morbidity. However, arthroscopic treatment of elbow contractures is a technically demanding procedure [8]. Ulnohumeral arthroplasty is successful at achieving its principal goal—pain relief at the extremes of motion. However, it is only marginally successful at actually improving motion, with an average improvement in extension of 7 to 12 degrees and an average improvement in flexion of 8 to 17 degrees in

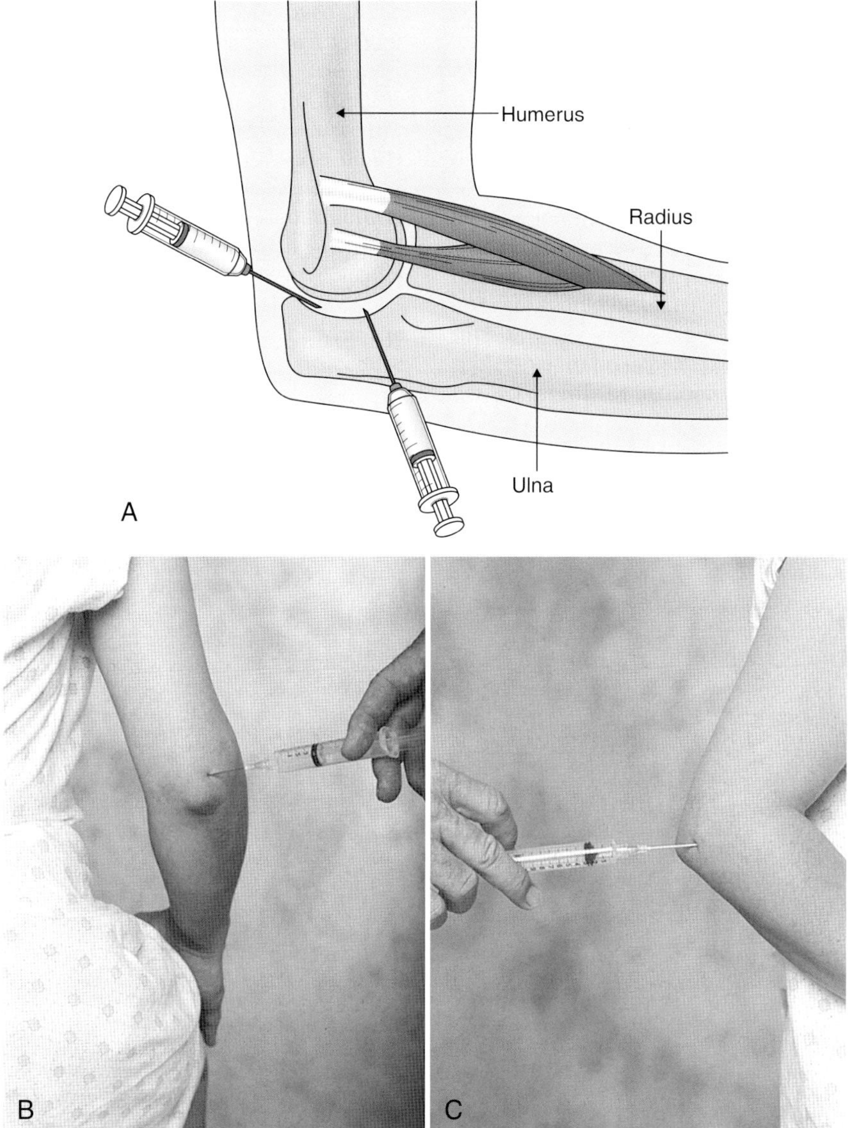

FIGURE 21.3 Internal anatomic (**A**) and approximate surface anatomic (**B**, lateral; **C**, posterior) sites for injection of the elbow laterally and posteriorly. *(From Lennard TA. Pain Procedures in Clinical Practice, 2nd ed. Philadelphia, Hanley & Belfus, 2000.)*

four reported series [4,9–11]. Overall, 85% of patients in these series were satisfied with the results. As expected, the results deteriorate with time as the arthritis progresses.

Less commonly, patients with primary arthritis complain of pain throughout the arc of motion. Their radiographs will probably demonstrate advanced arthritis with severe joint space narrowing. Simple removal of the osteophytes is not likely to be successful. Total elbow arthroplasty would seem to be a reasonable option. However, unlike their rheumatoid counterparts, most of these patients are otherwise healthy, vigorous people who would regularly stress their joint replacement. For this reason, total elbow arthroplasty in this setting is best reserved for the sedentary patient older than 65 years [12].

For the younger patient with advanced primary arthritis, a distraction interposition arthroplasty is recommended [13–15]. This procedure involves a radical débridement of the joint followed by a resurfacing of the joint surfaces with an interposition material, such as autologous fascia lata or allograft Achilles tendon. A hinged external fixator is then applied, which will protect the healing interposition material while simultaneously maintaining elbow stability and permitting motion. In the one relatively large series of distraction interposition arthroplasty [15], pain relief was satisfactory in 69% of patients at an average of 5 years postoperatively. An advantage of interposition arthroplasty is the potential for conversion to total elbow arthroplasty, ideally after the age of 60 years [16], but this procedure certainly does not produce a normal elbow.

Other nonimplant surgical options include elbow arthrodesis and resection arthroplasty. There is no ideal position for an elbow fusion. The elbow looks more cosmetically appealing when it is relatively straight. However, this position is relatively useless. Consequently, elbow arthrodesis is performed rarely, usually in the setting of intractable infection. Resection arthroplasty is an option for a failed total elbow arthroplasty. This procedure permits some elbow motion, although the elbow tends to be very unstable.

For the rheumatoid patient with elbow arthritis, elbow synovectomy and débridement provide predictable short-term pain relief [17]. Interestingly, the results do not necessarily correlate with the severity of the arthritis. The results do, however, deteriorate somewhat over time, drifting down from 90% success at 3 years to 70% success by 10 years as the synovitis recurs [18–20]. Elbow motion is not necessarily improved by synovectomy; only 40% of patients obtain better motion. A study comparing arthroscopic and open synovectomy demonstrated equivalent results with either technique if the preoperative arc of flexion is greater than 90 degrees [19]. For stiff rheumatoid elbows, arthroscopic synovectomy performed better than the open method did.

Total elbow arthroplasty is a reliable procedure for the rheumatoid patient with advanced elbow arthritis [21,22]. The Mayo Clinic has reported excellent results with a semi-constrained prosthesis [23], with pain relief in 92% of patients and an average arc of motion of 26 to 130 degrees, with 64 degrees of pronation and 62 degrees of supination. An outcomes study demonstrated good satisfaction of the patients, although the majority of patients continued to have some functional impairments, presumably due, in part, to rheumatoid involvement in other joints [24]. In spite of the excellent clinical results, the patient should be made aware that the complication rate for total elbow arthroplasty is significantly higher than that for the more conventional hip and knee replacements.

Potential Disease Complications

End-stage rheumatoid arthritis of the elbow can produce either severe stiffness or instability. Advanced primary arthritis invariably produces stiffness. Either outcome results in pain and limited function of the involved extremity. In addition, entrapment or traction neuritis of the ulnar nerve is not uncommon. Compressive injury to the posterior interosseous nerve from rheumatoid synovial hyperplasia has also been reported.

Potential Treatment Complications

The systemic complications of the disease-modifying agents used in treatment of rheumatoid arthritis are numerous and are beyond the scope of this chapter (see Chapters 34 and 41). Analgesics and nonsteroidal anti-inflammatory drugs have well-known side effects that most commonly affect the gastric, hepatic, and renal systems. Intra-articular steroid injections introduce the risk of iatrogenic infection and may produce transient chondrocyte damage.

Potential surgical complications include infection, wound problems, neurovascular injury, stiffness, recurrent synovitis, triceps disruption, periprosthetic lucency, fracture, and iatrogenic instability. In the primary and post-traumatic osteoarthritic elbow, motion-improving procedures such as ulnohumeral arthroplasty do not halt the inevitable radiographic progression of the disease. Similarly, synovectomy of the rheumatoid elbow, even if it is successful in alleviating pain and synovitis, does not reliably prevent further joint destruction. Preoperative ulnar nerve symptoms can occasionally be made worse by surgery, and simultaneous ulnar nerve transposition should be considered in such patients when the preoperative range of motion is limited [11]. In an analysis of 473 consecutive elbow arthroscopies, major and temporary minor complications occurred in 0.8% and 11% of patients, respectively [8]. The most significant risk factors for development of temporary nerve palsies were rheumatoid arthritis and contracture.

With total elbow arthroplasty, wound healing problems, infection, triceps insufficiency, and implant loosening are the principal complications, occurring in approximately 5% to 7% of patients. As a result, most surgeons place lifelong restrictions on high-impact loading (no golf, no lifting of more than 10 pounds) to minimize the need for revision surgery.

References

[1] Porter BB, Park N, Richardson C, Vainio K. Rheumatoid arthritis of the elbow: the results of synovectomy. J Bone Joint Surg Br 1974;56:427–37.
[2] Le TB, Mont MA, Jones LC, et al. Atraumatic osteonecrosis of the adult elbow. Clin Orthop 2000;373:141–5.
[3] Gramstad GD, Galatz LM. Management of elbow osteoarthritis. J Bone Joint Surg Am 2006;88:421–30.
[4] Morrey BF. Primary degenerative arthritis of the elbow: treatment by ulnohumeral arthroplasty. J Bone Joint Surg Br 1992;74:409–13.
[5] Ortner DJ. Description and classification of degenerative bone changes in the distal joint surface of the humerus. Am J Phys Anthropol 1968;28:139–55.
[6] Morrey BF, Askew L, An KN, et al. A biomechanical study of normal functional elbow motion. J Bone Joint Surg Am 1981;63:872–7.
[7] Morrey BF, Adams RA. Semi-constrained arthroplasty for the treatment of rheumatoid arthritis of the elbow. J Bone Joint Surg Am 1992;74:479–90.
[8] Kelly EW, Morrey BF, O'Driscoll SW. Complications of elbow arthroscopy. J Bone Joint Surg Am 2001;83:25–34.
[9] Oka Y. Debridement arthroplasty for osteoarthrosis of the elbow. Acta Orthop Scand 2000;71:185–90.
[10] Wada T, Isogai S, Ishii S, Yamashita T. Debridement arthroplasty for primary osteoarthritis of the elbow. J Bone Joint Surg Am 2004;86:233–41.
[11] Antuña SA, Morrey BF, Adams RA, O'Driscoll SW. Ulnohumeral arthroplasty for primary degenerative arthritis of the elbow. J Bone Joint Surg Am 2002;84:2168–73.
[12] Moro JK, King GJ. Total elbow arthroplasty in the treatment of posttraumatic conditions of the elbow. Clin Orthop Relat Res 2000;370:102–14.
[13] Gramstad GD, King GJ, O'Driscoll SW, Yamaguchi K. Elbow arthroplasty using a convertible implant. Tech Hand Up Extrem Surg 2005;9:153–63.
[14] Wright PE, Froimson AI, Morrey BF. Interposition arthroplasty of the elbow. In: Morrey BF, editor. The elbow and its disorders. 3rd ed. Philadelphia: WB Saunders; 2000. p. 718–30.
[15] Cheng SL, Morrey BF. Treatment of the mobile, painful, arthritic elbow by distraction interposition arthroplasty. J Bone Joint Surg Br 2000;82:223–8.
[16] Blaine TA, Adams R, Morrey BF. Total elbow arthroplasty after interposition arthroplasty for elbow arthritis. J Bone Joint Surg Am 2005;87:286–92.
[17] Ferlic DC, Patchett CE, Clayton ML, Freeman AC. Elbow synovectomy in rheumatoid arthritis. Clin Orthop 1987;220:119–25.
[18] Alexiades MM, Stanwyck TS, Figgie MP, Inglis AE. Minimum ten-year follow-up of elbow synovectomy for rheumatoid arthritis. Orthop Trans 1990;14:255.
[19] Tanaka N, Sakahashi H, Hirose K, et al. Arthroscopic and open synovectomy of the elbow in rheumatoid arthritis. J Bone Joint Surg Am 2006;88:521–5.
[20] Horiuchi K, Momohara S, Tomatsu T, et al. Arthroscopic synovectomy of the elbow in rheumatoid arthritis. J Bone Joint Surg Am 2002;84:342–7.
[21] Hargreaves D, Emery R. Total elbow replacement in the treatment of rheumatoid disease. Clin Orthop Relat Res 1999;366:61–71.
[22] Ferlic DC. Total elbow arthroplasty for treatment of elbow arthritis. J Shoulder Elbow Surg 1999;8:367–78.
[23] Gill DR, Morrey BF. The Coonrad-Morrey total elbow arthroplasty in patients with rheumatoid arthritis: a 10- to 15-year follow-up study. J Bone Joint Surg Am 1998;80:1327–35.
[24] Angst F, John M, Pap G, et al. Comprehensive assessment of clinical outcome and quality of life after total elbow arthroplasty. Arthritis Rheum 2005;53:73–82.

CHAPTER 22

Lateral Epicondylitis

Lyn D. Weiss, MD
Jay M. Weiss, MD

Synonyms

Tendinosis [1]
Lateral epicondylitis
Tennis elbow

ICD-9 Code

726.32 Lateral epicondylitis

ICD-10 Codes

M77.10 Lateral epicondylitis, unspecified elbow
M77.11 Lateral epicondylitis, right elbow
M77.12 Lateral epicondylitis, left elbow

Definition

Epicondylitis is a general term used to describe inflammation, pain, or tenderness in the region of the medial or lateral epicondyle of the humerus. The actual nidus of pain and pathologic change has been debated. Lateral epicondylitis implies an inflammatory lesion with degeneration at the tendinous origin of the extensor muscles (the lateral epicondyle of the humerus). The tendon of the extensor carpi radialis brevis muscle is primarily affected. Other muscles that can contribute to the condition are the extensor carpi radialis longus and the extensor digitorum communis.

Although the term *epicondylitis* implies an inflammatory process, inflammatory cells are not identified histologically. Instead, the condition may be secondary to failure of the musculotendinous attachment with resultant fibroplasia [2], termed tendinosis. Other postulated primary lesions include angiofibroblastic tendinosis, periostitis, and enthesitis [3]. Overall, the focus of injury appears to be the common extensor tendon origin. Symptoms may be related to failure of the repair process [4].

Repetitive stress has been implicated as a factor in this condition [5]. Overuse from a tennis backhand (especially a one-handed backhand with poor technique) can frequently lead to lateral epicondylitis (hence, the term *tennis elbow* is frequently used synonymously with lateral epicondylitis, regardless of its etiology). Repetitive computer use (especially with a mouse) as well as golf, swimming, and baseball can cause or exacerbate epicondylitis.

Symptoms

Patients usually report pain in the area just distal to the lateral epicondyle. The patient may complain of pain radiating proximally or distally. Patients may also complain of pain with wrist or hand movement, such as gripping a doorknob, carrying a briefcase, or shaking hands. Patients occasionally report swelling as well.

Physical Examination

On examination, the hallmark of epicondylitis is tenderness over the extensor muscle origin. The common origin of the extensor muscles can be located one fingerbreadth below the lateral epicondyle. With lateral epicondylitis, pain is increased with resisted wrist extension, especially with the elbow extended, the forearm pronated, the wrist radially deviated, and the hand in a fist. The middle finger test can also be used to assess for lateral epicondylitis. Here, the proximal interphalangeal joint of the long finger is resisted in extension, and pain is elicited over the lateral epicondyle. Swelling is occasionally present. In cases of recalcitrant lateral epicondylitis, the diagnosis of radial nerve entrapment should be considered. The radial nerve can become entrapped just distal to the lateral epicondyle where the nerve pierces the intermuscular septum (between the brachialis and brachioradialis muscles). There may be localized tenderness along the course of the radial nerve around the radial head. Motor and sensory findings are usually absent.

Functional Limitations

The patient may complain of an inability to lift or to carry objects on the affected side secondary to increased pain. Typing, using a computer mouse, or working on a keyboard may re-create the pain. Even handshaking or squeezing may be painful in lateral epicondylitis. Athletic activities may cause pain, especially with an acute increase in repetition, poor technique, and equipment changes (frequently with a new racket or stringing).

Diagnostic Studies

The diagnosis is usually made on clinical grounds. Magnetic resonance imaging, which is particularly useful for soft tissue definition, can be used to assess for tendinitis, tendinosis, degeneration, partial tears or complete tears, and detachment of the common extensor tendons at the lateral epicondyle [6]. Magnetic resonance imaging is rarely needed, however, except in recalcitrant epicondylitis, and it will not alter the treatment significantly in the early stages. The lateral collateral ligament complexes can be evaluated for tears as well as for chronic degeneration and scarring. Ultrasonography has been used to diagnose lateral epicondylitis [7]. Arthrography may be beneficial if capsular defects and associated ligament injuries are suspected. Barring evidence of trauma, early radiographs are of little help in this condition but may be useful in cases of resistant tendinitis and to rule out occult fractures, arthritis, and an osteochondral loose body.

Differential Diagnosis

Posterior interosseous nerve syndrome
Bone infection or tumors
Ulnar or median neuropathy around the elbow
Osteoarthritis
Acute calcification around the lateral epicondyle [8]
Osteochondral loose body
Anconeus compartment syndrome [9]
Triceps tendinitis
Degenerative arthrosis [10]
Elbow synovitis
Lateral ligament instability [11]
Radial head fracture
Bursitis
Collateral ligament tears
Hypertrophic synovial plica [12]

Treatment

Initial

Initial treatment consists of relative rest, avoidance of repetitive motions involving the wrist, activity modification to avoid stress on the epicondyle, anti-inflammatory medications, and thermal modalities such as heat and ice for acute pain. Patients who develop lateral epicondylitis from tennis should modify their stroke (especially improving the backhand stroke to ensure that the forearm is in midpronation and the trunk is leaning forward) and their equipment, usually by reducing string tension and enlarging the grip size [5]. Frequently, a two-handed backhand will relieve the stress sufficiently.

In addition, a forearm band (counterforce brace) worn distal to the extensor muscle group origin can be beneficial (Fig. 22.1). The theory behind this device is that it will dissipate forces over a larger area of tissue than the lateral attachment site. Alternatively, the use of wrist immobilization splints may be helpful. A splint set in neutral can be helpful for lateral epicondylitis by relieving the tension on the flexors and extensors of the wrist and fingers. A splint set in 30 to 40 degrees of wrist extension will relieve the tension on the extensor tendons, including the extensor carpi radialis brevis muscle as well as other wrist and finger extensors [13,14]. Dynamic extension bracing has also been proposed [15].

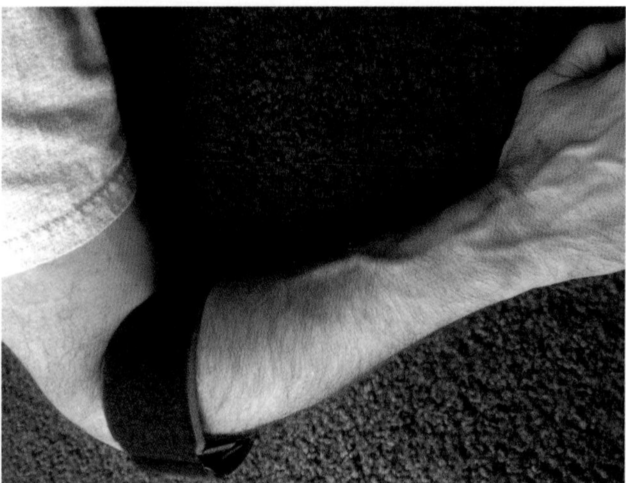

FIGURE 22.1 Forearm band (counterforce brace) used in patients with lateral epicondylitis.

Rehabilitation

Rehabilitation may include physical or occupational therapy. Therapy should include two phases. The first phase is directed at decreasing pain by physical modalities (ultrasound, electrical stimulation, phonophoresis, cortisone iontophoresis [16], myofascial release [17], heat, ice, massage) and decreasing disability (education, reduction of repetitive stress, and preservation of motion). When the patient is pain free, a gradual program is implemented to improve strength and endurance of wrist extensors and stretching. This program must be carefully monitored to permit strengthening of the muscles and work hardening of the tissues without itself causing an overuse situation. The patient should start with static exercises and advance to progressive resistive exercises (with an emphasis on the eccentric phase of the exercise). Thera-Band, light weights, and manual (self) resistance exercises can be used.

Work or activity restrictions or modifications may be required for a time.

Procedures

Injection of corticosteroid, usually with a local anesthetic, into the area of maximum tenderness (approximately 1 to 5 cm distal to the lateral epicondyle) has been shown to be effective in treatment of lateral epicondylitis (Fig. 22.2) [18]. To confirm the diagnosis, a trial of lidocaine alone may be given. An immediate improvement in grip strength should be noted after injection. Postinjection treatment includes icing of the affected area both immediately (for 5 to 10 minutes) and thereafter (a reasonable regimen is 20 minutes two or three times per day for 2 weeks) and wearing of a wrist splint (particularly for activities that involve wrist movement). The wrist splint should be set in slight extension for lateral

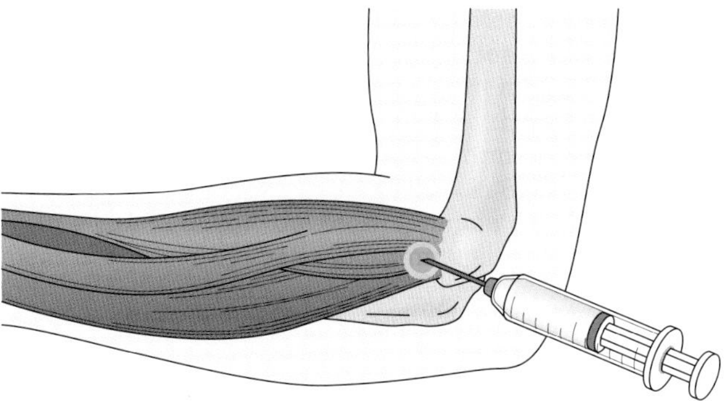

FIGURE 22.2 Under sterile conditions, with use of a 27-gauge needle and 1 to 2 mL of a local anesthetic combined with 1 to 2 mL of a corticosteroid preparation, inject the solution approximately 1 to 5 cm distal to the lateral epicondyle. The injected materials should flow smoothly. Resistance generally indicates that the solution is being injected directly into the tendon, and this should be avoided.

epicondylitis. Exacerbating activities are to be avoided. Platelet-rich plasma injections have been shown to reduce pain and to increase function in patients with lateral epicondylitis [19–21]. Injection of botulinum toxin into the extensor digitorum communis muscles to the third and fourth digits has been reported to be beneficial in chronic treatment–resistant lateral epicondylitis [22,23].

There are studies that support acupuncture as an effective modality in the short-term relief of lateral epicondylitis [24–26]. Extracorporeal shock wave treatment may also be beneficial in lateral epicondylitis [27].

Surgery

Surgery may be indicated in those patients with continued severe symptoms who do not respond to conservative management. For lateral epicondylitis, surgery is aimed at excision and revitalization of the pathologic tissue in the extensor carpi radialis brevis and release of the muscle origin [28]. Pinning may be done if the elbow joint is unstable [29].

Potential Disease Complications

Possible long-term complications of untreated epicondylitis include chronic pain, loss of function, and possible elbow contracture. In general, epicondylitis is more easily and successfully treated in the acute phase.

Potential Treatment Complications

Analgesics and nonsteroidal anti-inflammatory drugs have well-known side effects that most commonly affect the gastric, hepatic, and renal systems. Local steroid injections may increase the risk for disruption of tissue planes, create high-pressure tissue necrosis, rupture tendons [1], damage nerves, promote skin depigmentation or atrophy, or cause infection [30].

References

[1] Kraushaar BS, Nirschl RP. Tendinosis of the elbow (tennis elbow): clinical features and findings of histological, immunohistochemical, and electron microscopy studies. J Bone Joint Surg Am 1999;81:259–78.

[2] Nirschl RP, Pettrone FA. Tennis elbow. J Bone Joint Surg Am 1979;61:832–9.

[3] Nirschl RP. Elbow tendinosis/tennis elbow. Clin Sports Med 1992;11:851–70.

[4] Putnam MD, Cohen M. Painful conditions around the elbow. Orthop Clin North Am 1999;30:109–18.

[5] Cassvan A, Weiss LD, Weiss JM, et al. Cumulative Trauma Disorders. Boston: Butterworth-Heinemann; 1997, 123–125.

[6] Braddom RL. Physical Medicine and Rehabilitation. Philadelphia: WB Saunders; 1996, 222.

[7] Bodor M, Fullerton B. Ultrasonography of the hand, wrist, and elbow. Phys Med Rehabil Clin N Am 2010;21:509–31.

[8] Hughes E. Acute deposition of calcium near the elbow. J Bone Joint Surg Br 1950;32:30–4.

[9] Abrahamsson S, Sollerman C, Soderberg T, et al. Lateral elbow pain caused by anconeus compartment syndrome. Acta Orthop Scand 1987;58:589–91.

[10] Brems JJ. Degenerative joint disease of the elbow. In: Nicholas JA, Hershman EB, editors. The Upper Extremity in Sports Medicine. St. Louis: Mosby; 1995. p. 331–5.

[11] Morrey BF. Anatomy of the elbow joint. In: Morrey BF, et al., editors. The Elbow and Its Disorders. 2nd ed. Philadelphia: WB Saunders; 1993. p. 16.

[12] Kim DH, Gambardella RA, El Attrache NS, et al. Arthroscopic treatment of posterolateral elbow impingement from lateral synovial plicae in throwing athletes and golfers. Am J Sports Med 2006;34:438–44.

[13] Plancher KD. The athletic elbow and wrist, part I. Diagnosis and conservative treatment. Clin Sports Med 1995;15:433–5.

[14] Derebery VJ, Devenport JN, Giang GM, Fogarty WT. The effects of splinting on outcomes for epicondylitis. Arch Phys Med Rehabil 2005;86:1081–8.

[15] Faes M, van den Akker B, de Lint JA, et al. Dynamic extensor brace for lateral epicondylitis. Clin Orthop Relat Res 2006;442:149–57.

[16] Stefanou A, Marshall N, Holdan W, Siddiqui A. A randomized study comparing corticosteroid injection to corticosteroid iontophoresis for lateral epicondylitis. J Hand Surg [Am] 2012;37:104–9.

[17] Ajimsha MS, Chithra S, Thulasyammal RP. Effectiveness of myofascial release in the management of lateral epicondylitis in computer professionals. Arch Phys Med Rehabil 2012;93:604–9.

[18] Hay EH, Paterson SM, Lewis M, et al. Pragmatic randomized controlled trial of local corticosteroid injection and naproxen for treatment of lateral epicondylitis of elbow in primary care. BMJ 1999;319:964–8.

[19] Peerbooms JC, Sluimer J, Bruijn DJ, Gosens T. Positive effect of an autologous platelet concentrate in lateral epicondylitis in a double-blind randomized controlled trial: platelet-rich plasma versus corticosteroid injection with a 1-year follow-up. Am J Sports Med 2010;38:255–62.

[20] Gosens T. Ongoing positive effect of platelet-rich plasma versus corticosteroid injection in lateral epicondylitis: a double-blind randomized controlled trial with 2-year follow-up. Am J Sports Med 2011;39:1200–8.

[21] Hechtman KS, Uribe JW, Botto-vanDemden A, Kiebzak GM. Platelet-rich plasma injection reduces pain in patients with recalcitrant epicondylitis. Orthopedics 2011;34:92.

[22] Morre HH, Keizer SB, van Os JJ. Treatment of chronic tennis elbow with botulinum toxin. Lancet 1997;349:1746.

[23] Wong SM, Jui AC, Tong PY, et al. Treatment of lateral epicondylitis with botulinum toxin: a randomized, double-blind, placebo-controlled trial. Ann Intern Med 2005;143:793–7.

[24] Trinh KV, Phillips SD, Ho E, Damsma K. Acupuncture for the alleviation of lateral epicondyle pain: a systematic review. Rheumatology (Oxford) 2004;43:1085–90.

[25] Fink M, Wolkenstein E, Luennemann M, et al. Chronic epicondylitis: effects of real and sham acupuncture treatment: a randomised controlled patient- and examiner-blinded long-term trial. Forsch Komplementarmed Klass Naturheilkd 2002;9:210–5.

[26] Fink M, Wolkenstein E, Karst M, Gehrke A. Acupuncture in chronic epicondylitis: a randomized controlled trial. Rheumatology (Oxford) 2002;41:205–9.

[27] Gunduz R, Malas FU, Borman P, et al. Physical therapy, corticosteroid injection, and extracorporeal shock wave treatment in lateral epicondylitis. Clinical and ultrasonographical comparison. Clin Rheumatol 2012;31:807–12.

[28] Organ SW, Nirschl RP, Kraushaar BS, Guidi EJ. Salvage surgery for lateral tennis elbow. Am J Sports Med 1997;25:746–50.

[29] Brown D, Freeman E, Cuccurullo S. Elbow disorders. In: Cuccurullo S, editor. Physical Medicine and Rehabilitation Board Review. New York: Demos; 2004. p. 163–73.

[30] Nichols AW. Complications associated with the use of corticosteroids in the treatment of athletic injuries [review]. Clin J Sport Med 2005;15:370–5.

CHAPTER 23

Medial Epicondylitis

Lyn D. Weiss, MD
Jay M. Weiss, MD

Synonyms

Tendinosis [1]
Medial epicondylitis
Pitcher's elbow
Little Leaguer's elbow
Golfer's elbow

ICD-9 Code

726.31 Medial epicondylitis

ICD-10 Codes

M77.00 Medial epicondylitis, unspecified elbow
M77.01 Medial epicondylitis, right elbow
M77.02 Medial epicondylitis, left elbow

Definition

Epicondylitis is a general term used to describe inflammation, pain, or tenderness in the region of the medial or lateral epicondyle of the humerus. The actual nidus of pain and pathologic change has been debated. Medial epicondylitis implies an inflammatory lesion with degeneration at the origin of the flexor muscles (the medial epicondyle of the humerus). In medial epicondylitis, the tendon of the flexor muscle group is affected (flexor carpi radialis, flexor carpi ulnaris, flexor digitorum superficialis, and palmaris longus).

Although the term *epicondylitis* implies an inflammatory process, inflammatory cells are not identified histologically. Instead, the condition may be secondary to failure of the musculotendinous attachment with resultant fibroplasia [2], termed tendinosis. Other postulated primary lesions include angiofibroblastic tendinosis, periostitis, and enthesitis [3]. In children, medial elbow pain may result from repetitive stress on the apophysis of the medial epicondyle ossification center (Little Leaguer's elbow) [4]. Overall, the focus of injury appears to be the muscle origin. Symptoms may be related to failure of the repair process [5].

Repetitive stress has been implicated as a factor in this condition [6]. Poor throwing mechanics and excessive throwing have been implicated in Little Leaguer's elbow. Repetitive wrist flexion, as in the trailing arm in a golf swing, can cause medial epicondylitis (hence, the term *golfer's elbow* is frequently used for medial epicondylitis, regardless of etiology).

Symptoms

Patients usually report pain in the area just distal to the medial epicondyle. The patient may complain of pain radiating proximally or distally. Patients may also complain of pain with wrist or hand movement, such as gripping a doorknob, carrying a briefcase, or shaking hands. Patients occasionally report swelling as well.

Physical Examination

On examination, the hallmark of epicondylitis is tenderness over the flexor muscle origin (medial epicondylitis). The origin of the flexor muscles can be located one fingerbreadth below the medial epicondyle. With medial epicondylitis, pain is increased with resisted wrist flexion. There may be localized tenderness along the course of the radial nerve around the radial head. Motor and sensory findings are usually absent.

Functional Limitations

The patient may complain of an inability to lift or to carry objects on the affected side secondary to increased pain. Typing, using a computer mouse, or working on a keyboard may re-create the pain. Even handshaking or hand squeezing may be painful in medial epicondylitis. Athletic activities may cause pain, especially with an acute increase in repetition, poor technique, and equipment changes.

Diagnostic Studies

The diagnosis is usually made on clinical grounds. Magnetic resonance imaging, which is particularly useful for soft tissue definition, can be used to assess for tendinitis, tendinosis, degeneration, partial tears or complete tears, and detachment of the common flexor at the medial epicondyles [7]. Magnetic resonance imaging is rarely needed, however, except in recalcitrant epicondylitis, and it will not alter the treatment significantly in the early stages. The medial collateral ligament complexes can be evaluated for tears as well as for chronic degeneration and scarring. Ultrasonography has been used to diagnose medial epicondylitis [8,9]. Arthrography may be beneficial if capsular defects and associated ligament injuries are suspected. Barring evidence of trauma, early radiographs are of little help in this condition but may be useful in cases of resistant tendinitis and to rule out occult fractures, arthritis, and osteochondral loose body. Early radiographic studies (before commencing a rehabilitation program) may be considered in skeletally immature children with elbow pain to rule out growth plate disorders, osteochondritis dissecans, or ulnar collateral ligament tears [10].

Differential Diagnosis

Posterior interosseous nerve syndrome
Bone infection or tumors
Ulnar neuropathy around the elbow
Osteoarthritis
Osteochondral loose body
Anconeus compartment syndrome [11]
Triceps tendinitis
Degenerative arthrosis [12]
Elbow synovitis
Medial ligament instability [13]
Radial head fracture
Bursitis
Collateral ligament tears
Hypertrophic synovial plica [14]

Treatment

Initial

Initial treatment consists of relative rest, avoidance of repetitive motions involving the wrist, activity modification to avoid stress on the epicondyle, anti-inflammatory medications, and thermal modalities such as heat and ice for acute pain. Patients who develop medial epicondylitis from golf should consider modifying their swing to avoid excessive force on wrist flexor muscles. Biomechanical modifications may help reduce symptoms if the medial epicondylitis is thought to be due to poor pitching technique.

In addition, a forearm band (counterforce brace) worn distal to the flexor muscle group origin can be beneficial. The theory behind this device is that it will dissipate forces over a larger area of tissue than the medial attachment site [15]. Alternatively, the use of wrist immobilization splints may be helpful. A splint set in neutral can be helpful for medial epicondylitis by relieving the tension on the flexors and extensors of the wrist and fingers. Dynamic extension bracing has also been proposed [16].

Rehabilitation

Rehabilitation may include physical or occupational therapy. Therapy should include two phases. The first phase is directed at decreasing pain by physical modalities (ultrasound, electrical stimulation, phonophoresis, heat, ice, massage) and decreasing disability (education, reduction of repetitive stress, and preservation of motion). When the patient is pain free, a gradual program is implemented to improve strength and endurance of wrist flexors and should include stretching. This program must be carefully monitored to permit strengthening of the muscles and work hardening of the tissues without itself causing an overuse situation. The patient should start with static exercises and advance to progressive resistive exercises. Thera-Band, light weights, Kinesio taping [17], and manual (self) resistance exercises can be used.

Work or activity restrictions or modifications may be required for a time.

Procedures

Injection of corticosteroid, usually with a local anesthetic, into the area of maximum tenderness (approximately 1 to 5 cm distal to the medial epicondyle) has been shown to be effective in treatment of epicondylitis (Fig. 23.1) [18,19]. To confirm the diagnosis, a trial of lidocaine alone may be given. An immediate improvement in grip strength should be noted after injection. Postinjection treatment includes icing of the affected area both immediately (for 5 to 10 minutes) and thereafter (a reasonable regimen is 20 minutes two or three times per day for 2 weeks) and wearing of a wrist splint (particularly for activities that involve wrist movement). The wrist splint should be set in neutral for medial epicondylitis. Exacerbating activities are to be avoided. Platelet-rich plasma injections have been shown to reduce pain and to increase function in patients with recalcitrant epicondylitis [20], as have botulinum toxin injections [21].

Injections for medial epicondylitis must be used cautiously because of the risk of injury to the ulnar nerve (either by direct injection or by tissue changes that may promote nerve injury).

Surgery

Surgery may be indicated in those patients with continued severe symptoms who do not respond to conservative management. Surgery is aimed at excision and revitalization of the pathologic tissue and release of the muscle origin [22]. Pinning may be done if the elbow joint is unstable [4].

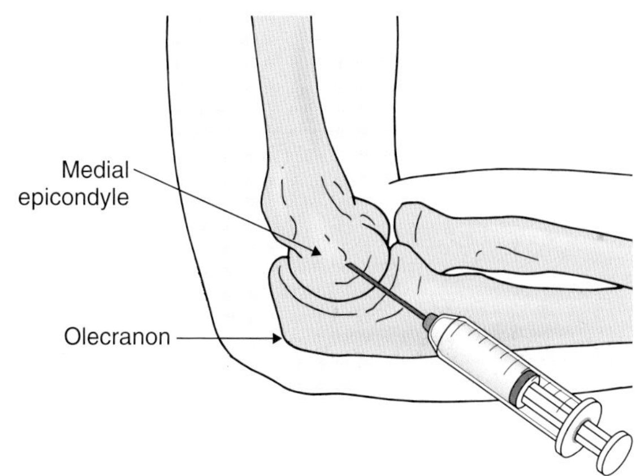

FIGURE 23.1 Medial epicondylitis injection.

Potential Disease Complications

Possible long-term complications of untreated epicondylitis include chronic pain, loss of function, and possible elbow contracture. Medial epicondylitis may lead to reversible impairment (neurapraxia) of the ulnar nerve [23]. In general, epicondylitis is more easily and successfully treated in the acute phase.

Potential Treatment Complications

Analgesics and nonsteroidal anti-inflammatory drugs have well-known side effects that most commonly affect the gastric, hepatic, and renal systems. Local steroid injections may increase the risk for disruption of tissue planes, create high-pressure tissue necrosis, rupture tendons [1], damage nerves, promote skin depigmentation or atrophy, or cause infection [24].

References

[1] Kraushaar BS, Nirschl RP. Tendinosis of the elbow (tennis elbow): clinical features and findings of histological, immunohistochemical, and electron microscopy studies. J Bone Joint Surg Am 1999;81:259–78.

[2] Nirschl RP, Pettrone FA. Tennis elbow. J Bone Joint Surg Am 1979;61:832–9.

[3] Nirschl RP. Elbow tendinosis/tennis elbow. Clin Sports Med 1992;11:851–70.

[4] Brown D, Freeman E, Cuccurullo S. Elbow disorders. In: Cuccurullo S, editor. Physical medicine and rehabilitation board review. New York: Demos; 2004. p. 163–73.

[5] Putnam MD, Cohen M. Painful conditions around the elbow. Orthop Clin North Am 1999;30:109–18.

[6] Cassvan A, Weiss LD, Weiss JM, et al. Cumulative trauma disorders. Boston: Butterworth-Heinemann; 1997, 123–125.

[7] Braddom RL. Physical medicine and rehabilitation. Philadelphia: WB Saunders; 1996, 222.

[8] Bodor M, Fullerton B. Ultrasonography of the hand, wrist, and elbow. Phys Med Rehabil Clin N Am 2010;21:509–31.

[9] Park GY, Lee SM, Lee MY. Diagnostic value of ultrasonography for clinical medial epicondylitis. Arch Phys Med Rehabil 2008;89:732–42.

[10] Emery KH. Imaging of sports injuries of the upper extremity in children. Clin Sports Med 2006;25:543–68.

[11] Abrahamsson S, Sollerman C, Soderberg T, et al. Lateral elbow pain caused by anconeus compartment syndrome. Acta Orthop Scand 1987;58:589–91.

[12] Brems JJ. Degenerative joint disease of the elbow. In: Nicholas JA, Hershman EB, editors. The upper extremity in sports medicine. Mosby: St. Louis; 1995. p. 331–5.

[13] Morrey BF. Anatomy of the elbow joint. In: Morrey BF, editor. The elbow and its disorders. 2nd ed, Philadelphia: WB Saunders; 1993. p. 16.

[14] Kim DH, Gambardella RA, El Attrache NS, et al. Arthroscopic treatment of posterolateral elbow impingement from lateral synovial plicae in throwing athletes and golfers. Am J Sports Med 2006;34:438–44.

[15] Walther M, Kirschner S, Koenig A, et al. Biomechanical evaluation of braces used for the treatment of epicondylitis. J Shoulder Elbow Surg 2002;11:265–70.

[16] Faes M, van den Akker B, de Lint JA, et al. Dynamic extensor brace for lateral epicondylitis. Clin Orthop Relat Res 2006;442:149–57.

[17] Chang HY, Wang CH, Chou KY, Cheng SC. Could forearm kinesio taping improve strength, force sense, and pain in baseball pitchers with medical epicondylitis? Clin J Sport Med 2012;22:327–33.

[18] Hay EH, Paterson SM, Lewis M, et al. Pragmatic randomized controlled trial of local corticosteroid injection and naproxen for treatment of lateral epicondylitis of elbow in primary care. BMJ 1999;319:964–8.

[19] Weiss LD, Silver JK, Lennard TA, Weiss JM. Easy injections. Philadelphia: Butterworth-Heinemann; 2007, 70.

[20] Hechtman KS, Uribe JW, Botto-vanDemden A, Kiebzak GM. Platelet-rich plasma injection reduces pain in patients with recalcitrant epicondylitis. Orthopedics 2011;34:92.

[21] Placzek R, Drescher W, Deuretzbacher G, et al. Treatment of chronic radial epicondylitis with botulinum toxin A. A double-blind, placebo-controlled, randomized multicenter study. J Bone Joint Surg Am 2007;89:255–60.

[22] Organ SW, Nirschl RP, Kraushaar BS, Guidi EJ. Salvage surgery for lateral tennis elbow. Am J Sports Med 1997;25:746–50.

[23] Barry NN, McGuire JL. Overuse syndromes in adult athletes. Rheum Dis Clin North Am 1996;22:515–30.

[24] Nichols AW. Complications associated with the use of corticosteroids in the treatment of athletic injuries [review]. Clin J Sport Med 2005;15:370–5.

CHAPTER 24

Median Neuropathy

Francisco H. Santiago, MD
Ramon Vallarino, Jr., MD

Synonyms

Pronator teres syndrome
Pronator syndrome
Anterior interosseous syndrome
Kiloh-Nevin syndrome

ICD-9 Code

354.1 Other lesion of median nerve (median nerve neuritis)

ICD-10 Codes

G56.10 Other lesion of median nerve, unspecified upper limb
G56.11 Other lesion of median nerve, right upper limb
G56.12 Other lesion of median nerve, procedure upper limb

Definition

There are three general areas in which the median nerve can become entrapped around the elbow and forearm. Because this chapter mainly deals with entrapment below the elbow and above the wrist, the most proximal and least frequent entrapment is not discussed but merely mentioned. Elbow median nerve entrapment is the compression of the nerve by a dense band of connective tissue called the ligament of Struthers, an aberrant ligament found immediately above the elbow. The topics discussed in this chapter are compression of the median nerve at or immediately below the elbow, where the pronator teres muscle compresses it, and compression distally of a branch of the median nerve—the anterior interosseous nerve.

Increased risk for pronator syndrome may be associated with individuals involved in repetitive elbow, wrist, and hand movements, such as chopping wood, playing racket sports, rowing, weightlifting, and throwing. However, pronator syndrome is four times more likely to affect women than men, suggesting that the dominant risk factor is an anatomic anomaly (structural variation) and not overuse. The dominant arm is most likely to be affected, particularly if the individual is heavily muscled (muscle hypertrophy). Pronator syndrome is most commonly diagnosed in individuals between the ages of 40 and 50 years [1]. Pronator syndrome is rare but is the second most common cause of medial nerve compression after carpal tunnel syndrome. Pronator syndrome is responsible for less than 1% of all median nerve entrapment disorders [2]. Anterior interosseous syndrome has a similar 1% occurrence rate in median nerve entrapment disorders [3].

Pronator Teres Syndrome

Pronator teres syndrome [4,5] is a symptom complex that is produced where the median nerve crosses the elbow and becomes entrapped as it passes first beneath the lacertus fibrosus—a thick fascial band extending from the biceps tendon to the forearm fascia—then between the two heads (superficial and deep) of the pronator teres muscle and under the edge of the flexor digitorum sublimis (Fig. 24.1). Compression may be related to a local process, such as pronator teres hypertrophy, tenosynovitis, muscle hemorrhage, fascial tear, postoperative scarring, anomalous median artery, or giant lipoma. The median nerve may also be injured by occupational strain, such as carrying a grocery bag or guitar playing, and by insertion of a catheter [4–13].

Anterior Interosseous Syndrome

The anterior interosseous nerve arises from the median nerve 5 to 8 cm distal to the lateral epicondyle [4,6,14]. Slightly distal to its course through the pronator teres muscle, the median nerve gives off the anterior interosseous nerve, a purely motor branch (Fig. 24.2). It contains no fibers of superficial sensation but does supply deep pain and proprioception to some deep tissues, including the wrist joint. This nerve may be damaged by direct trauma, forearm fractures, humeral fracture, injection into or blood drawing from the cubital vein, supracondylar fracture, and fibrous bands related to the flexor digitorum sublimis and flexor digitorum profundus muscles. In some patients, it is a component of brachial amyotrophy of the shoulder girdle (proximal fascicular lesion) or related to cytomegalovirus

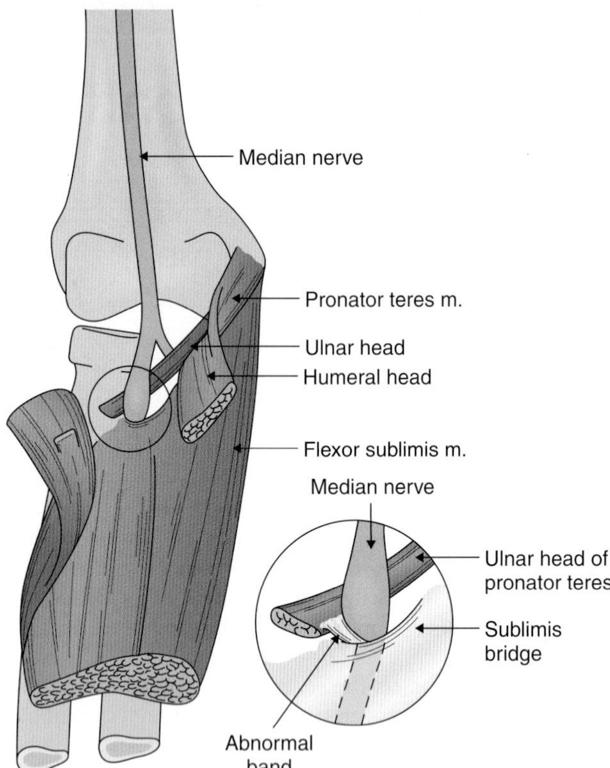

FIGURE 24.1 The median nerve is shown descending beneath the sublimis bridge after traversing the space between the two heads of the pronator teres. The nerve is compressed at the sublimis bridge. *(From Kopell HP, Thompson WA. Pronator syndrome: a confirmed case and its diagnosis. N Engl J Med 1958;259:713-715.)*

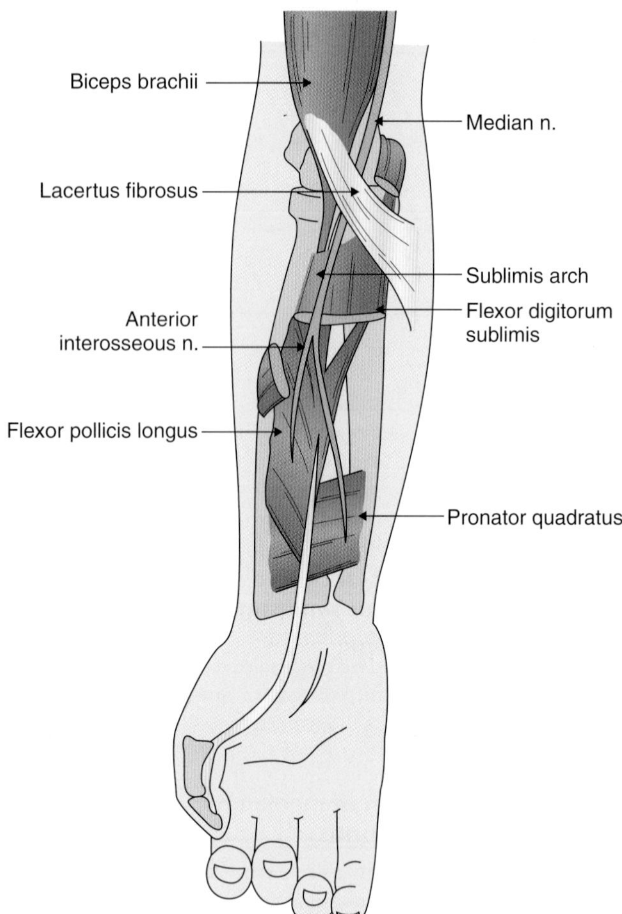

FIGURE 24.2 Course of the median nerve and its anterior interosseous branch.

infection or a bronchogenic carcinoma metastasis. The nerve may be partially involved, but in a fully established syndrome, three muscles are weak: flexor pollicis longus, flexor digitorum profundus to the second and sometimes the third digit, and pronator quadratus [4,6,12–18].

Symptoms

Pronator Teres Syndrome

In an acute compression, with unmistakable symptoms, the diagnosis is relatively simple to establish [5,14]. In many cases of intermittent, mild, or partial compression, the signs and symptoms are vague and nondescript. The most common symptom is mild to moderate aching pain in the proximal forearm, sometimes described as tiredness and heaviness. Use of the arm may cause a mild or dull aching pain to become deep or sharp. Repetitive elbow motions are likely to provoke symptoms. As the pain intensifies, it may radiate proximally to the elbow or even to the shoulder. Paresthesias in the distribution of the median nerve may be reported, but they are generally not as severe or well localized as the complaints in carpal tunnel syndrome. When numbness is a prominent symptom, the complaints may mimic carpal tunnel syndrome. However, unlike carpal tunnel syndrome, pronator teres syndrome rarely has nocturnal exacerbation, and the symptoms are not affected by a change of wrist position.

Anterior Interosseous Syndrome

The onset of anterior interosseous syndrome can be related to exertion, or it may be spontaneous. In classic cases of spontaneous anterior interosseous nerve paralysis, there is acute pain in the proximal forearm or arm lasting for hours or days. There may be a history of local trauma or heavy muscle exertion at the onset of pain. As mentioned, the patient may complain of weakness of the forearm muscles innervated by the anterior interosseous nerve. Theoretically, there should be no sensory complaints [6].

Physical Examination

Pronator Teres Syndrome

Findings may be ill-defined and difficult to substantiate in pronator teres syndrome [5,14]. The most important physical finding is tenderness over the proximal forearm. Pressure over the pronator teres muscle produces discomfort and may produce a radiating pain and digital numbness. The symptomatic pronator teres muscle may be firm to palpation compared with the other side. The contour of the forearm may be depressed, caused by the thickening of the lacertus fibrosus. Distinctive findings are weakness of both the intrinsic muscles of the hand supplied by the median nerve and the muscles proximal to the wrist and in the forearm with tenderness, Tinel sign over the point of entrapment, and absence of Phalen sign. Pain may be elicited by pronation of the forearm, elbow flexion, or even contraction of the superficial flexor of the second digit. Sensory examination findings are usually poorly defined but may involve not only the median nerve distribution of the digits but also the thenar region of the palm because of involvement of the palmar cutaneous branch of the median nerve. Deep tendon reflexes and cervical examination findings should be normal [7,12,13,15–19].

Anterior Interosseous Syndrome

To test the muscles that the anterior interosseous nerve innervates [5,14], the clinician braces the metacarpophalangeal joint of the index finger and the patient is asked to flex only the distal phalanx. This isolates the action of the flexor digitorum profundus on the terminal phalanx and eliminates the action of the flexor digitorum superficialis. There is no terminal phalanx flexion if the anterior interosseous nerve is injured.

Another useful test is to ask the patient to make the "OK" sign [20]. In anterior interosseous syndrome, the distal interphalangeal joint cannot be flexed, and this results in the index finger's remaining relatively straight during this test (Fig. 24.3). The patient is asked to forcefully approximate the finger pulps of the first and second digits. The patient with weakness of the flexor pollicis longus and digitorum profundus muscles cannot touch with the pulp of the fingers, but rather the entire volar surfaces of the digits are in contact. This is due to the paralysis of the flexor pollicis longus and flexor digitorum profundus of the second digit. The pronator quadratus is difficult to isolate clinically, but an attempt can be made by flexing the forearm and asking the patient to resist supination. Sensation and deep tendon reflexes should be normal [7,12,13,15–19].

Functional Limitations

Pronator Teres Syndrome

In pronator teres syndrome, there is clumsiness, loss of dexterity, and a feeling of weakness in the hand. This may lead to functional limitations both at home and at work. Repetitive elbow motions, such as hammering, cleaning fish, serving tennis balls, and rowing, are most likely to provoke symptoms.

Anterior Interosseous Syndrome

As weakness develops in anterior interosseous syndrome, there is loss of dexterity and pinching motion with difficulty in picking up small objects with the first two digits. Activities of daily living, such as buttoning shirts and tying shoelaces, can be impaired. Patients may have difficulty with typing, handwriting, cooking, and so on.

Diagnostic Studies

Pronator Teres Syndrome

Electrodiagnostic testing (nerve conduction studies and electromyography) is the "gold standard" for confirming pronator teres syndrome [4,21,22]. Results of nerve conduction studies may be abnormal in the median nerve distribution; however, the diagnosis may be best established by electromyographic studies demonstrating membrane instability (including increased insertional activity, fibrillation and positive sharp waves at rest, wide and high amplitude polyphasics on minimal contraction, and decreased recruitment pattern on maximal contraction) of the median nerve muscles below and above the wrist in the forearm but

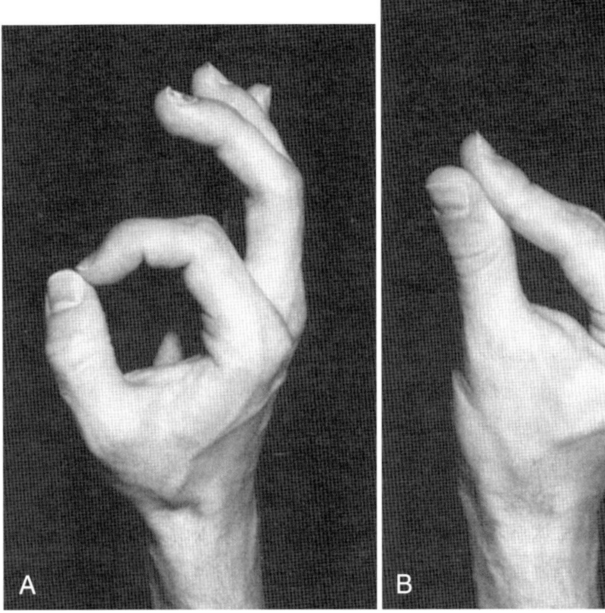

FIGURE 24.3 The anterior interosseous nerve innervates the flexor pollicis longus as well as the flexor digitorum profundus to the index and long fingers. **A,** It is responsible for flexion of the thumb interphalangeal joint and the index finger distal interphalangeal joint. **B,** An injury to the median nerve high in the forearm or to the anterior interosseous branch of the median nerve results in inability to forcefully flex these joints. *(From Concannon MJ. Common Hand Problems in Primary Care. Philadelphia, Hanley & Belfus, 1999.)*

with *sparing of the pronator teres* [22,23]. Imaging studies (e.g., radiography, computed tomography, hypoechoic swelling by ultrasonography, and magnetic resonance imaging) are used to exclude alternative diagnoses. Magnetic resonance imaging and high-resolution ultrasonography may be helpful in diagnosis, although there is no consensus on which is the preferred method [24–29].

Anterior Interosseous Syndrome

Electrodiagnostic studies may also help establish the diagnosis of anterior interosseous syndrome [5]. In general, the results of routine motor and sensory studies are normal. The most appropriate technique is surface electrode recording from the pronator quadratus muscle with median nerve stimulation at the antecubital fossa. On electromyography, findings of membrane instability are restricted to the flexor pollicis longus, flexor digitorum profundus (of the second and third digits), and pronator quadratus [9,21].

Imaging studies are useful in excluding other diagnoses. [25–29]

Differential Diagnosis

PRONATOR TERES SYNDROME
Carpal tunnel syndrome
Cervical radiculopathy, particularly lesions affecting C6 or C7
Thoracic outlet syndrome with involvement of the medial cord
Elbow arthritis
Epicondylitis

ANTERIOR INTEROSSEOUS SYNDROME
Paralytic brachial plexus neuritis
Entrapment or rupture of the tendon of the flexor pollicis longus
Rupture of the flexor pollicis longus and flexor digitorum profundus

Treatment

Initial

Pronator Teres Syndrome

Treatment is initially conservative, with rest and avoidance of the offending repetitive trauma [6,14]. A wrist immobilization splint is applied in 15 degrees of dorsiflexion for 4 to 6 weeks. The patient is instructed in friction massage. Ice and electrical stimulation are instituted three times a week for 10 treatments. The splint is discontinued at a time determined by the physician [30]. Nonsteroidal anti-inflammatory drugs may help with pain and inflammation. Analgesics may be used for pain. Low-dose tricyclic antidepressants may be used for pain and to help with sleep. Antiseizure medications are also often used for neuropathic pain (e.g., carbamazepine, gabapentin).

Anterior Interosseous Syndrome

Treatment of the anterior interosseous syndrome depends on the cause [5,14]. Penetrating wounds require immediate exploration and repair. Impending Volkmann contracture demands immediate decompression. In spontaneous cases associated with specific occupations, a trial of nonoperative therapy is indicated. If spontaneous improvement does not occur by 6 to 8 weeks, consideration should be given to surgical exploration. Conservative management includes avoiding the activity that exacerbates the symptoms. Pharmacologic treatment is similar to that for pronator teres syndrome.

Rehabilitation

Pronator Teres Syndrome

A splint that can put the thumb in an abducted, opposed position, such as a C bar or a thumb post–static orthosis, can be used (Fig. 24.4) [8,9,11]. Taping of the index and middle fingers in a buddy splint to stabilize the lack of distal interphalangeal flexion may be helpful [11].

Rehabilitation may include modalities such as ultrasound, electrical stimulation, iontophoresis, and phonophoresis. The patient can be instructed in ice massage as well. Once the acute symptoms have subsided, physical or occupational therapy can focus on exercises to improve forearm flexibility, muscle strength responsible for thumb abduction, opposition, and wrist radial flexion.

Anterior Interosseous Syndrome

Resting the arm by immobilization in a splint may be tried (Fig. 24.5) [31]. If the symptoms subside, conservative physical or occupational therapy, including physical modalities as previously described and exercises to improve strength and function of the pronator quadratus, flexor digitorum profundus, and flexor pollicis longus, can be initiated [11].

Procedures

In both anterior interosseous and pronator teres syndromes, a median nerve block may be attempted [32] (Figs. 24.6 and 24.7).

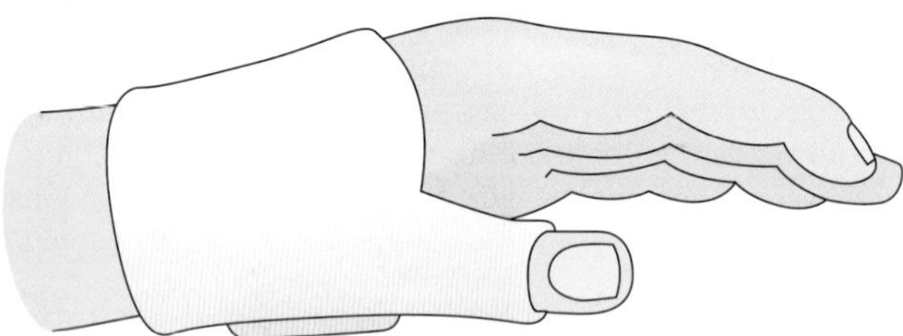

FIGURE 24.4 A typical splint used in pronator teres syndrome.

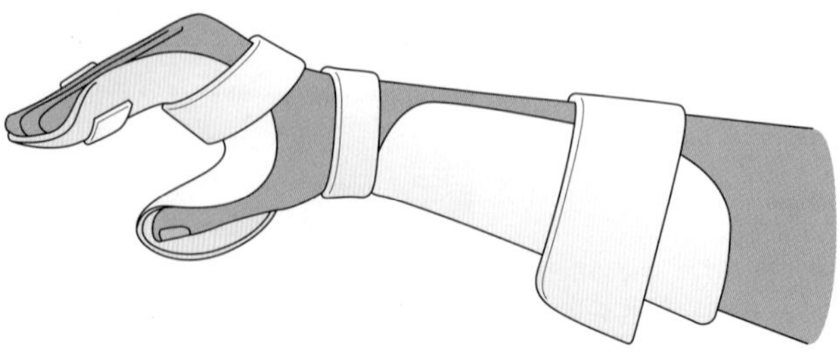

FIGURE 24.5 A typical splint used in anterior interosseous syndrome.

Surgery

Pronator Teres Syndrome

If symptoms fail to resolve, surgical release of the pronator teres muscle and any constricting bands (ligament of Struthers and lacertus fibrosus) should be considered with direct exploration of the area. Traditionally, an S-shaped incision is typically used to extensively expose the entire median nerve from the forearm to the hand [33]. Recent techniques have elucidated the possible advantage of using small-incision endoscopic procedures [34,35].

Anterior Interosseous Syndrome

If spontaneous improvement does not occur by 6 to 8 weeks, consideration should be given to surgical exploration. The surgical technique for exploration is exposure of the median nerve directly beneath the pronator teres or separation of this muscle from the flexor carpi radialis, identification of the anterior interosseous nerve, and release of the offending structures.

If surgical decompression was performed and failed to resolve the weakness, tendon transfers may be considered after a more proximal fascicular lesion is ruled out [33]. Endoscopically assisted technique has been tried but without much success at this point because of the depth of the surgical approach and limited view [36].

Postoperative Rehabilitation [30]

0 to 1 week

Postoperative dressing is removed. Active and gentle passive range of motion exercises are initiated for 15 minutes per hour. Desensitization and edema management are instituted. Pronation and elbow extension stretching exercises are instituted four times a day.

3 weeks

Strengthening is initiated in accordance with the patient's comfort level using putty, Hand Helper, and Thera-Band.

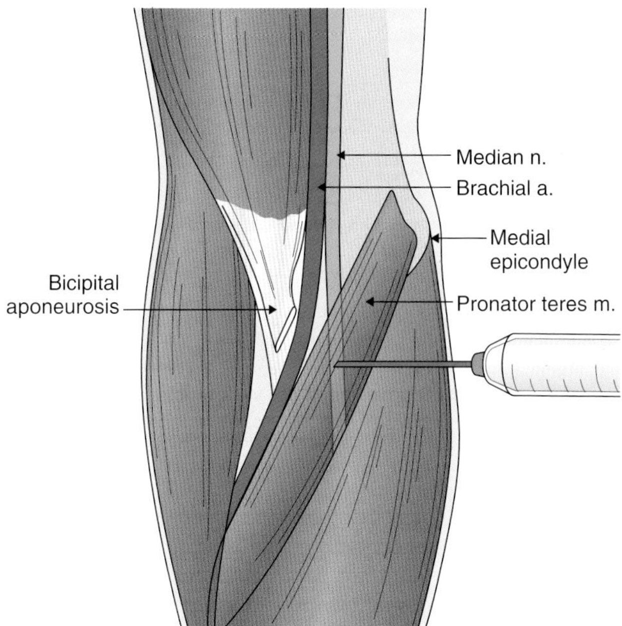

FIGURE 24.6 Pronator teres nerve block. At the elbow crease, make a mark at the midpoint between the medial epicondyle and the biceps tendon. Then, under sterile conditions, insert a 25-gauge, 1½-inch disposable needle into the pronator teres muscle approximately 2 cm below the mark or at the point of maximal tenderness in the muscle. Confirmation of needle placement can be made by a nerve stimulator. Then, inject 3 to 5 mL of a corticosteroid-anesthetic solution (e.g., 2 mL of methylprednisolone [40 mg/mL] combined with 2 mL of 1% lidocaine). Postinjection care may include icing for 10 to 15 minutes and splinting of the wrist and forearm in a functional position for a few days. Also, the patient should be cautioned to avoid aggressive use of the arm for at least 1 to 2 weeks. *(From Lennard TA. Pain Procedures in Clinical Practice, 2nd ed. Philadelphia, Hanley & Belfus, 2000.)*

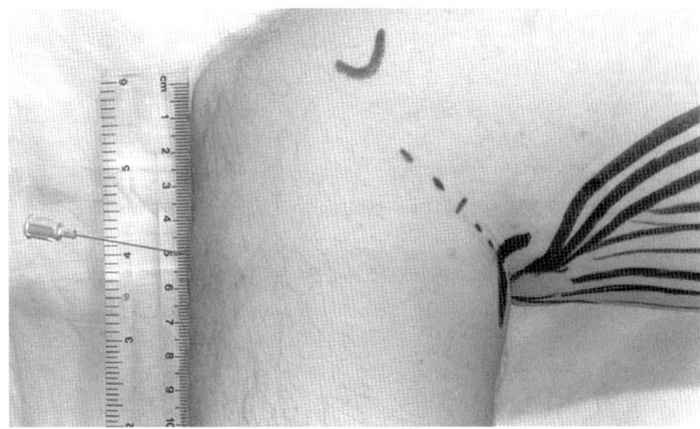

FIGURE 24.7 Anterior interosseous nerve block. The anterior interosseous nerve can be blocked by either an anterior or a posterior approach. For the posterior approach, the posterior elbow is exposed and the forearm is placed in neutral. Under sterile conditions with use of a 2-inch, 25-gauge disposable needle, inject 3 to 5 mL of a corticosteroid-anesthetic solution (e.g., 2 mL of methylprednisolone [40 mg/mL] combined with 2 mL of 1% lidocaine) approximately 5 cm distal to the tip of the olecranon. The needle should penetrate about 3.5 to 5 cm toward the biceps tendon insertion at the radius. A nerve stimulator is necessary to ensure proper placement. Postinjection care is similar to that of the pronator teres nerve block. *(From Lennard TA. Pain Procedures in Clinical Practice, 2nd ed. Philadelphia, Hanley & Belfus, 2000.)*

Potential Disease Complications

Pronator Teres Syndrome

Disease-related complications, if the condition is left unresolved, include permanent loss of the use of the pinch grasp, lack of wrist flexion, and incessant pain.

Anterior Interosseous Syndrome

If it is allowed to persist, this syndrome will cause inability to perform the pinch grasp, resulting in the functional deficits mentioned before.

Potential Treatment Complications

Use of anti-inflammatory medications such as nonsteroidal anti-inflammatory drugs can induce gastric, renal, and hepatic side effects. Local steroid injections can induce skin depigmentation, local atrophy, or infection. Surgical complications include infection, bleeding, and injury to surrounding structures.

References

[1] Lee MJ, LaStayo PC. Pronator syndrome and other nerve compressions that mimic carpal tunnel syndrome. J Orthop Sports Phys Ther 2004;34:601–9.

[2] Mercier LR. Pronator syndrome. Ferri's Clinical advisor. Philadelphia: Elsevier Mosby; 2010.

[3] Sotereanos DG, Sarris I, Gobel F. Pronator and anterior interosseous nerve compression syndromes. In: Berger RA, Weiss AC, editors. Hand surgery. Philadelphia: Lippincott Williams & Wilkins; 2004. p. 49.

[4] Liveson J. Peripheral neurology—case studies in electrodiagnosis. 2nd ed. Philadelphia: FA Davis; 1991, 23–26.

[5] Shapiro BE, Preston DC. Entrapment and compressive neuropathies. Med Clin North Am 2003;87:663–96.

[6] Lee MJ, La Stayo PC. Pronator syndrome and other nerve compressions that mimic carpal tunnel syndrome. J Orthop Sports Phys Ther 2004;34:601–9.

[7] Bilecenoglu B, Uz A, Karalezli N. Possible anatomic structures causing entrapment neuropathies of the median nerve: an anatomic study. Acta Orthop Belg 2005;71:169–76.

[8] Puhaindran ME, Wong HP. A case of anterior interosseous nerve syndrome after peripherally inserted central catheter (PICC) line insertion. Singapore Med J 2003;44:653–5.

[9] Rieck B. Incomplete anterior interosseous syndrome in a guitar player. Handchir Mikrochir Plast Chir 2005;37:418–22 [in German].

[10] Lederman RJ. Neuromuscular and musculoskeletal problems in instrumental music. Muscle Nerve 2003;27:549–61.

[11] Burke SL, Higgins J, Saunders R, et al. Hand and upper extremity rehabilitation: a practical guide. 3rd ed. St. Louis: Elsevier Churchill Livingstone; 2006, 87–95.

[12] Bromberg MB, Smith AG, editors. Handbook of peripheral neuropathy. Boca Raton, Fla: Taylor & Francis; 2005. p. 476–8.

[13] Valbuena SE, O'Toole GA, Roulot E. Compression of the median nerve in the proximal forearm by a giant lipoma: a case report. J Brachial Plex Peripher Nerve Inj 2008;3:17.

[14] Dawson D, Hallett M, Millender L. Entrapment neuropathies. 3rd ed. Boston: Little, Brown; 1999, 98–109.

[15] Stewart J, Jablecki C. Median nerve. In: Brown W, Boulton C, Aminoff J, editors. Neuromuscular function and disease, basic clinical and electrodiagnostic aspects. Philadelphia: WB Saunders; 2002. p. 873.

[16] Spinner RJ, Amadio PC. Compressive neuropathies of the upper extremities. Clin Plast Surg 2003;30:158–9.

[17] Campbell WW. Proximal median neuropathy. DeJong's The neurologic examination. 6th ed Philadelphia: Lippincott Williams & Wilkins; 2005, 553–554.

[18] Prescott D, Shapiro B. Proximal median neuropathy. In: Electromyography and neuromuscular disorders: clinical electrophysiologic correlations. 2nd ed. Philadelphia: Elsevier; 2005. p. 281–90.

[19] Dyck PJ, Thomas PK. Peripheral Neuropathy, vol. 2. Philadelphia: Elsevier Saunders; 2005, 1453–1454.

[20] Mackinnon SE. Pathophysiology of nerve compression. Hand Clin 2002;18:231–41.

[21] Bridgeman C, Naidu S, Kothari MJ. Clinical and electrophysiological presentation of pronator syndrome. Electromyogr Clin Neurophysiol 2007;47:89–92.

[22] Dumitru D. Electrodiagnostic medicine. Philadelphia: Hanley & Belfus; 1994, 864–867.

[23] Wilbourne AS. Electrodiagnostic examination with peripheral nerve injuries. Clin Plast Surg 2003;30:150–1.

[24] Kimura J. Electrodiagnosis in diseases of nerve and muscle: principles and practice. 3rd ed, New York: Oxford University Press; 2001, 14–15, 719-723.

[25] Martinoli C, Bianchi S, Pugliese F, et al. Sonography of entrapment neuropathies in the upper limb (wrist excluded). J Clin Ultrasound 2004;32:438–50.

[26] Jacobson JA, Fessell DP, Lobo Lda G, Yang LJ. Entrapment neuropathies I: upper limb (carpal tunnel excluded). Semin Musculskelet Radiol 2010;14:473–86.

[27] Peer S, Bodner G, editors. High-resolution sonography of the peripheral nervous system. New York: Springer; 2003.

[28] Andreisik G, Crook DW, Burg D, et al. Peripheral neuropathies of the median, radial, and ulnar nerves: MR imaging features. Radiographics 2006;26:1267–87.

[29] Kim S, Choi JY, Huh YM, et al. Role of magnetic resonance imaging in entrapment and compressive neuropathy—what, where, and how to see the peripheral nerves on the musculoskeletal magnetic resonance image: part 2. Upper extremity. Eur Radiol 2007;17:509–22.

[30] Pronator syndrome therapy. E-hand.com the electronic textbook of hand therapy. American Society for Surgery of the Hand.

[31] Trombly C, editor. Occupational therapy for physical dysfunction. 4th ed. Philadelphia: Lippincott Williams & Wilkins; 1997. p. 556–8.

[32] Hunter J, Mackin E, Callahan A, editors. Rehabilitation of the hand and upper extremity. 5th ed. St. Louis: Mosby–Year Book; 2002.

[33] Braddom R. Physical medicine and rehabilitation. Philadelphia: WB Saunders; 1996, 328–329.

[34] Zancolli 3rd. ER, Zancolli 4th EP, Perotto CJ. New mini-invasive decompression for pronator syndrome. J Hand Surg [Am] 2012;37:1706–10.

[35] Lee AK, Khorsandi M, Nurbhai N, et al. Endoscopically assisted decompression for pronator syndrome. J Hand Surg [Am] 2012;37:1173–9.

[36] Keiner D, Tschabitscher M, Welschehold S, Oertel J. Anterior interosseus nerve compression: is there a role for endoscopy? Acta Neurochir (Wien) 2011;153:2225–9.

CHAPTER 25

Olecranon Bursitis

Charles Cassidy, MD
Sarah Shubert, MD

Synonyms

Miner's elbow
Student's elbow
Draftsman's elbow
Dialysis elbow
Elbow bursitis

ICD-9 Code

726.23 Olecranon bursitis

ICD-10 Codes

M70.20 Olecranon bursitis, unspecified elbow
M70.21 Olecranon bursitis, right elbow
M70.22 Olecranon bursitis, left elbow

Definition

Olecranon bursitis is a swelling of the subcutaneous, synovium-lined sac that overlies the olecranon process. The bursa functions to cushion the tip of the olecranon and to reduce friction between the olecranon and the overlying skin during elbow motion. Because of the paucity of soft tissue covering the elbow, the olecranon bursa is susceptible to injury.

The causes of olecranon bursitis can be classified as traumatic, inflammatory, septic, and idiopathic [1]. Traumatic bursitis may result from a single, direct blow to the elbow or from repetitive stress. Football players, particularly those who play on artificial turf, are at risk for development of acute bursitis. More commonly, repeated minor trauma from direct pressure on the elbow or elbow motion is responsible for the problem. Trauma is thought to stimulate increased vascularity, resulting in bursal fluid production and fibrin coating of the bursal wall [2]. Persons engaged in certain occupations or certain activities are susceptible to olecranon bursitis, including auto mechanics, gardeners, plumbers, carpet layers, students, gymnasts, wrestlers, and dart throwers. Interestingly, approximately 7% of hemodialysis patients develop olecranon bursitis [3]. Repeated, prolonged positioning of the elbow and anticoagulation appear to be contributing factors.

Inflammatory causes include diseases that affect the bursa primarily, such as rheumatoid arthritis, gout, and chondrocalcinosis. Olecranon bursitis is commonly seen in rheumatoid patients, in whom the bursa may actually communicate with the affected elbow joint. Crystal-induced olecranon bursitis may be difficult to differentiate from septic bursitis.

Septic olecranon bursitis represents 20% of olecranon bursitis [4]. The source is most often transcutaneous, and about half have identifiable breaks in the skin. When culture samples are positive, the bursal fluid usually contains *Staphylococcus aureus* [5]. Sepsis is unusual. Both underlying bursal disease (gout, rheumatoid arthritis, chondrocalcinosis) and systemic conditions such as diabetes mellitus, uremia, alcoholism, injection drug use, and steroid therapy are considered predisposing factors. There appears to be a seasonal trend, with a peak of staphylococcal septic bursitis during the summer months [6].

In approximately 25% of cases, no identifiable cause of the olecranon bursitis is found. Presumably, repetitive, minor irritation is responsible for the bursal swelling.

Symptoms

Painless swelling is the chief complaint in noninflammatory, aseptic olecranon bursitis. When patients are symptomatic, they usually have discomfort when the elbow is flexed beyond 90 degrees and have trouble resting on the elbow. Moderate to severe pain is the predominant complaint of patients with septic or crystal-induced olecranon bursitis. These patients may also have fever, malaise, and limited elbow motion.

Physical Examination

The physical examination varies somewhat, depending on the underlying condition. With noninflammatory aseptic bursitis, a nontender fluctuant mass is present over the tip of the elbow (Fig. 25.1). Elbow motion is usually full and painless. With chronic bursitis, the fluctuance may be replaced with a thickened bursa (Fig. 25.2).

The distinction between crystal-induced and septic bursitis may be subtle. Both conditions may produce tender fluctuance, induration, swelling, warmth, and local erythema.

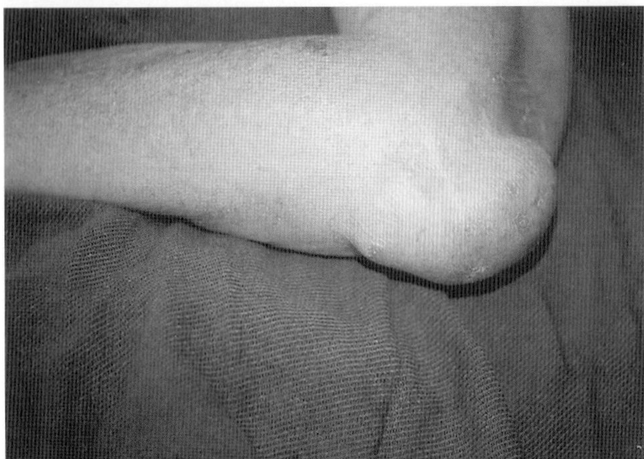

FIGURE 25.1 Atraumatic olecranon bursitis in a 55-year-old woman. A large, fluctuant mass is present.

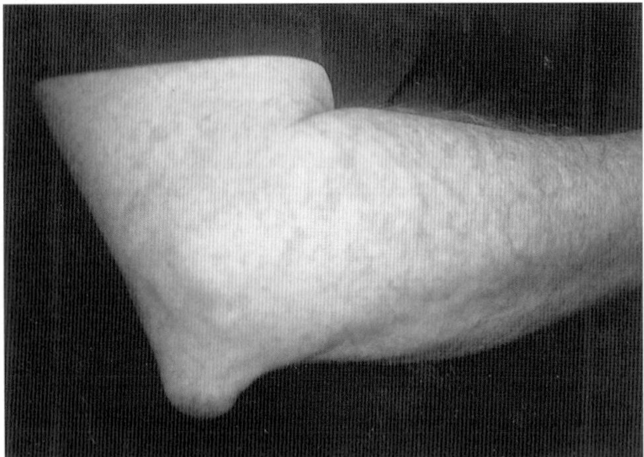

FIGURE 25.2 Chronic gouty olecranon bursitis. The prominence at the tip of the elbow is firm with thinning of the overlying skin.

Elbow flexion may be somewhat limited, although not as limited as with septic arthritis of the elbow joint. Fever and a break in the skin over the elbow are important clues to an underlying septic process (Fig. 25.3). Cellulitis extending distally along the forearm is also more likely to be due to an infection.

In inflammatory cases, pain inhibition may produce mild weakness of elbow flexion and extension. Sensation and distal pulses are unaffected. Examination findings of other joints should also be normal.

Functional Limitations

Functional limitations depend on the underlying diagnosis. Traumatic olecranon bursitis usually causes minimal functional limitation. Patients may note some mild discomfort with direct pressure over the tip of the elbow (e.g., when sitting at a desk or resting the arm on the armrest of a chair or in the car). With crystal-induced and septic bursitis, pain is the predominant issue. Patients may have trouble sleeping and have difficulty with most activities of daily living that involve the affected extremity (e.g., dressing, grooming, cleaning, shopping, and carrying packages).

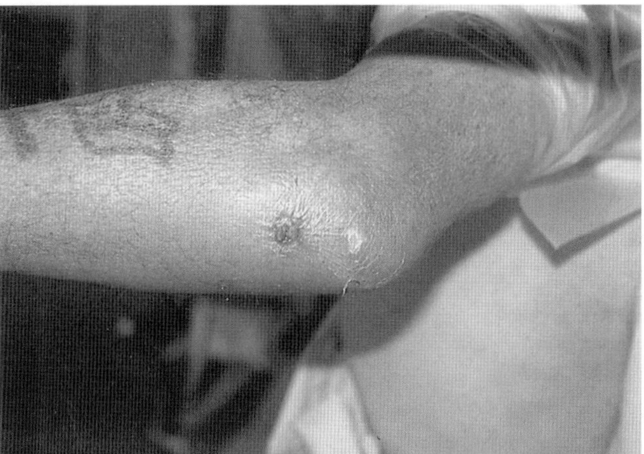

FIGURE 25.3 Septic olecranon bursitis. Cellulitis is present over a wide area. The white scab at the tip of the elbow represents the site of the penetrating injury. Distally, the draining area of granulation tissue developed at the site of needle aspiration. Aspiration of the bursa should be done by use of a long needle inserted well away from the fluctuant area.

Diagnostic Studies

The diagnosis of aseptic, noninflammatory olecranon bursitis is usually straightforward, based on a characteristic appearance on physical examination. In this setting, additional studies are not usually necessary. However, plain radiographs may demonstrate an olecranon spur in about one third of cases (Fig. 25.4). Because this is an extra-articular process, a joint effusion is not present.

If crystal-induced or septic bursitis is suspected, aspiration of the bursal fluid is usually indicated. The fluid should be sent for cell count, Gram stain and culture, and crystal analysis. Acute, traumatic bursal fluid typically has a serosanguineous appearance, containing fewer than 1000 white blood cells per high-power field, with a predominance of monocytes. Infected bursal fluid usually contains an increased white blood cell count, with a high percentage of polymorphonuclear cells. The Gram stain is positive in only 50% of septic cases. Even in the setting of infection, the fluid should be examined under a polarizing microscope because simultaneous infectious and crystal-induced arthritis can occur [7].

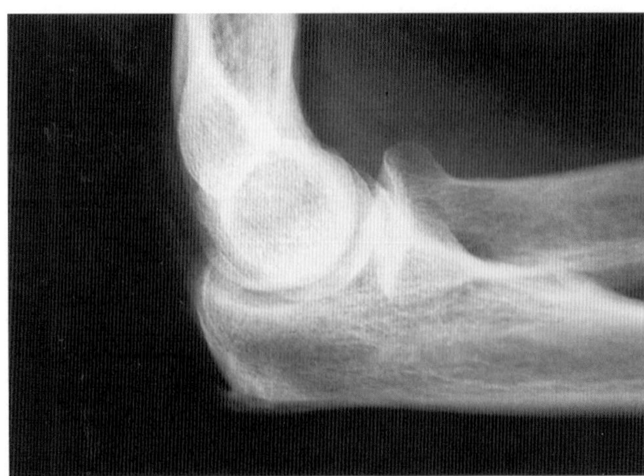

FIGURE 25.4 Lateral radiograph of the elbow in a patient with chronic olecranon bursitis. Note the olecranon spur.

A complete blood cell count and determination of serum uric acid level may provide supportive information in confusing cases, although a normal serum white blood cell count does not preclude septic bursitis.

Magnetic resonance imaging may be of some value to distinguish septic from nonseptic olecranon bursitis, although there is considerable overlap of findings [8]. Absence of bursal and soft tissue enhancement is consistent with nonseptic olecranon bursitis. Olecranon marrow edema is suggestive but not diagnostic of septic olecranon bursitis. The use of magnetic resonance imaging may also help clarify the diagnosis of unusual masses around the elbow.

Differential Diagnosis

Rheumatoid nodule
Lipoma
Tophus
Elbow synovitis
Olecranon spur

Treatment

Initial

Treatment of traumatic olecranon bursitis begins with prevention of further injury to the involved elbow. An elastic elbow pad provides compression and protects the bursa. The patient should be counseled in ways of protecting the elbow at work and during recreation. Nonsteroidal anti-inflammatory drugs are usually prescribed. Traumatic, noninflammatory bursitis usually resolves with this treatment [9]. On occasion, when the bursa is very large, aspiration of the bloody fluid will be a first-line treatment. This is followed by application of a compressive wrap and splint for several days.

In suspected cases of septic olecranon bursitis, it is important to palpate for fluctuance. If a fluid collection is appreciated, the bursa should be aspirated (see the section on procedures). When cellulitis over the tip of the elbow is present without an obvious collection, empirical treatment with antibiotic therapy to cover penicillin-resistant *S. aureus*, the most common offender, is recommended. (Less common organisms include group A streptococcus and *Staphylococcus epidermidis*.) The decision whether to use oral or intravenous antibiotics depends on the appearance of the elbow, the signs of systemic illness, and the general health of the patient. The elbow should be splinted in a semiflexed position (approximately 60 degrees) without pressure on the olecranon. Nonsteroidal anti-inflammatory drugs may be prescribed unless they are contraindicated for empirical treatment of gout and pseudogout. When final culture results return, the antibiotic therapy is adjusted appropriately. Outpatient cases are observed closely, with any changes in the size of the bursa and the quality of the overlying skin noted; oral antibiotic therapy should continue for at least 10 days.

Patients with extensive infection or underlying bursal disease, systemic disease, or immunosuppression and outpatients refractory to oral treatment should be treated with an intravenous cephalosporin. In one study, the average duration of intravenous therapy was 4.4 days if symptoms had been present for less than 1 week and 9.2 days if symptoms had been present for longer than 1 week [10]. The conversion to oral antibiotics should occur only after consistent improvement is seen in the appearance of the patient and the elbow. Serial aspirations may also constitute part of the therapy; alternatively, some clinicians use a suction irrigation system placed into the bursa. Surgical consultation is recommended if the bursitis has failed to improve within several days of appropriate management.

Rehabilitation

Because the process is extra-articular, permanent elbow stiffness is not usually a problem. Physical or occupational therapy for gentle range of motion may be indicated once the olecranon wound has clearly healed. Extreme flexion should be avoided early on because this position puts tension on the already compromised skin. If prolonged immobilization is necessary to permit the soft tissues to heal, therapy may include range of motion and strengthening of the arm and forearm.

Patients who have traumatic or recurrent olecranon bursitis should be counseled in ways to modify their home and work activities to eliminate irritation to the bursa. This might include the use of ergonomic equipment, such as forearm rests (also called data arms) that do not contact the elbow. In some instances, vocational retraining may be indicated.

Procedures

Needle aspiration is therapeutic as well as diagnostic and usually reduces symptoms (Fig. 25.5). It can be performed for patients with traumatic bursitis if they have symptoms compromising their regular activities and should be done (as previously described) for patients in whom inflammatory or septic causes are suspected.

The elbow is prepared in a sterile fashion. The skin is infiltrated locally with 1% lidocaine (Xylocaine). To minimize the risk of persistent drainage after aspiration, it is

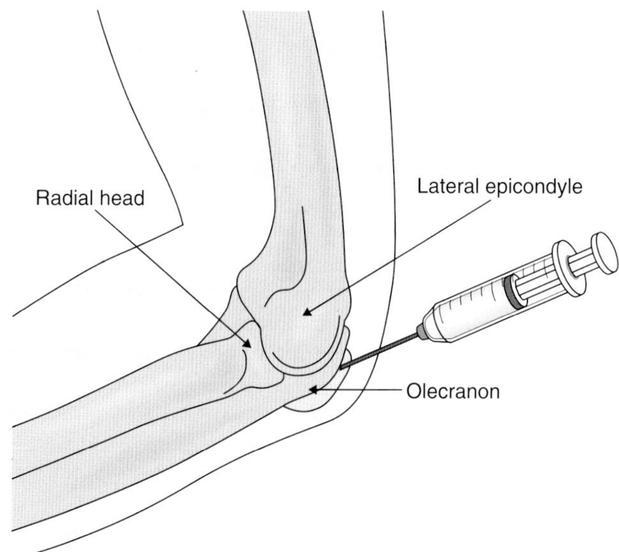

FIGURE 25.5 Approach for olecranon aspiration and injection.

recommended to insert a long 18-gauge needle at a point well proximal to the tip of the elbow. The bursa should be drained as completely as possible. The fluid should be sent for Gram stain, culture and sensitivity, cell count, and crystal analysis.

Postinjection care includes local icing for 10 to 20 minutes. A sterile compressive dressing is then applied, followed by an anterior plaster splint that maintains the elbow in 60 degrees of flexion.

Corticosteroid injections into the bursa have been shown to hasten the resolution of traumatic and crystal-induced olecranon bursitis [11]. However, the risk of complications is high, including infection, skin atrophy, and chronic local pain. Consequently, the routine use of steroid injections for olecranon bursitis is not recommended.

Surgery

Surgery is rarely indicated for traumatic olecranon bursitis. Chronic drainage of bursal fluid is the most common indication for surgery [1]. Bursectomy is conventionally done through an open technique, although a recently developed arthroscopic method has shown some promise. Surgery is usually curative for both traumatic and septic bursitis. However, the success rates are very different for patients with rheumatoid arthritis; surgery provides successful relief for 5 years in only 40% of patients with rheumatoid arthritis versus 94% of nonrheumatoid patients [12].

After surgery, suction drains are often placed for several days. Splinting of the elbow at 60 degrees of flexion or greater for 2 weeks is thought to help prevent recurrence.

Potential Disease Complications

Septic bursitis poses the greatest threat with regard to disease complications. If it is neglected, the infection may thin the overlying skin and eventually erode through it (Fig. 25.6). This complication is difficult to manage, often requiring extensive débridement and flap coverage. Persistent infection can also result in osteomyelitis of the olecranon process. Immunocompromised patients are at risk for sepsis from olecranon bursitis. Necrotizing fasciitis originating from a septic olecranon bursitis, although rare, may prove to be fatal.

Potential Treatment Complications

Analgesics and nonsteroidal anti-inflammatory drugs have well-known side effects on the gastric, hepatic, and renal systems. Persistent drainage from a synovial fistula is an uncommon complication of aspiration of the olecranon bursa; however, this problem is serious enough to discourage the routine aspiration of olecranon bursal fluid in noninflammatory conditions. Complications of steroid injection, as described earlier, can be serious. In addition, wound problems are the major complication associated with surgical treatment of olecranon bursitis. Because of the superficial location of the olecranon and the tenuous blood supply of the overlying skin, wound healing can be difficult. Malnourished and chronically ill patients are especially at risk for surgical complications.

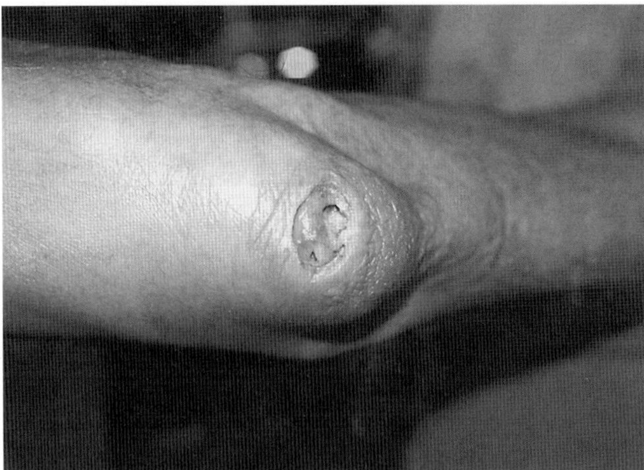

FIGURE 25.6 Untreated septic bursitis with a large olecranon ulcer. The periosteum of the olecranon is visible in the wound. This problem is difficult to manage and often requires flap coverage.

References

[1] Morrey BF. Bursitis. In: Morrey BF, editor. The elbow and its disorders. 3rd ed. Philadelphia: WB Saunders; 2000. p. 901–8.

[2] Canoso JJ. Idiopathic or traumatic olecranon bursitis. Clinical features and bursal fluid analysis. Arthritis Rheum 1977;20:1213–6.

[3] Irby R, Edwards WM, Gatter RJ. Articular complications of hemotransplantation and chronic renal hemodialysis. Rheumatology 1975;2:91–9.

[4] Jaffe L, Fetto JF. Olecranon bursitis. Contemp Orthop 1984;8:51–6.

[5] Zimmerman III B, Mikolich DJ, Ho Jr. G. Septic bursitis. Semin Arthritis Rheum 1995;24:391–410.

[6] Cea-Pereiro JC, Garcia-Meijide J, Mera-Varela A, Gomez-Reino JJ. A comparison between septic bursitis caused by *Staphylococcus aureus* and those caused by other organisms. Clin Rheumatol 2001;20:10–4.

[7] Gerster JC, Lagier R, Boivin G. Olecranon bursitis related to calcium pyrophosphate dihydrate deposition disease. Arthritis Rheum 1982;25:989–96.

[8] Floemer F, Morrison WB, Bongartz G, Ledermann HP. MRI characteristics of olecranon bursitis. AJR Am J Roentgenol 2004;183:29–34.

[9] Smith DL, McAfee JH, Lucas LM, et al. Treatment of nonseptic olecranon bursitis. A controlled, blinded prospective trial. Arch Intern Med 1989;149:2527–30.

[10] Ho G, Su EY. Antibiotic therapy of septic bursitis. Arthritis Rheum 1981;24:905–11.

[11] Weinstein PS, Canso JJ, Wohlgethan JR. Long-term follow-up of corticosteroid injection for traumatic olecranon bursitis. Ann Rheum Dis 1984;43:44–6.

[12] Stewart NJ, Manzanares JB, Morrey BF. Surgical treatment of aseptic olecranon bursitis. J Shoulder Elbow Surg 1997;6:49–54.

CHAPTER 26

Radial Neuropathy

Lyn D. Weiss, MD
Thomas E. Pobre, MD

Synonyms

Radial nerve palsy
Radial nerve compression
Wristdrop neuropathy
Finger or thumb extensor paralysis
Saturday night palsy
Supinator syndrome
Radial tunnel syndrome
Cheiralgia paresthetica

ICD-9 Code

354.3 Lesion of the radial nerve

ICD-10 Codes

G56.30 Lesion of radial nerve, unspecified upper limb
G56.31 Lesion of radial nerve, right upper limb
G56.32 Lesion of radial nerve, left upper limb

Definition

The radial nerve originates from the C5 to T1 roots. These nerve fibers travel along the upper, middle, and lower trunks. They continue as the posterior cord and terminate as the radial nerve.

The radial nerve is prone to entrapment in the axilla (crutch palsy), the upper arm (spiral groove), the forearm (posterior interosseous nerve), and the wrist (cheiralgia paresthetica). Radial neuropathies can result from direct nerve trauma, compressive neuropathies, neuritis, or complex humerus fractures [1].

In the proximal arm, the radial nerve gives off three sensory branches (posterior cutaneous nerve of the arm, lower lateral cutaneous nerve of the arm, and posterior cutaneous nerve of the forearm). The radial nerve supplies a motor branch to the triceps and anconeus before wrapping around the humerus in the spiral groove, a common site of radial nerve injury. The nerve then supplies motor branches to the brachioradialis, the long head of the extensor carpi radialis, and the supinator. Just distal to the lateral epicondyle, the radial nerve divides into the posterior interosseous nerve (a motor nerve) and the superficial sensory nerve (a sensory nerve). The posterior interosseous nerve supplies the supinator muscle and then travels under the arcade of Frohse (another potential site of compression) before coursing distally to supply the extensor digitorum communis, extensor digiti minimi, extensor carpi ulnaris, abductor pollicis longus, extensor pollicis longus, extensor pollicis brevis, and extensor indicis proprius. The superficial sensory nerve supplies sensations to the dorsum of the hand, excluding the fifth and ulnar half of the fourth digit, which is supplied by the ulnar nerve (Fig. 26.1). Radial neuropathy is relatively uncommon compared with other compressive neuropathies of the upper limb. A study in 2000 showed that the annual age-standardized rates per 100,000 of new presentations in primary care were 2.97 in men and 1.42 in women for radial neuropathy, 87.8 in men and 192.8 in women for carpal tunnel syndrome, and 25.2 in men and 18.9 in women for ulnar neuropathy [2].

Symptoms

Symptoms of radial neuropathy depend on the site of nerve entrapment [3] (Table 26.1). In the axilla, the entire radial nerve can be affected. This may be seen in crutch palsy if the patient is improperly using crutches in the axilla, causing compression. With this type of injury, the median, axillary, or suprascapular nerves may also be affected. All radially innervated muscles (including the triceps) as well as sensation in the posterior arm, forearm, and dorsum of the hand may be affected.

The radial nerve is especially prone to injury in the spiral groove (also known as Saturday night palsy or honeymooner's palsy). Symptoms include weakness of all radially innervated muscles except the triceps and sensory changes in the posterior arm and hand. In the forearm, the radial nerve is susceptible to injury as it passes through

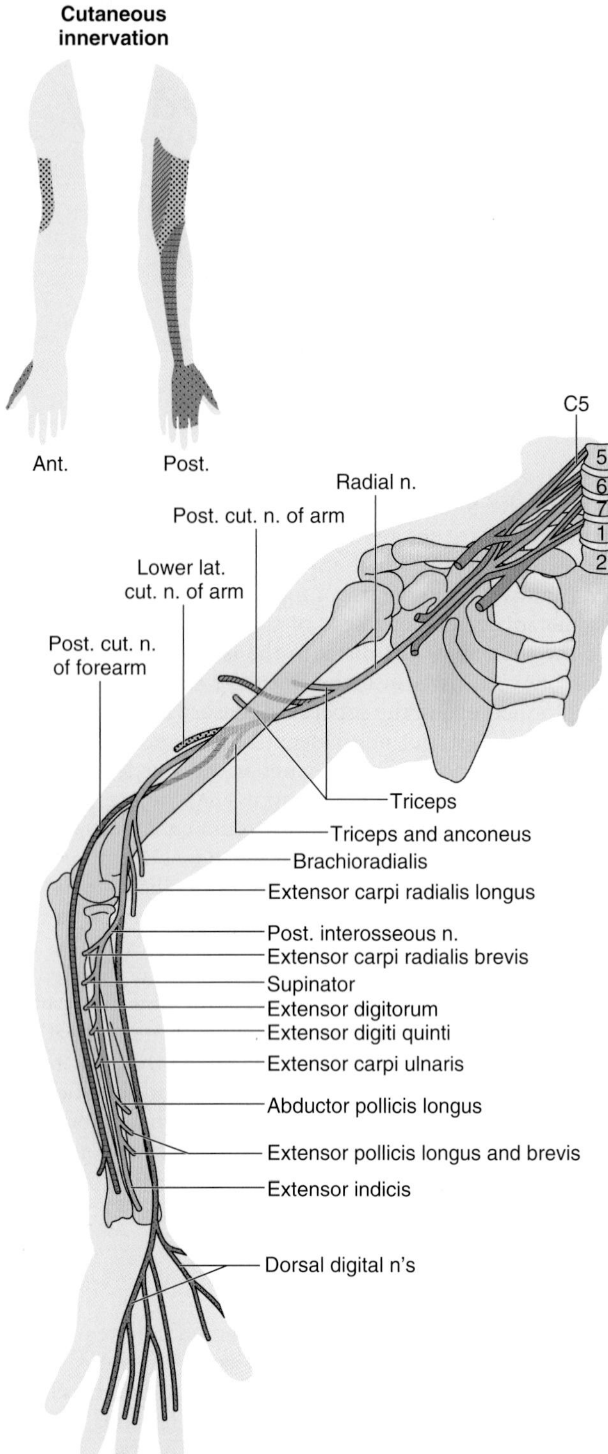

FIGURE 26.1 Neural branching of the radial nerve. Its origin in the axilla to the termination of its motor and sensory branches is shown. The inset demonstrates the cutaneous distribution of the various sensory branches of the radial nerve. *(From Haymaker W, Woodhall B. Peripheral Nerve Injuries. Philadelphia, WB Saunders, 1953.)*

the supinator muscle and the arcade of Frohse. Because the superficial radial sensory nerve branches before this area of impingement, sensation will be spared. The patient will complain of weakness in the wrist and finger extensors. On occasion, the superficial radial sensory nerve is entrapped at the wrist, usually as a result of lacerations at the wrist or a wristwatch that is too tight. In this situation, the symptoms will be sensory, involving the dorsum of the hand.

Physical Examination

The findings on physical examination depend on where the injury is along the anatomic course of the nerve. A Tinel sign may be present at the site of compression. Injury in the axilla will lead to weakness in elbow extension, wrist extension, and finger extension. The entire sensory distribution of the radial nerve will be affected. If the injury is in the spiral groove, the examination findings will be the same, except that *triceps function will be spared*. Radial neuropathy in the forearm will usually result in sparing of sensory functions. If the nerve is entrapped in the supinator muscle, supinator strength should be normal. This is because the branch to innervate the supinator muscle is given off proximal to the muscle. The patient will have radial deviation with wrist extension and weakness of finger extensors. Injury to the superficial radial sensory nerve will result in paresthesias or dysesthesias over the radial sensory distribution in the hand.

Functional Limitations

The prognosis for patients with acute compressive radial neuropathies is good [4]. Functional limitation depends on the extent of the injury and the level of the lesion. In high radial nerve palsy, wrist and finger extension are impaired. However, the inability to stabilize the wrist in extension leads to the main functional limitation. The loss of the power of the wrist and finger extensors destroys the essential reciprocal tenodesis action vital to the normal grasp and release pattern of the hand and results in ineffective finger flexion function. Activities such as gripping or holding objects will therefore be impaired. The sensory loss associated with radial nerve palsy is of lesser functional consequence compared with that of median or ulnar nerve lesions. Sensory loss is limited to the dorsoradial aspect of the hand, and this leaves the more functionally important palmar surface intact. Pain from posterior interosseous nerve entrapment can be disabling enough to limit the function of the involved extremity.

Diagnostic Studies

Electrodiagnostic testing (electromyography and nerve conduction studies) is the most useful test to assess for radial neuropathies. This test can be used to diagnose, to localize, to prognosticate, and to rule out other nerve injuries. The test is usually performed 3 weeks after the onset of clinical findings [5]. At this time, muscle denervation potentials will be observed if axonal injury is present. Radiography and magnetic resonance imaging can be used to rule out a mass (ganglion or tumor) [6] or fracture [7,8] as the reason for the radial neuropathy. Studies have used ultrasound (Fig. 26.2) to investigate the appearance of the radial nerve in the lateral aspect of the distal upper arm [9–11].

Table 26.1 Extensor Tendon Compartments—Wrist

Muscles	Insertion	Evaluation
Abductor pollicis longus	Dorsal base of thumb metacarpal	Bring thumb out to side
Extensor pollicis brevis	Proximal phalanx of the thumb	
Extensor carpi radialis longus	Dorsal base of index and middle metacarpals	Dorsiflex the wrist with the hand in a fist and apply resistance radially
Extensor carpi radialis brevis		
Extensor pollicis longus	Distal phalanx of the thumb	Hand flat on table Lift only thumb
Extensor digitorum communis	Extensor hood and base of proximal phalanges of the ulnar four digits	Extend fingers with wrist in neutral
Extensor indicis proprius		Extend index finger
Extensor digiti minimi	Proximal phalanx of the little finger	Straighten little finger with other fingers in fist
Extensor carpi ulnaris	Dorsal base of the fifth metacarpal	Wrist extension with ulnar deviation

From American Society for Surgery of the Hand. The Hand: Examination and Diagnosis. New York, Churchill Livingstone, 1983.

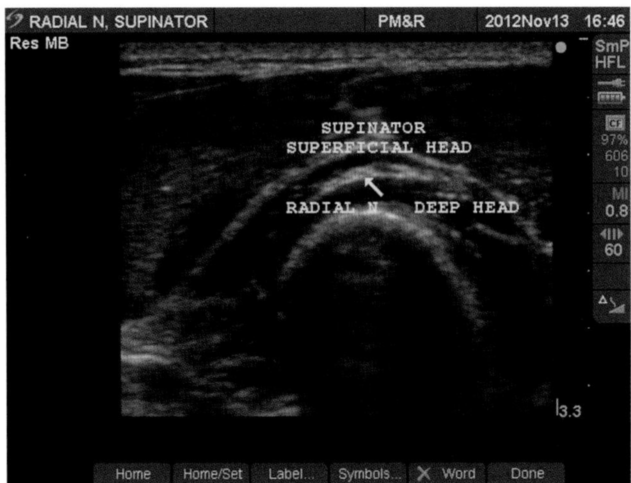

FIGURE 26.2 Short-axis ultrasound image of the radial nerve at the elbow between the heads of the supinator muscle.

Differential Diagnosis

Cervical radiculopathy (C6, C7)
Brachial neuritis
Posterior cord brachial plexopathy
Upper or middle trunk brachial plexopathy
Extensor tendon rupture
Epicondylitis
de Quervain tenosynovitis
Wristdrop secondary to lead polyneuropathy
Posterior interosseous nerve mononeuropathy
Peripheral neuropathy
Axillary nerve injury
Tumor
Chondroma [13]
Hematoma
Carpal tunnel syndrome
Upper extremity extensor compartment syndrome
Ulnar neuropathy
Entrapment neuropathy due to chronic injection-induced triceps fibrosis [14]
Superficial radial neuropathy caused by intravenous injection [15]
Neuropathy after vascular access cannulation for hemodialysis [12]

Treatment

Initial

Radial neuropathies from compression can be managed conservatively in nearly all cases. Elimination of offending factors, such as improper use of crutches, and avoidance of provocative activities are the first steps in the treatment of radial neuropathy. Medications, including tricyclic agents, anticonvulsants, antiarrhythmics, topical solutions, clonidine, and opioids, can be considered for pain management. Nonpharmaceutical treatments, including transcutaneous electrical nerve stimulation and acupuncture, may be considered as adjuvants to medication [12].

Rehabilitation

The main goal of rehabilitation is prevention of joint contractures, shortening of the flexor tendons, and overstretching of the extensors while waiting for nerve recovery. This can be achieved by exercises to maintain range of motion, passive stretching, and proper splinting. Functional splinting can make relatively normal use of the hand possible. Dynamic splints use elastic to passively extend the finger at the metacarpophalangeal joints with the wrist immobilized in slight dorsiflexion. This provides stability to the wrist joint, passive extension of the digits by the elastic band, and active flexion of the fingers. A splint designed at the Hand Rehabilitation Center in Chapel Hill, North Carolina, uses a static nylon cord rather than a dynamic rubber band to suspend the proximal phalanges (Fig. 26.3). The design simulates the tenodesis action of the normal grasp and release pattern of the hand.

Postsurgical release of compression should be immediately followed by exercises to increase or to maintain range of motion and a nerve gliding program to prevent adhesions. Overly aggressive strengthening should be avoided during reinnervation. In tendon transfers, preoperative strengthening of the muscle to be transferred and postoperative muscle reeducation are vital to the success of the procedure.

Procedures

Local anesthetic blocks or injections of hydrocortisone can be used [16] but are rarely necessary and have shown

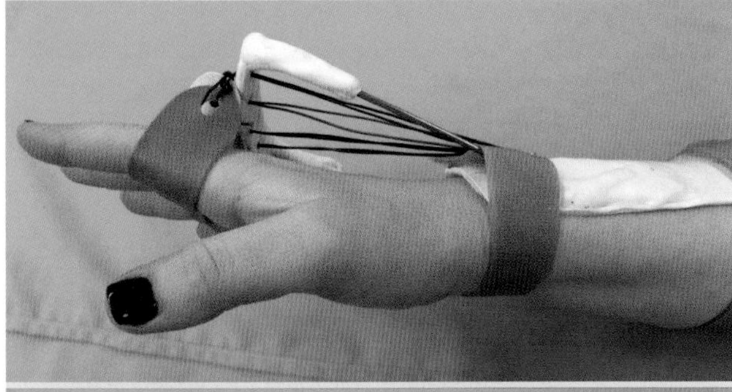

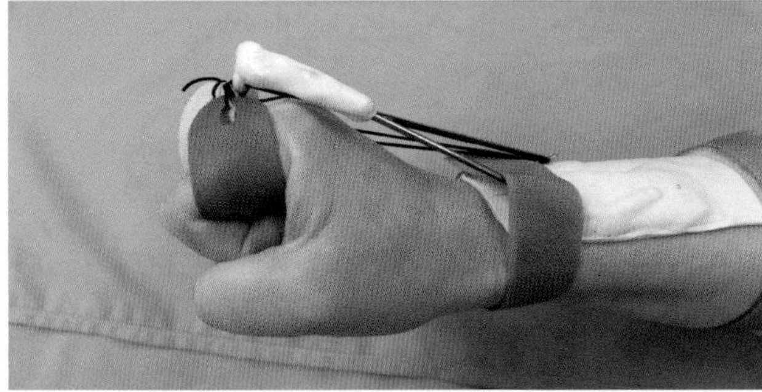

FIGURE 26.3 Radial palsy splint with metacarpophalangeal joint extended and flexed.

only temporary symptomatic relief. Lateral epicondylitis may mimic posterior interosseous nerve entrapment at the elbow. When lateral epicondylitis does not respond to conservative treatment, including injections of the lateral epicondyle, a diagnostic and therapeutic radial nerve injection at the elbow may be indicated [17].

Surgery

Surgical decompression may be required for patients who do not respond to conservative treatment or patients with severe nerve injury. Radial tunnel release has been advocated for compression neuropathies of the posterior interosseous nerve, but the results have been questionable [18]. Surgical intervention for anastomosis may be indicated in cases of complete radial injury (neurotmesis). Tendon transfers may be considered in these instances if the surgery is not performed or is not successful [19,20]. Care must be exercised to avoid the radial sensory branch during operations involving the wrist [16]. Surgery has been noted to be less successful if there are coexisting additional nerve compressions or lateral epicondylitis or if the patient is receiving workers' compensation [21].

Potential Disease Complications

Patients with incomplete recovery may suffer significant functional loss in the upper extremity. Like any patient with nerve injury, they are at risk for development of complex regional pain syndrome (reflex sympathetic dystrophy) [22]. Contractures and chronic pain may develop as well.

Potential Treatment Complications

There are inherent risks with any surgery, including failure to correct the problem, infection, additional deformity, and death. Any injection or surgery involving the wrist should avoid the superficial radial sensory nerve as this could cause additional paresthesias or dysesthesias.

References

[1] Lowe 3rd JB, Sen SK, Mackinnon SE. Current approach to radial nerve paralysis. Plast Reconstr Surg 2002;110:1099–113.
[2] Latinovic R, Guilliford MC, Hughes RA. Incidence of common compressive neuropathies in primary care. J Neurol Neurosurg Psychiatry 2006;77:263–5.
[3] Silver J. Radial neuropathy. In: Weiss L, Silver J, Weiss J, editors. Easy EMG. New York: Butterworth-Heinemann; 2004. p. 135–9.
[4] Arnold WD, Krishna VR, Freimer M, et al. Prognosis of acute compressive radial neuropathy. Muscle Nerve 2012;45:893.
[5] Weiss L, Weiss J, Johns J, et al. Neuromuscular rehabilitation and electrodiagnosis: mononeuropathy. Arch Phys Med Rehabil 2005;86(Suppl 1):S3–10.
[6] Bordalo-Rodrigues M, Rosenberg ZS. MR imaging of entrapment neuropathies at the elbow [review]. Magn Reson Imaging Clin N Am 2004;12:247–63, vi.
[7] Ring D, Chin K, Jupiter JB. Radial nerve palsy associated with high-energy humeral shaft fractures. J Hand Surg [Am] 2004;29:144–7.
[8] Larsen LB, Barfred T. Radial nerve palsy after simple fracture of the humerus. Scand J Plast Reconstr Surg Hand Surg 2000;34:363–6.
[9] Foxall GL. Ultrasound anatomy of the radial nerve in the distal upper arm. Reg Anesth Pain Med 2007;32:217–20.
[10] Cartwright MS, Yoon JS, Lee KH, et al. Diagnostic ultrasound for traumatic radial neuropathy. Am J Phys Med Rehabil 2011;90:342–3.
[11] McCartney CJ, Xu D, Constantinescu C, et al. Ultrasound examination of peripheral nerves in the forearm. Reg Anesth Pain Med 2007;32:434–9.
[12] Kalita J, Misra UK, Sharma RK, Rai P. Femoral and radial neuropathy following vascular access cannulation for hemodialysis. Nephron 1995;69:362.
[13] De Smet L. Posterior interosseous neuropathy due to compression by a soft tissue chondroma of the elbow. Acta Neurol Belg 2005;105:86–8.
[14] Midroni G, Moulton R. Radial entrapment neuropathy due to chronic injection-induced triceps fibrosis. Muscle Nerve 2001;24:134–7.
[15] Sheu JJ, Yuan RY. Superficial radial neuropathy caused by intravenous injection. Acta Neurol Belg 1999;99:138–9.
[16] Braidwood AS. Superficial radial neuropathy. J Bone Joint Surg Br 1975;57:380–3.
[17] Weiss L, Silver J, Lennard T, Weiss J. Easy injection. Philadelphia: Elsevier; 2007.
[18] De Smet L, Van Raebroeckx T, Van Ransbeeck H. Radial tunnel release and tennis elbow: disappointing results. Acta Orthop Belg 1999;65:510–3.
[19] Kozin SH. Tendon transfers for radial and median nerve palsies [review]. J Hand Ther 2005;18:208–15.
[20] Herbison G. Treatment of peripheral neuropathies. Plenary session. Neuropathy: from genes to function. Philadelphia: American Association of Electrodiagnostic Medicine; 2000.
[21] Lee JT. Long term results of radial tunnel release—the effect of co-existing tennis elbow, multiple compression syndromes and workers' compensation. J Plast Reconstr Aesthet Surg 2008;61:1095–9.
[22] Wasner G, Backonja MM, Baron R. Traumatic neuralgias: complex regional pain syndrome (reflex sympathetic dystrophy and causalgia): clinical characteristics, pathophysiological mechanism and therapy. Neurol Clin 1998;16:851–68.

CHAPTER 27

Ulnar Neuropathy (Elbow)

Lyn D. Weiss, MD
Jay M. Weiss, MD

Synonyms

Cubital tunnel syndrome
Tardy ulnar palsy
Ulnar neuritis
Compression of the ulnar nerve

ICD-9 Code

354.2 Lesion of ulnar nerve

ICD-10 Codes

G56.20 Lesion of ulnar nerve, unspecified upper limb
G56.21 Lesion of ulnar nerve, right upper limb
G56.22 Lesion of ulnar nerve, left upper limb

Definition

The ulnar nerve is derived predominantly from the nerve roots of C8 and T1 with a small contribution from C7. The C8 and T1 fibers form the lower trunk of the brachial plexus. The ulnar nerve is the continuation of the medial cord of the brachial plexus at the level of the axilla.

Ulnar neuropathy at the elbow is the second most common entrapment neuropathy. Only carpal tunnel syndrome (median neuropathy at the wrist) is more frequent. The ulnar nerve is susceptible to compression at the elbow for several reasons. First, the nerve has a superficial anatomic location at the elbow. Hitting the "funny bone" (ulnar nerve at the elbow) creates an unpleasant sensation that most people have experienced. If the ulnar nerve is susceptible to subluxation, further injury may result. Second, the nerve is prone to repeated trauma from leaning on the elbow or repetitively flexing and extending the elbow. Poorly healing fractures at the elbow may damage this nerve. Finally, and perhaps most important, the ulnar nerve can become entrapped at the arcade of Struthers, in the cubital tunnel (ulnar collateral ligament and aponeurosis between the two heads of the flexor carpi ulnaris; Fig. 27.1), or within the flexor carpi ulnaris muscle. The nerve lengthens and becomes taut with elbow flexion. In addition, there is decreased space in the cubital tunnel in this position. The volume of the cubital tunnel is maximal in extension and can decrease by 50% with elbow flexion [1]. The nerve may also become compromised after a distal humerus fracture, either as a direct result of the fracture or because of an altered carrying angle of the elbow and decreased elbow extension (tardy ulnar palsy). Repetitive or incorrect throwing can lead to damage of the ulnar nerve at the elbow [2]. Biomechanical risk factors (repetitive holding of a tool in one position), obesity, and other associated upper extremity work-related musculoskeletal disorders (especially medial epicondylitis and other nerve entrapment disorders) have also been associated with the development of ulnar neuropathy at the elbow [3].

Symptoms

If the ulnar nerve is entrapped at the elbow, both the dorsal ulnar cutaneous nerve (which arises just proximal to the wrist) and the palmar cutaneous branch of the ulnar nerve will be affected. Patients will therefore complain of numbness or paresthesias in the dorsal and volar aspects of the fifth and ulnar side of the fourth digits. Hand intrinsic muscle weakness may be apparent. In cases of severe ulnar neuropathy, clawing of the fourth and fifth digits (with attempted hand opening) and atrophy of the intrinsic muscles may be noted by the patient (Fig. 27.2). Symptoms may be exacerbated by elbow flexion. Pain may be noted and may radiate proximally or distally.

Physical Examination

The ulnar nerve may be palpable in the posterior condylar groove (posterior to the medial epicondyle) with elbow flexion and extension. A Tinel sign may be present at the elbow; however, it should be considered significant only if the Tinel sign is absent on the nonaffected side. The ulnar nerve may be felt subluxing with flexion and extension of the elbow. Sensory deficits may be noted in the fifth and ulnar half of the

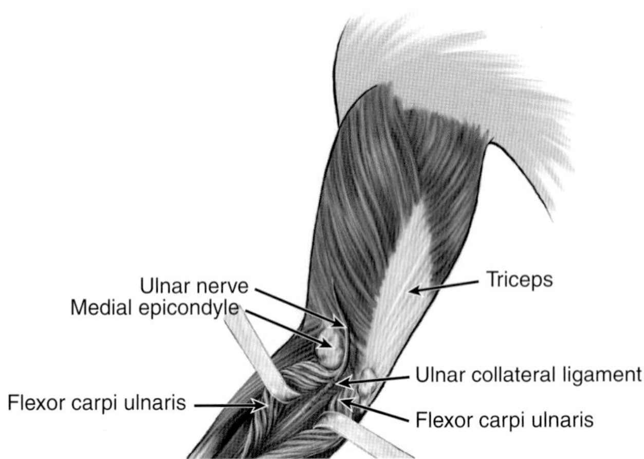

FIGURE 27.1 The cubital tunnel. *(From Bernstein J, ed. Musculoskeletal Medicine. Rosemont, Ill, American Academy of Orthopaedic Surgeons, 2003.)*

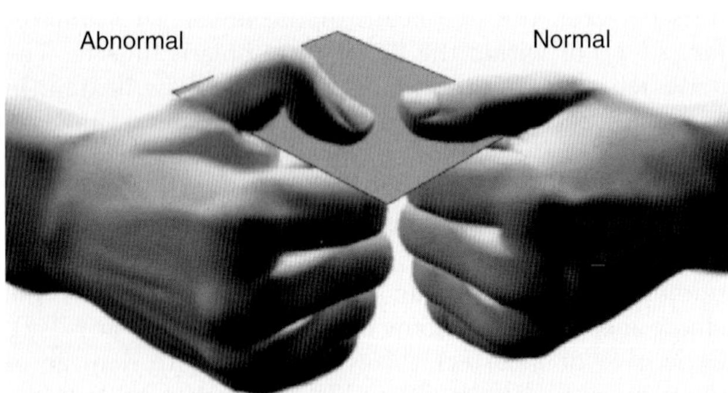

FIGURE 27.2 Froment sign. Note prominent atrophy of the intrinsic muscles. *(From Weiss L, Silver J, Weiss J, eds. Easy EMG. New York, Butterworth-Heinemann, 2004.)*

fourth digits. Atrophy of the intrinsic hand muscles and hand weakness may be noted as well (although this is generally seen in more advanced cases). Wartenberg sign (abduction of the fourth and fifth digits) may occur. The patient should be tested for Froment sign. Here, a patient is asked to grasp a piece of paper between the thumb and radial side of the second digit. The examiner tries to pull the paper out of the patient's hand. If the patient has injury to the adductor pollicis muscle (ulnar innervated), the patient will try to compensate by using the median-innervated flexor pollicis longus muscle (Fig. 27.2).

Functional Limitations

The patient with ulnar neuropathy at the elbow may have poor hand function and complain of dropping things or clumsiness. There may be difficulty with activities of daily living, such as dressing, holding a pen, or using keys.

Diagnostic Studies

Electrodiagnostic studies can help identify, localize, and gauge the severity of an ulnar nerve lesion at the elbow. The findings of abnormal spontaneous potentials (fibrillations and positive sharp waves) in ulnar innervated muscles on needle electromyographic study indicate axonal damage and portend a worse prognosis than with injury to the myelin only. Slowing of the ulnar nerve across the elbow or conduction block (a drop in compound motor action potential amplitude across the elbow) indicates myelin injury. These studies can also identify other areas of nerve compression that may accompany ulnar neuropathy at the elbow. Several studies using ultrasound have shown an increased cross-sectional area of the ulnar nerve in patients with ulnar neuropathy at the elbow [4,5]. Magnetic resonance neurography may play a role in the evaluation of ulnar neuropathy at the elbow [6]. Radiographs of the elbow with cubital tunnel views can be obtained if fractures, spurs, arthritis, and trauma are suspected. In rare cases, magnetic resonance imaging [7] with arthrography may be used to assess for tears in the ulnar collateral ligament or soft tissue disease.

Differential Diagnosis

Ulnar neuropathy at a location other than the elbow
C8-T1 radiculopathy
Brachial plexopathy (usually lower trunk)
Thoracic outlet syndrome
Elbow fracture
Elbow dislocation
Medial epicondylitis
Carpal tunnel syndrome
Ulnar collateral ligament injury
Soft tissue disorders at the elbow

Treatment

Initial

Treatment initially involves relative rest and protecting the elbow. Elbow pads or night splinting in mild flexion may be beneficial. Treatment should be directed at avoidance of aggravating biomechanical factors, such as leaning on the elbows, prolonged or repetitive elbow flexion, and repetitive valgus stress in throwing. Nonsteroidal anti-inflammatory drugs may also be prescribed.

Rehabilitation

Successful rehabilitation of ulnar neuropathy at the elbow includes identification and correction of biomechanical factors. This may include workstation modifications to decrease the amount of elbow flexion, substitution of headphones for telephone handsets, and use of forearm rests. Often, an elbow pad can be beneficial; the pad protects the ulnar nerve and keeps the elbow in relative extension. A rehabilitation program should include strengthening of forearm pronator and flexor muscles. Flexibility exercises should be instituted to maintain range of motion and to prevent soft tissue tightness. Advanced strengthening, including eccentric and dynamic joint stabilization exercises, can be added [8,9].

Procedures

Procedures are not typically performed to treat ulnar neuropathy at the elbow.

Surgery

If conservative management has failed or if significant damage to the ulnar nerve is evident, surgery may be considered [10–12]. The type of surgery depends on the area of ulnar nerve injury and may involve release of the cubital tunnel, ulnar nerve transposition [13], decompression of the ulnar nerve (open or arthroscopic) [14,15], subtotal medial epicondylectomy [16,17], or ulnar collateral ligament repair. Simple decompression and decompression with transposition have been shown to be equally effective in idiopathic ulnar neuropathy at the elbow [18].

Potential Disease Complications

If ulnar neuropathy at the elbow is left untreated, complications may include hand weakness, poor coordination, intrinsic muscle atrophy, sensory loss, and pain. In addition, flexion contractures and valgus deformity may develop at the elbow [8].

Potential Treatment Complications

The results of surgery depend on the extent of ulnar nerve compression, accuracy of identifying the site of compression, type of procedure, thoroughness of compression release, comorbid factors, degree of prior intrinsic muscle loss, and previous sensory loss [8,19–23]. Nonsteroidal anti-inflammatory drugs may cause gastric, hepatic, or renal complications.

References

[1] Weiss L. Ulnar neuropathy. In: Weiss L, Silver J, Weiss J, editors. Easy EMG. New York: Butterworth-Heinemann; 2004. p. 127–34.

[2] Aoki M, Takasaki H, Muraki T, et al. Strain on the ulnar nerve at the elbow and wrist during throwing motion. J Bone Joint Surg Am 2005;87:2508–14.

[3] Descatha A, Leclerc A, Chastang JF, Roquelaure Y, Study Group on Repetitive Work. Incidence of ulnar nerve entrapment at the elbow in repetitive work. Scand J Work Environ Health 2004;30:234–40.

[4] Beekman R. Ultrasonography in ulnar neuropathy at the elbow: a critical review. Muscle Nerve 2011;43:627–35.

[5] Thoirs K. Ultrasonographic measurements of the ulnar nerve at the elbow: role of confounders. J Ultrasound Med 2008;27:737–43.

[6] Keen NN. Diagnosing ulnar neuropathy at the elbow using magnetic resonance neurography. Skeletal Radiol 2012;41:401–7.

[7] Timmerman L, Schwartz M, Andrew J. Preoperative evaluation of the ulnar collateral ligament by magnetic resonance imaging and computed tomography arthrography: evaluation of 25 baseball players with surgical confirmation. Am J Sports Med 1994;22:26–32.

[8] Stokes W. Ulnar neuropathy (elbow). In: Frontera W, Silver J, editors. Essentials of physical medicine and rehabilitation. Philadelphia: Hanley & Belfus; 2002. p. 139–42.

[9] Wilk K, Chmielewski T. Rehabilitation of the elbow. In: Canavan P, editor. Rehabilitation in sports medicine. Stamford: Conn, Appleton & Lange; 1998. p. 237–56.

[10] Asamoto S, Boker DK, Jodicke A. Surgical treatment for ulnar nerve entrapment at the elbow. Neurol Med Chir (Tokyo) 2005;45:240–4, discussion 244–245.

[11] Nathan PA, Istvan JA, Meadows KD. Intermediate and long-term outcomes following simple decompression of the ulnar nerve at the elbow. Chir Main 2005;24:29–34.

[12] Beekman R, Wokke JH, Schoemaker MC, et al. Ulnar neuropathy at the elbow: follow-up and prognostic factors determining outcome. Neurology 2004;63:1675–80.

[13] Matei CI, Logigian EL, Shefner JM. Evaluation of patients with recurrent symptoms after ulnar nerve transposition. Muscle Nerve 2004;30:493–6.

[14] Nabhan A, Ahlhelm F, Kelm J, et al. Simple decompression or subcutaneous anterior transposition of the ulnar nerve for cubital tunnel syndrome. J Hand Surg [Br] 2005;30:521–4.

[15] Kovachevich R. Arthroscopic ulnar nerve decompression in the setting of elbow osteoarthritis. J Hand Surg [Am] 2012;37:663–8.

[16] Anglen J. Distal humerus fractures. J Am Acad Orthop Surg 2005;13:291–7.

[17] Popa M, Dubert T. Treatment of cubital tunnel syndrome by frontal partial medial epicondylectomy. A retrospective series of 55 cases. J Hand Surg [Br] 2004;29:563–7.

[18] Caliandro P, La Torre G, Padua R, et al. Treatment for ulnar neuropathy at the elbow. Cochrane Database Syst Rev 2012;7, CD006839.

[19] Dellon A. Review of treatment for ulnar nerve entrapment at the elbow. J Hand Surg [Am] 1989;14:688–700.

[20] Jobe F, Fanton G. Nerve injuries. In: Morrey B, editor. The Elbow and its disorders. Philadelphia: WB Saunders; 1985. p. 497.

[21] Efstathopoulos DG, Themistocleous GS, Papagelopoulos PJ, et al. Outcome of partial medial epicondylectomy for cubital tunnel syndrome. Clin Orthop Relat Res 2006;444:134–9.

[22] Davis GA, Bulluss KJ. Submuscular transposition of the ulnar nerve: review of safety, efficacy and correlation with neurophysiological outcome. J Clin Neurosci 2005;12:524–8.

[23] Gervasio O, Gambardella G, Zaccone C, Branca D. Simple decompression versus anterior submuscular transposition of the ulnar nerve in severe cubital tunnel syndrome: a prospective randomized study. Neurosurgery 2005;56:108–17.

SECTION IV
Hand and Wrist

CHAPTER 28

de Quervain Tenosynovitis

Carina J. O'Neill, DO

Synonyms

Washerwoman's sprain [1]
Stenosing tenosynovitis [2]
Tenovaginitis [3,4]
Tendinosis [5]
Tendinitis [6]
Peritendinitis [6]

ICD-9 Codes

727.0	**Synovitis and tenosynovitis**
727.04	**de Quervain tenosynovitis**
727.05	**Other tenosynovitis of hand and wrist**

ICD-10 Codes

M65.9	**Synovitis and tenosynovitis, unspecified**
M65.4	**de Quervain tenosynovitis**
M66.131	**Rupture of synovium and tendon, right wrist**
M66.132	**Rupture of synovium and tendon, left wrist**
M66.139	**Rupture of synovium and tendon, unspecified wrist**
M66.141	**Rupture of synovium and tendon, right hand**
M66.142	**Rupture of synovium and tendon, left hand**
M66.143	**Rupture of synovium and tendon, unspecified hand**
M67.20	**Other disorders of tendon and synovium, unspecified site**

Definition

Tenosynovitis is inflammation of a tendon and its enveloping synovial sheath [7]. de Quervain tenosynovitis is classically defined as a stenosing tenosynovitis of the synovial sheath of tendons of the abductor pollicis longus and extensor pollicis brevis muscles in the first compartment of the wrist due to repetitive use [2]. Fritz de Quervain first described this condition in 1895 [3]. Histologic studies have found that this disorder is characterized by degeneration and thickening of the tendon sheath and that it is not an active inflammatory condition [8].

In fact, de Quervain described thickening of the tendon sheath compartment at the distal radial end of the extensor pollicis brevis and abductor longus [3]. Extensor triggering, which is manifested by locking in extension, is rare but has also been reported in de Quervain tenosynovitis with a prevalence of 1.3% [1].

Overexertion related to household chores and recreational activities including piano playing, sewing, knitting, typing, bowling, golfing, and fly-fishing have been reported to cause de Quervain tenosynovitis. Workers involved with fast repetitive manipulations such as pinching, grasping, pulling, and pushing are also at risk [6]. Excessive use of the text messaging feature on a cellular phone has now also been linked to this painful condition [9].

For a majority of cases, the onset of de Quervain tenosynovitis is gradual and not associated with a history of acute trauma, although several authors have noted a traumatic etiology, such as falling on the tip of the thumb [6].

de Quervain tenosynovitis primarily affects women (gender ratio approximately 10:1) between the ages of 35 and 55 years. There is no predilection for right versus left side, and no racial differences have been observed [6].

Symptoms

Patients may complain of pain in the lateral wrist during grasp and thumb extension [3]. They may also describe pain with palpation over the lateral wrist [10]. Symptoms are often gradual in onset and persistent for several weeks or months, and there is often a history of chronic overuse of the wrist and the hand [11]. Pain is the most prominent symptom quality, but some patients report stiffness as well. Pain is often described as severe and may be sufficiently intense to render the hand useless [6]. Paresthesia in the distribution of the anterior terminal branch superficial radial nerve is uncommon [6].

Physical Examination

On examination, the findings of local tenderness and moderate swelling around the radial styloid are likely to be present [11]. A positive Finkelstein test result can confirm the diagnosis [12]. The Finkelstein test is performed by grasping the patient's thumb and quickly abducting the hand in ulnar deviation [4] (Fig. 28.1). Reproduction of pain is a positive test result. A similar test, described by Eichhoff in 1927, provides ulnar deviation while the patient is flexing the thumb and curling fingers around it. Pain should disappear the moment the thumb is again extended, even if the ulnar abduction is maintained [3]. The Eichhoff test is sometimes erroneously called the Finkelstein test. The Brunelli test maintains the wrist in radial deviation while forcibly abducting the thumb [3] (Fig. 28.2). Pain over the radial styloid from these provocative stretch maneuvers differentiates de Quervain tenosynovitis from arthritis of the first metacarpal joint [10]. Strength and sensation are expected to be normal in patients with de Quervain tenosynovitis. However, strength, particularly grip and pinch strength, may be decreased from pain or disuse secondary to pain [13]. A comprehensive examination of the neck and entire upper extremity should be performed before the wrist examination to rule out radiating pain from a more proximal problem, such as a herniated cervical disc [10]. Assessment of the first carpometacarpal joint, including range of motion, palpation for tenderness and crepitus, and radiographic investigation, should also be performed because injury to this joint can give a false-positive Finkelstein test result [14].

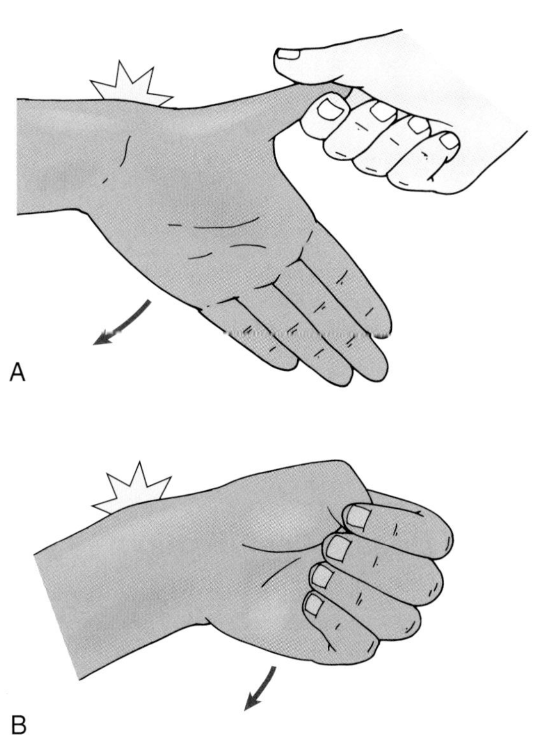

FIGURE 28.1 Finkelstein test (**A**) and Eichhoff test (**B**).

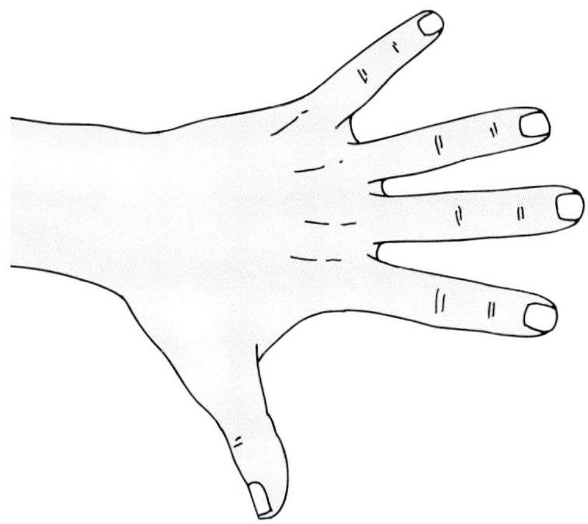

FIGURE 28.2 Brunelli test.

Functional Limitations

Functional impairment is believed to be caused by impaired gliding of the abductor pollicis longus or extensor pollicis brevis tendon through a narrowed fibro-osseous canal [6]. Functional impairment of the thumb is a result of mechanical impingement or pain. Activities of daily living, such as dressing, can be impaired. Fastening of buttons often causes significant pain. In addition, household chores can be limited secondary to pain. Limits in recreational activities, such as bowling, fly-fishing, sewing, and knitting, are also seen in de Quervain tenosynovitis. Workers with jobs requiring repetitive motions, such as pushing or pulling in a factory setting, are at risk for development of the condition. Thus pain from the condition can have a significant economic inpact [6].

Diagnostic Studies

Tenosynovitis of the wrist is a clinical diagnosis, but some authors recommend obtaining a wrist radiograph to rule out other potential causes of wrist pain [6]. Some clinicians report that relief of symptoms after injection of a local anesthetic into the first dorsal compartment is often helpful as a diagnostic tool [6]. When clinical findings are nondiagnostic, a bone scan can help confirm the diagnosis [2]. On ultrasound examination, tenosynovitis is characterized by hypoechoic fluid distending the tendon sheath with inflammatory changes within the tendon [15]. Newer studies use ultrasound to evaluate for subcompartmentalization within the first extensor compartment, which may complicate treatment.

Differential Diagnosis

Carpal joint arthritis
Triscaphoid arthritis
Rheumatoid arthritis
Intersection syndrome
Radial nerve injury
Ganglion cyst
Cervical radiculopathy
Scaphoid fracture
Carpal tunnel syndrome
Radioscaphoid arthritis
Kienböck disease
Extensor pollicis longus tenosynovitis

Treatment

Initial

Initial treatment of de Quervain tenosynovitis is injections. There is no evidence that conservative treatment is effective in reducing symptoms of de Quervain tenosynovitis. Some literature has evaluated effectiveness of ice, nonsteroidal anti-inflammatory drugs (NSAIDs), heat, orthoses, strapping, rest, and massage. Available research does not show these techniques to be effective in the treatment of de Quervain tenosynovitis [6]; however, no randomized controlled study has been performed. One study compared splinting with rest and NSAID therapy. Only 14% of patients who were splinted were cured versus 0% with rest and NSAIDs [16].

Rehabilitation

The goals of therapy are to reduce pain and to improve function of the affected hand. Classically, therapy includes physical modalities such as ice, heat, transcutaneous electrical nerve stimulation, ultrasound, and iontophoresis [8]. In addition, friction massage and active exercises have been employed [8]. A thumb spica splint has been used for immobilization as well [17]. A thumb spica splint is thought to be an effective way to manage symptoms because it inhibits gliding of the tendon through the abnormal fibro-osseous canal [6]. One small, randomized study demonstrated that patients with mild symptoms are more likely to improve with therapy and NSAIDs alone, with the majority of patients with moderate to severe symptoms not responding to therapy [17]. Although steroid injection is the treatment of choice for de Quervain tenosynovitis, because of the benign profile of physical therapy, it is reasonable to consider these less invasive approaches (such as ice, thumb spica splinting, and NSAIDs) as adjuvants when this disorder is mild and first treated [18].

Procedure

Injection of local anesthetics and corticosteroids, with or without immobilization, became popular in the 1950s [6]. It is currently the most frequent treatment modality for patients with de Quervain tenosynovitis. Injection into the first extensor compartment can relieve symptoms (Fig. 28.3). One study described an 83% cure rate with injection [16].

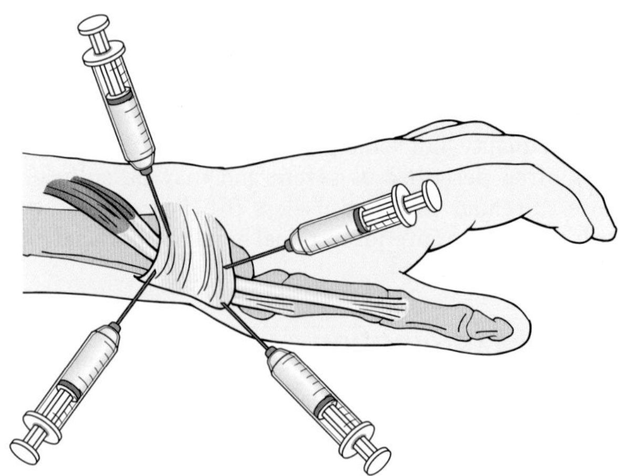

FIGURE 28.3 The four-point injection technique. The injection is divided into two pairs, with each pair including a proximal and distal injection point corresponding with paths of the extensor pollicis brevis and abductor pollicis longus tendons.

In recent years, multiple types of injection techniques have been compared. One study comparing a one-point injection (directed into the first compartment) versus a two-point injection technique (injection corresponding with the paths of both the extensor pollicis brevis and the abductor pollicis longus) showed the latter to be more beneficial [19]. A study evaluating treatment with a four-point injection technique (injecting both the proximal and distal locations for both extensor pollicis brevis and abductor pollicis longus) showed some benefit over the two-point procedure [14]. It is essential that corticosteroid enter the compartment of both the extensor pollicis brevis and abductor pollicis longus for the injection to be effective. Many patients have anatomic variations with a septum creating two subcompartments. Incidence of septation of the first compartment reportedly varies in cadaveric studies from 24% to 76% [20,21]. Ultrasound-guided injections have reportedly increased improvement after injection to 97% [20]. Given the success of injections over therapy, injections remain the first-line treatment of the condition [18].

Surgery

Before 1950, surgery was considered the treatment of choice for de Quervain tenosynovitis. Now, with the success of injections, it is reserved for those whose injection therapy fails [22]. Surgery involves release of the extensor retinaculum, and both open and endoscopic techniques can be used. Partial resection of the retinaculum can be used as well [23]. The patient returns to normal activities after 2 to 3 weeks. On average, surgical success rates range from 83% to 92% [6].

Potential Disease Complications

Because of friction, the tendon sheath becomes edematous, which can further increase friction. This can eventually lead to fibrosis of the tendon [6]. The condition is characterized not by inflammation [6] but by thickening of the tendon sheath and most notably by the accumulation of mucopolysaccharide, an indicator of myxoid degeneration. These changes are pathognomonic of the condition and are not seen in control tendon sheaths. The term *stenosing tenovaginitis* is a misnomer; de Quervain disease is the result of intrinsic, degenerative mechanisms rather than of extrinsic, inflammatory ones [24].

Potential Treatment Complications

NSAIDs have well-known side effects that most commonly affect the gastric, hepatic, and renal systems. The most common immediate adverse reaction reported with injection was pain at the injection site (35%), followed by immediate inflammatory flare reaction (10%), temporary radial nerve paresthesia (4%), and vasovagal reaction (4%); 31% had late adverse reactions ranging from minimal skin color lightening to subcutaneous fat atrophy [6]. In this study, no postinjection infection, bleeding, or tendon rupture was seen, although this could be possible with any injection. With any type of steroid injection, there is a risk of bleeding. Repeated steroid injections have the potential to weaken the tendon and may cause a tendon rupture. Surgical treatment complications include radial nerve injury, incomplete retinacular release, and tendon subluxation [22].

References

[1] Alberton GM, High WA, Shin AY, Bishop AT. Extensor triggering in de Quervain's stenosing tenosynovitis. J Hand Surg [Am] 1999;24:1311–4.

[2] Leslie WD. The scintigraphic appearance of de Quervain tenosynovitis. Clin Nucl Med 2006;31:602–4.

[3] Ahuja NK, Chung KC. Fritz de Quervain, MD (1868-1940): stenosing tendovaginitis at the radial styloid process. J Hand Surg [Am] 2004;29:1164–70.

[4] Finkelstein H. Stenosing tendovaginitis at the radial styloid process. J Bone Joint Surg 1930;12:509–40.

[5] Ashe MC, McCauley T, Khan KM. Tendinopathies in the upper extremity: a paradigm shift. J Hand Ther 2004;17:329–34.

[6] Moore JS. De Quervain's tenosynovitis: stenosing tenosynovitis of the first dorsal compartment. J Occup Environ Med 1997;39:990–1002.

[7] http://medical-dictionary.thefreedictionary.com/tenosynovitis.

[8] Walker MJ. Manual physical therapy examination and intervention of a patient with radial wrist pain: a case report. J Orthop Sports Phys Ther 1994;34:761–9.

[9] Ashurst JV, Turco DA, Lieb BE. Tenosynovitis caused by texting: an emerging disease. J Am Osteopath Assoc 2010;110:294–6.

[10] Forman TA, Forman SK, Rose NE. A clinical approach to diagnosing wrist pain. Am Fam Physician 2005;72:1753–8.

[11] Abe Y, Tsue K, Nagai E, et al. Extensor pollicis longus tenosynovitis mimicking de Quervain's disease because of its course through the first extensor compartment: a report of 2 cases. J Hand Surg [Am] 2004;29:225–9.

[12] Alexander RD, Catalano LW, Barron OA, Glickel SZ. The extensor pollicis brevis entrapment test in the treatment of de Quervain's disease. J Hand Surg [Am] 2002;27:813–6.

[13] Fournier K, Bourbonnais D, Bravo G, et al. Reliability and validity of pinch and thumb strength measurements in de Quervain's disease. J Hand Ther 2006;19:2–10.

[14] Pagonis T, Ditsios K, Toli P, et al. Improved corticosteroid treatment of recalcitrant de Quervain tenosynovitis with a novel 4-point injection technique. Am J Sports Med 2011;39:398–403.

[15] Torriani M, Kattapuram SV. Musculoskeletal ultrasound: an alternative imaging modality for sports-related injuries. Top Magn Reson Imaging 2003;14:103–11.

[16] Richie CA, Briner WW. Corticosteroid injection for treatment of de Quervain's tenosynovitis: a pooled quantitative literature evaluation. J Am Board Fam Pract 2003;16:102–6.

[17] Lane LB, Boretz RS, Stuchin SA. Treatment of de Quervain's disease: role of conservative management. J Hand Surg [Br] 2001;26:258–60.

[18] Slawson D. Best treatment for de Quervain's tenosynovitis uncertain. Am Fam Physician 2003;68:533.

[19] Peters-Veluthamaningal C, Winters JC, Groenier KH, Meyboom-De Jong B. Randomised controlled trial of local corticosteroid injections for de Quervain's tenosynovitis in general practice. BMC Musculoskelet Disord 2009;10:131.

[20] McDermott JD, Ilyas AM, Nazarian LN, Leinberry CF. Ultrasound-guided injections for de Quervain's tenosynovitis. Clin Orthop Relat Res 2012;470:1925–31.

[21] Mirzanli C, Ozturk K, Ezenyel CZ, et al. Accuracy of intrasheath injection techniques for de Quervain's disease: a cadaveric study. J Hand Surg Eur Vol 2012;37:155–60.

[22] Kent TT, Eidelman D, Thomson JG. Patient satisfaction and outcome of surgery for de Quervain's tenosynovitis. J Hand Surg [Am] 1999;24:1071–7.

[23] Altay MA, Erturk C, Isikan UE. De Quervain's disease treatment using partial resection of the extensor retinaculum: a short term results survey. Orthop Traumatol Surg Res 2011;97:489–93.

[24] Clark MT, Lyall HA, Grant JW, et al. The histopathology of de Quervain's disease. J Hand Surg [Br] 1998;23:732–4.

CHAPTER 29

Dupuytren Contracture

Michael F. Stretanski, DO

Synonyms

Dupuytren disease
Viking disease
Cooper contracture

ICD-9 Code

728.6 Dupuytren contracture

ICD-10 Code

M72.0 Dupuytren contracture (palmar fascial fibromatosis)

Definition

Dupuytren disease is a nonmalignant fibroproliferative disorder causing progressive and permanent contracture of the palmar fascia; subsequent flexion contracture usually begins with the fourth and fifth digits on the ulnar side of the hand (Fig. 29.1). The eponym Cooper contracture has been suggested for Astley Cooper, who first described and lectured on the entity in 1822. A nodule in the palm is the primary lesion in Dupuytren contracture. It is a firm, soft tissue mass fixed to both the skin and the deeper fascia. It is characterized histologically by dense, noninflammatory, chaotic cellular tissue and appears on the anterior aspect of the palmar aponeurosis.

The key cell response for tissue contraction in Dupuytren disease is thought to be the fibroblast and its differentiation into a myofibroblast [1]. This idiopathic activation happens in response to the fibrogenic cytokines interleukin-1, prostaglandin F_2, prostaglandin E_2, platelet-derived growth factor, connective tissue–derived growth factor, and, most important, transforming growth factor-β and fibroblast growth factor 2. In addition, microRNAs (miRNAs) identified in Dupuytren contracture samples, including miR-29c, miR-130b, miR-101, miR-30b, and miR-140-3p, were found to regulate important genes related to the β-catenin pathway: *WNT5A*, *ZIC1*, and *TGFB1* [2]. As the nodule extends slowly, it induces shortening and tension on the longitudinal fascial bands of the palmar aponeurosis, resulting in cords of hypertrophied tissue. It is unique among ailments of the hand, and one could conceive of it as a focal autoimmune collagen vascular phenomenon. Dupuytren disease is thought to begin in the overlying dermis. Unlike the nodule, the cord is strikingly different histologically; it contains few or no myofibroblasts and few fibroblasts in a dense collagen matrix with less vascularity. Skin changes are the earliest signs of Dupuytren disease, including thickening of the palmar skin and underlying subcutaneous tissue. Rippling of the skin can occur before the development of a digital flexion deformity [3].

A controversy exists as to whether there is a relationship between Dupuytren disease and repetitive microtrauma [4], but more recent meta-analysis does seem to suggest some degree of occupational correlation with manual work and vibration exposure [5]. It is now thought that microruptures of the palmar fascia are related to the contracture rather than a primary cause [6]. Cessation of manual labor and immobilization can lead to acceleration of the disease, which has been noted in laborers after retirement [7]. One study seems to suggest that there may be an association with rock climbing in men [8].

A genetic predisposition is thought to be inherited as an autosomal dominant trait with variable penetrance [9]. Family history is often unreliable as many individuals are unaware they have family members with the disease. Dupuytren disease has been termed Viking disease [10] because it has a high prevalence in areas that were populated by the Vikings and where the Vikings migrated. Global prevalence is 3% to 6% of the white population, and it is rare in nonwhite populations. Dupuytren disease occurs more commonly in the elderly but tends to be associated with greater functional compromise in younger patients. Women are affected half as often as men [11]. There is no relationship to handedness; however, affected individuals tend to complain more frequently about the dominant hand. Other associations with the condition include diabetes mellitus [12] (specifically with an increased risk from diet-controlled diabetes to sulfonylureas to metformin to insulin requiring), alcohol consumption [13], cigarette smoking [13,14], human immunodeficiency virus infection [15], and antecedent Colles fracture. Conflicting reports exist of an association with epilepsy, but antiepileptic drugs do not present an increased risk [12,16].

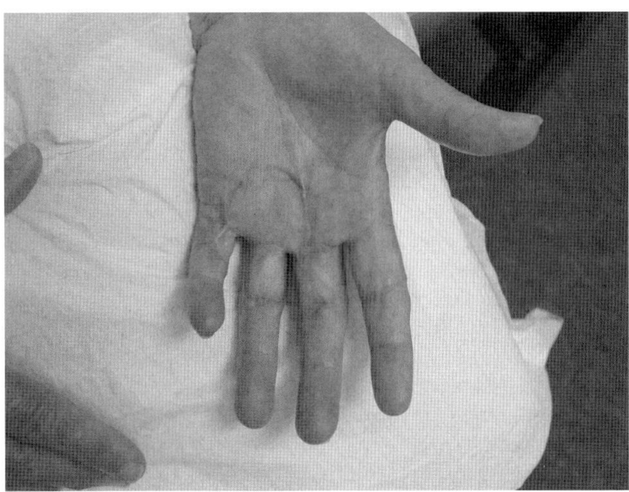

FIGURE 29.1 Typical appearance of ulnar palmar surface after surgical release; notice scarring and incomplete extension.

There are potential secondary findings in Dupuytren disease that are rarely seen but when present suggest a strong Dupuytren diathesis (genetic penetrance of the disease). These findings include knuckle pads (Garrod nodes), plantar fascial disease, and Peyronie disease. The contractile tissue in all of these conditions resembles the pathologic findings of Dupuytren disease in the palm [17], and alterations in the expression of certain gene families, fibroblast to myofibroblast differentiation among others, are similar [18]. However, these associated conditions are found in only an estimated 1% or less of patients with Dupuytren disease [19]. All patients with the disease have a diathesis. The association with these conditions as well as onset at an early age and family history suggests that the diathesis is strong. Recognition of a strong diathesis is important for planning an appropriate rehabilitation protocol, including long-term follow-up and awareness of possible poor prognosis and likelihood of recurrence with surgical treatment.

Symptoms

Dupuytren disease typically has a painless onset and progression. Decreased range of motion, loss of dexterity, and getting the hand "caught" when trying to place it in one's pant-pocket are common presenting symptoms. Pain can be a result of concomitant injuries to the hand and fingers that can precede the development or worsening of Dupuytren disease. Abrasions or ecchymosis to the distal interphalangeal and proximal interphalangeal joints of the affected digits may be seen and may be the reason for the initial consultation. With use of the relatively new Dupuytren disease scale of subjective well-being of patients questionnaire, which covers four areas of the quality of life, there were no differences in quality of life in patients affected in the left or right hand regardless of hand dominance of the patients [20].

The progression of the condition is generally considered to be a result of immobility after an injury in a predisposed individual rather than of the injury itself. Pure sensory symptoms in digits four and five may arise from palmar digital nerves against the relatively inelastic deep transverse metacarpal ligament.

Physical Examination

The most common first sign of Dupuytren disease is a lump in the palm close to the distal palmar crease and in the axis of the ray of the fourth digit (ring finger) (Fig. 29.2). It can also be manifested in the digit, generally over the proximal phalanx. The thumb and index finger are the least affected of the five digits. The nodule can be tender to palpation. In most cases, the skin is closely adherent to the nodule, and movement with tendon excursion often suggests other conditions, such as stenosing tenosynovitis. The condition is more readily apparent when it is manifested in a more advanced stage with palmar nodule, cord, and digital flexion contracture. Conditions associated with this disease include fat pads at the knuckles and evidence of the disease in the plantar fascia. "Swan-neck" deformity as a dorsal variant of Dupuytren disease has been suggested [21].

The examination should evaluate the range of motion and kinetic chain of the entire upper limb, including associated adhesive capsulitis, epicondylitis, and other tenosynovitis. Sensory, manual motor, and muscle stretch reflex components of the neurologic examination should be normal.

Functional Limitations

The majority of individuals with this condition have little functional limitation early on. With more advanced contracture, properly opening the palm and grasping can become difficult, making gripping activities such as activities of daily living, opening cans, buttoning shirts, and placing keys in automotive ignitions troublesome. In many cases, the insidious onset allows gradual compensation, and outside observers may notice irregularity during a simple hand shake.

Diagnostic Studies

The diagnosis of Dupuytren disease is generally made on a clinical basis. Biopsy is considered when a palmar soft tissue mass cannot be reliably differentiated from sarcoma [22]. The suspicion for sarcoma is higher in a younger individual with no strong evidence of Dupuytren disease because sarcoma is more likely in younger age groups. Unfortunately,

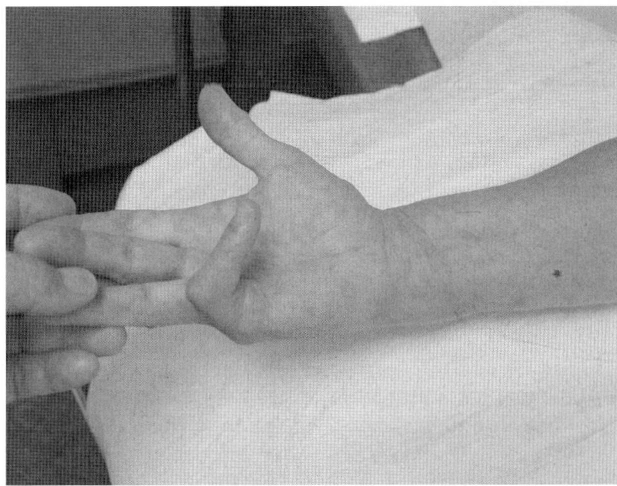

FIGURE 29.2 Dupuytren contracture of the ring finger.

histologic differentiation is not always easy because a Dupuytren nodule can appear cellular with mitotic figures and closely resemble an aggressive sarcoma. Blood work relevant to underlying secondary disease (e.g., hemoglobin A_{1c} level, human immunodeficiency virus testing, uric acid level, erythrocyte sedimentation rate) should be entertained. Electrodiagnostic studies are usually normal. However, concomitant median neuropathy at the wrist or spinal cord may cause sensory loss due to impingement of digital nerves, or Dupuytren tissue may compress the palmar digital nerves against the relatively inelastic deep transverse metacarpal ligament [23]. Sensory nerve action potentials should be recorded to digit four and not just digit five.

Differential Diagnosis

Fibroma
Lipoma
Epithelioid sarcoma
Giant cell tumor
Neurofibroma
Tendon nodules of stenosing tenosynovitis
Inclusion cysts
Dorsal Dupuytren disease
Retinacular ganglions at the A1 pulley
Non-Dupuytren palmar fascial disease
Tophi

Treatment

Initial

Many patients who seek consultation for Dupuytren disease are merely looking for reassurance that they do not have a malignant neoplasm and are satisfied to learn that the contracture is not a sign of a more ominous disease.

Conventional noninvasive treatment has generally been of little or no value in the prevention of contracture or recurrence in Dupuytren disease. This includes the use of steroid injections, splinting, ultrasound, and nonsteroidal anti-inflammatory medications. Radiotherapy, topical dimethyl sulfoxide, colchicine, and interferon have also been proposed but lack data demonstrating long-term efficacy. Topical 5-fluorouracil [24], topical imiquimod (Aldara) [25], and oral simvastatin [26] seem to target the underlying fibroblastic process, but long-term outcome studies do not exist. Traumatic rupture has never gained acceptance as a method of correcting flexion contracture; however, anecdotal reports of individuals correcting their deformity in such a fashion exist [27], but recurrence in true Dupuytren disease would be expected. Continuous passive traction has been proposed by some for severely flexed digit contractures [28]; however, this is used as a preoperative adjunctive procedure and not done in isolation.

Ergonomic assessment and equipment modification can be of use in some instances with laborers who are functionally limited by contracture. Tobacco abuse or excessive alcohol consumption should be addressed if applicable.

Rehabilitation

Rehabilitation efforts are minimal preoperatively and focus on adaptive equipment recommendations for work and home (e.g., large-handled tools for gripping). Splinting may be done by therapists with prefabricated or custom designs, but there is no evidence that this delays contracture or affects the underlying pathohistologic changes. Continuous passive traction has been proposed by some for severely flexed digit contractures [26]; however, this is used as a preoperative adjunctive procedure and not done in isolation.

Postoperative rehabilitation is needed to facilitate a satisfactory outcome. The length of the rehabilitation generally reflects the invasiveness of the surgical procedure; limited fasciotomies often involve a period of 4 to 6 weeks, whereas more extensive surgery may necessitate a formal rehabilitation process of up to 3 to 6 months. Stretching, splinting in palmar extension, and continuous passive traction in some individuals are used early postoperatively. Strengthening and functional activities are added later, after incision healing. Again, splinting may be an option to prevent recurrence, and adaptive equipment recommendations can help with resumption of functions that involve gripping or repetitive hand use.

Procedures

Closed needle fasciotomy has been used [29] but is prone to complications, including infection, nerve injury, and skin breakdown as well as recurrence.

Enzymatic fasciotomy with purified collagenase including injection into the central cord has greatly improved nonsurgical relief of contracture [30–32], with recurrence rates in the range of 14% for metacarpophalangeal joints to 23% for proximal interphalangeal joints at 2-year follow-up where initial collagenase treatment was successful [33]. Xiaflex consists of a 1:1 ratio of collagenases, collagenase AUX-I and AUX-II, isolated from the fermentation of *Clostridium histolyticum* bacteria. This agent has been used for débridement of burns and skin ulcers as well as for Peyronie disease [34]. Steroid injection into the palmar nodule can be a useful adjunct to flatten the nodule. Concern for potential adverse effect on the underlying flexor tendons should be noted. Thus, care must be taken to avoid injection into the underlying flexor tendons. Identification of unique miRNA expression in Dupuytren contracture may eventually lead to the development of novel molecular therapy.

Surgery

Appropriate selection is critical for patients considering surgical treatment. The potential for recurrence and worsening after surgery is higher in patients with a strong diathesis. Recurrence is defined as the development of nodules and contracture in the area of previous surgery. Extension is the development of lesions outside of the surgical area where there had previously been no disease. All patients should be made aware that surgery is not curative of this disease and that recurrence and extension are likely at some time. Extensive recurrence is more likely if surgery is performed during the proliferative phase of the condition.

Nevertheless, many individuals have improved hand function after surgical treatment, compared with their preoperative status, for years on follow-up [35]. The goals of surgical treatment, when it is indicated, are to improve function, to reduce deformity, and to prevent recurrence. Surgical indication is generally thought to include digital flexion contracture of the proximal interphalangeal and metacarpophalangeal joints and web space contracture. Metacarpophalangeal joint contractures are often fully correctable; however, proximal interphalangeal joint contractures often have residual deformity [36].

Multiple surgical procedures have been described for the treatment of Dupuytren contracture. Malingue's procedure is a modified Z-plasty, making use of Euclidean geometry and avoiding the use of skin grafts or flaps, and may potentially have a lower incidence of reoperation [37].

In addition, variations of subcutaneous fasciotomy, fasciectomy, and skin grafting have been used. A controlled randomized trial between the two most common approaches found no statistical difference at 2 years [38]. Fewer complications are seen with limited fasciectomy, and this is often the procedure of choice for higher risk patients, for whom temporary relief is a therapeutic goal. A diseased cord arising from the abductor digiti minimi is noted to be present in approximately 25% of cases [39], and it should be released at the time of surgery if it is present. Full-thickness skin grafting has been shown to prevent recurrence [40] and is considered in patients with a strong diathesis who have functionally limiting contracture.

Potential Disease Complications

In some individuals, the condition can become functionally limiting because of severe contracture. The thumb and index finger tend to be less affected than the other digits. Secondary contracture of the proximal interphalangeal joints can also develop in long-standing deformity. Vascular compromise is rare and more often part of complex regional pain syndrome after surgery. It appears that there is an advantage with axillary block or intravenous regional anesthesia with clonidine over lidocaine alone or general anesthesia in preventing complex regional pain syndrome in patients undergoing Dupuytren surgery [41].

Potential Treatment Complications

Overall, recurrence of the disease after surgery is common (approximately 31%) [42], which is unsurprising when one considers that surgery does not alter the underlying histopathologic process. Loss of flexion into the palm is particularly disturbing to patients. The presence of thickly calloused hands can result in increased postoperative swelling, leading to longer postoperative follow-up. "Flare reaction" is a postoperative complication in 5% to 10% of patients that occurs 3 to 4 weeks after surgery and is characterized by redness, swelling, pain, and stiffness [43]. Complication rates are higher with greater disease severity, in particular proximal interphalangeal joint flexion contracture of 60 degrees or more. Amputation and ray resections are reported complications more common in surgery for recurrences [43]. Although women with the disease less frequently meet operative criteria, they are thought to have a higher incidence of complex regional pain syndrome postoperatively [44]. Other potential surgical complications are digital hematoma, granulation, scar contracture, inadvertent division of a digital nerve or artery, infection, and graft failure in full-thickness grafting procedures. A potential complication of injection therapy is injury to nearby structures, including the digital artery, nerve, and flexor tendons. One study [31] reported 96.6% of the patients who received collagenase to have had at least one "treatment-related" adverse event (compared with 21.2% with placebo), but care should be taken in interpreting this number as events such as "ecchymosis" and "injection-site pain" are potentially subjective, to be expected with any needle entry, and should not necessarily be attributed to the collagenase.

References

[1] Cordova A, Tripoli M, Corradino B, et al. Dupuytren's contracture: an update of biomolecular aspects and therapeutic perspectives. J Hand Surg [Br] 2005;30:557–62.
[2] Mosakhani N, Guled M, Lahti L, et al. Unique microRNA profile in Dupuytren's contracture supports deregulation of β-catenin pathway. Mod Pathol 2010;23:1544–52.
[3] McFarlane RM. Patterns of the diseased fascia in the fingers in Dupuytren's contracture. Plast Reconstr Surg 1974;54:31–44.
[4] Skoog T. The pathogenesis and etiology of Dupuytren's contracture. Plast Reconstr Surg 1963;31:258.
[5] Descatha A, Jauffret P, Chastang JF, et al. Should we consider Dupuytren's contracture as work-related? A review and meta-analysis of an old debate. BMC Musculoskelet Disord 2011;12:96.
[6] Early P. Population studies in Dupuytren's contracture. J Bone Joint Surg Br 1962;44:602–13.
[7] Liss GM, Stock SR. Can Dupuytren's contracture be work-related? Review of the literature. Am J Ind Med 1996;29:521–32.
[8] Logan AJ, Mason G, Dias J, Makwana N. Can rock climbing lead to Dupuytren's disease? Br J Sports Med 2005;39:639–44.
[9] Ling RSM. The genetic factors in Dupuytren's disease. J Bone Joint Surg Br 1963;45:709.
[10] Hueston J. Dupuytren's contracture and occupation. J Hand Surg [Am] 1987;12:657.
[11] Yost J, Winters T, Fett HC. Dupuytren's contracture: a statistical study. Am J Surg 1955;90:568–72.
[12] Geoghegan JM, Forbes J, Clark DI, et al. Dupuytren's disease risk factors. J Hand Surg [Br] 2004;29:423–6.
[13] Godtfredson NS, Lucht H, Prescott E, et al. A prospective study linked both alcohol and tobacco to Dupuytren's disease. J Clin Epidemiol 2004;57:858–63.
[14] An JS, Southworth SR, Jackson T, et al. Cigarette smoking and Dupuytren's contracture of the hand. J Hand Surg [Am] 1994;19:442.
[15] Bower M, Nelson M, Gazzard BG. Dupuytren's contractures in patients infected with HIV. Br Med J 1990;300:165.
[16] Lund M. Dupuytren's contracture and epilepsy. Acta Psychiatr Neurol 1941;16:465–92.
[17] Hueston JT. Some observations on knuckle pads. J Hand Surg [Br] 1984;9:75.
[18] Qian A, Meals RA, Rajfer J, Gonzalez-Cadavid NF. Comparison of gene expression profiles between Peyronie's disease and Dupuytren's contracture. Urology 2004;64:399–404.
[19] Cavolo DJ, Sherwood GF. Dupuytren's disease of the plantar fascia. J Foot Surg 1982;21:12.
[20] Trybus M, Bednarek M. Psychologic aspects of Dupuytren's disease: a new scale of subjective well-being of patients. Ann Acad Med Stetin 2011;57:31–7, discussion 37.
[21] Boyce DE, Tonkin MA. Dorsal Dupuytren's disease causing a swan-neck deformity. J Hand Surg [Br] 2004;29:636–7.
[22] Monacelli G, Spagnoli AM, Rizzo MI, et al. Dupuytren's disease simulated by epithelioid sarcoma with atypical perineural invasion of the median nerve. Case report. G Chir 2008;29:149–51.
[23] Guney F, Yuruten B, Karalezli N. Digital neuropathy of the median and ulnar nerves caused by Dupuytren's contracture: case report. Neurologist 2009;15:217–9.

[24] Bulstrode NW, Mudera V, McGrouther DA. 5-Fluorouracil selectively inhibits collagen synthesis. Plast Reconstr Surg 2005;116:209–21.
[25] Namazi H. Imiquimod: a potential weapon against Dupuytren contracture. Med Hypotheses 2006;66:991–2.
[26] Namazi H, Emami MJ. Simvastatin may be useful in therapy of Dupuytren contracture. Med Hypotheses 2006;66:683–4.
[27] Sirotakova M, Elliot D. A historical record of traumatic rupture of Dupuytren's contracture. J Hand Surg [Br] 1997;22:198–201.
[28] Citron N, Mesina J. The use of skeletal traction in the treatment of severe primary Dupuytren's disease. J Bone Joint Surg Br 1998;80:126–9.
[29] Badois F, Lermusiaux J, Masse C, et al. Nonsurgical treatment of Dupuytren's disease using needle fasciotomy. Rev Rhum Engl Ed 1993;60:692–7.
[30] Holzer LA, Holzer G. Collagenase clostridium histolyticum in the management of Dupuytren's contracture. Handchir Mikrochir Plast Chir 2011;43:269–74.
[31] Hurst LC, Badalamente MA, Hentz VR, et al. Injectable collagenase clostridium histolyticum for Dupuytren's contracture. N Engl J Med 2009;361:968–79.
[32] Azzopardi E, Boyce DE. Clostridium histolyticum collagenase in the treatment of Dupuytren's contracture. Br J Hosp Med (Lond) 2012;73:432–6.
[33] Badalamente MA. Satisfactory recurrence rates for collagenase in hand contractures. Medscape Feb 23, 2011, American Academy of Orthopaedic Surgeons (AAOS) 2011 annual meeting, February 18, 2011. Abstract 568.
[34] Gelbard M, James K, Riach P, et al. Collagenase versus placebo in the treatment of Peyronie's disease: a double-blind study. J Urol 1993;149:56–8.
[35] Forgon M, Farkas G. Results of surgical treatment of Dupuytren's contracture. Handchir Mikrochir Plast Chir 1988;20:279–84.
[36] Riolo J, Young VL, Ueda K, Pidgeon L. Dupuytren's contracture. South Med J 1991;84:983–96.
[37] Apard T, Saint-Cast Y. Malingue's procedure for digital retraction in Dupuytren's contracture—principle, modelling and clinical evaluation. Chir Main 2011;30:31–4.
[38] Citron ND, Nunez V. Recurrence after surgery of Dupuytren's disease: a randomized trial of two skin incisions. J Hand Surg [Br] 2005;30:563–6.
[39] Meathrel KE, Thoma A. Abductor digiti minimi involvement in Dupuytren's contracture of the small finger. J Hand Surg [Am] 2004;29:510–3.
[40] Villani F, Choughri H, Pelissier P. Importance of skin graft in preventing recurrence of Dupuytren's contracture. Chir Main 2009;28: 349–51.
[41] Reuben SS, Pristas R, Dixon D, et al. The incidence of complex regional pain syndrome after fasciectomy for Dupuytren's contracture: a prospective observational study of four anesthetic techniques. Anesth Analg 2006;102:499–503.
[42] Bulstrode NW, Jemec B, Smith PJ. The complications of Dupuytren's contracture surgery. J Hand Surg [Br] 2005;30:1021–5.
[43] Del Frari B, Estermann D, Piza-Katzer H. Dupuytren's contracture—surgery of recurrences. Handchir Mikrochir Plast Chir 2005;37:309–15.
[44] Zemel NP, Balcomb TV, Stark HH, et al. Dupuytren's disease in women: evaluation of long-term results after operation. J Hand Surg [Am] 1987;12:1012.

CHAPTER 30

Extensor Tendon Injuries

Jeffrey S. Brault, DO

Synonyms

Mallet finger
Extensor hood injury
Central slip injury
Extensor sheath injury
Boutonnière deformity
Buttonhole deformity

ICD-9 Codes

727.63 Hand extensor injury
736.1 Mallet finger
736.21 Boutonnière deformity

ICD-10 Codes

S69.90 Injury of unspecified wrist, hand and finger(s)
S69.91 Injury of right wrist, hand and finger(s)
S69.92 Injury of left wrist, hand and finger(s)
Add seventh character for episode of care (A—initial, D—subsequent, S—sequela)
M20.011 Mallet of right finger(s)
M20.012 Mallet of left finger(s)
M20.019 Mallet of unspecified finger(s)
M20.021 Boutonnière deformity of right finger(s)
M20.022 Boutonnière deformity of left finger(s)
M20.029 Boutonnière deformity of unspecified finger(s)

Definition

Extensor tendon injuries occur to the extensor mechanism of the digits. They include the finger and the thumb extensors and abductors. These injuries are more common than flexor tendon injuries because of their superficial position and relative lack of soft tissue between them and the underlying bone. As a result, the extensor tendons are prone to laceration, abrasion, crushing, burns, and bite wounds [1]. Demographic data defining age, gender, and occupation for the development of extensor tendon injury are not well documented. However, in our clinical experience, extensor tendon injuries commonly occur from lacerations, fist to mouth injuries, and rheumatologic conditions.

Extensor tendon injuries result in the inability to extend the finger because of transection of the tendon itself, extensor lag, joint stiffness, and poor pain control [2,3]. There are eight zones to the extensor mechanism where injury can result in differing pathomechanics [4] (Fig. 30.1).

Symptoms

Patients typically lose the ability to fully extend the involved finger (Fig. 30.2). This lack of motion may be confined to a single joint or the entire digit. Pain in surrounding regions often accompanies the loss of motion because of abnormal tissue stresses. Diminished sensation may be present if there is concomitant injury to the digital nerves.

Physical Examination

Physical examination begins with observation of the resting hand position. If the extensor tendon is completely disrupted, the unsupported finger will assume a flexed posture. Range of motion, both active and passive, is evaluated for each finger joint. Grip strength is commonly measured by use of a hand-held dynamometer. Individual finger extension strength can be recorded by manual muscle testing or finger dynamometry. Sensation should be checked because of the proximity of the extensor mechanism to the digital nerves. The radial and ulnar sides of the digit should be checked to assess light touch, pinprick, and two-point discrimination.

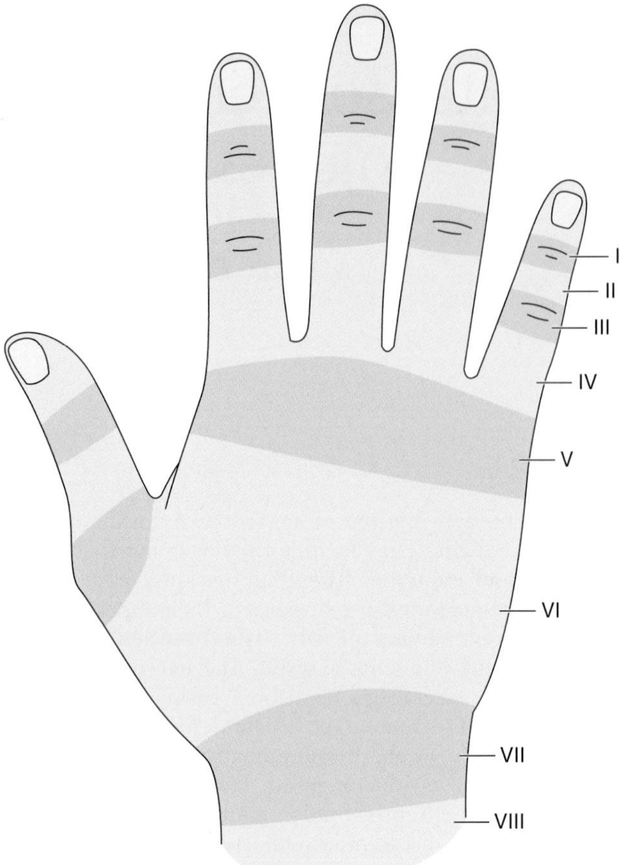

FIGURE 30.1 Zones of extensor tendons. Odd numbers overlie the respective joints, and even numbers overlie areas of intermediate tendon regions.

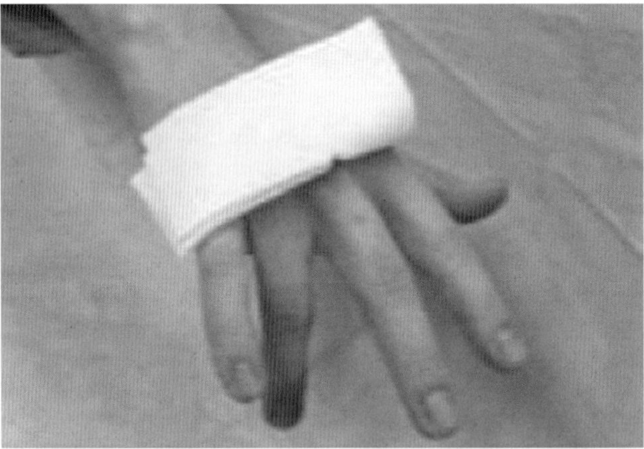

FIGURE 30.2 Extensor tendon disruption of the ring finger resulting in an inability to extend the ring finger. *(Modified from Daniels JM II, Zook EG, Lynch JM. Hand and wrist injuries: part I. Nonemergent evaluation. Am Fam Physician 2004;69:1941-1948.)*

Functional Limitations

The positioning of the hand in preparation for grip or pinch is occasionally more important and limiting than the inability to grasp. Functional limitations therefore are manifested as the inability to produce finger extension in preparation for grip or pinch. As a result, writing and manipulation of small objects can be problematic. Patients may also have difficulty reaching into confined areas, such as pockets, because of a flexed digit with the limited ability to extend.

Diagnostic Studies

Anteroposterior and lateral radiographs of the involved hand and fingers are obtained when there is a possibility of bone or soft tissue injury, such as fracture of a metacarpal from a bite wound, foreign body retention from glass or metal, or air in the soft tissues or joint space secondary to penetration of a foreign object. Ultrasonography is an inexpensive alternative to magnetic resonance imaging for the detection of foreign bodies and identification of traumatic lesions of tendons. However, ultrasonography and magnetic resonance imaging are generally not necessary but can be used to confirm clinical suspicion of chronic and partial extensor tendon injuries.

Differential Diagnosis

Fracture dislocation
Joint dislocation
Peripheral nerve injury
Osteoarthritis
Rheumatoid arthritis
Trigger finger (stenosing tenosynovitis)

Treatment

Initial

The treatment protocols for extensor tendon injuries vary by zone, mechanism, and time elapsed since the injury. If the disruption of the extensor mechanism is due to a laceration, crush injury, burn, or bite, surgical referral is warranted. In open injuries, if repair is not immediate, appropriate antibiotics should be initiated, the injured tendon should be promptly irrigated, and primary coverage by skin suturing should be performed to protect the tendon and to decrease the potential for infection. The surgeon who will be performing the definitive repair should be contacted before this, however [5]. Conservative splinting can be attempted for closed zone I and zone II extensor tendon injuries.

Rehabilitation

Conservative treatment and splinting have been recommended for zone I and zone II injuries. Conservative treatment of injuries involving zones III through VIII has limited success in restoring normal range of motion and function. Acute injuries in these zones usually require surgical repair, and chronic injuries often require surgical review.

Zone I (Mallet Deformity)

Disruption of continuity of the extensor tendon over the distal interphalangeal (DIP) joint produces the characteristic flexion deformity of the DIP joint [6]. Injury in this region is the result of a traumatic event, such as sudden forced hyperflexion of an extended DIP joint with tendinous disruption or avulsion fracture at the site of insertion. The digits most commonly involved are the long, ring, and small fingers of the dominant hand [7]. When it is left untreated for a prolonged time, hyperextension of the proximal interphalangeal (PIP) joint (swan-neck deformity) may develop because of proximal retraction of the central band [6].

In a closed injury, the most common method of treatment is 6 weeks of continuous immobilization of the DIP joint in full extension or slight hyperextension (0 to 15 degrees) [8–12]. The DIP joint should not be immobilized in excessive hyperextension because of compromise of the vascular supply to the dorsal skin [7]. Stack splints are commonly used to achieve extension at the DIP joint. The splint should be worn continuously, except during hygiene. When the splint is removed, the DIP joint should be maintained in extension. If no extensor lag is identified after 7 weeks, range of motion exercises consisting of 10 repetitions hourly of passive, pain-free motion of the DIP joint can be initiated. The splint should be worn during exercise and at night. Splinting may be discontinued and exercises progressed to active extension after 8 weeks. In chronic mallet deformities, in which no treatment is initiated for 3 weeks after injury, splinting is recommended for 8 weeks before beginning of range of motion exercises (Table 30.1) [9,11,12].

Zone II

Injuries in zone II are often due to a laceration or crush injury. Treatment involves routine wound care and splinting for 7 to 10 days, followed by active motion if less than 50% of the tendon width is cut. If more than 50% of the tendon is cut, it should be repaired primarily, followed by 6 weeks of splinting [6].

Zone III (Boutonnière Deformity)

Zone III injuries usually result from direct forceful flexion of an extended PIP joint, laceration, or bite. If the lateral bands slip volarly, a boutonnière deformity results. The boutonnière deformity develops gradually and usually appears 10 to 14 days after the initial injury. Diagnosis is best made after splinting of the finger straight for a few days and reexamination of the finger after swelling subsides. Absent or weak active extension of the PIP joint is a positive, confirmatory finding [6].

Closed injuries are initially treated with 4 to 6 weeks of splinting of the PIP joint in extension with the metacarpophalangeal (MCP) and wrist joints left free. The splint is reapplied for recurrence of deformity [6]. Displaced closed avulsion fractures at the base of the middle phalanx, axial and lateral instability of the PIP joint with loss of joint motion, and failed nonoperative treatment are indications for surgical intervention [6]. In addition, acute open injuries require primary surgical repair.

Postoperative rehabilitation has changed in recent years with the implementation of early protected motion [8–10,13]. Postoperatively, the finger is immobilized in a PIP joint gutter splint. This splint is removed hourly to perform guarded active motion exercises, which may consist of using two exercise braces that provide optimal gliding of the extensor mechanism (Table 30.2).

Zone IV

Injuries in zone IV usually spare the lateral bands. However, there is often considerable adhesion with resultant loss of motion that develops because of the intricate relationship of the tendon and bone in this area. Rehabilitation and splinting techniques are similar to those in zone III (see Table 30.2).

Table 30.1 Zone I and Zone II Injuries

	Splint	Exercises	Wound and Skin Care
Acute DIP Joint Injuries, Mallet Deformity (Less than 3 Weeks)			
0-5 weeks	Continuous DIP joint extension (stack)	Active flexion and extension of PIP and MCP joints (hourly)	Remove splint daily to check for skin integrity and hygiene (maintain DIP joint in extension)
6 weeks	Worn between exercises and at night	Active flexion and extension of DIP joint (hourly)	Remove splint daily to check for skin integrity and hygiene (maintain DIP joint in extension)
7 weeks	Worn between exercises and at night	Passive flexion and extension of DIP joint (hourly)	Remove splint daily to check for skin integrity and hygiene (maintain DIP joint in extension)
8 weeks	If no extensor lag, may gradually wean from splint	Continue with active and passive DIP joint exercises	Remove splint daily to check for skin integrity and hygiene (maintain DIP joint in extension)
Chronic DIP Joint Injuries, Mallet Deformity (More than 3 Weeks)			
0-7 weeks	Continuous DIP joint extension (stack)	Active flexion and extension of PIP and MCP joints (hourly)	Remove splint daily to check for skin integrity and hygiene (maintain DIP joint in extension)
8 weeks	Worn between exercises and at night	Active flexion and extension of DIP joint (hourly)	Remove splint daily to check for skin integrity and hygiene (maintain DIP joint in extension)
9 weeks	Worn between exercises and at night	Passive flexion and extension of DIP joint (hourly)	Remove splint daily to check for skin integrity and hygiene (maintain DIP joint in extension)
10 weeks	If no extensor lag, may gradually wean from splint	Continue with active and passive DIP joint exercises	Remove splint daily to check for skin integrity and hygiene (maintain DIP joint in extension)

From Brault J. Rehabilitation of extensor tendon injuries. Oper Tech Plast Reconstr Surg 2000;7:25-30.

Table 30.2 Zone III and Zone IV Injuries (Immediate Motion)

	Splint	Exercises	Wound and Skin Care
Start 24-48 hours	DIP joint and PIP joint neutral splint	Exercise hourly with two splints	Daily removal of splint for wound cleaning Edema control with compressive wrap
0-2 weeks		Splint 1: allows 30 degrees of PIP joint and 25 degrees of DIP joint range of motion Splint 2: PIP joint in neutral, DIP active flexion	Daily removal of splint for wound cleaning Edema control with compressive wrap
2-3 weeks	If no extensor lag noted	Splint 1: increase PIP joint in flexion to 40 degrees Splint 2: continue	Daily removal of splint for wound cleaning Edema control with compressive wrap
4-5 weeks	If no extensor lag noted	Splint 1: increase PIP joint in flexion to 40 degrees Splint 2: continue	Daily removal of splint for wound cleaning Edema control with compressive wrap
6 weeks	If no extensor lag noted, discontinue use of splints	Allow full active PIP joint and DIP joint flexion	Daily removal of splint for wound cleaning Edema control with compressive wrap

From Brault J. Rehabilitation of extensor tendon injuries. Oper Tech Plast Reconstr Surg 2000;7:25-30.

Zone V

Zone V is located over the MCP joints. This is the most common area of extensor tendon injuries resulting from bites, lacerations, or joint dislocation [1]. The injury more often occurs with the joint in flexion, so the tendon injury will actually be proximal to the dermal injury [6]. Acute open injuries are surgically repaired after thorough irrigation if they are not the result of a human bite or fist to mouth injury.

Many authors have recently recommended that dynamic splinting be initiated in the first week [8,9,11,12,14,15]. This is accomplished with a dorsal dynamic extension splint that has stop beads on the suspension line, which limits flexion (Fig. 30.3A). Patients are instructed to perform active flexion of the fingers hourly (Fig. 30.3B). The rubber band suspension provides passive extension. Therapy is initiated early by a skilled therapist by positioning the wrist in 20 degrees of flexion and passively flexing the MCP joint to 30 degrees. This provides for safe protected gliding of the extensor mechanism. At postoperative week 7, progressive strengthening exercises can be initiated. At week 9, all bracing may be discontinued if no extensor lag is present (Table 30.3).

When the wound is associated with a human bite, it is extensively inspected and débrided; culture specimens are obtained, and the wound is irrigated and left open. Broad-spectrum antibiotics are initiated. The hand is splinted with the wrist in approximately 45 degrees of extension and the MCP joint in 15 to 20 degrees of flexion. The wound typically heals within 5 to 10 days, and secondary repair is rarely needed [6].

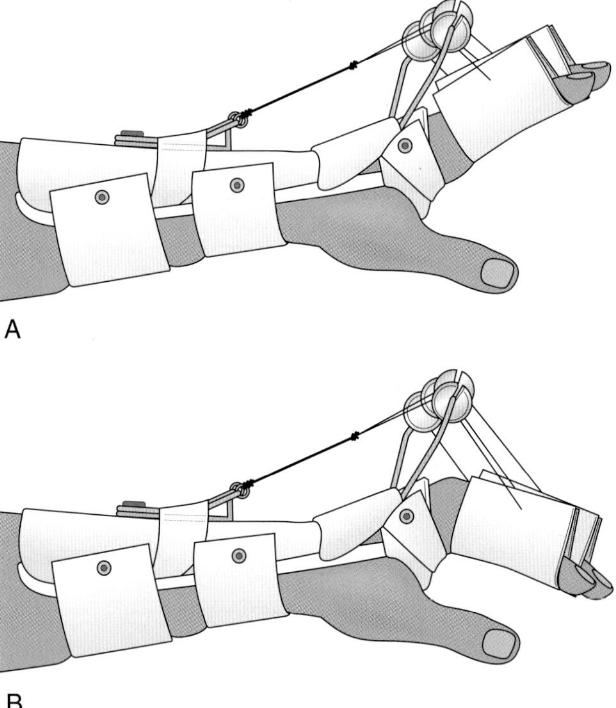

FIGURE 30.3 **A,** Splint allows 30 to 40 degrees of active MCP joint flexion with passive return to neutral. **B,** Flexion is limited by stop beads on the outrigger strings.

Zone VI

Zone VI is located over the metacarpals. Injuries to this area have a clinical picture similar to that of zone V injuries and are treated as such (see Table 30.3) [9,11,12,14,15].

Zone VII

Zone VII lies at the level of the wrist. Tendons in this region course through a fibro-osseous tunnel and are covered by the extensor retinaculum. Complete laceration of the tendons in this region is rare. Tendon retraction can be a significant problem in this region, and primary repair is warranted, with preservation of a portion of the retinaculum to prevent extensor bowstringing [6]. Rehabilitation is similar to that in zone V (see Table 30.3).

Zone VIII

Zone VIII lies at the level of the distal forearm. Multiple tendons may be injured in this area, making it difficult to

Table 30.3 Zone V, Zone VI, and Zone VII Injuries

	Splint	Exercises	Wound and Skin Care
Start 24-48 hours	Dorsal dynamic extension splint (see Fig. 30.3) Night splint: MCP joint	Exercise hourly in extension splint: allows 30-40 degrees of MCP joint flexion With skilled therapist: wrist at 20 degrees, passive MCP joint flexion to 30 degrees; patient performs active extension (daily to 3 times a week)	Daily removal of splint for wound cleaning Edema control with 0-3 compressive wrap
4 weeks	Continue with dynamic day splint, static night splint	Increase active range of motion to 50-60 degrees	Daily removal of splint for wound cleaning Edema control with 0-3 compressive wrap
5 weeks	Discontinue dynamic extension splint MCP joint block splint worn at night and between exercises	Increase active range of motion exercises to full motion	Daily removal of splint for wound cleaning Edema control with 0-3 compressive wrap
6 weeks	MCP joint block splint	Passive flexion exercises of MCP and IP joints (buddy tape)	Daily removal of splint for wound cleaning Edema control with 0-3 compressive wrap
7 weeks	MCP joint block splint	Progressive extension exercises, with mild resistance	Daily removal of splint for wound cleaning Edema control with 0-3 compressive wrap
9 weeks	If no extensor lag, discontinue all splints	Continue with active and passive DIP joint exercises	Daily removal of splint for wound cleaning Edema control with 0-3 compressive wrap

From Brault J. Rehabilitation of extensor tendon injuries. Oper Tech Plast Reconstr Surg 2000;7:25-30.

identify individual tendons. Restoration of independent wrist and thumb extension should be given priority [6]. Injuries in this location often require tendon retrieval for complete lacerations, and surgical intervention is warranted.

Postoperative rehabilitation consists of static immobilization of the wrist in 45 degrees of extension with the MCP joints in 15 to 20 degrees of flexion. Splinting is generally maintained for 4 to 5 weeks. However, early controlled motion with a dynamic extensor splint may help decrease adhesions and subsequent contractures. Dynamic motion of the MCP joints may be started at 2 weeks.

Procedures

Surgical repair is the mainstay for treatment of most extensor tendon injuries. Injections are typically not appropriate for the management of these conditions.

Surgery

Zone I and zone II injuries are typically treated nonoperatively, unless there is laceration of the terminal extensor slip (zone II injury), which may then require surgical repair. Surgical correction of zone I and zone II injuries usually results from failed conservative bracing, usually in a younger patient. In addition, patients may elect to have the terminal extensor tendon repaired or the DIP joint fused for cosmetic reasons. In older individuals with fixed deformities and painful arthritic conditions that limit function, joint arthrodesis is a reasonable approach.

Surgical intervention in zones III through VIII is usually primary repair of the injured extensor tendon mechanism. If primary repair is not possible, tendon grafting has been described [4,16].

Potential Disease Complications

Extensor tendon injury can result in permanent loss of finger extension, primarily due to adhesion formation or joint contracture. Painful degeneration of the affected joints can occur if normal motion is not restored.

Potential Treatment Complications

Analgesics and nonsteroidal anti-inflammatory drugs have well-known side effects that most commonly affect the gastric, hepatic, renal, and cardiovascular systems. Acute tendon ruptures as a result of aggressive therapy necessitate reoperation, which may include tendon grafting. Therapy programs that are not aggressive enough often result in reduced range of motion and strength. Surgical complications include infection, adhesion formation, and advanced joint degeneration.

References

[1] Hart R, Uehara D, Kutz J. Extensor tendon injuries of the hand. Emerg Med Clin North Am 1993;11:637–49.
[2] Evans R, Burkhalter W. A study of the dynamic anatomy of extensor tendons and implications for treatment. J Hand Surg [Am] 1986;11:774–9.
[3] Newport M, Blair W, Steyers C. Long-term results of extensor tendon repair. J Hand Surg [Am] 1990;15:961–6.
[4] Kleinert H, Verdan C. Report of the committee on tendon injuries. J Hand Surg [Am] 1983;8:794–8.
[5] Daniels II JM, Zook EG, Lynch JM. Hand and wrist injuries: part II. Emergent evaluation. Am Fam Physician 2004;69:1949–56.
[6] Rockwell WB, Butler PN, Byrne BA. Extensor tendon: anatomy, injury, and reconstruction. Plast Reconstr Surg 2000;106:1592–603.
[7] Bendre AA, Hartigan BJ, Kalainov DM. Mallet finger. J Am Acad Orthop Surg 2005;13:336–44.
[8] Evans R. An update on extensor tendon management. In: Hunter J, Mackin E, Callahan A, editors. 4th ed. Rehabilitation of the hand: surgery and therapy, vol. 1. St. Louis: Mosby; 1995. p. 656–706.

[9] Minamikawa Y. Extensor repair and rehabilitation. In: Peimer C, editor. Surgery of the hand and upper extremity, vol 1. New York: McGraw-Hill; 1996. p. 1163–88.
[10] Rosenthal E. The extensor tendon: anatomy and management. In: Hunter J, Mackin E, Callahan A, editors. 4th ed. Rehabilitation of the hand: surgery and therapy, vol. 1. St. Louis: Mosby; 1995. p. 519–64.
[11] Evans R. Managing the injured tendon: current concepts. J Hand Ther 2012;25:173–89.
[12] Evans RB. Clinical management of extensor tendon injuries; the therapist's perspective. In: Skirven TM, Osterman AL, Fedorczyk JM, Amadio PC, editors. Rehabilitation of the hand and upper extremity. 6th ed. Philadelphia: Elsevier; 2011. p. 521–54.
[13] Evans RB. Early short arc motion for the repaired central slip. J Hand Surg [Am] 1994;19:991–7.
[14] Brault J. Rehabilitation of extensor tendon injuries. Oper Tech Plast Reconstr Surg 2000;7:25–30.
[15] Thomas D. Postoperative management of extensor tendon repairs in zones V, VI, VII. J Hand Ther 1996;9:309–14.
[16] Rosenthal EA, Elhassan BT. The extensor tendons: evaluation and surgical management. In: Skirven TM, Osterman AL, Fedorczyk JM, Amadio PC, editors. Rehabilitation of the hand and upper extremity. 6th ed. Philadelphia: Elsevier; 2011. p. 487–520.

CHAPTER 31

Flexor Tendon Injuries

Jeffrey S. Brault, DO

Synonyms

Flexor tendon injury, laceration, or rupture
Jersey or sweater finger

ICD-9 Codes

727.64 Rupture of flexor tendons of hand and wrist, nontraumatic
842.1 Sprains and strains of the wrist and hand, unspecified site
848.9 Lacerated tendon (not specific to the hand)

ICD-10 Codes

M66.341 Spontaneous rupture of flexor tendons, right hand
M66.342 Spontaneous rupture of flexor tendons, left hand
M66.349 Spontaneous rupture of flexor tendons, unspecified hand
S63.90 Sprain of unspecified part of unspecified wrist and hand
S63.91 Sprain of unspecified part of right wrist and hand
S63.92 Sprain of unspecified part of left wrist and hand
The appropriate seventh character is added to each code of category 63 to determine episode of care.
S66.921 Laceration of unspecified muscle, fascia and tendon at wrist and hand level, right hand
S66.922 Laceration of unspecified muscle, fascia and tendon at wrist and hand level, left hand
S66.929 Laceration of unspecified muscle, fascia and tendon at wrist and hand level, unspecified hand
The appropriate seventh character is added to each code of category 66 to determine episode of care.

Definition

The flexor tendons of the hand are vulnerable to laceration and rupture. These injuries are most commonly seen in individuals who work around moving equipment, use knives, or wash glass dishes; in people with rheumatoid arthritis; and in athletes (jersey finger) [1]. The flexor digitorum profundus (FDP) of the ring finger is the most commonly involved [2]. Incomplete injuries to the flexor tendon are easily missed on physical examination and can progress to full ruptures.

Regions of potential tendon injury are divided into five zones (Fig. 31.1) [3]. Zone I is from the tendon insertion at the base of the distal phalanx to the midportion of the middle phalanx. Laceration or injury in this zone results in disruption of the FDP tendon and the inability to flex the distal interphalangeal (DIP) joint. Zone II extends from the midportion of the middle phalanx to the distal palmar crease. This zone is known as no man's land because of the poor functional results after tendon repair [4,5]. Tendon injury in this zone usually involves both FDP and flexor digitorum superficialis (FDS) tendons and results in inability to flex the DIP and proximal interphalangeal (PIP) joints. Zone III is located from the distal palmar crease to the distal portion of the transverse carpal ligament. This zone includes the intrinsic hand muscles and vascular arches. Zone IV overlies the transverse carpal ligament in the area of the carpal tunnel. In this zone, injuries usually involve multiple FDP and FDS tendons. Zone V extends from the wrist crease to the level of the musculotendinous junction of the flexor tendons. Injuries in this region most often result from self-inflicted laceration (suicide attempts).

The flexor tendons are held close to the bone in zone I and zone II by a complex series of pulleys and vincula. These structures are frequently injured with the tendons [1].

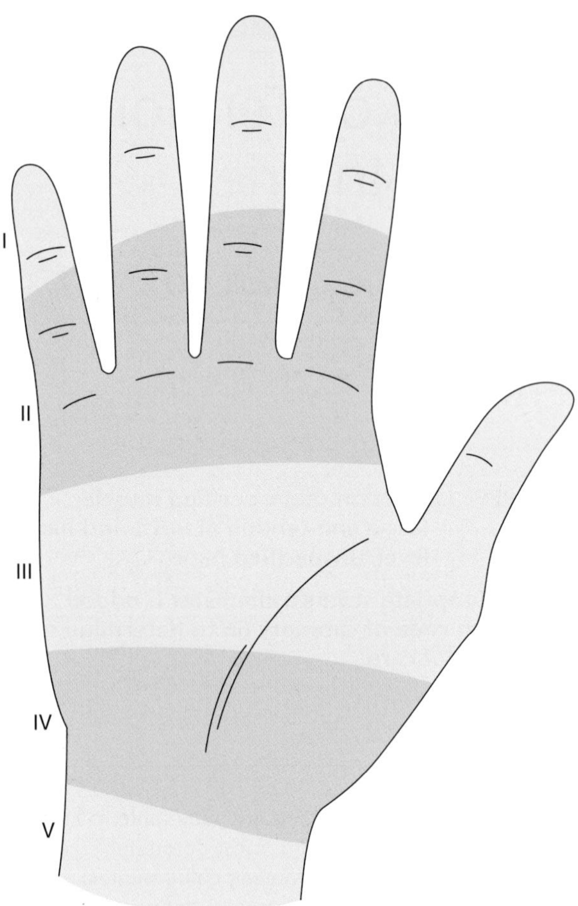

FIGURE 31.1 Zones of flexor tendons.

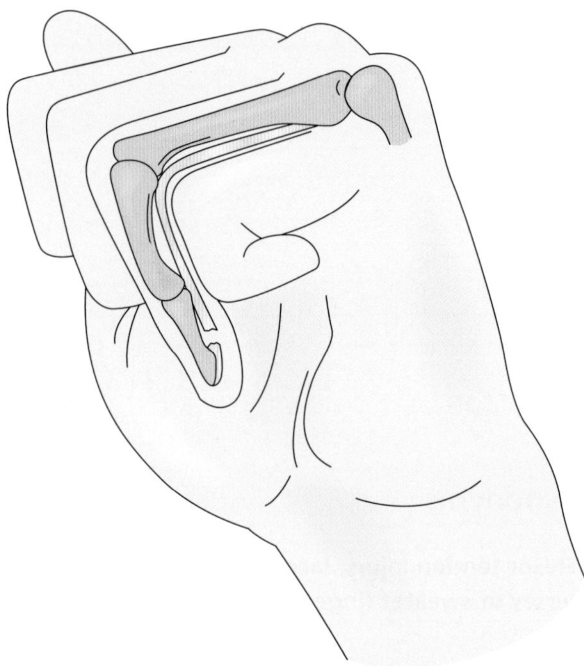

FIGURE 31.2 Jersey finger. The flexor profundus tendon is detached by a forced hyperextension of the DIP joint. *(Reprinted from Mellion MB. Office Sports Medicine, 2nd ed. Philadelphia, Hanley & Belfus, 1996.)*

Symptoms

On occasion, individuals may hear a popping sensation as the flexor tendon tears. This is followed by pain, swelling, and inability to flex the affected joint. Sensation of the involved finger is often affected because of the proximity of the flexor tendons to the neurovascular bundle.

Physical Examination

Obtaining a detailed history is important to outline the mechanism of injury. Evaluation begins with observation of the resting hand position. If the flexor tendon is completely severed, the unsupported finger will assume an extended position (Fig. 31.2) [1,6]. Active flexion of all finger joints needs to be assessed. If active finger flexion is not observed because of pain, tenodesis can be employed to determine whether the tendon is intact. The wrist is passively extended, and all fingers should assume a relatively flexed posture. If the flexor tendons are disrupted, the finger will remain in a relatively extended posture.

Flexion strength of each digit should be evaluated by manual muscle testing or finger dynamometry. Strength is evaluated by having the patient individually flex first the DIP joint and then the PIP joint against applied resistance. It is possible to have a complete laceration of the flexor tendons with preservation of peritendinous structures and active motion. In these cases, however, flexion will be weak [7].

For individual function of the FDP tendon to be checked, the patient is asked to flex the fingertip at the DIP joint while the PIP joint is maintained in extension. If there is injury to the FDP tendon, the patient will be unable to flex the DIP joint.

It is difficult to diagnose solitary injuries of the FDS tendon because of the FDP tendon's ability to perform flexion of all finger joints through intertendinous connections. For the integrity of the FDS tendon to be isolated, all the fingers are held straight, placing the FDP tendon in a biomechanically disadvantaged position. The patient actively attempts to flex the finger to be tested while the other fingers are held in relative extension. If the patient is unable to move the finger, injury most likely has occurred to the FDS tendon. This test is reliable only for the middle, ring, and small fingers.

Sensation of the finger should be evaluated because open tendon injuries often are accompanied by injuries of the nearby digital nerves. Two-point discrimination of radial and ulnar aspects of the digit should be assessed before injection of local anesthetic for wound care [1].

Functional Limitations

Functional limitations include difficulty with power grasp if the ulnarly sided tendons are involved and precision grasp problems if the radially sided tendons are involved. The patient may present with inability to button shirts, to pinch small objects, or to firmly grasp objects.

Diagnostic Studies

Radiographic evaluation includes anteroposterior and lateral views of the involved fingers. These assist in identification of joint dislocation, articular disruption, avulsion, long bone fractures, and potential for retained foreign bodies. Ultrasonography and magnetic resonance imaging are used to identify partially lacerated or ruptured tendons. Ultrasound provides dynamic studies of the tendons.

Differential Diagnosis

Partial tendon laceration
Anterior interosseous nerve injury
Trigger finger (stenosing tenosynovitis)
Median nerve injury

Treatment

Initial

Surgical intervention is almost always required for flexor tendon injuries [1,7]. Protection of the affected finger in a bulky dressing and meticulous wound care are recommended before surgical correction.

Cleaning and repair of superficial wounds should be performed if surgical referral is delayed. Optimally, surgical correction of the flexor tendon injury occurs within the first 12 to 24 hours. Delayed primary repair is performed in the first 10 days. If primary repair is not performed because of infection, secondary repair can be performed up to 4 weeks. If repair is not performed within 4 weeks, the tendon usually is retracted within the sheath, making surgical repair difficult [7].

Newer surgical repair and suture techniques have improved the strength of repaired flexor tendons, providing for earlier rehabilitation [7–9].

Rehabilitation

Postoperative rehabilitation of repaired tendons has changed greatly in the past three decades through initiation of early protected motion [10–14]. Historically, the repaired fingers were placed in an immobilization splint for up to 2 months. This often led to adhesion formation and ultimately the loss of motion and function [12].

The currently accepted rehabilitation schemes for repaired flexor tendons are essentially the same for all zones (Table 31.1).

Immediately postoperatively, the hand is placed in a protective dorsal splint with 20 to 30 degrees of wrist flexion. All metacarpophalangeal (MCP) joints are placed in 20 to 50 degrees of flexion, depending on zone [13–15]. A dorsal hood extends to the fingertip level, allowing PIP joint and DIP joint extension to 0 degrees. All of the fingers are held in flexion by dynamic traction applied by rubber bands originating from the proximal forearm with a pulley at the palm and attachment to the fingernails (Fig. 31.3A).

The patient is typically seen by the therapist 24 to 48 hours after surgical repair. Dressings are changed, edema control measures are initiated, and rehabilitation goals are discussed [12–14]. The patient is instructed to actively extend the fingers against the rubber band traction to the dorsal block, 10 repetitions hourly, to prevent flexion contractures (see Fig. 31.3B). The rubber band traction passively returns the fingers to a flexed position. At night, the traction is removed and the fingers are strapped to the dorsal hood with the PIP and DIP joints in extension.

The rehabilitation program may involve immediate short arc motion [12,13,16,17]. Under the supervision of a skilled therapist, the injured digit is placed in moderate flexion with the wrist in 30 to 40 degrees of extension, the MCP joints in 80 degrees of flexion, the PIP joints in 75 degrees of flexion, and the DIP joints in 30 to 40 degrees of flexion. The patient is then instructed to actively hold this position for 10 seconds. On completion of the static contraction, the therapist passively flexes the wrist. This allows natural tenodesis to extend the fingers. At day 21, the patient can initiate unsupervised active flexion exercises. At 35 days, the dorsal digital splint is removed and active tendon gliding exercises are initiated [12,14,15,17,18].

Modalities such as ultrasound, contrast or paraffin baths, whirlpool, and fluidized therapy may be used to promote wound healing and range of motion in the latter stages of therapy.

Table 31.1 Flexor Tendon Injuries (Immediate Motion)

	Splint	Exercises	Wound and Skin Care
Postoperatively to 21 days	Postoperative dynamic flexion splint with dorsal hood (see Fig. 31.3) Wrist flexion at 20-30 degrees MCP joint, 20-50 degrees; PIP and DIP joints, 0 degrees of extension	Patient actively extends each finger 10 times hourly (start postoperative day 2) Under the direction of a hand therapist, wrist flexion is used to produce less tension on the flexor tendon during passive exercises Initiate supervised active flexion exercises (postoperative day 14)	Daily removal of splint for wound cleaning Edema control with compressive wrap
21-35 days	Progressive reduction in use of splint	Patient may begin to perform active flexion exercises without therapist	Continue with wound care and edema control as needed
35 days	Discontinue splint	Progress to increased active and passive flexion exercises; grip strengthening	Continue with wound care and edema control as needed

Modified from Evans R. Early active motion after flexor tendon repair. In Berger RA, Weiss APC, eds. Hand Surgery. Lippincott Williams & Wilkins 2003:710-735; Groth GN. Current practice patterns of flexor tendon rehabilitation. J Hand Ther 2005;18:169-174; and Evans R. Managing the injured tendon: current concepts. J Hand Ther 2012;25:173-189.

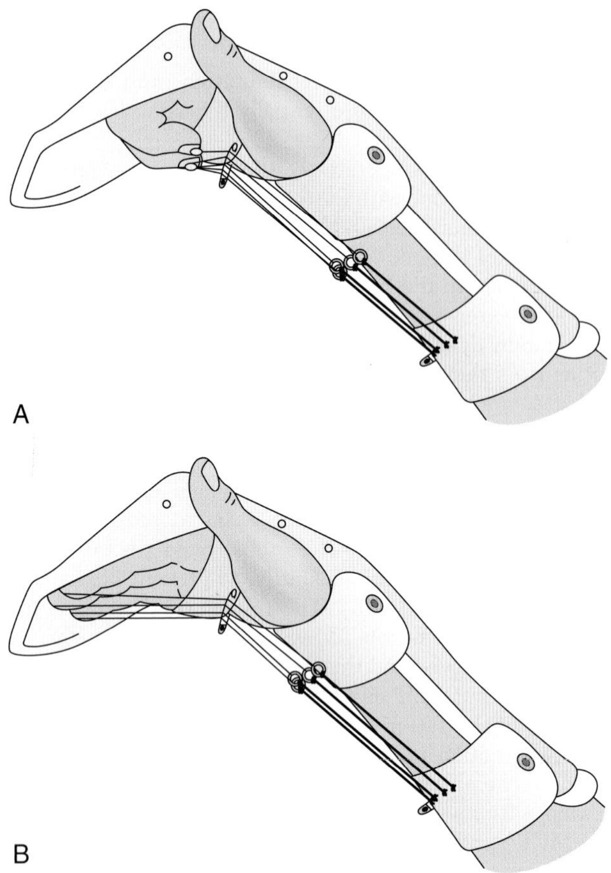

FIGURE 31.3 **A,** Dorsal dynamic protection splint; fingers in resting position. **B,** Dorsal dynamic protection splint; active extension exercises.

Procedures

Procedures are generally not indicated in flexor tendon injuries. Wound care is paramount to prevent infections of surgical incisions. Corticosteroid injections can be performed if stenosing tenosynovitis (triggering) develops at the flexor pulleys.

Surgery

Optimally, repair of the flexion tendon should occur within the first 48 hours after injury. Improper handling of tissues during repair can result in hematoma, damage to the pulley integrity, and damage to the vincula—the vascular supply of the tendons [19].

Potential Disease Complications

Injury to the flexor tendon mechanism can result in permanent loss of finger flexion. Partial tendon damage can easily be missed and result in either weakness or complete rupture.

Potential Treatment Complications

Analgesics and nonsteroidal anti-inflammatory drugs have well-known side effects that most commonly affect the gastric, hepatic, and renal systems. Postsurgical complications include adhesion formation and tendon rupture. Postsurgical tendon rupture is usually the result of aggressive motion, by either the patient or therapist, that results in failure of the repair. Reoperation is often required, which results in the greater propensity for adhesion formation. Adhesion formation and the loss of motion and strength complicate surgical repair, particularly in zone II [4,5].

Many other factors affect healing of the tendon and postoperative rehabilitation. Factors such as advanced age, poor circulation, tobacco and caffeine use, and generalized poor health can contribute to impaired healing. Scar formation can result in adhesion formation and decreased movement. Poor motivation and compliance with the therapy program result in less than optimal recovery.

References

[1] Mass DP. Early repairs of flexor tendon injuries. In: Berger RA, Weiss APC, editors. Hand surgery. Philadelphia: Lippincott Williams & Wilkins; 2003. p. 679–98.
[2] Amadio P. Epidemiology of hand and wrist injuries in sports. Hand Clin 1990;6:429–53.
[3] Kleinert H, Schepel S, Gill T. Flexor tendon injuries. Surg Clin North Am 1981;61:267–86.
[4] Chow J, Thomas L, Dovelle S, et al. A combined regimen of controlled motion following flexor tendon repair in "no man's land." Plast Reconstr Surg 1987;79:447–53.
[5] Hister GD, Kleinert HE, Kutz JE, Atasoy E. Primary flexor tendon repair followed by immediate controlled mobilization. J Hand Surg [Am] 1977;2:441–51.
[6] Idler R, Manktelow R, Lucus G, et al. The hand: examination and diagnosis. 3rd ed. New York: Churchill Livingstone; 1990, p. 59–62.
[7] Strickland J. Flexor tendons—acute injuries. In: Green D, Hotchkiss R, Peterson W, editors. Green's operative hand surgery. 4th ed. Philadelphia: Churchill Livingstone; 1999. p. 1851–97.
[8] Miller L, Mas DP. A comparison of four repair techniques for Camper's chiasma flexor digitorum superficialis lacerations: tested in an in vitro model. J Hand Surg [Am] 2000;25:1122–6.
[9] Angeles JG, Heminger H, Mass DP. Comparative biomechanical performances of 4-strand core suture repairs for zone II flexor tendon lacerations. J Hand Surg [Am] 2002;27:508–17.
[10] Strickland J. Biologic rationale, clinical application and result of early motion following flexor tendon repair. J Hand Ther 1989;2:71–83.
[11] Pettengill KM. The evolution of early mobilization of the repaired flexor tendon. J Hand Ther 2005;18:157–68.
[12] Evans R. Early active motion after flexor tendon repair. In: Berger RA, Weiss APC, editors. Hand surgery. Lippincott Williams & Wilkins; 2003. p. 710–35.
[13] Groth GN. Current practice patterns of flexor tendon rehabilitation. J Hand Ther 2005;18:169–74.
[14] Pettengill K, VanStrien G. Postoperative management of flexor tendon injuries. In: Skirven TM, Osterman AL, Fedorczyk JM, Amadio PC, editors. Rehabilitation of the hand and upper extremity. 6th ed. Philadelphia: Elsevier; 2011. p. 457–78.
[15] Evans R. Managing the injured tendon: current concepts. J Hand Ther 2012;25:173–89.
[16] Evans R. Immediate active short arc motion following tendon repair. In: Hunter J, Schneider L, Mackin E, editors. Tendon and nerve surgery in the hand—a third decade. Mosby: St. Louis; 1997. p. 362–93.
[17] Lund A. Flexor tendon rehabilitation: a basic guide. Operat Tech Plast Reconstr Surg 2000;7:20–4.
[18] Werntz J, Chesher S, Breiderbach W, et al. A new dynamic splint and postoperative treatment of flexor tendon injury. J Hand Surg [Am] 1989;14:559–66.
[19] Taras JS, Martyak GG, Steelman PJ. Primary care of flexor tendon injuries. In: Skirven TM, Osterman AL, Fedorczyk JM, Amadio PC, editors. Rehabilitation of the hand and upper extremity. 6th ed. Philadelphia: Elsevier; 2011. p. 445–56.

CHAPTER 32

Hand and Wrist Ganglia

Charles Cassidy, MD
Victor Chung, MD

Synonyms

Carpal cyst
Synovial cyst
Mucous cyst
Intraosseous cyst

ICD-9 Codes

727.41 Ganglion of joint
727.42 Ganglion of tendon sheath

ICD-10 Codes

M67.40 Ganglion of joint, unspecified site
M67.40 Ganglion of tenon sheath

Definition

Hand and wrist ganglia account for 50% to 70% of all hand masses. The ganglion is a benign, mucin-filled cyst found in relation to a joint, ligament, or tendon. It is typically filled from the joint through a tortuous duct or "stalk" that functions as a valve directing the flow of fluid. The mucin itself contains high concentrations of hyaluronic acid as well as glucosamine, albumin, and globulin [1]. When it is used to describe ganglia, the term *synovial cyst* is actually a misnomer because ganglion cysts do not contain synovial fluid and are not true cysts lined by epithelium but rather by flat cells. The etiology of ganglia remains a mystery, although many think that ligamentous degeneration or trauma plays an important role [1,2].

By far, the most common location for a ganglion is the dorsal wrist (Fig. 32.1), with the pedicle arising from the scapholunate ligament in virtually all cases. Only 20% of ganglia are found on the volar wrist (Fig. 32.2). This type may originate from either the radioscaphoid or scaphotrapezial joint. Alternatively, ganglia can occur near the joints of the finger. One subtype of hand-wrist ganglia is the "occult" cyst, which is not palpable on physical examination.

Ganglion cysts occur more commonly in women, usually between the ages of 20 and 30 years. However, they can develop in either sex at any age. Ganglia of childhood usually resolve spontaneously during the course of 1 year [3]. The most commonly seen ganglion of the elderly, the mucous cyst, arises from an arthritic distal interphalangeal joint (Fig. 32.3).

Other common types of ganglia in the hand include the retinacular cyst (flexor tendon sheath ganglion; Fig. 32.4), proximal interphalangeal joint ganglion, and first extensor compartment cyst associated with de Quervain tenosynovitis. Less common ganglia include cysts within the extensor tendons or carpal bones (intraosseous) and those associated with a second or third carpometacarpal boss (arthritic spur). Rarely, ganglia within the carpal tunnel or Guyon canal can produce carpal tunnel syndrome or ulnar neuropathy, respectively.

As noted, the cause of ganglion cyst formation is not known, but there may be a link to light, repetitive activity, demonstrated by an increased incidence in typists, musicians, and draftsmen. Interestingly, there is no increased risk in heavy laborers, who bear a greater load on their wrists. Wrist instability has also been discussed as both a possible cause and an effect of the disease. Overall, there is a history of trauma in 10% to 30% of people presenting with the disease [2].

Symptoms

Patients with a wrist ganglion usually present with a painless wrist or hand mass of variable duration. The cyst may fluctuate in size or disappear altogether for a time. Pain and weakness of grip are occasional presenting symptoms; however, an underlying concern about the appearance or seriousness of the problem is usually the reason for seeking medical attention. The pain, when present, is most often described as aching and aggravated by certain motions. With dorsal wrist ganglia, patients often complain of discomfort as the wrist is forcefully extended (e.g., when pushing up from a chair). Interestingly, dorsal wrist pain may be the principal complaint of patients with an occult dorsal wrist ganglion, which is not readily visible. The wrist pain usually subsides as the mass enlarges.

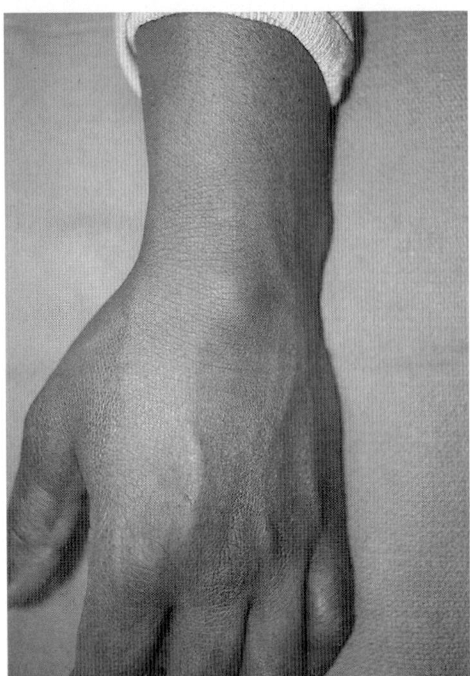

FIGURE 32.1 Dorsal wrist ganglion. The mass is typically found overlying the scapholunate area in the center of the wrist.

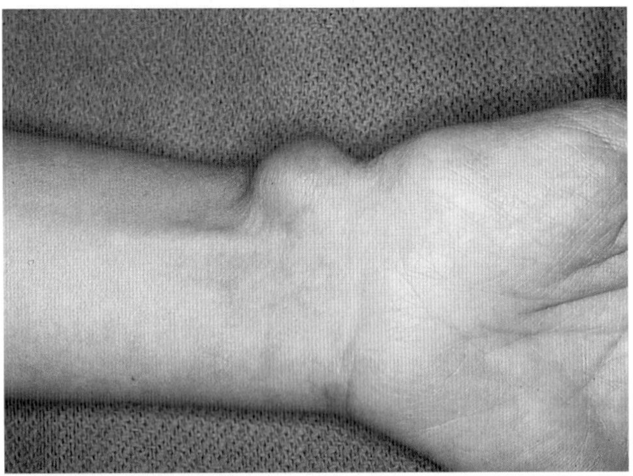

FIGURE 32.2 Clinical appearance of a volar wrist ganglion.

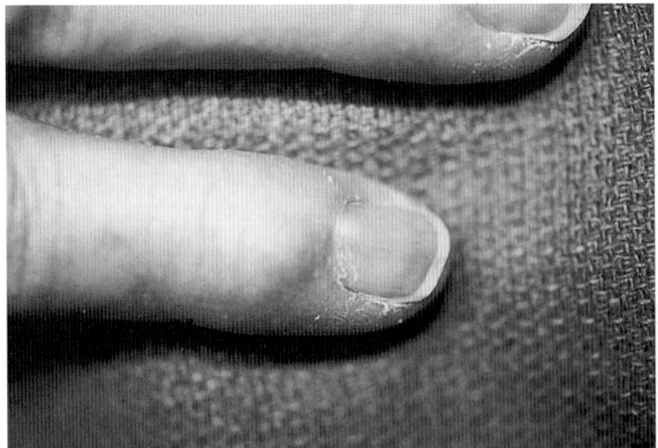

FIGURE 32.3 Mucous cyst. This ganglion originates from the distal interphalangeal joint. Pressure on the nail matrix by the cyst may produce flattening of the nail plate, as is seen here.

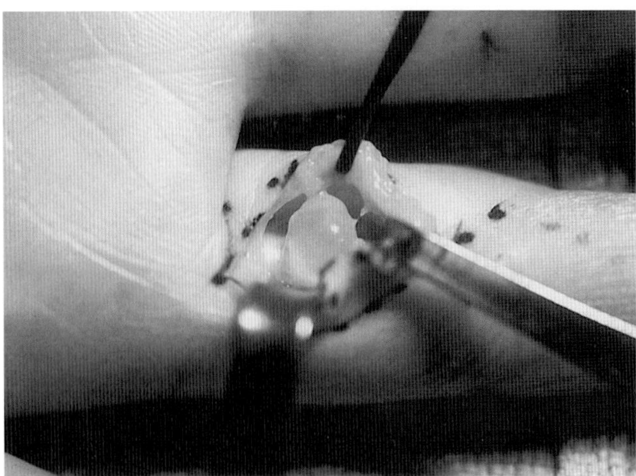

FIGURE 32.4 Retinacular cyst. This ganglion originates from the flexor tendon sheath.

With a retinacular cyst, patients usually complain of slight discomfort when gripping, for example, a racket handle or shopping cart. Patients whose complaints of pain are primarily related to de Quervain tenosynovitis (see Chapter 28) may notice a bump over the radial styloid area. Pain with grip is also a complaint of patients with a carpometacarpal boss. On occasion, the digital extensor tendons may jump over the cyst with radioulnar deviation. Mucous cysts can drain spontaneously and can also produce nail deformity, either of which may be a presenting complaint. Symptoms identical to those of carpal tunnel syndrome will be noted by patients with a carpal tunnel ganglion. A ganglion in the Guyon canal will produce hand weakness (due to loss of intrinsic function) and may produce numbness in the ring and small fingers.

Physical Examination

Ganglia are typically solitary cysts, although they are often found to be multiloculated on surgical exploration. They are usually mobile a few millimeters in all directions on physical examination. The mass may be slightly tender. When the cyst is large, transillumination (placing a penlight directly onto the skin overlying the mass) will help differentiate it from a solid tumor.

The classic location for a dorsal wrist ganglion is ulnar to the extensor pollicis longus, between the third and fourth tendon compartments, or directly over the scapholunate ligament [1]. However, these ganglia may have a long pedicle that courses through various tendon compartments and exits at different locations on the dorsal wrist or even the volar wrist. When the ganglion is small, it may be apparent only with wrist flexion. Wrist extension and grip strength may be slightly diminished. Dorsal wrist pain and tenderness with no obvious mass or instability should suggest an occult ganglion.

Volar ganglia occur most commonly at the wrist flexion crease on the radial side of the flexor carpi radialis tendon but may extend into the palm or proximally, or even dorsally, into the carpal tunnel. They can involve the radial artery, complicating their surgical removal. They may seem to be pulsatile, although careful inspection will demonstrate that the radial artery is draped over the mass.

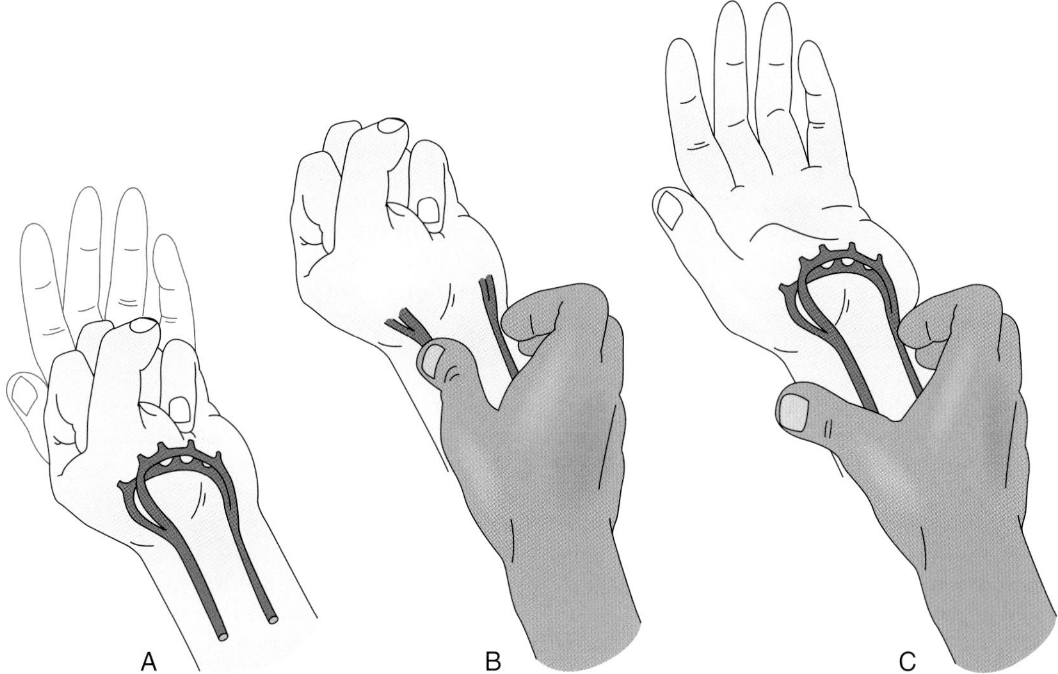

FIGURE 32.5 The Allen test is performed by asking the patient to open and close the hand several times as quickly as possible and then to make a tight fist (**A**). The examiner then compresses the radial and ulnar arteries as the hand is opened (**B**). One artery is tested by releasing the pressure over the artery to see whether the hand flushes (**C**). The other artery is tested in a similar fashion, and the opposite hand is tested for comparison.

Retinacular cysts are usually not visible but are palpable as pea-sized masses, typically located at the volar aspect of the digit at the palmar digital crease. They are adherent to the flexor tendon sheath and do not move with finger flexion. Alternatively, intratendinous ganglia are distinguished by the fact that they move with finger motion.

Mucous cysts are located over the distal interphalangeal joint, and the overlying skin may be quite thin. They are occasionally mistaken for warts. Spontaneous drainage and even septic distal interphalangeal joint arthritis are not uncommon. Nail plate deformity is an associated finding. Proximal interphalangeal joint ganglia are located on the dorsum of the digit, slightly off midline. Ganglia associated with carpometacarpal bosses produce tender prominences on the dorsum of the hand distal to the typical location for a wrist ganglion.

An important sign to look for on physical examination, especially in planning for surgery, is compression of the median or ulnar nerve or of the radial artery. An Allen test should be performed before surgery to evaluate radial and ulnar artery patency, particularly in the case of a volar cyst (Fig. 32.5).

Functional Limitations

Physical limitations due to ganglion cysts are rare. With dorsal wrist ganglia, fatigue and weakness are occasional findings. Patients may have difficulty with weight bearing on the affected extremity with the wrist extended (e.g., when pushing up from a chair).

Diagnostic Studies

The diagnosis of a ganglion cyst is usually straightforward, and ancillary studies are often unnecessary. With wrist ganglia, plain radiographs of the wrist are usually obtained preoperatively to evaluate the carpal relationships and to exclude the possibility of an intraosseous ganglion. With a mucous cyst, radiographs of the affected digit will usually demonstrate a distal interphalangeal joint osteophyte. Ultrasonography or magnetic resonance imaging may be useful in identifying deep cysts in cases of vague dorsal wrist pain. Specifically, magnetic resonance imaging is indicated to rule out Kienböck disease in patients with dorsal wrist pain and no obvious ganglion or wrist instability. In hand soft tissue masses when magnetic resonance imaging is nondiagnostic, the most common underlying diagnoses include giant cell tumor of tendon sheath, angioleiomyoma, fibroma, and peripheral nerve sheath tumor [4]. Cyst aspiration is the single best confirmatory study for ganglion. Aspiration characteristically yields a viscous, clear to yellowish fluid with the appearance and consistency of apple jelly. On occasion, the fluid will be blood tinged.

Differential Diagnosis

WRIST
Carpal boss
Extensor tenosynovitis
Wrist synovitis
Scapholunate ligament injury or sprain
Kienböck disease (avascular necrosis of the lunate)
Lipoma

DIGITS
Giant cell tumor of tendon sheath
Hemangioma
Angioleiomyoma
Peripheral nerve sheath tumor
Fibroma
Synovitis

Treatment

Initial

Reassurance is the single most important initial treatment. Many patients are satisfied to know that they do not have a serious illness. It is important to tell patients that the cyst often fluctuates in size and occasionally disappears on its own. Undoubtedly, observation is the most appropriate treatment of ganglia in children, as long as the diagnosis is certain. In adults, splinting is an appropriate initial treatment of cysts associated with discomfort. A cock-up wrist splint is prescribed for carpometacarpal and dorsal and volar wrist ganglia, whereas a radial gutter splint is prescribed for ganglia associated with de Quervain tenosynovitis. Traditional methods of crushing the cyst with a coin or a Bible, even though occasionally successful, are not recommended. Anecdotally, daily massage of mucous cysts by patients may be successful in resolving them as long as the overlying skin is healthy. Analgesics or nonsteroidal anti-inflammatory drugs may be used on a limited basis for discomfort but do little to treat the disorder.

Rehabilitation

Rehabilitation has a role primarily in the postsurgical setting. The usual course of treatment after dorsal ganglion excision involves 7 to 14 days of immobilization in slight wrist flexion to minimize loss of wrist flexion secondary to scarring. Frequent, active range of motion of the wrist should be started after splint removal, and the patient should be able to return to relatively normal activity approximately 3 weeks after surgery [1]. Most patients are able to carry out their own rehabilitation at home. Formal therapy can be ordered if patients have difficulty returning to normal functioning. Therapy may include modalities for pain control, active-assisted and passive range of motion exercises, and strengthening exercises. Therapists may also evaluate return to work issues, including adaptive equipment that may assist patients in their daily work functions.

Procedures

Aspiration of the cyst serves two purposes: it confirms the diagnosis, and it may be therapeutic. Unfortunately, the recurrence rate after ganglion aspiration is high. One study [5] demonstrated long-term success rates of 27% and 43% for dorsal and volar wrist ganglia, respectively, treated with aspiration, multiple puncture, and 3 weeks of immobilization. Importantly, cysts present for longer than 6 months almost uniformly recurred. The results for aspiration of retinacular cysts were somewhat better, averaging 69% successful.

However, a significant number of patients may elect to proceed with cyst aspiration despite the high likelihood of recurrence. Aspiration of volar wrist ganglia may cause displacement of the cyst and envelop the radial artery. Aspiration of proximal interphalangeal joint ganglia may be successful in eliminating the cyst [6]. Aspiration of mucous cysts is not recommended.

Steroids have not been shown to add any therapeutic benefit to ganglia aspiration.

Surgery

Many patients opt for surgical excision of the cyst, often for primarily cosmetic reasons. Surgery should be advised when the diagnosis is unclear. To minimize the likelihood of recurrence, the surgeon should not only remove the cyst but trace the stalk to its origin within the joint. For wrist ganglia, the surgeon often finds that the visible mass grossly underestimates its actual size and extent. Because these procedures require opening of the wrist joint, they cannot be performed with the use of local anesthesia. With proper technique, recurrence rates should be less than 5%. Volar ganglia are more difficult to access and more often variable in their shape and location, making for more complicated surgery. A prospective cohort study of volar wrist ganglion treatment by observation, aspiration, or surgery concluded that at 5 years, there were no significant differences in the recurrence rates with any of the treatments; 42% of the excised ganglia recurred, whereas 51% of the untreated ganglia had resolved spontaneously [7]. Clearly, it is important that the risks and benefits of surgical treatment of ganglion cysts be carefully discussed with the patient.

Arthroscopic resection of dorsal wrist ganglia has been advocated to be a safe and reliable procedure, with recurrence rates of less than 5% [8]. A small case series of arthroscopic débridement of volar wrist ganglia has demonstrated excellent results as well [9].

The surgical management of mucous cysts must include excision of the cyst stalk as well as the offending osteophyte, which originates from either the dorsal base of the distal phalanx or the head of the middle phalanx. The nail deformity should resolve during several months [10].

Potential Disease Complications

Chronic wrist pain as the result of an untreated wrist ganglion is rare. The cosmetic deformity, however, is obvious. The most important complication associated with a neglected cyst is septic arthritis of the distal interphalangeal joint resulting from spontaneous drainage of a mucous cyst. For that reason, we recommend mucous cyst excision when the overlying skin is thin or spontaneous drainage has occurred.

Potential Treatment Complications

Analgesics and nonsteroidal anti-inflammatory drugs have well-known side effects that most commonly affect the gastric, hepatic, and renal systems. The patient must understand that surgery will replace a bump with a scar. Slight limitation of wrist flexion after dorsal ganglion excision is not uncommon. Another risk is iatrogenic injury to the scapholunate ligament, extensor tendon, and cutaneous nerve. Recurrence is another possibility.

Surgery performed on the volar wrist carries a greater risk of injury to artery and nerve. The structures most at risk are the palmar cutaneous branch of the median nerve and the terminal branches of the lateral antebrachial cutaneous nerve as well as the radial artery, which is often intertwined with the cyst. Perhaps because of the more intricate nature of its surgical removal, the volar cyst is associated with a higher rate of recurrence after surgery.

References

[1] Athanasian EA. Bone and soft tissue tumors. In: Green DP, Hotchkiss RN, Pederson WC, et al., editors. Green's operative hand surgery. 5th ed Philadelphia: Churchill Livingstone; 2005.
[2] Peimer C, editor. Surgery of the hand and upper extremity, vol. 1. New York: McGraw-Hill; 1996. p. 837–52.
[3] Wang AA, Hutchinson DT. Longitudinal observation of pediatric hand and wrist ganglia. J Hand Surg [Am] 2001;26:599–602.
[4] Sookur PA, Saifuddin A. Indeterminate soft-tissue tumors of the hand and wrist: a review based on a clinical series of 39 cases. Skeletal Radiol 2011;40:977–89.
[5] Richman JA, Gelberman RH, Engber WD, et al. Ganglions of the wrist and digits: results of treatment by aspiration and cyst wall puncture. J Hand Surg [Am] 1987;12:1041–3.
[6] Cheng CA, Rockwell WB. Ganglions of the proximal interphalangeal joint. Am J Orthop 1999;28:458–60.
[7] Dias J, Buch K. Palmar wrist ganglion: does intervention improve outcome? A prospective study of the natural history and patient-reported treatment outcomes. J Hand Surg [Br] 2003;28:172–6.
[8] Rizzo M, Berger RA, Steinmann SP, Bishop AT. Arthroscopic resection in the management of dorsal wrist ganglions: results with a minimum 2-year follow-up period. J Hand Surg [Am] 2004;29:59–62.
[9] Ho PC, Lo WN, Hung LK. Arthroscopic resection of volar ganglion of the wrist: a new technique. Arthroscopy 2003;19:218–21.
[10] Kasdan ML, Stallings SP, Leis VM, Wolens D. Outcome of surgically treated mucous cysts of the hand. J Hand Surg [Am] 1994;19:504–7.

CHAPTER 33

Hand Osteoarthritis

David Ring, MD, PhD

Synonyms

Arthritis
Degenerative arthritis
Osteoarthritis
Degenerative joint disease
Joint destruction

ICD-9 Codes

715.14 Osteoarthritis, primary, localized to the hand
715.24 Osteoarthritis, secondary, localized to the hand
716.14 Traumatic arthropathy of the hand

ICD-10 Codes

M19.041 Primary osteoarthritis, right hand
M19.042 Primary osteoarthritis, left hand
M19.049 Primary osteoarthritis, unspecified hand
M19.241 Secondary osteoarthritis, right hand
M19.242 Secondary osteoarthritis, left hand
M19.279 Secondary osteoarthritis, unspecified hand
M12.541 Traumatic arthropathy, right hand
M12.542 Traumatic arthropathy, left hand
M12.549 Traumatic arthropathy, unspecified hand

Definition

Osteoarthritis of the hand is a degenerative condition of hyaline cartilage in diarthrodial joints. It is distinct from inflammatory arthropathies, such as rheumatoid arthritis, in which the primary component is an inflammatory or systemic pathophysiologic process. Idiopathic osteoarthritis excludes post-traumatic arthritis or arthritic conditions resulting from pyrophosphate deposition disease, infection, or other known causes. It is associated with aging, but variations in onset and severity seem genetically determined [1]. In particular, the early onset of osteoarthritis of the distal interphalangeal and trapeziometacarpal joints is genetically mediated separate from osteoarthritis at other joints; in other words, a 50-year-old person with severe hand arthritis is not at risk for early hip arthritis. The prevalence of osteoarthritis of the hand increases with age and is more common in men than in women until menopause. In individuals older than 65 years, osteoarthritis of the hand has been estimated to be as high as 78% in men and 99% in women [2]. The distal interphalangeal and proximal interphalangeal joints and the base of the thumb are the most affected joints.

Symptoms

Patients typically report pain, stiffness, and disability. Symptoms follow a waxing and waning course as the disease gradually and inevitably progresses. The correlation between radiographic findings and pain intensity and magnitude of disability is limited, most likely as a reflection of the psychosocial factors that mediate the difference between disease and illness and between impairment and disability. Psychological distress and ineffective coping strategies should be identified and addressed.

Physical Examination

Osteoarthritis is insidious. Although a joint "goes gray" during decades, patients often notice an acute onset of symptoms that can make it difficult for them to believe their problem is an expected slow deterioration. The hallmarks of physical examination are deformity, restriction of motion, pain, and crepitation. A careful examination of all of the joints notes any deformity, effusions, erythema, limitations in range of motion, and swelling. The findings on neurologic examination should be normal.

Interphalangeal Joints

Osteoarthritis of the distal interphalangeal joint is characterized by enlargement of the distal joint by osteophytes, forming the so-called Heberden node (Fig. 33.1). Angulatory and rotatory deformities of the terminal phalanx can develop (Fig. 33.2). Ganglion (or mucous) cysts are associated with osteoarthritis of the distal (and less commonly the proximal) interphalangeal joints. The pressure of these cysts on the germinal matrix can cause a groove in the fingernail. The proximal interphalangeal joint is less commonly

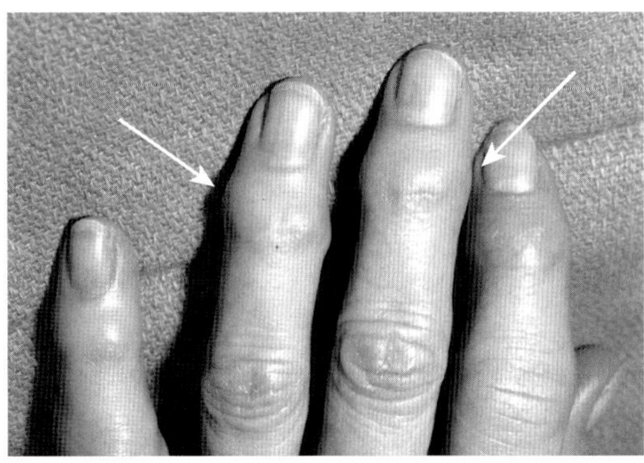

FIGURE 33.1 Patients with degenerative joint disease of the hands can present with Heberden nodes *(arrows)*. These nodules represent osteophytes at the distal interphalangeal joint. *(From Concannon MJ. Common Hand Problems in Primary Care. Philadelphia, Hanley & Belfus, 1999.)*

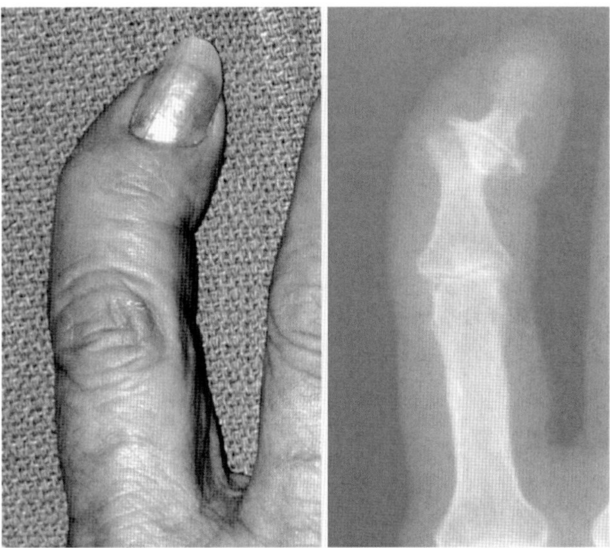

FIGURE 33.2 Severe osteoarthritis at the distal interphalangeal joint of the fifth finger. Osteophyte formation, joint destruction, and angulation are demonstrated. *(From Concannon MJ. Common Hand Problems in Primary Care. Philadelphia, Hanley & Belfus, 1999.)*

involved than the distal joint. The enlargement and deformity at the proximal interphalangeal joint is referred to as a Bouchard node.

Metacarpophalangeal Joints

It is relatively uncommon for the metacarpophalangeal joints to be involved in primary idiopathic osteoarthritis. The presentation at this joint is usually characterized by complaints of pain and stiffness rather than deformity.

Trapeziometacarpal Joint

Arthritis of the trapeziometacarpal joint is associated with aging. Among women aged 80 years and older, 94% have radiographic signs of arthritis; two thirds of these have severe joint destruction [3]. Men develop arthritis more slowly than women do, but by the age of 80 years, 85% have arthritis. The process progresses from subluxation and slight narrowing of the joint to osteophyte formation, deformity, and destruction of the joint [4]. As the disease progresses, the base of the metacarpal subluxates radially, there is an adduction contracture of the metacarpal toward the palm, and laxity and hyperextension of the metacarpophalangeal joint develop in compensation. Axial compression and rotation and shear (the compression test) will produce crepitation and reproduce symptoms [5,6]. Both active and passive movement is restricted. Grip and pinch strength gradually diminish. It is useful to screen for carpal tunnel syndrome and trigger thumb, both of which are common in this age group.

Functional Limitations

The classic forms of reported disability are activities that require a forceful grasp, such as opening a tight jar, turning a key, or opening a doorknob. Whereas fine motor tasks are often impaired by interphalangeal osteoarthritis, complaints of disability are far less common; perhaps because the disease is so gradual, most patients adapt.

Diagnostic Studies

Radiographs are rarely necessary to establish a diagnosis or to guide treatment; their chief use is for ruling out other pathologic processes and increasing the patient's understanding and acceptance of the disease process. Characteristic findings are joint space narrowing, subchondral sclerosis, osteophyte formation, and degenerative cyst formation in the subchondral bone. Eaton and Littler classified trapeziometacarpal arthritis into four radiographic stages [7]. In stage I, the articular contours are normal with no subluxation or joint debris. The joint space may be widened if an effusion is present. In stage II, there is slight narrowing of the thumb trapezial metacarpal joint, but the joint space and articular contours are preserved. Joint debris is less than 2 mm and may be present. In stage III, there is significant trapezial metacarpal joint destruction with sclerotic resistive changes and subchondral bone with osteophytes larger than 2 mm. Stage IV is characterized by pantrapezial arthritis in which both the trapezial metacarpal and scaphoid trapezial joints are affected.

Differential Diagnosis

Post-traumatic arthritis
Inflammatory arthritis (e.g., Lyme disease, gout, rheumatoid arthritis, psoriatic arthritis)
Calcium pyrophosphate deposition disease
Septic arthritis
Systemic lupus erythematosus
Scleroderma

Treatment

Initial

There are no proved disease-modifying treatments of osteoarthritis. All treatments take the form of either palliation (management) or salvage (e.g., arthrodesis or arthroplasty). Because osteoarthritis is so common (as people age, they all have some evidence of osteoarthritis to some degree) and at least annoying if not disabling, there is extensive marketing that suggests the disease can be modified, but there is no proof of this assertion. There is also no proof that exercise or activity accelerates osteoarthritis. Exercise and activity can improve muscle strength, proprioception, and range of motion. Physicians should be cautious about advising activity restriction because it can directly create or exacerbate disability in a patient who associates pain with joint damage. Activity restriction is a personal choice determined by desired comfort level; it is entirely appropriate to remain active in spite of painful, degenerated joints.

Non-narcotic analgesics (acetaminophen and nonsteroidal anti-inflammatory medications) are useful for pain relief and safe enough for routine use in most patients. Some patients find ice, heat, or topical creams useful. Splints that immobilize arthritic joints (for instance, a hand-based thumb spica with the interphalangeal joint free for trapeziometacarpal arthritis) can provide symptomatic relief, but it must be made clear to the patient that they will not cure the disease or prevent progression by wearing them and that splint wear is optional. The interphalangeal joints are rarely splinted because of the associated functional limitations as well as infrequent requests by patients. Intra-articular injections of corticosteroids or hyaluronate [8] inconsistently provide temporary relief, but patients need to understand that these injections cannot cure the disease and that they must either cultivate effective coping mechanisms or elect salvage reconstructive surgery.

Rehabilitation

Patients can be taught alternative ways to perform tasks that are hindered by arthritis (Table 33.1). For instance, they can get a device that helps them open jars and a larger grip for pens and pencils; they can change their doorknobs to levers. Prefabricated and custom hand- or forearm-based thumb spica splints can diminish the pain of trapeziometacarpal arthritis and may be most useful during certain tasks. Therapeutic modalities such as paraffin baths may be beneficial for some people. Contrast baths and ice massage are economical modalities that may provide some relief.

Minimal supervision is needed after simple trapeziectomy. Patients are allowed activities as tolerated, and motion returns with normal use over time. If the joint is immobilized with a Kirschner wire or ligament reconstruction is performed, the joint is protected in a cast or splint for at least 1 month. If the hand gets stiff, patients are instructed in active, self-assisted stretching exercises. Distal interphalangeal joint arthrodesis is protected with splinting until healing is apparent. Proximal interphalangeal joint arthroplasties start motion exercises as comfort allows with protection of healing ligaments as necessary.

Procedures

At best, an intra-articular injection of corticosteroids or hyaluronate will provide a few months of relief [9]. Serious complications, such as infection, are rare. The worst aspect of an injection is the disappointment felt by patients when their hoped-for miracle cure is not forthcoming or when the helpful injection (be it placebo or otherwise [10]) wears off after a few weeks to months. When the role of injections is accurately described, patients can make an informed decision. In my experience, patients do not find them very appealing. The number of corticosteroid injections at a single site is limited by the potential for skin discoloration, subcutaneous atrophy, and capillary fragility. I will not give more than three lifetime injections in the same area (Fig. 33.3).

Under sterile conditions, with use of a 25- to 27-gauge needle and a mixture of local anesthetic (e.g., 0.5 to 1 mL of 1% lidocaine) and corticosteroid (e.g., 0.5 to 1 mL of triamcinolone), the joint is injected. Small joints of the hand will not accommodate large volumes, so the total amount of fluid injected should typically be in the range of 1 to 2 mL. It is helpful to distract the joint by pulling on the finger.

Surgery

Osteoarthritis of the hand is a part of human development that all of us will experience if we are lucky to live long enough. Given the prevalence of arthritis, it is probably safe to assume that most patients adapt well to their arthritis, have effective coping skills, and never bring the arthritis to the attention of a physician. Among those who do bring the problem to a physician's attention, most are satisfied with an explanation of the disease process, the reassurance that it is normal and inevitable, an understanding that the disease cannot yet be modified, and suggestions for management

Table 33.1 Basic Principles of Arthritis Management

Understand pain	The pain does not reflect ongoing harm; it is the result of the existing, permanent disease process. Any rest or activity restriction is voluntary and intended to diminish pain. Patients should be encouraged to continue in painful activities that they value without feeling guilty, neglectful, or irresponsible.
Modify activities	Patients can be taught alternative, less painful, and easier ways to accomplish daily tasks that do not rely on painful joints. Jar openers, pen grips, and door levers rather than knobs can be useful modifications.
Maintain strength and range of motion	Patients are encouraged to continue both daily activities and sports and exercise as a means for preserving active range of motion and muscle conditioning. Daily activities may be supplemented with active range of motion exercises targeted for specific joints.
Use stronger muscles and larger joints	In addition, the patient can be taught to carry items close to the body or to cradle them in the entire arm to distribute loads, rather than relying on smaller muscles and joints of the hand to bear the entire load.
Use adaptive equipment or splints	The patient is provided with information on specific adaptive devices that are helpful in reducing or eliminating positions of deformity or stress on the smaller joints. Splints can be useful for limiting pain with specific activities.

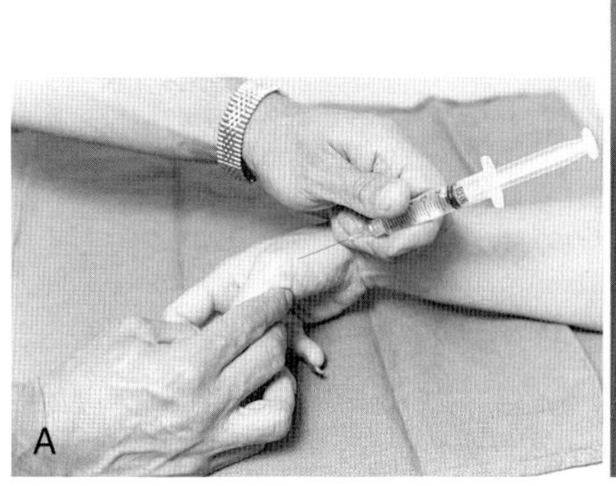
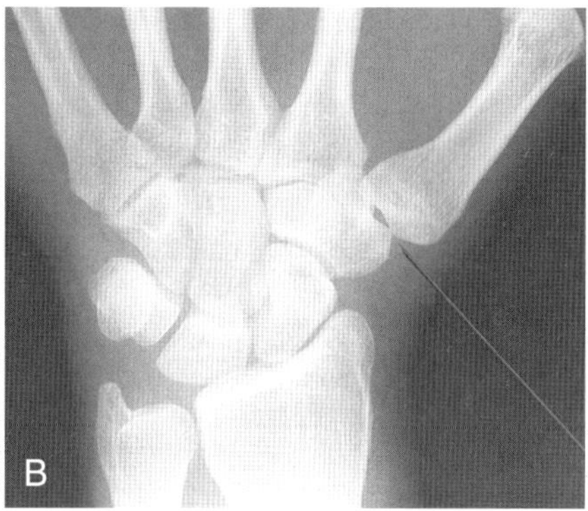
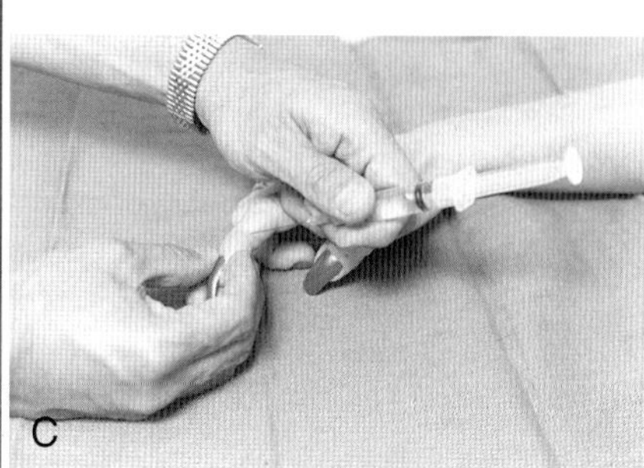

FIGURE 33.3 **A,** Needle placement into the carpometacarpal joint. **B,** Anteroposterior radiograph of the hand demonstrating needle placement into the first carpometacarpal joint. **C,** Needle placement into the interphalangeal joint. *(From Lennard TA. Pain Procedures in Clinical Practice, 2nd ed. Philadelphia, Hanley & Belfus, 2000.)*

and palliation. Surgery provides fairly predictable pain relief, but in my experience, an informed patient who is involved in the decision infrequently requests operative treatment to reconstruct or to salvage the arthritic joint.

Distal Interphalangeal Joint

Infected mucous cysts are typically effectively treated with oral antibiotics (cephalexin or the equivalent to treat *Staphylococcus aureus* infection). Operative treatment is necessary only for long-standing cases with potential osteomyelitis. Because the joint is already severely damaged, there is no need to be concerned about joint damage from the infection.

Aspiration of mucous cysts is not expected to be curative. Patients sometimes elect aspiration to reduce the size of a very large cyst or to improve skin cover when it has become thin and translucent. The recurrence rate is also high after surgery. Patients must choose between leaving the cyst alone and making an attempt to resolve it with surgery, being mindful of the discomfort, inconvenience, and risks of surgery as well as the high recurrence rate.

Patients usually request arthrodesis when there is substantial ulnar or radial deviation of the distal interphalangeal joint. It is more aesthetic than functional. Patients rarely request distal interphalangeal joint arthrodesis for pain or disability.

Proximal Interphalangeal Joint

It is uncommon to operate on idiopathic osteoarthritis of the proximal interphalangeal joint, probably a reflection of the relatively low incidence and severity of osteoarthritis at this joint compared with the distal interphalangeal joint and effective coping with an insidious, slowly progressive disease. Arthrodesis and arthroplasty are both options at this joint and the indication is usually pain relief.

Arthrodesis is more predictable. Arthroplasty is used only in patients who are motivated to retain some mobility at the sacrifice of pain relief and stability [11]. Newer arthroplasties made of pyrolitic carbon (PyroCarbon) or metal have not proved superior to conventional Silastic rubber arthroplasty [12].

Trapeziometacarpal Joint

The trapeziometacarpal joint is the most common upper extremity site of surgical reconstruction for osteoarthritis. Operative treatment consists of the salvage procedures arthrodesis and resection arthroplasty [13,14]. Arthrodesis is less used because of the need for protection, the risk of nonunion, and the inability to place the hand flat on the table that is often bothersome to patients. Some surgeons favor arthrodesis in younger patients who use the hand for strength, but this recommendation is not evidence based.

Reconstruction of the palmar oblique ligament without resection of the trapezium and extension osteotomy of the metacarpal are controversial treatments for a painful trapeziometacarpal joint in a relatively young patient with limited radiographic signs of arthritis. Neither procedure is known to affect the natural history of the disease, and until it is demonstrated to be better than sham surgery, it should be considered to be strongly subject to the placebo or meaning effect, in my opinion [13]. Patients with laxity related to a connective tissue disorder are not helped by ligament reconstruction; their only option is arthrodesis, and it is elective.

There are many variations of resection arthroplasty [7,14,15]. The sources of variation include the following: the amount of trapezium resected; whether the palmar oblique ligament is reconstructed and what technique and tendon are used; what, if anything, is placed in the space created by trapeziectomy (rolled up tendon, prosthesis, or other commercial spacers); operative approach (volar, direct radial, arthroscopic); pinning of the joint; and tendons used or included in the reconstruction. Simple trapeziectomy has been shown to be as effective as more sophisticated techniques in some prospective randomized trials [16], but many hand surgeons find this simple resection arthroplasty relatively unappealing. I favor simple trapeziectomy for its simplicity, safety, and quicker recovery [16].

Potential Disease Complications

Hand osteoarthritis is a chronic, progressive disease that is a nuisance and not a danger. The only potential complications are associated with treatments.

Potential Treatment Complications

Nonsteroidal anti-inflammatory drugs have well-known side effects that most commonly affect the gastric, hepatic, and renal systems. The newer nonsteroidal anti-inflammatory drugs (e.g., cyclooxygenase 2 inhibitors) have been associated with cardiovascular risks [17].

The primary risks associated with injections are infection and an allergic reaction to the medication used, but both are extremely rare. Some patients develop a hematoma or complain of substantial pain after an injection.

Potential surgical complications include wound infection, neuroma, and hematoma. The major source of dissatisfaction after surgery is persistent pain, and its sources are controversial.

References

[1] Kalichman L, Hernández-Molina G. Hand osteoarthritis: an epidemiological perspective. Semin Arthritis Rheum 2010;39:465–76.

[2] Chaisson CE, Zhang Y, McAlindon TE, et al. Radiographic hand osteoarthritis incidents, patterns, and influence of preexisting disease in a population based sample. J Rheumatol 1997;24:1337–43.

[3] Sodha S, Ring D, Zurakowski D, Jupiter JB. Prevalence of osteoarthrosis of the trapeziometacarpal joint. J Bone Joint Surg Am 2005;87:2614–8.

[4] Burton RI. Basal joint arthrosis of the thumb. Orthop Clin North Am 1973;4:331–48.

[5] Poulter RJ, Davis TR. Management of hyperextension of the metacarpophalangeal joint in association with trapeziometacarpal joint osteoarthritis. J Hand Surg Eur Vol 2011;36:280–4.

[6] Klinefelter R. Metacarpophalangeal hyperextension deformity associated with trapezial-metacarpal arthritis. J Hand Surg [Am] 2011;36:2041–2, quiz 2043.

[7] Eaton RG, Littler JW. A study of the basal joint of the thumb. Treatment of its disabilities by fusion. J Bone Joint Surg Am 1969;51:661–8.

[8] Towheed TE, Anastassiades TP. Glucosamine therapy for osteoarthritis. J Rheumatol 1999;26:2294–7.

[9] Wolf JM. Injections for trapeziometacarpal osteoarthrosis. J Hand Surg [Am] 2010;35:1007–9.

[10] Stahl S, Karsh-Zafrir I, Ratzon N, Rosenberg N. Comparison of intraarticular injection of depot corticosteroid and hyaluronic acid for treatment of degenerative trapeziometacarpal joints. J Clin Rheumatol 2005;11:299–302.

[11] Sweets TM, Stern PJ. Pyrolytic carbon resurfacing arthroplasty for osteoarthritis of the proximal interphalangeal joint of the finger. J Bone Joint Surg Am 2011;93:1417–25.

[12] Dovelle S, Heeter PK. Hand injuries: a rehabilitation perspective in orthopedic assessment and treatment of the geriatric patient. St. Louis: Mosby; 1993, p. 205.

[13] Lynn HH, Wyrick JD, Stern PJ. Proximal interphalangeal joint silicone replacement arthroplasty: clinical results using an interior approach. J Hand Surg [Am] 1995;20:123–32.

[14] Burton RI, Pellegrini Jr VD. Surgical management of basal joint arthritis of the thumb. Part 2. Ligament reconstruction with tendon interposition arthroplasty. J Hand Surg [Am] 1986;11:324–32.

[15] Thompson JS. Complications and salvage of trapezial metacarpal arthroplasties. Instr Course Lect 1989;38:3–13.

[16] Gangopadhyay S, McKenna H, Burke FD, Davis TR. Five- to 18-year follow-up for treatment of trapeziometacarpal osteoarthritis: a prospective comparison of excision, tendon interposition, and ligament reconstruction and tendon interposition. J Hand Surg [Am] 2012;37:411–7.

[17] McGettigan P, Henry D. Cardiovascular risk and inhibition of cyclooxygenase: a systematic review of the observational studies of selective and nonselective inhibitors of cyclooxygenase 2. JAMA 2006;296:1633–44.

CHAPTER 34

Hand Rheumatoid Arthritis

David Ring, MD, PhD
Jonathan Kay, MD

Synonyms

Rheumatoid arthritis
Rheumatism
Inflammatory arthritis

ICD-9 Code

714.0 Rheumatoid arthritis

ICD-10 Code

M06.9 Rheumatoid arthritis, unspecified

Definition

Rheumatoid arthritis is a systemic inflammatory disorder of unknown etiology. It is a progressive condition that results in deformity and dysfunction when synovial inflammation erodes cartilage, bone, and soft tissues. However, the widespread early use of methotrexate has transformed rheumatoid arthritis into a much less devastating disease [1]. The availability of targeted biologic therapies, such as the tumor necrosis factor (TNF) antagonists, has further improved the outcome of rheumatoid arthritis [2]. Surgery has become much less common and more straightforward in patients with rheumatoid arthritis. For a detailed discussion of rheumatoid arthritis, see Chapter 151.

Symptoms

Presenting symptoms in the hand include joint pain in the fingers as well as stiffness and swelling, typically involving the proximal interphalangeal and metacarpophalangeal joints but—in contrast to osteoarthritis—sparing the distal interphalangeal joints. Stiffness usually is most pronounced in the morning. If it is left untreated, rheumatoid arthritis may result in progressive deformity and disability.

Physical Examination

The evaluation of a rheumatoid arthritic hand should include the following: joint pain and inflammation; joint stability; limitations in active and passive range of motion for grip and pinch strength deficits; limitations in hand dexterity; and degree of disability with respect to self-care, vocational activities, and recreational activities.

Early in the course of disease, involved joints are usually stiff, painful, and swollen as synovitis predominates. In some patients, the first sign of rheumatoid arthritis may be extensor tenosynovitis on the dorsum of the hand and wrist (although this can also be an idiopathic condition). Chronic synovitis may destroy capsuloligamentous and tendinous structures, creating laxity and deformity. In rheumatoid arthritis, in contrast to the arthritis of systemic lupus erythematosus, this soft tissue damage is usually accompanied by destruction of bone with periarticular erosions evident on radiographs.

Typical hand deformities associated with advanced rheumatoid arthritis include boutonnière deformity (flexion deformity of the proximal interphalangeal joint and extension deformity of the distal interphalangeal joint) and swan-neck deformity (hyperextension of the proximal interphalangeal joint with flexion of the distal interphalangeal joint). It is not uncommon to see varying patterns on the fingers of one hand (Fig. 34.1).

Inability to extend the index through small fingers may be due to the following: deformity and subluxation or dislocation of the index through small finger metacarpophalangeal joints; ulnar translocation of the extensor tendons due to laxity and destruction of the radial sagittal bands; extensor tendon ruptures due to a combination of dorsal tenosynovitis and distal radioulnar joint deformity or abrasions; or posterior interosseous nerve compression by elbow synovitis. Ulnar drift of the fingers usually accompanies each of these deformities.

Rupture of the extensor tendons usually proceeds in a sequence from ulnar to radial, referred to as the Vaughn-Jackson syndrome [3]. Mannerfelt syndrome is the equivalent on the volar side, progressing from the thumb to the index and long fingers, producing tendon ruptures as a result of synovitis and scaphotrapezial trapezoid irregularity [4].

Synovitis in the wrist results in volar and ulnarward subluxation and supination of the hand in relation to the

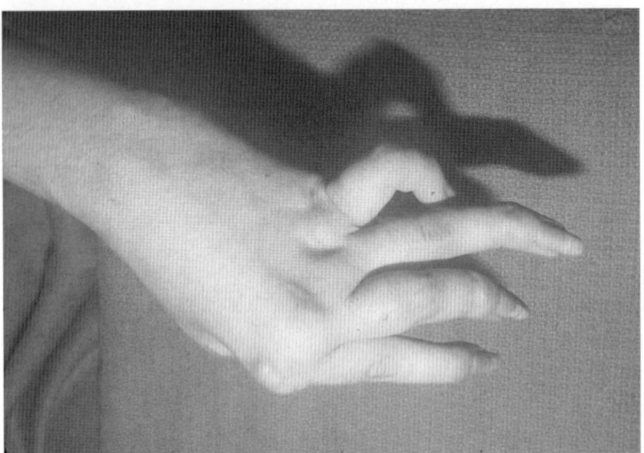

FIGURE 34.1 Rheumatoid hand. Note the multiple presentations in one hand: ulnar drift at the metacarpophalangeal joints, swan-neck deformities of the third and fourth fingers, boutonnière deformity of the fifth finger, volar subluxation at the metacarpophalangeal joint, and radial rotation of the metacarpals.

forearm. This wrist deformity can exacerbate the Vaughn-Jackson syndrome and ulnar drift.

Extensive synovitis or tenosynovitis can cause nerve compression, but, except for carpal tunnel syndrome, this is uncommon now that synovitis is controlled by effective medications.

Functional Limitations

Surgery is considered when correction of a deformity will improve function. Rheumatoid deformities typically progress slowly, and patients often adapt well. In some cases, realignment or stabilization of one joint or finger will actually decrease function because it will interfere with an adaptive mechanism. For this reason, surgery for rheumatoid deformity must carefully match the functional desires and goals of the patient with the risks and benefits of operative intervention. Many severe deformities are left untreated when patients have adapted well.

Diagnostic Studies

The diagnosis of rheumatoid arthritis is based predominantly on its clinical presentation. Laboratory testing is used to monitor disease activity and toxicity of drug therapy. Acute phase reactants, such as C-reactive protein and erythrocyte sedimentation rate, may be elevated in the setting of active joint inflammation. Most patients with rheumatoid arthritis have circulating rheumatoid factor or anti-citrullinated protein antibodies. The presence of one of these serologic markers suggests a more aggressive and destructive disease course.

Diffuse periarticular osteopenia is the earliest radiographic sign of rheumatoid arthritis. Joint space narrowing and periarticular erosions may be observed in more than half of patients with rheumatoid arthritis during the first 2 years of disease [5]. If left untreated, joints involved by rheumatoid arthritis may be destroyed by chronic synovitis.

Diagnostic ultrasonography is often used to detect early erosions and joint swelling in patients with rheumatoid arthritis [6]. Magnetic resonance imaging of the hand may reveal synovitis and erosions early in the course of rheumatoid arthritis. However, radiographs remain the reference standard for diagnostic imaging of rheumatoid arthritis.

Differential Diagnosis

Septic arthritis
Psoriatic arthritis
Systemic lupus erythematosus
Gout
Lyme disease
Calcium pyrophosphate dihydrate deposition disease (pseudogout)

Treatment

Initial

Nonsteroidal anti-inflammatory drugs decrease pain and inflammation by inhibiting prostaglandin synthesis; they do not inhibit synovial proliferation and thus do not slow the progression of bone erosion and joint destruction. Low-dose corticosteroids also reduce symptoms of joint inflammation; but unlike nonsteroidal anti-inflammatory drugs, low-dose corticosteroids retard the progression of joint destruction. However, the widespread use of corticosteroids is limited by their many deleterious side effects, including osteoporosis, osteonecrosis of bone, cataracts, cushingoid features, and hyperglycemia.

Since the mid-1980s, the widespread and early use of low-dose weekly methotrexate has transformed rheumatoid arthritis into a much less destructive disease than it had been previously. Leflunomide also may be used to suppress synovial proliferation and joint destruction [7]. Other disease-modifying antirheumatic drugs (DMARDs) that have been used to treat rheumatoid arthritis include antimalarial drugs such as hydroxychloroquine, sulfasalazine, intramuscular and oral gold, D-penicillamine, immunosuppressive agents (azathioprine and cyclophosphamide), and cyclosporine.

Since the late 1990s, targeted biologic therapies have been used to treat rheumatoid arthritis and other inflammatory diseases. TNF antagonists, such as adalimumab, certolizumab pegol, etanercept, golimumab, and infliximab result in the rapid and marked improvement of signs and symptoms of joint inflammation and dramatically slow the rate of joint destruction [8–12]. Abatacept (an inhibitor of T-cell costimulation), tocilizumab (a monoclonal anti-IL-6 receptor antibody), and rituximab (a monoclonal anti–B-cell antibody) have also been approved by the U.S. Food and Drug Administration to treat patients with rheumatoid arthritis; tocilizumab and rituximab are each approved to treat patients who have had an inadequate response to one or more TNF antagonists, whereas abatacept is approved to treat patients who have had an inadequate response to one or more DMARDs, such as methotrexate or TNF antagonists. TNF antagonists, abatacept, and rituximab are each effective when used in combination with methotrexate [9,13-15]. Tofacitinib (an oral Janus kinase 3 [JAK3] inhibitor), has recently been approved by the U.S. Food and Drug Administration, either as monotherapy or in combination with methotrexate or other nonbiologic DMARDs, to treat patients with rheumatoid arthritis who have had an inadequate response or intolerance to methotrexate [16].

Rehabilitation

Rehabilitation of the rheumatoid hand involves adaptation and work simplification instructions (refer to Table 33.1), splinting regimens, heat modalities, active range of motion exercise, and resistive exercise (see also Chapter 33).

Flexor and Extensor Tendon Reconstruction Postoperative Rehabilitation

The rehabilitation protocol after flexor and extensor tendon reconstruction varies according to the injury, operative technique, and preferences of the surgeon. Most surgeons protect repairs with cast or splint immobilization for 4 to 6 weeks. Active and active-assisted motion is then encouraged.

Metacarpophalangeal Joint Postoperative Rehabilitation

There is also substantial variation in the preferences of surgeons for rehabilitation after metacarpophalangeal arthroplasty. However, continuous passive motion and dynamic splinting have not proved better than a month of cast immobilization with active-assisted motion exercises thereafter [17].

Interphalangeal Joint Postoperative Rehabilitation

Interphalangeal joint arthrodesis is usually performed with internal fixation that allows the patient to be splint free and to work on active motion of the metacarpophalangeal joints immediately. Rehabilitation after implant arthroplasty of the proximal interphalangeal joint varies according to operative exposure. Patients treated through a volar exposure begin active exercises within a few days, but patients in whom the extensor tendon or a collateral ligament was taken down and repaired during surgery are immobilized for about 4 weeks initially.

Procedures

Injection of intra-articular steroids may reduce the activity of the synovitis in a given joint. A good rule of thumb is no more than three injections spaced at least 3 months apart (refer to Chapter 33 for procedure details).

Surgery

Indications for surgery include pain relief and functional restoration. Another benefit—and the source of patients' satisfaction—of hand surgery in rheumatoid arthritis is improvement in the appearance of the hand [18]. The goals may be different when both hands have severe deformities. One may be addressed in a way that enhances fine motor skills, whereas the other is prepared for gross functional tasks requiring strength.

Some have advocated advancement from proximal to distal in rheumatoid hand reconstruction, arguing that if the hand cannot be placed in useful positions in space, postoperative rehabilitation will be hindered. Wrist deformity affects hand deformity and is usually corrected first or simultaneously [19].

Extensor Tendon Surgery

Patients with extensor tenosynovitis present with a painless dorsal wrist mass distal to the retinaculum of the wrist. Tenosynovectomy is indicated to establish diagnosis and to prevent tendon rupture, which is uncommon after this surgery. Treatment of tendon rupture involves transfer of the distal end of the ruptured tendon to an adjacent tendon. In the event of multiple tendon ruptures, tendon transfer of the extensor indicis proprius or the flexor digitorum superficialis of the long or ring finger may be indicated. When both wrist extensor tendons are ruptured on the radial side, arthrodesis is preferred [20].

Flexor Tendon Surgery

Flexor tenosynovitis can contribute to pain, morning stiffness, volar swelling, and median nerve compression. A tenosynovitis may be diffuse or create discrete nodules that can limit tendon excursion. At the wrist, tenosynovectomy and biopsy are indicated for median nerve compression, painful tenosynovial mass, or tendon rupture. The tendon most commonly ruptured is the flexor pollicis longus. A tendon bridge graft can be used if the rupture is relatively recent, but tendon transfer or arthrodesis of the interphalangeal joint is more commonplace. A ruptured flexor digitorum profundus tendon is sutured to an adjacent intact profundus tendon to another finger. The presence of one tendon rupture is an indication to promptly perform surgery to prevent further tendon damage.

The palm is the most common location of flexor tenosynovitis. Indications for flexor tenosynovectomy in the palm include pain with use, triggering, tendon rupture, and passive flexion of the fingers that is greater than active flexion.

Metacarpophalangeal Joint Surgery

The most common deformities of the metacarpophalangeal joint are palmar dislocation of the proximal phalanx and ulnar deviation of the fingers. As the inflammatory process disrupts the digit stabilizers, anatomic forces during use of the hand propel the digits into ulnar deviation. Metacarpophalangeal synovectomy is rarely performed in patients with rheumatoid arthritis. Silicone implant arthroplasty is indicated in patients with diminished range of motion, marked flexion contractures, and severe ulnar drift. Arthroplasty does not improve motion, it just places it in a more functional and aesthetic range. Deformities recur over time [21].

Interphalangeal Joint Surgery

There are two types of proximal interphalangeal joint deformities, the boutonnière deformity and the swan-neck deformity. Surgical intervention, such as flexor sublimis tenodesis or oblique retinacular ligament reconstruction, is designed to prevent hyperextension. On occasion, there is a mallet of the distal interphalangeal joint that can be corrected by partial extension. In later disease, intrinsic tightness requires release. In late swan-neck deformity with loss of proximal interphalangeal movement, implant arthroplasty of the proximal interphalangeal joint as well as sufficient soft tissue immobilization and release to achieve movement in flexion once again can help. In late deformities, especially in the index and middle fingers, arthrodesis may be preferred. Implant arthroplasties are recommended for the proximal interphalangeal joints of the ring and small fingers. No advantage has been demonstrated for newer implant designs (e.g., pyrolytic carbon [PyroCarbon]), which are not clearly better than traditional silicone arthroplasty [22].

For boutonnière deformity, extensor tenotomy over the middle phalanx (Fowler) can gain distal interphalangeal joint flexion. In late disease, fixed flexion contracture with inability to passively extend the proximal interphalangeal joint may be present. Treatment options are proximal interphalangeal arthrodesis and arthroplasty with a Silastic implant [23].

The thumb presents with two types of deformities. One is the boutonnière deformity with flexion of the metacarpophalangeal joint and extension of the interphalangeal joint. These are usually treated with metacarpophalangeal arthrodesis. The other is the swan-neck deformity with abduction subluxation of the base of the thumb metacarpal, hyperextension of the metacarpophalangeal joint, and flexion deformity of the interphalangeal joint of the thumb. For severe swan-neck deformity, carpometacarpal arthrodesis or arthroplasty may help.

Potential Disease Complications

Complications of rheumatoid disease in the hand include severe loss of function with complete joint destruction, severe flexion and ulnar deviation deformities of the digits, and severe swan-neck and boutonnière deformities.

Potential Treatment Complications

Complications of operative treatment include infection, hardware breakage, nonunion, Silastic implant breakage, silicone synovitis, and progression of deformity [24]. All of these eventually lead to loss of function of the hand.

Nonsteroidal anti-inflammatory drugs have associated toxicities that most commonly affect the gastric, hepatic, renal, and cardiovascular systems. Methotrexate may cause liver, hematologic, and, less frequently, lung toxicity. Thus, all patients receiving low-dose weekly methotrexate therapy should have complete blood count and liver function monitoring at least every 8 weeks [25].

The efficacy of targeted biologic therapies and of small molecule kinase inhibitors is tempered by potential toxicities. Because treatment with a TNF antagonist, tocilizumab, or tofacitinib each increases the risk for reactivation of latent tuberculosis, all patients for whom one of these medications is considered should undergo purified protein derivative (PPD) testing or an interferon-γ–release assay (IGRA). If the PPD test result is reactive or if the IGRA result is positive, treatment of latent tuberculosis should be initiated before treatment is begun with any of these drugs. Also, because the severity of bacterial infections may be increased in patients receiving treatment with rituximab, a TNF antagonist, tocilizumab, or tofacitinib, all patients taking these medications should be warned to seek immediate medical attention if signs or symptoms of infection develop [2].

References

[1] Kremer JM. Safety, efficacy, and mortality in a long-term cohort of patients with rheumatoid arthritis taking methotrexate: followup after a mean of 13.3 years. Arthritis Rheum 1997;40:984–5.

[2] Furst DE, Keystone EC, Braun J, et al. Updated consensus statement on biological agents for the treatment of rheumatic diseases, 2011. Ann Rheum Dis 2012;71(Suppl. 2):i2–i45.

[3] Vaughan-Jackson OJ. Attrition ruptures of tendons in the rheumatoid hand [abstract]. J Bone Joint Surg Am 1958;40:1431.

[4] Mannerfelt LG, Norman O. Attrition ruptures of flexor tendons in rheumatoid arthritis caused by bony spurs in the carpal tunnel. A clinical and radiological study. J Bone Joint Surg Br 1969;51:270–7.

[5] Wolfe F, Sharp JT. Radiographic outcome of recent-onset rheumatoid arthritis: a 19-year study of radiographic progression. Arthritis Rheum 1998;41:1571–82.

[6] Ostergaard M, Szkudlarek M. Ultrasonography: a valid method for assessing rheumatoid arthritis? Arthritis Rheum 2005;52:681–6.

[7] O'Dell JR. Therapeutic strategies for rheumatoid arthritis. N Engl J Med 2004;350:2591–602.

[8] Keystone EC, Kavanaugh AF, Sharp JT, et al. Radiographic, clinical, and functional outcomes of treatment with adalimumab (a human anti-tumor necrosis factor monoclonal antibody) in patients with active rheumatoid arthritis receiving concomitant methotrexate therapy: a randomized, placebo-controlled, 52-week trial. Arthritis Rheum 2004;50:1400–11.

[9] Klareskog L, van der Heijde D, de Jager JP, et al. Therapeutic effect of the combination of etanercept and methotrexate compared with each treatment alone in patients with rheumatoid arthritis: double-blind randomised controlled trial. Lancet 2004;363:675–81.

[10] Lipsky PE, van der Heijde DM, St. Clair EW, et al. Infliximab and methotrexate in the treatment of rheumatoid arthritis. Anti-Tumor Necrosis Factor Trial in Rheumatoid Arthritis with Concomitant Therapy Study Group. N Engl J Med 2000;343:1594–602.

[11] Keystone E, van der Heijde D, Mason Jr D, et al. Certolizumab pegol plus methotrexate is significantly more effective than placebo plus methotrexate in active rheumatoid arthritis: findings of a fifty-two-week, phase III, multicenter, randomized, double-blind, placebo-controlled, parallel-group study. Arthritis Rheum 2008;58:3319–29.

[12] Weinblatt ME, Westhovens R, Mendelsohn AM, et al. Radiographic benefit and maintenance of clinical benefit with intravenous golimumab therapy in patients with active rheumatoid arthritis despite methotrexate therapy: results up to 1 year of the phase 3, randomised, multicentre, double blind, placebo controlled GO-FURTHER trial. Ann Rheum Dis 2013 Sep 3.doi:10.1136/annrheumdis-2013-203742. [Epub ahead of print].

[13] Emery P, Fleischmann R, Filipowicz-Sosnowska A, et al. The efficacy and safety of rituximab in patients with active rheumatoid arthritis despite methotrexate treatment: results of a phase IIB randomized, double-blind, placebo-controlled, dose-ranging trial. Arthritis Rheum 2006;54:1390–400.

[14] Kremer JM, Genant HK, Moreland LW, et al. Effects of abatacept in patients with methotrexate-resistant active rheumatoid arthritis: a randomized trial. Ann Intern Med 2006;144:865–76.

[15] Emery P, Keystone E, Tony HP, et al. IL-6 receptor inhibition with tocilizumab improves treatment outcomes in patients with rheumatoid arthritis refractory to anti-tumour necrosis factor biologicals: results from a 24-week multicentre randomised placebo-controlled trial. Ann Rheum Dis 2008;67:1516–23.

[16] Fleischmann R, Kremer J, Cush J, et al. Placebo-controlled trial of tofacitinib monothaerapy in rheumatoid arthritis. N Engl J Med 2012;367:495–507.

[17] Ring D, Simmons BP, Hayes M. Continuous passive motion following metacarpophalangeal joint arthroplasty. J Hand Surg [Am] 1998;23:505–11.

[18] Mandl LA, Galvin DH, Bosch JP, et al. Metacarpophalangeal arthroplasty in rheumatoid arthritis: what determines satisfaction with surgery? J Rheumatol 2002;29:2488–91.

[19] Millender LH, Phillips C. Combined wrist arthrodesis and metacarpophalangeal joint arthroplasty in rheumatoid arthritis. Orthopedics 1978;1:43–8.

[20] Millender LH, Nalebuff EA. Arthrodesis of the rheumatoid wrist. An evaluation of sixty patients and a description of a different surgical technique. J Bone Joint Surg Am 1973;55:1026–34.

[21] Goldfarb CA, Stern PJ. Metacarpophalangeal joint arthroplasty in rheumatoid arthritis. A long-term assessment. J Bone Joint Surg Am 2003;85:1869–78.

[22] Sweets TM, Stern PJ. Pyrolytic carbon resurfacing arthroplasty for osteoarthritis of the proximal interphalangeal joint of the finger. J Bone Joint Surg Am 2011;93:1417–25.

[23] El-Sallakh S, Aly T, Amin O, Hegazi M. Surgical management of chronic boutonniere deformity. Hand Surg 2012;17:359–64.

[24] Ono S, Entezami P, Chung KC. Reconstruction of the rheumatoid hand. Clin Plast Surg 2011;38:713–27.

[25] Kremer JM, Alarcon GS, Lightfoot Jr RW, et al. Methotrexate for rheumatoid arthritis. Suggested guidelines for monitoring liver toxicity. American College of Rheumatology. Arthritis Rheum 1994;37:316–28.

CHAPTER 35

Kienböck Disease

Charles Cassidy, MD
Vivek M. Shah, MD

Synonyms

Lunatomalacia
Osteonecrosis of the lunate
Avascular necrosis of the lunate

ICD-9 Codes

715.23	**Osteoarthrosis of the wrist, secondary**
732.3	**Kienböck's disease**

ICD-10 Codes

M19.231	**Secondary osteoarthritis, right wrist**
M19.232	**Secondary osteoarthritis, left wrist**
M19.239	**Secondary osteoarthritis, unspecified wrist**
M93.1	**Kienböck's disease of adults**

Definition

Kienböck disease is avascular necrosis of the lunate, unrelated to acute fracture, often leading to fragmentation and collapse. Although the precise etiology and natural history of this disorder remain unknown, interruption of the blood supply to the lunate is undoubtedly a part of the process. Trauma has been implicated as a cause [1–3]. This disease occurs most often in the dominant hand of men in the age group of 20 to 40 years. Many of these patients are manual laborers who report a history of a major or repetitive minor injury. Associations have also been made between Kienböck disease and corticosteroid use, cerebral palsy, systemic lupus erythematosus, sickle cell disease, gout, and streptococcal infection.

An important radiographic observation has been made regarding the radius-ulna relationship at the wrist and the development of Kienböck disease [4]. In these patients, the ulna is generally shorter than the radius, a finding termed ulnar negative (or minus) variance. Normally, the lunate rests on both the radius and the triangular fibrocartilage complex covering the ulnar head. It has been speculated that when the ulna is significantly shorter than the radius, a shearing effect occurs in the lunate, which can make it more susceptible to injury.

Symptoms

Presenting symptoms include chronic wrist pain, decreased range of motion, and weakness [5]. The pain is usually deep within the wrist, although the patient often points to the dorsum of the wrist, and is aggravated by activity. Some patients complain of a pressure-like pain that may awaken them. A history of recent trauma is often provided; however, many patients report having had long-standing mild wrist pain preceding the recent injury. Symptoms may often be present for months or years before the patient seeks medical attention.

Physical Examination

Mild dorsal wrist swelling and tenderness in the mid-dorsal aspect of the wrist may be present. Wrist flexion and extension are limited. Forearm rotation is usually preserved. Grip strength is often considerably less on the affected side because of pain.

Neurologic and vascular examination findings are normal.

Functional Limitations

Functional limitations include difficulty with heavy lifting, gripping, and activities involving the extremes of wrist motion. Many heavy laborers are unable to perform the essential tasks required of their occupation.

Diagnostic Studies

The initial diagnostic imaging for suspected Kienböck disease includes standard wrist radiographs. Early in the disease process, the radiographs may be normal. With time, a characteristic pattern of deterioration occurs, beginning with sclerosis of the lunate, followed by fragmentation, collapse, and finally arthritis [6,7] (Fig. 35.1). A radiographic staging system for Kienböck disease, proposed by Lichtman, is helpful in describing the extent of the disease and guiding treatment [1] (Table 35.1).

For clinical suspicion of Kienböck disease with normal radiographs, a technetium bone scan or magnetic resonance

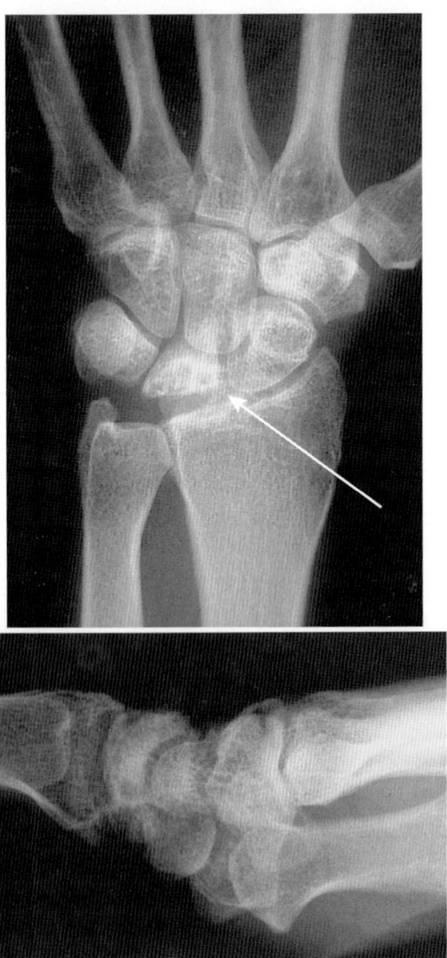

FIGURE 35.1 Advanced Kienböck disease. Cystic and sclerotic changes are present within the collapsed lunate *(arrow)*.

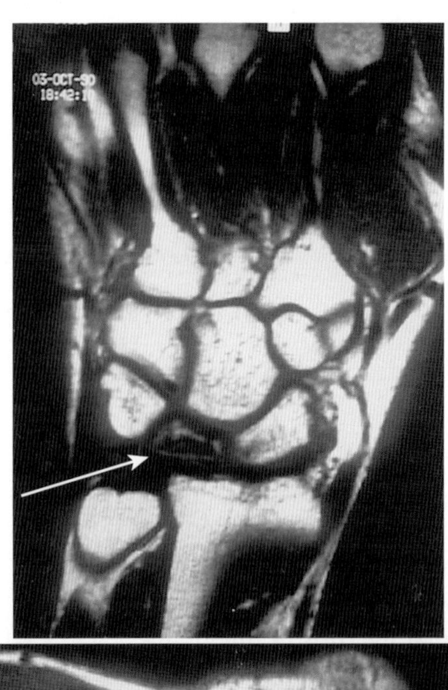

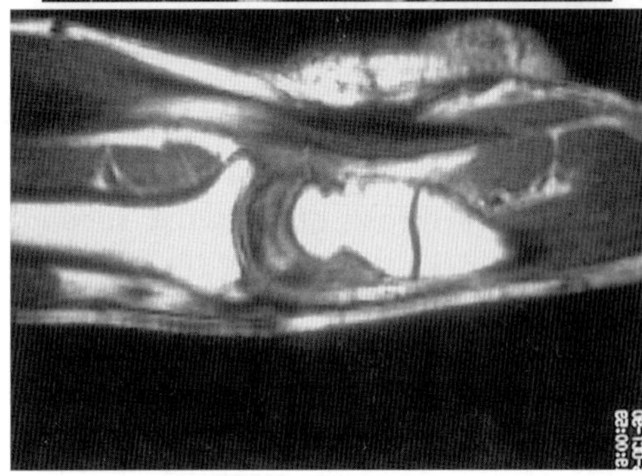

FIGURE 35.2 MRI in Kienböck disease. T1-weighted images demonstrate diffuse low signal within the lunate *(arrow)*.

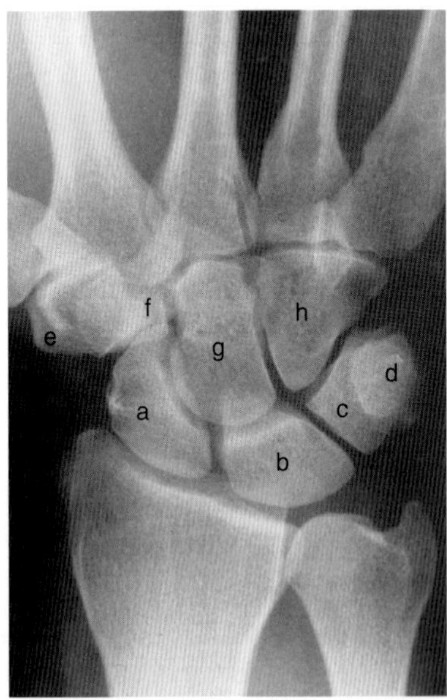

FIGURE 35.3 Posteroanterior view of the wrist demonstrating the proximal and distal carpal rows. *a,* scaphoid; *b,* lunate; *c,* triquetrum; *d,* pisiform; *e,* trapezium; *f,* trapezoid; *g,* capitate; and *h,* hamate. *(From Jebson PJL, Kasdan ML, eds. Hand Secrets. Philadelphia, Hanley & Belfus, 1998:220.)*

Table 35.1 Stages of Kienböck Disease

Stage I	Normal radiographs or linear fracture
Stage II	Lunate sclerosis, one or more fracture lines with possible early collapse on the radial border
Stage III	Lunate collapse
IIIA	Normal carpal alignment and height
IIIB	Fixed scaphoid rotation (ring sign), carpal height decreased, capitate migrates proximally
Stage IV	Severe lunate collapse with intra-articular degenerative changes at the midcarpal joint, radiocarpal joint, or both

imaging (MRI) may be helpful. In fact, MRI has supplanted plain radiography for the detection and evaluation of the early stages of Kienböck disease when there has been no trabecular bone destruction. Characteristic signal changes include decreased signal on T1-weighted and increased signal on T2-weighted images (Fig. 35.2). Computed tomography is more effective than MRI in assessing for fracture of the lunate, but it provides limited information about its vascularity (Figs. 35.3 and 35.4).

Differential Diagnosis

Wrist sprain
Scapholunate ligament tear
Osteoarthritis
Ganglion
Inflammatory arthritis (e.g., rheumatoid arthritis)
Preiser disease (avascular necrosis of the scaphoid)
Tendinitis
Scaphoid fracture

Treatment

Initial

Given the limited information about the etiology and natural history of this uncommon disease, it is not surprising that the treatment has not been standardized. Without surgery, progressive radiographic collapse and radiographic arthritis almost invariably occur [5]. However, symptoms correlate only weakly with the radiographic appearance, and many patients maintain good long-term function even without

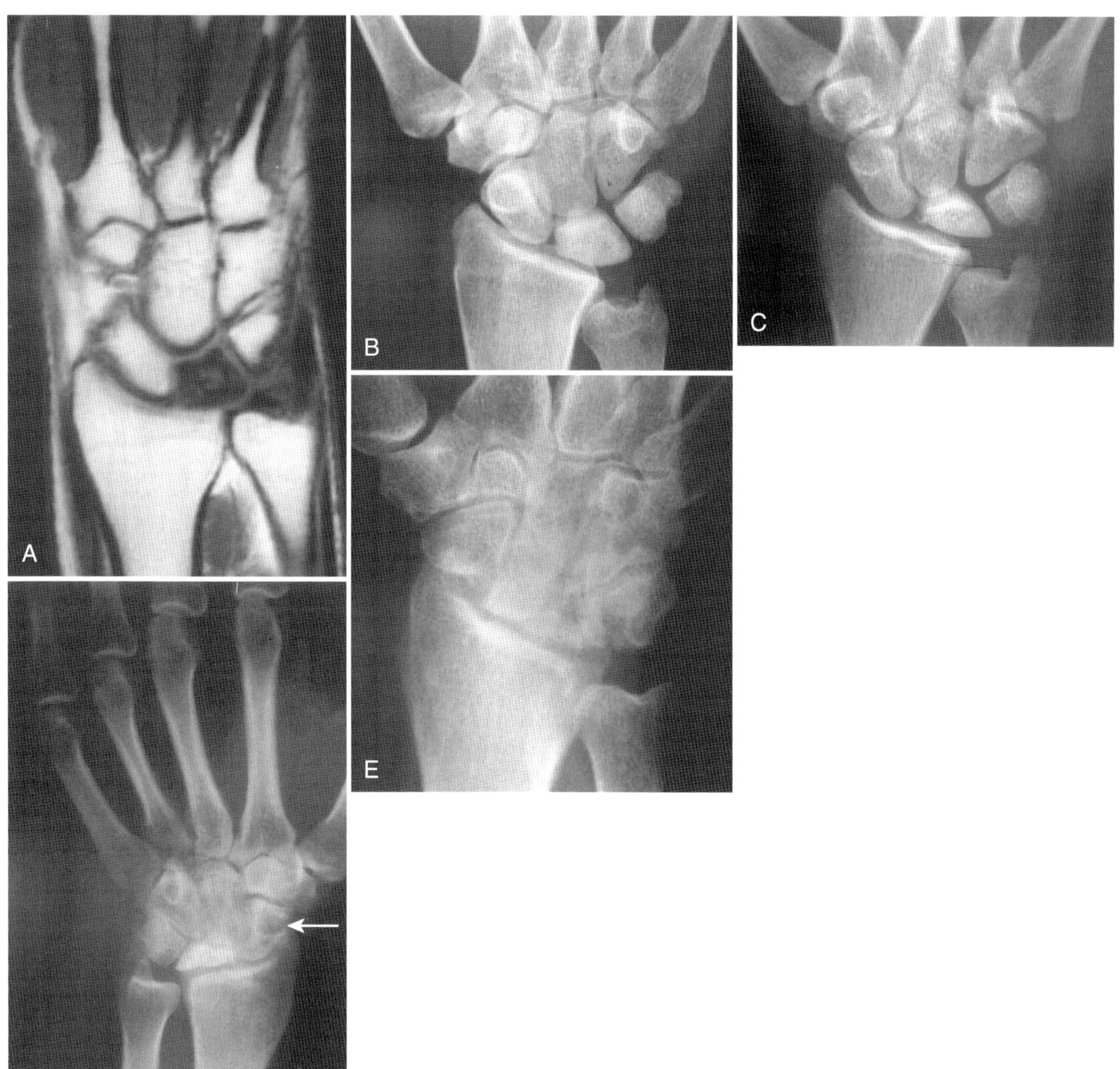

FIGURE 35.4 The stages of Kienböck disease. **A,** Stage I. T1-weighted MRI shows marked signal reduction in the lunate, compatible with loss of blood supply. **B,** Stage II. Density changes in the lunate as indicated by sclerosis. Note the ulnar minus variance. **C,** Stage IIIA. Collapse of the lunate. There are no fixed carpal derangements. **D,** Stage IIIB. Decreased carpal height and proximal migration of the capitate. Note the scaphoid cortical ring sign *(arrow)*. **E,** Stage IV. Generalized degenerative changes in the carpus. *(From Weinzweig J, ed. Plastic Surgery Secrets. Philadelphia, Hanley & Belfus, 1999:605-606.)*

surgery [8]. The goals of surgery ideally would be to relieve the pain and to halt the progression of the disease. Surgical interventions appear to be relatively effective in achieving the first goal but have not as yet reliably altered the radiographic deterioration of the lunate. Consequently, treatment options range from simple splints to external fixation and from radial shortening to vascularized grafts to fusions. Factors taken into consideration in assigning treatment include stage of the disease; ulnar variance; and age, occupation, pain, and functional impairment of the patient [9]. An argument can be made to treat young, active patients with early-stage disease more aggressively in an effort to prevent progression; however, intra-articular procedures invariably result in some permanent loss of motion.

Many clinicians prefer to begin with symptomatic treatment. Depending on the situation, this may involve a splint and activity modification or a short arm cast. However, an appropriate length of immobilization has not been established. Some clinicians have attempted this treatment for as long as 1 year, but most clinicians prescribe a cast for 6 to 12 weeks. The immobilization probably helps the pain associated with synovitis and with wrist activity and motion; however, it does nothing to alter the vascularity of the bone or the shear stresses across the lunate. The patient should be informed that the radiographs will, in all likelihood, demonstrate worsening of the disease over time.

Pain can be treated with analgesics, including nonsteroidal anti-inflammatory drugs. Narcotic medications are generally not recommended because of the chronicity of this condition.

Rehabilitation

Rehabilitation does not play a major role early in conservative treatment. Once the pain has subsided, gentle range of motion and strengthening may be initiated. Therapy is important for the postoperative patient, particularly if an intra-articular procedure has been performed or an external fixator has been applied. The wrist is typically immobilized postoperatively until the vascularized graft or fusion has healed (about 6 weeks). At that point, occupational or physical therapy can effectively begin with gentle range of motion exercises, gradually progressing to strengthening exercises.

Procedures

Intra-articular steroids are of no proven benefit in the management of Kienböck disease.

Surgery

Some authors think that most patients treated nonoperatively do well [6], whereas others think that surgery is indicated for most patients with Kienböck disease [10–12]. The surgical treatment options for this disease may be divided into stress reduction (unloading), revascularization, lunate replacement, and salvage procedures [9]. Radial shortening of 2 to 3 mm is currently the most popular procedure for early-stage Kienböck disease in the setting of ulnar minus variant [10,13]. The goal is to make the radius and ulna lengths the same and thus to reduce shear forces on the lunate. Other unloading procedures include limited wrist fusion, capitate shortening, and external fixation [14]. Revascularization procedures have shown promise in the management of avascular necrosis of the lunate [15,16]. The most popular of the pedicled bone grafts, based on the extensor compartmental arteries of the wrist, is transplanted from the distal radius into the lunate. In one series with relatively short-term follow-up, significant pain relief was observed in 92% of patients, and actual lunate revascularization was seen in 60% on follow-up MRI [15]. An intriguing method of indirect revascularization of the lunate has been proposed by Illarramendi and colleagues [17], who perform a metaphyseal drilling of the radius and ulna, without violating the wrist joint. In their series, 16 of 20 patients were pain free at an average of 10 years postoperatively. Silastic lunate replacement has been abandoned because of implant dislocation and synovitis.

When the lunate has collapsed to the point that it is not reconstructable, salvage procedures such as proximal row carpectomy and partial or total wrist arthrodesis are considered. Obviously, these procedures sacrifice motion in an effort to provide pain relief. The results of the various procedures are dependent, to some extent, on the stage of the disease. Wrist arthroscopy may be of some benefit in determining the extent of the disease and in selecting the appropriate salvage procedure [18]. Regardless of the specific type of salvage procedure, most authors report 70% to 100% satisfaction of patients. Advanced arthritis (stage IV) is generally best treated with a total wrist arthrodesis.

Potential Disease Complications

Without surgery, progressive radiographic collapse of the lunate and arthritis of the wrist invariably occur.

Potential Treatment Complications

Analgesics and nonsteroidal anti-inflammatory drugs have well-known side effects that most commonly affect the gastric, hepatic, and renal systems. Infection is uncommon after hand surgery. Complications such as nerve injury, painful hardware, and stiffness of the wrist and digits are inherent in hand surgery. A radial shortening osteotomy or partial wrist fusion may fail to heal (nonunion). Secondary wrist arthritis can develop after partial wrist fusions or proximal row carpectomy. Grip strength virtually never returns to normal. Finally, and most important, whether surgery favorably alters the natural history of this rare condition remains unproven.

References

[1] Fredericks TK, Fernandez JE, Pirela-Cruz MA. Kienböck's disease. I. Anatomy and etiology. Int J Occup Med Environ Health 1997;10:11–7.
[2] Fredericks TK, Fernandez JE, Pirela-Cruz MA. Kienböck's disease. II. Risk factors, diagnosis, and ergonomic interventions. Int J Occup Med Environ Health 1997;10:147–57.
[3] Watson HK, Guidera PM. Aetiology of Kienböck's disease. J Hand Surg [Br] 1997;22:5–7.
[4] Hulten O. Über anatomische Variationen der Handgelenkknochen. Acta Radiol 1928;9:155–68.
[5] Beckenbaugh RD, Shives TS, Dobyns JH, Linscheid RL. Kienböck's disease: the natural history of Kienböck's disease and considerations of lunate fractures. Clin Orthop 1980;149:98–106.

[6] Stahl F. On lunatomalacia (Kienböck's disease): clinical and roentgenological study, especially on its pathogenesis and late results of immobilization treatment. Acta Chir Scand Suppl 1947;126:1–133.
[7] Lichtman DM, Mack GR, MacDonald RI, et al. Kienböck's disease: the role of silicon replacement arthroplasty. J Bone Joint Surg Am 1977;59:899–908.
[8] Mirabello SC, Rosenthal DI, Smith RJ. Correlation of clinical and radiographic findings in Kienböck's disease. J Hand Surg [Am] 1987;12:1049–54.
[9] Cassidy C, Ruby LK. Carpal fractures and dislocations. In: Browner BD, Levine AM, Jupiter JB, Trafton P, editors. Skeletal trauma: fractures, dislocations, ligamentous injuries. 4th ed. Philadelphia: WB Saunders; 2008.
[10] Salmon J, Stanley JK, Trail IA. Kienböck's disease: conservative management versus radial shortening. J Bone Joint Surg Br 2000;82:820–3.
[11] Mikkelsen SS, Gelineck J. Poor function after nonoperative treatment of Kienböck's disease. Acta Orthop Scand 1987;58:241–3.
[12] Delaere O, Dury M, Molderez A, Foucher G. Conservative versus operative treatment for Kienböck's disease. J Hand Surg [Br] 1998;23:33–6.
[13] Almquist EE. Kienböck's disease. Hand Clin North Am 1987;3:141–8.
[14] Zelouf DS, Ruby LK. External fixation and cancellous bone grafting for Kienböck's disease. J Hand Surg [Am] 1996;21:743–53.
[15] Moran SL, Cooney WP, Berger RA, et al. The use of the 4+5 extensor compartmental vascularized bone graft for the treatment of Kienböck's disease. J Hand Surg [Am] 2005;30:50–8.
[16] Daecke W, Lorenz S, Wieloch P, et al. Vascularized os pisiform for reinforcement of the lunate in Kienböck's disease: an average of 12 years of follow-up study. J Hand Surg [Am] 2005;30:915–22.
[17] Illarramendi AA, Schulz C, De Carli P. The surgical treatment of Kienböck's disease by radius and ulna metaphyseal core decompression. J Hand Surg [Am] 2001;26:252–60.
[18] Bain GI, Begg M. Arthroscopic assessment and classification of Kienböck's disease. Tech Hand Up Extrem Surg 2006;10:8–13.

CHAPTER 36

Median Neuropathy (Carpal Tunnel Syndrome)

Meijuan Zhao, MD
David T. Burke, MD, MA

Synonyms

Median nerve entrapment at the wrist or carpal tunnel syndrome
Median nerve compression

ICD-9 Code

354.0 Carpal tunnel syndrome

ICD-10 Codes

G56.00 Carpal tunnel syndrome, unspecified upper limb
G56.01 Carpal tunnel syndrome, right upper limb
G56.02 Carpal tunnel syndrome, left upper limb

Definition

Carpal tunnel syndrome (CTS), an entrapment neuropathy of the median nerve at the wrist, is the most common compression neuropathy of the upper extremity. This syndrome produces paresthesias, numbness, pain, subjective swelling, and, in advanced cases, muscle atrophy and weakness of the areas innervated by the median nerve. The condition is often bilateral, although the dominant hand tends to be more severely affected.

CTS is thought to result from a compression of the median nerve as it passes through the carpal tunnel. The clinical presentation is variable. Whereas there is some variation as to what should be included in this definition, CTS is most often thought to involve sensory changes in the radial 3½ digits of the hand with burning, tingling, numbness, and a subjective sense of swelling. Those affected often first note symptoms at night. In the later stages, complaints include motor weakness in the thenar eminence.

It is helpful to think of the carpal tunnel as a structure with four sides, three of which are defined by the carpal bones and the fourth, the "top" of the tunnel, by the transverse carpal ligament (Figs. 36.1 and 36.2). Passing through the tunnel are the median nerve and nine tendons with their synovial sheaths; these include the flexor pollicis longus, the four flexor digitorum superficialis, and the four flexor digitorum profundus tendons. None of the sides of the tunnel yields well to expansion of the fluid or structures within. Because of this, swelling will increase pressure within the tunnel and may result in compression of the median nerve. CTS occurs more commonly in women than in men, with a prevalence in the general adult population ranging from 2.7% to 5.8% [1,2]. It is most common in middle-aged persons between the ages of 30 and 60 years. The older adults may have objective clinical and electrophysiologic evidence of a more severe median nerve entrapment [3]. Most cases of CTS are idiopathic with congenital predisposition. Some focal or systemic conditions, such as wrist injury, arthritis, diabetes, thyroid disease, rheumatoid arthritis, and pregnancy, can increase pressure on the median nerve in the carpal tunnel and contribute to the development of CTS. Prolonged postures in extremes of wrist flexion or extension, repetitive use of the flexor muscles, and exposure to vibration are the primary exposures that have been reported [4–7]. The pathophysiologic mechanism of CTS involves a combination of mechanical trauma, increased pressure, and ischemic injury to the median nerve within the carpal tunnel [8].

Symptoms

The classic symptoms of CTS include numbness and paresthesias in the radial 3½ fingers (Fig. 36.3). A typical early complaint is awakening in the night with numbness or pain in the fingers. Symptoms during the day are often brought out by activities placing the wrist in substantial flexion or extension or requiring repetitive motion of the structures that traverse the carpal tunnel. Many patients report symptoms outside the distribution of the median nerve as well [9].

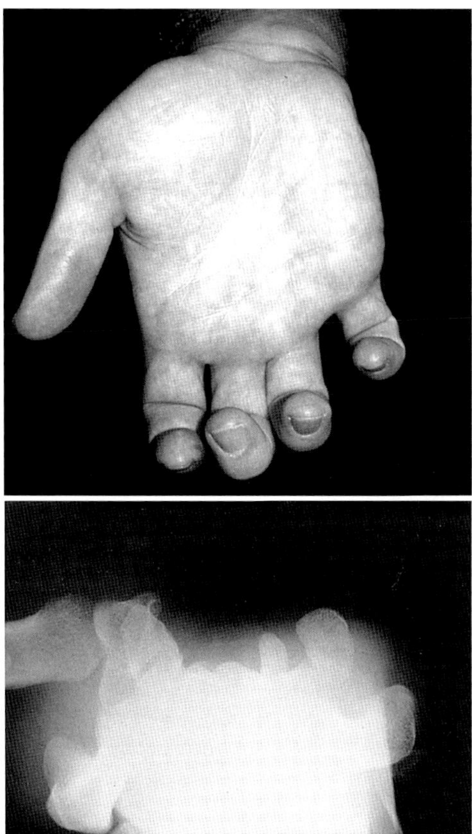

FIGURE 36.1 Radiographic demonstration of the carpal tunnel (for orientation, the hand is in the same position in the radiograph). The carpal tunnel is formed radially, ulnarly, and dorsally by the carpal bones. *(From Concannon M. Common Hand Problems in Primary Care. Philadelphia, Hanley & Belfus, 1999.)*

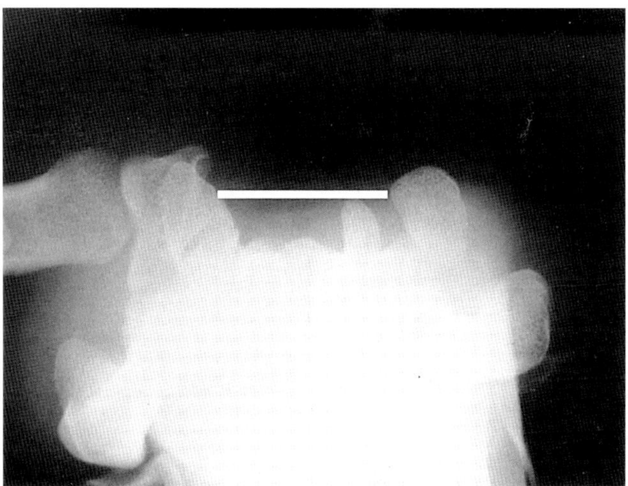

FIGURE 36.2 The volar carpal ligament *(line)* forms the roof of the carpal tunnel. This thick, fibrous structure does not yield to expansion, and increased pressure within the carpal tunnel can cause impingement of the median nerve. *(From Concannon M. Common Hand Problems in Primary Care. Philadelphia, Hanley & Belfus, 1999.)*

Numbness and pain in the hand may also be accompanied by volar wrist pain and aching at the forearm. The patient may describe the symptoms as being positional, with symptoms relieved by the shaking of a hand, often referred to as the flick sign [10].

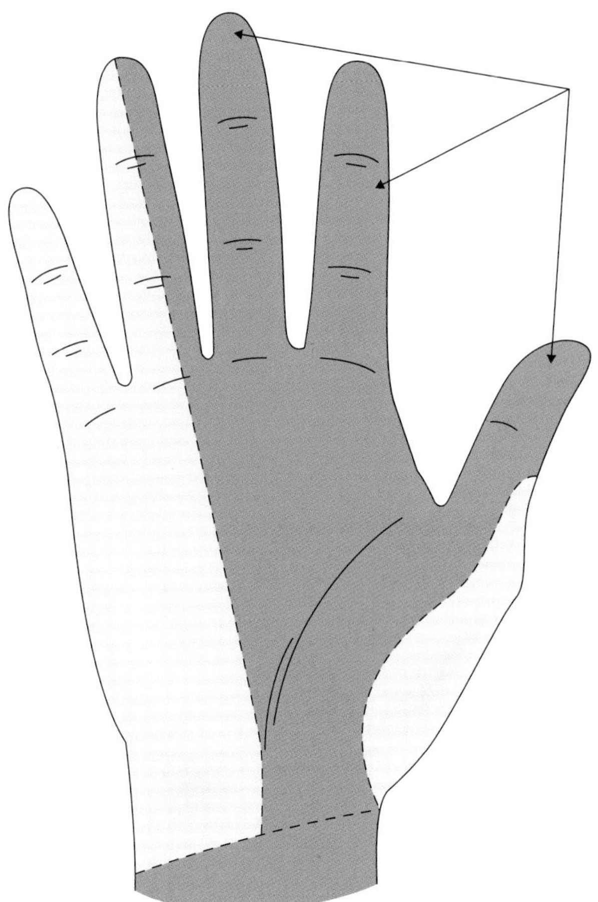

FIGURE 36.3 Patients with carpal tunnel syndrome complain of numbness or paresthesia within the median nerve distribution *(orange area, arrows). (From Concannon M. Common Hand Problems in Primary Care. Philadelphia, Hanley & Belfus, 1999.)*

Patients may complain of a sense of swelling in the hands, often noting that they have difficulty wearing jewelry or watches, with this sensation fluctuating throughout the day or week. Some patients also report dry skin and cold hands. In the later stages of CTS, the numbness may become constant and motor disturbances more apparent, with complaints of weakness manifested by a functional decrease of strength. Patients may then report dropping objects.

Physical Examination

A two-point sensory discrimination test is thought to be the most sensitive of the bedside examination techniques. This involves a comparison of the two-point discriminating sensory ability of the median with that of the ulnar nerve distribution of the hand. Careful observation of the hands, comparing the affected side with the unaffected side and comparing the thenar and hypothenar eminences of the same hand, may reveal an increasing asymmetry. Weakness of the thenar intrinsic muscles of the hand can be tested with a dynamometer or clinically by testing abduction of the thumb against resistance. The more common special tests include the Phalen, the Tinel, and the nerve compression tests. The Phalen test involves a forced flexion at the wrist to 90 degrees for a period of 1 minute; a positive test result

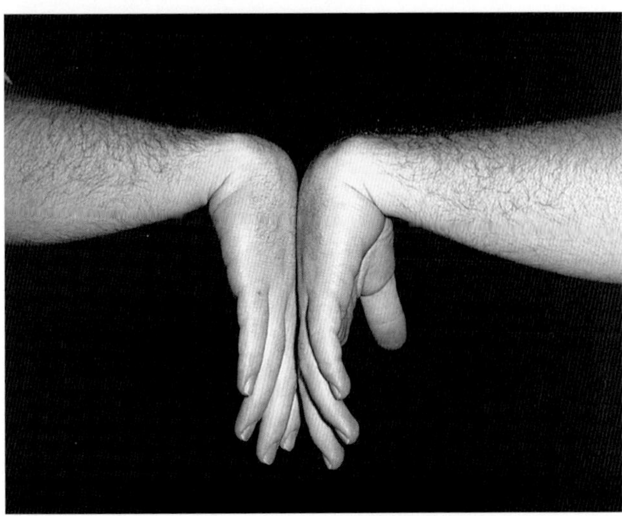

FIGURE 36.4 Phalen test. Patients maximally flex both wrists and hold the position for 1 to 2 minutes. If symptoms of numbness or paresthesia within the median nerve distribution are reproduced, the test result is positive. *(From Concannon M. Common Hand Problems in Primary Care. Philadelphia, Hanley & Belfus, 1999.)*

reproduces the symptoms of CTS (Fig. 36.4). The reverse Phalen maneuver is the same test completed with forced extension. The Tinel test involves tapping sharply over the volar aspect of the wrist just distal to the distal wrist crease. The test result is positive when a sensory disturbance radiates down the region of the distribution of the median nerve. The nerve compression test involves the placement of two thumbs over the roof of the carpal tunnel, with pressure maintained for 1 minute. The test result is positive if symptoms are reproduced in the area of the distribution of the median nerve. A review showed an overall estimate of 68% sensitivity and 73% specificity for the Phalen test, 50% sensitivity and 77% specificity for the Tinel test, and 64% sensitivity and 83% specificity for the carpal compression test [11]. Two-point discrimination and testing of atrophy or strength of the abductor pollicis brevis proved to be specific but not very sensitive. [11].

Functional Limitations

Functional limitations of CTS often include difficulty with sleep due to frequent awakenings by the symptoms. Because certain sustained or repetitive motions are difficult, tasks that often become more difficult include driving a car and sustained computer keyboard or mouse use at work. The later symptom of weakness in the thenar eminence may result in difficulty maintaining grip. Profound CTS may result in functional limitations, such as the inability to tie one's shoes, to button shirts, and to put a key in a lock.

Diagnostic Studies

Whereas CTS is a syndrome rather than a singular finding, it is often suggested that the "gold standard" test of CTS is electrodiagnostic testing. Electromyography and nerve conduction studies can confirm the diagnosis, determine the severity (if any) of nerve damage, guide and measure the effect of treatment, and rule out other conditions such as radiculopathy and brachial plexopathy. Ultrasound studies, which reveal an enlarged median nerve, may assist with the diagnosis [12]. Typically, the ultrasound examination may show flattening of the nerve within the tunnel and enlargement of the nerve proximal and distal to the tunnel. Pooling of recent articles seems to confirm that sonography using cross-sectional area of the median nerve could not be an alternative to electrodiagnostic testing for diagnosis of CTS but could give complementary results. Ultrasound examination should be considered in doubtful cases or secondary cases of CTS [13].

Others have advocated the injection of corticosteroids or bupivacaine into the carpal tunnel. If the injection is accompanied by a relief of symptoms, it provides diagnostic evidence of CTS [14].

A wrist radiograph may be helpful if a fracture or degenerative joint disease is suspected.

Blood tests should be ordered if underlying rheumatologic disease or endocrine disturbance is suspected. These include fasting blood glucose concentration, erythrocyte sedimentation rate, thyroid function, and rheumatoid factor.

Differential Diagnosis

Cervical radiculopathy in C5 to T1 distribution
Brachial plexopathy
Proximal median neuropathy
Ulnar or radial neuropathy
Generalized neuropathy
Arthritis of carpometacarpal joint of thumb
de Quervain tenosynovitis
Tendinitis of the flexor carpi radialis
Raynaud phenomenon
Hand-arm vibration syndrome
Arthritis of the wrist
Gout

Treatment

Initial

Once the diagnosis is established, treatment should begin with conservative management in patients with mild disease. Nighttime wrist splinting (Fig. 36.5) in a neutral

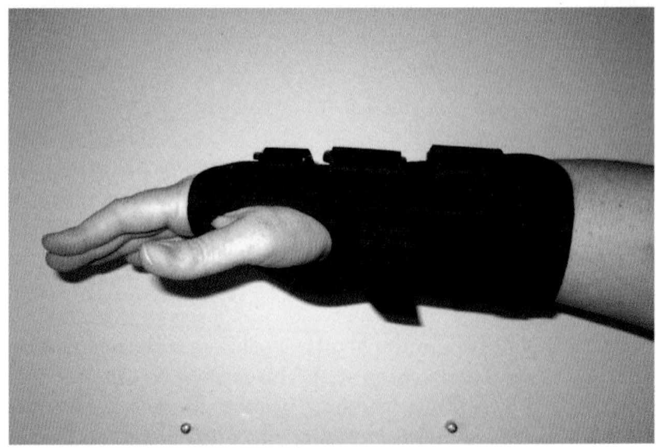

FIGURE 36.5 Wrist splint in neutral position.

position may help reduce or completely relieve CTS symptoms. Wrist splinting in neutral position may be more effective than in 20-degree extension in the short term [15]. Full-time use, if tolerable, has been shown to provide greater improvement of symptoms and electrophysiologic measures than night-only use [16]. Compliance with full-time use is more difficult [16]. Most patients will achieve maximal symptom relief through splinting within 2 to 3 weeks. If current treatment fails to resolve symptoms within 2 to 7 weeks, another nonsurgical treatment or surgery is suggested [17]. Nonsteroidal anti-inflammatory drugs are frequently prescribed as an adjunct to wrist splinting. However, studies have demonstrated that nonsteroidal anti-inflammatory drugs, vitamin B_6, and diuretics are often no more effective than placebo in relieving the symptoms of CTS [15].

The use of oral steroids (prednisone in doses of 20 mg daily for the first week and 10 mg daily for the second week [18], or prednisolone at 25 mg daily for 10 days [19]) has proved to be of some benefit, although not as impressive as the results noted through injection (see later) [19]. However, the effectiveness of oral or injected steroids was not maintained in the long term [15].

Underlying conditions, such as hypothyroidism, rheumatoid arthritis, or diabetes, should be treated. Frequent periods of rest of the wrist should be prescribed, especially when vocational activities involve sustained positioning or repetitive and forceful flexion or extension of the wrist. Ice after periods of use may be effective for symptom relief. Positioning of the body while a task is being performed should be reviewed to relieve unnecessary strain as necessary motions are performed.

Rehabilitation

Rehabilitation must address the patterns of hand use, which exacerbates the symptoms of CTS in many individuals. Lifestyle modifications, including decreasing repetitive activity and using ergonomic devices, have been traditionally advocated but have inconsistent evidence to support their effectiveness. Occupational therapists can be helpful in instructing flexion and extension stretching of the wrist and forearm. Although many therapists advocate strengthening as part of a treatment program, aggressive strengthening exercises should be avoided until symptom relief is nearly complete.

Icing after long periods of use has been advocated to reduce the pain and swelling. In addition, it is important that patients be instructed in a program of general physical conditioning; generalized deconditioning exacerbates the symptoms of CTS [20].

There is no evidence for the effectiveness of postoperative splinting [15]. It is suggested that the wrist not be immobilized postoperatively after routine carpal tunnel surgery [17]. Active motion of the hand and wrist should start immediately postoperatively to prevent joint stiffness and to ensure adequate glide of the tendons and median nerve in the carpal tunnel. Passive range of motion should be initiated at least 4 weeks postoperatively for mobilization of stiff joints and tendons. Strengthening is initiated at 3 to 4 weeks as wounds heal and inflammation resolves [21].

On average, postsurgical patients were able to return to driving in 9 days, to activities of daily living in 13 days, and to work in 17 days [22].

Procedures

The patient can also be treated with corticosteroid injections into the carpal tunnel. A number of authors have suggested various injection techniques to avoid direct injury to the median nerve [23–26].

For injection into the carpal tunnel (Fig. 36.6), 1 mL of steroid (triamcinolone, 40 mg/mL) can be injected under sterile conditions. For delivery, one should use a ⅝-inch, 27-gauge needle, placing the needle proximal to the distal wrist crease and ulnar to the palmaris longus tendon. The needle should be directed dorsally and angled at 30 degrees to a depth of about ⅝ inch (the length of the needle) or contact with a flexor tendon. Slowly inject 1 mL of the corticosteroid. Anesthetics are not typically used in this injection unless for diagnostic verification. In individuals lacking a palmaris longus tendon (about 2% to 20% of the population), the needle can be placed midpoint between the ulna and radial styloid process. The injection will increase the volume of fluid within the carpal tunnel and thus may exacerbate the discomfort for a few hours; relief is expected within the 24 to 48 hours after injection. Although effectiveness is primarily short term, corticosteroid injection may be particularly useful to control the pain and to reduce symptoms for patients wishing to delay surgical treatment.

It has been reported that ultrasound-guided carpal tunnel injection improves the performance, clinical outcomes, and cost-effectiveness of injection of the carpal tunnel compared with conventional blind, palpation-guided injection

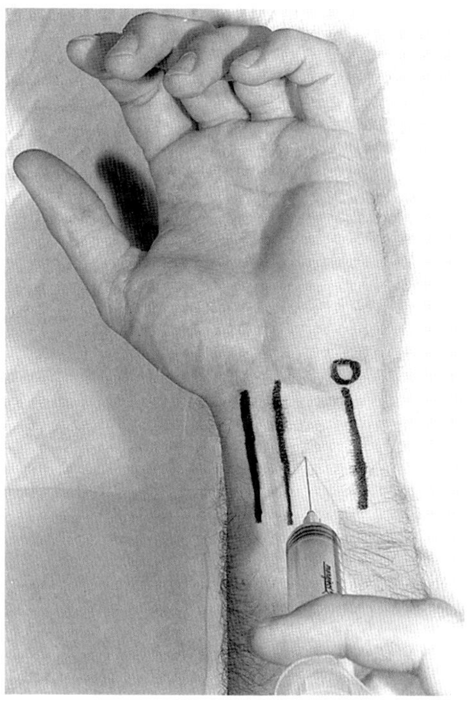

FIGURE 36.6 Preferred method for ulna bursa injection. Needle puncture is just ulnar to the palmaris longus tendon. The circle is over the pisiform bone. *(From Lennard TA. Pain Procedures in Clinical Practice, 2nd ed. Philadelphia, Hanley & Belfus, 2000.)*

in a single randomized controlled trial [27]. However, the exact role of ultrasound guidance for carpal tunnel injection is still arguable [28].

Surgery

Carpal tunnel release surgery should be considered in patients with symptoms that do not respond to conservative measures and for whom electrodiagnostic testing clearly confirms median neuropathy at the wrist. Surgery or another nonsurgical treatment is suggested when the current treatment fails to resolve symptoms within 2 to 7 weeks [17]. Six weeks to 3 months of conservative treatment is reasonable in patients with mild disease [29].

Early surgery is indicated when there are signs of atrophy or muscle weakness. The optimal timing of surgery in the natural history of CTS has not been established, although timing is an important factor for total recovery after surgery. A long-lasting compression could result in irreversible axonal damage, which would not improve despite surgical intervention [15]. Surgical treatment has been shown to lead to better outcome than nonsurgical treatment [30]. The primary reason for a poor result is an error in diagnosis.

The open release of the transverse carpal ligament represents the standard procedure and can be performed by dividing the transverse carpal ligament through a small open wrist incision. The reliability of and good visualization provided by the open technique continue to make it the preferred operation for many hand surgeons [31]. The endoscopic techniques were introduced in the late 1980s to be minimally invasive and to prevent the palmar scarring. Both methods have equal efficacy and provide excellent outcomes in relieving symptoms of CTS [32], with satisfaction rates up to 90%. Potential benefits of the endoscopic technique, including a more rapid functional recovery, must be weighed against the technique's increased cost and higher complication rate [32].

Potential Disease Complications

As with any insult to a peripheral nerve, untreated CTS may result in chronic sensory disturbance or motor impairment in the area serviced by the median nerve. It is important that the clinician be wary of this and not allow the nerve disturbance to progress to permanent nerve damage.

Potential Treatment Complications

Although oral analgesics may be important for symptomatic relief early in the stages of CTS, gastric, renal, and hepatic complications of nonsteroidal anti-inflammatory drugs should be monitored. Complications from local corticosteroid injections include infection, bleeding, skin depigmentation, skin and fat atrophy, potential for tendon rupture, and potential for injury to the median nerve at the time of injection.

Surgical complications have been noted to be few in the literature. These include accidental transection of the median nerve, with permanent loss of function distal to the transection. In addition, some have suggested that endoscopic surgery might damage the Berrettini branch of the median nerve, a sensory branch [33]. Whereas complications of surgical intervention are thought to be relatively infrequent, a number have been reported. The most common complication of surgical intervention is the incomplete sectioning of the transverse carpal ligament. Other potential complications include injury to the median nerve, palmar cutaneous branch, recurrent motor branch, and superficial palmar arch; hypertrophied or thickened scar due to inappropriate incision; tendon adhesions because of wound hematoma; recurrence because of repair of the ligament; bowstringing of flexor tendons; malposition of the median nerve; inappropriate separation of the nerve fibers from surrounding scars; pillar pain; and reflex sympathetic dystrophy.

References

[1] de Krom MC, Knipschild PG, Kester AD, et al. Carpal tunnel syndrome, prevalence in the general population. J Clin Epidemiol 1992;45:373–6.
[2] Atroshi I, Gummesson C, Johnsson R, et al. Prevalence of carpal tunnel syndrome in a general population. JAMA 1999;282:153–8.
[3] Blumenthal S, Herskovitz S, Verghese J. Carpal tunnel syndrome in older adults. Muscle Nerve 2006;34:78–83.
[4] Chell J, Stevens A, Davis TR. Work practices and histopathological changes in the tenosynovium and flexor retinaculum in carpal tunnel syndrome in women. J Bone Joint Surg Am 1999;81:868–70.
[5] Martin S. Carpal tunnel syndrome: a job-related risk. Am Pharm 1991;31:21–4.
[6] Nathan PA, Meadows KD, Doyle LS. Occupation as a risk factor for impaired sensory conduction of the median nerve at the carpal tunnel. J Hand Surg [Br] 1988;13:167–70.
[7] Pelmear PL, Taylor W. Carpal tunnel syndrome and hand-arm vibration syndrome. A diagnostic enigma. Arch Neurol 1994;51:416–20.
[8] Ibrahim I, Khan WS, Goddard N, Smitham P. Carpal tunnel syndrome: a review of the recent literature. Open Orthop J 2012;6:69–76.
[9] Stevens JC, Smith BE, Weaver AL, et al. Symptoms of 100 patients with electromyographically verified carpal tunnel syndrome. Muscle Nerve 1999;22:1448–56.
[10] Pryse-Phillips WE. Validation of a diagnostic sign in carpal tunnel syndrome. J Neurol Neurosurg Psychiatry 1984;47:870–2.
[11] MacDermid JC, Wessel J. Clinical diagnosis of carpal tunnel syndrome: a systematic review. J Hand Ther 2004;17:309–19.
[12] Cartwright MS, Hobson-Webb LD, Boon AJ, et al. Evidence-based guideline: neuromuscular ultrasound for the diagnosis of carpal tunnel syndrome. Muscle Nerve 2012;46:287–93.
[13] Descatha A, Huard L, Aubert F, et al. Meta-analysis on the performance of sonography for the diagnosis of carpal tunnel syndrome. Semin Arthritis Rheum 2012;41:914–22.
[14] Phalen GS. The carpal tunnel syndrome—clinical evaluation of 598 hands. Clin Orthop 1972;83:29–40.
[15] Huisstede BM, Hoogvliet P, Randsdorp MS, et al. Carpal tunnel syndrome. Part I: effectiveness of nonsurgical treatments—a systemic review. Arch Phys Med Rehabil 2010;91:981–1004.
[16] Walker WC, Metzler M, Cifu DX, et al. Neutral wrist splinting in carpal tunnel syndrome: a comparison of night-only versus full-time wear instruction. Arch Phys Med Rehabil 2000;81:424–9.
[17] Keith MW, Masear V, Chung KC, et al American Academy of Orthopaedic Surgeons. American Academy of Orthopaedic Surgeons clinical practice guideline on the treatment of carpal tunnel syndrome. J Bone Joint Surg Am 2010;92:218–9.
[18] Herskovitz S, Berger AR. Low-dose, short-term oral prednisone in the treatment of carpal tunnel syndrome. Neurology 1995;45:1923–5.
[19] Wong SM, Hui AC, Tang A. Local vs systemic corticosteroids in the treatment of carpal tunnel syndrome. Neurology 2001;56:1565–7.
[20] Nathan PA, Keniston RC. Carpal tunnel syndrome and its relation to general physical condition. Hand Clin 1993;9:253–61.
[21] Hayes EP, Carney K, Wolf J, et al. Carpal tunnel syndrome. In: Hunter JM, Mackin EJ, Callahan AD, editors. Rehabilitation of the hand and upper extremity. 5th ed St. Louis: Mosby; 2002. p. 643.
[22] Acharya AD, Auchincloss JM. Return to functional hand use and work following open carpal tunnel surgery. J Hand Surg [Br] 2005;30:607–10.
[23] Frederick HA, Carter PR, Littler T. Injection injuries to the median and ulnar nerves at the wrist. J Hand Surg [Am] 1992;17:645–7.

[24] Kay NR, Marshall PD. A safe, reliable method of carpal tunnel injection. J Hand Surg [Am] 1992;17:1160–1.
[25] Racasan O, Dubert T. The safest location for steroid injection in the treatment of carpal tunnel syndrome. J Hand Surg [Br] 2005;30:412–4.
[26] Hui AC, Wong S, Leung CH, et al. A randomized controlled trial of surgery vs steroid injection for carpal tunnel syndrome. Neurology 2005;64:2074–8.
[27] Chavez-Chiang NR, Delea SL, Sibbitt Jr WL, et al. Outcomes and cost-effectiveness of carpal tunnel injections using sonographic needle guidance. Arthritis Rheum 2010;62:S677, 1626.
[28] Goldberg G, Wollstein R, Chimes GP. Carpal tunnel injection: with or without ultrasound guidance? PM R 2011;3:976–81.
[29] Shrivastava N, Szabo RM. Decision making in upper extremity entrapment neuropathies. J Musculoskelet Med 2008;25:278–89.
[30] Jarvik JG, Comstock BA, Kliot M, et al. Surgery versus non-surgical therapy for carpal tunnel syndrome: a randomised parallel-group trial. Lancet 2009;374:1074–81.
[31] Leinberry CF, Rivlin M, Maltenfort M, et al. Treatment of carpal tunnel syndrome by members of the American Society for Surgery of the Hand: a 25-year perspective. J Hand Surg [Am] 2012;37:1997–2003.
[32] Mintalucci DJ, Leinberry Jr. CF. Open versus endoscopic carpal tunnel release. Orthop Clin North Am 2012;43:431–7.
[33] Stancic MF, Micovic V, Potocnjak M. The anatomy of the Berrettini branch: implications for carpal tunnel release. J Neurosurg 1999;91:1027–30.

CHAPTER 37

Trigger Finger

Keith A. Bengtson, MD
Julie K. Silver, MD

Synonyms

Stenosing tenosynovitis
Digital flexor tenosynovitis
Locked finger

ICD-9 Code

727.03 Trigger finger

ICD-10 Code

M65.30 Trigger finger, unspecified finger

Definition

Trigger finger is the snapping, triggering, or locking of a finger as it is flexed and extended. This is due to hypertrophy and fibrocartilaginous metaplasia at the tendon-pulley interface that does not allow the tendon to glide normally back and forth under the pulley. Trigger finger is thought to arise from high pressures at the proximal edge of the A1 pulley when there is a discrepancy in the diameter of the flexor tendon and its sheath at the level of the metacarpal head [1] (Fig. 37.1). The thumb (33%) and the ring finger (27%) are most commonly affected in adults, but 90% of pediatric trigger fingers involve the thumbs, 25% of which are bilateral [1]. It is often encountered in patients with diabetes and rheumatoid arthritis [2,3]. The relationship of trigger finger to repetitive trauma has been cited frequently in the literature [3–5]; however, the exact mechanism of this correlation is still open to debate [6]. Rarely, it is due to acute trauma or space-occupying lesions [7–9].

Symptoms

Patients typically complain of pain in the proximal interphalangeal joint of the finger, rather than in the true anatomic location of the problem—at the metacarpophalangeal joint. Some individuals may report swelling or stiffness in the fingers, particularly in the morning. Patients may also have intermittent locking in flexion of the digit, which is overcome with forceful voluntary effort or passive assistance. Involvement of multiple fingers can be seen in patients with rheumatoid arthritis or diabetes [2,3]. In one study, the perioperative symptoms differed for trigger thumbs versus trigger fingers [10]. In this study, patients complained of pain with motion with trigger thumb; with trigger finger, they complained primarily of triggering and loss of range of motion.

Physical Examination

The essential element in the physical examination is the localization of the disorder at the level of the metacarpophalangeal joint. There is palpable tenderness and sometimes a tender nodule or crepitus over the volar aspect of the metacarpal head. Swelling of the finger may also be noted. Opening and closing of the hand actively produces a painful clicking as the inflamed tendon passes through a constricted sheath. With chronic triggering, the patient may have interphalangeal joint flexion contractures [11]. Therefore it is important to determine whether there is normal passive range of motion in the metacarpophalangeal and interphalangeal joints. Neurologic examination findings, including muscle strength, sensation, and reflexes, should be normal, with the exception of severe cases associated with disuse weakness or atrophy. Comorbidities can affect the neurologic examination findings as well (e.g., patients with diabetic neuropathy or carpal tunnel syndrome may have impaired sensation).

Functional Limitations

Functional limitations include difficulty with grasping and fine manipulation of objects due to pain, locking, or both. Fine motor problems may include difficulty with inserting a key into a lock, typing, or buttoning a shirt. Gross motor skills may include limitation in gripping a steering wheel or in grasping tools at home or at work.

Diagnostic Studies

This is a clinical diagnosis. Patients without a history of injury or inflammatory arthritis do not need routine radiographs [12]. Magnetic resonance imaging can confirm tenosynovitis of the flexor sheath, but this offers minimal advantage over clinical diagnosis [13]. Alternatively, a diagnostic ultrasound examination can show tendon nodules, tenosynovitis, and active triggering at the level of the A1 pulley.

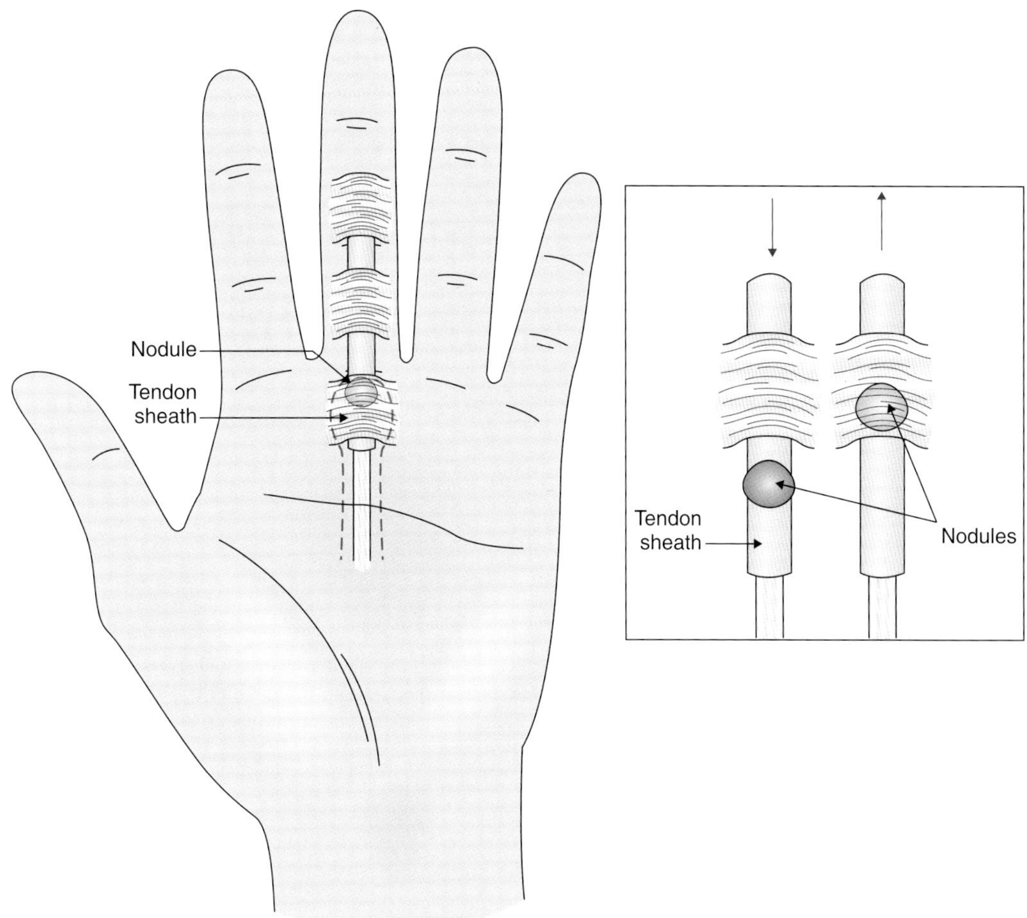

FIGURE 37.1 The flexor tendon nodule catches under the annular ligament and produces the snapping or triggering sensation.

Differential Diagnosis

Dupuytren disease
Ganglion of the tendon sheath (retinacular cyst)
Tumor of the tendon sheath (giant cell tumor or space-occupying lesion, such as an amyloidosis)
Rheumatoid arthritis

Treatment

Initial

The goal of treatment is to restore the normal gliding of the tendon through the pulley system. This can often be achieved with conservative treatment. Typically, the first line of treatment is a local steroid injection [14]. The determination of whether to inject first or to try noninvasive measures is often based on the severity of the patient's symptoms (more severe symptoms generally respond better to injections), the level of activity of the patient (e.g., someone who needs to return to work as quickly as possible), and the patient's and clinician's preferences.

Noninvasive measures generally involve splinting of the metacarpophalangeal joint at 10 to 15 degrees of flexion with the proximal interphalangeal and distal interphalangeal joints free, for up to 6 weeks continuously [15]. This has been reported to be effective, although less so in the thumbs [16,17]. Also, splinting provides a reliable and functional means of treating work-related trigger finger without loss of time from work [18]. Additional conservative treatment includes nonsteroidal anti-inflammatory drugs and avoidance of exacerbating activities, such as typing and repetitive gripping. Wearing padded gloves provides protection and may help decrease inflammation by avoiding direct trauma.

Rehabilitation

Rehabilitation may include treatment with an occupational or physical therapist experienced in the treatment of hand problems. Supervised therapy is generally not necessary but may be useful in the following scenarios: when a patient has lost significant strength, range of motion, or function from not using the hand or from prolonged splinting; when modalities such as ultrasound and iontophoresis are recommended to reduce inflammation; and when a customized splint is deemed to be necessary.

Therapy should focus on increasing function and decreasing inflammation and pain. This can be done by techniques such as ice massage, contrast baths, ultrasound, and iontophoresis with local steroid use. For someone with a very large or small hand or other anatomic variations (e.g., arthritic joints), a custom splint may fit better and allow him or her to function at work more easily than with a prefabricated splint. Range of motion and strength can be improved through supervised therapy either before surgery or postoperatively.

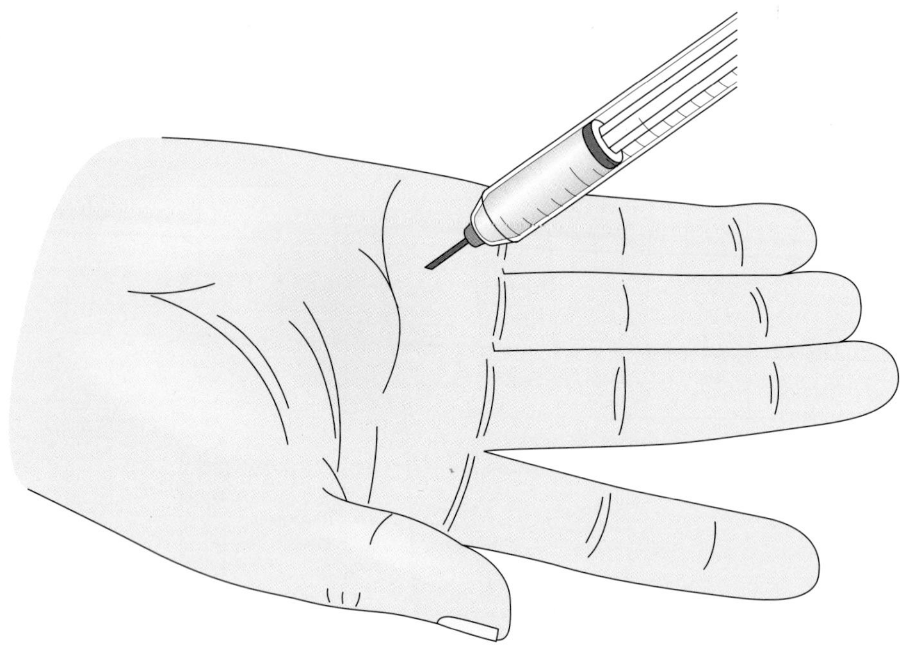

FIGURE 37.2 Under sterile conditions with use of a 27-gauge, ⅝-inch needle, a 2- to 3-mL aliquot of a local anesthetic and steroid mixture (e.g., 1 mL of 1% lidocaine mixed with 1 mL [40 mg] of methylprednisolone) is injected into the palm at the level of the distal palmar crease, which directly overlies the tendon. Before cleaning of the area to be injected, palpate for the nodule to localize exactly where the injection should be placed.

Procedures

A local corticosteroid injection combined with local anesthetic (Fig. 37.2) can be used as an alternative or in addition to other management [19,20]. A splint can be worn after the injection for a few days, purportedly to help protect the injected area. Because it may take 3 to 5 days for the medication to take effect, the patient should be advised to avoid activities with the affected hand as much as possible for 1 week after the injection.

The injections are usually beneficial and frequently curative [21,22]. Although the most recent Cochrane review found a clear benefit of corticosteroid injection over placebo [23], the reported success rates have varied widely. One study reported a treatment success of 54% and improvement rate of 88% at 1 year after a single injection [24]. This procedure is less effective with involvement of multiple digits (such as in patients with diabetes or rheumatoid arthritis) or when the condition has persisted longer than 4 months [22].

Surgery

In adults, steroid injections should be tried for most trigger finger cases before surgery is considered. However, surgical intervention is highly successful for conservative treatment failures and should be considered for patients desiring quick and definitive relief from this disability [25]. Individuals with diabetes, rheumatoid arthritis, multiple joint involvement, and younger age at onset are more likely to require surgery [2,26].

There are two general types of surgery for this condition: the standard open operative release of the A1 pulley and the percutaneous A1 pulley release procedure. In one study using a percutaneous trigger finger release technique, the success rate was 100% at 12 weeks of follow-up [27]. Both surgical procedures are generally effective and carry a relatively low risk of complications [25,28].

Potential Disease Complications

Disease-related complications are rare and could include permanent loss of range of motion from development of a contracture in the affected finger, most commonly at the proximal interphalangeal joint [11]. More rarely, chronic intractable pain may develop despite treatment.

Potential Treatment Complications

Treatment-related complications from nonsteroidal anti-inflammatory drugs are well known and include gastric, renal, and hepatic side effects. Complications from local corticosteroid injections include skin depigmentation, dermatitis, subcutaneous fat atrophy, tendon rupture, digital sensory nerve injury, and infection [29,30]. Individuals with rheumatoid arthritis are more likely to have a tendon rupture [31]; therefore repeated injections are not recommended in these cases. Possible surgical complications include infection, nerve injury, and flexor tendon bowstringing [32–34].

References

[1] Akhtar S, Bradley MJ, Quinton DN, Burke FD. Management and referral for trigger finger/thumb. BMJ 2005;331:30–3.

[2] Stahl S, Kanter Y, Karnielli E. Outcome of trigger finger treatment in diabetes. J Diabetes Complications 1997;11:287–90.

[3] Gray RG, Gottlieb NL. Hand flexor tenosynovitis in rheumatoid arthritis. Prevalence, distribution, and associated rheumatic features. Arthritis Rheum 1977;20:1003–8.

[4] Bonnici AV, Spencer JD. A survey of 'trigger finger' in adults. J Hand Surg [Br] 1988;13:202–3.
[5] Verdon ME. Overuse syndromes of the hand and wrist. Prim Care 1996;23:305–19.
[6] Trezies AJ, Lyons AR, Fielding K, Davis TR. Is occupation an etiological factor in the development of trigger finger? J Hand Surg [Br] 1998;23:539–40.
[7] Tohyama M, Tsujio T, Yanagida I. Trigger finger caused by an old partial flexor tendon laceration: a case report. Hand Surg 2005;10:105–8.
[8] Lee SJ, Pho RW. Report of an unusual case of trigger finger secondary to phalangeal exostosis. Hand 2005;10:135–8.
[9] Fujiwara M. A case of trigger finger following partial laceration of flexor digitorum superficialis and review of the literature. Arch Orthop Trauma Surg 2005;125:430–2.
[10] Moriya K, Uchiyama T, Kawaji Y. Comparison of the surgical outcomes for trigger finger and trigger thumb: preliminary results. Hand Surg 2005;10:83–6.
[11] Lapidus PW. Stenosing tenovaginitis. Surg Clin North Am 1953;1317–47.
[12] Katzman BM, Steinberg DR, Bozentka DJ, et al. Utility of obtaining radiographs in patients with trigger finger. Am J Orthop 1999;28:703–5.
[13] Gottlieb NL. Digital flexor tenosynovitis: diagnosis and clinical significance. J Rheumatol 1991;18:954–5.
[14] Nimigan AS, Ross DC, Gan BS. Steroid injections in the management of trigger fingers. Am J Phys Med Rehabil 2005;85:36–43.
[15] Ryzewicz M, Wolf JM. Trigger digits: principles, management, and complications. J Hand Surg [Am] 2006;31:135–46.
[16] Patel MR, Bassini L. Trigger fingers and thumb: when to splint, inject, or operate. J Hand Surg [Am] 1992;17:110–3.
[17] Valdes K. A retrospective review to determine the long-term efficacy of orthotic devices for trigger finger. J Hand Ther 2012;25:89–95, quiz 96.
[18] Rodgers JA, McCarthy JA, Tiedeman JJ. Functional distal interphalangeal joint splinting for trigger finger in laborers: a review and cadaver investigation. Orthopedics 1998;21:305–9, discussion 309–310.
[19] Lambert MA, Morton RJ, Sloan JP. Controlled study of the use of local steroid injection in the treatment of trigger finger and thumb. J Hand Surg [Br] 1992;17:69–70.
[20] Benson LS, Ptaszek AJ. Injection versus surgery in the treatment of trigger finger. J Hand Surg [Am] 1997;22:138–44.
[21] Anderson B, Kaye S. Treatment of flexor tenosynovitis of the hand ('trigger finger') with corticosteroids. A prospective study of the response to local injection. Arch Intern Med 1991;151:153–6.
[22] Newport ML, Lane LB, Stuchin SA. Treatment of trigger finger by steroid injection. J Hand Surg [Am] 1990;15:748–50.
[23] Peters-Veluthamaningal C, van der Windt DA, Winters JC, Meyboom-de Jong B. Corticosteroid injection for trigger finger in adults. Cochrane Database Syst Rev 2009;1, CD005617.
[24] Peters-Veluthamaningal C, Winters JC, Groenier KH, Jong BM. Corticosteroid injections effective for trigger finger in adults in general practice: a double-blinded randomised placebo controlled trial. Ann Rheum Dis 2008;67:1262–6.
[25] Turowski GA, Zdankiewicz PD, Thomson JG. The results of surgical treatment of trigger finger. J Hand Surg [Am] 1997;22:145–9.
[26] Rozental TD, Zurakowski D, Blazar PE. Trigger finger: prognostic indicators of recurrence following corticosteroid injection. J Bone Joint Surg Am 2008;90:1665–72.
[27] Dierks U, Hoffmann R, Meek MF. Open versus percutaneous release of the A1-pulley for stenosing tendovaginitis: a prospective randomized trial. Techn Hand Up Extrem Surg 2008;12:183–7.
[28] Luan TR, Chang MC, Lin CF, et al. Percutaneous A1 pulley release for trigger digits. Zhonghua Yi Xue Za Zhi (Taipei) 1999;62:33–9.
[29] Fitzgerald BT, Hofmeister EP, Fan RA, Thompson MA. Delayed flexor digitorum superficialis and profundus ruptures in a trigger finger after a steroid injection: a case report. J Hand Surg [Am] 2005;30:479–82.
[30] Sawaizumi T, Nanno M, Ito H. Intrasheath triamcinolone injection for the treatment of trigger digits in adult. Hand Surg 2005;10:37–42.
[31] Ertel AN. Flexor tendon ruptures in rheumatoid arthritis. Hand Clin 1989;5:177–90.
[32] Thorpe AP. Results of surgery for trigger finger. J Hand Surg [Br] 1988;13:199–201.
[33] Heithoff SJ, Millender LH, Helman J. Bowstringing as a complication of trigger finger release. J Hand Surg [Am] 1988;13:567–70.
[34] Carrozzella J, Stern PJ, Von Kuster LC. Transection of radial digital nerve of the thumb during trigger release. J Hand Surg [Am] 1989;14:198–200.

CHAPTER 38

Ulnar Collateral Ligament Sprain

Sheila Dugan, MD

Sol M. Abreu Sosa, MD, FAAPMR

Synonyms

Skier's thumb
Ulnar collateral ligament tear or rupture
Gamekeeper's thumb
Break-dancer's thumb
Stener lesion [1] (ruptured, displaced ulnar collateral ligament with interposed adductor aponeurosis)

ICD-9 Code

842.00 Sprains and strains of hand and wrist

ICD-10 Codes

S63.90 Sprain of unspecified part of unspecified wrist and hand
S63.91 Sprain of unspecified part of right wrist and hand
S63.92 Sprain of unspecified part of left wrist and hand

Definition

The ulnar collateral ligament (UCL) complex includes the ulnar proper collateral ligament and the ulnar accessory collateral ligament [1]. These ligaments are located deep to the adductor aponeurosis of the thumb and stabilize the first metacarpophalangeal (MCP) joint. Tears can occur if a valgus force is applied to an abducted first MCP joint [2]. A lesion of the UCL is commonly called skier's thumb.

Acute injuries can occur when the strap on a ski pole forcibly abducts the thumb. In the United States, estimates for skiing injuries are 3 or 4 per 1000 skier-hours; thumb injuries account for about 10% of skiing injuries [3]. A study of downhill skiing found that thumb injuries accounted for 17% of skiing injuries, second only to knee injuries [4]. Three fourths of the thumb injuries were UCL sprains. UCL injury in football players may be related to falls or blocking. Other sports involving ball handling or equipment with repetitive abduction forces to the thumb, like basketball or lacrosse, can cause injury to the UCL.

UCL injuries may be accompanied by avulsion fractures. Complete tears can fold back proximally when they are ruptured distally and become interposed between the adductor aponeurosis [1]. This injury is known as the Stener lesion and has been described as a complication of complete UCL tears, with a frequency ranging from 33% to 80% [5].

Chronic ligamentous laxity is more common in occupational conditions associated with repetitive stresses to the thumb. The term *gamekeeper's thumb* was coined in the mid-1950s to describe an occupational injury of Scottish gamekeepers [6]. The term is also used for acute injuries to the UCL.

Rupture of the thumb MCP joint UCL represents one of the most common ligamentous injuries of the hand. Failure to recognize these injuries or to treat them appropriately can lead to instability, pain, and weakness of the joint [7].

Symptoms

Patients report pain and instability of the thumb joint. In the acute injury setting, patients can often recall the instant of injury. If the UCL is ruptured, patients report swelling and hematoma formation; pain may be minimal with complete tears. When pain is present, it can cause thumb weakness and reduced function. Numbness and paresthesias are not typical findings.

Physical Examination

The physical examination begins with the uninvolved thumb, noting the individual's normal range of motion and stability. Palpate to determine the point of maximal tenderness, assessing for distal tenderness; if the ligament is torn, it tears distally off the proximal phalanx. Initially, the examiner may be able to detect a knot at the site of ligament disruption. Laxity of the UCL is the key finding on examination. Ligament injuries are graded as follows: grade I sprains, local injury without loss of integrity; grade II sprains, local injury with partial loss of integrity, but end-feel is present; and grade III sprains, complete tear with loss of integrity and end-feel (Fig. 38.1). Passive abduction can be painful, especially in acute grade I and grade II sprains.

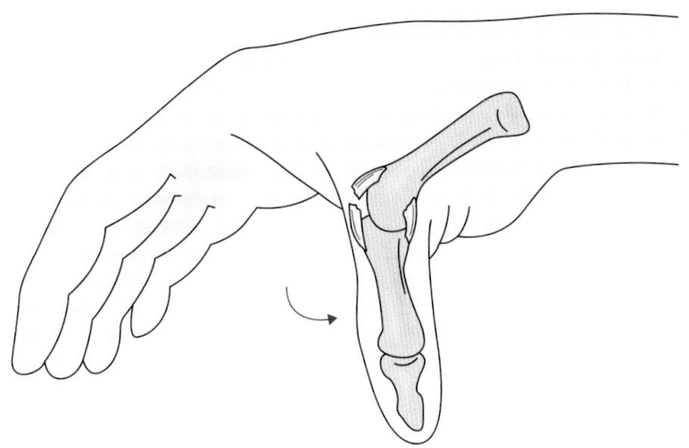

FIGURE 38.1 Skier's thumb. The ulnar collateral ligament to the metacarpophalangeal joint is disrupted by an abduction force. *(From Mellion MB. Office Sports Medicine, 2nd ed. Philadelphia, Hanley & Belfus, 1996.)*

The UCL should be tested with the first MCP joint in extension and flexion to evaluate all bands. The excursion is compared with the uninjured side. Testing for disruption of the ulnar proper collateral ligament is done with the thumb flexed to 90 degrees [1]. With the thumb in extension, a false-negative finding may result. The stability of the joint will not be impaired even if the ulnar proper collateral ligament is torn because of the taut ulnar accessory ligament in extension.

To avoid a false interpretation, the examiner must prevent MCP rotation by grasping the thumb proximal to the joint. If there is more than 30 degrees of laxity (or 15 degrees more laxity than on the noninjured side), rupture of the proper collateral ligament is likely. The thumb is then positioned in extension for repeated valgus stress testing. If valgus laxity is less than 30 degrees (or 15 degrees less than on the non-injured side), the accessory collateral ligament is intact. If valgus laxity is greater than 30 degrees (or 15 degrees more than on the noninjured side), the accessory collateral ligament is also ruptured [8].

A displaced fracture is a contraindication to stress testing. The fracture is manifested with swelling or discoloration on the ulnar side of the first MCP joint and tenderness along the base of the proximal phalanx. Some authors recommend that conventional radiographs be obtained before stressing of the UCL to determine whether a large undisplaced fracture is present because stress testing could cause displacement [9]. More than 3 mm of volar subluxation of the proximal phalanx indicates gross instability. The patient may be unable to pinch. Pain may limit the complete examination and lead to under-estimation of injury extent. Infiltration of local anesthetic around the injury site can reduce discomfort and improve the accuracy of the examination [10].

Avulsion fracture represents a special class of collateral ligament injury. It cannot be graded I to III because technically the ligament is not torn. However, it still deserves mention because fracture can compromise the bone-ligament-bone stabilization complex and lead to chronic symptoms [11].

Functional Limitations

Individuals describe difficulty with pinching activities (e.g., turning a key in a lock). Injuries affecting the dominant hand can have an impact on many fine motor manipulations, such as buttoning or retrieving objects from one's pocket. Injuries affecting the nondominant hand can impair bilateral hand activities requiring stabilization of small objects. Sports performance can be reduced with dominant hand injuries, and skiing, ball handling, or equipment use may be contraindicated in the acute stage of injury or on the basis of the extent of injury. In the setting of high-level or professional sports competition, the clinical decision to allow an athlete to compete with appropriate splinting or casting is based on severity of symptoms, with the caveat that the potential for worsening of the injury exists.

Diagnostic Studies

Whereas clinical examination is the mainstay of diagnosis, imaging studies are useful in the setting of uncertain diagnosis [12]. A plain radiograph is essential to rule out an avulsion fracture of the base of the ulnar side of the proximal phalanx. A stress film with the thumb in abduction is occasionally useful and should be compared with the uninjured side. UCL rupture presents with an angle greater than 35 degrees. Magnetic resonance imaging has greater than 90% sensitivity and specificity for UCL tears but is expensive and not always required [13].

Ultrasonography has been used as a less expensive means for diagnosis of UCL tears, but controversy exists as to whether it is useful or fraught with pitfalls [12,14–16]. However, a retrospective review of ultrasound studies from 17 surgically proven displaced full-thickness UCL tears identified the following ultrasound criteria for 100% accuracy in the diagnosis of a displaced full-thickness UCL tear: lack of UCL fibers and presence of a heterogeneous mass-like abnormality proximal to the MCP joint of the thumb. Such displaced UCL tears were most often located proximal to the leading edge of the adductor aponeurosis rather than superficially. Standardized ultrasound technique, which includes dynamic imaging, should be a consideration when the ultrasound examination is performed for this diagnosis [17].

Differential Diagnosis

Radial collateral ligament sprain or rupture
First MCP joint dislocation with or without volar plate injury
Thumb fracture-dislocation (Bennett fracture)

Treatment

Initial

Pain and edema are managed with ice, nonsteroidal anti-inflammatory drugs, and rest. Initial treatment of a first-degree (grade I) UCL sprain is taping for activity. Initial treatment of an incomplete (grade II) UCL sprain involves immobilization in a thumb spica cast for 3 to 6 weeks with the thumb slightly abducted. Injuries involving nondisplaced or small avulsion fractures associated with an incomplete UCL tear can also be managed nonsurgically and may require a longer course of immobilization. The cast may be extended to include the wrist for greater stability [18]. An alpine splint allows interphalangeal flexion while prohibiting abduction and extension of the first MCP joint [19]. A study of 63 cases of nonoperative and postsurgical patients compared short arm plaster cast immobilization with functional splinting that prevented ulnar and radial deviation of the thumb; there was no difference between the two groups in regard to stability, thumb range of motion or strength, and length of sick leave after an average follow-up of 15 months [20]. Even slightly displaced avulsion fractures without complete UCL rupture tended to do well with immobilization in a study of 30 patients; those with larger bone fragments and larger initial rotation of the fragment were more likely to have residual symptoms [21].

Grade III injuries require surgical repair unless surgery is contraindicated for other reasons. Prompt referral for surgical consultation is recommended to maximize ligament positioning for reattachment. Failure to refer promptly or misdiagnosis of a complete tear can result in a less favorable outcome, including a Stener lesion [5].

Rehabilitation

Physical or occupational therapy is important in the rehabilitation management of UCL sprains. Therapists who have completed special training and are certified hand therapists (often called CHTs) can be great resources. Range of motion of the unaffected joints of the arm, especially the interphalangeal joint of the thumb, must be maintained. In the setting of a grade I sprain, after a short course of relative rest and taping, therapy may be required to restore strength to the preinjury level. In grade II sprains, a volar splint replaces the cast after 3 to 6 weeks. Splints may be custom molded by the therapist. They can be removed for daily active range of motion exercises. Passive range of motion and isometric strength training are initiated once pain at rest has resolved, and the patient is progressed to concentric exercise after about 8 weeks for nonsurgical lesions and 10 to 12 weeks for postsurgical lesions. Prophylactic taping is appropriate for transitioning back to sports-specific activity (Fig. 38.2). Postsurgical rehabilitation is less aggressive, with avoidance of strengthening, especially a power pinch, for 8 weeks postoperatively [22]. Protected early postoperative range of motion is indicated [23]. Full activity after grade II tears with or without nondisplaced avulsion fractures begins at 10 to 12 weeks compared with 12 to 16 weeks for surgically repaired injuries [24].

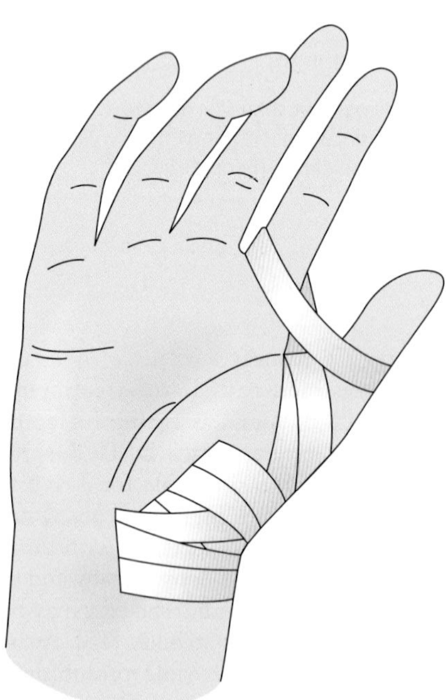

FIGURE 38.2 Taping technique to protect the ulnar collateral ligament.

Procedures

There are no specific nonsurgical procedures performed for this injury.

Surgery

Early direct repair is required in the setting of a ruptured UCL (grade III) injury. Grade II and grade III injuries resulting in severe instability, displaced fractures, or intra-articular fragments are also surgical candidates. Surgery is indicated in the setting of gross instability [25]. Surgery is also indicated if the thumb is unstable in extension (more than 30 degrees of laxity or 15 degrees more laxity than on the noninjured side), which indicates a complete rupture, and ligament displacement is likely [8]. Tension wiring is used to fixate avulsions; open reduction may be required for large displaced avulsion defects. Surgical approaches that improve stability are the focus of new techniques [26,27]. However, postoperative immobilization is being reconsidered. A cadaver study concluded that a controlled active motion therapy protocol after suture anchor repair of a ruptured UCL is safe from a biomechanical point of view [28]. Reconstruction may be necessary for a chronic tear, including bone-retinaculum-bone reconstruction [29].

The techniques for reconstruction of chronic UCL injuries or gamekeeper's thumb involve either dynamic or static procedures. Dynamic procedures use musculotendinous units to stabilize the MCP joint by pulling the proximal phalanx ulnarward. Static procedures use free tendon grafts through bone tunnels or pull-out sutures to reconstruct the proper and accessory collateral ligaments. Static procedures have gained in popularity as they allow ligament reconstruction and preservation of existing thumb function, whereas dynamic procedures require the removal of existing muscle units and do not restore the anatomy of the ulnar collateral ligament [30].

Potential Disease Complications

Disease complications include chronic laxity with associated functional limitations, pain, and inability to pinch [31]; premature arthritis and persistent pain in the first MCP joint; and decreased range of motion of the thumb.

Potential Treatment Complications

Analgesics and nonsteroidal anti-inflammatory drugs have well-known side effects that most commonly affect the gastric, renal, and hepatic systems. Prolonged splinting can lead to loss of range of motion of the joint and weakness and atrophy of the surrounding joints, depending on the extent of the injury and the length of time spent in a splint. Surgical risks include nonunion of avulsed fragments and the typical infrequent surgical complications, such as infection and bleeding. Surgery can result in persistent numbness on the ulnar aspect of the thumb. A neurapraxia secondary to injury of the radial sensory nerve from either swelling or intraoperative traction is the most common nerve injury and usually resolves spontaneously [8,32].

References

[1] Stener B. Displacement of the ruptured ulnar collateral ligament of the metacarpophalangeal joint of the thumb. A clinical and anatomical study. J Bone Joint Surg Br 1962;44:869–79.
[2] McCue FC, Hussamy OD, Gieck JH. Hand and wrist injuries. In: Zachazewski JE, Magee DJ, Quillen WS, editors. Athletic injuries and rehabilitation. Philadelphia: WB Saunders; 1996. p. 589–99.
[3] Schneider T. Snow skiing injuries. Aust Fam Physician 2003;32:499–502.
[4] Enqkvist O, Balkfors B, Lindsjo U. Thumb injuries in downhill skiing. Int J Sports Med 1982;3:50–5.
[5] Louis DS, Huebner JJ, Hankin FM. Rupture and displacement of the ulnar collateral ligament of the metacarpophalangeal joint of the thumb. Preoperative diagnosis. J Bone Joint Surg Am 1986;68:1320–6.
[6] Campbell CS. Gamekeeper's thumb. J Bone Joint Surg Br 1955;37:148–9.
[7] Rhee PC, Jones DB, Kakar S. Management of thumb metacarpophalangeal ulnar collateral ligament injuries. J Bone Joint Surg Am 2012;94:2005–12.
[8] Heyman P. Injuries to the ulnar collateral ligament of the thumb metacarpophalangeal joint. J Am Acad Orthop Surg 1997;5:224–9.
[9] Kibler WB, Press JM. Rehabilitation of the wrist and hand. In: Kibler WB, Herring SA, Press JM, editors. Functional rehabilitation of sports and musculoskeletal injuries. Gaithersburg, Md: Aspen; 1998. p. 186–7.
[10] Cooper JG, Johnstone AJ, Hider P, Ardagh MW. Local anaesthetic infiltration increases the accuracy of assessment of ulnar collateral ligament injuries. Emerg Med Australas 2005;17:132–6.
[11] Patel S, Potty A, Taylor EJ, et al. Collateral ligament injuries of the metacarpophalangeal joint of the thumb: a treatment algorithm. Strategies Trauma Limb Reconstr 2010;5:1–10.
[12] Koslowsky TC, Mader K, Gausepohl T, et al. Ultrasonographic stress test of the metacarpophalangeal joint of the thumb. Clin Orthop Relat Res 2004;427:115–9.
[13] Plancher KD, Ho CP, Cofield SS, et al. Role of MR imaging in the management of "skier's thumb" injuries. Magn Reson Imaging Clin N Am 1999;7:73–84.
[14] Hergan K, Mittler C, Oser W. Pitfalls in sonography of the gamekeeper's thumb. Eur Radiol 1997;7:65–9.
[15] Susic D, Hansen BR, Hansen TB. Ultrasonography may be misleading in the diagnosis of ruptured and dislocated ulnar collateral ligaments of the thumb. Scand J Plast Reconstr Surg Hand Surg 1999;33:319–20.
[16] Schnur DP, DeLone FX, McClellan RM, et al. Ultrasound: a powerful tool in the diagnosis of ulnar collateral ligament injuries of the thumb. Ann Plast Surg 2002;49:19–22.
[17] Melville D, Jacobson JA, Haase S, et al. Ultrasound of displaced ulnar collateral ligament tears of the thumb: the Stener lesion revisited. Skeletal Radiol 2013;42:667–73.
[18] Reid DC, editor. Sports injury assessment and rehabilitation. New York: Churchill Livingstone; 1992. p. 1089–92.
[19] Moutet F, Guinard D, Corcella D. Ligament injuries of the first metacarpophalangeal joint. In: Bruser P, Gilbert A, editors. Finger bone and joint injuries. London: Martin Dunitz; 1999. p. 207–11.
[20] Kuz JE, Husband JB, Tokar N, McPherson SA. Outcome of avulsion fractures of the ulnar base of the proximal phalanx of the thumb treated nonsurgically. J Hand Surg [Am] 1999;24:275–82.
[21] Sollerman C, Abrahamsson SO, Lundborg G, Adalbert K. Functional splinting versus plaster cast for ruptures of the ulnar collateral ligament of the thumb. A prospective randomized study of 63 cases. Acta Orthop Scand 1991;62:524–6.
[22] Neviaser RJ. Collateral ligament injuries of the thumb metacarpophalangeal joint. In: Strickland JW, Rettig AC, editors. Hand injuries in athletes. Philadelphia: WB Saunders; 1992. p. 95–105.
[23] Firoozbakhsh K, Yi IS, Moneim MS, et al. A study of ulnar collateral ligament of the thumb metacarpophalangeal joint. Clin Orthop Relat Res 2002;403:240–7.
[24] Brown AP. Ulnar collateral ligament injury of the thumb. In: Clark GL, Wilgis EF, Aiello B, et al., editors. Hand rehabilitation: a practical guide. 2nd ed New York: Churchill Livingstone; 1997. p. 369–75.
[25] Jackson M, McQueen MM. Gamekeeper's thumb: a quantitative evaluation of acute surgical repair. Injury 1994;25:21–3.
[26] Lee SK, Kubiak EN, Liporace FA, et al. Fixation of tendon grafts for collateral ligament reconstructions: a cadaveric biomechanical study. J Hand Surg [Am] 2005;30:1051–5.
[27] Lee SK, Kubiak EN, Lawler E, et al. Thumb metacarpophalangeal ulnar collateral ligament injuries: a biomechanical simulation study of four static reconstructions. J Hand Surg [Am] 2005;30:1056–60.
[28] Harley BJ, Werner FW, Green JK. A biomechanical modeling of injury, repair, and rehabilitation of ulnar collateral ligament injuries of the thumb. J Hand Surg [Am] 2004;29:915–20.
[29] Guelmi K, Thebaud A, Werther JR, et al. Bone-retinaculum-bone reconstruction for chronic posttraumatic instability of the metacarpophalangeal joint of the thumb. J Hand Surg [Am] 2003;28:685–95.
[30] Carlsen BT, Moran SL. Thumb trauma: Bennett fractures, Rolando fractures, and ulnar collateral ligament injuries. J Hand Surg [Am] 2009;34:945–52.
[31] Smith RJ. Post-traumatic instability of the metacarpophalangeal joint of the thumb. J Bone Joint Surg Am 1977;59:14–21.
[32] Ritting AW, Baldwin PC, Rodner CM. Ulnar collateral ligament injury of the thumb metacarpophalangeal joint. Clin J Sport Med 2010;20:106–12.

CHAPTER 39

Ulnar Neuropathy (Wrist)

Ramon Vallarino, Jr., MD
Francisco H. Santiago, MD

Synonym

Guyon canal entrapment

ICD-9 Code

354.2 Lesion of ulnar nerve

ICD-10 Codes

G56.20 Lesion of ulnar nerve, unspecified upper limb
G56.21 Lesion of ulnar nerve, right upper limb
G56.22 Lesion of ulnar nerve, left upper limb

Definition

Entrapment neuropathy of the ulnar nerve can be encountered at the wrist in a canal formed by the pisiform and the hamate and its hook (the pisohamate hiatus). These are connected by an aponeurosis that forms the ceiling of Guyon canal (Fig. 39.1). This canal generally contains the ulnar nerve and the ulnar artery and vein. The following three types of lesions can be encountered [1].

Type I affects the trunk of the ulnar nerve proximally in Guyon canal and involves both the motor and sensory fibers. This is the most commonly seen lesion.

Type II affects only the deep (motor) branch distally in Guyon canal and may spare the abductor digiti quinti, depending on the location of its branching. A further classification is type IIa (still pure motor), in which all the hypothenar muscles are spared because of a lesion distal to their neurologic branching.

Type III affects only the superficial branch of the ulnar nerve, which provides sensation to the volar aspect of the fourth and fifth fingers and the hypothenar eminence. There is sparing of all motor function, although the palmaris brevis is affected in some cases. This is the least common lesion encountered.

This injury is commonly seen in bicycle riders and people who use a cane improperly because they place excessive weight on the proximal hypothenar area at the canal of Guyon and therefore are predisposed to distal ulnar nerve traumatic injury, especially affecting the deep ulnar motor branch (type II) [2,3]. Entrapment at Guyon canal has also been associated with prolonged, repetitive occupational use of tools, such as pliers and screwdrivers [2]. With the advancement of endoscopic carpal tunnel release during the past few years, there have been reports of both adverse and favorable consequences to the ulnar nerve at Guyon canal, which is very close anatomically. There have been inadvertent injuries to the ulnar nerve as well as documented decompression and improvement of nerve conduction [4,5].

Other rare causes have been reported in the literature. These include fracture of the hook of the hamate, ganglion cyst formation, tortuous or thrombosed ulnar artery aneurysm (hypothenar hammer syndrome), osteoarthritis or osteochondromatosis of the pisotriquetral joint, anomalous variation of abductor digiti minimi, schwannomas, aberrant fibrous band, and idiopathic [6–9].

Of 250 wrists studied by 3T magnetic resonance imaging assessment, it was noted that anatomy of the Guyon canal was normal in 168 (67.2%) wrists; 73 (29.2%) wrists presented with anatomic variations, and 9 (3.6%) wrists had derangements with clinical and radiologic features attributed to Guyon canal syndrome [10].

Symptoms

Signs and symptoms can vary greatly and depend on which part of the ulnar nerve and its terminal branches are affected and where along Guyon canal itself (Table 39.1). It is of great importance to be able to differentiate entrapment of the ulnar nerve at the wrist from entrapment at the elbow, which occurs far more commonly. The two clinical findings that confirm the diagnosis of Guyon canal entrapment instead of ulnar entrapment at the elbow are (1) sparing of the dorsal ulnar cutaneous sensory distribution in the hand and (2) sparing of function of the flexor carpi ulnaris and the two medial heads of the flexor digitorum profundus (Figs. 39.2 and 39.3). Otherwise, the symptoms in both conditions are generally similar and may include hand intrinsic muscle weakness and atrophy, numbness in the fourth and fifth fingers, hand pain, and sometimes severely decreased function.

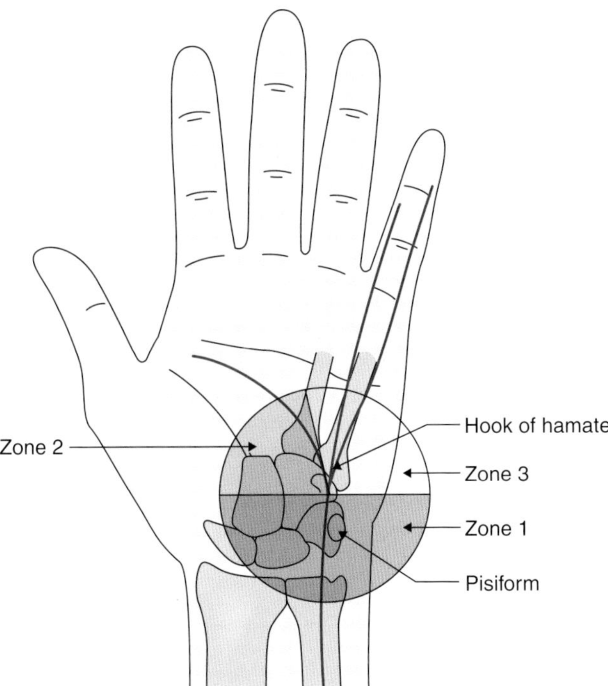

FIGURE 39.1 Distal ulnar tunnel (Guyon canal) showing the three zones of entrapment. Lesions in zone 1 give motor and sensory symptoms, lesions in zone 2 cause motor deficits, and lesions in zone 3 create sensory deficits.

Table 39.1 Volar Forearm and Hand: Ulnar Nerve

Muscle	Action
Flexor carpi ulnaris	Flexes wrist, ulnarly deviates
Flexor digitorum profundus	Flexes distal interphalangeal joint (fourth and fifth)
Abductor digiti quinti*	Analogous to dorsal interosseous
Flexor digiti quinti*†	Analogous to dorsal interosseous
Opponens digiti quinti*†	Flexes and supinates fifth metacarpal
Volar interossei*	Adduct fingers, weak flexion metacarpophalangeal
Dorsal interossei*†	Abduct fingers, weak flexion metacarpophalangeal
Lumbricals (ring and fifth)*†	Coordinate movement of fingers; extend interphalangeal joints; flex metacarpophalangeal joints
Adductor pollicis*	Adducts thumb toward index finger
Lumbricals (ring, small)*	Coordinate movement of fingers; extend interphalangeal joints; flex metacarpophalangeal joints

*Hand intrinsic muscles.
†Hypothenar mass.

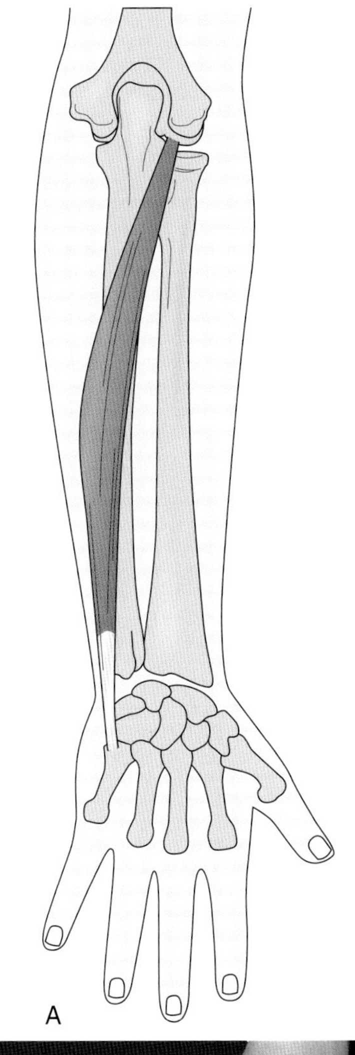

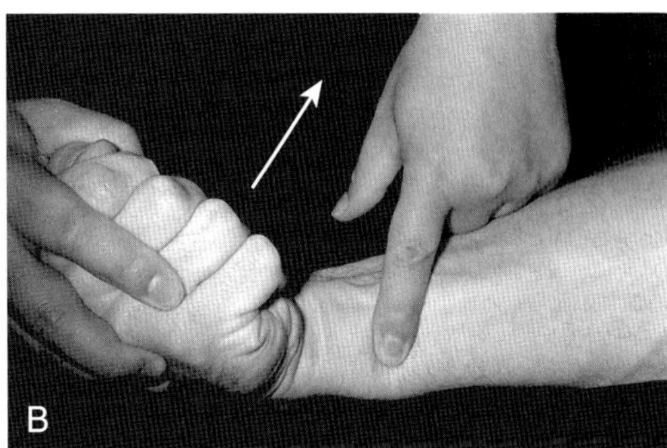

FIGURE 39.2 **A,** The flexor carpi ulnaris functions as a wrist flexor and an ulnar deviator. **B,** It can be tested by the patient's forcefully flexing *(arrow)* and ulnarly deviating the wrist. The clinician palpates the tendon while the patient performs this maneuver. *(From Concannon MD: Common Hand Problems in Primary Care. Philadelphia, Hanley & Belfus, 1999.)*

Physical Examination

Careful examination of the hand and a thorough knowledge of the anatomy of motor and sensory distribution of ulnar nerve branches are required to determine the location of the lesion. Except for the five muscles innervated by the median nerve (abductor pollicis brevis, opponens pollicis, flexor pollicis brevis superficial head, and first two lumbricals), the ulnar nerve supplies every other intrinsic muscle in the hand. Classically, there is notable atrophy of the first web space due to denervation of the first dorsal interosseous muscle (Fig. 39.4). In lesions involving the motor branches where the compression is in the proximal aspect of Guyon canal, there will be weakness and eventually atrophy of the interossei, the adductor pollicis, the fourth and fifth lumbricals, and the deep head of the flexor

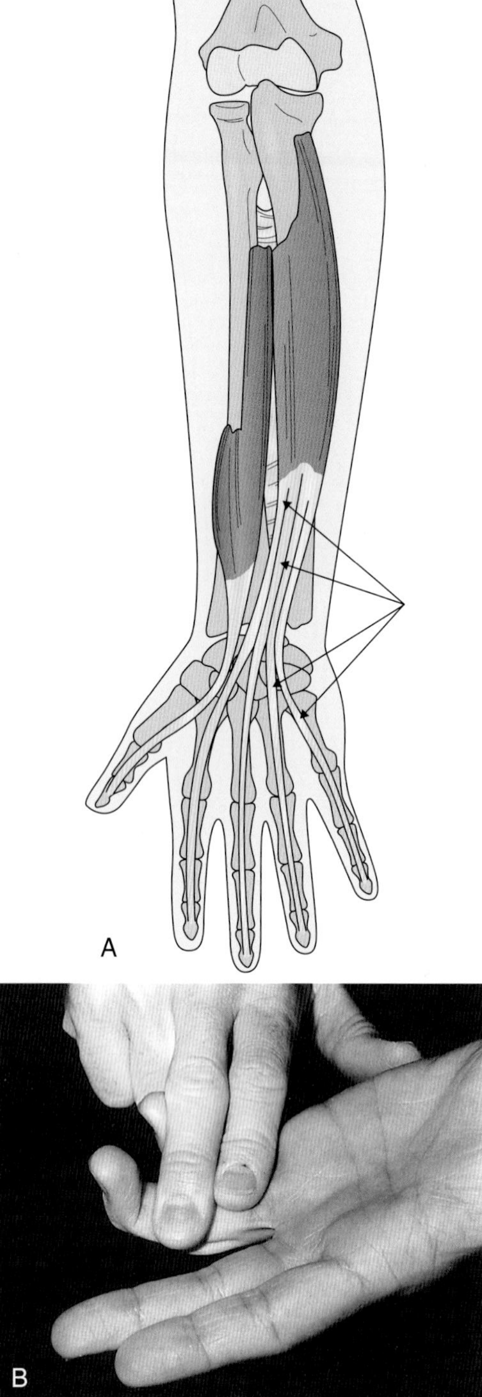

FIGURE 39.3 **A,** Flexor digitorum profundi *(arrows)*. **B,** These tendons can be tested by the patient's flexing the distal phalanx while the clinician blocks the middle phalanx from flexing. *(From Concannon MD: Common Hand Problems in Primary Care. Philadelphia, Hanley & Belfus, 1999.)*

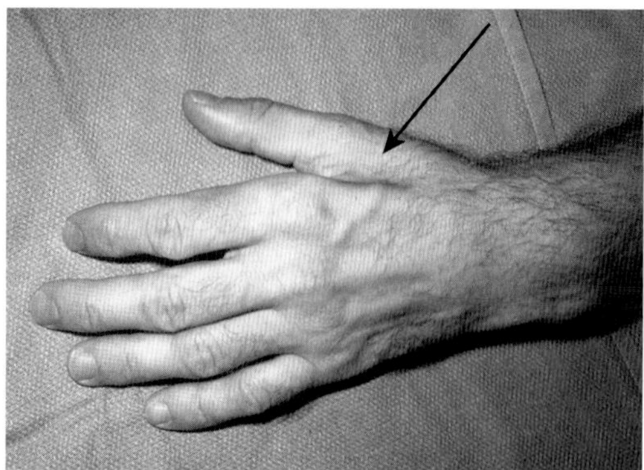

FIGURE 39.4 It is not unusual for patients with ulnar neuropathy to present with signs of muscle atrophy. It is most noticeable at the first web space, where atrophy of the first dorsal interosseous muscle leaves a hollow between the thumb and the index rays *(arrow)*. *(From Concannon MD. Common Hand Problems in Primary Care. Philadelphia, Hanley & Belfus, 1999.)*

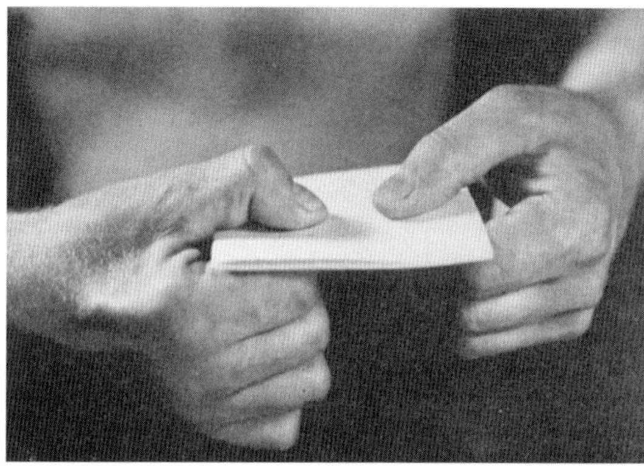

FIGURE 39.5 Ulnar nerve lesion. A patient with an ulnar nerve lesion is asked to pull a piece of paper apart with both hands. Note that the affected side (right hand) uses the flexor pollicis longus muscle to prevent the paper from slipping out of the hand, thus substituting for the adductor pollicis muscle and generating the Froment sign. *(From Haymaker W, Woodhall B. Peripheral Nerve Injuries. Philadelphia, WB Saunders, 1953.)*

pollicis brevis. The palmaris brevis, abductor digiti quinti, opponens digiti quinti, and flexor digiti quinti may be involved or spared, depending on the level of the lesion.

Sensory examination in all but type II, in which the compression of the ulnar nerve is at the level of the lower wrist, reveals decreased sensation of the volar aspect of the hypothenar eminence and the fourth and fifth fingers (with splitting of the fourth in most patients). There is always sparing of the sensation of the dorsum of the hand medially because it is innervated by the dorsal ulnar cutaneous branch of the ulnar nerve, which branches off the forearm proximal to Guyon canal [1]. The ulnar claw (hyperextension of the fourth and fifth metacarpophalangeal joints with flexion of the interphalangeal joints) seen in more proximal lesions may be more pronounced because of preserved function of the two medial heads of the flexor digitorum profundus. This creates flexion that is unopposed by the weakened interossei and lumbricals [1,11]. The flexor carpi ulnaris has normal strength. All the signs of intrinsic hand muscle weakness that are seen in more proximal ulnar nerve lesions, such as the Froment paper sign, are also found in Guyon canal entrapment affecting the motor nerve fibers (Fig. 39.5) [12]. Grip strength is invariably reduced in these patients when the motor branches of the ulnar nerve are affected [13].

Type III is the least common and involves pure sensory loss from the compression of the superficial branch at the distal aspect of Guyon canal.

Functional Limitations

Functional loss can vary from isolated decreased sensation in the affected region to severe weakness and pain with impaired hand movement and dexterity. As can be anticipated, lesions affecting motor nerve fibers are functionally more severe than those affecting only sensory nerve fibers. The patient may have trouble holding objects and performing many activities of daily living, such as occupation, daily household chores, grooming, and dressing. Vocationally, individuals may not be able to perform the basic requirements of their jobs (e.g., operating a computer or cash register, carpentry work). This can be functionally devastating.

Diagnostic Studies

The cause of the clinical lesion suspected after careful history and physical examination can be investigated with the use of imaging techniques. Plain radiographs could reveal a fracture of the hamate or other carpal bones as well as of the metacarpals and the distal radius, especially if there has been a traumatic injury. Magnetic resonance imaging [10] and computed tomography (multislice spiral computed tomographic angiography, multidetector computed tomography) can be helpful if a fracture, angioleiomyoma, tortuous ulnar artery, pseudoaneurysm of the ulnar artery, lipoma, or ganglion cyst is suspected [14–17]. As technology and accuracy of ultrasound equipment have advanced, there are now reports of the use of conventional and color duplex sonography to diagnose conditions such as thrombosed aneurysm of the ulnar artery [18,19].

Nerve conduction study and electromyography are helpful in confirming the diagnosis and the classification as well as in determining the severity of the lesion and the prognosis for functional recovery. Ulnar nerve entrapment in Guyon canal may be due to recurrent carpal tunnel syndrome [4]. As a rule, the dorsal ulnar cutaneous sensory nerve action potential is normal compared with the unaffected side [4]. Abnormalities in both sensory and motor conduction studies are seen in type I. The ulnar sensory nerve action potential recorded from the fifth finger is normal in type II, and an isolated abnormality is encountered in type III. The compound muscle action potential of the abductor digiti quinti is normal in types IIa and III. For this reason, it is important to perform motor studies recording from more distal muscles, such as the first dorsal interosseous [20]. Motor conduction studies should include stimulation across the elbow to rule out a lesion there, as it is far more common. Furthermore, ulnar nerve stimulation at the palm, after the traditional stimulation at the wrist and across the elbow, can be useful in sorting out the location of the compression and which fascicles are affected [21]. Care must be taken not to overstimulate because median nerve–innervated muscles are very close (i.e., lumbricals 1 and 2), and their volume-conducted compound muscle action potentials could confuse the diagnosis. A "neurographic" palmaris brevis sign has been described in type II ulnar neuropathy at the wrist [22]. This consists of a positive wave preceding the delayed abductor digiti minimi motor response, presumably caused by volume-conducted depolarization of a spared palmaris brevis muscle. Needle electromyography helps in documenting axonal loss, determining severity of the lesion to allow prognosis for recovery, and more precisely localizing a lesion for an accurate classification. The flexor carpi ulnaris and the ulnar heads of the flexor digitorum profundus should be completely spared in a lesion at Guyon canal [23].

Differential Diagnosis [24]

Ulnar neuropathy at the elbow (or elsewhere)
Thoracic outlet syndrome (typically lower trunk or medial cord)
Cervical radiculopathy at C8-T1
Motor neuron disease
Superior sulcus tumor (affecting the medial cord of the plexus)
Camptodactyly (an unusual developmental condition with a claw deformity)

Treatment

Initial

Initial treatment involves rest and avoidance of trauma (especially if occupational or repetitive causes are suspected). Ergonomic and postural adjustments can be effective in these cases. The use of nonsteroidal anti-inflammatory drugs in cases in which an inflammatory component is suspected can also be beneficial. Analgesics may help control pain. Low-dose tricyclic antidepressants may be used both for pain and to help with sleep. More recently, the use of antiepileptic medications for neuropathic pain syndromes has been increasing because of good efficacy. Prefabricated wrist splints may be beneficial and are often prescribed for night use. For individuals who continue their sport or work activities, padded, shock-absorbent gloves may be useful (e.g., for cyclists, jackhammer users).

Rehabilitation

A program of physical or occupational therapy performed by a skilled hand therapist can help obtain functional range of motion and strength of the interossei and lumbrical muscles. Instruction of the patient in a daily routine of home exercises should be done early in the diagnosis. Static splinting (often done as a custom orthosis) with an ulnar gutter will ensure rest of the affected area. In more severe cases, the use of static or dynamic orthotic devices may be considered to improve the patient's functional level. Weakness in the ulnar claw deformity can be corrected to improve grasp with the use of a dorsal metacarpophalangeal block (lumbrical bar) to the fourth and fifth fingers with a soft strap over the palmar aspect [25].

A work site evaluation may be beneficial as well. Ergonomic adaptations can prove helpful to individuals with ulnar nerve entrapment at the wrist (e.g., switching to a foot computer mouse or voice-activated computer software).

Procedures

Injections into Guyon canal may be tried if a compressive entrapment neuropathy is suspected and generally provide symptomatic relief (Fig. 39.6) [2].

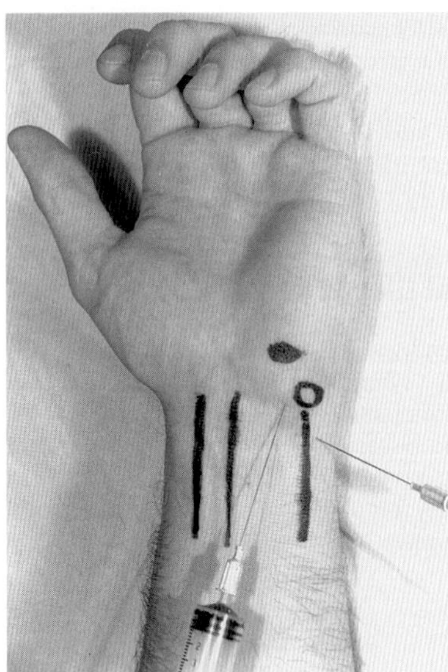

FIGURE 39.6 Approaches for two ulnar nerve blocks. The needle with syringe attached demonstrates the puncture for block at Guyon canal. The circle is over the pisiform bone, and the solid mark is over the hook of the hamate. The second needle demonstrates the puncture site for an ulnar nerve block at the wrist, ulnar approach. *(From Lennard TA. Pain Procedures in Clinical Practice, 2nd ed. Philadelphia, Hanley & Belfus, 2000.)*

Under sterile conditions, with use of a 25-gauge, 1½-inch disposable needle, a mixture of corticosteroid and 1% or 2% lidocaine totaling no more than 1 mL is injected into the distal wrist crease to the radial side of the pisiform bone; the needle is angled sharply distally so that its tip lies just ulnar to the palpable hook of the hamate [2,26]. Postinjection care includes ensuring hemostasis immediately after the procedure, local icing for 5 to 10 minutes, and instructions to the patient to rest the affected limb during the next 48 hours.

Surgery

Surgery is recommended when there is a fracture of the hook of the hamate or of the pisiform or a tortuous ulnar artery that causes neurologic compromise. Ganglion cyst and pisohamate arthritis are also indications for surgical treatment. Surgery in general involves exploration, excision of the hook of hamate or pisiform (if fractured), repair of the ulnar artery as necessary, decompression, and neurolysis of the ulnar nerve [2,6]. Experience and a sound knowledge of the possible anatomic variations (i.e., muscles, fibrous bands) and the arborization patterns of the ulnar artery in Guyon canal are of great importance in promoting a positive outcome when surgery is medically necessary [8,27].

Preoperatively, the patient is educated about the expected clinical course after nerve release. The patient is warned about incisional tenderness for 8 to 12 weeks postoperatively. Nighttime numbness, weakness, or clumsiness will resolve gradually, and recovery may be incomplete.

For days 0 to 5, the patient is instructed in isolated tendon glide exercises for all digits. No heavy resistance activities are permitted for 6 weeks after surgery. From 1 to 6 weeks, active range of motion of the wrist, edema control, scar massage, and desensitization are initiated when the incision is made accessible. From 6 to 12 weeks, progressive strengthening exercises are initiated [28].

Potential Disease Complications

The severity and type of lesion of the ulnar nerve at the wrist will ultimately determine the complications. Severe motor axon loss will cause profound weakness and atrophy of ulnar-innervated muscles in the hand and render the patient unable to perform even simple tasks because of lack of vital grip strength. Some patients also have chronic pain in the affected hand, which can be severely debilitating, perhaps inciting a complex regional pain syndrome, and it can predispose them to further problems, such as depression and drug dependency.

Potential Treatment Complications

The use of nonsteroidal anti-inflammatory drugs should be carefully monitored because there are potential side effects, including gastrointestinal distress and cardiac, renal, and hepatic disease. Low-dose tricyclic antidepressants are generally well tolerated but may cause fatigue, so they are usually prescribed for use in the evening. Injection complications include injury to a blood vessel or nerve, infection, and allergic reaction to the medication used. Complications after surgery include infection, wound dehiscence, recurrence, and, rarely, complex regional pain syndrome.

References

[1] Dumitru D. Electrodiagnostic medicine. Philadelphia: Hanley & Belfus; 1995, p. 887–891.

[2] Dawson D, Hallet M, Millender L. Entrapment neuropathies. 2nd ed. Boston: Little, Brown; 1990, p. 193–195.

[3] Akuthota V, Plastaras C, Lindberg K, et al. The effect of long-distance bicycling on ulnar and median nerves: an electrodiagnostic evaluation of cyclist palsy. Am J Sports Med 2005;33:1224–30.

[4] Ozdemir O, Calisaneller T, Gulsen S, Caner H. Ulnar nerve entrapment in Guyon's canal due to recurrent carpal tunnel syndrome: case report. Turk Neurosurg 2011;21:435–7.

[5] Mondelli M, Ginanneschi F, Rossi A. Evidence of improvement in distal conduction of ulnar nerve sensory fibers after carpal tunnel release. Neurosurgery 2009;65:696–700.

[6] Murata K, Shih JT, Tsai TM. Causes of ulnar tunnel syndrome: a retrospective study of 31 subjects. J Hand Surg [Am] 2003;28:647–51.

[7] Harvie P, Patel N, Ostlere SJ. Prevalence of epidemiological variation of anomalous muscles at Guyon's canal. J Hand Surg [Br] 2004;29:26–9.

[8] Bozkurt MC, Tajil SM, Ozcakal L, et al. Anatomical variations as potential risk factors for ulnar tunnel syndrome: a cadaveric study. Clin Anat 2005;18:274–80.

[9] Jose RM, Bragg T, Srivata S. Ulnar nerve compression in Guyon's canal in the presence of a tortuous ulnar artery. J Hand Surg [Br] 2006;31:200–2.

[10] Pierre-Jerome C, Moncayo V, Terk MR. The Guyon's canal in perspective: 3-T MRI assessment of the normal anatomy, the anatomical variations and Guyon's canal syndrome. Surg Radiol Anat 2011;33:897–903.

[11] Liveson JA, Spielholz NI. Peripheral neurology: case Studies in electrodiagnosis. Philadelphia: FA Davis; 1991, p. 162–165.

[12] Haymaker W, Woodhall B. Peripheral nerve injuries. Philadelphia: WB Saunders; 1953.

[13] Snider RK. Essentials of musculoskeletal care. Rosemont, Ill: American Academy of Orthopaedic Surgeons; 1997, p. 260–262.

[14] Jeong C, Kim HN, Park IJ. Compression of the ulnar nerve in Guyon's canal by an angioleiomyoma. J Hand Surg Eur Vol 2010;35:594–5.

[15] Stocker RL, Kosak D. Compression of the ulnar nerve at Guyon's canal by a pseudoaneurysm of the ulnar artery. Handchir Mikrochir Plast Chir 2012;44:51–4.

[16] Ozdemir O, Calisaneller T, Genimez A, et al. Ulnar nerve entrapment in Guyon's canal due to lipoma. J Neurosurg Sci 2010;54:125–7.

[17] Blum AG, Zabel JP, Kohlman R, et al. Pathologic conditions of the hypothenar eminence: evaluation with multidetector CT and MR imaging. Radiographics 2006;26:1021–44.
[18] Coulier B, Goffin D, Malbecq S, Mairy Y. Colour duplex sonographic and multislice spiral CT angiographic diagnosis of ulnar artery aneurysm in hypothenar hammer syndrome. JBR-BTR 2003;86:211–4.
[19] Peeters EY, Nieboer KH, Osteaux MM. Sonography of the normal ulnar nerve at Guyon's canal and of the common peroneal nerve dorsal to the fibular head. J Clin Ultrasound 2004;32:375–80.
[20] Witmer B, DiBenedetto M, Kang CG. An improved approach to the evaluation of the deep branch of the ulnar nerve. Electromyogr Clin Neurophysiol 2002;42:485–93.
[21] Wee AS. Ulnar nerve stimulation at the palm in diagnosing ulnar nerve entrapment. Electromyogr Clin Neurophysiol 2005;45:47–51.
[22] Morini A, Della Sala WS, Bianchini G, et al. 'Neurographic' palmaris brevis sign in type II degrees ulnar neuropathy at the wrist. Clin Neurophysiol 2005;116:43–8.
[23] Kim DJ, Kalantri A, Guha S, Wainapel SF. Dorsal cutaneous nerve conduction: diagnostic aid in ulnar neuropathy. Arch Neurol 1981;38:321–2.
[24] Patil JJP. Entrapment neuropathy. In: O'Young BJ, Young MA, Stiens SA, editors. Physical medicine and rehabilitation secrets. 2nd ed. Philadelphia: Hanley & Belfus; 2002. p. 144–50.
[25] Irani KD. Upper limb orthoses. In: Braddom RL, editor. Physical medicine and rehabilitation. Philadelphia: WB Saunders; 1996. p. 328–30.
[26] Mauldin CC, Brooks DW. Arm, forearm, and hand blocks. In: Lennard TA, editor. Physiatric procedures. Philadelphia: Hanley & Belfus; 1995. p. 145–6.
[27] Murata K, Tamaj M, Gupta A. Anatomic study of arborization patterns of the ulnar artery in Guyon's canal. J Hand Surg [Am] 2006;31:258–63.
[28] Ulnar nerve Guyon's canal therapy. E-hand.com The electronic textbook of hand therapy. American Society for Surgery of the Hand.

CHAPTER 40

Wrist Osteoarthritis

Anna Babushkina, MD

Chaitanya S. Mudgal, MD, MS (Orth), MCh (Orth)

Synonyms

Degenerative arthritis of the wrist
Osteoarthritis of the wrist
Post-traumatic arthritis of the wrist
SLAC wrist
SNAC wrist

ICD-9 Codes

715.1 **Osteoarthrosis, localized, primary, wrist**
715.2 **Osteoarthrosis, localized, secondary, wrist**
716.1 **Traumatic arthropathy, wrist**
718.83 **Other joint derangement, not elsewhere classified, wrist**
719.03 **Joint effusion, wrist**
719.13 **Pain in joint, wrist**
842.01 **Wrist sprain**

ICD-10 Codes

M19.031 **Primary osteoarthrosis, right wrist**
M19.032 **Primary osteoarthrosis, left wrist**
M19.039 **Primary osteoarthrosis, unspecified wrist**
M19.231 **Secondary osteoarthrosis, right wrist**
M19.232 **Secondary osteoarthrosis, left wrist**
M19.239 **Secondary osteoarthrosis, unspecified wrist**
M12.531 **Traumatic arthropathy, right wrist**
M12.532 **Traumatic arthropathy, left wrist**
M12.539 **Traumatic arthropathy, unspecified wrist**
M24.831 **Other specific joint derangement of right wrist, not elsewhere classified**
M24.832 **Other specific joint derangement of left wrist, not elsewhere classified**
M24.839 **Other specific joint derangement, unspecified wrist, not elsewhere classified**
M25.431 **Effusion, right wrist**
M25.432 **Effusion, left wrist**
M25.439 **Effusion, unspecified wrist**
M25.531 **Pain in right wrist**
M25.532 **Pain in left wrist**
M25.539 **Pain in unspecified wrist**
S63.501 **Unspecified sprain of right wrist**
S63.502 **Unspecified sprain of left wrist**
S63.509 **Unspecified sprain of unspecified wrist**
Add the appropriate seventh character to category 63 for the episode of care

Definition

Osteoarthritis of the wrist refers to the painful degeneration of the articular surfaces that make up the wrist due to noninflammatory arthritides. It commonly affects the joints between the distal radius and the proximal row of carpal bones. Symptoms include pain, swelling, stiffness, and crepitation. Radiographs will reveal different degrees of joint space narrowing, cyst formation, subchondral sclerosis, and osteophyte formation.

Secondary osteoarthritis resulting from post-traumatic conditions, as can be seen after distal radius fractures, carpal fractures, and carpal instability, is the most common form [1]. Primary osteoarthritis in the wrist is rare. The Framingham study showed a 9-year incidence of only 1% of radiographically significant wrist osteoarthritis in women and 1.7% in men. These rates are significantly lower than the rates of thumb basal joint osteoarthritis (30%), distal interphalangeal joint arthritis (28%-35% in patients older than 40 years), and radiographic hand osteoarthritis in patients 80 years and older (90%-100%) [2]. Rare conditions that may cause wrist osteoarthritis include idiopathic osteonecrosis of the lunate (Kienböck disease) and the scaphoid (Preiser disease). Distal radius fractures that have healed inappropriately (malunited) can also be the cause (Fig. 40.1). In considering malunited fractures of the distal radius, abnormal parameters that have been shown to

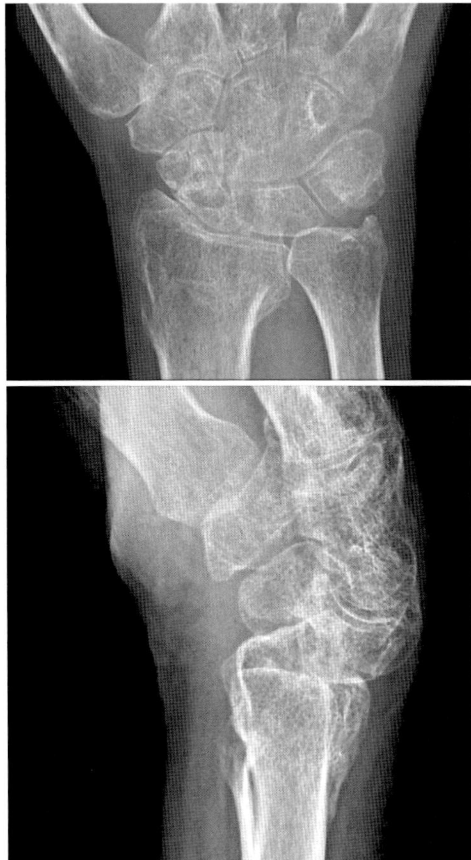

FIGURE 40.1 Wrist osteoarthritis secondary to a malunited wrist fracture. Note the dorsal angulation of the distal articular surface and the reduced joint space. This patient also had significant osteopenia secondary to pain-induced lack of use.

be associated with wrist arthritis include the following: on an anteroposterior radiograph, an intra-articular step-off of more than 2 mm and radial shortening of more than 5 mm; and on the lateral radiograph, a dorsal angulation of more than 10 degrees [3–5].

Carpal fractures that fail to heal, particularly of the scaphoid, can also be the cause of arthritis [6]. This bone is predisposed to nonunions biologically because of its fragile vascular supply and biomechanically on account of the shear forces it encounters [7,8]. Other factors associated with nonunions include fracture displacement, fracture location, and delay in initiation of treatment [9,10]. Features of a scaphoid nonunion that appear to be associated with arthritis are the displacement of the cartilaginous surfaces and the loss of carpal stability [11,12]. Both of these lead to abnormal loading of the cartilage and consequently to ensuing arthritis. This pattern of arthritis is known as scaphoid nonunion advanced collapse (SNAC) (Fig. 40.2).

Carpal instability can also result in uneven loading of the articular surfaces and subsequent arthritis [13] (Figs. 40.3 and 40.4). The most common form of carpal instability is scapholunate dissociation [14]. It consists of a disruption of the interosseous ligament between the scaphoid and lunate. The resultant abnormal biomechanics lead to abnormal loading and subsequent arthritis, a pattern known as scapholunate advanced collapse [1] (SLAC).

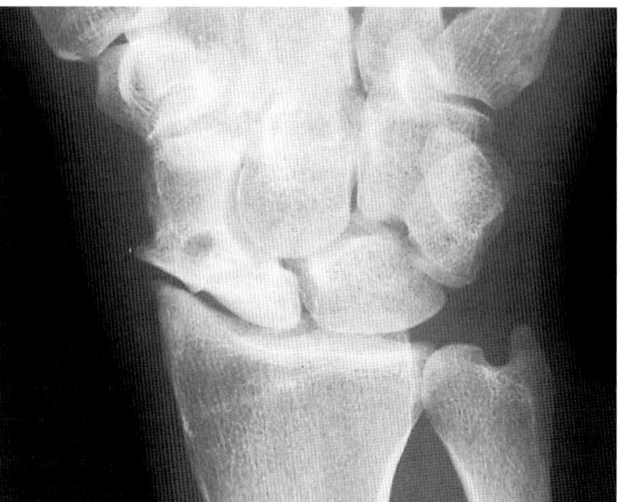

FIGURE 40.2 Osteoarthritic change of a wrist with a scaphoid nonunion (SNAC), stage 2. Notable features include the "beaked" appearance of the radial styloid, cystic change along with a nonunion in the scaphoid, and "kissing" osteophytes on adjoining surfaces of the radius and scaphoid.

Symptoms

Wrist pain is the presenting symptom in the overwhelming majority of patients. For the most part, this pain is of insidious onset, although many patients will recall a particular event that brought it to their attention. It is diffusely located across the dorsum of the wrist. It may be activity related and may bear little correlation to radiographic findings. Patients may also report inability to do their daily activities because of weakness, but on further questioning, this weakness is often secondary to pain.

Another presenting symptom is stiffness, particularly in flexion and extension of the wrist. Pronation and supination are usually not affected, unless the arthritic process is extensive and also involves the distal radioulnar joint. Motion may also be associated with a clicking sensation or with audible crepitation.

Complaints about cosmetic deformity are also common, particularly after distal radius fractures that have healed with an inappropriate alignment. Swelling is also commonly noted by the patients. This swelling is essentially a representation of the malunited fracture, but in patients with advanced arthritis irrespective of the etiology, it may represent synovial hypertrophy or osteophyte formation. In this situation, the swelling tends to be located in the dorsoradial region of the wrist (Fig. 40.5).

Physical Examination

Examination of the wrist includes a thorough examination of the entire upper limb. Comparison with the opposite side is useful to determine the degree of motion loss, if any. In wrist osteoarthritis, the most obvious finding may be loss of motion. Normal range of motion includes approximately 80 degrees of flexion, 60 degrees of extension, 20 degrees of radial deviation, and 40 degrees of ulnar deviation [15]. Comparison with the opposite side, if it is not involved, is useful to determine the degree of motion loss.

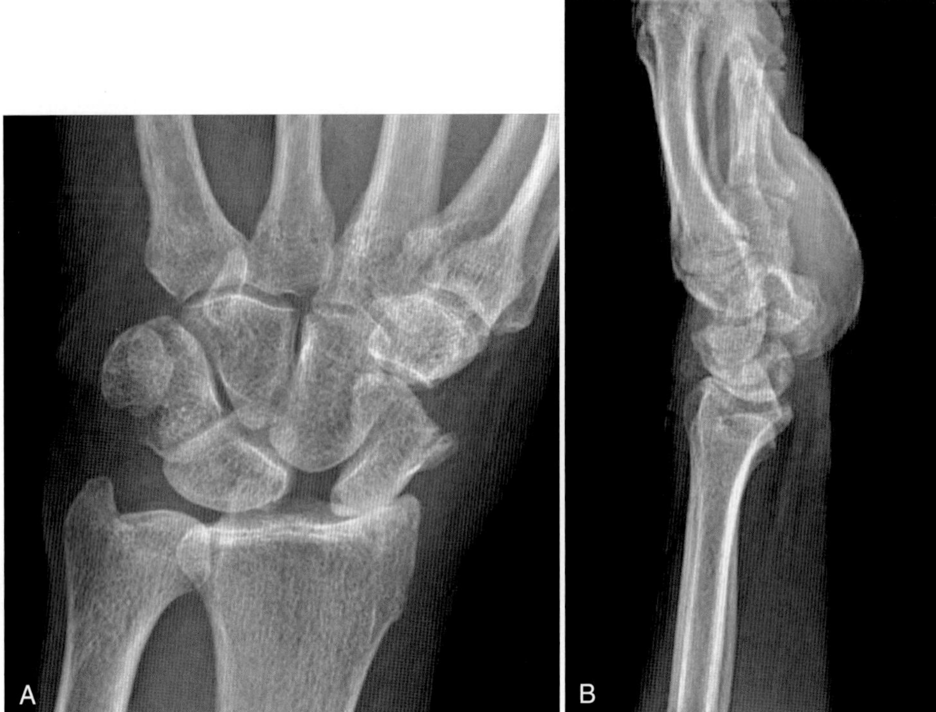

FIGURE 40.3 **A** and **B,** Wrist osteoarthritis secondary to scapholunate advanced collapse (SLAC), stage 2. Note the increased scapholunate space and the sclerosis of the radioscaphoid joint. Early osteophytes are clearly seen on the radial border of the scaphoid. The lateral view shows dorsal osteophytes as well as the dorsally angled lunate.

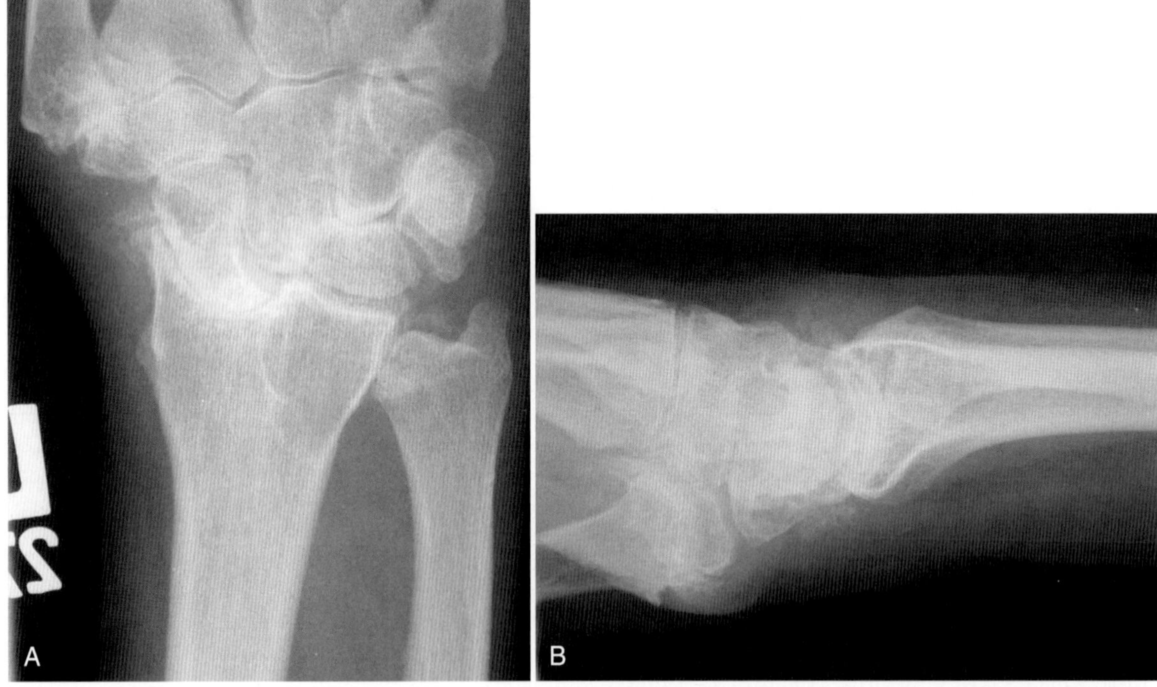

FIGURE 40.4 **A** and **B,** Advanced wrist osteoarthritis secondary to SLAC (stage 3). Note the increased scapholunate space, the sclerosis in the radioscaphoid and lunocapitate joints, and the proximal migration of the capitate. Most notable in both views is the complete loss of normal wrist alignment.

The wrist is palpated for evidence of cysts or tenderness. Tenderness just distal to Lister tubercle may be a sign of pathologic change at the scapholunate joint, including scapholunate dissociation, Kienböck disease, or synovitis of the radiocarpal joint. Tenderness at the anatomic snuffbox may indicate a scaphoid fracture or nonunion and, in early SNAC wrists, may be the site of radioscaphoid degeneration. In the presence of pancarpal arthritis, the tenderness is usually diffuse.

Provocative maneuvers should also be performed to check for signs of carpal instability. The scaphoid shift test

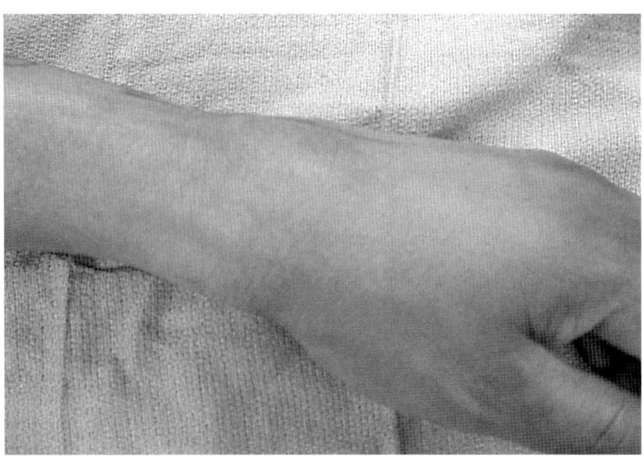

FIGURE 40.5 Clinical appearance of an osteoarthritic wrist that in this particular instance was secondary to a scaphoid nonunion. The diffuse radiodorsal swelling indicates some degree of synovitis.

of Watson evaluates for scapholunate instability [16]. In this test, the examiner places a thumb volarly on the patient's scaphoid tubercle, and the rest of the fingers wrap around the wrist to lie dorsally over the proximal pole of the scaphoid. As the wrist is taken from ulnar deviation to radial deviation, the thumb will apply pressure on the scaphoid tubercle and force the scaphoid to sublux out of its fossa dorsally in ligamentously lax patients as well as in those with frank scapholunate instability. Once pressure from the thumb is released, the scaphoid will then shift back into its fossa. This finding is best demonstrated in those who have ligamentous laxity or those with recent injuries. Patients who have chronic injuries often develop sufficient fibrosis to prevent subluxation of the scaphoid out of its fossa. However, they often still have pain that is reproduced with this maneuver. Comparison with the unaffected side is essential, especially if the patient has evidence of generalized ligamentous laxity.

The strength of the abductor pollicis brevis is tested by asking the patient to palmar abduct the thumb against resistance, and it should be compared with the opposite side. Similarly, the strength of the first dorsal interosseus should be checked by asking the patient to radially deviate the index finger against resistance. These tests evaluate for motor deficits of the median nerve and ulnar nerve, respectively. Sensation should also be compared with the opposite side. Whereas static two-point discrimination is an excellent way to test sensation in the office, a more precise evaluation of early sensory deficits can be performed by graduated Semmes-Weinstein monofilaments. Frequently, this test requires a referral to occupational therapists who perform it.

Functional Limitations

The majority of the limitations in wrist arthritis arise from a lack of motion. A range of motion from 10 degrees of flexion to 15 degrees of extension is required for activities involving personal care [17]. The loss of motion mainly affects activities of daily living such as washing one's back, fastening a brassiere, and writing. Eating, drinking, and using a telephone require 35 degrees of extension. However, learned compensatory maneuvers can allow most activities of daily living to be accomplished with as little as 5 degrees of flexion and 6 degrees of extension [18].

Diagnostic Studies

The initial evaluation of the arthritic wrist includes standard posteroanterior, lateral, and pronated oblique radiographs. In the posteroanterior view, any evidence of arthritis between the radius and proximal row of carpal bones or between the proximal and distal rows should be noted. Radiographic features that indicate an arthritic process include reduction or loss of joint space, osteophyte formation, cyst formation in periarticular regions, and loss of normal bone alignment (see Figs. 40.2 to 40.4).

Injury to the scapholunate ligament is evidenced by a space between the scaphoid and the lunate greater than 2 mm and a cortical ring sign of the scaphoid [14]. Sclerosis or collapse of the lunate is consistent with Kienböck disease [19]. The lateral view can reveal signs of carpal instability, such as a dorsally or palmarly oriented lunate. An angle between the scaphoid and the lunate in excess of 60 degrees is also consistent with scapholunate dissociation. The oblique view will often demonstrate the site of a scaphoid nonunion. Although it may be possible to make a diagnosis of scapholunate dissociation on plain radiographs, some patients can often have bilateral scapholunate distances and angles in excess of normal limits. It is therefore critical to obtain contralateral radiographs before a diagnosis of scapholunate injury is made.

Patterns of arthritic progression in SLAC and SNAC wrists have been classified into three stages. In a SLAC wrist, stage 1 involves arthritis between the radial styloid and the distal pole of the scaphoid; stage 2 results in reduction or loss of joint space between the radius and the proximal pole of the scaphoid (see Fig. 40.3), and stage 3 indicates capitolunate degeneration with proximal migration of the capitate between the scaphoid and lunate (see Fig. 40.4). In a SNAC wrist, stage 1 and stage 3 are similar to those in a SLAC wrist. However, in stage 2, there is degenerative change between the distal pole of the scaphoid and capitate (see Fig. 40.2).

Other imaging modalities are not necessary for the diagnosis of osteoarthritis. Computed tomography is sometimes used to evaluate the alignment of the scaphoid fragments in cases of nonunion and the amount of collapse of the lunate in Kienböck disease. Magnetic resonance imaging is occasionally used to evaluate the vascularity of the scaphoid proximal pole and lunate in scaphoid nonunions and Kienböck disease, respectively [19,20]. Wrist arthroscopy offers the optimal ability to assess the condition of the articular cartilage; however, this assessment can be made from plain radiographs or at the time of surgical reconstruction of the wrist.

Differential Diagnosis

Acute fracture
Septic arthritis
Crystalline arthritis
Carpal tunnel syndrome
Rheumatoid arthritis
de Quervain tenosynovitis

Treatment

Initial

Osteoarthritis of the wrist is a condition that has usually been present for a significant amount of time. However, it is not uncommon for symptoms to be of a short duration, and they can often be manifested after seemingly trivial trauma. It is important for the physician to establish good rapport with the patient during several visits so that the pathophysiologic changes of the process can be emphasized to the patient. This becomes even more important in situations involving workers' compensation or litigation or both. It is also important for the patient to understand that the condition cannot be reversed and that the symptoms are likely to be cyclic. Patients must understand that over time, the condition may worsen radiographically; however, it is impossible to predict the rate of progression or severity of symptoms that might ensue.

Many patients present with symptoms of wrist osteoarthritis that are not severe enough to be limiting but enough to be noticed. These patients are often looking for reassurance about their condition. If they are able to do all the activities that they want to do, intervention is not needed. They should not refrain from doing their activities in fear that they may accelerate the condition; there is no scientific evidence to substantiate this concern. This approach offers the least amount of risk to the patient.

Other patients may prefer to have some symptom reduction, particularly during episodes of acute worsening, despite some inconvenience or small risks. An over-the-counter wrist splint with a volar metal stabilizing bar (cock-up splint) can be a small inconvenience; however, by virtue of immobilizing the wrist, it can provide great symptom relief during daily activities. This metal bar can be contoured to place the wrist in the neutral position rather than in extension, as most splints of this nature tend to do. The neutral position appears to be better tolerated by patients and affords better compliance with splint wear. Both over-the-counter and custom leather splints have been shown to relieve pain and to improve function and grip strength. Custom splints, however, provided more of these improvements and were better liked by patients in one study [21]. Nonsteroidal anti-inflammatory drugs can also provide significant pain relief, particularly during periods of acute exacerbation of symptoms. A long-term use of nonsteroidal anti-inflammatory drugs is not indicated. Periodic application of ice, especially during periods of acute symptom exacerbation, can be of help. On occasion, in patients with radioscaphoid arthritis (SNAC), inclusion of the thumb in a custom-made orthoplast splint may provide better pain relief. Use of magnetic and copper bracelets has not been shown to be effective in clinical trials [22].

Rehabilitation

Once the acute inflammation phase has passed, most patients are able to resume most activities. Some may complain of persistent lack of motion or strength. These patients may benefit from a home exercise program for range of motion and strengthening directed by an occupational therapist. Modalities such as fluidized therapy may help with range of motion. Static progressive splinting is usually not recommended to improve range of motion because there is often a bone block to motion. It is always important to understand that therapy itself may worsen symptoms, especially passive stretching exercises. Active range of motion and active-assisted range of motion exercises are better tolerated by patients, and some patients may be better off without any formal rehabilitation.

Procedures

Nonsurgical procedures, including corticosteroid injections, may be indicated for wrist osteoarthritis, although they appear to have a greater use in crystalline and inflammatory arthritides. Hyaluronan injections for osteoarthritis have been studied in other joints, including the thumb carpometacarpal joint, with beneficial results; however, their use in the wrist is still considered experimental [23]. Typically, all injections around the wrist should be done by aseptic technique with a 25-gauge, 1½-inch needle and a mixture of a nonprecipitating, water-soluble steroid preparation that is injected along with 2 mL of 1% lidocaine.

The radiocarpal joint can be injected from the dorsal aspect approximately 1 cm distal to Lister tubercle, with the needle angled proximally about 10 degrees to account for the slight volar tilt of the distal radius articular surface. This is done with the wrist in the neutral position. Gentle longitudinal traction by an assistant can help widen the joint space, which may be reduced on account of the disease. An alternative radiocarpal injection site is the ulnar wrist, just palmar to the extensor carpi ulnaris tendon at the level of the ulnar styloid process. With strict aseptic technique, a 25-gauge, 1½-inch needle is inserted into the ulnocarpal space, just distal to the ulnar styloid, just dorsal or volar to the easily palpable tendon of the extensor carpi ulnaris. The needle must be angled proximally by 20 to 30 degrees to enter the space between the ulnar carpus and the head of the ulna. It is important to ascertain that the injectate flows freely. Any resistance indicates a need to reposition the needle appropriately. Alternatively, the injection may be performed by fluoroscopic guidance with the help of a mini image intensifier, if one is available in the office.

If a midcarpal injection is required, this is done through the dorsal aspect, under fluoroscopic guidance, with injection into the space at the center of the lunate-triquetrum-hamate-capitate region.

Surgery

The goal of surgery in an osteoarthritic wrist is pain relief. Surgical procedures for osteoarthritis can be divided into motion-sparing procedures and fusions (arthrodesis). However, even motion-sparing procedures often result in significant loss of motion. This is very important in patients who have almost no motion preoperatively. These patients will not benefit from motion-sparing procedures and are better served with total wrist fusions. The decision to proceed with surgery should not be made until nonsurgical means have been tried for an adequate time, which usually amounts to a period of 3 to 6 months. In some patients who are going to have a total wrist fusion, before a decision is made about surgery, it is useful to apply a well-molded fiberglass short arm cast for 2 weeks to accustom the patient to the lack of wrist motion.

Motion-sparing procedures include proximal row carpectomy, total wrist arthroplasty, and limited intercarpal fusions with scaphoid excision. The excision of the scaphoid is essential because 95% of wrist arthritis involves the scaphoid [1]. Proximal row carpectomy involves removal of the scaphoid, lunate, and triquetrum. The capitate then articulates with the radius through the lunate fossa (Fig. 40.6). Wrist stability is maintained by preserving the volar wrist ligaments. As a prerequisite for this procedure, the lunate fossa of the radius and the articular surface over the head of the capitate must be healthy and free of degenerative change (Fig. 40.7). The main advantage of this procedure is that it does not involve any fusions. After a short period of postoperative casting, patients are allowed to start moving the wrist as early as 3 weeks after surgery. Most people are able to attain a flexion-extension arc of 60 to 80 degrees and 60% to 80% of the grip strength of the uninvolved side [24,25] (Fig. 40.8). This procedure is appropriate for the early stages of SLAC and SNAC arthritis. Some surgeons have attempted to

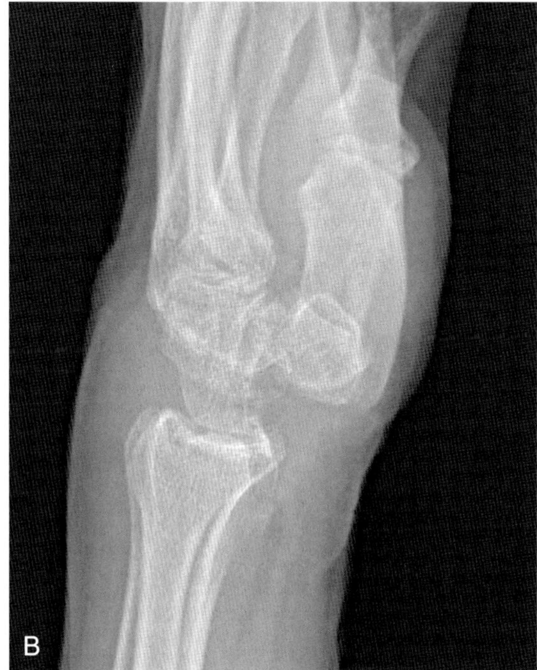

FIGURE 40.6 **A** and **B**, Plain radiographs of the patient seen in Figure 40.3 after she underwent a proximal row carpectomy. A terminal radial styloidectomy has also been performed to reduce impingement of the trapezium on the tip of the radius. Note how well the capitate articulates with the lunate fossa of the distal radius.

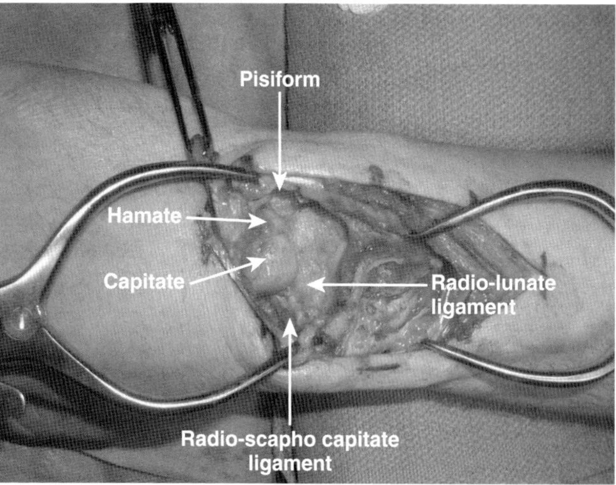

FIGURE 40.7 An intraoperative photograph of the patient seen in Figures 40.3 and 40.6, during a proximal row carpectomy, to show healthy articular cartilage over the head of the capitate.

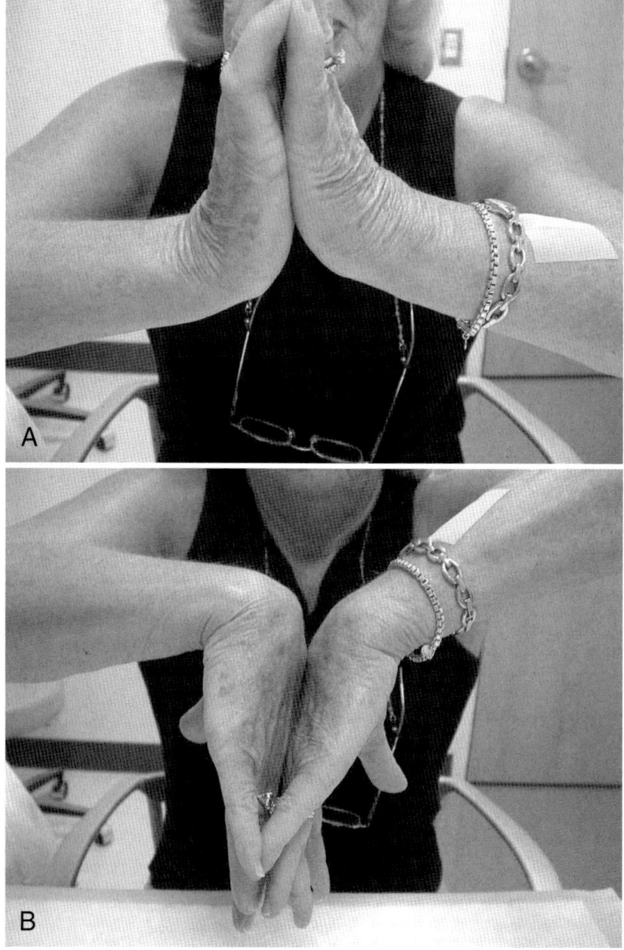

FIGURE 40.8 **A** and **B**, Postoperative function 6 months after a proximal row carpectomy. The patient has recovered nearly a 100-degree arc of motion and has no pain.

extend the indications for proximal row carpectomy in the setting of capitate head cartilage loss or lunate fossa arthrosis by suggesting interposition of soft tissue allograft or autograft or osteochondral autograft to the capitate from the excised carpal bones [26–28].

Indications for total wrist arthroplasty have expanded from end-stage rheumatoid arthritis to include post-traumatic osteoarthritis, end-stage primary osteoarthritis, and Kienböck disease. Patients are discouraged from heavy lifting after arthroplasty surgery but can otherwise return to full activity after a 2- to 3-month period of splinting in 30 to 40 degrees of extension to prevent flexion contracture. Short-term results have been encouraging with significant pain relief, maintenance of grip strength of 60% of the uninvolved side, preservation of motion, and even an increase in radial deviation in one study [29,30]. Total wrist arthroplasty is not recommended in people younger than 50 years, heavy laborers, or those dependent on walking aids.

The most common limited intercarpal fusion is known as the four-corner or four-bone fusion. It involves creating a fusion mass between the lunate, triquetrum, capitate, and hamate. The scaphoid is excised. The prerequisite for this procedure is an intact joint between the radius and the lunate. A theoretical advantage of this procedure over a proximal row carpectomy is that it maintains carpal height, leading to a better grip strength (Fig. 40.9). However, this has not been shown to be the case in larger studies comparing these two procedures. The flexion-extension arc of wrist motion is also not significantly different between these two procedures [31]. Theoretical disadvantages of a four-corner fusion include protracted immobilization until fusion is confirmed (usually 8 weeks) and the possibility of needing a secondary operative procedure to remove hardware (Fig. 40.10). This procedure is also appropriate for the early stages of SLAC and SNAC arthrosis.

Patients with severe arthrosis that involves not only the radiocarpal joint but also the joint between the proximal and distal carpal rows (midcarpal joint) are better served with total wrist fusion. This procedure is also beneficial in patients who present preoperatively with minimal or no wrist motion. It involves a fusion between the radius, proximal row, and distal row of carpal bones. The wrist is

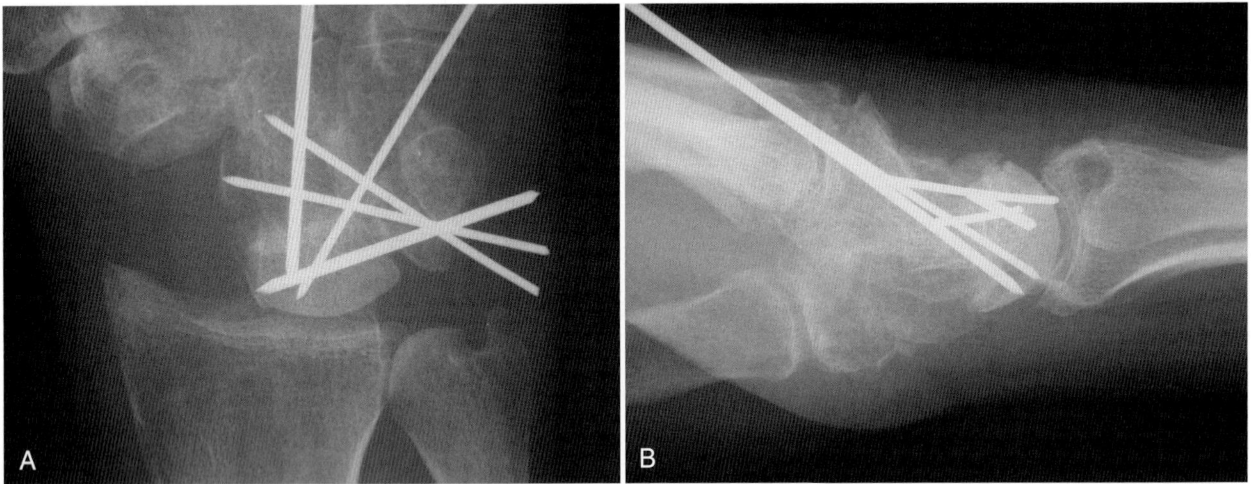

FIGURE 40.9 **A** and **B,** Postoperative radiographs after scaphoid excision and four-bone fusion have been performed.

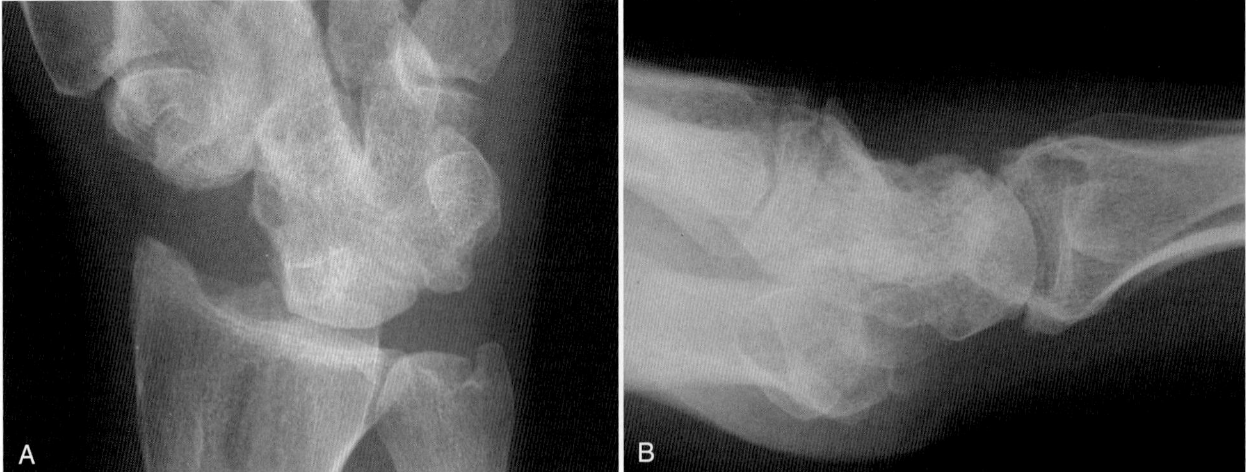

FIGURE 40.10 **A** and **B,** A mature four-bone fusion after a secondary procedure to remove the pins seen in Figure 40.9. To avoid the second operative procedure, some may elect to leave the pins percutaneous and to remove them during an office visit.

protected with a splint for 4 to 6 weeks. Most patients are able to attain a grip strength that is 60% to 80% of the opposite side [32]. A successful fusion abolishes the flexion-extension arc of wrist motion and, more important, can be effective in obtaining pain relief. However, the lost motion makes it difficult for patients to position the hand in tight spaces and can affect perineal care [31]. In these patients, the loss of motion does not appear to have an adverse functional impact because most of these patients have significant reduction of motion at the time of presentation. The pain relief provided by this procedure, however, can have a positive impact on functional outcome to a significant degree. Pronation and supination are unaffected. This procedure is appropriate for the advanced stages of SLAC and SNAC arthritis (Fig. 40.11).

Wrist denervation, which does not address the osteoarthritis directly but acts as a palliative option, was proposed in 1965 by Wilhelm [33]. The procedure involves ablation of sensory branches of local nerves to the wrist capsule without addressing any bone deformity. Since then, others have modified the approach and have also suggested partial denervations. Pain relief can be as high as 80% to 100%. The major benefit of denervation is that all the other options remain at the surgeon's disposal should bone procedures become necessary. Despite early concerns, the wrist does not undergo Charcot arthropathy after denervation [34,35].

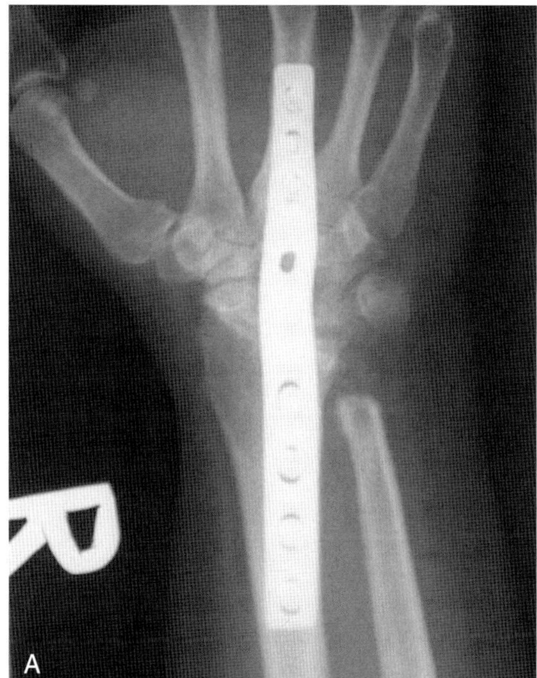

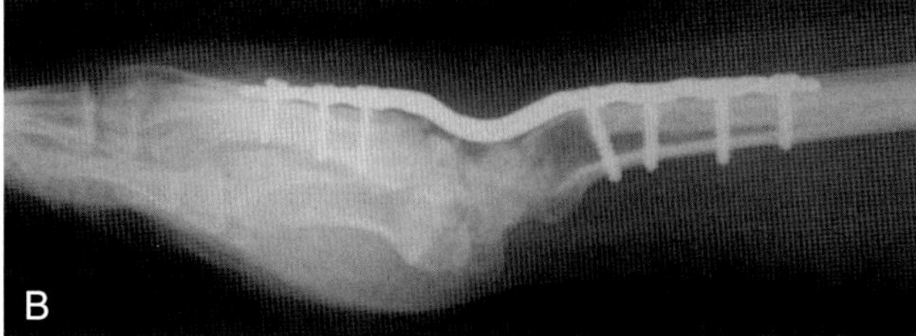

FIGURE 40.11 **A** and **B**, A total wrist arthrodesis with a contoured plate and screws. In the anteroposterior radiograph, it is evident that the wrist is in mild ulnar deviation; in the lateral radiograph, the wrist appears to be in mild dorsiflexion. This is the optimal position for hand function in such patients. The patient also underwent excision of the distal ulna.

Potential Disease Complications

Wrist osteoarthritis that progresses to advanced stages results in severely painful limitation of motion. Patients are unable to do their activities of daily living because any load across the arthritic wrist joint results in pain. The pain and stiffness can also inhibit the ability of the patient to position the hand in space. Rarely, osteophytes occurring over the dorsal aspect of the distal radius and the distal radioulnar joint can cause attritional ruptures of extensor tendons.

Potential Treatment Complications

Nonsteroidal anti-inflammatory medicines carry risks to the cardiovascular, gastric, renal, and hepatic systems. For these reasons, these medications are typically used for short periods. Surgery exposes the patient to significant risks from anesthesia, infection, nerve injury, and tendon injury. Fusions carry the risk of nonunion and malunion as well as that of hardware complications, such as prominence of the hardware, tendon irritation, and metal sensitivity. Motion-sparing procedures can eventually lead to further degenerative disease (Fig. 40.12) and in the presence of symptoms may require further surgery, which most commonly consists of a total wrist fusion. Total wrist arthroplasties can be complicated by infection, loosening, wound issues, hardware failure, instability, dislocation, tendon rupture, and impingement, with complication rates varying from 9% to 75%. Survival rates of total wrist arthroplasty in a Norwegian study ranged from 57% to 78% at 5 years and were as high as 71% at 10 years, depending on the implant and preoperative diagnosis [30].

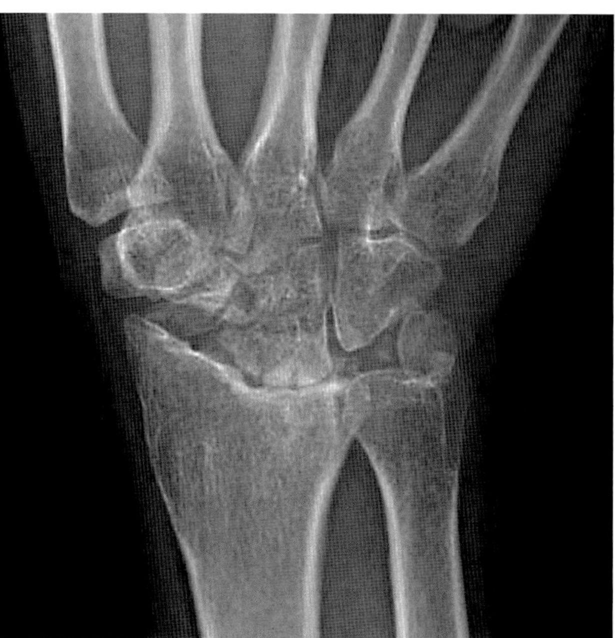

FIGURE 40.12 Advanced degenerative disease in a patient who underwent a proximal row carpectomy a few years before. Despite the radiographic appearance, the patient reported only mild pain.

References

[1] Watson HK, Ballet FL. The SLAC wrist: scapholunate advanced collapse pattern of degenerative arthritis. J Hand Surg [Am] 1984;9:358–65.
[2] Haugen IK, Englund M, Aliabadi P, et al. Prevalence, incidence and progression of hand osteoarthritis in the general population: the Framingham Osteoarthritis Study. Ann Rheum Dis 2011;70:1581–6.
[3] Knirk JL, Jupiter JB. Intra-articular fractures of the distal end of the radius in young adults. J Bone Joint Surg Am 1986;68:647–59.
[4] Aro HT, Koivunen T. Minor axial shortening of the radius affects outcome of Colles' fracture treatment. J Hand Surg [Am] 1991;16:392–8.
[5] Gliatis JD, Plessas SJ, Davis TR. Outcome of distal radial fractures in young adults. J Hand Surg [Br] 2000;25:535–43.
[6] Ruby LK, Stinson J, Belsky MR. The natural history of scaphoid non-union. A review of fifty-five cases. J Bone Joint Surg Am 1985;67:428–32.
[7] Gelberman RH, Menon J. The vascularity of the scaphoid bone. J Hand Surg [Am] 1980;5:508–13.
[8] Slade 3rd. JF, Dodds SD. Minimally invasive management of scaphoid nonunions. Clin Orthop Relat Res 2006;445:108–19.
[9] Cooney WP, Linscheid RL, Dobyns JH. Scaphoid fractures. Problems associated with nonunion and avascular necrosis. Orthop Clin North Am 1984;15:381–91.
[10] Osterman AL, Mikulics M. Scaphoid nonunion. Hand Clin 1988;4:437–55.
[11] Lindstrom G, Nystrom A. Incidence of post-traumatic arthrosis after primary healing of scaphoid fractures: a clinical and radiological study. J Hand Surg [Br] 1990;15:11–3.
[12] Mack GR, Bosse MJ, Gelberman RH, Yu E. The natural history of scaphoid non-union. J Bone Joint Surg Am 1984;66:504–9.
[13] O'Meeghan CJ, Stuart W, Mamo V, et al. The natural history of an untreated isolated scapholunate interosseous ligament injury. J Hand Surg [Br] 2003;28:307–10.
[14] Walsh JJ, Berger RA, Cooney WP. Current status of scapholunate interosseous ligament injuries. J Am Acad Orthop Surg 2002;10:32–42.
[15] Ryu J, Cooney III WP, Askew LJ, et al. Functional ranges of motion of the wrist joint. J Hand Surg [Am] 1991;16:409–19.
[16] Watson HK, Weinzweig J. Physical examination of the wrist. Hand Clin 1997;13:17–34.
[17] Brumfield RH, Champoux JA. A biomechanical study of normal functional wrist motion. Clin Orthop Relat Res 1984;187:23–5.
[18] Nissen KL. Symposium on cerebral palsy (orthopaedic section). Proc R Soc Med 1951;44:87–90.
[19] Allan CH, Joshi A, Lichtman DM. Kienböck's disease: diagnosis and treatment. J Am Acad Orthop Surg 2001;9:128–36.
[20] Simonian PT, Trumble TE. Scaphoid nonunion. J Am Acad Orthop Surg 1994;2:185–91.
[21] Thiele J, Nimmo R, Rowell W, et al. A randomized single blind crossover trial comparing leather and commercial wrist splints for treating chronic wrist pain in adults. BMC Musculoskelet Disord 2009;10:129–36.
[22] Richmond SJ, Brown SR, Campion PD, et al. Therapeutic effects of magnetic and copper bracelets in osteoarthritis: a randomized placebo-controlled crossover trial. Complement Ther Med 2009;17:249–56.
[23] Fuchs S, Monikes R, Wohlmeiner A, Heyse T. Intra-articular hyaluronic acid compared with corticoid injections for the treatment of rhizarthrosis. Osteoarthritis Cartilage 2006;14:82–8.
[24] Imbriglia JE, Broudy AS, Hagberg WC, McKernan D. Proximal row carpectomy: clinical evaluation. J Hand Surg [Am] 1990;15:426–30.
[25] Cohen MS, Kozin SH. Degenerative arthritis of the wrist: proximal row carpectomy versus scaphoid excision and four-corner arthrodesis. J Hand Surg [Am] 2001;26:94–104.
[26] Kwon BC, Choi SJ, Shin J, Baek GH. Proximal row carpectomy with capsular interposition arthroplasty for advanced arthritis of the wrist. J Bone Joint Surg Br 2009;91:1601–6.
[27] Carneiro Rrdos S, Dias CE, Baptista CM. Proximal row carpectomy with allograft scaffold interposition arthroplasty. Tech Hand Up Extrem Surg 2011;15:253–6.
[28] Dang J, Nydick J, Polikandriotis JA, Stone J. Proximal row carpectomy with capitate osteochondral autograft transplantation. Tech Hand Up Extrem Surg 2012;16:67–71.
[29] Nydick JA, Greeberg SM, Stone JD, et al. Clinical outcomes of total wrist arthroplasty. J Hand Surg [Am] 2012;37:1580–4.
[30] Krukhaug Y, Lie SA, Havelin LI, et al. Results of 189 wrist replacements. A report from the Norwegian Arthroplasty Register. Acta Orthop 2011;82:405–9.
[31] Weiss AC, Wiedeman Jr G, Quenzer D, et al. Upper extremity function after wrist arthrodesis. J Hand Surg [Am] 1995;20:813–7.
[32] Bolano LE, Green DP. Wrist arthrodesis in post-traumatic arthritis: a comparison of two methods. J Hand Surg [Am] 1993;18:786–91.
[33] Wilhelm A. Denervation of the wrist. Hefte Unfallheilkd 1965;81:109–14.
[34] Schweizer A, von Kanel O, Kammer E, Meuli-Simmen C. Long-term follow-up evaluation of denervation of the wrist. J Hand Surg [Am] 2006;31:559–64.
[35] Braga-Silva J, Roman JA, Padoin AV. Wrist denervation for painful conditions of the wrist. J Hand Surg [Am] 2011;36:961–6.

CHAPTER 41

Wrist Rheumatoid Arthritis

Melissa A. Klausmeyer, MD

Chaitanya S. Mudgal, MD, MS (Orth), MCh (Orth)

Synonyms

Rheumatoid wrist
Synovitis of the wrist
Tenosynovitis of the wrist
Rheumatoid synovial hypertrophy

ICD-9 Codes

714.0	**Rheumatoid arthritis**
718.93	**Joint derangement, wrist**
719.43	**Joint pain, wrist**
727.00	**Synovitis, wrist**
727.05	**Tenosynovitis**
736.00	**Joint deformity**

ICD-10 Codes

M06.831	**Rheumatoid arthritis, right wrist**
M06.832	**Rheumatoid arthritis, left wrist**
M06.839	**Rheumatoid arthritis, unspecified wrist**
M24.831	**Other specific joint derangement of right wrist, not elsewhere classified**
M24.832	**Other specific joint derangement of left wrist, not elsewhere classified**
M24.839	**Other specific joint derangement of unspecified wrist, not elsewhere classified**
M25.531	**Pain in right wrist**
M25.532	**Pain in left wrist**
M25.539	**Pain in unspecified wrist**
M67.331	**Transient synovitis, right wrist**
M67.332	**Transient synovitis, left wrist**
M67.339	**Transient synovitis, unspecified wrist**
M65.9	**Synovitis and tenosynovitis, unspecified**
M21.90	**Unspecified acquired deformity of unspecified limb**

Definition

Rheumatoid arthritis is a systemic autoimmune disorder involving the synovial joint lining and is characterized by chronic symmetric erosive synovitis. It has been estimated that 1% to 2% of the world's population is affected by this disorder. Women are affected more frequently with a ratio of 2.5:1. The cause of rheumatoid arthritis is thought to be multifactorial, including both genetic and environmental factors. The diagnostic criteria for rheumatoid arthritis include symptoms (morning stiffness, symmetric joint swelling, and skin nodules), laboratory test results, and radiographic findings. The wrist is among the most commonly involved peripheral joints; more than 65% of patients have some wrist symptoms within 2 years of diagnosis, increasing to more than 90% by 10 years. Of patients with wrist involvement, 95% have bilateral involvement [1–5].

The inflamed and hypertrophied synovial tissue is responsible for the destruction of adjacent tissues and resultant deformities. The cascade of events that lead to articular cartilage damage is a T cell–mediated autoimmune process mediated by the HLA class II locus [4,5]. The synovium is infiltrated by destructive molecules, resulting in thickening and proliferation of the synovium, chemotactic attraction of polymorphonuclear cells, and release by the polymorphonuclear cells of lysosomal enzymes and free oxygen radicals, which destroy joint cartilage.

The wrist articulation can be divided into three compartments, all of which are lined by synovium and therefore involved in rheumatoid arthritis: the radiocarpal, midcarpal, and distal radioulnar joints. Cartilage loss from both degradation and synovial proliferation contributes to ligamentous laxity of the extrinsic and intrinsic wrist ligaments. The laxity around the wrist leads to the classic rheumatoid deformities of carpal supination and ulnar translocation. The normally stout volar radioscaphocapitate ligament and the dorsal radiotriquetral ligament, which are important stabilizers of the carpus in relation to the distal radius, are stretched, resulting in ulnar translocation of the carpus. Laxity of the volar radioscaphocapitate ligament leads to loss of the ligamentous support to the waist of the scaphoid as well as weakening of the intrinsic scapholunate ligament. The scaphoid responds by adopting a flexed posture, and this is accompanied by radial deviation of the hand at the radiocarpal articulation. The bony carpus supinates and subluxes palmarly and ulnarly; thus, the ulna is left relatively prominent on the dorsal aspect of the wrist, a condition sometimes referred to as the caput ulnae syndrome [5–7]. The secondary effect of carpal supination is subluxation of the extensor carpi ulnaris tendon in a volar direction to the point that it no longer functions effectively as a wrist extensor. The bony architecture of the wrist is affected secondarily, in that the inflammatory cascade also stimulates bone-resorbing osteoclasts, which cause subchondral and periarticular osteopenia.

Areas of the wrist that display vascular penetration into bone or contain significant synovial folds, such as the radial attachment of the radioscaphocapitate ligament (the most radial of the volar radiocarpal ligaments), the waist of the scaphoid, and the base of the ulnar styloid (prestyloid recess), are the most common sites of progressive synovitis. The results of chronic erosive changes in these areas are bone spicules that can abrade and weaken tendons passing in their immediate vicinity, ultimately causing tendon rupture and functional deterioration. The extensor tendons to the small finger and ring finger (Vaughn-Jackson syndrome) [8], which rupture at the level of the ulnar head (see caput ulnae syndrome earlier), and the flexor tendon of the thumb at the level of the scaphoid (Mannerfelt syndrome) [9] are the most commonly involved. In addition to mechanical abrading, the extensor tendons are enclosed in a sheath of synovium at the wrist, which makes them susceptible to the damaging changes of synovial hypertrophy that is commonly seen in rheumatoid arthritis. The synovial proliferation causes changes in tendons of both an ischemic and inflammatory nature, which make them susceptible to weakening and eventual rupture.

Symptoms

Three distinct areas of the wrist can be the source of symptoms from rheumatoid disease: the distal radioulnar joint, the radiocarpal joint, and the extensor tendons. However, symptoms can originate as far proximal as the cervical spine or involve the shoulder and the elbow. Joint-related symptoms in early disease include swelling and pain, with morning stiffness as a classic characteristic. Loss of motion in the early stages usually results from synovial hypertrophy and pain. Progressive loss of motion is seen with disease progression and represents articular destruction. The distal radioulnar joint can be painful because of inflammation within the joint, and it can be a source of decreased forearm rotation (Figs. 41.1 and 41.2). Later stages of the disease usually are manifested with complaints of severe pain, decreased motion, significant cosmetic concerns, and difficulties in performing activities of daily living. Erosive changes are more strongly associated with changes in subjective disability than joint space narrowing is [10].

Tenosynovitis of the tendons traversing the dorsal wrist can often be manifested as a painless swelling. Patients with advanced rheumatoid disease in the wrist or those unresponsive to medical management may present with loss of

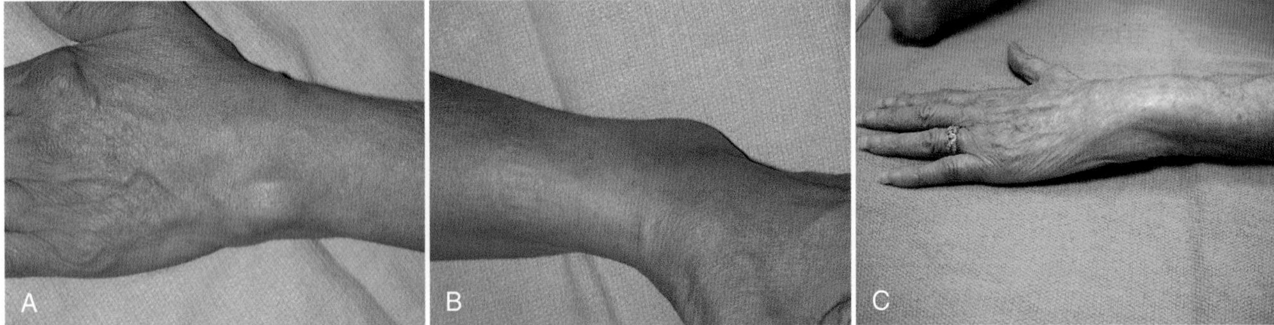

FIGURE 41.1 **A,** Appearance of the wrist in early rheumatoid arthritis. Note the swelling around the ulnar head. **B,** The synovial hypertrophy around the head of the ulna and distal radioulnar joint is appreciated in profile. There is also an early radial deviation of the hand at the wrist. **C,** The prominence of the ulnar head is compounded by the subluxation and supination of the carpus, creating an appearance of an abrupt change in contour from the wrist to the hand.

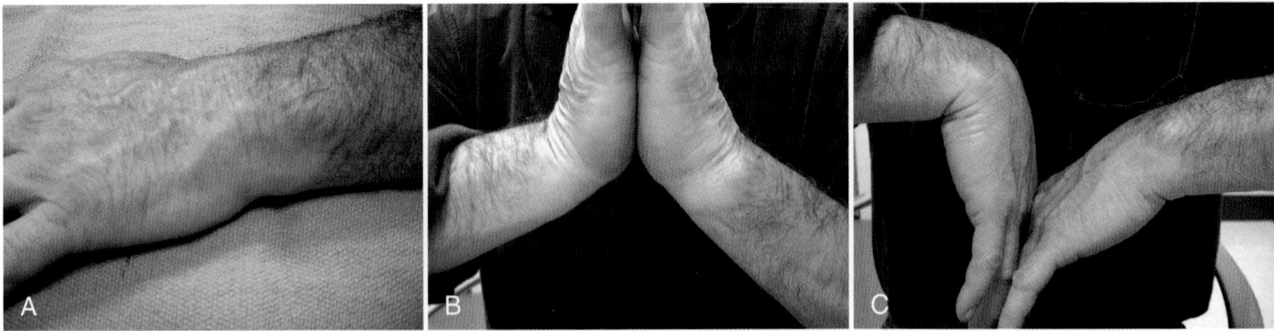

FIGURE 41.2 **A,** Synovitis around the distal end of the ulna may be manifested with swelling just volar to the ulnar styloid, as in this patient. **B** and **C,** Loss of motion in early rheumatoid disease of the wrist, as in this patient, is often a manifestation of the synovitis and pain associated with it rather than a true joint destruction.

extension of the digits at the metacarpophalangeal joints or with inability to flex the thumb at the interphalangeal articulation. These findings result from extensor digitorum communis tendon ruptures over the dorsal aspect of the wrist or a rupture of the flexor pollicis longus over the volar scaphoid as described before. Deformity of the wrist and hand is often the most concerning factor for patients and is attributable to the progressive carpal rotation and translocation discussed earlier, coupled with the extensor tendon imbalance accentuated at the metacarpophalangeal joints of the hand, which causes ulnar drift of the digits. The compensatory ulnar deviation occurs at the metacarpophalangeal joints, and it can often be the presenting symptom in undiagnosed or untreated patients.

Symptoms of median nerve compression and dysfunction (altered or absent sensation primarily in the radially sided digits and night pain and paresthesias in the hand) can be associated with rheumatoid arthritis as well. This is primarily due to hypertrophy of the tenosynovium around the flexor tendons within the confined space of the carpal canal, with resulting compression of the median nerve. Vascular damage of the peripheral nerve (rheumatoid neuropathy) may also contribute to symptoms [11].

Physical Examination

Keeping in mind the three primary locations of rheumatoid involvement in the wrist, careful physical examination can help identify the sources of pain and dysfunction and plan a course of treatment. Swelling around the ulnar styloid and loss of wrist extension secondary to extensor carpi ulnaris subluxation indicate early wrist involvement. Dorsal wrist swelling is commonly present and can be due to radiocarpal synovitis, tenosynovitis, or a combination of the two processes. An inflamed synovial membrane surrounding the radiocarpal joint is usually tender to palpation, but there can be surprisingly little swelling on examination if it is confined only to the dorsal capsule. Swelling that is related to the joint usually does not display movement with passive motion of the digits. Tenosynovitis, however, is typically painless and nontender and moves with tendon excursion as the digits are moved.

Distal radioulnar joint involvement is confirmed with tenderness to palpation, pain, crepitation, limitation of forearm rotation, and prominence of the ulnar head indicating subluxation or dislocation. If the ulnar border of the hand and carpus are in straight alignment with the ulna, it is indicative of radial deviation and carpal supination. As mentioned previously, ulnar drift of the digits at the metacarpophalangeal joints often accompanies this. It is important to examine the function and integrity of the tendons of the digits, primarily the extensor tendons and flexor pollicis longus tendon, to identify any attritional ruptures that may be present.

Examination for provocative signs of carpal tunnel syndrome includes eliciting of Tinel sign over the carpal canal, reproduction or worsening of numbness in the digits with compression over the proximal edge of the canal at the distal wrist crease (Durkan test), and flexion of the wrist (Phalen test). A careful neurologic examination may detect decreased light touch sensibility in the thumb, index, middle, and radial aspects of the ring finger if there is advanced median nerve dysfunction. Consideration should be given to the possibility of more proximal (cervical neuropathy) causes of symptoms.

If there is significant synovitis of the radiocapitellar joint proximally, there can be posterior interosseous nerve dysfunction as well. This is manifested during the wrist and hand examination as the inability to extend the thumb and digits and, to some extent, the wrist. This finding, however, needs to be differentiated from tendon rupture or subluxation at the level of the metacarpophalangeal joints. Strength testing may be diminished because of pain from synovitis, muscle atrophy, or the inability to contract a muscle secondary to tendon rupture.

Functional Limitations

Rheumatoid patients often have shoulder, elbow, and hand involvement and an abnormal wrist, which leads to significant limitations in activities of daily living. Because the distal radioulnar joint is important in allowing functional forearm rotation and in helping to position the hand in space, advanced synovitis of this joint causing pain and fixed deformity can have a severe impact on a patient's daily functional activity. Functional difficulties that are commonly experienced by these patients include activities of lifting, carrying, and sustained or repetitive grasp. Whereas a loss of pronation may be compensated for by shoulder abduction and internal rotation, supination loss is very difficult to compensate. This can lead to difficulty in opening doors and turning keys. Simple acts such as receiving change during shopping can be compromised by reduced supination. Furthermore, in patients with shoulder involvement, the freedom of compensatory motion at the shoulder can be severely limited, compounding the limitations imposed on the patient's function by limitation of forearm rotation.

Diagnostic Studies

In patients in whom rheumatoid arthritis is suspected clinically, appropriate diagnostic serologic tests may include rheumatoid factor, antinuclear antibody, HLA-B27, sedimentation rate, and anticitrulline antibody assay. These tests are performed in conjunction with a consultation by a rheumatologist or an internist experienced in the care of rheumatoid disease.

Plain radiographs of the wrist that include posterior-anterior, lateral, and oblique views allow thorough examination of the radiocarpal, midcarpal, and distal radioulnar joints. Specifically, a supinated oblique view [12] should be closely inspected for early changes consistent with rheumatoid synovitis. The earliest of these changes are symmetric soft tissue swelling and juxta-articular osteoporosis. Radiographic staging can be performed as well [13] (Table 41.1).

Although most patients already have a diagnosis of rheumatoid arthritis, radiographic examination occasionally detects the earliest signs of the disease by changes in areas of the wrist where there is a concentration of synovitis. These changes include erosions at the base of the ulnar styloid, the sigmoid notch of the distal radius, and the waist of the scaphoid and isolated joint space narrowing of the capitolunate joint seen on the posteroanterior view (Figs. 41.3 and 41.4). Ulnar translocation of the carpus can also be

Table 41.1 Larsen Radiographic Staging of Rheumatoid Arthritis

Larsen Score	Radiographic Status
0	No changes, normal joint
1	Periarticular swelling, osteoporosis, slight narrowing
2	Erosion and mild joint space narrowing
3	Moderate destructive joint space narrowing
4	End-stage destruction, preservation of articular surface
5	Mutilating disease, destruction of normal articular surfaces

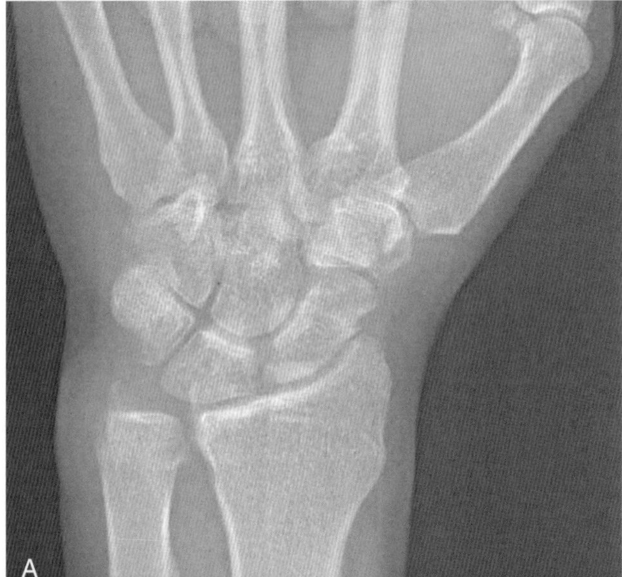

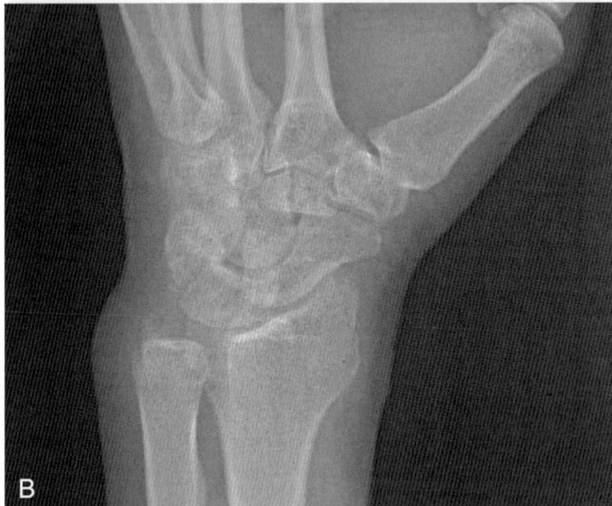

FIGURE 41.3 **A** and **B**, Radiographs (of the patient in Figure 41.2) in early rheumatoid disease of the wrist show bone erosions in areas of synovitis, such as around the ulnar styloid and distal radioulnar joint. There are also early erosive changes in the scapholunate articulation. The soft tissue swelling and deformity around the distal ulna are easily appreciated. These radiographs represent Larsen stage 2 disease.

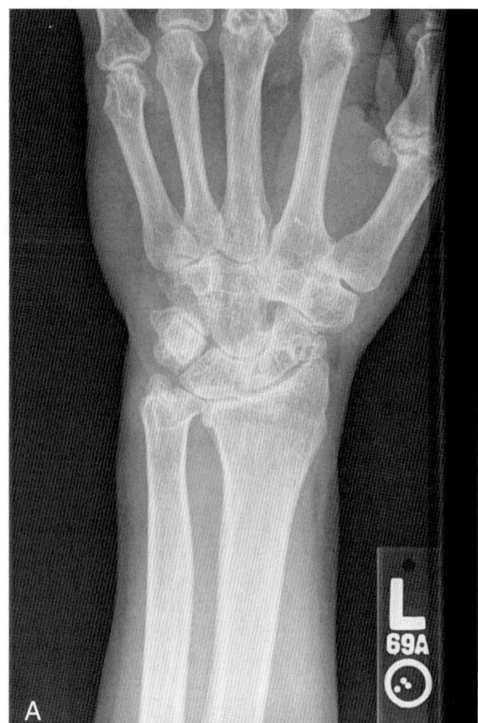

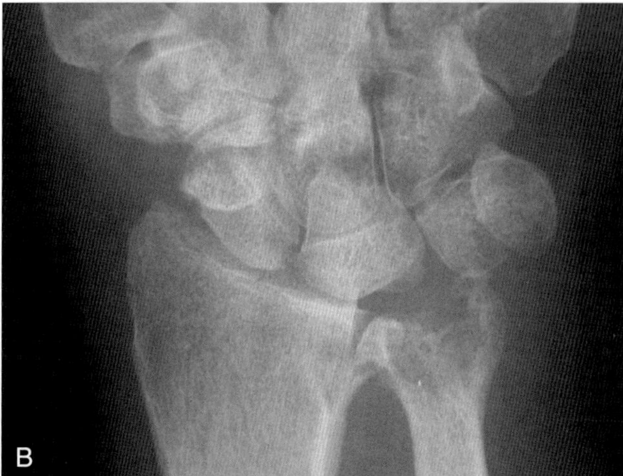

FIGURE 41.4 **A,** As the disease advances, cystic changes in the radioscaphoid articulation, reduction in joint space, and osteophyte formation are clearly seen in this radiograph of stage 3 disease. **B,** Radiographic appearance in stage 3 of persistent synovitis around the ulnar head and distal radioulnar joint, which leads to destruction of the ulnar head and osteophyte formation, both of which can contribute to extensor tendon attrition and rupture. There is ulnar translocation of the carpus best appreciated by the ulnar displacement of the lunate.

seen on this view. The lateral radiograph can show small bone spikes protruding palmarly, usually from the scaphoid. Late radiographic changes include pancompartmental loss of joint spaces and large subchondral erosions [14] (Fig. 41.5). Although radiographic findings may not always correlate well with clinical findings, the information gained from plain radiographs can be important in influencing which procedures will be of most benefit in patients with poor medical disease control. Significant joint subluxation,

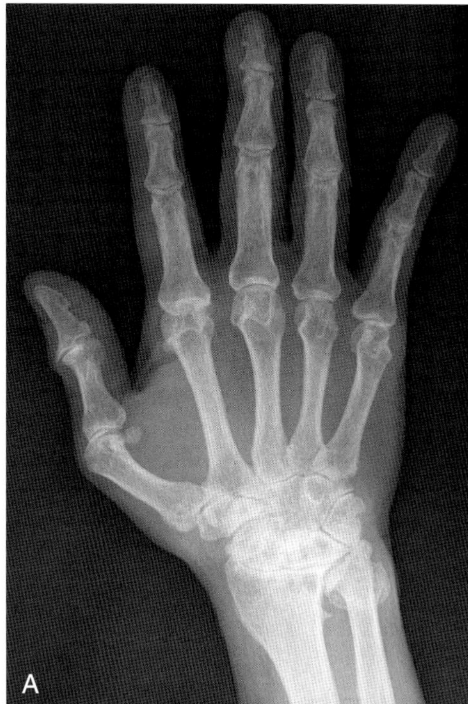

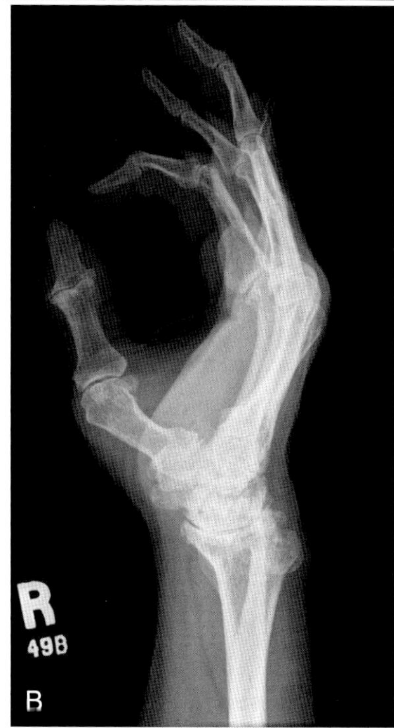

FIGURE 41.5 **A** and **B**, In advanced disease (stage 4), there is complete loss of joint space affecting the entire wrist, profuse osteophyte formation best appreciated in the lateral view, and deformation and dorsal dislocation of the ulnar head.

bone loss, relative ulnar length, and ulnar translocation can help determine which procedure best serves a patient.

Advanced imaging techniques, such as magnetic resonance imaging and computed tomography, are not usually helpful in evaluation or planning for surgery. Electrodiagnostic studies are recommended if neurologic symptoms are present.

Differential Diagnosis

Post-traumatic arthritis
Chronic scapholunate advanced collapse
Septic arthritis
Septic tenosynovitis
Wrist instability
Carpal tunnel syndrome
Gout

Treatment

Initial

The monitored use of disease-modifying agents has dramatically improved control of the disease, especially with early, aggressive treatment. The medical treatment consists of three categories of drugs: nonsteroidal anti-inflammatory agents; corticosteroids; and disease-modifying drugs, both nonbiologic (i.e., methotrexate) and biologic (i.e., tumor necrosis factor inhibitors) [4]. The details of medical treatment are beyond the scope of this chapter.

Management of local disease depends on several factors, such as severity of disease, functional limitations, pain, and cosmetic deformity. The patient's education, nutrition, and psychological health should be maximized.

Acutely painful, inflamed wrists are best managed with rest and immobilization and oral anti-inflammatory agents. Splints available over-the-counter may be ill-suited for this population of patients because the material cannot mold to altered anatomic contours. In such cases, a custom-made, forearm-based, volar resting splint that holds the wrist in the neutral position will provide support and comfort and is likely to be worn with greater compliance. Splints serve to stabilize joints that are subjected to subluxation forces and to improve grip when it is impaired by pain. However, splinting should be treated as a comfort measure and is not effective for preventing deformity as a result of progression of the disease [15].

Rehabilitation

Occupational therapy can provide potential pain control measures, activity modification education, custom splinting (see Initial Treatment), and exercises for range of motion tendon gliding and strengthening. A home exercise program can be developed to improve function and strength if the disease is also under adequate medical control [15].

In patients affected with local tenosynovitis of the extensor aspect and unwilling to have an injection, a trial of iontophoresis may prove beneficial. In patients with large amounts of subcutaneous adipose tissue, iontophoresis may be of limited efficacy in joints or periarticular structures. Studies on the effects of hot and cold in patients with rheumatoid arthritis show benefits in pain, joint stiffness, and strength but do not prove the superiority of one modality over the other [16]. Paraffin baths and moist heat packs are used to improve joint motion and pain, allowing increased activity tolerance. The results with paraffin baths are superior when they are combined with exercise programs [17]. Hydrotherapy can be an adjunct to many treatment programs, primarily for the purpose of decreasing muscle tension and reducing pain. Physical therapy particularly focusing on shoulder and elbow range of motion to position the hand in space may be of benefit if multiple joints are affected and symptomatic. Improvement of shoulder and elbow function is important because it is difficult to position a hand in space with a painful, stiff joint proximal to it.

Potentially the most critical role of therapy is in the postoperative period. It is then that patients particularly require monitored splinting, improvement in range of motion and strength, and edema control.

Procedures

Intra-articular cortisone injections are effective in alleviating wrist pain due to synovitis. Typically, all injections around the wrist should be done by aseptic technique with a 25-gauge, 1½-inch needle and a mixture of a steroid preparation, which is injected along with 1% lidocaine. The radiocarpal joint can be injected from the dorsal aspect approximately 1 cm distal to Lister tubercle, with the needle angled proximally about 10 degrees to account for the slight volar tilt of the distal radius articular surface. This is done with the wrist in the neutral position. Gentle longitudinal traction by an assistant can help widen the joint space, which may be reduced on account of the disease.

An alternative radiocarpal injection site is the ulnar wrist, just dorsal or volar to the easily palpable extensor carpi ulnaris tendon at the level of the ulnar styloid process. The needle must be angled proximally by 20 to 30 degrees to enter the space between the ulnar carpus and the head of the ulna. It is important to ascertain that the injectate flows freely. Any resistance indicates a need to reposition the needle appropriately. Alternatively, the injection may be performed with imaging guidance, such as a mini image intensifier or ultrasound, if it is available in the office.

If a midcarpal injection is required, this is done through the dorsal aspect, under fluoroscopic guidance, with injection into the space at the center of the lunate-triquetrum-hamate-capitate region.

Injections into the carpal tunnel are usually performed at the level of the distal wrist crease with the needle introduced just ulnar to the palmaris longus, which in most patients is just palmar to the median nerve and therefore protects it at this level. In patients who do not display clinical evidence of a palmaris longus, we do not recommend carpal tunnel injections. For treatment of associated carpal tunnel syndrome, patients should be issued a wrist splint primarily for nighttime use. Steroid injection into the carpal canal is an option, but the risks of possible attritional tendon rupture need to be discussed with the patient. Thorough knowledge of local anatomy is essential before an injection into the carpal tunnel is attempted. More important, alteration of local anatomy (and therefore altered location of the median nerve) must be considered very carefully before a carpal tunnel injection.

Patients must be counseled about the postinjection period. It is not uncommon for patients to experience some increase in local discomfort for 24 to 36 hours after the injection. Use of the splint is recommended during this time, and icing of the area may also be of benefit. In our experience, most steroid injections take a few days to have a therapeutic effect. As is the case with any joint, because of the deleterious effect that corticosteroids can have on articular cartilage by transient inhibition of chondrocyte synthesis, repeated injections should be minimized if there is no radiographic sign of advanced cartilage wear, but there is no specific maximum number of injections. On the other hand, in advanced disease, when joint surgery in inevitable, there is no contraindication to repeated injections that have proved beneficial to a patient.

Surgery

The indications for operative treatment of the rheumatoid wrist include one or more of the following: disabling pain and chronic synovitis not relieved by a minimum of 4 to 6 months of adequate medical and nonoperative measures; deformity and instability that limit hand function; tendon rupture; and nerve compression. Deformity alone is rarely an indication for surgery. It is not uncommon to see patients with significant deformities demonstrate excellent function with the use of compensatory maneuvers in the absence of pain. Corrective surgery in these patients is ill-advised.

Surgical procedures can be divided into those involving bone and those involving soft tissue (Table 41.2) [18]. On occasion, a bone procedure will be combined with a soft tissue procedure in the same setting. Synovectomy involves the removal of the inflamed, thickened joint lining from the radiocarpal and distal radioulnar joints and is best performed for the painful joint that demonstrates little or no radiographic evidence of joint destruction. Tenosynovectomy involves débridement of the tissue around involved tendons in the hope of avoiding future attritional tendon ruptures. Patients best suited for these procedures have relatively good medical disease control, no fixed joint deformity, and minimal radiographic changes. If tendon rupture has already occurred, most commonly over the distal ulna, the procedure of choice is some form of tendon transfer, usually combined with resection of the ulnar head (Darrach procedure) [19].

Table 41.2 Wrightington Classification of Rheumatic Disease

Wrightington Grade	Radiographic Findings	Surgical Therapy
1	Preservation of wrist architecture Periarticular cysts, osteoporosis	Synovectomy
2	Preservation of radioscaphoid joint Ulnar translocation, flexion of lunate or scaphoid, or radiolunate joint involvement	Darrach procedure, tendon rebalancing, partial arthrodesis
3	Preservation of radius architecture Intracarpal arthritis, radioscaphoid joint arthritis, or volar subluxation of carpus	Arthroplasty versus arthrodesis
4	Loss of radius bone stock	Arthrodesis

Repair is not indicated or possible in most cases because of the poor tissue quality and extensive loss of tendon tissue in the zone of rupture. Depending on the number of tendons ruptured, it is possible to transfer the ruptured distal tendon into a neighboring healthier tendon or to transfer a more distant tendon, such as the extensor indicis proprius or superficial flexor tendon, into the affected tendon. The distal end of a ruptured extensor tendon may also be sutured to its unaffected neighboring extensor in some cases.

Bone procedures include resection arthroplasty, resurfacing arthroplasty, and limited or complete wrist fusions. Resection arthroplasty, such as the Darrach procedure, in which the distal ulna is resected, is beneficial in the setting of distal ulnar impingement on the carpus or for distal radioulnar joint disease. It may also prevent tendon rupture of the extensor tendons on the dorsum of the ulnar head. However, it may further ulnar translocation of the carpus and therefore should be combined with a radiolunate arthrodesis in patients with weak ligamentous support where this is a concern (see later). An alternative treatment for debilitating distal radioulnar joint pain is the Sauvé-Kapandji procedure, in which the distal ulna is fused to the distal radius along with a distal ulnar osteotomy. This osteotomy is essentially a resection of a small segment of bone proximal to the fused distal radioulnar joint to construct a "false joint," or pseudarthrosis, through which the patient may be able to rotate the forearm. Excellent pain relief has been demonstrated in rheumatoid patients with this procedure [20,21]. Although this procedure is better at preventing ulnar translocation, nonunion of the arthrodesis site is an issue, particularly in rheumatoid arthritis patients with poor bone stock.

To address the radiocarpal joint, two options exist: wrist resurfacing arthroplasty or fusion. The arthroplasty requires the resection of a portion of the distal radius and carpus and insertion of an implant usually made of a metallic component with a polyethylene spacer. It is generally restricted to patients with low functional demands who have bilateral rheumatoid wrist disease and require some motion in one wrist if the other is fused. It is most effective in patients who have good bone stock, relatively good alignment, and intact extensor tendons. The benefits of the arthroplasty include maintenance of range of motion and pain relief. Although some studies show promising results with wrist arthroplasty [22–26], other long-term studies show loosening in half to two thirds of the population [27,28], with removal in 25% to 40%.

Fusion, or arthrodesis, procedures to eliminate pain due to significantly degenerative joints are well described [29–34]. However, depending on the nature of the fusion, these lead to a partial or complete loss of wrist motion. Limited fusions are described of the radiolunate joint (Chamay arthrodesis) or the radioscapholunate joint. The potential benefit of limited fusions is some sparing of wrist motion, which can occur through the articulations that remain unfused, and this sparing of some motion can be critical to overall function in this group of patients. In each of these procedures, the midcarpal joint must be well preserved.

Total wrist fusion is a reliable, safe, and well-established procedure for relieving pain and providing a stable wrist that improves hand function but without range of motion of the radiocarpal joint [29,30,32]. Success rates of 65% to 85% have been shown in terms of eliminating or significantly improving wrist pain [32]. For advanced wrist rheumatoid disease, it has become the most common bone procedure. Fusion can be accomplished either with a contoured dorsal plate fixed to the wrist by screws or with one or more large intraosseous pins placed across the wrist (Fig. 41.6). The intraosseous pins

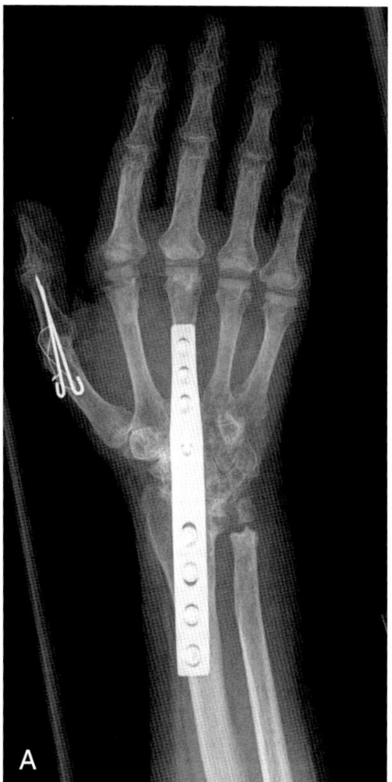

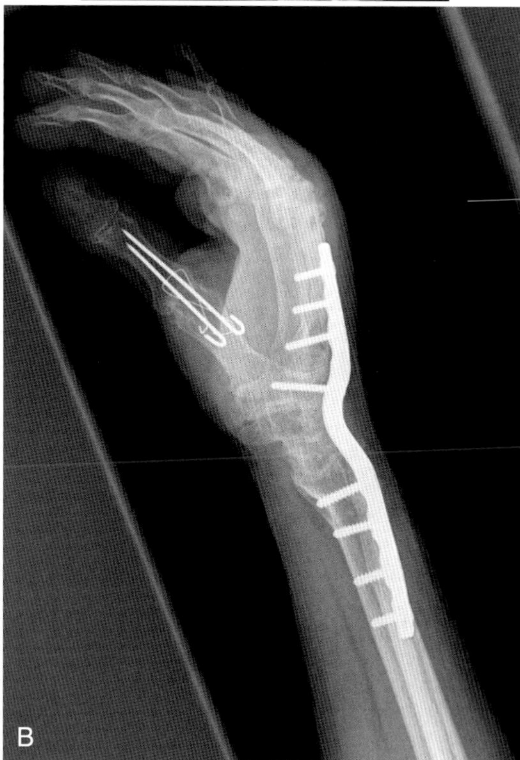

FIGURE 41.6 **A** and **B,** Radiographs depicting a total wrist arthrodesis with use of a contoured plate and screws. Note that the distal end of the ulna has also been excised (Darrach procedure). The polyarthritic nature of the disease process is emphasized by the metacarpophalangeal joint arthroplasties in the fingers and a metacarpophalangeal arthrodesis of the thumb.

are usually placed through the second or third metacarpal or through both, across the wrist into the medullary canal of the radius. Ideally, the wrist is fused in slight extension to allow improved grip strength. However, if both wrists are to be fused, one may consider fusing one in slight flexion and the other in slight extension to allow functional differences [5]. High rates of fusion and a 15% rate of symptomatic hardware removal have been described [31]. Consideration of the quality of the overlying soft tissue is necessary in deciding on a fusion technique, as more soft tissue dissection is necessary for the plate and may result in wound complications.

If significant median nerve compression exists, an extended open carpal tunnel release with flexor tenosynovectomy is typically performed through a palmar incision.

Potential Disease Complications

Rheumatoid arthritis is a chronic, progressive disease that can cause significant upper extremity disability at many locations by stiffness or instability from the shoulder to the hand. If wrist involvement becomes advanced, this contributes to problems with motion, pain, stiffness, and nerve compression. Extensor and flexor tendon rupture is a common scenario in rheumatoid disease and can complicate management. During the course of their disease, most patients with rheumatoid disease will lose some functional capacity, and about half will have disabling disease that requires significant physical dependence on adaptive measures for performance of the activities of daily living. Occupational therapists and social workers play roles in obtaining and using aids and appliances, such as special grips and alterations of household appliances, to maximize the patient's function.

Potential Treatment Complications

Systemic complications from the medical treatment of rheumatoid arthritis with current disease-modifying agents are beyond the scope of this chapter. Analgesics and nonsteroidal anti-inflammatory medications have well-known side effects that can affect the cardiac, gastric, renal, and hepatic systems. Intra-articular corticosteroid injections involve a very small risk of infection as well as cumulative cartilage injury from repeated exposure to steroid.

Surgical complications can result from wound healing problems, infection, neurovascular injury, recurrent synovitis, recurrent tendon rupture, persistent joint instability, and implant loosening or failure. To some extent, meticulous surgical technique and judicious management of medications affecting wound healing and immunity, such as methotrexate and systemic steroids, may reduce the frequency of complications.

References

[1] Hämäläinen M, Kammonen M, Lehtimäki M, et al. Epidemiology of wrist involvement in rheumatoid arthritis. Rheumatology 1992;17:1–7.

[2] Lee SK, Hausman MR. Management of the distal radioulnar joint in rheumatoid arthritis. Hand Clin 2005;21:577–89.

[3] Papp SR, Athwal GS, Pichora DR. The rheumatoid wrist. J Am Acad Orthop Surg 2006;14:65–77.

[4] Chung K, Pushman G. Current concepts in the management of rheumatoid hand. J Hand Surg [Am] 2011;36:736–47.

[5] Trieb K. Treatment of the wrist in rheumatoid arthritis. J Hand Surg [Am] 2008;33:113–23.

[6] Bäckdahl M. The caput ulnae syndrome in rheumatoid arthritis. A study of morphology, abnormal anatomy and clinical picture. Acta Rheumatol Scand Suppl 1963;5:1–75.

[7] Wilson RL, DeVito MC. Extensor tendon problems in rheumatoid arthritis. Hand Clin 1996;12:551–9.

[8] Vaughan-Jackson OJ. Rupture of extensor tendons by attrition at the inferior radio-ulnar joint: report of two cases. J Bone Joint Surg Br 1948;30:528–30.

[9] Mannerfelt L, Norman O. Attrition ruptures of flexor tendons in rheumatoid arthritis caused by bony spurs in the carpal tunnel: a clinical and radiological study. J Bone Joint Surg Br 1969;51:270–7.

[10] Koevoets R, Dirven L, Klarenbeek NB, et al. Insights in the relationship of joint space narrowing versus erosive joint damage and physical functioning of patients with RA. Ann Rheum Dis 2013;72:870–4.

[11] Muramatsu K, Tanaka H, Taguchi T. Peripheral neuropathies of the forearm and hand in rheumatoid arthritis: diagnosis and options for treatment. Rheumatol Int 2008;28:951–7.

[12] Nørgaard F. Earliest roentgenological changes in polyarthritis of the rheumatoid type: rheumatoid arthritis. Radiology 1965;85:325–9.

[13] Larsen A, Dale K, Eek M, et al. Radiographic evaluation of rheumatoid arthritis by standard reference films. J Hand Surg [Am] 1983;8:667–9.

[14] Resnick D. Rheumatoid arthritis of the wrist: the compartmental approach. Med Radiogr Photogr 1976;52:50–88.

[15] Heine PJ, Williams MA, Williamson E, et al. Development and delivery of an exercise intervention for rheumatoid arthritis; strengthening and stretching for rheumatoid arthritis of the hand (SARAH) trial. Physiotherapy 2012;90:121–30.

[16] Adams J, Burridge J, Mullee M, et al. The clinical effectiveness of static resting splints in early rheumatoid arthritis: a randomized controlled trial. Rheumatology 2008;47:1548–53.

[17] Michlovitz SL. The use of heat and cold in the management of rheumatic diseases. In: Michlovitz S, editor. Thermal agents in rehabilitation. 2nd ed. Philadelphia: FA Davis; 1990. p. 158–74.

[18] Hodgson SP, Stanley JK, Muirhead A. The Wrightington classification of rheumatoid wrist x-rays: a guide to surgical management. J Hand Surg [Br] 1989;14:451–5.

[19] Darrach W. Partial excision of lower shaft of ulna for deformity following Colles's fracture. Ann Surg 1913;57:764–5.

[20] Vincent KA, Szabo RM, Agee JM. The Sauvé-Kapandji procedure for reconstruction of the rheumatoid distal radioulnar joint. J Hand Surg [Am] 1993;18:978–83.

[21] Fujita S, Masada K, Takeuchi E, et al. Modified Sauvé-Kapandji procedure for disorders of the distal radioulnar joint in patients with rheumatoid arthritis. J Bone Joint Surg Am 2005;87:134–9.

[22] Cobb TK, Beckenbaugh RD. Biaxial total-wrist arthroplasty. J Hand Surg [Am] 1996;21:1011–21.

[23] Bosco JA, Bynum DK, Bowers WH. Long-term outcome of Volz total wrist arthroplasties. J Arthroplasty 1994;9:25–31.

[24] Anderson MC, Adams BD. Total wrist arthroplasty. Hand Clin 2005;21:621–30.

[25] Nydick JA, Greenberg SM, Stone JD, et al. Clinical outcomes of total wrist arthroplasty. J Hand Surg [Am] 2012;37:1580–4.

[26] Ferreres A, Lluch A, del Valle M. Universal total wrist arthroplasty: midterm follow-up study. J Hand Surg [Am] 2011;36:967–73.

[27] Ward C, Kuhl T, Adams BD. Five to ten year outcomes of the Universal total wrist arthroplasty in patients with rheumatoid arthritis. J Bone Joint Surg Am 2011;93:914–9.

[28] van Harlingen D, Heesterbeek PJC, de Vos MJ. High rate of complications and radiographic loosening of the biaxial total wrist arthroplasty in rheumatoid arthritis. Acta Orthop 2011;82:721–6.

[29] Barbier O, Saels P, Rombouts JJ, et al. Long-term functional results of wrist arthrodesis in rheumatoid arthritis. J Hand Surg [Br] 1999;24:27–31.

[30] Jebson PJ, Adams BD. Wrist arthrodesis: review of current technique. J Am Acad Orthop Surg 2001;9:53–60.

[31] Meads BM, Scougall PJ, Hargreaves IC. Wrist arthrodesis using a Synthes wrist fusion plate. J Hand Surg [Br] 2003;28:571–4.

[32] Ishikawa H, Murasawa A, Nakazono K. Long-term follow-up study of radiocarpal arthrodesis for the rheumatoid wrist. J Hand Surg [Am] 2005;30:658–66.

[33] Solem H, Berg NJ, Finsen V. Long term results of arthrodesis of the wrist: a 6-15 year follow up of 35 patients. Scand J Plast Reconstr Surg Hand Surg 2006;40:175–8.

[34] Rauhaniemi J, Tiusanen H, Sipola E. Total wrist fusion: a study of 115 patients. J Hand Surg [Br] 2005;30:217–9.

SECTION V
Mid Back

CHAPTER 42

Thoracic Compression Fracture

Toni J. Hanson, MD

Synonyms

Thoracic compression fracture
Dorsal compression fracture
Wedge compression
Vertebral crush fracture

ICD-9 Codes

733.19 Pathologic fracture of other specified site
733.13 Pathologic fracture of vertebrae

ICD-10 Codes

M84.40 Pathological fracture, unspecified site
S22.009 Unspecified fracture of unspecified thoracic vertebra
Add seventh character (A—Initial encounter closed fracture, B—initial encounter open fracture, D—subsequent encounter fracture with routine healing, G—subsequent encounter fracture with delayed healing, K—subsequent encounter fracture with nonunion, S—sequela)

Definition

A compression fracture is caused by forces transmitted along the vertebral body. The ligaments are intact, and compression fractures are usually stable [1] (Fig. 42.1). Compression fractures in the thoracic vertebrae are commonly seen in osteoporosis with decreased bone mineral density. They may be asymptomatic and diagnosed incidentally on radiography. Such fractures may occur with trivial trauma and are usually stable [2,3]. Pathologic vertebral fractures may occur with metastatic cancer (commonly from lung, breast, or prostate) as well as with other processes affecting vertebrae. Trauma, such as a fall from a height or a motor vehicle accident, can also result in thoracic compression fracture. Considerable force is required to fracture healthy vertebrae, which are resistant to compression. In such cases, the force required to produce a fracture may cause extension of fracture components into the spinal canal with neurologic findings. There may be evidence of additional trauma, such as calcaneal fractures from a fall. Multiple thoracic compression fractures, as seen with osteoporosis, can produce a kyphotic deformity [4–6]. An estimated 1.5 million vertebral compression fractures occur annually in the United States, with 25% of postmenopausal women affected in their lifetime. Estimates indicate that there are 44 million persons with osteoporosis and 34 million with low bone mass in the United States [7]. Existence of vertebral compression fracture increases the risk of future vertebral compression fractures (with 1 fracture, there is a 5-fold increase; with 2 or more fractures, there is a 12-fold increase) [8].

Symptoms

Pain in the thoracic spine over the affected vertebrae is the usual hallmark of the presentation. It may be severe, sharp, exacerbated with movement, and decreased with rest. Severe pain may last 2 to 3 weeks and then decrease during 6 to 8 weeks, but pain may persist for months. Acute fractures in osteoporosis, however, may result in little discomfort or poor localization [9]. In osteoporotic fractures, the mid and lower thoracic vertebrae are typically affected. A good history and physical examination

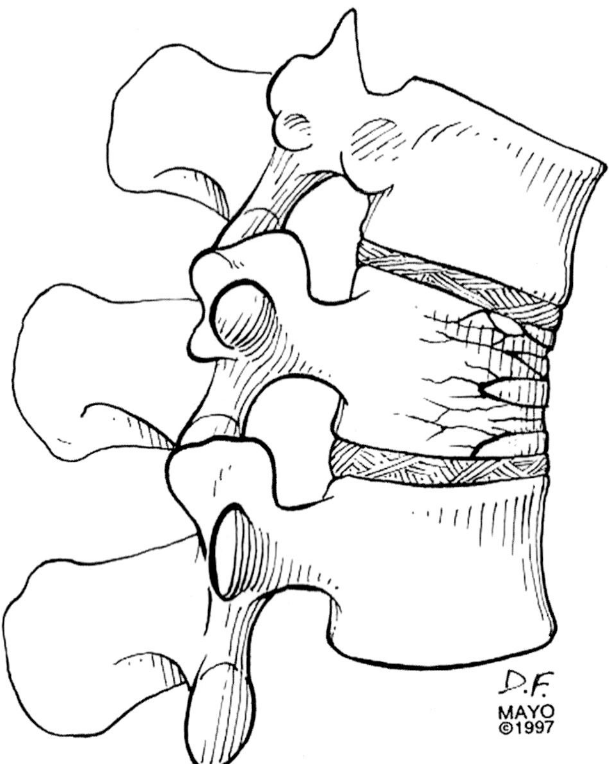

FIGURE 42.1 Thoracic compression fracture with reduction in anterior vertebral height and wedging of the vertebrae.

are essential as there may be indicators of a more ominous underlying pathologic process [10,11].

Physical Examination

Tenderness with palpation or percussion over the affected region of the thoracic vertebrae is the primary finding on physical examination. Spinal movements also produce pain. Kyphotic deformity, loss of height, and impingement of the lower ribs on the superior iliac crest may be present in the patient who has had multiple prior compression fractures. Neurologic examination below the level of the fracture is recommended to assess for presence of reflex changes, pathologic reflexes such as Babinski sign, and sensory alterations. Sacral segments can be assessed through evaluation of rectal tone, volitional sphincter control, anal wink, and pinprick if there is concern about bowel and bladder function [12]. It is also important to assess the patient's gait for stability. Comorbid neurologic and orthopedic conditions may contribute to gait dysfunction and fall risk [13,14].

Functional Limitations

Functional limitations in a patient with an acute painful thoracic compression fracture can be significant. The patient may experience loss of mobility and independence in activities of daily living and household activities, and there may be an impact on social, avocational, vocational, and psychological functioning. In patients with severe symptoms, hospitalization may be necessary [15].

Diagnostic Testing

Anteroposterior and lateral radiographs of the thoracic spine can confirm the clinical impression of a thoracic compression fracture. On radiographic examination in a thoracic compression fracture, the height of the affected vertebrae is reduced, generally in a wedge-shaped fashion, with anterior height less than posterior vertebral height. In osteoporosis, biconcave deformities can also be noted on spinal radiographs (Fig. 42.2A). A bone scan may help localize (but not necessarily determine the etiology of) processes such as metastatic cancer, occult fracture, and infection. Spinal imaging, such as computed tomography or magnetic resonance imaging, may also elucidate further detail [16] (Fig. 42.2B). Percutaneous needle biopsy of the affected vertebral body can be helpful diagnostically in selected cases. Laboratory tests are obtained as appropriate. These include a complete blood count and sedimentation rate or C-reactive protein level (which are nonspecific but sensitive indicators of an occult infection or inflammatory disease). Serum alkaline phosphatase, serum and urine protein electrophoresis, and other laboratory tests are beneficial when a malignant neoplasm is suspected. Diagnostic testing is directed, as appropriate, on the basis of the entire clinical presentation, including secondary causes of osteoporosis. Bone densitometry can be performed when the patient is improved clinically.

Differential Diagnosis

Thoracic sprain
Thoracic radiculopathy
Thoracic disc herniation
Metastatic malignant disease
Primary spine malignant neoplasm (uncommon, most frequently multiple myeloma) [17]
Benign spinal tumors
Infection, osteomyelitis (rare) [18]
Inflammatory arthritis
Musculoskeletal pain, other
Referred pain (pancreatic cancer, abdominal aortic aneurysm)

Treatment

Initial

Initial treatment consists of activity modification, including limited bed rest. Cushioning with use of a mattress overlay (such as an egg crate) can also be helpful. Pharmacologic agents, including oral analgesics, muscle relaxants, and anti-inflammatory medications, as appropriate to the patient, are helpful. Agents such as tramadol 50 mg (one or two every 4 to 6 hours, not exceeding eight per day), acetaminophen 300 mg/codeine 30 mg (one or two every 4 to 6 hours), and controlled-release oxycodone CR (10 mg or 20 mg every 12 hours) may be considered. Acetaminophen dose should not exceed 3 g/day. Muscle relaxants such as cyclobenzaprine, 10 mg three times daily, may be helpful initially with muscle spasm. A variety of nonsteroidal anti-inflammatory drugs, including celecoxib (Celebrex, a cyclooxygenase 2 inhibitor),

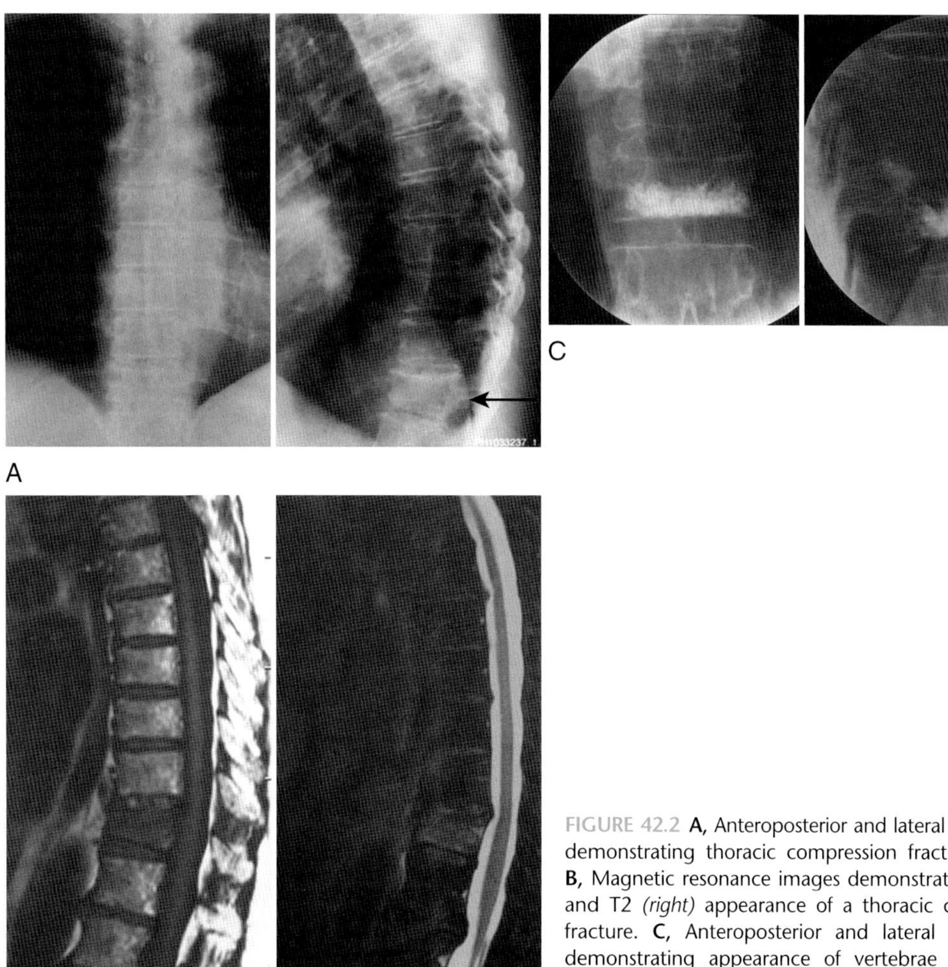

FIGURE 42.2 **A,** Anteroposterior and lateral radiographs demonstrating thoracic compression fracture *(arrow)*. **B,** Magnetic resonance images demonstrating T1 *(left)* and T2 *(right)* appearance of a thoracic compression fracture. **C,** Anteroposterior and lateral radiographs demonstrating appearance of vertebrae after vertebroplasty. *(Courtesy Kent R. Theilen, MD, Mayo Clinic, Rochester, Minn.)*

can be considered, depending on the patient. Calcitonin (one spray daily, alternating nostrils, providing 200IU per spray) has also been used for painful osteoporotic fractures [19]. Stool softeners and laxatives may be necessary to reduce strain with bowel movements and constipation, particularly with narcotic analgesics. Selection of pharmacologic agents must factor in the age, comorbidities, and clinical status of the patient. Avoidance of spinal motion, especially flexion, by appropriate body mechanics (such as log rolling in bed) and spinal bracing is helpful. There are a variety of spinal orthoses that reduce spinal flexion (Fig. 42.3). They must be properly fitted [20,21]. A lumbosacral orthosis may be sufficient for a low thoracic fracture. A thoracolumbosacral orthosis is used frequently (Fig. 42.3A-D). If a greater degree of fracture immobilization is required, an off-the-shelf orthosis (Fig. 42.3E) or a custom-molded body jacket may be fitted by an orthotist. Proper diagnosis and treatment of underlying contributors to the thoracic compression fracture are necessary [22,23]. Most thoracic compression fractures will heal with symptomatic improvement in 4 to 6 weeks [24,25].

Rehabilitation

Physical therapy is helpful to assist with gentle mobilization of the patient by employing proper body mechanics, optimizing transfer techniques, and training with gait aids (such as a wheeled walker) to reduce biomechanical stresses on the spine and to ensure gait safety [26]. Pain-relieving modalities, such as therapeutic heat or cold, and transcutaneous electrical stimulation may also be employed. Exercise should not increase spinal symptoms and should be implemented at the appropriate juncture. In addition to proper body mechanics and postural training emphasizing spinal extension and avoidance of flexion, spinal extensor muscle strengthening, limb muscle strengthening, stretching to muscle groups (such as the chest, hips, and lower extremity muscles), and deep breathing exercises may also be indicated. Weight-bearing exercises for bone health, balance, and fall prevention are also important [27]. Proper footwear, with cushioning inserts, can also be helpful. Occupational therapy can help the patient with activities of daily living, reinforce proper spinal ergonomics, address equipment needs, and prevent falls. Successful rehabilitation is targeted at increasing the patient's comfort, decreasing deformity, and decreasing resultant disability and is individualized to address specific patient needs [28–30].

Procedures

Invasive procedures are generally not necessary. Percutaneous vertebroplasty or kyphoplasty with use of polymethyl

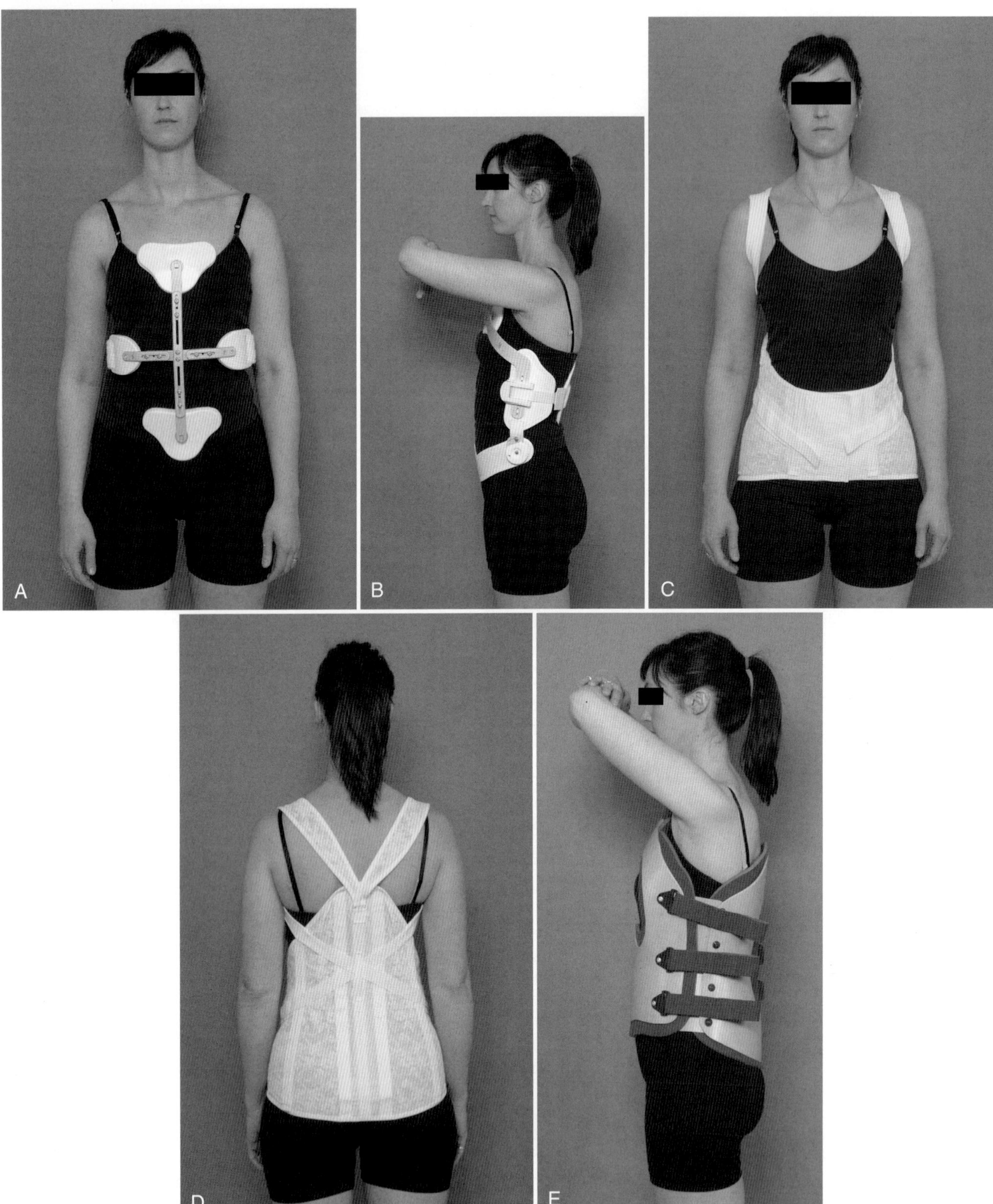

FIGURE 42.3 **A,** Cruciform anterior spinal hyperextension brace (to limit flexion). **B,** Three-point sagittal hyperextension brace (to limit flexion). **C,** Thoracolumbosacral orthosis, anterior view. **D,** Thoracolumbosacral orthosis, posterior view. **E,** Off-the-shelf molded spinal orthosis with Velcro closures.

methacrylate may be helpful to reduce fracture pain, to reinforce thoracic vertebral strength, and to improve function; with kyphoplasty, some potential restoration of vertebral height has been reported [26,31] (Fig. 42.2C). Patients with imaging evidence of an acute or a subacute thoracic fracture who have correlating pain, who fail to improve with conservative management, and who are without contraindications may be candidates for such interventional procedures [32,33]. In two randomized controlled trials, no beneficial effect was noted in vertebroplasty versus sham [32,34].

Surgery

Surgery is rarely necessary. Surgical stabilization can be considered in patients with continued severe pain after compression fracture as a result of nonunion of the fracture, in patients with spinal instability, or if neurologic complications occur. Referral to a spine surgeon is recommended in these cases for further assessment [35].

Potential Disease Complications

Neurologic complications, including nerve or spinal cord compromise, as well as orthopedic complications with continued pain, nonunion, and instability can occur. Underlying primary disease, for example, metastatic thoracic compression, needs to be addressed. Patients with severe kyphosis may experience cardiopulmonary dysfunction. Severe kyphosis may also result in rib impingement on the iliac bones, producing further symptoms. Severe pain accompanying a fracture may further limit deep breathing and increase the risk of pulmonary complications, such as pneumonia. Progressive spinal deformity may produce secondary pain generators. The patient may have progressive levels of dependency as a result.

Potential Treatment Complications

Side effects with medications, particularly nonsteroidal anti-inflammatory drugs as well as narcotic medications, can occur. It is important to select medications appropriate for individual patients. There may be difficulty with the use of spinal orthotics, such as intolerance in patients with gastroesophageal reflux disease. Kyphotic patients frequently do not tolerate orthoses and fitting is a problem. Complications of vertebroplasty or kyphoplasty can include infection, bleeding, fracture (in the treated or adjacent vertebrae), and systemic issues such as embolism. Cement leaks into surrounding tissues with spinal cord, spinal nerve, or vascular compression can occur [36]. Surgery can result in many complications, not only from general anesthesia risks but also from infection, bleeding, or thromboembolism. Poor mechanical strength of bone, as in osteoporosis with paucity of dense lamellar and cortical bone, may result in suboptimal surgical outcome.

Acknowledgments

The author thanks Dr. Kent Thielen for use of the case study; Sara Harstad for orthotic modeling; and Pamela Harders for secretarial support.

References

[1] Bezel E, Stillerman C. The thoracic spine. St. Louis: Quality Medical Publishers; 1999, p. 20.
[2] Toh E, Yerby S, Bay B. The behavior of thoracic trabecular bone during flexion. J Exp Clin Med 2005;30:163–70.
[3] Toyone T, Tanaka T, Wada Y, Kamikawa K. Changes in vertebral wedging rate between supine and standing position and its association with back pain: a prospective study in patients with osteoporotic vertebral compression fractures. Spine 2006;31:2963–6.
[4] Kesson M, Atkins E. The thoracic spine. In: Kesson M, Atkins E, editors. Orthopaedic medicine: a practical approach. Boston: Butterworth-Heinemann; 1998. p. 262–81.
[5] McRae R. The thoracic and lumbar spine. In: Parkinson M, editor. Pocketbook of orthopaedics and fractures, vol 1. London: Churchill Livingstone/Harcourt; 1999. p. 79–105.
[6] Dandy D, Edwards D. Disorders of the spine. In: Dandy D, Edwards D, editors. Essential orthopaedics and trauma. New York: Churchill Livingstone; 1998. p. 431–51.
[7] Qaseem A, Snow V, Shekelle P, et al. Pharmacologic treatment of low bone density or osteoporosis to prevent fractures: a clinical practice guideline from the American College of Physicians. Ann Intern Med 2008;149:404–15.
[8] Marshall D, Johnell O, Wedel H. Meta-analysis of how well measures of bone mineral density predict occurrence of osteoporotic fractures. BMJ 1996;18:1254–9.
[9] Bonner F, Chesnut C, Fitzsimmons A, Lindsay R. Osteoporosis. In: DeLisa J, Gans BM, editors. Rehabilitation medicine: principles and practice. 3rd ed. Philadelphia: Lippincott-Raven; 1998. p. 1453–75.
[10] Van de Velde T. Disorders of the thoracic spine: non-disc lesions. In: Ombregt L, editor. A system of orthopaedic medicine. Philadelphia: WB Saunders; 1995. p. 455–69.
[11] Errico T, Stecker S, Kostuik J. Thoracic pain syndromes. In: Frymoyer J, editor. The adult spine: principles and practices. 2nd ed. Philadelphia: Lippincott-Raven; 1997. p. 1623–37.
[12] Huston C, Pitt D, Lane C. Strategies for treating osteoporosis and its neurologic complications. Appl Neurol 2005;1.
[13] Hu S, Carlson G, Tribus C. Disorders, diseases, and injuries of the spine. In: Skinner H, editor. Current diagnosis and treatment in orthopedics. 2nd ed. New York: Lane Medical Books/McGraw-Hill; 2000. p. 177–246.
[14] Pattavina C. Diagnostic imaging. In: Hart R, editor. Handbook of orthopaedic emergencies. Philadelphia: Lippincott-Raven; 1999. p. 32–47, 116–126; 127–140.
[15] Goldstein T. Treatment of common problems of the spine. In: Goldstein T, editor. Geriatric orthopaedics: rehabilitative management of common problems. 2nd ed. Gaithersburg, Md: Aspen Publications; 1999. p. 211–32.
[16] Bisese J. Compression fracture secondary to underlying metastasis. In: Bolger E, Ramos-Englis M, editors. Spinal MRI: a teaching file approach. New York: McGraw-Hill; 1992. p. 73–129.
[17] Heller J, Pedlow F. Tumors of the spine. In: Garfin S, Vaccaro AR, editors. Orthopaedic knowledge update. Spine. Rosemont, Ill: American Academy of Orthopaedic Surgeons; 1997. p. 235–56.
[18] Levine M, Heller J. Spinal infections. In: Garfin S, Vaccaro A, editors. Orthopaedic knowledge update. Spine. Rosemont, Ill: American Academy of Orthopaedic Surgeons; 1997. p. 257–71.
[19] Kim D, Vaccaro A. Osteoporotic compression fractures of the spine; current options and considerations for treatment. Spine 2006;6:479–87.
[20] Saunders H. Spinal orthotics. In: Saunders R., editor. Evaluation, treatment and prevention of musculoskeletal disorders, vol. 1. Bloomington, Minn: Educational Opportunities; 1993. p. 285–96.
[21] Bussel M, Merritt J, Fenwick L. Spinal orthoses. In: Redford J, editor. Orthotics clinical practice and rehabilitation technology. New York: Churchill Livingstone; 1995. p. 71–101.
[22] Khosla S, Bilezikian J, Dempster D, et al. Benefits and risks of bisphosphonate therapy for osteoporosis. J Clin Endocrinol Metab 2012;97:2272–82.
[23] Mura M, Drake M, Mullan R, et al. Clinical review. Comparative effectiveness of drug treatments to prevent fragility fractures: a systematic review and network meta-analysis. J Clin Endocrinol Metab 2012;97:1871–80.
[24] Brunton S, Carmichael B, Gold D. Vertebral compression fractures in primary care. J Fam Pract 2005;54:781–8.
[25] Old J, Calvert M. Vertebral compression fractures in the elderly. Am Fam Physician 2004;69:111–6.

[26] Rehabilitation of patients with osteoporosis-related fractures. Washington, DC: National Osteoporosis Foundation; 2003, p. 4.
[27] Sinaki M. Critical appraisal of physical rehabilitation measures after osteoporosis vertebral fracture. Osteoporos Int 2003;14:773–9.
[28] Browngoehl L. Osteoporosis. In: Grabois M, Garrison SJ, Hart KA, Lehmkuhl LD, editors. Physical medicine and rehabilitation: the complete approach. Malden, Mass: Blackwell Science; 2000. p. 1565–77.
[29] Eilbert W. Long-term care and rehabilitation of orthopaedic injuries. In: Hart R, Rittenberry TJ, Uehara DT, editors. Handbook of orthopaedic emergencies. Philadelphia: Lippincott-Raven; 1999. p. 127–38.
[30] Barr J, Barr M, Lemley T, McCann R. Percutaneous vertebroplasty for pain relief and spinal stabilization. Spine 2000;25:923–8.
[31] Kostuik J, Heggeness M. Surgery of the osteoporotic spine. In: Frymoyer J, editor. The adult spine: principles and practice. 2nd ed. Philadelphia: Lippincott-Raven; 1997. p. 1639–64.
[32] Kallmes D, Comstock B, Heagerty P, et al. A randomized controlled trial of vertebroplasty for osteoporotic spine fractures. N Engl J Med 2009;361:569–79.
[33] Rad A, Gray L, Sinaki M, Kallmes D. Role of physical activity in new onset fractures after percutaneous vertebroplasty. Acta Radiol 2011;52:1020–3.
[34] Buchbinder R, Osborne R, Ebeling P, et al. A randomized trial of vertebroplasty for painful osteoporotic vertebral fractures. N Engl J Med 2009;361:557–68.
[35] Snell E, Scarponc M. Orthopaedic issues in aging. In: Baratz M, Watson AD, Imbriglia JE, editors. Orthopaedic surgery: the essentials. New York: Thieme; 1999. p. 865–70.
[36] Khosla A, Diehn F, Rad A, Kallmes D. Neither subendplate cement deposition nor cement leakage into the disk space during vertebroplasty significantly affects patient outcomes. Radiology 2012;264:180–6.

CHAPTER 43

Thoracic Radiculopathy

Darren Rosenberg, DO

Daniel C. Pimentel, MD

Synonyms

Thoracic radiculitis
Thoracic disc herniation

ICD-9 Code

724.4 Thoracic or lumbosacral neuritis or radiculitis, unspecified

ICD-10 Code

M54.14 Radiculopathy, thoracic region

Definition

Thoracic radiculopathy is a painful syndrome caused by mechanical compression, chemical irritation, or metabolic abnormalities of the thoracic spinal nerve root. Thoracic disc herniation accounts for less than 5% of all disc protrusions [1,2]. It accounts for less than 2% of all spinal disc surgeries and 0.15% to 4% of all symptomatic spinal disc herniations [3]. The majority of thoracic disc herniations (35%) occur between the levels of T8 and T12, with a peak (20%) at T11-12. Most patients (90%) present clinically between the fourth and seventh decades of life; 33% present between the ages of 40 and 49 years. Approximately 33% of thoracic disc protrusions are lateral, preferentially encroaching on the spinal nerve root. The remainder are central or central lateral, resulting primarily in various degrees of spinal cord compression. Synovial cysts, although rare in the thoracic spine (0.06% of patients requiring decompressive surgery), may also be responsible for foraminal encroachment. These tend to be more common at the lower thoracic levels [4].

Natural degenerative forces and trauma are generally thought to be the most important factors in the etiology of mechanical thoracic radiculopathy. Foraminal stenosis from bone encroachment may also cause compression of the exiting nerve root and radicular symptoms. Perhaps one of the most common metabolic causes of thoracic radiculopathy is diabetes, often resulting in multilevel disease [4]. This may occur at any age but often appears with other neuropathic symptoms due to injury to the blood supply to the nerve root. Finally, another etiology that should be considered a possible cause of thoracic radiculopathy is neoplastic compression. Primary spine tumors are rare, although the spine is a frequent metastasis site (4%-15%) of primary solid tumors, such as breast, lung, and prostate cancer [5]. Regarding spine metastasis, the thoracic spine is the most commonly affected (70%), followed by lumbar (20%) and cervical (10%) [6].

Symptoms

Most patients (67%) present with complaints of "band-like" chest pain (Fig. 43.1). The second most common symptom (16%) is lower extremity pain [7]. Injury to nerve roots T2-3 may be manifested as axillary or midscapular pain. Injury to nerve roots T7-12 may be manifested as abdominal pain [8]. Unlike thoracic radiculopathy, spinal cord compression produces upper motor neuron signs and symptoms consistent with myelopathy. Therefore examiners should pay close attention to the presence of motor impairment, hyperreflexia and spasticity, sensory impairment, and bowel and bladder dysfunction. The last may be caused by T11-12 lesions damaging the conus medullaris or cauda equina [9].

Thus, in thoracic radiculopathy, pain—localized, axial, or radicular—is the primary complaint in 76% of patients. It is also important to include in the history any trauma (present in 37% of patients) [10] or risk factors for nonneurologic causes of chest wall or abdominal pain. Thoracic compression fractures that may mimic the symptoms of thoracic radiculopathy may be seen in young people with acute trauma, particularly falls, regardless of whether they land on their feet. In older people (particularly women with a history of osteopenia or osteoporosis) or in individuals who have prolonged history of steroid use, a compression fracture should be considered. Because thoracic radiculopathy is not common, it is important in nontraumatic cases to be suspicious of more serious pathologic processes, such as malignant disease. Therefore a history of weight loss, decreased appetite, and previous malignant disease should be elicited.

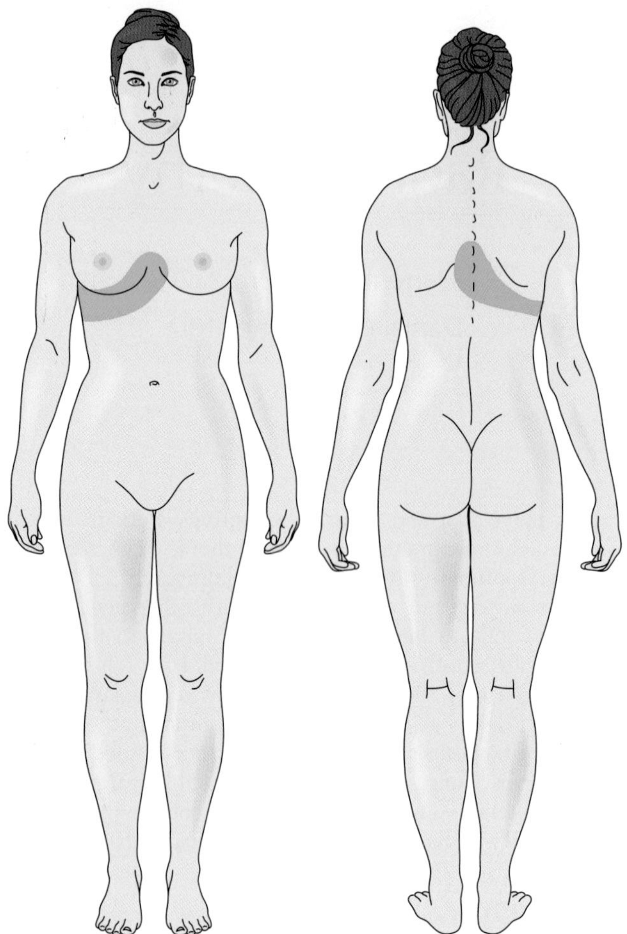

FIGURE 43.1 Typical pain pattern in a thoracic radiculopathy.

Physical Examination

The physical examination may show only limitations of range of motion—particularly trunk rotation, flexion, and extension—generally due to pain. In traumatic cases, location of ecchymosis or abrasions should be noted. Range of motion testing should not be done repeatedly if an acute spinal fracture is suspected. Careful palpation for tenderness over the thoracic spinous and transverse processes as well as over the ribs and intercostal spaces is critical in localizing the involved level. Pain with percussion over the vertebral bodies should alert the clinician to the possibility of a vertebral fracture.

On the other hand, uncommon symptoms in the lower limbs, such as pain, reflex changes, spasticity, and weakness, can be a result of spinal cord compression by thoracic disc herniation [11], although this phenomenon is seldom observed.

Physical examination in diagnosis of thoracic radiculopathy has a modest accuracy and reliability because there is difficulty in testing strength of possibly affected muscles (such as paraspinal, intercostal, and abdominal muscles) isolatedly [12], although it is crucial for ruling out other possible causes of pain or neurologic abnormalities. In addition, sensation may be abnormal in a dermatomal pattern. This will direct the examiner to more closely evaluate the involved level. Any abnormalities of the spine should be noted, including scoliosis, which is best detected when the patient flexes forward. A thorough examination of the cardiopulmonary system, abdominal organs, and skin should be performed, particularly in individuals who have sustained trauma or relevant comorbidities.

Functional Limitations

The pain produced by thoracic radiculopathy often limits an individual's movement and activity. Patients may be limited in activities such as dressing and bathing and other activities that include trunk movements, such as putting on shoes. Work activities may be restricted, such as lifting, climbing, and stooping. Even sedentary workers may be so uncomfortable that they are not able to perform their jobs. Anorexia may result from pain in the abdominal region.

Diagnostic Studies

Because of the low incidence of thoracic radiculopathy and the possibility of serious disease (e.g., tumor), the clinician should have a low threshold for ordering imaging studies in patients with persistent (more than 2 to 4 weeks) thoracic pain of unknown origin. Magnetic resonance imaging remains the imaging study of choice to evaluate the soft tissue structures of the thoracic spine. Computed tomography and computed tomographic myelography are alternatives if magnetic resonance imaging cannot be obtained.

The electromyographic evaluation of thoracic radiculopathy can be challenging because of the limited techniques available and the lack of easily accessible muscles representing a myotomal nerve root distribution. The muscles most commonly tested are the paraspinals, intercostals, and abdominals. The clinician must investigate multiple levels of the thoracic spine to best localize the lesion. Techniques for intercostal somatosensory evoked potentials have also been shown to isolate individual nerve root levels [8].

In patients who have sustained trauma, plain radiographs are advised to rule out fractures and spinal instability.

Differential Diagnosis

SPINAL DIAGNOSES

Compression fracture
Malignant neoplasm (primary or metastatic)
Pott disease (tuberculosis of the spine)

EXTRASPINAL DIAGNOSES

Intercostal neuralgia
Postherpetic neuralgia
Myofascial trigger point
Enthesopathy (ligament or tendon)
Costovertebral joint dysfunction
Costotransverse ligament sprain
Rib fracture
Angina
Myocardial infarction
Aortic aneurysm
Cholecystitis
Pyelonephritis
Peptic ulcer disease
Esophageal disorders
Mastalgia
Pleuritis
Pulmonary embolism
Adiposis dolorosa

Treatment

Initial

Pain control is important early in the disease course. Patients should be advised to avoid activities that cause increased pain and to avoid heavy lifting. Nonsteroidal anti-inflammatory drugs are often the first line of treatment and help control pain and inflammation. Oral steroids can be powerful anti-inflammatory medications and are typically used in the acute stages. This is generally done by starting at a moderate to high dose and tapering during several days. For example, a methylprednisolone (Medrol) dose pack is a prepackaged prescription that contains 21 pills. Each pill is 4 mg of Solu-Medrol. The pills are taken during the course of 6 days. On the first day, six tablets are taken, and then the dose is decreased by one pill each day. Both non-narcotic and narcotic analgesics may be used to control pain. In subacute or chronic cases, other medications may be tried, such as tricyclic antidepressants and anticonvulsants (e.g., gabapentin and carbamazepine), which have been effective in treating symptoms of neuropathic origin [13,14]. Moist heat or ice can be used, as tolerated, for pain. Transcutaneous electrical nerve stimulation units may also help with pain [15].

Rehabilitation

Physical therapy can be used initially to assist with pain control. Modalities such as ultrasound and electrical stimulation may reduce pain and improve mobility [16]. Physical therapy can then progress with spine stabilization exercises, back and abdominal strengthening [17], and a trial of mechanical spine traction [18]. Some patients may benefit from a thoracolumbar brace to reduce segmental spine movement [19], although it should be carefully used because of possible postural muscle weakness that can result from its long-term use. Patients with significant spinal instability documented by imaging studies should be referred to a spine surgeon.

In addition, physical therapy should address postural retraining, particularly for individuals with habitually poor posture. Work sites can be evaluated, if indicated. All sedentary workers should be counseled on proper seating, including use of a well-fitting adjustable chair with a lumbar support. More active workers should be advised on appropriate lifting techniques and avoidance of unnecessary trunk rotation.

Finally, physical therapy can focus on improving biomechanical factors that may play a role in abnormal loads on the thoracic spine. These include flexibility exercises for tight hamstring muscles and orthotics for pes planus (flat feet).

Procedures

Transforaminal injections can have both diagnostic and therapeutic purposes [20]. They have been shown to significantly reduce radiating pain [21]. This is done under fluoroscopic guidance to minimize risk of injury to the lung and to ensure the accuracy of the level of injection.

Surgery

Thoracoscopic microsurgical excision of herniated thoracic discs has been shown to have excellent outcomes with less surgical time, less blood loss, fewer postoperative complications, and shorter hospitalizations than more traditional and invasive surgical approaches [22,23]. Traditionally, mechanical causes of thoracic radiculopathy have been treated with posterior laminectomy, lateral costotransversectomy, or anterior discectomy by a transthoracic approach. In a cohort study with 167 patients who underwent thoracoscopic discectomy, 79% reported a good or excellent outcome regarding pain improvement, and 80% reported good or excellent outcome for motor function [24].

Potential Disease Complications

If it is left untreated, thoracic radiculopathy can result in chronic pain and its associated comorbidities. Progressive thoracic spinal cord compression, if unrecognized, can lead to paraparesis, neurogenic bowel and bladder, and spasticity.

Potential Treatment Complications

Analgesics and nonsteroidal anti-inflammatory drugs have well-known side effects that most commonly affect the gastric, hepatic, and renal systems. Care should be taken with use of steroids in diabetic patients because they may elevate blood glucose levels. In patients with uncontrolled diabetes who present with thoracic radiculopathy, glucose control should be attempted, although extremely elevated serum glucose levels have not been proved to cause the diabetic form of thoracic radiculopathy. Because of the risk of gastric ulceration, steroids are not typically used simultaneously with nonsteroidal anti-inflammatory drugs. Rarely, short-term oral steroid use may produce avascular necrosis of the hip. Tricyclic antidepressants may cause dry mouth and urinary retention. Along with anticonvulsants, they may also cause sedation. On occasion, physical therapy may exacerbate symptoms. The risks of invasive pain procedures and surgery, including bleeding, infection, and further neurologic compromise, are well documented.

References

[1] Arce CA, Dohrmann GJ. Herniated thoracic disks. Neurol Clin 1985;3:383–92.

[2] Brown CW, Deffer Jr PA, Akmakjian J, et al. The natural history of thoracic disc herniation. Spine (Phila Pa 1976) 1992;17:S97–102.

[3] Leininger B, Bronfort G, Evans R, Reiter T. Spinal manipulation or mobilization for radiculopathy: a systematic review. Phys Med Rehabil Clin N Am 2011;22:105–25.

[4] Cohen-Gadol AA, White JB, Lynch JJ, et al. Synovial cysts of the thoracic spine. J Neurosurg Spine 2004;1:52–7.

[5] Hayat MJ, Howlader N, Reichman ME, Edwards BK. Cancer statistics, trends, and multiple primary cancer analyses from the Surveillance, Epidemiology, and End Results (SEER) Program. Oncologist 2007;12:20–37.

[6] Spinazze S, Caraceni A, Schrijvers D. Epidural spinal cord compression. Crit Rev Oncol Hematol 2005;56:397–406.

[7] Bicknell J, Johnson S. Widespread electromyographic abnormalities in spinal muscles in cancer, disc disease, and diabetes. Univ Mich Med Center J 1976;42:124–7.

[8] Rubin DI, Shuster EA. Axillary pain as a heralding sign of neoplasm involving the upper thoracic root. Neurology 2006;66:1760–2.

[9] Tokuhashi Y, Matsuzaki H, Uematsu Y, Oda H. Symptoms of thoracolumbar junction disc herniation. Spine (Phila Pa 1976) 2001;26:E512–8.

[10] Stillerman CB, Chen TC, Couldwell WT, et al. Experience in the surgical management of 82 symptomatic herniated thoracic discs and review of the literature. J Neurosurg 1998;88:623–33.
[11] Ueda Y, Kawahara N, Murakami H, et al. Thoracic disk herniation with paraparesis treated with transthoracic microdiskectomy in a 14-year-old girl. Orthopedics 2012;35:e774–7.
[12] O'Connor RC, Andary MT, Russo RB, DeLano M. Thoracic radiculopathy. Phys Med Rehabil Clin N Am 2002;13:623–44, viii.
[13] Kasimcan O, Kaptan H. Efficacy of gabapentin for radiculopathy caused by lumbar spinal stenosis and lumbar disk hernia. Neurol Med Chir (Tokyo) 2010;50:1070–3.
[14] Selph S, Carson S, Fu R, et al. Drug class review: neuropathic pain: final update 1 report [Internet]. Drug Class Reviews 2011;.
[15] Plastaras CT, Schran S, Kim N, et al. Complementary and alternative treatment for neck pain: chiropractic, acupuncture, TENS, massage, yoga, Tai Chi, and Feldenkrais. Phys Med Rehabil Clin N Am 2011;22:521–37.
[16] Iversen MD. Rehabilitation interventions for pain and disability in osteoarthritis. Am J Nurs 2012;112:S32–7.
[17] Kennedy DJ, Noh MY. The role of core stabilization in lumbosacral radiculopathy. Phys Med Rehabil Clin N Am 2011;22:91–103.
[18] Hahne AJ, Ford JJ, McMeeken JM. Conservative management of lumbar disc herniation with associated radiculopathy: a systematic review. Spine (Phila Pa 1976) 2010;35:E488–504.
[19] Agabegi SS, Asghar FA, Herkowitz HN. Spinal orthoses. J Am Acad Orthop Surg 2010;18:657–67.
[20] Manchikanti L, Boswell MV, Singh V, et al. Comprehensive evidence-based guidelines for interventional techniques in the management of chronic spinal pain. Pain Physician 2009;12:699–802.
[21] Richardson J, Jones J, Atkinson R. The effect of thoracic paravertebral blockade on intercostal somatosensory evoked potentials. Anesth Analg 1998;87:373–6.
[22] Wait SD, Fox Jr DJ, Kenny KJ, Dickman CA. Thoracoscopic resection of symptomatic herniated thoracic discs: clinical results in 121 patients. Spine (Phila Pa 1976) 2012;37:35–40.
[23] Rosenthal D, Dickman CA. Thoracoscopic microsurgical excision of herniated thoracic discs. J Neurosurg 1998;89:224–35.
[24] Quint U, Bordon G, Preissl I, et al. Thoracoscopic treatment for single level symptomatic thoracic disc herniation: a prospective followed cohort study in a group of 167 consecutive cases. Eur Spine J 2012;21:637–45.

CHAPTER 44

Thoracic Sprain or Strain

Darren Rosenberg, DO

Daniel C. Pimentel, MD

Synonyms

Thoracic sprain
Pulled upper back
Benign thoracic pain

ICD-9 Codes

721.2 Thoracic spondylosis, aggravated
724.1 Thoracalgia (thoracic–mid back pain)
847.1 Sprains and strains of other unspecified parts of back (thoracic)
847.2 Thoracic strain

ICD-10 Codes

M47.814 Spondylosis, thoracic region
M54.6 Pain in thoracic spine
S23.3 Sprain of the thoracic spine
S39.012 Strain of muscle, fascia and tendon of lower back

Definition

Thoracic strain or sprain refers to the acute or subacute onset of pain in the region of the thoracic spine due to soft tissue injury, including muscles, ligaments, tendons, and fascia, of an otherwise normal back. Sprain relates to injury in ligament fibers without total rupture, whereas strain is an overstretching or overexertion of some part of the musculature [1]. Because the thoracic cage is unified by the overlying fascia, thoracic sprain or strain can translate into pain throughout the thoracic spine.

Epidemiology

Although the scientific literature on musculoskeletal pain in the cervical and lumbar spine is abundant, similar information about the thoracic region is sparse because of its lower prevalence [2]. The lifetime prevalence in the general population of having a musculoskeletal complaint in the thoracic spine is 17% in contrast to 57% in the low back and 40% in the neck [3]. Therefore observation and characterization of such lesions are minimal, subsequently limiting the potential to improve treatment methods for thoracic sprain and strain disorders. Moreover, pain felt in the thoracic spine is often referred from the cervical spine, mistakenly giving the impression that the incidence is higher [4].

Thoracic strain or sprain may be the indirect result of disc lesions, which have been reported to be evenly distributed in incidence between the sexes and are most common in patients from the fourth to sixth decades of life [5]. Muscles adjacent to the injured disc tend to become tight in response to the local inflammatory process, which may jeopardize the local muscle equilibrium, possibly leading to ligament strains and muscle sprains in the thoracic region. Other structures that may lead to strain or sprain in the mid back due to the same inflammatory rationale are the thoracic facet joints and the nerve roots [6].

As with most nonspecific mechanical disorders of the cervical and lumbar regions, the natural history of the majority of patients with nonspecific thoracic strain or sprain is resolution within 1 to 6 months [7].

Mechanisms

The thoracic spine is considered to be the least mobile area of the vertebral column secondary to the length of the transverse processes, the presence of costovertebral joints, the decrease in disc height compared with the lumbar spine, and the presence of the rib cage. Movements that occur in the thoracic spine include rotation with flexion or extension.

Thoracic sprain and strain injuries can occur in all age groups, but there is an increased prevalence among patients of working age [8]. Intrinsic mechanisms include bone disease as well as alteration of normal spine or upper extremity biomechanics. This includes cervical or thoracic deformity from neuromuscular or spinal disease as well as shoulder or scapular dysfunction. The most common intrinsic cause of thoracic strain, however, is poor posture or excessive sitting. Poor posture may be related to development of Scheuermann disease in the young and osteoporosis in the elderly that leads to kyphosis and compression deformities seen in those patients.

Poor posture is often manifested as excessive protraction or drooping of the neck and shoulders as well as decreased lumbar lordosis or "flat back." With the classic "slouched position" encountered in children and adolescents and often carried on through adulthood, there is excessive flexion of the thoracic spine with a decrease in rotation and extension.

Postural alterations promote increased thoracic kyphosis, resulting in the "flexed posture." Excessive flexion results in excessive strain on the "core," including the small intrinsic muscles of the spine, the long paraspinal muscles, and the abdominal and rib cage muscles. Excessive flexion can increase the risk of rib stress fractures as well as costovertebral joint irritation. This can cause referral of pain to the chest wall with subsequent development of trigger points in the erector spinae, levator scapulae, rhomboids, trapezius, and latissimus dorsi. Poor motion in extension and rotation can place an increased load on nearby structures, such as the lumbar or cervical spine and shoulders.

Extrinsic or environmental mechanisms include repetitive strain, trauma, and obesity. Risk factors include occupational and recreational activities characterized by repetitive motions, such as lifting, twisting, and bending. Occupations requiring manual labor or extended periods in a sitting position are predisposed to a higher incidence of such disorders [9]. Traumatic causes include falls, violence, and accidents leading to vertebral fractures, chest wall contusions, or flail chest.

Symptoms

Patients typically report pain in the mid back, which may be related to upper extremity or neck movements. Symptoms may be exacerbated by deep breathing, coughing, rotation of the thoracic spine, or prolonged standing or sitting. The pain can be generalized in the mid back area or focal. If it is focal, it is usually described as a "knot," which is deep and aching. It may radiate to the anterior chest wall, abdomen, upper limb, cervical spine, or lumbosacral spine and may be accentuated with movement of the upper extremity or neck. As described by McKenzie [4], the location of pain in mechanical disorders of the thoracic spine is either central (symmetric) or unilateral (asymmetric).

Other symptoms include muscle spasm, tightness, and stiffness as well as pain or decreased range of motion in the mid back, low back, neck, or shoulder.

Physical Examination

The essential finding in the physical examination of thoracic sprain or strain is thoracic muscle spasm with normal neurologic examination findings. Pain may be exacerbated when the patient lifts the arms overhead, extends backward, or rotates. Rib motion may be restricted and may be assessed by examining excursion of the chest wall. This is accomplished by laying hands on the upper and lower chest wall and looking for symmetry and rhythm of movement. The upper ribs usually move in a bucket-handle motion, whereas the lower ribs move in a pump-handle motion. Restriction of specific ribs can be assessed by examining individual rib movements with respiration.

The position of comfort is usually flexion, but this is the position that should be avoided. Sensation and reflex examination findings should be normal. A finding of lower extremity weakness or neurologic deficit on physical examination suggests an alternative diagnosis and may warrant further investigation [10].

As the thoracic cage and spine are the anchors for the upper limbs, the thoracic spine influences and is influenced by active and resisted movement of the extremities, cranium, and lumbar and cervical spine [11]. Therefore, a careful spinal and shoulder examination is essential to rule out restrictive movements, obvious deformity, soft tissue asymmetry, and skin changes (that may be seen in infection or tumor). Detailed examination of other organ systems is important because thoracic pain can be referred.

Examination includes static and dynamic assessment of posture. The patient should be observed in relaxed stance with the shirt removed. Viewing is from the posterior, lateral, and anterior perspectives, and deviations from an ideal posture are noted [11]. With dynamic assessment, it is important to provoke the patient's symptoms by moving and stressing the structures from which pain is thought to originate.

In addition, the presence of deformities and the site of pain and tenderness are noted. Pain is often felt between the scapulae, around the lower border of the scapula, and centrally in the area between T1 and T7. Much of the pain felt in the thoracic area, however, has been shown to originate in the cervical spine. Pain in the region above an imaginary line drawn between the inferior borders of the scapulae is most likely secondary to the cervical region, mainly lower cervical facet joints [12].

Functional Limitations

Functional limitations include difficulty with bending, lifting, and overhead activities, such as throwing and reaching. These limitations affect both active and sedentary workers. Activities of daily living, such as upper extremity bathing and dressing, might be affected. General mobility may be impaired. As most sports-related or leisure activities involve use of the upper extremity, extension, or rotation of the thorax, athletic participation and functional capacity may be limited as well.

Diagnostic Studies

Thoracic sprain and strain injuries are typically diagnosed on the basis of the history and physical examination. No tests are usually necessary during the first 4 weeks of symptoms if the injury is nontraumatic. If there is suspicion of tumor (night pain, constitutional symptoms), infection (fever, chills, malaise), or fracture (focal tenderness with history of trauma or fall), earlier and more complete investigation is warranted.

Plain films are indicated as an initial image diagnostic approach if the injury is associated with recent trauma or malignant disease. Magnetic resonance imaging is the study of choice in considering thoracic malignant neoplasia and osteoporotic compression fracture or when the patient has unilateral localized thoracic pain with sensory-motor deficits to rule out a thoracic disc herniation with consequent radiculopathy [13]. A computed tomographic scan or triple-phase bone scan can identify bone abnormalities if magnetic resonance imaging is contraindicated. Magnetic resonance imaging, however, can detect abnormalities unrelated to the patient's symptoms because many people who do not have pain have abnormal imaging findings [14]. This fact emphasizes the importance of a meticulous clinical evaluation of patients with thoracic pain.

Differential Diagnosis

SPINAL DIAGNOSES
Thoracic radiculopathy
Facet joint arthropathy
Structural rib dysfunction
Spinal stenosis
Scheuermann disease
Ankylosing spondylosis
Discitis
Vertebral fracture (trauma, insufficiency, pathologic)
Scoliosis or kyphosis

EXTRASPINAL DIAGNOSES
Peptic ulcer disease
Pancreatitis
Cholecystitis
Nephrolithiasis
Shingles

Treatment

Initial

The initial treatment of a thoracic sprain or strain injury generally involves the use of cold packs to decrease pain and edema during the first 48 hours after the injury. Thereafter, the application of moist heat to reduce pain and muscle spasm is indicated. Bed rest for up to 48 hours may be beneficial, but prolonged bed rest is discouraged because it can lead to muscle weakness. Relative rest by avoidance of activities that exacerbate pain is preferable to complete bed rest. Temporary use of a rib binder or elastic wrap may reduce pain as well as increase activity tolerance and mobility. A short course of nonsteroidal anti-inflammatory drugs, acetaminophen, muscle relaxants, or topical anesthetics such as Lidoderm patches may be beneficial. Narcotics are generally not necessary.

Rehabilitation

Most acute thoracic sprain or strain injuries will heal spontaneously with rest and physical modalities used at home, such as ice, heating pad, and massage. Body mechanics and postural training are important aspects of the rehabilitation program for thoracic sprain or strain [15,16]. A focus on correct posture at work, at leisure, and while driving is important. In the car, patients can use a lumbar roll to promote proper posture; at work, patients are advised to sit upright at the computer in an adjustable, comfortable chair with an adequate monitor adjustment. The monitor should be adjusted to be aligned with the keyboard and in a height that aligns the first row of text with eye level. Finally, the correct depth should be achieved in a way that the user does not need to lean forward to comfortably read [17]. Other workplace modifications include forearm seat rests to support the arms, foot rests, and the use of a telephone earpiece or headset to prevent neck and upper thoracic strain.

For patients with abnormally flexed or slouched posture, household modifications can be made that might help encourage extension and subsequently decrease pain. These include pillows or lumbar rolls on chairs and replacement of sagging mattresses with firm bedding. Also, use of paper plates and lightweight cookware in the kitchen and reassignment of objects in overhead cabinets to areas that are more accessible can help if lifting or reaching is painful.

If pain persists beyond a couple of weeks, physical therapy may be indicated. In general, physical therapy will apply movements that centralize, reduce, or diminish the patient's symptoms while discouraging movements that peripheralize or increase the patient's symptoms [4]. In most cases, an active approach that encourages stretching and strengthening exercises is preferred to a more passive approach. To correct sitting posture, patients are advised to continue to use the lumbar roll in all sitting environments. To correct standing posture, patients are shown how to normalize lumbar curvature and to move the lower part of the spine backward while at the same time moving the upper spine forward, raising the chest and retracting the head and neck. To correct lying posture, patients should use a firm mattress as previously indicated. In the case of patients who experience more pain in the thoracic spine when lying in bed, this advice often leads to worsening of the symptoms rather than a resolution. In these patients, advice should be given to deliberately sag the mattress by placing pillows under each end of the mattress so that it becomes dished. In this manner, the thoracic kyphosis is not forced into the extended range in lying supine, and the removal of this stress allows a comfortable night's sleep. Long-term goals, however, still include improvement in extension range of motion [4].

After a formal physical therapy program is completed, a home exercise or gym regimen is essential and should be prescribed and individualized for all patients to maintain gains made during physical therapy. Exercises at home are aimed at improvement in flexibility of the thoracic spine and may include extension in lying, standing, and sitting performed six to eight times throughout the day. In addition, alternating arm and leg lifts and active trunk extension in the prone position should be performed. Finally, regular stretching to improve extension and rotation with trigger pointing can decrease muscle tension over the affected muscles. A thoracic wedge, which is designed to increase extension range of motion, can be used. The wedge is a hard piece of molded plastic or rubber with a wedge cut out to accommodate the spine. The patient lies on the ground with the wedge placed in between the shoulder blades. The patient is instructed to arch over it. Alternatively, two tennis balls can be taped together for the same effect. These exercises can be done before regular stretching to increase excursion. Regular massage therapy can maintain flexibility and prevent tightening from more regular exercise.

At the gym, progressive dynamic movements such as rowing, latissimus pull-downs, pull-ups, and an abdominal crunch strengthening program should be emphasized. Instruction in proper positioning and technique should be provided to prevent further injury. Use of a "physioball" at home or at the gym can facilitate trunk extension as well as abdominal stretching and strengthening to increase overall conditioning of the thoracic cage and core musculature. This can be done in conjunction with use of Thera-Bands with progressive resistance to facilitate stretching of the arms and shoulders with mild strengthening of the shoulder, arm, and core muscles. Finally, a pool program can be prescribed. Swimming strokes such as the crawl, backstroke, and butterfly emphasize extension and can be very useful to prevent or to correct a flexion bias. With the crawl, patients are instructed to breathe on both sides to prevent unilateral strain in the neck and upper thoracic spine.

Procedures

Trigger point injections may help reduce focal pain caused by taut bands of muscle, allowing the patient to exercise to restore range of motion, to correct postural imbalance, and to increase strength and balance of the dysfunctional segment [18]. Acupuncture can be used for local as well as for systemic treatment. Finally, botulinum toxin type A (Botox) has been used for specific muscles, including rhomboids, trapezius, levator scapulae, and serratus, that often contribute to thoracic strain and sprain.

Although there are no studies specifically looking at the use of botulinum toxin type A for treatment of thoracic strain, there are studies that looked at treatment of regional myofascial pain disorders. One study showed effective pain relief for generalized myofascial pain syndrome [19]. In another study, there was no statistically significant improvement in pain with direct trigger point injections of patients with cervicothoracic myofascial pain syndrome [20]. A recent comprehensive review found inconclusive evidence on the use of botulinum toxin type A for muscle treatment, although some encouraging data are available [21].

Another possible treatment of myofascial pain syndrome that can be applied in thoracic sprain or strain cases is extracorporeal shock wave therapy. This may be an effective alternative to needling or medication infusion [22].

Surgery

Surgery is not usually indicated unless focal disc herniation with neurologic abnormalities such as radiculopathy (see Chapter 43) has occurred or there is instability of particular spinal segments from fracture or dislocation.

Potential Disease Complications

Thoracic sprain and strain injuries can occasionally develop into myofascial pain syndromes.

Potential Treatment Complications

Possible complications include gastrointestinal side effects from nonsteroidal anti-inflammatory drugs. Other possible complications include somnolence or confusion from muscle relaxants; addiction from narcotics; bleeding, infection, postinjection soreness, and pneumothorax from trigger point injections; excessive weakness and development of antibodies from botulinum toxin; and temporary post-treatment exacerbation of pain from manual medicine or extracorporeal shock wave therapy [23].

References

[1] Sprains and strains, MeSH (Medical Subject Headings). National Center for Biotechnology Information, U.S. National Library of Medicine; 2012. Available at http://www.ncbi.nlm.nih.gov/mesh/68013180 [accessed 2012].

[2] Edmondston SJ, Singer KP. Thoracic spine: anatomical and biomechanical considerations for manual therapy. Man Ther 1997;2:132–43.

[3] Leboeuf-Yde C, Nielsen J, Kyvik KO, et al. Pain in the lumbar, thoracic or cervical regions: do age and gender matter? A population-based study of 34,902 Danish twins 20-71 years of age. BMC Musculoskelet Disord 2009;10:39.

[4] McKenzie RA. The cervical and thoracic spine: mechanical diagnosis and therapy. Waikanae, NZ: Spinal Publications Ltd; 1990.

[5] Love JG, Schorn VG. Thoracic-disk protrusions. JAMA 1965;191:627–31.

[6] Manchikanti L, Helm S, Singh V, et al. An algorithmic approach for clinical management of chronic spinal pain. Pain Physician 2009;12:E225–64.

[7] Malmivaara A, Hakkinen U, Aro T, et al. The treatment of acute low back pain—bed rest, exercises, or ordinary activity? N Engl J Med 1995;332:351–5.

[8] Choi BC, Levitsky M, Lloyd RD, Stones IM. Patterns and risk factors for sprains and strain in Ontario, Canada 1990: an analysis of the Workplace Health and Safety Agency data base. J Occup Environ Med 1996;38:379–89.

[9] Manchikanti L, Singh V, Datta S, et al. Comprehensive review of epidemiology, scope, and impact of spinal pain. Pain Physician 2009;12:E35–70.

[10] Acute low back problems in adults: assessment and treatment. Acute Low Back Problems Guideline Panel. Agency for Health Care Policy and Research. Am Fam Physician 1995;51:469–84.

[11] Kendall FP, McCreary EK, Provance PG. Muscles: testing and function. 4th ed. Philadelphia: Lippincott Williams & Wilkins; 1993.

[12] Isaac Z, Slipman CW. Cervical radicular pain: an algorithmic methodology. In: Slipman CW, Derby R, Simeone FA, Mayer TG, editors. Interventional spine: an algorithmic approach. Philadelphia: Saunders Elsevier; 2008. p. 613–5.

[13] Dietze Jr DD, Fessler RG. Thoracic disc herniations. Neurosurg Clin N Am 1993;4:75–90.

[14] Wood KB, Garvey TA, Gundry C, Heithoff KB. Magnetic resonance imaging of the thoracic spine. Evaluation of asymptomatic individuals. J Bone Joint Surg Am 1995;77:1631–8.

[15] Richmond J. Multi-factorial causative model for back pain management; relating causative factors and mechanisms to injury presentations and designing time- and cost effective treatment thereof. Med Hypotheses 2012;79:232–40.

[16] Guccione AA. Physical therapy for musculoskeletal syndromes. Rheum Dis Clin North Am 1996;22:551–62.

[17] Bleecker ML, Celio MA, Barnes SK. A medical-ergonomic program for symptomatic keyboard/mouse users. J Occup Environ Med 2011;53:562–8.

[18] Hong CZ. New trends in myofascial pain syndrome. Zhonghua Yi Xue Za Zhi (Taipei) 2002;65:501–12.

[19] Graboski CL, Gray DS, Burnham RS. Botulinum toxin A versus bupivacaine trigger point injections for the treatment of myofascial pain syndrome: a randomised double blind crossover study. Pain 2005;118:170–5.

[20] Ferrante FM, Bearn L, Rothrock R, King L. Evidence against trigger point injection technique for the treatment of cervicothoracic myofascial pain with botulinum toxin type A. Anesthesiology 2005;103:377–83.

[21] Soares A, Andriolo RB, Atallah AN, da Silva EM. Botulinum toxin for myofascial pain syndromes in adults. Cochrane Database Syst Rev 2012;4: CD007533.

[22] Gleitz M, Hornig K. Trigger points—diagnosis and treatment concepts with special reference to extracorporeal shockwaves. Orthopade 2012;41:113–25.

[23] Rompe JD, Segal NA, Cacchio A, et al. Home training, local corticosteroid injection, or radial shock wave therapy for greater trochanter pain syndrome. Am J Sports Med 2009;37:1981–90.

SECTION VI
Low Back

CHAPTER 45

Lumbar Degenerative Disease

Michael K. Schaufele, MD
Jordan L. Tate, MD, MPH

Synonyms

Osteoarthritis of the spine
Spondylosis
Lumbar arthritis
Degenerative joint disease of the spine
Degenerative disc disease

ICD-9 Codes

721.3 **Lumbosacral spondylosis without myelopathy**
721.90 **Spondylosis of unspecified site (spinal arthritis)**
722.52 **Degeneration of lumbar or lumbosacral intervertebral disc**
724.2 **Low back pain**

ICD-10 Codes

M47.817 **Spondylosis without myelopathy or radiculopathy, lumbosacral region**
M47.899 **Other spondylosis, site unspecified**
M51.36 **Other intervertebral disc degeneration, lumbar region**
M51.37 **Other intervertebral disc degeneration, lumbosacral region**
M54.5 **Low back pain**

Definition

Degeneration of the anatomic structures of the lumbar spine is a process associated with aging. Degenerative processes may affect several anatomic structures, resulting in different clinical syndromes, or may be entirely asymptomatic. Approximately one third of asymptomatic and one half of symptomatic younger adults show degenerative changes on lumbar spine magnetic resonance imaging [1,2]. At ages older than 60 years, degenerative changes are found in more than 90% of adults [3]. Degeneration may be accelerated in patients with previous trauma or injury to the lumbar spine. Factors such as diabetes mellitus, smoking, and obesity have been associated with increased rates of lumbar spine degeneration. L4-L5 and L5-S1 are the most commonly involved lumbar levels, given that they undergo the greatest torsion and compressive loads during activity. There has not been a proven gender predominance; however, some studies suggest that disc degeneration may affect more men, whereas facet arthropathy may be more prevalent in women [4]. Genetic factors have been suggested to play a major role in determining presence and extent of spine degeneration [5]. Twin studies have shown heritabilities ranging from 52% to 68% for various lumbar disc degeneration phenotypes [6].

The intervertebral disc experiences progressive dehydration as part of the normal aging process. In certain patients, fissures in the anulus fibrosus may develop, causing an inflammatory response. Nociceptive pain fibers may grow into these fissures [7]. Further degeneration may result in progression of the disease or complete annular tears, which may be the source of discogenic low back pain, also referred to as internal disc disruption syndrome. Up to 39% of patients with chronic low back pain may suffer from internal disc disruption [8]. The loss of segmental integrity may lead to further degeneration of the disc, which results in narrowing of the intervertebral disc space. Because of increased loads on the posterior elements, facet degeneration may develop.

The facet (zygapophyseal) joints and sacroiliac joints, like other synovial joints in the body, may develop osteoarthritis [9].

Facet arthropathy may be an independent or concurrent source of low back pain. Further disc degeneration and subsequent loss of disc height may cause subluxation of the facet joints, resulting in degenerative spondylolisthesis, most commonly at the L4-L5 level [10].

Other conditions seen with lumbar degeneration include spondylosis deformans and diffuse idiopathic skeletal hyperostosis. Spondylosis deformans is a degenerative condition marked by formation of anterolateral osteophytes and is mainly a radiologic diagnosis. In spondylosis deformans, the intervertebral spaces are usually well preserved, unlike in degenerative disc disease. The initiating factor in the development of this condition may be degeneration of the anulus fibrosus, primarily in the anterolateral disc space [11]. Spondylosis deformans may become clinically symptomatic if excessive osteophyte formation leads to neural compression, such as in spinal stenosis. Diffuse idiopathic skeletal hyperostosis involves ossification of the ligamentous attachments to the vertebral bones (entheses). Radiologic features consist of multilevel excessive anterior osteophyte formation. Diffuse idiopathic skeletal hyperostosis affects 5% to 10% of patients older than 65 years [12]. This diagnosis is typically an incidental finding on radiologic studies [13].

Other factors associated with lumbar degeneration include environmental, occupational, and psychosocial influences. Environmental influences include cigarette smoking and occupational activities that involve repetitive bending and prolonged exposures to stooping, sitting, or vibrational stresses. These repetitive actions may result in degeneration of the lumbosacral motion segments [12]. Psychosocial factors are well known to contribute to significant disability in low back pain, often in patients with only minimal structural impairment [14].

Symptoms

Lumbar degenerative symptoms range from minor to debilitating. Common complaints include chronic back pain and stiffness. Patients may also report limited range of motion, especially with extension in the case of facet arthropathy or spinal stenosis. Pain with lumbar flexion, coughing, sneezing, or Valsalva maneuver is often associated with disc disease. Should the degenerative changes result in compression of neural structures, patients may develop radicular symptoms into the leg. This can be seen in conditions such as lumbar disc herniations and spinal stenosis.

Lumbar degenerative disease is probably entirely asymptomatic in the majority of cases. Approximately one third of subjects have substantial abnormalities on magnetic resonance imaging despite being clinically asymptomatic [1]. Because of factors not well understood, such as leakage of inflammatory factors from the disc, a chronic pain syndrome may develop in some patients, possibly from repetitive sensitization of nociceptive fibers in the anulus fibrosus [15].

Clinicians should inquire about atypical symptoms of back pain, including night pain, fever, and recent weight loss. These may lead to the diagnosis of malignant neoplasm or infection.

Clinicians should also inquire about symptoms of chronic pain, including sleep disturbances and depression.

Physical Examination

The purpose of the physical examination is to direct further evaluation and therapy toward one of the five most common sources of low back pain: discogenic, facet arthropathy or instability, radiculopathy or neural compression, myofascial or soft tissue, and psychogenic. Combinations of these sources of back pain often exist. A diagnosis based on physical findings will allow the use of advanced diagnostic tests and therapeutic options in the most cost-effective approach.

A standardized low back examination should include assessment of flexibility (lumbosacral flexion, extension, trunk rotation, finger-floor distance, hamstring and iliopsoas range of motion, and hip range of motion). An inclinometer (Fig. 45.1) may assist in standardizing lumbar range of motion measurements [16]. A complete examination includes inspection of lower extremities for atrophy and vascular insufficiency, muscle strength testing, and assessment for sensory abnormalities and their distribution. It is important to note asymmetries in deep tendon reflexes (patellar tendon [L4], hamstring tendon [L5], and Achilles tendon [S1]), which may be the most objective finding. Upper motor neuron signs, such as Babinski and ankle clonus, should also be tested. Functional strength testing should include heel to toe walking, calf and toe raises, single-leg knee bends, and complete gait evaluation. Specific testing for lower back

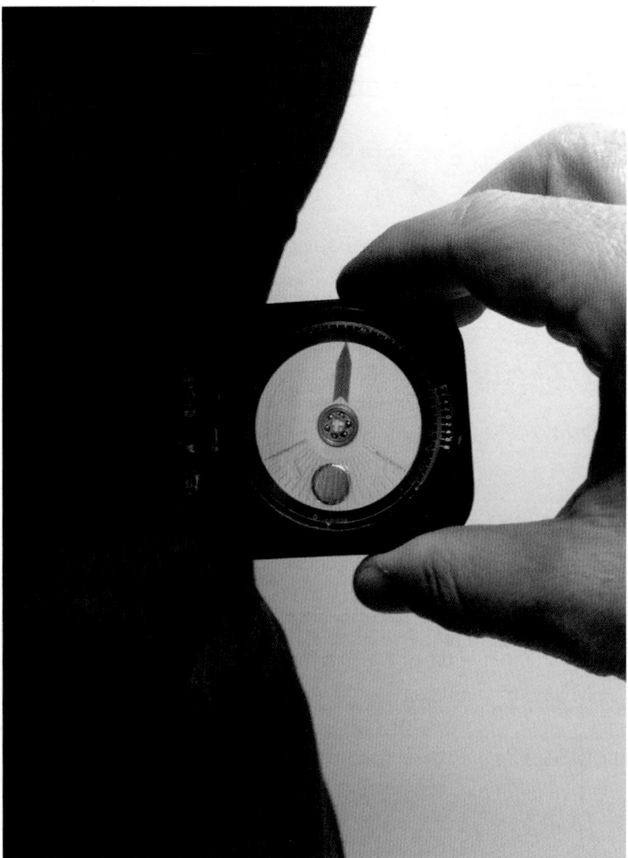

FIGURE 45.1 Inclinometers can be used for true lumbar spine range of motion measurements (neutral position demonstrated).

Table 45.1 Waddell Signs

Five nonorganic physical signs are described by Waddell.

Tenderness	Nonorganic tenderness may be either superficial or nonanatomic. Superficial tenderness can be elicited by lightly pinching over a wide area of lumbar skin. Nonanatomic pain is described as deep tenderness felt over a wide area rather than localized to one structure.
Simulation test	This is usually based on movement that produces pain. Two examples are axial loading, in which low back pain is reported on vertical loading over the standing patient's skull by the clinician's hands, and rotation, in which back pain is reported when the shoulder and pelvis are passively rotated in the same plane as the patient stands relaxed with feet together.
Distraction test	If a positive physical finding is demonstrated in a routine manner, this finding is checked while the patient's attention is distracted. Straight-leg raising is the most useful distraction test. There are several variations to this test; most commonly, however, straight-leg raise is done in the supine position and then, while the patient is distracted, in the sitting position. This is commonly referred to as the flip test. However, one should keep in mind that biomechanically, the two positions are very different.
Regional disturbances	Regional disturbances involve a widespread area, such as an entire quarter or half of the body. The essential feature of this nonorganic physical sign is divergence of the pain beyond the accepted neuroanatomy. Examples include give-away weakness in many muscle groups manually tested and sensory disturbances, such as diminished sensation to light touch, pinprick, or vibration, that do not follow a dermatomal pattern. Again, care must be taken not to mistake multiple root involvement for regional disturbance.
Overreaction	Waddell reported that overreaction during the examination may take the form of disproportionate verbalization, facial expression, muscle tension, tremor, collapsing, and even profuse sweating. Analysis of multiple nonorganic signs showed that overreaction was the single most important nonorganic physical sign. However, this sign is also the most influenced by the subjectivity of the observer.

Modified from Geraci MC Jr, Alleva JT. Physical examination of the spine and its functional kinetic chain. In Cole AJ, Herring SA, eds. The Low Back Pain Handbook. Philadelphia, Hanley & Belfus, 1997.

syndromes includes straight-leg raising, femoral stretch sign, dural tension signs, and sacroiliac joint provocative maneuvers (e.g., FABER, Gillet, Yeoman, and Gaenslen tests) as well as specific evaluation techniques, such as the McKenzie technique. Assessment of the patient for nonorganic signs of back pain (Waddell signs; Table 45.1) will help the clinician to recognize patients in whom psychological factors may contribute to the pain syndrome [17].

Functional Limitations

Functional limitations in degenerative diseases of the lumbar spine depend on the anatomic structures involved. All aspects of daily living, including self-care, work, sports activities, and recreation, may be affected.

Symptoms are typically exacerbated during bending, twisting, stooping, and forward flexion in patients with primary discogenic pain. Patients with facet arthropathy or instability report increased pain with extension-based activity, including standing and walking. Pain is often relieved with sitting and other similar forward-flexed positions. Patients with myofascial or soft tissue syndromes report pain that is worsened with static and prolonged physical activity. Symptomatic improvement may be associated with rest and modalities including heat, cold, and pressure. Patients with contributing psychological factors, such as depression and somatization disorders, typically report pain out of proportion to the underlying pathologic process, poor sleep, and significant disability in their daily activities.

Diagnostic Studies

Diagnostic testing is directed by the history and physical examination and should be ordered only if the therapeutic plan will be significantly influenced by the results. Anteroposterior and lateral lumbar spine radiographs are helpful for identifying loss of disc height as a result of disc degeneration, spondylosis or osteophyte formation, spondylolisthesis, scoliosis, and facet arthropathy (Fig. 45.2). Oblique views are helpful to identify spondylolysis. Flexion-extension films are necessary to identify dynamic instability and can assist in the selection of appropriate surgical candidates for fusion procedures. Significant degenerative instability usually does not occur before the age of 50 years, but it should be included in the differential diagnosis in patients with clinical symptoms suggestive of advanced facet arthropathy and disc degeneration [11]. Magnetic resonance imaging of the lumbar spine is used because of its sensitivity for identification of abnormalities of the soft tissues and neural structures. It is particularly helpful in identifying various stages of degenerative disc disease as well as annular tears and disc herniation. Other significant sources of back pain, such as neoplasms, osteomyelitis, and fractures, can also be identified with magnetic resonance imaging. Computed tomography is a valuable diagnostic tool in assessing fractures and other osseous abnormalities of the lumbar spine. Computed tomographic imaging in combination with myelography (computed tomographic myelography) aids in presurgical planning by allowing identification of osseous structures causing neural compression, especially in spinal stenosis.

Discography is currently the only technique to correlate structural abnormalities of the intervertebral disc seen on advanced imaging studies with a patient's pain response. Reproduction of painful symptoms with intradiscal injection of radiopaque contrast material aids in the localization of specific disc levels as pain generators and can be useful in separating painful disc degeneration from painless degeneration. Exploratory studies on blockade of the sinuvertebral nerve, which is thought to carry nociceptive sensation to the intervertebral disc, have been undertaken as an alternative means for diagnosis of discogenic pain [18]. Electrodiagnostic studies may become necessary in cases of peripheral neurologic deficits not clarified by physical examination or imaging. They allow identification of compression neuropathy, radiculopathy, or systemic motor and sensory diseases.

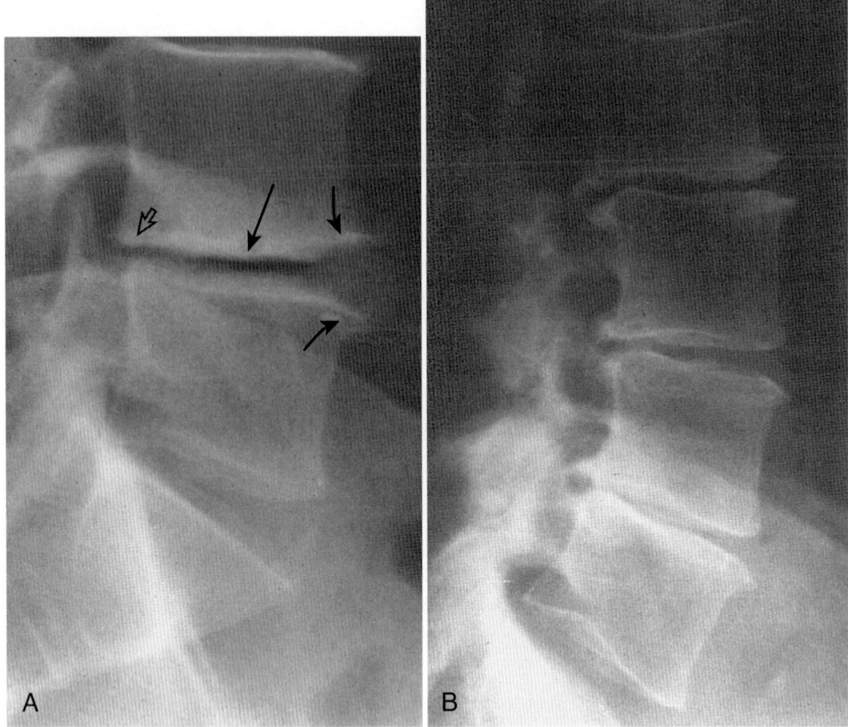

FIGURE 45.2 Chronic degenerative changes—plain film. **A,** On a coned down lateral film, the L4-5 motion segment shows a vacuum phenomenon in the disc *(large arrow),* end-plate remodeling with large anterior spurs *(curved arrows),* and grade I retrolisthesis *(open arrow).* **B,** A standing lateral film shows multilevel degenerative disc disease with large posterior spurs, small anterior osteophytes, end-plate remodeling, and moderately severe disc space narrowing at L2-3, L3-4, and L4-5. *(From Cole AJ, Herzog RJ. The lumbar spine: imaging options. In Cole AJ, Herring SA, eds. The Low Back Pain Handbook. Philadelphia, Hanley & Belfus, 1997.)*

Differential Diagnosis (see also Table 45.2)

Radiculopathy
Spondylolysis, spondylolisthesis
Spinal stenosis
Tumors
Fractures (e.g., osteoporotic compression fractures)
Osteomyelitis of the spine, discitis

Treatment

Initial

The most important treatment of any low back pain condition is education and reassurance of the patient. Most of the acute low back symptoms are self-limited and typically resolve within 4 to 6 weeks. The mostly benign nature of degenerative conditions of the spine should be emphasized as well as the fact that acute exacerbations tend to improve over time regardless of therapy. Therapy is directed toward management of the symptoms rather than "cure" of the disease. Initial therapy for lumbar degenerative disease should consist of anti-inflammatory medications, muscle relaxants (Table 45.3), occasionally opioid medications for severe symptom exacerbation, and a functionally oriented physical therapy program. Most patients do well with these measures and do not require any invasive procedures. Other useful initial treatments may include trigger point injections as well as physical modalities such as heat and cold. Low-dose tricyclic antidepressants can help with improvement of sleep.

Rehabilitation

Rehabilitation of lumbar degenerative disc disease includes a detailed assessment of functional limitations and functional goals for every patient. A full assessment of occupational and leisure activity demands and goals should also be obtained. For example, patients with advanced degenerative disc disease may benefit from early vocational rehabilitation and counseling with the goal of avoiding future occupational disability and surgical procedures.

On occasion, lumbar orthotics are prescribed, but these are generally not thought to be beneficial in the treatment of degenerative low back pain unless there is significant spondylolisthesis or some other specific indication.

Therapy goals focus on normalization of impairments in flexibility, strength, and endurance and should emphasize healthy lifestyle modifications. A basic lumbar stabilization program with a focus on posture, footwear modifications (if necessary), workplace modifications (if appropriate), and general conditioning works for most patients. Modalities such as ultrasound and electrical stimulation can be used for acute low back pain; however, the focus of supervised therapy should be on an active program rather than the passive treatment that modalities provide.

In patients whose condition does not improve with the outlined initial therapeutic measures, a more intensive, functional restoration approach may be helpful. This commonly

Table 45.2 Pseudospine Pain: Diagnostic Keys

	Condition	Diagnostic Keys
Vascular	Abdominal aortic aneurysm	Older than 50 years Abdominal and back pain Pulsatile abdominal mass
Gynecologic	Endometriosis	Woman of reproductive age Cyclic pelvic and back pain
	Pelvic inflammatory disease	Young, sexually active woman Systemically ill (fever chills) Discharge, dysuria
	Ectopic pregnancy	Missed period Abdominal or pelvic pain Positive pregnancy test result
Genitourinary	Prostatitis	Men older than 30 years Dysuria Low back and perineal pain
	Nephrolithiasis	Flank and groin pain Hematuria
Gastrointestinal	Pancreatitis	Abdominal pain radiating to back Systemic signs (fever, nausea, vomiting) Elevated serum amylase
	Penetrating or perforated duodenal ulcer	Abdominal pain radiating to back
Rheumatologic	Fibromyalgia	Young to middle-aged woman Widespread pain Multiple tender points Disrupted sleep, fatigue Normal radiographs and laboratory values
	Polymyalgia rheumatica	Older than 50-60 years Hip or shoulder girdle pain and stiffness Elevated erythrocyte sedimentation rate Dramatic response to low-dose prednisone
	Seronegative spondyloarthropathies (ankylosing spondylitis, Reiter syndrome, psoriatic, enteropathic)	Younger man (ankylosing spondylitis, Reiter syndrome) Lower lumbosacral pain Morning stiffness ("gel") Improvement with activity Radiographic sacroiliitis
	Diffuse idiopathic skeletal hyperostosis (Forestier disease)	Older than 50-60 years Thoracolumbar stiffness or pain Flowing anterior vertebral calcification
	Piriformis syndrome	Buttock and leg pain Pain on resisted hip external rotation and abduction Transgluteal or transrectal tenderness
	Scheuermann kyphosis	Age 12-15 years Thoracic or thoracolumbar pain Increased fixed thoracic kyphosis 3 or more wedged vertebrae with end-plate irregularities
	Trochanteric bursitis, gluteal fasciitis	Pain or tenderness over greater trochanter
	Adult scoliosis	Back pain Uneven shoulders, scapular prominence Paravertebral hump with forward flexion
Metabolic	Osteoporosis	Woman older than 60 years Severe acute thoracic pain (fracture) Severe weight-bearing pelvic pain (fracture) Aching, dull thoracic pain; relieved in supine position (mechanical) Loss of height, increased thoracic kyphosis
	Osteomalacia	Diffuse skeletal pain or tenderness Increased alkaline phosphatase
	Paget disease	Bone pain: low back, pelvic, tibia Increased alkaline phosphatase Characteristic radiographic appearance
	Diabetic polyradiculopathy	Older than 50 years Diffuse leg pain, worse at night Proximal muscle weakness
Malignant neoplasia		Older than 50 years Back pain unrelieved by positional change—night pain Previous history of malignant disease Elevated erythrocyte sedimentation rate

Modified from Mazanec D. Pseudospine pain: conditions that mimic spine pain. In Cole AJ, Herring SA, eds. The Low Back Pain Handbook. Philadelphia, Hanley & Belfus, 1997.

Table 45.3 Commonly Used Drugs for Muscle Relaxation

Generic Name	Brand Name	Common Doses
Cyclobenzaprine	Flexeril	5-20 mg po tid
Carisoprodol	Soma	350 mg po tid
Baclofen	Lioresal	10-20 mg po q6h
Methocarbamol	Robaxin	500-750 mg po tid
Chlorzoxazone	Parafon Forte	250-500 mg po tid
Orphenadrine	Norflex	100 mg po bid
Metaxalone	Skelaxin	800 mg tid-qid

Modified from Schofferman J. Medications for low back pain. In Cole AJ, Herring SA, eds. The Low Back Pain Handbook. Philadelphia, Hanley & Belfus, 1997.

includes comprehensive physical rehabilitation with psychological support. These programs can be called many things (e.g., comprehensive spine program, chronic pain program, work conditioning program). Although most of these programs are traditionally considered later in the course of degenerative diseases, early referral may be helpful in decreasing related disability [19]. Another common functional rehabilitation technique is the dynamic lumbar stabilization approach [20]. This muscle stabilization program uses static and dynamic postural exercises to improve the patient's overall function. It includes education about proper body mechanics during activities of daily living, improved extremity strength and endurance, and muscle stabilization through gym training and healthy lifestyle activities. The hallmark of this program is that postural control is attained through pelvic tilting to control the degree of lumbar lordosis in a pain-free range. The program is designed to advance the patient toward increasingly demanding exercises and to incorporate these exercises into activities of daily living. The program progresses through the building of static strength into dynamic stabilization for patients with more physically demanding athletic activities and occupational demands. This program is supported by a home exercise program.

Core strengthening expands on the concept of lumbar stabilization and has become a key component of rehabilitation programs for all patients, not only for athletes. Core stability is the ability of the lumbo-pelvic-hip complex to prevent buckling and to return to equilibrium after perturbation. Although bone and soft tissues contribute, core stability is predominantly maintained by the dynamic function of the trunk musculature. Decreased core stability may predispose to injury, and appropriate training may reduce injury [21,22].

Postoperative rehabilitation should focus on strength retraining with increasing aerobic exercise while maintaining neutral spine alignment. There is no consensus on when to initiate rehabilitation after surgery, but strong evidence exists for enrolling patients in intensive programs within 6 weeks of surgery to improve functional outcomes and rates of return to work [23].

Procedures

Spinal injection procedures have become an increasingly important part of the overall treatment program for lumbar degenerative disease. These procedures have diagnostic, therapeutic, and even prognostic benefits. It is now commonly agreed that injections should ideally be performed with x-ray guidance and contrast enhancement [24]. The most commonly used procedures are epidural steroid injections, which are beneficial primarily for temporary relief of radicular symptoms [25]. Injection techniques, such as the transforaminal approach, ensure that the medication, usually a corticosteroid, is delivered into the anterior epidural space [26]. Theoretically, medication delivery to the anterior epidural space would decrease inflammatory processes in local structures, such as degenerative discs. However, recent meta-analyses have found good evidence for epidural steroid injections for radicular pain but only fair evidence for axial pain. Moreover, studies have suggested that epidural injections with local anesthesia but without steroid have rates of efficacy similar to those of injections with steroid [27]. Facet (zygapophyseal joint) anesthesia can be obtained through injections done intra-articularly or by blocking the innervating nerves (medial branches) to these joints. Intra-articular facet injections may allow temporary pain relief in cases of synovitis and facet joint cysts. Medial branch injections are used to establish the diagnosis of facet-mediated pain by temporary blockade of the supplying nerve branches of the affected joint [28]. Medial branch neurotomies ("facet rhizotomies") by radiofrequency ablation may provide longer symptomatic relief for patients with clearly identified facet pain [29]. On occasion, intradiscal steroid injections are applied, but their use is debated because intradiscal steroid may cause discitis, progression of disc degeneration, and calcification of the intervertebral disc [30,31].

Minimally invasive intradiscal therapies (e.g., chemonucleolysis, laser, percutaneous disc decompression) have been used since the 1970s with various clinical successes. Treatment techniques including intradiscal electrothermal therapy involve controlled thermal application to the posterior anulus through an intradiscal catheter. Research data show conflicting results about the therapeutic efficacy of these treatment modalities [32]. There are promising biologic agents currently being studied (e.g., bone morphogenetic protein, mesenchymal stem cell, fibrin adhesive, juvenile chondrocytes) for injection into discs that aim to reverse degenerative and inflammatory changes. Animal studies have revealed augmentation of disc height on imaging studies after intradiscal administration of stem cells [33].

Surgery

The surgical indications for degenerative disc disease of the lumbar spine are highly debated and evolving. Some U.S. insurance companies have recently declared lumbar spine fusion surgery to not be medically necessary if the sole indication is degenerative disc disease. Most insurance carriers require prior authorization of lumbar spine fusion and will consider approval for surgery only when intensive nonsurgical therapy, including physical therapy, injection procedures, and semi-invasive procedures, have failed and the patient continues to have functionally limiting pain. Confounding psychological factors and mental disorders should be excluded before any surgical procedure [34]. Current data are incomplete to judge the scientific validity of spinal fusion for low back pain syndromes [35]. However, if the intervertebral disc is clearly identified as the source of low back pain, interbody fusion with excision of the diseased disc appears to have favorable results. In general, surgical options include posterior fusion procedures with or without pedicle screw instrumentation, anterior interbody fusion with or without pedicle screws, and a combination of these procedures. In case of neural compression, additional decompression procedures may be required. Disc arthroplasty ("artificial disc") became available in the United States after more than a decade of positive experience in Europe [36,37]. The indication for this surgery is chronic low back pain due to symptomatic degenerative disc disease without significant radiographic instability, neural compression, and facet joint arthropathy. Current outcome studies do not show a clear benefit in pain and functional improvement over fusion surgeries, and questions about the longevity of the implants remain.

Recent developments in endoscopic and minimally invasive surgical techniques have expanded surgical management options. Current research maintains insufficient data for firm conclusions to be drawn about the therapeutic efficacy of these surgical techniques [38].

Potential Disease Complications

In general, degenerative lumbar disease is a benign condition. However, increasing functional limitations can occur, especially if advanced segmental degeneration leads to neural compression and symptoms of spinal stenosis, neural claudication, and segmental instability develop. Persistent neurologic deficits from these conditions are rare and can be avoided if the conditions are diagnosed early and appropriate treatment is begun. A small number of patients may develop chronic pain syndromes. Low back pain is the most common cause of the chronic pain syndrome. Not surprisingly, the incidence of mental disorders, such as depression and somatoform disorders, is high, and these disorders commonly respond better to a behavioral psychology approach than to disease-oriented medical treatment approaches. Early detection of patients with mental disorders will help avoid unnecessary medical treatment and allow appropriate psychological and psychiatric interventions.

Potential Treatment Complications

As with any medications, clinicians must be fully aware of their risks and unwanted side effects. Analgesics and nonsteroidal anti-inflammatory drugs have well-known side effects that most commonly affect the gastric, hepatic, and renal systems. Muscle relaxants can cause sedation. Low-dose tricyclic antidepressants can cause sedation and urinary retention in men with benign prostatic hypertrophy. Some patients require chronic opioid therapy, and issues of constipation and dependence arise. Risks associated with spinal injection include cortisone flare, hyperglycemia, dural puncture, and, rarely, hematoma, infection, and neurologic damage. All potential complications should be thoroughly discussed with the patient before treatment. Potential surgical complications, including nerve damage, malpositioned hardware, wound infection, and medical complications (pulmonary embolism, pneumonia, acute kidney injury), will vary with the procedure but can be as high as 17% for lumbar fusion procedures for degenerative disc disease [39].

References

[1] Boden SD, Davis DO, Dina TS, et al. Abnormal magnetic-resonance scans of the lumbar spine in asymptomatic subjects: a prospective investigation. J Bone Joint Surg Am 1990;72:403–8.

[2] Takatalo J, Karppinen J, Niinimäki J, et al. Prevalence of degenerative imaging findings in lumbar magnetic resonance imaging among young adults. Spine (Phila Pa 1976) 2009;34:1716–21.

[3] Lotz JC, Haughton V, Boden SD, et al. New treatments and imaging strategies in degenerative disease of the intervertebral disks. Radiology 2012;264:6–19.

[4] Ha K, Chang C, Kim K, et al. Expression of estrogen receptor of the facet joints in degenerative spondylolisthesis. Spine (Phila Pa 1976) 2005;30:562–6.

[5] Kao PY, Chan D, Samartzis D, et al. Genetics of lumbar disk degeneration: technology, study designs, and risk factors. Orthop Clin North Am 2011;42:479–86, vii.

[6] MacGregor A, Andrew T, Sambrook P, et al. Structural, psychological, and genetic influences on low back and neck pain: a study of adult female twins. Arthritis Rheum 2004;51:160–7.

[7] Freemont AJ, Peacock TE, Goupille P, et al. Nerve ingrowth into diseased intervertebral disc in chronic back pain. Lancet 1997;350:178–81.

[8] Schwarzer AC, Aprill CN, Derby R, et al. The prevalence and clinical features of internal disc disruption in patients with chronic low back pain. Spine (Phila Pa 1976) 1995;20:1878–83.

[9] Schwarzer AC, Aprill CN, Bogduk N. The sacroiliac joint in chronic low back pain. Spine (Phila Pa 1976) 1995;20:31–7.

[10] Kirkaldy-Willis WH. Managing low back pain. New York: Churchill Livingstone; 1999.

[11] Schmorl G, Junghanns H. The human spine: health and disease. 2nd ed. New York: Grune & Stratton; 1971.

[12] Fraser RD, Bleasel JF, Moskowitz RW. Spinal degeneration: pathogenesis and medical management. In: Frymoyer JW, editor. The adult spine: principles and practice. 2nd ed. Philadelphia: Lippincott-Raven; 1997. p. 735–59.

[13] Helms CA. Fundamentals of skeletal radiology. 2nd ed. Philadelphia: WB Saunders; 1995.

[14] Rainville J, Ahern DK, Phalen L, et al. The association of pain with physical activities in chronic low back pain. Spine (Phila Pa 1976) 1992;17:1060–4.

[15] Saal JS. The role of inflammation in lumbar pain [see comments]. Spine (Phila Pa 1976) 1995;20:1821–7.

[16] Rainville J, Sobel JB, Hartigan C. Comparison of total lumbosacral flexion and true lumbar flexion measured by a dual inclinometer technique. Spine (Phila Pa 1976) 1994;19:2698–701.

[17] Waddell G, McCulloch JA, Kummel E, Venner RM. Nonorganic physical signs in low-back pain. Spine (Phila Pa 1976) 1980;5:117–25.

[18] Schliessbach J, Siegenthaler A, Heini P, et al. Blockade of the sinuvertebral nerve for the diagnosis of lumbar diskogenic pain: an exploratory study. Anesth Analg 2010;111:204–6.

[19] Mayer TG, Gatchel RJ, Mayer H, et al. A prospective two-year study of functional restoration in industrial low back injury. An objective assessment procedure [published erratum appears in JAMA 1988;259:220]. JAMA 1987;258:1763–7.

[20] Saal JA. Dynamic muscular stabilization in the nonoperative treatment of lumbar pain syndromes. Orthop Rev 1990;19:691–700.

[21] Bliss LS, Teeple P. Core stability: the centerpiece of any training program. Curr Sports Med Rep 2005;4:179–83.

[22] Willson JD, Dougherty CP, Ireland ML, Davis IM. Core stability and its relationship to lower extremity function and injury. J Am Acad Orthop Surg 2005;13:316–25.

[23] Ostelo RW, de Vet HC, Waddell G, et al. Rehabilitation following first-time lumbar disc surgery: a systematic review within the framework of the Cochrane Collaboration. Spine (Phila Pa 1976) 2003;28:209–18.

[24] O'Neill C, Derby R, Kenderes L. Precision injection techniques for diagnosis and treatment of lumbar disc disease [review]. Semin Spine Surg 1999;11:104–18.

[25] Carette S, Leclaire R, Marcoux S, et al. Epidural corticosteroid injections for sciatica due to herniated nucleus pulposus. N Engl J Med 1997;336:1634–40.

[26] Lutz GE, Vad VB, Wisneski RJ. Fluoroscopic transforaminal lumbar epidural steroids: an outcome study. Arch Phys Med Rehabil 1998;79:1362–6.

[27] Benyamin RM, Manchikanti L, Parr AT, et al. The effectiveness of lumbar interlaminar epidural injections in managing chronic low back and lower extremity pain. Pain Physician 2012;15:E363–404.
[28] Carette S, Marcoux S, Truchon R, et al. A controlled trial of corticosteroid injections into the facet joints for chronic low back pain. N Engl J Med 1998;325:1002–7.
[29] Dreyfuss P, Halbrook B, Pauza K, et al. Efficacy and validity of radiofrequency neurotomy for chronic lumbar zygapophysial joint pain. Spine 2000;25:1270–7.
[30] Darmoul M, Bouhaouala MH, Rezgui M. Calcification following intradiscal injection, a continuing problem? [in French]. Presse Med 2005;34:859–60.
[31] Carragee EJ, Tanner CM, Khurana S, et al. The rates of false-positive lumbar discography in select patients without low back symptoms. Spine (Phila Pa 1976) 2000;25:1373–80.
[32] Saal JA, Saal JS. Intradiscal electrothermal treatment for chronic discogenic low back pain: a prospective outcome study with minimum 1-year follow-up. Spine (Phila Pa 1976) 2000;25:2622–7.
[33] Hiyama A, Mochida J, Sakai D. Stem cell applications in intervertebral disc repair. Cell Mol Biol (Noisy-le-grand) 2008;54:24–32.
[34] Cheng JS, Lee MJ, Massicotte E, et al. Clinical guidelines and payer policies on fusion for the treatment of chronic low back pain. Spine (Phila Pa 1976) 2011;36(Suppl.):S144–63.
[35] Bigos SJ. A literature-based review as a guide for generating recommendations to patients acutely limited by low back symptoms. In: Garfin SR, Vaccaro AR, editors. Orthopaedic knowledge update. Spine. Rosemont, Ill: American Academy of Orthopaedic Surgeons; 1997. p. 15–25.
[36] Tropiano P, Huang RC, Girardi FP, et al. Lumbar total disc replacement. Seven- to eleven-year follow-up. J Bone Joint Surg Am 2005;87:490–6.
[37] Jacobs WC, der Gaag NA Van, Kruyt MC, et al. Total disc replacement for chronic discogenic low-back pain: a Cochrane review. Spine (Phila Pa 1976) 2013;38:24–36.
[38] Yousefi-Nooraje R, Schonstein E, Heidari K, et al. Low level laser therapy for nonspecific low back pain. Cochrane Database Syst Rev 2007;2, CD005107.
[39] Fritzell P, Hagg O, Wessberg P, et al. Volvo award winner in clinical studies: lumbar fusion versus nonsurgical treatment for chronic low back pain. Spine (Phila Pa 1976) 2001;26:2521–34.

CHAPTER 46

Lumbar Facet Arthropathy

Ted A. Lennard, MD

Synonyms

Facet joint pain
Facet joint arthritis
Z-joint pain
Zygapophyseal joint pain
Apophyseal joint pain
Facet syndrome
Posterior element disorder

ICD-9 Codes

721.3	**Lumbosacral spondylosis without myelopathy**
721.90	**Spondylosis of unspecified site (spinal arthritis)**
724.2	**Low back pain**

ICD-10 Codes

M47.817	**Spondylosis without myelopathy or radiculopathy, lumbosacral region**
M47.899	**Other spondylosis, site unspecified**
M54.5	**Low back pain**

Definition

Lumbar facet joints are formed by the articulation of the inferior and superior articular facets of adjacent vertebrae (Fig. 46.1). These joints, located posteriorly in the spinal axis, are lined with synovium and have highly innervated joint capsules. Lumbar facet arthropathy refers to any acquired, traumatic, or degenerative process that changes the normal function or anatomy of a lumbar facet joint. These changes often disrupt the normal biomechanics of the joint, resulting in hyaline cartilage damage and ultimately periarticular hypertrophy. When they are painful, these joints may limit activities of daily living, work, and recreational sports. Lumbar facet joints may be a primary source of pain, but they are often painful concomitantly with a degenerative or injured lumbar disc, fracture, or ligamentous injury.

Lumbar facet arthropathy is more severe at the L4-L5 level and is common with advancing age and progressive intervertebral disc disease. These findings are independent of race and sex [1,2]. Postsurgical facet joint pain appears to be associated with advancing age, prolonged intraoperative time, intraoperative complications, discectomy, history of recurrent disc prolapse, and lack of rehabilitation [3,4].

Symptoms

Patients often complain of generalized or lateralized spinal pain, sometimes well localized. Pain may be provoked with spinal extension and rotation, from either a standing or a prone position. Relief with partial lumbar flexion is common. In the lumbar spine, these joints may refer pain into the buttock or posterior thigh but rarely below the knee [5–7]. Neurologic symptoms, such as lower extremity weakness, numbness, and paresthesias, would be unexpected from a primary facet joint disorder.

Physical Examination

A detailed examination of the lumbar spine and a lower extremity neurologic examination are considered standard procedure for those thought to have facet arthropathy. Although no portion of the examination has been shown to definitively correlate with the diagnosis of a facet joint disorder, the physical examination can be helpful in elevating the clinician's level of suspicion for this diagnosis [8,9]. The examination starts with simple observation of the patient's gait, posture, movement patterns, and range of motion. Generalized and segmental spinal palpation is followed by a detailed neurologic examination for sensation, reflexes, tone, and strength. In the absence of coexisting pathologic processes, such as lumbar radiculopathy, strength, sensation, and deep tendon reflexes should be normal.

Provocative maneuvers and nerve tension tests, including straight-leg raising, should accompany the evaluation to rule out any superimposed nerve root injury that might accompany a facet disorder. The clinician notes the patient's response when the lower extremity is raised with the hip flexed and the knee extended. This "tension" placed on inflamed or injured lower lumbosacral nerve roots will provoke pain, paresthesias, or numbness down the extremity.

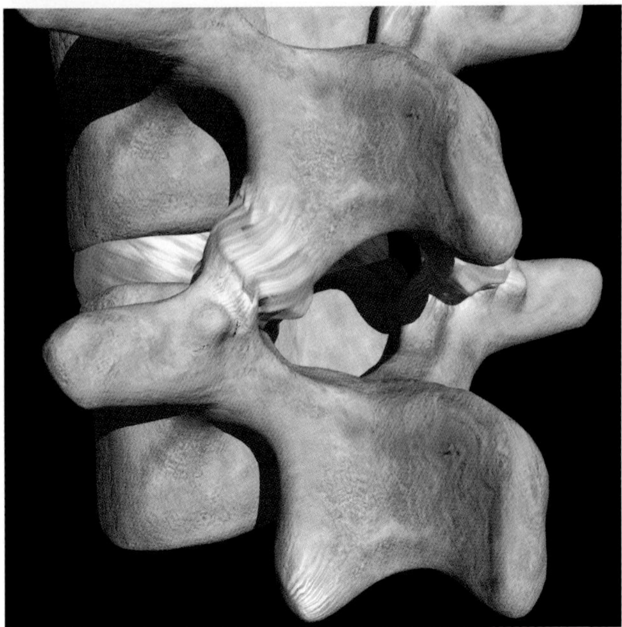

FIGURE 46.1 Posterior view of the lumbar spine demonstrating the paired facet joints. Note the thick capsule surrounding the facet joint. *(Reprinted from OrthoClick.com.)*

Typically, in isolated cases of lumbar facet disorders, this maneuver does not provoke radiating symptoms into the lower extremity, but it may cause lower back pain. Some physicians find that facet pain can be reproduced with prone extension with rotation, hip extension, lumbar extension while standing on a single leg, and standing spinal extension.

Functional Limitations

Patients with lumbar facet joint arthropathy may experience difficulty with prolonged walking, stair climbing, twisting, standing, and prone lying. Because facet problems are common with underlying disc disease, patients often have difficulty with lumbar flexion activities, such as lifting, stooping, and bending.

Diagnostic Studies

Fluoroscopy-guided, contrast-enhanced, anesthetic intra-articular or medial branch blocks are considered the "gold standard" for the diagnosis of a painful lumbar facet joint (Figs. 46.2 and 46.3) [10–12]. Clinical history, examination findings, radiographic changes, computed tomography, magnetic resonance imaging, and bone scan have not been shown to correlate with facet joint pain [8,9,13].

Differential Diagnosis

Internal disc disruption
Myofascial pain syndrome
Nerve root compression
Radiculopathy
Spondylolysis or spondylolisthesis
Lumbar stenosis
Spondylosis
Sacroiliac joint dysfunction

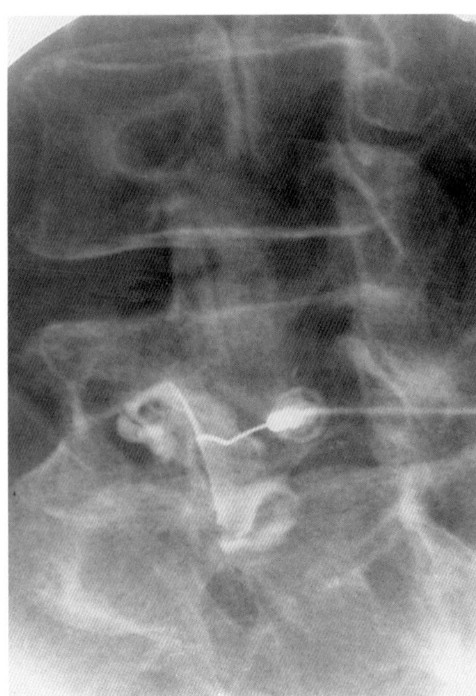

FIGURE 46.2 Oblique radiograph of an L5-S1 facet joint arthrogram. Superior and inferior capsular recesses are demonstrated. *(From Lennard TA. Pain Procedures in Clinical Practice. Philadelphia, Hanley & Belfus, 2000.)*

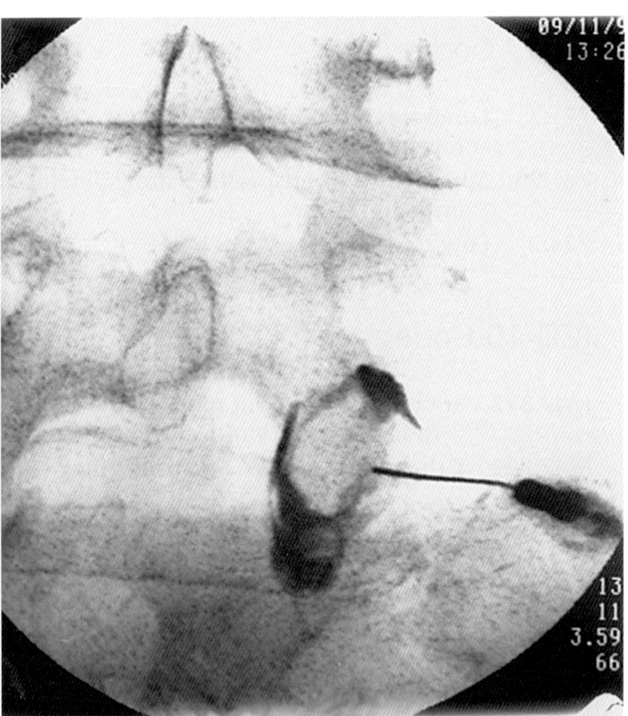

FIGURE 46.3 Anteroposterior radiograph of a needle placed into the L5-S1 facet joint with an arthrogram. *(From Lennard TA. Pain Procedures in Clinical Practice. Philadelphia, Hanley & Belfus, 2000.)*

Treatment

Initial

Initial treatment emphasizes local pain control with oral analgesics and nonsteroidal anti-inflammatory drugs, ice, topical creams, local blind periarticular corticosteroid injections, and avoidance of exacerbating activities. Spinal manipulations and acupuncture may also reduce local pain. Temporary wearing of corsets and limited activity may be used.

Rehabilitation

Physical therapy may include modalities to control pain (e.g., ice, heat, ultrasound), traction, instruction in body mechanics, flexibility training (including hamstring stretching), articular mobilization techniques, core strengthening, generalized conditioning, and restoration of normal movement patterns. Critical assessment of the biomechanics of specific activities that may be job related (e.g., sitting at a desk, carpentry work, driving) or sports related (e.g., running, cycling) is important. This assessment can result in prevention of recurrent episodes of pain because changes in a technique or activity may reduce the underlying forces at the joint level. Simple ergonomic measures that act to support the lumbar spine during sitting and standing may reduce the occurrence of low back pain from the facet joints. These measures include proper chair height and design, properly designed work table, and adjustable chair supports. While standing, the addition of a footrest, pads, and the ability to change body position routinely may reduce low back pain.

Procedures

Intra-articular, fluoroscopy-guided, contrast-enhanced facet injections are considered essential in the proper diagnosis and treatment of a painful facet joint [10,11,14–17]. Ultrasound guidance for these procedures is an emerging option [18–21]. Patients can be evaluated before and after injection to determine what portion of their pain can be attributed to the joints injected. After confirmation with contrast material, 1 to 2 mL of an anesthetic-corticosteroid mix is injected directly into the joint. An alternative approach is to perform anesthetic medial branch blocks with small volumes (0.1 to 0.3 mL) of anesthetic. Recent data suggest that medial branch blocks may be the preferred method for diagnosis of facet joint pain [16,22,23]. If the facet joint is found to be the putative source of pain, a medial branch neurotomy may be desirable [24–26].

Surgery

Surgery is rare in primary and isolated facet arthropathies. Surgical spinal fusion may be performed for discogenic pain, which may affect secondary cases of facet arthropathies.

Potential Disease Complications

Because a common cause of facet arthropathy is degenerative in nature, this disorder is often progressive, resulting in chronic, intractable spinal pain [26]. It often coexists with spinal disc abnormalities, further leading to chronic pain. This subsequently results in diminished spinal motion and weakness.

Potential Treatment Complications

Treatment-related complications may be caused by medications; nonsteroidal anti-inflammatory drugs may cause gastrointestinal and renal problems, and analgesics may result in liver dysfunction and constipation. Local periarticular injections and acupuncture may cause local transient needle pain. Local manual treatments or injections will often cause transient exacerbation of symptoms. Intra-articular facet injections will cause transient local spinal pain and swelling and possibly bruising. More serious injection-related complications include an allergic reaction to the medications, injury to a blood vessel or nerve, trauma to the spinal cord, and infection. When more serious injection complications occur, they can usually be attributed to poor procedure technique [10].

References

[1] Li J, Muehleman C, Abe Y, Masuda K. Prevalence of facet joint degeneration in association with intervertebral joint degeneration in a sample of organ donors. J Orthop Res 2011;29:1267–74.

[2] Master DL, Eubanks JD, Ahn NU. Prevalence of concurrent lumbar and cervical arthrosis: an anatomic study of cadaveric specimens. Spine (Phila Pa 1976) 2009;15:E272–5.

[3] Steib K, Proescholdt M, Brawanski A, et al. Predictors of facet joint syndrome after lumbar disc surgery. J Clin Neurosci 2012;19:418–22.

[4] Manchikanti L, Pampati V, Rivera J, et al. Role of facet joints in chronic low back pain in the elderly: a controlled comparative prevalence study. Pain Pract 2001;1:332–7.

[5] Dreyer SJ, Dreyfuss P. Low back pain and the zygapophyseal joints. Arch Phys Med Rehabil 1996;77:290–300.

[6] Dreyer S, Dreyfuss P, Cole A. Posterior elements and low back pain. Phys Med Rehabil State Art Rev 1999;13:443–71.

[7] Fukui S, Ohseto K, Shiotani M, et al. Distribution of referred pain from the lumbar zygapophyseal joints and dorsal rami. Clin J Pain 1997;13:303–7.

[8] Dolan AL, Ryan PJ, Arden NK, et al. The value of SPECT scans in identifying back pain likely to benefit from facet joint injection. Br J Rheumatol 1996;35:1269–73.

[9] Schwarzer AC, Scott AM, Wang S, et al. The role of bone scintigraphy in chronic low back pain: comparison of SPECT and planar images and zygapophyseal joint injection. Aust N Z J Med 1992;22:185.

[10] Bogduk N. International Spinal Injection Society Guidelines for the performance of spinal injection procedures. Part I: zygapophysial joint blocks. Clin J Pain 1997;13:285–302.

[11] Dreyfuss P, Kaplan M, Dreyer SJ. Zygapophyseal joint injection techniques in the spinal axis. In: Lennard TA, editor. Pain procedures in clinical practice. Philadelphia: Hanley & Belfus; 2000. p. 332–69.

[12] Schutz U, Cakir B, Dreinhofer K, et al. Diagnostic value of lumbar facet joint injection: a prospective triple cross-over study. PLoS One 2011;6:e27991.

[13] Pneumaticos SG, Chatziioannou SN, Hipp JA, et al. Low back pain: prediction of short term outcomes of facet joint injection with bone scintigraphy. Radiology 2006;238:693–8.

[14] Boswell MV, Colson JD, Spillane WF. Therapeutic facet joint interventions in chronic spinal pain: a systematic review of effectiveness and complications. Pain Physician 2005;8:101–14.

[15] Sehgal N, Dunbar EE, Shah RV, Colson J. Systematic review of diagnostic utility of facet (zygapophysial) joint injections in chronic spinal pain: an update. Pain Physician 2007;10:213–28.

[16] Lindner R, Sluijter ME, Schleinzer W. Pulsed radiofrequency treatment of the lumbar medial branch for facet pain: a retrospective analysis. Pain Med 2006;7:435–9.

[17] Kennedy DJ, Shokat M, Visco CJ. Sacroiliac joint and lumbar zygapophysial joint corticosteroid injections. Phys Med Rehabil Clin N Am 2010;21:835–42.

[18] Galiano K, Obwegeser AA, Bodner G, et al. Ultrasound guidance for facet joint injections in the lumbar spine: a computed tomography–controlled feasibility study. Anesth Analg 2005;101:579–83.

[19] Shim JK, Moon JC, Yoon KB, et al. Ultrasound guided lumbar medial branch block: a clinical study with fluoroscopy control. Reg Anesth Pain Med 2006;32:451–4.

[20] Gofeld M, Bristow SJ, Chiu S. Ultrasound-guided injection of lumbar zygapophyseal joints: an anatomic study with fluoroscopy validation. Reg Anesth Pain Med 2012;37:228–31.

[21] Loizides A, Peer S, Plaikner M, et al. Ultrasound-guided injections in the lumbar spine. Med Ultrason 2011;13:4–8.

[22] Bogduk N. Lumbar medial branch. In: Bogduk N, editor. Practice guidelines, spinal diagnostic and treatment procedures. San Francisco: International Spinal Intervention Society; 2004. p. 47–65.
[23] Birkenmaier C, Veihelmann A, Trouillier HH, et al. Medial branch blocks versus pericapsular blocks in selecting patients for percutaneous cryodenervation of lumbar facet joints. Reg Anesth Pain Med 2007;32:27–33.
[24] Dreyfuss P, Halbrook B, Pauza K, et al. Lumbar radiofrequency neurotomy for chronic zygapophyseal joint pain: a pilot study using dual medial branch blocks. Int Spinal Injection Soc Sci Newslett 1999;3:13–31.
[25] Dreyfuss P, Halbrook B, Pauza K, et al. Efficacy and validity of radiofrequency neurotomy for chronic lumbar zygapophyseal joint pain. Spine 2000;25:1270–7.
[26] van Kleef M, Barendse G, Kessels A, et al. Randomized trial of radiofrequency lumbar facet denervation for chronic low back pain. Spine (Phila Pa 1976) 1999;24:1937–42.

CHAPTER 47

Lumbar Radiculopathy

Maury Ellenberg, MD

Michael J. Ellenberg, MD

Synonyms

Lumbar radiculitis
Sciatica
Pinched nerve
Herniated nucleus pulposus with nerve root irritation

ICD-9 Codes

724.4 Lumbar radiculopathy
722.22 Disc herniation

ICD-10 Codes

M54.16 Radiculopathy, lumbar region
M51.9 Unspecified thoracic, thoracolumbar, lumbosacral intervertebral disc disorder

Definition

Lumbar radiculopathy refers to a pathologic process involving the lumbar nerve roots. Lumbar radiculitis refers to an irritation or inflammation of a nerve root. These terms should not be confused with disc herniation, which is a displacement of the lumbar disc from its anatomic location between the vertebrae (often into the spinal canal) (Fig. 47.1). Although lumbar radiculopathy is often caused by a herniated lumbar disc, this is not invariably the case. Many pathologic processes, such as bone encroachment, tumors, and metabolic disorders (e.g., diabetes), can also result in lumbar radiculopathy. It is of utmost significance that disc herniation is often an incidental finding on imaging of the lumbar spine of asymptomatic individuals [1,2]. Therefore, without a clear correlation with the history and physical examination, imaging studies alone can be more misleading than beneficial. When disc herniation results in radiculopathy, the precise cause of the pain is not fully understood. The two possibilities are mechanical compression and inflammation. It has been demonstrated that in a "nonirritated" nerve, mechanical stimulus rarely leads to pain. In contrast, an "irritated" nerve usually results in pain. Furthermore, inflammatory mediators have experimentally been shown to cause radicular pain in the absence of compression [3–5]. It is likely that both factors may be at work individually or together in any given patient. As a result of the imaging findings in asymptomatic individuals and the various causes of pain in radiculopathy, it should be no surprise that disc herniations and nerve root compression can be present in asymptomatic patients [2] and that patients can have radiculopathy without visible disc herniations or nerve root compression [6].

The prevalence of lumbar radiculopathy in the general population varies from 2.2% to 8%, depending on the study, and the incidence ranges from 0.7% to 9.6% [7,8]. One study found a higher incidence in men (67%), with the highest prevalence in individuals 45 to 65 years old [9], and an association with obesity and smoking as well as a correlation with occupations requiring very heavy physical activity.

Symptoms

The most common symptom in lumbar radiculopathy is pain, which may vary in severity and location. The pain may be severe and is often exacerbated or precipitated by standing, sitting, coughing, and sneezing. The location of the pain depends on the nerve root involved, with a great deal of overlap among the dermatomes. Most commonly, S1 radiculopathy produces posterior thigh and calf pain; L5, buttocks and anterolateral leg pain; L4, anterior thigh, anterior or medial knee, and medial leg pain; and L3, groin pain. The patient usually cannot pinpoint the precise onset of pain. Location of pain at onset may be in the back; however, by the time the patient is evaluated, the pain may be present only in the buttocks or limb.

Paresthesias are also common and occur in the dermatomal distribution of the involved nerve root (rarely is the sensory loss complete). On occasion, the patient may present with complaints of weakness. Rarely, there is bladder and bowel involvement, which may be manifested as urinary retention or bowel incontinence.

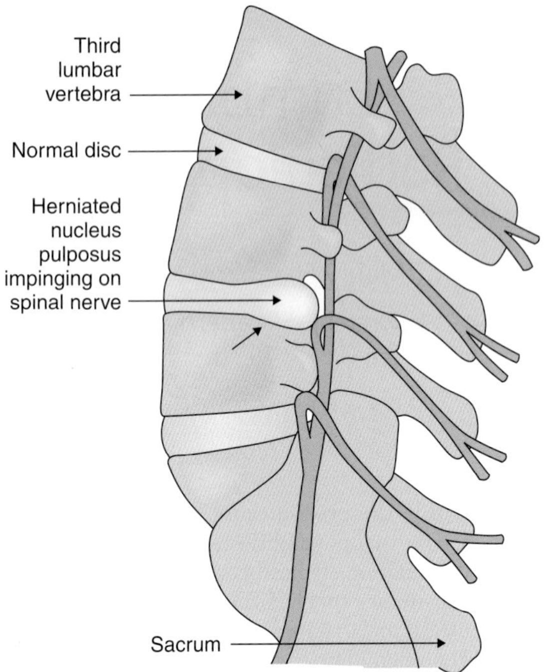

FIGURE 47.1 A herniated disc.

Physical Examination

The most important elements in the evaluation of lumbar radiculopathy are the history and physical examination [10].

A thorough musculoskeletal and peripheral neurologic examination should be performed. Examine the back for asymmetry or a shift over one side of the pelvis. Evaluate back motion and see whether radicular symptoms (pain radiating to an extremity) in the distribution of the patient's complaints are produced. In an L5 or S1 radiculopathy, forward flexion of the back while standing is equivalent to a straight-leg raising test and may produce pain in the buttock or posterior thigh. In an L4 or L3 radiculopathy, extension may produce groin or anterior thigh pain.

Manual muscle testing is a vital part of the examination for radiculopathy. The major muscle weakness in relation to the nerve root involved is as follows: L3, hip flexors; L4, knee extensors and hip adductors; L5, hip abductors, knee flexors, ankle dorsiflexors, foot evertors, foot inverters, and great toe extensor; S1, ankle plantar flexors (Table 47.1). Try to detect weakness in the distribution of two peripheral nerves arising from the same nerve root. Proximal muscle weakness in the appropriate nerve root distribution is useful in distinguishing bilateral radiculopathy from peripheral neuropathy.

The straight-leg raising test can be performed with the patient sitting or supine. The leg is raised straight up by the examiner, and the test result is positive if the patient complains of pain in the extremity (not the back), typically in a specific nerve root distribution. If pain occurs only in the back, this is not an indicator of radiculopathy and is most often seen with nonspecific low back pain. On occasion, the process of lumbar radiculopathy may start with low back pain, and several days or weeks later, the symptom will occur in the leg. It is possible that the initial process of nucleus pulposus rupture through the anulus may result in the initial back pain, but the pathogenesis is not completely known at this time. Compare side to side to confirm a positive response to the straight-leg raise as opposed to the pain associated with passive hamstring stretch. Rectal examination and perianal and inguinal sensory testing should be done if there is history of bowel or bladder incontinence or retention or recent onset of erectile dysfunction.

Waddell signs are a group of indicators that a nonorganic process is interfering with the accuracy of the physical examination. The signs are superficial—nonanatomic tenderness; simulation—axial loading or rotation of the head causes complaints of back pain; distraction—sitting straight-leg raising versus supine; regional disturbance—weakness or sensory loss in a region of the body that is in a nonanatomic distribution; and overreaction—what is described commonly as excessive pain behavior. These signs are often present in patients with compensation, litigation, or psychoemotional issues [11]. Evaluation for presence of Waddell signs should be a routine part of the examination in patients with pain complaints, particularly if they are long-standing or the history reveals that some of these issues are present.

Functional Limitations

The functional limitations depend on the severity of the symptoms and weakness. Limitations usually occur because of pain but may occasionally occur because of weakness. Standing and walking may be limited, and sitting tolerance is often decreased. Patients with an L4 radiculopathy are at risk of falling down stairs if the involved leg is their "trailing"

Table 47.1 Diagnosis of Lumbar Radiculopathy

Nerve Root	Pain Radiation	Gait Deviation	Motor Weakness	Sensory Loss	Reflex Loss
L3	Groin and inner thigh	Sometimes antalgic	Hip flexion	Anteromedial thigh	Patellar (variable)
L4	Anterior thigh or knee, or upper medial leg	Sometimes antalgic Difficulty rising onto a stool or chair with one leg	Knee extension, hip flexion and adduction	Lateral or anterior thigh, medial leg, and knee	Patellar
L5	Buttocks, anterior or lateral leg, dorsal foot	Difficulty heel walking; if more severe, then foot slap or steppage gait Trendelenburg gait	Ankle dorsiflexion, foot eversion and inversion, toe extension, hip abduction	Posterolateral thigh, anterolateral leg, and mid-dorsal foot	Medial hamstring (variable)
S1	Posterior thigh, calf, plantar foot	Difficulty toe walking or cannot rise on toes 20 times	Foot plantar flexion	Posterior thigh and calf, lateral and plantar foot	Achilles

(power) leg on the stairs. They would also have difficulty ascending stairs or rising from a seated position, depending on the degree of weakness (although that is not as dangerous as descending stairs). Patients with a severe S1 radiculopathy will be unable to run because of calf weakness, even when the pain resolves. Patients with L5 radiculopathy may catch the foot on curbs or, if weakness is severe, on the ground. They may require a brace (ankle dorsiflexion assist). In patients with acute radiculopathy that is severe, the pain will usually preclude them from a whole range of activities—household, recreation, and work. In the majority of patients, once the acute process is ameliorated, they can return to most activities except for heavy household and work activity. After about 3 to 6 months, they can return to all activities unless there is residual weakness, in which case they would be functionally limited as noted before, depending on the radiculopathy level.

Diagnostic Studies

Diagnostic testing takes two forms: one to corroborate the diagnosis and the second to determine the etiology. For simple cases, despite the current "rush toward imaging," diagnostic testing is usually not needed and the clinical picture can guide the treatment. A history that includes trauma, cancer, bacterial infection, human immunodeficiency virus infection, or diabetes would be an indication for earlier diagnostic testing.

Electromyography

Electromyography and nerve conduction studies, when performed by an individual well versed in the diagnosis of neuromuscular disorders, can be valuable in the diagnosis of lumbar radiculopathy. They can also help with differential diagnoses and in clarifying the diagnosis in patients whose physical examination is not reliable. Electromyography has the advantage over imaging techniques of high specificity, and recordings will rarely be abnormal in asymptomatic individuals [12]. Electrodiagnostic studies, however, do not give direct information about the *cause* of the radiculopathy.

Imaging

Imaging techniques in relation to lumbar radiculopathy usually refer to lumbosacral spine radiography, computed tomography (CT) scan, and magnetic resonance imaging (MRI).

Plain radiography can be useful to exclude traumatic bone injury or metastatic disease. It allows visualization of the disc space but not the contents of the spinal canal or the nerve roots. CT and MRI allow visualization of the disc, spinal canal, and nerve roots (Fig. 47.2). There is a high incidence of abnormal findings in asymptomatic people, with rates of disc herniation ranging from 21% in the 20- to 39-year age group to 37.5% in the 60- to 80-year age group [2]. In fact, in one study, only 36% of asymptomatic individuals had normal discs at all levels. In other words, it is "normal" to have some disc abnormality, which occurs as part of normal aging [1]. To be meaningful, CT and MRI must clearly correlate with the clinical findings. Perform these studies if tumor is suspected or surgery is contemplated. They also may be useful in precisely locating pathologic changes for transforaminal epidural steroid injection. The most accurate study is MRI, and gadolinium enhancement is not needed unless a tumor is suspected or the patient has undergone prior surgery. Gadolinium enhancement is useful postsurgically to distinguish disc herniation from scar tissue.

Differential Diagnosis

Trochanteric bursitis
Anserine bursitis
Hamstring strain
Lumbosacral plexopathy
Diabetic amyotrophy
Sciatic neuropathy
Tibial neuropathy
Peroneal neuropathy
Femoral neuropathy
Hip osteoarthritis
Sacroiliitis
Avascular necrosis of the hip
Pelvic stress fracture
Occult hip fracture
Shin splints
Lateral femoral cutaneous neuropathy (meralgia paresthetica)
Spinal stenosis
Cauda equina syndrome
Demyelinating disorder
Lumbar facet syndrome
Piriformis syndrome
Transient migratory regional osteoporosis

Treatment

Initial

The treatment goal is to reduce inflammation and thereby relieve the pain and allow resolution of the radiculopathy regardless of the underlying anatomic abnormalities. Bed rest, which had been the mainstay of nonoperative treatment, is now recommended only for symptom control. In previous studies, bed rest has not been shown to have an effect on the final outcome of the disorder [13]. As long as patients avoid aggravating activities or bending or lifting, which tend to increase intradiscal pressure, they can carry on most everyday activities.

Use nonsteroidal anti-inflammatory drugs (NSAIDs) to help reduce inflammation and to provide pain relief. NSAIDs have been shown to be effective in acute low back pain [14]. However, a review that included pooling of three randomized clinical trials using NSAIDs showed no effectiveness over placebo [15]. It is still reasonable to give NSAIDs a short trial in acute lumbar radiculopathy for pain relief, although they will not shorten the course of the disorder. The use of oral steroids remains controversial and has not passed the scrutiny of well-controlled studies, even in acute low back pain. In a recent meta-analysis of the use of NSAIDS, corticosteroids, tricyclic antidepressants, and anticonvulsants, although the pooled data showed no efficacy with any of these medications over placebo in chronic radiculopathy [16], there was one study that found short-term efficacy for gabapentin [17]. There were two studies

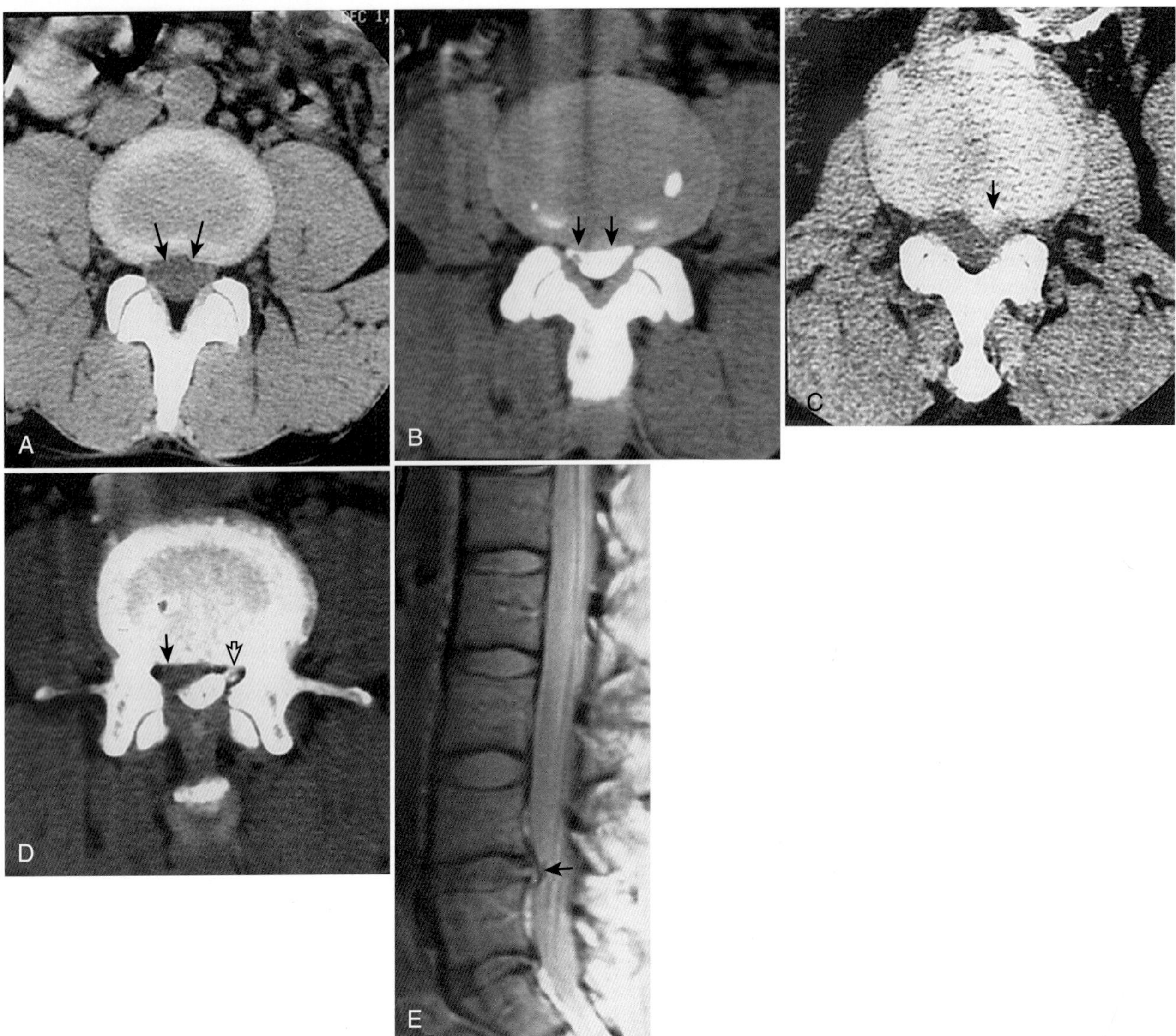

FIGURE 47.2 **A,** Normal disc. Note the concave posterior margin of the disc *(arrows)*. **B,** Bulging disc. Image from a CT myelogram shows the broad-based margin of the bulging disc *(arrows)* pushing on the anterior thecal sac. **C,** Left posterior disc herniation *(arrow)*. **D,** Right posterior disc herniation. The abnormal soft tissue from the herniated disc is seen in the right lateral recess on this CT myelogram *(arrow)*. Note the normally opacified nerve root sheath on the contralateral side *(open arrow)*. **E,** Herniated discs L4-L5 and L5-S1; the L4-L5 herniation is the larger of the two. There is posterior displacement of the low-signal posterior longitudinal ligament *(arrow)*. *(From Barckhausen RR, Math KR. Lumbar spine diseases. In Katz DS, Math KR, Groskin SA, eds. Radiology Secrets. Philadelphia, Hanley & Belfus, 1998.)*

in patients with acute radiculopathy in which oral corticosteroids seemed to be effective in the short-term treatment of radicular pain [16]. Other medications, such as cyclobenzaprine, metaxalone, methocarbamol, and chlorzoxazone, some of which may have effectiveness in acute low back pain, have not been shown to be effective in acute radiculopathy [18].

Clinically, for acute radiculopathy, there are several options. If the pain is severe, early epidural steroid injection (see the section on procedures) and testing with imaging and electromyography are reasonable. Another option is oral steroids, such as methylprednisolone (Medrol) dose pack, and the use of opioids for short-term pain control. For more chronic radicular pain, it would be reasonable to try anticonvulsants, such as gabapentin, or a combination of gabapentin and a tricyclic antidepressant, such as amitriptyline or nortriptyline. Start treatment with a low dose and titrate up gradually to determine the minimally effective dose.

Opioids may be used for pain relief, although their effectiveness is suboptimal in neuropathic pain, with some suggestion that they should be used only in severe cases [19]. There is no major concern for addiction in acute care of patients who have not demonstrated past addictive behavior. The needs range from none to relatively high doses, such as the equivalent of 60 to 100 mg of morphine (e.g., MS Contin) a day. Start with hydrocodone or oxycodone and titrate up as needed. For more severe pain, use a long-acting opioid, such as oxycodone (OxyContin) or MS Contin, and for breakthrough pain, use a shorter acting opioid, such as hydrocodone, oxycodone, or short-acting morphine. These treatments should be short term to avoid the risks of dependency or addiction. There seems to be no efficacy of opioids versus placebo for symptom relief or decrease in disability in chronic radiculopathy [20].

Rehabilitation

With an acute painful radiculopathy, it is generally best to wait for some of the acute stage to subside before ordering physical therapy. In a longer standing problem, therapy may be the best first approach.

Physical methods are a useful adjunct to the medication treatment. Various methods, which include flexion and extension exercises (often called a lumbosacral stabilization program), have been tried. Whatever method is used, if radicular pain is produced, the exercises should be stopped. After the radiculopathy resolves, the patient should be prescribed a proper exercise regimen to improve flexibility and muscle strength. Lumbar stabilization exercises, core muscle strengthening, and remaining active may be the most effective of the various methods studied carefully in lumbar radiculopathy. One study showed no effectiveness of lumbar traction [21]. Other modalities, such as transcutaneous electrical nerve stimulation, acupuncture, massage, and manipulation, are not well studied with randomized clinical trials in lumbar radiculopathy [6]. Because they are not likely to cause injury, they can be given a short trial. The manipulation should be done cautiously.

Procedures

Epidural steroid injections are beneficial in acute radiculopathy in patients with or without disc herniation [21,22]. The results in chronic radiculopathy are less convincing. The most effective technique and material to be used for epidural steroid injection are controversial [23,24]. Some literature suggests that either steroid preparations or local anesthetics are superior to placebo for long-term effects. Short-term effects, however, favored the steroid group [24,25]. Some studies show that transforaminal epidural steroid injections have a marginally greater improvement in pain scores compared with lumbar epidural steroid injections. However, on the basis of the preferred safety profile, greater procedural comfort of lumbar epidural steroid injections, and nearly equal functional gains of the two procedures, a reasonable clinical approach is to attempt a lumbar epidural steroid injection initially and then, in the absence of significant improvement or resolution in 2 weeks, to attempt a transforaminal epidural steroid injection [22,23].

Whereas the scientific literature shows that the effects of these interventions are relatively short-lived [21,23], the intervention is beneficial because it limits opiate use [23] and referral for surgical management.

These procedures should be performed under fluoroscopic guidance [26]. It is advisable to perform one injection and to re-evaluate the patient in 1 or 2 weeks to determine whether further injections are required. It is not appropriate to perform a "series of three injections." On the other hand, a maximum of three injections should be performed for any one episode of radiculopathy. It is reasonable to repeat this procedure for recurrent episodes of radiculopathy after 3 to 6 months.

Nonoperative treatment allows resolution of the radiculopathy in up to 90% of cases [15,27,28]. More interestingly, studies have demonstrated that when radiculopathy is the result of disc herniation, the actual herniation will resolve in the majority of cases, and even when the herniation remains, the symptoms often will still abate [29–31].

Surgery

Surgery is appropriate under two conditions. First, surgery is performed on an emergency basis when a patient presents with a central disc herniation with bowel and bladder incontinence or retention and bilateral lower extremity weakness. In this very rare condition, a neurosurgeon or orthopedic spine surgeon must be consulted immediately and the patient operated on, preferably within 6 hours. Second, surgery is an option if a patient continues to have pain that limits function after an adequate trial of nonoperative treatment.

Patient selection is extremely important to achieve a good surgical outcome. The best outcomes occur in patients with single-level root involvement; with pain experienced more in the limb than in the back; and when an anatomic abnormality on imaging corresponds to the patient's symptoms, physical examination findings, and electromyographic findings in patients without psychological or secondary gain issues [32,33].

A recent update of a Cochrane review on the subject of surgery versus conservative care concluded that in selected patients, surgery can provide faster relief, but there remains no convincing evidence of a difference in long-term outcomes [34].

The type of surgery depends on the cause of the radiculopathy. For cases of disc herniation, simple laminectomy and discectomy suffice; there seems to be no difference between the standard, microdiscectomy, and newer minimally invasive procedures on outcome or time to return to activity [35]. Fusion should be avoided in these instances. With spinal stenosis, a more extensive laminectomy with foraminotomy may be needed. Fusion should be reserved for the relatively infrequent case of well-demonstrated spinal instability together with radiculopathy or if the surgical procedure will result in spinal instability. One study [36] suggested that fusion is needed in the case of spondylolisthesis, but this has not been confirmed with any randomized clinical trials.

Potential Disease Complications

Complications relate to involvement of the nerve roots in the cauda equina. The most serious is the "paraplegic disc." In this case, the herniated disc can cause paralysis, but this is very rare. More common, but still unusual, is a disc that causes lower limb weakness and involvement of bowel and bladder function. Residual lower limb weakness may occur either spontaneously or after surgery. Patients may progress to a chronic low back pain syndrome; this is particularly likely to occur in patients with secondary gain issues.

Potential Treatment Complications

NSAIDs can cause gastrointestinal bleeding, mouth ulcers, and renal and hepatic complications. Newer cyclooxygenase 2 inhibitors may avoid gastrointestinal bleeding. There have been associations attributed to the use of cyclooxygenase 2 inhibitors and other NSAIDs with cardiovascular disease. These medications should always be used cautiously, in proper doses, and for limited periods.

Corticosteroids, when used long term, have myriad complications, including weight gain, fat redistribution, osteoporosis, and diabetes mellitus, among others. The short-term use should cause few complications in healthy individuals. Those with diabetes will experience a rise in blood glucose concentration, and some patients may experience mental and emotional difficulties that can include psychosis. Steroids may also lead to gastrointestinal bleeding.

Use of opioids can lead to dependency in some patients. Although they may be of use in patients with lumbar radiculopathy, their use with low back pain and chronic nonmalignant pain, in which effectiveness is questionable [37], has led to an epidemic of the use and abuse of these drugs [38,39].

Epidural steroid injections can (rarely) result in epidural abscess and epidural hematoma. Patients should not take aspirin for 7 days before the injection. Some centers recommend that NSAIDs not be taken for 3 to 5 days before the procedure, although there is no literature documenting an increased incidence of bleeding complications from epidural or spinal injections when patients are taking NSAIDs. Warfarin should be discontinued, and if in doubt, the international normalized ratio should be checked. Clopidogrel (Plavix) and similar antiplatelet agents should be discontinued for a week before injection. The injection can produce local pain, and if it is performed without fluoroscopy, it can often result in spinal headache from piercing of the dura and a resultant spinal fluid leak. This occurs considerably less often when fluoroscopic guidance is used. Contamination of injectable material from a compounding pharmacy, has led to central nervous system infections, primarily with *Exserohilum rostratum*, and *Aspergillus*. Twenty-two other pathogens have also been identified. As of June 2013 this has resulted in 745 confirmed infections and 58 deaths. Currently the scope of regulatory oversight within the compounding industry is under review [40].

Surgical complications include infection, nerve root injury, paralysis, local back pain, and the usual postoperative complications (e.g., thrombophlebitis, bladder infection). More serious surgical complications include nerve root or cauda equine injury, arachnoiditis, and post-laminectomy pain syndromes. These complications may lead to repeated surgery, which may be more extensive.

References

[1] Jensen MC, Brant-Zawadzki MN, Obuchowski N, et al. Magnetic resonance imaging of the lumbar spine in people without back pain. N Engl J Med 1994;331:69–73.

[2] Boden SD, Davis DO, Dina TS, et al. Abnormal magnetic-resonance scans of the lumbar spine in asymptomatic subjects. J Bone Joint Surg Am 1990;72:403–8.

[3] Murata Y, Olmarker K, Takahashi I, et al. Effects of selective tumor necrosis factor-alpha inhibition to pain-behavioral changes caused by nucleus pulposus–induced damage to the spinal nerve in rats. Neurosci Lett 2005;382:148–52.

[4] Mulleman D, Mammou S, Griffoul I, et al. Pathophysiology of disk-related sciatica. I. Evidence supporting a chemical component. Joint Bone Spine 2006;73:151–8.

[5] Valat JP, Genevay S, Marty M, et al. Sciatica. Best Pract Res Clin Rheumatol 2010;24:241–52.

[6] Rhee JM, Schaufele M, Abdu W. Radiculopathy and the herniated lumbar disc. Controversies regarding the pathophysiology and management. J Bone Joint Surg Am 2006;88:2070–80.

[7] Younes M, Bejia I, Aguir Z, et al. Prevalence and risk factors of disk-related sciatica in an urban population in Tunisia. Joint Bone Spine 2006;72:538–42.

[8] Tarulli AW, Raynor EM. Lumbosacral radiculopathy. Neurol Clin 2007;25:387–405.

[9] Praemer A, Furner S, Rice DP. Musculoskeletal conditions in the United States. 2nd ed. Rosemont, Ill: American Academy of Orthopaedic Surgeons; 2011.

[10] Deyo RA, Rainville J, Kent DL. What can the history and physical examination tell us about low back pain? JAMA 1992;268:760–5.

[11] Waddell G, McCulloch JA, Kummel E, Venner RM. Nonorganic physical signs in low-back pain. Spine (Phila Pa 1976) 1980;5:117–25.

[12] Robinson LR. Electromyography, magnetic resonance imaging, and radiculopathy: it's time to focus on specificity. Muscle Nerve 1999;22:149–50.

[13] Vroomen P, de Krom M, Wilmink JT, et al. Lack of effectiveness of bed rest for sciatica. N Engl J Med 1999;340:418–23.

[14] van Tulder MW, Scholten RJ, Koes BW, Deyo RA. Nonsteroidal anti-inflammatory drugs for low back pain. A systematic review within the framework of the Cochrane Collaboration Back Review Group. Spine (Phila Pa 1976) 2000;25:2501–13.

[15] Vroomen PC, de Krom MC, Slofstra PD, Knottnerus JA. Conservative treatment of sciatica: a systematic review. J Spinal Disord 2000;13: 463–9.

[16] Pinto RZ, Maher CG, Ferreira ML, et al. Drugs for relief of pain in patients with sciatica: systematic review and meta-analysis. BMJ 2012;344:e497.

[17] Yildirim K, Sisecioglu M, Karatay S, et al. The effectiveness of gabapentin in patients with chronic radiculopathy. Pain Clin 2003;15:213–8.

[18] van Tulder MW, Touray T, Furlan AD, et al Cochrane Back Review Group. Muscle relaxants for nonspecific low back pain: a systematic review within the framework of the Cochrane Collaboration. Spine (Phila Pa 1976) 2003;28:1978–92.

[19] Chou R. Treating sciatica in the face of poor evidence. BMJ 2012;344:e487.

[20] Khoromi S, Cui L, Nackers L, Max MB. Morphine, nortriptyline and their combination vs placebo in patients with chronic lumbar root pain. Pain 2007;130:66–75.

[21] Carette S, Leclaire R, Marcoux S, et al. Epidural corticosteroid injections for sciatica due to herniated nucleus pulposes. N Engl J Med 1997;336:1634–7.

[22] Lutz GE, Vad VB, Wisneski RJ. Fluoroscopic transforaminal lumbar epidural steroids: an outcome study. Arch Phys Med Rehabil 1998;79:1362–6.

[23] Gharibo CG, Varlotta GP, Rhame EE, et al. Interlaminar versus transforaminal epidural steroids for the treatment of subacute lumbar radicular pain: a randomized, blinded, prospective outcome study. Pain Physician 2011;14:499–511.

[24] Quraishi N. Transforaminal injection of corticosteroids for lumbar radiculopathy: systemic review and meta-analysis. Eur Spine J 2012;21:214–9.

[25] Riew KD, Park JB, Cho YS, et al. Nerve root blocks in the treatment of lumbar radicular pain. A minimum five-year follow-up. J Bone Joint Surg Am 2006;88:1722–5.

[26] Thomas E, Cytevak C, Abiad L, et al. Efficacy of transforaminal versus interspinous corticosteroid injection in discal radiculalgia—a prospective randomized, double-blind study. Clin Rheumatol 2003;22:229–304.

[27] Saal JA, Saal JS. Nonoperative treatment of herniated lumbar intervertebral disc with radiculopathy: an outcome study. Spine (Phila Pa 1976) 1997;14:431–7.

[28] Legrand E, Bouvard B, Audran M, et al. Sciatica from disk herniation: medical treatment or surgery? Joint Bone Spine 2007;74:530–5.

[29] Ellenberg M, Reina N, Ross M, et al. Regression of herniated nucleus pulposus: two patients with lumbar radiculopathy. Arch Phys Med Rehabil 1989;70:842–4.

[30] Ellenberg M, Ross M, Honet JC, et al. Prospective evaluation of the course of disc herniations in patients with proven radiculopathy. Arch Phys Med Rehabil 1993;74:3–8.

[31] Saal JA, Saal JS, Herzog J. The natural history of intervertebral disc extrusions treated nonoperatively. Spine (Phila Pa 1976) 1990;7:683–6.

[32] Finneson BE, Cooper VR. A lumbar disc surgery predictive scorecard. A retrospective evaluation. Spine (Phila Pa 1976) 1979;4:141–4.

[33] Nguyen TH, Randolph DC, Talmage J, et al. Long-term outcomes of lumbar fusion among workers' compensation subjects. Spine (Phila Pa 1976) 2011;36:320–31.

[34] Gibson JN, Waddell G, et al. Surgical interventions for lumbar disc prolapse: updated cochrane review. Spine (Phila Pa 1976) 2007;32:1735–47.
[35] Jacobs WC, Arts MP, van Tulder MW, et al. Surgical techniques for sciatica due to herniated disc, a systematic review. Eur Spine J 2012;21:2232–51.
[36] Herkowitz H, Kurz L. Degenerative lumbar spondylolisthesis with spinal stenosis. J Bone Joint Surg Am 1991;73:802–8.
[37] Martell BA, O'Connor PG, Kerns RD, et al. Systematic review: opioid treatment for chronic back pain: prevalence, efficacy, and association with addiction. Ann Intern Med 2007;146:116–27.
[38] Dunn KM, Saunders KW, Rutter CM, et al. Opioid prescriptions for chronic pain and overdose: a cohort study. Ann Intern Med 2010;152:85–92.
[39] McLellan AT. Chronic noncancer pain management and opioid overdose: time to change prescribing practices. Ann Intern Med 2010;152:123–4.
[40] Ritter JA, Muehlenbachs A, Blau DM, et al. Exserohilum infections associated with contaminated steroid injections: a clinicopathologic review of 40 cases. Am J Pathol 2013;183:881–92.

CHAPTER 48

Low Back Strain or Sprain

Omar El Abd, MD

Joao E.D. Amadera, MD, PhD

Synonyms

Acute low back pain ("preferred terminology")
"Pulled muscle" in the low back

ICD-9 Codes

722.10 Degenerative disc disease, lumbar spine
724.2 Low back pain
724.6 Sacroiliac joint disorder
724.8 Facet joint arthropathy

ICD-10 Codes

M51.36 Other intervertebral disc degeneration, lumbar region
M54.5 Low back pain
M12.88 Other specified arthropathies, not elsewhere classified, vertebrae

Definition

Lumbar strain or sprain is a term used by clinicians to describe an episode of acute low back pain. The patients report pain in the low back at the lumbosacral region accompanied by contraction of the paraspinal muscles (hence, the expression "muscle sprain" or "strain"). The definite cause is unknown in most cases. It most likely is secondary to a chemical or mechanical irritation of the sensory nociceptive fibers in the intervertebral discs, facet joints, sacroiliac joints, or muscles and ligaments at the lumbosacral junction area.

Low back pain is a prevalent condition associated with work absenteeism, disability, and large health care costs [1]. Episodes of low back pain constitute the second leading symptom prompting patients to seek evaluation by a physician [2]. It is estimated that 50% to 80% of adults experience at least one episode of acute low back pain in their lives [3,4]. The incidence of radiculopathy is reported to be much lower than the incidence of axial back pain at 2% to 6% [5]. Patients who experience acute back pain usually see improvements and are able to return to work within a month [6,7]. However, 2% to 7% of patients have chronic back pain [8,9]. Several studies suggest that 90% of patients with an acute episode of low back pain recover within 6 weeks [10–12]. In contrast, some well-conducted cohort studies demonstrate a less optimistic picture, providing short-term estimates of recovery ranging from 39% to 76% [13,14]. Pengel and colleagues [6] published a meta-analysis investigating the course of acute low back pain, concluding that both pain and disability improve rapidly within weeks (58% reduction of initial scores in the first month) and recurrences are common. On the other hand, more recently, Menezes and associates [1] demonstrated that the typical course of acute low back pain is initially favorable, with a marked reduction in mean pain and disability in the first 6 weeks. After 6 weeks, improvement slows, and only small reductions in mean pain and disability are apparent for up to 1 year. By 1 year, the average measures of pain and disability for acute low back pain were very low, suggesting that patients can expect to have minimal pain or disability at 1 year.

Clinicians encounter a number of patients who convert from acute pain to chronic pain. In a recent review involving 10 studies and more than 4000 participants, Hallegraef and coworkers [15] investigated adults with acute and subacute nonspecific low back pain. The odds that patients with negative recovery expectations will remain absent from work because of progression to chronic low back pain was two times greater than for those with more positive expectations.

Consequently, the goals of the clinician evaluating patients with an episode of acute low back pain are to have a working differential diagnosis of the condition and its etiology, to rule out radiculopathy or other serious medical causes, to have a rehabilitation plan that aims to prevent recurrence of this episode, to educate the patient about the pathologic process, and to formulate a management plan if the condition does not improve promptly.

Symptoms

The pain develops spontaneously or acutely after traumatic or strenuous events such as sports participation, repetitive bending, lifting, motor vehicle accidents, and falls. Pain is

Table 48.1 Red Flags

Symptom	Concern
Pain in the lower extremities (including the buttocks) more than pain in the lower back	Radiculopathy
Weakness or sensory deficit in one or both lower extremities	Radiculopathy and the possibility of cauda equina syndrome (especially if there is bilateral involvement of the lower extremities)
Bowel or bladder changes; saddle anesthesia	Cauda equina
Severe pain in the low back, including pain while lying down	Malignant neoplasm
Fever, chills, night sweats, recent loss of weight	Infection and malignant neoplasm
Injury related to a fall from a height or motor vehicle crash in a young patient or from a minor fall or heavy lifting in a patient with osteoporosis or possible osteoporosis	Fracture
History of cancer metastatic to bone	Malignant neoplasm

predominantly located in the lumbosacral area (axial) overlying the lumbar spinous processes and along the paraspinal muscles. There may be an association with pain in the lower extremities; however, the lower extremity pain is less intense than the low back pain. Pain is usually described as sharp and shooting in character accompanied by paraspinal muscle tightness.

Trunk rotation, sitting, and bending forward usually exacerbate pain. Lying down with application of modalities (heat or ice) usually mitigates it.

Red flags that require prompt medical response are outlined in Table 48.1.

Etiology

Axial Pain (Pain Overlying the Lumbosacral Area)

Discogenic pain due to degenerative disc disease is the most common known cause of axial pain. The pain from the intervertebral discs is located in proximity to the degenerated disc. Multiple inflammatory products are found in the painful disc tissue that may increase the excitability of the sensory neurons. The pain is referred from the disc to the surrounding paraspinal and pelvic girdle muscles.

Facet (zygapophyseal) joint arthropathy is another source of axial pain, present in about 30% to 50% of patients describing axial pain in the lumbar as well as in the cervical spine [16–18]. The facets are paired synovial joints adjacent to the neural arches. Pain is predominantly in the paraspinal area and is accompanied by contractions of the muscles that guard around the facet joints. The pain from the facet joints can be unilateral or bilateral.

Sacroiliac joint arthropathy is a cause of axial back pain as well. The pain is located in the lumbosacral-buttock junction with referral to the lower extremity and to the groin area. Painful conditions of the sacroiliac joint are known to result from spondyloarthropathies, infection, malignant neoplasms, pregnancies, and trauma and even to occur spontaneously.

Radicular Pain

Predominant buttocks area pain is a common presentation of lumbar radicular pain. Nerve roots can be affected secondary to mechanical pressure and inflammation. Mechanical pressure is usually secondary to disc protrusion (herniation) or due to spinal stenosis. Disc herniations involve all age groups, with predominance in the young and middle aged. Spinal stenosis, on the other hand, predominantly affects the elderly; it is a combination of disc degeneration, ligamentum hypertrophy, and facet arthropathy or spondylolisthesis. In radiculopathy, symptoms are present along a nerve root distribution. Sensory symptoms include pain, numbness, and tingling that follow the distribution of a particular nerve root. The symptoms may be accompanied by motor weakness in a myotomal distribution. Diagnosis and treatment of radiculopathy are discussed in Chapter 47.

Myofascial Pain

There are different theories explaining muscular reasons for acute low back pain, but they remain unproved [19,20]. These theories include inflammation—failure at the myotendinous junction and the production of an inflammatory repair response; ischemia—postural abnormalities causing chronic muscle activation and ischemia; trigger points secondary to repetitive strain of muscles (this theory remains the most attractive) [20]; and muscle imbalance.

The currently most accepted theory for muscle pain is related to the myofascial pain syndrome, which is a common reported disorder in chronic conditions but can be present in the acute conditions as well [21]. It is characterized by myofascial trigger points—hard, palpable, discrete, localized nodules located within taut bands of skeletal muscle and painful on compression. An active myofascial trigger point is associated with spontaneous pain, in which pain is present without palpation. This spontaneous pain can be at the site of the myofascial trigger points or remote from it. The current diagnostic standard for myofascial pain is based on palpation for the presence of trigger points in a taut band of skeletal muscle and an associated symptom cluster that includes referred pain patterns [22]. Treatment of myofascial pain involves massage, needling of the myofascial trigger points (with or without anesthetic injections), acupuncture, and stretching [23].

Referred Pain

Musculoskeletal structures in proximity to the spine and organs in the abdomen and pelvis are potential sources of pain with referral to the spine and the paraspinal area.

Occult Lesions

These lesions may be manifested with axial or radicular symptoms or with both. Spine metastasis [24] and spine and paraspinal infections are considered a rare possibility.

Skilled history taking and physical examination are necessary in diagnosis of these dangerous conditions.

Physical Examination

The physical examination starts with a thorough history to ascertain the pain's onset, character, location, and aggravating and mitigating factors. Inquiry about associated symptoms, such as weakness, bowel or bladder symptoms, fever, and abnormal loss of weight, and past medical history are important. Examination includes inspection of the lower back and the lower extremities. Palpation of the paraspinal muscles, lumbar facet joints, inguinal lymph nodes, and lower extremity pulses is performed. Hip examination, root tension signs, discogenic provocative maneuvers, and sacroiliac joint maneuvers are performed (Table 48.2). Gait examination, with heel and toe walking, is assessed. Sensory examination and thorough manual muscle testing are performed. Deep tendon reflexes are examined.

Table 48.2 Spine Physical Examination Maneuvers

Maneuver	Description	Significance
Pelvic rock	In a supine position, flex the patient's hips until the flexed knees approximate to the chest; then, rotate the lower extremities from one side to the other.	Lumbar discogenic pain provocation
Sustained hip flexion	In a supine position, raise the patient's extended lower extremities to approximately 60 degrees. Ask the patient to hold the lower extremities in that position and release. The test result is positive on reproduction of low lumbar or buttock pain. Then lower the extremities successively approximately 15 degrees and, at each point, note the reproduction and intensity of pain.	Lumbar discogenic pain provocation
Root tension signs—upper extremity	Contralateral neck lateral bending and abduction of the ipsilateral upper extremity	Reproduces cervical radicular pain in the periscapular area or in the upper extremity
Spurling maneuver	Passively perform cervical extension, lateral bending toward the side of symptoms, and axial compression.	Reproduces cervical radicular pain in the periscapular area or in the upper extremity
Straight-leg raise	While the patient is lying supine, the involved lower extremity is passively flexed to 30 degrees with the knee in full extension.	Reproduces pain in the buttock, posterior thigh, and posterior calf in conditions with S1 radicular pain
Reverse straight-leg raise	While the patient is lying prone, the involved lower extremity is passively extended, the knee flexed.	Reproduces pain in the buttock and anterior thigh in conditions with high lumbar (such as L3 and L4) radicular pain
Crossed straight-leg raise	While the patient is lying supine, the contralateral lower extremity is passively flexed to 30 degrees with the knee in full extension.	Reproduces pain in the ipsilateral buttock, posterior thigh, and posterior calf in conditions with S1 radicular pain
Sitting root test	While the patient is sitting, the involved lower extremity is passively flexed with the knee extended.	Reproduces pain in the buttock, posterior thigh, and posterior calf in conditions with S1 radicular pain
Lasègue sign	While the patient is lying supine, the involved lower extremity is passively flexed to 90 degrees.	Reproduces pain in the buttock, posterior thigh, and posterior calf in conditions with S1 radicular pain
Bragard sign	While the patient is lying supine, the involved lower extremity is passively flexed to 30 degrees, with dorsiflexion of the foot.	Reproduces pain in the buttock, posterior thigh, and posterior calf in conditions with S1 radicular pain
Gaenslen maneuver	The patient is placed in a supine position with the affected side flush with the edge of the examination table. The hip and knee on the unaffected side are flexed, and the patient clasps the flexed knee to the chest. The examiner then applies pressure against the clasped knee, extends the lower extremity on the ipsilateral side, and brings it under the surface of the examination table.	Reproduces pain in patients with sacroiliac joint syndrome
Sacroiliac joint compression	Apply compression to the joint with the patient lying on the side.	Reproduces pain in patients with sacroiliac joint syndrome
Pressure at sacral sulcus	Apply pressure on the posterior superior iliac spine (dimple).	Reproduces pain in patients with sacroiliac joint syndrome
Patrick test (FABER test)	While the patient is supine, the knee and hip are flexed. The hip is abducted and externally rotated.	Reproduces pain in patients with sacroiliac joint syndrome, facet joint arthropathy (pain is reproduced in the low back), and degenerative joint disease of the hip (pain is reproduced in the groin)
Yeoman test	While the patient is in the prone position, the hip is extended and the ilium is externally rotated.	Reproduces pain in patients with sacroiliac joint syndrome
Iliac gapping test	Distraction can be performed to the anterior sacroiliac ligaments by applying pressure to the anterior superior iliac spines.	Reproduces pain in patients with sacroiliac joint syndrome

Diagnostic Studies

Without clinical signs of serious disease, diagnostic imaging and laboratory testing are not required [25,26]. However, imaging is recommended in the presence of red flags (such as history of trauma, constitutional symptoms, suspicion of radiculopathy, history of cancer, or persistent symptoms lasting longer than 1 month without improvement), in rheumatologic conditions, with prolonged use of steroids, and in the case of litigations.

The "gold standard" for evaluation of painful spine conditions is magnetic resonance imaging (MRI), which allows good visualization of discs and nerves as well as provides valuable information necessary for further management if the condition does not improve. MRI evaluation is required only if symptoms persist for longer than 1 month or at the onset of radicular pain or weakness. It is also used in the workup for back pain accompanied by constitutional symptoms.

Differential Diagnosis

Degenerative disc disease
Facet joint arthropathy
Lumbar radiculopathy
Sacroiliac joint syndrome
Acute vertebral compression fracture
Sacral stress fracture
Referred pain from abdomen or pelvis
Occult lesions in the spine, such as metastasis or infection

Treatment

Initial

Although there are numerous treatments for lumbar sprain and strain, most have little evidence of benefit. Inflammation is a major culprit of pain. Nonsteroidal anti-inflammatory drugs (NSAIDs) are a cornerstone of pain management and should be provided in adequate doses. The selective cyclooxygenase 2 (COX-2) inhibitors show fewer gastric side effects compared with traditional NSAIDs; however, studies have shown that COX-2 inhibitors are associated with increased cardiovascular risks in specific patient populations [27].

Muscle relaxants are beneficial [26] and commonly used for pain management along with NSAIDs. These medications do not target a particular pathologic process and should be used in conjunction with NSAIDs. They are particularly helpful in improving sleep and relieving muscle "spasms" or "tightness" in patients with low back pain. Tramadol and opioid medications can be used in cases of severe pain, but an association between early receipt of opioids for acute low back pain and poor outcomes such as need for surgery and risk of receiving late opioids was found in a large cohort study [28]. If there is a need for extended use of these medicines, imaging studies should be performed and other management modalities should be considered. Modalities such as heat and ice can also be used.

Bed rest is not recommended in management of acute low back pain. It is advisable to remain active as much as possible [29].

In a recent review, no substantial benefit was shown with oral steroids, acupuncture, massage, traction, lumbar supports, or regular exercise programs in management of acute low back pain. Manipulative therapy, such as spinal manipulation and chiropractic techniques, is no more effective than established medical treatments, and adding it to established treatments does not improve outcomes [26].

Rehabilitation

The cornerstone for a complete recovery and the prevention of a recurrence of lumbar strain or sprain or the transformation to chronic low back pain is participation in a regular spine stabilization program. The program should begin immediately after the pain starts to improve. Initiation of an exercise program while the patient is experiencing severe symptoms is not helpful because the patient's ability to participate is limited by pain. Exercises directed by a physical therapist, such as spine stabilization exercises, may decrease recurrent pain and need for further health care services and expenses [30,31]. A lumbar stabilization exercise program consists of stretching the lower extremities, pelvis, and lumbosacral muscles as well as performing exercises to strengthen the lumbosacral muscles. Postural training and learning proper body mechanics are essential. Patients are taught to perform these exercises and are advised to incorporate them into their daily routine.

Acupuncture

Acupuncture is widely used to treat patients with low back pain. A systematic review of the literature concluded that acupuncture is effective for pain relief and functional improvement in chronic back pain for a short term, but for acute back pain, no evidence of the effectiveness of acupuncture was found [32].

Procedures

Spinal injections are not considered a first-line management of acute low back pain. If progressive radiculopathy is suspected and the MRI study is consistent with this diagnosis, therapeutic spinal nerve root blocks should be promptly considered. In axial acute low back pain, if conservative management fails in 4 weeks, MRI is performed. If the MRI findings and the clinical findings suggest intervertebral disc disease, transforaminal epidural steroid injections or interlaminar epidural steroid injections are used. In this context, if MRI findings are unremarkable and pain persists, therapeutic facet joint injections or sacroiliac joint injections are used.

Surgery

Surgical intervention is not indicated in the management of acute low back pain without radiculopathy causing progressive neurologic deficits.

Potential Disease Complications

Most patients will recover within 2 weeks. However, if symptoms change from axial low back pain to radicular pain, weakness develops in one or both lower extremities, or pain persists, the clinician should promptly order imaging studies. Further management is required as soon as possible to prevent deterioration of the patient's condition.

Potential Treatment Complications

Traditional NSAIDs used in management have resulted in gastrointestinal complications, such as peptic ulcer disease. Patients must take the medications with food, antacids, or ulcer-preventing medications. COX-2 inhibitors are associated with increased cardiovascular risks and should be taken for only short periods.

Muscle relaxants, tramadol, and opioids have sedative side effects. Patients are advised to refrain from driving and operating machinery while taking these medications.

References

[1] Menezes Costa L da C, Maher CG, Hancock MJ, et al. The prognosis of acute and persistent low-back pain: a meta-analysis. CMAJ 2012;184:E613–24.

[2] Cypress BK. Characteristics of physician visits for back symptoms: a national perspective. Am J Public Health 1983;73:389–95.

[3] Waddell G. The epidemiology of low back pain. In: Waddell G, editor. The back pain revolution. New York: Churchill Livingstone; 1998. p. 69–84.

[4] Rubin DI. Epidemiology and risk factors for spine pain. Neurol Clin 2007;25:353–71.

[5] Deyo RA, Tsui-Wu YJ. Descriptive epidemiology of low back pain and its related medical care in the United States. Spine (Phila Pa 1976) 1987;12:264–8.

[6] Pengel LH, Herbert RD, Maher CG, Refshauge KM. Acute low back pain: systematic review of its prognosis. BMJ 2003;327:323.

[7] Shin JS, Ha IH, Lee TG, et al. Motion style acupuncture treatment (MSAT) for acute low back pain with severe disability: a multicenter, randomized, controlled trial protocol. BMC Complement Altern Med 2011;11:127.

[8] Woolf AD, Pfleger B. Burden of major musculoskeletal conditions. Bull World Health Organ 2003;81:646–56.

[9] Koes BW, van Tulder MW, Thomas S. Diagnosis and treatment of low back pain. BMJ 2006;332:1430–4.

[10] Shekelle PG, Markovich M, Louie R. An epidemiologic study of episodes of back pain care. Spine (Phila Pa 1976) 1995;20:1668–73.

[11] Manchikanti L. Epidemiology of low back pain. Pain Physician 2000;3:167–92.

[12] van Tulder M, Becker A, Bekkering T, et al., COST B13 Working Group on Guidelines for the Management of Acute Low Back Pain in Primary Care. Chapter 3. European guidelines for the management of acute nonspecific low back pain in primary care. Eur Spine J 2006;15(Suppl 2):S169–91.

[13] Grotle M, Brox JI, Veierød MB, et al. Clinical course and prognostic factors in acute low back pain: patients consulting primary care for the first time. Spine (Phila Pa 1976) 2005;30:976–82.

[14] Henschke N, Maher CG, Refshauge KM, et al. Prognosis in patients with recent onset low back pain in Australian primary care: inception cohort study. BMJ 2008;337:a171.

[15] Hallegraeff JM, Krijnen WP, van der Schans CP, de Greef MH. Expectations about recovery from acute non-specific low back pain predict absence from usual work due to chronic low back pain: a systematic review. J Physiother 2012;58:165–72.

[16] Aprill C, Bogduk N. The prevalence of cervical zygapophyseal joint pain. A first approximation. Spine (Phila Pa 1976) 1992;17:744–7.

[17] Bogduk N, Marsland A. The cervical zygapophyseal joint as a source of neck pain. Spine (Phila Pa 1976) 1988;13:610–7.

[18] Schwarzer AC, Wang S, Bogduk N, et al. Prevalence and clinical features of lumbar zygapophysial joint pain: a study in an Australian population with chronic low back pain. Ann Rheum Dis 1995;54:100–6.

[19] Bogduk N. Low back pain. In: Bogduk N, editor. Clinical anatomy of the lumbar spine and sacrum. 3rd ed. New York: Churchill Livingstone; 1997. p. 187–214.

[20] Manchikanti L, Singh V, Fellows B. Structural basis of chronic low back pain. In: Manchikanti L, Slipman CW, Fellows B, editors. Low back pain: diagnosis and treatment. Paducah, Ky: American Society of Interventional Pain Physicians; 2002. p. 77–95.

[21] Ketenci A, Basat H, Esmaeilzadeh S. The efficacy of topical thiocolchicoside (Muscoril) in the treatment of acute cervical myofascial pain syndrome: a single-blind, randomized, prospective, phase IV clinical study. Agri 2009;21:95–103.

[22] Simons DG, Travell JG, Simons PT. Travell and Simons' myofascial pain and dysfunction: the trigger point manual. 2nd ed. Upper Half of Body. vol 1. Baltimore: Williams & Wilkins; 1999.

[23] Sikdar S, Shah JP, Gebreab T, et al. Novel applications of ultrasound technology to visualize and characterize myofascial trigger points and surrounding soft tissue. Arch Phys Med Rehabil 2009;90:1829–38.

[24] Slipman CW, Patel RK, Botwin K, et al. Epidemiology of spine tumors presenting to musculoskeletal physiatrists. Arch Phys Med Rehabil 2003;84:492–5.

[25] Deyo RA, Diehl AK. Lumbar spine films in primary care: current use and effects of selective ordering criteria. J Gen Intern Med 1986;1:20–5.

[26] Casazza BA. Diagnosis and treatment of acute low back pain. Am Fam Physician 2012;85:343–50.

[27] Roelofs PD, Deyo RA, Koes BW, et al. Non-steroidal anti-inflammatory drugs for low back pain. Cochrane Database Syst Rev 2008;1, CD000396.

[28] Webster BS, Verma SK, Gatchel RJ. Relationship between early opioid prescribing for acute occupational low back pain and disability duration, medical costs, subsequent surgery and late opioid use. Spine (Phila Pa 1976) 2007;32:2127–32.

[29] Hagen KB, Jamtvedt G, Hilde G, Winnem MF. The updated Cochrane review of bed rest for low back pain and sciatica. Spine 2005;30:542–6.

[30] Kriese M, Clijsen R, Taeymans J, Cabri J. Segmental stabilization in low back pain: a systematic review. Sportverletz Sportschaden 2012;24:17–25.

[31] Gellhorn AC, Chan L, Martin B, Friedly J. Management patterns in acute low back pain: the role of physical therapy. Spine (Phila Pa 1976) 2012;37:775–82.

[32] Furlan AD, van Tulder M, Cherkin D, et al. Acupuncture and dry-needling for low back pain: an updated systematic review within the framework of the Cochrane collaboration. Spine (Phila Pa 1976) 2005;30:944–63.

CHAPTER 49

Lumbar Spondylolysis and Spondylolisthesis

Jennifer L. Earle, MD
Imran J. Siddiqui, MD
James Rainville, MD
John C. Keel, MD

Synonyms

Slipped vertebra

ICD-9 Codes

738.4 Lumbar spondylolisthesis
756.11 Lumbar spondylolysis

ICD-10 Codes

M43.07 Spondylolysis (lumbosacral)
Q76.2 Spondylolisthesis (congenital)
M43.10 Spondylolisthesis (acquired)
S33.100 Lumbar vertebral slippage (subluxation)
Add seventh character to S33 for the episode of care (A—initial encounter, D—subsequent encounter, S—sequela)
Q67.5 Congenital spine defect
S32.009 Unspecified fracture of unspecified lumbar vertebra
Add seventh character to S32 for the episode of care (A—initial encounter closed fracture, B—initial encounter open fracture, D—subsequent encounter fracture with routine healing, G—subsequent encounter fracture with delayed healing, K—subsequent encounter fracture with nonunion, S—sequela)
M53.2X7 Spinal instability, lumbar region

Definition

Spondylolysis refers to a bone defect in the pars interarticularis. *Pars interarticularis* translates to "bridge between the joints" and as such is the isthmus or bone bridge between the inferior and superior articular surfaces of the neural arch of a single vertebra (Figs. 49.1 and 49.2). When bilateral spondylolysis is present, the posterior aspect of the neural arch, including the inferior articular surfaces, is no longer connected by bone to the rest of the vertebra.

Spondylolysis is an acquired condition; it has never been found at birth [1]. Spondylolysis is most commonly acquired early in life [2,3] and is identified by lumbar radiographs in 4.4% of children 5 to 7 years of age [2,4]. By 18 years of age, 6% of the population has spondylolysis [2], with few additional cases thought to occur thereafter. The prevalence remains steady at approximately 6% in radiographic screening of adult spines [5,6]. Community population prevalence ranges from 5.7% to 11.5% when screening is performed by computed tomography (CT) scan [6,7].

Spondylolysis most commonly occurs at the L5 vertebrae, where about 90% of the cases are found. It is found with decreasing frequency at progressively higher lumbar levels [2,8,9]. It is more common in males than in females with roughly a 2:1 ratio (7.7%-9% vs 3.1%-4.6%) [6–8,10], can be unilateral (less common) or bilateral (more common), and has a suspected genetic predisposition [2,10,11].

The most likely cause of spondylolysis is a stress fracture of the pars that persists as a nonunion [12]. This is consistent with the higher incidence of spondylolysis suspected in adolescents and young adults who aggressively participate in sports requiring repetitive flexion-extension movements, such as gymnastics, throwing sports, football, wrestling, rugby, judo, dance, and swimming breast and butterfly strokes. Specifically among gymnasts, those with spondylolysis tend to be heavier, older, or training with more intensity. The incidence of spondylolysis is as high as 30% in professional soccer and baseball players in Japan [5].

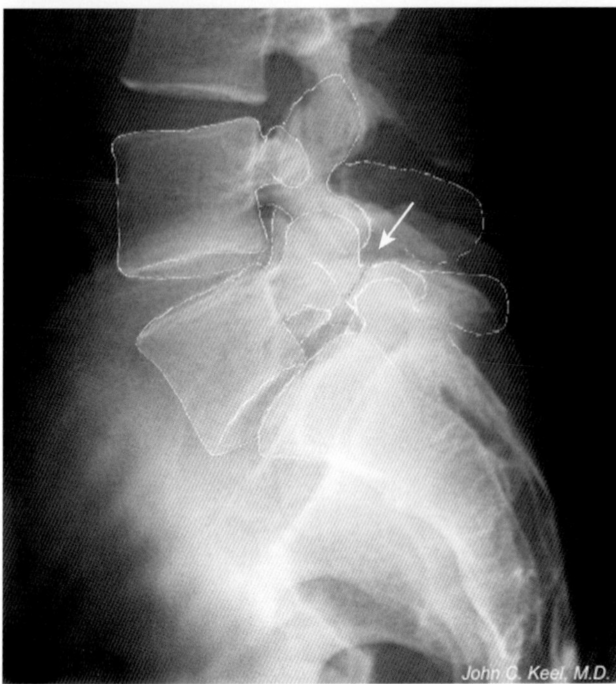

FIGURE 49.1 Spondylolysis of L5 with L5-S1 spondylolisthesis *(arrow)*.

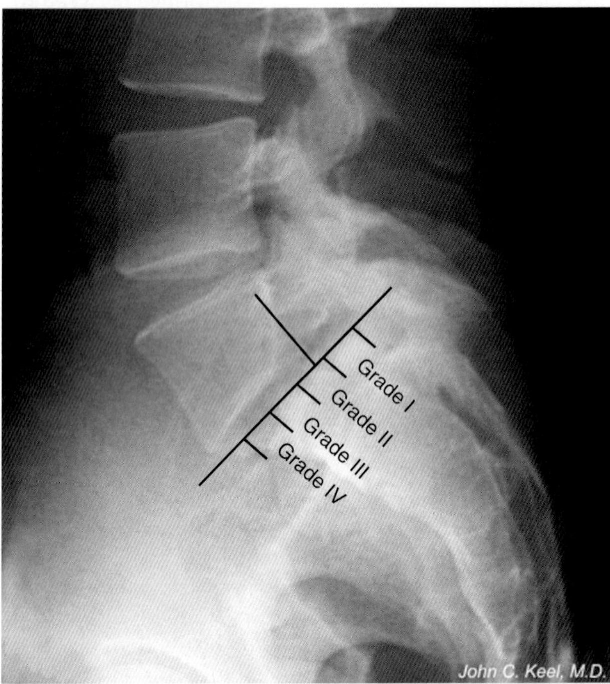

FIGURE 49.2 Meyerding classification of spondylolisthesis into grades based on the amount of slippage of the superior vertebral body on the vertebral body below.

Further supporting an acquired stress fracture as the cause is the lack of spondylolysis in the lumbar spines of individuals who have never walked [13].

Spondylolisthesis refers to displacement of a vertebral body in relation to the one below it. The most common type of spondylolisthesis, and the alignment abnormality that is implied when the term is used in this chapter, is an anterior displacement, also called anterolisthesis. Spondylolisthesis can also occur in a posterior direction, called retrolisthesis, or laterally, called laterolisthesis. Spondylolisthesis is an abnormal finding. Whenever spondylolisthesis is present, it is pathognomonic of structural and functional failure of the neural arch and facet joints, which are responsible for maintaining normal vertebral alignment.

Table 49.1 Etiology of Spondylolisthesis

Type	Etiology
Dysplastic	Congenital dysplasia of one or more facet joints
Isthmic (spondylolytic)	Bilateral pars defects (bilateral spondylolysis)
Degenerative	Degeneration of the facet joints and intervertebral discs
Traumatic	Fractures of posterior elements other than the pars
Pathologic	Malignant neoplasm, infection, or primary bone disease

Spondylolisthesis is classified by etiology and grade. There are five etiologic types (Table 49.1):

Dysplastic spondylolisthesis results from congenital dysplasia of one or more facet joints.

Isthmic or spondylolytic spondylolisthesis results from bilateral pars defects (bilateral spondylolysis).

Degenerative spondylolisthesis results from degeneration of the facet joints and intervertebral discs (most common at L4-L5 and with advancing age).

Traumatic spondylolisthesis results from fractures of posterior elements other than the pars, such as facet joints, laminae, or pedicles.

Pathologic spondylolisthesis results from pathologic changes in posterior elements due to malignant neoplasm, infection, or primary bone disease.

Isthmic spondylolisthesis is male predominant, whereas degenerative spondylolisthesis is more common in females [7]. This chapter is limited to discussion of spondylolytic (isthmic) spondylolisthesis.

The grade of spondylolisthesis is rated by the percentage of slippage of the posterior corner of the vertebral body above over the superior surface of the vertebral body below. At least 5% slippage must be present for a diagnosis of spondylolisthesis to be conferred. Slippage can be further categorized into five grades: grade I indicates slippage from 5% to 25%; grade II is 26% to 50%; grade III is 51% to 75%; grade IV is more than 75% [14]; and grade V is complete dislocation of adjacent vertebrae, also called spondyloptosis. Most cases (60%-75%) are classified as grade I; 20% to 38% are classified as grade II; and less than 2% of all cases are graded III, IV, and V [8,15]. Slip of 15% or more is associated with increased risk of radicular pain or weakness [16] and is always associated with moderate to severe degeneration of the lumbosacral disc [10].

In children and adolescents with bilateral spondylolysis, spondylolisthesis is already present in 50% to 75% at the time of initial diagnosis of the spondylolysis [10,11,17,18]. The incidence of spondylolisthesis increases with age. After diagnosis, concern about the progression of spondylolisthesis is common but prognostic factors are lacking, making it difficult to predict which patients are at risk for progression [10,18]. However, participation in competitive sports has not been found to influence the progression of spondylolisthesis [10]. In addition, unilateral spondylolysis almost never progresses to spondylolisthesis [10]. Whereas spondylolysis is male predominant [7], spondylolisthesis and slippage are more common in females when bilateral spondylolisthesis is present on CT [19]. Typically, progression occurs before and during the early teenage years [2], and only minor progression occurs after skeletal maturity [10]. Advancing age may lead to slight additional progression of spondylolytic spondylolisthesis, which is usually attributed to progressive degeneration of the disc and facet joints [20]. There is a positive correlation between the percentage of slip and the degree of degenerative change but no correlation with disc herniation [10].

Symptoms

Most people with spondylolysis and spondylolisthesis are asymptomatic. Less than 5% of children diagnosed with spondylolysis or spondylolisthesis have back pain before the age of 18 years [10]. Whereas the incidence of back pain increases with age, the incidence of back pain in those with spondylolysis or spondylolisthesis is similar to that of the general population [2,8,10,16]. In addition, the reverse is true: those with and without back pain have nearly an identical incidence of spondylolysis [21]. Furthermore, the degree of spondylolytic spondylolisthesis is not associated with the prevalence of back pain [10], and no study has linked progression of spondylolisthesis with pain symptoms. Disability because of back pain is no more prevalent in the population with spondylolysis and spondylolisthesis than in the general public [10,17]. Ultimately, in patients with established spondylolysis, with or without spondylolisthesis, it is difficult to attribute pain symptoms to these abnormalities.

One exception is the child or adolescent who initially presents with acute back pain, in whom reactive changes to the bone marrow from spondylolysis or spondylolisthesis likely contribute to the patient's symptoms. For these patients and others with back pain from associated spondylolysis or spondylolisthesis, no distinct pain characteristics have been found to distinguish their pain from that experienced by others with common degenerative back disorders [2,17]. The back pain can range from mild to severe and is frequently described as a dull, aching pain in the back, buttocks, and posterior thigh [2].

Spondylolysis with spondylolisthesis combined with disc degeneration may result in significant narrowing of the neuroforamina at the affected level. This can cause compression or irritation of the exiting spinal nerve, resulting in radiating pain and neurologic sequelae in the lower limb, often in dermatomal or myotomal distribution. Because spondylolytic spondylolisthesis most commonly involves the L5-S1 level, the L5 nerve is most often affected by this problem.

Physical Examination

The physical examination in spondylolysis and spondylolisthesis has few specific or sensitive findings. Painful trunk range of motion is often noted with children and adolescents with symptoms from acute spondylolysis. It is suspected that pain with trunk extension may be common in acute spondylolysis as this motion shifts load to the posterior vertebral elements and thus through the region of the pars [22]. Indeed, limited range of motion for trunk extension has been observed [15,23]. However, the precision of painful trunk extension has not been determined, and these findings are common to other spinal disorders. Palpation of the back may reveal local tenderness at the lumbosacral junction, the level at which spondylolysis is most common [15].

Detection of spondylolisthesis on physical examination is difficult except in the rare cases of grade III or greater slips. Here, a "step-off" of the spinous processes can be seen or palpated at the level of the spondylolisthesis. In grade I and II spondylolisthesis, the step-off is much more difficult to detect and has never been shown to be a reliable finding. Neurologic deficits and positive results of straight-leg raising tests are rarely found in cases of spondylolytic spondylolisthesis, including cases with sciatica [15]. When neurologic deficits are noted, they usually involve the L5 roots, which can become irritated within their neuroforamina, presenting as an L5 radiculopathy (weakness of the extensor hallucis longus and hip abductors as well as sensory loss on the dorsum of the great toe) [15,24,25].

Diagnostic Studies

The lateral oblique radiograph may reveal the classic "collar on the Scottie dog" finding of spondylolysis (Fig. 49.3). This represents the bone defect between the inferior and superior articulating processes. The sensitivity of this view approaches only 33% because the plane of the pars defect must be close to the plane of the radiographic image to be

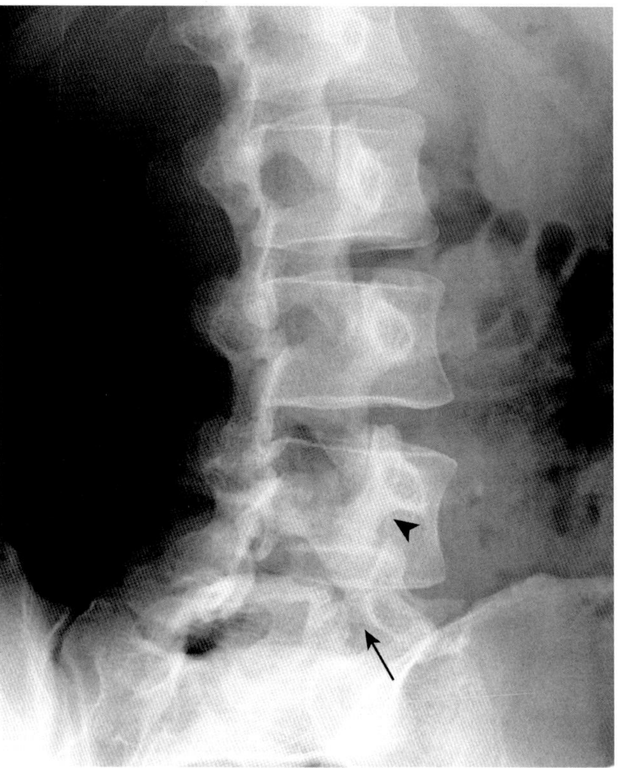

FIGURE 49.3 Spondylolysis defect of L5 noted on oblique radiograph. *(arrow)*. Compare the intact pars at L4. *(arrowhead)*. *(From Slipman CW, Derby R, Simeone FA, Mayer TG. Interventional Spine: An Algorithmic Approach. Philadelphia, WB Saunders, 2008.)*

clearly visualized [26]. The lateral radiograph reveals the presence and grade of spondylolisthesis.

Because of its ability to clearly visualize bone, CT is considered superior to magnetic resonance imaging (MRI) for direct visualization of the pars interarticularis, and some advocate CT axial images as the test of choice (Fig. 49.4) for identifying spondylolysis [27]. Even with CT, pars defects can be difficult to identify because they can simulate the adjacent facet joints. However, they usually lack the regular cortical surfaces of the facets [28]. Also useful is trying to identify an intact cortical ring for each vertebra, including the vertebral body, the pedicles, the pars, and the posterior neural arch. If the intact ring is not found in any of the cuts through the levels of the pedicles, a defect in the ring at the appropriate position suggests diagnosis of spondylolysis [29]. If spondylolysis is suspected when CT is ordered, scanning can be done with thin sections or reverse gantry angle to ensure optimum visualization of the pars [27].

For children and adolescents with acute spondylolysis, MRI with fat saturation technique can identify subtle bone marrow edema of early stress injury to the pars interarticularis [30]. Identifying the bone defect of the pars is more challenging with MRI. Defects are most commonly noted as a lack of bone continuity between the superior and inferior articulating process on sagittal T1 images. MRI has a sensitivity of 57% to 86% (Fig. 49.5) [31]. Axial T2 MRI demonstrating increased fluid in the facet joints is also sensitive for early detection of spondylolisthesis (Fig. 49.6) [32]. Combining both of these MRI methods increases the sensitivity for detection of spondylolisthesis to 94%. MRI is also useful for grading spondylolisthesis and for visualizing the neuroforamina. As spondylolisthesis progresses, the neuroforamina become horizontally oriented, resulting in a position of the exiting spinal nerve that is between the pedicle above and the uncovered disc below. As the disc degenerates and loses height, foraminal narrowing is exacerbated, which may entrap the exiting spinal nerve. This is well visualized on T1 sagittal and axial images as the high fat signal that normally surrounds the spinal nerve becomes obliterated [25].

Bone scintigraphy uses radioisotopes that accumulate in metabolically hyperactive bone. Acute spondylolysis will reveal the bone activity of attempted healing. Longstanding spondylolysis with an established nonunion reveals no such activity [33]. Single-photon emission computed

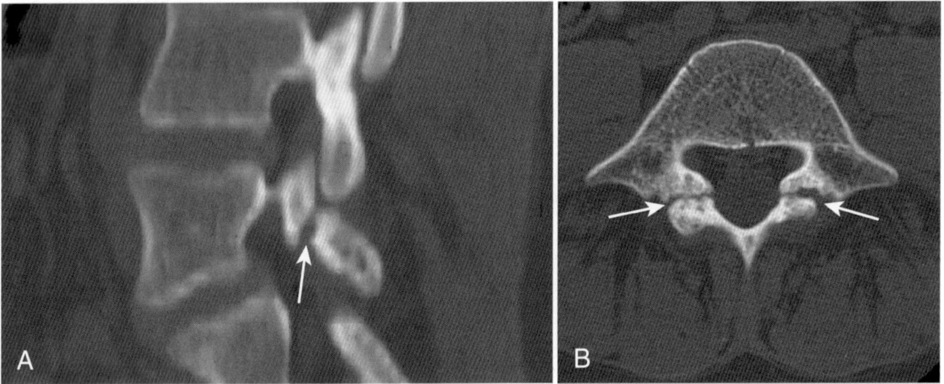

FIGURE 49.4 Spondylolysis defects of L5 as seen on parasagittal (**A**) and axial (**B**) computed tomographic scans. *(arrows)*. Note the lack of complete vertebral ring on axial view. *(From Slipman CW, Derby R, Simeone FA, Mayer TG. Interventional Spine: An Algorithmic Approach. Philadelphia, WB Saunders, 2008.)*

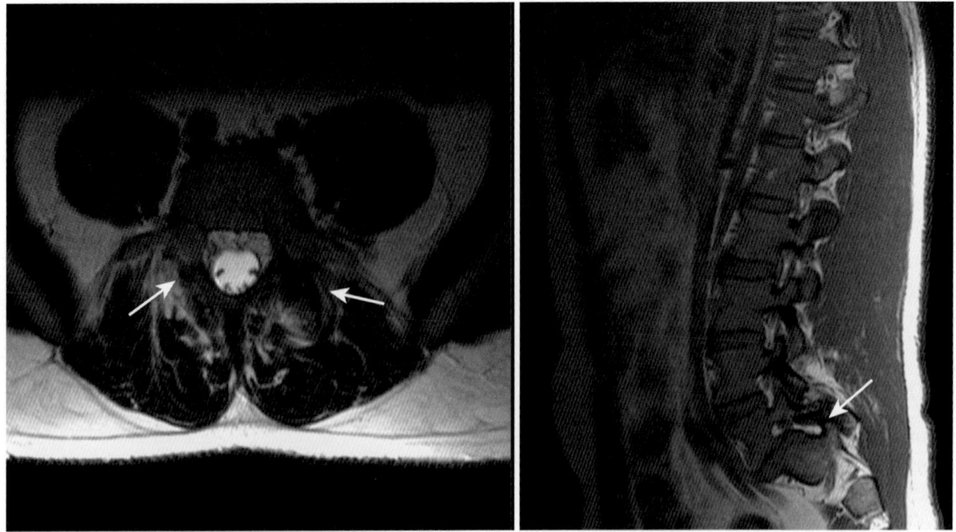

FIGURE 49.5 MRI of spondylolytic spondylolisthesis. Discontinuity of the vertebral ring is demonstrated *(arrows)* on the axial T2 image *(left)*, and discontinuity of the pars is seen *(arrow)* on the parasagittal T1 image *(right)*. Compare the elongated, horizontally oriented neuroforamina at L5-S1.

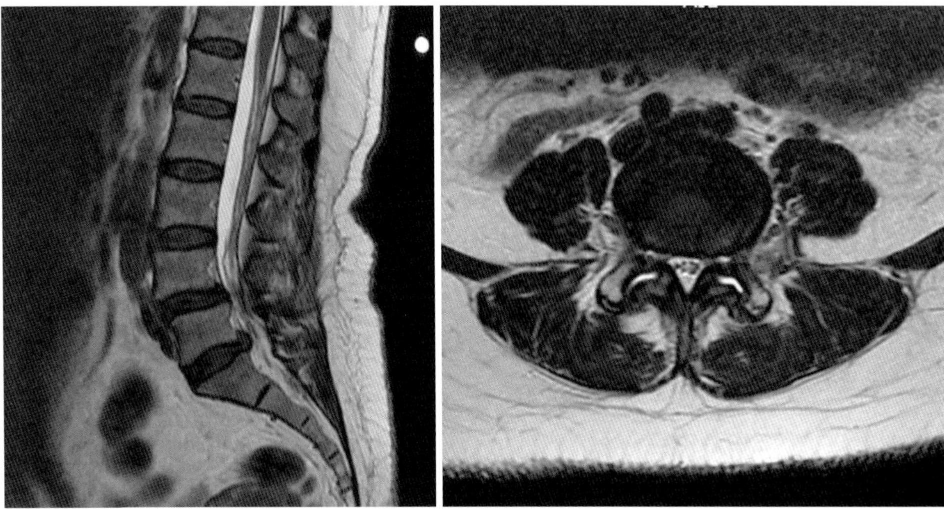

FIGURE 49.6 MRI of degenerative spondylolisthesis at L4-L5 *(left)*. Increased T2 signal is demonstrated in axial view of the L4-L5 facet joints *(right)*.

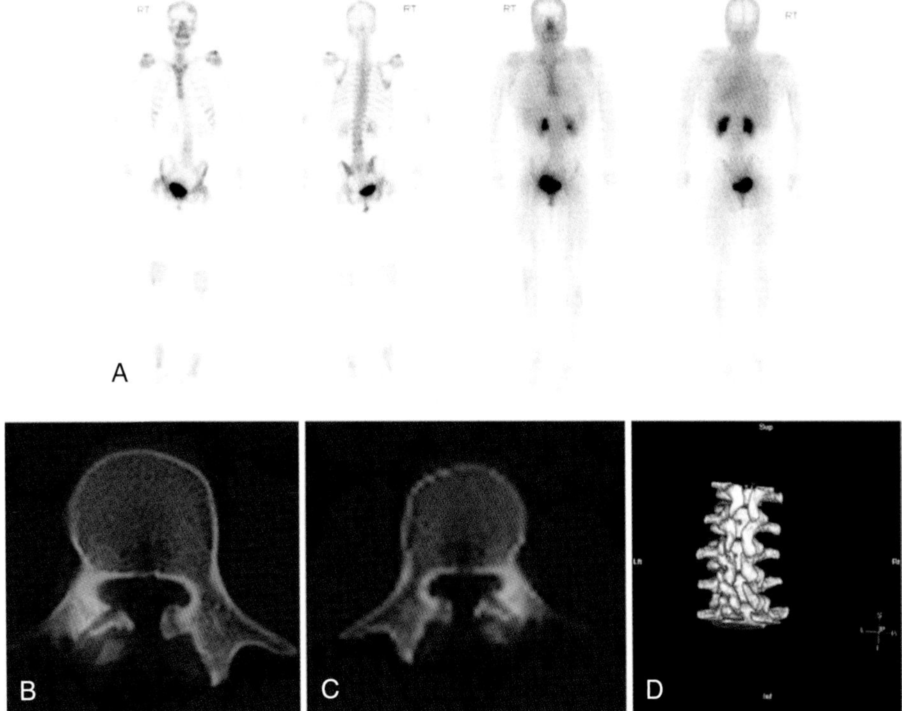

FIGURE 49.7 Child with back pain. **A,** Whole-body imaging shows scoliosis and a focal lesion at the right side of mid lumbar spine. SPECT/CT confirmed bilateral spondylolysis with increased activity. **B,** Fused SPECT/CT shows a spondylolysis with focal increased activity in the right L3 pars. **C,** Fused SPECT/CT shows a spondylolysis with focal increased activity in the left L4 pars. **D,** Three-dimensional CT image shows deficiency of posterior spinous processes in the lumbar spine from previous laminectomy that may have produced the altered stress that led to development of the bilateral spondylolysis. *(From Nadel H. Pediatric bone scintigraphy update. Semin Nucl Med 2010;40:31-40.)*

tomography (SPECT) improves the localizing ability of bone scintigraphy (Fig. 49.7). SPECT creates a series of slices through the target structure, permitting spatial separation of overlapping bone. Because of these abilities, SPECT imaging has established its place for the evaluation of adolescent athletes with back pain [34,35]. Nonetheless, MRI is considered a first-line imaging modality, given that it demonstrates a high level of agreement with SPECT in diagnosis of juvenile spondylolysis [36] without exposing the patient to radiation.

Differential Diagnosis

Degenerative low back pain
Lumbar disc herniation
Discitis
Lumbar radiculopathy
Spinal stenosis (central vs neuroforaminal)
Vertebral fracture (by compression, tumor, infection)
Lumbar sprain or strain

Treatment

Initial

In children or adolescents with acute symptomatic spondylolysis as suggested by bone scintigraphy, SPECT, or MRI, attempts to induce or to aid healing are warranted. Nonoperative treatments for spondylolysis include bracing, activity restriction, and therapeutic exercises [37]. Rigid antilordotic bracing for 3 to 6 months (often for 23 hours a day) has been advocated to reduce stress on the pars interarticularis [38]; however, a more recent meta-analysis found that although 83.9% of nonoperatively treated patients clinically improve, there is not a difference between those treated with and without bracing [37]. Activity modification is usually recommended until symptoms subside, and physical therapy for trunk muscle strengthening has been used. With this approach, symptoms improve in about 75% of children, and many lytic defects are noted to heal [38]. Unilateral defects are more likely to heal than bilateral defects [37]. With nonoperative treatment of spondylolysis, children and young adults return to a pain-free or nearly pain-free state in unrestricted activities 84% of the time [37].

A similar approach is advocated in children and adolescents with concurrent spondylolisthesis. However, once spondylolisthesis is present, healing of the pars defect becomes improbable. In this situation, the goal is symptom reduction, and good results are observed in many patients. Nonoperative treatment does not specifically lead to a bone union in terminal defects but may alleviate symptoms [37]. To date, there is no evidence to support bracing for the prevention of slip progression. In cases of incidental findings of spondylolisthesis, there is no need for treatment or restriction of activities, including aggressive sports [12,39].

In adults with spondylolysis, with or without spondylolisthesis, back pain complaints are treated like other nonspecific back pain disorders. Such treatment includes education, analgesics, nonsteroidal anti-inflammatory drugs, exercise, avoidance of bed rest, and rapid return to activities [40–42].

Rehabilitation

Exercise has received some study as a treatment of symptomatic spondylolysis and spondylolisthesis. One study has advocated flexion over extension exercise [43], although methodologic shortcomings limit the strength of these recommendations. A spinal stabilization exercise program was found to be superior to uncontrolled treatment at short- and long-term follow-up [44]. Aggressive physical therapy programs for those with back pain including spondylolysis or spondylolisthesis have been shown to provide significant short-term benefit in terms of flexibility, strength, endurance, pain tolerance, and level of disability. This type of program consists of stretching and high-intensity, progressively resistive exercise training, performed in a non–pain-contingent manner [45,46]. Stretching targets the hip flexors, hamstrings, quadriceps, and gastrocnemius-soleus muscles. Strengthening targets the abdominal and various back muscles. Active individual therapy and functional restoration program participation both improve work ability and hasten return to sports and leisure activities; the functional restoration program participation improves endurance in treatment of chronic low back pain [47].

A randomized controlled trial comparing fusion surgery with intensive rehabilitation for chronic low back pain, including patients with spondylolisthesis, found that both approaches led to symptom improvement and suggested there was no clear evidence that surgery is more beneficial [48]. With the complications and cost of surgery, this minimal difference is worth considering in choosing a treatment approach [48].

For lumbosacral pain in general, in addition to exercise, cognitive interventions allowing patients to feel safe while being active lead to improvements in fear-avoidance beliefs and forward bending ability in patients with chronic back pain [49]. It has been suggested that the specific type of exercise may be less important than the general message exercise conveys—that normal use of the back is not harmful [50]. A randomized trial of rehabilitation methods after spinal fusion has demonstrated that early postoperative implementation of a combination of motor training exercise and cognitive-behavioral therapy is safe and results in superior functional outcomes compared with a customary exercise program of strength, flexibility, and cardiovascular exercises, including in patients with spondylolisthesis [51].

Alternative therapies such as massage [52] and therapeutic horseback riding [53] have been considered potentially beneficial treatments at the case report level. Modalities including ultrasound and electrical stimulation have not been shown to improve symptoms and are generally of limited value.

Procedures

Various types of spinal injections are given with use of fluoroscopy to ensure proper needle placement (Fig. 49.8). Anesthetic agents may be used for short-term pain relief, usually for diagnostic purposes. Injection of steroids may be tried for longer term therapeutic purposes in adults with

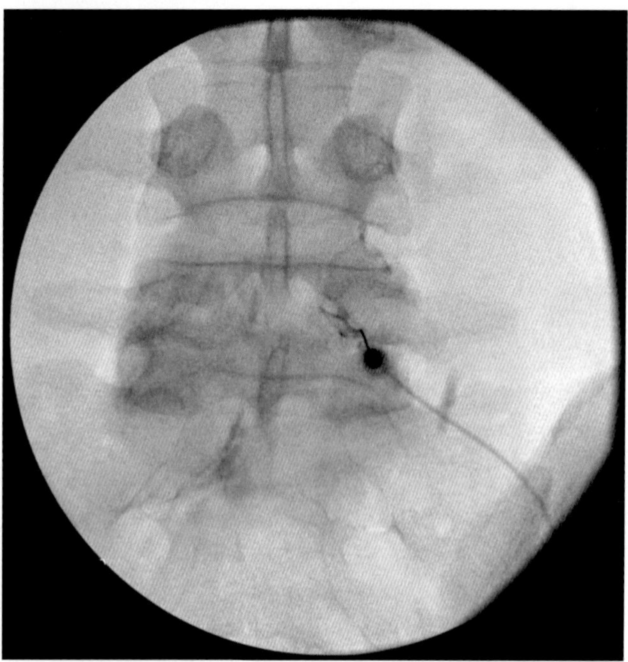

FIGURE 49.8 Fluoroscopic injection of pars interarticularis defect, with contrast material filling the pseudojoint capsule.

symptomatic spondylolysis or spondylolisthesis. For radicular pain, epidural injections may be used if the site of nerve root compression lies within the spinal canal, whereas selective nerve root blocks may be used if compression lies within the transforaminal space. For axial pain, facet injections may be used if the facet joints themselves are thought to be the source of pain.

Surgery

Referral to a surgeon is indicated in cases of spondylolisthesis causing progressive neurologic deficit; cauda equina compression with leg weakness, sensory loss, or bladder or bowel incontinence; neurogenic claudication; and persistent and severe back and leg pain despite aggressive conservative treatment. However, the patient's preference, age, and comorbidities must be considered before surgery because rates of reoperation range from 7% to 15% with a perioperative mortality of 0.5% to 1.3% [54–56]. In general, lumbar spinal decompression or fusion is usually indicated only when imaging studies correlate well with the history and physical examination findings. Surgical outcomes are generally favorable [57].

Potential Disease Complications

Most cases of spondylolysis and spondylolisthesis are asymptomatic and remain that way [58]. The intervertebral disc and facet degeneration that occurs naturally with age is accelerated in the presence of spondylolysis. Because of this, spondylolytic spondylolisthesis can progress and result in spinal nerve compression or spinal stenosis [59].

Potential Treatment Complications

Nonsteroidal anti-inflammatory drugs can cause gastric bleeding and renal and hepatic toxicity. Acetaminophen, in large amounts, can cause hepatic toxicity. Narcotic analgesics are potentially addictive, and because studies of the low back pain population have not found significant differences between narcotics and nonsteroidal anti-inflammatory drugs in terms of pain relief, extreme caution should be used beyond the short term [60]. Exercise can irritate spinal tissue already inflamed. Spinal injections may result in a temporary increase in pain, spinal headache, infection, spinal nerve damage, or spinal cord damage. Surgical decompression or fusion can lead to infection, failed fusion, persistent back pain, spinal nerve damage, or spinal cord damage. Lumbar stabilization can accelerate adjacent level degeneration [61].

References

[1] Lonstein J. Spondylolisthesis in children: cause, natural history, and management. Spine (Phila Pa 1976) 1999;24:2640–8.
[2] Fredrickson B, Baker D, McHolick WJ, et al. The natural history of spondylolysis and spondylolisthesis. J Bone Joint Surg Am 1984;66:699–707.
[3] Wertzberger K, Peterson H. Acquired spondylolysis and spondylolisthesis in the young child. Spine (Phila Pa 1976) 1980;5:437–42.
[4] Baker D, McHolick WJ. Spondyloschisis and spondylolisthesis in children. J Bone Joint Surg Am 1956;38:933–4.
[5] Sakai T, Sairyo K, Suzue N, et al. Incidence and etiology of lumbar spondylolysis: review of the literature. J Orthop Sci 2010;15:281–8.
[6] Belfi L, Ortiz O, Katz D. Computed tomography evaluation of spondylolysis and spondylolisthesis. Spine (Phila Pa 1976) 2006;31:E907–10.
[7] Kalichman L, Kim DH, Li L, Guermazi A, et al. Spondylolysis and spondylolisthesis: prevalence and association with low back pain in the adult community-based population. Spine (Phila Pa 1976) 2009;34:199–205.
[8] Osterman K, Schlenzka D, Poussa M, et al. Isthmic spondylolisthesis in symptomatic and asymptomatic subjects, epidemiology, and natural history with special reference to disk abnormalities and mode of treatment. Clin Orthop Relat Res 1993;297:65–70.
[9] Rothman S, Glenn W. CT multiplanar reconstruction in 253 cases of lumbar spondylolysis. AJNR Am J Neuroradiol 1984;5:81–90.
[10] Beutler W, Fredrickson BE, Murtland A, et al. The natural history of spondylolysis and spondylolisthesis: 45-year follow-up evaluation. Spine (Phila Pa 1976) 2003;28:1027–35.
[11] Shahriaree H, Sajadi K, Rooholamini S. A family with spondylolisthesis. J Bone Joint Surg Am 1979;61:1256–8.
[12] Wiltse L, Widell E, Jackson D. Fatigue fracture: the basic lesion in isthmic spondylolisthesis. J Bone Joint Surg Am 1975;57:17–22.
[13] Rosenberg N, Bargar W, Friedman B. The incidence of spondylolysis and spondylolisthesis in nonambulatory patients. Spine (Phila Pa 1976) 1981;6:35–8.
[14] Meyerding H. Spondylolisthesis. Surg Gynecol Obstet 1932;54:371–7.
[15] Möller H, Hedlund R. Surgery versus conservative management in adult "isthmic spondylolisthesis"—a prospective randomized study: part I. Spine (Phila Pa 1976) 2000;25:1711–5.
[16] Denard P, Holton KF, Miller J, et al. Back pain, neurogenic symptoms, and physical function in relation to spondylolisthesis among elderly men. Spine J 2010;10:865–73.
[17] Frennered A, Danielson B, Nachemson A. Natural history of symptomatic isthmic low-grade spondylolisthesis in children and adolescents: a seven-year follow-up study. J Pediatr Orthop 1991;11:209–13.
[18] Danielson B, Frennered A, Irstam L. Radiologic progression of isthmus lumbar spondylolisthesis in young patients. Spine (Phila Pa 1976) 1991;16:422–5.
[19] Takao S, Sakai T, Sairyo K, et al. Radiographic comparison between male and female patients with lumber spondylolysis. J Med Invest 2010;57:133–7.
[20] Fredrickson B, et al. The natural history of spondylolysis and spondylolisthesis: 45-year follow-up. In: North American Spine Society 15th annual meeting; New Orleans, La; October 25-28, 2000.
[21] Rauch R, Jinkins J. Lumbosacral spondylolisthesis associated with spondylolysis. Neuroradiol Clin N Am 1993;3:543–53.
[22] Yamane T, Yosida T, Mimatsu K. Early diagnosis of lumbar spondylolysis by MRI. J Bone Joint Surg Br 1993;75:764–8.
[23] McGregor A, Cattermole H, Hughes S. Global spinal motion in subjects with lumbar spondylolysis and listhesis. Does the grade or type of slip affect global spinal motion? Spine (Phila Pa 1976) 2001;26:282–6.
[24] Jinkins J, Matthes JC, Sener RN, et al. Spondylolysis, spondylolisthesis, and associated nerve entrapment in the lumbosacral spine: MR evaluation. AJR Am J Roentgenol 1992;159:799–803.
[25] Jinkins J, Rauch A. Magnetic resonance imaging of entrapment of lumbar nerve roots in spondylolytic spondylolisthesis. J Bone Joint Surg Am 1994;76:1643–8.
[26] Saifuddin A, White J, Tucker S. Orientation of lumbar pars defects: implications for radiological detection and surgical management. J Bone Joint Surg Br 1998;80:208–11.
[27] Harvey C, Richenberg J, Saifuddin A. The radiological investigation of lumbar spondylolysis. Clin Radiol 1998;53:723–8.
[28] Grogan J, Hemminghytt S, Williams AL, et al. Spondylolysis studied with computer tomography. Radiology 1982;145:737–42.
[29] Langston J, Gavant M. "Incomplete ring" sign; a simple method for CT detection of spondylolysis. J Comput Assist Tomogr 1985;9:728–9.
[30] Hollenberg G, Beattie PF, Meyers SP, et al. Stress reaction of the lumbar pars interarticularis: the development of a new MRI classification system. Spine (Phila Pa 1976) 2002;27:181–6.
[31] Saifuddin A, Burnett S. The value of lumbar spine MRI in the assessment of the pars interarticularis. Clin Radiol 1997;52:666–71.
[32] Schinnerer K, Katz L, Grauer J. MR findings of exaggerated fluid in facet joints predicts instability. J Spinal Disord Tech 2008;21:468–72.
[33] Lowe J, Schachner E, Hirschberg E, et al. Significance of bone scintigraphy in symptomatic spondylolysis. Spine (Phila Pa 1976) 1984;9:653–5.
[34] Bellar RD, Summerville DA, Treves ST, Micheli LJ. Low-back pain in adolescent athletes: detection of stress injuries to the pars interarticularis with SPECT. Radiology 1991;180:509–12.
[35] Itol K, Hashimoto T, Shigenobu K. Bone SPECT of symptomatic lumbar spondylolysis. Nucl Med Commun 1996;17:389–96.

[36] Campbell R, Grainger AJ, Hide IG, et al. Juvenile spondylolysis: a comparative analysis of CT, SPECT and MRI. Skeletal Radiol 2005;34:63–73.

[37] Klein G, Mehlman C. Nonoperative treatment of spondylolysis and grade I spondylolisthesis in children and young adults: a meta-analysis of observation studies. J Pediatr Orthop 2009;29:146–56.

[38] Morita T, Ikata T, Katoh S, Miyake R. Lumbar spondylolysis in children and adolescents. J Bone Joint Surg Br 1995;77:620–5.

[39] Semon R, Spengler D. Significance of lumbar spondylolysis in college football players. Spine (Phila Pa 1976) 1981;6:172–4.

[40] Deyo R, Diehl A, Rosenthal M. How many days of bed rest for acute low back pain? A randomized clinical trial. N Engl J Med 1986;315:1064–70.

[41] Gilbert J, Taylor DW, Hildebrand A, Evans C. Clinical trial of common treatments for low back pain in family practice. Br Med J (Clin Res Ed) 1995;291:789–94.

[42] Malmivaara A, Häkkinen U, Aro T, et al. The treatment of acute low back pain—bed rest, exercises or ordinary activity? N Engl J Med 1995;332:351–5.

[43] Sinaki M, Lutness MP, Ilstrup DM, et al. Lumbar spondylolisthesis: retrospective comparison and three year follow-up of two conservative treatment programs. Arch Phys Med Rehabil 1989;70:594–8.

[44] O'Sullivan P, Twomey L, Allison G. Evaluation of specific stabilizing exercises in the treatment of chronic low back pain with radiologic diagnosis of spondylolysis and spondylolisthesis. Spine (Phila Pa 1976) 1997;22:2959–67.

[45] Rainville J, Sobel JB, Hartigan C, Wright A. The effect of compensation involvement on the reporting of pain and disability by subjects referred for rehabilitation of chronic low back pain. Spine (Phila Pa 1976) 1997;22:2016–24.

[46] Rainville J, Mazzaferro R. Evaluation of outcomes of aggressive spine rehabilitation in patients with back pain and sciatica from previously diagnosed spondylolysis and spondylolisthesis. Arch Phys Med Rehabil 2001;82:1309.

[47] Roche G, Ponthieux A, Parot-Shinkel E, et al. Comparison of a functional restoration program with active individual physical therapy for patients with chronic low back pain: a randomized controlled trial. Arch Phys Med Rehabil 2007;88:1229–35.

[48] Fairbank J, Frost H, Wilson-MacDonald J, et al. Randomised controlled trial to compare surgical stabilisation of the lumbar spine with an intensive rehabilitation programme for patients with chronic low back pain: the MRC spine stabilisation trial. BMJ 2005;330:1233.

[49] Brox J, Sørensen R, Friis A, et al. Randomized clinical trial of lumbar instrumented fusion and cognitive intervention and exercise in patients with chronic low back pain and disc degeneration. Spine (Phila Pa 1976) 2003;28:1913–21.

[50] Rainville J, Nguyen R, Suri P. Effective conservative treatment for chronic low back pain. Semin Spine Surg 2009;21:257–63.

[51] Abbott A, Tyni-Lenné R, Hedlund R. Early rehabilitation targeting cognition, behavior, and motor function after lumbar fusion: a randomized controlled trial. Spine (Phila Pa 1976) 2010;35:848–57.

[52] Halpin S. Case report: the effects of massage therapy on lumbar spondylolisthesis. J Bodyw Mov Ther 2012;16:115–23.

[53] Ungermann C, Gras L. Therapeutic riding followed by rhythmic auditory stimulation to improve balance and gait in a subject with orthopedic pathologies. J Altern Complement Med 2011;17:1191–5.

[54] Atlas S, Keller RB, Robson D, et al. Surgical and nonsurgical management of lumbar spinal stenosis: four year outcomes from the Maine lumbar spine study. Spine (Phila Pa 1976) 2000;25:556–62.

[55] Deyo R, Ciol MA, Cherkin DC, et al. Lumbar spinal fusion: a cohort study of complications, reoperations and resources use in the Medicare population. Spine (Phila Pa 1976) 1993;18:1463–70.

[56] Weinstein J, Lurie JD, Tosteson TD, et al. Surgical compared with nonoperative treatment for lumbar degenerative spondylolisthesis: four-year results in the Spine Patient Outcomes Research Trial (SPORT) randomized and observational cohorts. J Bone Joint Surg Am 2009;91:1295–304.

[57] Swan J, Hurwitz E, Malek F, et al. Surgical treatment for unstable low-grade isthmic spondylolisthesis in adults: a prospective controlled study of posterior instrumented fusion compared with combined anterior-posterior fusion. Spine J 2006;6:606–14.

[58] Torgerson W, Dotter W. Comparative roentgenographic study of the asymptomatic and symptomatic lumbar spine. J Bone Joint Surg Am 1976;56:850–3.

[59] Floman Y. Progression of lumbosacral spondylolisthesis in adults. Spine (Phila Pa 1976) 2000;25:342–7.

[60] Rathmell J. A 50-year-old man with chronic low back pain. JAMA 2008;299:2066–77.

[61] Heo D, Cho YJ, Cho SM, et al. Adjacent segment degeneration after lumbar dynamic stabilization using pedicle screws and a nitinol spring rod system with 2-year minimum follow-up. J Spinal Disord Tech 2012;25:409–14.

CHAPTER 50

Lumbar Spinal Stenosis

Zacharia Isaac, MD

Edrick Lopez, MD, JD

Synonyms

Pseudoclaudication
Neurogenic claudication
Spinal claudication
Low back pain

ICD-9 Code

724.02 Spinal stenosis, lumbar region

ICD-10 Code

M48.06 Spinal stenosis, lumbar region

Definition

Lumbar spinal stenosis is classically defined as narrowing of the spinal canal, nerve root canals, or tunnels of the intervertebral foramina at the lumbar level [1]. A significant portion of the general population may have anatomic spinal stenosis without symptoms. Studies have indicated that 20% to 25% of asymptomatic people older than 40 years have significant narrowing of the lumbar spinal canal [2]. Stenosis causes symptoms only when there is sufficient impingement on neural structures, including the cauda equina or exiting nerve roots. Therefore spinal stenosis as a clinical entity is considered significant only if it results in symptomatic pain and compromised function.

The significant anatomic elements of the lumbosacral spine include the five lumbar vertebrae L1 to L5, the sacrum, the intervertebral discs, the ligamentum flavum, the zygapophyseal joints, the lumbar spinal nerve rootlets, the spinal nerve roots, and the cauda equina (Fig. 50.1).

Various schemes for classification of spinal stenosis have been devised and are listed in Table 50.1.

Congenital lumbar spinal stenosis is less common, representing 9% of cases [3]; symptoms first appear in patients during their 30s. Achondroplastic dwarves often have stenosis secondary to hypoplasia of the pedicles. Acromegaly may cause spinal stenosis by enlargement of the synovium and cartilage, which results in decreased cross-sectional area of the canal. Symptomatic spinal stenosis secondary to purely isolated congenital causes is rare. More commonly, patients will have a combination of congenital and acquired stenosis; a developmentally smaller canal predisposes them to symptoms once acquired changes occur to the surrounding anatomy. Developmental factors that lead to a small canal include statistically significantly shorter pedicles and a trefoil-shaped canal.

The acquired types of spinal stenosis are numerous, but degenerative is the most common. The first stage in the degenerative process is generally degradation of the hydrophilic proteoglycans within the intervertebral disc, attendant disc desiccation, and loss of disc height. This causes a shift of load onto the posterior structures of the canal, in particular the facet joints, which normally provide 3% to 25% of the support during axial loading but may bear up to 47% with degeneration of the disc [4]. As the facets bear more of the burden, they undergo degeneration, one aspect of which is osteophyte formation. This further diminishes the cross-sectional area of the canal and can also result in stenosis of the neural foramina (termed *foraminal stenosis*). The ligamentum flavum undergoes buckling with decreased intervertebral disc height, leading to further encroachment of the canal. Epidural fat may contribute to reduced canal space in some patients [5]. Patients can have degenerative facet synovial cysts that focally can encroach on the spinal canal and nerve rootlets and cause radicular pain.

Spinal stenosis can be differentiated by anatomic location, including central canal, lateral recess, foraminal, and extraforaminal (Table 50.2). Additional subcategorization includes division of the lateral canal into three regions: entrance zone, mid-zone, and exit zone.

Canal Measurements

The normal adult central canal has a midsagittal diameter of at least 13 mm. Relative stenosis is defined as a canal

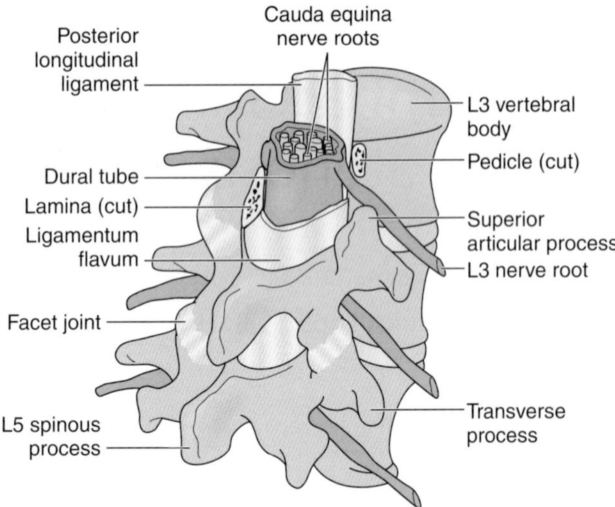

FIGURE 50.1 Normal anatomic structures of the lumbar spine at the third through the fifth lumbar levels. Note the close association between the nerve roots and the dural tube, the ligamentum flavum, the facet joints, the pedicles, and the lamina. The ligamentum (interlaminar ligament) attaches laterally to the facet capsules.

Table 50.1 Etiologic Classification of Spinal Stenosis

Congenital
Achondroplastic
Acromegaly
Acquired
Degenerative
Post-traumatic
Spondylolytic (isthmic spondylolisthesis)
Iatrogenic
Metabolic (Paget disease, chlorosis, fluorosis, diffuse interstitial skeletal hypertrophy, pseudogout, oxalosis)
Combined congenital and acquired

Table 50.2 Anatomic Classification of Spinal Stenosis

Central canal
Lateral canal
Entrance zone (lateral recess)
Mid-zone (underneath pars interarticularis and pedicle)
Exit zone (intervertebral foramen)
Foraminal
Extraforaminal

diameter between 10 and 13 mm; patients may or may not be symptomatic. Absolute stenosis occurs at a diameter of less than 10 mm, and patients are usually symptomatic. Extraforaminal nerve root compression can occur with disc herniation, degenerative scoliosis, or isthmic spondylolisthesis. Far-out syndrome, described by Wiltse and colleagues [6], involves L5 root impingement between the L5 transverse process and sacral ala in patients with spondylolisthesis. Extension of the spine can reduce foraminal cross-sectional area by 20% and central canal volume by up to 67% [7].

Finally, spinal stenosis has been categorized according to the patient's presenting pain syndrome of mechanical back pain, radicular pain, or neurogenic claudication. The pain pattern can be an indication of the anatomic and pathophysiologic mechanism of the patient's particular case of spinal stenosis.

Symptoms

Patients with acquired lumbar spinal stenosis usually have symptoms during their 50s and 60s. Symptomatic lumbar spinal stenosis may result in both back pain (from axial components, such as facet degeneration) and leg pain (from radicular components of nerve root compression, either central or lateral). Leg pain is often greater than back pain, and depending on which nerve roots are impinged, leg pain can be unilateral or bilateral and monoradicular or polyradicular. Patients with acquired, degenerative lumbar spinal stenosis tend to have a history of chronic low back pain and develop leg pain later in their course. In a study of 100 patients with lumbar spinal stenosis, back pain had been present for an average of 14 years and leg pain for an average of 2 years [8]. The classic symptom of lumbar spinal stenosis is neurogenic claudication, also known as pseudoclaudication, which typically is manifested as buttock, thigh, and calf pain exacerbated with walking, standing, or lumbar extension and alleviated with sitting, lying, or lumbar flexion. Symptoms also commonly involve cramping, numbness, tingling, heaviness, and spasms. Because the spinal canal and neural foramina widen with flexion and become narrower with extension, pain often improves with squatting and walking tolerance increases with a flexed posture, such as while walking uphill or on an inclined treadmill or while pushing a shopping cart. From a diagnostic point of view, neurogenic claudication was found in one study to have a sensitivity of 63% and a specificity of 71% compared with a combination of clinical, radiologic, and imaging test findings [9].

Symptoms that have been reported to have high sensitivity for lumbar spinal stenosis are as follows: best posture with regard to symptoms is sitting (89%) [10], worst posture with regard to symptoms is standing or walking (89%) [10], pain below buttocks (88%) [11], pain in legs worsened by walking and relieved by sitting (81%) [10], radiating leg pain (81%) [9], and age older than 65 years (77%) [11]. Symptoms with high specificity for lumbar spinal stenosis include no pain when seated (93%) and symptoms improved when seated (83%) [11]. A systematic review of the accuracy of the clinical history (the information in this sentence is about symptoms and not about findings in clinical examination) for the diagnosis of lumbar spinal stenosis, encompassing four studies and 741 patients, found that having no pain when seated (likelihood ratio [LR], 7.4; 95% confidence interval [CI], 1.9-30), improvement of symptoms when bending forward (LR, 6.4; 95% CI, 4.1-9.9), presence of bilateral buttock or leg pain (LR, 6.3; 95% CI, 3.1-13), and neurogenic claudication (LR, 3.7; 95% CI, 2.9-4.8) were the most useful individual findings for identifying the syndrome of lumbar spinal stenosis.

Physical Examination

Unlike the history, no physical examination findings are considered classic for lumbar spinal stenosis. Abnormal findings in lumbar spinal stenosis are similar to those in other disorders that cause peripheral neurologic deficits, but they are often not present. On physical examination, having a wide-based gait (LR, 13; 95% CI, 1.9-95) and an abnormal Romberg test result (LR, 4.2; 95% CI, 1.4-13) also increased the likelihood of the clinical syndrome of lumbar spinal stenosis. On the other hand, absence of neurogenic claudication (LR, 0.23; 95% CI, 0.17-0.31) decreased the likelihood of the diagnosis [12]. In the study by Amundsen and colleagues [8], abnormal findings within the 100-subject cohort included sensory dysfunction (51%), diminished deep tendon reflexes (47%), positive Lasègue test result (24%), and leg weakness (23%), among others. Physical and functional findings with high sensitivity include longer recovery time after level versus inclined treadmill walking (82%) [10] and no pain with lumbar flexion (79%) [11]. Highly specific aspects of examination and testing include improved walking tolerance on inclined versus level treadmill (92%), earlier onset of symptoms on level versus inclined treadmill (83%) [10], absent Achilles reflex (78%), lower extremity weakness (78%), pinprick or vibration deficit (>75%), wide-based gait (>75%), and presence of Romberg sign (>75%) [11]. Checking arterial pulses is important and necessary in patients thought to have lumbar spinal stenosis, but it is not sufficient to rule out arterial disease. A prospective study examining the rate of peripheral arterial disease in patients with intermittent claudication with concurrent lumbar spinal canal stenosis found that peripheral arterial disease was present in 26% of the subjects. Screening for peripheral arterial disease by ankle-brachial index and toe-brachial index tests should be considered in patients with intermittent claudication and lumbar spinal stenosis [13].

Functional Limitations

Worsening leg and back pain from walking, back extension, and prolonged standing is the primary contributor to activity limitation. As such, patients with lumbar spinal stenosis tend to have difficulties with walking long distances, going down stairs, and household or yard work (e.g., dishwashing, lawn mowing, and vacuuming) as well as with tasks that require overhead work (which may induce spinal extension). Balance deficits from sensory deficits may increase fall risk.

Diagnostic Studies

Diagnostic studies can provide useful information on structural and neurologic changes associated with spinal stenosis, but they must be interpreted in the context of the patient's clinical presentation. Several studies have demonstrated that there is no correlation between radiologic findings and clinical or functional outcomes [14]. However, another study found that severity of lumbar spinal stenosis as measured on functional myelography predicted long-term disability independent of therapeutic intervention [15]. The various qualities of the diagnostic tests are summarized in Table 50.3.

Differential Diagnosis

Lumbar spondylosis without spinal stenosis
Cervical and thoracic spinal stenosis
Herniated nucleus pulposus
Lumbar facet syndrome
Vertebral fracture with significant deformity or retropulsed fragments
Peripheral vascular disease
Venous claudication after thrombosis
Myxedema claudication
Inferior vena caval obstruction
Sacroiliac dysfunction
Osteoarthritis of the hips and knees
Trochanteric bursitis
Anterior tibial compartment syndrome
Spinal tumors
Conus medullaris and cauda equina neoplasms
Neurofibromas, ependymomas, hemangioblastomas, dermoids, epidermoids, lipomas
Metastatic spread of tumor
Peripheral neuropathy
Peripheral nerve entrapment
Restless legs syndrome
Stroke
Myofascial pain syndrome
Epidural abscess
Inflammatory arachnoiditis

Treatment

Initial

There is an overall lack of high-quality prospective controlled studies examining the efficacy of various noninvasive treatments of lumbar spinal stenosis. Moreover, many of the existing recommendations are in regard to back pain in general, without differentiation of pain associated specifically with lumbar spinal stenosis. Therefore much of clinical practice is based on extrapolation of recommendations, anecdotal experience, and expert opinion.

The oral analgesics used in lumbar spinal stenosis are acetaminophen, nonsteroidal anti-inflammatory drugs, muscle relaxants, anti–neuropathic pain medications including anticonvulsants and antidepressants, tramadol, and opioids. However, a number of systematic reviews have evaluated the use of pain medications in nonspecific low back pain. The review by Mens [23] stated that acetaminophen, nonsteroidal anti-inflammatory drugs, and mild opioids are potential first-line drugs, but there is no evidence that one is more effective than another. Nonbenzodiazepine muscle relaxants were listed as second-line drugs for acute low back pain. The efficacy of these medications for the treatment of symptomatic lumbar spinal stenosis is still unclear, and the sedating quality of these medications poses an increased risk of adverse events in elderly patients. Antidepressants with mixed-receptor or predominantly noradrenergic activity, including tricyclics, bupropion, venlafaxine, and duloxetine, are somewhat effective [24]. First-generation (e.g., carbamazepine and phenytoin) and second-generation (e.g., gabapentin and pregabalin) antiepileptic drugs are also somewhat effective.

Table 50.3 Comparison of Various Diagnostic Tests for Lumbar Spinal Stenosis

Imaging Method	Pertinent Findings	Advantages	Disadvantages	Accuracy
Plain radiography	Anteroposterior view: narrow interpedicular distance (normally 23-30 mm) [8] Lateral view: decreased canal width Ferguson view: far-out syndrome [18] Facet degeneration, cyst formation Ligamentum flavum ossification Intervertebral disc space narrowing Vertebral body end-plate osteophyte	Inexpensive Easy to obtain Can rule out gross bone disease	Poor soft tissue visualization	Sensitivity 66% and specificity 93% compared with plain CT as reference [18]
Plain myelography	Ventral extradural defects: caused by disc protrusions and vertebral end-plate osteophytes Lateral or posterior extradural defects: caused by facet osteophytes Hourglass constriction: indicates central stenosis	Shows sagittal plane	Invasive May need several dye injections for high-grade stenosis Limited view of foramen Contraindicated in patients with contrast allergy, alcoholism, seizures, phenothiazine intake [18]	71.8% correlation with surgical findings [16] Sensitivity 54%-100%; equivocal compared with CT or MRI Specificity slightly higher than that of CT or MRI
Plain computed tomography (CT)	Fat plane obliteration at exiting root Canal shape (trefoil vs round or ovoid) Pedicle length—direct measurement	Relatively inexpensive Axial view Superior bone detail	Poor soft tissue visualization Higher radiation exposure vs other imaging techniques	83% correlation with surgical findings [16] Sensitivity 74%-100%
Computed tomographic myelography	As above Useful in degenerative scoliosis or history of prior instrumentation	Visualization of central and lateral canals	Invasive Higher radiation exposure vs other imaging techniques	Sensitivity 87% [17] Comparable to MRI
Magnetic resonance imaging (MRI)	Disc degeneration: dark on T2 Annular tears: bright on T2 Stenosis and herniations in central and foraminal zones well visualized Evaluation of spine and spinal cord tumors	Noninvasive Shows sagittal plane Good soft tissue visualization	Interference from ferromagnetic implants Limitations on patient's body size, need to lie still, claustrophobia Expensive and time-consuming	83% correlation with surgical findings [16] Sensitivity 77%-87% Three-dimensional magnetic resonance myelography sensitivity 100% As accurate as CT myelography [19]
Electrodiagnostics	Bilateral multilevel lumbosacral radiculopathy is most common diagnosis Paraspinal mapping electromyography score >4 [20] Tibial F wave and soleus H reflex latencies after exercise [21,22]	Can evaluate for peripheral neuropathy and entrapments as well as progression of neurologic impairment Can rule out other neuromuscular disease	Significant interpretation bias May be difficult to differentiate lumbar spinal stenosis from other multiroot diseases (e.g., arachnoiditis) Patient discomfort or pain Expensive and time-consuming	Abnormal study in 78%-97% of patients with stenosis Paraspinal mapping electromyography score >4: specificity 100% and sensitivity 30%

Rehabilitation

To our knowledge, there are no randomized controlled trials in which the effectiveness of physical or manual therapies in the treatment of patients specifically with lumbar spinal stenosis is evaluated. General recommendations include relative rest (avoidance of pain-exacerbating activities while staying active to minimize deconditioning) and a flexion-biased exercise program, including inclined treadmill and exercise bicycle. Flexion biasing increases the cross-sectional area of the spinal canal compared with exercises performed in neutral or extension, thereby maximizing activity tolerance [25]. Whitman and associates [26] reported a case series of three patients who demonstrated significant improvements in pain and function at 18 months after undergoing specialized physical therapy programs that included spinal manipulation, flexion and rotation spine mobilization exercises, hip joint mobilization, hip flexor stretching, muscle retraining (lower abdominal, gluteal, and calf muscles), body weight–supported ambulation, and daily walking with properly prescribed orthotics. Body weight–supported ambulation acts to decrease the axial loading of the spine to increase the cross-sectional area of the neural foramina, and studies have provided some support of this strategy [27]. Physical modalities such as cold or hot packs, ultrasound, iontophoresis, and transcutaneous electrical nerve stimulation may be helpful, but data of clinical efficacy are lacking. Physicians and therapists must be aware of any medical comorbidities, such as cardiovascular and pulmonary disease, osteoporosis, cognitive deficits, and other musculoskeletal or neuromuscular conditions, that may have an impact on therapy tolerance. A retrospective analysis of predictors of walking performance and walking capacity showed that body mass index, pain, female sex, and age predict walking performance and capacity in people with lumbar spinal stenosis, those with low back pain, and asymptomatic control subjects. The authors of this analysis concluded that obesity and pain are modifiable predictors of walking deficits that could be targets for future intervention studies aimed at increasing walking performance and capacity in both the low back pain and lumbar spinal stenosis populations [28].

Procedures

Recommendations for the use of nonsurgical interventional procedures in the symptomatic control of lumbar spinal stenosis, particularly fluoroscopically guided epidural steroid injections, are somewhat controversial. A systematic review by Abdi and colleagues [29] concluded that for interlaminar, transforaminal, and caudal epidural steroid injections, there is strong evidence for short-term relief and limited to moderate evidence for long-term relief of lumbar radicular pain. A number of studies have cited short-term success rates of 71% to 80% [30,31] and long-term success rates of 32% to 75% [30,32]. Furthermore, symptomatic management with epidural steroid injections may delay surgery an average of 13 to 28 months [33,34]. A randomized controlled trial found that patients with lumbar central spinal stenosis received significant pain relief and improved their Oswestry disability scores after receiving lumbar interlaminar injections with or without steroids [35]. A study looking at the effects of fluoroscopic transforaminal epidural steroid injections in patients with degenerative lumbar scoliosis combined with spinal stenosis and radicular pain found them to be a more effective short-term option compared with lidocaine injections [36]. In general, epidural steroid injections can be considered a safe and reasonable therapeutic option for symptomatic management before surgical intervention is pursued.

Surgery

Patients with persistent symptoms despite conservative measures may benefit from surgical treatment. There are no universally accepted indications for and contraindications to surgery. A key feature in the selection of patients is ensuring that the symptoms indeed arise from nerve root compression. It is also important to screen for depression. A prospective clinical study of lumbar spinal stenosis patients who underwent surgery found at 2-year follow-up that patients with depressive symptoms had poorer surgical outcomes than those with normal mood [37]. Surgery generally consists of decompressive laminectomy with medial facetectomy. The decompression relieves central canal stenosis; the medial facetectomy and attendant dissection along the lateral recesses decompress areas of foraminal stenosis.

The Maine Lumbar Spine Study [38] prospectively examined the outcome of initial surgical versus nonsurgical treatment in 148 patients at 1, 4, and 8 to 10 years. Rates of improvement in predominant symptom, low back pain, and leg pain at 1 year ranged from 77% to 79% in the surgery group and 42% to 45% in the nonsurgical group. At 8- to 10-year follow-up, the rates dropped to 53% to 67% in the surgery group and remained essentially stable at 41% to 50% in the nonsurgical group. As such, the benefits from surgery diminished over time, although improvements in leg pain and back-related functional status were maintained. A time-dependent decrease in benefit among older patients was evident in another study by Yamashita and colleagues [39]. In patients requiring surgery, earlier intervention is associated with improved long-term outcomes [38,40].

The Spine Patient Outcomes Research Trial compared the outcomes of patients who underwent surgical management of lumbar spinal stenosis with the outcomes of those who underwent conservative treatment. They found that at 2-year follow-up and at 4-year follow-up, intention-to-treat analysis showed significant improvement in SF-36 bodily pain and Oswestry disability index from baseline in the surgical group compared with the nonsurgical group. In addition, comparative effectiveness evidence for defined diagnostic groups from the Spine Patient Outcomes Research Trial showed good value for surgery compared with nonoperative care during 4 years. They also found that patients with predominant leg pain improved significantly more with surgery than did patients with predominant low back pain. However, patients with predominant low back pain still improved significantly more with surgery than with nonoperative treatment [41]. Patients often will have residual back pain at some point after surgical intervention. Once the patient is cleared by the operating spine surgeon, a lumbar core stabilization exercise program that emphasizes general core strength, postural education, hip girdle flexibility and strength, and cardiovascular reconditioning is important postoperatively.

Two key controversies in the surgical management of lumbar spinal stenosis are the appropriate role for a concomitant arthrodesis (lumbar fusion) and the utility of instrumentation. A comprehensive multipart systematic review by Resnick and colleagues [42,43] concluded that the literature consistently supports the addition of arthrodesis, particularly posterior lumbar fusion, to decompression surgery only in patients with lumbar spinal stenosis secondary to spondylolisthesis.

Potential Disease Complications

The natural history of lumbar spinal stenosis is not well understood, but existing literature seems to indicate that most cases do not lead to significant deterioration. Johnsson and coworkers [44] examined the symptomatic and functional outcomes of 19 patients with moderate stenosis who did not undergo surgery. Average follow-up was 31 months, at which time 26% were worse, 32% unchanged, and 42% improved. Another study by Johnsson and colleagues [45] observed 32 patients with spinal stenosis who did not receive treatment, 75% of whom had neurogenic claudication. At a mean follow-up period of 49 months, 70% were unchanged, 15% were worse, and 15% were better. In patients with worsening symptomatic stenosis, there may be a progressive increase in back or leg pain and a decrease in walking tolerance. Severe stenosis may lead to a neurogenic bladder, especially in patients with narrowed dural sac anteroposterior diameter. Cauda equina syndrome is a rare but serious complication, in which case emergent surgical decompression is generally required.

Potential Treatment Complications

Exacerbation of symptoms is possible, particularly with functional restoration programs that may attempt to condition patients to painful activities through safe repetition of pain-inducing motions. In addition, patients with significant comorbidities, such as cardiopulmonary disease, are at risk for activity-induced adverse events. Complications from medication use include liver toxicity with acetaminophen; gastritis, gastrointestinal bleeds, renal toxicity, and platelet inhibition with nonsteroidal anti-inflammatory drugs; increased risk of cardiovascular events with some cyclooxygenase 2 inhibitors; nausea and lowering of seizure threshold with tramadol; anticholinergic effects including dry mouth and urinary retention with tricyclic antidepressants; sedation, ataxia, and other cognitive side effects with anticonvulsants (although gabapentin and pregabalin are relatively safe); and sedation, constipation, urinary retention, tolerance, and central pain sensitization with opioids. Adverse gastrointestinal events related to nonsteroidal anti-inflammatory drugs can be minimized with the use of a cyclooxygenase 2 inhibitor or concomitant use of a gastroprotective agent, such as a proton pump inhibitor or H_2 blocker [46].

Quantified data on complications associated with nonsurgical interventional procedures, including epidural steroid injections, are limited. A retrospective study of 207 patients receiving transforaminal epidural steroid injections [47] reported the following adverse events: transient nonpositional headaches that resolved within 24 hours (3.1%), increased back pain (2.4%), facial flushing (1.2%), increased leg pain (0.6%), vasovagal reaction (0.3%), increased blood glucose concentration in an insulin-dependent diabetic (0.3%), and intraoperative hypertension (0.3%). Other potential complications are infection at the injection site, dural puncture potentially with associated spinal headache, chemical or infectious meningitis, epidural hematoma, intravascular penetration, anaphylaxis, and nerve root or spinal cord injury leading to paresis or paralysis [48].

Complications of decompressive surgery include infection (0.5% to 3%), epidural hematoma, vascular injury (0.02%), thromboembolism including pulmonary embolism (0.5%), dural tears (<1% to 15%), nerve root injury, postsurgical spinal instability, nonunion or hardware failure, adjacent segment degeneration, recurrence of symptoms (10% to 15%), and death (0.35% to 2%) [49].

References

[1] Arnoldi CC, Brodsky AE, Cauchoix J, et al. Lumbar spinal stenosis and nerve root entrapment syndromes: definition and classification. Clin Orthop Relat Res 1976;115:4–5.
[2] Boden SD, Davis DO, Dina TS, et al. Abnormal magnetic-resonance scans of the lumbar spine in asymptomatic subjects: a prospective investigation. J Bone Joint Surg Am 1990;72:403–8.
[3] Getty CJ. Lumbar spinal stenosis: the clinical spectrum and the results of operation. J Bone Joint Surg Br 1980;62:481–5.
[4] Yang KH, King AI. Mechanism of facet load transmission as a hypothesis for low-back pain. Spine (Phila Pa 1976) 1984;9:557–65.
[5] Herzog RJ, Kaiser JA, Saal JA, Saal JS. The importance of posterior epidural fat pad in lumbar central canal stenosis. Spine (Phila Pa 1976) 1991;16(Suppl):S227–33.
[6] Wiltse LL, Guyer RD, Spencer CW, et al. Alar transverse process impingement of the L5 spinal nerve: the far-out syndrome. Spine (Phila Pa 1976) 1984;9:31–41.
[7] Sortland O, Magnaes B, Hauge T. Functional myelography with metrizamide in the diagnosis of lumbar spinal stenosis. Acta Radiol Suppl 1977;355:42–54.
[8] Amundsen T, Weber H, Lilleas F, et al. Lumbar spinal stenosis: clinical and radiologic features. Spine (Phila Pa 1976) 1995;20:1178–86.
[9] Roach KE, Brown MD, Albin RD, et al. The sensitivity and specificity of pain response to activity and position in categorizing patients with low back pain. Phys Ther 1997;77:730–8.
[10] Fritz JM, Erhard RE, Delitto A, et al. Preliminary results of the use of a two-stage treadmill test as a clinical diagnostic tool in the differential diagnosis of lumbar spinal stenosis. J Spinal Disord 1997;10:410–6.
[11] Katz JN, Dalgas M, Stucki G, et al. Degenerative lumbar spinal stenosis: diagnostic value of the history and physical examination. Arthritis Rheum 1995;38:1236–41.
[12] Suri P, Rainville J, Kalichman L, et al. Does this older adult with lower extremity pain have the clinical syndrome of lumbar spinal stenosis? JAMA 2010;304:2628–36.
[13] Imagama S, Matsuyama Y, Sakai Y, et al. An arterial pulse examination is not sufficient for diagnosis of peripheral arterial disease in lumbar spinal canal stenosis: a prospective multicenter study. Spine (Phila Pa 1976) 2011;36:1204–10.
[14] Haig AJ, Tong HC, Yamakawa KS, et al. Spinal stenosis, back pain, or no symptoms at all? A masked study comparing radiologic and electrodiagnostic diagnoses to the clinical impression. Arch Phys Med Rehabil 2006;87:897–903.
[15] Hurri H, Slatis P, Soini J, et al. Lumbar spinal stenosis: assessment of long-term outcome 12 years after operative and conservative treatment. J Spinal Disord 1998;11:110–5.
[16] Modic MT, Masaryk T, Boumphrey F, et al. Lumbar herniated disk disease and canal stenosis: prospective evaluation by surface coil MR, CT, and myelography. AJR Am J Roentgenol 1986;147:757–65.
[17] Bischoff RJ, Rodriguez RP, Gupta K, et al. A comparison of computed tomography–myelography, magnetic resonance imaging, and myelography in the diagnosis of herniated nucleus pulposus and spinal stenosis. J Spinal Disord 1993;6:289–95.
[18] Truumees E. Spinal stenosis: pathophysiology, clinical and radiologic classification. Instr Course Lect 2005;54:287–302.
[19] Schnebel B, Kingston S, Watkins R, Dillin W. Comparison of MRI to contrast CT in the diagnosis of spinal stenosis. Spine (Phila Pa 1976) 1989;14:332–7.
[20] Haig AJ, Tong HC, Yamakawa KS, et al. The sensitivity and specificity of electrodiagnostic testing for the clinical syndrome of lumbar spinal stenosis. Spine (Phila Pa 1976) 2005;30:2667–76.
[21] Adamova B, Vohanka S, Dusek L. Dynamic electrophysiological examination in patients with lumbar spinal stenosis: is it useful in clinical practice? Eur Spine J 2005;14:269–76.
[22] Bal S, Celiker R, Palaoglu S, Cila A. F wave studies of neurogenic intermittent claudication in lumbar spinal stenosis. Am J Phys Med Rehabil 2006;85:135–40.
[23] Mens JM. The use of medication in low back pain. Best Pract Res Clin Rheumatol 2005;19:609–21.
[24] Maizels M, McCarberg B. Antidepressants and antiepileptic drugs for chronic non-cancer pain. Am Fam Physician 2005;71:483–90.
[25] Sikorski JM. A rationalized approach to physiotherapy for low-back pain. Spine 1985;10:571–9.

[26] Whitman JM, Flynn TW, Fritz JM. Nonsurgical management of patients with lumbar spinal stenosis: a literature review and a case series of three patients managed with physical therapy. Phys Med Rehabil Clin N Am 2003;14:77–101, vi-vii.
[27] Fritz JM, Erhard RE, Vignovic M. A nonsurgical treatment approach for patients with lumbar spinal stenosis. Phys Ther 1997;77:962–73.
[28] Tomkins-Lane CC, Holz SC, Yamakawa KS, et al. Predictors of walking performance and walking capacity in people with lumbar spinal stenosis, low back pain, and asymptomatic controls. Arch Phys Med Rehabil 2012;93:647–53.
[29] Abdi S, Datta S, Lucas LF. Role of epidural steroids in the management of chronic spinal pain: a systematic review of effectiveness and complications. Pain Physician 2005;8:127–43.
[30] Delport EG, Cucuzzella AR, Marley JK, et al. Treatment of lumbar spinal stenosis with epidural steroid injections: a retrospective outcome study. Arch Phys Med Rehabil 2004;85:479–84.
[31] Papagelopoulos PJ, Petrou HG, Triantafyllidis PG, et al. Treatment of lumbosacral radicular pain with epidural steroid injections. Orthopedics 2001;24:145–9.
[32] Botwin KP, Gruber RD, Bouchlas CG, et al. Fluoroscopically guided lumbar transformational epidural steroid injections in degenerative lumbar stenosis: an outcome study. Am J Phys Med Rehabil 2002;81:898–905.
[33] Riew KD, Yin Y, Gilula L, et al. The effect of nerve-root injections on the need for operative treatment of lumbar radicular pain: a prospective, randomized, controlled, double-blind study. J Bone Joint Surg Am 2000;82:1589–93.
[34] Narozny M, Zanetti M, Boos N. Therapeutic efficacy of selective nerve root blocks in the treatment of lumbar radicular leg pain. Swiss Med Wkly 2001;131:75–80.
[35] Manchikanti L, Cash KA, McManus CD, et al. Lumbar interlaminar epidural injections in central spinal stenosis: preliminary results of a randomized, double-blind, active control trial. Pain Physician 2012;15:51–63.
[36] Nam HS, Park YB. Effects of transforaminal injection for degenerative lumbar scoliosis combined with spinal stenosis. Ann Rehabil Med 2011;35:514–23.
[37] Sinikallio S, Aalto T, Airaksinen O, et al. Depression is associated with a poorer outcome of lumbar spinal stenosis surgery: a two-year prospective follow-up study. Spine (Phila Pa 1976) 2011;36:677–82.
[38] Atlas SJ, Keller RB, Wu YA, et al. Long-term outcomes of surgical and nonsurgical management of lumbar spinal stenosis: 8 to 10 year results from the Maine Lumbar Spine Study. Spine (Phila Pa 1976) 2005;30:936–43.
[39] Yamashita K, Ohzono K, Hiroshima K. Five-year outcomes of surgical treatment for degenerative lumbar spinal stenosis: a prospective observational study of symptom severity at standard intervals after surgery. Spine (Phila Pa 1976) 2006;31:1484–90.
[40] Niggemeyer O, Strauss JM, Schulitz KP. Comparison of surgical procedures for degenerative lumbar spinal stenosis: a meta-analysis of the literature from 1975 to 1995. Eur Spine J 1997;6:423–9.
[41] Tosteson AN, Tosteson TD, Lurie JD, et al. Comparative effectiveness evidence from the spine patient outcomes research trial: surgical versus nonoperative care for spinal stenosis, degenerative spondylolisthesis, and intervertebral disc herniation. Spine (Phila Pa 1976) 2011;36:2061–8.
[42] Resnick DK, Choudhri TF, Dailey AT, et al. Guidelines for the performance of fusion procedures for degenerative disease of the lumbar spine. Part 10: fusion following decompression in patients with stenosis without spondylolisthesis. J Neurosurg Spine 2005;2:686–91.
[43] Resnick DK, Choudhri TF, Dailey AT, et al. Guidelines for the performance of fusion procedures for degenerative disease of the lumbar spine. Part 9: fusion in patients with stenosis and spondylolisthesis. J Neurosurg Spine 2005;2:679–85.
[44] Johnsson KE, Uden A, Rosen I. The effect of decompression on the natural course of spinal stenosis: a comparison of surgically treated and untreated patients. Spine (Phila Pa 1976) 1991;16:615–9.
[45] Johnsson KE, Rosen I, Uden A. The natural course of lumbar spinal stenosis. Clin Orthop Relat Res 1992;279:82–6.
[46] Physicians' desk reference. 59th ed. Montvale, NJ: Thomson Healthcare; 2005.
[47] Botwin KP, Gruber RD, Bouchlas CG, et al. Complications of fluoroscopically guided transforaminal lumbar epidural injections. Arch Phys Med Rehabil 2000;81:1045–50.
[48] Huntoon MA, Martin DP. Paralysis after transforaminal epidural injection and previous spinal surgery. Reg Anesth Pain Med 2004;29:494–5.
[49] Jansson KA, Blomqvist P, Granath F, Nemeth G. Spinal stenosis surgery in Sweden 1987-1999. Eur Spine J 2003;12:535–41.

CHAPTER 51

Sacroiliac Joint Dysfunction

Zacharia Isaac, MD
Richard Feeney, DO

Synonyms

Sacroiliac joint syndrome
Sacroiliac joint pain
Sacroiliac joint injury
Sacroiliac subluxation
Sacroiliac joint instability
Sacroiliac joint ankylosis
Sacroiliac joint sprain and strain

ICD-9 Codes

724.6 Disorders of sacrum
846.1 Sprain and strain of sacroiliac ligament
846.8 Sprain and strain of sacroiliac region

ICD-10 Code

S33.6 Sprain of sacroiliac joint or ligament
Add seventh character to S33 for episode of care (A—initial encounter, D—subsequent encounter, S—sequela)

Definition

Although chronic low back pain is more commonly attributed to the lumbar intervertebral disc and the zygapophyseal joints, the sacroiliac joint remains a significant cause of low back and buttock pain. However, diagnosis and treatment of sacroiliac joint dysfunction are a clinical challenge. The diagnosis of sacroiliac dysfunction should be considered only after careful exclusion of many separate distinct pathologic entities. Sacral fractures, sacroiliac joint inflammation (such as is seen with various seronegative spondyloarthropathies), metastatic disease, and even infectious seeding of the sacroiliac joint are but a few known pathologic conditions that deserve investigation. Imaging studies are often unhelpful and nonspecific in sacroiliac joint dysfunction. In addition, because of its redundant and variable innervation, sacroiliac joint dysfunction can be manifested with a variable pain referral pattern [1]. Thus, one must consider pathologic changes of neighboring structures sharing pain referral regions with the sacroiliac joint before deciding on the diagnosis of sacroiliac joint dysfunction.

The prevalence of sacroiliac joint dysfunction in those with low back pain complaints is thought to be between 10% and 25%, although during pregnancy the sacroiliac joint is the source of low back or posterior pelvic pain in 20% to 80% of cases [2]. As such, sacroiliac joint dysfunction may be more common in women than in men, and various studies demonstrate a female-to-male ratio of approximately 3:1 to 4:1 [1,3,4]. Moreover, in comparing causes of chronic low back pain, female gender and low body mass index are associated with sacroiliac joint dysfunction [5].

Adjoining the axial and appendicular skeleton, the sacroiliac joint occupies a critical biomechanical position (Fig. 51.1). It is thought that joint dysfunction occurs with structural change to the joint or positional changes relative to the sacrum and pelvis [6]. One can appreciate such changes in pregnancy-related instability [7] or with joint misalignment in adolescents, both of which are known sources of sacroiliac joint pain and dysfunction [8]. Pain associated with changes in position or the joint anatomy itself may be mediated by intra-articular, capsular, and ligamentous structures.

The sacroiliac joints are the bilateral weight-bearing joints that connect the articular surface of the sacrum with the ilium. The anterior and inferior third of the joint is synovial; the remainder of the joint space is syndesmotic. The sacroiliac joint is bordered on its ventral and superior edges by the ventral sacroiliac ligament and on its dorsal and inferior surfaces by the interosseous and dorsal sacroiliac ligaments. The articular capsule of the sacroiliac joint is thin and stabilized anteriorly by the ventral sacroiliac ligament. The strong extracapsular fibers of the dorsal sacroiliac and interosseous ligaments contribute principally to the stability of the joint. Further anchoring of the sacroiliac joint is conferred by the sacrotuberous and sacrospinous ligaments, which provide additional connections between the pelvis and sacrum. Innervation of the sacroiliac joint remains an area of active study, and differing descriptions of sacroiliac joint innervation exist. Anatomic studies have described innervation primarily through dorsal rami of spinal nerve roots

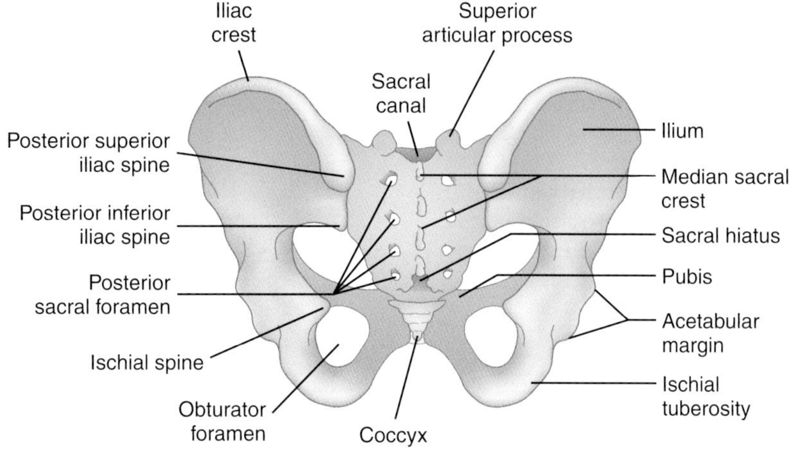

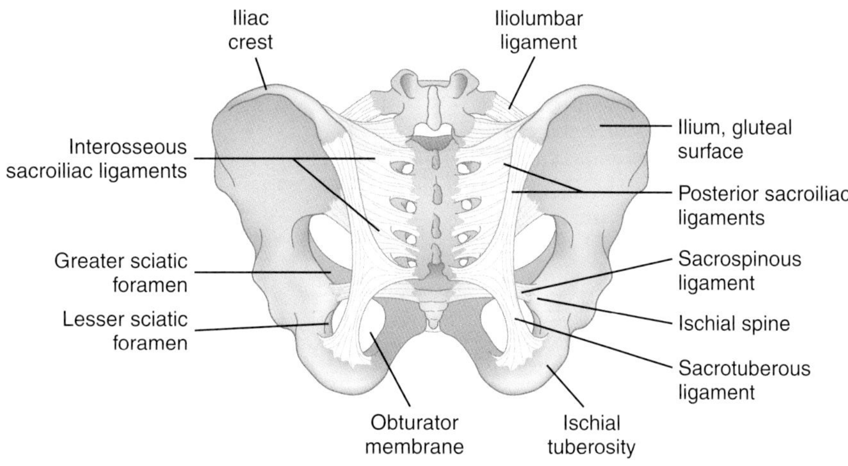

FIGURE 51.1 Sacroiliac joint and ligamentous structures. *(From Huntoon M, Benzon H, Nauroze S. Spinal Injections and Peripheral Nerve Blocks. Philadelphia, WB Saunders, 2012. Interventional and Neuromodulatory Techniques for Pain Management, vol 4.)*

L5-S4. However, recent studies indicate that the sacroiliac joint receives its innervation from the ventral rami of L4 and L5, the superior gluteal nerve, and the dorsal rami of L5, S1, and S2 or that it is almost exclusively derived from the sacral dorsal rami [9]. Yet others suggest that dorsal innervation to the sacroiliac joint is from the L5 dorsal ramus and the S1-S3 lateral branches, whereas the ventral innervation derives from the ventral rami of L4 and L5 [10].

The sacroiliac joint undergoes changes throughout life that affect the biomechanics of the joint. During childhood and adolescence, the joint is more mobile, absorbing forces throughout the gait cycle. With normal aging, the joints develop uneven opposing surfaces, and the joints are thought to gradually fuse in later years [11]. Movements around the sacroiliac joints are small in magnitude yet complex in nature. As body weight is transmitted downward through the first sacral vertebra, the sacrum is pushed downward and forward, causing its lower end to rotate upward and backward. Although there are no muscles that directly control movements around the joint, imbalance of the musculature surrounding the sacroiliac joint can affect stresses through the joint. Muscles anterior to the sacroiliac joint, including the psoas and iliacus, can influence movement of the sacrum [12]. Weakness in posterior muscles, such as the gluteus maximus and medius, can affect pelvic posture during weight bearing, thereby altering stresses through the joint.

Symptoms

By far the most common presenting symptom of sacroiliac joint dysfunction is low back and gluteal pain, which can be indolent and refractory to traditional interventions and therapies. Pain referral from sacroiliac joint dysfunction is not limited to the lumbosacral region or buttocks, however. Presenting complaints often include pain that is aggravated by prolonged standing, asymmetric weight bearing, or stair climbing. Pain can also stem from running, large strides, or extreme postures [13]. Because of the complex and extensive innervation of the sacroiliac joint as detailed before, dysfunction within the joint may be manifested with pain localizing to several rather removed regions, such as the thigh, groin, and leg. Sacroiliac joint dysfunction does not cause pain by neural compression. However, because of the anatomic proximity of spinal nerve roots to the lumbar and sacral plexuses, pain referral patterns can mimic a variety of neurologic pathologic processes. In a retrospective study of 50 patients with positive diagnostic response to fluoroscopically guided sacroiliac joint injection, investigators sought to characterize the most common presenting symptoms experienced by the cohort. The most common symptoms were buttock pain (94%), lower lumbar pain (72%), and lower extremity pain (50%). Pain in the distal leg and pain in the foot were also reported, as was low abdominal pain and groin pain [1]. Interestingly, the sacroiliac joint is recognized as the most likely source of low back pain after lumbar fusion [14].

Physical Examination

A thorough assessment of the low back, hips, and pelvis, including musculoskeletal and neurologic testing, is essential in isolating back pain caused by sacroiliac joint dysfunction and to exclude other common diagnoses. Examination should include measurement of leg length and assessment of pelvic symmetry by inspection of the posterior superior iliac spine, anterior superior iliac spine, gluteal folds, pubic tubercles, ischial tuberosities, and medial malleoli. The sacral sulcus is palpated and inspected with the patient prone, and any muscle atrophy in the gluteal muscles or distal extremity is noted. Atrophy in the limb implicates a lumbar radiculopathy more than sacroiliac joint syndrome. Palpation of the bony sacrum, subcutaneous tissues, muscles, and ligaments also helps to complete the examination.

Provocative tests have long been used by clinicians to differentiate sacroiliac joint–derived back pain from other regional pain generators. However, repeated clinical studies have suggested that when they are considered separately, the most commonly used provocative tests have low specificity for sacroiliac dysfunction [15–18]. One possible explanation for this is poor inter-rater reliability. Others suggest that both the minimal range of motion around the joints and the difficulty in simulating physiologic stresses through the joints make it more likely that provocative tests will elicit pain from surrounding structures [13]. Such structures include the lumbar intervertebral disc, zygapophyseal joint, and hip joint. Several investigators have shown that in the diagnosis of sacroiliac joint disease, a multitest regimen is more clinically useful than any isolated finding. Recent research suggests that three or more positive findings on provocative tests are 82% to 85% sensitive and 57% to 79% specific for sacroiliac joint disease [18,19]. There is some evidence, in fact, that patients with low back pain who point to the posterior superior iliac spine or within 2 cm from this landmark are more likely to respond to periarticular sacroiliac joint blockade, thus making the patient's ability to pinpoint the pain a potentially useful tool.

Provocative Tests

Gaenslen Test

With the patient supine, lying close to the edge of the examination table with the buttock of the tested side over the edge of the table, the patient's leg is dropped off the table such that the thigh and hip are in hyperextension. The contralateral knee is then maximally flexed. Pain or discomfort with this maneuver suggests sacroiliac joint disease, although a false-positive result can be seen in patients with an L2-L4 nerve root lesion [20], spondylolisthesis, sacral fractures, lumbar compression fractures, or spinal stenosis (Fig. 51.2).

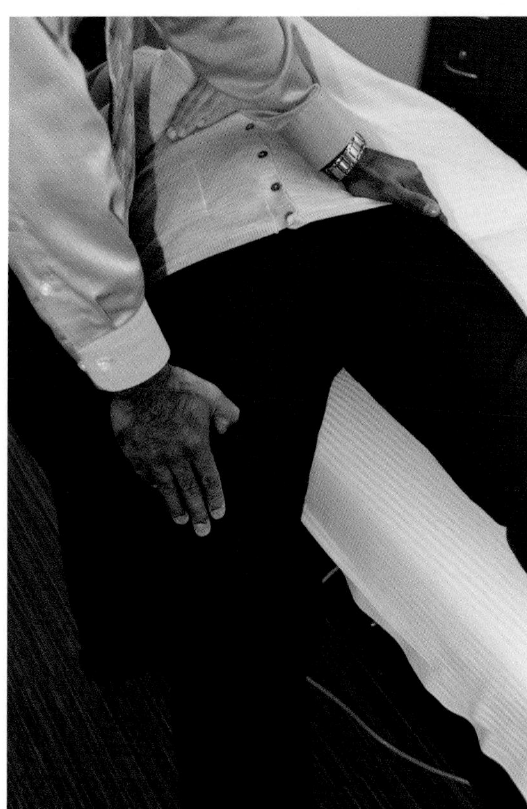

FIGURE 51.2 Gaenslen test. The patient lies supine and moves toward the edge of the examination table. The examiner presses on the contralateral anterior superior iliac spine and the ipsilateral thigh. The result is considered positive if the test reproduces familiar gluteal pain.

Patrick Test (also called FABER Test)

With the patient supine on a level surface, the thigh is flexed and the ankle placed above the patella of the opposite extended leg. Downward pressure is applied simultaneously to the flexed knee and the opposite anterior superior iliac spine as the ankle maintains its position above the knee. Pain or discomfort in the gluteal region reflects sacroiliac disease; pain in the groin or thigh may be suggestive of hip disease (Fig. 51.3).

Gillet Test

With the patient standing, the examiner palpates both the spinous process of the second sacral vertebra and the posterior superior iliac spine of the affected side. The patient is asked to maximally flex the hip on the involved side. A positive test result is indicated by a reproduction of pain and the failure of the palpated posterior superior iliac spine to move inferiorly in relation to the second sacral vertebra [2].

POSH Test (Posterior Shear Test)

With the patient supine, the examiner flexes the hip of the involved side to 90 degrees and adducts the thigh toward midline, providing axial pressure along the femur, directed into the table. This maneuver produces a shear force across the sacroiliac joint and reproduces pain in a symptomatic patient [2].

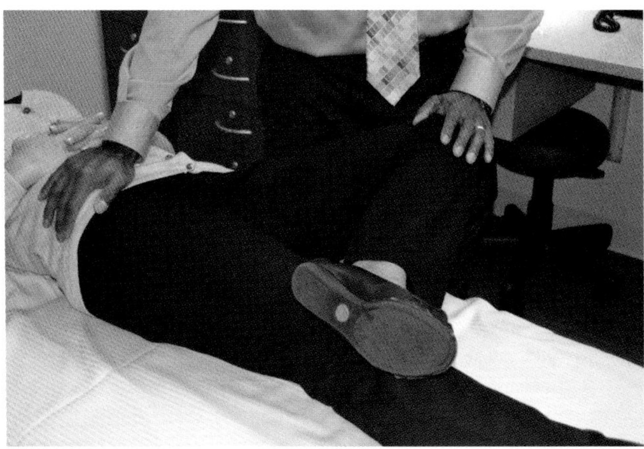

FIGURE 51.3 FABER (flexion, abduction, external rotation), also known as Patrick test. The patient's thigh is put into position while the examiner presses on the contralateral anterior superior iliac spine and ipsilateral thigh. The test result is considered positive if familiar gluteal pain is produced.

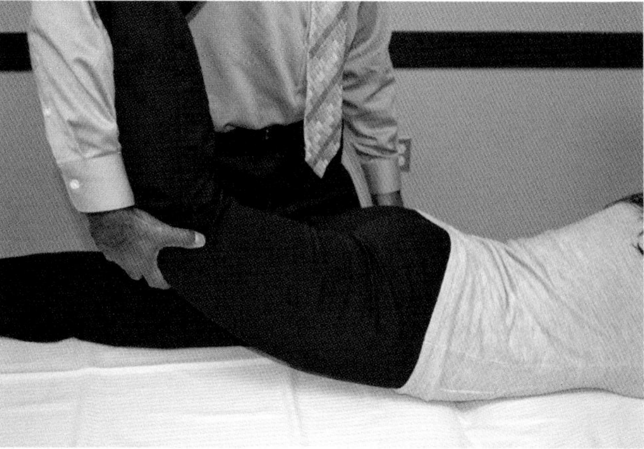

FIGURE 51.4 Yeoman test. The patient is positioned prone and the ipsilateral hip is passively extended by the examiner while the knee is at a 90-degree angle. The test result is considered positive if familiar gluteal pain is provoked.

REAB Test (Resisted Abduction)

With the patient supine, the hip of the involved side is placed in 30 degrees of abduction with the knee extended. The patient is asked to provide an isometric abduction contraction while the examiner resists at the lateral ankle. Reproduction of pain in the region of the sacroiliac joint is a positive test result. The test is thought to stress the cephalad aspect of the joint [2].

Distraction Test (also called the Gapping Test)

With the patient supine, pressure is applied downward and laterally to the bilateral anterior superior iliac spines. This maneuver stretches the ventral sacroiliac ligaments and joint capsule while placing pressure on the dorsal sacroiliac ligaments.

Compression Test

With the patient lying in the lateral recumbent position, the examiner stands behind the patient and applies pressure downward on the uppermost iliac crest, compressing the pelvis. This stretches the dorsal sacroiliac ligaments and compresses the ventral sacroiliac ligaments.

Yeoman Test

With the patient positioned prone, the knee is flexed to approximately 90 degrees and the hip is extended by the examiner. The sacroiliac joint ipsilateral to the extended hip is being tested. Reproduction of familiar gluteal or pelvic pain is considered a positive test result (Fig. 51.4).

Pressure over the Sacral Sulcus

Application of pressure to the gluteal region causing familiar gluteal pain can be suggestive of sacroiliac joint dysfunction. This is commonly seen and is a nonspecific finding; it is often seen in discogenic axial pain, radicular pain, sacral fractures, facet syndrome, and piriformis syndrome.

Active Straight-Leg Raise

While lying supine, the patient lifts the lower extremity, one at a time with the knee extended, approximately 20 cm above the horizontal surface. Pain over the posterior pelvic girdle on either side represents a positive test result suggestive of sacroiliac joint dysfunction. This test has been validated against a prior test of posterior pelvic pain after pregnancy, in which excessive motion at the sacroiliac joint is thought to play a role [21].

Functional Limitations

Patients with sacroiliac joint dysfunction can have a range of functional limitations. There can often be difficulty with sitting, standing, walking, lying, bending, lifting, or sustaining any one position. Thus, their ability to work certain jobs will be limited. These functional limitations can be mild or incapacitating. Known sequelae of chronic pain conditions, including sacroiliac joint dysfunction, are insomnia, depression, globalization of pain syndrome, psychological pain behavior, and symptom magnification. These sequelae can have additional or disproportionate associated functional limitations.

Diagnostic Studies

Sacroiliac joint dysfunction has no valid or reliable diagnostic imaging studies. The purpose of obtaining imaging is to evaluate for alternative diagnoses. Plain radiography can reveal osteologic causes of sacroiliac joint–mediated pain, such as infection and inflammatory or degenerative arthritis. Plain radiographic views, including Ferguson views and anteroposterior views, can help identify sacroiliac joint erosions. Bone scan and computed tomography can detect bone changes caused by entities such as fracture, infection, tumor, sacroiliac joint erosions, and arthritis. Magnetic resonance imaging can reveal these entities as well as show soft tissue disease and marrow changes in sacroiliitis with its associated erosions. Recently, ultrasound has emerged as a modality capable of not only detecting pathologic changes within posterior ligamentous structures of the sacroiliac joint but also providing guidance for accurate intra-articular needle placement for diagnostic or therapeutic purposes [22]. However, true sacroiliac joint dysfunction can often be seen in the presence of normal imaging, and thus it is often defined clinically.

Fluoroscopically guided diagnostic intra-articular injection of anesthetics is considered by some the "gold standard" for diagnosis of sacroiliac joint–derived low back pain [4,17,23,24]. However, numerous investigators have shown anesthetic leakage from the joint space after injection, and there is speculation that overlap to adjacent neural structures may yield erroneous diagnoses of sacroiliac dysfunction. A placebo effect and other nonspecific factors also can lead to improper diagnosis. For these reasons, confirmatory studies should be performed after informed consent has been obtained and the patient is educated about the reasons for confirmatory studies. These confirmatory studies include a patient-blinded, placebo versus anesthetic injection and a variable-duration anesthetic time-dependent block. Despite these measures, reviews of the American Pain Society guidelines suggest that there is only fair to poor evidence for sacroiliac joint blocks to diagnose sacroiliac joint pain [25]. Recent evidence suggests that extracapsular structures, the dense ligamentous network comprising the sacroiliac joint complex, may be a principal cause of persistent pain. In a 2009 study by Dreyfuss and coworkers [10], anesthetic injections performed on asymptomatic individuals provided a strong case for comparative, multisite, multidepth lateral branch blocks as a diagnostic tool before radiofrequency neurotomy, a promising technique for refractory sacroiliac joint pain.

Differential Diagnosis

Discogenic low back pain
Lumbar radicular pain
Lumbar facet syndrome
Spondylolisthesis
Spinal stenosis
Bertolotti syndrome
Hip osteoarthritis
Piriformis syndrome
Sacral fractures
Multiple myeloma
Metastatic disease
Gout
Pseudogout
Seronegative spondyloarthropathy or sacroiliitis
Septic joint
Pelvic abscess
SAPHO (synovitis, acne, pustulosis, hyperostosis, osteitis) syndrome
Osteochondritis dissecans
Osteitis condensans ilii

Treatment

Initial

Sacroiliac joint dysfunction is treated initially with relative rest and avoidance of provocative activities. Local modalities, such as ice and heat, or topical analgesics, such as lidocaine in patch form, can be applied for symptomatic relief. Manipulative therapy can alleviate pain and help with muscle spasms but does not change joint alignment significantly. Approximately only 2 degrees of rotation and 0.77 mm of translation occur with stress or manipulation [26,27]. Despite this, there is some evidence that the combination of high-velocity low-amplitude manipulation to both the sacroiliac joint and lumbar spine may provide improvements in pain and functional disability 1 month after intervention for those with sacroiliac dysfunction [28].

Commonly used pharmacologic interventions include acetaminophen, nonsteroidal anti-inflammatory medications, and muscle relaxants. Chronic use of nonsteroidal anti-inflammatory drugs should be avoided because of gastric, renal, and possibly cardiac side effects. Opiates in rare instances can be considered for short-term use but carry potential risks of sedation, constipation, physical dependence, and addiction. Patients with true sacroiliitis related to a seronegative spondyloarthropathy may be candidates for the use of biologic tumor necrosis factor-α inhibitor drugs or other disease-modifying agents.

Rehabilitation

Physical therapy is directed toward lumbar core muscle strength and hip girdle flexibility. Modalities such as ice massage, heat, electrical stimulation for the alleviation of pain or muscle spasm, sacroiliac joint mobilization techniques, and postural education exercises may be employed. Sacroiliac joint belts can be helpful and are worth an initial trial to address symptoms. Addressing hip girdle muscle strength, hip range of motion, tight iliotibial band, hip or knee osteoarthritis, trochanteric bursitis, leg length discrepancy, or pelvic obliquity can have adjunctive benefit. Given that most patients undergo rehabilitation for their low back pain without a specific diagnosis, it is difficult to determine whether physical therapy outcomes for sacroiliac joint dysfunction are any more or less effective than for other causes of low back pain. It stands to reason that exercise therapy aimed at improving strength, range of motion, and cardiovascular endurance can only benefit the patient overall and prevent the inherent trend toward deconditioning and activity avoidance behavior.

Procedures

Fluoroscopically guided intra-articular steroid injection can have therapeutic benefit. One study has suggested that up to two thirds of patients with sacroiliac joint dysfunction may attain significant pain relief [29], although the American Pain Society still regards the current evidence behind this therapy as poor [30]. Whenever possible, injection therapy should be complemented with a therapeutic exercise regimen.

Radiofrequency neurotomy has also been described as an effective treatment of sacroiliac joint dysfunction [31]. Interest and study have grown tremendously in this area of late. A recent meta-analysis endorses radiofrequency ablation as beneficial for sacroiliac joint pain for up to 6 months [32]. It is generally accepted that cooled rather than conventional or pulsed radiofrequency ablation is more effective at achieving pain relief [33,34]. Furthermore, recent evidence suggests that multisite, multidepth lateral branch blocks are physiologically effective at a rate of 70%, making this a valuable technique in diagnosis and in deciding to proceed with radiofrequency ablation to manage extra-articular sacroiliac joint pain [10].

Neuromodulatory therapies with an electrical stimulator implanted at the third sacral nerve root in a limited number of subjects with sacroiliac joint pain have also been effective in the management of refractory cases [35]. Prolotherapy has also been described for the treatment of sacroiliac joint dysfunction [16]. Well-designed randomized controlled trials are lacking for nearly all sacroiliac joint dysfunction treatments.

Surgery

Surgery is very rarely performed for sacroiliac joint dysfunction. A thorough workup is required before surgery with minimally invasive diagnostic anesthetization of the sacroiliac joint and to exclude discogenic, facet, radicular, and hip-mediated pain. Surgical intervention involves fusion of the sacroiliac joint with hardware.

Potential Disease Complications

Sacroiliac joint dysfunction, like other causes of chronic pain, can produce pain-related insomnia, depression, anxiety, globalization of pain, and disability. Older patients with gluteal pain should be evaluated for fracture or tumor, and younger patients should be evaluated for seronegative spondyloarthropathy. Degenerative causes of sacroiliac pain are more prevalent in women, whereas inflammatory causes predominate in men.

Potential Treatment Complications

Pharmacologic measures can have numerous side effects. Acetaminophen can be hepatotoxic in large doses. Nonsteroidal anti-inflammatory drug therapy is well known to be associated with gastrointestinal and renal side effects along with increased cardiac risk. Manipulation therapy or therapeutic exercise can increase pain in some patients. Intra-articular steroid injection can be associated with temporary increase in pain and local bleeding. Potential systemic steroid effects include increase in serum blood glucose concentration, hypertension, psychosis, and fluid retention. Local steroid injection can cause fatty atrophy, potential infection, and skin depigmentation.

References

[1] Slipman CW, Jackson HB, Lipetz JS, et al. Sacroiliac joint pain referral zones. Arch Phys Med Rehabil 2000;81:334–8.

[2] Zelle BA, Gruen GS, Brown S, et al. Sacroiliac joint dysfunction: evaluation and management. Clin J Pain 2005;5:446–55.

[3] Broadhurst N, Bond MJ. Pain provocation tests for the assessment of sacroiliac joint dysfunction. J Spinal Disord 1998;11:341–5.

[4] van der Wurff P, Buijs EJ, Groen GJ. A multitest regimen of pain provocation tests as an aid to reduce unnecessary minimally invasive sacroiliac joint procedures. Arch Phys Med Rehabil 2006;87:10–4.

[5] DePalma MJ, Ketchum JM, Saulio TR. What is the source of chronic low back pain and does age play a role? Pain Med 2011;12:224–33.

[6] Dreyfuss P, Dryer S, Griffin J, et al. Positive sacroiliac screening tests in asymptomatic adults. Spine (Phila Pa 1976) 1994;19:1138–43.

[7] Osterhoff G, Ossendorf C, Ossendorf-Kimmich N, et al. Surgical stabilization of postpartum symphyseal instability: two cases and a review of the literature. Gynecol Obstet Invest 2012;73:1–7.

[8] Stoev I, Powers AK, Puglisi JA, et al. Sacroiliac joint pain in the pediatric population. J Neurosurg Pediatr 2012;9:602–7.

[9] Forst SL, Wheeler MT, Fortin JD, et al. The sacroiliac joint: anatomy, physiology, and clinical significance. Pain Physician 2006;9:61–7.

[10] Dreyfuss P, Henning T, Malladi N, et al. The ability of multi-site, multi-depth sacral lateral branch blocks to anesthetize the sacroiliac joint complex. Pain Med 2009;10:679–88.

[11] Rosse C, Gaddum-Rosse P. Hollinshead's textbook of anatomy. In: 5th ed. Philadelphia: Lippincott-Raven; 1997. p. 312–3.

[12] Greenman PE. Principles of manual medicine. 2nd ed. Baltimore: Williams & Wilkins; 1996. p. 305–67, 530–532.

[13] Dreyfuss P, Dreyer SJ, Cole A, Mayo K. Sacroiliac joint pain. J Am Acad Orthop Surg 2004;12:255–65.

[14] DePalma MJ, Ketchum JM, Saullo TR. Etiology of chronic low back pain in patients having undergone lumbar fusion. Pain Med 2011;12:732–9.

[15] Berthelot JM, Labat JJ, Le Goff B, et al. Provocative sacroiliac joint maneuvers and sacroiliac joint block are unreliable for diagnosing sacroiliac joint pain. Joint Bone Spine 2006;73:17–23.

[16] Linetsky FS, Manchikanti L. Regenerative injection therapy for axial pain. Tech Reg Anesth Pain Manage 2005;9:40–9.

[17] Dreyfuss P, Michaelsen M, Pauza K, et al. The value of medical history and physical examination in diagnosing sacroiliac joint pain. Spine 1996;21:2594–602.

[18] van der Wurff P, Meyne W, Hagmeijer RH. Clinical tests of the sacroiliac joint. Man Ther 2000;5:89–96.

[19] Stanford G, Burham RS. Is it useful to repeat sacroiliac joint provocative tests post-block? Pain Med 2010;11:1774–6.

[20] Magee DJ. Orthopedic physical assessment. 3rd ed. Philadelphia: WB Saunders; 1997. p. 434–59.

[21] Mens JM, Vleeming A, Snijders CJ, et al. Reliability and validity of the active straight leg raise test in posterior pelvic pain since pregnancy. Spine 2001;26:1167–71.

[22] Le Goff B, Berthelot JM, Maugars Y. Ultrasound assessment of the posterior sacroiliac ligaments. Clin Exp Rheumatol 2011;29:1014–7.

[23] Broadhurst N, Bond MJ. Pain provocation tests for the assessment of sacroiliac joint dysfunction. J Spinal Disord 1998;11:341–5.

[24] Slipman CW, Sterenfeld EB, Chou LH, et al. The predictive value of provocative sacroiliac joint stress maneuvers in the diagnosis of sacroiliac joint syndrome. Arch Phys Med Rehabil 1998;79:288–92.

[25] Manchikanti L, Datta S, Derby R, et al. A critical review of the American Pain Society clinical practice guidelines for interventional techniques: part 1. Diagnostic interventions. Pain Physician 2010;13:E141–74.

[26] Egund N, Olsson TH, Schmid H, Selvik G. Movements in the sacroiliac joints demonstrated with roentgen stereophotogrammetry. Acta Radiol Diagn (Stockh) 1978;19:833–46.

[27] Sturesson B, Selvik G, Uden A. Movements of the sacroiliac joints. A roentgen stereophotogrammetric analysis. Spine 1989;14:162–5.

[28] Kamali F, Shokri E. The effect of two manipulative therapy techniques and their outcome in patients with sacroiliac joint syndrome. J Bodyw Mov Ther 2012;16:29–35.

[29] Liliang PC, Lu K, Weng HC, et al. The therapeutic effect of sacroiliac joint blocks with triamcinolone acetonide in the treatment of sacroiliac joint dysfunction without spondyloarthropathy. Spine (Phila Pa 1976) 2009;34:896–900.

[30] Manchikanti L, Datta S, Gupta S, et al. A critical review of the American Pain Society clinical practice guidelines for interventional techniques: part 2. Therapeutic interventions. Pain Physician 2010;13:E215–64.

[31] Yin W, Willard F, Carreiro J, Dreyfuss P. Sensory stimulation–guided sacroiliac joint radiofrequency neurotomy: technique based on neuroanatomy of the dorsal sacral plexus. Spine (Phila Pa 1976) 2003;28:2419–25.

[32] Aydin SM, Gharibo CG, Mehnert M, et al. The role of radiofrequency ablation for sacroiliac joint pain: a meta-analysis. PM R 2010;2:842–51.

[33] Vanelderen P, Szadek K, Cohen SP, et al. Sacroiliac joint pain. Pain Pract 2010;10:470–8.

[34] Cohen SP, Strassels SA, Kurihara C, et al. Outcome predictors for sacroiliac joint (lateral branch) radiofrequency denervation. Reg Anesth Pain Med 2009;34:206–14.

[35] Calvillo O, Esses SI, Ponder C, et al. Neuroaugmentation in the management of sacroiliac joint pain: report of two cases. Spine (Phila Pa 1976) 1998;23:1069–72.

SECTION VII Pelvis, Hip, and Thigh

CHAPTER 52

Adhesive Capsulitis of the Hip

Peter M. McIntosh, MD

Synonyms

Adhesive capsulitis of the hip
Frozen hip
Contracture of the hip joint
Ankylosis of the hip joint

ICD-9 Codes

718.45	**Contracture of hip joint**
718.55	**Ankylosis of hip**
719.55	**Limitation of motion of hip**
719.95	**Hip joint disorder**
726.0	**Adhesive capsulitis of hip**
726.90	**Capsulitis NOS**

ICD-10 Codes

M24.551	**Contracture, right hip joint**
M24.552	**Contracture, left hip joint**
M24.559	**Contracture, unspecified hip joint**
M24.651	**Ankylosis, right hip**
M24.652	**Ankylosis, left hip**
M24.659	**Ankylosis, unspecified hip**
M25.851	**Joint disorder, right hip**
M25.852	**Joint disorder, left hip**
M23.859	**Joint disorder, unspecified hip**
M76.891	**Enthesopathies of right lower limb excluding foot**
M76.892	**Enthesopathies of left lower limb excluding foot**
M76.899	**Enthesopathies of unspecified lower limb excluding foot**
M77.9	**Enthesopathy or capsulitis, unspecified**

Definition

Adhesive capsulitis of the hip joint is a condition of unknown etiology characterized by the gradual loss of passive and active hip motion, which is a result of retraction of the fibrous joint capsule.

Lequesne and colleagues [1] classified adhesive capsulitis into primary and secondary forms. Primary adhesive capsulitis is characterized by idiopathic, progressive, painful loss of both active and passive range of motion. Secondary adhesive capsulitis results from known intrinsic or extrinsic causes. Hannafin [2] reported that secondary adhesive capsulitis has a histopathologic appearance similar to that of primary adhesive capsulitis but can be associated with any one of multiple medical conditions (Table 52.1).

The hip joint is functionally and structurally complex, consisting of the femoral articulation, acetabulum, supporting soft tissue, muscles, and cartilaginous structures (Fig. 52.1). It is a multiaxial synovial ball-and-socket joint [3,4].

The femoral articulation forms roughly two thirds of a sphere, approximately 40% of which is covered by the acetabulum. Articular (hyaline) cartilage covers the femoral articulation except at the fovea capitis, a depression on the central surface.

The acetabulum is formed by fusion of the ilium, ischium, and pubis. It is hemispheric in shape and projects anterolaterally and inferiorly. The lunate surface is the articular portion, and the nonarticular portion constitutes the floor (acetabular fossa). The acetabular fossa (covered by synovium) is continuous with the acetabular notch, which lies between the ends of the lunate surface. The acetabular fossa lies in the inferomedial portion, close to the ligamentum teres (round ligament), which attaches to the fovea capitis. The depth of the acetabulum is increased by the dense fibrocartilaginous labrum, which attaches to the rim of the acetabulum except at the acetabular notch.

The transverse ligament bridges the acetabular notch and in combination with the acetabular labrum forms a complete ring around the acetabulum. It converts the acetabular notch into a foramen through which the intra-articular vessels pass to supply the head of the femur [3,4].

The fibrous capsule of the hip joint attaches to the labrum to form a circular recess, which encloses the joint and most of the femoral neck (Fig. 52.1). Medially, it attaches to the base of the acetabulum and extends to the innominate. Inferiorly, it attaches to the transverse acetabular ligament. Laterally, it attaches to the femur anteriorly and extends along the intertrochanteric line and along the femoral neck

Table 52.1 Medical Conditions Associated with Adhesive Capsulitis

Thyroid dysfunction [15,37]
Recurrent minor trauma [12,38]
Diabetes mellitus (juvenile and adult onset) [39–41]
Female gender (>70%) [18]
Age (>40 years) [38]
Prolonged immobilization of a joint [23]
Coronary artery disease [25]
Autoimmune disorders [17]
After hip surgery
Intra-articular loose bodies
Osteoid osteoma
Synovial chondromatosis
Osteoarthritis
Dupuytren contracture
Elevated C-reactive protein level, positive HLA-B27/serum IgA level
Myocardial infarction
Pulmonary tuberculosis
Bronchitis
Stroke with hemiparesis

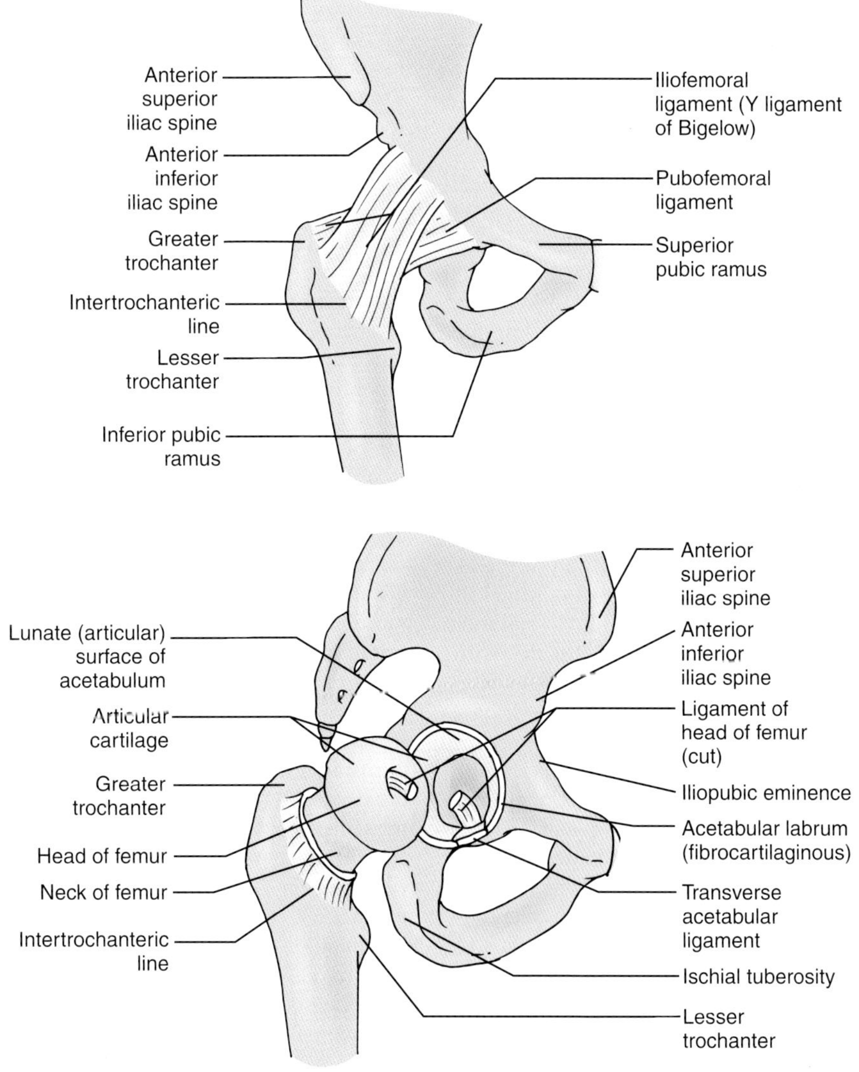

FIGURE 52.1 Hip joint. Normal anatomy and fibrous capsule.

posteriorly and inferiorly. The fibrous capsule is reinforced by the pubofemoral, ischiofemoral, and iliofemoral ligaments, which are considered thickening of the fibrous capsule and help to stabilize the hip joint. The capsular fiber consists of both superficial bands and deep bands. The deep circular bands from the iliofemoral ligament form the zona orbicularis, which divides the synovial cavity into medial and lateral recesses. The hip joint is dynamically stabilized by numerous muscles.

Neviaser introduced the term *adhesive capsulitis* and described pathologic changes in the synovium and subsynovium [5,6]. Evidence supports the hypothesis that the underlying pathologic process involves synovial inflammation with reactive capsular fibrosis, thus making adhesive capsulitis both an inflammatory and a fibrosing condition [2,5–9].

The histologic changes of adhesive capsulitis seen in the hip are similar to those in the shoulder. There is chronic inflammatory reaction in the capsule and synovium with subsequent adherence to the femoral neck [2,8,10,11]. Biopsy tissue shows evidence of edematous, fibrotic synovial tissue with partial or complete loss of synovial lining [2,12].

Many authors acknowledge that adhesive capsulitis is a relatively common clinical syndrome when it occurs in the shoulders (2% to 5% of the general population) but is infrequently described in other joints, such as the wrist, hip, and ankles [2,12–14].

Symptoms

The diagnosis of hip adhesive capsulitis is based on clinical findings of decreased passive and active range of motion in all planes of the hip joint, with no abnormal radiographic findings [5,15]. The patient may describe gradual onset of stiffness with hip movements, resulting in difficulty in crossing the leg or sitting in certain positions. Patients may describe difficulty with lower extremity dressing, such as putting on socks, or with hygiene, such as clipping of toenails.

Pain is usually a presenting symptom, especially with extreme external rotation or abduction, and is usually the reason for seeking medical evaluation. Gait difficulty may or may not be present, but it is usually not to the severity that a gait aid is required.

The diagnosis of hip adhesive capsulitis is rarely made, possibly because the hip joint can sustain range of motion loss without significant disability, whereas even a mild loss of motion in the shoulders can result in significant difficulty with performance of routine activities of daily living [12,13,15].

Physical Examination

Hip pain can be caused by different intra-articular and extra-articular structures. Differentiating the specific pathologic structures can be challenging, but it is critical for appropriate medical management. The history, physical examination, and adjuvant imaging are crucial in identifying the source of pain. In patients with adhesive capsulitis of the hip, the clinical examination findings may be minimal. The patient may or may not exhibit an antalgic gait pattern. The neuromuscular and neurovascular examination findings are usually unremarkable. The back examination is usually benign unless there is a concomitant spinal condition. Provocative maneuvers of the hip joint (i.e., Stinchfield and FABERE tests) may generate nonspecific groin discomfort. The hallmark finding on physical examination is limitation of range of motion of the hip joint in all planes (flexion-extension, internal and external rotation, and abduction-adduction) [16].

Functional Limitations

Functional limitations may differ, depending on the severity of pain and range of motion deficits. Difficulty with activities of daily living are limited to the lower extremities. This can be manifested as difficulty with lower extremity dressing, such as donning or doffing pants, socks, or shoes. There is difficulty in crossing one leg over the other or sitting in a tailor's position. There may be difficulty in sleeping on one side or the other or standing with the hip externally rotated and abducted. There may be difficulty with prolonged sitting or driving a car, especially if a manual shift is used.

The onset of pain and inflammation causes reflex inhibition of the muscles around the joint, which can subsequently lead to loss of mobility and compensatory abnormal movement of the joint. If gait pattern is affected, recreational and vocational activities that require prolonged ambulation can be affected (i.e., golfing, tennis, or power walking for exercise). With time, there is resolution of pain, but residual range of motion deficits and limitation of function can remain. This persistent loss of mobility and dysfunction can lead to psychosocial issues, such as irritability, depression and anxiety, and disordered sleep patterns.

Diagnostic Studies

Laboratory studies are important in the initial evaluation of intra-articular hip abnormalities. They help assess for autoimmune and rheumatologic conditions. The results of laboratory studies, including blood cell counts, electrolyte values, chemistry panels, acute phase reactants, and rheumatologic screening studies (such as antinuclear antibodies, double-stranded DNA, rheumatoid factor, and HLA-B27 antibodies), are usually normal in patients with adhesive capsulitis of the hip [17,18].

Multiple imaging modalities are available to assess the pelvis and hip joint and surrounding soft tissues. Conventional radiography including anteroposterior views remains the initial imaging modality of choice in assessing patients with groin pain and dysfunction. These studies, however, are of limited value if there is internal derangement as the cause of hip pain because findings are typically normal in those circumstances. In hip adhesive capsulitis, results of these studies are usually normal except for possible diffuse osteopenia, most likely related to pain and decreased range of motion from underlying disease [19]. Griffiths and colleagues [12] reported on a series of patients who had adhesive capsulitis of the hips related to mild trauma or repetitive activity. In all of the patients, the conventional radiographs were unremarkable.

Bone scans can show increased uptake in the areas of osteopenia, but this is usually nonspecific. Focal accumulation of radionuclide reflects an alteration of balanced bone turnover due to changes in bone blood flow and can occur in several conditions [20].

Ultrasonography of the hip has been widely accepted as a useful diagnostic tool in patients with hip pain or limited range of motion. It allows evaluation of different anatomic and pathologic structures, such as joint recess, bursa, tendons, and muscles. It also allows evaluation of the osseous structures of the joint, ischial tuberosity, and greater trochanter. It is useful for guided procedures in the hip joint and periarticular soft tissue under direct visualization.

Ultrasonography has considerable advantages over computed tomography (CT) and magnetic resonance imaging (MRI); these include absence of radiation, good visualization of the joint cavity, quantification of soft tissue abnormalities, multiple joint scanning, and rapid side-to-side anatomic comparison. It also has relatively low cost, good patient compliance, and dynamic real-time study of multiple planes. Direct contact with the patient allows maneuvers that elicit symptoms to be evaluated while the study is being performed. Direct ultrasonographic visualization offers the possibility of guided procedures in the hip joint and periarticular soft tissues. The limited size and number of acoustic windows make detailed examination of some structures extremely difficult (i.e., femoral cartilage and hip capsule) [21]. It is not recommended for evaluation of hip adhesive capsulitis, in which there is retraction of the fibrous joint capsule with little or no fluid in the synovial space.

Supplemental imaging with CT or MRI is often used to further evaluate the pelvis and hip to rule out the presence of simple, nondisplaced avulsion to complex fractures and to assess for displacement, comminution, and locations of fragments. MRI is helpful in diagnosis of occult injuries and stress fractures and in the evaluation of the soft tissue and musculature of the pelvis and hip [19,22]. In adhesive capsulitis, CT scans are usually unremarkable and MRI shows capsular thickening with little or no fluid in the synovial space. If the clinical examination or a nonarthrographic CT or MRI study suggests a possible labral or intra-articular hip disease, direct magnetic resonance arthrography is performed [4,23].

Computed tomographic or magnetic resonance arthrography is the preferred examination for evaluation of the joint capsule, labrum, and articular cartilage. Intra-articular needle placement is confirmed under fluoroscopic guidance before 15 mL of 1:200 dilution of a gadolinium contrast agent and normal saline is injected into the joint [4]. Characteristic arthroscopic findings show a hip joint with low volume and loss of normal recesses, high intracapsular pressure, and a thick capsule (Figs. 52.2 and 52.3). There is usually reduction of intra-articular capacity of at least one third (<10 mL). In the series reported by Griffiths, the patients who underwent arthrography all had small-volume joint space (<8 mm) with a thick capsule and increased intra-articular pressure. Cone and associates [24] prospectively monitored intracapsular pressure during arthrographic evaluation of 10 patients with a painful hip prosthesis and radiographic evidence of loosening. Fifty percent of patients had restriction of the intra-articular space around the neck of the femoral component during arthroscopy. The contrast agent exhibited irregular appearance related to fibrosis and scarring of the capsule consistent with adhesive capsulitis. In those patients in whom an arthrographic abnormality was demonstrated, the intra-articular pressure was three times greater than normal.

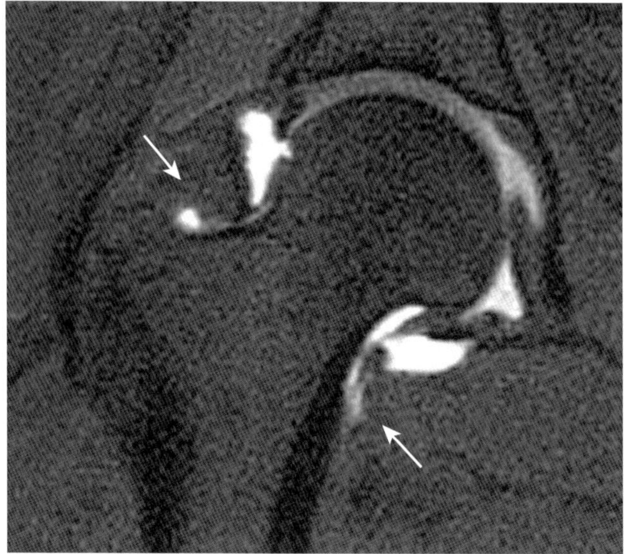

FIGURE 52.2 Coronal image from magnetic resonance arthrography of the hip depicting a small-volume joint with tight joint capsule. Very small recesses of the hip joint, compatible with adhesive capsulitis, are demonstrated *(arrows)*.

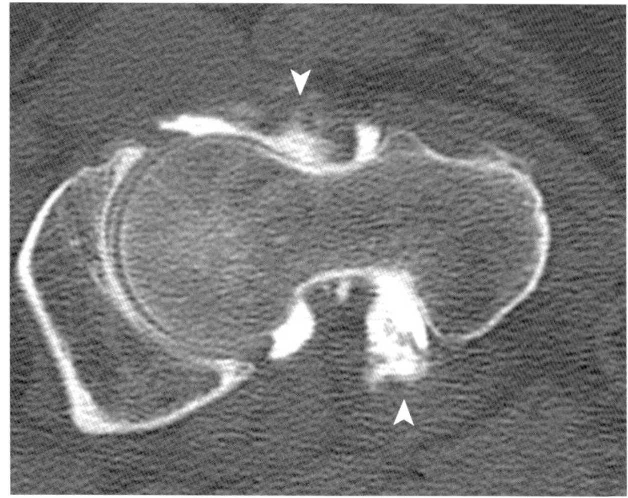

FIGURE 52.3 Coronal image from computed tomographic arthrography of the hip showing a small-volume joint with tight joint capsule. Areas of capsule rupture and extra-articular contrast material are demonstrated *(arrowheads)*.

Lequesne described seven patients with pain and limitation of movement in the hip, which he called idiopathic capsular constriction of the hip [1]. Plain radiographs were unremarkable, but hip arthrography suggested diminished articular volume. There was absence of filling of the normal recesses, and the joint had a smaller capacity (<10 mL) than a normal joint (14-20 mL) [12]. It has been said that if an experienced radiologist has difficulty entering the hip joint, adhesive capsulitis is often the cause [25].

Differential Diagnosis

Osteoarthritis of the hip joint (mild or early onset)
Intra-articular loose bodies [32]
Irritable hip syndrome (pain with little or no restriction of movement)
Iliopsoas bursitis or tendinosis [4]
Snapping hip syndrome (iliotibial band, iliopsoas tendon) [19]
Greater trochanteric pain syndrome, trochanteric bursitis, iliotibial band tendinitis
Ischiofemoral impingement [33]
Femoroacetabular impingement [4,32]
Osteitis pubis [19]
Athletic pubalgia [19]
Subtle hip fractures or stress fracture [4]
Synovial osteochondromatosis
Osteonecrosis of femoral head, avascular necrosis
Labral disease [32]
Osteoid osteoma [4]
Neoplastic infiltration (whether it is metastatic disease or primary pelvic tumor)
Pyogenic arthritis
Hemochromatosis
Spondyloarthropathy (ankylosing spondylitis) [34]
Diffuse idiopathic skeletal hyperostosis
Diabetic cheiroarthropathy (syndrome of limited joint mobility)
Lumbar radiculopathy
Tumoral calcinosis [35]
Complex regional pain syndrome type [3,7,36]

Treatment

Treatment of adhesive capsulitis of the hip is controversial. There are many studies, in both the rheumatologic and orthopedic literature, regarding treatment of the shoulder, but not much is written about treatment of the hips. Neviaser [6–9] and Hannafin [2] have stressed the importance of an individualized program in the treatment of adhesive capsulitis of the shoulder based on the understanding of the clinical stages of the disease. The same should apply to the treatment of the hip. However, the diagnosis of hip capsulitis is rarely made, and when it is made, it is usually in the latter stages of the disease based on the time interval. It is exceedingly difficult to accurately quantify stages of the disease in the hip and therefore to correlate a treatment plan based on those stages.

Conservative treatment is recommended as the disease is self-limited. Spontaneous recovery time on average is approximately 13 months, with a range of 5 to 18 months [1,13,26,27]. Chard and Jenner [13] described three middle-aged patients with pain and stiffness in the hips. No evidence of systemic disease, local infection, or lumbar spine disease was found. Bone scan indicated increased uptake in two patients, but the results of hip arthrography and laboratory studies were normal. The patients recovered spontaneously after a few months.

Initial

Pain control can be achieved early with use of a nonsteroidal anti-inflammatory drug or oral steroid. If this is not beneficial, an analgesic can be tried. Activity modification is recommended to prevent irritation of the involved extremity. Physical modalities, such as ice massage, superficial moist heat, transcutaneous nerve stimulation, interferential current therapy, and ultrasound, can be applied to help with pain control, swelling, and facilitation of physical therapy.

Rehabilitation

Physical therapy is the treatment of choice. The goal of treatment is primarily to restore mobility. Passive mobilization techniques are used to restore the optimal joint kinematics. These techniques can involve lateral translation, distraction, and anteroposterior glide. These maneuvers are done with the patient lying supine; the proximal thigh is palpated while the distal leg rests over the therapist's shoulder. The hip joint is distracted by the application of various forces parallel to the neck of the femur. Initially, the mobilization techniques should be gentle, keeping within the range of pain and reactive muscle spasm. The intensity of the exercises can be adjusted according to the irritability of the joint. Ultimately, stronger passive mobilization techniques may be required in which the joint is taken strongly and specifically to the physiologic limit of range to restore the full function of the hip joint. Stretching of the muscles around the hip joint, which tend to shorten, is important. Active mobilization techniques can be used to restore the optimal length of the erector spinae, quadratus lumborum, hamstrings, rectus femoris, iliopsoas, tensor fascia lata, hip adductors, piriformis, and deep external rotators of the hip. Strengthening of the core muscles, gluteals, and hip groups should be done to address strength, endurance, and timing of recruitment of those muscle groups. Miller and coworkers [28] reviewed the cases of 50 patients in a 10-year period and found that the majority of the patients regained motion with minimal residual deficits after conservative treatment with physical therapy and oral medications. In contrast, Shaffer and colleagues [29] reported that 50% of patients had pain or residual stiffness at 7 years after treatment. A specific home exercise program should be included with continued range of motion and flexibility exercises to prevent recurrence of hip adhesive capsulitis.

Procedures

Trigger point injection and intra-articular injection can be tried in recalcitrant cases not responding to conservative treatment. Trigger point injection can be helpful if there is associated muscle pain and spasm. Ultrasound-guided intra-articular injection with long-acting local anesthetic and corticosteroid has been used for pain control. Several randomized, placebo-controlled clinical trials have shown improvement of pain and hip disability after intra-articular injection of corticosteroids [30]. Fluoroscopically guided hip injection with contrast material to confirm intra-articular needle placement has been tried; alternatively, the hip joint can be injected during computed tomographic or magnetic resonance arthroscopy.

Manipulation under anesthesia is widely used for adhesive capsulitis of the shoulder but is rarely used in treatment of hip adhesive capsulitis. Luukkainen and associates [31] reported the case of a man with adhesive capsulitis of the hip treated successfully with manipulation under anesthesia and pressure dilation of the joint space by use of isotonic sodium chloride. The patient failed to respond to physical therapy, pharmacotherapy, and intra-articular hip injection with triamcinolone and lidocaine during a period of 3 years.

Surgical intervention may be deemed appropriate if conservative treatment fails and the symptoms persist for more than 15 months with interference of activities of daily living. Arthroscopic release is rarely performed. Mont and colleagues [27] described a patient with adhesive capsulitis who failed to respond to conservative treatment with oral medications, physical therapy, and injection trials. The patient underwent hip capsulectomy through an anterolateral approach 1 year after initial presentation. Continuous passive motion was used during the early postoperative period to maintain range of motion. The anterior approach was used to preserve femoral head vascularity and to limit postoperative bleeding.

Potential Disease Complications

Disease complications are usually related to the range of motion deficits and associated pain that accompanies hip adhesive capsulitis. Functional limitations, which vary from patient to patient, may develop. The loss of mobility at the hip joint can result in difficulties with prolonged stance, ambulation, and sitting. Sleeping postures can also be affected as the patient may not be able to sleep on either side.

Potential Treatment Complications

Pharmacotherapy can lead to treatment complications. Nonsteroidal anti-inflammatory drugs have well-documented side effects related to the gastrointestinal and renal systems. Oral steroids, if they are used at high doses for a prolonged time, can have systemic effects, such as easy bruising, weight gain, and osteoporosis. The pharmacotherapy complications can be minimized by closely observing the patient's ongoing medical issues, medication use, and response and potential for drug interactions.

Local injections can cause allergic reactions, infection at the injection site, hematoma, nerve damage, or tendon rupture with inadvertent injection into a nerve or tendon. Physical therapy can result in increased pain and dysfunction if it is not supervised by a well-trained, board-certified physical therapist. Manipulation under anesthesia can lead to an increased risk for chondrolysis and vascular and neurologic insult. Surgical complications are numerous and can include excessive blood loss and postsurgical infection. Compromise of the vascular supply to the femoral head can lead to avascular necrosis and the need for additional surgical procedures. Surgery can result in a cosmetically unpleasant incision around the hip.

References

[1] Lequesne M, Becker J, Bard M, et al. Capsular constriction of the hip: arthrographic and clinical considerations. Skeletal Radiol 1982;6:1–10.

[2] Hannafin JA, Chiaia TA. Adhesive capsulitis. A treatment approach. Clin Orthop Relat Res 2000;372:95–109.

[3] Williams PL, Warwick R, editors. Arthrology: the joints of the lower limb—the hip joint. Gray's Anatomy. 36th ed. New York: Churchill Livingstone; 1980. p. 477–82.

[4] Hodnett PA, Shelly MJ, MacMahon PJ, et al. MRI imaging of overuse injuries of the hip. Magn Reson Imaging Clin N Am 2009;17:667–79.

[5] Neviaser JS. Adhesive capsulitis of the shoulder. Study of pathological findings in periarthritis of the shoulder. J Bone Joint Surg 1945;27:211–22.

[6] Neviaser RJ, Neviaser JS. The frozen shoulder. Diagnosis and management. Clin Orthop 1987;223:59–64.

[7] Neviaser JS. Arthrography of the shoulder joint. J Bone Joint Surg Am 1942;44:1321–6.

[8] Neviaser JS. Adhesive capsulitis and the stiff and painful shoulder. Orthop Clin North Am 1980;11:327–31.

[9] Neviaser RJ. Painful conditions effecting the shoulder. Clin Orthop 1983;173:63–9.

[10] Rizk TE, Pinals RS. Frozen shoulder. Semin Arthritis Rheum 1982;11:440–52.

[11] Modesto C, Crespo E, Villas C, et al. Adhesive capsulitis. Is it possible in childhood? Scand J Rheumatol 1995;24:255–6.

[12] Griffiths HJ, Utz R, Burke J, Bonfiglio T. Adhesive capsulitis of the hip and ankle. AJR Am J Roentgenol 1985;144:101–5.

[13] Chard MD, Jenner JR. The frozen hip: an underdiagnosed condition. BMJ 1988;297:596–7.

[14] Luukkainen R, Asikainen E. Frozen hip. Scand J Rheumatol 1992;21:97.

[15] McGrory BJ, Endrizzi DP. Adhesive capsulitis of the hip after bilateral adhesive capsulitis of the shoulder. Am J Orthop (Belle Mead NJ) 2000;29:457–60.

[16] Thomas-Byrd JW, Jones KS. Adhesive capsulitis of the hip. Arthroscopy 2006;22:89–94.

[17] Bulgen DY, Binder A, Hazleman BL, Park JR. Immunological studies in frozen shoulder. J Rheumatol 1982;9:893–8.

[18] Binder A, Bulgen DY, Hazleman BL, Roberts S. Frozen shoulder: a long term prospective study. Ann Rheum Dis 1984;43:361–4.

[19] Guanche CA. Clinical update: MR imaging of the hip. Sports Med Arthrosc 2009;17:49–55.

[20] Hoffer PB, Genant HK. Radionuclide joint imaging. Semin Nucl Med 1976;6:121–33.

[21] Nestorova R, Vlad V, Petranova T, et al. Ultrasonography of the hip. Med Ultrason 2012;14:217–24.

[22] Bogost GA, Lizerbram EK, Crues JV. MRI in evaluation of suspected hip fracture: frequency of unsuspected bone and soft tissue injury. Radiology 1997;197:263–7.

[23] Conway WF, Totty WG, McErney KW. CT and MR imaging of the hip. Radiology 1996;198:297–307.

[24] Cone RO, Yaru N, Resnick D, et al. Intracapsular pressure monitoring during arthrographic evaluation of painful hip prosthesis. AJR Am J Roentgenol 1983;14:885–9.

[25] Murphy WA, Siegel MJ, Gilula LA. Arthrography in the diagnosis of unexplained chronic hip pain with regional osteopenia. AJR Am J Roentgenol 1977;129:283–7.

[26] Caroit M, Djian A, Hubault A, et al. 2 Cases of retractile capsulitis of the hip. Rev Rhum Mal Osteoartic 1963;30:784–9.

[27] Mont MA, Lindsey JM, Hungerford DS. Adhesive capsulitis of the hip. Orthopedics 1999;22:343–5.

[28] Miller MD, Wirth MA, Rockwood Jr. CA. Thawing the frozen shoulder: the "patient" patient. Orthopedics 1996;19:849–53.

[29] Shaffer B, Tibone JE, Kerlan RK. Frozen shoulder: a long term follow-up study. J Bone Joint Surg Am 1992;74:738–46.

[30] Micu MC, Bogdan GD, Fodor D. Steroid injection for hip osteoarthritis: efficacy under ultrasound guidance. Rheumatology 2010;49:1490–4.

[31] Luukkainen R, Sipola E, Varjo P. Successful treatment of frozen hip with manipulation and pressure dilation. Open Rheumatol J 2008;2:31–2.

[32] Tibor LM, Sekiya JK. Differential diagnosis of pain around the hip joint. Arthroscopy 2008;24:1407–21.

[33] Stafford GH, Villar RN. Ischiofemoral impingement. J Bone Joint Surg Br 2011;93:1300–2.

[34] Jordan CL, Rhon DI. Differential diagnosis and management of ankylosing spondylitis masked as adhesive capsulitis: a resident's case problem. J Orthop Sports Phys Ther 2012;42:842–52.

[35] Croock AD, Silver RM. Tumoral calcinosis presenting as adhesive capsulitis: case report and literature review. Arthritis Rheum 1987;30:455–9.

[36] Joassin R, Vandemeulebroucke M, Nisolle JF, et al. Adhesive capsulitis of the hip: three case reports. Ann Readapt Med Phys 2008;51:301–14.

[37] Bowman CA, Jeffcoate WJ, Patrick M. Bilateral adhesive capsulitis, oligoarthritis and proximal myopathy as presentation of hypothyroidism. Br J Rheumatol 1988;27:62–4.

[38] Lloyd-Roberts GG, French PR. Periarthritis of the shoulder: a study of the disease and its treatment. Br Med J 1959;1:1569–71.

[39] Kapoor A, Sibbitt Jr. WL. Contractures in diabetes mellitus: the syndrome of limited joint mobility. Semin Arthritis Rheum 1989;18:168–80.

[40] Dihlmann W, Höpker WW. Adhesive (retractile) capsulitis of the hip joint in diabetes mellitus. Rofo 1992;157:235–8.

[41] Bridgman JF. Periarthritis of the shoulder and diabetes mellitus. Ann Rheum Dis 1972;31:69–71.

CHAPTER 53

Hip Adductor Strain

Ricardo Colberg, MD

Synonyms

Groin strain
Hip adductor tendinitis or tendinopathy

ICD-9 Codes

719.45 **Pain hip/pelvis**
843 **Sprains and strains of hip and thigh**
843.8 **Sprains and strains of other specified sites of hip and thigh**
843.9 **Sprains and strains of hip and thigh, unspecified site; hip NOS; thigh NOS**

ICD-10 Codes

M25.551 **Pain in right hip**
M25.552 **Pain in left hip**
M25.559 **Pain in unspecified hip**
S76.211 **Strain of adductor muscle, fascia and tendon of right thigh**
S76.212 **Strain of adductor muscle, fascia and tendon of left thigh**
S76.219 **Strain of adductor muscle, fascia and tendon of unspecified thigh**
Add seventh character to S76 for episode of care

Definition

Hip adductor strain refers to an injury of the hip adductor muscles at the muscle belly, myotendinous junction, or tendon. It can be an acute or chronic injury. The hip adductor muscles include the adductor magnus, adductor brevis, adductor longus, pectineus, and gracilis muscles (Fig. 53.1). All of these muscles are innervated by the obturator nerve with the exception of the pectineus muscle, which is innervated by the femoral nerve. Their functions include hip adduction and hip flexion. Adductor strain is the most common cause of acute groin pain in athletes [1]. The adductor longus myotendinous junction is the most commonly injured site [2].

A prospective cohort study of the incidence of groin injuries during a 1-year period among Swedish male club soccer players reported that 8% of all injuries were in the groin area, and 52% of these were attributed to adductor muscle or tendon injuries [3]. A similar incidence was reported in a study of Norwegian female elite soccer players, in which 9% of all injuries were hip or groin strains; 83% of these were acute injuries and 17% were secondary to overuse [4]. For male ice hockey players of a single National Hockey League team, Tyler and colleagues [5] reported 3.2 strains per 1000 player-game exposures. Orchard and Seward [6] monitored all the injuries that occurred in the Australian Football League during 4 consecutive years. In total, more than 660 elite male athletes played 22 matches per season among 16 teams. There was an incidence of 3.3 groin strains per team per season, the second most common musculoskeletal injury after hamstring strain, and a recurrence rate of 21%. In addition, it was the third most prevalent injury after hamstring strain and anterior cruciate ligament tear, with 11.9 matches missed per team per season. A retrospective cohort study of 500 Australian Football League players indicated that 17% sustained a hip or groin injury during their junior years. Of these, 31% were secondary to a hip adductor strain or tear, and 17% were recurrent injuries [7]. Recurrence of hip adductor strains has been reported to be as high as 32% to 44% in ice hockey and Australian football athletes [5,8]. Adductor strains in elderly athletes older than 70 years occur at a slightly decreased incidence of 5% [9]. The incidence and prevalence of hip adductor strains in sedentary patients are unknown.

Athletes who participate in sports that require cutting and sudden change of direction (e.g., soccer, ice hockey, Australian-rules football) are at increased risk for this injury [10]. Adductor strains may also occur from an eccentric contraction of the adductor muscles opposing the abductor muscles, as may be seen with an explosive lateral propulsion in ice hockey [11]. Hip adductor strains have been attributed to low strength or flexibility of this muscle group [12]. There is usually poor conditioning of the trunk and lower extremities characterized by muscle imbalance among the pelvic stabilizing muscles, including the hip abductor and adductor muscles, as well as the core muscles and hip flexors [10]. In addition, poor technique and overuse are risk factors for adductor strains. In rare instances, sacroiliac dysfunction may be associated with adductor injuries [13].

Adductor strains may be classified according to functional limitation on physical examination or pathologic injury on radiographic imaging (Table 53.1). The functional classification

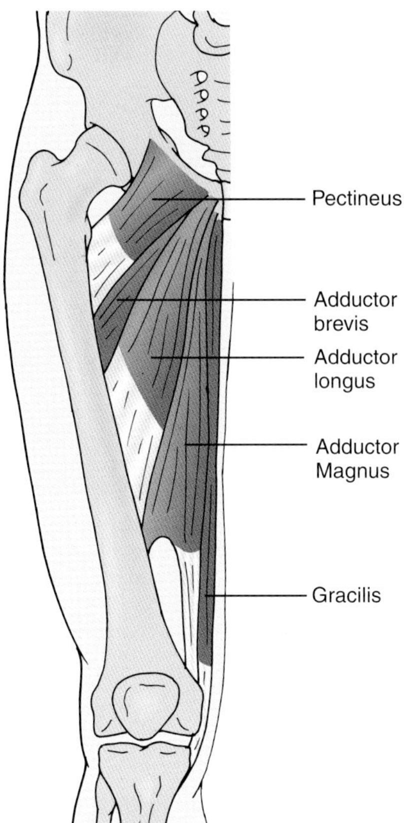

FIGURE 53.1 Hip adductor muscles.

Table 53.1 Functional and Radiographic Classifications

Grade	Functional Classification	Radiographic Classification
1	No loss or minimal loss of function or mobility	Inflammation at the injured site with no tear
2	Partial loss of strength and mobility	Partial tear of the adductor muscle or tendon
3	Complete loss of function	Full tear of the adductor muscle or tendon

may or may not directly correlate with the pathologic change of the tissue seen on radiographic imaging. If the injury is localized at the tendon or myotendinous junction, it may also be described as an adductor tendinitis, referring to an acute injury with active inflammatory process, or as an adductor tendinosis, referring to a chronic injury that is causing functional limitations and does not have an ongoing inflammatory reaction. Because it may be difficult to classify the presence of an inflammatory process, tendinopathy is used frequently to refer to an adductor tendon or myotendinous injury with partial or complete loss of function that may be acute or chronic.

Symptoms

Patients with hip adductor strains complain of sharp, stinging, or aching pain in the groin area that may radiate down to the anteromedial thigh. Symptoms are worse when they adduct and flex the leg at the hip, such as when they move the outside leg into a car. They usually report tightness in the groin or anteromedial pelvic girdle region. In injuries involving a partial or complete tear of the muscle or tendon, they complain of soft tissue swelling and bruising in the medial thigh. Chronic injuries may hurt only during physical activity or sports participation.

Physical Examination

The patient presents with tenderness to palpation in the groin region, most commonly over the adductor longus tendon or myotendinous junction distal to the origin of the muscle at the anterior surface of the pubis between the crest and the symphysis. In severe injuries, a defect may be palpated in the muscle representing a tear in the muscle or tendon. There can be associated ecchymosis, swelling, and tenderness of the surrounding soft tissue. Antalgic gait may be noted with ambulation secondary to pain or dysfunction. Single-leg standing and squatting may reveal Trendelenburg sign, excessive hip internal or external rotation, or genu valgus or varus.

Pain or weakness of the hip adductor muscle may be elicited with active resisted hip adduction, hip adduction and flexion, and hip flexion. Groin pain may also be reproduced with passive forced hip abduction as well as with passive flexion, abduction, and external rotation of the hip (FABER test). The cross-over sign may be used to determine if the adductor strain is moderate to severe and likely to cause functional impairment. This maneuver consists of reproducing the typical groin pain while performing any of the provocative maneuvers mentioned before on the contralateral side (i.e., FABER test, active resisted hip adduction, or passive hip abduction). The squeeze test and the static resisted hip adduction test are specific examinations for hip adductor muscles. During the squeeze test, the patient is in the supine position with feet on the table, hips flexed to 45 degrees, and knees flexed to 90 degrees. The examiner places the fist between the knees and asks the patient to squeeze the fist by adducting the hips bilaterally. The resisted hip adduction test consists of laying the patient supine with legs straight, positioning each leg at 15 degrees of abduction, and bilaterally resisting active hip adduction.

Functional Limitations

Patients usually have difficulty with walking, running, doing pivot turns, going up and down stairs, and standing up from a sitting position and vice versa. As mentioned before, getting in and out of a car is particularly painful. Sexual intimacy is frequently avoided because of the proximity of the injury to the sexual organs and groin pain experienced as the adductor muscles contract to stabilize the pelvis.

Hip adductor strains present with significant functional limitations during sports participation and interfere with athletes' optimal performance. They may report difficulty with propulsion in the lateral direction due to the eccentric contraction of the hip adductor muscles attempting to decelerate the leg stride, tightness in the groin region despite stretching, and loss of maximal sprinting speed, among other complaints [10,14]. The biomechanics of movements involving the hip joint are consequently altered as the athlete tries to avoid experiencing pain. If it is left uncorrected, this adaptation eventually leads to other injuries, such as contralateral hip adductor strain, osteitis pubis, and sports hernia.

Diagnostic Studies

Initial evaluation of groin pain should include plain films to rule out bone disease, such as hip osteoarthritis and neoplasm. Avulsion injuries of the symphysis pubis and inferior pubic ramus may also occur from chronic overuse and be manifested with adductor enthesopathy and osteitis pubis [15]. Magnetic resonance imaging is the optimal imaging tool to evaluate for groin and hip disease because it provides visualization of a large field and gives a three-dimensional view of the region with excellent soft tissue contrast resolution [16]. It is particularly effective for diagnosis of adductor muscle and tendon disease. Fat-saturated, fluid-sensitive magnetic resonance sequences in the axial-oblique and coronal planes are best for evaluating hip adductor strains [17] (Figs. 53.2 and 53.3). Magnetic resonance imaging also helps differentiate hip adductor injuries from other pelvic disease, such as acetabular labrum tears and osteitis pubis.

Ultrasound can be used to evaluate the adductor muscles under dynamic conditions, to compare the asymptomatic side, and specifically to image the area of maximal tenderness to detect tissue injury such as a partial or full tear [18] (Fig. 53.4). Ultrasound imaging can be as sensitive as magnetic resonance imaging in the acute setting; however, it has limited visualization in patients with large thighs and is less useful when prognostic indicators are required [19,20].

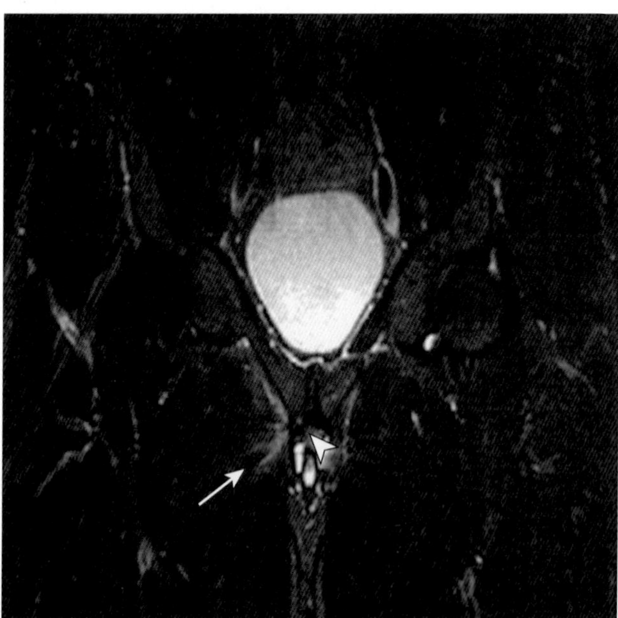

FIGURE 53.2 Coronal T2-weighted fat-suppressed magnetic resonance image of a right grade 1 adductor longus strain shows edema within the proximal tendon *(arrow)* and capsular injury to the pubic symphysis *(arrowhead)*. *(From Kavanagh EC, Koulouris G, Ford S, et al. MR imaging of groin pain in the athlete. Semin Musculoskelet Radiol 2006;10:197-207.)*

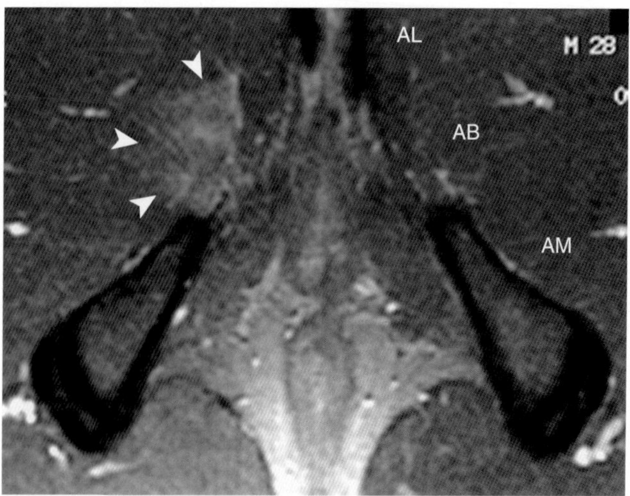

FIGURE 53.3 Axial T2-weighted fat-saturated magnetic resonance image of a right grade 2 adductor brevis tear shows edema within the myotendinous region of the right adductor brevis *(arrowheads)*. *AL*, left adductor longus; *AB*, left adductor brevis; *AM*, left adductor magnus. *(From Brittenden J, Robinson P. Imaging of pelvic injuries in athletes. Br J Radiol 2005;78:457-468.)*

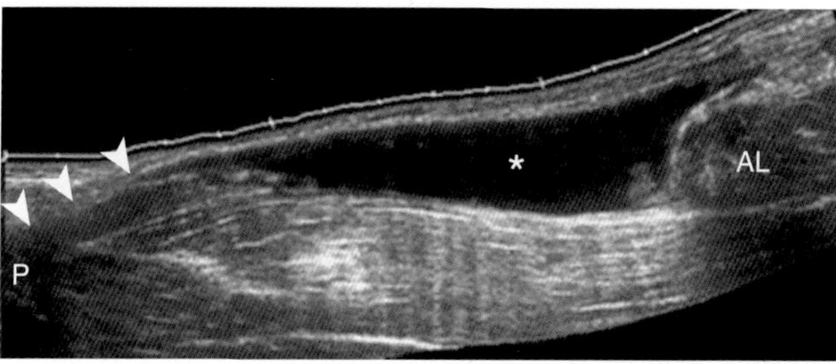

FIGURE 53.4 Extended longitudinal ultrasound view of a grade 3 tear of the adductor longus at the myotendinous junction with associated muscle retraction. *AL*, adductor longus; *P*, pubic bone; proximal tendon *(arrowheads)*; hematoma *(asterisk)*. *(From Brittenden J, Robinson P. Imaging of pelvic injuries in athletes. Br J Radiol 2005;78:457-468.)*

Differential Diagnosis

Athletic pubalgia or sports hernia
Osteitis pubis
Acetabular labrum tear
Stress fracture of the femoral neck or pubic ramus
Osteoarthritis
Iliopsoas muscle strain
Rectus femoris muscle strain
Hip joint toxic synovitis
Slipped capital femoral epiphysis
Avascular necrosis of the femoral head
Inguinal or femoral hernia
Genitourinary causes, including testicular torsion
Lymphadenopathy
Obturator nerve entrapment
Sacroiliac joint pain

Treatment

Initial

Hip adductor strains are managed initially with rest, ice, compression, elevation, and nonsteroidal anti-inflammatory drugs (NSAIDs) to decrease swelling and inflammation. Athletes with acute hip adductor strains are requested to stop competitive participation and training to avoid further injury. The initial treatment (first phase of rehabilitation) should focus on tissue protection using an elastic wrap or compression shorts, reducing the local inflammation with cryotherapy and NSAIDs, and minimizing excessive motion of the injured site as well as weight bearing as tolerated with crutches. This is especially important in the presence of an apophyseal injury or tendon tear. Other causes of groin pain should be ruled out (see differential diagnosis) before a comprehensive rehabilitation program is implemented.

Rehabilitation

When the acute inflammatory phase subsides, usually within 48 hours, the second phase of rehabilitation is started to facilitate tissue healing and proper collagen deposition. Any increased muscle tone guarding the injured site should be addressed with various therapeutic modalities, including soft tissue massage and gentle passive range of motion. The appropriate time to commence stretching is debated. Some experts suggest that stretching should be done early to promote proper lengthening of the injured tissue as it remodels. Others suggest that early stretching may expose the athlete to development of chronic tendinopathy and should not start until at least 4 days after the injury [14].

A gradual muscle strengthening program is implemented, initially focusing on gentle active range of motion of the hip and strengthening of adjacent regions including core stabilization exercises. After full pain-free passive range of motion is achieved, exercises specifically focusing on hip adductor strengthening are initiated, starting with static exercises and progressing to concentric exercises. Neuromuscular electrical stimulation may be used to assist proper muscle activation. Once the patient is pain free with concentric exercises, on average 2 to 4 weeks after the initial injury, eccentric exercises are started for strengthening of the injured site. In an example of a hip adductor eccentric exercise, the patient lies supine, places the feet together against a wall with knees at full extension and hips at 60 degrees of flexion, and then slowly opens the legs symmetrically into hip abduction. If pain is experienced during any of the stages of the gradual strengthening program, the specific painful activity should be modified or stopped until the exercises can be completed pain free.

The third phase of the rehabilitation program involving functional training can be implemented once strength and flexibility are recovered. Proprioceptive training and plyometric exercises on unbalanced surfaces are done to continue strengthening of the hip adductor muscles and to reeducate proper neuromuscular activation of the various pelvic stabilizing agonist and antagonist muscles. In addition, dynamic strengthening exercises that incorporate the entire body are started (e.g., cable cross-over pull while standing on unstable surface).

At some point between the second and third phase of rehabilitation, the patient may start doing straight-line aerobic exercises, such as jogging or cycling, as long as muscle guarding is eliminated, there is no cross-over sign, and there is no pain experienced with the strengthening program. Distance, intensity, and time should be gradually increased as tolerated, ensuring that the athlete does not experience pain during or after the activity. Once the athlete tolerates straight-line running exercises at more than 75% of maximum performance, drills involving lateral movements and change of directions can be implemented. The last stage of functional training focuses on sports-specific exercises and drills that simulate actual playing.

The ultimate objective of the rehabilitation protocol is to improve the pelvic stability by balancing the strength between the opposing pelvic stabilizing muscles and, in the case of athletes, gradually return them to peak performance. Specifically, hip adductor muscles should have at least 80% of the strength of the ipsilateral hip abductor muscles before return to play [21]. The length of the rehabilitation program varies according to the severity of the injury and the athlete's demand on the pelvic stabilizing muscles for participation in his or her sport. Severe injuries may take up to 12 weeks for full recovery and return to play.

Procedures

Patients may have trigger points along the muscle belly of one or more of the adductor muscles. These may be managed by trigger point injections with a local anesthetic such as lidocaine. In chronic cases in which pain is severely interfering with the rehabilitation program, a corticosteroid injection under ultrasound guidance may be placed in the peritendinous area, avoiding direct injection into the adductor tendon. This will decrease any residual inflammatory reaction, reduce pain, and facilitate the athlete's completion of the rehabilitation protocol. In cases that have been recalcitrant to conservative measures, the patient may benefit from needling the tendon under ultrasound guidance to reactivate the tissue healing cascade [22]. A regenerative injectate such as platelet-rich plasma may be used; nonetheless, there is limited evidence of the benefits with use of these injectates [23,24]. Extracorporeal shock wave therapy may also be considered for recalcitrant cases [25].

Surgery

Referral to a sports medicine orthopedic surgeon should be considered with a significant avulsion fracture, complete adductor tendon tear, or chronic recalcitrant cases that failed the rehabilitation program. Depending on the chronicity of the injury, the patient may benefit from a partial or complete adductor tendon release. Most athletes who undergo adductor longus tenotomy return to competitive sports within 3 months [26].

Potential Disease Complications

Early diagnosis and treatment usually lead to successful outcomes and complete recovery. Continued activity or sports participation without proper rehabilitation frequently causes worsening pain, weakness, and functional limitations. Signs of mild hip adductor strains include recurrent tightness during or after activity with no relief from stretching and a decrease in sports-specific performance. Mild injuries may become severe if they are not treated accordingly. In addition, the injured adductor muscle will cause pelvic instability and may lead to further injury of the suprapubic muscles or the contralateral hip adductor muscles.

Potential Treatment Complications

Early return to play may lead to recurrent hip adductor strains [27]. Management of a hip adductor strain with only rest or NSAIDs will provide symptom relief but will not address the original cause of the injury, which in most cases is attributed to poor conditioning and imbalance of the pelvic stabilizing muscles. Athletes who complete an active training program are more likely to have excellent outcomes and pain-free successful return to sports in the first 6 months as well as to maintain significant improvement in symptoms up to 12 years after the injury compared with athletes who undergo a physiotherapy program without an active strengthening program [28,29]. Inadequate rehabilitation may lead to chronic injury, especially if there is concomitant pelvic dysfunction that is left untreated.

One of the most frequently used treatments for the pain associated with tendinopathies is prescription-strength anti-inflammatory drugs such as NSAIDs, selective cyclooxygenase 2 inhibitors, and corticosteroid injections. However, these treatment options carry potential risks for complications. A study of the effect of ibuprofen over rat Achilles tendon cells showed increased activity of the collagen-degrading enzymes, suggesting a detrimental effect of ibuprofen on the mechanism for tendon healing [30]. In vitro and in vivo experiments showed that NS-398, a specific cyclooxygenase 2 inhibitor, inhibited the proliferation and maturation of differentiated myogenic precursor cells, suggesting a detrimental effect on skeletal muscle healing [31]. Studies of corticosteroid injections for lateral epicondylitis show positive short-term results but frequent relapses and no significant difference from placebo or physiotherapy in the long term [32,33]. In addition, corticosteroid injections have resulted in tendon rupture in several cases of Achilles tendinopathy [34]. Surgery also carries significant risks. In addition to the risk of infection or nerve injury seen with most surgeries, adductor longus tenotomy may leave patients with decreased hip adduction strength [26]. Patients should be educated on the corresponding risks versus benefits of the chosen treatment plan.

Acknowledgment

The author thanks Michael T. Ellerbusch, MD, for his contribution to this chapter.

References

[1] Bradshaw C, Holmich P. Acute hip and groin pain. In: Brukner P, Khan K, editors. Clinical sports medicine. revised 3rd ed. New York: McGraw-Hill; 2009. p. 394–404.

[2] Morelli V, Weaver V. Groin injuries and groin pain in athletes, part 1. Prim Care 2005;32:163–83.

[3] Ekstrand J, Hilding J. The incidence and differential diagnosis of acute groin injuries in male soccer players. Scand J Med Sci Sports 1999;9:98–103.

[4] Tegnander A, Olsen OE, Moholdt TT, et al. Injuries in Norwegian female elite soccer: a prospective one-season cohort study. Knee Surg Sports Traumatol Arthrosc 2008;16:194–8.

[5] Tyler TF, Nicholas SJ, Campbell RJ, et al. The association of hip strength and flexibility on the incidence of groin strains in professional ice hockey players. Am J Sports Med 2001;29:124–8.

[6] Orchard J, Seward H. Epidemiology of injuries in the Australian Football League, seasons 1997–2000. Br J Sports Med 2002;36:39–45.

[7] Gabbe BJ, Bailey M, Cook JL, et al. The association between hip and groin injuries in the elite junior football years and injuries sustained during elite senior competition. Br J Sports Med 2010;44:799–802.

[8] Seward H, Orchard J, Hazard H, et al. Football injuries in Australia at the elite level. Med J Aust 1993;159:298–301.

[9] Kallinen M, Alen M. Sports-related injuries in elderly men still active in sports. Br J Sports Med 1994;28:52–5.

[10] Maffey L, Emery C. What are the risk factors for groin strain injury in sport? A systematic review of the literature. Sports Med 2007;37:881–94.

[11] Nicholas SJ, Tyler TF. Adductor muscle strains in sport. Sports Med 2002;32:339–44.

[12] Hrysomallis C. Hip adductors' strength, flexibility, and injury risk. J Strength Cond Res 2009;23:1514–7.

[13] Macintyre JG. Kinetic chain dysfunction in ballet injuries. Med Probl Perform Art 1994;9:39–42.

[14] Bradshaw C, Holmich P. Longstanding groin pain. In: Brukner P, Khan K, editors. Clinical sports medicine. revised 3rd ed. New York: McGraw-Hill; 2009. p. 405–26.

[15] Stevens MA, El-Khoury GY, Kathol MH, et al. Imaging features of avulsion injuries. Radiographics 1999;19:655–72.

[16] Ansede G, English B, Healy JC. Groin pain: clinical assessment and the role of MR imaging. Semin Musculoskelet Radiol 2011;15:3–13.

[17] Kavanagh EC, Koulouris G, Ford S, et al. MR imaging of groin pain in the athlete. Semin Musculoskelet Radiol 2006;10:197–207.

[18] Jansen JA, Mens JM, Backx FJ, et al. Diagnostics in athletes with long-standing groin pain. Scand J Med Sci Sports 2008;18:679–90.

[19] McSweeney S, Naraghi A, Salonen D, et al. Hip and groin pain in the professional athlete. Can Assoc Radiol J 2012;63:87–99.

[20] Brittenden J, Robinson P. Imaging of pelvic injuries in athletes. Br J Radiol 2005;78:457–68.

[21] Tyler TF, Nicholas SJ, Campbell R, et al. The effectiveness of a preseason exercise program on the prevention of adductor strains in professional ice hockey players. Am J Sports Med 2002;30:680–3.

[22] McShane JM, Nazarian LN, Harwood MI. Sonographically guided percutaneous needle tenotomy for treatment of common extensor tendinosis in the elbow. J Ultrasound Med 2006;25:1281–9.

[23] Nguyen R, Borg-Stein J, McInnis K. Applications of platelet-rich plasma in musculoskeletal and sports medicine: an evidence-based approach. PM R 2011;3:226–50.

[24] Mautner K, Colberg R, Borg-Stein J, et al. Outcomes following ultrasound-guided platelet-rich plasma injections for chronic tendinopathies: a multicenter retrospective review. PM R 2013;5:169–75.

[25] Wang CJ. Extracorporeal shockwave therapy in musculoskeletal disorders. J Orthop Surg Res 2012;7:1–8.

[26] Akemark C, Johansson C. Tenotomy of the adductor longus tendon in the treatment of chronic groin pain in athletes. Am J Sports Med 1992;20:640–3.

[27] Macintyre J, Johson C, Schroeder EL. Groin pain in athletes. Curr Sports Med Rep 2006;5:293–9.

[28] Hölmich P, Uhrskou P, Ulnits L, et al. Effectiveness of active physical training as treatment for long-standing adductor-related groin pain in athletes: a randomized trial. Lancet 1999;353:439–43.

[29] Hölmich P, Nyvold P, Larsen K. Continued significant effect of physical training as treatment for overuse injury: 8- to 12-year outcome of a randomized clinical trial. Am J Sports Med 2011;39:2447–51.

[30] Tsai WC, Hsu CC, Chang HN, et al. Ibuprofen upregulates expressions of matrix metalloproteinase-1, -8, -9, and -13 without affecting expressions of types I and III collagen in tendon cells. J Orthop Res 2010;28:487–91.

[31] Shen W, Li Y, Tang Y, et al. NS-398, a cycloxoygenase-2–specific inhibitor, delays skeletal muscle healing by decreasing regeneration and promoting fibrosis. Am J Pathol 2005;167:1105–17.

[32] Smidt N, Assendelft WJ, van der Windt DA, et al. Corticosteroid injections for lateral epicondylitis; a systematic review. Pain 2002;96:23–40.

[33] Smidt N, van der Windt DA, Assendelft WJ, et al. Corticosteroid injections, physiotherapy, or a wait-and-see policy for lateral epicondylitis: a randomised controlled trial. Lancet 2002;359:657–62.

[34] Kleinman M, Gross AE. Achilles tendon rupture following steroid injection: report of three cases. J Bone Joint Surg Am 1983;65:1345–7.

CHAPTER 54

Femoral Neuropathy

Earl J. Craig, MD
Daniel M. Clinchot, MD

Synonym

Diabetic amyotrophy

ICD-9 Codes

355.2	**Other lesion of femoral nerve**
355.8	**Mononeuritis of lower limb, unspecified**
355.9	**Mononeuritis of unspecified site**
782.0	**Disturbance of skin sensation**

ICD-10 Codes

G57.20	**Lesion of femoral nerve, unspecified lower limb**
G57.21	**Lesion of femoral nerve, right lower limb**
G57.22	**Lesion of femoral nerve, left lower limb**
G57.90	**Mononeuropathy of unspecified lower limb**
G57.91	**Mononeuropathy of right lower limb**
G57.92	**Mononeuropathy of left lower limb**
G58.9	**Mononeuropathy, unspecified**
R20.9	**Disturbance of skin sensation**

Definition

Femoral neuropathy is the focal injury of the femoral nerve causing various combinations of pain, weakness, and sensory loss in the anterior thigh. The exact incidence of femoral neuropathy is not clear. However, the most common etiology is iatrogenic followed by tumor-related injury [1]. Hemorrhage, most often due to anticoagulation therapy, also is common. Table 54.1 lists other possible causes of femoral neuropathy.

The femoral nerve arises from the anterior rami of the lumbar nerve roots 2, 3, and 4. After forming, the nerve passes on the anterolateral border of the psoas muscle, between the psoas and iliacus muscles, down the posterior abdominal wall, and through the posterior pelvis until it emerges under the inguinal ligament lateral to the femoral artery (Fig. 54.1) [2–4]. The course continues down the anterior thigh, innervating the anterior thigh muscles. The sensory-only saphenous nerve branches off the femoral nerve distal to the inguinal ligament and courses through the thigh until the Hunter (subsartorial) canal, where the nerve dives deep. The femoral nerve innervates the psoas and iliacus muscles in the pelvis and the sartorius, pectineus, rectus femoris, vastus medialis, vastus lateralis, and vastus intermedius muscles in the anterior thigh. The femoral nerve provides sensory innervation to the anterior thigh. The saphenous nerve provides sensory innervation to the anterior patella, anteromedial leg, and medial foot (Fig. 54.2).

Symptoms

The symptoms depend on how acute the injury is and what caused the injury. A patient will often first complain of a dull, aching pain in the inguinal region, which may intensify within hours. Shortly thereafter, the patient may note difficulty with ambulation secondary to leg weakness. The patient may or may not complain of weakness in the hip or thigh but will often notice difficulty with functional activities, such as getting out of a chair and traversing stairs or inclines. Numbness over the anterior thigh and medial leg is common. The numbness may extend into the anteromedial leg and the medial aspect of the foot.

Physical Examination

The examination includes a complete neuromuscular evaluation of the low back, hips, and both lower limbs. This should include inspection for asymmetry or atrophy, manual muscle testing, muscle stretch reflexes, and sensory testing for light touch and pinprick.

In the case of femoral neuropathy, the clinician may see atrophy or asymmetry of the quadriceps muscles. Weakness of hip flexion or knee extension may be present. Strength testing may be limited because of pain. Quadriceps strength should be compared with adductor strength, which typically is normal. Palpation over the inguinal ligament may reveal a

Table 54.1 Possible Causes of Focal Femoral Neuropathy [1,2]

Open Injuries

Retraction during abdominal-pelvic surgery [3,4]
Hip surgery—heat used by methyl methacrylate, especially in association with leg lengthening [5,6]
Penetration trauma (e.g., gunshot and knife wounds, glass shards)

Closed Injuries

Retroperitoneal bleeding after femoral vein or artery puncture [7]
Cardiac angiography
Central line placement
Retroperitoneal fibrosis
Injury during femoral nerve block
Diabetic amyotrophy
Infection
Cancer [8]
Pregnancy
Radiation
Acute stretch injury due to a fall or other trauma
Hemorrhage after a fall or other trauma
Spontaneous hemorrhage—typically due to anticoagulant therapy
Idiopathic
Hypertrophic mononeuropathy [9]

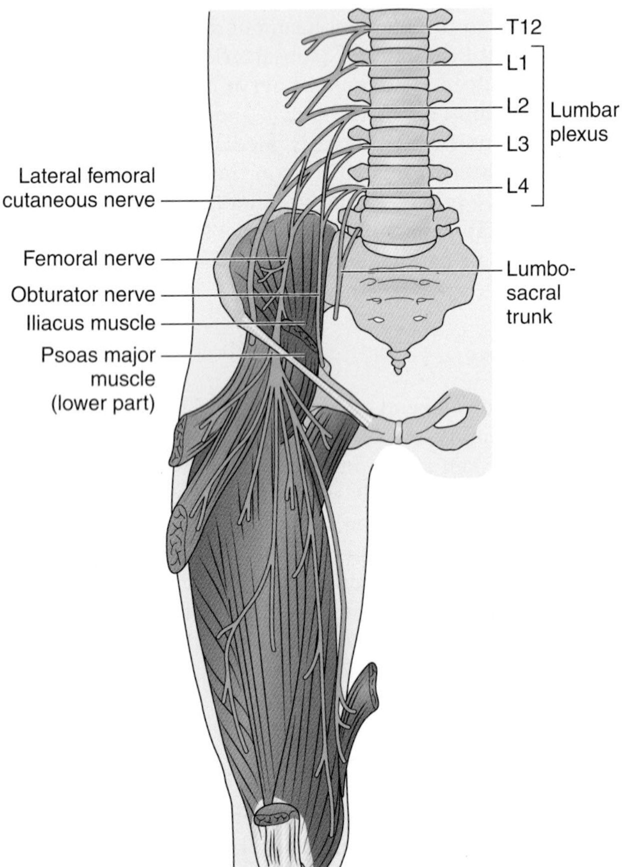

FIGURE 54.1 Anatomy of the femoral nerve.

fullness or exacerbate the patient's pain symptoms. There is often a decreased or loss of quadriceps reflex and decreased sensation to the anterior thigh and anterior and medial leg. The thigh and groin may be tender to palpation. Pain may be exacerbated with hip extension (Fig. 54.3) [2,3].

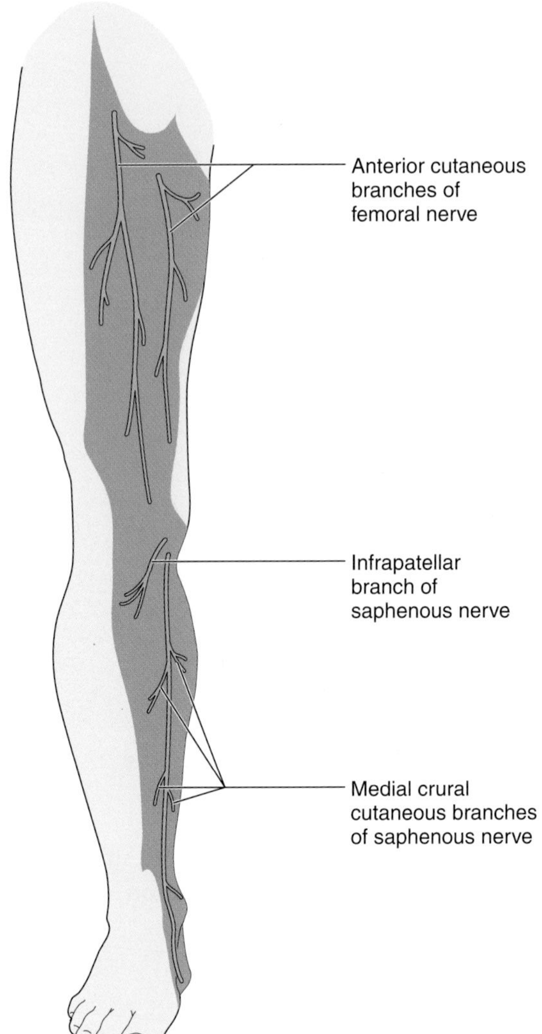

FIGURE 54.2 Sensory innervation of the femoral nerve.

Functional Limitations

Functional limitations due to femoral neuropathy are generally a result of weakness and vary according to the severity of the injury and the functional reserve of the patient. Individuals may have difficulty in getting up from a seated position and walking without falling. Inclines and stairs often magnify the limitations. Recreational and work-related activities are often affected, such as running, climbing, and jumping.

Diagnostic Studies

Electrodiagnostic studies (nerve conduction studies and electromyography) are the "gold standard" to confirm the presence of a femoral nerve injury. These should be performed no earlier than 3 to 4 weeks after the injury. Obviously, in cases of suspected hemorrhage, imaging studies should be done immediately. Imaging studies may include magnetic resonance imaging or computed tomography of the pelvis to look for a hemorrhage or a mass causing impingement [4–7]. Ultrasound has been found

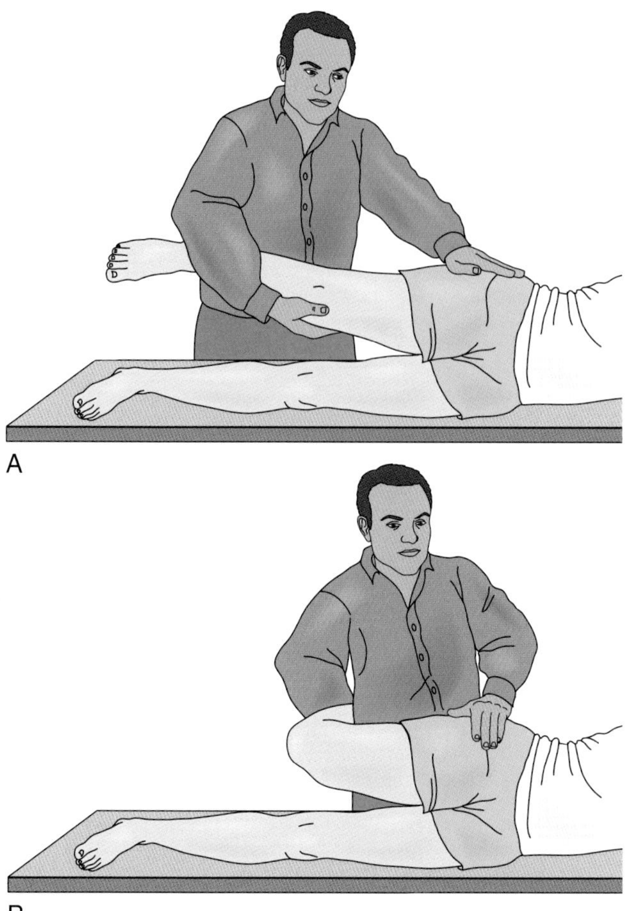

FIGURE 54.3 Traction on the femoral nerve may be accomplished with hip and knee extension initially (**A**) and then gentle knee flexion (**B**).

to be a valuable tool in needle localization for femoral nerve blocks as well as in the identification of femoral nerve injury [8,9].

In terms of electrodiagnostic studies, nerve conduction studies of the femoral motor component are routinely used. Sensory conduction studies of the medial femoral cutaneous nerve can be useful in the localization of femoral neuropathy [10]. Saphenous nerve sensory evaluation is available but is often technically difficult and unreliable [3]. The needle electromyography should evaluate muscles innervated by the femoral, obturator, tibial, and peroneal nerves. The needle evaluation therefore should include evaluation of the iliopsoas, at least two of the four quadriceps femoris muscles, one or two adductor muscles, gluteus minimus, three muscles between the knee and the ankle, and paraspinal muscles. Electromyography should be performed to rule out other causes of neuropathic thigh pain, including upper and mid lumbar radiculopathy, polyradiculopathy, and plexopathy. Serial electromyographic studies may help with evaluation of the recovery process. High-resolution magnetic resonance neurography is useful in the evaluation of femoral neuropathy, providing insight into pathologic causes including compressive lesions, as can be found in retroperitoneal hemorrhage or cancer [11].

Differential Diagnosis

Lumbar radiculopathy
Lumbar polyradiculopathy
Lumbar plexopathy
Avascular necrosis of the femoral head
Polymyalgia rheumatica

Treatment

Initial

Treatment of femoral neuropathy is focused on three separate areas: relief of symptoms, facilitation of nerve healing, and restoration of function. In acute cases in which hemorrhage or trauma is the cause, surgical intervention may be the initial treatment. This is also the case when the injury is due to a mass lesion, such as a tumor.

Acute, subacute, and chronic relief of the pain and numbness is attempted with modalities and medications. Ice may be helpful acutely, and heat may be helpful in the subacute stage. If an inflammatory component is suspected, nonsteroidal anti-inflammatory drugs may help both pain and inflammation. Alternatively, oral corticosteroids may be used. Narcotics are used when acetaminophen and nonsteroidal anti-inflammatory drugs do not control the pain. Antiseizure medications, such as carbamazepine and gabapentin, are also of benefit for the neuropathic pain in some individuals [12,13]. Transcutaneous electrical nerve stimulation may also help with pain control.

Facilitation of healing depends on the cause of the injury to the nerve. In the case of diabetes, improved blood glucose control may help recovery [14]. Injury due to impingement may be improved by removal of the mass. Too often, little can be done to facilitate healing. Nerves that have sustained a less severe injury (neurapraxia injury) often heal within hours to weeks once the irritant is removed. Nerves that have sustained a more serious injury (neurotmesis or axonotmesis) typically have a much longer healing course because of the time required for wallerian degeneration and regeneration. It is important to educate the patient about the potential for a prolonged (sometimes more than 1 year) course of healing. Also, it is important to counsel patients that healing may not be complete and that there may be permanent loss of strength and sensation as well as continued pain symptoms.

Rehabilitation

Once the damage has been stopped or reversed, the focus turns to improvement of hip flexion and knee extension strength by maximizing the function of the available neuromuscular components. This is accomplished with physical therapy instruction and a home exercise program. Improvement of strength in all lower extremity muscle groups is important. Aggressive strengthening should be limited in a nerve that is acutely injured because it may promote further injury and delay healing [15].

It is also essential to work on proper gait mechanics. The physical therapist can help the patient with gait training and gait aids to prevent falls and to improve energy use. Range of motion in all lower extremity joints should be addressed. Neuromuscular electrical stimulation may be of benefit in improving strength in some individuals.

Procedures

Procedures are not indicated for this disease process.

Surgery

In the case of femoral nerve injury due to impingement, mass lesion, or hemorrhage, surgery may be required to remove the pressure. Early surgical evacuation in patients with femoral nerve compression secondary to retroperitoneal hemorrhage can reduce the likelihood of prolonged neurologic impairment [16]. In the case of a penetrating injury to the femoral nerve, surgery to align the two ends of the nerve and to remove scar tissue may be required. Successful transfer of the obturator nerve to the femoral nerve has also been reported in cases in which the lesion of the femoral nerve is complete [17].

Potential Disease Complications

Potential complications include continued pain, numbness, and weakness despite treatment. In addition, the weakness in the hip and knee increases the risk for falls.

Potential Treatment Complications

Analgesics and nonsteroidal anti-inflammatory drugs have well-known side effects that most commonly affect the gastric, hepatic, and renal systems. Narcotics have the potential for addiction and sedation. Carbamazepine can cause sedation and aplastic anemia. The patient taking carbamazepine should be evaluated with serial complete blood counts and checking of carbamazepine level. Gabapentin can cause sedation. The potential risks of surgical intervention include bleeding, infection, and adverse reaction to the anesthetic agent.

References

[1] Campbell AA, Eckhauser FE, Belzberg A, Campbell JN. Obturator nerve transfer as an option for femoral nerve repair: case report. Neurosurgery 2010;66(ONS Suppl 2):onsE375.

[2] Chhabra A, Faridian-Aragh N. High-resolution 3-T MR neurography of femoral neuropathy. AJR Am J Roentgenol 2012;198:3–10.

[3] Dumitru D. Electrodiagnostic medicine. Philadelphia: Hanley & Belfus; 1995.

[4] Eaton RP, Qualls C, Bicknell J, et al. Structure-function relationships within peripheral nerves in diabetic neuropathy: the hydration hypothesis. Diabetologia 1996;39:439–46.

[5] Finnerup NB, Sindrup SH, Jensen TS. The evidence for pharmacological treatment of neuropathic pain. Pain 2010;150:573–81.

[6] Flack S, Anderson C. Ultrasound guided lower extremity blocks. Paediatr Anaesth 2012;22:72–80.

[7] Geiger D, Mpinga E, Steves MA, Sugarbaker PH. Femoral neuropathy: unusual presentation for recurrent large-bowel cancer. Dis Colon Rectum 1998;41:910–3.

[8] Kim DH, Murovic JA, Tiel RL, Kline DG. Intrapelvic and thigh-level femoral nerve lesions: management and outcomes in 119 surgically treated cases. J Neurosurg 2004;100:989–96.

[9] Kimura J. Electrodiagnosis in diseases of nerve and muscle: principles and practice. 2nd ed. Philadelphia: FA Davis; 1989.

[10] Moore KL. Clinically oriented anatomy. 2nd ed. Williams & Wilkins: Baltimore; 1985.

[11] Oh SJ, Hatanaka Y, Ohira M, et al. Clinical utility of sensory nerve conduction of medial femoral cutaneous nerve. Muscle Nerve 2012;45:195–9.

[12] Oldenburg M, Muller RT. The frequency, prognosis and significance of nerve injuries in total hip arthroplasty. Int Orthop 1997;21:1–3.

[13] Parmer SS, Carpenter JP, Fairman RM, et al. Femoral neuropathy following retroperitoneal hemorrhage: case series and review of the literature. Ann Vasc Surg 2006;20:536–40.

[14] Robinson MD, Shannon S. Rehabilitation of peripheral nerve injuries. Phys Med Rehabil Clin N Am 2002;13:109–35.

[15] Schafhalter-Zoppoth I, Zeitz ID, Gray AT. Inadvertent femoral nerve impalement and intraneural injection visualized by ultrasound [letter to the editor]. Anesth Analg 2004;99:627.

[16] Takao M, Fukuuchi Y, Koto A, et al. Localized hypertrophic mononeuropathy involving the femoral nerve. Neurology 1999;52:389–92.

[17] Vorobeychik Y, Gordin V, Mao J, Chen L. Combination therapy for neuropathic pain. CNS Drugs 2011;25:1023–34.

CHAPTER 55

Hip Osteoarthritis

Patrick M. Foye, MD
Todd P. Stitik, MD

Synonyms

Hip osteoarthritis
Hip degenerative joint disease
Degenerative hip joint
Coxarthrosis

ICD-9 Codes

715.15 **Primary (idiopathic) osteoarthritis of the hip**
715.25 **Secondary osteoarthritis of the hip**
716.15 **Traumatic osteoarthritis of the hip**

ICD-10 Codes

M16.10 **Unilateral primary osteoarthritis, unspecified hip**
M16.11 **Unilateral primary osteoarthritis, right hip**
M16.12 **Unilateral primary osteoarthritis, left hip**
M16.7 **Secondary unilateral osteoarthritis, hip**
M16.50 **Post-traumatic osteoarthritis, unspecified hip**
M16.51 **Post-traumatic osteoarthritis, right hip**
M16.52 **Post-traumatic osteoarthritis, left hip**

Definition

Hip osteoarthritis (OA, also called degenerative joint disease) is the most prevalent pathologic condition at the hip joint. The hip joint (femoroacetabular joint) is a ball-and-socket joint, with the femoral head situated within the concavity formed by the acetabulum and labrum. This anatomic arrangement allows movements in multiple planes, including flexion, extension, adduction, abduction, internal rotation, and external rotation. Significant mechanical forces (three to eight times body weight) [1,2] are exerted on the hip joint during weight-bearing activities such as walking, running, jumping, and lifting. Additional stresses are created by recreational activities (e.g., impacts and falls during sports) and severe trauma (e.g., motor vehicle collisions). Hip trauma is significantly associated with unilateral but not bilateral hip OA, whereas obesity is associated with bilateral but not unilateral hip OA [3]. Occupational heavy lifting and frequent stair climbing seem to increase the risk of hip OA [4].

In a study of 2490 subjects aged 55 to 74 years, the prevalence of hip OA was 3.1%; 58% of hip OA cases were unilateral and 42% were bilateral [3]. The prevalence of hip OA is about 3% to 6% in the white population, but by contrast, it is far lower in Asian, black, and East Indian populations [5]. Total hip replacement in patients with hip OA is twice as common in women [6].

A central feature of hip OA is cartilage breakdown, thus compromising the femoroacetabular articulation. In addition to cartilage, other tissues affected by the disease process include subchondral bone, synovial fluid, ligaments, synovial membrane, joint capsule, and adjacent muscles. Eventually, the joint develops osteophytes (exostosis), joint space narrowing, bone sclerosis adjacent to the joint, and potentially even joint fusion (arthrosis). OA can be classified as either primary (idiopathic) or secondary [7]. The most common form of hip OA is primary [8], which represents the "wear and tear" degenerative changes that occur over time. Hip OA is considered secondary if a specific underlying cause can be identified, such as significant prior hip trauma, joint infection, or preexisting congenital or other deformities [7]. Among patients undergoing total hip replacement, the likelihood that the hip OA was primary (rather than secondary) is highest among white individuals (66%), followed by black subjects (54%), Hispanics (53%), and Asians (28%) [9]. Unlike rheumatoid arthritis, OA is relatively noninflammatory during most stages of the disease process. Symptomatic acetabular structural abnormalities can occur in patients with hip instability from classic developmental dysplasia or post-traumatic acetabular dysplasia as well as with retroversion of the acetabulum [10].

Symptoms

Groin pain is the classic manifesting symptom for hip OA. Other presenting symptoms of hip OA include hip pain, stiffness, and associated functional limitations. Many patients report "hip" pain when really they are referring to the superior lateral thigh region (e.g., greater trochanteric bursitis rather than hip joint disease). Hip joint pain typically presents as groin pain, perhaps with some referred pain down toward (and even beyond) the medial knee. Questioning the patient about lumbosacral, sacroiliac, or coccyx pain may reveal that the "hip" symptoms are actually referred from the spine. Hip OA pain usually has an insidious onset, is worse with activity (particularly weight bearing and rotational loading of the joint), and is somewhat relieved with rest [7]. Advanced OA may be painful even at rest [7]. The physician should specifically ask about any constitutional symptoms that might suggest infection or malignant disease and also about any history of hip trauma [11] (recent or remote).

Physical Examination

Antalgic gait is characterized by a limp with decreased single-limb stance time on the painful limb, a shortened stride length for the contralateral limb, and an increased double support time.

Range of motion should be evaluated not only at both hip joints (in multiple planes) but also at the lumbosacral spine, knees, and ankles to more thoroughly evaluate the kinetic chain. The earliest sign of hip OA is loss of hip internal rotation [12,13]. Limping, groin pain, or limited hip internal rotation supports a diagnosis of a hip (rather than spine) disorder [14], but it still remains prudent also to perform a lumbosacral physical examination when lumbosacral pain generators are being considered. Whereas no one physical examination maneuver is diagnostic of hip OA or other form of intra-articular hip disease, assessment for painful range of motion about the hip, palpation, manual muscle testing, screening for radiculopathy and neuropathy, observation for systemic signs of OA, and performance of a provocative maneuver known as the Patrick test represent a reasonable evaluation. The Patrick test is performed by having the patient supine with the ipsilateral heel on the contralateral knee, thus forming the figure four position, also referred to by the acronym FABER (hip flexed, abducted, and externally rotated) maneuver (Fig. 55.1). The physician pushes the raised leg toward the table, producing groin pain that suggests intra-articular hip disease or back or buttock pain that suggests sacroiliac joint disease.

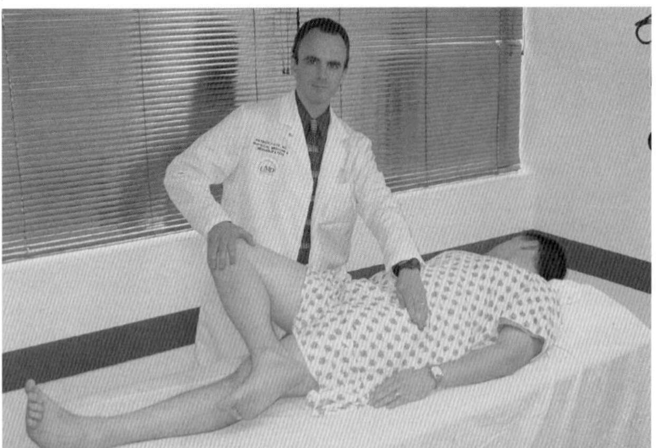

FIGURE 55.1 FABER maneuver (Patrick test). Pain produced in the groin suggests intra-articular disease, such as hip OA; pain produced in the back or buttock suggests sacroiliac disease.

Palpation of the tissues about the greater trochanteric region, proximal iliotibial bands, sacroiliac joints, gluteal muscles, underlying piriformis and obturator internus muscles, and ischial bursae may reveal pain generators other than the hip joint itself.

Weak hip girdle muscles may be due to pain or disuse, but radiculopathy and neuropathy can also be considered. Hip abductor weakness may be manifested with a Trendelenburg gait [13]. With hip OA, the remainder of the neurologic examination in the lower limbs is normal (e.g., muscle stretch reflexes and sensory testing).

On inspection of the fingers, hypertrophic degenerative changes (exostoses), such as Heberden nodes at the distal interphalangeal joints [12], are independent risk factors for hip OA [11]. Their presence thus increases the likelihood of similar findings at the hip joint.

Functional Limitations

Patients with hip OA often report functional limitations in weight-bearing activities such as walking, running, and climbing stairs. The hip range of motion restrictions may cause difficulties with activities such as donning or doffing socks and shoes, picking up clothing from the floor [15], and getting in and out of cars. Hip pain and weakness may necessitate use of the upper limbs to arise from a chair [15]. A careful history can elicit details of occupational, recreational, and other functional activities that the patient has decreased or ceased because of the hip OA.

Diagnostic Studies

Plain radiography is the primary diagnostic study for hip OA [16] (Fig. 55.2). The severity of radiographic hip OA findings can be categorized on the basis of the minimal joint space (MJS), defined as the shortest distance on the radiograph between the femoral head margin and the acetabular edge [15]. MJS is determined by four joint space measurements (medial, lateral, superior, and axial). Croft's MJS grades are 0 (MJS $>$ 2.5 mm), 1 (MJS $>$ 1.5 mm and $\leq$ 2.5 mm), and 2 (MJS $\leq$ 1.5 mm) [15]. MJS is predictive of hip pain, is strongly associated with other radiographic features of hip OA, and has a high inter-rater reliability [17]. Alternatively, the Kellgren-Lawrence grading system of hip OA is a scale of 0 to 5 that considers not only joint space narrowing but also three additional factors: presence of osteophytes, subchondral sclerosis, and subchondral cysts [15]. Both MJS and Kellgren-Lawrence grade are associated with clinical symptoms of hip OA [15].

Magnetic resonance imaging is generally not needed to diagnose hip OA, but it is superior to radiography or bone scan when the differential diagnosis includes avascular necrosis or hip labral tear [18]. Hip joint arthrography is also generally unnecessary for the diagnosis of hip OA but may help define labral tears. Diagnostic musculoskeletal ultrasound can assist in early detection of hip OA, can sometimes demonstrate gross evidence of bone and cartilage damage, can detect associated synovitis [19], and can detect concomitant iliopsoas bursitis [20]. Hip pain that is relieved through intra-articular diagnostic injection of local anesthetic (e.g., with ultrasound [21] or fluoroscopic guidance)

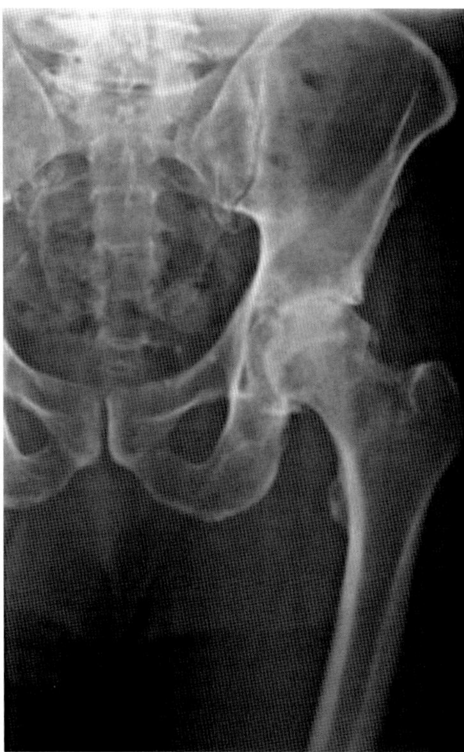

FIGURE 55.2 Radiograph demonstrating hip OA, including joint space narrowing, superior migration of the femur within the acetabulum, and subchondral sclerosis.

can help confirm that the patient's symptoms are arising from the hip joint and predicts a good surgical outcome with joint replacement [21]. Patients who fail to obtain adequate relief with image-guided anesthetic injection tend to have alternative pathologic processes at the spine (61%) or knee (16%) [21].

Electrodiagnostic studies should be considered when the differential diagnosis includes lumbosacral radiculopathy or peripheral nerve disease.

Differential Diagnosis

INTRA-ARTICULAR
Avascular necrosis
Protrusio acetabuli
Hip labral (cartilage) tear
Hip joint infection
Acetabular fracture
Inflammatory arthropathy, such as rheumatoid arthritis

EXTRA-ARTICULAR
Femur fracture
Trochanteric bursitis
Iliotibial band tendinitis
Iliopsoas bursitis
Piriformis myofascial pain
Snapping hip syndrome
Muscle or tendon groin strain
Lumbosacral radiculopathy
Sacroiliac pain
Coccydynia

Treatment

Initial

Patients with OA should be educated about their diagnosis, prognosis, and available treatments. Patients are encouraged to take an active role in managing their OA and maximizing their outcomes [22].

Weight loss is important because body weight is an independent risk factor for the development and progression of hip OA [23,24], although this relationship is less clearly established at the hip than at the knee [12]. Forces on the hip joint are roughly three to five times the patient's body weight during ambulation [2] and up to eight times body weight during jogging [1]. Loss of even modest amounts of excess body weight can significantly decrease lower extremity joint forces, OA progression, and related symptoms [23,24].

The initial medication of choice for OA is acetaminophen [25,26], at a maximum dose of 1000 mg three times a day, depending on the presence or absence of hepatic dysfunction. Although OA is primarily considered a noninflammatory arthritis (at least in early stages), prescription of nonsteroidal anti-inflammatory drugs in addition to the acetaminophen can provide further analgesic benefit [12]. Diagnostic musculoskeletal ultrasound offers the clinician a practical way of quickly assessing for evidence of inflammation and thus potentially influencing medication selection. In appropriately selected patients, tramadol or more traditional opioid analgesics may also be used for pain relief and associated functional benefits [12].

Rehabilitation

The American College of Rheumatology guidelines for the medical management of hip and knee OA recommend exercise as an important component of treatment [24,25]. These guidelines recommend an exercise program consisting of range of motion, muscle strengthening, and aerobic conditioning by walking or aquatic therapy [24,25]. Water-based exercise for lower limb OA decreases pain and increases function in the short term and also at 1 year [27].

Stretching programs can address the range of motion restrictions in patients with hip OA, which are, in order of severity, extension, internal rotation, abduction, external rotation, adduction, and flexion [22]. Flexibility programs often begin with patients gently moving their joints through the available range of motion (to maintain range of motion) and then progress to regaining of lost range of motion. [12] Proper stretching should be sustained for at least 30 seconds while avoiding the sudden, jerky, or ballistic stretching that would be likely to exacerbate OA [12].

Muscle strengthening programs should address all planes of hip movement [22]. OA patients may begin with static strengthening exercises [12] to minimize joint movements that could exacerbate the OA symptoms [12]. Eventually, incorporation of dynamic exercises can maximize strength and function [12]. Patients with hip OA are often deconditioned, thus suggesting a role for aerobic exercises [22]. Because OA particularly affects the elderly, it is especially important to screen for cardiovascular or other precautions before an exercise program is begun. Many patients with hip OA may have difficulty tolerating high-impact aerobics, such as jogging and stair climbing [22], so activities such as cycling (perhaps using a high-seat bike or recumbent bike, depending on the patient's symptoms) and aquatic exercises may be substituted. It is important to encourage ongoing exercise compliance [8,12].

There is little clinical scientific evidence supporting passive modalities (e.g., cryotherapy, thermotherapy, transcutaneous electrical nerve stimulation) for hip OA [22], although theoretically they may facilitate better tolerance of the active therapy program [12]. A recent literature review by a European multispecialty panel of experts concluded that massage, therapeutic ultrasound, electrotherapy, electromagnetic field, and low-level laser therapy cannot be recommended in hip OA [28].

Hip OA pain may be decreased by use of a cane in the contralateral hand [8,13], presumably by shifting the center of gravity medially, away from the involved hip. In cases of bilateral hip OA, the cane can be used contralateral to the more severely involved hip. A shoe lift can correct a leg length discrepancy [8] caused by hip joint space narrowing or superior migration of the femoral head within the acetabulum.

An occupational therapy evaluation of activities of daily living may identify difficulties with hand activities (e.g., due to hand OA) and difficulties with donning and doffing footwear (due to restricted hip range of motion). Adaptive equipment (e.g., reachers, sock donners, long-handled shoe horns, elastic shoelaces) may help maximize independence despite persistent physical impairments [12].

Procedures

Nonsurgical procedures for hip OA primarily include intra-articular injections with corticosteroids or viscosupplements.

Corticosteroid Injections

Although early OA is considered relatively noninflammatory, end-stage OA may have an inflammatory component [7], which may provide a basis for anti-inflammatory intra-articular injections with corticosteroids. It is difficult to obtain true intra-articular hip joint injection without fluoroscopy [8,12] or other image guidance such as ultrasound [21,29], particularly because the hip joint cannot be palpated and is adjacent to important neurovascular structures [29]. Also, OA can decrease the targeted joint space and osteophytes can obstruct needle entry [30]. A randomized controlled trial of fluoroscopically guided intra-articular hip joint injections has shown that compared with local anesthetic, corticosteroids decrease hip OA pain (at 3- and 12-week follow-up), improve hip range of motion in all directions, and significantly improve functional abilities [31]. Ultrasound-guided hip joint corticosteroid injection for hip OA has shown significant relief of pain during walking compared with saline injection [32]. Another prospective study of ultrasound-guided corticosteroid injection for hip OA showed that compared with baseline, there is significantly decreased walking pain at 1 and 3 months after injection [33] and 75% of the hips show decreased synovial hypertrophy at 1 and 3 months after injection [33]. Even in patients with advanced hip OA waiting for total hip replacement, image-guided intra-articular steroid injection can provide months of improved pain and function [34].

Despite the benefits shown in prospective, randomized controlled trials [31,32], it is notable that one retrospective study seems to show that combined injections of corticosteroid, contrast agent, and anesthetic before total hip arthroplasty may increase the risk of postoperative infection and surgical revision [35]. Despite the limitations of that study (inherent flaws of a retrospective review and data lacking statistical power to determine the role of the time interval between steroid injection and subsequent total hip arthroplasty) [35], the possibility of infection should be discussed with patients before corticosteroid injection. Hip joint injection under fluoroscopic guidance is shown in Figure 55.3.

Viscosupplementation Injections

True intra-articular placement is even more important with viscosupplementation than with corticosteroids because viscosupplements have high molecular weights and are unlikely to permeate to the joint capsule [30]. Thus, when it is available, image guidance with fluoroscopy [30] or ultrasonography seems prudent for viscosupplementation injections [35].

At the time of this writing, viscosupplements are approved by the Food and Drug Administration only for use at the knee. Some initial studies indicate that image-guided hip joint viscosupplementation injections are well tolerated, safe, and beneficial for hip OA [36]. Image-guided intra-articular hip viscosupplementation injections in symptomatic hip OA patients seems to effectively delay the need for total hip replacement surgery, thus decreasing OA-related financial costs and decreasing mortality related to total hip replacement [37]. A literature review concluded that viscosupplementation is as effective for hip OA as for knee

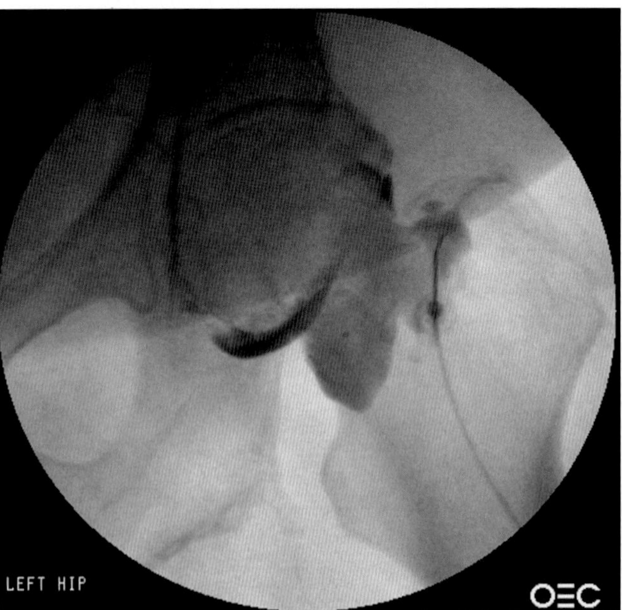

FIGURE 55.3 Fluoroscopic image showing intra-articular injection of contrast material (before corticosteroid), which can be seen spreading within the joint capsule along the proximal aspect of the femoral neck and also up into the space between the femoral head and the acetabulum. The image guidance helps ensure appropriate intra-articular placement of the injectate.

OA, appears to be a reasonable and safe alternative to oral nonsteroidal anti-inflammatories, and appears to work best in patients with milder radiographic findings of OA [38].

Surgery

Surgical treatment of hip OA (see Chapter 61) includes joint realignment (realignment osteotomy, such as for hip dysplasia [13]), joint fusion (arthrodesis), and, most commonly, joint replacement (arthroplasty) [26]. Hip joint arthroplasty can be categorized as either hemiarthroplasty (prosthetic replacement of the proximal femur while the acetabulum is left intact) or total hip arthroplasty (also called total hip replacement, with surgical replacement of both the acetabulum and the proximal femur) [26]. Hip hemiarthroplasty is often performed after proximal femur fractures, when the acetabulum is relatively intact. Conversely, in OA, there is usually degeneration of both the acetabulum and the femur; thus, the definitive surgery is to replace both of these through total hip arthroplasty. An arthroplasty can also be categorized on the basis of the specific prosthetic hardware used (e.g., unipolar or bipolar) and whether cement is used to hold the hardware in place [26]. Comparisons of the posterior and direct lateral surgical approaches for total hip arthroplasty show similar rates of postoperative dislocation (1% to 4%), postoperative Trendelenburg gait, and sciatic nerve injury [39].

Customized preoperative exercises are well tolerated even in patients with end-stage hip OA and improve early recovery of physical function after eventual total hip arthroplasty is performed [40]. Postoperative rehabilitation with physical therapy (and perhaps occupational therapy) generally includes therapeutic exercise, transfer training, gait training, and instruction in activities of daily living [41]. After total hip arthroplasty, early ambulation (even within the first 1 to 2 days postoperatively) [8] may maximize recovery and minimize complications such as deep venous thrombosis and symptomatic thromboembolism [41].

The patient is taught how to follow the weight-bearing status specified by the orthopedic surgeon [8], which depends on factors such as whether the prosthesis was cemented in place [41]. Many patients may safely bear weight as tolerated [41]. A cane or walker should be used until hip abductors are strong enough that the patient no longer limps during unassisted gait [8]. After a posterior approach total hip arthroplasty, prevention of hip dislocation often involves "hip precautions" (e.g., teaching the patient to carefully avoid positions of hip adduction, flexion, and internal rotation) [8]. Patients are taught to use elevated chair seats and elevated toilet seats and to avoid crossing the legs [8]. The recommended duration for hip precautions varies widely from 6 weeks to 6 months. Postoperative patients with a significant fall or sudden onset of pain should undergo radiography for evaluation of dislocation.

Prophylaxis against deep venous thrombosis and related venous thromboembolism may include early ambulation, intermittent pneumatic compression stockings, inferior vena cava filters, and pharmacologic methods (such as unfractionated heparin, low-molecular-weight heparin, warfarin, or synthetic pentasaccharides) [41]. The optimal duration of thromboprophylaxis is not known, but a 4- to 6-week course has been suggested after total hip arthroplasty [41].

After the acute care hospital, total hip arthroplasty patients are discharged to either inpatient rehabilitation (acute or subacute) or directly home, depending on postoperative pain, functional status, and home environment [8,41].

Potential Disease Complications

Hip OA is a degenerative process characterized by gradual progressive worsening of femoroacetabular joint destruction and resultant symptoms. Hip OA can produce severe pain, stiffness, functional limitations, and associated compromise of quality of life. The decrease in mobility can subsequently result in weakness, osteoporosis, obesity, and cardiovascular deconditioning.

Potential Treatment Complications

Acetaminophen can cause hepatic side effects; nonsteroidal anti-inflammatory drugs are associated with gastrointestinal, renal, and cardiovascular risks. Tramadol can cause sedation and dizziness. Hip injections carry risks of infection and postprocedure exacerbation of symptoms. Hip replacement surgeries can be complicated by infection, nerve injury, dislocation, hardware loosening, deep venous thrombosis, and anesthesia-related side effects [41].

References

[1] Anderson K, Strickland SM, Warren R. Hip and groin injuries in athletes. Am J Sports Med 2001;29:521–33.

[2] Hashimoto N, Ando M, Yayama T, et al. Dynamic analysis of the resultant force acting on the hip joint during level walking. Artif Organs 2005;29:387–92.

[3] Tepper S, Hochberg MC. Factors associated with hip osteoarthritis: data from the First National Health and Nutrition Examination Survey (NHANES-I). Am J Epidemiol 1993;137:1081–8.

[4] Coggon D, Kellingray S, Inskip H, et al. Osteoarthritis of the hip and occupational lifting. Am J Epidemiol 1998;147:523–8.

[5] Hoaglund FT, Steinbach LS. Primary osteoarthritis of the hip: etiology and epidemiology. J Am Acad Orthop Surg 2001;9:320–7.

[6] Croft P, Lewis M, Wynn Jones C, et al. Health status in patients awaiting hip replacement for osteoarthritis. Rheumatology (Oxford) 2002;41:1001–7.

[7] Stitik TP, Kaplan RJ, Kamen LB, et al. Rehabilitation of orthopedic and rheumatologic disorders. 2. Osteoarthritis assessment, treatment, and rehabilitation. Arch Phys Med Rehabil 2005;86(Suppl 1):S48–55.

[8] Nicholas JJ. Rehabilitation of patients with rheumatic disorders. In: Braddom RL, editor. Physical medicine and rehabilitation. Philadelphia: WB Saunders; 1996. p. 711–27.

[9] Hoaglund FT, Oishi CS, Gialamas GG. Extreme variations in racial rates of total hip arthroplasty for primary coxarthrosis: a population-based study in San Francisco. Ann Rheum Dis 1995;54:107–10.

[10] Trousdale RT. Acetabular osteotomy: indications and results. Clin Orthop Relat Res 2004;429:182–7.

[11] Cooper C, Inskip H, Croft P, et al. Individual risk factors for hip osteoarthritis: obesity, hip injury, and physical activity. Am J Epidemiol 1998;147:516–22.

[12] Stitik TP, Foye PM, Stiskal D, Nadler RR. Osteoarthritis. In: DeLisa JA, editor. 4th ed. Physical Medicine and Rehabilitation: Principles and Practice, vol 1. Philadelphia: Lippincott Williams & Wilkins; 2005. p. 765–86.

[13] Lieberman JR, Berry DJ, Bono JV, Mason JB. Hip and thigh. In: Snider RJ, editor. Essentials of musculoskeletal care. Rosemont, Ill: American Academy of Orthopaedic Surgeons; 1998. p. 264–303.

[14] Brown MD, Gomez-Marin O, Brookfield KF, Li PS. Differential diagnosis of hip disease versus spine disease. Clin Orthop Relat Res 2004;419:280–4.
[15] Reijman M, Hazes JM, Pols HA, et al. Validity and reliability of three definitions of hip osteoarthritis: cross sectional and longitudinal approach. Ann Rheum Dis 2004;63:1427–33.
[16] Boegard T, Jonsson K. Hip and knee osteoarthritis. Conventional X-ray best and cheapest diagnostic method. Lakartidningen 2002;99:4358–60 [in Swedish].
[17] Croft P, Cooper C, Wickham C, Coggon D. Defining osteoarthritis of the hip for epidemiologic studies. Am J Epidemiol 1990;132:514–22.
[18] Bluemke DA, Zerhouni EA. MRI of avascular necrosis of bone. Top Magn Reson Imaging 1996;8:231–46.
[19] Moller I, Bong D, Naredo E, et al. Ultrasound in the study and monitoring of osteoarthritis. Osteoarthritis Cartilage 2008;16(Suppl 3):S4–7.
[20] Tormenta S, Sconfienza LM, Iannessi F, et al. Prevalence study of iliopsoas bursitis in a cohort of 860 patients affected by symptomatic hip osteoarthritis. Ultrasound Med Biol 2012;38:1352–6.
[21] Yoong P, Guirguis R, Darrah R, et al. Evaluation of ultrasound-guided diagnostic local anaesthetic hip joint injection for osteoarthritis. Skeletal Radiol 2012;41:981–5.
[22] Arokoski JP. Physical therapy and rehabilitation programs in the management of hip osteoarthritis. Eura Medicophys 2005;41:155–61.
[23] Foye PM. Weight loss in the treatment of osteoarthritis. Phys Med Rehabil State Art Rev 2001;15:33–41.
[24] Foye PM, Stitik TP, Chen B, Nadler SF. Osteoarthritis and body weight. Nutrition Res 2000;20:899–903.
[25] Recommendations for the medical management of osteoarthritis of the hip and knee: 2000 update. American College of Rheumatology Subcommittee on Osteoarthritis Guidelines. Arthritis Rheum 2000;43:1905–15.
[26] Stitik TP, Foye PM. Osteoarthritis. Physical medicine and rehabilitation: arthritis and connective tissue disorders. eMedicine April 8, 2005;. http://www.emedicine.com/PMR/topic93.htm, Accessed June 26, 2005.
[27] Cochrane T, Davey RC, Matthes Edwards SM. Randomised controlled trial of the cost-effectiveness of water-based therapy for lower limb osteoarthritis. Health Technol Assess 2005;9:iii–iv, ix–xi, 1–114.
[28] Peter WF, Jansen MJ, Hurkmans EJ, et al. Physiotherapy in hip and knee osteoarthritis: development of a practice guideline concerning initial assessment, treatment and evaluation. Acta Reumatol Port 2011;36:268–81.
[29] Dorleijn DM, Luijsterburg PA, Reijman M, et al. Effectiveness of intramuscular corticosteroid injection versus placebo injection in patients with hip osteoarthritis: design of a randomized double-blinded controlled trial. BMC Musculoskelet Disord 2011;12:280.
[30] Foye PM, Stitik TP. Fluoroscopic guidance during injections for osteoarthritis. Arch Phys Med Rehabil 2006;87:446–7.
[31] Kullenberg B, Runesson R, Tuvhag R, et al. Intraarticular corticosteroid injection: pain relief in osteoarthritis of the hip? J Rheumatol 2004;31:2265–8.
[32] Qvistgaard E, Christensen R, Torp-Pedersen S, Bliddal H. Intra-articular treatment of hip osteoarthritis: a randomized trial of hyaluronic acid, corticosteroid, and isotonic saline. Osteoarthritis Cartilage 2006;14:163–70.
[33] Micu MC, Bogdan GD, Fodor D. Steroid injection for hip osteoarthritis: efficacy under ultrasound guidance. Rheumatology (Oxford) 2010;49:1490–4.
[34] Atchia I, Kane D, Reed MR, et al. Efficacy of a single ultrasound-guided injection for the treatment of hip osteoarthritis. Ann Rheum Dis 2011;70:110–6.
[35] Kaspar S, de V de Beer J. Infection in hip arthroplasty after previous injection of steroid. J Bone Joint Surg Br 2005;87:454–7.
[36] Pourbagher MA, Ozalay M, Pourbagher A. Accuracy and outcome of sonographically guided intra-articular sodium hyaluronate injections in patients with osteoarthritis of the hip. J Ultrasound Med 2005;24:1391–5.
[37] Migliore A, Bella A, Bisignani M, et al. Total hip replacement rate in a cohort of patients affected by symptomatic hip osteoarthritis following intra-articular sodium hyaluronate (MW 1,500-2,000 kDa) ORTOBRIX study. Clin Rheumatol 2012;31:1187–96.
[38] Mulvaney SW. A review of viscosupplementation for osteoarthritis of the hip and a description of an ultrasound-guided hip injection technique. Curr Sports Med Rep 2009;8:291–4.
[39] Jolles BM, Bogoch ER. Posterior versus lateral surgical approach for total hip arthroplasty in adults with osteoarthritis. Cochrane Database Syst Rev 2004;1, CD003828.
[40] Gilbey HJ, Ackland TR, Wang AW, et al. Exercise improves early functional recovery after total hip arthroplasty. Clin Orthop Relat Res 2003;408:193–200.
[41] Bitar AA, Kaplan RJ, Stitik TP, et al. Rehabilitation of orthopedic and rheumatologic disorders. 3. Total hip arthroplasty rehabilitation. Arch Phys Med Rehabil 2005;86(Suppl 1):S56–60.

CHAPTER 56

Hip Labral Tears

Matthew M. Diesselhorst, MD
Jonathan T. Finnoff, DO

Synonyms

None

ICD-9 Code

726.5 Enthesopathy of hip region

ICD-10 Codes

M76.891 Enthesopathies of right lower limb excluding foot
M76.892 Enthesopathies of left lower limb excluding foot
M76.899 Enthesopathies of unspecified lower limb excluding foot

Definition

A hip labral tear is a tear of the fibrocartilaginous labrum that attaches to the periphery of the acetabulum. The acetabular labrum is a horseshoe-shaped fibrocartilaginous structure that attaches to the peripheral rim of the acetabulum, contacts the articular surface of the femoral head, and blends inferiorly with the transverse acetabular ligament. The labrum plays a major biomechanical role in hip joint stabilization and function. It increases the effective depth of the acetabulum, increasing static stability; it contributes to hydrostatic pressurization of the intra-articular space, joint lubrication, and load distribution; and it has proprioceptive and nociceptive nerve function [1].

The labrum can be divided into two distinct zones: the well-vascularized extra-articular side consisting of dense connective tissue; and the intra-articular side, which is largely avascular [2]. The chondrolabral junction is not uniform and has lower biomechanical strength at its anterosuperior acetabular attachment, which contributes to the higher incidence of labral tears in this area [3,4].

Hip injuries account for 3.1% to 8.4% of sports injuries, and labral tears are present in 22% to 55% of athletes with hip complaints [3,4]. Labral tears may be due to hip instability, iliopsoas impingement, trauma, and osteoarthritis. Many labral tears are associated with a condition called femoroacetabular impingement (FAI) [5,6]. FAI is characterized by abnormal contact between the femoral head-neck junction and the acetabular rim caused by abnormal bone morphology. Ganz and colleagues [7] described two types of FAI: pincer and cam. Pincer-type FAI is due to excessive femoral head coverage by the acetabulum (Fig. 56.1), whereas cam-type FAI results from a decrease in the femoral head-neck offset distance (Fig. 56.1). Pincer-type FAI typically occurs in middle-aged women; cam-type FAI is more common in men in their fourth decade. Most cases of FAI have components of both pincer and cam types.

Whereas labral tears associated with both types of FAI tend to occur in the anterosuperior region, the bone abnormalities in cam-type and pincer-type FAI cause different patterns of labral tears. In pincer-type impingement, repeated contact between the femoral neck and the prominent anterior aspect of the acetabular rim leads to labral degeneration, tears, intrasubstance ganglion formation, and, occasionally, labral ossification. In cam-type impingement, abnormal contact between the femoral head-neck junction and the acetabulum produces an outside-in abrasion of the acetabular cartilage and delamination between the acetabular cartilage and the adjacent labrum and subchondral bone [2]. The labral tears tend to occur on the articular rather than on the capsular surface. Although the bone patterns of FAI may differ, more commonly the osseous dysmorphism is a combined pattern.

Symptoms

Patients with labral tears complain of anterior groin pain made worse by long periods of standing, sitting, or walking. The pain can also be referred to the gluteal area or the trochanteric region. The onset of pain is usually insidious, with the patient often unable to recall a specific inciting event [2]. On occasion, the labral tear is due to trauma. Mechanical symptoms of clicking, locking, and instability are highly variable and not always indicative of intra-articular disease. A thorough history is critical, including inquiry about childhood diseases such as hip dysplasia, Legg-Calvé-Perthes disease, and slipped capital femoral epiphysis.

Physical Examination

The hip examination should begin by observing the patient's gait for antalgia. Palpation of the hip girdle may

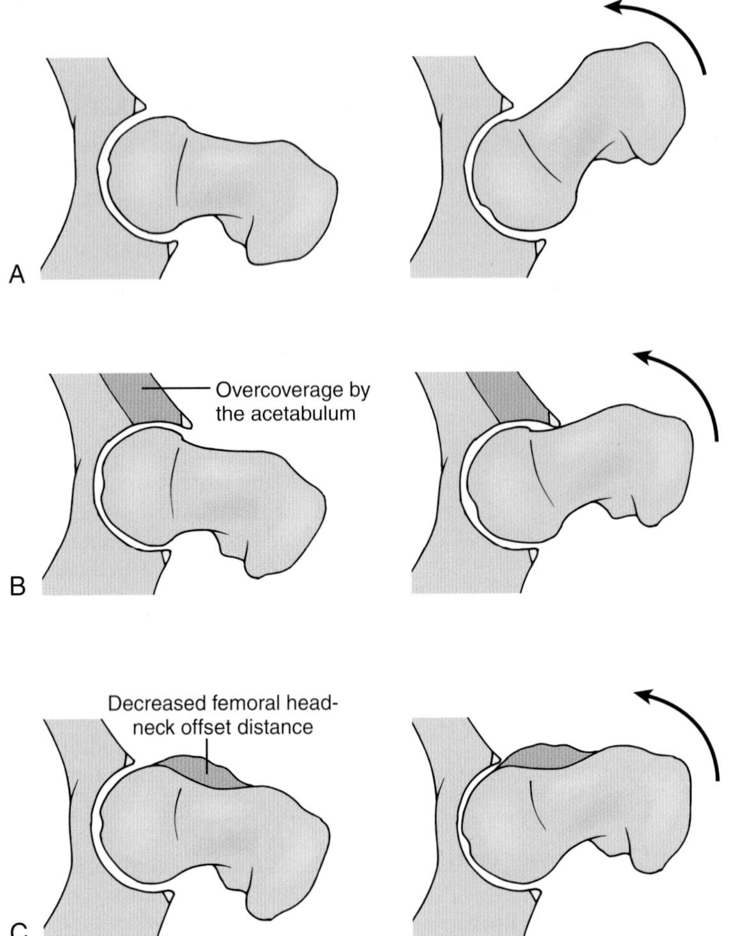

FIGURE 56.1 **A,** Normal hip joint, which allows unrestricted hip motion. **B,** Pincer-type femoroacetabular impingement due to excessive coverage of the femoral head by the acetabulum. **C,** Cam-type femoroacetabular impingement secondary to a decreased femoral head-neck offset distance. *(Modified from Tannast M, Siebenrock KA, Anderson SE. Femoroacetabular impingement: radiographic diagnosis—what the radiologist should know. AJR Am J Roentgenol 2007;188:1540-1552.)*

reveal some tenderness in the groin region, but this is a nonspecific finding. Lumbar spine, hip, and knee range of motion should be assessed. Frequently, pain will be provoked with hip internal rotation during the hip range of motion assessment. A neurologic examination of the lower extremities should be completed, including evaluation of strength, sensation, and reflexes. The neurologic examination findings are typically normal. The most reliable test for FAI and a labral tear is the anterior hip impingement test, which is done by flexing the hip beyond 90 degrees, then adducting and internally rotating the hip (Fig. 56.2). The result is considered positive if the test elicits anterior groin pain [8]. A hip scouring maneuver, in which the hip is taken from an abducted and externally rotated position, through a flexed and neutral rotation position, and finally into adduction and internal rotation, may produce pain and possibly a "click" if a labral tear is present. Passive hip extension and external rotation may cause pain if a labral tear is present. This is commonly referred to as the posterior impingement test. Hip disease can also be provoked by placing the patient's leg in a figure four position. This test is referred to as the Patrick test or FABER test because the hip is in a flexed, abducted, and externally rotated position. Intra-articular hip disease can also be elicited by a resisted straight-leg raise in the supine position. Although a detailed physical examination assists the clinician in determining that the patient's pain is coming from the hip joint, it is nonspecific and cannot differentiate between the various causes of hip pain.

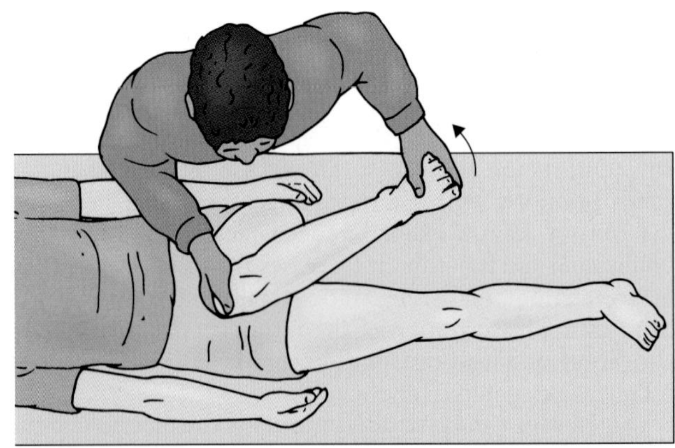

FIGURE 56.2 The anterior impingement test involves flexing the patient's hip to 90 degrees and adducting and internally rotating the hip. A positive test result is characterized by hip pain.

Functional Limitations

Although it is uncommon, a patient with a labral tear may have a limp or a Trendelenburg gait and rarely may require an assistive device to walk. A labral tear may also cause pain that limits activities, such as gymnastics or construction work, that involve repetitive hip loading, pivoting, and deep flexion.

Diagnostic Studies

Plain radiographs remain the mainstay in evaluating hip pain. A minimum of two radiographic views must be obtained. Proper patient positioning is critical to correctly assess the osseous anatomy. Commonly, an anteroposterior pelvis view and a cross-table (false profile) lateral view of the affected hip are used. Wenger and colleagues [9] reviewed hip radiographs of patients with labral tears and found that 87% had at least one bone abnormality consistent with FAI.

Pincer-type FAI may be due to generalized overcoverage of the femoral head from an excessively deep acetabulum or focal overcoverage related to acetabular retroversion. On the anteroposterior radiograph of the pelvis, the normal acetabulum should cover at least 75% of the femoral head. A deep acetabulum is present if the acetabular fossa or the femoral head projects medial to the ilioischial line. Focal acetabular retroversion is suggested by the cross-over sign, in which the cephalad portion of the anterior acetabular wall is lateral to the posterior acetabular wall. The cross-table lateral radiograph may demonstrate posteroinferior joint space narrowing.

Cam-type FAI can be evaluated with anteroposterior pelvis and cross-table lateral radiographs [10]. The primary radiologic finding of cam-type FAI is a decrease in the anterior or superior femoral head-neck offset distance, which causes the femoral head-neck junction to appear flattened or convex rather than concave. The asphericity of the femoral head-neck junction caused by cam-type FAI is commonly referred to as a pistol grip deformity (Fig. 56.3).

Magnetic resonance imaging is the preferred imaging modality for intra-articular hip disease as it provides high-resolution images of the acetabular labrum, hip joint cartilage, and joint space [2]. Magnetic resonance arthrography is the combination of magnetic resonance imaging with intra-articular injection of a gadolinium-based contrast agent and is the test of choice for evaluation of the acetabular labrum (Fig. 56.4) [11].

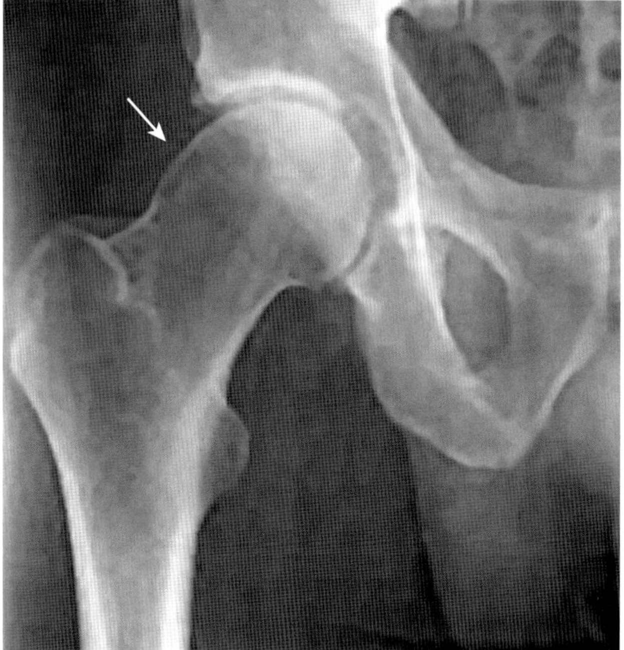

FIGURE 56.3 Anteroposterior right hip radiograph in a patient with cam-type femoroacetabular impingement. The arrow is pointing to the cam lesion. This femoral head-neck configuration is commonly referred to as a pistol grip deformity.

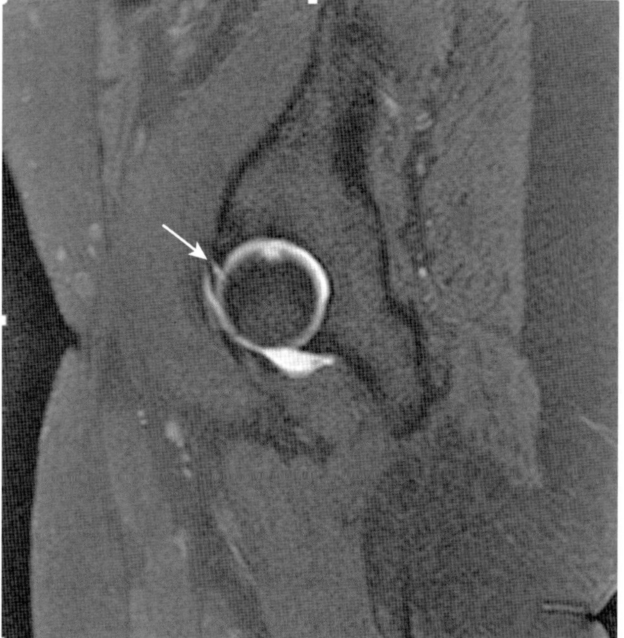

FIGURE 56.4 Sagittal T2-weighted magnetic resonance arthrogram of the hip. The arrow is pointing to a labral tear.

Differential Diagnosis

Legg-Calvé-Perthes disease
Slipped capital femoral epiphysis
Hip dysplasia
Hip septic arthritis, inflammatory arthritis, or osteoarthritis
Hip malignant neoplasm
Snapping hip syndrome
Coxa profunda
Protrusio acetabuli
Avascular necrosis of femoral head
Stress fracture of femoral neck
Trochanteric bursitis
Lumbar radiculopathy
Inguinal or femoral hernia
Iliopsoas tendinitis
Psoas bursitis
Peripheral nerve entrapment (e.g., genitofemoral nerve)
Femoral artery thrombosis or dissection
Femoral vein thrombosis

Treatment

Initial

The initial treatment of labral tears should be conservative and may include local application of physical modalities, mild oral analgesics such as acetaminophen or nonsteroidal anti-inflammatory drugs, and rehabilitation. If the patient's symptoms persist despite these measures, an intra-articular corticosteroid injection could be considered [12]. Patients should be instructed to avoid aggravating activities.

Rehabilitation

The rehabilitation program for acetabular labral tears should progress through three phases. The first phase should focus on pain reduction through physical modalities, activity modification, and mild analgesics. The patient should work on reestablishing full pain-free range of motion and perform static strengthening exercises of the hip girdle musculature. Core strengthening exercises should be introduced, and the patient should maintain aerobic fitness through pain-free forms of nonimpact aerobic conditioning exercises. Kinetic chain deficits should be identified and addressed. Proprioceptive exercises such as single-leg stance on a stable surface or double-leg stance on an unstable surface should be included in the program. The second phase of rehabilitation should gradually introduce nonpainful, dynamic hip girdle strengthening exercises and low- to moderate-impact aerobic conditioning. Core stability and proprioceptive exercises should be advanced according to the patient's tolerance during this phase of rehabilitation. The final rehabilitation phase should transition the patient to sports-specific exercises (or work-specific exercises if the patient is not an athlete) and a home exercise program to maintain hip girdle strength and flexibility, core stability, aerobic fitness, and neuromuscular coordination [12].

An appropriate postsurgical rehabilitation program is necessary to maximize the patient's recovery [13]. Immediately after surgery, measures should be taken to reduce the patient's discomfort, including oral medications and local physical modalities. Compression should be applied at regular intervals to reduce postoperative edema. Frequently, a postoperative brace is used for the first 1 to 2 weeks during waking hours to prevent hip flexion beyond 80 degrees. At night, the patient may be required to wear an immobilizing brace to prevent hip external rotation, which places excessive tension on the anterior capsular structures. Gentle passive hip range of motion and active knee and ankle range of motion should be initiated. For the first 2 weeks after surgery, the patient should avoid excessive hip flexion, internal rotation, and abduction. As the pain resolves, the patient can begin working on reestablishing full pain-free range of motion. This usually takes place approximately 2 to 4 weeks after surgery. At 4 weeks after surgery, stretching exercises of the hip girdle and thigh musculature can be initiated.

Isometric hip girdle and thigh muscle strengthening can begin immediately after surgery but should be performed in a pain-free manner. Progression to isotonic hip girdle strengthening can begin after 2 to 4 weeks, with a focus on the hip abductors. Weight-bearing strengthening exercises typically can begin approximately 4 to 6 weeks after surgery. Exercises should include transverse plane movements but should always be pain free.

Partial weight bearing is continued for the first 2 to 6 weeks postoperatively, depending on the type of surgery performed and the surgeon's preference. The patient is weaned off of crutches after that time is complete.

Functional rehabilitation exercises usually begin approximately 6 to 8 weeks after surgery. Aerobic conditioning can progress from a limited weight-bearing environment (e.g., pool), to nonimpact full weight bearing (e.g., elliptical machine), to walking and jogging. Most individuals are unable to progress to impact-type aerobic conditioning (e.g., running) and cutting or pivoting activities until 12 to 24 weeks after surgery. In general, manual laborers can return to unrestricted work approximately 12 to 24 weeks after surgery, whereas athletes can return to competitive sports after 12 to 32 weeks, depending on the type of surgery performed and their ability to progress through the rehabilitation program.

Procedures

Some patients with acetabular labral tears may benefit symptomatically from an intra-articular corticosteroid injection. Hip injections should be performed with image guidance, such as ultrasound or fluoroscopy, to ensure accurate placement of the injectate into the hip joint, to minimize potential complications, and to maximize the therapeutic efficacy of the injection. Hip injections are typically considered as a treatment option after the patient has failed to respond to other nonoperative measures, such as local physical modalities, medications, and rehabilitation. However, if the patient is in significant pain and cannot participate in a rehabilitation program because of the severity of the pain, an intra-articular corticosteroid injection could be considered early in treatment to reduce pain and to facilitate the rehabilitation program.

Surgery

Surgical treatment should be considered in patients who have failed to respond to nonoperative measures or have significant mechanical symptoms. Originally, hip labral tears were treated surgically with open labral débridement. More recently, the advent of hip arthroscopy has allowed access to the labrum with significantly less morbidity. Short-term good to excellent results have been achieved with arthroscopic labral débridement. However, most of these studies included subjects with additional hip disease (e.g., articular cartilage injury) and were performed before the recognition of FAI [14]. Recently, it has been suggested that the optimal surgical treatment of hip labral tears is to repair rather than to débride the labrum to restore normal labral function [8]. The most commonly used labral repair technique involves placement of simple stitches. Comparison studies between labral débridement and labral repair surgeries are lacking. Thus, future investigations are required to answer the question of which surgical technique results in the best clinical outcomes [14].

When surgically treating a labral tear, many surgeons advocate addressing bone dysmorphisms that cause FAI (e.g., acetabuloplasty for pincer-type FAI or femoroplasty for cam-type FAI). Although there is a recent trend toward addressing the bone abnormality, there is no definitive evidence that the clinical outcome achieved with combined treatment of the osseous abnormality and the labral tear will be more favorable than that provided by isolated treatment of the labral tear [2].

Potential Disease Complications

If left untreated, labral tears can cause pain, mechanical symptoms (e.g., snapping, popping, locking), functional limitations, and potentially osteoarthritis. If the patient also has FAI, the morphologic abnormalities of the femoral head or acetabulum result in abnormal contact between the femoral neck or head and the acetabulum. This leads to damage of the labrum and underlying cartilage. Theoretically, continued abnormal contact results in further deterioration and wear of the cartilage, with eventual onset of arthritis [15].

Potential Treatment Complications

Most nonoperative treatments have limited risk. The patient could have an allergic reaction to a medication, experience medication side effects such as dyspepsia, or have a medication complication such as gastric ulceration. Potential complications of intra-articular injections include infection, allergic reaction, and injury to adjacent neurovascular structures.

Potential complications of hip arthroscopy are mostly related to patient position and surgical technique. Traction is required for hip arthroscopy, which can cause nerve injury. This type of injury is minimized by avoidance of excessive traction and use of a wide post in the perineum. Adequate portal placement is of paramount importance in hip arthroscopy; inappropriate portal placement can lead to neurovascular injury and inadequate joint visibility, which can lead to iatrogenic structural damage [8].

References

[1] Rakhra KS. Magnetic resonance imaging of acetabular labral tears. J Bone Joint Surg Am 2011;93(Suppl 2):28–34.

[2] Beaulé PE, O'Neill M, Rakhra K. Acetabular labral tears. J Bone Joint Surg Am 2009;91:701–10.

[3] McCarthy JC. The Otto E. Aufranc award: the role of labral lesions to development of early degenerative hip disease. Clin Orthop Relat Res 2001;393:25–37.

[4] Smith CD. A biomechanical basis for tears of the human acetabular labrum. Br J Sports Med 2009;43:574–8.

[5] Seldes RM, Tan V, Hunt J, et al. Anatomy, histologic features, and vascularity of the adult acetabular labrum. Clin Orthop Relat Res 2001;382:232–40.

[6] Lage LA, Patel JV, Villar RN. The acetabular labral tear: an arthroscopic classification. Arthroscopy 1996;12:269–72.

[7] Ganz R, Parvizi J, Beck M, et al. Femoroacetabular impingement: a cause for osteoarthritis of the hip. Clin Orthop Relat Res 2003;417:112–20.

[8] Ejnisman L, Philippon MJ, Lertwanich P. Acetabular labral tears: diagnosis, repair, and a method for labral reconstruction. Clin Sports Med 2011;30:317–29.

[9] Wenger DE, Kendell KR, Miner MR, et al. Acetabular labral tears rarely occur in the absence of bony abnormalities. Clin Orthop Relat Res 2004;426:145–50.

[10] Eijer H, Leunig M, Mahomed MN, et al. Cross-table lateral radiograph for screening of anterior femoral head-neck offset in patients with femoro-acetabular impingement. Hip Int 2001;11:37–41.

[11] Chan YS, Lien LC, Hsu HL, et al. Evaluating hip labral tears using magnetic resonance arthrography: a prospective study comparing hip arthroscopy and magnetic resonance arthrography diagnosis. Arthroscopy 2005;21:1250.

[12] Yazbeck PM, Ovanessian V, Martin RL, et al. Nonsurgical treatment of acetabular labrum tears: a case series. J Orthop Sports Phys Ther 2011;41:5.

[13] Enseki KR, Martin R, Kelly BT. Rehabilitation after arthroscopic decompression for femoroacetabular impingement. Clin Sports Med 2010;29:247–55.

[14] Safran MR. The acetabular labrum: anatomic and functional characteristics and rationale for surgical intervention. J Am Acad Orthop Surg 2010;18:338–45.

[15] Parvizi J, Leunig M, Ganz R. Femoroacetabular impingement. J Am Acad Orthop Surg 2007;15:561–70.

CHAPTER 57

Lateral Femoral Cutaneous Neuropathy

Earl J. Craig, MD
Daniel M. Clinchot, MD

Synonyms

Meralgia paresthetica
Bernhardt-Roth syndrome

ICD-9 Codes

355.1	**Meralgia paresthetica**
355.8	**Mononeuritis of lower limb, unspecified**
355.9	**Mononeuritis of unspecified site**
782.0	**Disturbance of skin sensation**

ICD-10 Codes

G57.10	**Meralgia paresthetica, unspecified lower limb**
G57.11	**Meralgia paresthetica, right lower limb**
G57.12	**Meralgia paresthetica, left lower limb**
G57.90	**Unspecified mononeuritis of unspecified lower limb**
G57.91	**Unspecified mononeuritis of right lower limb**
G57.92	**Unspecified mononeuritis of left lower limb**
G58.9	**Mononeuropathy, unspecified**
R20.9	**Disturbance of skin sensation**

Definition

Lateral femoral cutaneous neuropathy, commonly called meralgia paresthetica, is the focal injury of the lateral femoral cutaneous nerve causing pain and sensory loss in the lateral thigh of the affected individual. The incidence of lateral femoral cutaneous neuropathy in the general population is 4.3 per 10,000 person-years. In addition, van Slobbe and colleagues [1] found that this neuropathy is more common in patients with carpal tunnel syndrome.

The lateral femoral cutaneous nerve is a pure sensory nerve that receives fibers from lumbar nerve roots L2-L3 (Fig. 57.1; see also Fig. 54.1). After forming, the nerve passes through the psoas major muscle and around the pelvic brim to the lateral edge of the inguinal ligament, where it passes out of the pelvis in a tunnel created by the inguinal ligament and the anterior superior iliac spine [2–4]. A number of anatomic variations have described the exit of the lateral femoral cutaneous nerve from the pelvis [5]. Approximately 25% of the population has an anomalous course of the lateral femoral cutaneous nerve out of the pelvis [6]. Approximately 12 cm below the anterior superior iliac spine, the nerve splits into anterior and posterior branches. The nerve provides cutaneous sensory innervation to the lateral thigh. The size of the area innervated varies among individuals.

The nerve may be injured as a result of a number of causes, as outlined in Table 57.1. Lateral femoral cutaneous neuropathy is more commonly seen in overweight individuals because of compression of the nerve (due to abdominal girth) when the thigh is flexed in a seated position.

Symptoms

Patients typically complain of lateral thigh pain and numbness. The numbness may be described as tingling or a decrease in sensation. The pain is often burning in quality but may be sharp, dull, or aching. The patient may also complain of an itching sensation. In some instances, there will be a precipitating event, such as a long car ride in which the patient was seated for a prolonged period, putting stress on the nerve. This is especially true in individuals who wear the seat belt snuggly. The patient should not complain of weakness in the lower extremities. The diagnosis requires a high index of suspicion by the evaluating clinician.

Physical Examination

Because the lateral femoral cutaneous nerve is purely sensory, the only finding typical of this condition is decreased

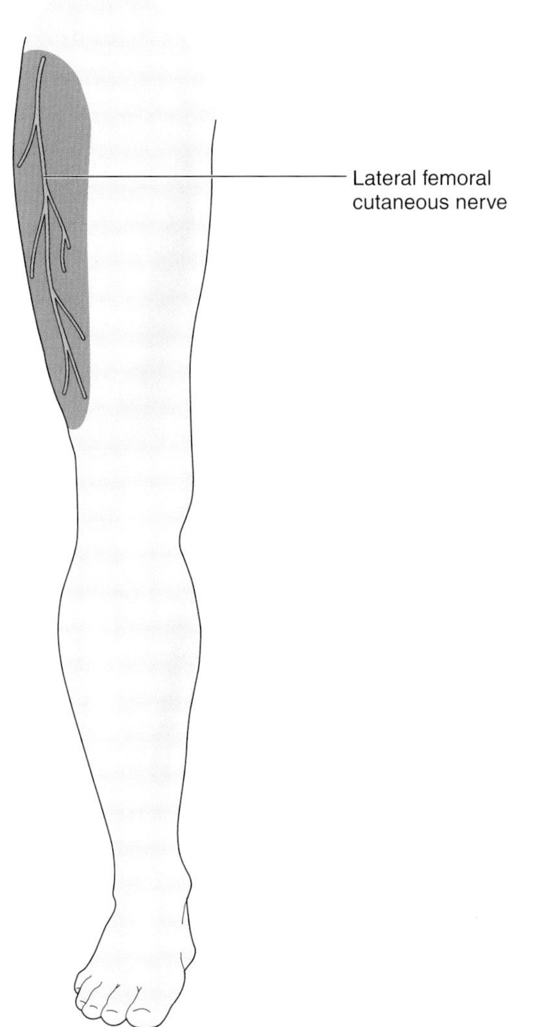

FIGURE 57.1 The lateral femoral cutaneous nerve is purely sensory and innervates the anterolateral thigh.

Table 57.1 Causes of Lateral Femoral Cutaneous Neuropathy

Operative and postoperative complications and scarring
Retroperitoneal tumor
Retroperitoneal fibrosis
Spinal tumor
Infection
Pregnancy
Penetrating injury
Iliac bone graft
Pressure injury
Tight clothing
Seat belt
Obesity
Idiopathic

sensation, which should be limited to an area of variable diameter in the lateral thigh. In adult men, the clinician may also see an area on the lateral thigh in which the hair has rubbed off. Palpation over the anterior superior iliac spine may exacerbate symptoms.

The physical examination is also used to exclude other possible causes of pain and weakness of the hip, thigh, and knee. A complete neuromuscular evaluation of the low back, the hips, and the entire lower extremities is needed. This examination should include inspection for asymmetry or atrophy, manual muscle testing, muscle stretch reflexes, and sensory testing for light touch and pinprick. In the case of lateral femoral cutaneous neuropathy, the clinician should not see muscle atrophy or asymmetry or weakness of lower extremities. Reflexes should remain intact, and sensory testing outside of the lateral thigh should reveal intact function.

Functional Limitations

Typically, there are no functional limitations because this injury is more an annoyance than truly disabling. No true weakness is seen, although prolonged standing and extension at the hip may exacerbate the pain and thus limit the patient in performing tasks such as standing and walking. The nerve may be further compressed and the symptoms exacerbated when the patient is seated, so long car or plane rides may be difficult. Similarly, individuals who are sedentary at work may experience painful symptoms that limit their ability to function.

Diagnostic Studies

History and physical examination are the most important diagnostic tools, and all other testing should be used as an extension of these. Electromyography is the primary diagnostic tool and should include lateral femoral cutaneous sensory nerve conduction studies and needle electromyography of the lower extremity [3,4]. Although routine lateral femoral cutaneous nerve conduction studies have standard normal values with which an individual's study result can be compared, it is generally recommended to do comparison studies on the unaffected side, as the studies are technically difficult [4,7–9]. The side-to-side amplitude ratio has been shown to be a better way to confirm the diagnosis [10]. Shin and colleagues [11] documented the utility of recording from two sites within the lateral femoral cutaneous dermatome. This technique facilitates use of a more realistic amplitude in the side-to-side comparison. Controversy exists in regard to the best site of stimulation of the lateral femoral cutaneous nerve. Classically, the stimulation electrode is placed 1 cm medial to the anterior superior iliac spine. Recently, a stimulation site of 4 cm distal to the anterior superior iliac spine has been suggested as a means to obtain a more reliable response [12]. The needle electromyography is done to rule out other pathologic processes, and the recording should be normal. Serial electromyographic studies may help with evaluation of the recovery process.

Somatosensory evoked potentials may also be used, but a study reported that sensory conduction studies are a more reliable method of evaluation of the lateral femoral cutaneous nerve [13]. High-resolution ultrasound has also been advocated for the assessment of lateral femoral cutaneous neuropathy and has been found to highly correlate with electrodiagnostic findings [14]. Once the diagnosis is made, magnetic resonance imaging or computed tomography of the pelvis may be required to look for a mass causing impingement.

Differential Diagnosis

Lumbar radiculopathy
Lumbar polyradiculopathy
Lumbar plexopathy
Lumbar facet syndrome
Retroperitoneal mass
Femoral neuropathy

Treatment

Initial

Treatment of lateral femoral cutaneous neuropathy is focused on symptom relief and facilitation of nerve healing.

Both early and late symptomatic relief of the pain and numbness is attempted with modalities and medications. If an inflammatory component is suspected, nonsteroidal anti-inflammatory drugs or corticosteroids may be used. Narcotics are used when acetaminophen and anti-inflammatory medications do not control the pain. Acting as membrane stabilizers, antiseizure medications, such as carbamazepine and gabapentin, are also of benefit in some individuals [15,16].

Facilitation of healing varies according to the cause of the injury to the nerve. For most individuals, this entails removal of the cause of the pressure over the anterior iliac region. The pressure may be caused by tight clothing, belts, seat belts, or excess weight. Elimination of the pressure may include weight loss or clothing adjustment. Nerves that have sustained a less serious (neurapraxic) injury often heal within hours to weeks once the irritant is removed. Nerves that have sustained a more severe injury (neurotmesis or axonotmesis) typically have a much longer healing course because of the time required for wallerian degeneration and regeneration. The use of anti-inflammatory medications may also be of benefit in the healing process.

Rehabilitation

Physical therapy may facilitate healing of the injured nerve. Gentle stretching of the anterior thigh and groin is indicated to prevent contracture of the hip flexor muscles. The application of hot packs or ultrasound often facilitates the stretching process. Ice may be helpful when the patient continues to have swelling and inflammation around the pelvic brim. In some individuals, a general conditioning program to help with weight loss may also be useful. A dietitian can assist the patient with weight loss. A skilled therapist may be able to use soft tissue mobilization to help free an impinged and inflamed nerve. Augmented soft tissue mobilization is one of several techniques that may be useful. Electrical stimulation and transcutaneous nerve stimulation may be helpful in reducing the perception of pain by the patient during therapy treatments. Transcutaneous electrical nerve stimulation can be used on a daily basis for pain control.

Procedures

When conservative treatment fails, injection of the nerve at or near the anterior superior iliac spine with steroids and local anesthetic may be helpful (Fig. 57.2). If the steroid injection is helpful but short lasting, the nerve can be injected with phenol or other neurotoxic agents as a last resort.

Under sterile conditions, the pelvis is palpated and the anterior superior iliac spine and inguinal ligament are identified. A 25-gauge, 2-inch needle is placed perpendicular to the skin approximately 1 inch medial to the anterior superior iliac spine and inferior to the inguinal ligament. The needle is advanced into the soft tissue approximately 1 inch (this depends on the patient's size and amount of excess subcutaneous tissue). At times, paresthesias may be elicited, thereby verifying needle placement; however, it is important not to inject directly into the nerve. Once the area to be injected is located, inject a 5- to 10-mL solution of local anesthetic and steroid (e.g., 2.5 mL of triamcinolone, 40 mg/mL, mixed with 2.5 mL of 0.5% bupivacaine). Ultrasound guidance of perineural lateral femoral cutaneous injection can significantly decrease failure rates by ensuring adequate needle localization [17].

Postinjection care may include icing of the injected area for 10 to 15 minutes and counseling of the patient to avoid pressure on the nerve.

Surgery

In the case of lateral femoral cutaneous nerve injury due to impingement, surgery may be required to remove the pressure. Surgical removal of neuroma or neurectomy proximal to the neuroma may also be helpful if a neuroma is found.

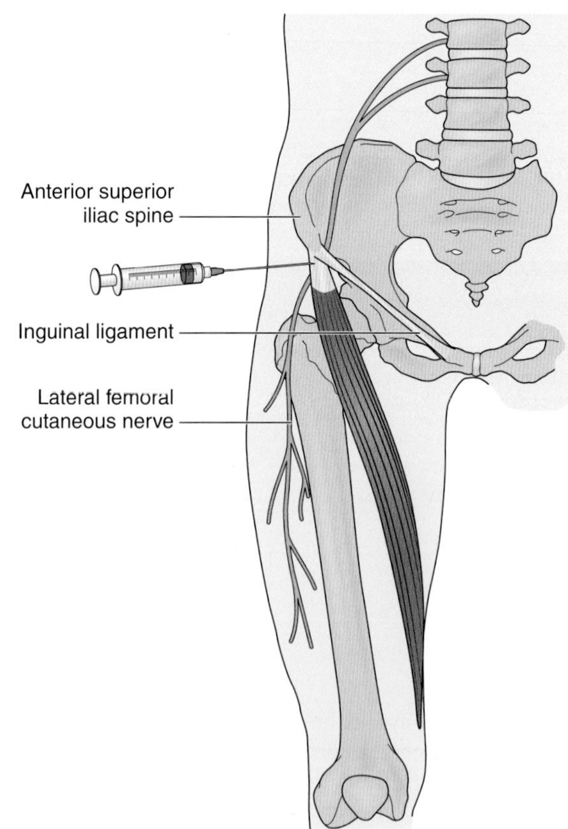

FIGURE 57.2 The nerve injection site for steroids and local anesthetic is at or near the anterior superior iliac spine.

In individuals with severe symptoms, neurolysis has been shown to result in a good outcome. This holds true even for individuals with prolonged symptoms. However, obesity has been associated with a poorer outcome when neurolysis is performed [18].

Potential Disease Complications

Potential complications include continued pain and numbness despite treatment.

Potential Treatment Complications

Complications of treatment are well recognized. Each medication has potential adverse side effects. Nonsteroidal anti-inflammatory drugs have the potential of gastric bleeding, decreased renal blood flow, and decreased platelet function. Narcotics have the potential for addiction and sedation. Carbamazepine can cause sedation and aplastic anemia. The patient taking carbamazepine should be evaluated with serial complete blood counts. Gabapentin can cause sedation. The injection of the nerve also has potential risks, which include bleeding, infection, and worsening of the pain. The potential risks of surgical intervention include bleeding, infection, and adverse reaction to the anesthetic agent.

References

[1] van Slobbe AM, Bohnen AM, Bernsen RM, et al. Incidence rates and determinants in meralgia paresthetica in general practice. J Neurol 2004;251:294–7.

[2] Moore KL. Clinically oriented anatomy. 2nd ed. Baltimore: Williams & Wilkins; 1985.

[3] Kimura J. Electrodiagnosis in diseases of nerve and muscle: principles and practice. 2nd ed. Philadelphia: FA Davis; 1989.

[4] Dumitru D. Electrodiagnostic medicine. Philadelphia: Hanley & Belfus; 1995.

[5] Williams PH, Trzil KP. Management of meralgia paresthetica. J Neurosurg 1991;74:76–80.

[6] de Ridder VA, de Lange S, Popta JV. Anatomic variations of the lateral femoral cutaneous nerve and the consequences for surgery. J Orthop Trauma 1999;13:207–11.

[7] Butler ET, Johnson EW, Kaye ZA. Normal conduction velocity in the lateral femoral cutaneous nerve. Arch Phys Med Rehabil 1974;55:31–2.

[8] Lagueny A, Deliac MM, Deliac P, et al. Diagnostic and prognostic value of electrophysiologic tests in meralgia paresthetica. Muscle Nerve 1991;14:51–6.

[9] Sarala PK, Nishihara T, Oh SJ. Meralgia paresthetica: electrophysiologic study. Arch Phys Med Rehabil 1979;60:30–1.

[10] Seror P, Seror R. Meralgia paresthetica: clinical and electrophysiological diagnosis in 120 cases. Muscle Nerve 2006;33:650–4.

[11] Shin YB, Park JH, Kwon DR, Park BY. Variability in conduction of the lateral femoral cutaneous nerve. Muscle Nerve 2006;33:645–9.

[12] Russo MJ, Firestone LB, Mandler RN, Kelly JJ. Nerve conduction studies of the lateral femoral cutaneous nerve. Implications in the diagnosis of meralgia paresthetica. Am J Electroneurodiagnostic Technol 2005;45:180–5.

[13] Seror P. Lateral femoral cutaneous nerve conduction v somatosensory evoked potentials for electrodiagnosis of meralgia paresthetica. Am J Phys Med Rehabil 1999;78:313–6.

[14] Aravindakannan T, Wilder-Smith EP. High-resolution ultrasonography in the assessment of meralgia paresthetica. Muscle Nerve 2012;45:434–5.

[15] Vorobeychik Y, Gordin V, Mao J, Chen L. Combination therapy for neuropathic pain. CNS Drugs 2011;25:1023–34.

[16] Finnerup NB, Sindrup SH, Jensen TS. The evidence for pharmacologic treatment of neuropathic pain. Pain 2010;150:573–81.

[17] Tagliafico A, Serafini G, Lacelli F, et al. Ultrasound-guided treatment of meralgia paresthetica (lateral femoral cutaneous neuropathy). J Ultrasound Med 2011;30:1341–6.

[18] Siu TL, Chandran KN. Neurolysis for meralgia paresthetica: an operative series of 45 cases. Surg Neurol 2005;63:19–23.

CHAPTER 58

Piriformis Syndrome

Rathi L. Joseph, DO
Joseph T. Alleva, MD, MBA
Thomas H. Hudgins, MD

Synonyms

Hip pocket neuropathy
Wallet neuritis

ICD-9 Codes

719.45	**Pain in joint, pelvic region, and thigh**
729.1	**Piriformis pain (musculoskeletal pain)**

ICD-10 Codes

M25.551	**Pain in right hip**
M25.552	**Pain in left hip**
M25.559	**Pain in unspecified hip**
M79.1	**Piriformis pain (musculoskeletal pain)**

Definition

Piriformis syndrome describes a clinical variations of this relationship have been well documented (Fig. 58.1). Cadaver studies have described situation whereby the piriformis muscle is compressing the sciatic nerve, resulting in a sciatic neuropathy. The piriformis muscle and sciatic nerve both exit the pelvis through the greater sciatic notch. Numerous anatomic the sciatic nerve passing below the piriformis muscle, through the muscle belly, as a divided nerve above and through the muscle, and as a divided nerve through and below the muscle [1,2]. More recently, a case report of piriformis syndrome described a fifth variation of an undivided nerve passing above an undivided piriformis muscle [3]. Yeoman [4] was the first to describe the relationship of these two structures in 1928, and Robinson [5] first coined the term *piriformis syndrome* in 1947.

Although the anatomic relation of these two structures is well documented, this remains a controversial diagnosis. There is no consensus among clinicians on the validity of this entity and therefore no documentation of the incidence [6]. Some authors suggest that piriformis syndrome is responsible for up to 36% of low back pain and "sciatica" cases, whereas others found the piriformis to be culpable in less than 1% of sciatica cases [7,8]. Nevertheless, Goldner [9] estimated an incidence of less than 1% in an orthopedic practice. Prevalence is difficult to identify because the diagnosis is one of exclusion and based on clinical findings [10].

Sciatic neuropathy related to piriformis syndrome may be a result of intrinsic injury to the piriformis muscle (primary syndrome) or a compression at the pelvic outlet (secondary syndrome) [11]. Secondary causes of piriformis syndrome can include superior and inferior gluteal artery aneurysm, benign pelvic tumor, endometriosis, and myositis ossificans. Often, a history of minor trauma may be described, such as falling onto the buttock [12].

Symptoms

The patient with piriformis syndrome will complain of buttock pain with or without radiation into the leg. Sitting on hard surfaces will exacerbate the symptoms of pain and occasional numbness and paresthesias without weakness. This may be seen in chronic as well as in acute situations. Activities that produce a motion of hip adduction and internal rotation, such as cross-country skiing and the overhead serve in tennis, may also exacerbate the symptoms [13,14]. Because of the relationship of the piriformis muscle with the lateral pelvic wall, patients may also experience pain with bowel movements, and women may complain of dyspareunia [15].

Physical Examination

The physical examination will reveal normal neurologic findings with symmetric strength and reflexes. Tenderness to palpation is experienced from the sacrum to the greater trochanter, representing the area of the piriformis muscle [16]. A palpable taut band is tender with both rectal and pelvic examination because the piriformis muscle sits in the deep pelvic floor [14]. Passive hip abduction and internal rotation may compress the sciatic nerve, reproducing pain (a Freiberg sign). Contraction of the piriformis with resistance to active hip external rotation and abduction may also reproduce pain or asymmetric weakness (a Pace sign) [17]. A positive result of the straight-leg test may also be appreciated [18]. Rectal examination may be performed to palpate a taut band. See Table 58.1.

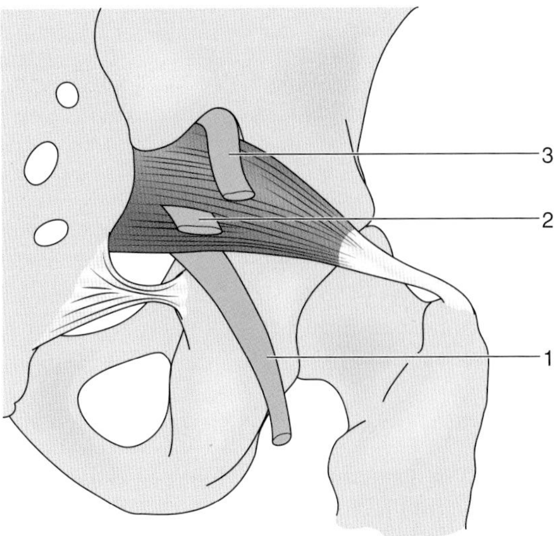

FIGURE 58.1 Three variations in the course of the sciatic nerve as related to the piriformis muscle. The sciatic nerve is shown above *(3)*, through *(2)*, and below *(1)* the piriformis muscle.

Table 58.1 Examination

Examination	Findings
Pace sign	Pain with resisted active hip external rotation and abduction with knee and hip flexed
Freiberg sign	Pain with passive hip abduction and internal rotation
Lasègue sign or straight-leg raise	Pain at greater sciatic notch with knee extension while hip is flexed to 90 degrees
Piriformis sign	Pain with tonic external rotation at the hip
FAIR testing	Pain with flexion, adduction, and internal rotation in lateral recumbent position with affected side up

Functional Limitations

The patient with piriformis syndrome will experience pain with prolonged sitting and with activities that produce hip internal rotation and adduction. This may include cross-country skiing and one-legged motions, such as the overhead serve in tennis and the kicking motion in soccer. Sitting on hard surfaces such as benches, church pews, or wallets kept in a back pocket ("wallet neuritis") may exacerbate symptoms. Driving or sitting as a passenger in a car or other form of transportation may limit someone's ability to get to work or to travel.

Diagnostic Testing

Piriformis syndrome is a clinical diagnosis. Magnetic resonance imaging and computed tomography are primarily reserved to rule out other disorders associated with sciatic neuropathy. A few case reports have demonstrated hypertrophy of the piriformis muscle on both computed tomography and magnetic resonance imaging [19]. Electrodiagnostic testing may reveal a prolonged H reflex in symptomatic cases [20]. This was validated by demonstration of a prolongation of the H reflex with hip flexion, adduction, and internal rotation (the FAIR test) in symptomatic cases. Patients diagnosed with piriformis syndrome by this FAIR test demonstrated successful treatment outcomes with physical therapy and injections in 70% of the cases [21]. Electrodiagnosis is also helpful in excluding piriformis syndrome during an evaluation for lumbosacral radiculopathy. Direct magnetic resonance imaging can be useful to diagnose secondary causes of piriformis syndrome, although no radiographic criteria have been established [22].

Differential Diagnosis

Lumbar facet syndrome
L5-S1 radiculopathy [17]

Treatment

Initial

Nonsteroidal anti-inflammatory drugs and analgesic medications are prescribed to reduce local prostaglandin-mediated inflammation, pain, and spasm [14]. Judicious use of modalities, such as heat therapy, may be beneficial to increase collagen distensibility and compliance with a physical therapy program. Avoidance of exacerbating activities and use of soft cushions for prolonged sitting are also advocated initially.

Rehabilitation

The use of heat therapy, such as ultrasound, is followed by a gentle stretch of the piriformis muscle. The piriformis is stretched with hip internal rotation above 90 degrees of hip flexion and with external rotation below 90 degrees of hip flexion [21]. Strengthening of the hip abductors, in particular the gluteus medius, should be emphasized. This is performed with Thera-Band around the ankles and walking sideways. The gluteus medius may also be isolated with lunges in a transverse and coronal plane. Correction of biomechanical imbalances that may predispose the individual to piriformis syndrome should also be initiated; these include increased pronation, hip abductor weakness, lower lumbar spine dysfunction, sacroiliac joint hypomobility, and hamstring tightness [13,14]. These imbalances may lead to a gait with hip in external rotation, shortened stride length, and functional leg length discrepancy.

Procedures

Recalcitrant cases may require a perisciatic injection of corticosteroid [18]. An approach of 1 cm caudal and 2 cm lateral to the lower border of the sacroiliac joint, as seen in Figures 58.2 and 58.3, correlated to successful distribution of the injectate near the sciatic nerve area confirmed by fluoroscopic guidance and nerve stimulator [23]. A cadaveric study comparing the accuracy of fluoroscopic guidance to ultrasound guidance for piriformis injection showed ultrasound guidance to be more accurate in contrast-controlled injection. This study showed 30% accuracy in fluoroscopically guided injections versus 95%

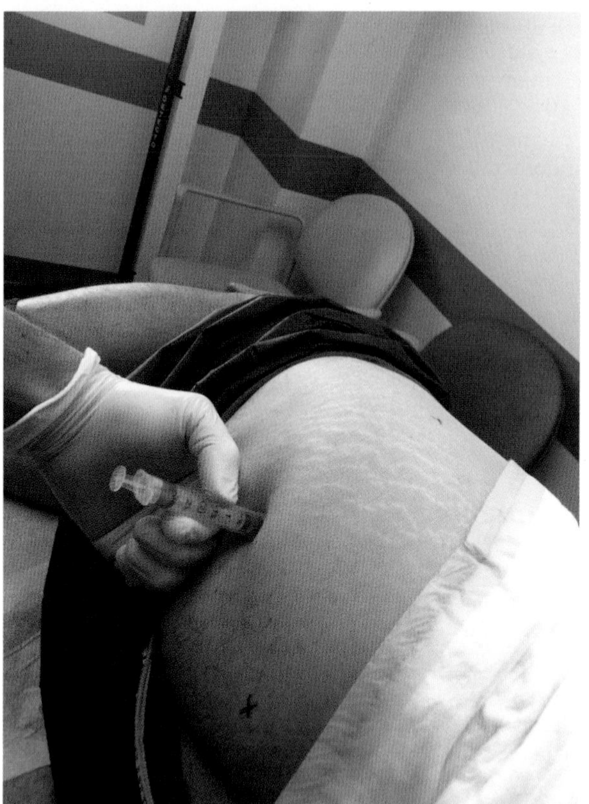

FIGURE 58.2 With the patient in a prone, or side-lying position (shown above), the sacroiliac joint is identified with fluoroscopy (*X*) and the needle is inserted 1 cm caudal and 2 cm lateral to the lower border of the sacroiliac joint.

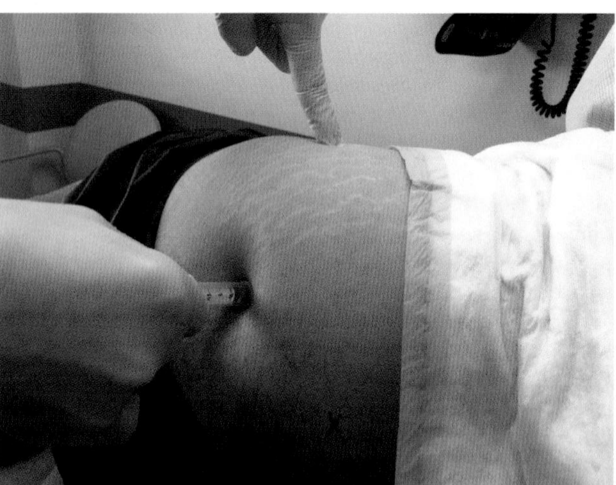

FIGURE 58.3 The needle is inserted at approximately the level of the greater trochanter (identified here with the gloved finger). A nerve stimulator is used to ensure proper placement near the sciatic nerve before introduction of the steroid solution.

accuracy in ultrasound-guided injections into the piriformis muscle [24]. Caudal epidural steroid injection to bathe the lower sacral nerve roots in corticosteroid has been described with mixed results. Injection of botulinum toxin type A (150 units) into the piriformis muscle under computed tomography guidance relieved pain and improved quality of life in a group of 20 patients with refractory symptoms. This pain relief was significant 12 weeks after injection, much longer than a corticosteroid injection is thought to last. No head-to-head studies comparing corticosteroids to botulinum toxin have been performed [25].

Surgery

Rarely, surgical release of the piriformis muscle is performed to relieve the compression [16]. Piriformis syndrome carries a favorable prognosis; most patients will respond to a nonoperative approach [13].

Potential Disease Complications

This is a clinical diagnosis that is often overlooked. The primary complication is chronic sciatica.

Potential Treatment Complications

Bleeding and gastrointestinal and renal side effects of nonsteroidal anti-inflammatory drugs are well documented. Complications of local corticosteroid injections include infection, hematoma or bleeding, and soft tissue atrophy at the site. Surgical techniques must be careful to avoid inadvertent injury to the nerves in the buttock. The functional loss of sectioning of the piriformis muscle is inconsequential as the other hip abductors may compensate for this movement [16,23].

References

[1] Pecina M. Contribution to the etiological explanation of the piriformis syndrome. Acta Anat (Basel) 1979;105:181–7.

[2] Beaton LE, Anson BJ. Sciatic nerve and the piriformis muscle: their interrelation as a possible cause of coccydynia. J Bone Joint Surg 1938;20:686–8.

[3] Ozaki S, Hamabe T, Muro T. Piriformis syndrome resulting from an anomalous relationship between the sciatic nerve and piriformis muscle. Orthopedics 1999;22:771–2.

[4] Yeoman W. The relation of arthritis of the sacroiliac joint to sciatica. Lancet 1928;2:1119–22.

[5] Robinson D. Piriformis syndrome in relation to sciatic pain. Am J Surg 1947;73:355–8.

[6] Silver JK, Leadbetter WB. Piriformis syndrome: assessment of current practice and literature review. Orthopedics 1998;21:1133–5.

[7] Boyajian-O'Neill LA, McClain RL, Coleman MK, Thomas PP. Diagnosis and management of piriformis syndrome: an osteopathic approach. J Am Osteopath Assoc 2008;108:657–64.

[8] Jawish RM, Assoum HA, Khamis CF. Anatomical, clinical and electrical observations in piriformis syndrome. J Orthop Surg Res 2010;5:3.

[9] Goldner JL. Piriformis compression causing low back and lower extremity pain. Am J Orthop 1997;26:316–8.

[10] Kirschner JS, Foye PM, Cole JL. Piriformis syndrome, diagnosis and treatment. Muscle Nerve 2009;40:10–8.

[11] Papadopoulos EC, Khan SN. Piriformis syndrome and low back pain: a new classification and review of the literature. Orthop Clin North Am 2004;35:65–71.

[12] Childers MK, Wilson DJ, Gnatz SM, et al. Botulinum toxin type A use in piriformis muscle syndrome: a pilot study. Am J Phys Med Rehabil 2002;81:751–9.

[13] Douglas S. Sciatic pain and piriformis syndrome. Nurse Pract 1997;22:166–80.

[14] Parziale JR, Hudgins TH, Fishman LM. The piriformis syndrome. Am J Orthop 1996;25:819–23.

[15] Barton PM. Piriformis syndrome: a rational approach to management. Pain 1991;47:345–52.

[16] McCrory P, Bell S. Nerve entrapment syndromes as a cause of pain in the hip, groin and buttock. Sports Med 1999;27:261–74.

[17] Yuen EC, So YT. Sciatic neuropathy. Neurol Clin 1999;17:617–31.
[18] Hanania M, Kitain E. Perisciatic injection of steroid for the treatment of sciatica due to piriformis syndrome. Reg Anesth Pain Med 1998;23:223–8.
[19] Jankiewicz JJ, Hennrikus WL, Hookum JA. The appearance of the piriformis muscle syndrome in computed tomography and magnetic resonance imaging. A case report and review of the literature. Clin Orthop 1991;262:205–9.
[20] Fishman LM, Zybert PA. Electrophysiologic evidence of piriformis syndrome. Arch Phys Med Rehabil 1992;73:359–64.
[21] Fishman LM, Dombi GW, Michaelsen C, et al. Piriformis syndrome: diagnosis, treatment, and outcome—a 10-year study. Arch Phys Med Rehabil 2002;83:295–301.
[22] Petchprapa EN, Rosenberg ZS, Sconfienza LM, et al. MR Imaging of entrapment neuropathies of the lower extremity. Part 1. The pelvis and hip. Radiographics 2010;30:983–1000.
[23] Benzon HT, Katz JA, Benzon HA, Iqbal MS. Piriformis syndrome: anatomic considerations, a new injection technique, and a review of the literature. Anesthesiology 2003;98:1442–8.
[24] Finnoff JT, Hurdle MF, Smith J. Accuracy of ultrasound-guided versus fluoroscopically guided contrast-controlled piriformis injections. J Ultrasound Med 2008;27:1157–63.
[25] Yoon SJ, Ho J, Kang HY, et al. Low-dose botulinum toxin type A for the treatment of refractory piriformis syndrome. Pharmacotherapy 2007;27:657–65.

CHAPTER 59

Pubalgia

Atul T. Patel, MD, MHSA

Synonyms

Athletic hernia
Athletic pubalgia
Gilmore's groin
Gracilis syndrome
Groin pain
Groin pull
Groin strain
Osteitis pubis
Pectineus syndrome
Sports hernia

ICD-9 Codes

727.09 Adductor tendinitis
959.19 Groin injury
789.00 Groin pain
848.8 Groin strain
848.8 Ilioinguinal strain
848.8 Inguinal muscle strain
733.5 Osteitis pubis

ICD-10 Codes

M77.9 Tendinitis NOS
S39.91 Groin injury (abdomen)
Use seventh character for the episode of care
R10.30 Groin pain (lower abdomen)
S39.011 Groin strain (abdominal muscle)
S39.011 Ilioinguinal strain (abdominal muscle)
S39.011 Inguinal muscle strain (abdominal muscle)
M85.38 Osteitis, other sites

Definition

Although there is no universally accepted definition of this condition, pubalgia is pain in the groin area that is due to musculoskeletal causes. Despite the prevalence of the condition, the literature is filled with varying causes, anatomy involved, and terminology. Pubalgia usually refers to pain in the groin or lower abdominal area, typically in athletes who engage in activities involving repetitive sprinting, kicking, or twisting movements. Most of the published studies include athletes involved in soccer, rugby, ice hockey, running, or football. It is typically a multifactorial condition initially thought to be due to weakness of the posterior wall of the inguinal canal (Fig. 59.1). These patients have no obvious hernias or symptoms, such as numbness, clicking, a lump, or dysuria, to suggest other causes. However, medical causes need to be considered and recognized before it is concluded that the pain is due to a musculoskeletal cause [1,2]. The majority of the conditions resulting in chronic groin pain in athletes are musculoskeletal in origin [3,4]. There is ample evidence that this condition is much more common in amateur and professional athletes than in the general population [5–7].

Symptoms

The symptoms are often vague and diffuse and in the area of the lower abdomen, groin, or medial thigh. The pain is often insidious in onset and a chronic aching type [8]. Most athletes cannot remember how or when the pain started. The symptoms are worse during and after strenuous activity and exacerbated by an increase in abdominal pressure, such as coughing or sneezing. The pain may limit the ability to stand or to sit. In men, the pain can radiate into the testicle on the involved side and to the surrounding areas of the abdomen and lower back. Women may complain of a dull ache in the groin aggravated by physical exertion or intermittent neurologic pain in the distribution of the ilioinguinal nerve [9].

Physical Examination

The findings on examination can be tenderness in the area of the pubic symphysis [10,11] and pain on contraction of the hip flexors, hip adductors, or abdominal muscles [12]. Pain and tenderness at the external inguinal ring without a frank lump may be associated with pubalgia, but the presence of a lump would indicate an inguinal hernia [13]. Tenderness and dilation of the external inguinal ring can be found in up to 94% of patients with an athletic hernia [14]. Reduced range of motion of the short adductors of the hip may indicate injury to these muscles. Decreased internal hip range of motion can be due to osteitis pubis, whereas generalized

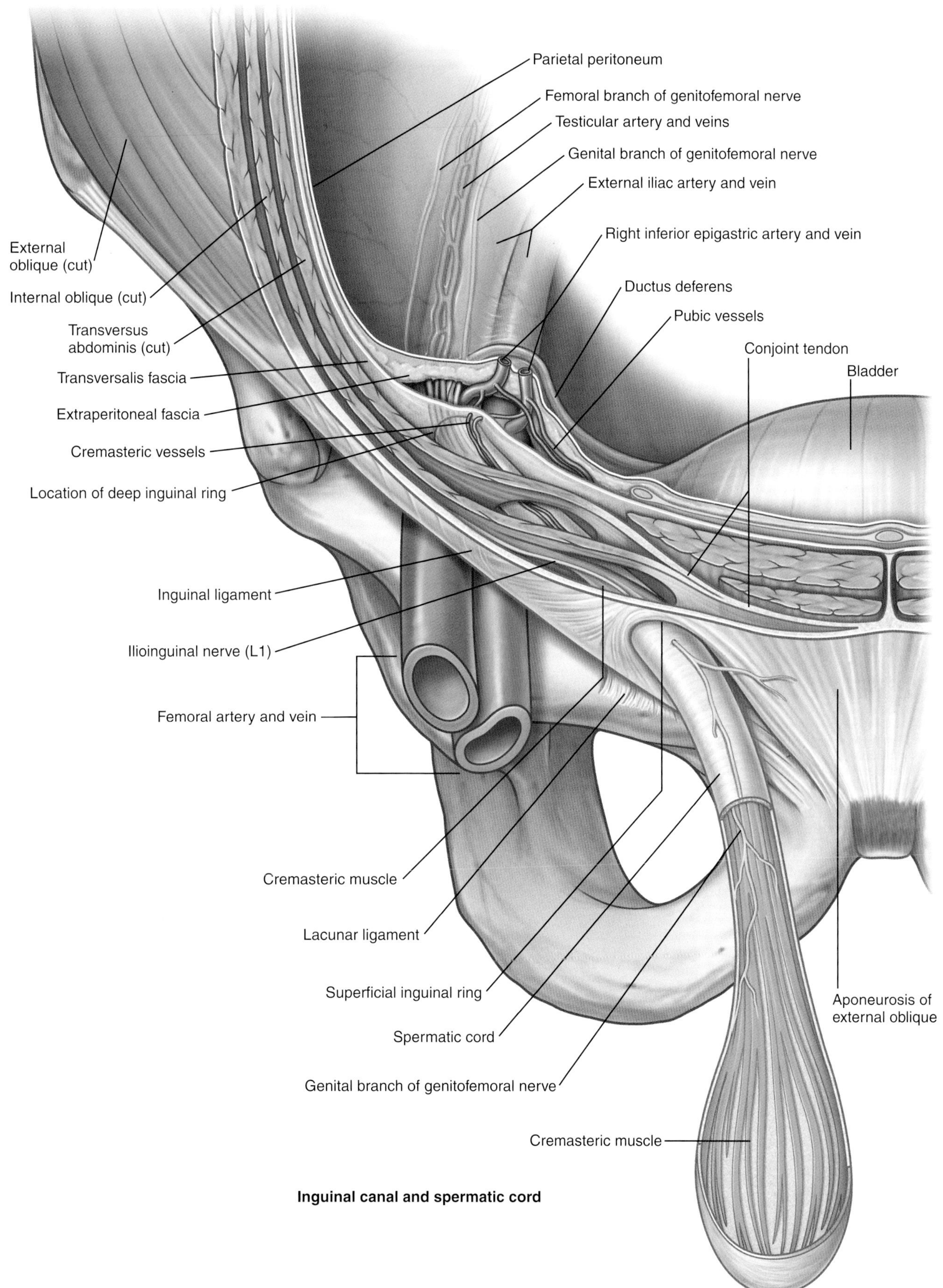

FIGURE 59.1 The anatomic layers of the groin showing the various muscles and other structures. The rectus abdominis is seen medially. *(From Drake R. Gray's Atlas of Anatomy. New York, Churchill Livingstone, 2008.)*

reduction in hip range of motion is suggestive of hip joint disease. The muscles originating from the pubic area should be palpated to assess for possible strain (adductors, sartorius, rectus femoris, and rectus abdominis). A general examination of the region should be carried out to assess for other potential causes of the symptoms. This should include examination of the testis in men and the rectum in both sexes. A gynecologic examination may be indicated in a female patient. A multidisciplinary approach to the evaluation should be considered in these patients, given the spectrum of potential diagnoses and various areas involved (abdomen, genitourinary system, musculoskeletal system) [15,16].

Functional Limitations

Pubalgia can limit activities that require repetitive hip flexion or abduction on the side of the injury. Because the pain is usually brought on by activity, it can limit athletic activities such as kicking, sprinting, or twisting.

Diagnostic Studies

Plain radiography of the pelvis can be helpful in assessing for degenerative changes involving the hips, sacroiliac joints, and lower spine. In addition, it can be helpful in assessing for other bone disease, such as stress fractures or tumors. Osteitis pubis typically produces symmetric bone resorption and sclerosis and may show widening of the symphysis [17]. Magnetic resonance imaging can be helpful in assessing the soft tissues of the pelvis and proximal thigh. It can also detect bone marrow edema about the pubic symphysis and tendon injuries [18]. Magnetic resonance imaging can help with identifying hip joint disease, such as labral tears, which too can be manifested with activity-related groin pain of insidious onset in young to middle-aged patients [18]. Selective injections can have diagnostic value in differentiating the source of pain, for example, the symphysis pubis or hip joint [19]. These are usually performed with guidance by fluoroscopy or ultrasonography. Herniography can be a sensitive way to diagnose hernias [20]. Ultrasound examination is becoming an inexpensive and noninvasive way of assessing for hernias in the groin area and tendinopathy [21].

Differential Diagnosis

Adductor tendinopathy
Osteitis pubis
Sports (occult, incipient) hernias
Conjoint tendon lesions
Rectus abdominis tendinopathy
Inguinal canal disease

Treatment

Initial

The patient usually presents with chronic symptoms. However, when the patient does present with an acute groin injury or groin pain, the treatment should include rest, use of nonsteroidal anti-inflammatory drugs (NSAIDs), analgesic medications, and ice. The patient may benefit from a muscle relaxant if there are muscle spasms.

Rehabilitation

There are limited studies in the literature on the treatment of pubalgia or adductor muscle strain and no specific protocols for therapy after surgery. Clinical experience dictates that the acute treatment consist of interventions to prevent further injury and inflammation. After the acute phase, the goals are to restore range of motion of the hip and to prevent muscle atrophy and deconditioning. The muscles that tend to be weak are the ipsilateral adductors, lower abdominals, ipsilateral gluteus medius and minimus, and contralateral tensor fascia lata. The patient may require stretching of surrounding muscles and need to learn techniques to transfer with less pain. The postoperative patient can have similar deficits and may benefit from the same therapies once wound healing is stable. Friction massage of the adductors may be needed. The stretching of the adductors should start in non–weight-bearing positions and then progress to weight bearing. Finally, functional training is a crucial component of the rehabilitation program [22].

Procedures

Patients with osteitis pubis can receive relief with fluoroscopically or sonographically guided corticosteroid injections [19]. Ultrasonography is gaining in popularity to aid in the diagnosis and treatment with corticosteroid injections around the nerves (ilioinguinal, iliohypogastric, and genitofemoral) and muscle origins (adductors, rectus femoris, sartorius, and rectus abdominis) in the inguinal region.

Surgery

Many patients continue to have symptoms despite conservative treatment; therefore surgery is often an option to eliminate the pain and return them to prior activities, including sports participation. However, most of the studies are case series without comparison to nonsurgical treatment. The surgical options fall into two categories: open versus laparoscopic. However, they are not compared in any of the studies. Only one prospective, randomized study is found that involved 66 soccer players with failed conservative treatment of groin pain. The patients were randomized into four groups: open surgical repair and neurotomy, individual training, physical therapy and NSAIDs, and controls [22]. Only the surgical group was found to have a statistically significant improvement in symptoms and ability to return to sport. Other surgeries include open repair of the posterior wall deficiencies [8,23]. More recently, laparoscopic procedures have become more popular. They tout quicker recovery and good responses [14,24–26].

Potential Disease Complications

In any condition that results in chronic pain, there is the risk of secondary complications of disuse atrophy, stiffening, and reduction in the range of motion of the affected joints and continued impact on the patient's function and quality of life.

Potential Treatment Complications

Analgesics and NSAIDs have well-known side effects that most commonly affect the gastric, hepatic, and renal systems. Aggressive stretching of the adductor muscles should be avoided in the acute phase as this may cause further pain and possible strain. Herniography is an invasive diagnostic study and there can be a risk for self-resolving bowel punctures.

References

[1] Macintyre J, Johnson C, Schroeder EL. Groin pain in athletes. Curr Sports Med Rep 2006;5:293–9.
[2] Morelli V, Smith V. Groin injuries in athletes. Am Fam Physician 2001;64:1405–14.
[3] Anderson K, Strickland SM, Warren R. Hip and groin injuries in athletes. Am J Sports Med 2001;29:521–33.
[4] Orchard J, Read JW, Verrell GM, Slavotinek JP. Pathophysiology of chronic groin pain in the athlete (online). Int SportMed J 2000;1(Suppl):1, Accessed Dec 9, 2012.
[5] Zoga AC, Kavanagh EC, Omar IM, et al. Athletic pubalgia and "sport's hernia": MR imaging findings. Radiology 2008;247:797–807.
[6] Hammoud S, Bedi A, Magennis E, et al. High incidence of athletic pubalgia symptoms in professional athletes with symptomatic femoroacetabular impingement. Arthroscopy 2012;28:1388–95.
[7] Robertson BA, Barker PJ, Fahrer M, Schache G. The anatomy of the pubic region revisited. Sports Med 2009;39:225–34.
[8] Polgase AL, Frydman GM, Farmer KC. Inguinal surgery for debilitating chronic groin pain in athletes. Med J Aust 1991;155:674–7.
[9] Grant T, Neuschler E, Hartz III W. Groin pain in women: use of sonography to detect occult hernia. J Ultrasound Med 2011;30:1701–7.
[10] Hackney RG. The sports hernia: a cause of chronic groin pain. Br J Sports Med 1993;27:58–62.
[11] Meyers WC, Foley DP, Garrett WE, et al. Management of severe abdominal or inguinal pain in high-performance athletes. Am J Sports Med 2000;28:2–8.
[12] Ekstrand J, Ringborg S. Surgery versus conservative treatment in soccer players with chronic groin pain: a prospective randomized study in soccer players. Eur J Sports Traumatol Relat Res 2001;23:141–5.
[13] Williams P, Foster ME. Gilmore's groin—or is it? Br J Sports Med 1995;29:206–8.
[14] Genitsaris M, Goulimaris I, Sikas N. Laparoscopic repair of groin pain in athletes. Am J Sports Med 2004;32:1238–42.
[15] Ekberg O, Persson NH, Abrahamsson P, et al. Longstanding groin pain in athletes: a multidisciplinary approach. Sports Med 1988;6:56–61.
[16] Martin HD, Kelly BT, Leunig M, et al. The pattern and technique in the clinical evaluation of the adult hip: the common physical examination tests of hip specialists. Arthroscopy 2010;26:161–72.
[17] Harris NH, Murray RO. Lesions of the symphysis pubis in athletes. BMJ 1974;4:211–4.
[18] Mintz DN, Hooper T, Connell D, et al. Magnetic resonance imaging of the hip: detection of labral and chondral abnormalities using noncontrast imaging. Arthroscopy 2005;21:385–93.
[19] O'Connell MJ, Powell T, McCaffrey NM, et al. Symphyseal cleft injection in the diagnosis and treatment of osteitis pubis in athletes. AJR Am J Roentgenol 2002;79:955–9.
[20] Eames N, Deans GT, Lawson JT, Irwin ST. Herniography for occult hernia and groin pain. Br J Surg 1994;81:1529–30.
[21] Brandon CJ, Jacobson JA, Fessell D, et al. Groin pain beyond the hip: how anatomy predisposes to injury as visualized by musculoskeletal ultrasound and MRI. AJR Am J Roentgenol 2011;197:1190–7.
[22] Hertling D, Kessler RM. Hip. In: Hertling D, Kessler RM, editors. Management of common musculoskeletal disorders: physical therapy principles and methods. 4th ed. Philadelphia: Lippincott Williams & Wilkins; 2006. p. 468–70.
[23] Malycha P, Lovell G. Inguinal surgery in athletes with chronic groin pain: the "sportsman's" hernia. Aust N Z J Surg 1992;62:123–5.
[24] Susmallian S, Ezri T, Elis M, et al. Laparoscopic repair of "sportsman's hernia" in soccer players as treatment of chronic inguinal pain. Med Sci Monit 2004;10:52–4.
[25] Minnich JM, Hanks JB, Muschaweck U, et al. Sports hernia: diagnosis and treatment highlighting a minimal repair surgical technique. Am J Sports Med 2011;39:1341–9.
[26] Larson CM, Pierce BR, Giveans MR. Treatment of athletes with symptomatic intra-articular hip pathology and athletic pubalgia/sports hernia: a case series. Arthroscopy 2011;27:768–75.

CHAPTER 60

Quadriceps Contusion

J. Michael Wieting, DO, MEd, FAOCPMR, FAAPMR
Michael Slesinski, DO

Synonym

Traumatic quadriceps strain

ICD-9 Codes

924.00 Contusion of lower limb (thigh)
924.9 Contusion of lower limb (unspecified site)

ICD-10 Codes

S70.00 Contusion of unspecified hip
S70.01 Contusion of right hip
S70.02 Contusion of left hip
S70.10 Contusion of unspecified thigh
S70.11 Contusion of right thigh
S70.12 Contusion of left thigh
S80.10 Contusion of unspecified lower leg
S80.11 Contusion of right lower leg
S80.12 Contusion of left lower leg
Add seventh character for episode of care (A—initial encounter, D—subsequent encounter, S—sequela)

Definition

Muscle contusions and strains account for 90% of contact sport–related injuries [1,2]. Quadriceps muscle contusions result from blunt trauma to the anterior thigh and are encountered most commonly in contact sports such as football, soccer, basketball, and wrestling. Injury is caused by a direct hit from a helmet, shoulder pad, elbow, or knee or being struck by a puck while playing hockey [3]. The acute trauma damages muscle tissue, causing hemorrhage and subsequent inflammation. A contracted muscle will absorb more force and this will result in a less severe injury [4]. At 12 to 24 hours after the injury, quadriceps contusions are graded mild, moderate, or severe. A mild contusion has more than 90 degrees of knee flexion with normal gait; moderate, between 45 and 90 degrees of knee flexion with antalgic gait; and severe, less than 45 degrees of knee flexion with severely antalgic gait [4,5].

Symptoms

Quadriceps contusions may not be immediately evident after the contact injury. Pain, swelling, and decreased range of motion of the knee, particularly flexion, are seen within 24 hours. Symptoms may worsen with active muscle contraction and with passive stretch. Loss of knee range of motion can be the result of muscle and articular edema as well as of physiologic inhibition of the quadriceps muscle group and "splinting" due to pain. After injury, the quadriceps muscle group often becomes stiff, and the patient may have difficulty bearing weight on the affected extremity, resulting in an antalgic gait. Hemorrhage and resultant hematoma are described as either intermuscular (between the muscles) or intramuscular (within a muscle).

Physical Examination

Visual inspection of quadriceps contusion shows a variable amount of swelling and discoloration over the anterior thigh due to hematoma formation and intramuscular bleeding. Pain of varying intensity is present on palpation of the quadriceps muscle group. A firm palpable mass may be noted in the anterior thigh and is usually due to hematoma formation; if the hematoma formation is large, a knee effusion may also be present. Bone incongruity and tenderness may indicate fracture of the femur, patella, or tibial plateau. Check for the presence of distal pulses and capillary refill and assess range of motion of adjacent joints to be sure that the injury is localized to the anterior thigh.

Evaluation of range of motion reveals decreased knee flexion, especially past 90 degrees; knee extension will be less painful than flexion [6]. Extension lag or complete lack of extension is noted in partial or complete quadriceps rupture. With quadriceps tendon rupture, a palpable defect may be present. However, quadriceps rupture is a relatively rare injury more common in patients older than 50 years, and it is typically associated with underlying metabolic or inflammatory disease [7]. Muscle stretch reflexes of the patellar tendon may be inhibited, and serial measurements of thigh circumferences should be made during the initial 24- to 72-hour postinjury period to assess for possible compartment syndrome. Paresthesias, loss of pulses, distal pallor, intense pain, and decreased temperature should alert the clinician to consider this diagnosis (see Chapter 67). Sensory testing should include the femoral and saphenous nerve distribution of the distal leg.

An intermuscular hematoma with septal or fascial sheath hemorrhage may be more likely to disperse and to result in distal ecchymosis. If the contusion is in the distal third of the quadriceps, discoloration and swelling will often track into the knee region because of gravity. An intramuscular hematoma may resolve more slowly and may be associated with myositis ossificans and scar contracture.

Functional Limitations

Initially, gait will be antalgic and weight bearing difficult on the involved extremity. Rehabilitation typically occurs in three phases. In the first phase (first 24 hours), pain usually limits activity, and the patient may require crutches [8]. During a period of days to weeks, climbing stairs, running, and "kicking" activities will be limited secondary to knee stiffness and pain associated with terminal knee flexion and extension. Most patients recover uneventfully.

Diagnostic Studies

Plain radiographs are initially obtained in moderate to severe quadriceps contusions to rule out a coexisting fracture. Magnetic resonance imaging is the diagnostic imaging study of choice and allows visualization of the involved quadriceps muscles. Resolution of the injury, as detected by magnetic resonance imaging, lags behind functional recovery [9]. Ultrasonography may be helpful if tendon injury is suspected [10]. Nuclear bone scan may be ordered in the days to weeks after injury to assess for the development of myositis ossificans traumatica, heterotopic bone formation that may develop in up to 20% of injuries. Bone scans are more sensitive than plain films for detection of heterotopic bone formation and can be useful in monitoring its resolution. Suspicion of compartment syndrome warrants consideration of intracompartmental pressure monitoring, although conservative management in cases without concomitant fracture has been reported [9,11]. Compartment syndrome may be more likely in a patient with associated fracture or suspected large-vessel injury. For severe contusions or in a patient who appears ill, laboratory work is indicated, including creatine kinase activity, hematocrit determination, and possibly coagulation studies [12].

Differential Diagnosis

Quadriceps tear or strain
Quadriceps tendon rupture
Soft tissue tumors
Compartment syndrome
Fracture of femur, patella, or tibial plateau
Referred pain from hip or knee
Metabolic abnormalities leading to tendon injuries (hypocalcemia, steroid use)
Morel-Lavallée lesion of the knee

Treatment

Initial

Immediately, the patient should cease activity. The knee is gently elevated and flexed to 120 degrees, and ice is applied to the anterior thigh (for 20 minutes at a time every 2 or 3 hours). A brace or elastic bandage should be placed around the injured leg and thigh to maintain 120 degrees of knee flexion as soon as possible after the injury and gentle compression applied to reduce hematoma formation for the initial 24-hour postinjury period [13]. After the initial 24 hours, the brace or bandage should be removed and active, pain-free range of motion of the knee should be initiated with static quadriceps strengthening and stretching [4]. If the injury is mild, icing is repeated for 2 or 3 days; the patient should ambulate with crutches, either non–weight bearing or partial weight bearing. In between icing, a thigh pad is applied. Temporary bed rest may be appropriate if the injury is severe. However, rehabilitation should be aggressive to the limit of pain tolerance. Avoid massage for the first 1 to 2 weeks after injury to lessen the chance of additional hemorrhage. Whirlpool, heat, and ultrasound modalities are avoided for the same reason until the edema stabilizes. If edema persists or becomes severe or warning signs of compartment syndrome develop, surgical referral is made to evaluate the possibility of compartment syndrome or ongoing hemorrhage. Needle aspiration of a formed hematoma may be indicated to relieve pressure and pain [14].

Determination of the appropriate time to progress the amount of activity performed and readiness for return to activity is important for recovery from injury. Animal models of muscle contusion suggest that continued use of the extremity promotes circulation and venous drainage, minimizing postinjury swelling. Because of the risk of hematoma formation, nonsteroidal anti-inflammatory drugs (NSAIDs) are avoided in the first 24 hours after injury. The role of NSAIDs in the treatment of muscle injuries is unclear because inflammatory cells are an important part of clearing away necrotic muscle followed by the regeneration and scar formation phase, leading to the question of whether NSAIDs help or delay the healing process [15]. The inflammatory response may be a necessary phase in soft tissue healing. Clinically, NSAIDs are used, but alternative analgesics like acetaminophen may be considered. However, in the animal model of quadriceps contusion, continued use of the contused muscle was more predictive of recovery than whether the animal received acetaminophen or NSAIDs [15]. Steroids should be avoided [1,4]. Medication use should facilitate continued rehabilitation and tolerance of activity progression.

Rehabilitation

Rehabilitation consists of three phases. The goals of the first phase are to limit bleeding, to immobilize the knee in full flexion, to elevate the leg for 24 hours, and to prescribe relative rest. Excessive activity or alcohol ingestion, which could aggravate the injury, is avoided. Phase two involves restoration of motion, the use of therapeutic modalities, and return to weight bearing. Crutches and partial weight bearing are used during this phase and until the patient has at least 90 degrees of knee flexion, good quadriceps control, and limited limp. After 48 hours from the injury and for the next 2 to 5 days, test range of motion with the patient in the prone position. Perform knee flexion exercises in the "pain-free range" with associated hip flexion. This can be followed with active-assisted range of motion exercises. It is important to avoid forced stretching because this may aggravate the injury and slow healing. Static quadriceps exercises can be instituted. Animal models of muscle contusion demonstrate that early mobilization increases tensile strength of muscle compared with immobilization [16]. Proprioceptive neuromuscular facilitation exercises using reciprocal inhibition of the quadriceps and hamstrings can be done as well [17]. Modalities may include pulsed ultrasound or high-velocity galvanic stimulation, with continuous pulses of 80 to 120 per second, at the patient's level of sensory perception for 20- to 25-minute periods. Interferential electrical stimulation may assist in further edema resolution, but both ultrasound and electrical stimulation should be used once edema has stabilized. Cautious use of ultrasound can help increase blood resorption [17]. Cold compression may be useful to decrease pain and swelling.

Phase three starts when the patient has 120 degrees of pain-free range of motion and excellent quadriceps control. Noncontact sports and other vigorous physical activities involving the lower limbs may be resumed at this point, along with active knee range of motion, progressive resistive exercises, and cycling. Pain-free knee range of motion within 10 degrees of the unaffected extremity should be the goal before return to activity is considered. Jumping, sprinting, and cutting activities should be incorporated into the rehabilitation program, at which point functional testing to assess safe return to activity can be done. In the case of athletes, a protective pad larger than the original contusion should be worn during play for 3 to 6 months after injury. Most quadriceps contusions resolve within a few weeks, and complications are rare. If the patient does not have painless, full range of motion 3 to 4 weeks after injury, radiographic imaging should be performed to detect whether myositis ossificans is present. Time to return to activity is variable and depends on severity of injury; with severe contusions, full recovery is expected within by 5 to 8 weeks.

Procedures

On occasion, needle aspiration of a formed hematoma is performed to alleviate pressure and pain. This can be done at initial diagnosis or if symptoms are not responding to the measures outlined earlier.

Surgery

Surgery is rarely indicated with these injuries, except in association with a concomitant compartment syndrome or fracture. Untreated compartment syndrome may lead to muscle necrosis, fibrosis, scarring, and contractures. However, even in severe quadriceps muscle contusion, there is some indication that treatment should be conservative with pain management and maintenance of knee range of motion [9].

Potential Disease Complications

If the quadriceps region becomes extremely warm with marked increased edema and the patient complains of paresthesias with abnormal findings on neurovascular examination and significant quadriceps weakness, consideration must be given to the development of a potential compartment syndrome. A case of osteomyelitis has been reported in an otherwise healthy athlete who sustained a quadriceps contusion [18].

Myositis ossificans traumatica usually stabilizes and is resorbed spontaneously by 6 months after injury with conservative care [19]. Plain films may show ectopic bone formation 2 to 4 weeks after injury; the most common location is in the midshaft of the femur. Serial bone scans can be performed to monitor resolution of ectopic bone in a symptomatic athlete. Surgical removal of ectopic bone is rarely indicated and should not be performed for at least 12 months after injury to allow adequate maturation; this is to prevent enlargement of ectopic bone and recurrence. NSAIDs are the treatment of choice for prevention and initial treatment of myositis ossificans based on studies performed in hip replacements and related heterotopic ossification [4].

Potential Treatment Complications

Analgesics and NSAIDs have well-known side effects that most commonly affect the gastric, hepatic, and renal systems. Avoid vigorous soft tissue massage and passive stretch in the acute postinjury period to prevent further bleeding and hematoma formation (this occurs frequently in a field setting after hamstring injury).

References

[1] Beiner JM, Jokl P, Cholewicki J, Panjabi MM. The effect of anabolic steroids and corticosteroids on healing of muscle contusion injury. Am J Sports Med 1999;27:2–9.

[2] Canale ST, Cantler Jr ED, Sisk TD, Freeman 3rd BL. A chronicle of injuries of an American intercollegiate football team. Am J Sports Med 1981;9:384–9.

[3] LaPrade RF, Wijdicks CA, Griffith CJ. Division I intercollegiate ice hockey team coverage. Br J Sports Med 2009;43:1000–5.

[4] Kary JM. Diagnosis and management of quadriceps strains and contusions. Curr Rev Musculoskelet Med 2010;3:26–31.

[5] Reid D. Sports injury assessment and rehabilitation. New York: Churchill Livingstone; 1992.

[6] Ryan JB, Wheeler JH, Hopkinson WJ, et al. Quadriceps contusions. West Point update. Am J Sports Med 1991;19:299–304.

[7] Katz T, Alkalay D, Rath E, et al. Bilateral simultaneous rupture of the quadriceps tendon in an adult amateur tennis player. J Clin Rheumatol 2006;12:32–3.

[8] Schenck Jr RC. Athletic Training and Sports Medicine. 3rd ed. Rosemont, Ill: American Academy of Orthopaedic Surgeons; 1999.

[9] Diaz JA, Fischer DA, Rettig AC, et al. Severe quadriceps muscle contusions in athletes. A report of three cases. Am J Sports Med 2003;31:289–93.

[10] Heyde CE, Mahlfeld K, Stahel PF, Kayser R. Ultrasonography as a reliable diagnostic tool in old quadriceps tendon ruptures: a prospective multicentre study. Knee Surg Sports Traumatol Arthrosc 2005;13:564–8.

[11] Robinson D, On E, Halperin N. Anterior compartment syndrome of the thigh in athletes—indications for conservative treatment. J Trauma 1992;32:183–6.

[12] DeBerardino T, Milne L, DeMaio M. Quadriceps injury. http://www.emedicine.com [accessed 21.06.06].

[13] Aronen JG, Garrick JG, Chronister RD, McDevitt ER. Quadriceps contusions: clinical results of immediate immobilization in 120 degrees of knee flexion. Clin J Sport Med 2006;16:383–7.

[14] DeLee JC, Drez D. Orthopaedic Sports Medicine: Principles and Practice. Philadelphia: WB Saunders; 1994.
[15] Rahusen FT, Weinhold PS, Almekinders LC. Nonsteroidal anti-inflammatory drugs and acetaminophen in the treatment of an acute muscle injury. Am J Sports Med 2004;32:1856–9.
[16] Jarvinen MJ, Lehto MU. The effects of early mobilisation and immobilisation on the healing process following muscle injuries. Sports Med 1993;15:78–89.
[17] Geraci M. Rehabilitation of the hip, pelvis, and thigh. In: Kibler WB, Herring SA, Press JM, editors. Functional rehabilitation of sports and musculoskeletal injuries. Gaithersburg, Md: Aspen; 1998.
[18] Bonsell S, Freudigman PT, Moore HA. Quadriceps muscle contusion resulting in osteomyelitis of the femur in a high school football player. A case report. Am J Sports Med 2001;29:818–20.
[19] Young JL, Laskowski ER, Rock MG. Thigh injuries in athletes. Mayo Clin Proc 1993;68:1099–106.

CHAPTER 61

Total Hip Replacement

Juan A. Cabrera, MD
Alison L. Cabrera, MD

Synonyms

Total hip replacement
Bipolar hemiarthroplasty
Unipolar hemiarthroplasty
Revision arthroplasty

ICD-9 Codes

715.95	Osteoarthritis, hip
733.42	Aseptic necrosis of bone, head and neck of femur
820.09	Fracture of neck of femur, other (head of femur, subcapital)
820.8	Fracture of neck of femur, unspecified part of neck of femur, closed
835.00	Dislocation of hip
996.59	Loosening of total hip replacement
V43.64	Total hip replacement

ICD-10 Codes

M16.0	Bilateral primary osteoarthritis of hip
M16.10	Unilateral primary osteoarthritis, unspecified hip
M16.11	Unilateral primary osteoarthritis, right hip
M16.12	Unilateral primary osteoarthritis, left hip
M87.050	Idiopathic aseptic necrosis of pelvis
M87.051	Idiopathic aseptic necrosis of right femur
M87.052	Idiopathic aseptic necrosis of left femur
M87.059	Idiopathic aseptic necrosis of unspecified femur
S72.011	Unspecified intracapsular fracture of right femur
S72.012	Unspecified intracapsular fracture of left femur
S72.019	Unspecified intracapsular fracture of unspecified femur
S72.001	Fracture of unspecified part of neck of right femur
S72.002	Fracture of unspecified part of neck of left femur
S72.009	Fracture of unspecified part of neck of unspecified femur
S73.004	Unspecified dislocation of right hip
S73.005	Unspecified dislocation of left hip
S73.006	Unspecified dislocation of unspecified hip
T84.030	Mechanical loosening of internal right hip prosthetic joint
T84.031	Mechanical loosening of internal left hip prosthetic joint
Z96.641	Presence of right artificial hip joint
Z96.642	Presence of left artificial hip joint
Z96.643	Presence of artificial hip joint, bilateral

Add seventh character for categories S72, S73, and T84 for episode of care

Definition

Total hip arthroplasty (THA), commonly called hip replacement surgery, involves the reconstruction of a diseased, damaged, or ankylosed hip joint. The most common causes of adult hip disease are osteoarthritis, inflammatory arthritides, avascular necrosis, post-traumatic degenerative joint disease, congenital hip disease, oncologic bone disease, and infection involving the hip joint. The surgical treatment of hip arthritides has evolved from the first excisional arthroplasty by Anthony White in

1821 into the modern THA [1]. The modern era of hip joint replacement began in the late 1960s when Sir John Charnley combined a stainless steel femoral component with a polyethylene socket fixed to the adjacent acetabulum with polymethyl methacrylate (cement). Since that time, arthroplasty of the hip joint has become an accepted and standard treatment of common adult hip joint disease. Modern hip arthroplasty surgery has resulted in the restoration of pain-free motion and improved quality of life for millions [2]. Total joint arthroplasty, including hip and knee, has become the most common elective surgical procedure performed in the United States, with more than one million performed in 2009 [3]. The Centers for Disease Control and Prevention reported that 327,000 total hip replacements were performed in the United States in 2009 [3].

Hip joint arthroplasty can be divided into either THA, which provides a prosthetic replacement of the proximal femur and acetabulum, or hemiarthroplasty, which replaces the proximal femur while leaving the native acetabulum intact. Hip hemiarthroplasty is reserved for patients with a healthy articular surface in the acetabulum and is most commonly seen after proximal femur fractures. The focus of this chapter is on THA, which is the preferred surgical option for patients with degenerative changes affecting both the femur and acetabulum. Further categorization for hip arthroplasty can be made by prosthetic hardware components, surgical approach, or fixation method of the prosthesis (cement versus biologic or "press-fit" integration). Surgical decision-making for hardware type, approach, and prosthetic fixation is beyond the scope of this chapter, but it is important to note that there are no published consensus guidelines on best prostheses, approach, or fixation method among surgeons performing total hip arthroplasties.

Symptoms

The primary symptom of hip disease is groin pain, but patients may also have associated back and knee pain. Patients may describe a decline in mobility, self-care, and activities of daily living. They may present with an abnormal gait or may describe difficulty in walking long distances and need for an assistive device. Donning their shoes or socks and taking them off and getting in and out of the seated position may be difficult daily activities. Inability to participate in recreational activities or light sports may be a presenting complaint.

Physical Examination

Patients with hip disease are likely to have physical examination findings that will require continued attention postoperatively (Table 61.1). The examiner should examine both hips, knees, and back for range of motion. Decreased range of motion of the affected hip will be found and may be the first physical examination finding in cases of mild disease. Also, a thorough neurovascular examination of all extremities should be performed. One of the most commonly observed examination findings is an antalgic (painful) gait pattern representing a combination of pain that inhibits motion, structural loss of joint motion, avoidance behavior, and weakness. Hip pain or weakness of the hip abductors can result in contralateral pelvic tilt or drop (Trendelenburg sign) with ipsilateral weight bearing (Fig. 61.1). Muscle weakness is typically not true neurologic weakness but rather represents a disuse weakness associated with pain and avoidance. A hip flexion contracture may be observed with the Thomas test (Fig. 61.2), and accentuated lumbar lordosis may be seen in those with a hip flexion contracture, which may result in secondary mechanical low back pain due to alteration of normal spine mechanics. A limb length discrepancy may be observed, with the affected hip being the shorter limb.

Table 61.1 Goals of Rehabilitation after Total Hip Arthroplasty

Successful postoperative pain management
Maintain medical stability
Achieve successful surgical incision healing
Guard against dislocation of the implant
Prevent bed rest hazards (e.g., thrombophlebitis, pulmonary embolism, decubiti, pneumonia)
Obtain pain-free range of motion within precaution limits
Strengthen hip and knee musculature
Gain functional strength
Teach transfers and ambulation with assistive devices
Successful progression to prior living situation

Modified from Cameron H, Brotzman SB, Boolos M. Rehabilitation after total joint arthroplasty. In Brotzman SB, ed. Clinical Orthopaedic Rehabilitation. St. Louis, Mosby, 1996.

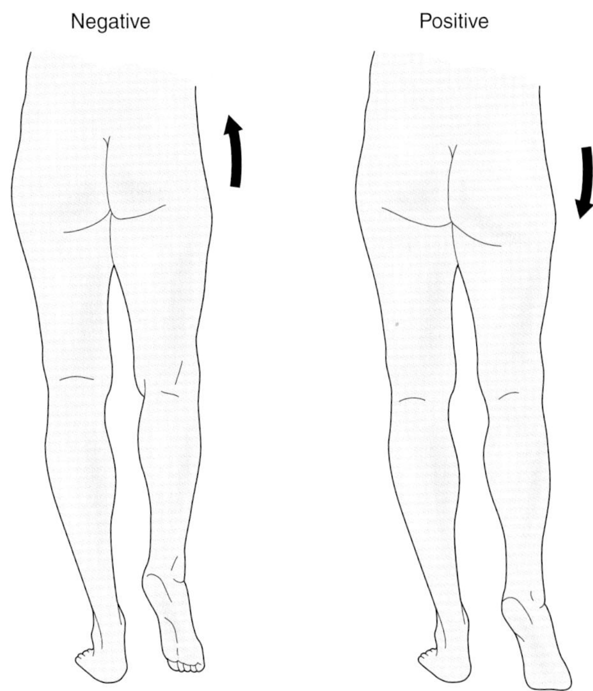

FIGURE 61.1 Trendelenburg sign. *(From Goldstein B, Chavez F. Applied anatomy of the lower extremities. Phys Med Rehabil State Art Rev 1996;10:601-630.)*

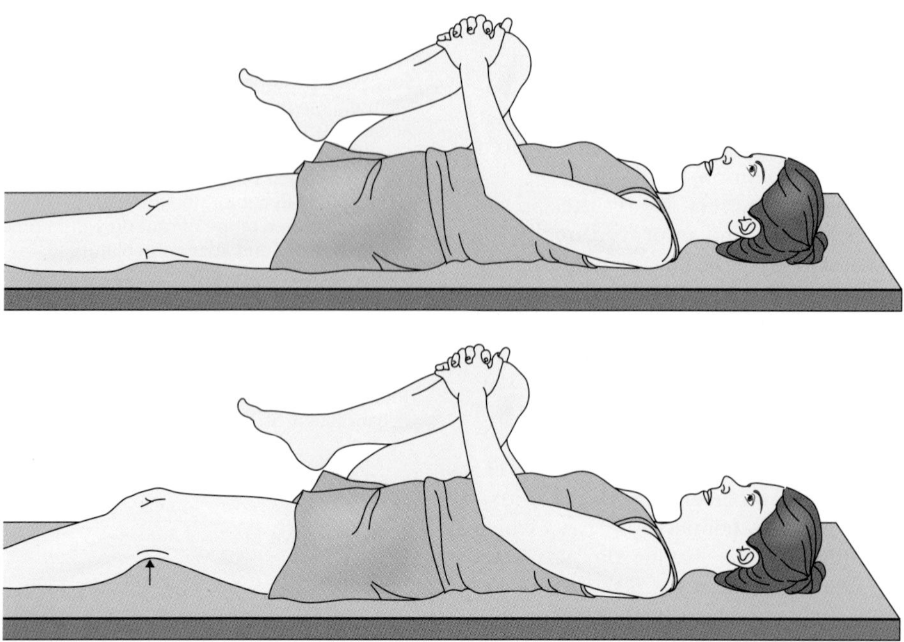

FIGURE 61.2 Thomas test to assess a hip flexion contracture. The patient lies supine while a hip is flexed, bringing the knee to the chest and flattening the lumbar spine. The patient holds the flexed knee and hip against the chest. If there is a flexion contracture of the hip, the patient's other leg will rise off the table.

Functional Limitations

Functional limitations from severe hip disease include difficulty in walking and with all mobility, even rising from a seated position, because of pain and weakness. This may affect a patient's ability to dress, to bathe, to perform household chores, to participate in recreational activities, and to work outside the home. The goal of THA is to improve pain and consequently to improve function with activities of daily living.

Diagnostic Studies

Plain radiography remains the primary imaging tool for evaluation of hip disease and for postoperative assessment of THA. On radiographic examination, significant loss of joint cartilage as demonstrated by joint space narrowing, joint incongruity, osteophyte formation, subchondral cysts, and sclerosis are seen in individuals being considered for THA (Fig. 61.3). Many postoperative complications after THA can be evaluated by plain radiography. In patients thought to have a dislocation after THA, radiographs should be obtained urgently because a true dislocation must be relocated expediently (Fig. 61.4). Plain radiographs are also obtained in patients thought to have prosthetic loosening or periprosthetic fracture (Fig. 61.5). If plain radiographs do not show pathologic changes in a patient with enigmatic hip pain after THA, magnetic resonance imaging can be done with minimal artifact and can demonstrate disease in the periprosthetic soft tissues, including synovitis, periprosthetic inflammation, osteolysis, and iliopsoas tendinitis [4]. A computed tomography scan or bone scan may be part of the evaluation for osteolysis or loosening and infection.

Differential Diagnosis

Infection
Loosening of acetabular component
Stress fracture
Iliopsoas tendinitis with impingement
Occult fractures
Pelvic osteolysis
Synovitis from metal or polyethylene debris
Vascular disease
Inguinal hernia
Metastatic cancer
Dissecting retroperitoneal disease
Neurologic disease (including radiculopathy or spinal cord lesions)

Treatment

Treatment protocols after THA can be broadly divided into an initial (acute postoperative) phase and a rehabilitation phase. All patients will have weight-bearing and activity restrictions for approximately 6 weeks postoperatively. These restrictions are not universally accepted, are influenced by surgical technique (cemented versus uncemented fixation of the prosthesis), and can vary by surgeon preference. Ultimately, postoperative restrictions should be clarified by communication with the surgeon.

Initial

The initial phase (acute postoperative) usually includes up to 4 days after surgery and is performed on an inpatient

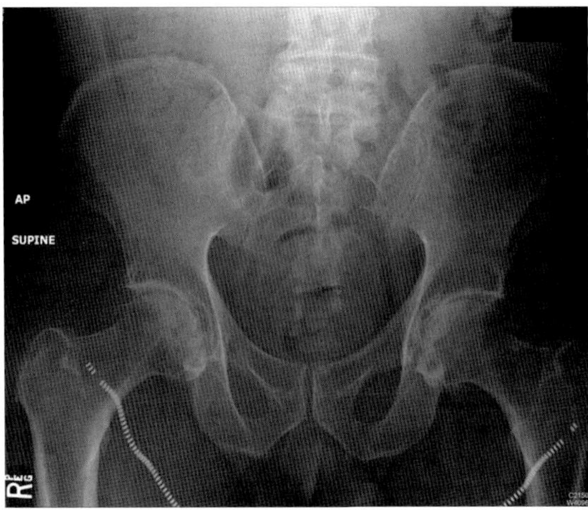

FIGURE 61.3 Anteroposterior pelvis radiograph showing moderate to severe degenerative changes of the hips. Notice the sclerotic changes at the acetabular and femoral heads. Note the loss of joint space, especially inferiorly, and osteophytes.

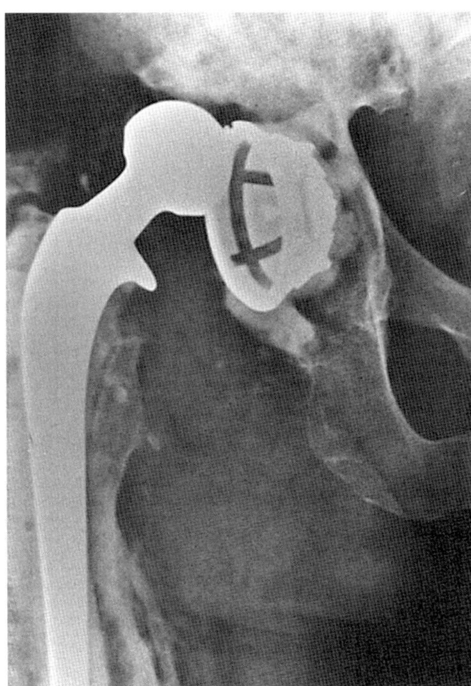

FIGURE 61.4 Total hip replacement—dislocation. The femur has dislocated superiorly and laterally relative to the acetabulum. This dislocation is due to abnormal (vertical) position of the acetabular cup that occurred from loosening (see widened cement-bone interface). *(From Katz DS, Math KR, Groskin SA. Radiology Secrets. Philadelphia, Hanley & Belfus, 1998.)*

basis. Therapy typically begins on postoperative day 1 and focuses on getting the patient out of bed; education is provided on safe transfers, and static exercises are performed for gluteal muscles, quadriceps, and ankle pumps. Pain control strategies frequently begin with intravenous narcotics (patient-controlled analgesic pumps), cryotherapy, and appropriate education to reduce anxiety. Rehabilitation strategies on postoperative day 2 through the day of discharge should stress education on hip precautions, compliance with weight-bearing restrictions, early mobilization

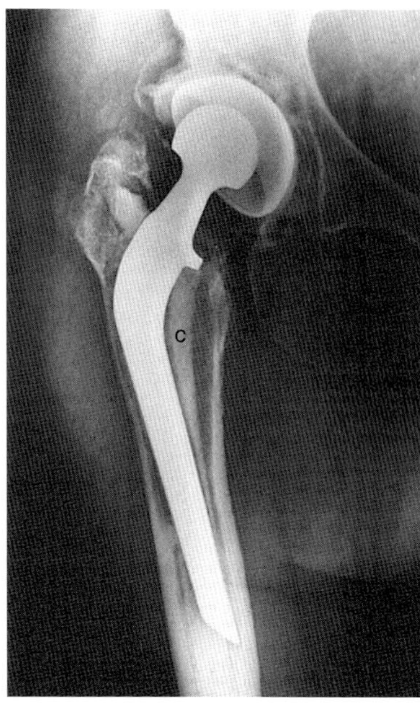

FIGURE 61.5 Total hip replacement—loose femoral component. There is a wide area of lucency between the opaque cement *(C)* and the adjacent bone at the medial aspect of the proximal femur in addition to the area of lucency at the metal-bone interface surrounding the acetabular prosthesis. These were new findings indicative of loosening of both components. *(From Katz DS, Math KR, Groskin SA. Radiology Secrets. Philadelphia, Hanley & Belfus, 1998.)*

with use of an assistive device, instruction on the use of adaptive equipment for functional independence (bathing, grooming), and continued pain control [5]. Pain control should be transitioned to oral medications and may require any combination of non-narcotic analgesics, nonsteroidal anti-inflammatory drugs, long-acting narcotics, or short-acting narcotics. Recently, intravenous acetaminophen has been shown to be a safe and effective pain medication in patients after joint replacement, which is of paramount importance considering the many side effects of narcotics in the elderly population [6]. Other interventions during the initial phase after THA include administration of perioperative prophylactic antibiotics, autologous blood transfusions for blood loss–induced anemia, and initiation of deep venous thrombosis prophylaxis. The patient may be receiving pharmacologic or mechanical deep venous thrombosis prophylaxis based on current clinical practice guidelines and individual patient factors [7]. By the third postoperative day, the patient should be able to tolerate 2 to 3 hours of therapy a day unless severe anemia or other medical problems result in further functional limitations. If the patient's condition is stable, the patient is ready for discharge from the acute care hospital by the third or fourth postoperative day.

Rehabilitation

Once the initial (acute postoperative) phase is complete, a decision needs to be made for the most appropriate environment for the rehabilitation phase. This decision is based on physical and social factors and should be made with the patient, the patient's primary caregiver, surgeon, physiatrist, therapists, nursing staff, and social worker. Goals for rehabilitation after THA should be to restore maximal range of motion, to minimize pain, to improve muscle strength, to promote ambulation, and to facilitate functional independence (Table 61.1).

Hip precautions should be followed and are taught to patients to minimize the possibility of hip dislocation. Patients with weak periarticular tissues, revision surgeries, or previous dislocations are at the highest risk for a dislocation, which is greatest during the first postoperative week. Most surgeons use a posterolateral approach to the hip joint and dislocate the joint by hyperflexion (greater than 90 degrees), adduction, and internal rotation. After hip replacement, that combination of movements increases the risk of dislocation. Therefore, an abduction pillow or wedge can be placed between the legs to maintain a safe position. Patients are taught not to use low chairs or to reach forward by flexing at the hip. Many surgeons who perform THA by anterior and anterolateral approaches are advocates for these approaches because of a lessened risk of dislocation. There is level II evidence suggesting that the risk of hip dislocation is reduced with a direct anterior or anterolateral approach, and strict hip precautions are not necessary [8]. There is little information in the literature to guide the duration of hip precautions. Most surgeons encourage strict precautions for at least 6 weeks and some encourage these precautions indefinitely. The performing surgeon should clarify the prescription of hip precautions, including restricted movements and duration of precautions, before initiating any rehabilitation protocol.

Active-assisted range of motion and strengthening exercises are progressed as tolerated. Resisted hip exercises should be avoided in the first 4 to 6 weeks to prevent excessive torsional forces on the implant [5]. Strengthening exercises for knee extension are encouraged. Quadriceps weakness can persist for up to 1 year after THA if it is not addressed during rehabilitation [5]. Electrical stimulation can be used for patients with atrophy of the quadriceps. Range of motion including stretching exercises for the hip flexor and adductor muscles should be included to prevent gait abnormalities. Subjective leg length discrepancy (typically longer on the side of THA) is commonly corrected with improved posture and stretching of hip abductor muscles [5].

Early protected ambulation progresses toward independent mobility as tolerated on the basis of the individual's response and weight-bearing restrictions. Ambulation training after THA begins with appropriate assistive devices, such as a rolling walker. Weight-bearing restrictions in the postoperative phase are used to prevent "out of plane" or torsional forces on the implant. Patients should be taught to ascend stairs one step at a time and should lead with the contralateral limb to avoid torsional forces on the implant [5]. Determination of weight-bearing restrictions is made by surgeon preference and surgical technique; little literature exists to support consensus guidelines for weight-bearing restrictions after THA. However, there is some evidence to support early rehabilitation with unrestricted weight bearing after uncemented THA with a reciprocating gait pattern [9]. These patients should use protected weight bearing with stair climbing during the first weeks after surgery because of excessive forces through the hip [9]. Most patients should be able to ambulate community distances, initially with a walker or a cane, and then advance to ambulation without an assistive device or return to their presurgical baseline within 4 to 12 weeks after hip arthroplasty. The rate of advancement in gait training is usually limited by the weight-bearing status established at the time of surgery.

Postoperative gait changes include decreased velocity, decreased stride length, decreased sagittal hip range of motion, reduced peak hip abduction, and increased peak hip flexion and extension moments [10]. Gait symmetry and velocity at 1 year after THA were most improved with supervised rehabilitation focusing on muscle strengthening and motor relearning [11].

The existing literature does not allow us to draw definitive conclusions on sports in general or high-risk activity after THA [12]. Most surgeons agree that patients should avoid contact or high-impact athletic activity after THA. Some patients can return to noncontact, low-impact athletic activity between 3 and 6 months after surgery; however, the true relationship between athletic activity and rate of revision surgery remains unclear [12]. Patients should be counseled of the details of possible complications, prosthesis failure, and revision surgery before resuming athletic activity [12].

Activities of daily living are assessed, and each individual's unique needs and goals drive the specific, individualized plan of care and treatments given. Upper and lower body bathing and dressing within hip and weight-bearing precautions are essential components of the rehabilitation program. Appropriate adaptive equipment including sock aids, reachers, and dressing sticks to perform lower body self-care should be provided. Bathroom transfers and kitchen activities are also incorporated into the rehabilitation program. Often, raised toilet seats or commodes and tub transfer benches are helpful and necessary to prevent excessive hip flexion and dislocation in the sitting position.

Discharge planning to the next level of care, including durable medical equipment, medical follow-up, and follow-up rehabilitation services (either in the home or in the community), must be communicated to the patient and family. Discharge to an inpatient rehabilitation facility has been influenced by the Centers for Medicare and Medicaid Services, which has determined that hospitals are eligible for payment of rehabilitation after total joint arthroplasty if (1) it is a bilateral procedure, (2) age is older than 85 years, or (3) body mass index is above 50. A typical total hip replacement clinical pathway or protocol for inpatient rehabilitation is now a 7- to 10-day program [13]. Many published sources outline the benefits as well as the elements of the total hip replacement clinical pathway; however, there is a need to update the literature, given the changes in surgical technique [14–16]. There is also a shift toward rapid discharge to home from acute care with an outpatient rehabilitation program, especially in the era of minimally invasive surgery [17]. A Cochrane review with silver level of evidence showed that early multidisciplinary rehabilitation can improve outcomes with regard to activity levels and postoperative participation [18]. There is a paucity of literature discussing the optimal intensity, frequency, cost-effectiveness, and long-term effects of early multidisciplinary rehabilitation.

Individuals who undergo THA revision surgery have a more difficult postoperative rehabilitation experience; they often show less progress in functional independence measures, longer rehabilitation length of stay, and greater hospital charges compared with patients undergoing primary hip replacement surgery. These differences in outcomes are even more pronounced if an infected prosthesis is the cause of the revision arthroplasty [19].

Procedures

Wound care, staple or suture removal, and Steri-Strip application are typically performed after THA.

Surgery

Most surgeons will consider THA if a patient is having severe pain that is affecting the patient's quality of life, there are signs of degenerative joint disease on radiographs, and the patient has maximized conservative treatment options. However, there are no minimum standards or universally accepted criteria for patient selection. Patient selection may also be influenced by the patient's ability to cooperate with the rehabilitation program after surgery, serious comorbid medical conditions, morbid obesity, high levels of activity, high fall risk, or younger age [20]. These factors can contribute to early failure and complications. Contraindications include local or systemic infection, neuromuscular compromise, dementia, poor bone quality, and poor vascular supply.

The THA components include a femoral stem, a femoral neck, a femoral head, and an acetabular shell or cup with a polyethylene liner (Fig. 61.6). This allows resurfacing of both sides of the hip joint and permits the highest degree of "customization" for each individual. Surgical technique and decision-making are beyond the scope of this text; however, there are some considerations that will have implications for rehabilitation.

Rehabilitation of THA will be affected by fixation techniques: cemented versus uncemented. The cemented technique is used only on the femoral component. After a cement restrictor plug is placed in the distal femoral canal, polymethyl methacrylate cement is freshly made and inserted into the femoral canal by pressurized cementing technique. Insertion of the femoral stem creates an intimate fit of the prosthesis to the intramedullary canal with a small circumferential cement mantle. Cement polymerization rigidly fixates the femoral component. Frequently, the patient with a cemented prosthesis is allowed to bear weight as tolerated immediately, whereas the individual with a noncemented press-fit prosthesis often must wait for 6 to 8 weeks before fully bearing weight to allow stability by bone ingrowth. Rehabilitation will also be affected if surgical technique includes trochanteric osteotomy. If a trochanteric osteotomy is performed during the surgery, hip abduction resistance exercises are usually restricted.

The changing population of patients undergoing THA is driving the current trends in THA. The high-demand, younger patient population with hip disease has led to the use of alternative bearing surfaces (ceramic-ceramic articulations, metal-on-metal articulations, and improved polyethylene surfaces). These alternative bearing surfaces are intended to improve durability and wear for highly active patients. There is growing interest in the orthopedic literature on the safety and outcomes of these alternative surfaces; however, there is no superior articulation at this time. Less invasive and minimally invasive approaches have been developed to facilitate rehabilitation and to decrease rehabilitation time. Navigation technology has been used in total knee arthroplasty but is now being considered to assist with implant positioning in hip replacement (particularly with the use of minimally invasive approaches). Bone-preserving techniques, including resurfacing techniques and short-stemmed femoral implants, have also been considered for the younger and more active patients undergoing THA. The long-term effects and outcomes of these trends have yet to be determined in the literature but are currently being studied.

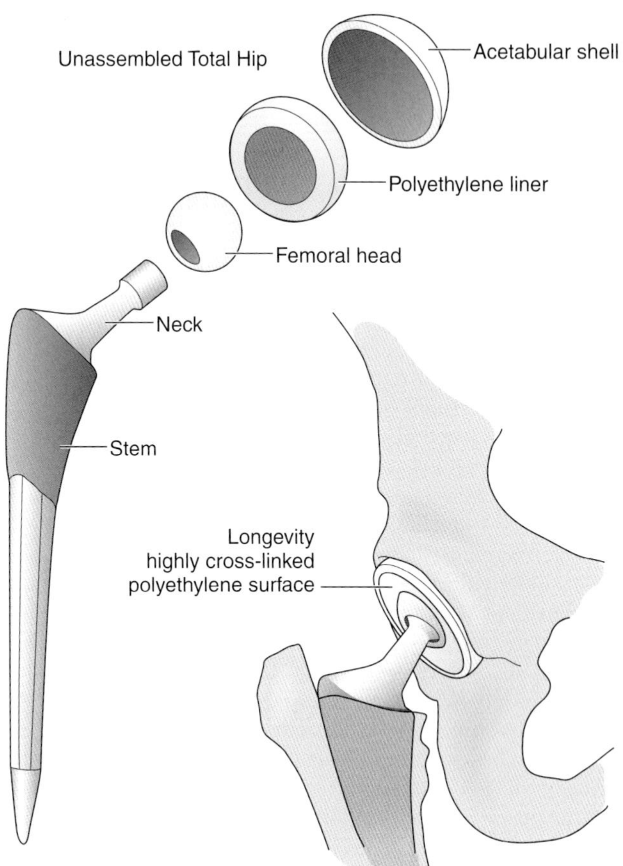

FIGURE 61.6 The components of a total hip replacement.

Whereas all patient subgroups have demonstrated functional improvements from joint arthroplasty, younger age and male sex are associated with the increased risk of revision surgery. In one systematic review, older age and male sex are associated with increased mortality, and older age (particularly in women) is related to worse function after arthroplasty [21].

Potential Disease Complications

Common physical impairments of hip disease after THA include decreased muscle strength, limited hip range of motion, limited flexibility, and abnormalities of gait. Hip joint weakness has been shown to persist at 2 years after surgery, indicating a need for prolonged exercise. Current data suggest that THA patients continue to experience physical and functional limitations lasting at least 1 year postoperatively. Persistent groin pain after an otherwise successful surgery has been documented in as high as 18% of total hip arthroplasties [22]. Therefore it is reasonable to have patients continue with therapeutic exercises to address these limitations well beyond the early recovery period (first 12 weeks) [23,24].

Potential Treatment Complications

Perioperative and postoperative complications after THA include infection, deep venous thrombosis, pulmonary embolism, dislocation, periprosthetic fracture, nerve injury, iliopsoas impingement, limb length inequality, anemia, bleeding, myocardial infarction, and death.

The incidence of deep venous thrombosis after total hip implantation without prophylactic anticoagulation is 45% to 57%; the incidence of proximal clot (defined as any thrombosis in the popliteal vein or more proximal) is between 23% and 36%; and the incidence of fatal pulmonary embolism is between 0.7% and 30% [25]. Clinical practice guidelines encourage surgeons to assess the thrombosis and bleeding risk for each individual patient and help guide which prophylactic treatment is indicated [6]. Postoperative limb swelling should trigger deep venous thrombosis surveillance screening with venous ultrasonography and Doppler wave signal analysis (commonly referred to as duplex scanning). If pulmonary embolism is suspected in a patient with hypoxia or shortness of breath, chest radiography, electrocardiography, and ventilation/perfusion scanning or computed tomographic pulmonary angiography are included as part of the evaluation.

Careful attention is given to treatment of anemia because patients with adequate hemoglobin levels generally tolerate activity well and progress in rehabilitation more readily than do those with low hemoglobin levels. Adequate nutrition, iron supplements, vitamins, and, if needed, erythropoietin can be used. Blood transfusions may be necessary if the hemoglobin level continues to drift downward and there is concern of hemodynamic instability or if the patient has symptoms or physical examination findings indicative of low perfusion status.

A hip dislocation is not subtle and should be suspected if the patient cannot endure weight bearing, the limb is acutely shortened and internally rotated, or the patient is intolerant of gentle hip motion because of excessive pain. A patient can usually give an exact moment or event that led to the dislocation. A dislocation often results in a significant functional setback as the patient is often more cautious and fearful of performing activities of daily living and mobility training. Reduction typically requires sedation and muscle relaxation and may require a return trip to the operating room.

Wound care of the incision line is accomplished with dry sterile dressing changes once or twice a day. Once wound drainage ceases, a dressing is no longer essential. Tape burns around the surgical incision are a common problem and can be treated with a hydrogel pad such as DuoDerm for approximately 1 week. Serous drainage without signs of erythema or induration is commonplace for 3 or 4 days postoperatively, but persistent drainage beyond 7 days should trigger clinical suspicion for wound infection. Wound problems should be communicated to the operative surgeon for collaboration on additional management including cultures, antibiotics, and more invasive intervention if necessary.

Late prosthetic hip infection by a hematogenous source can be a serious complication, often requiring extensive hospitalization, intravenous administration of antibiotics, and removal of the hip prosthesis. Eventual reimplantation is done after the infection is eradicated. Currently, there is no consensus for antibiotic prophylaxis before invasive procedures (dental work, colonoscopy). Most surgeons do recommend antibiotic prophylaxis for their patients after THA, but there is no consensus on how long after THA, if not indefinitely, they should have antibiotic prophylaxis.

Iliopsoas impingement can cause significant pain in the otherwise successful THA patient. Typically, the culprit is iatrogenic, from an oversized acetabulum component with anterior overhang, relative retroversion of the components, or protrusion of fixation screws, which results in iliopsoas tendinitis from tendon impingement.

References

[1] Gomez PF, Morcuende JA. Early attempts at hip arthroplasty. Iowa Orthop J 2005;25:25–9.
[2] Jones CA, Pohar S. Health-related quality of life after total joint arthroplasty: a scoping review. Clin Geriatr Med 2012;28:395–429.
[3] U.S. Department of Health and Human Services, Centers for Disease Control and Prevention, National Center for Health Statistics. http://www.cdc.gov/nchs/; 2009 [accessed November 2012].
[4] Cooper HJ, Ranawat AS, Potter HG, et al. Magnetic resonance imaging in the diagnosis and management of hip pain after total hip arthroplasty. J Arthroplasty 2009;24:661–7.
[5] Bhave A. Rehabilitation after total hip and total knee arthroplasty. In: Barrack RL, editor. American Academy of Orthopaedic Surgeons' orthopaedic knowledge update. Hip and knee reconstruction. 3rd ed. Rosemont, Ill: American Academy of Orthopaedic Surgeons; 2006. p. 295–308.
[6] Jahr JS, Breitmeyer JB, Pan C, et al. Safety and efficacy of intravenous acetaminophen in the elderly after major orthopaedic surgery: subset data analysis from 3, randomized, placebo-controlled trials. Am J Ther 2012;19:66.
[7] The American Academy of Orthopaedic Surgeons. Preventing venous thromboembolic disease in patients undergoing elective hip and knee arthroplasty; Sept. 2011. http://www.aaos.org/research/guidelines/VTE/VTE_guideline.asp [accessed November 2012].
[8] Restrepo C, Mortazavi SM, Brothers J, et al. Hip dislocation: are hip precautions necessary in anterior approaches? Clin Orthop Relat Res 2011;469:417–22.
[9] Hol AM, van Grinsven S, Lucas C, et al. Partial versus unrestricted weight bearing after an uncemented femoral stem in total hip arthroplasty: recommendation of a concise rehabilitation protocol from a systematic review of the literature. Arch Orthop Trauma Surg 2010;130:547–55.
[10] Ewen AM, Stewart S, St Clair Gibson A, et al. Post-operative gait analysis in total hip replacement patients—a review of current literature and meta-analysis. Gait Posture 2012;36:1–6.
[11] Hodt-Billington C, Helbostad JL, Vervaat W, et al. Changes in gait symmetry, gait velocity and self-reported function following total hip replacement. J Rehabil Med 2011;43:787–93.
[12] Vogel LA, Carotenuto G, Basti JJ, et al. Physical activity after total joint arthroplasty. Sports Health 2011;3:441–50.
[13] Wang A, Hall S, Gilbey H, et al. Patient variability and the design of clinical pathways after primary total hip replacement surgery. J Qual Clin Pract 1997;17:123–9.
[14] Aspen Reference Group. Clinical pathways for medical rehabilitation. Gaithersburg, Md: Aspen; 1998.
[15] Cameron H, Brotzman SB, Boolos M. Rehabilitation after total joint arthroplasty. In: Brotzman SB, editor. Clinical orthopaedic rehabilitation. St. Louis: Mosby; 1996. p. 284–311.
[16] Dowsey MM, Kilgour ML, Santamaria NM, Choong PF. Clinical pathways in hip and knee arthroplasty: a prospective randomized controlled study. Med J Aust 1999;170:59–62.
[17] Berger RA, Jacobs JJ, Meneghini RM, et al. Rapid rehabilitation and recovery with minimally invasive total hip arthroplasty. Clin Orthop Relat Res 2004;429:239–47.

[18] Khan F, Ng L, Gonzalez S, et al. Multidisciplinary rehabilitation programmes following joint replacement at the hip and knee in chronic arthropathy [review]. Cochrane Database Syst Rev 2008;2, CD004957.
[19] Vincent KR, Vincent HK, Lee LW, et al. Outcomes after inpatient rehabilitation of primary and revision total hip arthroplasty. Arch Phys Med Rehabil 2006;87:1026–32.
[20] Mancuso CA, Ranawat CS, Esdaile JM, et al. Indications for total hip and total knee arthroplasties: results of orthopaedic surveys. J Arthroplasty 1996;11:34–46.
[21] Santaguida PL, Hawker GA, Hudak PL, et al. Patient characteristics affecting the prognosis of total hip and knee joint arthroplasty: a systematic review. J Can Chir 2008;51:428–36.
[22] Henderson RA, Lachiewicz PF. Groin pain after replacement of the hip. J Bone Joint Surg Br 2012;94:145–51.
[23] Long WT, Dorr LD, Healy B, Perry J. Functional recovery of noncemented total hip arthroplasty. Clin Orthop Relat Res 1993;228: 73–7.
[24] Brander VA, Stulberg SD, Chang RW. Rehabilitation following hip and knee arthroplasty. Phys Med Rehabil Clin N Am 1994;5: 815–36.
[25] Colwell CW, Hardwick ME. Venous thromboembolic disease and prophylaxis in total joint arthroplasty. In: Barrack RL, editor. American Academy of Orthopaedic Surgeons' orthopaedic knowledge update. Hip and knee reconstruction. 3rd ed. Rosemont, Ill: American Academy of Orthopaedic Surgeons; 2006. p. 233–40.

CHAPTER 62

Greater Trochanteric Pain Syndrome

Michael Fredericson, MD
Cindy Lin, MD
Kelvin Chew, MBBCh, MSpMed

Synonyms

Trochanteric bursitis
Hip bursitis
Gluteus medius tendinopathy

ICD-9 Codes

719.45	**Pain in hip joint**
726.5	**Trochanteric bursitis**
843.8	**Tear/sprain of gluteus muscle (hip and thigh)**
726.5	**Tendinitis of hip region**

ICD-10 Codes

M25.551	**Pain in right hip**
M25.552	**Pain in left hip**
M25.559	**Pain in unspecified hip**
M70.60	**Trochanteric bursitis of hip, unspecified hip**
S76.001	**Injury of muscle, fascia and tendon of right hip**
S76.002	**Injury of muscle, fascia and tendon of left hip**
S76.009	**Injury of muscle, fascia and tendon of unspecified hip**

Add seventh character to S76 for episode of care (A—initial encounter, D—subsequent encounter, S—sequela)

M70.61	**Trochanteric bursitis of hip, right hip**
M70.62	**Trochanteric bursitis of hip, left hip**
M76.00	**Gluteal tendinitis, unspecified hip**
M76.01	**Gluteal tendinitis, right hip**
M76.02	**Gluteal tendinitis, left hip**

Definition

Greater trochanteric pain syndrome (GTPS) is a common cause of lateral extra-articular hip pain. GTPS is clinically characterized by peritrochanteric pain and focal tenderness [1]. GTPS describes a continuum of disorders with causes ranging from gluteus medius and minimus tears, tendinitis, or tendinopathy to trochanteric bursitis and external coxa saltans [2]. Previously, it was thought that excessive gluteal tendon friction at the greater trochanter attachment led to subgluteus maximus bursal inflammation; hence, it was called greater trochanteric bursitis [3]. However, histopathologic and imaging studies have not identified bursal inflammation as a consistent finding, thus leading to the current clinical description of this entity as GTPS [2].

The peak incidence of GTPS is between the fourth and sixth decades of life. It occurs four times more frequently in women than in men, which may be due to gender differences in pelvic and lower limb biomechanics [4,5]. It affects up to 10% of the general population and has been reported in up to 20% of patients with low back pain [5,6]. GTPS can result from direct macrotrauma after contusions from falls or contact sports [7]. However, it is more often due to cumulative microtrauma and abnormal loading forces on the gluteus medius and minimus tendons inserting on the greater trochanter. It has been suggested that gluteal tendon degeneration and tears at the greater trochanter attachment may induce secondary reactive inflammation in the bursae [4]. Contributing factors include hip or knee osteoarthritis, lumbar spine degenerative disorders, obesity, true or functional leg length discrepancies, gait abnormalities, and iliotibial band tightness [5,6,8]. GTPS can also occur after hip surgery, such as femoral osteotomy [9], hip joint replacement, or arthroscopic surgery, and from postoperative hip abductor weakness. Less common causes to consider in the differential diagnosis include infection and inflammatory arthritis if there are systemic symptoms and signs, lateral hip swelling, redness, or heat [10–12].

The greater trochanter of the femur is the insertion site of the gluteus medius, gluteus minimus, piriformis, and obturator internus muscles, and it is also the origin of the vastus lateralis muscle [13]. Three main bursae surround the greater trochanter, including the subgluteal maximus, medius, and minimus bursae [14]. The subgluteus maximus bursa is the largest bursa and lies lateral to the greater trochanter beneath the gluteus maximus and iliotibial tract. The subgluteus medius bursa lies deep beneath the gluteus medius tendon and posterosuperior to the lateral facet of the greater trochanter. The subgluteus minimus bursa lies beneath the gluteus minimus tendon at the anterosuperior edge of the greater trochanter. The subgluteus maximus bursa is most often involved in cases of trochanteric bursitis [3].

Symptoms

The main clinical symptom is lateral hip pain at the greater trochanteric region. The pain can radiate down the lateral aspect of the thigh as a pseudoradiculopathy that does not extend past the knee. Symptoms are exacerbated by hip movements, in particular external rotation and abduction. Pain may also be provoked by standing, walking, stair climbing, crossing the legs, running, or running on banked surfaces. Recent changes in physical activity or sports training programs may precede symptoms. Sleep may be affected with pain aggravated by lying in the lateral decubitus position directly on the affected side or from lying with the affected side up and in passive hip adduction.

Physical Examination

In GTPS, localized tenderness is found on direct palpation of the greater trochanter. Lateral hip pain may be reproduced on examination with resisted hip abduction with the patient in a side-lying position. Pain can also be elicited with active hip internal or external rotation at 45 degrees of hip flexion [15].

Evaluation for gait, hip, or spine disorders and leg length discrepancy is important as abnormal motion and joint loading in one region of the kinetic chain can contribute to the development of GTPS. The Trendelenburg sign can be seen in GTPS as a result of weakness or inhibition of the hip abductor muscles [16]. The gluteus medius and minimus play an important role in hip abduction and pelvic stabilization during gait. In GTPS, with weight bearing on the affected limb during single-leg stance, the hip abductors are unable to stabilize the pelvis, resulting in contralateral pelvic drop [17]. Activity-related pain, particularly in the anterior groin, or restricted hip range of motion may indicate intra-articular hip disease, such as osteoarthritis, femoroacetabular impingement, or labral disorders that warrant further investigation. Lumbosacral radiculitis or radiculopathy should be ruled out with detailed history and neurologic examination; the neurologic examination findings should be normal in GTPS.

Functional Limitations

GTPS can limit activity and mobility and cause further weakness of the lateral hip rotator muscles and deconditioning. This can have an impact on basic activities of daily life, including walking, running, and stair climbing. Pain may also interrupt sleep.

Diagnostic Studies

Laboratory studies, although seldom required, should be performed if an infectious or rheumatologic process is suspected. The diagnosis of GTPS can usually be made by history and physical examination. Imaging studies are used mainly to exclude other underlying causes of lateral hip pain or when symptoms do not respond to conservative treatments.

Magnetic resonance imaging can be useful in cases in which there is clinical concern for other causes of lateral hip pain. Magnetic resonance imaging or ultrasonography can be used to detect tendinopathy, muscle tears, cortical irregularity, bursal fluid or thickening, or muscle atrophy [18,19]. The identification of bursal fluid on magnetic resonance imaging or ultrasound examination is thought to be a secondary manifestation of local disease rather than the primary process in most cases of GTPS [18].

Ultrasound examination can be helpful in visualizing the muscle insertions on the facets of the greater trochanter to localize the pathologic process. The insertion for the gluteus minimus tendon is the anterior facet; for the gluteus medius tendon, the lateral and superolateral facets; and for the subgluteal maximus and trochanteric bursa, the posterior facet (Fig. 62.1) [20]. A "bald" facet, with absence of the tendinous insertion, suggests a complete tear. Anechoic defects within the tendon suggest partial tears. Gluteal tendinosis on ultrasound examination is identified by tendon thickening, heterogeneous signal, and decreased echogenicity [18].

Hip plain films may demonstrate calcifications in the region of the bursa or in the gluteal tendon insertions related to calcific tendinosis [2,18].

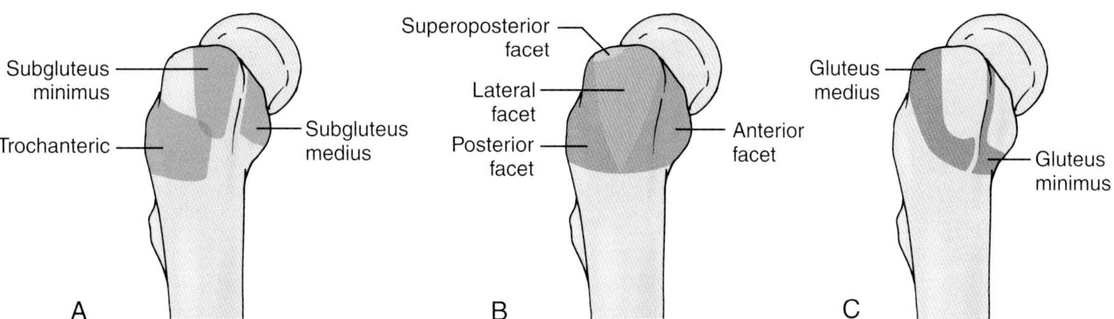

FIGURE 62.1 Anatomy of greater trochanter with tendinous insertion sites and bursae. **A,** The three main bursae and their positions. **B,** Geometry of greater trochanter with different facets. **C,** Footprints of gluteus medius and minimus tendon insertions. *(Modified from Domb BG, Nasser RM, Botser IB. Partial-thickness tears of the gluteus medius: rationale and technique for trans-tendinous endoscopic repair. Arthroscopy 2010;26:1697-1705.)*

Differential Diagnosis

Osteoarthritis of the hip
Lumbosacral radiculopathy
Lumbosacral radiculitis
Leg length discrepancy
Avascular necrosis of the femoral head
Iliotibial band syndrome
Hip stress fracture
Acetabular labral disease
Tumors

Treatment

Initial

Initial treatment is to provide acute pain relief through icing, analgesic pain medications, and sports and activity modification, such as avoidance of stair climbing and other exacerbating activities. Direct pressure on the painful lateral hip should be avoided; as such, recommendations on sleep positioning can be given. Gentle stretching of the iliotibial band, tensor fascia lata, and gluteal muscles is encouraged with avoidance of end-range hip motion in the acute phase.

Rehabilitation

Physical therapy entails a combination of strengthening, stretching, and correction of identifiable underlying spine or hip disorders that precipitated GTPS. Strengthening should focus on the core and hip abductors, extensors, and external rotators with progression to eccentric loading of the gluteal muscles in cases of tendinopathy. Myofascial soft tissue release, stretching, or therapeutic ultrasound may be helpful for the tensor fascia lata–iliotibial band complex.

Focal ice massage may be useful at the outset of the injury. Extracorporeal shock wave therapy can be beneficial for pain relief during the subacute to chronic phases [21]. Addressing gait abnormalities through orthotics or assistive devices, such as walkers or canes, should also be considered. Weight loss is advised in obesity.

Procedures

For cases unresponsive to noninvasive treatments, corticosteroid injections combined with local anesthetic can be used. Whereas some studies have found corticosteroid injections to be effective in the short term in improving pain and activity, other studies report incomplete long-term relief and symptom recurrence [21–24]. The injection technique involves the patient's lying in the lateral decubitus position with the affected side up and the knees flexed comfortably. The point of maximal tenderness over the greater trochanter is identified and marked. Under sterile conditions, a syringe with a 25-gauge needle, containing triamcinolone (40 mg) with 1% lidocaine (3 to 4 mL), is advanced until contact is made with the greater trochanter bone; the needle is then withdrawn 3 or 4 mm. Once negative aspiration has verified that the needle is not intravascular, the solution is introduced after a lack of resistance is detected. Patients are reevaluated within a month after injection to assess therapeutic response.

Ultrasound or fluoroscopic guidance may be used to enhance precise injection placement. However, fluoroscopically guided trochanteric injections have not been found to be superior to blind injections in terms of patient outcomes and are associated with increased cost [24]. Caution must be exercised with repeated injection because it may be associated with muscle and tendon weakening or rupture [25].

Surgery

In refractory cases and if significant functional limitations are present, surgery can be considered. Depending on the underlying pathologic process, this may involve arthroscopic bursectomy [26], iliotibial band release or lengthening, or open or endoscopic gluteal tendon repair [20,27,28].

Potential Disease Complications

GTPS should be a self-limited condition. If symptoms persist, consider other underlying causes. If the underlying predisposing factors are not appropriately addressed, the syndrome may progress to chronic pain, which can lead to muscle deconditioning, hip abductor muscle weakness, functional decline, and increased risk of falls in elderly or frail patients.

Potential Treatment Complications

Complications from anti-inflammatory medications include drug hypersensitivity, gastric ulceration, and renal toxicity. Complications from corticosteroid injections include bleeding, bruising, infection, drug hypersensitivity reactions, tendon ruptures, nerve injury, fat atrophy, and skin hypopigmentation [23,25].

References

[1] Karpinski MR, Piggott H. Greater trochanteric pain syndrome. A report of 15 cases. J Bone Joint Surg Br 1985;67:762–3.
[2] Silva F, Adams T, Feinstein J, Arroyo RA. Trochanteric bursitis: refuting the myth of inflammation. J Clin Rheumatol 2008;14:82–6.
[3] Dunn T, Heller CA, McCarthy SW, Dos Remedios C. Anatomical study of the "trochanteric bursa." Clin Anat 2003;16:233–40.
[4] Ferber R, Davis IM, Williams DS. Gender differences in lower extremity mechanics during running. Clin Biomech (Bristol, Avon) 2003;18:350–79.
[5] Segal NA, Felson DT, Torner JC, et al. Greater trochanteric pain syndrome: epidemiology and associated factors. Arch Phys Med Rehabil 2007;88:988–92.
[6] Tortolani PJ, Carbone JJ, Quartararo LG. Greater trochanteric pain syndrome in patients referred to orthopedic spine specialists. Spine J 2002;2:251–4.
[7] Haller CC, Coleman PA, Estes NC, Grisolia A. Traumatic trochanteric bursitis. Kans Med 1989;90:17–8, 22.
[8] Shbeeb ML, Matteson EL. Trochanteric bursitis (greater trochanteric pain syndrome). Mayo Clin Proc 1996;71:565–9.
[9] Glassman AH. Complications of trochanteric osteotomy. Orthop Clin North Am 1992;23:321–33.
[10] Jaovisidha S, Chen C, Ryu KN, et al. Tuberculous tenosynovitis and bursitis: imaging findings in 21 cases. Radiology 1996;201:507–13.
[11] Yamamoto T, Iwasaki Y, Kurosaka M. Tuberculosis of the greater trochanteric bursa occurring 51 years after tuberculous nephritis. Clin Rheumatol 2002;21:397–400.
[12] Tanaka H, Kido K, Wakisaka A, et al. Trochanteric bursitis in rheumatoid arthritis. J Rheumatol 2002;29:1340–1.

[13] Jenkins DB. Hollinshead's functional anatomy of the limbs and back. 9th ed. St. Louis: Saunders Elsevier; 2009.
[14] Bencardino JT, Palmer WE. Imaging of hip disorders in athletes. Radiol Clin North Am 2002;40:267–87.
[15] Ho GW, Howard TM. Greater trochanteric pain syndrome: more than bursitis and iliotibial tract friction. Curr Sports Med Rep 2012;11:232–8.
[16] Bird PA, Oakley SP, Shnier R. Prospective evaluation of magnetic resonance imaging and physical examination findings in patients with greater trochanteric pain syndrome. Arthritis Rheum 2001;44:2138–45.
[17] Hardcastle P, Nade S. The significance of the Trendelenburg test. J Bone Joint Surg Br 1985;67:741–6.
[18] Kong A, Van der Vliet A, Zadow S. MRI and US of gluteal tendinopathy in greater trochanteric pain syndrome. Eur Radiol 2007;17:1772–83.
[19] Kingzett-Taylor A, Tirman PF, Feller J, et al. Tendinosis and tears of the gluteus medius and minimus muscles as a cause of hip pain. AJR Am J Roentgenol 1999;173:1123–6.
[20] Domb BG, Nasser RM, Botser IB. Partial-thickness tears of the gluteus medius: rationale and technique for trans-tendinous endoscopic repair. Arthroscopy 2010;26:1697–705.
[21] Rompe JD, Segal NA, Cacchio A, et al. Home training, local corticosteroid injection, or radial shock wave therapy for greater trochanter pain syndrome. Am J Sports Med 2009;37:1981–90.
[22] Shbeeb MI, O'Duffy JD, Michet Jr CJ, et al. Evaluation of glucocorticosteroid injection for the treatment of trochanteric bursitis. J Rheumatol 1996;23:2104–6.
[23] Brinks A, van Rijn RM, Willemsen SP, et al. Corticosteroid injections for greater trochanteric pain syndrome: a randomized controlled trial in primary care. Ann Fam Med 2011;9:226–34.
[24] Cohen SP, Strassels SA, Foster L, et al. Comparison of fluoroscopically guided and blind corticosteroid injections for greater trochanteric pain syndrome: multicentre randomised controlled trial. BMJ 2009;338:b1088.
[25] Speed CA. Fortnightly review; corticosteroid injections in tendon lesions. BMJ 2001;323:382–6.
[26] Fox JL. The role of arthroscopic bursectomy in the treatment of trochanteric bursitis. Arthroscopy 2002;18:E34.
[27] Slawski DP, Howard RF. Surgical management of refractory trochanteric bursitis. Am J Sports Med 1997;25:86–9.
[28] Bradley DM, Dillingham MF. Bursoscopy of the trochanteric bursa. Arthroscopy 1998;14:884–7.

SECTION VIII
Knee and Leg

CHAPTER 63

Anterior Cruciate Ligament Tear

William Micheo, MD
Eduardo Amy, MD
Fernando Sepúlveda, MD

Synonyms

Anterior cruciate ligament (ACL) tear
ACL sprain
ACL-deficient knee

ICD-9 Codes

717.83	**Old disruption of anterior cruciate ligament**
844.2	**Cruciate injury, acute**

ICD -10 Codes

M23.611	**Spontaneous disruption of anterior cruciate ligament of right knee**
M23.612	**Spontaneous disruption of anterior cruciate ligament of left knee**
M23.619	**Spontaneous disruption of anterior cruciate ligament of unspecified knee**
S83.104	**Dislocation of right knee**
S83.105	**Dislocation of left knee**
S83.106	**Dislocation of unspecified knee**

Definition

The anterior cruciate ligament (ACL) is an intra-articular structure essential for the normal function of the knee. It is commonly injured during activities that involve complex movements, such as cutting and pivoting. It is estimated that 1 in 3000 individuals sustains an ACL injury each year in the United States, corresponding to an overall injury rate of approximately 100,000 injuries annually [1]. The injury usually results from a sudden deceleration during high-velocity movements in which a forceful contraction of the quadriceps muscle is required. Other mechanisms of injury are valgus stress, hyperextension, and external rotation, as in landing from a jump, and severe internal rotation of the knee with varus or hyperextension [1]. Approximately 70% of the acute ACL injuries are sports related and affect women more than men, particularly in sports such as basketball and soccer [2]. Non–sports-related injuries might include a patient slipping on ice or falling from considerable height and landing with the knee in hyperextension and valgus. In the last two decades, there has also been an increase in the incidence and appropriate diagnosis of ACL injuries in children associated with more participation in high-demand contact and noncontact sports, increased awareness of the injury, and better imaging techniques [3]. Risk factors associated with ACL injuries can be classified as anatomic, hormonal, environmental, biomechanical, and neuromuscular. Some of the modifiable risk factors include proprioception, core strength, decreased hamstring strength (relative to quadriceps strength), conditioning, footwear, playing surface, weather conditions, training techniques, and biomechanical variations in landing from a jump or cutting. Nonmodifiable factors include gender, reduced femoral intercondylar notch size, increased slope of the tibial plateau, knee hyperextension, physiologic rotatory laxity, small ACL size, and familial predisposition [1,4–6].

The ACL may be partially or completely torn. It also may be injured in combination with other structures, most commonly tears of the medial collateral ligament and medial meniscus.

The ACL is a collagenous structure approximately 38 mm in length and 10 mm in width. The ligament arises from a wide base in the tibia anterolateral to the anterior tibial spine. It then traverses the knee in a posterolateral direction, attaching in a broad fan-like fashion at the posterolateral corner of the intercondylar notch of the femur. According to Fu and collaborators, it is organized in two major bundles named after their insertion sites on the tibia [7]. The anteromedial bundle, which tightens in flexion and is the longer of the two, controls anterior translation of the tibia on the femur. The posterolateral bundle, which tightens in extension and internal rotation, controls rotation [8–10].

Biomechanical studies, with use of cadaver specimens, have evaluated the forces that affect the ACL [11]. These forces are highest in the last 30 degrees of extension, in hyperextension, and under other load conditions, including anterior tibial translation, internal rotation, and varus. The ACL is a static stabilizer of the knee with a primary function of resisting hyperextension and anterior tibial translation in flexion and providing rotatory control. It is also a secondary restraint to valgus and varus forces in all degrees of flexion.

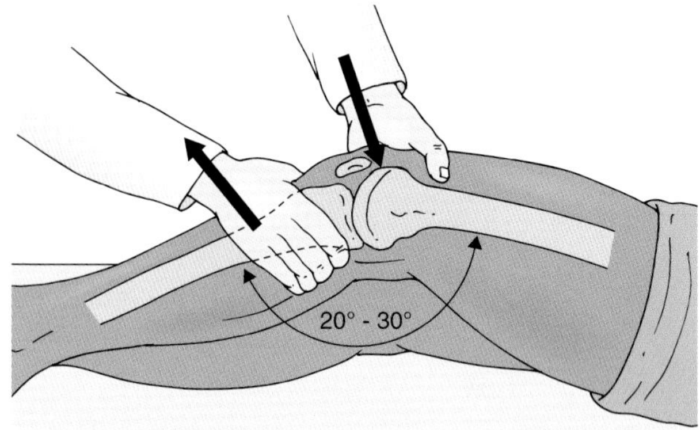

FIGURE 63.1 Position for the Lachman test. The knee is flexed at 20 to 30 degrees. The distal femur is stabilized with one hand while the other hand pulls the proximal tibia anteriorly.

Symptoms

Individuals usually present with pain, immediate swelling, and limited range of motion. They may give a history of hearing a "pop." In an acute injury, the individual will have severe pain and difficulty with walking. In a chronic injury, a patient may have a history of recurrent episodes of knee instability associated with swelling and limited motion. Patients may describe locking or a "giving way" phenomenon. They may also give a history of a remote injury to the knee that was not rehabilitated.

Physical Examination

The physical examination has been found to be sensitive and specific in the diagnosis of ACL tears and correlates with arthroscopically documented knee injuries [1]. The clinician should observe the knee for asymmetry, palpate for areas of tenderness, measure active and passive range of motion, and document muscle atrophy. The apprehension test to rule out patellar instability, valgus and varus testing with the knee in full extension and 30 degrees of flexion to evaluate the collateral ligaments, and joint line palpation as well as the McMurray test to evaluate the meniscus are all important tests to look for injury of associated structures.

The key physical examination maneuver for evaluating the integrity of the ACL in the patient with an acute injury is the Lachman test, in which an anterior force is applied to the tibia with the knee in 30 degrees of flexion while the clinician tries to reproduce anterior migration of the tibia on the femur (Fig. 63.1). Another important test in the acute setting is the lateral pivot shift maneuver, in which the examiner attempts to reproduce anterolateral instability by internally rotating the leg, applying a valgus stress to the knee as it is flexed, and feeling for anterior migration of the tibia on the femur (Fig. 63.2). After injury, the Lachman test is most important for acute diagnosis, whereas the lateral pivot shift test has shown a better correlation to future sports participation and functional stability [1,12]. In the patient who is able to flex the knee to 90 degrees, particularly in chronic or recurrent injury, the anterior drawer test, in which an anterior force is applied to the tibia, should be performed (Fig. 63.3). In acute injury, this test may provide a false-negative result because the secondary stabilizers may reduce anterior tibial displacement with the knee in 90 degrees of flexion [13]. It is important to complete the examination by performing the posterior drawer test, which evaluates the posterior cruciate ligament; a torn posterior cruciate ligament with posterior tibial subluxation may give a false-positive result of the anterior drawer maneuver as the tibia is reduced. In general, findings should be normal on the neurologic examination, including muscle strength, sensation, and reflexes; however, there may be some associated weakness (particularly of the knee extensors) due to pain inhibition or disuse.

Functional Limitations

Limitations include reduced knee motion, muscle weakness, and pain that interferes with activities involving pivoting and jumping. Recurrent episodes of instability may limit participation in strenuous sports, such as basketball, soccer, tennis, and volleyball [14,15]. These episodes of the knee's giving way may result in increased ligamentous laxity, leading to limitations with activities of daily living, such as going down stairs and changing directions while walking.

Diagnostic Studies

Diagnostic studies include plain radiographs to rule out intra-articular fractures (tibial spine avulsion, Segond fracture), loose bodies, and arthritic changes. These include the standing anteroposterior view, lateral view, tunnel view, standing posteroanterior 45-degree flexion view, and Merchant view of the patella. Magnetic resonance imaging may be indicated in the acute setting to evaluate associated pathologic changes, such as bone bruises, meniscal tears, and other ligamentous injuries, and to aid in treatment planning of combined injuries. In the pediatric and adolescent athlete, magnetic resonance imaging may also give information about physeal injuries that may otherwise go unnoticed.

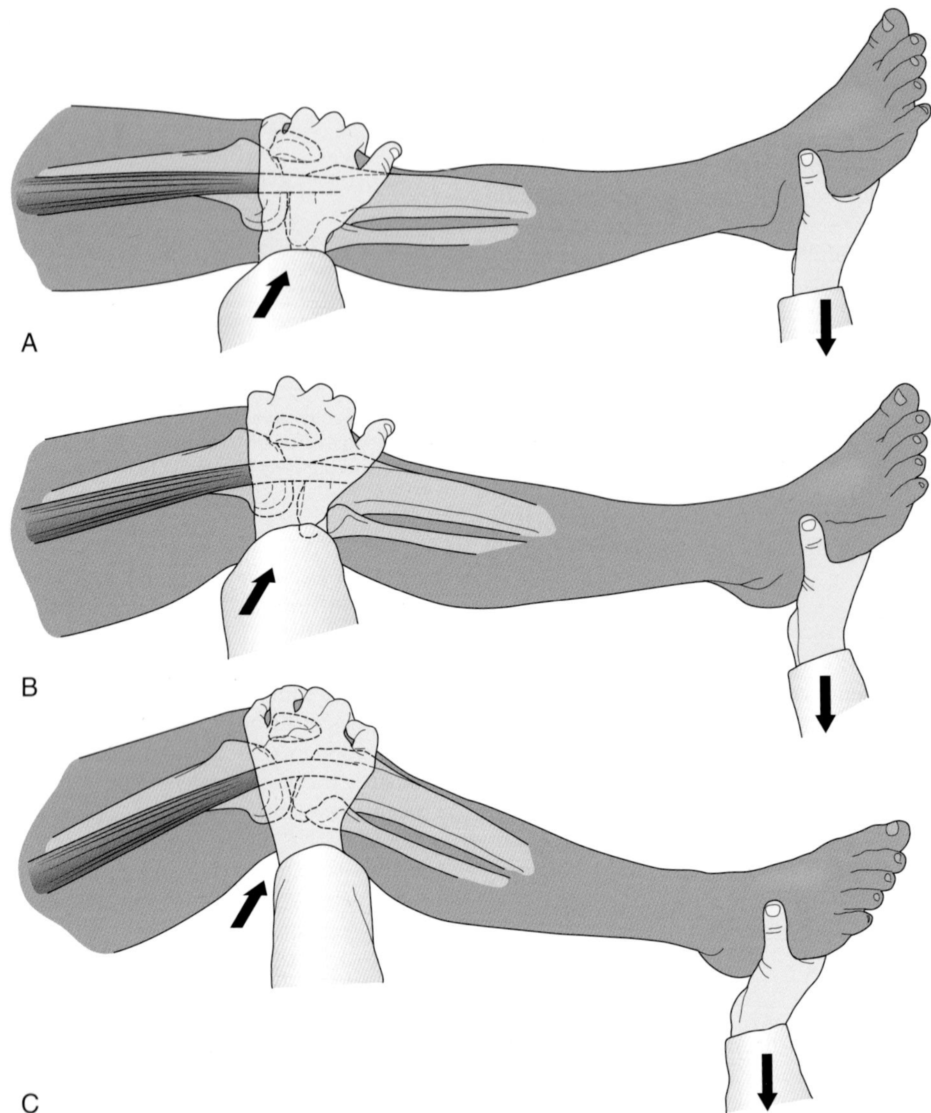

FIGURE 63.2 Position for the lateral pivot shift test. **A,** Note that the patient's knee is fully extended. Internally rotate the leg and apply a valgus stress. **B,** As you flex the knee between 20 and 45 degrees, the lateral tibial plateau is subluxed. **C,** As tension in the iliotibial band is less ened at 45 degrees of flexion, a pivot shift is felt as the tibia is reduced. This test identifies a rupture of the anterior cruciate ligament.

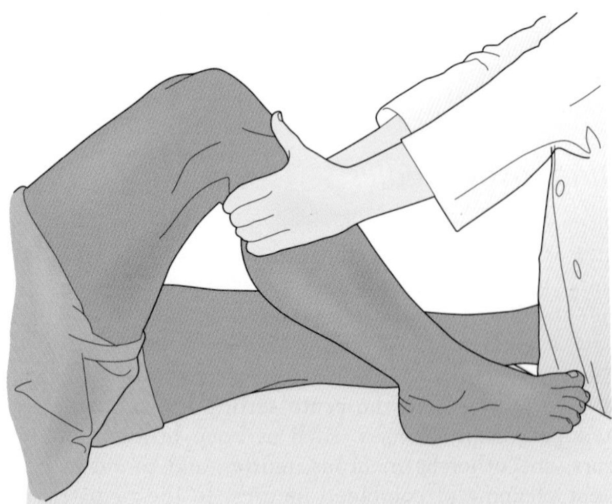

FIGURE 63.3 Position for the anterior drawer test. The hip is flexed 45 degrees, the knee is flexed 90 degrees, and the tibia is in neutral rotation. Anterior pull can be applied to the proximal tibia with both hands.

Differential Diagnosis

Isolated ACL tear
Combined lesions
  Posterolateral ligamentous complex tear
  Medial collateral ligament and medial meniscus
Intra-articular fracture
Patellar dislocation
Meniscal tear

Treatment

Initial

Immediately after injury, the management of an ACL tear includes relative rest, ice, compression, elevation, and analgesic or anti-inflammatory medication. Many patients will initially benefit from use of a knee immobilizer and crutches. If the knee is very swollen and painful with limited motion that restricts participation in treatment, arthrocentesis may be performed. It is important to establish an accurate diagnosis and the presence of associated injuries as these may necessitate prompt surgery. These include chondral or osteochondral fractures, meniscal tears, and other injured capsular structures. In general, in the absence of associated injuries, the acute management can be conservative with early protected rehabilitation.

Treatment of ACL injuries depends on a number of factors, including the patient's age, level of activity, presence of associated injuries, and importance of returning to athletic activities that involve acceleration and deceleration and cutting moves. Surgery is the only definitive treatment of complete ACL injuries, but it is generally not necessary for older individuals who do not complain of knee instability with recreational activities or work.

In general, younger patients and those with a high activity level should be considered for ACL reconstruction. Surgical referral is not necessary in the immediate postinjury period but should be facilitated as soon as it is clear that an individual desires surgery as a definite treatment measure. When associated injuries are present, especially if these cause mechanical symptoms, or in the case of the elite competitive athlete, surgical treatment should be considered as soon as the initial inflammatory phase has passed (Fig. 63.4) [16].

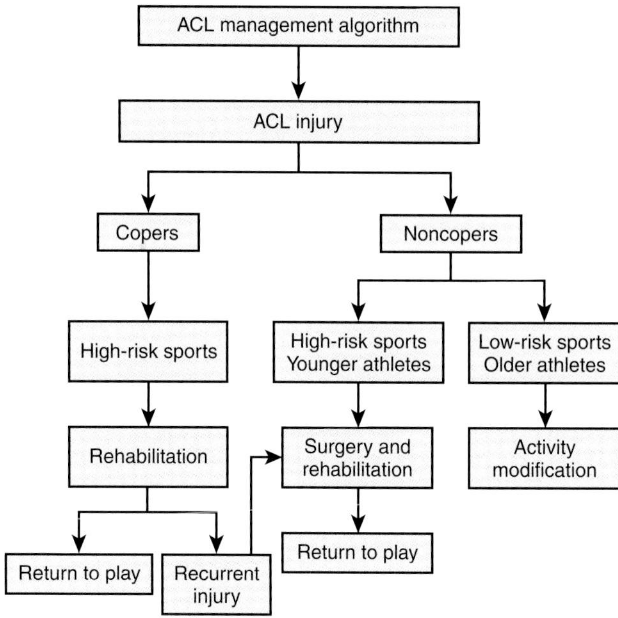

FIGURE 63.4 University of Puerto Rico Center for Sports Health anterior cruciate ligament (ACL) injury management algorithm. *(From Micheo WM, Hernandez L, Seda C. Evaluation, management, and prevention of anterior cruciate ligament injury: current concepts. PM R 2010;2:935-944.)*

Rehabilitation

The rehabilitation of an ACL tear begins as soon as the injury occurs. Rehabilitation management focuses on reducing pain, restoring full motion, correcting muscle strength deficits, achieving muscle balance, and returning the patient to full activity free of symptoms [17]. The rehabilitation program consists of acute, recovery, and functional phases.

Anterior Cruciate Ligament Injury

The patient with an ACL-deficient knee may present with an acute or a recurrent injury. In the acutely injured knee, protection of secondary structures is of paramount importance, and progression of rehabilitation will depend on the extent of damage to other knee structures. Early use of closed kinetic chain exercises, in which the distal segment of the extremity is fixed and the proximal segments are free to move, has allowed functional progression of strengthening. These exercises allow quadriceps strengthening with hamstring muscle co-contraction, which reduces the strain in the ACL and minimizes patellofemoral joint reaction forces (Table 63.1) [17,18].

The individual with a recurrently unstable knee will benefit from a trial of rehabilitation. Correction of muscle weakness and proprioceptive deficits and functional retraining in combination with activity modification could reduce

Table 63.1 Anterior Cruciate Ligament Tear Rehabilitation

	Acute Phase	Recovery Phase	Functional Phase
Therapeutic intervention	Modalities: cryotherapy, high-voltage galvanic stimulation, electrical stimulation Active-assisted flexion and extension Static quadriceps and hamstring exercise General conditioning: bicycle and pool exercises Ambulation with crutches	Modalities: superficial heat, pulsed ultrasound, electrical stimulation Range of motion, flexibility exercises Dynamic lower extremity strengthening Closed kinetic chain exercises, multiplanar lower extremity joint exercises General conditioning Gradual return to sports-specific training with functional bracing	General flexibility, strengthening training Power and endurance of lower extremities: diagonal and multiplanar motions, plyometrics Neuromuscular control, proprioceptive training Return to sports-specific participation with functional bracing
Criteria for advancement	Pain reduction Recovery of pain-free motion Adequate knee muscle control Tolerance for strengthening exercises	Full nonpainful motion Symmetric quadriceps and hamstring strength Correction of inflexibility Symptom-free progression in a sports-specific program	No clinical symptoms Normal running and jumping mechanics Normal kinetic chain integration Completed sports-specific program

episodes of instability and should be considered before surgery in the individual with low activity levels.

Acute Phase

This phase focuses on treatment of tissue injury, clinical signs, and symptoms. The goal in this stage is to allow tissue healing while reducing pain and inflammation. Reestablishment of nonpainful range of motion, prevention of muscle atrophy, and maintenance of general fitness should be addressed. This phase may last 1 to 2 weeks.

Recovery Phase

This phase focuses on obtaining normal passive and active knee motion, improving knee muscle function, achieving normal hamstrings and quadriceps muscle balance, and working on proprioception. Biomechanical and functional deficits, including inflexibilities and inability to run or jump, should begin to be addressed. This phase may last 2 to 8 weeks after the injury occurs.

Functional Phase

This phase focuses on increasing power and endurance of the lower extremities while improving neuromuscular control. Rehabilitation at this stage works on the entire kinetic chain, addressing specific functional deficits. This program should be continuous with the ultimate goal of prevention of recurrent injury and safe return to competition. The functional phase may last 8 weeks to 6 months after the injury occurs.

If the patient completes a rehabilitation program and is willing to modify the activity level, including the limitation of sports activity that involves cutting and pivoting maneuvers, the functional prognosis for daily living activities is good [11,19]. In this group of patients, functional braces may be used for sports participation that involves changes of direction. These braces may reduce symptoms of instability in individuals who use them, improve proprioception, and appear to reduce some strain in the ACL in low-demand activities.

Postsurgical Rehabilitation

In the patient who is a candidate for ACL reconstruction, rehabilitation should start before surgery. Reduction of pain and swelling, achievement of full range of motion, voluntary muscle activation, and finally achievement of normal muscle strength should be attempted before reconstruction. After surgery, rehabilitation should begin on the first postoperative day. Early use of cryotherapy, compression, and elevation has been shown to reduce swelling postoperatively. It is important to achieve full extension and to initiate early active flexion in the first few days after surgery. Weight bearing with crutches is usually started immediately after the operation [20].

Rapid progression of the rehabilitation program has reduced complications usually associated with ACL knee surgery, which included stiffness, muscle atrophy, muscle weakness, and patellofemoral pain. In the early rehabilitation period, special precautions need to be taken to avoid excessive strain of the reconstructed ligament with terminal (0 to 30 degrees) extension-resisted quadriceps exercises. Early use of closed kinetic chain exercises, such as mini-squats, steps, and leg press, has allowed quadriceps strengthening with tolerable shear forces to the graft [17,18,20] (Table 63.2). Aquatic exercises that allow progressive weight bearing with benefit from the effects of buoyancy can be started as soon as the sutures are removed.

Individuals will vary in the rate in which they achieve full motion, normal strength, normal proprioception, and adequate sports-specific skills. Achievement of these goals should be accomplished before the individual is allowed to return to sports activity. With accelerated rehabilitation programs, patients usually return to activity in 6 to 8 months after surgery. These accelerated rehabilitation programs do not lead to an increase in anterior knee

Table 63.2 Postsurgical Anterior Cruciate Ligament Tear Rehabilitation

	Acute Phase	Recovery Phase	Functional Phase
Therapeutic intervention	Modalities: cryotherapy, electrical stimulation Active-assisted flexion, passive extension Static quadriceps (90 to 45 degrees), dynamic hamstrings exercises, straight-leg raise exercises General conditioning: upper extremity ergometer Ambulation with crutches	Modalities: superficial heat, pulsed ultrasound, electrical stimulation Active flexion and extension exercises Dynamic quadriceps (90 to 30 degrees), hamstring strengthening Closed kinetic chain exercises, multiplanar lower extremity joint exercises General conditioning: bicycle, swimming, aquatic exercises Gradual return to sports-specific training with optional functional brace use	General flexibility training, strengthening exercise program Power and endurance of lower extremities: diagonal and multiplanar motions with tubings, light weights, medicine balls, plyometrics Neuromuscular control, proprioceptive training Return to sports-specific participation Optional functional brace use
Criteria for advancement	Pain reduction Recovery of 90 degrees of flexion, full extension Adequate knee muscle control Tolerance for strengthening exercises	Full flexion, knee hyperextension Symmetric quadriceps and hamstring strength Symptom-free progression in a sports-specific program	No clinical symptoms Normal running and jumping mechanics Normal kinetic chain integration Completed sports-specific program

laxity compared with nonaccelerated rehabilitation, and both accelerated and nonaccelerated rehabilitation appear to have the same effect in terms of clinical assessment, satisfaction of patients, functional performance, proprioception, and isokinetic thigh muscle strength [21,22]. The use of postoperative functional bracing does not improve outcome compared with no bracing [23].

Procedures

Knee joint aspiration may be attempted in the first 24 to 48 hours after the injury to document hemarthrosis and to assist in the diagnosis. If the injured individual is not progressing in treatment because of swelling and significant limitation of motion, aspiration may be performed at later stages of treatment for symptom relief. Under sterile conditions, with a 25-gauge, 1-inch sterile disposable needle, infiltrate the skin with a local anesthetic approximately 2 cm proximal and lateral (or medial) to the patella. Follow this injection with a second injection by use of an 18-gauge, 1½-inch needle into the joint capsule. Aspirate any fluid and note the color and consistency. Without withdrawal of the needle, take off the syringe and empty it. Repeat this until all of the fluid is aspirated. Use one hand to compress the suprapatellar area to be sure all of the fluid is out before the procedure is completed.

After aspiration, icing of the knee for 15 minutes after the procedure and then for 20 minutes two or three times daily for several days is recommended.

Surgery

Surgery is indicated in patients with recurrent episodes of instability in activities of daily living and in active recreational athletes who are symptomatic and do not wish to modify their activities. Surgery is definitely indicated in the high-demand competitive athlete.

The surgical procedure of choice is the arthroscopically assisted autograft by full endoscopic or two-incision techniques, with use of either patellar bone–tendon–bone graft or four strands of hamstring tendon graft. A debate exists between the proponents of each graft source and fixation, although both seem to be fairly equal in long-term studies [24,25]. The hamstring tendon group tends to recover faster initially and to have less pain and swelling. However, although the graft strength is good, the fixation of the graft as well as the incorporation of the graft to bone seems to be weaker than with the patellar tendon [15,26,27].

The patellar tendon group, on the other hand, has better fixation and incorporation because it heals bone to bone and behaves biomechanically like a single unit; the sum of these gives it a more reproducible result, making it the preferred graft for the high-demand athlete [3,28]. The downside of its use is that it tends to produce more morbidity, such as swelling, pain, and difficulty in gaining motion initially. It also has a higher incidence of postoperative patellofemoral pain. Other grafts used are the quadriceps tendon and contralateral patellar tendon. Allograft tendon material, such as patellar tendon and tibialis anterior tendon, has also gained popularity. The advantages of these are clear and include less donor site morbidity. The disadvantages are the possibility of disease transmission, slower graft incorporation, potential for stretching of the graft, and higher cost.

A new modality of reconstruction, the anatomic ACL reconstruction, has been popularized by Fu and coworkers [15]. This procedure tries to reconstruct both the anteromedial and the posterolateral bundles of the ACL. Fu and others have shown in vitro that this double-bundle anatomic ACL reconstruction better controls the important aspect of rotational instability of ACL deficiency. A study showed that the anatomic single- and double-bundle technique resulted in better anteroposterior and rotational stability than conventional single-bundle reconstruction [15,29,30]. The use of the ligament augmentation reconstruction system (LARS) synthetic ligament has gained popularity, with fewer graft failures and cases of synovitis compared with previous generations of synthetic grafts. However, longer follow-up studies should be undertaken to evaluate for possible complications [31].

Increased participation in competitive sports has caused an upsurge in pediatric ACL tears. The management of such injuries in the skeletally immature population is controversial. Whereas some advocate conservative management, this could cause damage to secondary structures and subsequent early osteoarthritis. Therefore surgical management has been advocated in patients with ACL deficiency returning to high-risk activities. Multiple techniques have been described in this population, including physeal-sparing, partial transphyseal, and complete transphyseal procedures. Good functional outcomes have been obtained with all techniques; however, the physeal-sparing approach has been promoted as a way to reduce the risk of growth retardation [32].

Potential Disease Complications

An untreated ACL injury can produce changes in the knee joint that may lead to significant alterations in the patient's lifestyle. The patients who continue participation in strenuous sports have recurrent episodes of pain and giving out secondary to anterior laxity and rotatory instability. These may lead to damage of associated structures, such as the menisci and other secondary restraints. A significant number of patients develop joint space narrowing with evidence of osteoarthritis. Risk factors associated with osteoarthritis after initial injury and surgical treatment include injury to the articular cartilage, meniscal tears, loss of range of motion (particularly in extension), high body mass index, and possibly arthrogenic muscle inhibition resulting in quadriceps weakness. The prevalence of radiographic knee osteoarthritis after surgical reconstruction ranges from 29% to 51%, with no statistically significant difference compared with conservative management (24%-48%). However, the prevalence of tibiofemoral osteoarthritis in isolated ACL injury has been reported to be lower (0%-13%) than in combined ACL and meniscal injuries (21%-48%), which highlights the role of meniscal injury in associated morbidity [1,11,19,33,34].

After surgical reconstruction, the incidence of ipsilateral graft tear is 5.8%; the risk of contralateral rupture is 11.8% [35]. Attention has recently been given to prevention of initial or recurrent ACL injury by modifying neuromuscular risk factors, such as muscle weakness and muscle imbalance and proprioceptive deficits, and working on sports-specific techniques, such as cutting and jumping. These programs combine strengthening, balance, and plyometric exercises with apparent improved dynamic stability and a reduction in the incidence of injury [35–37].

Potential Treatment Complications

Medication complications include gastric, cardiovascular, and renal toxicity with nonsteroidal anti-inflammatory drugs. Injections carry the risk of infection (in approximately 1% to 2% of cases). Surgery has the risks of venous thrombosis and complications from the anesthesia. Fibrous ankylosis and significant loss of motion can be seen in the early rehabilitation stages secondary to poor progression of therapy or compliance of the patient [35].

Poor graft placement and fixation can lead to loss of motion and subsequent graft failure with recurrent instability. In patients in whom chondral lesions or meniscal tears are identified at the time of surgery, long-term sequelae include the development of arthritis even after the reconstruction [4,6,30,33,34,38].

References

[1] Micheo W, Hernandez L, Seda C. Evaluation, management, and prevention of anterior cruciate ligament injury: current concepts. PM R 2010;2:935–44.

[2] Arendt E, Dick R. Knee injury patterns among men and women in collegiate basketball and soccer: NCAA data and review of literature. Am J Sports Med 1995;23:694–701.

[3] Utukuri MM, Somayaji HS, Khanduja V, et al. Update on paediatric ACL injuries. Knee 2006;13:345–52.

[4] Huston LJ, Greenfield ML, Wotjys EM. Anterior cruciate ligament injuries in the female athlete: potential risk factors. Clin Orthop 2002;372:50–63.

[5] Smith H, Vacek P, Johnson R, et al. Risk factors for anterior cruciate ligament injury: a review of the literature—part 1: neuromuscular and anatomic risk. Sports Health 2012;4:69–78.

[6] Smith H, Vacek P, Johnson R, et al. Risk factors for anterior cruciate ligament injury: a review of the literature—part 2: hormonal, genetic, cognitive function, previous injury and extrinsic risk factors. Sports Health 2012;4:155–61.

[7] Thore Z, Petersen W, Fu F. Anatomy of the anterior cruciate ligament: a review. Oper Tech Orthop 2005;15:20–8.

[8] Amis A, Bull A, Denny T, et al. Biomechanics of rotational instability and anterior cruciate reconstruction. Oper Tech Orthop 2005;15:29–35.

[9] Yasuda K, Kondo E, Ichiyama H, et al. Surgical and biomechanical concepts of anatomic ACL reconstruction. Oper Tech Orthop 2005;15:96–102.

[10] Yagi M, Kuroda R, Yoshiya S, et al. Anterior cruciate ligament reconstruction: the Japanese experience. Oper Tech Orthop 2005;15:116–22.

[11] Fithian DC, Paxton LW, Goltz DH. Fate of the anterior cruciate ligament-injured knee. Orthop Clin North Am 2002;33:621–36.

[12] Kocher MS, Steadman JR, Briggs KK, et al. Relationships between objective assessment of ligament stability and subjective assessment of symptoms and function after anterior cruciate ligament reconstruction. Am J Sports Med 2004;32:629–34.

[13] Amy E, Micheo WM. Anterior cruciate ligament tear. In: Micheo WM, editor. Musculoskeletal, sports, and occupational medicine. New York: Demos; 2011. p. 25–7.

[14] Boden BP, Griffin LY, Garrett WE. Etiology and prevention of noncontact ACL injury. Phys Sports Med 2000;28:53–62.

[15] Fu F, Bennett CH, Ma B, et al. Current trends in anterior cruciate ligament reconstruction. Part 2. Operative procedures and clinical correlations. Am J Sports Med 2000;28:124–30.

[16] Shelbourne KD, Foulk DA. Timing of surgery in acute anterior cruciate ligament tears on the return of quadriceps muscle strength after reconstruction using an autogenous patellar tendon graft. Am J Sports Med 1995;23:686–9.

[17] Gotlin RS, Huie R. Anterior cruciate ligament injuries: operative and rehabilitative options. Phys Med Rehabil Clin N Am 2000;11:895–924.

[18] Escamilla RF, Fleisig GS, Zheng N, et al. Biomechanics of the knee during closed kinetic chain and open kinetic chain exercises. Med Sci Sports Exerc 1998;30:556–69.

[19] Daniel DM, Stone ML, Dobson BE, et al. Fate of the ACL-injured patient: a prospective outcome study. Am J Sports Med 1994;22:632–44.

[20] Arnold T, Shelbourne KD. A perioperative rehabilitation program for anterior cruciate ligament surgery. Phys Sports Med 2000;28:31–49.

[21] Beynnon BD, Uh BS, Johnson RJ, et al. Rehabilitation after anterior cruciate ligament reconstruction: a prospective, randomized, double-blind comparison of programs administered over 2 different time intervals. Am J Sports Med 2005;33:347–59.

[22] Beynnon BD, Johnson RJ, Naud S. Accelerated versus nonaccelerated rehabilitation after anterior cruciate ligament reconstruction: a prospective, randomized, double-blind investigation evaluating knee joint laxity using roentgen stereophotogrammetric analysis. Am J Sports Med 2011;39:2536–48.

[23] Spindler KP, Wright RW. Clinical practice. Anterior cruciate ligament tear. N Engl J Med 2008;359:2135–42.

[24] Cha P, Chhabra A, Harner C. Single bundle anterior cruciate ligament reconstruction using the medial portal technique. Oper Tech Orthop 2005;15:89–95.

[25] Herrington L, Wrapson C, Matthews M, et al. Anterior cruciate ligament reconstruction, hamstrings versus bone–patella tendon–bone grafts: a systematic literature review of outcome from surgery. Knee 2005;12:41–50.

[26] Roe J, Pinczewski LA, Russell VJ, et al. A 7-year follow-up of patella tendon and hamstring tendon grafts for arthroscopic anterior cruciate ligament reconstruction: differences and similarities. Am J Sports Med 2005;33:1337–45.

[27] Freedman KB, D'Amato MJ, Nedeff DD, et al. Arthroscopic anterior cruciate ligament reconstruction: a metaanalysis comparing patellar tendon and hamstring tendon autografts. Am J Sports Med 2003;31:2–11.

[28] Foster MC, Foster IW. Patella tendon or four-strand hamstring? A systematic review of autografts for anterior cruciate ligament reconstruction. Knee 2005;12:225–30.

[29] Hussein M, Van Eck CF, Cretnik A, et al. Prospective randomized clinical evaluation of conventional single-bundle, anatomic single-bundle, and anatomic double-bundle anterior cruciate ligament reconstruction. Am J Sports Med 2012;40:512–20.

[30] Aglietti P, Cuomo P, Giron F, et al. Double bundle ACL reconstruction. Oper Tech Orthop 2005;15:111–5.

[31] Newman SD, Atkinson HD, Willis-Owen CA. Anterior cruciate ligament reconstruction with the ligament augmentation and reconstruction system: a systematic review. Int Orthop 2013;37:321–6.

[32] McConkey MO, Bonasia DE, Amendola A. Pediatric anterior cruciate ligament reconstruction. Curr Rev Musculoskelet Med 2011;4:37–44.

[33] Shelbourne DK, Freeman H, Gray T. Osteoarthritis after anterior cruciate ligament reconstruction: the importance of regaining and maintaining full range of motion. Sports Health 2012;4:79–85.

[34] Oiestad BE, Engebretsen L, Storheim K, et al. Knee osteoarthritis after anterior cruciate ligament injury: a systematic review. Am J Sports Med 2009;37:1434–43.

[35] Wright RW, Magnussen RA, Dunn WR, et al. Ipsilateral graft and contralateral ACL rupture at five years or more following ACL reconstruction: a systematic review. J Bone Joint Surg Am 2011;93:1159–65.

[36] Wilk KE, Reinhold MM, Hooks TR. Recent advances in the rehabilitation of isolated and combined anterior cruciate ligament injuries. Orthop Clin North Am 2003;34:107–37.

[37] Wilk KE, Macrina LC, Cain EL, et al. Recent advances in the rehabilitation of anterior cruciate ligament injuries. J Orthop Sports Phys Ther 2012;42:153–71.

[38] Brown CH, Carson EW. Revision anterior cruciate ligament surgery. Clin Sports Med 1999;18:109–71.

CHAPTER 64

Baker Cyst

Darren Rosenberg, DO

Joao E.D. Amadera, MD, PhD

Synonym

Popliteal cyst

ICD-9 Code

727.51 Synovial cyst of popliteal space (Baker cyst)

ICD-10 Codes

M71.20 Synovial cyst of popliteal space (Baker), unspecified knee

M71.21 Synovial cyst of popliteal space (Baker), right knee

M71.22 Synovial cyst of popliteal space (Baker), left knee

Definition

Baker cyst, the most common cyst in the posterior knee, was first described more than a century and a half ago by Adams [1] and later by Baker [2]. It affects approximately 19% of asymptomatic adults (especially adults older than 50 years) [3] and 6.3% of children [4]. It is more common in boys and in children with arthritic knees or hypermobility syndrome [5]. Two age incidence peaks exist: 4 to 7 years and 35 to 70 years [6,7]. Three factors are key to the formation of Baker cyst: (1) communication between the knee joint and popliteal bursae, (2) one-way valve effect, and (3) unequal pressure between the joint and bursae during varying angles of knee movement [7].

Chronic irritation in the knee joint may increase production of synovial fluid, which may flow from the knee joint into the bursae under higher intra-articular pressure until the one-way valve formed by the gastrocnemius-soleus complex "closes," trapping the fluid in one of the popliteal bursae. This bursa then distends and forms a palpable mass, more commonly in the posteromedial aspect of the popliteal fossa [8]. Anatomically, the lack of supporting structures in this area may predispose this region of the popliteal space to cyst formation [8]. Most commonly, the source of this chronic irritation is an inflammatory or degenerative joint disease, such as rheumatoid arthritis or osteoarthritis. Furthermore, conditions like infectious arthritis, polyarthritis, villonodular synovitis, connective tissue diseases, chondromalacia patellae, and persistent capsulitis are also commonly associated with Baker cysts [9,10]. In a study of 40 patients with radiographic evidence of primary osteoarthritis of the knee, 22% had Baker cyst diagnosed by ultrasonography [11]. Popliteal cysts are associated with meniscal tears in 71% to 82% of the cases, anterior cruciate ligament insufficiency in 30%, and degenerative cartilage lesions in 30% to 60% of the cases [9,10]. Noncommunicating cysts are rare in adults, often have no associated knee disease, and may be primary bursal enlargements from repeated trauma to the bursa itself related to muscle activation. Direct trauma is the most common cause of these cysts in children [4].

Symptoms

Baker cysts are often nonpainful and may be manifested as a fluctuant mass in the popliteal fossa (Fig. 64.1). Typical symptoms, if present, include swelling, pain, and stiffness exacerbated by activity such as walking. Symptoms are most readily elicited when knee flexion compresses the fluid-filled cyst, although knee extension may also cause tension on the cyst by the extended gastrocnemius-soleus muscles. The mass is often accompanied by leg swelling or diffuse calf tenderness. Numbness and tingling in the posterior aspect of the calf and plantar aspect of the foot may be present if there is neural or vascular involvement.

Physical Examination

Baker cysts are often visible or at least palpable along the medial aspect of the popliteal fossa. The cyst may be identified with the patient prone with the knee first extended and then flexed while the popliteal fossa is inspected and palpated. The round, smooth, fluctuant, and often tender cyst will be firm on palpation with knee extension and may soften or disappear with 45 degrees of knee flexion, a phenomenon known as Foucher sign [12]. The cyst can extend into the thigh or leg, or it can have multiple satellites

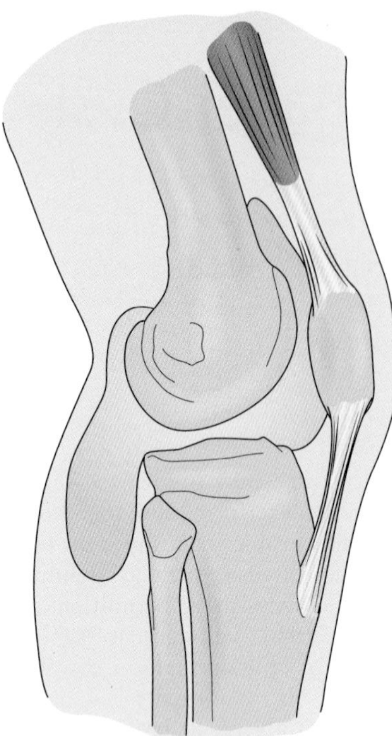

FIGURE 64.1 Schematic diagram of Baker cyst.

along the calf and even into the foot. These satellite cysts may or may not be connected to the primary cyst through channels. When a joint effusion accompanies the cyst, it is worthwhile to search for the source of chronic irritation. Examine the knee's range of motion, test for ligamentous laxity, and evaluate for potential patellofemoral pain and meniscal tears [9]. Furthermore, because of the proximity of the sciatic nerve and its branches to the popliteal region where cysts may be present, in rare cases nerve compression may be manifested as decreased sensation along the plantar aspect of the foot and muscle atrophy in the tibialis posterior, flexor digitorum longus, and flexor hallucis longus [13–15].

Functional Limitations

The degree of impairment produced by the cyst depends on its size and amount of tenderness. Baker cysts are usually painless and limit movement minimally, if at all, unless there is an underlying meniscal injury. However, larger cysts may be associated with moderate limitations in physical activity, particularly walking.

Diagnostic Studies

Plain films of the knee can be used to diagnose underlying degenerative joint disease but are rarely necessary to diagnose Baker cyst. Ultrasonography distinguishes solid from cystic masses and is therefore especially helpful in detecting Baker cysts when extensive joint deformities, such as those present with rheumatoid arthritis, obscure the cyst [16]. Furthermore, ultrasonography is an economical and helpful method of differentiating thrombophlebitis from Baker cysts if there is diagnostic uncertainty. Arthrography, through the injection of contrast dye into the knee joint or bursa, may clearly demonstrate the enlarged bursal structure. In addition, computed tomography may differentiate cysts from lipomas and malignant neoplasms and may show noncommunicating cysts or cysts that are not in the typical locations. Magnetic resonance imaging outlines the anatomy of the entire joint and is a sensitive test to identify Baker cyst as well as its likely cause. Magnetic resonance imaging also helps in ruling out suspected solid tumors and defining pathologic changes for possible surgical excision. On magnetic resonance imaging, Baker cysts appear as well-circumscribed masses with low signal intensity on T1-weighted images and high signal intensity on T2-weighted images (Fig. 64.2). Ultrasonography and magnetic resonance imaging are the two most common radiologic methods for evaluation of suspected Baker cysts, each with its strengths and drawbacks [17]. Testing of the erythrocyte sedimentation rate may also be helpful if an inflammatory process is suspected. In cases in which there is doubt about the cyst's etiology, analysis and culture of aspirated fluid can help differentiate between infectious, inflammatory, and mechanical processes.

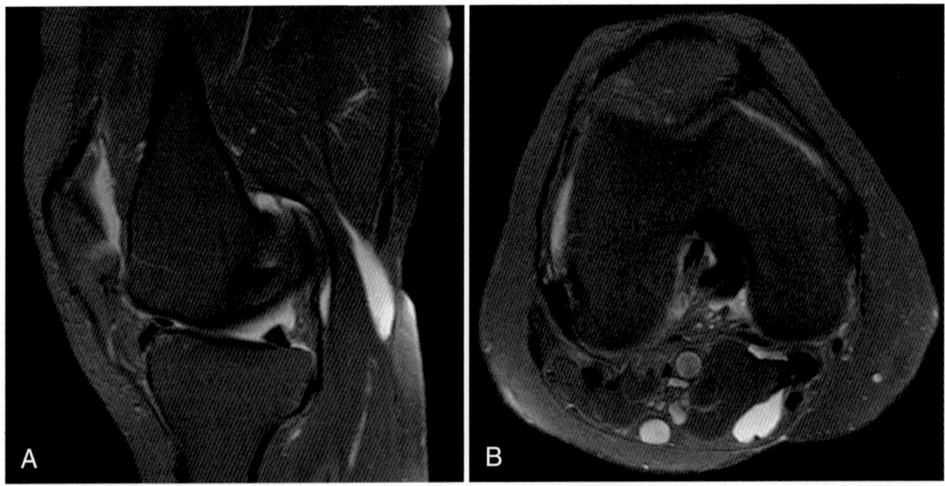

FIGURE. 64.2 Magnetic resonance imaging of a Baker cyst. Sagittal (**A**) and axial (**B**) T2-weighted images. *(Courtesy Dr. Jader José da Silva, Hospital do Coração.)*

Differential Diagnosis

Venous complexes
Inflammatory arthritis (rheumatoid)
Fat pads
Liposarcoma
Hematoma
Ganglionic cysts
Synovial hemangioma
Abscess
Malignant fibrous histiocytoma
Neoplasms (sarcoma, schwannoma)
Thrombophlebitis
Arterial aneurysms
Pseudothrombophlebitis
Compartment syndrome

Treatment

Initial

Intervention is needed only when a Baker cyst is symptomatic. The simplest treatment is to aspirate the fluid because aspiration collapses the cyst, and the symptoms consequently disappear. However, treatment of the cyst alone may not be adequate, and treatment of the underlying joint disease may be necessary. Ice and anti-inflammatory agents (nonsteroidal anti-inflammatory drugs) can reduce the inflammatory effusions produced by degenerative joint disease. Quadriceps strengthening exercises can be used for an associated patellofemoral syndrome. In some cases, venous sclerosants are used to prevent recurrence [12]. The cysts tend to involute spontaneously in children.

Rehabilitation

Rehabilitation may include compression and range of motion exercises as a means of decreasing swelling in addition to physical modalities (such as ice) and pharmacotherapy (such as nonsteroidal anti-inflammatory drugs, mentioned before). Furthermore, in cases of degenerative joint disease, cruciate ligament tears, and meniscal injuries, resistance exercises to maintain and to improve lower extremity muscle strength may be helpful. A comprehensive rehabilitation program may lead to progress in gait and in function to perform daily activities.

Procedures

Needle aspiration of the cyst is the most effective therapy, and provided the predisposing cause of the cyst resolves, it generally results in improvement of symptoms and function. Furthermore, if knee joint effusion is present, joint aspiration, accompanied by intra-articular corticosteroid injection, may be beneficial. In cases of noncommunicating cysts, corticosteroid injection directly into the cyst may help decrease swelling. The effect of this intervention may be followed serially through ultrasonography [18]. On the other hand, there is evidence that direct cyst infiltration with steroids has better results in patients with knee osteoarthritis compared with intra-articular injection [19]. The possibility of a vascular malformation must be eliminated either by auscultation of the mass with a stethoscope to listen for bruits or by palpation of it to feel for a pulse before cyst aspiration [20]. In addition, imaging techniques such as ultrasonography may assist in detecting cysts.

Surgery

Surgical excision is attempted only after all other methods have failed and the cyst is sufficiently large and remains symptomatic [21]. In the past, open excision was an option if the cyst remained symptomatic, but the associated recurrence rate was high (up to 63%) [22]. On occasion, surgery was necessary to correct the underlying pathologic process (e.g., arthroscopic surgery for meniscal tears or total knee replacement for intractable degenerative joint disease). Because of that, arthroscopic treatment of popliteal cysts has been the current option. Recently, the arthroscopic approach has been used to simultaneously correct both the valvular opening, by reestablishing a normal bidirectional communication, and the associated intra-articular disease responsible for the persistence of the cyst. Also, large open wounds can be avoided [23,24].

Potential Disease Complications

The most common complications of Baker cysts are dissection into the calf and rupture, leading to calf, ankle, and foot ecchymoses [12]. When the cyst ruptures, it produces a "pseudothrombophlebitis syndrome," meaning that it results in intense calf pain and swelling without associated deep venous thrombosis. Less commonly, Baker cyst produces compartment syndrome [25], peripheral neuropathy [13,14], or lower extremity claudication [26]. Rarely, if the cyst is infected, it can result in septic arthritis of the knee if an intra-articular–bursal communication exists [27]. Moreover, a possible sequela of Baker cysts may be intramuscular dissection, both distally [28] and less commonly proximally [29].

Potential Treatment Complications

Analgesics and nonsteroidal anti-inflammatory drugs have well-known side effects that most commonly affect the gastric, hepatic, and renal systems. Aspiration can result in recurrence, infection, bleeding, and neurovascular compromise. Surgery can result in local neurovascular complications and recurrence of the cysts [22,30].

References

[1] Adams R. Chronic rheumatic arthritis of the knee joint. Dublin J Med Sci 1840;17:520–2.
[2] Baker WM. On the formation of the synovial cysts in the leg in connection with disease of the knee joint. St Barth Hosp Rep 1877;13:245–61.
[3] Tshirch F, Schmid M, Pfirrmann C, et al. Prevalence of size of meniscal cysts, ganglionic cysts, synovial cysts of the popliteal space, fluid-filled bursae, and other fluid collections in asymptomatic knees on MR imaging. AJR Am J Roentgenol 2003;180:1431–6.
[4] De Maeseneer M, Debaere C, Desprechins B, Osteaux M. Popliteal cysts in children: prevalence, appearance and associated findings at MR imaging. Pediatr Radiol 1999;29:605–9.
[5] Neubauer H, Morbach H, Schwarz T, et al. Popliteal cysts in paediatric patients: clinical characteristics and imaging features on ultrasound and MRI. Arthritis 2011;2011:751593.
[6] Gristina A, Wilson P. Popliteal cysts in adults and children. Arch Surg 1964;88:357–63.

[7] Handy J. Popliteal cysts in adults: a review. Semin Arthritis Rheum 2001;31:108–18.

[8] Labropoulos N, Shifrin DA, Paxinos O. New insights into the development of popliteal cysts. Br J Surg 2004;91:1313–8.

[9] Tinker R. Orthopaedics in Primary Care. Baltimore: Williams & Wilkins; 1979.

[10] Fritschy D, Fasel J, Imbert JC, et al. The popliteal cyst. Knee Surg Sports Traumatol Arthrosc 2006;14:623–8.

[11] Naredo E, Cabero F, Palop M, et al. Ultrasonographic findings in knee osteoarthritis: a comparative study with clinical and radiographic assessment. Osteoarthritis Cartilage 2005;13:568–74.

[12] Langsfeld M, Matteson B, Johnson W, et al. Baker's cysts mimicking the symptoms of deep vein thrombosis: diagnosis with venous duplex scanning. J Vasc Surg 1997;25:658–62.

[13] Ginanneschi F, Rossi A. Lateral cutaneous nerve of calf neuropathy due to peri-popliteal cystic bursitis. Muscle Nerve 2006;34:503–4.

[14] Willis JD, Carter PM. Tibial nerve entrapment and heel pain caused by a Baker's cyst. J Am Podiatr Med Assoc 1998;88:310–1.

[15] Dash S, Bheemreddy SR, Tiku ML. Posterior tibial neuropathy from ruptured Baker's cyst. Semin Arthritis Rheum 1998;27:272.

[16] Katz WA. Diagnosis and Management of Rheumatic Diseases. 2nd ed. Philadelphia: JB Lippincott; 1988.

[17] Jacobson J. Musculoskeletal ultrasound and MRI: which do I choose? Semin Musculoskelet Radiol 2005;9:135–49.

[18] Acebes JC, Sanchez-Pernaute O, Diaz-Oca A, Herrero-Beaumont G. Ultrasonographic assessment of Baker's cysts after intra-articular corticosteroid injection in knee osteoarthritis. Clin Ultrasound 2006;34:113–7.

[19] Bandinelli F, Fedi R, Generini S, et al. Longitudinal ultrasound and clinical follow-up of Baker's cysts injection with steroids in knee osteoarthritis. Clin Rheumatol 2012;31:727–31.

[20] Birnbaum J. The Musculoskeletal Manual. New York: Academic Press; 1982.

[21] Takahashi M, Nagano A. Arthroscopic treatment of popliteal cyst and visualization of its cavity through the posterior portal of the knee. Arthroscopy 2005;21:638.e1–4.

[22] Rauschning W, Lindgren PG. Popliteal cysts (Baker's cysts) in adults. 1. Clinical and roentgenological results of operative excision. Acta Orthop Scand 1979;50:583–91.

[23] Malinowski K, Synder M, Sibinski M. Selected cases of arthroscopic treatment of popliteal cyst with associated intra-articular knee disorders primary report. Ortop Traumatol Rehabil 2011;13:573–82.

[24] Lie CW, Ng TP. Arthroscopic treatment of popliteal cyst. Hong Kong Med J 2011;17:180–3.

[25] Schimizzi A, Jamali A, Herbst K, Pedowitz R. Acute compartment syndrome due to ruptured Baker cyst after nonsurgical management of an anterior cruciate ligament tear: a case report. Am J Sports Med 2006;34:657–60.

[26] Zhang W, Lukan J, Dryjski M. Nonoperative management of lower extremity claudication caused by a Baker's cyst: case report and review of the literature. Vascular 2005;13:244–7.

[27] Izumi M, Ikeuchi M, Tani T. Septic arthritis of the knee associated with calf abscess. J Orthop Surg (Hong Kong) 2012;20:272–5.

[28] Fang CS, McCarthy CL, McNally EG. Intramuscular dissection of Baker's cysts: report on three cases. Skeletal Radiol 2004;33:367–71.

[29] Abdelrahman MH, Tubeishat S, Hammoudeh M. Proximal dissection and rupture of a popliteal cyst: a case report. Case Rep Radiol 2012;2012:292414.

[30] Kp V, Yoon JR, Nha KW, et al. Popliteal artery pseudoaneurysm after arthroscopic cystectomy of a popliteal cyst. Arthroscopy 2009;25:1054–7.

CHAPTER 65

Knee Chondral Injuries

Alison L. Cabrera, MD
Kurt Spindler, MD

Synonyms

Loose body of the knee
Chondromalacia of the patella
Articular cartilage disorder
Derangement, internal, knee, unspecified
Osteochondritis dissecans
Chondromalacia of medial or lateral compartments of the knee

ICD-9 Codes

717.6	Loose body of the knee
717.7	Chondromalacia of the patella
718.0	Articular cartilage disorder
719.9	Derangement, internal, knee, unspecified
732.7	Osteochondritis dissecans
733.92	Chondromalacia of medial or lateral compartments of the knee

ICD-10 Codes

M23.40	Loose body in knee, unspecified knee
M23.41	Loose body in knee, right knee
M23.42	Loose body in knee, left knee
M22.40	Chondromalacia patellae, unspecified knee
M22.41	Chondromalacia patellae, right knee
M22.42	Chondromalacia patellae, left knee
M24.10	Other articular cartilage disorders, unspecified site
M23.90	Unspecified internal derangement of unspecified knee
M23.91	Unspecified internal derangement of right knee
M23.92	Unspecified internal derangement of left knee
M93.20	Osteochondritis dissecans of unspecified site
M94.261	Chondromalacia, right knee
M94.262	Chondromalacia, left knee
M94.269	Chondromalacia, unspecified knee

Definition

Chondral injuries are any degree of loss of the normal thickness and structure of articular hyaline cartilage. Chondral damage can occur in any joint, but most of the literature has focused on the knee, which is the focus of this chapter. Outerbridge [1] classified cartilage lesions in 1961, and this remains the current classification used to date (Fig. 65.1). Partial-thickness articular cartilage injuries do not heal but are rarely associated with significant clinical symptoms [2]. Full-thickness cartilage injuries, in which the injury extends to the depth of subchondral bone, may heal in with fibrocartilage, but this type of cartilage has shown inferior biomechanical and biochemical properties compared with hyaline cartilage [2,3]. Large, full-thickness cartilage defects are less likely to benefit from the healing fibrocartilaginous response and frequently will lead to symptoms [2].

The exact incidence of acute cartilage injury is unknown. In young, active patients who present with a hemarthrosis of the knee after a traumatic event, 5% to 10% are found to have cartilage injury [4]. Many studies have retrospectively reviewed the incidence of cartilage injury after arthroscopy for other injury and found rates ranging from 5% to 11% for full-thickness lesions [5,6]. A study looking retrospectively at 25,124 arthroscopies found a 60% incidence of cartilage lesions [7]. Regarding age differences, the incidence of a localized grade III or grade IV cartilage lesion in patients undergoing arthroscopy ranged from 5% to 7% for patients younger than 40 years and 7% to 9% for patients younger than 50 years [6,7]. These studies included both acute and chronic cartilage lesions. Grade II was the most frequent lesion, seen in 42% [7]. The most common locations were the patellar articular surface (36%) and medial femoral

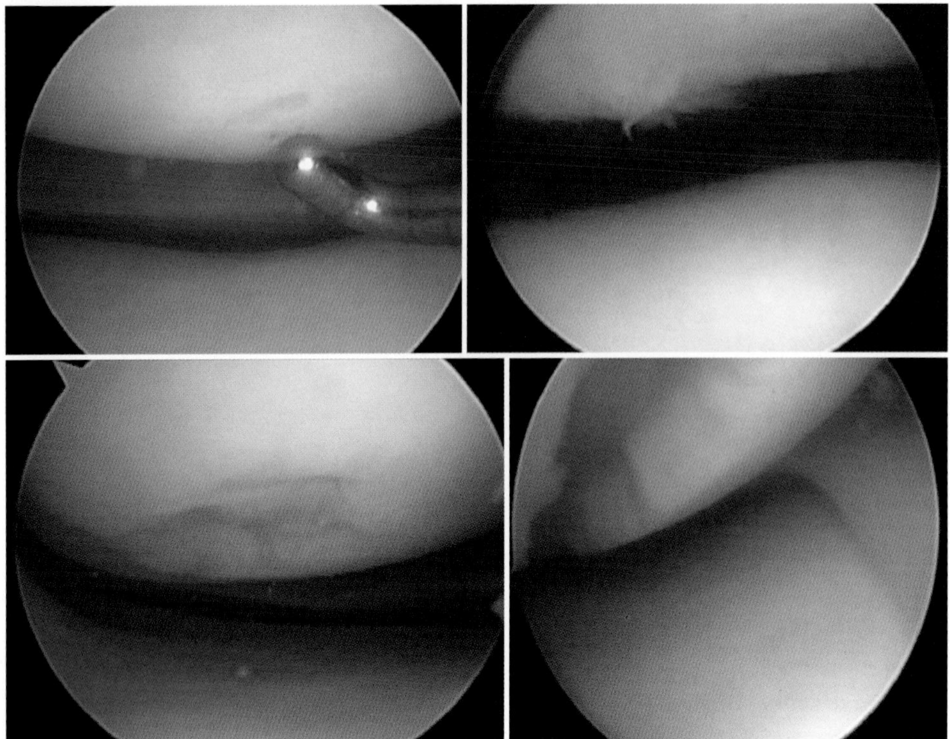

FIGURE 65.1 Outerbridge classification depicted by arthroscopic examples: grade I *(upper left):* cartilage softening and swelling; grade II *(upper right):* a partial-thickness defect with fissures on the surface that do not reach subchondral bone or exceed 1.5 cm in diameter; grade III *(bottom left):* fissuring to the level of subchondral bone in an area with a diameter of more than 1.5 cm; grade IV *(bottom right):* exposed subchondral bone.

condyle (34%) [7]. Seventy percent of the chondral lesions seen were associated with other injury, with medial meniscus tear (37%) and injury of the anterior cruciate ligament (36%) being the most common [7].

Most authors would agree that progression to osteoarthritis is a concern; however, there is little evidence to date that quantifies the incidence or severity of osteoarthritis after chondral injury. More natural history and outcomes research is needed to better predict a patient's likelihood of progression to symptomatic osteoarthritis according to the characteristics of the cartilage injury.

Symptoms

Patients may present with effusion, localized pain, and possible mechanical symptoms. If a full-thickness fragment has detached partially or completely, a patient may have locking or a "loose body" sensation as the fragment moves within the knee joint (Fig. 65.2). If the injury extends to subchondral bone, a hemarthrosis will be present. Some patients may have more vague symptoms without large effusion and a more generalized pain, making the diagnosis less clear.

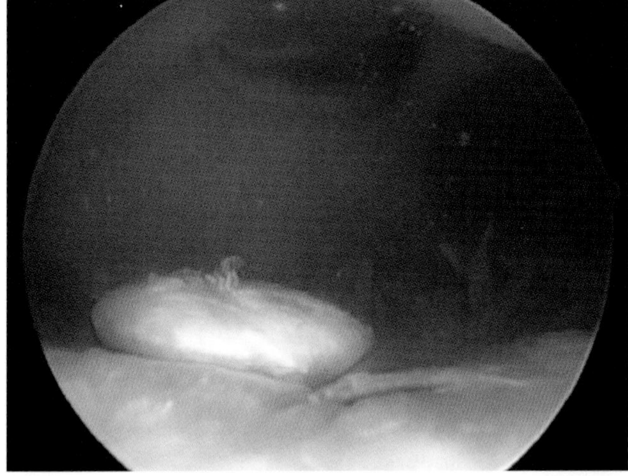

FIGURE 65.2 Arthroscopic image of a free articular cartilage fragment in the suprapatellar pouch.

Physical Examination

The practitioner should evaluate the patient for joint effusion and any tenderness to palpation. The patient will likely have tenderness to palpation over the anatomic region with chondral injury. The patient may have tenderness along the joint line, but more detail in examination will show that the area of maximal tenderness is over the site of chondral damage. Active and passive range of motion should be assessed. Crepitus or clunk may be present with range of motion with significant cartilage defects. It is important to perform a thorough ligamentous laxity examination to rule out any concomitant injuries [7].

Functional Limitations

The patient may have difficulty with ambulation and may walk with a limp. Activities such as climbing stairs and household chores may be limited by knee pain and swelling.

Most often, patients will be unable to return to the activity they were participating in immediately after the acute injury.

Diagnostic Studies

Plain films including standing anteroposterior, lateral, and sunrise views are obtained initially to rule out osteochondral fracture, osseous loose body, osteoarthritis, osteochondritis dissecans, and Segond fracture. Magnetic resonance imaging (MRI) is currently the standard of care in evaluating the morphology of an articular cartilage injury and can also assess for ligamentous or meniscal injuries. Even with current MRI protocols, cartilage evaluation requires expertise to characterize lesions accurately. New biochemical imaging techniques including T2 mapping, T1rho imaging, sodium MRI, and delayed gadolinium-enhanced MRI of cartilage have been used primarily for research purposes but are gaining support for their use in the clinical setting to improve detection and management of cartilage lesions [8].

Differential Diagnosis

Meniscus tear
Anterior cruciate ligament tear
Osteoarthritis
Plica syndrome
Osteochondral fracture
Osteochondritis dissecans

Treatment

Initial

Initial treatment is focused on pain control and resolving any effusion. Anti-inflammatories will usually suffice for pain relief. Aspiration of any effusion present will help alleviate pain and can be combined with injection of an anesthetic. Animal studies represent most of the literature on chondrolysis after intra-articular injection of anesthetic and primarily have evaluated bupivacaine toxicity [9]. However, a study using human chondrocytes has shown improved viability of chondrocytes after 0.5% ropivacaine versus 0.5% bupivacaine [9]. An intact matrix has been shown to offer a chondroprotective effect [9]. With our current knowledge of the chondrotoxicity of 0.5% bupivacaine, it should be used judiciously. A better alternative may be 0.5% ropivacaine, but longer term studies in humans are needed.

Rehabilitation

Early physical therapy is recommended to regain joint range of motion and muscle strength. Focus should be on quadriceps and hamstrings exercises. Most cartilage injuries will be associated with other injuries (e.g., anterior cruciate ligament injury), and therefore the rehabilitation protocol will vary. Numerous animal studies show an improved cartilage healing response with continuous passive motion after cartilage injury [10,11]. However, currently there are only few level III studies and no randomized controlled trials regarding this topic [12]. Nevertheless, most surgeons agree on using continuous passive motion as well as keeping the patient non–weight bearing after cartilage restoration surgery. Patients are kept non–weight bearing ranging from 6 to 12 weeks, depending on the surgeon's protocol and any patient comorbidities.

Surgery

Most authors agree that cartilage defects to be considered for surgical treatment include full-thickness lesions (i.e., Outerbridge grade III or grade IV) larger than 2 cm^2 in a patient younger than 40 years [13,14]. Without taking the grade of the chondral lesion into consideration, the incidence of chondral injuries larger than 2 cm^2 was only 7% in one study [7]. Microfracture, osteochondral autograft transfer or transplantation (i.e., OAT), and autologous chondrocyte implantation (ACI) are the principal cartilage restoration procedures available that have been evaluated in randomized clinical trials.

Microfracture involves arthroscopic débridement of the cartilage lesion to stable squared off edges. The zone of calcified cartilage is removed, and cortical penetration with an awl is performed, allowing medullary bleeding and clot formation [13] (Fig. 65.3). Osteochondral autograft transplantation or mosaicplasty involves harvesting of viable, structurally intact cartilage and bone plugs from a "dispensable" portion of a joint and transplanting the autograft to the chondral defect. ACI involves the harvest of chondrocytes from a nonessential portion of the knee during the first-stage surgery. The specimen undergoes expansion of chondrocytes in a laboratory. The chondrocytes are then placed in a medium, which is implanted on the defect with an overlying periosteal patch or collagen scaffold during the second-stage surgery. Given limitations of available comparative studies, no clear outcome benefit can be confirmed for either OAT or ACI over microfracture [13,15]. Only one level I study indicates better outcomes in athletes with initial arthroscopic OAT versus microfracture [16]. For cartilage lesions larger than 2 cm^2, Gudas and colleagues [16] showed worse clinical outcomes with microfracture. Currently, the literature lacks any level I study with a natural history control

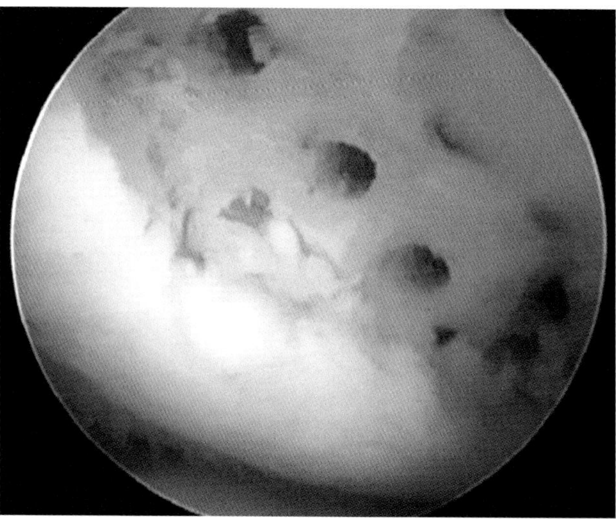

FIGURE 65.3 Arthroscopic image of the microfracture technique showing medullary bleeding after cortical penetration with an awl.

group, which makes outcomes after current surgical procedures difficult to interpret. With lack of superiority of any one surgical treatment, microfracture has been considered the first-line therapy, given its technical ease, lack of donor site graft morbidity, and affordability [13,15].

Potential Disease Complications

Most clinicians assume that traumatic articular cartilage lesions will continue to progress to osteoarthritis. However, the true natural history of these lesions has yet to be formally studied and remains unknown. Messner and Maletius [17] looked at radiographs 14 years after diagnosis of severe chondral injury in 28 patients to find that 22 had joint space narrowing of less than 50% in the compartment with injury.

Potential Treatment Complications

Common complications encountered after cartilage restoration surgery include arthrofibrosis, superficial wound infections, and tissue hypertrophy [15]. Lower incidences of deep venous thrombosis, hemarthrosis, and graft malpositioning occur [15]. Arthrofibrosis appears to occur with equal frequency with microfracture, ACI, and the OAT procedure [15]. Tissue hypertrophy surrounding the lesion and reactive synovitis are associated more commonly with ACI [15]. Proud or recessed graft is limited to the OAT procedure [15]. Reoperation is another complication and appears to be higher with ACI versus microfracture [15,18]. Newer all-arthroscopic, second-generation ACI techniques with a collagen membrane patch may show lower reoperation rates and decreased arthrofibrosis over the first-generation periosteal ACI techniques [18].

References

[1] Outerbridge RE. The etiology of chondromalacia patellae. J Bone Joint Surg Br 1961;43:752–7.
[2] Mankin HJ. The response of articular cartilage to mechanical injury. J Bone Joint Surg Am 1982;64:460–6.
[3] Furukawa T, Eyre DR, Koide S, et al. Biochemical studies on repair cartilage resurfacing experimental defects in the rabbit knee. J Bone Joint Surg Am 1980;62:79–89.
[4] Noyes FR, Basset RW, Grood ES, et al. Arthroscopy in acute traumatic hemarthrosis of the knee: incidence of anterior cruciate tears and other injuries. J Bone Joint Surg Am 1980;62:687–95.
[5] Aroen A, Loken S, Heir S, et al. Articular cartilage lesions in 993 consecutive knee arthroscopies. Am J Sports Med 2004;32:211–5.
[6] Hjelle K, Solheim E, Strand T, et al. Articular cartilage defects in 1000 knee arthroscopies. Arthroscopy 2002;18:730–4.
[7] Widuchowski W, Widuchowski J, Trzaska T. Articular cartilage defects: study of 25,124 knee arthroscopies. Knee 2007;14:177–82.
[8] Jazrawi LM, Alaia MJ, Chang G, et al. Advances in magnetic resonance imaging of articular cartilage. J Am Acad Orthop Surg 2011;19:420–9.
[9] Piper SL, Kim HT. Comparison of ropivacaine and bupivacaine toxicity in human articular chondrocytes. J Bone Joint Surg Am 2008;90:986–91.
[10] Salter RB, Simmonds DF, Malcom BW, et al. The biological effect of continuous passive motion on the healing of full-thickness defects in articular cartilage. An experimental investigation in the rabbit. J Bone Joint Surg Am 1980;62:1232–51.
[11] Martin-Hernandez C, Cebamanos-Celma J, Molina-Ros A, et al. Regenerated cartilage produced by autogenous periosteal grafts: a histologic and mechanical study in rabbits under the influence of continuous passive motion. Arthroscopy 2010;26:76–83.
[12] Fazalare JA, Griesser MJ, Siston RA, et al. The use of continuous passive motion following knee cartilage defect surgery: a systematic review. Orthopedics 2010;33:878.
[13] Safran MR, Seiber K. The evidence for surgical repair of articular cartilage in the knee. J Am Acad Orthop Surg 2010;18:259–66.
[14] Mandelbaum BR, Browne JE, Fu F, et al. Articular cartilage lesions of the knee. Am J Sports Med 1998;26:853–61.
[15] Magnussen RA, Dunn WR, Carey JL, et al. Treatment of focal articular cartilage defects in the knee: a systematic review. Clin Orthop Relat Res 2008;466:952–62.
[16] Gudas R, Kalesinskas RJ, Kimtys V, et al. A prospective randomized clinical study of mosaic osteochondral autologous transplantation versus microfracture for the treatment of osteochondral defects in the knee joint in young athletes. Arthroscopy 2005;21:1066–75.
[17] Messner K, Maletius W. The long-term prognosis for severe damage to weight-bearing cartilage in the knee: a 14-year clinical and radiographic follow-up in 28 young athletes. Acta Orthop Scand 1996;67:165–8.
[18] Harris JD, Siston RA, Brophy RH, et al. Failures, re-operations, and complications after autologous chondrocyte implantation—a systematic review. Osteoarthritis Cartilage 2011;19:779–91.

CHAPTER 66

Collateral Ligament Sprain

Paul Lento, MD

Venu Akuthota, MD

Synonyms

Knee ligamentous injuries
Medial or lateral collateral knee injury
Knee valgus or varus instability or insufficiency

ICD-9 Codes

717.81 Old disruption of lateral collateral ligament
717.82 Old disruption of medial collateral ligament
844.0 Sprains and strains of knee and leg (lateral collateral ligament)
844.1 Sprains and strains of knee and leg (medial collateral ligament)

ICD-10 Codes

M23.641 Spontaneous disruption of lateral collateral ligament of right knee
M23.642 Spontaneous disruption of lateral collateral ligament of left knee
M23.649 Spontaneous disruption of lateral collateral ligament of unspecified knee
M23.631 Spontaneous disruption of medial collateral ligament of right knee
M23.632 Spontaneous disruption of medial collateral ligament of left knee
M23.639 Spontaneous disruption of medial collateral ligament of unspecified knee
S83.421 Sprain of lateral collateral ligament of right knee
S83.422 Sprain of lateral collateral ligament of left knee
S83.429 Sprain of lateral collateral ligament of unspecified knee
S83.411 Sprain of medial collateral ligament of right knee
S83.412 Sprain of medial collateral ligament of left knee
S83.419 Sprain of medial collateral ligament of unspecified knee
Add seventh character for episode of care

Definition

The medial collateral ligament (MCL) and lateral collateral ligament (LCL) are important structures that predominantly prevent valgus and varus forces, respectively, through the knee (Fig. 66.1). Like other ligamentous injuries, knee collateral ligament sprains can be defined by three grades of injury. With a grade I sprain, there is localized tenderness without frank laxity. Anatomically, only a minimal number of fibers are torn. On physical examination, the joint space opens less than 5 mm (i.e., 1+ laxity). With a moderate, or grade II, sprain, there is more generalized tenderness without frank laxity. Grade II sprains can cover the gamut from a few fibers torn to nearly all fibers torn [1]. The joint may gap 5 to 10 mm (i.e., 2+ laxity) when force is applied. A severe, or grade III, sprain, by definition, is a complete disruption of all ligamentous fibers with a joint space gap of more than 10 mm (i.e., 3+ laxity) on stressing of the ligament [2].

Medial Complex Injury and Resultant Instability

The MCL is the most commonly injured ligament of the knee [3]. In fact, injury to this structure has been estimated to occur in 0.24 per 1000 people in the United States in any given year and to be twice as high in males (0.36) compared with females (0.18) [4]. This ligament is usually injured when valgus forces are applied to the knee [5]. Contact injuries produce grade III MCL deficits; noncontact MCL injuries typically result in lower grade injuries. Although MCL injury can occur in isolation, valgus forces typically instigate injury to other medial structures [6]. Findings of a rotational component to medial joint instability should prompt

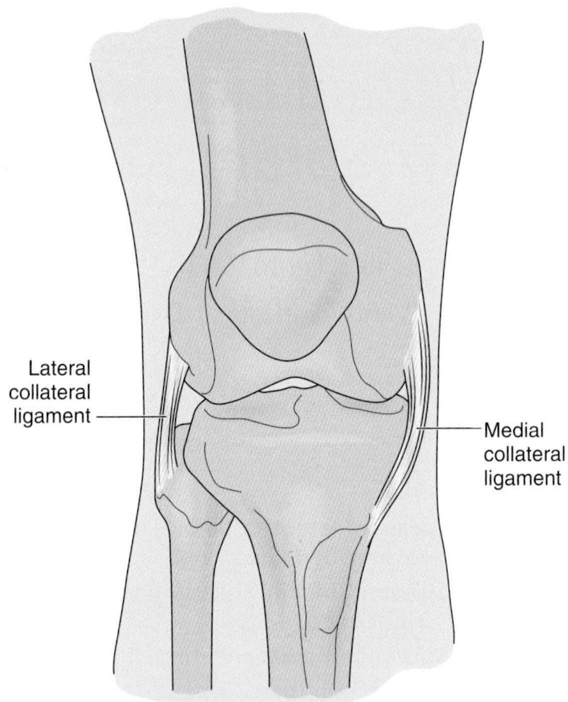

FIGURE 66.1 Medial and lateral collateral ligaments.

a search for cruciate ligament, meniscal, or posterior oblique ligament involvement [7,8].

Lateral Complex Injury and Resultant Instability

The LCL is much less frequently injured than the MCL. True isolated injury to the LCL is rare. True straight lateral instability requires a large vector force. Thus, a complete knee dislocation with possible damage to neurovascular structures should be suspected if straight lateral instability is present [9]. Posterolateral rotatory instability appears to be a more frequent cause of lateral instability than of straight lateral instability. Most authors believe that posterolateral rotatory instability requires disruption of the arcuate complex, the posterior cruciate ligament, and the LCL. The usual mechanism of posterolateral rotatory instability is forcing of the knee into hyperextension and external rotation [6,9].

Symptoms

Medial or lateral knee pain is the most common symptom related to knee collateral ligament injury. Interestingly, grade I and grade II injuries cause more pain than grade III injuries do [3,10]. Pain is often accompanied by a sensation of knee locking [8]. This may be due to hamstring muscle contraction or concomitant meniscal injury. Patients may also report an audible pop, although this is more common with anterior cruciate ligament injuries [3]. A giving way sensation or a feeling of instability is often reported with high-grade injuries. Moreover, patients with high-grade injuries may also have neurovascular damage [11]. Therefore these individuals may complain of a loss of sensation or muscle strength below the level of the knee [9].

Physical Examination

Physical examination begins with the uninjured knee to obtain a baseline. Palpatory examination can be as important as ligamentous laxity testing. Palpation can reveal tenderness along the length of the collateral ligament, localized swelling, or a tissue defect [8]. Localized swelling correlates well with the area of injury to the MCL [10]. With pure joint line tenderness, an underlying meniscal injury should be suspected. A true knee joint effusion may also be present with collateral ligament injuries; however, it is more prevalent with meniscal or cruciate ligament injury [12].

Laxity of the medial joint ligaments is determined by the abduction stress test (Fig. 66.2A), performed by examination of the knee at 0 and 30 degrees of joint flexion. If the test result is negative, a firm endpoint will be reached. If the test result is grossly positive, the femur and tibia will gap with valgus stress and "clunk" back when the stress is removed [13]. Although it is controversial, increased medial joint laxity of the fully extended knee with a valgus force not only implies damage to the superficial and deep fibers of the MCL but also indicates rupture of the posterior cruciate ligament or posterior oblique ligament [14–16]. If laxity occurs at 30 degrees of flexion but not at 0 degrees, one may confidently conclude that MCL injury is present with sparing of the posterior capsule and posterior cruciate ligament [10,13]. The soft endpoint during valgus stress with the knee at 30 degrees of flexion is the intact cruciate ligament [16]. Although the anterior drawer test is classically used for chronic anterior

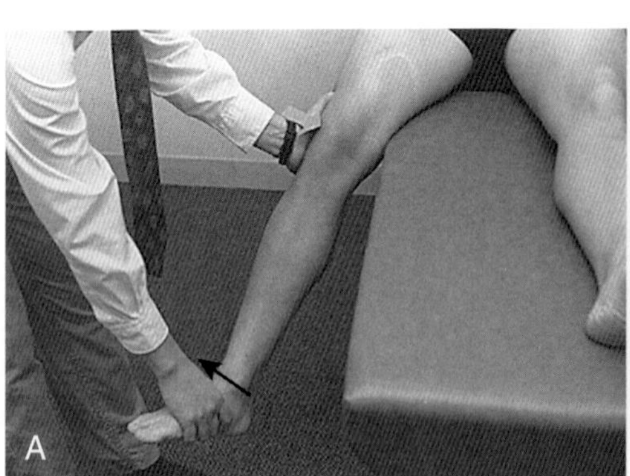

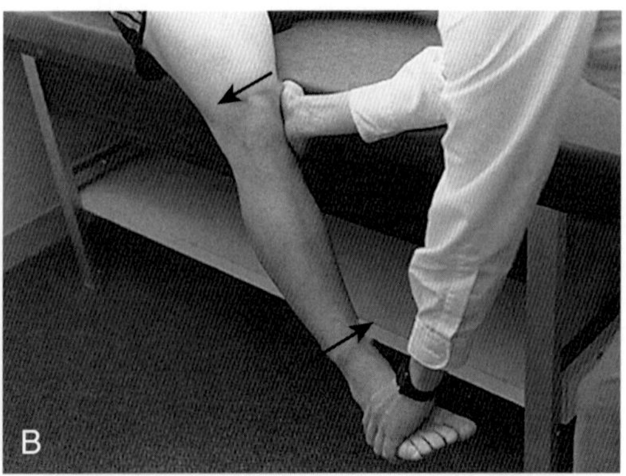

FIGURE 66.2 **A,** Abduction stress of the knee at 30 degrees tests for medial collateral ligament injury. **B,** Adduction stress of the knee at 30 degrees tests for lateral collateral ligament injury. *(From Mellion MB, Walsh WM, Shelton GL. The Team Physician's Handbook, 2nd ed. Philadelphia, Hanley & Belfus, 1997.)*

cruciate ligament tears, it can be a useful adjunctive test for detection of MCL or posterior oblique ligament injury [10].

Laxity of the lateral knee joint ligaments is determined by the adduction stress test, which is also performed at 0 and 30 degrees of knee flexion and compared with the opposite "normal" knee (Fig. 66.2B). Gapping of the lateral joint line at 30 degrees of knee flexion indicates damage to the LCL and arcuate ligament complex [12,15]. However, joint opening with the knee in full extension indicates damage not only to the LCL but also to the middle third of the capsular ligament, cruciate ligaments, iliotibial band, or arcuate ligament complex [6,17]. When LCL injury is associated with rotational instability, the reverse pivot shift may be helpful [18]. This maneuver is performed by application of a varus force to an initially flexed knee. A positive test result reveals a clunk as the knee is passively extended from a flexed position. The clunk is a result of the relocation with extension of a knee subluxed in flexion [11,15]. Rotational instability may also be detected by the external rotation recurvatum test (Fig. 66.3).

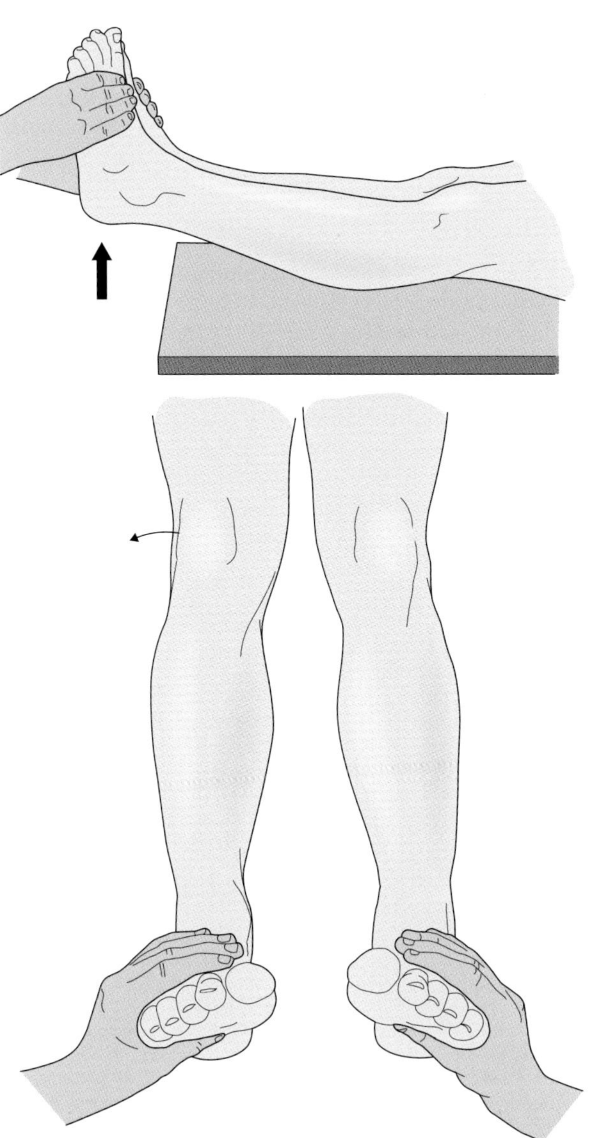

FIGURE 66.3 External rotation recurvatum test. Both knees are passively held in extension by holding the forefoot. If the tibia on the affected side externally rotates more than the normal side, the test result is considered positive and indicates damage to the posterolateral knee structures.

Functional Limitations

The functional limitations for patients with MCL and LCL injuries result from instability. In general, sagittal plane movements are better tolerated than frontal or transverse plane motions. Most patients with grade III tears of the MCL are able to walk comfortably without an assistive device. Few, however, are able to traverse steps or to do a full knee squat [10]. Patients may also report difficulty with transfers and "cutting" sports activities. Some individuals with posterolateral ligament injuries may have pain with prolonged standing or knee hyperextension. This posterolateral laxity may eventually result in significant genu recurvatum as well as tibia vara, producing pain with even basic activities such as walking and standing [6].

Diagnostic Testing

Plain radiographs are usually normal in acute sprains of the collateral ligaments. Radiographs may be particularly useful to detect avulsion and tibial plateau fractures [7]. For example, an avulsion fracture of the proximal fibula can be detected after a varus-type injury and is associated with posterolateral corner injury, the so-called arcuate sign [19]. Stress views may be indicated in skeletally immature patients for evaluation of physeal injuries [20]. The current "gold standard" diagnostic test is magnetic resonance imaging. Magnetic resonance imaging can detect concomitant injury as well as the severity of collateral ligament damage [21]. Bone bruises not evident on plain films may be detected by magnetic resonance imaging. This can be an important finding, particularly in patients who are experiencing persistent pain. Diagnostic musculoskeletal ultrasound has been used to diagnose and prognosticate injuries of the collateral ligaments and posterolateral corner of the knee [22–24].

Differential Diagnosis

MEDIAL KNEE PAIN

Medial meniscus injury
Anterior cruciate ligament injury
Medial compartment osteoarthritis
Pes anserine bursitis
Medial tibial plateau fracture
Vastus medialis obliquus injury
Medial plica band syndrome

MEDIAL OR LATERAL KNEE PAIN

Patella subluxation or dislocation
Bone bruise
Osteochondral injury
Referred or radicular pain

LATERAL KNEE PAIN

Lateral meniscus tear
Iliotibial band syndrome
Lateral compartment osteoarthritis
Popliteus or biceps tendinitis
Lateral gastrocnemius strain

Treatment

Initial

After it has been determined whether concomitant injury is present, all grades of collateral ligament injuries are treated initially in the same manner. The basic principles of PRICE (*p*rotect, *r*est, *i*ce, *c*ompression, *e*levation) apply. Immobilization can be used if pain is a significant issue but typically only for a limited time in grade II MCL and LCL injuries [25]. Alternatively, patients with grade II and grade III injuries may need crutches or a hinged knee brace locked between 20 and 60 degrees to provide additional support for an unstable knee, but there is no consensus regarding this [26]. Allowable brace range of motion is increased as tolerated to prevent arthrofibrosis [7,12,27]. Nonsteroidal anti-inflammatory medications may be prescribed to provide pain relief as well as to reduce local inflammation associated with acute injury [28].

Rehabilitation

The goals of rehabilitation for the knee with a collateral ligament injury are to restore range of motion, to increase stability, and to return pain-free activity. Rehabilitation protocols have been described even for grade III MCL injuries [25]. Within the first 24 to 48 hours after injury, static isometric quadriceps contractions and electrical stimulation can be instituted to reduce local tissue swelling and to retard muscle atrophy [13,27]. Range of motion exercises and gentle stretching activities are introduced after the first day [7]. Early weight bearing is also encouraged. Aerobic conditioning can be maintained by use of upper body ergometry, stationary bicycle, or swimming with gentle flutter kicks. Maintenance-phase rehabilitation should emphasize exercise in multiple planes. Rehabilitation should eventually progress to functional or sport-specific activity [25]. A combination of closed and open kinetic chain exercises is used [25,29]. Typically, individuals with mild collateral ligament injuries return to activity after 3 to 4 weeks; patients with grade II and grade III injuries may be able to return to activity after 8 to 12 weeks [30]. Prophylactic hinged knee brace use has been advocated, although effectiveness remains controversial [31–33]. Postsurgical rehabilitation for grade III LCL and MCL injuries with concomitant anterior cruciate ligament, posterior cruciate ligament, or meniscal repair should be at the discretion of the individual surgeon. Variability occurs with each surgeon in respect to immediate weight bearing, protected range of motion, and return to full activity [34].

Procedures

Procedures such as corticosteroid injections have not been studied in acute collateral ligament injuries and typically are not indicated [35]. Needling of symptomatic calcifications within the MCL has been reported [36].

Surgery

The treatment of grade I and grade II injuries of the MCL and LCL is nonsurgical. Grade III injuries, especially when they are associated with concomitant injuries, may be treated surgically. However, most practitioners treat isolated grade III MCL injuries nonsurgically secondary to the high healing rates [3,13,27,37]. Repair of an MCL tear without repair of an associated anterior cruciate ligament injury may lead to a high failure rate [8]. In contrast, grade III LCL injuries or posterolateral complex tears with or without associated cruciate ligament injuries have been shown to heal poorly with nonsurgical measures [7,38,39]. In this case, surgical intervention within 2 weeks, addressing deficits of the arcuate ligament complex, lateral meniscus, and cruciates, provides optimal outcomes [7].

Potential Disease Complications

The most significant disease complication is chronic knee instability. This most commonly occurs with undetected injury to the posterolateral joint complex. Another cited complication is an increased risk of osteoarthritis. Osteoarthritis occurs more frequently with combined MCL and anterior cruciate ligament ruptures than with pure MCL injury [40]. Pellegrini-Stieda disease may also be a rare complication [41]. This condition consists of focal calcium deposition in the area of the injured ligament, typically on the femoral insertion of the MCL. Massage or manipulation may worsen this condition. Instead, calcium reabsorption may be stimulated by dry needling [7,12,36].

Potential Treatment Complications

Analgesics and nonsteroidal anti-inflammatory drugs have well-known side effects that most commonly affect the gastric, hepatic, and renal systems. If the injured knee is immobilized for too long or if range of motion does not proceed in an appropriate fashion, stiffness may result with possible loss of full extension. Similarly, if a surgeon reattaches the deep or superficial components of the MCL to the femoral condyle as opposed to the epicondyle, ankylosis of the joint may result, restricting flexion as well as extension [8].

References

[1] Wijdicks CA, Griffith CJ, Johansen S, et al. Injuries to the medial collateral ligament and associated medial structures of the knee. J Bone Joint Surg Am 2010;92:1266–80.

[2] Committee on the Medical Aspects of Sports, American Medical Association. Standard Nomenclature of Athletic Injuries. Chicago: American Medical Association; 1966, 99-101.

[3] Linton RC, Indelicato P. Medial ligament injuries. In: DeLee JC, Drez D, editors. Orthopaedic sports medicine: principles and practice, vol 2. Philadelphia: WB Saunders; 1994. p. 1261–74.

[4] Daniel DM, Pedowitz RA, O'Connor JJ, Akeson WH, editors. Daniel's knee injuries: ligament and cartilage structure, function, injury, and repair. 2nd ed. Philadelphia: Lippincott Williams & Wilkins; 2003.

[5] Wijdicks CA, Ewart DT, Nuckley DJ, et al. Structural properties of the primary medial knee ligaments. Am J Sports Med 2010;38:1638–46.

[6] Hughston JC, Andrews JR, Cross MJ, et al. Classification of knee ligament instabilities. Part II. The lateral compartment. J Bone Joint Surg Am 1976;58:173–83.

[7] LaPrade RF. Medial ligament complex and the posterolateral aspect of the knee. In: Arendt EA, editor. Orthopaedic knowledge update. Rosemont, Ill: American Academy of Orthopedic Surgeons; 1999. p. 327–47.

[8] Bocell JR. Medial collateral ligament injuries. In: Baker CL, editor. The hughston clinic sports medicine book. Baltimore: Williams & Wilkins; 1995. p. 516–25.

[9] Jakob RP, Warner JP. Lateral and posterolateral rotatory instability of the knee. In: DeLee JC., Drez D, editors. Orthopaedic sports medicine: principles and practice, vol 2. Philadelphia: WB Saunders; 1994. p. 1275–312.

[10] Hughston JC, Andrews JR, Cross MJ, et al. Classification of knee ligament instabilities. Part I. The medial compartment and cruciate ligaments. J Bone Joint Surg Am 1976;58:159–72.
[11] Delee JC, Riley MB, Rockwood CA. Acute posterolateral rotatory instability of the knee. Am J Sports Med 1983;11:199–207.
[12] Simon RR, Koenigsknecht SJ. The knee. In: Simon RR, Koenigsknecht SJ, editors. Emergency orthopedics: the extremities. 3rd ed. Norwalk, Conn: Appleton & Lange; 1995. p. 437–62.
[13] Reider B. Medial collateral ligament injuries in athletes. Sports Med 1996;21:147–56.
[14] Swenson TM, Harner CD. Knee ligament and meniscal injuries. Orthop Clin North Am 1995;26:529–46.
[15] Magee DJ. Knee. In: Magee DJ, editor. Orthopedic physical examination. 2nd ed. Philadelphia: WB Saunders; 1992. p. 372–447.
[16] Chen L, Kim PD, Ahmad CS, Levine WN. Medial collateral ligament injuries of the knee: current treatment concepts. Curr Rev Musculoskelet Med 2008;1:108–13.
[17] Grood E, Noyes F, Butler D, Suntay W. Ligamentous and capsular restraints preventing straight medial and lateral laxity in intact human cadaver knees. J Bone Joint Surg Am 1981;63:1257.
[18] LaPrade RF, Terry GC. Injuries to the posterolateral aspect of the knee. Association of anatomic injury patterns with clinical instability. Am J Sports Med 1997;25:433–8.
[19] Huang GS, Joseph SY, Munshi M, et al. Avulsion fracture of the head of the fibula (the "arcuate" sign): MR imaging findings predictive of injuries to the posterolateral ligaments and posterior cruciate ligament. AJR Am J Roentgenol 2003;180:381–7.
[20] Zionts LE. Fractures around the knee in children. J Am Acad Orthop Surg 2002;10:345–55.
[21] Stoller DW, Cannon WD, Anderson LJ. The knee. In: Stoller DW, editor. Magnetic resonance imaging in orthopaedics and sports medicine. 2nd ed. Philadelphia: JB Lippincott; 1997. p. 203–442.
[22] Finlay K, Friedman L. Ultrasonography of the lower extremity. Orthop Clin North Am 2006;37:245–75, v.
[23] Lee JI, Song IS, Jung YB, et al. Medial collateral ligament injuries of the knee: ultrasonographic findings. J Ultrasound Med 1996;15:621–5.
[24] Sekiya JK, Swaringen JC, Wojtys EM, Jacobson JA. Diagnostic ultrasound evaluation of posterolateral corner knee injuries. Arthroscopy 2010;26:494–9.
[25] Giannotti BF, Rudy T, Graziano J. The non-surgical management of isolated medial collateral ligament injuries of the knee. Sports Med Arthrosc 2006;14:74–7.
[26] LaPrade R, Wijdicks CA. The management of injuries to the medial side of the knee. J Orthop Sports Phys Ther 2012;42:221–30.
[27] Richards DB, Kibler BW. Rehabilitation of knee injuries. In: Kibler BW, Herring SA, Press JM, editors. Functional rehabilitation of sports and musculoskeletal injuries. Gaithersburg, Md: Aspen; 1998. p. 244–53.
[28] Mehallo CJ, Drezner JA, Bytomski JR. Practical management: nonsteroidal antiinflammatory drug (NSAID) use in athletic injuries. Clin J Sport Med 2006;16:170–4.
[29] Shelbourne K, Patel D, Adsit W, Porter D. Rehabilitation after meniscal repair. Clin Sports Med 1996;15:595–612.
[30] Brukner PKK. Acute knee injuries. In: Brukner PKK, editor. Clinical sports medicine. 2nd ed. New York: McGraw-Hill; 2001. p. 426–63.
[31] Rovere GD, Haupt HA, Yates CS. Prophylactic knee bracing in college football. Am J Sports Med 1987;15:111–6.
[32] Teitz CC, Hermanson B, Kronmal R, Diehr P. Evaluation of the use of braces to prevent injury to the knee in collegiate football players. J Bone Joint Surg Am 1987;69:2–9.
[33] Hewson GF, Mendini RA, Wang JB. Prophylactic knee bracing in college football. Am J Sports Med 1986;14:262–6.
[34] Marchant MH, Tibor LM, Sekiya JK, et al. Management of medial-sided knee injuries, part 1: medial collateral ligament. Am J Sports Med 2011;39:1102–13.
[35] Cole BJ, Schumacher HR. Injectable corticosteroids in modern practice. J Am Acad Orthop Surg 2005;13:37–46.
[36] Muschol M, Müller I, Petersen W, Hassenpflug J. Symptomatic calcification of the medial collateral ligament of the knee joint: a report about five cases. Knee Surg Sports Traumatol Arthrosc 2005;13:598–602.
[37] Reider B, Sathy MR, Talkington J, et al. Treatment of isolated medial collateral ligament injuries in athletes with early functional rehabilitation. A five-year follow-up study. Am J Sports Med 1994;22:470–7.
[38] LaPrade RF, Hamilton CD, Engebretsen L. Treatment of acute and chronic combined anterior cruciate ligament and posterolateral knee ligament injuries. Sports Med Arthrosc Rev 1997;5:91.
[39] Kannus P. Nonoperative treatment of grade II and III sprains of the lateral ligament compartment of the knee. Am J Sports Med 1989;17:83–8.
[40] Lundberg M, Messner K. Ten-year prognosis of isolated and combined medial collateral ligament ruptures. A matched comparison in 40 patients using clinical and radiographic evaluations. Am J Sports Med 1997;25:2–6.
[41] Schein A, Matcuk G, Patel D, et al. Structure and function, injury, pathology, and treatment of the medial collateral ligament of the knee. Emerg Radiol 2012;19:489–98.

CHAPTER 67

Compartment Syndrome of the Leg

Joseph E. Herrera, DO
Mahmud M. Ibrahim, MD

Synonyms

Acute compartment syndrome
- **Volkmann ischemia**
- **Traumatic tension in muscles**
- **Calf hypertension**
- **Well leg compartment syndrome**

Chronic compartment syndrome
- **Chronic exertional compartment syndrome**
- **Exercise-induced compartment syndrome**
- **Anterior or medial tibial pain syndrome**

ICD-9 Codes

728.9 Unspecified disorder of muscle, ligament, and fascia
958.8 Other early complications of trauma (compartment syndrome)

ICD-10 Codes

M62.9 Disorder of muscle, unspecified
T79.A0 Compartment syndrome, unspecified

Definition

Compartment syndrome can be either an acute or chronic condition caused by increased tissue pressure within an enclosed fascial space. The focus of this chapter is compartment syndrome of the leg, although it can also affect the thighs or upper extremities.

Acute Compartment Syndrome

Acute compartment syndrome (ACS) is a serious condition caused by a rapid rise in pressure in an enclosed space, which can lead to necrosis of the muscles and nerves in the involved compartment. Untreated, ACS can progress to contractures, paralysis, infection, and gangrene in the limb as well as systemic problems, such as myoglobinuria and kidney failure [1]. ACS, most commonly occurring in males younger than 35 years, is most often caused by trauma such as fractures, crush injuries, muscle rupture, direct blow to a muscle, and circumferential burns. Direct pressure from a cast or antishock garment can increase the risk for compartment syndrome [2]. ACS can occur in as many as 17% of tibial fractures [3]. The anterior compartment is most commonly affected, although multiple compartments are often involved.

Nontraumatic causes of ACS are more rare. These include hemorrhage into a compartment, as can occur in anticoagulated patients [2], and compartment syndrome after diabetic muscle infarction [4]. In patients with decreased mental status with prolonged limb compression, such as with alcohol or drug abuse, ACS can also develop from soft tissue injury and swelling [5].

Another nontraumatic cause of compartment syndrome is ischemia and then hyperperfusion caused by prolonged surgery in the lithotomy position. This is also known as well leg compartment syndrome and is most often seen after pelvic and perineal surgery. Risk factors include the length of the procedure, the amount of leg elevation, the amount of perioperative blood loss, and the presence of peripheral vascular disease and obesity. The overall incidence in complex pelvic surgeries may be as high as 1 in 500 [6].

Chronic Compartment Syndrome

Chronic compartment syndrome (CCS) occurs when the fascia in the lower leg does not accommodate to the increase in blood flow and fluid shifts that may occur with heavy exercise [7]. An increase in compartmental pressure then interferes with blood flow, leading to ischemia and pain when the metabolic demands cannot be met [8]. The risk of CCS is increased by anabolic steroids, which can induce muscle hypertrophy, thereby causing an increase in intracompartmental pressure and decreasing fascial elasticity [9]. CCS is most commonly seen in runners [10], cyclists, and other athletes in sports that demand running, jumping, and cutting, such as basketball and soccer. The true incidence is unknown as most people suffering from early symptoms will decrease or modify their activity [11]. With normal physical activity, muscle volume can increase up to 20% [12]. The anterior compartment is most commonly involved, followed by the deep posterior compartment [11].

Symptoms

The area in which symptoms occur and the type of complaints depend on which compartment is involved.

Acute Compartment Syndrome

Patients may present with pain out of proportion to the injury and swelling or tenseness in the area. Other symptoms include severe pain with passive movement of the muscles within the compartment, loss of voluntary movement of the muscles involved, and sensory changes and paresthesias in the area supplied by the nerve involved [3,7]. The classic findings associated with arterial insufficiency are often described as signs of ACS, but this is incorrect. Of the five classic signs (pain, pallor, pulselessness, paresthesias, paralysis), only pain is commonly associated with compartment syndrome, particularly in its early stages [12].

Chronic Compartment Syndrome

In CCS, pain has a gradual onset that usually coincides with an increase in exercise training load or training on hard surfaces. It is described as aching, burning, or cramping and occurs with repetitive movements in a specific muscle region. The pain usually occurs around the same time each time the patient participates in the activity (e.g., after 15 minutes of running) and increases or stays constant if the activity continues. The pain disappears or dramatically lessens after a few minutes of rest. Symptoms can occur bilaterally [8].

As symptoms progress, a dull aching pain may persist. Pain may be localized to a particular compartment, although multiple compartments can often be involved. Numbness and tingling may occur in the nerves that travel within the involved lower limb compartment. CCS can be seen with other overuse syndromes (e.g., concurrent with tibial stress fractures).

Physical Examination

The examination is focused on the following four compartments of the leg (Fig. 67.1).

Anterior compartment contains the tibialis anterior, which dorsiflexes the ankle; the long toe extensors, which dorsiflex the toes; the anterior tibial artery; and the deep peroneal nerve, which supplies sensation to the first web space.

Lateral compartment contains the peroneus longus and brevis, which evert the foot, and the superficial peroneal nerve, which supplies sensation to the dorsum of the foot.

Superficial posterior compartment contains the gastrocnemius and soleus muscles, which plantar flex the foot, and part of the sural nerve, which supplies sensation to the lateral foot and distal calf [1,8,12].

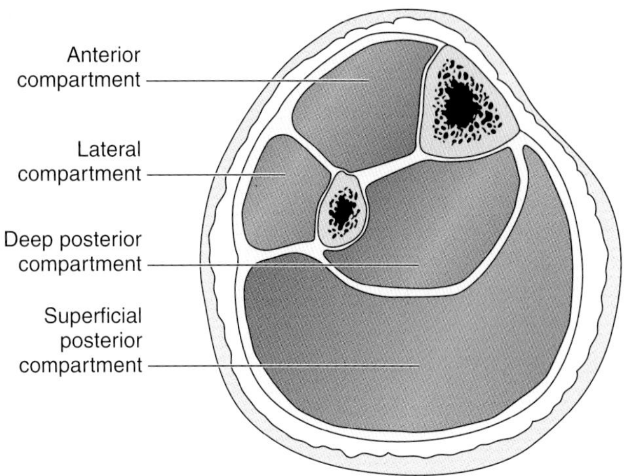

FIGURE 67.1 The focus of the physical examination in compartment syndrome is the anterior, lateral, superficial posterior, and deep posterior compartments.

Deep posterior compartment contains the tibialis posterior, which plantar flexes and inverts the foot; the long toe flexors, which plantar flex the toes; the peroneal artery; and the tibial nerve, which supplies sensation to the plantar surface of the foot. This compartment may contain several subcompartments [13].

Acute Compartment Syndrome

In ACS, inspection reveals a swollen, tense limb. Motor testing reveals weakness or paralysis of the muscles involved in the affected compartment. Sensory testing may show numbness in the area supplied by the nerve involved in the affected compartment. Two-point discrimination is a better diagnostic test for compartment syndrome than pinprick [13]. Pulses and capillary refills are generally normal as these are involved only with extremely high pressures [3,7,14,15].

Chronic Compartment Syndrome

In CCS, inspection is usually unremarkable, but fascial defects have been observed in up to 40% of individuals. These defects may represent the body's attempt to accomplish an autorelease [11]. Palpation of the affected area will reveal a firm compartment and tender muscle group. There may also be tenderness along the posteromedial surface of the tibia [16]. In approximately 40% of cases, muscle herniation in the compartment can be palpated, especially in the anterior and lateral compartments where the superficial peroneal nerve pierces the fascia [6]. In severe cases, sensory testing will show numbness in the area supplied by the nerve involved, but this is usually normal at rest [7]. Motor testing may reveal weakness, depending on the compartment involved: dorsiflexion weakness if the anterior compartment is involved, foot eversion weakness if the lateral compartment is involved, and plantar flexion weakness if one of the posterior compartments is involved. Pain is reproduced by repetitive activity, such as toe raises, or running in place. Compartment syndrome occurs more commonly in patients who pronate during running; thus, pronation is a common finding on physical examination [1,7,17].

Functional Limitations

Acute Compartment Syndrome

The sequelae of ACS may be nerve and muscle injury with resulting footdrop, severe muscle weakness, and contractures. This can lead to an abnormal gait and all the limitations that this can cause, including difficulties with stairs, sports participation, and activities of daily living. In addition, it can lead to muscle necrosis, thereby causing long-term disability [18].

Chronic Compartment Syndrome

With CCS, functional limitations usually occur around the same point each time during exercise, at that individual's ischemic threshold. For example, symptoms may start to develop each time a runner reaches the half-mile mark or each time a cyclist climbs a large hill. This may significantly limit sports participation and occasionally even interferes with activities of daily living, such as prolonged walking.

Diagnostic Studies

Compartmental tissue pressure measurement is the "gold standard" for diagnosis. The devices most commonly used to measure intracompartmental pressures were traditionally the slit and wick catheters (Fig. 67.2) [7]. Newer devices, such as the transducer-tipped probe (Fig. 67.3), are now gaining popularity [19]. Ultrasound-guided transducer placement is especially helpful in patients receiving anticoagulation, patients with a large body habitus, and patients with distorted anatomy, such as after surgery or trauma [11].

Acute Compartment Syndrome

Normal compartment pressure is less than 10 mm Hg. Traditionally, absolute tissue pressure above 30 mm Hg was considered the cutoff value for fasciotomy to be performed [7,19]. However, it is likely that many unnecessary fasciotomies were performed by use of this measure alone. Currently, continuous monitoring of compartment pressures is used in high-risk cases, such as leg trauma with tibial fractures. The differential pressure, calculated as the intramuscular pressure subtracted from the diastolic blood pressure, determines the treatment course. If the differential pressure is less than 30 mm Hg, fasciotomy is indicated [20]. Studies have shown that if this differential pressure remains consistently above 30 mm Hg, even with markedly

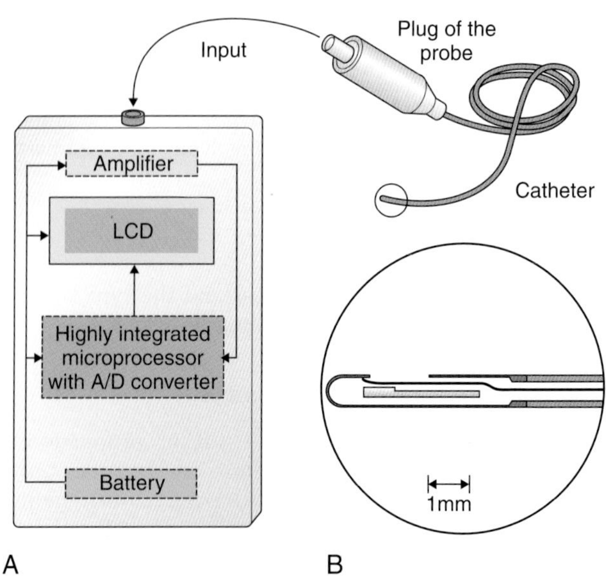

FIGURE 67.3 Transducer-tipped probe. **A,** Hand-held device. **B,** Catheter tip with pressure-sensing mechanics. *(From Willy C, Gerngross H, Sterk J. Measurement of intracompartmental pressure with use of a new electronic transducer-tipped catheter system. J Bone Joint Surg Am 1999;81:158-168.)*

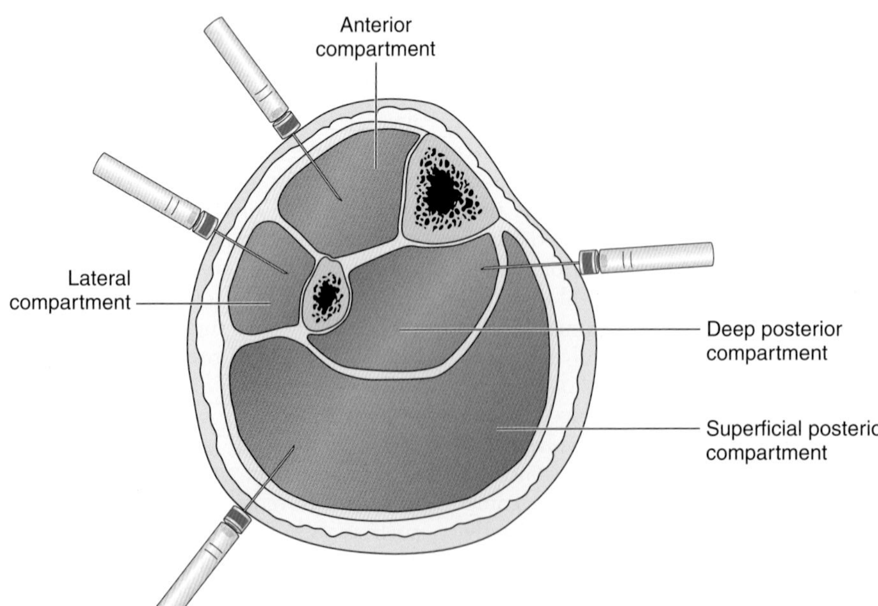

FIGURE 67.2 Compartmental tissue pressure measurements for the diagnosis of compartment syndrome with the use of slit and wick catheters.

elevated tissue pressures, patients have excellent clinical outcomes and fasciotomy is not necessary [20,21].

Because of the invasive nature of compartmental pressure measurements, other diagnostic tools have been sought. Magnetic resonance imaging may be helpful in making the diagnosis. Magnetic resonance imaging findings may include loss of normal muscle architecture on T1-weighted images, edema within the compartment, and strong enhancement of the affected compartment with the contrast agent gadolinium-DTPA [22].

Chronic Compartment Syndrome

For CCS, absolute pressure measurements obtained at rest, during exercise, and after exercise are used to make the diagnosis. Interestingly, there does not seem to be a particular threshold compartmental pressure at which symptoms occur, and patients with higher pressures do not necessarily have worse symptoms than those of patients with less abnormal pressures [23]. The average time from the onset of symptoms to the time that the diagnosis is made is 22 months [7].

The following is one set of values [7,15] commonly used to diagnose *anterior compartment* syndrome:

- Pre-exercise pressure >15 mm Hg
- 1 minute after exercise >30 mm Hg
- 5 minutes after exercise >20 mm Hg

It is important that the patient's symptoms correlate with the compartment in which there is elevated pressure. Pressure should increase in the symptomatic compartment with exercise and remain elevated for an abnormal time [8,23]. Values for *posterior compartments* are more controversial. Normal resting pressures are less than 10 mm Hg, and values should return to resting levels after 1 to 2 minutes of exercise [15].

Drawbacks to measurement of pressures include the following:

- They are invasive and can be complicated by bleeding or infection.
- Because of the anatomy, it is difficult to test the deep posterior compartment.
- Pressures are dependent on the position of the leg and the technique used, so strict standards should be followed.
- It is time-consuming because each compartment must be tested separately, and all compartments should be tested because multiple areas are often involved.
- It is often difficult for patients to exercise with the catheter in place [17,24].

Because of these drawbacks, alternative tests to confirm the diagnosis are sometimes used. Magnetic resonance imaging done before and after exercise can show increased signal intensity throughout the affected compartment in the T2-weighted images after exercise in patients with compartment syndrome [25,26]. Alternatively, near-infrared spectroscopy has been used as well. This method measures the hemoglobin saturation of tissues [9]. In cases of CCS, there is deoxygenation of muscle during exercise and delayed reoxygenation after exercise. Failure of the compartment to return to baseline within 25 minutes after exercise is diagnostic of CCS [11]. Although near-infrared spectroscopy seems to be helpful in patients with anterior compartment syndrome, light absorption may be altered in deeper compartments, and therefore it is more difficult to monitor the pressure in these deeper compartments [9]. Other methods include thallium stress testing and nuclear magnetic resonance spectroscopy, which may also be helpful in the diagnosis of CCS [9]. Triple-phase bone scan and single-photon emission computed tomography scans can be used to rule out other conditions in the differential diagnosis, such as medial tibial stress syndrome or stress fractures [11].

Differential Diagnosis

ACUTE COMPARTMENT SYNDROME

Arterial occlusion
Severe muscle trauma
Neurapraxia of the common, deep, or superficial peroneal or tibial nerve
Deep venous thrombosis
Cellulitis
Fracture

CHRONIC COMPARTMENT SYNDROME

Tibial or fibular stress fractures
Shin splints
Atherosclerosis with vascular claudication
Popliteal artery compression from aberrant insertion of the medial gastrocnemius
Muscle hyperdevelopment causing compression of the popliteal artery
Cystic adventitial disease [27]

Treatment

Initial

Acute Compartment Syndrome

If the differential pressure is less than 30 mm Hg, treatment of ACS is surgical fasciotomy, which is described later [20]. In cases in which the differential pressure remains above 30 mm Hg, it has been shown to be safe to observe those patients with serial pressure measurements [21].

Chronic Compartment Syndrome

For CCS, the initial treatment consists of rest, ice, and nonsteroidal anti-inflammatory drugs. Counseling the patient to avoid running on hard surfaces, to use orthotics to control pronation, and to wear running shoes with the appropriate amount of cushion and a flared heel is important [7]. Surgery is usually reserved for symptoms persisting beyond 6 to 12 weeks, despite conservative therapy [13].

Rehabilitation

Acute Compartment Syndrome

The rehabilitation of ACS is limited to the postfasciotomy stage. Rehabilitation depends on the extent of the injury. Proper skin care for either the open area left to close by secondary intent or the skin grafts that have been applied is imperative. An ankle-foot orthotic to correct footdrop is often needed. Physical therapy is needed for gentle range of motion exercises to prevent contractures and should begin as soon after surgery as possible and as allowed by wound healing issues. Other measures include strengthening of muscles that may be only partially affected and gait training, possibly with an assistive device. There is no scientific literature to support any specific rehabilitation protocols, and so programs should be individualized on the basis of the particular patient's needs. If the patient has deficits in activities of daily living, such as dressing or transfers, occupational therapy may be helpful in addressing these areas.

Chronic Compartment Syndrome

Controversy exists about the success of conservative treatment of CCS [7]. Current recommendations are based on the initial use of PRICE (*p*rotection, *r*est, *i*ce, *c*ompression, and *e*levation), with progression to reestablishing range of motion and soft tissue mobility, incorporating stretching, nerve gliding techniques, strengthening exercises, and incorporating biomechanical analysis of the patient during sport-specific activity [28]. Evaluating and identifying the underlying cause, such as excessive pronation, is important in considering the rehabilitation course. Treatment of excessive pronation includes establishing normal muscle lengths throughout the kinetic chain, especially stretching the gastrocnemius and posterior tibialis, and strengthening the anterior tibialis [29]. Shoe orthoses to address excessive pronation may also be helpful. Training errors, such as rapid increases in intensity or duration, are addressed and corrected. In addition, soft tissue mobilization and manipulation techniques, including massage, myofascial stretching, and taping, may increase fascial compliance. This would address the proposed pathophysiologic process involving increased facial thickness, stiffness, and increased pressure [28].

If fasciotomy is done for CCS, postsurgical rehabilitation should follow. Weight bearing is permitted as tolerated, and gentle range of motion exercises are begun 1 to 2 days postoperatively. Strengthening and gradual return to activity begin at 1 to 2 weeks. Full return to activity such as running usually takes 8 to 12 weeks [30].

Procedures

Procedures are not typically done in compartment syndrome except as stated earlier to measure compartmental pressures as a diagnostic procedure.

Surgery

Acute Compartment Syndrome

Fasciotomy should be performed for ACS as soon as possible. Large longitudinal incisions are made in the affected compartment. These incisions are left open to be closed gradually, or split-thickness skin grafts are applied. Results of the surgery are variable and depend on the length of time of ischemia and other injuries involved [31]. Newer techniques allow fasciotomy to be performed with endoscopy and minimally invasive incisions [11,13]. Controversy exists as to whether all four compartments need to be released in cases of ACS. One study showed that release of only the anterior compartment had equivalent results to release of the anterior and lateral compartments [32]. If treatment is delayed for more than 12 hours, it is assumed that permanent damage has occurred to the muscles and nerves in the involved compartment. Late reconstruction procedures can be done, if necessary, to correct muscle contractures or to perform tendon transfers for footdrop [31].

Chronic Compartment Syndrome

Fasciotomy is also the mainstay for surgical treatment of CCS [7]. Different techniques for fasciotomy have been described. Most consist of making a small incision in the skin and then releasing the fascia as far proximally and distally as possible while avoiding nerves and vessels. Results of surgery are usually good, with average success rates of 80% to 90% as defined by a decrease in symptoms and a return to sports [30].

Potential Disease Complications

Acute Compartment Syndrome

In ACS, ischemia of less than 4 hours usually does not cause permanent damage. If ischemia lasts more than 12 hours, severe damage is expected. Ischemia of 4 to 12 hours can also cause significant damage, including muscle necrosis, muscle contractures, loss of nerve function, infection, gangrene, myoglobinuria, and renal failure. Amputation of the affected limb is sometimes necessary, and even death may occur from the systemic effects of necrosis or infection [1,3,7]. Recurrence has also been known to develop. Calcific myonecrosis can also be a late side effect [33].

Chronic Compartment Syndrome

If CCS is left untreated, it may become acute in presentation and result in irreversible sequelae [13].

Potential Treatment Complications

ACS fasciotomy has serious complications. Mortality rates are 11% to 15%, and serious morbidity is common, including amputation rates of 10% to 20% and diminished limb function in 27% [34].

CCS fasciotomy is a less extensive surgery on a healthier population. Complications are uncommon but can include bleeding, infection, deep venous thrombosis, wound infection, lymphocele, and nerve injury, particularly to the superficial peroneal nerve. Case series report a recurrence rate of 3% to 20%. The most common reasons for recurrence are excessive scar tissue formation, causing the compartment to become tight again, and inadequate fascial release. A case series exploring the outcome of repeated fasciotomy for recurrence of symptoms reported that 70% of patients had good or excellent outcomes [35].

One potential long-term complication of fasciotomy is an increased risk for development of chronic venous insufficiency caused by the loss of the calf musculovenous pump [36].

References

[1] Swain R, Ross D. Lower extremity compartment syndrome. When to suspect acute or chronic pressure buildup. Postgrad Med 1999;105:159–62, 165, 168.

[2] Horgan AF, Geddes S, Finlay IG. Lloyd-Davies position with Trendelenburg—a disaster waiting to happen? Dis Colon Rectum 1999;42:916–9, discussion 919–920.
[3] Gulli B, Templeman D. Compartment syndrome of the lower extremity. Orthop Clin North Am 1994;25:677–84.
[4] Woolley SL, Smith DR. Acute compartment syndrome secondary to diabetic muscle infarction: case report and literature review. Eur J Emerg Med 2006;13:113–6.
[5] Beraldo S, Dodds SR. Lower limb acute compartment syndrome after colorectal surgery in prolonged lithotomy position. Dis Colon Rectum 2006;49:1772.
[6] Detmer DE. Diagnosis and management of chronic compartment syndrome of the leg. Semin Orthop 1988;3:223.
[7] DeLee JC, Drez D. Orthopaedic sports medicine: principles and practice. Philadelphia: WB Saunders; 2002, 1612–1619.
[8] Styf JR, Körner LM. Diagnosis of chronic anterior compartment syndrome in the lower leg. Acta Orthop Scand 1987;58:139–44.
[9] Aweid O, Buono A, Malliaras P, et al. Systematic review and recommendations for intracompartmental pressure monitoring in diagnosing chronic exertional compartment syndrome of the leg. Clin J Sport Med 2012;22:356–70.
[10] Edwards Jr PH, Wright ML, Hartman JF. A practical approach for the differential diagnosis of chronic leg pain in the athlete. Am J Sports Med 2005;33:1241–9.
[11] George C, Hutchinson M. Chronic exertional compartment syndrome. Clin Sports Med 2012;31:307–19.
[12] Newton EJ, Love J. Acute complications of extremity trauma. Emerg Med Clin North Am 2007;25:751.
[13] Murdock M, Murdock M. Compartment syndrome: a review of the literature. Clin Podiatr Med Surg 2012;29:301–10.
[14] Mars M, Hadley GP. Failure of pulse oximetry in the assessment of raised limb intracompartmental pressure. Injury 1994;25: 379–81.
[15] Mubarak SJ, Hargens AR, Owen CA, et al. The wick catheter technique for measurement of intramuscular pressure. A new research and clinical tool. J Bone Joint Surg Am 1976;58:1016–20.
[16] Blackman PG. A review of chronic exertional compartment syndrome in the lower leg. Med Sci Sports Exerc 2000;32(Suppl):S4–S10.
[17] Hayes AA, Bower GD, Pitstock KL. Chronic (exertional) compartment syndrome of the legs diagnosed with thallous chloride scintigraphy. J Nucl Med 1995;36:1618–24.
[18] Bong MR, Polatsch DB, Jazrawi LM, Rokito AS. Chronic exertional compartment syndrome: diagnosis and management. Bull Hosp Jt Dis 2005;62:77.
[19] Elliott KG, Johnstone AJ. Diagnosing acute compartment syndrome. J Bone Joint Surg Br 2003;85:625–32.
[20] White TO, Howell GE, Will EM, et al. Elevated intramuscular compartment pressures do not influence outcome after tibial fracture. J Trauma 2003;55:1133–8.
[21] McQueen MM, Court-Brown CM. Compartment monitoring in tibial fractures. The pressure threshold for decompression. J Bone Joint Surg Br 1996;78:99–104.
[22] Rominger MB, Lukosch CJ, Bachmann GF. MR imaging of compartment syndrome of the lower leg: a case control study. Eur Radiol 2004;14:1432–9.
[23] Mannarino F, Sexson S. The significance of intracompartmental pressures in the diagnosis of chronic exertional compartment syndrome. Orthopedics 1989;12:1415–8.
[24] Takebayashi S, Takazawa H, Sasaki R, et al. Chronic exertional compartment syndrome in lower legs: localization and follow-up with thallium-201 SPECT imaging. J Nucl Med 1997;38:972–6.
[25] Lauder TD, Stuart MJ, Amrami KK, Felmlee JP. Exertional compartment syndrome and the role of magnetic resonance imaging. Am J Phys Med Rehabil 2002;81:315–9.
[26] Van den Brand JG, Nelson T, Verleisdonk EJ, van der Werken C. The diagnostic value of intracompartmental pressure measurement, magnetic resonance imaging, and near-infrared spectroscopy in chronic exertional compartment syndrome: a prospective study in 50 patients. Am J Sports Med 2005;33:699–704.
[27] Ni Mhuircheartaigh N, Kavanagh E, O'Donohoe M, Eustace S. Pseudo compartment syndrome of the calf in an athlete secondary to cystic adventitial disease of the popliteal artery. Br J Sports Med 2005;39:e36.
[28] Schubert A. Exertional compartment syndrome: review of the literature and proposed rehabilitation guidelines following surgical release. Int J Sports Phys Ther 2011;6:126–41.
[29] Blackman PG, Simmons LR, Crossley KM. Treatment of chronic exertional anterior compartment syndrome with massage: a pilot study. Clin J Sport Med 1998;8:14–7.
[30] Schepsis AA, Gill SS, Foster TA. Fasciotomy for exertional anterior compartment syndrome: is lateral compartment release necessary? Am J Sports Med 1999;27:430–5.
[31] Finkelstein JA, Hunter GA, Hu RW. Lower limb compartment syndrome: course after delayed fasciotomy. J Trauma 1996;40:342–4.
[32] Schepsis AA, Martini D, Corbett M. Surgical management of exertional compartment syndrome of the lower leg. Long-term followup. Am J Sports Med 1993;21:811–7.
[33] Snyder BJ, Oliva A, Buncke HJ. Calcific myonecrosis following compartment syndrome: report of two cases, review of the literature, and recommendations for treatment. J Trauma 1995;39:792–5.
[34] Heemskerk J, Kitslaar P. Acute compartment syndrome of the lower leg: retrospective study on prevalence, technique, and outcome of fasciotomies. World J Surg 2003;27:744–7.
[35] Schepsis AA, Fitzgerald M, Nicoletta R. Revision surgery for exertional anterior compartment syndrome of the lower leg: technique, findings, and results. Am J Sports Med 2005;33:1040–7.
[36] Singh N, Sidawy AN, Bottoni CR, et al. Physiological changes in venous hemodynamics associated with elective fasciotomy. Ann Vasc Surg 2006;20:301–5.

CHAPTER 68

Hamstring Strain

Omar M. Bhatti, MD
Beth M. Weinman, DO
Anne Z. Hoch, DO

Synonyms

Hamstring contusion
Hamstring pull
Hamstring tear
Hamstring avulsion
Delayed-onset muscle soreness of the posterior thigh
Stretch-induced injury to the hamstring

ICD-9 Codes

843.8 Sprains and strains of hip and thigh, other specified site
843.9 Sprains and strains of hip and thigh, unspecified site

ICD-10 Codes

S73.101 Unspecified sprain of right hip
S73.102 Unspecified sprain of left hip
S73.109 Unspecified sprain of unspecified hip

Definition

Hamstring strains are among the most common muscle injuries, particularly in athletes. Hamstring strains increase in incidence with age and are most common in football, soccer, and sports that require sprinting. The hamstrings consist of three muscles: the semimembranosus and semitendinosus muscles medially and the long and short heads of the biceps femoris muscle laterally.

Hamstring strains constitute a range of injuries from delayed-onset muscle soreness to partial tears to complete rupture of the muscle-tendon unit [1]. Injuries can occur from direct or indirect forces. Direct forces refer to lacerations and contusions. Complete avulsion of the proximal hamstring origin from the ischial tuberosity has been described, most commonly in water-skiers [2,3]. These injuries occur when forced hip flexion is sustained while the knee remains in complete extension.

Most hamstring injuries, however, occur from indirect forces with exertional use of the muscles, such as running, sprinting, and hurdling. Most hamstring injuries occur at the myotendinous junction during eccentric actions when the muscle lengthens while developing force, most commonly in the lateral hamstrings [4]. The biceps femoris has two heads with different origins and dual innervation and is therefore considered a "hybrid" muscle [5]. Dyssynergic contraction of the muscles is one of many proposed etiologic factors predisposing the hamstrings to strain. Other proposed etiologic factors include the hamstring's being a two-joint muscle, insufficient hamstring flexibility (Fig. 68.1), insufficient warm-up and stretching before activity, strength imbalance between the hamstrings and quadriceps, strength imbalances between the right and left hamstrings, previous injury to the hamstring, higher running speeds, and poor strength or endurance of the hamstrings. Hamstring strains can occur in a variety of patients from young to old and in any level of athletics from the "weekend warrior" to the elite athlete.

The hamstrings function over two joints. Like other biarticular muscle groups, such as the quadriceps femoris, the gastrocnemius, and the biceps brachii, the hamstrings are more susceptible to injury. The hamstrings cross the hip and knee joint (with the exception of the short head of the biceps femoris). During the latter part of the swing phase of gait, the hamstrings act eccentrically to decelerate knee extension; and at heel strike, the hamstrings act concentrically to extend the hip. During running, this rapid change in function puts the muscle at risk for injury; the higher the running speed and angular velocity, the greater the forces at heel strike [6,7]. Any large strength imbalance between the larger and stronger quadriceps and the hamstrings will put the hamstrings at a disadvantage. If the synergy of antagonists is altered, a vigorous contraction of the weaker muscle may result in injury. Any factor that adversely affects the neuromuscular coordination during running, such as lack of proper

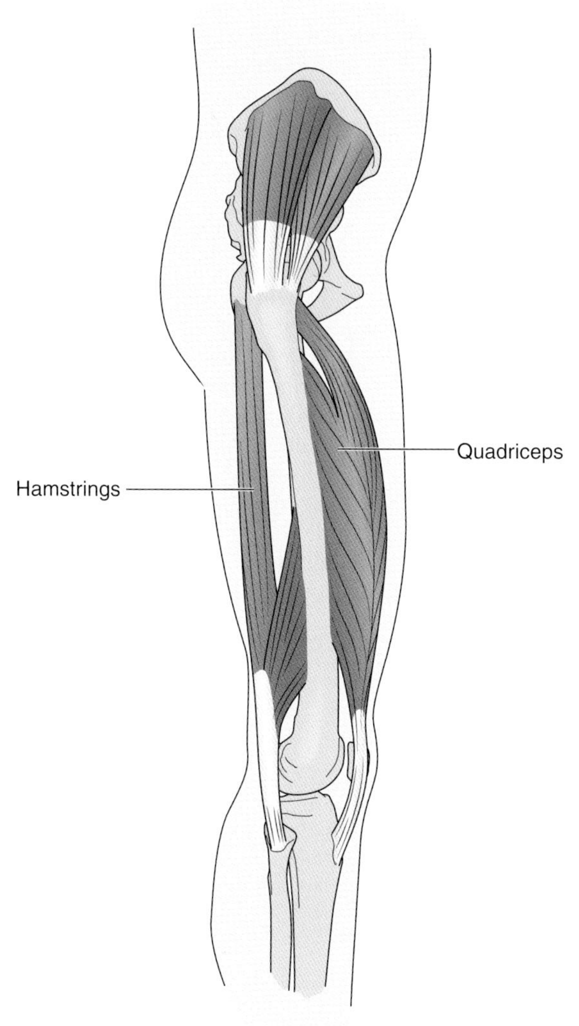

FIGURE 68.1 Tight hamstring muscles may lead to an imbalance between the quadriceps and hamstring muscles, placing an athlete at increased risk for injury.

warm-up, poor training, or muscle fatigue, may result in a strain injury.

Hamstring strains can be divided into three grades according to their severity:

1. Grade I, or first-degree, strain: mild strain with minimal muscle damage (less than 5% of muscle fiber disruption). There is associated pain but little or no loss of muscle strength.
2. Grade II, or second-degree, strain: moderate strain with more severe partial tearing of the muscle but no complete disruption of the myotendinous unit. Pain is present with loss of knee flexion strength.
3. Grade III, or third-degree, strain: severe strain involving complete tearing of the myotendinous unit. This injury presents with severe pain and marked loss of knee flexion strength [1,8].

Avulsion of the hamstrings tendon from its origin on the ischium or distally from the tibia or fibula is not graded like the classic myotendinous strains. These injuries are usually complete or partial avulsion injuries and described as such.

Symptoms

At the time of injury, patients typically report a sudden, sharp pain in the back of the thigh. Some describe a "popping" or tearing sensation. There is generalized pain and point tenderness at the site of injury. The patient may complain of tightness, weakness, and impaired range of motion. Depending on the severity of the injury, the individual may or may not be able to continue the activity and occasionally is unable to bear weight on the affected limb. Swelling and ecchymosis are variable and may be delayed for several days. The ecchymosis may descend to the thigh and be manifested at the distal thigh or back of the knee, calf, or ankle. The injury may occur in the early or late stages of activity, and patients may give a history of inadequate warm-up or fatigue.

Rarely the patient may complain of symptoms of numbness, tingling, and distal extremity weakness. If these are present, further investigation into a sciatic nerve irritation is warranted. Complete tears and proximal hamstring avulsion injuries can cause a large hematoma or scar tissue to form around the sciatic nerve [9,10].

Alternatively, any change in training patterns and increased eccentric exercise in a previously untrained subject can lead to hamstring injury with delayed-onset muscle soreness. This is thought to be the result of microscopic damage followed by a local inflammatory response [11].

Physical Examination

The physical examination begins with assessment of gait abnormalities. Patients with hamstring injuries often have a shortened walking gait or running stride associated with a limp. Swelling and ecchymosis may not be detectable for several days after the initial injury, and the amount of bleeding depends on the severity of the strain. Unlike direct muscle contusions, in which the ecchymosis remains confined to the muscle proper, the bleeding in a hamstring strain can escape through the ruptured fascia with resultant ecchymosis into interfascial spaces, explaining the common finding of ecchymosis distal to the site of injury [12].

The posterior thigh is inspected for visible defects and deformity, asymmetry, swelling, and ecchymosis (Fig. 68.2). The entire length of the hamstrings should be palpated, including the proximal origin near the ischial tuberosity and distal insertions at the posterior knee. A palpable defect in the posterior thigh indicates a more severe injury with possible complete rupture of the muscle.

Active and passive range of motion of the hamstrings should be tested and compared with the contralateral side. Range of motion of the knee can be measured with the hip at 90 degrees in the supine position or sitting position. Deficits in knee and hip range of motion are common, and the point at which pain limits range of motion should be noted (Fig. 68.3). Concentric and eccentric muscle strength testing of the hamstrings should also be performed with the patient both sitting and prone. Weakness of knee flexion and hip extension is common. Asymmetry of the hamstrings can sometimes be accentuated with active-resisted static muscle contraction. A soft tissue defect with distal bulging of the retracted muscle belly indicates a partial or complete rupture.

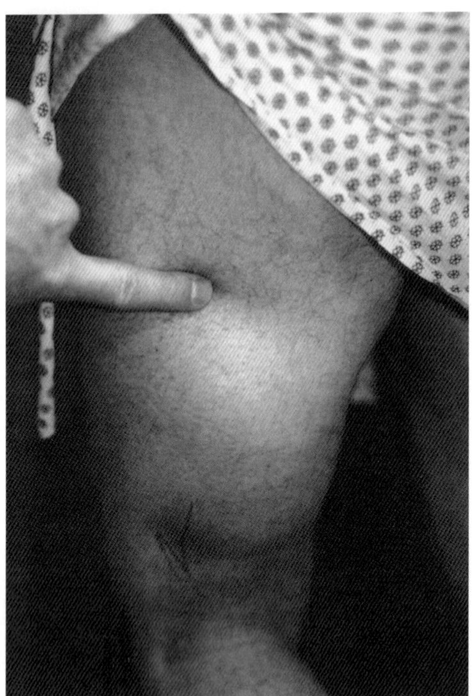

FIGURE 68.2 Clinical photograph of posterior thigh deformity after complete tear of the hamstrings.

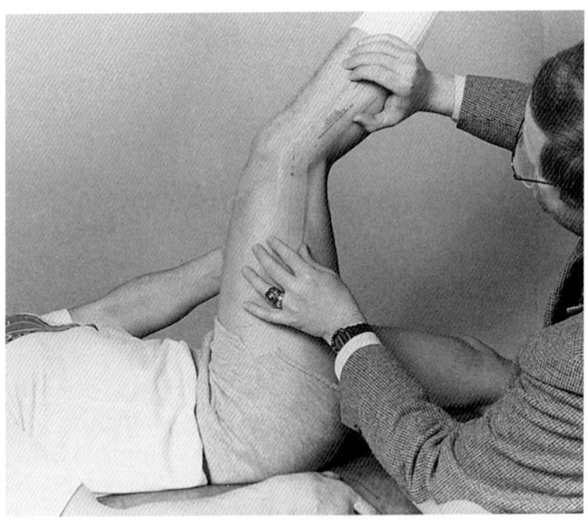

FIGURE 68.3 Measurement of hamstring tightness. With the patient supine and the hip flexed 90 degrees, the knee should extend fully if the hamstrings are flexible. If the knee will not extend completely, the residual knee flexion angle is measured and recorded as hamstring tightness. *(From Mellion MB. Office Sports Medicine, 2nd ed. Philadelphia, Hanley & Belfus, 1996.)*

Neurologic examination findings should be normal except for strength testing of the hamstring group and in rare cases when there is an associated sciatic nerve irritation. In these cases, there may be weakness, particularly notable in plantar flexion, and loss of the affected Achilles reflex.

Functional Limitations

Most patients sustaining a hamstring strain have no residual deficits and return to their previous level of function. However, others may experience difficulty with walking or running, time lost from occupation, and delayed return to sports. Hamstring strains heal slowly and are at high risk for reinjury if return to activities is too early. With severe injuries, it may take up to 1 year for patients to resume preinjury activities; in some cases of complete ruptures, patients never return to the previous level of function [13].

Diagnostic Studies

The common hamstring strain usually requires no additional testing because the diagnosis is made by history and clinical examination. However, more severe cases may warrant diagnostic imaging. If the injury localizes near the origin of the hamstrings, plain radiographs may help identify irregularities of the ischial tuberosity, such as a bone avulsion of the ischial tuberosity (especially in the adolescent). Other radiographic findings may include ectopic calcification consistent with chronic myositis ossificans [4,8]. Magnetic resonance imaging may be used to determine the degree of injury and to identify complete proximal avulsion injuries (Fig. 68.4). Ultrasound imaging, in the hands of an experienced practitioner, may also be used as a diagnostic tool.

Differential Diagnosis

S1 radiculopathy
Piriformis syndrome
Referred pain from sacroiliac joint or lumbar spine
Bone avulsion or apophysitis of the ischial tuberosity
Ischial bursitis (weaver's bottom)
Stress fracture in the pelvis, femoral neck, or femoral shaft
Adductor magnus strain
Hip osteoarthritis
Pelvic floor dysfunction

Treatment

Initial

Initial management of a hamstring strain consists of the PRICE principle (*p*rotection, *r*est, *i*ce, *c*ompression, and *e*levation). Relative rest and protection may involve weight bearing as tolerated or, with higher grade injuries (grade II or grade III injuries), cane or crutch walking. Ambulatory aids help prevent tissue irritation and the resulting inflammation, both of which prolong recovery. Assistive devices should be used until the patient can walk without a limp in a normal heel-toe gait. The application of ice as often as every 2 or 3 hours for 20 minutes the first few days is indicated to limit the amount of pain and swelling. Ice provides an anti- inflammatory effect and helps reduce swelling. Icing is continued through the recovery to inhibit inflammation and to allow muscle healing. Compression by taping or elastic wrapping of the thigh combined with elevation reduces hemorrhage, thereby helping control edema and pain. Nonsteroidal anti-inflammatory drugs and other analgesics are commonly used to limit the inflammatory reaction and for pain control in the first few days. Soft tissue mobilization to the site of pain should be avoided for at least 5 days because this may exacerbate the inflammatory response.

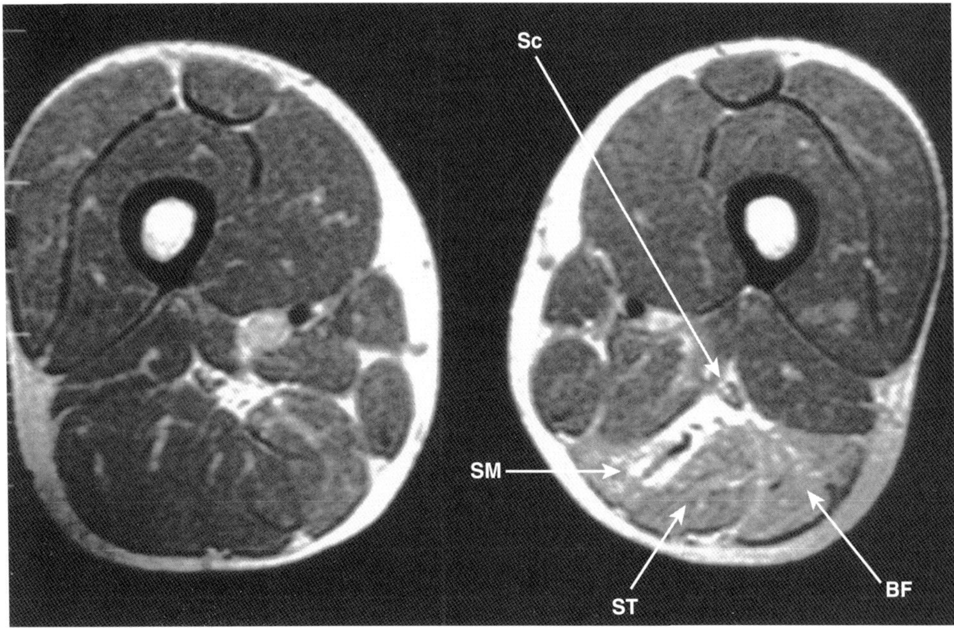

FIGURE 68.4 Axial magnetic resonance image demonstrating injury to the semitendinosus (*ST*), semimembranosus (*SM*), and biceps femoris (*BF*) muscles. The sciatic nerve (*Sc*) is shown anterior to the muscles and within the hematoma of injury.

Rehabilitation

The elements of a hamstring rehabilitation program involve a pain-free progression of stretching, strengthening, and sports-specific activities. In the acute phase, pain-free range of motion should be achieved as soon as possible to prevent adhesions and scarring in the muscle tissue. Patients should start with pain-free active range of motion and progress to pain-free passive range of motion and gentle stretching. For a full stretch of the hamstring muscle to be achieved, the hip must be flexed to 90 degrees and the knee fully extended. This stretch is best achieved in the supine position; a towel can facilitate hamstring lengthening (Fig. 68.5). It is also critical to improve flexibility throughout the spine and lower extremities. Strengthening can begin when the patient achieves full active extension without pain. It is best to start with static contractions, such as multiple-angle submaximal isometric exercises [14]. Once these are performed at 100% effort without pain, the patient may progress to isotonic exercise, such as prone hamstring strengthening and isokinetic exercise. These concentric strength exercises are followed by eccentric strength exercises and sports-specific activities as tolerated. Examples of eccentric training include Nordic hamstring exercises, straight-leg windmills, straight-leg dead lift, and flywheel training [15]. Return to sport is allowed when full motion is restored, strength is at least 90% that of the uninjured side, and hamstring-quadriceps strength ratio is symmetric [6]. Hamstring flexibility must be maintained throughout the rehabilitation process to prevent reinjury. Aerobic conditioning should continue throughout the rehabilitation process. Bicycling *without* toe clips (toe clips increase use of hamstrings), swimming or jogging in a pool, and upper body ergometry are recommended. Rehabilitation programs incorporating progressive agility and trunk stabilization exercising have been shown to decrease reinjury rates [16].

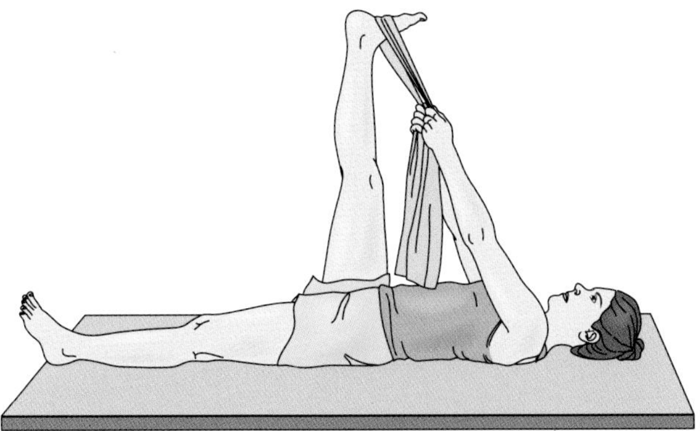

FIGURE 68.5 Stretching the hamstring fully requires the hip to be at 90 degrees with the ankle dorsiflexed. However, forceful stretching should be avoided.

It is critical to educate patients about how to prevent recurrent hamstring injuries. This includes a good warm-up period before engaging in sports. Full return to play must be gradual because the risk of recurrent injury is high. In addition, training errors, such as an abrupt switch to a hard surface or an increase in training intensity, should be avoided.

Procedures

Procedures are not typically performed in hamstring strain injuries. However, the use of platelet-rich plasma to aid in the recovery of high hamstring strains has been gaining popularity [17]. Given the increased use of autologous blood injections and dry needling techniques, further clinical and laboratory research is warranted.

Surgery

Routine hamstring strains do not require surgical intervention and respond well to a conservative rehabilitation program. However, in the case of complete hamstring avulsion from the ischial tuberosity, surgical repair is recommended because of the residual loss of power and function in nonoperatively treated patients [2,3,18]. Surgical neurolysis is also recommended for the rare complication of symptomatic scarring around the sciatic nerve [9,10].

Potential Disease Complications

The most common complication of hamstring strain is recurrent injury. Loss of hamstring flexibility and strength as well as neuromuscular coordination puts the patient at risk for reinjury, especially if the return to activity is before full recovery. The high injury recurrence rate is believed to be due to return to play before full strength is regained in the lengthened hamstring position [19].

Two cases of posterior thigh compartment syndrome have been reported with complete hamstring tears, one resulting from injury alone and one complicated by anticoagulation therapy [20,21]. Complete hamstring tears can also result in substantial scar formation around the sciatic nerve within the posterior thigh. Patients may present with radicular-type symptoms ranging from sensory paresthesias to footdrop.

Patients with chronic complete hamstring avulsion off the ischial tuberosity may complain of pain, weakness, and cramping as well as difficulty in running and walking and poor leg control, especially walking downhill [3].

Potential Treatment Complications

Nonsteroidal anti-inflammatory drugs are known to have gastrointestinal, renal, and liver side effects. Ultrasound therapy should be avoided in the acute treatment of high-degree strains, especially if hematoma formation is suspected, because it may extend the hematoma [21]. Potential complications of surgical repair of an avulsion fracture include sensation loss along the incision site and postoperative sciatica [22].

References

[1] Kujala UM, Orava S, Järvinen M. Hamstring injuries: current trends in treatment and prevention. Sports Med 1997;23:397–404.
[2] Brewer BJ. Athletic injuries; musculotendinous unit. Clin Orthop 1962;23:30–8.
[3] Blasier RB, Morawa LG. Complete rupture of the hamstring origin from a water skiing injury. Am J Sports Med 1990;18:435–7.
[4] Morris AF. Sports medicine: prevention of athletic injuries. Dubuque: William C. Brown Publishers; 1984, 162–163.
[5] Burkett LN. Investigation into hamstring strains: the case of the hybrid muscle. J Sports Med 1976;3:228–31.
[6] Young JL, Laskowski ER, Rock M. Thigh injuries in athletes. Mayo Clin Proc 1993;68:1099–106.
[7] Agre JC. Hamstring injuries: proposed aetiological factors, prevention, and treatment. Sports Med 1985;2:21–33.
[8] Zarins B, Ciullo JV. Acute muscle and tendon injuries in athletes. Clin Sports Med 1983;2:167–82.
[9] Street CC, Burks RT. Chronic complete hamstring avulsion causing foot drop. Am J Sports Med 2000;28:1–3.
[10] Hernesman SC, Hoch AZ, Vetter CS, Young CC. Foot drop in a marathon runner from chronic complete hamstring tear. Clin J Sport Med 2003;13:365–8.
[11] Brockett CL, Morgan DL, Proske U. Predicting hamstring strain injury in elite athletes. Med Sci Sports Exerc 2004;36:379–87.
[12] Best TM. Soft-tissue injuries and muscle tears. Clin Sports Med 1997;16:419–34.
[13] Salley PI, Friedman RL, Coogan PG, et al. Hamstring muscle injuries among water skiers: functional outcome and prevention. Am J Sports Med 1996;24:130–6.
[14] Worrel TW. Factors associated with hamstring injuries: an approach to treatment and preventative measures. Sports Med 1994;17:338–45.
[15] Opar D, Williams M, Shield A. Hamstring strain injuries. Sports Med 2012;42:209–26.
[16] Ali K, Leland M. Hamstring strains and tears in the athlete. Clin Sports Med 2012;31:263–72.
[17] Sherry MA, Best TM. A comparison of 2 rehabilitation programs in the treatment of acute hamstring strains. J Orthop Sports Phys Ther 2004;34:116–25.
[18] Cross MG, Vandersluis R, Wood D, Banff M. Surgical repair of chronic complete hamstring tendon rupture in the adult patient. Am J Sports Med 1998;26:785–8.
[19] Schmitt B, Tim T, McHugh M. Hamstring injury rehabilitation and prevention of reinjury using lengthened state eccentric training: a new concept. Int J Sports Phys Ther 2012;7:333–41.
[20] Oseto MC, Edwards JC, Acus RW. Posterior thigh compartment syndrome associated with hamstring avulsion and chronic anticoagulation therapy. Orthopedics 2004;27:229–30.
[21] Kwong Y, Patel J. Spontaneous complete hamstring avulsion causing posterior thigh compartment syndrome. Br J Sports Med 2006;40:723–4.
[22] Birmingham P, Muller M, Wickiewicz T, et al. Functional outcome after repair of proximal hamstring avulsions. J Bone Joint Surg Am 2011;93:1819–26.

CHAPTER 69

Iliotibial Band Syndrome

Venu Akuthota, MD
Sonja K. Stilp, MD
Paul Lento, MD
Peter Gonzalez, MD
Alison R. Putnam, DO

Synonyms

Iliotibial band friction syndrome
Iliotibial tract friction syndrome
Snapping hip

ICD-9 Codes

719.65 Snapping hip
728.89 Iliotibial band syndrome

ICD-10 Codes

M24.851 Joint derangement of right hip, not elsewhere classified (snapping hip)
M24.852 Joint derangement of left hip, not elsewhere classified (snapping hip)
M24.859 Joint derangement of unspecified hip, not elsewhere classified (snapping hip)
M76.30 Iliotibial band syndrome, unspecified leg
M76.31 Iliotibial band syndrome, right leg
M76.32 Iliotibial band syndrome, left leg

Definition

The iliotibial band (ITB) is a dense fascia on the lateral aspect of the knee and hip. Traditionally, the gluteus maximus and tensor fascia lata were thought to be the proximal origin of the ITB. Further anatomic dissections have demonstrated that the gluteus medius also has direct and indirect contributions to the ITB (Fig. 69.1) [1]. Proximal attachment includes the iliac tubercle or iliac crest [2,3]. In the distal thigh, the ITB attaches to the linea aspera and the upper edge of the lateral femoral epicondyle [3,4]. According to Terry [5], after passing over the lateral femoral epicondyle, it separates into two components. The iliotibial tract of the distal ITB attaches to Gerdy tubercle of the anterolateral proximal tibia. The iliopatellar band of the ITB has aponeurotic connections to the patella and the vastus lateralis [5]. Other distal attachments include the biceps femoris, the lateral patellar retinaculum, and the patellar tendon [5,6]. An anatomic pouch can be found underlying the posterior ITB at the level of the lateral femoral epicondyle [7]. Controversy exists as to whether this pouch is a bursa, a synovial extension of the knee joint, or degenerative tissue [7,8]. Others have reported that a highly innervated fat pad overlies the lateral femoral epicondyle [9].

Iliotibial band syndrome (ITBS) or iliotibial band friction syndrome is an overuse injury typically referring to lateral knee pain as a result of impingement of the distal ITB over the lateral femoral epicondyle. Less commonly, ITBS may refer to hip pain associated with movement of the ITB across the greater trochanter. This chapter deals primarily with distal ITBS. The suspected pain generator in ITBS is as controversial as the anatomy around the lateral epicondyle. It has been postulated to be bursitis, synovitis, or irritation of the fat pad, posterior fibers of the ITB, or periosteum [3,6,9–12]. Although the anatomic pain generator may not be fully known, pain at the distal aspect of the ITB is thought to be caused by the fibers of the ITB passing over the lateral femoral epicondyle with knee flexion and extension [6,11].

Friction has been implicated as the most important factor in ITBS [8,11]. Maximum friction occurs when the posterior fibers of the ITB pass over the lateral femoral epicondyle at 20 to 30 degrees of knee flexion, the putative "impingement zone." [8] Repeated knee flexion and extension, particularly with increased running mileage per week, creates friction and has been shown to predispose an individual to lateral knee pain [8,11]. Friction has been shown to play a role in cycling activities as well. Cycling-induced ITBS is thought to result

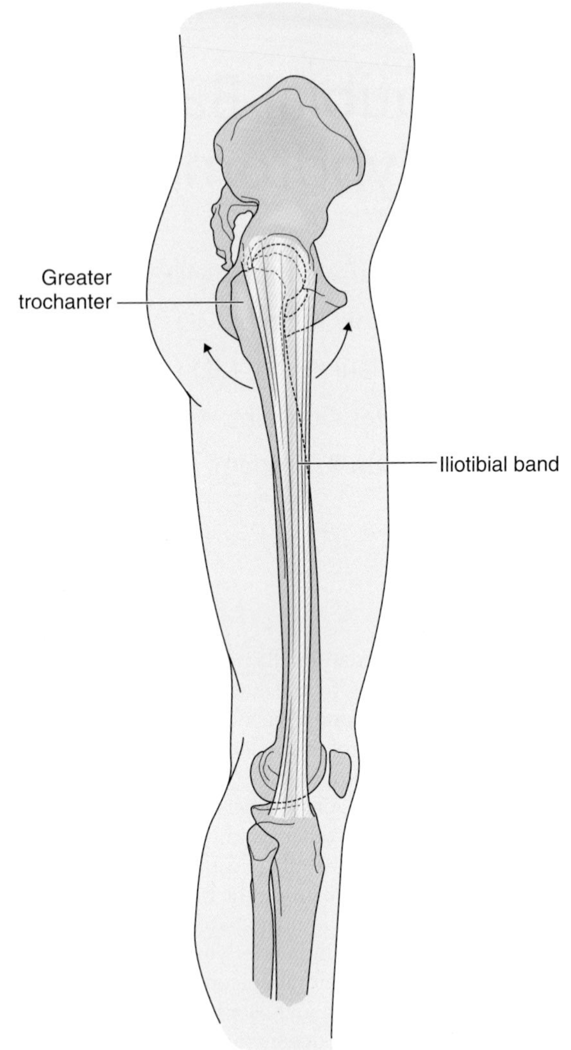

FIGURE 69.1 Anatomy of the iliotibial band, which can cause "snapping" as it slips anteriorly and posteriorly over the prominent greater trochanter.

from the repetitive activity of cycling, as less time is spent in the impingement zone than during running activities [11]. Other authors have theorized that pain is due not only to friction but also to compression of the fat pad between the ITB and the lateral femoral epicondyle. The compression of the fat pad was found to be greatest at 30 degrees of flexion, similar to previous reports, and increased with internal rotation of the tibia during knee flexion [6,9].

Several factors may increase the risk for development of ITBS. Although it has not been extensively studied, poor neuromuscular control appears to be an important *modifiable* risk factor for ITBS. Weakness of hip abductors has been implicated in ITBS [6]. However, difference in strength of hip abduction was not found in a study of 10 runners with ITBS compared with controls [13]. Specifically, neuromuscular control is needed to attenuate the valgus–internal rotation vectors at the knee after heel strike. If appropriate control is not available, the ITB may have an abrupt increase in tension at its insertion site [10,14,15]. Increased hip adduction and knee internal rotation have been noted in female runners, suggesting increased ITB strain as a mechanism of injury [15]. Increased foot inversion, maximum knee flexion, and knee internal rotation were noted during an exhaustive run in recreational runners with history of ITBS [16]. Peak rearfoot eversion, knee internal rotation angle, and hip adduction angle were increased in 35 female runners with history of ITBS compared with matched controls [17]. Contradictory results were found in a study of 18 runners with ITBS compared with controls. Results indicated decreased hip adduction in those with ITBS, although they were found to have a lack of "coordination" defined as earlier hip flexion and knee flexion [18]. Hamill and colleagues [19] noted that the strain rate of the ITB during stance phase was increased in female runners who developed ITBS compared with healthy age-matched controls, and Miller and coworkers [16] noted increased ITB strain in recreational runners with history of ITBS. Strengthening of the gluteus medius and tensor fascia lata, decelerators of the valgus–internal rotation vectors at the knee, has been shown to reduce symptoms of ITBS [10,20]. Lack of dynamic flexibility, particularly of the ITB, has been implicated with ITB injury susceptibility [6,15,21,22]. No research study to date, though, has revealed a correlation between ITB tightness and ITB injury. Theoretically, however, tightness of the ITB or its constituent muscles increases impingement of the ITB on the lateral femoral epicondyle [8]. Other risk factors that may be attenuated with proper shoe wear or foot orthoses include excessive foot-ankle pronation and supination [6,16]. Training errors, such as rapid changes in training routine, hill training, striding, and excessive mileage, have also been highlighted as increasing the risk of ITBS [6,12]. Increased ground reaction force, as with running in old shoes, may also increase frictional forces at the knee and exacerbate symptoms [8]. Intrinsic or nonmodifiable factors, such as bone malalignment or a wide distal ITB, may contribute to the development of ITBS [22,23]. Finally, repeated direct trauma to the lateral knee, particularly with soccer goalies, appears to be injurious to the ITB impingement area [23].

Symptoms

Symptoms of ITBS occur typically at the lateral femoral epicondyle but may emanate from the distal attachment of the ITB at Gerdy tubercle on the tibia [6,12]. ITBS is the most common cause of lateral knee pain in runners [6]. Individuals present with sharp or burning lateral knee pain that is aggravated during repetitive activity. This pain may radiate up into the lateral thigh or down to Gerdy tubercle [24]. Runners often describe a specific, reproducible time when the symptoms commence [25]. Pain usually subsides after a run; however, in severe cases, persistent pain may cause restriction in distance [26,27]. Runners also note more pain with downhill running because of the increased time spent in the impingement zone [8]. Paradoxically, runners state that faster running and sprinting often do not produce pain. Fast running allows the athlete to spend more time in knee angles greater than 30 degrees [8]. Cyclists present with rhythmic, stabbing pain with pedaling. Specifically, they complain of pain at the end of the downstroke or the beginning of the upstroke. Bikers with improper saddle height and cleat position may experience greater symptoms [28,29].

ITBS symptoms may also occur as a lateral snapping hip. An external or lateral snapping hip occurs as the ITB rapidly passes anteriorly over the greater trochanter as the femur passes from extension to flexion [30]. Athletes, particularly dancers, sometimes experience an audible painful snap on landing in poor turnout (decreased external rotation at the hip) and with excessive anterior pelvic tilt [31].

Physical Examination

Physical examination begins with a screening examination of the joints above and below the site of injury. Hip girdle examination includes an assessment for joint range of motion, asymmetries [32], muscle strength (particularly hip abductors) [10], and lumbopelvic somatic dysfunctions [33]. The modified Thomas and Ober tests are used to assess flexibility of the ITB and related musculature at the hip and knee (Figs. 69.2 and 69.3) [6,12,34].

The knee examination includes palpation, patellar accessory motion [35], and the Noble compression test (Fig. 69.4) [8]. Knee tenderness is noted either at the lateral femoral epicondyle (above the lateral joint line) or at Gerdy tubercle. Palpatory examination should also include a thorough assessment for myofascial restrictions and trigger points along the lateral thigh musculature [25,26]. On rare occasion, ITB swelling and crepitus accompany tenderness. Pain can also be elicited by the Noble compression test [6]. Other conditions are effectively ruled out by performing a relevant physical examination.

The foot and ankle examination is particularly useful in the determination of gastrocnemius-soleus inflexibility, subtalar motion restrictions, and specific foot type (e.g., hindfoot varus). Finally, a biomechanical assessment of sports-specific activity can be done. Walkers and runners are observed for abnormalities such as excessive foot-ankle pronation, inability to attenuate shock at the knee, Trendelenburg frontal plane gait at the pelvis, and forward trunk lean [33,36]. Bicyclers are observed for proper foot placement on the pedal, saddle height, and knee angles with pedaling revolution [28,29]. Dancers can be observed performing *rond de jambe* or *grand plié* for proper turnout and pelvic stabilization [31].

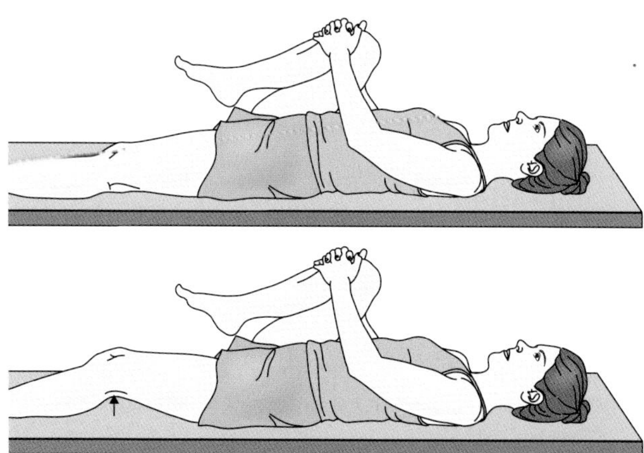

FIGURE 69.2 Thomas test to assess hip flexion contracture. The patient lies supine while the clinician flexes one of the patient's hips, bringing the knee to the chest to flatten the lumbar spine. The patient holds the flexed knee and hip against the chest. If there is a flexion contracture of the hip, the patient's other leg will rise off the table.

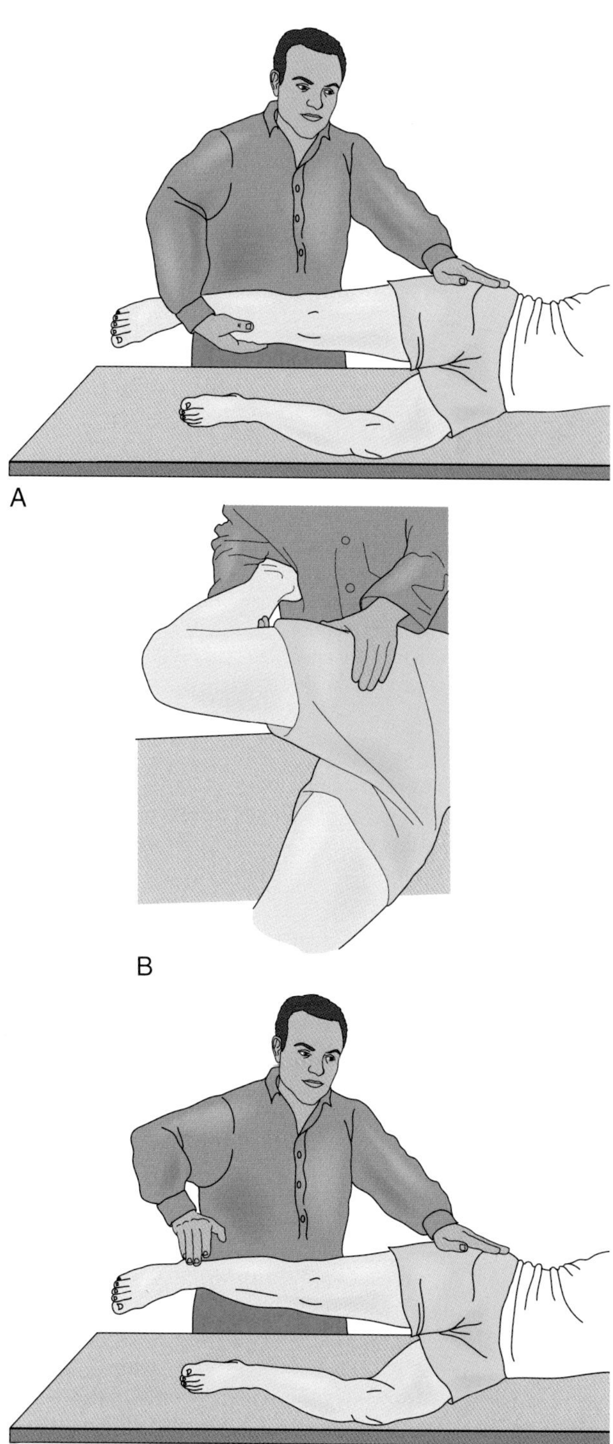

FIGURE 69.3 Ober test to assess contracture of the iliotibial band. The patient is side-lying with the lower leg flexed at the hip and knee. The clinician passively abducts and extends the patient's upper leg with the knee straight (**A**) or flexed to 90 degrees (**B**). The test result is positive if the leg remains abducted and does not fall to the table (**C**).

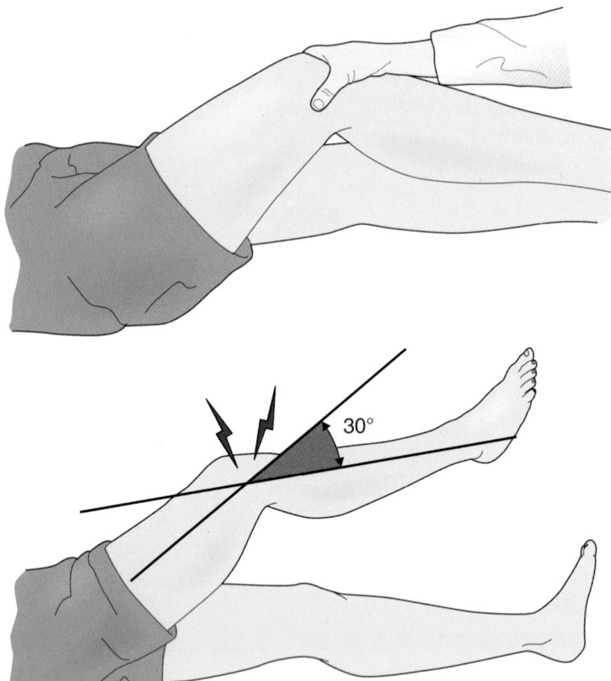

FIGURE 69.4 Noble compression test to determine whether there is iliotibial band friction at the knee. The patient lies supine, and the knee is flexed to 90 degrees (the hip flexes as well). The clinician applies pressure with the thumb at the lateral femoral epicondyle while the patient slowly extends the knee. The test result is positive if the patient complains of severe pain over the lateral femoral epicondyle at 30 degrees.

The findings of the neurologic examination, including strength, sensation, and reflexes, are typically normal. Strength may be affected by disuse or guarding due to pain, particularly in the hip abductors and external rotators.

Functional Limitations

ITBS pain usually restricts athletes from their sports activity but does not typically cause limitations of daily activities. Yet, a vicious circle is set forth in which biomechanical deficits (e.g., gluteal weakness and ITB tightness) cause ITB tissue injury with resultant functional adaptations to avoid the pain of the tissue injury (e.g., external rotation of the hip) [32].

Diagnostic Studies

Imaging has a limited role in ITBS because it is usually a clinical diagnosis. Radiographs are rarely helpful [12]. Diagnostic ultrasonography has been used in some centers to confirm injuries [37]. Diagnostic ultrasound examination can measure ITB thickness for which normal values have been determined in uninjured subjects [38]. Dynamic sonography may also be helpful in identifying abnormal motion of the proximal ITB in diagnosis of external snapping hip syndrome [39]. When definitive diagnosis is needed or other diagnoses need to be excluded, magnetic resonance imaging has emerged as a potentially useful test. Magnetic resonance imaging may show a thickened ITB or high intensity on axial T2-weighted images [40].

Differential Diagnosis

ILIOTIBIAL BAND: HIP

Hip joint disease
Meralgia paresthetica
Trochanteric bursitis
Internal snapping hip
Referred or radicular pain from lumbar spine
Primary myofascial pain

ILIOTIBIAL BAND: KNEE

Popliteus tendinitis
Lateral collateral ligament injury
Lateral hamstring strain
Lateral meniscus tear
Patellofemoral pain
Common peroneal nerve injury
Fabella syndrome
Lateral plica
Stress fracture
Primary myofascial pain

Treatment

Initial

Acute phase treatment is akin to that of other musculoskeletal injuries. Relative rest consists of activity modification, particularly with restriction of those activities that exacerbate the pain symptoms [6,26]. In most instances, this does not mean a complete cessation of activity. The clinician needs to emphasize the positive aspects of relative rest and provide alternative training regimens. The ITB can be relatively off-loaded if an individual can keep his or her activity below the threshold of pain. Frequently, this can be achieved by simply decreasing intensity or training duration. Medications such as nonsteroidal anti-inflammatory drugs may help reduce pain and inflammation in the first few weeks of injury. If swelling is present, some authors advocate a local corticosteroid injection in the initial stages [25,26]. As well, modalities such as ice, ice massage, ultrasound, iontophoresis, and phonophoresis can be helpful in the early period to reduce early inflammation and pain [6,11,26]. It is critical early on to address the biomechanical cause of ITB injury [26].

Rehabilitation

Ultrasound, phonophoresis, iontophoresis, and electrical stimulation may also be used to reduce early inflammation and pain [26]. The subacute phase of rehabilitation addresses the biomechanical deficits found on physical examination. Typically, flexibility deficits are seen in the ITB, iliopsoas, quadriceps, and gastrocnemius-soleus [25,26]. Incorporation of flexibility and strengthening into the rehabilitation treatment is often recommended [6,13,26]. Proper stretching addresses all three planes and incorporates proximal and distal musculotendinous fibers.

Fredericson and colleagues [21] studied the relative effectiveness of three commonly prescribed standing ITB stretches. The authors concluded that when overhead arm extension is added to the standing ITB stretch, the ITB length and average external adduction moments could be increased [21]. This stretch is performed standing with the symptomatic leg extended and adducted across the uninvolved leg. The subject laterally flexes the trunk toward the contralateral side and extends both arms overhead (Fig. 69.5). A study evaluated the effectiveness of the Ober test (see Fig. 69.3) and the modified Ober test in stretching the ITB and the most distal component, the iliotibial tract. The modified test is performed the same as the Ober test except the knee remains extended at 0 degrees. The investigators used ultrasonography to assess the soft tissue changes of the iliotibial tract and concluded that both tests are effective in the initial stages of stretching. However, the modified Ober test may afford a greater stretch of the iliotibial tract of the ITB when additional adduction of the hip is allowed [41]. In a cadaveric study, Falvey and colleagues [3] found limited ability to lengthen the ITB by the modified Ober test and by hip flexion, adduction, and external rotation with knee flexion (hip test) compared with control (straight-leg raise), although the hip test had significantly greater strain. In another limb of the same study, they found minimal change in length with isometric contraction of the tensor fascia lata, concluding that focus should be on stretching the muscle component of the ITB complex. Some muscle groups do not respond to stretch unless myofascial and joint restrictions are concomitantly addressed by experienced therapists or by self-administered techniques [25,26]. In a systematic review by Ellis and coworkers [11], one study of transverse friction massage was not found to be beneficial. Proper facilitation of hip girdle musculature can be achieved by addressing antagonistic tight structures, such as tight hip flexors or anterior hip capsule [34]. Subtalar mobilizations are often needed to prevent excessive valgus–internal rotation forces from transferring to the knee and ITB [36]. In conjunction with a flexibility and joint mobilization program, strengthening of weak or inhibited muscles can be started. Strengthening regimens ultimately need to move away from the plinth to more functional activities, such as single squats and lunges, with an emphasis on proper pelvic and core stabilization [26,33].

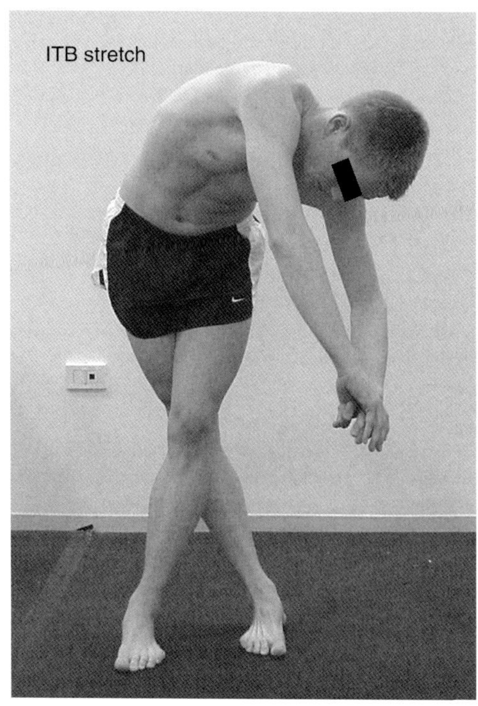

FIGURE 69.5 Iliotibial band (*ITB*) stretch.

Finally, the maintenance phase focuses on returning patients to their respective activities with confidence in their functional abilities. In this phase, athletes are ideally observed or videotaped in their sporting environment. Frequently, runners have form deviations that lead to uncontrolled valgus–internal rotation of the knee. These abnormalities include excessive pronation, inability to shock attenuate at the knee, and Trendelenburg frontal plane gait at the pelvis [33,36]. A change to shock-absorbing or motion-control shoes can accommodate supination and overpronation, respectively [36]. Foot orthoses have also been advocated for runners with lower limb injuries. Their benefit is as yet empirical. Cyclists can often correct their ITB problems with equipment and bicycle adjustments [24,28]. Dancers performing *rond de jambe* or *grand plié* can be cued on maintaining turnout and neutral pelvic position [34]. After sports-specific adjustments have been made, athletes need to be reintroduced to activity gradually and individually.

Procedures

Corticosteroid injections may be performed at different locations along the ITB. Injection into the anatomic pouch at the lateral femoral epicondyle is a relatively simple procedure and is advocated for patients with persistent pain and swelling (Fig. 69.6) [25]. A mixture of anesthetic (e.g., 1 mL of 1% lidocaine) and long-acting steroid (e.g., 1 mL of betamethasone) is instilled to the affected site. A randomized controlled study evaluating the efficacy of corticosteroid injections in runners with acute symptoms of ITB-mediated pain showed that runners in the injection group experienced less pain during running activities [42]. Steroid injections should be repeated only if adequate relief is obtained after the initial injection. Patients can return to play as their pain allows.

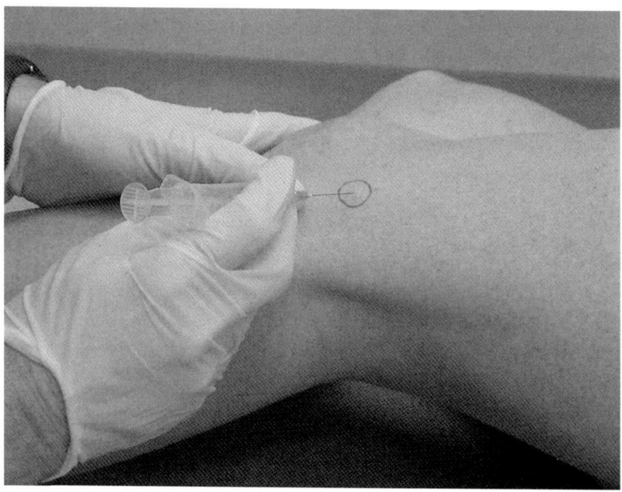

FIGURE 69.6 Distal iliotibial band injection technique at the lateral epicondyle of the femur.

Surgery

Surgical treatment of ITBS is rarely needed. Surgery involves excision of the posterior half of the ITB where it passes over the lateral femoral epicondyle, Z lengthening, or removal of the underlying putative bursa by open or endoscopic techniques [12,43,44]. These procedures appear to have mixed results and should be contemplated only for patients who have exhausted all other options, including a comprehensive rehabilitation program as previously outlined.

Potential Disease Complications

If ITBS is not properly addressed, biomechanical adaptations can occur [32]. Chronic pain, leading to progressive disability, is a potential complication.

Potential Treatment Complications

Rehabilitation complications are rare. Nonsteroidal anti-inflammatory drugs and analgesics have well-known side effects that may affect gastrointestinal, hepatic, or renal function. Corticosteroid injections have the potential complications of infection, depigmentation of skin, and flare of symptoms at the site of injection. Surgical procedures for ITBS carry inherent risks. Postoperative infection and other standard risks should be explained to patients before surgical interventions. Overall, interventional procedures for the ITB carry few risks or complications.

References

[1] Gottschalk F, Kourosh S, Leveau B. The functional anatomy of tensor fasciae latae and gluteus medius and minimus. J Anat 1989;166:179–89.

[2] Sher I, Umans H, Downie SA, et al. Proximal iliotibial band syndrome: what is it and where is it? Skeletal Radiol 2011;40:1553–6.

[3] Falvey EC, Clark RA, Franklyn-Miller A, et al. Iliotibial band syndrome: an examination of the evidence behind a number of treatment options. Scand J Med Sci Sports 2010;20:580–7.

[4] Vieira EL, Vieira EA, da Silva RT, et al. An anatomic study of the iliotibial tract. Arthroscopy 2007;23:269–74.

[5] Terry G. The anatomy of the iliopatellar band and iliotibial tract. Am J Sports Med 1986;14:39–45.

[6] Baker RL, Souza RB, Fredericson M. Iliotibial band syndrome: soft tissue and biomechanical factors in evaluation and treatment. PM R 2011;3:550–61.

[7] Nemeth WC, Sanders BL. The lateral synovial recess of the knee: anatomy and role in chronic iliotibial band friction syndrome. Arthroscopy 1996;12:574–80.

[8] Orchard JW, Fricker PA, Abud AT, Mason BR. Biomechanics of iliotibial band friction syndrome in runners. Am J Sports Med 1996;24:375–9.

[9] Fairclough J, Hayashi K, Toumi H, et al. The functional anatomy of the iliotibial band during flexion and extension of the knee: implications for understanding iliotibial band syndrome. J Anat 2006;208:309–16.

[10] Fredericson M, Cookingham CL, Chaudhari AM, et al. Hip abductor weakness in distance runners with iliotibial band syndrome. Clin J Sport Med 2000;10:169–75.

[11] Ellis R, Hing W, Reid D. Iliotibial band friction syndrome—a systematic review. Man Ther 2007;12:200–8.

[12] Strauss E, Kim S, Calcei J, Park D. Iliotibial band syndrome: evaluation and management. J Am Acad Orthop Surg 2011;16:728–36.

[13] Grau S, Krauss I, Maiwald C, et al. Hip abductor weakness is not the cause for iliotibial band syndrome. Int J Sports Med 2008;29:579–83.

[14] Powers CM. The influence of abnormal hip mechanics on knee injury: a biomechanical perspective. J Orthop Sports Phys Ther 2010;40:42–51.

[15] Noehren B, Davis I, Hamill J. ASB clinical biomechanics award winner 2006 prospective study of the biomechanical factors associated with iliotibial band syndrome. Clin Biomech (Bristol, Avon) 2007;22:951–6.

[16] Miller RH, Lowry JL, Meardon SA, Gillette JC. Lower extremity mechanics of iliotibial band syndrome during an exhaustive run. Gait Posture 2007;26:407–13.

[17] Ferber R, Noehren B, Hamill J, Davis IS. Competitive female runners with a history of iliotibial band syndrome demonstrate atypical hip and knee kinematics. J Orthop Sports Phys Ther 2010;40:52–8.

[18] Grau S, Krauss I, Maiwald C, et al. Kinematic classification of iliotibial band syndrome in runners. Scand J Med Sci Sports 2011;21:184–9.

[19] Hamill J, Miller R, Noehren B, Davis I. A prospective study of iliotibial band strain in runners. Clin Biomech (Bristol, Avon) 2008;23:1018–25.

[20] Beers A, Ryan M, Kasubuchi Z, et al. Effects of multi-modal physiotherapy, including hip abductor strengthening, in patients with iliotibial band friction syndrome. Physiother Can 2008;60:180–8.

[21] Fredericson M, White JJ, MacMahon JM, Andriacchi TP. Quantitative analysis of the relative effectiveness of 3 iliotibial band stretches. Arch Phys Med Rehabil 2002;83:589–92.

[22] Lavine R. Iliotibial band friction syndrome. Curr Rev Musculoskelet Med 2010;3:18–22.

[23] Xethalis J, Lorei M. Soccer injuries. In: Nicholas J, Hershman E, editors. The lower extremity and spine in sports medicine. St. Louis: Mosby; 1995. p. 1509–57.

[24] Holmes J, Pruitt A, Whalen N. Cycling injuries. In: Nicholas J, Hershman E, editors. The lower extremity and spine in sports medicine. St. Louis: Mosby; 1995. p. 1559–79.

[25] Fredericson M, Guillet M, Debenedictis L. Innovative solutions for iliotibial band syndrome. Phys Sportsmed 2000;28:53–68.

[26] Fredericson M, Wolf C. Iliotibial band syndrome in runners: innovations in treatment. Sports Med 2005;35:451–9.

[27] Lindenberg G, Pinshaw R, Noakes T. Iliotibial band friction syndrome in runners. Phys Sportsmed 1984;12:118–30.

[28] Wanich T, Hodgkins C, Columbier JA, et al. Cycling injuries of the lower extremity. J Am Acad Orthop Surg 2007;15:748–56.

[29] Holmes J, Pruitt A, Whalen N. Lower extremity overuse in bicycling. Clin Sports Med 1994;13:187–205.

[30] Allen W, Cope R. Coxa saltans: the snapping hip revisited. J Am Acad Orthop Surg 1995;3:303–8.

[31] Khan K, Brown J, Way S. Overuse injuries in classical ballet. Sports Med 1995;19:341–57.

[32] Press J, Herring S, Kibler W. Rehabilitation of the combatant with musculoskeletal disorders. In: Dillingham T, Belandres P, editors. Rehabilitation of the injured combatant. Washington, DC: Office of the Surgeon General; 1999. p. 353–415.

[33] Geraci MC, Brown W. Evidence-based treatment of hip and pelvic injuries in runners. Phys Med Rehabil Clin N Am 2005;16:711–47.

[34] Geraci MC. Rehabilitation of the hip, pelvis, and thigh. In: Kibler W, Herring S, Press J, editors. Functional rehabilitation of sports and musculoskeletal injuries. Gaithersburg, Md: Aspen; 1998. p. 216–43.

[35] Puniello MS. Iliotibial band tightness and medial patellar glide in patients with patellofemoral dysfunction. J Orthop Sports Phys Ther 1993;17:144–8.

[36] Barber F, Sutker A. Iliotibial band syndrome. Sports Med 1992;14:144–8.

[37] Martens M, Libbrecht P, Burssens A. Surgical treatment of the iliotibial band friction syndrome. Am J Sports Med 1985;17:651–4.

[38] Gyaran IA, Spiezia F, Hudson Z, Maffulli N. Sonographic measurement of iliotibial band thickness: an observational study in healthy adult volunteers. Knee Surg Sports Traumatol Arthrosc 2011;19:458–61.

[39] Choi Y, Lee S. Dynamic sonography of external snapping hip syndrome. J Ultrasound Med 2002;21:753–8.

[40] Bergman A, Fredericson M. MR imaging of stress reactions, muscle injuries, and other overuse injuries in runners. Magn Reson Imaging Clin N Am 1999;7:151–74.

[41] Wang TG, Jan MH, Lin KH, Wang HK. Assessment of stretching of the iliotibial tract with Ober and modified Ober tests: an ultrasonographic study. Arch Phys Med Rehabil 2006;87:1407–11.

[42] Gunter P, Schwellnus MP. Local corticosteroid injection in iliotibial band friction syndrome in runners: a randomised controlled trial [commentary]. Br J Sports Med 2004;38:269–72.

[43] Hariri S, Savidge ET, Reinold MM, et al. Treatment of recalcitrant iliotibial band friction syndrome with open iliotibial band bursectomy: indications, technique, and clinical outcomes. Am J Sports Med 2009;37:1417–24.

[44] Ilizaliturri Jr VM, Camacho-Galindo J. Endoscopic treatment of snapping hips, iliotibial band, and iliopsoas tendon. Sports Med Arthrosc Rev 2010;18:120–7.

CHAPTER 70

Knee Osteoarthritis

Michael Sein, MD
Allen N. Wilkins, MD
Edward M. Phillips, MD

Synonyms

Degenerative joint disease of the knee joint
Degenerative arthritis
Joint destruction of the knee
Osteoarthrosis

ICD-9 Codes

715.16 **Osteoarthrosis, localized, primary, lower leg**
715.26 **Osteoarthrosis, localized, secondary, lower leg**
716.16 **Traumatic arthropathy, lower leg**

ICD-10 Codes

M17.0 **Bilateral primary osteoarthritis of knee**
M17.10 **Unilateral primary osteoarthritis, unspecified knee**
M17.11 **Unilateral primary osteoarthritis, right knee**
M17.12 **Unilateral primary osteoarthritis, left knee**
M17.4 **Other bilateral secondary osteoarthritis of knee**
M17.5 **Other unilateral secondary osteoarthritis of knee**
M12.561 **Traumatic arthropathy, right knee**
M12.562 **Traumatic arthropathy, left knee**
M12.569 **Traumatic arthropathy, unspecified knee**

Definition

Osteoarthritis is steadily becoming the most common cause of disability for the middle-aged and has become the most common cause of disability for those older than 65 years [1]. The knee joint is the most common site for lower extremity osteoarthritis [2]. It is estimated that nearly half of all adults will have symptomatic knee osteoarthritis in their lifetimes [3]. In addition to the growing population of elderly patients with knee osteoarthritis, an increasing number of former athletes with previous knee injuries may experience post-traumatic knee osteoarthritis. Osteoarthritis of the knee results from mechanical and idiopathic factors. Osteoarthritis alters the balance between degradation and synthesis of articular cartilage and subchondral bone.

Osteoarthritis can involve any or all of the three major knee compartments: medial, patellofemoral, or lateral. The medial compartment is most often involved, leading to medial joint space collapse and thus to a genu varum (bowleg) deformity. Lateral compartment involvement may lead to a genu valgum (knock-knee) deformity. Isolated disease of the patellofemoral joint occurs in up to a quarter of patients with osteoarthritis of the knee [4]. Arthritis in one compartment may, through altered biomechanical stress patterns, eventually lead to involvement of another compartment.

Osteoarthritis affects all structures within and around a joint. Hyaline articular cartilage is lost. Bone remodeling occurs, with capsular stretching and weakness of periarticular muscles. Synovitis is present in some cases and ligamentous laxity occurs. Lesions in the bone marrow may also develop, which may suggest trauma to bone [5]. Osteoarthritis involves the joint in a nonuniform and focal manner. Localized areas of loss of cartilage can increase focal stress across the joint, leading to further cartilage loss. With a large enough area of cartilage loss or with bone remodeling, the joint becomes tilted, and malalignment develops.

The threat of knee osteoarthritis is not only a concern for elderly populations. Malalignment is the most potent risk factor for structural deterioration of the knee joint [6]. By further increasing the degree of focal loading, malalignment creates a vicious circle of joint damage that ultimately can lead to joint failure. The role of obesity as a risk factor for knee osteoarthritis has been well documented. A large, population-based prospective study found that the risk for knee osteoarthritis was seven times greater for people with a body mass index of 30 or higher compared with those with a body mass index below 25 [7]. Moreover, women (of average height) who lost 5 kg of weight reduced their risk of symptomatic knee osteoarthritis by 50% [8].

Sports injuries and vigorous physical activity are considered to be important risk factors in knee osteoarthritis. Elite athletes who take part in high-impact sports, such as soccer and ice hockey, have an increased risk of knee osteoarthritis [9]. It is unclear whether the increased risk in this particular study was directly related to traumatic injury. However, it has been suggested in another study that subjects with a history of knee injury are at a five-fold to sixfold increased risk for development of knee osteoarthritis [10]. Knee osteoarthritis is common in those performing heavy physical work, especially if this involves knee bending, squatting, kneeling, or repetitive use of joints [11]. It is unclear if the association of knee osteoarthritis with these work-related activities is secondary to the nature of the work or the increased likelihood of injury.

Symptoms

Knee osteoarthritis is characterized by joint pain, tenderness, decreased range of motion, crepitus, occasional effusion, and often inflammation of varying degrees. Initial osteoarthritis symptoms are generally minimal, given the gradual and insidious onset of the condition. Pain typically occurs around the knee, particularly during weight bearing, and decreases with rest. With progression of the disease, pain can persist even at rest. Activities associated with osteoarthritic pain are climbing stairs, getting out of a chair, getting in and out of a car, and walking long distances. Pain may also radiate to adjacent sites as osteoarthritis indirectly alters the biomechanics of other anatomic structures, such as ligaments, muscles, nerves, and veins.

Joint stiffness may occur after periods of inactivity, such as after awakening in the morning or prolonged sitting. Patients often report higher pain levels in the morning but usually for less than 30 minutes. Patients often experience limitation of movement because of joint stiffness or swelling. Many patients report a "locking" or a "catching" sensation, which is probably due to a variety of causes, including debris from degenerated cartilage or meniscus in the joint, increased adhesiveness of the relatively rough articular surfaces, muscle weakness, and even tissue inflammation. Stiffness can discourage mobility. This initiates a cycle that results in deconditioning, decreased function, and increased pain.

Barometric changes, such as those associated with damp, rainy weather, will often increase pain intensity. Patients often note that their knees "give way" or feel unstable at times.

Physical Examination

Examination of the patient includes testing for various possible causes of knee pain (see section on differential diagnosis). Therefore the entire limb, from the hip to the ankle, is examined. It is important to identify findings such as quadriceps weakness or atrophy and knee and hip flexion contractures. Gait should be observed for presence of a limp, functional limb length discrepancy, or buckling. Genu varum or valgum is often better appreciated when the patient is standing.

Table 70.1 Typical Physical Examination Findings in Knee Osteoarthritis

Inspection	Bone hypertrophy Varus deformity from preferential medial compartment involvement
Palpation	Increased warmth Joint effusion Joint line tenderness
Range of motion	Painful knee flexion Decreased joint flexion secondary to pain Crepitus (coarse)
Joint stability	Mediolateral instability

The affected knee should be compared with the contralateral uninvolved knee. Knee examination may reveal decreased knee extension or flexion secondary to effusion or osteophytes (both of which may be palpable). Osteophytes along the femoral condyles may be palpated, especially along the medial distal femur. Palpation may reveal patellar or parapatellar tenderness. Crepitation, resulting from juxtaposition of roughened cartilage surfaces, may be appreciated along the joint line when the knee is flexed or extended. A mild effusion and tenderness may be appreciated along the medial joint line or at the pes anserine bursa. Ligament testing may reveal laxity of one or both of the collateral ligaments. Lateral subluxation of the patella may be found in patients with genu valgum (Table 70.1). Another clue on examination that the patient probably has knee osteoarthritis is the finding of visible bone enlargements (exostoses) of the fingers. At the distal interphalangeal joints, these are referred to as Heberden nodes; at the proximal interphalangeal joints, they are known as Bouchard nodes, usually a slightly later finding.

The findings of the neurologic examination are typically normal, with the exception of decreased muscle strength, particularly in the quadriceps, due to disuse or guarding secondary to pain.

Diagnostic Studies

Osteoarthritis is diagnosed clinically on the basis of history and physical examination. Imaging, however, can be used to confirm the diagnosis and to rule out other conditions. Radiographic abnormalities can be found both in joint areas subjected to excessive pressure and in joint areas subjected to diminished pressure. These changes include joint space narrowing, subchondral sclerosis, and bone cysts in weight-bearing regions of the joint and osteophytes in low-pressure areas, especially along the marginal regions of the joint. Joint space narrowing is the initial finding, followed by subchondral sclerosis, then by osteophytes, and finally by cysts with sclerotic margins (known as synovial cysts, subchondral cysts, subarticular pseudocysts, or necrotic pseudocysts).

Radiographic evidence of osteoarthritis is not well correlated with symptoms [12]. Results have been conflicting, probably because of the differences in populations studied and radiographic and clinical criteria used. The presence of osteophytes had a strong association with knee pain, whereas the absence or presence of joint space narrowing was not associated with pain [13].

Knee pain severity was a more important determinant of functional impairment than radiographic severity of osteoarthritis [14,15]. There was no correlation between joint space narrowing and a disability score (Western Ontario and McMaster Universities Osteoarthritis index, WOMAC) at a single time point [15].

Osteophytes *alone* are associated with aging rather than with osteoarthritis. Indications for plain x-ray films include trauma, effusion, symptoms not readily explainable by physical examination findings, severe pain, presurgical planning, and failure of conservative management. Recommended films are weight-bearing (standing) anteroposterior, lateral, and patellar views. Radiographs taken during weight bearing with the knee in full extension and partial flexion may reveal a constellation of findings associated with osteoarthritis, including asymmetric narrowing of the joint space (typically medial compartment), osteophytes, sclerosis, and subchondral cysts (Fig. 70.1). A Merchant view specifically evaluates the patellofemoral space. Non–weight-bearing lateral views may help in the evaluation of the patellofemoral and tibiofemoral joint spaces. Tunnel views can help visualize loose osteochondral bodies.

Magnetic resonance imaging usually adds little but cost to the entire evaluation of osteoarthritis of the knee. It may reveal changes that suggest the presence of osteoarthritis. However, it is not indicated in the initial evaluation of older persons with chronic knee pain. Magnetic resonance imaging may detect incidental findings, such as meniscal tears, that are common in middle-aged and older adults with and without knee pain. Musculoskeletal ultrasonography has potential for detecting bone erosions, synovitis, tendon disease, and enthesopathy. It has a number of distinct advantages over magnetic resonance imaging, including good patient tolerability and ability to scan multiple joints in a short time. However, there are scarce data about its validity, reproducibility, and responsiveness to change, making interpretation and comparison of studies difficult. In particular, there are limited data describing standardized scanning methodology and standardized definitions of ultrasound pathologic changes [16].

Laboratory test results are typically normal, but analysis may be undertaken, especially for elderly patients, to establish a baseline (e.g., blood urea nitrogen concentration, creatinine concentration, or liver function tests before use of nonsteroidal anti-inflammatory drugs or acetaminophen) or to exclude other conditions such as rheumatoid arthritis. Synovial fluid analysis should not be undertaken unless destructive, crystalline, or septic arthritis is suspected.

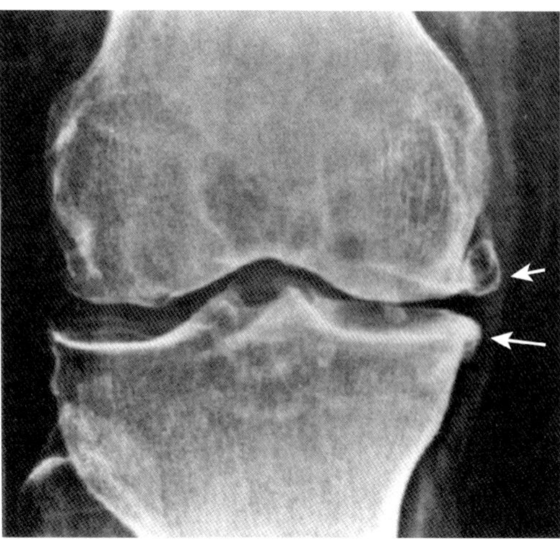

FIGURE 70.1 Knee radiograph demonstrating osteophytes *(arrows)* and medial joint space narrowing consistent with degenerative arthritis. *(From West SG. Rheumatology Secrets. Philadelphia, Hanley & Belfus, 1997.)*

Differential Diagnosis

COMMON CAUSES OF KNEE PAIN BY AGE GROUP

Children and adolescents	Patellar subluxation
	Osgood-Schlatter disease
	Patellar tendinitis
	Referred pain (e.g., slipped capital femoral epiphysis)
	Osteochondritis dissecans
	Subchondral fracture
	Genetic or congenital defect
	Septic arthritis
	Tumor
Adults	Patellofemoral pain syndrome (chondromalacia patellae)
	Medial plica syndrome
	Pes anserine bursitis
	Trauma: ligamentous sprains
	Meniscal tear
	Inflammatory arthropathy: rheumatoid arthritis, Reiter syndrome
	Septic arthritis
	Midlumbar radiculopathy
	Tumor
Older adults	Osteoarthritis
	Crystal-induced inflammatory arthropathy: gout, pseudogout
	Rheumatoid arthritis
	Popliteal cyst
	Tumor

DIFFERENTIAL DIAGNOSIS OF KNEE PAIN BY ANATOMIC SITE

Anterior knee pain	Patellar subluxation or dislocation
	Tibial apophysitis (Osgood-Schlatter lesion)
	Jumper's knee (patellar tendinitis)
	Patellofemoral pain syndrome (chondromalacia patellae)
Medial knee pain	Medial collateral ligament sprain
	Medial meniscal tear
	Pes anserine bursitis
	Medial plica syndrome
Lateral knee pain	Lateral collateral ligament sprain
	Lateral meniscal tear
	Iliotibial band tendinitis
Posterior knee pain	Popliteal cyst (Baker cyst)
	Posterior cruciate ligament injury

Treatment

Initial

The PRICE regimen may help provide initial relief for patients in pain: *p*rotection with limited weight bearing by use of a cane or modification of exercise to reduce stress; relative

Table 70.2 Pharmacologic and Supplemental Nutrition Treatment Options

Medication	Related Details
Acetaminophen	The maximum dosage is 4 g/day in patients with normal hepatic function.
Oral NSAIDs	Studies show almost equal efficacy among traditional NSAIDs [18]. A randomized prospective study demonstrated equal efficacy between selective cyclooxygenase 2 inhibitors and traditional NSAIDs [19].
Tramadol-acetaminophen	American Pain Society guidelines recommend tramadol-acetaminophen for treatment of osteoarthritis pain when NSAIDs alone cannot provide adequate relief. It is considered safe and effective in a subset of elderly patients [20].
Oxycodone	Patients with moderate to severe pain from osteoarthritis can achieve effective pain relief without deterioration in function when opioids are included as part of a comprehensive pain management program [21].
Topical NSAIDs	A quantitative systematic review of 86 trials evaluating the efficacy of topical NSAIDs in osteoarthritis and tendinitis found them significantly more effective than placebo [22].
Topical capsaicin	Limited data from controlled trials have shown improvements with capsaicin [23].
Glucosamine sulfate (1500 mg orally qd) and chondroitin sulfate (1200 mg orally qd)	One large randomized clinical trial found that glucosamine and chondroitin sulfate alone or in combination did not reduce pain effectively in the overall group of patients with osteoarthritis of the knee. However, the combination of glucosamine and chondroitin sulfate was effective in the subgroup of patients with moderate to severe knee pain [24].

NSAIDs, nonsteroidal anti-inflammatory drugs.

*r*est (or taking adequate rests throughout the day, avoiding prolonged standing, climbing of stairs, kneeling, deep knee bending); *i*ce (applied while the skin is protected with a towel for up to 15 minutes at a time several times a day; note, however, that some patients with chronic pain may find better relief with moist heat); *c*ompression (if swelling exists, wrapping with an elastic bandage or a sleeve may help); and *e*levation (may help diminish swelling, if it is present). There are a wide variety of initial treatment options for knee arthritis. Current guidelines put forth by the American College of Rheumatology emphasize the use of acetaminophen as a first-line therapy for osteoarthritis [17]. Other options include oral and topical nonsteroidal anti-inflammatory drugs; topical capsaicin cream; and nutritional intervention, such as glucosamine sulfate and chondroitin sulfate (Table 70.2). Orthotics and footwear are also included in the list of treatment options and are discussed further in the next section.

Rehabilitation

Exercise

Exercises are likely to be most effective if they train muscles for the activities a person performs daily [25]. Randomized studies support the benefits of exercise, even if it is home based, on pain and function in patients with osteoarthritis [26]. Because there is currently no cure for osteoarthritis, most research continues to evaluate the use of exercise as a treatment to alleviate symptoms of the disease and to enhance functional capacity. Two meta-analyses published in 2004 focus specifically on the efficacy of strengthening [27] and aerobic exercise [28] for osteoarthritis.

With regard to muscle strengthening, improvements in strength, pain, function, and quality of life were noted. However, there was no evidence that the type of strengthening exercise influences outcome. Static or dynamic strengthening exercises can maintain or improve periarticular muscle strength, thereby reversing or preventing biomechanical abnormalities and their contribution to joint dysfunction and degeneration.

With regard to aerobic exercise, results indicated that aerobic exercise alleviates pain and joint tenderness and promotes functional status and respiratory capacity. Aerobic exercise improves activity tolerance, increases pain threshold, and can have positive effects on mood and motivation for participation in other activities. Whereas strengthening appears superior to aerobic exercise in the short term for specific impairment-related outcomes (e.g., pain), aerobic exercise appears more effective for functional outcomes in the longer term. There is also evidence that exercise can improve proprioception [27], thus improving biomechanics and protective responses.

Attempts to maintain function can be helped through non–weight-bearing strengthening, especially of the quadriceps. For patients with greater pain, this can be done with static exercise or through water aerobics, which allows motion at the knee with reduced joint loads. Exercise bicycles and walking should be recommended to enhance aerobic capacity. Deep knee bends in the presence of effusion should be avoided. Particular attention must be paid to strengthening of the medial quadriceps in patients with genu valgum who have lateral subluxation of the patella. Maintaining activity is critical to maintaining function. Even those patients scheduled for total knee arthroplasty should pursue static and dynamic strengthening as well as cardiovascular conditioning preoperatively to ease the postoperative rehabilitation [29].

Therapeutic Modalities

Transcutaneous electrical nerve stimulation (TENS), the application of an electrical current through the skin with the aim of pain modulation, is a frequently used modality in knee osteoarthritis. Although this is a popular treatment option, research supporting its efficacy is lacking. The treatment is supported only by a few small, short-term trials. In a small-scale, randomized, double-blind crossover trial comparing active and placebo TENS for symptomatic knee osteoarthritis in subjects who were considered to be candidates for total knee replacement, patients reported significantly more pain relief and less medication use with active TENS therapy than with the placebo [30]. For most patients, pain relief was experienced only during periods of active use of the device, although the beneficial effect was sustained for several hours in a few. Despite the positive results in these small trials, a meta-analysis could not confirm this modality's effectiveness. The systematic review attributed inconclusive results to questionable methodologic quality and a high degree of heterogeneity among trials [31].

Additional therapeutic modalities, such as electrical stimulation or massage, may also be used. Therapists may also review postural alignment and joint positioning techniques, especially for when the patient is sleeping. In particular, the use of a pillow under bent knees, much favored by many patients when they are supine, should be avoided because resulting knee flexion contractures, even if small, can significantly increase stresses on the knee during gait. Stretching of the hamstrings and quadriceps may also prove beneficial. Patients should be counseled against prolonged wearing of high heels, which is associated with medial knee osteoarthritis [32].

Adaptive Equipment

Adaptive equipment, such as a cane or walker, can reduce hip or knee loading, thereby reducing pain. It may also prevent falls in patients with impaired balance. Proper training in the use of a cane is important because it reduces joint loading in the contralateral hip but amplifies forces in the ipsilateral hip.

Bracing and Footwear

The basic rationale for a knee brace for unicompartmental knee osteoarthritis is to improve function by reducing the patient's symptoms. This can be accomplished, in theory, by reducing the biomechanical load on the affected compartment of the knee. Clinical trials are generally small and difficult to control adequately because of the nature of knee braces and the difficulty in designing a trial with a true placebo. Also, each brace has a unique design and may have features that make it more or less acceptable to the patient. Therefore clinical trials done with one brace design may not be applicable to all osteoarthritis knee braces.

A review of the published literature on knee bracing for osteoarthritis points out some of the limitations of the clinical trials to date but acknowledges the limited evidence for improvement in pain and function in patients using osteoarthritis braces compared with medical treatment or neoprene sleeves [33].

In patients with osteoarthritis and varus malalignment of the knees, a shoe wedge (thicker laterally) moves the center of loading laterally during walking, a change that extends from foot to knee, lessening medial load across the knee. Although such modifications to footwear decrease varus malalignment [34], one randomized trial [35] showed no reduction in pain compared with a neutral insert. However, a review of the published literature on the efficacy of laterally wedged foot orthotics for improving these symptoms does indicate a strong scientific basis for applying wedged insoles in an attempt to reduce pain in patients with medial compartment knee osteoarthritis [36].

Tilting or malalignment of the patella may cause patellofemoral pain. Patellar realignment with the use of braces or tape to pull the patella back into the trochlear sulcus of the femur or to reduce its tilt may lessen pain. In clinical trials with tape to reposition the patella into the sulcus without tilt, knee pain was reduced compared with placebo [37,38]. However, patients may find it difficult to apply tape, and skin irritation is common. Commercial patellar braces are also available, but their efficacy has not been studied formally.

Heel lifts or built-up shoes may be required in the presence of leg length discrepancy to prevent compensatory knee flexion gait on the longer side. In the presence of knee deformity, therapists can also evaluate for altered biomechanics (e.g., genu varum may lead to femoral internal torsion, resulting in compensatory external rotation of the tibia, which predisposes the patient to increased arthritic changes). Therapists can also visit the homes and workplaces of patients to suggest adjustments, such as raised toilet seats, grab bars, reachers, and the like.

Acupuncture

Acupuncture, a technique in existence for thousands of years, has gained renewed interest as a treatment of osteoarthritis. A multicenter, 26-week National Institutes of Health–funded randomized controlled trial found acupuncture to be effective as adjunctive therapy for reducing pain and improving function in patients with knee osteoarthritis [39].

Procedures

Intra-articular corticosteroid injections may help in reduction of local inflammation and improvement of symptoms. The response is generally rapid but may not be sustained in the longer term. A systematic review of intra-articular corticosteroid injections demonstrated evidence of pain reduction at 2 weeks and at 3 weeks after intervention. At 4 to 24 weeks after injection, evidence of an effect on pain and function was lacking [40]. Because the corticosteroid is delivered directly, systemic toxicity is minimized. Intra-articular corticosteroid injections should be given no more than two or three times a year to reduce potential damage to cartilage from the steroids. Given the short-term effect and limitation on injection frequency, corticosteroid injection is most often used as an adjunctive therapy for acute or severe symptom flares (Fig. 70.2). Table 70.3 lists potential systemic side effects of corticosteroid injections. Administration of steroids through iontophoresis may be an alternative for patients hesitant to undergo injections.

The authors' preferred technique for intra-articular injection of the knee is as follows. With the patient supine, under sterile conditions with use of a 25-gauge needle, 2 or 3 mL of local anesthetic (e.g., 1% lidocaine) is injected just posterior to the upper lateral pole of the patella. Alternatively, ethyl chloride spray can be used. Then, by use of a 1½-inch, 22- to 25-gauge needle, either local steroid (e.g., methylprednisolone, 20 to 40 mg/mL) or hyaluronic acid is injected in the same region (these products are available in 2-mL vials or prefilled syringes, one injection per vial). If a knee effusion exists, it may be necessary to drain the effusion to avoid dilution of the medications. This is ideally done with an 18- to 20-gauge needle. Switching of

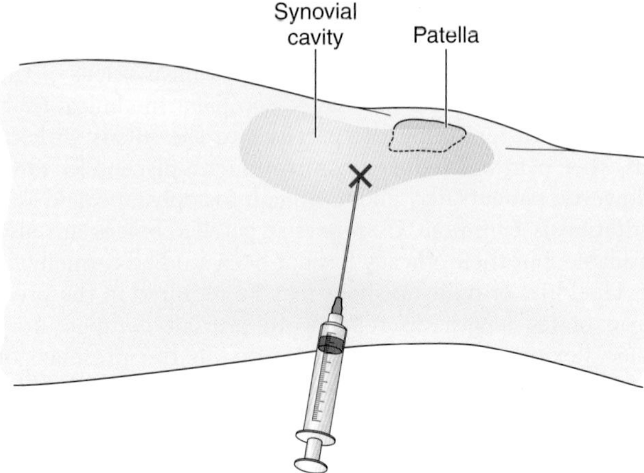

FIGURE 70.2 Location for needle insertion.

Table 70.3 Minimizing Potential Side Effects of Intra-articular Corticosteroid Injection

Side Effect	Ways to Minimize Risk
Systemic effects	Avoid high doses and multiple simultaneous injections; use accurate injection techniques
Tendon rupture, fat atrophy, muscle wasting, skin pigment changes	Avoid misdirected injections
Septic arthritis	Use sterile technique; withhold therapy in at-risk patients
Nerve and blood vessel damage	Use accurate injection techniques
Postinjection symptom flare or synovitis	Avoid the same preparation for future injections
Flushing	Avoid high doses
Anaphylaxis	Take careful drug allergy history
Steroid arthropathy	Avoid high doses and overly frequent injections

the syringes while the needle remains in place prevents additional trauma. Postinjection care includes local icing for 5 to 10 minutes. Patients are advised to avoid excessive weight bearing for 24 to 48 hours after an injection.

Viscosupplementation with hyaluronic acid, available as naturally occurring hyaluronan or synthetic hylan G-F 20, may be helpful. The rationale for using viscosupplementation is to impart protective properties to synovial fluid, including shock absorption, energy dissipation, and lubrication of the articular cartilage surface [41]. Hyaluronan is administered in a series of five weekly injections; hylan G-F 20 is given in three weekly injections. Treatments are typically repeated two to four times per year. Clinical trials of viscosupplementation have demonstrated limited efficacy in pain relief [42]. Compared with corticosteroid injection, the effect of hyaluronic acid appears to be less dramatic but more durable. In a meta-analysis comparing both interventions, hyaluronic acid was less effective for pain relief in the first 4 weeks after injection [43]. By week 4, the two approaches had equal efficacy. Beyond week 8, hyaluronic acid had a greater effect [43]. Side effects included local inflammation and increased pain at the injection site. There is no evidence that hyaluronan injection in humans alters biologic processes or progression of cartilage damage. The hyaluronic acid is injected into the knee in the same manner as the intra-articular steroid is administered.

Surgery (Table 70.4)

Most would agree that the term *arthroscopic débridement* includes lavage and the removal of loose bodies, debris, mobile fragments of articular cartilage, unstable torn menisci, and impinging osteophytes. However, it is clear from the literature that drilling, abrasion chondroplasty, microfracture, saucerization, notchplasty, osteophyte removal, synovectomy, and arthrolysis are also performed simultaneously in many clinical series. Patients who have a short history and a sudden onset of mechanical symptoms and also have knee effusions are likely to do best [44]. Meniscal symptoms and signs, synovitis or synovial impingement, osteophytic impingement, and catching or locking caused by loose bodies favor a good

Table 70.4 Surgical Options for Osteoarthritis of the Knee

Established Techniques	Indications	Outcome
Arthroscopic débridement	Knee effusions Meniscal signs and symptoms Synovitis Osteophytic impingement Catching or locking caused by loose bodies	Most reports show improvement in 50% to 80% of patients; however, results deteriorate with time
Osteotomy of the proximal tibia or distal femur	Predominantly medial compartment involvement	Recovery is prolonged Relief of symptoms often incomplete
Unicompartmental knee replacement	Predominantly medial compartment involvement Minimal lateral compartment disease No major anterior knee pain Stable knee joint Correctable varus deformity Fixed flexion deformity of less than 10 degrees	Survivorship rate for implants of 90% at 20 years
Patellofemoral replacement	Isolated patellofemoral joint involvement	Results have been variable
Total knee replacement	Tricompartmental disease	Survival rates of between 84% and 98% at 15 years

outcome. Significant instability and malalignment are poor prognostic factors. Patients who have radiographic signs of advanced degeneration are unlikely to benefit [45].

Although arthroscopic surgery has been widely used for osteoarthritis of the knee, scientific evidence to support its efficacy is lacking. Most of the orthopedic literature supporting its use is based on retrospective studies, with authors reporting improvement in 50% to 80% of patients [46,47]. However, in a randomized, controlled trial, arthroscopic surgery for osteoarthritis of the knee provided no additional benefit to optimized physical and medical therapies [48].

Up to a quarter of patients with osteoarthritis of the knee have predominantly arthritis of the medial compartment. The surgical options for such patients are medial unicompartmental knee replacement, proximal tibial or distal femoral osteotomy, and total knee replacement (see Chapter 80). Osteotomy is a less drastic measure than knee replacement and is often favored by younger, active patients with unicompartmental symptoms. In osteotomy, a wedge-shaped piece of bone is removed from either the femur or tibia to bring the knee joint back into a more physiologic alignment. This procedure moves the weight-bearing axis to the less damaged compartment. Recovery is prolonged and relief of symptoms often incomplete, but osteotomy may delay the need for total knee replacement for 5 to 10 years [49,50]. Successful treatment could allow a return to sport. The risks specific to this surgery depend on the technique and include nonunion at the osteotomy site, common peroneal nerve injury, pain from the proximal tibiofibular joint, and overcorrection or undercorrection of the deformity. Part of an ongoing debate within the orthopedic community concerns the relative merits of high tibial osteotomy compared with unicompartmental knee replacement in younger patients. Unicompartmental knee replacement requires a smaller surgical approach than for total knee replacement, leading to less blood loss and quicker rehabilitation. The range of knee motion after unicompartmental knee replacement is generally superior to that after total knee replacement. Finally, revision of a unicompartmental knee replacement to a total knee replacement is potentially more straightforward than revision of a total knee replacement [51]. The prerequisites for a unicompartmental knee replacement include stability of the joint, correctable varus deformity, fixed flexion deformity of less than 10 degrees, and minimal lateral compartment disease. Radiographic evidence of patellofemoral osteoarthritis is not necessarily a problem, provided patients do not have major anterior knee pain. Survivorship rates for implants are estimated at 93% and 90% at 15 and 20 years, respectively [52]. These rates are comparable to the best reported for total knee replacement and are an improvement on rates previously reported for unicompartmental knee replacement.

The relative merits of unicompartmental knee replacement over total knee replacement or proximal tibial osteotomy in young (<60 years) active patients continue to be debated. Unicompartmental knee replacement has now become an accepted treatment for older patients with medial compartment arthritis. The results of unicompartmental knee replacement in lateral compartment disease have yet to be fully determined. Total knee replacements, with a quarter-century track record, have generally provided most patients with good pain relief. Whereas joint replacement surgery has been found in numerous studies to provide pain relief, it paradoxically may lead to increase of services as patients become more mobile [53].

Patients considered for patellofemoral replacement must be assessed for degenerative changes in the rest of the knee joint. Several types of patellofemoral arthroplasties are available, but the results have been variable, highlighting the need for careful selection of patients [54–56]. The most common problems are maltracking of the patella, excessive wear of the polyethylene implant, and disease progression in the rest of the knee joint. Severe chondromalacia may necessitate patellectomy (patella excision). Knee arthrodesis today is generally reserved for patients in whom knee replacement surgery fails. Other less commonly used surgical options, such as synovectomy and small prostheses (to correct deformity), are also possible.

Potential Disease Complications

Progressive knee osteoarthritis may result in reduced mobility and the general systemic complications of immobility and deconditioning. Antalgic gait can result in contralateral hip disease (e.g., greater trochanteric bursitis). The risk of falls will be increased by decreased mobility at the knee. Complaints of chronic pain may result from the initial knee osteoarthritis if it is inadequately treated.

Potential Treatment Complications

Complications of anti-inflammatory medication and steroid injections are well known. Repeated steroid injections can lead to further cartilage destruction as well as to sepsis. Infection is a rare but possible result of joint injection or surgery. Cryotherapy or heat therapy can, of course, lead to frostbite or burns. Hyaluronic acid injections may result in localized transient pain or effusion.

Arthroscopy may damage the articular surface membrane, thus initiating damage to uninvolved cartilage. Excessive arthroscopic scraping has sometimes been associated with persistent pain. The possibility of infection and deep venous thrombosis and the small but real possibility of intraoperative mortality limit the use of surgery to a last-line option. One series of patients *not* taking anticoagulants experienced a 50% rate of deep venous thrombosis, 14.5% of which was proximal deep venous thrombosis [57], thus indicating the importance of anticoagulation, which reduces the risk to less than 5%. In any case, mechanical wear and prosthesis loosening, especially for cemented prostheses, often lead to the need for revision after a decade or so.

References

[1] Bashaw RT, Tingstad EM. Rehabilitation of the osteoarthritic patient: focus on the knee. Clin Sports Med 2005;24:101–31.

[2] Hootman J, Bolen J, Helmick C, Langmaid G. Prevalence of doctor-diagnosed arthritis and arthritis-attributable activity limitation—United States, 2003-2005. MMWR Morb Mortal Wkly Rep 2006;55:1089–92.

[3] Murphy L, Schwartz TA, Helmick CG, et al. Lifetime risk of symptomatic knee osteoarthritis. Arthritis Rheum 2008;59:1207–13.

[4] Duncan RC, Hay EM, Saklatvala J, et al. Prevalence of radiographic osteoarthritis—it all depends on your point of view. Rheumatology (Oxford) 2006;45:757–60.

[5] Felson DT, McLaughlin S, Goggins J, et al. Bone marrow edema and its relation to progression of knee osteoarthritis. Ann Intern Med 2003;139:330–6.

[6] Sharma L, Song J, Felson DT, et al. The role of knee alignment in disease progression and functional decline in knee osteoarthritis. JAMA 2001;286:188–95.
[7] Toivanen AT, Heliövaara M, Impivaara O, et al. Obesity, physically demanding work and traumatic knee injury are major risk factors for knee osteoarthritis—a population-based study with a follow-up of 22 years. Rheumatology (Oxford) 2010;49:308–14.
[8] Pai Y-C, Rymer WZ, Chang RW, et al. Effect of age and osteoarthritis on knee proprioception. Arthritis Rheum 1997;40:2260–5.
[9] Tveit M, Rosengren BE, Nilsson JA, et al. Former male elite athletes have a higher prevalence of osteoarthritis and arthroplasty in the hip and knee than expected. Am J Sports Med 2012;40:527–33.
[10] Felson DT, Zhang Y, Hannan MT, et al. The incidence and natural history of knee osteoarthritis in the elderly: the Framingham Osteoarthritis Study. Arthritis Rheum 1995;38:1500–5.
[11] Hunter DJ, March L, Sambrook PN. Knee osteoarthritis: the influence of environmental factors. Clin Exp Rheumatol 2002;20:93–100.
[12] Lawrence J, Bremner J, Bier F. Osteo-arthrosis. Prevalence in the population and relationships between symptoms and x-ray changes. Ann Rheum Dis 1966;25:1–24.
[13] Cicuttini F, Baker J, Hart D, et al. Association of pain with radiological changes in different compartments and views of the knee joint. Osteoarthritis Cartilage 1996;4:143–7.
[14] Bruyere O, Honore A, Giacovelli G, et al. Radiologic features poorly predict clinical outcomes in knee osteoarthritis. Scand J Rheumatol 2002;31:13–6.
[15] McAlindon T, Cooper C, Kirwan J, et al. Determinants of disability in osteoarthritis of the knee. Ann Rheum Dis 1993;52:258–62.
[16] Wakefield RJ, Balint PV, Szkudlarek M, et al. Musculoskeletal ultrasound including definitions for ultrasonographic pathology. J Rheumatol 2005;32:2485–7.
[17] Hochberg MC, Altman RD, Brandt KD, et al. Guidelines for the medical management of osteoarthritis. Part II. Osteoarthritis of the knee. American College of Rheumatology. Arthritis Rheum 1995;38:1541–6.
[18] Goldberg SH, Von Feldt JM, Lonner JH. Pharmacologic therapy for osteoarthritis. Am J Orthop 2002;31:673–80.
[19] Cannon GW, Caldwell JR, Holt P, et al. Rofecoxib, a specific inhibitor of cyclooxygenase 2, with clinical efficacy comparable with that of diclofenac sodium: results of a one-year, randomized, clinical trial in patients with osteoarthritis of the knee and hip. Rofecoxib Phase III Protocol 035 Study Group. Arthritis Rheum 2000;43:978–87.
[20] Rosenthal NR, Silverfield JC, Wu SC, et al. CAPSS-105 Study Group. Tramadol/acetaminophen combination tablets for the treatment of pain associated with osteoarthritis flare in an elderly patient population. J Am Geriatr Soc 2004;52:374–80.
[21] Apgar B. Controlled-release oxycodone for osteoarthritis-related pain. Am Fam Physician 2000;62:1405–6.
[22] Moore RA, Tramer MR, Carroll D, et al. Quantitative systematic review of topically applied non-steroidal anti-inflammatory drugs. BMJ 1998;316:333–8.
[23] Zhang WY, Li Wan Po A. The effectiveness of topically applied capsaicin: a meta-analysis. Eur J Clin Pharmacol 1994;46:517–22.
[24] Clegg DO, Reda DJ, Harris CL, et al. Glucosamine, chondroitin sulfate, and the two in combination for painful knee osteoarthritis. N Engl J Med 2006;354:795–808.
[25] Felson D. Osteoarthritis of the knee. N Engl J Med 2006;354:841–8.
[26] Roddy E, Zhang W, Doherty M. Aerobic walking or strengthening exercise for osteoarthritis of the knee? A systematic review. Ann Rheum Dis 2005;64:544–8.
[27] Pelland L, Brosseau L, Wells G, et al. Efficacy of strengthening exercises for osteoarthritis. Part I: a meta-analysis. Phys Ther Rev 2004;9:77–108.
[28] Brosseau L, Pelland L, Wells G, et al. Efficacy of aerobic exercises for osteoarthritis. Part II: a meta-analysis. Phys Ther Rev 2004;9:125–45.
[29] Swank AM, Kachelman JB, Bibeau W, et al. Prehabilitation before total knee arthroplasty increases strength and function in older adults with severe osteoarthritis. J Strength Cond Res 2011;25:318–25.
[30] Puett DW, Griffin MR. Published trials of nonmedicinal and noninvasive therapies for hip and knee osteoarthritis. Ann Intern Med 1994;121:133–40.
[31] Rutjes AW, Nuesch E, Sterchi R, et al. Transcutaneous electrostimulation for osteoarthritis of the knee. Cochrane Database Syst Rev 2009;4, CD002823.
[32] Kerrigan D, Todd M, O'Reilly P. Knee osteoarthritis and high heeled shoes. Lancet 1998;351:1399–401.
[33] Brouwer R, Jakma T, Verhagen A, et al. Braces and orthoses for treating osteoarthritis of the knee. Cochrane Database Syst Rev 2005;1, CD004020.
[34] Kerrigan DC, Lelas JL, Goggins J, et al. Effectiveness of a lateral-wedge insole on knee varus torque in patients with knee osteoarthritis. Arch Phys Med Rehabil 2002;83:889–93.
[35] Maillefert JF, Hudry C, Baron G, et al. Laterally elevated wedged insoles in the treatment of medial knee osteoarthritis: a prospective randomized controlled study. Osteoarthritis Cartilage 2001;9:738–45.
[36] Marks R, Penton L. Are foot orthotics efficacious for treating painful medial compartment knee osteoarthritis? A review of the literature. Int J Clin Pract 2004;58:49–57.
[37] Hinman RS, Crossley KM, McConnell J, Bennell KL. Efficacy of knee tape in the management of osteoarthritis of the knee: blinded randomised controlled trial. BMJ 2003;327:135.
[38] Cushnaghan J, McCarthy C, Dieppe P. Taping the patella medially: a new treatment for osteoarthritis of the knee joint? BMJ 1994;308:753–5.
[39] Hochberg M, Lixing L, Bausell B, et al. Traditional Chinese acupuncture is effective as adjunctive therapy in patients with osteoarthritis of the knee [abstract]. Arthritis Rheum 2004;50:S644.
[40] Bellamy N, Campbell J, Welch V, et al. Intraarticular corticosteroid for treatment of osteoarthritis of the knee. Cochrane Database Syst Rev 2009;2, CD005328.
[41] Balazs EA, Denlinger JL. Viscosupplementation: a new concept in the treatment of osteoarthritis. J Rheumatol Suppl 1993;39:3–9.
[42] Rutjes AW, Jüni P, da Costa BR, et al. Viscosupplementation for osteoarthritis of the knee: a systematic review and meta-analysis. Ann Intern Med 2012;157:180–91.
[43] Bannuru RR, Natov NS, Obadan IE, et al. Therapeutic trajectory of hyaluronic acid versus corticosteroids in the treatment of knee osteoarthritis: a systematic review and meta-analysis. Arthritis Rheum 2009;61:1704–11.
[44] Day B. The indications for arthroscopic débridement for osteoarthritis of the knee. Orthop Clin North Am 2005;36:413–7.
[45] Felson DT, Buckwalter J. Débridement and lavage for osteoarthritis of the knee. N Engl J Med 2002;347:132–3.
[46] Jackson RW, Dieterichs C. The results of arthroscopic lavage and débridement of osteoarthritic knees based on the severity of degeneration: a 4- to 6-year symptomatic follow-up. Arthroscopy 2003;19:13–20.
[47] Fond J, Rudin D, Ahmad S, et al. Arthroscopic débridement of osteoarthritis of the knee: 2- and 5-year results. Arthroscopy 2002;18:829–34.
[48] Kirkley A, Birmingham TB, Litchfield RB, et al. A randomized trial of arthroscopic surgery for osteoarthritis of the knee. N Engl J Med 2008;359:1097–107.
[49] Naudie D, Bourne RB, Rorabeck CH, Bourne TJ. The Install Award. Survivorship of the high tibial valgus osteotomy. A 10- to 22-year followup study. Clin Orthop Relat Res 1999;367:18–27.
[50] Billings A, Scott DF, Camargo MP, et al. High tibial osteotomy with a calibrated osteotomy guide, rigid internal fixation, and early motion. Long-term follow-up. J Bone Joint Surg Am 2000;82:70–9.
[51] Deshmukh RV, Scott RD. Unicompartmental knee arthroplasty: long-term results. Clin Orthop Relat Res 2001;392:272–8.
[52] Murray DW, Goodfellow JW, O'Connor JJ. The Oxford medial unicompartmental arthroplasty: a ten-year survival study. J Bone Joint Surg Br 1998;80:983–9.
[53] Orbell S, Espley A, Johnston M, Rowley D. Health benefits of joint replacement surgery for patients with osteoarthritis. J Epidemiol Community Health 1998;52:564–70.
[54] Svard UC, Price AJ. Oxford medial unicompartmental knee arthroplasty. A survival analysis of an independent series. J Bone Joint Surg Br 2001;83:191–4.
[55] Smith AM, Peckett WR, Butler-Manuel PA, et al. Treatment of patellofemoral arthritis using the Lubinus patellofemoral arthroplasty: a retrospective review. Knee 2002;9:27–30.
[56] Tauro B, Ackroyd CE, Newman JH, Shah NA. The Lubinus patellofemoral arthroplasty. A five- to ten-year prospective study. J Bone Joint Surg Br 2002;84:696–701.
[57] Fujita S, Hirota S, Oda T, et al. Deep venous thrombosis after total hip or total knee arthroplasty in patients in Japan. Clin Orthop Relat Res 2000;375:168–74.

CHAPTER 71

Knee Bursitis

Ed Hanada, MD
Florian S. Keplinger, MD
Navneet Gupta, MD

Synonyms

Prepatellar bursitis (housemaid's knee)
Infrapatellar bursitis (vicar's knee)
Anserine bursitis
Medial (tibial) collateral ligament bursitis
Semimembranosus bursitis

ICD-9 Codes

726.60	Enthesopathy of knee, unspecified bursitis of knee
726.61	Pes anserinus tendinitis or bursitis
726.62	Tibial collateral ligament bursitis
726.63	Fibular collateral ligament bursitis
726.65	Prepatellar bursitis
726.69	Other bursitis: infrapatellar; subpatellar

ICD-10 Codes

M76.891	Enthesopathies of right lower limb, excluding foot
M76.892	Enthesopathies of left lower limb, excluding foot
M76.899	Enthesopathies of unspecified lower limb, excluding foot
M71.561	Bursitis, not elsewhere classified, right knee
M71.562	Bursitis, not elsewhere classified, left knee
M71.569	Bursitis, not elsewhere classified, unspecified knee
M76.40	Tibial collateral bursitis, unspecified leg
M76.41	Tibial collateral bursitis, right leg
M76.42	Tibial collateral bursitis, left leg
M70.40	Prepatellar bursitis, unspecified knee
M70.41	Prepatellar bursitis, right knee
M70.42	Prepatellar bursitis, left knee
M70.50	Other bursitis of knee, unspecified knee
M70.51	Other bursitis of knee, right knee
M70.52	Other bursitis of knee, left knee

Definition

Knee bursitis is an inflammation of any bursa in the region of the knee joint and is a common clinical disorder that may lead to functional difficulties. Eleven bursae are found within this region (Fig. 71.1) [1]. Three bursae communicate with the knee joint: quadriceps or suprapatellar, popliteus, and medial gastrocnemius. Four bursae are associated with the patella: superficial and deep prepatellar, and superficial and deep infrapatellar. Two are related to the semimembranosus tendons, and two are related to the collateral ligaments of the knee (one of which is under the pes anserinus, or the conjoined tendons of the sartorius, gracilis, and semitendinosus muscles) [1].

In the popliteal fossa, a bursa is located between the medial head of the gastrocnemius and semimembranosus tendon. Swelling in this area is also called Baker cyst and may actually be due to other inflammatory or degenerative conditions (see Chapter 64). For this chapter's purpose, discussion is limited to knee bursitis arising from inflammation of the previously mentioned bursae.

The most common knee bursitis conditions are the following.

Prepatellar bursitis (housemaid's knee) is caused by direct trauma, such as falling on a bent knee or frequent kneeling on a hard surface [1]. A case of a massive prepatellar bursitis from chronic crawling as a means of household ambulation in an adult man with cerebral palsy has been reported [2]. In 376 subjects with knee pain and radiographic evidence of knee osteoarthritis, 3.1% had evidence of prepatellar bursitis on magnetic resonance imaging [3].

Infrapatellar bursitis (vicar's knee) is usually due to repetitive knee flexion in weight bearing, such as deep knee bends, squatting, or jumping; it can be associated with patellar-quadriceps tendinitis [4,5]. In 376 subjects undergoing routine magnetic resonance imaging who had

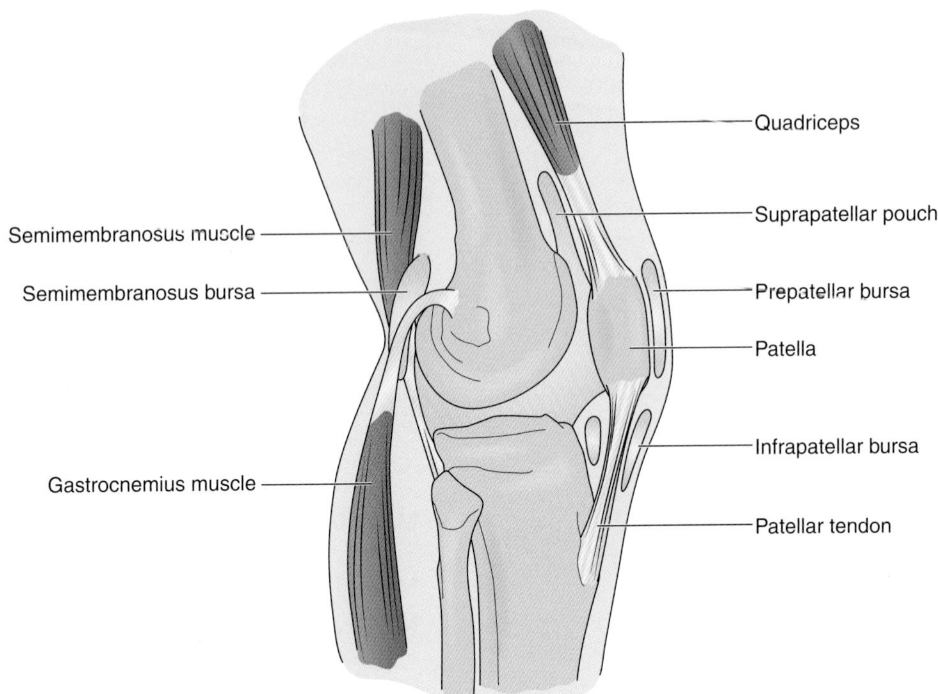

FIGURE 71.1 Bursae around knee joint.

knee pain and radiographic evidence of knee osteoarthritis, 10.6% had evidence of superficial infrapatellar bursitis [3].

Anserine bursitis is commonly seen in overweight older women who also have osteoarthritis of the knees and in individuals who participate in sports that require running, side-to-side movement, and cutting [5,6]. In a study involving persons with a symptomatic knee presenting to an orthopedic clinic with suspected internal knee derangement who had magnetic resonance imaging, only 2.5% of these patients had radiologic evidence of pes anserine bursitis, with no gender preference [7].

Medial collateral ligament bursitis refers to inflammation of a bursa located between the deep and superficial parts of the medial collateral ligament [5]. It has been associated with degenerative disease of the medial joint compartment, with marginal osteophytic spur formation [8]. Furthermore, this bursitis may be seen in equestrian and motorcycle athletes because of the friction applied to the medial side of the knee [8].

Semimembranosus bursitis is usually seen in runners and may be associated with hamstring tendinitis [4]. This was seen in 4.4% of symptomatic subjects undergoing routine magnetic resonance imaging [3].

Symptoms

The patient will usually complain of local pain, tenderness, or swelling in the affected site. The pain is worse with flexion and usually occurs at night or after activity. The pain also may be more prominent and accompanied by stiffness on waking in the morning. Limping may or may not be present.

Physical Examination

The patient may have an antalgic gait, with a shortened stance phase on the affected side. There is discrete tenderness to palpation associated with fullness at the site of the bursa involved, and there may be associated redness and increased temperature. If the bursa connects with the knee joint, there may be an associated effusion. There is often limited range of motion in the knee. Neurologic examination findings should be normal.

Functional Limitations

The patient may have difficulty with prolonged walking. Decreased balance is often seen in older patients, sometimes necessitating assistive devices (e.g., walker, crutches, cane, or wheelchair). If there is limitation in knee range of motion, patients may have difficulty bending the knees to drive or sitting at a desk at work. They will also have problems stooping, kneeling, crawling, or climbing, which may interfere with vocational and recreational activities. Athletes such as runners may have diminished performance or may be sidelined altogether.

Diagnostic Studies

The diagnosis is based mainly on history and clinical examination. Aspiration is rarely needed but may be necessary if an infection is suspected. Radiologic studies are usually performed to rule out other diagnoses but may show exostosis in areas related to the bursa. Ultrasound imaging may be helpful to visualize the swelling in the bursal sac and may be augmented by use of an air-steroid-saline mixture as a contrast medium [9]. Plain radiographs should be obtained if a bone tumor is suspected, particularly in patients with night pain. Arthrography, which is rarely done, may show the connection to the knee joint, if it is involved. Magnetic resonance imaging may be needed to rule out a tumor or malignant neoplasm and may show a fluid collection in the involved bursa [1,4].

Differential Diagnosis

Infection (e.g., septic knee)
Arthritis (osteoarthritis, rheumatoid arthritis, psoriatic arthritis)
Tumor
Patellar fracture
Meniscal tear
Collateral ligament sprain or tear
Saphenous nerve entrapment

Treatment

Initial

Restriction of activity that provokes or aggravates symptoms is important [1,4–6,10]. In athletes, this may mean a substitution of the usual athletic activities while the healing process proceeds. Local application of ice helps decrease pain and inflammation. The patient can be taught to use superficial heat for chronic bursitis. This can be done with moistened warm compresses or with a microwaveable or electric heating pad. Precautions should be observed and given to the patient to prevent burns and other complications (see section on potential treatment complications). Nonsteroidal anti-inflammatory drugs can be prescribed to decrease pain and inflammation. Oral steroids are generally not indicated as initial treatment.

Rehabilitation

Use of an orthosis in the affected knee may assist in preventing painful movement and further inflammation as well as provide comfort. Shoe inserts unilaterally or bilaterally, depending on the pathologic process, may also lead to positively altered biomechanics of the lower extremities to improve symptoms. For example, for those individuals with associated medial compartment knee osteoarthritis, a lateral wedge insole may improve symptoms and function [11].

Formal physical therapy may address stretching of the quadriceps, hamstrings, iliotibial band, and hip adductor muscles if these muscles are tight. Strengthening exercises are often needed in chronic knee bursitis because of disuse weakness. Correction of gait abnormalities (e.g., leg length discrepancy with a heel lift, or pes planus with orthotic inserts) is also important. Patients should also be counseled to protect their knees from further trauma (e.g., by avoidance of bending or kneeling or by use of knee pads).

Modalities such as ultrasound have not been proved to be more effective than a combination of the aforementioned measures. Ultrasound should be avoided when an effusion is present because it can worsen the effusion. Phonophoresis and iontophoresis may have merit, but they are still controversial [12].

Procedures

Intrabursal corticosteroid injection is appropriate if there is no response to conservative management or if the patient demonstrates significant functional limitations (Fig. 71.2). Typically, no more than three injections are done in a 6- to 12-month period. Alternative diagnoses should be considered for patients with refractory symptoms.

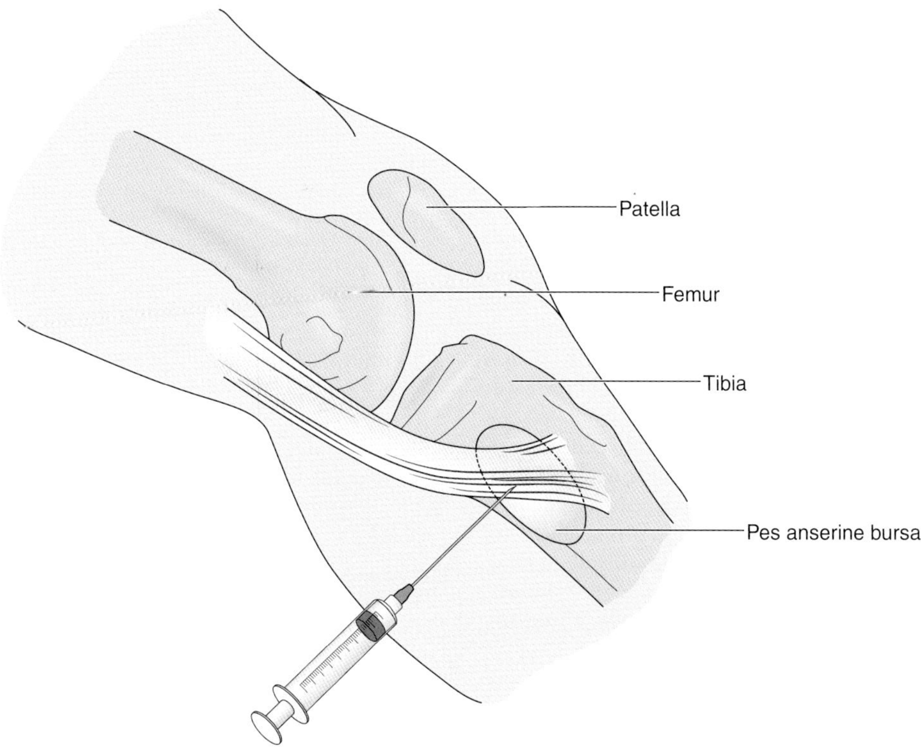

FIGURE 71.2 Under sterile conditions, with use of a 1½-inch, 22-gauge needle, inject the bursa at the point of maximal tenderness. A 1- to 3-mL combination of local anesthetic and corticosteroid is used (e.g., 1 mL of 1% lidocaine mixed with 1 mL of 40 mg/mL triamcinolone acetonide). Local anesthetics may be injected just before the steroid to diminish pain and to prevent postinjection steroid flare [1,4–6,13]. Application of ice is helpful in decreasing pain at the site after injection.

The patient is generally advised to avoid activity involving the area injected for approximately 2 weeks to promote retention of the corticosteroid in the bursa and to avoid systemic absorption [13]. There is some evidence to suggest that persons who have pes anserine bursitis that is demonstrated with ultrasonography may have the best outcome after corticosteroid injection [14,15].

With use of a high-frequency linear ultrasound transducer along the medial aspect of the knee, a mixture of anesthetic and long-acting corticosteroid may be injected through a 25-gauge needle [16]. However, a study demonstrated that there is no additional benefit after an injection with methylprednisolone [17].

As an alternative to surgery, in cases of persistent prepatellar bursitis, chemical ablation has been used, although no robust clinical trials exist to provide evidence for its efficacy [18].

Surgery

Surgery is generally not indicated and should be undertaken only in refractory cases. Excision of a bursa can be considered if the disease does not respond to conservative measures, despite treatment, and it greatly limits the patient's activities. Successful surgical resection of bursae has been reported in the literature [19–22]. Outpatient endoscopic bursectomy under local anesthesia has been reported in a case series as an effective treatment of post-traumatic prepatellar bursitis after failed conservative management [23].

Potential Disease Complications

Possible complications include chronic pain, deconditioning, disuse muscle atrophy, and knee flexion contracture. Furthermore, this may lead to decreased walking ability and postural instability over time, especially in older adults.

Potential Treatment Complications

Potential complications from medications include drug hypersensitivity and prolonged bleeding; nonsteroidal anti-inflammatory drugs have gastric, renal, and hepatic side effects. Hyperglycemia, electrolyte imbalance, and gastric irritation or ulceration from intrabursal steroid injection are not as common as with orally administered corticosteroids but can still occur from systemic absorption of the injectant. Local ice application may produce hypersensitivity and vasoconstriction in patients with Raynaud disease and peripheral vascular disease, and local heat application may produce burns, sedation, skin discoloration, and vascular compromise. Moreover, injections may result in drug hypersensitivity, sterile abscess, infection, nerve injury, tendon rupture, and lipoatrophy from intralesional steroids [13,14]. Furthermore, a case of patella tendon rupture has been reported after arthroscopic resection of the prepatellar bursa [24].

References

[1] Cailliet R. Knee pain and disability. 3rd ed. Philadelphia: FA Davis; 1992.
[2] Thompson T, Simpson B, Burgess D, Wilson R. Massive prepatellar bursa. J Natl Med Assoc 2006;98:90–2.
[3] Hill CL, Gale DR, Chaisson CE, et al. Periarticular lesions detected on magnetic resonance imaging: prevalence in knees with and without symptoms. Arthritis Rheum 2003;48:2836–44.
[4] Larson R, Grana W. The knee: form, function, pathology, and treatment. Philadelphia: WB Saunders; 1993.
[5] Biundo J. Regional rheumatic pain syndromes. 10th ed. Atlanta: Arthritis Foundation; 1993.
[6] Alvarez-Nemegyei J, Canosa JJ. Evidence-based soft tissue rheumatology IV: anserine bursitis. J Clin Rheumatol 2004;10:205–6.
[7] Rennie WJ, Saifuddin A. Pes anserine bursitis: incidence in symptomatic knees and clinical presentation. Skeletal Radiol 2005;34:395–8.
[8] McCarthy CL, McNally EG. The MRI appearance of cystic lesions around the knee. Skeletal Radiol 2004;33:187–209.
[9] Koski J, Saarakkala S, Heikkinen J, Hermunen H. Use of air-steroid-saline mixture as contrast medium in greyscale ultrasound imaging: experimental study and practical applications in rheumatology. Clin Exp Rheumatol 2005;23:373–8.
[10] Kang I, Han S. Anserine bursitis in patients with osteoarthritis of the knee. South Med J 2000;93:207–9.
[11] Toda Y, Tsukimura N. A six-month followup of a randomized trial comparing the efficacy of a lateral-wedge insole with subtalar strapping and an in-shoe lateral wedge insole in patients with varus deformity osteoarthritis of the knee. Arthritis Rheum 2004;50:3129–36.
[12] Basford J. Physical agents. In: Delisa J, Gans B, editors. Rehabilitation medicine: principles and practice. Philadelphia: JB Lippincott; 1993. p. 404–24.
[13] Neustadt D. Intra-articular corticosteroids and other agents: aspiration techniques. In: Katz W, editor. The diagnosis and management of rheumatic disease. Philadelphia: JB Lippincott; 1988. p. 812–25.
[14] Yoon H, Kim S, Suh Y, et al. Correlation between ultrasonographic findings and the response to corticosteroid injection in pes anserinus tendinobursitis syndrome in knee osteoarthritis patients. J Korean Med Sci 2005;20:109–12.
[15] Handy J. Anserine bursitis: a brief review. South Med J 1997;90:376–7.
[16] Jose J, Schallert E, Lesniak B. Sonography guided therapeutic injection for primary medial (tibial) collateral bursitis. J Ultrasound Med 2011;30:257–61.
[17] Vega-Morales D, Esquivel-Valerio JA, Negrete-López R, et al. Safety and efficacy of methylprednisolone infiltration in anserine syndrome treatment. Reumatol Clin 2012;8:63–7.
[18] Ike RW. Chemical ablation as an alternative to surgery for treatment of persistent prepatellar bursitis. J Rheumatol 2009;36:1560.
[19] Yamamoto T, Akisue T, Marui T, et al. Isolated suprapatellar bursitis: computed tomographic and arthroscopic findings. Arthroscopy 2003;19:E10.
[20] Klein W. Endoscopy of the deep infrapatellar bursa. Arthroscopy 1996;12:127–31.
[21] Kerr DR, Carpenter CW. Arthroscopic resection of olecranon and prepatellar bursae. Arthroscopy 1990;6:86–8.
[22] Dillon JP, Freedman I, Tan JS, et al. Endoscopic bursectomy for the treatment of septic pre-patellar bursitis: a case series. Arch Orthop Trauma Surg 2012;132:921–5.
[23] Huang YC, Yeh WL. Endoscopic treatment of prepatellar bursitis. Int Orthop 2011;35:355–8.
[24] Epstein DM, Capeci CM, Rokito AS. Patella tendon rupture after arthroscopic resection of the prepatellar bursa—a case report. Bull NYU Hosp Jt Dis 2010;68:307–10.

CHAPTER 72

Meniscal Injuries

Paul Lento, MD
Venu Akuthota, MD

Synonyms

Cartilage tears
Locked knee

ICD-9 Codes

717.3 Other and unspecified derangement of medial meniscus
717.4 Derangement of lateral meniscus
717.40 Derangement of lateral meniscus, unspecified
717.41 Bucket-handle tear of lateral meniscus
717.42 Derangement of anterior horn of lateral meniscus
717.43 Derangement of posterior horn of lateral meniscus
717.49 Derangement of lateral meniscus, other
717.5 Derangement of lateral meniscus, not elsewhere classified
717.9 Unspecified internal derangement of the knee
836.0 Acute tear of medial meniscus of knee
836.1 Acute tear of lateral meniscus of knee

ICD-10 Codes

M23.300 Other meniscus derangements, unspecified lateral meniscus, right knee
M23.301 Other meniscus derangements, unspecified lateral meniscus, left knee
M23.302 Other meniscus derangements, unspecified lateral meniscus, unspecified knee
M23.303 Other meniscus derangements, unspecified medial meniscus, right knee
M23.304 Other meniscus derangements, unspecified medial meniscus, left knee
M23.305 Other meniscus derangements, unspecified medial meniscus, unspecified knee
M23.306 Other meniscus derangements, unspecified meniscus, right knee
M23.307 Other meniscus derangements, unspecified meniscus, left knee
M23.309 Other meniscus derangements, unspecified meniscus, unspecified knee
S83.251 Bucket-handle tear of lateral meniscus, current injury, right knee
S83.252 Bucket-handle tear of lateral meniscus, current injury, left knee
S83.259 Bucket-handle tear of lateral meniscus, current injury, unspecified knee
Add seventh character to S83 for episode of care
M23.341 Meniscus derangements, anterior horn of lateral meniscus, right knee
M23.342 Meniscus derangements, anterior horn of lateral meniscus, left knee
M23.349 Meniscus derangements, anterior horn of lateral meniscus, unspecified knee
M23.351 Meniscus derangements, posterior horn of lateral meniscus, right knee
M23.352 Meniscus derangements, posterior horn of lateral meniscus, left knee
M23.359 Meniscus derangements, posterior horn of lateral meniscus, unspecified knee
M23.361 Other meniscus derangements, other lateral meniscus, right knee
M23.362 Other meniscus derangements, other lateral meniscus, left knee
M23.369 Other meniscus derangements, other lateral meniscus, unspecified knee

S83.241 Other tear of medial meniscus, current injury, right knee
S83.242 Other tear of medial meniscus, current injury, left knee
S83.249 Other tear of medial meniscus, current injury, unspecified knee
S83.281 Other tear of lateral meniscus, current injury, right knee
S83.282 Other tear of lateral meniscus, current injury, left knee
S83.289 Other tear of lateral meniscus, current injury, unspecified knee

Definition

The menisci serve important roles in maintaining proper joint health, stability, and function [1]. The anatomy of the medial and lateral menisci helps explain functional biomechanics. Viewed from above, the medial meniscus appears C shaped and the lateral meniscus appears O shaped (Fig. 72.1)[1]. Each meniscus is thick and convex at its periphery (the horns) but becomes thin and concave at its center. This contouring serves to provide a larger area for the rounded femoral condyles and the relatively flat tibia. Menisci do not move in isolation. They are connected by ligaments to each other anteriorly and to the anterior cruciate ligament, the patella, the femur, and the tibia [2,3].

The medial meniscus is less mobile than the lateral meniscus. This is due to its firm connections to the knee joint capsule and the medial collateral ligament. This decreased mobility, in conjunction with the fact that the medial meniscus is wider posteriorly, is cited as the usual reason for the higher incidence of tears within the medial meniscus than within the lateral meniscus [1]. The semimembranosus muscle (through attachments from the joint capsule) helps retract the medial meniscus posteriorly, serving to avoid entrapment and injury to the medial meniscus as the knee is flexed [3]. The lateral meniscus is not as adherent to the joint capsule. Unlike the medial meniscus, the lateral meniscus does not attach to its respective collateral ligament. The posterolateral aspect of the lateral meniscus is separated from the capsule by the popliteus tendon. Therefore the lateral meniscus is more mobile than the medial meniscus [1,3]. The attachment of the popliteus tendon to the posterolateral meniscus ensures dynamic retraction of the lateral meniscus when the knee internally rotates to return out of the screw-home mechanism [2]. Therefore both the medial and the lateral menisci, by having attachments to muscle structures, share a common mechanism that helps avoid injury.

The architecture of the vascular supply to the meniscus has important implications for healing [1,4]. Capillaries penetrate the menisci from the periphery to provide nourishment. After 18 months of age, as weight bearing increases, the blood supply to the central part of the menisci recedes. In fact, research has shown that eventually only the peripheral 10% to 30% of the menisci, or the red zone, receives this capillary network (Fig. 72.2) [5]. Therefore the central and internal portion or white zone of these fibrocartilaginous structures becomes avascular with age, relying on nutrition received through diffusion from the synovial fluid. Because of this vascular arrangement, the peripheral meniscus is more likely to heal than are the central and posterolateral aspects [4].

The primary but not sole function of the menisci is to distribute forces across the knee joint and to enhance stability [1,6–8]. Multiple studies have shown that the ability of the joint to transmit loads is significantly reduced if the meniscus is partially or wholly removed [1,6,7,9]. Fairbank [10] published a seminal article in 1948 suggesting that the menisci are vital in protecting the articular surfaces. He reported that individuals who had undergone total meniscectomies demonstrated premature osteoarthritis.

Meniscal tears are classified by their complexity, plane of rupture, direction, location, and overall shape. Tears are commonly defined as vertical, horizontal, longitudinal, or oblique in relation to the tibial surface (Fig. 72.3)[11]. Most meniscal tears in young patients will be vertical-longitudinal,

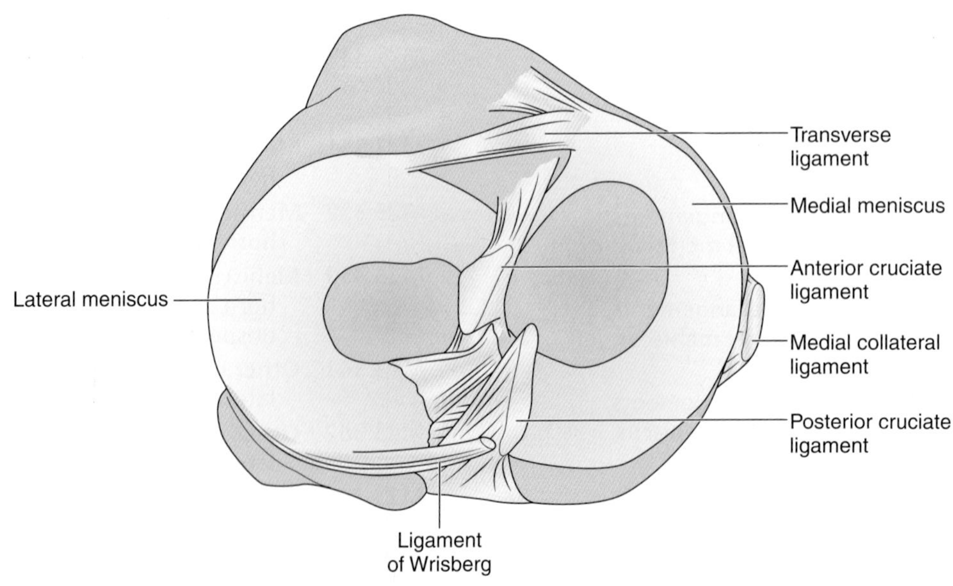

FIGURE 72.1 Superior view of medial and lateral menisci.

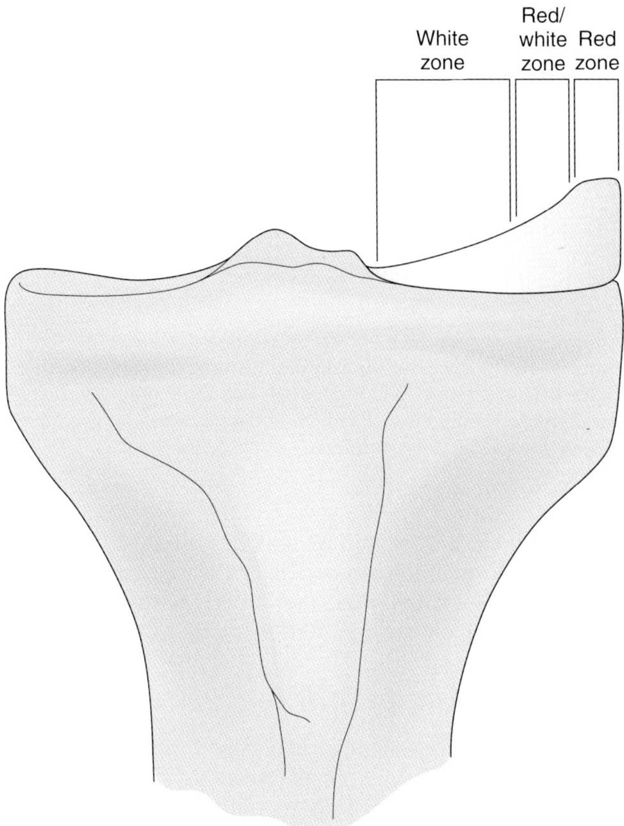

FIGURE 72.2 Vascular zones of the meniscus. Tears within the red zone have a higher healing potential.

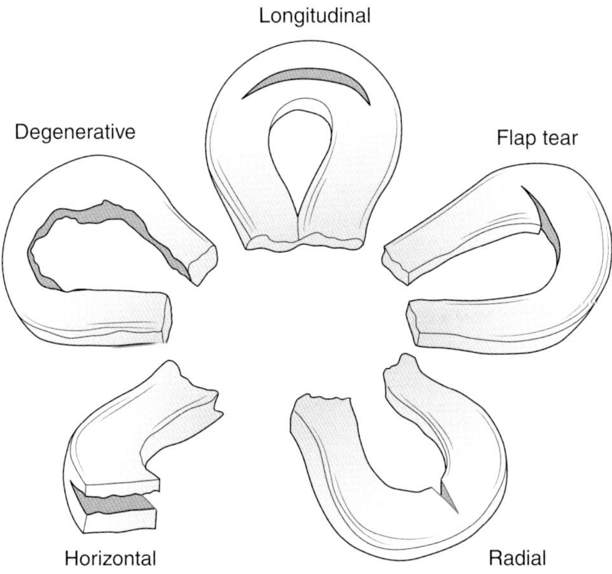

FIGURE 72.3 Types of meniscal tears.

whereas horizontal cleavage tears are more commonly found in older patients [12]. The bucket-handle tear is the most common type of vertical (or longitudinal) tear [13] (Fig. 72.4). Tears are also described as complete, full-thickness or partial tears. Complete, full-thickness tears are so named as they extend from the tibial to femoral surfaces. In addition, medial meniscus tears outnumber lateral meniscus tears from 2:1 to 5:1 [14,15].

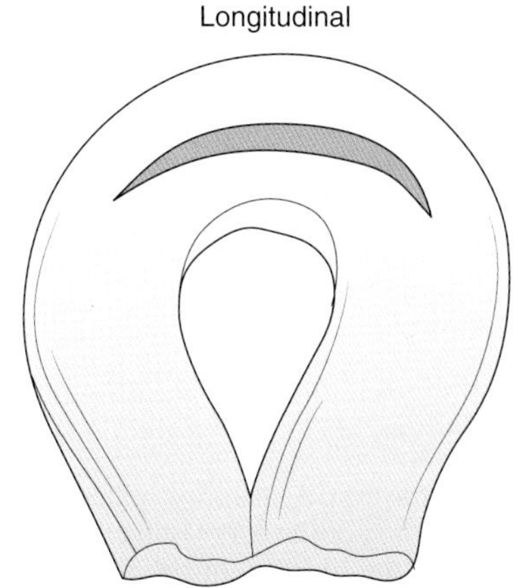

FIGURE 72.4 Bucket-handle type of meniscal tear.

Meniscal injuries may result from an acute injury or from gradual degeneration with aging [16]. Vertical tears (e.g., bucket-handle tears) tend to occur acutely in individuals 20 to 30 years of age and are usually located in the posterior two thirds of the meniscus [13,17]. Sports commonly associated with meniscal injuries are soccer, football, basketball, baseball, wrestling, skiing, rugby, and lacrosse. Injury commonly occurs when an axial load is transmitted through a flexed or extended knee that is simultaneously rotating [16]. Degenerative tears, in contrast, are usually horizontal and are seen in older individuals with concomitant degenerative joint changes [13,18].

On the basis of arthroscopic examination, the majority of acute peripheral meniscal injuries are associated with some degree of occult anterior cruciate ligament laxity [19]. In addition, true anterior cruciate ligament tears are associated with lesions of the posterior horns of the menisci [19]. Lateral meniscal tears appear to occur with more frequency with acute anterior cruciate ligament injuries, whereas medial meniscal tears have a higher incidence with chronic anterior cruciate ligament injuries. With chronic anterior cruciate ligament injuries, the medial meniscus may be more frequently damaged because its posterior horn serves as an important secondary stabilizer of anterior-posterior instability [20].

Symptoms

The history will help diagnose a meniscal injury 75% of the time [12,21]. Young patients who experience meniscal tears will recall the mechanism of injury 80% to 90% of the time and may report a "pop" or a "snap" at the time of injury. Deep knee bending activities are often painful, and mechanical locking may be present in 30% of patients [22]. Bucket-handle tears should be suspected in cases of mechanical locking with loss of full extension [16]. If locking is reported approximately 1 day after the injury, this may be due to "pseudolocking," which results from hamstring contracture [14]. Knee hemarthrosis may also occur acutely, especially if the vascularized, peripheral portion of the meniscus is involved. In fact, 20% of all acute traumatic knee hemarthroses are caused by isolated meniscal injury [23]. More typically, however, knee swelling occurs approximately 1 day later as the meniscal tear causes mechanical irritation within the intra-articular space, creating

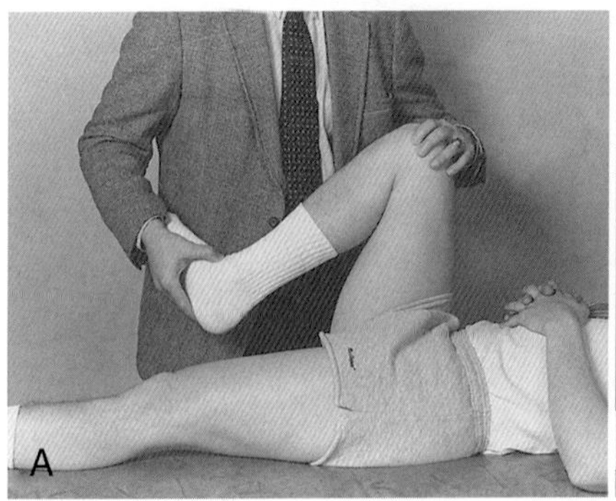

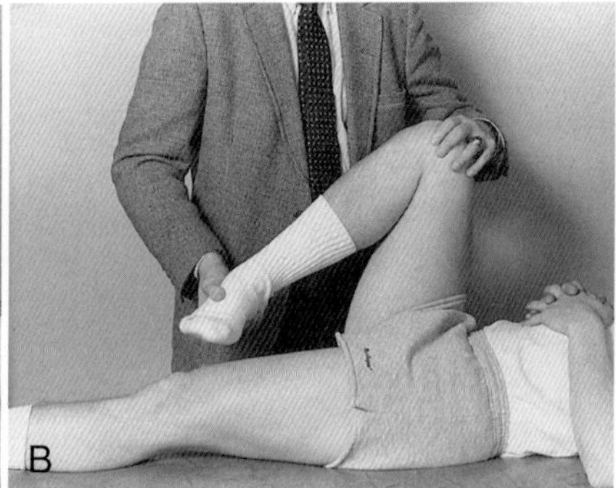

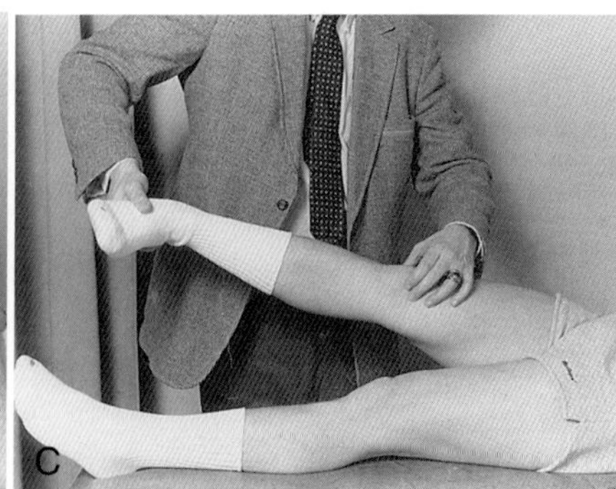

FIGURE 72.5 McMurray test. **A,** Starting position for testing of the medial meniscus. The knee is acutely flexed, with the foot and tibia in external rotation. **B,** Starting position for testing of the lateral meniscus. The knee is acutely flexed, and the foot and tibia are internally rotated. **C,** Ending position for the lateral meniscus. The knee is brought into extension while rotation is maintained. Ending position for the medial meniscus is the same but with the external rotation. If pain or a "clunk" is elicited, the test result is considered positive. *(From Mellion MB. Office Sports Medicine, 2nd ed. Philadelphia, Hanley & Belfus, 1996.)*

a reactive effusion. Typically, this effusion is secondary to a lesion in the central portion of the meniscus [16].

In contrast, degenerative meniscal tears are not usually associated with a history of trauma. In fact, the mechanism of injury, which may not be reported by the patient, can be simple daily activities, such as rising from a chair and pivoting on a planted foot [16]. Patients with degenerative tears often also report recurrent knee swelling, particularly after activity.

Physical Examination

Physical examination aids the accurate diagnosis of a meniscal injury in 70% of patients [24]. Gait evaluation may reveal an antalgic gait with decreased stance phase and knee extension on the symptomatic side [23]. A knee effusion is observed in about half of individuals with a known meniscal tear [25]. Quadriceps atrophy may be noted a few weeks after injury. Palpation of the joint line frequently results in tenderness. Posteromedial or lateral tenderness is most suggestive of a meniscal tear [12]. The result of a "bounce home" test may be positive. This test result is positive when pain or mechanical blocking is appreciated as the patient's knee is passively forced into full extension [14]. The result of the McMurray test is positive 58% of the time in the presence of a tear but is also reported to be positive in 5% of normal individuals (Fig. 72.5) [13]. The Apley compression test is an insensitive indicator of meniscal injury. With this test, the prone knee is flexed to 90 degrees and an axial load is applied (Fig. 72.6). A painful response is considered a confirmatory test result with a reported sensitivity of 45% [23]. A dynamic functional test known as the Thessaly maneuver can detect a meniscal tear [26]. This maneuver is performed while the patient stands with the affected knee flexed at either 5 degrees or 20 degrees and internally or externally rotates the body. The test result is considered suggestive of a meniscal tear if there is reproduction of joint line discomfort or if clicking or locking is noted [26]. No singular meniscal provocation test has been shown to be predictive of meniscal injury compared with findings on arthroscopy. Physical examination findings become even less reliable in patients with concomitant anterior cruciate ligament deficiencies [14,27]. Neurologic examination findings, including sensation and deep tendon reflexes, should be normal unless there is associated guarding due to pain or diffuse weakness, particularly with knee extension (quadriceps muscle inhibition).

Functional Limitations

Patients with meniscal injuries may have difficulty with deep knee bending activities, such as traversing stairs, squatting, or toileting. In addition, jogging, running, and even walking may become problematic, particularly if any rotational component is involved. Laborers who repetitively squat may report mechanical locking with loss of full knee extension on rising.

Diagnostic Studies

Standing plain radiographs are usually normal in isolated meniscal injuries. Presence of osteoarthritis, as with degenerative meniscal tears, can be detected with weight-bearing anteroposterior and lateral knee films. With nondegenerative tears, magnetic resonance imaging (MRI) has largely replaced plain radiographic examination in detecting injury;

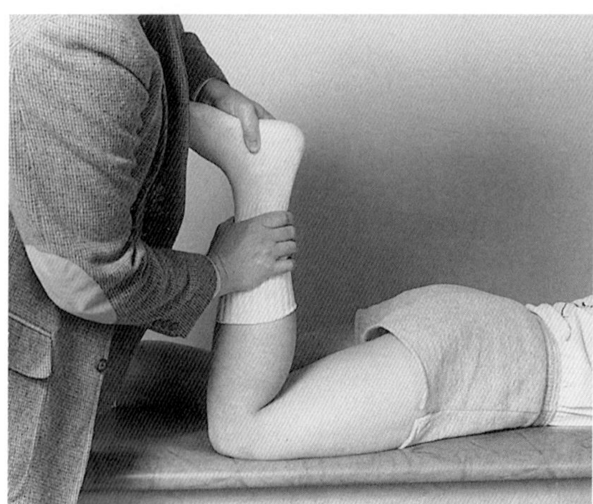

FIGURE 72.6 Apley compression test. The patient is prone. The examiner applies pressure on the sole of the foot toward the examination table. The tibia is internally and externally rotated. *(From Mellion MB. Office Sports Medicine, 2nd ed. Philadelphia, Hanley & Belfus, 1996.)*

however, meniscal tears can be present in asymptomatic individuals [12,28]. Sagittal views demonstrate the anterior and posterior horns of the menisci; coronal images can be vital in diagnosis of bucket-handle and parrot-beak tears [1,14]. There are three grades of meniscal injury as determined by the location of T2 signal intensity within the black cartilage. By definition, only grade 3 tears qualify as true meniscal tears; however, a few grade 2 lesions seen on MRI will be found to be true tears on arthroscopy (Fig. 72.7)[29]. With use of arthroscopy as the "gold standard," the sensitivity of MRI varies from 64% to 95%, with an accuracy of 83% to 93% [16]. MRI appears to have a false-positive rate of 10% [1,24]. A 5% false-negative rate is also reported and may be due to missed tears at the meniscosynovial junction [30]. Ultrasonography has also been used to diagnose meniscal tears but with lower specificity compared with MRI [31].

Interestingly, despite the recent accessibility and advancement in ultrasonography and MRI, clinical examination by experienced physicians is cheaper and appears to be as accurate as MRI for the diagnosis of meniscal tears [29,32]. However, MRI may be particularly helpful when history and physical examination findings are equivocal and the physician is required to establish an expedient diagnosis [13,23].

Differential Diagnosis

Anterior or posterior cruciate ligament tear
Medial collateral ligament tear
Osteoarthritis
Plica syndromes
Popliteal tendinitis
Osteochondritic lesions
Loose bodies
Patellofemoral pain
Fat pad impingement syndrome
Inflammatory arthritis
Physeal fracture
Tumors

Treatment

Initial

The truly locked knee resulting from a meniscal tear should be reduced within 24 hours of injury. Otherwise, acute tears of the meniscus may initially be treated with rest, ice, and compression, with weight bearing as tolerated. Patients may need to use crutches acutely. A knee splint may be applied for comfort of the patient, particularly in unstable knees with underlying ligamentous injury [22].

Analgesics such as acetaminophen or opioids can be used for pain. Nonsteroidal anti-inflammatory drugs can be used for pain and inflammation.

Arthrocentesis can be performed (ideally in the first 24 to 48 hours) for both diagnostic and treatment purposes when there is a significant effusion.

Rehabilitation

Not all meniscal injuries necessitate surgical intervention or resection. In fact, some meniscal lesions have gradual resolution of symptoms during a 6-week period and may have normal function by 3 months [11]. Types of tears that may be treated with nonsurgical measures include partial-thickness longitudinal tears, small (<5 mm) full-thickness peripheral tears, and minor inner rim or degenerative tears [33]. Healing potential is greatest for tears within the red zone [34]. In general, only meniscal injuries that are persistently symptomatic should be referred for surgical intervention.

Both nonsurgical and partial meniscectomy patients undergo similar rehabilitation protocols. Crutches may be used to off-load the affected limb. These can usually be discontinued when patients are ambulating without a limp [35]. The goal during the first week is to decrease pain and swelling while increasing range of motion and muscle strength and endurance. Institution of static strengthening in conjunction with electrical stimulation can retard quadriceps atrophy [30]. Aerobic conditioning can begin as long as the patient can tolerate bicycle training or aqua jogging. As time progresses,

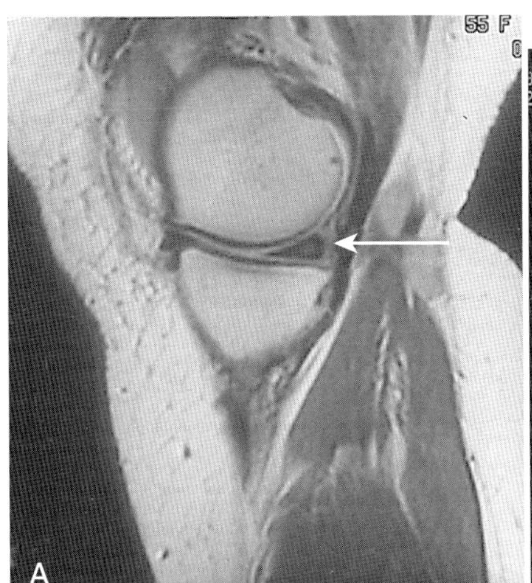

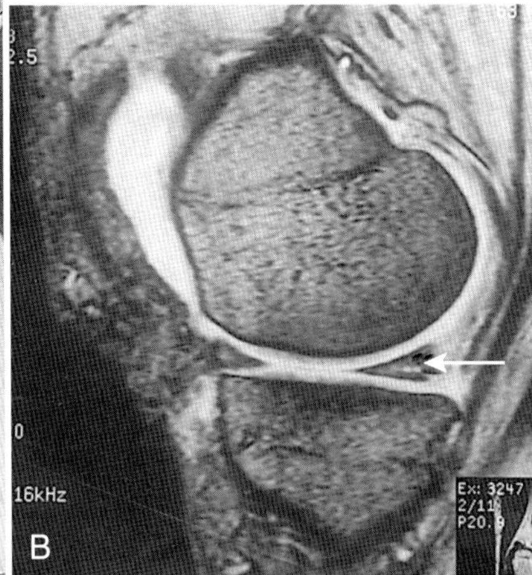

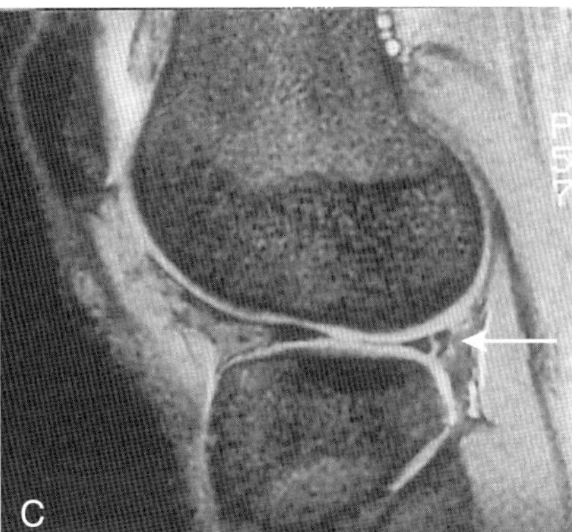

FIGURE 72.7 MRI grading of meniscal tears. **A**, Poorly defined "globular" zone of increased signal intensity *(arrow)*, corresponding to grade 1 change. **B**, Linear zone of hyperintensity *(arrow)* not communicating with the articular surfaces, corresponding to grade 2 change. **C**, Linear band of hyperintensity *(arrow)* communicating with both articular surfaces, corresponding to grade 3 change, that is, a complete tear. *(From Mellion MB. Office Sports Medicine, 2nd ed. Philadelphia, Hanley & Belfus, 1996.)*

a combination of open and closed kinetic chain exercises in all three planes (sagittal, coronal, and transverse) can be performed in conjunction with stretching of the lower limb. Gradually, during the ensuing weeks, more functional activities are introduced. More challenging proprioceptive and balancing activities also can be started as deemed appropriate. Finally, plyometric training is begun, and the individual is gradually introduced back into sport-specific activities.

Multiple rehabilitation protocols for the surgically repaired meniscus have been described. Rehabilitation programs ideally need to be individualized to the specific type of repair performed. In addition, there has been considerable controversy among physicians about the patient's weight-bearing and immobilization status soon after surgical repair [30,36–39]. In general, however, initial exercises are nonaggressive, avoiding dynamic shear forces that may occur from joint active range of motion. Therefore, exercises are initially static, targeting hip abductors, adductors, and extensors. Static quadriceps exercises are performed with care to avoid terminal knee extension. While superior and medial patella mobilization is begun, stretching of the lower limb musculature in multiple planes is emphasized. After 2 to 3 weeks, goals are to increase range of motion and to advance weight-bearing status while a resistance exercise program is introduced. With the absence of effusion and significant pain, improved knee range of motion from 5 to 110 degrees should be achieved. More aggressive active range of motion may be started, particularly if the repair was to the outer peripheral or vascular zone of the meniscus because the success rate for healing here is higher [30]. Gradually, more functional activities with use of resistive bands may be introduced. With time and success of the patient, resistance can be increased and proprioceptive neuromuscular facilitation activities can be implemented, ensuring that the individual is rehabilitated in the coronal, transverse, and sagittal planes [40].

Brace protection, if it was initially employed, may be discontinued, particularly when the patient demonstrates success with proprioceptive testing. Running, cutting, and rotational activities are avoided. However, sport-specific exercises can be initiated when no effusion exists, knee strength is at least 70% of normal, and the knee can attain full range of motion [39]. Athletes may be able to return to their individual activities at about 16 weeks for those with repairs in the vascular zone and 24 weeks for those with repairs in the nonvascular zone.

Procedures

Patients presenting after an acute injury with an effusion may benefit from a joint aspiration, not only to help relieve discomfort and stiffness but also to aid in discerning whether a hemarthrosis or marrow fat (to rule out an occult fracture) is present.

Surgery

Specific types of tears may not require surgical repair; these include longitudinal partial-thickness tears, stable full-thickness peripheral tears (<5 mm long), and short (<5 mm) radial tears [35]. These are usually stable and may not require either suture fixation or immobilization. However, arthroscopy may still be necessary to determine stability and to stimulate healing through perimeniscal abrasion [11].

Some larger longitudinal, radial, and degenerative meniscal tears are less likely to heal without surgical intervention. Although first-line treatment of these lesions is aggressive rehabilitation, recalcitrant cases may require a partial meniscectomy that preserves as much of the meniscus as possible [37]. In addition, the inner aspect of the cartilage, which may be ragged, may be rasped or shaved, providing a smooth surface that eliminates mechanical symptoms.

On occasion, other tears of the menisci, because of their size and location, are best treated by primary approximation with sutures and primary repair [41]. Typically, longitudinal tears longer than 5 mm in the periphery of the meniscus are best suited for this because they have a high rate of successful healing [35]. In older individuals, the mere presence of a horizontal or degenerative cleavage tear is insufficient to justify removal because these meniscal portions may still participate in significant load transmission but not necessarily cause symptoms [11]. Treatment of these degenerative tears is usually nonsurgical; however, unstable portions may be removed during arthroscopy. Good outcomes have been documented after patients with degenerative tears have been treated with aggressive rehabilitation [42].

Potential Disease Complications

Once a meniscal tear occurs, the joint inherently becomes less stable. This instability may promote further extension of the initial tear, turning a nonsurgical lesion into one in which arthroscopic repair may be necessary. Chronically, the resultant increased abnormal motion that occurs secondary to the meniscal injury may also lead to damage of the articular surface and predispose to premature osteoarthritis [12].

Potential Treatment Complications

Analgesics such as acetaminophen and nonsteroidal anti-inflammatory drugs have well-known side effects that may affect the gastric, hepatic, and renal systems. An overly aggressive regimen may lead to extension of the tear or failure of the meniscus to heal. A rehabilitative program that is too conservative, in contrast, may also lead to a significant loss of strength with muscle atrophy and decreased range of motion. If the surgical approach resulted in a significant amount of cartilage removed, the knee may be predisposed to development of osteoarthritis as originally described by Fairbank [10]. Saphenous nerve injuries as well as infections are also common complications after meniscal repair surgery and arthroscopy [12].

References

[1] Renström P, Johnson R. Anatomy and biomechanics of the menisci. Clin Sports Med 1990;9:523–38.

[2] Norkin C, Levangie P. The knee complex. In: Norkin C, Levangie P, editors. Joint structure and function. 2nd ed. Philadelphia: FA Davis; 1992. p. 337–78.

[3] Maitra RS, Miller MD, Johnson DL. Meniscal reconstruction. Part I: indications, techniques, and graft considerations. Am J Orthop 1999;28:213–8.

[4] Gray J. Neural and vascular anatomy of the menisci of the human knee. J Orthop Sports Phys Ther 1999;29:23.
[5] Arnoczky SP, Warren RF. The microvasculature of the meniscus and its response to injury. An experimental study in the dog. Am J Sports Med 1983;11:131–41.
[6] Seedholm BB. Transmission on the load in the knee joint with special reference to the role of the menisci: I. Anatomy, analysis and apparatus. Eng Med 1979;8:207–19.
[7] Walker PS, Erkiuan MJ. The role of the menisci in force transmission across the knee. Clin Orthop 1975;109:184.
[8] Ahmed A, Burke D. In-vitro measurement of static pressure distribution in synovial joints—part I: tibial surface of the knee. J Biomech Eng 1983;105:216.
[9] Krause W, Pope M, Johnson R, Wilder D. Mechanical changes in the knee after meniscectomy. J Bone Joint Surg Am 1976;58:599.
[10] Fairbank T. Knee joint changes after meniscectomy. J Bone Joint Surg Br 1948;30:664–70.
[11] Newman AP, Daniels A, Burks RT. Principles and decision making in meniscal surgery. Arthroscopy 1993;9:33–51.
[12] Fu FH, Baratz M. Meniscal injuries. In: DeLee JC, Drez D, editors. Orthopaedic sports medicine: principles and practice, vol. 2. Philadelphia: WB Saunders; 1994. p. 1146–62.
[13] Oberlander MA, Pryde J. Meniscal injuries. In: Baker CL, editor. The hughston clinic sports medicine book. Baltimore: Williams & Wilkins; 1995. p. 465–72.
[14] Hardin GT, Farr J, Bach Jr BR. Meniscal tears: diagnosis, evaluation, and treatment. Orthop Rev 1992;21:1311–7.
[15] Metcalf RW. The torn medial meniscus. In: Parisien JS, editor. Arthroscopic surgery. New York: McGraw-Hill; 1988. p. 93–110.
[16] Tuerlings L. Meniscal injuries. In: Arendt EA, editor. Orthopaedic knowledge update. Sports medicine 2. Rosemont, Ill: American Academy of Orthopaedic Surgeons; 1999. p. 349–54.
[17] Baker BE, Peckham AC, Pupparo F, Sanborn JC. Review of meniscal injury and associated sports. Am J Sports Med 1985;13:1–4.
[18] Rodkey W. Basic biology of the meniscus and response to injury. Instr Course Lect 2000;49:189–93.
[19] Poehling G, Ruch D, Chabon S. The landscape of meniscal injuries. Clin Sports Med 1990;9:539–49.
[20] Bellabarba C, Bush-Joseph C, Bach B. Patterns of meniscal injury in the anterior cruciate-deficient knee: a review of the literature. Am J Orthop 1997;26:18–24.
[21] Casscells SW. The place of arthroscopy in the diagnosis and treatment of internal derangement of the knee: an analysis of 1000 cases. Clin Orthop Relat Res 1980;151:135–42.
[22] Simon RR, Koenigsknecht SJ. The knee. In: Simon RR, Koenigsknecht SJ, editors. Emergency orthopedics: the extremities. 3rd ed. Norwalk, Conn: Appleton & Lange; 1995. p. 437–62.
[23] Muellner T, Nikolic A, Vécsei V. Recommendations for the diagnosis of traumatic meniscal injuries in athletes. Sports Med 1999;27:337–45.
[24] Rose NE, Gold SM. A comparison of accuracy between clinical examination and magnetic resonance imaging in the diagnosis of meniscal and anterior cruciate ligament tears. Arthroscopy 1996;12:398–405.
[25] Anderson AF, Lipscomb AB. Clinical diagnosis of meniscal tears. Description of a new manipulative test. Am J Sports Med 1986;14:291–3.
[26] Karachalios T, Hantes M, Zibis AH, et al. Diagnostic accuracy of a new clinical test (the Thessaly test) for early detection of meniscal tears. J Bone Joint Surg Am 2005;87:955–62.
[27] Mirzatolooei F, Yekta Z, Bayazidchi M, et al. Validation of the Thessaly test for detecting meniscal tears in anterior cruciate deficient knees. Knee 2010;17:221–3.
[28] Boden SD, Davis DO, Dina TS, et al. A prospective and blinded investigation of magnetic resonance imaging of the knee: abnormal findings in asymptomatic subjects. Clin Orthop 1992;282:177.
[29] Baratz ME, Rehak DC, Fu FH, Rudert M. Peripheral tears of the meniscus. The effect of open versus arthroscopic repair on intraarticular contact stresses in the human knee. Am J Sports Med 1988;16:1–6.
[30] Auberger SS, Mangine RE. Innovative approaches to surgery and rehabilitation. In: Mangine RE, editor. Physical therapy of the knee. 2nd ed. New York: Churchill Livingstone; 1995. p. 233–49.
[31] Shetty A, Tindall A, James K, et al. Accuracy of hand-held ultrasound scanning in detecting meniscal tears. J Bone Joint Surg Br 2008;90:1045–8.
[32] Ercin E, Kaya I, Sungur I, et al. History, clinical findings, magnetic resonance imaging, and arthroscopic correlation in meniscal lesions. Knee Surg Sports Traumatol Arthrosc 2012;20:851–6.
[33] DeHaven KE. Injuries to the menisci of the knee. In: Nicholas JA, Hershman EB, editors. The lower extremity and spine in sports medicine. St. Louis: Mosby; 1986. p. 905–28.
[34] Urquhart MW, O'Leary JA, Griffin JR, Fu FH. Meniscal injuries in the adult. In: DeLee JC, Drez D, editors. Orthopedic sports medicine: principles and practice. 2nd ed. Philadelphia: WB Saunders; 2003. p. 1668–86.
[35] Dehaven K, Bronstein RD. Injuries to the menisci of the knee. In: Nicholas JA, Hershman EB, editors. The lower extremity and spine in sports medicine. 2nd ed. St. Louis: Mosby; 1995. p. 813–23.
[36] Brukner P, Khan K. Acute knee injuries. In: Brukner P, Khan K, editors. Clinical sports medicine. 2nd ed. New York: McGraw-Hill; 2001. p. 426–63.
[37] Rispoli DM, Miller MD. Options in meniscal repair. Clin Sports Med 1999;18:77.
[38] Shelbourne K, Patel D, Adsit W, Porter D. Rehabilitation after meniscal repair. Clin Sports Med 1996;15:595–612.
[39] Kozlowski EJ, Barcia AM, Tokish JM. Meniscus repair: the role of accelerated rehabilitation in return to sport. Sports Med Arthrosc 2012;20:121.
[40] Gray G. Lunge tests. In: Gray GW, editor. Lower extremity functional profile. Adrian, Mich: Wynn Marketing; 1995. p. 100–8.
[41] Swenson TM, Harner CD. Knee ligament and meniscal injuries. Orthop Clin North Am 1995;26:529–46.
[42] Stensrud S, Roos EM, Risberg MA. A 12-week exercise therapy program in middle-aged patients with degenerative meniscus tears: a case series with 1 year follow up. J Orthop Sports Phys Ther 2012;42:919–31.

CHAPTER 73

Patellar Tendinopathy (Jumper's Knee)

Rathi L. Joseph, DO
Joseph T. Alleva, MD, MBA
Thomas H. Hudgins, MD

Synonyms

Patellar tendinitis
Quadriceps tendinitis
Patellar tendinosis
Patellar apicitis
Partial rupture of patellar ligament

ICD-9 Code

726.64 Patellar tendinitis

ICD-10 Codes

M76.50 Patellar tendinitis, unspecified knee
M76.51 Patellar tendinitis, right knee
M76.52 Patellar tendinitis, left knee

Definition

Patellar tendinopathy or "jumper's knee," first described by Blazina and colleagues [1] in 1973, is primarily a chronic overuse injury of the patellar tendon resulting from excessive stress on the knee extensor mechanism. Athletes involved in sports requiring repetitive jumping, running, and kicking (e.g., volleyball, basketball, tennis, track) are at greatest risk. For example, volleyball players have an increased incidence compared with other sports of 22% to 39% [2]. Acceleration, deceleration, takeoff, and landing generate eccentric forces that can be three times greater than conventional concentric and static forces. These eccentric forces may exceed the inherent strength of the patellar tendon, resulting in microtears anywhere along the bone-tendon interface [2–4]. With continued stress, a cycle of microtearing, degeneration, and regeneration weakens the tendon and may lead to tendon rupture.

As in other overuse injuries, the predisposing factors in jumper's knee include extrinsic causes, such as errors in training, and intrinsic causes, such as biomechanical flaws. Training errors include improper warm-up or cool-down, rapid increase in frequency or intensity of activity, and training on hard surfaces [3,4]. Biomechanical imbalances, such as tight hamstrings and excess femoral anteversion [3], and jumping mechanics [2,5] have been implicated as increased risk factors for development of patella tendinopathy (jumper's knee). Finally, an increased incidence of Osgood-Schlatter disease and idiopathic anterior knee pain during adolescence has been identified in patients with jumper's knee [3].

Because histologic studies of the patellar tendon reveal collagen degeneration with little or no evidence of acute inflammation, many authors argue that "patellar tendinopathy or tendinosis" is a more accurate description than "patellar tendinitis." [6–8] This distinction has important implications for rehabilitation. In treatment of patellar tendinosis and other chronic overuse tendinopathies, the treatment team should emphasize restoration of function rather than control of inflammation. This is an overuse syndrome that has no age or gender predilection.

Symptoms

Patients typically report a dull, aching anterior knee pain, initially noted after a strenuous exercise session or competition, that is insidious in onset and well localized [7]. The bone-tendon junction at the inferior pole of the patella is most frequently affected (65% of cases), followed by the superior pole of the patella (25%) and the tibial tubercle (10%) [6]. Other symptoms may include stiffness or pain after prolonged sitting or climbing stairs [3], a feeling of swelling or fullness over the patella, and knee extensor weakness [1]. Mechanical symptoms of instability, such as locking, catching, and give-way weakness, are uncommon.

Four phases have been described in the progression of jumper's knee: phase 1, pain is present after activity only and is not associated with functional impairment; phase 2, pain is present during and after activity but does not limit performance and resolves with rest; phase 3, pain is present continually and is associated with progressively impaired performance; and phase 4, complete tendon rupture [1].

As the disease progresses, the pain becomes sharper, more severe, and constant (present not only with athletic endeavor but also with walking and other everyday activities). If it is not treated, the disorder may result in tendon rupture, a sudden painful event associated with immediate inability to extend the knee [7].

Physical Examination

The hallmark of jumper's knee is tenderness at the site of involvement, usually the inferior pole of the patella [7]. This sign is best elicited on palpation of the knee in full extension [7], and the pain typically increases when the knee is extended against resistance [3]. On occasion, there may be swelling of the tendon or the fat pad, although a frank knee joint effusion is not typically present [3]. Mild patellofemoral crepitus and pain with compression of the patellofemoral joint have been noted [3]. In advanced disease, patients may have quadriceps atrophy without detectable weakness on manual muscle testing and hamstring tightness [3,7]. Test results for knee ligamentous laxity are negative. The examiner should also expect normal findings on neurologic examination.

Functional Limitations

Most patients experience little functional limitation in the early stages of jumper's knee. As the disease progresses, however, increasing disability from persistent pain and inhibition of knee extension impairs athletic performance. Eventually, walking and the ability to perform basic activities of living, such as ascending or descending stairs, may be compromised. In the event of patellar tendon rupture, complete functional impairment with inability to extend the affected knee, limiting weight bearing and ambulation, necessitates surgical repair.

Diagnostic Testing

Radiographic changes are rarely present during the first 6 months of patellar tendinopathy, limiting the usefulness of radiographs during initial evaluation [4]. When radiography is performed, the examination generally includes anteroposterior, lateral, intercondylar, and skyline (or sunrise) tracking patellar views [3]. Documented findings include radiolucency at the site of involvement, elongation of the involved pole, and occasionally a fracture at the junction of the elongation with the main portion of the patella. On occasion, calcification of the involved tendon and irregularity or even avulsion of the involved pole may be seen [1].

Ultrasonography has the advantage of allowing early diagnosis and dynamic imaging of the tendon while remaining inexpensive, noninvasive, reproducible, and sensitive to changes as small as 0.1 mm [4]. Some authors believe ultrasonography to be the preferred method for evaluation of jumper's knee. It has been used to confirm the diagnosis, to guide steroid injections, and to observe tendons after surgery [4]. It should be considered in cases that do not respond to a trial of conservative treatment after 4 to 6 weeks and when the diagnosis is questioned. Findings on ultrasound examination include thickening of the tendon [4,9]. A hypoechoic focal lesion at the area of greatest thickening correlates well with the lesion on magnetic resonance imaging (MRI), computed tomography, and histologic examination [3,10]. However, critics of ultrasonography have noted abnormalities in asymptomatic athletes. This phenomenon may be explained by a preclinical or postclinical stage of the disease [4]. Plain MRI, MRI with intravenous administration of gadolinium, and MRI arthrography with gadolinium have been used to corroborate the clinical diagnosis of jumper's knee. Increased thickening of the patellar tendon on MRI is present in all patients resistant to conservative therapy [11,12]. MRI is also advantageous in excluding other intrinsic joint disease. MRI arthrography is particularly useful in examining the chondral surfaces of the patella and femur when osteochondritis dissecans or other pathologic processes in these areas are suspected. Before advanced imaging, we recommend simple radiographic examination with three views of the knee to rule out bone pathologic changes and to evaluate joint space. If patients do not respond to physical therapy in 4 to 6 weeks, ultrasound examination is the preferred study at that time to confirm the diagnosis.

Differential Diagnosis

Patellofemoral maltracking
Retinacular pain
Fat pad lesion
Lipoma arborescens
Infrapatellar bursitis
Partial anterior cruciate ligament tear
Meniscal injuries
Chondromalacia patellae
Plica syndrome
Entrapment of the saphenous nerve
Osgood-Schlatter lesion
Sinding-Larsen-Johansson syndrome [3,4,7]

Treatment

Initial

Because the syndrome is progressive and associated with difficult and slow rehabilitation, the importance of early diagnosis and treatment cannot be overemphasized [13]. Initial interventions include control of pain with nonsteroidal anti-inflammatory drugs, ice, and relative rest. Passive modalities such as ultrasound and iontophoresis with corticosteroid preparation are also used judiciously to control pain.

Rehabilitation

A comprehensive rehabilitation program should address the biomechanical flaws found on the musculoskeletal examination. These include the functional deficits (inflexibilities that lead to altered biomechanics) and subclinical adaptations (substitution patterns that compensate for the functional deficits) [14]. This approach may be used in addressing all overuse syndromes. In patellar tendinopathy, hamstring and quadriceps tightness and weakness need to be addressed [14]. As the rehabilitation program advances and pain abates, eccentric strengthening exercises should be emphasized. This type of strengthening exercise is optimal for rehabilitation of tendinopathies because it places maximal tensile load on the muscle and tendon unit (Fig. 73.1) [15]. There is a paucity of randomized controlled studies supporting this type of exercise; however, eccentric strengthening is commonly recommended [16]. This type of exercise may provoke pain initially, given the increased load placed on the muscle-tendon unit. The final phase of rehabilitation should also encompass sports-specific drills and training. Knee supports and counterforce straps have been used to alleviate pain and to change the force dynamics through the patellar tendon with good results [4,17].

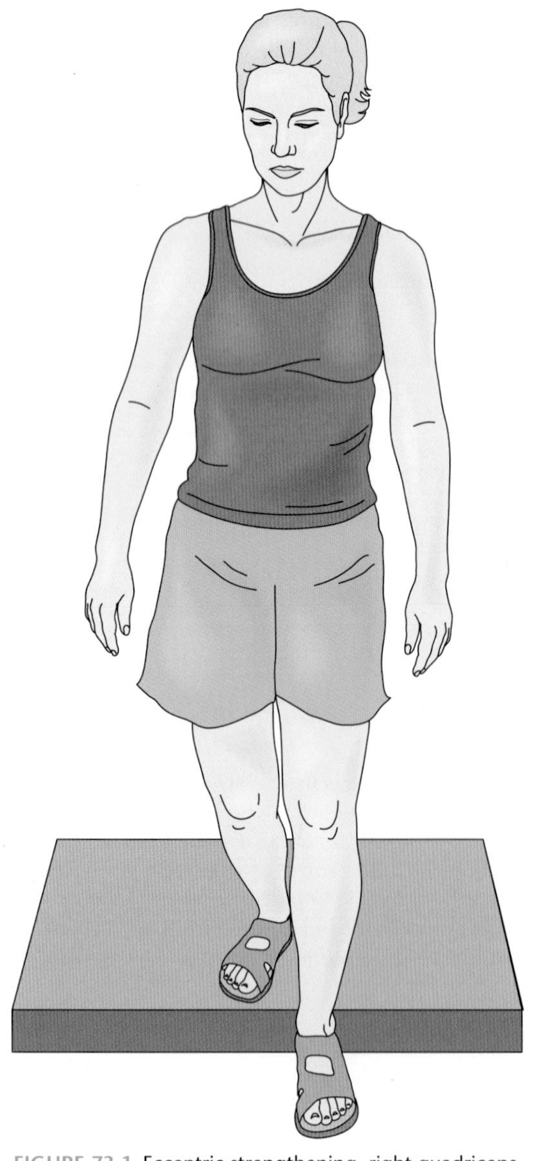

FIGURE 73.1 Eccentric strengthening, right quadriceps.

Procedures

Some authors recommend a peritendinous injection of steroid if noninvasive conservative therapy fails [3,4]. This is performed with ultrasound guidance to ensure accurate placement of the needle. Decreased pain with injection of the fat pad rather than of the tendon itself has been documented [3]. Because histologic studies have shown a minimal inflammatory component in surgical specimens, the mechanism of action of these approaches is unknown [4]. In addition, studies have associated tendon ruptures with steroid injection [4,18]. The efficacy of prolotherapy (10% dextrose) in patellar tendinopathy has not been studied [19]. Some anecdotal evidence supports the use of protein-rich plasma therapy [20].

Surgery

In the advanced stage of jumper's knee, if a well-documented conservative therapy trial has failed or if the tendon ruptures, surgery is indicated. Several approaches have had mixed success; resection of the tendon disease with resuturing of the tendon is most often cited, and authors report 77% to 93% good or excellent results [21,22].

However, when more invasive treatments, such as injections or surgery, are contemplated, it is incumbent on the practitioner to ensure that a comprehensive rehabilitation program has been followed thoroughly, as outlined earlier, before one declares a "conservative management failure." Criteria for conservative management failure are often ill-defined in the literature. In our experience, invasive procedures are rarely necessary for the management of jumper's knee. Postoperative rehabilitation begins with isometric strengthening of the quadriceps, restoring range of motion and advancing to eccentric strengthening in 6 to 12 weeks.

Potential Disease Complications

Stress reaction of the patella, stress fracture, and patellar tendon rupture are some of the advanced complications. Others include formation of accessory ossicles, avulsion apophysis, and bone growth acceleration or arrest in adolescents [23].

Potential Treatment Complications

Gastrointestinal bleeding and renal side effects of nonsteroidal anti-inflammatory drugs are well documented. Complications of corticosteroid injections include bleeding, infection, and soft tissue atrophy at the site of injection. Tendon weakening with possible increased incidence of tendon rupture has also been cited. Surgery can lead to inadvertent tibial or peroneal nerve injury.

References

[1] Blazina ME, Kerlan RK, Jobe FW, et al. Jumper's knee. Orthop Clin North Am 1973;4:665–78.
[2] Ferretti A, Puddu G, Mariani PP, Neri M. The natural history of jumper's knee. Int Orthop 1985;8:239–42.
[3] Duri ZA, Aichroth PM, Wilkins R, Jones J. Patellar tendonitis and anterior knee pain. Am J Knee Surg 1999;12:99–108.
[4] Fredberg U, Bolvig L. Jumper's knee. Scand J Med Sci Sports 1999;9:66–73.

[5] Colosimo AJ, Bassett FH. Jumper's knee diagnosis and treatment. Orthop Rev 1990;19:139–49.
[6] Popp JE, Yu JS, Kaeding CC. Recalcitrant patellar tendinitis. Am J Sports Med 1997;25:218–22.
[7] Lian O, Engebretsen L, Ovrebo RV, Bahr R. Characteristics of the leg extensors in male volleyball players with jumper's knee. Am J Sports Med 1996;24:380–5.
[8] Richards DP, Ajemian SV, Wiley JP, Zernicke RF. Knee joint dynamics predict patellar tendinitis in elite volleyball players. Am J Sports Med 1996;24:676–83.
[9] Visentini PJ, Khan KM, Cook JL, et al. The VISA score: an index of severity of symptoms in patients with jumper's knee (patellar tendinosis). J Sci Med Sport 1998;1:22–8.
[10] Khan KM, Cook JL, Kiss ZS, et al. Patellar tendon ultrasonography and jumper's knee in female basketball players: a longitudinal study. Clin J Sport Med 1997;7:199–206.
[11] Davies SG, Baudouin CJ, King JB, Perry JD. Ultrasound, computed tomography, and magnetic resonance imaging in patellar tendinitis. Clin Radiol 1991;43:52–6.
[12] Khan KM, Bonar F, Desmond PM, et al. Patellar tendinosis (jumper's knee): findings at histopathologic examination, US, and MRI Imaging. Radiology 1996;200:821–7.
[13] Jensen K, Di Fabio R. Evaluation of eccentric exercise in treatment of patellar tendinitis. Phys Ther 1989;69:211–6.
[14] Gotlin RS. Effective rehabilitation for anterior knee pain. J Musculoskelet Med 2000;17:421–32.
[15] Stanish WD, Rubinovich RM, Curwin S. Eccentric exercise in chronic tendinitis. Clin Orthop Relat Res 1985;285:65–8.
[16] Rabin A. Is there evidence to support the use of eccentric strengthening exercises to decrease pain and increase function in patients with patellar tendinopathy? Phys Ther 2006;86:450–6.
[17] Palumbo PM. Dynamic patellar brace: a new orthosis in the management of patellofemoral disorders. Am J Sports Med 1981;9:45–9.
[18] Ismail AM, Balakrishnan R, Rajakumar MK, Lumpur K. Rupture of patellar ligament after steroid infiltration. J Bone Joint Surg Br 1969;51:503–5.
[19] Reeves KD, Hassanein K. Randomized prospective double-blind placebo-controlled study of dextrose prolotherapy for knee osteoarthritis with or without ACL laxity. Altern Ther Health Med 2000;6(68–74):77–80.
[20] Ackermann PW, Renstrom P. Tendinopathy in sport. Sports Health 2012 May;4(3):193–201.
[21] Verheyden F, Geens G, Nelen G. Jumper's knee: results of surgical treatment. Acta Orthop Belg 1997;63:102–5.
[22] Pierets K, Verdonk R, De Muynck M, Lagast J. Jumper's knee: postoperative assessment. Knee Surg Sports Traumatol Arthrosc 1999;7:239–42.
[23] Cook JL, Khan KM, Harcourt PR, et al. A cross sectional study of 100 athletes with jumper's knee managed conservatively and surgically. Br J Sports Med 1997;31:332–6.

CHAPTER 74

Patellofemoral Syndrome

Rathi L. Joseph, DO
Joseph T. Alleva, MD, MBA
Thomas H. Hudgins, MD

Synonyms

Anterior knee pain
Chondromalacia patellae
Patellofemoral arthralgia
Patellar pain
Maltracking
Patellalgia [1,2]

ICD-9 Codes

715.36	**Patellofemoral degenerative joint disease**
716.96	**Arthritis, patellofemoral**
718.86	**Patellofemoral instability**
719.46	**Patellofemoral pain syndrome**

ICD-10 Codes

M17.9	**Osteoarthritis of knee, unspecified**
M13.861	**Other specified arthritis, right knee**
M13.862	**Other specified arthritis, left knee**
M13.869	**Other specified arthritis, unspecified knee**
M23.50	**Chronic instability of knee, unspecified knee**
M23.51	**Chronic instability of knee, right knee**
M23.52	**Chronic instability of knee, left knee**
M25.561	**Pain in right knee**
M25.562	**Pain in left knee**
M25.569	**Pain in unspecified knee**
M22.2X1	**Patellofemoral disorders, right knee**
M22.2X2	**Patellofemoral disorders, left knee**
M22.2X9	**Patellofemoral disorders, unspecified knee**
M22.3X1	**Other derangement of patella, right knee**
M22.3X2	**Other derangement of patella, left knee**
M22.3X9	**Other derangement of patella, unspecified knee**
M22.40	**Chondromalacia patellae, unspecified knee**
M22.41	**Chondromalacia patellae, right knee**
M22.42	**Chondromalacia patellae, left knee**

Definition

Patellofemoral syndrome is the most common ailment involving the knee in both the athletic and the nonathletic population [3–5]. In sports medicine clinics, 25% of patients complaining of knee pain are diagnosed with this syndrome, and it affects women twice as often as men [3]. Yet despite the common occurrence of this disorder, there is no clear consensus on the definition, etiology, and pathophysiology [6]. The most common theory is that the syndrome is an overuse injury from repetitive overload at the patellofemoral joint. This increased stress results in physical and biomechanical changes of the patellofemoral joint [6]. The literature has focused on identification of risk factors leading to altered biomechanics that produce poor patellar tracking in the femoral trochlear groove and thus stress at the patellofemoral joint. Possible pain generators include the subchondral bone, retinacula, capsule, and synovial membrane [7]. Historically, the histologic diagnosis of chondromalacia, or deterioration of the cartilage, had been associated with patellofemoral syndrome. However, chondromalacia is poorly associated with the incidence of patellofemoral syndrome [5]. Electromyographic comparison of vastus medialis oblique (VMO) to vastus lateralis activation has shown delayed VMO activation in those patients with patellofemoral syndrome [8]. A pilot investigation has been done with 64-channel surface electromyography and motion capture to evaluate activation of the four heads of the quadriceps muscle in three dimensions. That study showed increased variability in the pattern of activation in the patellofemoral group compared with controls, resulting in altered patellar kinematics and loading of the patellar facets [9].

Symptoms

The patient with patellofemoral syndrome will complain of diffuse, vague ache of insidious onset [3]. The anterior knee is the most common location for pain, but some patients describe posterior knee discomfort in the popliteal fossa [4]. The discomfort is aggravated by prolonged sitting with knees flexed ("theater" sign) as well as on ascending or descending of stairs and squatting because these positions place the greatest force on the patellofemoral joint [10]. The patient may also experience pseudolocking when the knee momentarily locks in an extended position [11,12].

Physical Examination

The examination focuses on identification of risk factors that contribute to malalignment and rules out other pathologic processes associated with anterior knee pain. Tenderness to palpation at the medial and lateral borders of the patella may be appreciated [3]. A minimal effusion may also be present. The results of manual testing for intra-articular disease, such as the Lachman (anterior cruciate ligament) and McMurray (meniscal) maneuvers, will be negative.

The presence of femoral anteversion, tibia internal rotation, excessive pronation at the foot, increased Q angle, and inflexibility of the hip flexors, quadriceps, iliotibial band, and gastrocnemius-soleus should be determined [13]. The patella position (baja or alta, internal or external rotation) should also be assessed with the patient sitting and standing. Each of these factors has either a direct or an indirect influence on the tracking of the patella with the femur (Fig. 74.1).

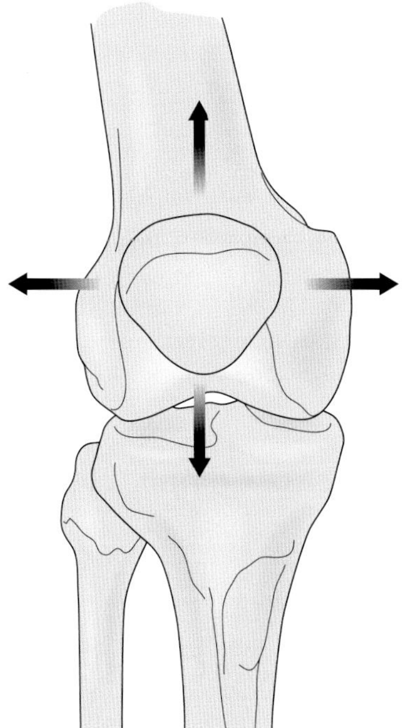

FIGURE 74.1 Forces on the patella in patellofemoral syndrome.

The Q angle is the intersection of a line from the anterior superior iliac spine to the patella with a line from the tibial tubercle to the patella (Fig. 74.2). This angle is typically less than 15 degrees in men and less than 20 degrees in women. An increased angle is associated with increased femoral anteversion and thus patellofemoral joint torsion [11]. However, a consensus on the importance of an increased Q angle is lacking [6]. Tight hip flexors, quadriceps, hamstrings, and gastrocnemius-soleus will increase knee flexion and thus patellofemoral joint reaction force. A tight iliotibial band will increase the lateral pull of the patella through the lateral retinacular fibers [14,15]. Static hip strength was not shown to be a predisposing component of patellofemoral syndrome pain in women [16]. It is imperative to assess each of these components in the lower extremity kinetic chain to prescribe a tailored physical therapy program for each individual (Table 74.1).

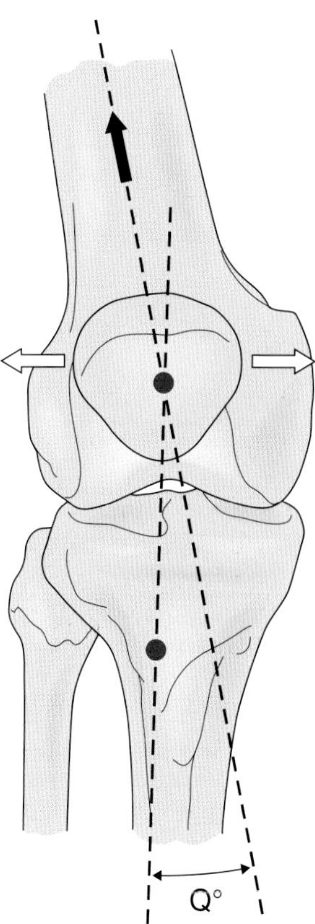

FIGURE 74.2 Measurement of Q angle. A line is drawn from the anterior iliac spine to the center of the patella. A second line is drawn from the center of the patella to the tibial tubercle. An angle between these two lines is called the Q angle.

Table 74.1 Causes of Altered Biomechanics

Altered Biomechanics	Etiology
Increased knee flexion	Tight hip flexors, quadriceps, hamstrings, gastrocnemius-soleus
Lateral pull of patella	Tight iliotibial band, weak vastus medialis oblique
Femoral anteversion	Increased Q angle
Tibial internal rotation	Excessive foot pronation

Functional Limitations

The patient with the patellofemoral syndrome will avoid activities that provoke the discomfort initially, such as stair climbing. Prolonged sitting in a car may be difficult. In chronic, progressive cases, ambulation may be enough to incite the pain, making all activities of daily living difficult.

Diagnostic Testing

Patellofemoral syndrome is a clinical diagnosis. Plain films may be used to evaluate Q angle and patella alta or baja. Advanced imaging, such as magnetic resonance imaging, is reserved for recalcitrant cases that do not respond to conservative care to rule out intra-articular disease. Bone scintigrams revealed diffuse uptake in the patellofemoral joint in 50% of patients diagnosed with patellofemoral syndrome [17].

Differential Diagnosis

Patella fracture
Patella dislocation
Quadriceps rupture
Patella tendinitis
Peripatellar bursitis
Osgood-Schlatter disease
Meniscal lesions
Ligamentous lesions
Plica syndromes
Osteochondritis dissecans

Treatment

Initial

As in other overuse injuries, the initial treatment focuses on decreasing pain. Icing is beneficial, particularly after activities. Nonsteroidal anti-inflammatory drugs may be used in a judicious manner. Relative rest with non–weight-bearing aerobic activity may also be necessary. A neoprene knee sleeve with patella cutout is helpful to increase proprioceptive feedback. McConnell's taping method can be used during the acute phase to reduce pain and to increase tolerance of a therapeutic exercise program, although it was less effective in patients with higher body mass index, larger lateral patellofemoral angle, and smaller Q angles [15,18–21]. Patella bracing was shown to reduce pain and to improve function in patients with patellofemoral syndrome but no more successfully than therapeutic exercise [22]. Of patients who had lower pain levels, wore less supportive footwear, had decreased ankle dorsiflexion range of motion, and reported an immediate reduction in pain when performing a single-leg squat with a foot orthosis, 78% found relief using foot orthoses at 12 weeks. In the same study, immediate pain relief while performing a single-leg squat with orthosis use was the greatest predictor of noncustomized prefabricated foot orthosis–related pain relief at 12 weeks [23].

Rehabilitation

With no consensus on the etiology and pathophysiology of patellofemoral syndrome, numerous treatment protocols and therapies have been proposed in the literature [24]. Nevertheless, most patients respond to a directed rehabilitation approach with therapeutic exercise [14,15]. The rehabilitation program should address deficiencies in strength, flexibility, and proprioception. Strength training can be achieved with both open kinetic chain and closed kinetic chain exercises. Open kinetic chain exercises occur when the distal link, the foot, is allowed to move freely in space, as in leg extensions. During closed kinetic chain exercises, the foot maintains contact with the ground, resulting in a multiarticular closed kinetic exercise, as in squatting or leg press [15]. Closed kinetic chain exercises are also less stressful than open chain exercises at the patellofemoral joint in the functional range of 0 to 45 degrees of knee flexion [25].

These exercises can be performed in multiple planes in a "functional" rehabilitation program (Figs. 74.3 and 74.4). This may entail having the patient perform a lunge (a closed kinetic chain exercise) in the coronal, sagittal, and transverse planes, simulating positions applied during activities. These exercises can also stress the patient's balance by performance of the lunges with eyes closed. Through this functional or skill training, the patient is being prepared for all functional tasks by achieving efficient nerve-muscle interactions [10].

Many studies have focused on selective strengthening of the VMO as a dynamic medial stabilizer on the patella. Selective VMO strengthening may be achieved with combined hip adduction because the fibers of the VMO originate on the adductor magnus tendon and, to a lesser extent, the adductor longus. However, attempts at proving isolated recruitment of the VMO in relation to the vastus lateralis have failed [3]. Biofeedback and comprehensive McConnell-based physical therapy have been shown to improve motor control of the VMO as evidenced by altered firing patterns [26,27]. Nevertheless, quadriceps strengthening in general should be incorporated in the rehabilitation program through closed kinetic chain and functional exercises, which need to be incorporated in a long-term maintenance program.

Procedures

Injections are not indicated because this is primarily a maltracking phenomenon without a clear consensus on the pain generator.

Surgery

Surgery is rarely indicated, and a directed rehabilitation program is often successful [4]. However, several techniques have been illustrated in the literature. These include lateral retinacular release to decrease the lateral force, proximal and distal realignment procedures, and elevation of the tibial tubercle [1].

Potential Disease Complications

Recalcitrant chronic cases of anterior knee pain may show progressive degenerative changes at the patellofemoral joint, such as severe (grade IV) chondromalacia patellae.

Potential Treatment Complications

Risks of chronic use of nonsteroidal anti-inflammatory drugs include gastrointestinal bleeding, renal toxicity, hypertension, and other cardiovascular complications; thus, duration should

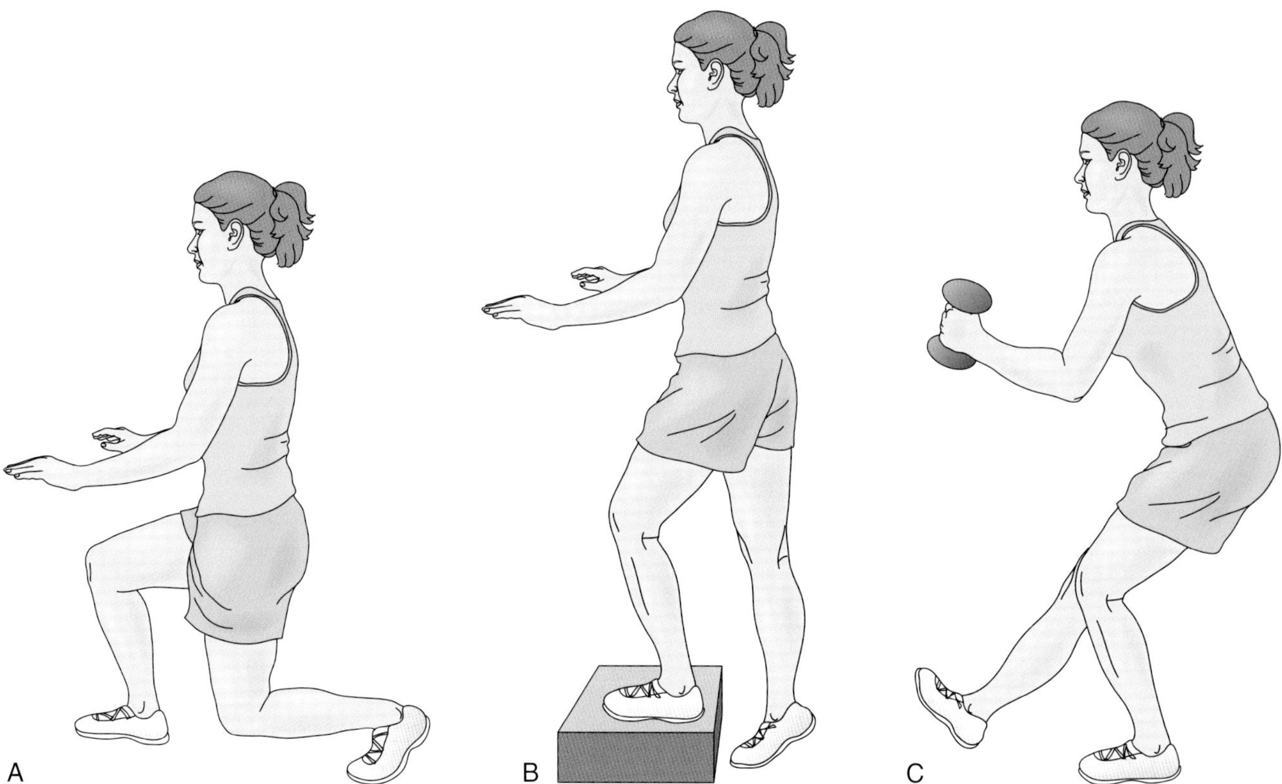

FIGURE 74.3 Skill training can help resolve anterior knee pain by improving strength and neuromuscular coordination. The lunge (**A**), step-down (**B**), and knee bend (**C**) are examples of force-absorbing skill-training exercises that are particularly valuable for improving strength, which in turn promotes stability. For the most benefit during the knee bend, the patient's knee should be aligned with the shoelaces.

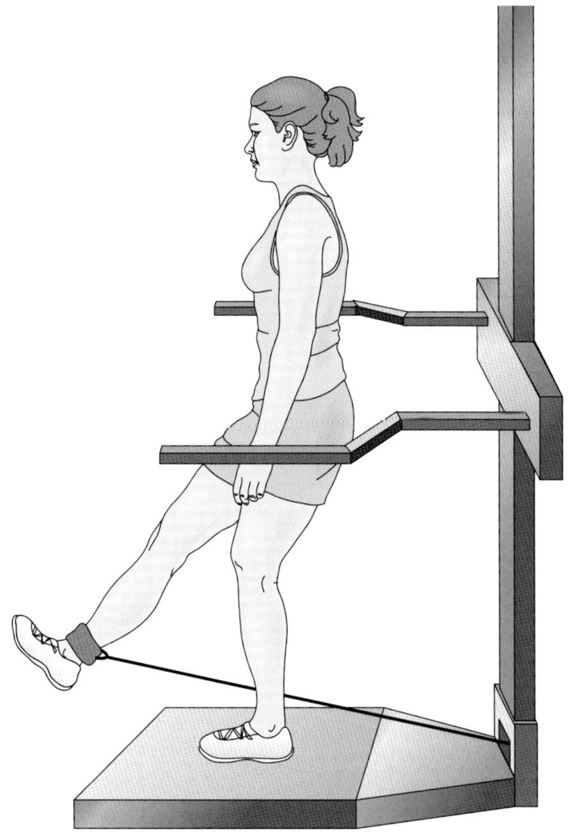

FIGURE 74.4 The standing cable column is an example of a skill-training exercise. The patient uses strength to exercise against resistance offered by a cable and simultaneously refines balancing skills.

be kept to a minimum. Systemic complication risk may be lessened by application of topical nonsteroidal anti-inflammatory drugs to the affected area only.

Overcompensation for the malalignment may occur with surgical techniques such as the lateral retinacular release. The surgeon may lyse too many fibers, leading to increased medial tracking. Many of the realignment procedures should also be reserved for the skeletally mature patient [1].

References

[1] Thomee R, Augustsson J, Karlsson J. Patellofemoral pain syndrome: a review of current issues. Sports Med 1999;28:245–62.

[2] Beckman M, Craig R, Lehman RC. Rehabilitation of patellofemoral dysfunction in the athlete. Clin Sports Med 1989;8:841–60.

[3] Powers CM. Rehabilitation of patellofemoral disorders: a critical review. J Orthop Sports Phys Ther 1998;5:345–54.

[4] Goldberg B. Patellofemoral malalignment. Pediatr Ann 1997;26:32–5.

[5] Sanchis-Alfonso V. Pathogenesis of anterior knee pain syndrome and functional patellofemoral instability in the active young. Am J Knee Surg 1999;12:29–40.

[6] Baker MM, Juhn MS. Patellofemoral pain syndrome in the female athlete. Clin Sports Med 2000;19:314–29.

[7] Papagelopoulos PJ, Sim FH. Patellofemoral pain syndrome: diagnosis and management. Orthopedics 1997;20:148–57.

[8] Cowan SM, Bennell KL, Hodges PW, et al. Delayed onset of electromyographic activity of vastus medialis obliquus relative to vastus lateralis in subjects with patellofemoral pain syndrome. Arch Phys Med Rehabil 2001;82:183–9.

[9] Balachandar V, Twycross-Lewis R, Morrissey D, et al. EMG mapping of the quadriceps in patellofemoral pain syndrome during functional activities: a pilot study. Br J Sports Med 2011;45:A14–5.

[10] Gotlin RS. Effective knee rehabilitation for anterior knee pain. J Musculoskelet Med 2000;17:421–32.

[11] Hilyard A. Recent developments in the management of patellofemoral pain. Physiotherapy 1990;76:559–65.

[12] Kannus P, Niittymaki S. Which factors predict outcome in the non-operative treatment of patellofemoral pain syndrome? A prospective follow-up study. Med Sci Sports Exerc 1993;26:289–96.
[13] Insall J, Falvo KA, Wise DW. Chondromalacia patellae. J Bone Joint Surg Am 1976;58:1–8.
[14] Juhn MS. Patellofemoral pain syndrome: a review and guidelines for treatment. Am Fam Physician 1999;60:2012–8.
[15] Press JM, Young JA. Rehabilitation of patellofemoral pain syndrome. In: Kibler WB, Herring SA, Press JM, editors. Functional rehabilitation of sports and musculoskeletal injuries. Gaithersburg, Md: Aspen; 1998. p. 254–64.
[16] Thijs Y, Pattyn E, Tiggelen DV, et al. Is hip muscle weakness a predisposing factor for patellofemoral pain in female novice runners? A prospective study. Am J Sports Med 2011;39:1877.
[17] Naslund JE. Diffusely increased bone scintigraphic uptake in patellofemoral syndrome. Br J Sports Med 2005;39:162–5.
[18] McConnell J. The management of chondromalacia patellae: a long term solution. Aust J Physiother 1986;32:215–33.
[19] Kowall MG, Kolk G, Nuber GW. Patellar taping in the treatment of patellofemoral pain. Am J Sports Med 1996;24:61–5.
[20] Larsen B. Patellar taping: a radiographic examination of the medial glide technique. Am J Sports Med 1995;23:465–71.
[21] Lan TY, Lin WP, Jiang CC, et al. Immediate effect and predictors of effectiveness of taping for patellofemoral syndrome: a prospective cohort study. Am J Sports Med 2010;38:1626.
[22] Lun VM, Wiley JP, Meeuwisse WH, Yanagawa TL. Effectiveness of patellar bracing for treatment of patellofemoral pain syndrome. Clin J Sport Med 2005;15:235–40.
[23] Barton CJ, Menz HB, Crossley KM. Clinical predictors of foot orthoses efficacy in individuals with patellofemoral pain. Med Sci Sports Exerc 2011;43:1603–10.
[24] Arroll B. Patellofemoral pain syndrome. Am J Sports Med 1997;25:207–12.
[25] Steinkamp LA. Biomechanical considerations in patellofemoral joint rehabilitation. Am J Sports Med 1993;21:438–42.
[26] Ng GY, Zhang AQ, Li CK. Biofeedback exercise improved the EMG activity ratio of the medial and lateral vasti muscles in subjects with patellofemoral pain syndrome. J Electromyogr Kinesiol 2008;18:128–33.
[27] Cowan SM, Bennell KL, Crossley KM, et al. Physical therapy alters recruitment of the vasti in patellofemoral pain syndrome. Med Sci Sports Exerc 2002;34:1879–85.

CHAPTER 75

Peroneal Neuropathy

John C. King, MD

Synonyms

Peroneal mononeuropathy
Compression neuropathy of the peroneal nerve
Peroneal palsy
Footdrop palsy
Lateral popliteal neuropathy

ICD-9 Codes

355.3	**Common peroneal neuropathy**
355.8	**Mononeuritis of lower limb, unspecified**
736.79	**Deformity of ankle and foot, also known as footdrop**

ICD-10 Codes

G62.9	**Polyneuropathy, unspecified**
G57.90	**Mononeuropathy of unspecified lower limb**
G57.91	**Mononeuropathy of right lower limb**
G57.92	**Mononeuropathy of left lower limb**
M21.371	**Foot drop, right foot**
M21.372	**Foot drop, left foot**
M21.379	**Foot drop, unspecified foot**

Definition

Peroneal neuropathy, the most common entrapment neuropathy of the lower extremity [1], is compromise of any portion of the peroneal nerve. This can be from its origins within the sciatic nerve, in which it remains distinct from the tibial portion, throughout the course of the sciatic nerve, to its terminations in the leg and foot. The common peroneal nerve completely separates from the tibial nerve in the upper popliteal fossa and then traverses laterally to curve superficially around the fibular head. Before the fibular head, the lateral cutaneous nerve of the calf branches off to supply cutaneous sensation to the upper lateral leg. Near the fibular head, the common peroneal nerve bifurcates into the superficial peroneal nerve and deep peroneal nerve, which describes their relative locations as they wrap around the fibular head. Because the deep portion is immediately adjacent to the hard bony surface, it is more susceptible to compression injuries at the fibular head, which is the most common site of peroneal nerve compromise [2,3].

The common peroneal nerve provides the lateral cutaneous nerve of the calf and the motor branch to the short head of the biceps femoris above the fibular head. The superficial peroneal nerve is predominantly sensory, providing cutaneous sensation to the lateral lower leg and most of the foot dorsum. The superficial peroneal nerve also innervates the foot evertors, peroneus longus and brevis. The deep peroneal nerve is predominantly motor, innervating the foot and toe dorsiflexors, but it has a small cutaneous representation at the dorsal first web space of the foot.

Predisposing factors for peroneal mononeuropathy at the fibular head, the most common site of compromise, include weight loss [2,4–7], diabetes [2,8], peripheral polyneuropathy [2], and positioning and localized prolonged pressure [9], such as habitual leg crossing [1] or prolonged squatting [2,10]. A history of such sustained pressure should be elicited.

Figure 75.1 shows the most common causes of acute and nonacute lesions. Iatrogenic causes should be considered. These include anesthesia for surgery, leading to immobility and possible positioning issues [9,11,12]; surgery about the hip [13–15], knee [16], or ankle [17]; prolonged imposed bed rest with decreased sensorium due to sepsis or coma [2,18]; intermittent sequential pneumatic compression [19]; acupuncture [20]; and plaster casts [2], braces, sports icing and compression wraps [21], and, ironically, ankle-foot orthoses [5,22]. A history of severe inversion ankle sprain or blunt trauma to the ankle, leg, or fibular head can be helpful in identifying likely pathophysiologic mechanisms.

Stretch injury commonly occurs at the hip region and may be associated with hip surgery (e.g., total hip arthroplasty, especially if the limb is lengthened) [13] or traumatic hip dislocation. The peroneal portion of the sciatic nerve is more susceptible to stretch injuries than the tibial portion because of its lateral position and the shorter distance between the piriformis and the fibular head than between

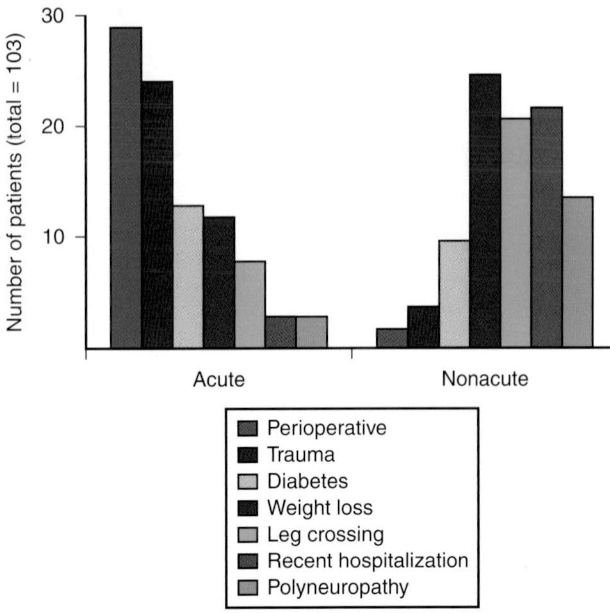

FIGURE 75.1 Predisposing factors in 103 patients with peroneal mononeuropathy divided between acute onset and nonacute onset. *(From Katirji MB, Wilbourn AJ. Common peroneal mononeuropathy: a clinical and electrophysiologic study of 116 lesions. Neurology 1988;38:1723-1728.)*

the piriformis and the tarsal tunnel (e.g., the sites of relative fixation of these two nerves). Distal peroneal nerve stretch injury can also occur at the point where it passes through the peroneus longus muscle. In addition, peroneal nerve injury is proposed to occur after stroke by equinovarus footdrop posturing [23].

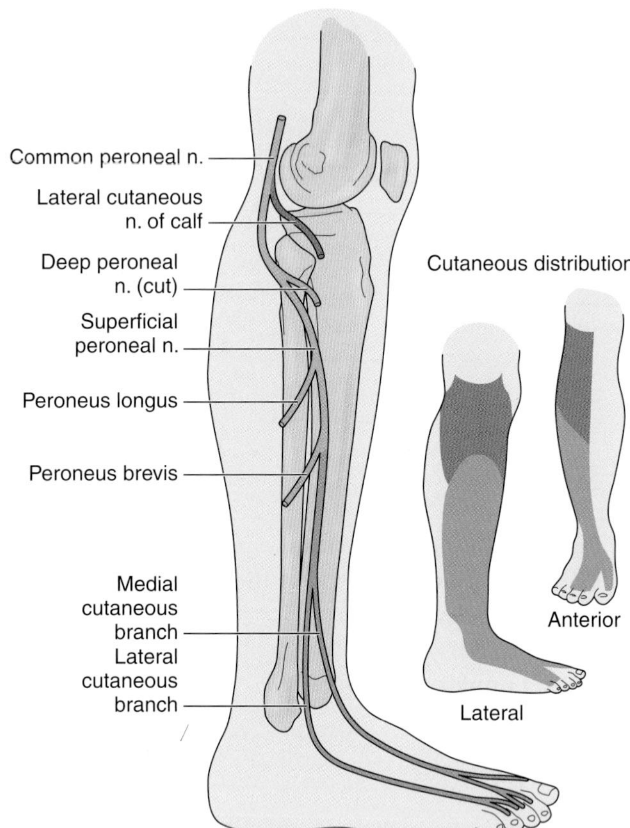

FIGURE 75.2 Common *(blue)* and superficial *(purple)* peroneal nerve branch cutaneous distributions and motor branches. *(From Haymaker W, Woodhall B. Peripheral Nerve Injuries: Principles of Diagnosis. Philadelphia, WB Saunders, 1953.)*

Symptoms

Peroneal neuropathy typically is manifested with acute footdrop, but this can sometimes occur insidiously during several days to weeks. The footdrop can be complete or partial, often with increased tripping or falls as the primary complaint. Numbness or dysesthesias frequently occur in the lower lateral leg and dorsum of the foot, although pain is uncommon. When pain is present, it is usually located around the knee and felt as deep and ill-defined [2]. When pain is prominent and neuropathic in character, stretch injury of the peroneal portion of the sciatic nerve should be considered.

Physical Examination

The examination should be guided by a close understanding of the relevant anatomy, with focused study of the elements of each component of the peroneal nerve.

Sensory deficits in the upper lateral leg (Fig. 75.2) suggest a lesion proximal to the fibular head. Testing of foot inversion, to rule out concomitant tibial nerve compromise and therefore sciatic nerve as the likely site of injury, must be performed with the foot passively slightly dorsiflexed for optimal strength testing (often the foot will initially, at rest, be in a plantar flexed position during examination as a result of the existing footdrop) because inversion is normally weak when the foot is relatively plantar flexed [1]. With the long head of the biceps femoris intact, knee flexion strength will test normal despite a compromise to the short head of the biceps femoris strength. Palpation may reveal a lack of tissue tensing where the short head of the biceps femoris should be located. This is, however, challenging to discern and helpful only in the case of acute complete proximal peroneal nerve compromise with relative sparing of the tibial-innervated hamstring muscles. The function and innervation of the long and short heads of the biceps femoris can be more accurately determined electrodiagnostically. If both are compromised, knee flexion will be weak, as will plantar flexion and toe flexion, suggesting a sciatic nerve lesion. Hip abduction strength testing has been found helpful in distinguishing peroneal neuropathy from L5 radiculopathy in patients with footdrop [24]. Muscle stretch reflexes will usually be normal unless the sciatic nerve is severely compromised, when the medial hamstring and Achilles reflexes could be reduced or absent.

Sensory deficit or dysesthesia in the lower lateral leg and over most of the dorsum of the foot suggests involvement of the superficial peroneal or this portion of the sciatic nerve (see Fig. 75.2). Eversion weakness is consistent with superficial peroneal nerve compromise. If the superficial peroneal nerve lesion is isolated, then Achilles, quadriceps, and medial hamstring muscle stretch reflexes will be normal.

If eversion is strong but dorsiflexion is very weak, a more focal deep peroneal nerve compromise is suggested. There may be sensory deficits or dysesthesias along the isolated area of the dorsum of the first web space of the foot on the affected side (Fig. 75.3). A combination of deep and

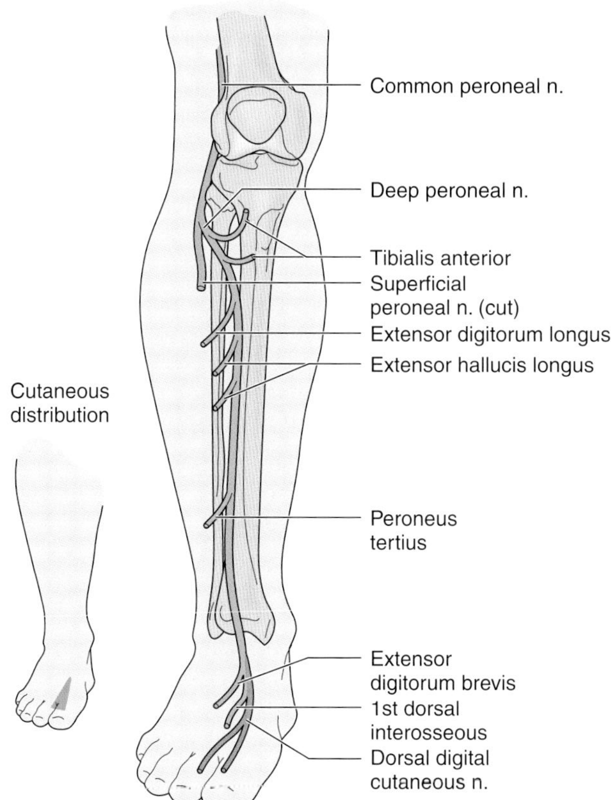

FIGURE 75.3 Deep *(blue area)* peroneal nerve cutaneous distribution and motor branches. *(From Haymaker W, Woodhall B. Peripheral Nerve Injuries: Principles of Diagnosis. Philadelphia, WB Saunders, 1953.)*

superficial peroneal nerve branch compromise often occurs, usually affecting the deep branch more severely than the superficial branch, especially with lesions at the fibular head.

Functional Limitations

The most common limitation is due to footdrop. This can lead to frequent tripping or falls and altered gait with foot slapping, circumduction, or hip hiking. These gait compensations require more energy per distance for walking and place one at a greater fall risk than if they are corrected by an ankle-foot orthosis. Any task requiring dynamic foot eversion or dorsiflexion muscle activity, such as walking and running or balance activities such as occur during lower extremity dressing, bathing, sports activities, or driving (especially when the right side is affected) [25], can be impaired.

Diagnostic Studies

Electrophysiologic studies are the "gold standard" for diagnosis of suspected peroneal neuropathy [1,26–29]. These studies can help distinguish site and severity of compromise from other possible causes of footdrop (see the section on differential diagnosis) [1,2,26]. This includes both sensory nerve conduction studies of the superficial peroneal nerve and motor nerve conduction studies of the common, deep, and superficial peroneal nerve to the functionally deficient muscles, such as the tibialis anterior or peroneus longus. Although the peroneal motor nerve is commonly studied to the extensor digitorum brevis for polyneuropathy screening, this is not the targeted muscle to evaluate footdrop, or dorsiflexion weakness, as the tibialis anterior is the more relevant and germane motor conduction study [2,26]. Needle electromyography, especially of the short head of the biceps femoris, can help determine if the lesion is proximal to the fibular head. Additional prognostic and severity data can be obtained by needle study as well as by comparison nerve conduction studies between the involved and uninvolved sides.

If the etiology cannot be determined with reasonable certainty, imaging studies can help identify less common, nontraumatic causes of peroneal neuropathy. These include ganglia [30], nerve tumors (primary nerve sheath, benign or malignant, or metastatic tumors with invasion or compression) [29], hematomas (especially with anticoagulation or bleeding dyscrasias) [2], aneurysms [31], venous thromboses [32,33], and knee osteoarthritis [34,35]. The most common imaging study is magnetic resonance imaging along the course of the nerve [13,36–38], but imaging studies could include plain radiography or ultrasonography, which is becoming more widely available and used [30,39–42].

Differential Diagnosis

Cerebral lesions, especially midline cortical
Spinal cord lesions, Brown-Séquard syndrome
Lumbosacral radiculopathy, especially L5
Lumbosacral plexopathy
Compartment syndromes in the leg (especially anterior compartment)
Acute or subacute polyneuropathy
Motor neuron disease

Treatment

Initial

Treatment depends on lesion site and prognostic factors found on electrophysiologic studies. If a good prognosis is predicted, watchful waiting is indicated with temporary adaptations and preventive measures to minimize functional impact until complete recovery occurs. Removal of pressure to the involved area is important, and this may require bed rail modifications or protective padding around the knees, especially for sleep. Work or sports activities and clothing that could result in pressure to the involved areas should be assessed and modified to eliminate any unnecessary pressure or padding added to minimize blunt trauma effects. Habitual leg crossers must modify this behavior. With pressure relief, neurapraxic injuries often significantly improve by 6 weeks. If the lesion is more axon stretch, recovery can take much longer, as much as a day for each millimeter that the axon must regrow. Completely denervated muscles need reinnervation by 18 months for recovery; the higher the lesion, the more likely a poor outcome will result for distal muscles. If prognosis is poor, such as with a severe high sciatic nerve injury, longer term adaptations and home preventive programs should be planned, as well as possible surgical considerations, especially in children [43].

If pain is neuropathic in nature (burning, tingling, or associated with hyperpathia), neuropathic pain medications such as the anticonvulsants or tricyclic antidepressants should be considered. These must be started in low dosage, taken routinely, and slowly titrated up; a steady-state level is needed to help block the new aberrant sodium channels of injured nerves, which is one mechanism by which these medications decrease neuropathic pain. These medications are not used on an as-needed basis like other more typical analgesics. When they are effective, the neuropathic pain medications tend to continue to be effective chronically and are often needed 6 months to 2 years, if not indefinitely [44].

Rehabilitation

Adaptive devices include an ankle-foot orthosis, which can be a simple, fixed-ankle, off-the-shelf model if no other comorbidities exist. This brace helps with footdrop and improves foot clearance during the leg swing-through phase of gait. If the peroneal neuropathy occurs in isolation, then no plantar sensory loss is present, and concerns for contact pressure of skin to orthosis are lessened. If the patient presents with comorbid tibial nerve deficits, custom molding of the ankle-foot orthosis to minimize contact pressures to the skin should be considered. If the prognosis is poor or recovery not forthcoming, the addition of dorsiflexion assist to the ankle-foot orthosis may help restore an even more normal gait than is achievable with a fixed ankle. With significant obesity or edema or in the face of severe polyneuropathy requiring special accommodative shoe wear, a dual upright ankle-foot orthosis may be indicated. The addition of dorsiflexion assist can easily be accomplished by adding springs to the posterior channels of a dual upright ankle-foot orthosis. The addition of dorsiflexion assist may be mandatory if the patient is having difficulty driving and right foot involvement is the cause. Most patients will have a stable and safe gait with an ankle-foot orthosis without additional gait aids, such as walkers, crutches, or canes; but when needed, gait training with any necessary gait aids should be ordered through physical therapy.

Because of the unbalanced weakness of the dorsiflexors, the lesser or unopposed plantar flexors must be actively stretched on a daily basis to prevent contracture development, which can occur in a matter of weeks. Similarly, the inverters may also need to be stretched in a home exercise program if the eversion function has been compromised. Splinting can also assist with contracture prevention and treatment.

As the muscle recovers function, which may occur during a few months if it is due to axonotmetic compression at the fibular head, strengthening can be initiated once manual muscle strength greater than 3/5 (antigravity strength but unable to take any resistance) returns. It is probably not prudent to exercise the newly reinnervated muscle to exhaustion, but moderate strengthening can be well tolerated. Patients may begin household ambulation without their ankle-foot orthoses before going long community distances. Patients should be advised to use their ankle-foot orthoses whenever prolonged walking is anticipated, even when manual muscle testing initially reveals 5/5 strength, because of early fatigue on initial strengthening.

Procedures

Although common peroneal neuropathy at the fibular head is rarely complicated by severe pain, sciatic or more distal superficial peroneal nerve stretch with axonotmesis can result in neuropathic pain. Medications focused on neuropathic pain are the mainstays of treatment, but additional nerve block is occasionally needed to resolve the associated pain adequately [44].

Surgery

When expected improvement does not occur or imaging studies reveal structures creating possible compromise of the nerve's function, surgical exploration, compression relief, or neurotomy or resection of compromising tumors, synovial cysts or ganglia, or other structures may be needed [45–47]. For poor-prognosis, high sciatic near-complete or complete peroneal lesions, a new technique of transplanting some tibial nerve elements into the denervated tibialis anterior muscle has been successful, especially in children, in restoring function where previous footdrop existed [43]. Tendon transfers have also been used with variable success [45].

Potential Disease Complications

A common complication of peroneal neuropathy is footdrop and its deleterious effects on gait and balance, leading to falls and additional trauma. The sensory impairments place portions of the lateral leg and foot dorsum at risk for pressure ulcers or acute injuries that are not adequately treated because of lack of pain and sensation in those areas. If range of motion of the ankle is not adequately addressed, ankle contractures can result, further impairing gait and ankle-foot orthosis use.

Potential Treatment Complications

Any surgical treatment has the potential for infection, excessive bleeding, anesthetic death, and making the condition worse. Procedures likewise could worsen the condition and are used only when pain is intolerable and recalcitrant to medication interventions. Pain medications are most typically neuropathic pain–focused medications, such as tricyclic antidepressants (e.g., amitriptyline) and anticonvulsants (e.g., gabapentin). These have unique contraindications and side effect profiles. These medications must be initiated at a low dose and built up over time to minimize the occurrence of side effects. They are not used in an as-needed fashion like the more typical analgesics (such as nonsteroidal anti-inflammatory drugs) or opioids. Opioids tend to be less often used because of the chronic and neuropathic nature of most associated pain. Nonsteroidal anti-inflammatory and opioid drugs also have unique side effect profiles. Physical dependence and development of tolerance with opioids must be considered because the neuropathic pain from peroneal nerve lesions is most often a chronic issue.

References

[1] Masakado Y, Kawakami M, Suzuki K, et al. Clinical neurophysiology in the diagnosis of peroneal nerve palsy. Keio J Med 2008;57:84–9.
[2] Katirji B. Peroneal neuropathy. Neurol Clin 1999;17:567–91.
[3] Baima J, Krivickas L. Evaluation and treatment of peroneal neuropathy. Curr Rev Musculoskelet Med 2008;1:147–53.
[4] Cruz-Martinez A, Arpa J, Palau F. Peroneal neuropathy after weight loss. J Peripher Nerv Syst 2000;5:101–5.

[5] Elias WJ, Pouratian F, Oskouian RJ, et al. Peroneal neuropathy following successful bariatric surgery: case report and review of the literature. J Neurosurg 2006;105:631–5.

[6] Weyns FJ, Beckers F, Vanormelingen L, et al. Foot drop as a complication of weight loss after bariatric surgery: is it preventable? Obes Surg 2007;17:1209–12.

[7] Milants C, Lempereur S, Dubuisson A. Bilateral peroneal neuropathy following bariatric surgery. Neurochirurgie 2013;59:50–2.

[8] Stamboulis E, Vassilopoulos D, Kalfakis N. Symptomatic focal mononeuropathies in diabetic patients: increased or not? J Neurol 2005;252:448–52.

[9] Tacconi P, Manca D, Tamburini G, et al. Bed footboard peroneal and tibial neuropathy. A further unusual type of Saturday night palsy. J Peripher Nerv Syst 2004;9:54–6.

[10] Toğrol E. Bilateral peroneal nerve palsy induced by prolonged squatting. Mil Med 2000;165:240–2.

[11] Wang J, Wong T, Chen J, et al. Bilateral sciatic neuropathy as a complication of craniotomy performed in the sitting position: localization of nerve injury by using magnetic resonance imaging. Childs Nerv Syst 2012;28:159–63.

[12] Lederman RJ, Breuer AC, Hanson MR, et al. Peripheral nervous system complications of coronary artery bypass graft surgery. Ann Neurol 1982;12:297–301.

[13] Edwards BN, Tullos HS, Noble PC. Contributory factors and etiology of sciatic nerve palsy in total hip arthroplasty. Clin Orthop Relat Res 1987;218:136.

[14] Justice PE, Bashar K, Preston DC, Grossman GE. Piriformis syndrome surgery causing severe sciatic nerve injury. J Clin Neuromuscul Dis 2012;14:45–7.

[15] Mall NA, Schoenecker PL, Goldfarb CA. Bilateral peroneal nerve palsy after bilateral hip osteotomy in a patient with multiple hereditary exostosis: a case report and review of the literature. JBJS Case Connector 2012;2:1–4.

[16] Asp L, Jonathan P, Rand J. Peroneal nerve palsy after total knee arthroplasty. Clin Orthop Relat Res 1990;261:233–7.

[17] Lui TH, Chan V. Deep peroneal nerve injury following external fixation of the ankle: case report and anatomic study. Foot Ankle Int 2011;32:S550–5.

[18] Aprile I, Padua L, Padua R, et al. Peroneal mononeuropathy: predisposing factors, and clinical and neurophysiological relationships. Neurol Sci 2000;21:367–71.

[19] McGrory BJ, Burke DW. Peroneal nerve palsy following intermittent sequential pneumatic compression. Orthopedics 2000;23:1103–5.

[20] Sato M, Katsumoto H, Kawamura K, et al. Peroneal nerve palsy following acupuncture treatment. J Bone Joint Surg Am 2003;85:916–8.

[21] Babwah T. Common peroneal neuropathy related to cryotherapy and compression in a footballer. Res Sports Med 2010;19:66–71.

[22] Ryan MM, Darras BT, Soul JS. Peroneal neuropathy from ankle-foot orthoses. Pediatr Neurol 2003;29:72–4.

[23] Tsur A. Common peroneal neuropathy in patients after first-time stroke. Isr Med Assoc J 2007;9:866–9.

[24] Jeon C, Chung N, Lee Y, et al. Assessment of hip abductor power in patients with foot drop: a simple and useful test to differentiate lumbar radiculopathy and peroneal neuropathy. Spine (Phila Pa 1976) 2013;38:257–63.

[25] Fann AV. Peroneal neuropathy. In: Frontera WR, Silver JK, editors. Essentials of physical medicine and rehabilitation. Philadelphia: Hanley & Belfus; 2002. p. 363–6.

[26] Wilbourn AJ. AAEE case report #12: common peroneal mononeuropathy at the fibular head. Muscle Nerve 1986;9:825–36.

[27] Marciniak C, Armon C, Wilson J, Miller R. Practice parameter: utility of electrodiagnostic techniques in evaluating patients with suspected peroneal neuropathy: an evidence-based review. Muscle Nerve 2005;31:520–7.

[28] Marciniak C. Fibular (peroneal) neuropathy: electrodiagnostic features and clinical correlates. Phys Med Rehabil Clin N Am 2013;24:121–37.

[29] Aregawi DG, Sherman JH, Douvas MG, et al. Neuroleukemiosis: case report of leukemic nerve infiltration in acute lymphoblastic leukemia. Muscle Nerve 2008;38:1196–2000.

[30] Visser LH. High resolution sonography of the common peroneal nerve: detection of intraneural ganglia. Neurology 2006;67:1473–5.

[31] Jan SH, Lee H, Seung Hoon H. Common peroneal nerve compression by a popliteal venous aneurysm. Am J Phys Med Rehabil 2009;88:947–50.

[32] Yamamoto N, Koyano K. Neurovascular compression of the common peroneal nerve by varicose veins. Eur J Vasc Endovasc Surg 2004;28:335–8.

[33] Bendszus M, Reiners K, Perez J, et al. Peroneal nerve palsy caused by thrombosis of crural veins. Neurology 2002;58:1675–7.

[34] Flores LP, Koerbel A, Tatagiba M. Peroneal nerve compression resulting from fibular head osteophyte-like lesions. Surg Neurol 2005;64:249–52.

[35] Fetzer GB, Prather H, Gelberman RH, Clohisy JC. Progressive peroneal nerve palsy in a varus arthritic knee. J Bone Joint Surg Am 2004;86:1538–40.

[36] Iverson DJ. MRI detection of cysts of the knee causing common peroneal neuropathy. Neurology 2005;65:1829–31.

[37] Vieira RLR, Rosenberg ZS, Kiprovski K. MRI of the distal biceps femoris muscle: normal anatomy, variants, and association with common peroneal entrapment neuropathy. AJR Am J Roentgenol 2007;189:549–55.

[38] Lee PP, Chalian M, Bizzell C, et al. Magnetic resonance neurography of common peroneal (fibular) neuropathy. J Comput Assist Tomogr 2012;36:455–61.

[39] Gruber H, Peer S, Meirer R, Bodner G. Peroneal nerve palsy associated with knee luxation: evaluation by sonography—initial experiences. AJR Am J Roentgenol 2005;185:1119–25.

[40] Padua L, Aprile I, Pazzaglia C, et al. Contribution of ultrasound in a neurophysiological lab in diagnosing nerve impairment: a one-year systematic assessment. Clin Neurophysiol 2007;118:1410–6.

[41] Lo YL, Fook-Chong S, Leoh TH, et al. High resolution ultrasound as a diagnostic adjunct in common peroneal neuropathy. Arch Neurol 2007;64:1798–800.

[42] Visser LH, Hens V, Soethout M, et al. The diagnostic value of high-resolution sonography in common fibular neuropathy at the fibular head. Muscle Nerve 2013;48:171–8.

[43] Gousheh J, Babaei A. A new surgical technique for the treatment of high common peroneal nerve palsy. Plast Reconstr Surg 2002;109:994–8.

[44] Menefee Pujol LA, Katz NP, Zacharoff KL. Pain syndromes from peripheral nerve injury and neurolysis. PainEDU.org Manual. Newton, Mass: Inflexxion; 2007, 78, 79, 141.

[45] Kim DH, Murovic JA, Tiel RL, Kline DG. Management and outcomes in 318 operative common peroneal nerve lesions. Neurosurgery 2004;54:1421–8.

[46] Thoma A, Fawcett S, Ginty M, Veltri K. Decompression of the common peroneal nerve. Plast Reconstr Surg 2001;107:1183–8.

[47] Hersekli MA, Akpinar S, Demirors H, et al. Synovial cysts of proximal tibiofibular joint causing peroneal nerve palsy: report of three cases and review of the literature. Arch Orthop Trauma Surg 2004;124:711–4.

CHAPTER 76

Posterior Cruciate Ligament Sprain

Farshad Adib, MD
Christine Curtis, MD
Peter Bienkowski, MD
Lyle J. Micheli, MD

Synonym

Posterior cruciate ligament tear

ICD-9 Codes

717.84 Old disruption of posterior cruciate ligament
844.2 Acute posterior cruciate ligament tear

ICD-10 Codes

M23.621 Spontaneous disruption of posterior cruciate ligament of right knee
M23.622 Spontaneous disruption of posterior cruciate ligament of left knee
M23.629 Spontaneous disruption of posterior cruciate ligament of unspecified knee
S83.521 Sprain of posterior cruciate ligament of right knee
S83.522 Sprain of posterior cruciate ligament of left knee
S83.529 Sprain of posterior cruciate ligament of unspecified knee
Add seventh character to category S83 for episode of care (A—initial encounter, D—subsequent encounter, S—sequela)

Definition

Posterior cruciate ligament (PCL) tears represent 5% to 38% of all knee ligament injuries [1,2]. The PCL is an intra-articular but extrasynovial structure that arises from the posterior aspect of the tibial plateau (about 1 cm distal to the joint line), crosses ("cruciate") behind the anterior cruciate ligament (ACL), and inserts into the lateral portion of the medial femoral condyle (Fig. 76.1). The main function of the PCL is to resist posterior displacement of the tibia on the femur. It also acts as a secondary restraint to external tibial rotation. The PCL also has some restraint against varus and valgus forces. The larger and stronger anterolateral bundle is tight in flexion, whereas the posteromedial bundle is tight in extension. The anterior meniscofemoral ligament (Humphry) and posterior meniscofemoral ligament (Wrisberg) make a Y-shaped sling around the PCL [3]. The average distance between the center of the femoral attachments of anterolateral and posteromedial bundles is 12.1 ± 1.3 mm; this distance on the tibial side is 8.9 ± 1.2 mm [4].

Together with the ACL, the PCL functions in the "screw-home" mechanism of the knee by which the tibia glides to its exact position at terminal knee extension. In general, PCL tears occur in a flexed knee when the tibia is displaced posteriorly. This can occur in a motor vehicle accident (dashboard injury) or during a fall on a flexed knee with the foot in plantar flexion. The PCL may also rupture from hyperextension and rotation on a planted foot or on forced hyperflexion. PCL injuries may occur in isolation, but they generally occur with other injuries (e.g., ACL tear, collateral ligament tear, and meniscal injuries).

In a chronic PCL-deficient knee, an increase of force on the medial and patellofemoral compartments might lead to development of early degenerative arthritis [5]. In contrast to ACL injuries, most series of PCL injuries have reported a higher incidence of injury to men [6]. Fewer studies have been done about PCL injuries in comparison to ACL injuries.

Symptoms

It is important to obtain information about the nature of the injury. Typically, patients report that they have fallen on a flexed knee or have sustained a blow to the anterior knee when it was flexed (e.g., on the dashboard of a car). Rarely, patients may recall feeling or hearing a "pop" at the time of injury (more common in ACL tear). Patients may

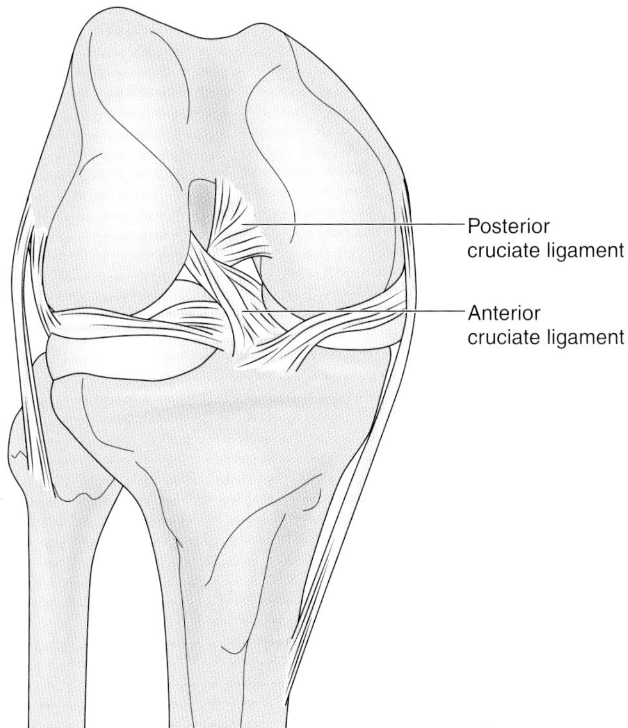

FIGURE 76.1 Anterior and posterior cruciate ligament structures.

Table 76.1 Classification of Posterior Cruciate Ligament Injuries

Grade	Definition	Laxity (mm)
I	PCL partially torn	<5
II	PCL partially torn	5-9
III	PCL completely torn	>10
IVa	PCL and LCL, posterolateral injury	>12
IVb	PCL and MCL, posteromedial injury	>12
IVc	PCL and ACL injury	>15

Note: grades I to III are isolated injuries; grade IV is a combined injury. *ACL*, anterior cruciate ligament; *LCL*, lateral collateral ligament; *MCL*, medial collateral ligament; PCL, posterior cruciate ligament.
Modified from Janousek AT, Jones DG, Clatworthy M, et al. Posterior cruciate ligament injuries of the knee joint. Sports Med 1999;28:429-441.

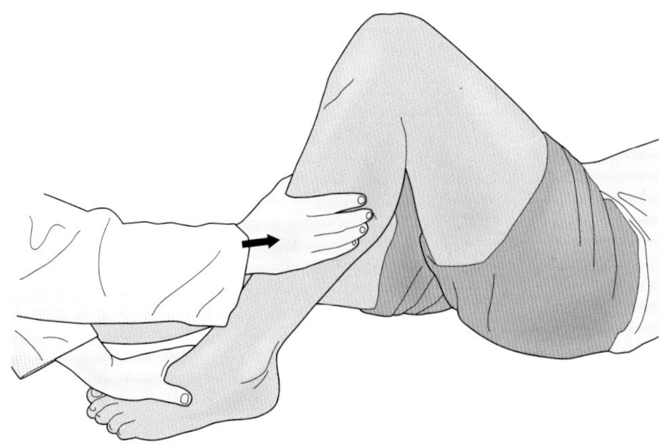

FIGURE 76.2 Posterior drawer test.

have pain in the posterior aspect of the knee in the acute cases or along the medial or patellofemoral region in the chronic cases.

Patients may report instability, stiffness, and an inability to bear weight and to walk. Swelling can range from insignificant to very swollen.

Physical Examination

In an acute injury, there may be contusion of the anterior tibia, and popliteal ecchymosis may be present. Swelling and effusion will vary and may not be present at all. Limb alignment, gait pattern, and range of motion should be evaluated. See Table **76.1** for the general classifications of PCL injuries. It has been shown that a grade III on posterior drawer testing and posterior tibial translation on stress radiography of more than 10 mm correlate with the presence of a posterolateral corner injury in addition to a complete disruption of the PCL [7].

It is essential during the examination of the knee to evaluate all knee ligaments thoroughly to identify combined ligamentous injuries. The goal of PCL evaluation is to identify posterior subluxation of the tibia, which occurs with PCL insufficiency.

The "gold standard" of PCL examination is the posterior drawer test (Fig. 76.2). During this test, the knee is flexed at 90 degrees with the hip held at 45 degrees of flexion. It is essential to appreciate a normal 1-cm step-off of the medial tibial plateau anterior to the medial femoral condyle. The absence of the step-off should alert the clinician to a possibility of PCL injury. Posterior pressure is applied to the tibia while the amount of displacement of the medial tibial step-off and the quality of the endpoint in comparison with the contralateral knee are noted. Posterolateral instability may be evaluated by the posterior drawer test with the foot externally rotated 15 degrees. Similarly, posteromedial instability is assessed by the posterior drawer test with the foot internally rotated 15 degrees.

The posterior Lachman test involves positioning of the knee at 30 degrees of flexion with posterior pressure applied to the proximal tibia (Fig. 76.3). The extent of displacement and the quality of the endpoint are evaluated and compared with the contralateral knee.

The posterior sag test is performed with the patient supine with the hips and knees at 90 degrees of flexion (Fig. 76.4). The clinician grasps both heels and inspects for posterior tibial translation consistent with an insufficient PCL.

The reverse pivot shift includes a valgus-loaded, externally rotated knee moved from 90 degrees of flexion to full extension (Fig. 76.5). A positive test result is indicated by a pivot shift felt at 20 to 30 degrees when the posteriorly subluxated tibia is reduced.

The dynamic posterior shift test is implemented by extending the knee from 90 degrees of flexion to full extension with 90 degrees of hip flexion. A positive result is indicated if the tibia is reduced with a "clunk" near full extension.

The quadriceps active test is achieved with the knee flexed at 60 degrees while the foot is secured by the clinician.

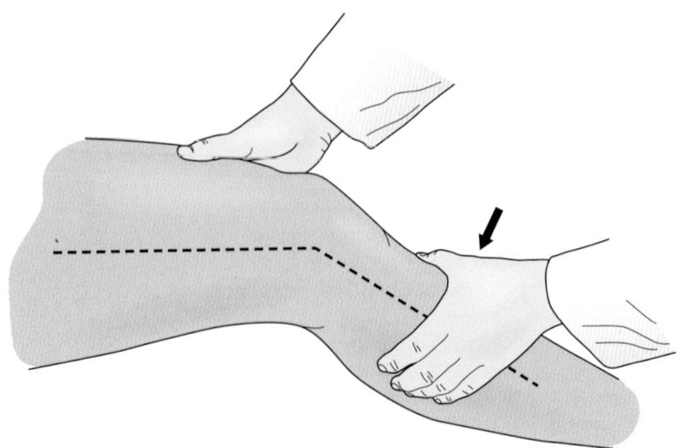

FIGURE 76.3 Correct position for posterior Lachman test.

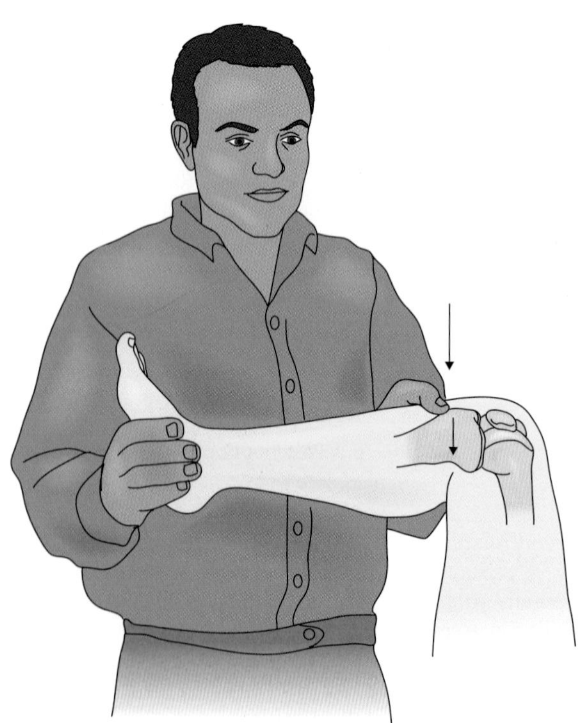

FIGURE 76.4 Posterior tibial sag test.

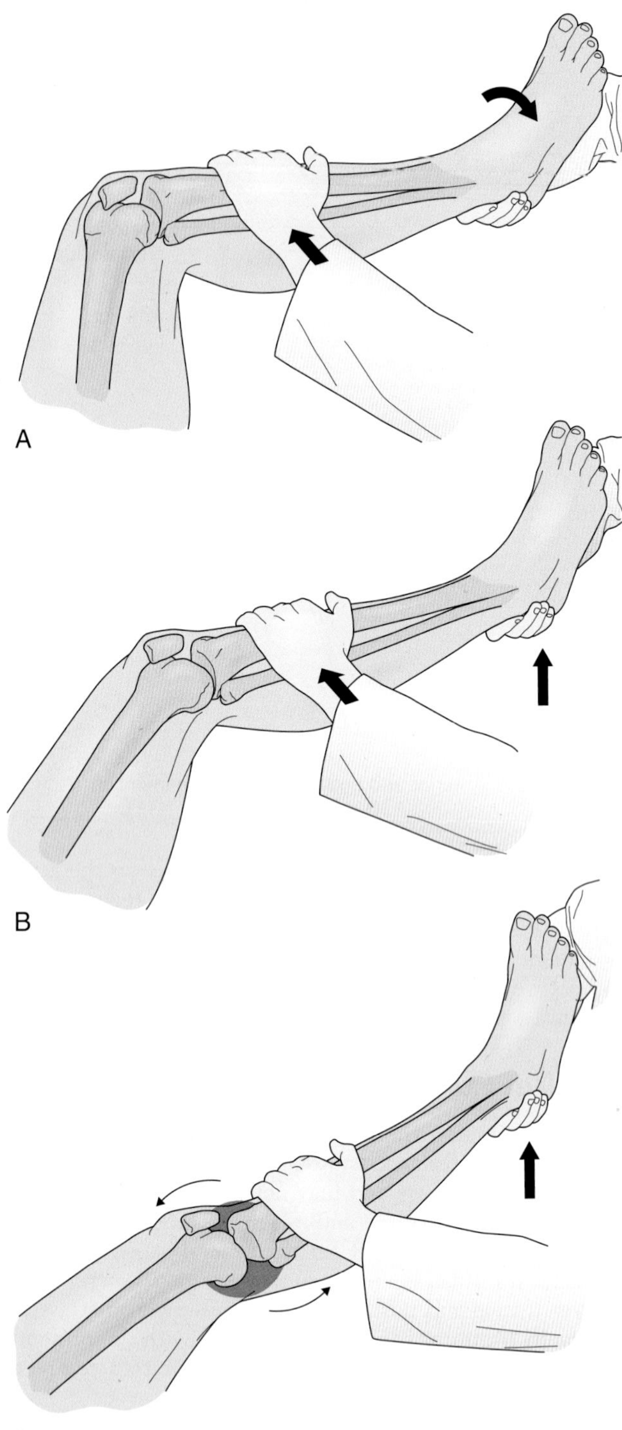

FIGURE 76.5 Reverse pivot shift test. **A,** The knee is flexed to 90 degrees. A valgus, external rotation force is applied to the knee. **B,** The knee is extended while the valgus, external rotation is maintained. **C,** Near full extension, the lateral tibia shifts forward, reducing the knee and confirming PCL deficiency.

The patient attempts to extend the knee statically. PCL insufficiency is demonstrated by anterior tibial translation from a subluxated position.

A careful neurovascular examination should be performed to rule out any injury to the popliteal artery and tibial and peroneal nerves. Some weakness of muscle may be detected because of pain or inactivity. Physical examination under anesthesia is a critical step before reconstruction.

Functional Limitations

Functional limitations of PCL tears may include difficulty with walking and a decrease in the level of functioning because of pain as well as apprehension of instability. Athletes may be unable to complete cutting movements. However, PCL injury is often less debilitating than ACL injury, and many athletes are still able to participate effectively in running sports. Return to sport after treatment of PCL injury is common, but in the majority of cases, development of degenerative changes is inevitable [8].

Diagnostic Studies

Diagnostic testing is useful as an adjunct to the clinical examination. The KT-1000 arthrometer is highly specific in the detection of high-grade (grade II, grade III) PCL tears [9]. Stress radiographs may document the extent of posterior instability but are rarely obtained in settings where magnetic resonance imaging is readily available. After an acute injury, plain radiographs must be performed to rule out fractures, including PCL avulsions (the tunnel view is best to visualize this). Magnetic resonance imaging assessment is highly specific and sensitive in assessment of PCL injuries, particularly when newer fat suppression and "fast spin" techniques are used [10–12]. Finally, diagnostic arthroscopy allows direct visualization of the PCL.

Differential Diagnosis

Anterior cruciate ligament tear
Collateral ligament tear
Meniscal tear
Osteochondral fracture
Patellar tendon rupture
Patellofemoral dislocation
Tibial plateau fracture

Treatment

Initial

Initial treatment consists of *p*rotection, *r*est, *i*ce, *c*ompression, and *e*levation (PRICE), crutches, an extension brace, and short-term nonsteroidal anti-inflammatory drugs. Analgesics may be used to control pain if this is an issue. Currently, nonoperative treatment is advocated for those with isolated PCL injuries with mild (grade I or grade II) laxity [9]. Some recommend conservative treatment for acute, isolated PCL injury as well as for chronic, isolated, asymptomatic PCL injury when it is newly diagnosed with no history of prior rehabilitation [13]. Subjective scores of patients with acute, isolated PCL injuries were independent of grade of PCL laxity, and mean scores did not decrease with time from injury [14].

Rehabilitation

Nonoperative rehabilitation begins after the signs and symptoms of acute injury have subsided (7 to 10 days). Range of motion and progressive resistance exercise for the quadriceps is initiated while posterior tibial sag is prevented. The use of a PCL functional brace has not been proved to be effective, although some patients may find it useful [15]. After acute symptoms have subsided, or immediately in dealing with a chronic tear, daily stationary bicycle exercises can be initiated. After 3 months, closed chain exercises are started, with the exception of isolated hamstring strengthening, which is done later in the course [16].

Postoperative PCL rehabilitation includes initial bracing in full extension to prevent posterior tibial translation. Continuous passive motion, straight-leg raising, and quadriceps static exercises are initiated immediately after surgery. The day after surgery, partial weight bearing with crutches is initiated as tolerated. In the early phase of rehabilitation, gravity-assisted flexion exercises to 90 degrees and closed chain exercises emphasizing quadriceps muscle strengthening are pursued. The progression to more than 90 degrees of flexion is delayed until 6 weeks after surgery. Rehabilitation after PCL reconstruction is more conservative than after ACL reconstruction.

Two studies by Italian investigators have documented the frequent clinical observation that the PCL, in contrast to the ACL, can undergo in situ healing of partial lesions, with improved stability and function [17–19]. This has been attributed to the capsular contiguity of the ligament, with better opportunity for revascularization than in the ACL [1]. It is thus imperative that the ligament be protected from undue stress during the rehabilitative phase of treatment. Intact meniscofemoral ligaments may support the injured PCL during the healing phase. This scaffold effect of meniscofemoral ligaments could be another reason for the healing potential of PCL injuries. At 9 to 12 months after surgical intervention, the patient with full range of motion, equal strength compared with the contralateral leg, and a stable knee is allowed to return to full activity.

Procedures

Arthrocentesis is performed for painful effusions (hemarthrosis). As mentioned earlier, KT-1000 arthrometer testing is done for diagnostic purposes and to document the degree of instability [9].

Surgery

Surgical intervention is advocated for patients with bone avulsion fractures, combined ligament injuries, and chronic symptomatic PCL laxity, particularly if this interferes with athletic participation in elite athletes [15]. In a high percentage of cases, athletic participation is still possible with PCL insufficiency [6]. Management includes immobilization in extension with a Velcro knee immobilizer and avoidance of hamstring exercise. It is important to keep in mind that grade III PCL injury almost always is associated with the posterolateral corner injury, which must be addressed at the time of PCL reconstruction to obtain a good clinical result.

Bone avulsions are best treated with anatomic repair, either by open technique with screws or by an arthroscopic method with anchor sutures [20]. Various surgical techniques have been developed for the reconstruction of the PCL. Controversy exists as to the most effective procedure [16]. The aim of surgery is to replace the PCL with a graft inserted into a tunnel drilled through the tibia and femur. Allograft or autograft tissue is most commonly used. Donor sites include the patellar tendon, the hamstring tendons, and, rarely, the quadriceps tendon [21]. Achilles tendon allograft is also useful. A mixed graft consisting of a hamstring (semitendinosus and gracilis) autograft plus tibialis anterior allograft tendon has been used with good results [22]. PCL reconstruction with artificial ligament is an alternative treatment option [23]. PCL reconstruction is performed arthroscopically, arthroscopically assisted, or open [13]. In the presence of significant bone malalignment, it should be addressed simultaneously or as the first step before the reconstruction. Proximal tibial slope should be considered in treating combined PCL and posterolateral corner injuries of the knee. It has been shown that increasing posterior tibial slope may improve sagittal stability in the PCL- and posterolateral corner–deficient knee [24].

Potential Disease Complications

Potential disease complications include pain, limitation of function and activity, and onset of degenerative arthritis. Patients with isolated PCL tears tend to fare better than do patients with combined ligamentous injuries [25]. Studies suggest that nonoperatively treated PCL injuries allow many athletes to return to their sport independent of level of laxity [25]. However, late degenerative arthritis has been reported as a consequence of PCL instability [26].

Potential Treatment Complications

Treatment complications include the well-known side effects of nonsteroidal anti-inflammatory drugs. Prolonged bracing or immobilization can lead to significant muscle weakness and atrophy. The risks of surgery, although uncommon, are also well known. These include the risks of anesthesia. In addition, bleeding is controlled with a tourniquet and surgical hemostasis. Infection is limited with diligent sterile technique as well as with antibiotics. Damage to nerve and vascular structures, the popliteal vessels in particular, is a slight risk. Postoperative laxity of the PCL graft may occur. The theoretical risk of disease transmission with the use of allograft tissues is extremely low.

References

[1] Kannus P, Bergfeld J, Jarvinen M, et al. Injuries to the posterior cruciate ligament of the knee. Sports Med 1991;12:110–31.
[2] Fanelli GC, Edson CJ. Posterior cruciate ligament injuries in trauma patients: part II. Arthroscopy 1995;1:526–9.
[3] Amis AA, Gupte CM, Bull AM, Edwards A. Anatomy of the posterior cruciate ligament and the meniscofemoral ligaments. Knee Surg Sports Traumatol Arthrosc 2006;14:257–63.
[4] Anderson CJ, Ziegler CG, Wijdicks CA, et al. Arthroscopically pertinent anatomy of the anterolateral and posteromedial bundles of the posterior cruciate ligament. J Bone Joint Surg Am 2012;94:1936–45.
[5] Janousek AT, Jones DG, Clatworthy M, et al. Posterior cruciate ligament injuries of the knee joint. Sports Med 1999;28:429–41.
[6] Parolie JM, Bergfeld JA. Long-term results of nonoperative treatment of isolated posterior cruciate ligament injuries in the athlete. Am J Sports Med 1986;14:35–8.
[7] Sekiya JK, Whiddon DR, Zehms CT, Miller MD. A clinically relevant assessment of posterior cruciate ligament and posterolateral corner injuries. Evaluation of isolated and combined deficiency. J Bone Joint Surg Am 2008;90:1621–7.
[8] Rosenthal MD, Rainey CE, Tognoni A, Worms R. Evaluation and management of posterior cruciate ligament injuries. Phys Ther Sport 2012;13:196–208.
[9] Rubinstein Jr RA, Shelbourne KD, McCarroll JR, et al. The accuracy of the clinical examination in the setting of posterior cruciate ligament injuries. Am J Sports Med 1994;22:550–7.
[10] Gross ML, Grover JS, Bassett LW, et al. Magnetic resonance imaging of the posterior cruciate ligament: clinical use to improve diagnostic accuracy. Am J Sports Med 1992;20:732–7.
[11] Schaefer F, Schaefer P, Brossmann J, et al. Value of fat-suppressed PD-weighted TSE-sequences for detection of anterior and posterior cruciate ligament lesions—comparison to arthroscopy. Eur J Radiol 2006;58:411–5.
[12] Ilaslan H, Sundaram M, Miniaci A. Imaging evaluation of the postoperative knee ligaments. Eur J Radiol 2005;54:178–88.
[13] Margheritini F, Mariani PF, Mariani PP. Current concepts in diagnosis and treatment of posterior cruciate ligament injury. Acta Orthop Belg 2000;66:217–28.
[14] Shelbourne KD, Muthukaruppan Y. Subjective results of nonoperatively treated, acute, isolated posterior cruciate ligament injuries. Arthroscopy 2005;21:457–61.
[15] St. Pierre P, Miller MD. Posterior cruciate ligament injuries. Clin Sports Med 1999;18:199–221.
[16] Barber FA, Fanelli GC, Matthews LS, et al. The treatment of complete posterior cruciate ligament tears. Arthroscopy 2000;16:725–31.
[17] Bellelli A, Mancini P, Polito M, et al. Magnetic resonance imaging of posterior cruciate ligament injuries: a new classification of traumatic tears. Radiol Med (Torino) 2006;111:828–35.
[18] Mariani P, Margheritini F, Christel P, et al. Evaluation of posterior cruciate ligament healing: a study using magnetic resonance imaging and stress radiography. Arthroscopy 2005;21:1354–61.
[19] Margheritini F, Mancini L, Mauro CS, et al. Stress radiography for quantifying posterior cruciate ligament deficiency. Arthroscopy 2003;19:706–11.
[20] Chen SY, Cheng CY, Chang SS, et al. Arthroscopic suture fixation for avulsion fractures in the tibial attachment of the posterior cruciate ligament. Arthroscopy 2012;28:1454–63.
[21] Wu CH, Chen AC, Yuan LJ, et al. Arthroscopic reconstruction of the posterior cruciate ligament by using a quadriceps tendon autograft: a minimum 5-year follow-up. Arthroscopy 2007;23:420–7.
[22] Yang JH, Yoon JR, Jeong HI, et al. Second-look arthroscopic assessment of arthroscopic single-bundle posterior cruciate ligament reconstruction: comparison of mixed graft versus Achilles tendon allograft. Am J Sports Med 2012;40:2052–60.
[23] Chen CP, Lin YM, Chiu YC, et al. Outcomes of arthroscopic double-bundle PCL reconstruction using the LARS artificial ligament. Orthopedics 2012;35:e800–6.
[24] Petrigliano FA, Suero EM, Voos JE, et al. The effect of proximal tibial slope on dynamic stability testing of the posterior cruciate ligament– and posterolateral corner–deficient knee. Am J Sports Med 2012;40:1322–8.
[25] Shelbourne KD, Davis TJ, Patel DV. The natural history of acute, isolated, nonoperatively treated posterior cruciate ligament injuries. Am J Sports Med 1999;27:276–83.
[26] Boynton MD, Tietjens BR. Long-term follow-up of untreated isolated posterior cruciate deficient knees. Am J Sports Med 1996;24:306–10.

CHAPTER 77

Quadriceps Tendinopathy and Tendinitis

Farshad Adib, MD
Christine Curtis, MD
Peter Bienkowski, MD
Lyle J. Micheli, MD

Synonym

Quadriceps tendinosis

ICD-9 Codes

726.60 Enthesopathy of knee, unspecified
844.8 Sprains and strains of knee and leg, other specified sites
959.7 Injury, other and unspecified, knee, leg, ankle, and foot

ICD-10 Codes

M76.891 Enthesopathies of right lower limb, excluding foot
M76.892 Enthesopathies of left lower limb, excluding foot
M76.899 Enthesopathies of unspecified lower limb, excluding foot
S83.90 Sprain of unspecified site of unspecified knee
S83.91 Sprain of unspecified site of right knee
S83.92 Sprain of unspecified site of left knee
S89.90 Injury of unspecified lower leg
S89.91 Injury of right lower leg
S89.92 Injury of left lower leg
S99.911 Injury of right ankle
S99.912 Injury of left ankle
S99.919 Injury of unspecified ankle
S99.921 Injury of right foot
S99.922 Injury of left foot
S99.929 Injury of unspecified foot
Add seventh character to categories S83, S89, and S99 for episode of care

Definition

The quadriceps tendon is located at the insertion of the quadriceps muscle into the patella and functions as part of the knee extensor mechanism. Quadriceps tendinitis (or, as named in the more recent literature, tendinosis or tendinopathy) is an overuse syndrome characterized by repetitive overloading of the quadriceps tendon. The common mechanism of injury is microtrauma, in which the basal ability of the tissue to repair itself is outpaced by the repetition of insult [1]. Quadriceps tendinopathy often occurs in athletes participating in running and jumping sports as well as in persons who perform frequent kneeling, squatting, and stair climbing [2]. The superior strength, mechanical advantage, and better vascularity of the quadriceps tendon make quadriceps tendinopathy much less frequent than patellar tendinopathy [3].

Symptoms

Patients usually report an insidious onset of knee pain and may note painful clicking. Their chief complaint is usually "knee pain." A burning sensation at the bone-tendon junction may be experienced [4]. The pain is aggravated by activity that challenges the extensor mechanism, including bending, stair climbing, running, and jumping. Reports of severe weakness, an inability to extend the knee, or the report of acute trauma with a "pop" should alert the clinician to the possibility of a quadriceps tendon partial or complete rupture. On occasion, a single episode of overload may elicit symptoms.

Physical Examination

On examination of the knee, point tenderness is localized along the superior pole of the patella and the quadriceps tendon. Quadriceps tendon pain may be elicited with extreme knee flexion and by resisted knee extension. The clinician should also be on the lookout for a palpable defect, suggesting partial rupture of the quadriceps tendon. Neurologic examination findings should be normal, with the possible exception of strength testing, which may be limited by pain or partial tendon rupture. Ligamentous examination of the knee is normal unless there is an internal derangement of the knee associated with trauma.

Functional Limitations

Quadriceps tendinopathy may interfere with activities of daily living. Pain is usually felt with stair climbing, kneeling, and rising from a chair. Athletes may be unable to participate in running and jumping activities.

Diagnostic Studies

Quadriceps tendinopathy is a clinical diagnosis, and diagnostic investigations are not generally necessary. If a partial tear of the quadriceps tendon is suspected but not apparent clinically, magnetic resonance imaging may be of assistance in confirming the diagnosis. Ultrasonography and Doppler study have also been found to be helpful [5].

Differential Diagnosis

Patellar tendinitis
Patellar fracture
Patellofemoral syndrome
Prepatellar bursitis
Apophysitis
Anterior fat pad syndrome
Chondromalacia patellae
Osteochondritis dissecans
Plica
Quadriceps tendon rupture
Quadriceps strain
Quadriceps contusion
Quadriceps tear

Treatment

Initial

Initial treatment includes rest from aggravating activities. Activity modification should include protection from eccentric or high-load knee extension (e.g., going up and down stairs, bending, jumping). Proper warm-up and stretching should be conducted before activity. Also, the application of ice to the injured area for 20 minutes, two or three times daily and before and after athletics, can be useful. Nonsteroidal anti-inflammatory drugs may be used for pain and inflammation. In some instances, knee immobilizers are used but may promote weakness and disuse atrophy.

Rehabilitation

The main rehabilitation modality includes muscle strengthening and stretching. All muscle strengthening exercises are conducted in the pain-free range. Static exercises may be used to minimize compressive forces across the patellofemoral joint [2]. Eccentric strengthening exercises may be useful [6]. Therapeutic modalities including ultrasound, phonophoresis, and iontophoresis may be used [2]. The use of icing immediately after activity or work has been advocated [7]. A general conditioning program is recommended.

Procedures

Local corticosteroid injections are not typically done because of the risk of tendon rupture, but they may be necessary in some cases unresponsive to treatment. Care should be taken to inject circumferential to the tendon and not in the tendon itself.

Surgery

Quadriceps tendinopathy is mostly managed nonoperatively. Surgical intervention may be necessary in rare cases of partial rupture. Tendocalcinosis may reflect a chronic partial tear [8]. If partial tendon rupture is suspected, surgical consultation is advised.

Potential Disease Complications

Functional deterioration with the development of chronic symptoms may occur. A high level of functioning in patients with quadriceps tendinopathy is usually regained and maintained [2]. In rare cases of progressive microtrauma to the injured area, rupture of tendon may result.

Potential Treatment Complications

The complications related to the use of nonsteroidal anti-inflammatory drugs include the development of gastritis as well as renal and hepatic involvement. Corticosteroid injection may predispose the tendon to rupture. Repeated injections of corticosteroids may increase the risk for mucoid degeneration, fibrinoid necrosis, mineralization, fibroblastic degeneration, and capillary proliferation within the tendon [9].

References

[1] Micheli LJ, Fehlandt Jr AF. Overuse injuries to tendons and apophyses in children and adolescents. Clin Sports Med 1992;11:713–26.
[2] Westrich GH, Haas SB, Bono JV. Occupational knee injuries. Orthop Clin North Am 1996;27:805–14.
[3] Won J, Maffulli N. Tendinopathy of the extensor apparatus of the knee. In: Micheli LJ, Kocher MS, editors. The pediatric and adolescent knee. Philadelphia: WB Saunders; 2006. p. 181–97.
[4] Yost Jr JG, Ellfeldt HJ. Basketball injuries. In: Nicholas JA, Hershman EB, editors. The lower extremity and spine in sports medicine. St. Louis: Mosby; 1986. p. 1440–66.
[5] Silvestri E, Biggi E, Molfetta L, et al. Power Doppler analysis of tendon vascularization. Int J Tissue React 2003;25:149–58.
[6] Stanish WD, Curwin S, Mandel S. Exercise and the muscle tendon unit. In: Stanish WD, Curwin S, editors. Tendinitis: etiology and treatment. New York: Oxford University Press; 2000. p. 43–7.
[7] Antich TJ, Randall CC, Westbrook RA, et al. Treatment of knee extensor mechanism disorders: comparison of four treatment modalities. J Orthop Sports Phys Ther 1986;8:225–59.
[8] Varghese B, Radcliffe GS, Groves C. Calcific tendonitis of the quadriceps. Br J Sports Med 2006;40:652–4.
[9] Key J, Johnson D, Jarvis G, Ponsonby D. Knee and thigh injuries. In: Subotnick SI, editor. Sports medicine of the lower extremity. New York: Churchill Livingstone; 1989. p. 297–310.

CHAPTER 78

Shin Splints

Michael F. Stretanski, DO

Synonyms

Medial tibial stress syndrome
Periostitis
Medial tibial periostalgia

ICD-9 Codes

730.3 Periostitis without mention of osteomyelitis
844.9 Sprains and strains of knee and leg, unspecified site

ICD-10 Codes

M89.9 Disorders of bone, unspecified
S83.90 Sprain of unspecified site of unspecified knee
S83.91 Sprain of unspecified site of right knee
S83.92 Sprain of unspecified site of left knee
Add seventh character for category S83 for episode of care (A—initial encounter, D—subsequent encounter, S—sequela)

Definition

"Shin splints" is best thought of as a clinical syndrome defined in terms of pain and discomfort in the anterior portion of the leg from repetitive activity on hard surfaces or from forcible, excessive use of the foot flexors. The diagnosis should be limited to musculoskeletal inflammations, excluding stress fractures, diet-related diseases [1], and ischemic disorders [2], although it may coexist with such disorders.

Shin splints most commonly occur in athletes who have sudden increases or changes in their training activity. This disorder occurs in runners and in athletes who participate in high-impact court or field sports as well as in gymnasts and particularly ballet dancers, alone or in conjunction with other overuse syndromes [3], but it has also been well documented and studied in military personnel [4–6]. The etiology of shin splints is not clearly defined, but it is likely to be multifactorial with biomechanical abnormalities of the foot and ankle, poor footwear and shock absorption, hard playing surfaces, and training errors. Other contributing factors may include weakness of anterior and posterior compartment musculature, inadequate warm-up, leg length discrepancy, tibial torsion, excessive femoral anteversion, and increased Q angle [7,8], as is seen in women.

One prospective study [6] in military cadets looked at seven anatomic variables and identified greater internal and external hip range of motion and lower mean calf girth to be associated with a higher incidence of exertional medial tibial pain in men. It also showed a high rate of injury among women, but no intrinsic factor was specifically identified. Nutritional and endocrine factors are more likely to play an etiologic role in stress reactions. In school-age athletes and adults who participate in seasonal sports, shin splints can occur when they resume their sport or start a new land-based sport (e.g., high-school or college athletes who go from playing basketball to cross-country or track).

It is important for the clinician to differentiate shin splints, a fairly benign condition, from acute compartment syndrome (a potential emergency) and from the different types of stress fractures that can occur in this region. The anterior lower leg is especially predisposed to compartment syndrome because of its high vulnerability to injury and its relatively limited compartment compliance [9]. It is most common to study these diagnoses together because many may coexist and symptoms overlap. Further discussion of these other diagnoses may be found in their respective chapters. Tibial periostitis has been described as an initial manifestation of polyarteritis nodosa [10]. Primary adamantinoma [11], a rare low-grade primary bone tumor, and hydatid bone disease [12] have also been reported in this region.

Symptoms

Patients presenting with shin splints usually complain of a dull and aching pain near the junction of the mid and distal thirds of the posteromedial or anterior tibia (Fig. 78.1). Clinicians should be aware of the wide differential diagnosis of pain in this region; not all anterior tibial pains are shin splints. Symptoms are commonly bilateral, occur with exercise, and are relieved with rest [13]. Initially the pain may

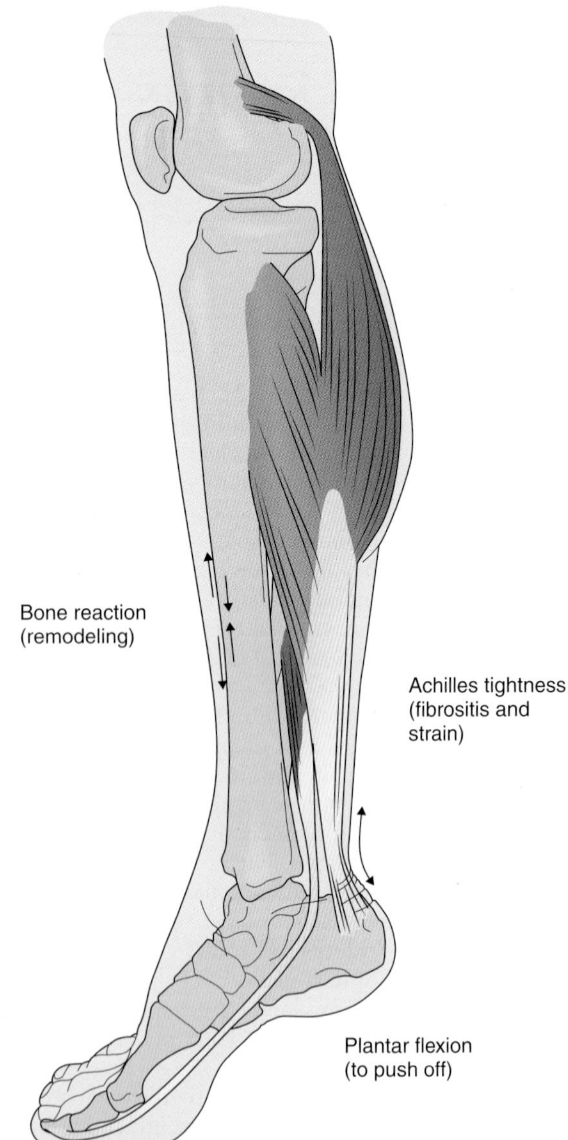

FIGURE 78.1 Repetitive microtrauma and overuse in running lead to soft tissue and even bone breakdown, a process commonly called shin splints. Muscle overpull can lead to periostitis, strain, or trabecular breakdown. The area approximately 13 cm proximal to the tip of the medial malleolus along the posterior tibial cortex appears to be maximally at risk.

ease with continued running and recur after prolonged activity. Those with more severe shin splints may have persistent pain with normal walking, with activities of daily living, or at rest.

Physical Examination

Physical examination typically reveals generalized tenderness along the medial tibia. Mild swelling may be present. Resisted plantar flexion, toe flexion, or toe raises may aggravate symptoms, and pain-inhibitory weakness may be evident. Striking a 128-Hz tuning fork and placing it on the tibia may reproduce the pain associated with stress fractures. Patients with stress fractures will usually have point tenderness over the bone at the site of stress fracture. Lower extremity idiopathic osteonecrosis is most common in the fifth decade of life at the medial tibial plateau [14], whereas those with shin splints will have more widespread tenderness to palpation that is more distal than these other pathologic processes. However, longitudinal tibial stress reactions may share a common anatomic pain distribution, and one study [15] showed tibial stress reactions in this same distal-third region.

The lower extremity examination focuses on static and dynamic components of the kinetic chain to uncover signs of coexisting lower extremity issues that may be contributing factors. These include forefoot pronation, pes cavus, pes planus, and excessive heel valgus or varus. Comparatively tight or weak lower extremity muscle groups should be noted for later rehabilitation goals. In particular, relative ankle plantar flexion, dorsiflexion, inversion, and eversion strength should be examined. Careful review of systems should be negative for fever, chills, night sweats, unintentional weight loss, and loss of bowel or bladder control. The neurologic portion of the examination, including sensation and muscle stretch reflexes, should be normal.

Functional Limitations

In early stages of shin splints, activity limitations occur most often during running or participation in ballistic activities. When symptoms are more severe, they may occur with walking or at rest, thus causing further functional limitations. Athletes may be unable to participate in their sport, and attempts to cross-train into other sports may result in worsening of symptoms.

Diagnostic Studies

Plain radiographs are typically normal early in the disease process but may be of use in ruling out more ominous disease, especially if symptoms are manifested unilaterally. Later, there may be evidence of periosteal thickening. Radionuclide bone scanning helps differentiate shin splints from stress fracture. Diffuse radioisotopic uptake along the medial or posteromedial tibia on the delayed phase is the pattern usually seen with shin splints. A focal defined area of uptake in all phases is more consistent with a stress fracture [16]. Fat-suppressed magnetic resonance imaging may also be useful for discrimination between stress fracture and shin splints before plain radiography shows detectable periosteal reaction [17]. Exertional compartment syndrome is uncommon, but if clinical suspicion is high, compartment pressure measurements must be done to rule it out. Magnetic resonance imaging of the lumbar spine may be indicated if lumbar radiculopathy is in the differential diagnosis or lumbar spinal stenosis is suspected in older athletes or younger athletes with a congenitally narrow spinal canal. Electrodiagnostic studies should be essentially normal, but membrane irritability manifested as positive sharp waves or fibrillations may be seen in any inflamed muscle. Nerve conductions should be normal in the absence of any concomitant nerve entrapment as may be seen in compartment syndrome.

Differential Diagnosis

Stress fracture
Chronic exertional compartment syndrome
Tendinitis
Muscle strain
Muscle herniation
Vascular and muscular abnormalities
Longitudinal tibial fatigue fracture
Hematoma
Primary muscle disease
Peroneal nerve entrapment
Fascial defect
Deep venous thrombosis
Sarcoma or osteosarcoma
Hydatid bone disease

Treatment

Initial

As with many overuse syndromes, relative rest—that is, participation only in those activities that can be done without pain—is the key to initial management. If reducing mileage, court time, or studio time or just reducing intensity allows the athlete to remain pain free, continuation of the activity may be acceptable. In general, however, even in mild cases, the athlete should avoid repetitive lower extremity stress for at least 1 to 2 weeks. In more serious cases, athletes may need to stop running entirely for a longer time. If walking is painful, crutches are indicated. A variety of commercially available off-the-shelf braces may decrease pain associated with weight bearing. Wearing of an elastic compression bandage may prevent additional swelling when compartment syndrome has been ruled out as compression may worsen vascular symptoms.

Stretching and ice or ice massage to the involved areas can be helpful. Nonsteroidal anti-inflammatory drugs can reduce inflammation and help manage pain. Analgesics can be taken for pain, but caution should be used to not enable further overtraining. Whirlpool, phonophoresis, iontophoresis, and therapeutic ultrasound are traditionally attempted and may have a role in symptomatic management or inflammatory phase reduction. Electrical stimulation should probably be considered contraindicated in this diagnosis, in which the pathoetiology points to excessive muscle contraction and a reactive periostitis in the first place.

In addressing malalignments of the lower extremities, orthoses, such as longitudinal arch supports with or without a medial heel wedge, may be indicated in select patients. Although a review of the literature fails to yield any objective evidence for the widespread use of any of these interventions, the most encouraging evidence seems to be for the use of shock-absorbing insoles [4,18]. Custom orthotic inserts, in one study of healthy female runners, have been shown to decrease rearfoot eversion angle and velocity and internal inversion moment as well as to decrease ankle dynamics in the frontal and sagittal planes. Whereas the particular relevance to shin splints is unclear, the ability to affect these measurements seems promising [19].

Rehabilitation

In individuals who continue to have pain despite initial conservative treatment, physical therapy may be indicated to decrease pain and further educate the patient about the disorder. Although pathophysiologically distinct from chronic exertional compartment syndrome, shin splints were once thought to be a form of chronic exertional compartment syndrome and vice versa [20], and the two entities are seldom discussed outside the context of each other. Ice, passive modalities (except electrical stimulation), and nonsteroidal anti-inflammatory drugs before exercise may help in enabling the rehabilitation program.

Once the symptoms have diminished, the rehabilitation program focuses on improving muscle strength, flexibility, and endurance and preventing recurrence of injury [21]. "Writing" the alphabet with the great toe moves the ankle through full range of motion in all planes and may be started early.

The primary muscles thought to be involved in shin splints are the flexor digitorum longus and the soleus. Others have implicated the tibialis posterior, but its attachment is more posterior than the area of typical shin splint symptoms, and it actually attaches to the interosseous membrane more than to the medial tibia [22]. The deep crural fascia also attaches to the posteromedial tibia. Long-term rehabilitation for shin splints involves improvement of the flexibility, strength, and endurance of the involved muscles and avoidance of contributing factors. Anterior compartment stretching exercises, Achilles tendon stretching, and overall lower extremity flexibility exercises are important. Eccentric strengthening of antagonistic muscle groups is also useful. Pain can be a guide in the advancement of the rehabilitation program.

Athletes should have full range of motion that is symmetric to the uninvolved side and have nearly full strength before returning to their prior activity or to competition. Plyometrics should be avoided until a high level of strength, endurance, and flexibility has been attained. Cardiovascular fitness should be maintained if possible through lower impact activities, such as stationary biking, swimming, or water running. Return to previous activity level should be a gradual process, individualized, and based on the athlete's response to increasing intensity of training. Proper footwear for the sport is thought to be essential. Running shoes lose more than 60% of their shock absorption after 250 miles of use [7]. Orthotic devices are often necessary in those individuals with foot abnormalities such as pes planus. More specifically, custom orthotics or shoe inserts can help align and stabilize the foot and ankle, taking stress off the lower leg. A plyometric program of strengthening and conditioning has been suggested as early as the third phase of rehabilitation [23], but return to sport outcomes have not been reported.

Procedures

There is no proven benefit noted in the literature to support any injection-based procedure, such as local exogenous glucocorticoid injection. Limited empirical opinions exist on a role for sclerotherapeutic solutions. Great care must be taken in ensuring the correct diagnosis, as potentially disastrous results may occur in dealing with a coexistent compartment syndrome. Theoretically, a palliative role may exist for either in chronic recalcitrant cases with functional decline. Compartment pressure measurement has no absolute contraindications and can be performed with relative simplicity [24]. Avoidance of areas with overlying cellulitis is recommended. The procedure itself carries some risk of infection, but this can usually be avoided with appropriate technical practices.

Surgery

Surgery is rarely indicated but involves a posteromedial fasciotomy with release of the fascial bridge of the medial soleus and the fascia of the deep posterior compartment, with periosteal cauterization [16]. Surgery is effective in relieving pain, but it frequently leaves the patient with persistent strength deficits, and full return to sports is not always achieved [25].

Potential Disease Complications

If shin splints are not treated and biomechanical malalignments are not addressed, stress fractures and potentially true fractures may occur. This would result in further morbidity and more time lost from the desired physical activity as well as potential function decline. Any chronic tendinopathy can theoretically lead to weakening of the tendon and subsequent rupture [26].

Potential Treatment Complications

Complications involving the gastrointestinal and renal systems may result from treatment with nonsteroidal anti-inflammatory drugs. Fasciotomy may result in residual weakness. Overly aggressive rehabilitation or rehabilitation of the incorrect diagnosis may progress the injury, cause secondary injury, or delay diagnosis of more ominous disease. The author has experience with a case of severe reflex sympathetic dystrophy and peripheral nerve injury after sclerotherapy.

References

[1] Lowdon J. Rickets: concerns over the worldwide increase. J Fam Health Care 2011;21:25–9.
[2] Subcommittee on Classification of Injuries in Sports and Committee on the Medical Aspects of Sports. Standard nomenclature of athletic injuries. Chicago: American Medical Association; 1966.
[3] Stretanski MF, Weber GJ. Medical and rehabilitation issues in classical ballet. Am J Phys Med 2002;81:383–91.
[4] Johnston E, Flynn T, Bean M, et al. A randomized controlled trial of a leg orthosis versus traditional treatment for soldiers with shin splints: a pilot study. Mil Med 2006;171:40–4.
[5] Larsen K, Weidich F, Leboeuf-Yde C. Can custom-made biomechanic shoe orthoses prevent problems in the back and lower extremities? A randomized, controlled intervention trial of 146 military conscripts. J Manipulative Physiol Ther 2002;25:326–31.
[6] Burne SG, Khan KM, Boudville PB, et al. Risk factors associated with exertional medial tibial pain—a 12 month prospective clinical study. Br J Sports Med 2004;38:441–5.
[7] Touliopolous S, Hershman EB. Lower leg pain: diagnosis and treatment of compartment syndromes and other pain syndromes of the leg. Sports Med 1999;27:193–204.
[8] Reid DC. Sports injury assessment and rehabilitation. New York: Churchill Livingstone; 1992; 269–300.
[9] Simon RR, Koenigsknecht SJ. Emergency orthopedics of the extremities. 4th ed. New York: McGraw-Hill; 2001.
[10] Vedrine L, Rault A, Debourdeau P, et al. Polyarteritis nodosa manifesting as tibial periostitis [in French]. Ann Med Interne (Paris) 2001;152:213–4.
[11] Ulmar B, Delling G, Werner M, et al. Classical and atypical location of adamantinomas—presentation of two cases. Onkologie 2006;29:276–8.
[12] Kalinova K, Proichev V, Stefanova P, et al. Hydatid bone disease: a case report and review of the literature. J Orthop Surg (Hong Kong) 2005;13:323–5.
[13] Andrish JA. The leg. In: DeLee JC, Drez D, editors. Orthopaedic sports medicine: principles and practice. Philadelphia: WB Saunders; 1994. p. 1603–7.
[14] Valenti JR, Illescas JA, Bariga A, Dlöz R. Idiopathic osteonecrosis of the medial tibial plateau. Knee Surg Sports Traumatol Arthrosc 2005;13:293–8.
[15] Ruohola JS, Kiuru MJ, Pihlajamaki HK. Fatigue and bone injuries causing anterior lower leg pain. Clin Orthop Relat Res 2006;444:216–23.
[16] Barry NN, McGuire JL. Acute injuries and specific problems in adult athletes. Rheum Dis Clin North Am 1996;22:531–49.
[17] Aoki Y, Yasuda K, Tohyama H, et al. Magnetic resonance imaging in stress fractures and shin splints. Clin Orthop Relat Res 2004;421:260–7.
[18] Thacker SB, Gilchrist J, Stroup DF, Kimsey CD. The prevention of shin splints in sports: a systematic review of the literature. Med Sci Sports Exerc 2002;34:32–40.
[19] MacLean C, Davis IM, Hamill J. Influence of a custom foot orthotics intervention on lower extremity dynamics in healthy runners. Clin Biomech 2006;21:623–30.
[20] Whitesides TE, Haney TC, Morimoto K, Harada H. Tissue pressure measurements as a determinant for the need of fasciotomy. Clin Orthop Relat Res 1975;113:43–51.
[21] Windsor RE, Chambers K. Overuse injuries of the leg. In: Kibler WB, Herring SA, Press JM, editors. Functional rehabilitation of sports and musculoskeletal injuries. Gaithersburg, Md: Aspen; 1998. p. 265–7.
[22] Beck BR, Osternig LR. Medial tibial stress syndrome: the location of muscles in the leg in relation to symptoms. J Bone Joint Surg Am 1994;76:1057–61.
[23] Herring KM. A plyometric training model used to augment rehabilitation from tibial fasciitis. Curr Sports Med Rep 2006;5:147–54.
[24] Whitesides Jr TE, Haney TC, Harada H, et al. A simple method for tissue pressure determination. Arch Surg 1975;110:1311–3.
[25] Yates B, Allen MJ, Barnes MR. Outcome of surgical treatment of medial tibial stress syndrome. J Bone Joint Surg Am 2003;85:1974–80.
[26] Wang JH, Iosifidis MI, Fu FH. Biomechanical basis for tendinopathy. Clin Orthop Relat Res 2006;443:320–32.

CHAPTER 79

Stress Fractures of the Lower Limb

Sheila Dugan, MD
Sol M. Abreu Sosa, MD, FAAPMR

Synonyms

Insufficiency fractures
Fatigue fractures
March fractures

ICD-9 Codes

821.0 Fracture of other and unspecified parts of femur, shaft or unspecified part, closed
823.8 Fracture of tibia and fibula, unspecified part, closed
824.8 Fracture of ankle, unspecified, closed
825.2 Fracture of tarsal and metatarsal bones, closed

ICD-10 Codes

S72.301 Unspecified fracture of shaft of right femur
S72.302 Unspecified fracture of shaft of left femur
S72.309 Unspecified fracture of shaft of unspecified femur

Add seventh character for S72 (A—initial encounter for closed fracture; B—initial encounter for open fracture type I or II; C—initial encounter for open fracture type IIIA, IIIB, or IIIC; D—subsequent encounter for closed fracture with routine healing; E—subsequent encounter for open fracture type I or II with routine healing; F—subsequent encounter for open fracture type IIIA, IIIB, or IIIC with routine healing; G—subsequent encounter for closed fracture with delayed healing; H—subsequent encounter for open fracture type I or II with delayed healing; J—subsequent encounter for open fracture type IIIA, IIIB, or IIIC with delayed healing; K—subsequent encounter for closed fracture with nonunion; M—subsequent encounter for open fracture type I or II with nonunion; N—subsequent encounter for open fracture type IIIA, IIIB, or IIIC with nonunion; P—subsequent encounter for closed fracture with malunion; Q—subsequent encounter for open fracture type I or II with malunion; R—subsequent encounter for open fracture type IIIA, IIIB, or IIIC with malunion; S—sequela)

S82.201 Unspecified fracture of shaft of right tibia
S82.202 Unspecified fracture of shaft of left tibia
S82.209 Unspecified fracture of shaft of unspecified tibia
S82.401 Unspecified fracture of shaft of right fibula
S82.402 Unspecified fracture of shaft of left fibula
S82.409 Unspecified fracture of shaft of unspecified fibula

Add seventh character for S82 (A—initial encounter for closed fracture, D—subsequent encounter for closed fracture with routine healing, G—subsequent encounter for closed fracture with delayed healing, K—subsequent encounter for closed fracture with nonunion, P—subsequent encounter for closed fracture with malunion, S—sequela)

M84.471 Pathological fracture, right ankle
M84.472 Pathological fracture, left ankle
M84.473 Pathological fracture, unspecified ankle
S92.201 Fracture of unspecified tarsal bone(s) of right foot
S92.202 Fracture of unspecified tarsal bone(s) of left foot
S92.209 Fracture of unspecified tarsal bone(s) of unspecified foot
S92.301 Fracture of unspecified metatarsal bone(s), right foot

S92.302 Fracture of unspecified metatarsal bone(s), left foot

S92.309 Fracture of unspecified metatarsal bone(s), unspecified foot

Add seventh character for S92
(A—initial encounter for closed fracture, B—initial encounter for open fracture, D—subsequent encounter for fracture with routine healing, G—subsequent encounter for fracture with delayed healing, K—subsequent encounter for fracture with nonunion, P—subsequent encounter for fracture with malunion, S—sequela)

Definition

Stress fractures are complete or partial bone fractures caused by the accumulation of microtrauma [1]. Normal bone accommodates to stress through ongoing remodeling. If this remodeling system does not keep pace with the force applied, stress reaction (microfractures) and, finally, stress fracture can result. Stress fracture is the end result of a continuum of biologic responses to stress placed on bone. Adolescent, young adult, and premenopausal women athletes have a higher incidence of stress injuries to bone than men do [2,3]. Stress fractures in juveniles are rare [4]. Both extrinsic and intrinsic factors have been implicated in this imbalance between bone resorption and bone deposition [5]. Malalignment and poor flexibility of the lower extremities (intrinsic factors) and inadequate footwear, changes in training surface, and increases in training intensity and duration without an adequate ramp-up period (extrinsic factors) can lead to stress fractures [6].

Stress fractures in athletes vary by sports and are most common in the lower extremities [2,7]. The most common sites are the tibia, metatarsals, and fibula, and they affect most commonly runners and dancers. The fracture site is the area of greatest stress, such as the origin of lower leg muscles along the medial tibia [8]. A narrower mediolateral tibial width was a risk factor for femoral, tibial, and foot stress fractures in a study of military recruits [9]. Studies of female runners demonstrated greater loading rates in those with history of tibial stress fractures compared with those without injury [10,11]. In contrast, in comparison of runners with and without history of tibial stress fracture, no difference in ground reaction forces, bone density, or tibial bone geometric parameters was found between groups [12].

Military recruits have been extensively studied in regard to lower extremity stress fractures. In a study of 179 Finnish military recruits aged 18 to 20 years, tall height, poor physical conditioning, low hip bone mineral content and density, and high serum parathyroid hormone level were risk factors for stress fractures [13]. The authors postulated that given the poor vitamin D status, intervention studies of vitamin D supplementation to lower serum parathyroid hormone levels and possibly to reduce the incidence of stress fractures are warranted. Prospective studies of vitamin D and calcium in stress fracture prevention, one in female young athletes and the second in female military recruits, were the focus of a recent review paper. A longitudinal study of female athletes aged 18 to 26 years showed that greater baseline intakes of dietary calcium, dairy products, and milk were linked to significant reductions in fracture incidence; fracture risk decreased by 62% per additional cup of skim milk consumed per day, and women who consumed less than 800 mg of calcium per day had nearly six times the stress fracture rate of women who consumed more than 1500 mg of calcium and more than double the rate for women who consumed between 800 and 1500 mg [14]. The second study of female military recruits who were prescribed an 8-week trial of supplementation with 2000 mg of calcium and 800 IU of vitamin D demonstrated a statistically significant 20% reduction in fracture injuries compared with women given a placebo [14]. The study concluded that evaluation of age-appropriate dietary guidelines for calcium and vitamin D levels is needed to promote bone health, to reduce the risk of stress fracture injury in the young athlete, and to achieve peak bone density that will promote lifelong bone health [14].

A database of systematic reviews, including 13 randomized prevention trials, concluded that shock-absorbing insert use in footwear probably reduces the incidence of stress fractures in military personnel [15]. There was insufficient evidence to determine the best design of such inserts.

Stress fractures may be related to abnormalities of the bone, such as in female athletes with low bone density due to exercise-induced menstrual abnormalities [16–19]. Premature osteoporosis leads to an increased risk for stress fractures. One study looked at premenopausal women runners and collegiate athletes and concluded that those with absent or irregular menses were at increased risk for musculoskeletal injuries while engaged in active training [17]. Muscle deficits in the gastrocnemius-soleus complex in jumping athletes have also been implicated in causing tibial stress fractures. Bone injury may be a secondary event after a primary failure of muscle function [20].

Recent literature review of the influence of sports participation on bone health in the young athlete concluded that high-impact and weight-bearing activities enhance bone density, particularly in anatomic locations directly loaded by those sports [21]. It also showed that participation in sports during the age range in which growth and skeletal maturity occur may result in a higher peak bone density [21]; in particular, athletes aged 10 to 30 years who participate in impact sports (particularly high-impact or odd-impact sports) may enjoy enhanced bone density and improvements in bone geometry. Nonimpact sports such as cycling and swimming are not associated with improvements in bone health, and prolonged participation in endurance sports, including long-distance running and cycling, may be associated with decreased peak bone density [21].

During the last few years, researchers have shown a link between stress fractures and long-term bisphosphonate use. Bisphosphonate medications are indicated for patients with postmenopausal osteoporosis, and it has been shown that bisphosphonate use improves bone mineral density, prevents bone loss, and reduces the number of fractures [22,23]. Bisphosphonates inhibit osteoclastic bone resorption, and therefore bone turnover, by inducing osteoclast apoptosis.

The combined and coordinated action of resorbing damaged bone and laying down new bone is fundamental to the process of bone remodeling [23]. If this coupling is impaired, the microdamage that occurs under physiologic conditions that normally is repaired may accumulate, resulting in a major reduction in the energy required to cause fracture [23]. These fractures are low-energy injuries and have characteristic findings observed on femoral radiographs: a transverse fracture line originating from the lateral tension side of the cortex and lateral cortical thickening adjacent to the fracture [23,24]. In addition, prodromal thigh pain from the insufficiency changes may be present. The subsequent minimal trauma that often is required to complete the fracture is characteristic, with patients often sustaining a spontaneous nontraumatic fracture during activities of daily living [23].

Individuals who are nonambulatory or have limited ambulation due to disability represent another population with abnormal bone and premature osteoporosis. In stroke patients, there is significant bone loss on the paretic side, which is greatest in those patients with the most severe functional deficits [25]. Spinal cord injury may not only cause bone loss but also alter bone structure and microstructure [26]. Practitioners caring for individuals with limited mobility should consider stress fracture in the differential diagnosis of overuse injuries.

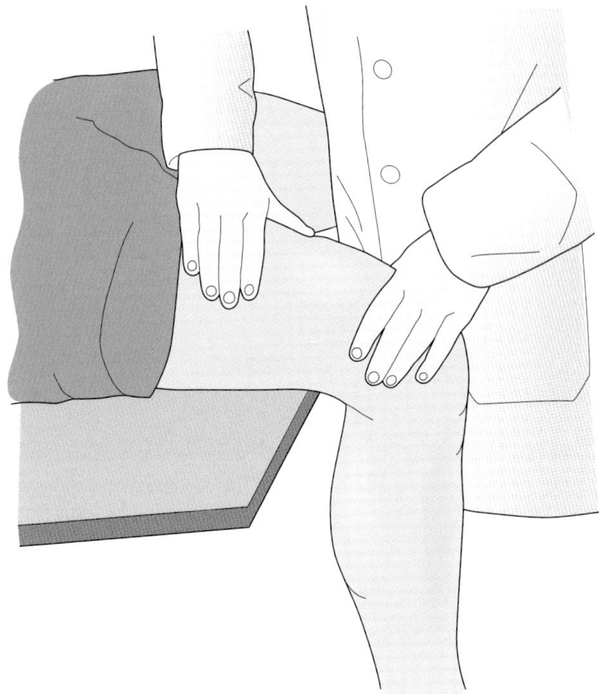

FIGURE 79.1 Physical examination technique to evaluate for femoral stress fracture. The examiner applies a downward pressure on the distal femur, using the examination table as a fulcrum, to increase the force across the fracture site. A positive test result reproduces the individual's pain.

Symptoms

Patients may report an increase in training or activity level or a change in training conditions preceding the onset of symptoms. Because of pain in the affected region of the bone, patients may seek medical attention during the microfracture or stress reaction phase of injury. Should they forego relative rest (avoidance of the pain-provoking activity), they can progress to stress fracture or even complete fracture. The pain will gradually increase with activity and may occur with less intense exercise, such as walking, or even at rest. In general, however, the pain will improve with rest. The pain can lead to a decline in performance. The individual may also note swelling in the affected region of the bone. Symptoms of paresthesias and numbness should alert the clinician to consider an alternative diagnosis.

Physical Examination

On physical examination, the clinician will find an area of exquisite, well-localized tenderness, warmth, and edema over the affected region of the bone. Ecchymosis along the plantar aspect may be present with foot involvement. Percussion of the nearby region can cause pain. Placement of a vibrating tuning fork over the fracture site intensifies the pain [27]. In the tibia, stress fractures primarily occur along the medial border; the frequency, in order, is upper, lower, and mid shaft. In the fibula, they usually occur one handbreadth proximal to the lateral malleolus [5]. Tarsal or metatarsal stress fractures are manifested with localized foot tenderness. Weight-bearing activity, such as a one-legged hop test, can provoke the pain by increasing the ground reaction forces. For a presumed femoral stress fracture, the clinician can provoke pain by applying a downward force on the distal femur while the affected individual is seated with the distal femur extending beyond the edge of the seat (Fig. 79.1).

The physical examination must include an examination of the lumbar spine and lower limbs to evaluate for any anatomic malalignment or biomechanical abnormalities. For instance, an individual with rigid supinated feet or weak foot intrinsic muscles may transmit more ground reaction forces to the tibia. On physical examination, one can identify problems that must be addressed in treatment planning.

Strength should be normal but occasionally limited by pain. Sensation and muscle stretch reflexes should also be normal.

Functional Limitations

Recreational and athletic activities requiring weight bearing through the affected lower limb may be limited by pain. For instance, running results in the transmission of increased ground reaction forces through the leg. These forces can increase if one runs on a concrete surface versus an all-weather track. In acute cases, ambulation can be painful.

Diagnostic Studies

Plain films may take as long as 6 weeks to demonstrate fracture, and films are initially normal in up to two thirds of patients [28]. Technetium Tc 99 m diphosphonate bone scanning will yield the earliest confirmatory data for stress fractures, demonstrating a "hot spot" 1 to 4 days after

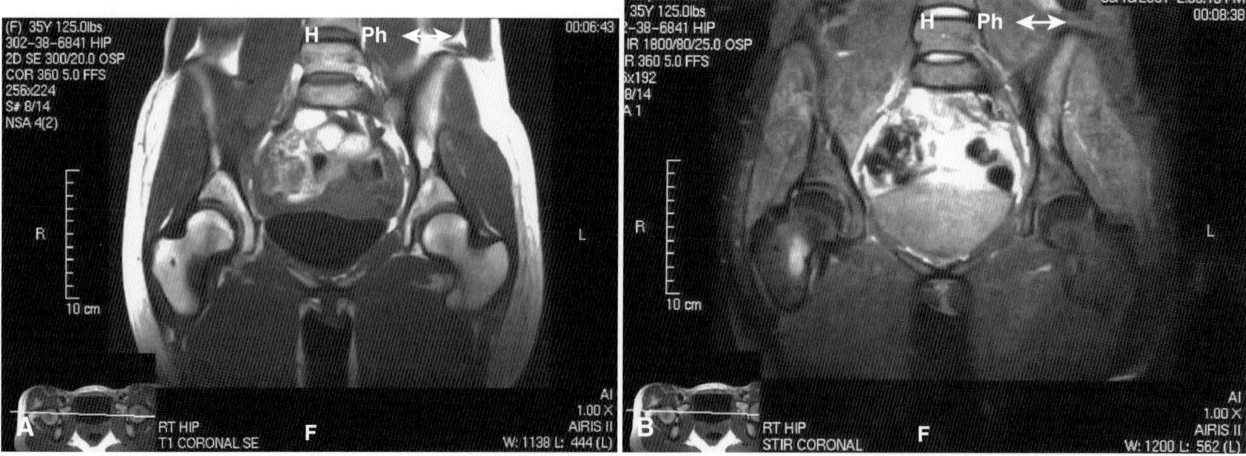

FIGURE 79.2 Femoral stress fracture on the compression side of the right femoral neck in a 35-year-old female marathon runner demonstrated on T1 (**A**) and STIR (**B**) coronal magnetic resonance images. *(Images courtesy David A. Turner, MD, Chairman, Department of Radiology, Rush University Medical Center, Chicago.)*

fracture [18]. The fracture site may not return to normal on a bone scan for 5 months or longer, so it is not clinically useful to assess recovery. Computed tomography is necessary to differentiate stress fractures of the sacrum and the tarsal navicular bone [29]. Magnetic resonance imaging (MRI) delineates the fracture location and status of healing (Fig. 79.2). MRI provides soft tissue definition, which can be helpful in the setting of stress reaction or tendinitis. Although it can confirm the diagnosis in the acute phase, it is generally not indicated initially. MRI findings can help with clinical decision-making about return to activity or play. A retrospective review of military recruits presenting with anterior lower leg pain showed that only 56% had positive findings on MRI testing, implicating tissues other than bone as the pain generator [30]. In a study, 12% of asymptomatic feet in male college basketball players demonstrated bone marrow edema on MRI; the authors noted that this early detection might lead to preventive strategies to avoid injury [31].

MRI grading systems have been developed with short T1 inversion recovery (STIR) sequences. Four grades of abnormality have been described from grade 1 (demonstration of periosteal edema on STIR or T2-weighted images) through grade 4 (visible injury line on T1- or T2-weighted images) [32,33]. Radiographic grading scales of stress injuries to bone can be useful in clinical trials to more specifically delineate response to management. One should consider bone density testing in a female patient with a history of amenorrhea [3].

Differential Diagnosis

Medial tibial stress syndrome
Osteoid osteoma
Compartment syndromes
Deep venous thrombosis
Knee disease (e.g., pes anserine bursitis)
Bone neoplasm
Osteomyelitis

Treatment

Initial

Pain and edema should be managed initially with PRICE (*p*rotection, *r*est, *i*ce, *c*ompression, and *e*levation). Use of nonsteroidal anti-inflammatory drugs (NSAIDs) is discouraged by several authors because of the negative impact of NSAIDs on tissue healing; in addition, masking of pain can compromise healing by reducing symptomatic feedback [34–37]. Acetaminophen may be helpful in patients who are resting but still have pain. Activities that provoke pain are eliminated. If ambulation is painful, athletes are placed on non–weight-bearing status or full crutch walking to eliminate painful weight bearing [38]. In non–weight-bearing subjects, a trial of walking is performed every 2 days, and once walking is pain free, full ambulation with crutches is begun. Fractures with the propensity to progress to nonunion, such as midshaft tibial stress fractures and tarsal navicular fractures, may require immediate immobilization with a bivalved orthotic boot. Femoral neck fractures on the tension (superior) aspect can become displaced and require strict non–weight-bearing status with axillary crutches initially [39]. Metatarsal stress fractures can be treated with a stiff shoe and a straight cane or a rigid orthosis. Navicular fractures may require immobilization in a short leg cast [34].

In the setting of female athletes with exercise-induced amenorrhea, nutritional counseling and correction of any energy debt must be included in the stress fracture treatment program. If the menstrual cycle does not return with these interventions, there is controversy about the use of an oral contraceptive pill to restore menses. Fewer athletes with fractures were using oral contraceptive pills than were athletes without fractures in one study [40]. In addition, women without stress fractures had a higher intake of calcium than did those with stress fractures. Nine elite runners with stress fractures were compared with matched control subjects without stress fractures, and significant differences in the number of menses per year (less in the fracture group) and the age at onset of menses (delayed in the fracture group) were identified [41].

In the setting of bisphosphonate-related stress fracture in the femoral subtrochanteric or high diaphyseal region, there is still debate as to whether it should be treated nonoperatively or operatively. A study suggested prophylactic fixation because eventually these fractures may become complete and displaced, requiring an eventual fixation [22].

Rehabilitation

Physical therapy modalities such as heat and interferential electrical stimulation are used to increase local blood flow and to promote healing; however, there is a lack of controlled studies to prove their efficacy. Deep soft tissue massage, including transverse friction massage, may be indicated and complement stretching for the muscles that originate along the medial tibia. Ongoing cardiovascular and strengthening activities should continue if they produce no pain; aqua jogging, stationary bicycling, or use of the elliptical machine can be substituted for running. Athletes can return to running once they are pain free with ambulation and cross-training activities; however, training schedules should be modified, and pain should be used as the guide to progression of the program [42]. In the setting of low-risk stress fractures, athletes may continue to participate if activity can be modified to minimize stress at the fracture site [43]. Sports-specific training must be addressed before return to play.

Careful attention to the training surface and equipment is mandatory. In the setting of significant forefoot or rearfoot biomechanical abnormalities, custom foot orthotics may be indicated. Taping may be used temporarily to provide stability of the ankle and foot. Local lower extremity strengthening is progressed from static exercises to concentric to eccentric training on the basis of symptoms. Plyometric (weight-bearing eccentric) training should precede return to play. Shock-absorbing insoles and running on shock absorbing surfaces are recommended and thought to decrease the ground reaction forces transmitted to the bones of the lower extremity [15,44]. In a prospective study of athletes without control subjects, immobilization with a pneumatic leg brace was used to allow participation in a modified training schedule earlier. The authors concluded that the brace promoted healing and limited the forces across the fracture site [45].

Rocker-bottom shoes and steel shanks can be used to prevent and to treat lower extremity stress fractures in susceptible disabled individuals.

Procedures

There is no specific nonsurgical procedure for this injury.

Surgery

Conservative management successfully treats lower extremity stress fractures with a few exceptions. Femoral neck stress fractures on the tensile (superior) aspect may require pinning if they do not heal after a course of non–weight bearing. Midshaft tibial fractures are at risk for nonunion and must be immobilized and observed closely; an open bone grafting procedure may be indicated in the setting of nonunion. Tarsal navicular stress fractures that do not respond to conservative treatment and demonstrate displacement, comminution, or nonunion may require open reduction with internal fixation [46]. In 26 subjects with 32 fractures treated for 2 years or more, surgical fixation of navicular stress fractures appears to be as effective as conservative management in the longer term [47].

Potential Disease Complications

If biomechanical and training principles are not addressed during treatment, stress fractures can recur. In female athletes with menstrual abnormalities and premature osteoporosis, failure to treat these conditions might also lead to recurrent stress fractures.

Potential Treatment Complications

Immobilization can lead to loss of joint range of motion and reduced muscle strength. Treatment risks with NSAIDs include gastrointestinal, hepatic, and renal side effects; in addition, detrimental effects on bone healing must be considered. A large retrospective study found that use of NSAIDs is associated with a 1.47 relative risk of fractures (nonvertebral) compared with control subjects who did not receive NSAIDs [48]. Treatment of amenorrhea with oral contraceptive pills involves increased risk for blood clots and their sequelae. Treatment of premature osteoporosis with bisphosphonates includes risk for esophageal erosion or ulceration. Complications of surgery include nonunion and other typical infrequent complications (e.g., infection, bleeding). Subjects who underwent surgical treatment for tarsal navicular stress fracture were more likely to continue to be tender over the navicular than were nonoperative subjects [47].

References

[1] McBryde AM. Stress fractures in runners. Clin Sports Med 1985;4:737–52.

[2] Bennell KL, Brukner PD. Epidemiology and site specificity of stress fractures. Clin Sports Med 1997;16:179–96.

[3] Nattiv A, Armsey TD. Stress injury to bone in the female athlete. Clin Sports Med 1997;16:197–219.

[4] Niemeyer P, Weinberg A, Schmitt H, et al. Stress fractures in the juvenile skeletal system. Int J Sports Med 2006;27:242–9.

[5] Reid DC. Exercise induced leg pain. In: Reid DC, editor. Sports injury assessment and rehabilitation. New York: Churchill Livingstone; 1992. p. 269.

[6] Sullivan D. Stress fractures in 51 runners. Clin Orthop 1984;187:188.

[7] Sanderlin BW, Raspa RF. Common stress fractures. Am Fam Physician 2003;68:1527–32.

[8] Markey KL. Stress fractures. Clin Sports Med 1987;6:405–25.

[9] Giladi M, Milgrom C, Simkin A, et al. Stress fractures: identifiable risk factors. Am J Sports Med 1991;19:647–52.

[10] Grimston SK, Engsberg JR, Kloiber R, Hanley DA. Bone mass, external loads and stress fractures in female runners. Int J Sports Biomech 1991;7:292–302.

[11] Milner CE, Ferber R, Pollard CD, et al. Biomechanical factors associated with tibial stress fracture in female runners. Med Sci Sports Exerc 2006;38:323–8.

[12] Bennell K, Crossley K, Jayarajan J, et al. Ground reaction forces and bone parameters in females with tibial stress fracture. Med Sci Sports Exerc 2004;36:397–404.

[13] Valimaki VV, Alfthan H, Lehmuskallio E, et al. Risk factors for clinical stress fractures in male military recruits: a prospective cohort study. Bone 2005;37:267–73.

[14] Tenforde AS, Sayres LC, Sainani KL, Fredericson M. Evaluating the relationship of calcium and vitamin D in the prevention of stress fracture injuries in the young athlete: a review of the literature. PM R 2010;2:945–9.

[15] Rome K, Handoll HH, Ashford R. Interventions for preventing and treating stress fractures and stress reactions of bone of the lower limbs in young adults. Cochrane Database Syst Rev 2005;2, CD000450.

[16] Barrow G, Saha S. Menstrual irregularity and stress fracture in collegiate female distance runners. Am J Sports Med 1988;16:209–16.

[17] Lloyd T, Triantafyllou SJ, Baker ER, et al. Women athletes with menstrual irregularity have increased musculoskeletal injuries. Med Sci Sports Exerc 1986;18:374–9.

[18] Marcus R, Cann C, Madvig P, et al. Menstrual function and bone mass in elite women distance runners: endocrine and metabolic factors. Ann Intern Med 1985;102:158–63.

[19] Myburgh KH, Bachrach LK, Lewis B, et al. Low bone mineral density at axial and appendicular sites in amenorrheic athletes. Med Sci Sports Exerc 1993;25:1197–202.

[20] Keats TE. Radiology of musculoskeletal stress injury. Chicago: Year Book; 1990.

[21] Tenforde AS, Fredericson M. Influence of sports participation on bone health in the young athlete: a review of the literature. PM R 2011;3:861–7.

[22] Banffy MB, Vrahas MS, Ready JE, et al. Nonoperative versus prophylactic treatment of bisphosphonate-associated femoral stress fractures. Clin Orthop Relat Res 2011;469:2028–34.

[23] Isaacs JD, Shidiak L, Harris IA, et al. Femoral insufficiency fractures associated with prolonged bisphosphonate therapy. Clin Orthop Relat Res 2010;468:3384–92.

[24] Kwek EB, Goh SK, Koh JS, et al. An emerging pattern of subtrochanteric stress fractures: a long-term complication of alendronate therapy? Injury 2008;39:224–31.

[25] Beaupre GS, Lew HL. Bone-density changes after stroke. Am J Phys Med Rehabil 2006;85:464–72.

[26] Jiang SD, Dai LY, Jiang LS. Osteoporosis after spinal cord injury. Osteoporos Int 2006;17:180–92.

[27] Young JL, Press JM. Rehabilitation of running injuries. In: Buschbacher R, Braddom R, editors. Sports medicine and rehabilitation: a sport-specific approach. Philadelphia: Hanley & Belfus; 1994. p. 123–34.

[28] Hersman EB, Mally T. Stress fractures. Clin Sports Med 1990;9: 183–214.

[29] Pavlov H, Torg JS, Freiberger JH. Tarsal navicular stress fractures: radiographic evaluation. Radiology 1983;148:641–5.

[30] Ruohola JP, Kiuru MJ, Pihlajamaki HK. Fatigue bone injuries causing anterior lower leg pain. Clin Orthop Relat Res 2006;444:216–23.

[31] Major NM. Role of MRI in prevention of metatarsal stress fractures in collegiate basketball players. AJR Am J Roentgenol 2006;186:255–8.

[32] Arendt EA, Griffith HJ. The use of MR imaging in the assessment and clinical management of stress reactions of bone in high- performance athletes. Clin Sports Med 1997;16:291–306.

[33] Fredericson M, Bergman AG, Hoffman KL, et al. Tibial stress reaction in runners. Correlation of clinical symptoms and scintigraphy with a new magnetic resonance imaging grading system. Am J Sports Med 1995;23:472–81.

[34] Snider RK, editor. Essentials of musculoskeletal care. Rosemont, Ill: American Academy of Orthopaedic Surgery; 1997. p. 485–6.

[35] Stovitz SD, Arendt EA. NSAIDs should not be used in treatment of stress fractures [comment]. Am Fam Physician 2004;70:1452–4.

[36] Ho ML, Chang JK, Chuang LY, et al. Effects of nonsteroidal anti-inflammatory drugs and prostaglandins on osteoblastic functions. Biochem Pharmacol 1999;58:983–90.

[37] Wheeler P, Batt ME. Do non-steroidal anti-inflammatory drugs adversely affect stress fracture healing? A short review. Br J Sports Med 2005;39:65–9.

[38] Arendt E, Agel J, Heikes C, Griffith H. Stress injuries to bone in college athletes: a retrospective review of experience at a single institution. Am J Sports Med 2003;31:959–68.

[39] Windsor RE, Chambers K. Overuse injuries of the leg. In: Kibler WB, Herring SA, Press JM, editors. Functional rehabilitation of sports and musculoskeletal injuries. Gaithersburg, Md: Aspen; 1998. p. 186–7.

[40] Myburgh KH, Hutchins J, Fataar AB, et al. Low bone density is an etiologic factor for stress fracture in athletes. Ann Intern Med 1990;113:754–9.

[41] Carbon R, Sambrook PN, Deakin V, et al. Bone density of elite female athletes with stress fractures. Med J Aust 1990;153:373–6.

[42] Brody DM. Techniques in the evaluation and treatment of the injured runner. Orthop Clin North Am 1982;13:541.

[43] Kaeding CC, Yu JR, Wright R, et al. Management and return to play of stress fractures. Clin J Sport Med 2005;15:442–7.

[44] Brukner P, Khan K. Clinical sports medicine. New York: McGraw-Hill; 1997, 412.

[45] Whitelaw GP, Wetzler MJ, Levy AS, et al. A pneumatic leg brace for the treatment of tibial stress fractures. Clin Orthop 1991;207:301–5.

[46] Coris EE, Lombardo JA. Tarsal navicular stress fractures. Am Fam Physician 2003;67:85–90.

[47] Potter N, Brukner P, Makdissi M, et al. Navicular stress fractures: outcomes of surgical and conservative management. Br J Sports Med 2006;40:692–5.

[48] Van Staa TP, Leufkens HG, Cooper C. Use of nonsteroidal anti-inflammatory drugs and risk of fractures. Bone 2000;27:563–8.

CHAPTER 80

Total Knee Replacement

Thomas E. Groomes, MD

Synonyms

Total knee arthroplasty
Total knee implant
Unicompartmental knee arthroplasty
Revision knee arthroplasty

ICD-9 Codes

715.16 Osteoarthrosis, localized, primary, lower leg
715.26 Osteoarthrosis, localized, secondary, lower leg

ICD-10 Codes

M17.10 Unilateral primary osteoarthritis, unspecified knee
M17.11 Unilateral primary osteoarthritis, right knee
M17.12 Unilateral primary osteoarthritis, left knee
M17.5 Other unilateral secondary osteoarthritis of knee

Definition

Arthroplasty involves the reconstruction by natural modification or artificial replacement of a diseased, damaged, or ankylosed joint. The knee joint functions as a complex hinge, allowing flexion, extension, rotation, and gliding. The knee joint itself is made up of three compartments, lateral, medial, and patellofemoral. Disease processes that cause damage to the cartilage of any or all of the three compartments may lead to the need for total knee arthroplasty (TKA). Examples of these diseases include osteoarthritis (idiopathic or traumatic), inflammatory arthritis (e.g., rheumatoid, psoriatic), avascular necrosis, tumors, and congenital abnormalities. The principal diagnoses most commonly associated with total knee replacement procedures are osteoarthrosis and allied disorders (90.9%), followed by rheumatoid arthritis and other inflammatory polyarthropathies (3.4%) [1].

TKA is a procedure that is widely performed for advanced arthropathies of the knee; it consistently alleviates pain, improves function, and enhances quality of life [2]. As the elderly population in the United States grows and indications for the procedure broaden, it is projected that an increasing number of patients will undergo TKA. The most common age group for total knee replacements is 65 to 84 years. Women in this age range are more likely to undergo TKA than are their male counterparts.

Approximately 700,000 TKAs are performed annually in the United States. With the aging of the U.S. population, this number is projected to increase to more than 3 million yearly by 2030 [3]. Younger and more active patients are electing to proceed with TKA.

TKA consists of resection of abnormal articular surfaces of the knee with resurfacing predominantly using metal and polyethylene components. The surgical use of a total condylar prosthesis (replaces all three compartments of the knee) dates to the early 1970s. There are three basic types of TKA: totally constrained, semiconstrained, and totally unconstrained. The amount of constraint built into an artificial joint reflects the amount of stability the hardware provides. As such, a totally constrained joint has the femoral portion physically attached to the tibial component and requires no ligamentous or soft tissue support. The semiconstrained TKA has two separate components that glide on each other, but the physical characteristics of the tibial component prevent excessive femoral glide. The totally unconstrained device relies completely on the body's ligaments and soft tissues to maintain the stability of the joint. The semiconstrained and totally unconstrained knee implants are most often used. In general, the totally unconstrained implants afford the most normal range of motion and gait.

In unicompartmental knee arthroplasty, only the joint surfaces on one side of the knee (usually the medial compartment) are replaced. Unicompartmental knee arthroplasty provides better relief than does a tibial osteotomy and greater range of motion than does a TKA as well as improved ambulation velocity. More recently, the concept of minimally invasive TKA has evolved from the procedures and investigations of unicompartmental knee arthroplasty. The distinctive features include decreased skin incision length, inferior and superior patellar capsular releases (necessary to gain exposure of the entire joint and to mobilize the patella), lack of patellar eversion (reducing risk of permanent dysfunction of the quadriceps muscle), and no tibiofemoral joint dislocation (minimizing capsular damage and postoperative pain).

The need for longer lasting TKAs continues, given the more active and anticipated longer living patient population. Efforts to design a better, longer lasting knee are focusing on alternative bearings and surfaces to reduce osteolysis. Areas being studied include the use of cross-linked ultrahigh-molecular-weight polyethylene inserts, alternative metal and ceramic bearing surfaces, and different mobile bearing designs. The goals of new designs are to minimize wear debris and to decrease risk of loosening and implant failure. The most important determinant of TKA long-lasting success remains a well-balanced, well-aligned, and well-fixed implantation procedure [4].

The increasing use of TKA has raised several public and clinical policy issues, including apparent racial and ethnic disparities in TKA use [5], broadening indications for TKA to include younger and older patients, and evidence that outcomes are better when TKA is performed in higher volume centers [6]. These issues were partially addressed in the Agency for Healthcare Research and Quality report [7]. That report concluded that there is no evidence that age, gender, or obesity is a strong predictor of functional outcomes. Patients with rheumatoid arthritis show more improvement than those with osteoarthritis, but this may be related to their poorer functional scores at the time of treatment and hence the potential for more improvement. The underlying indication, though, is consistent across all these groups, namely, that advanced osteoarthrosis of the knee compromises functional activities as the patient's knee pain becomes recalcitrant and unresponsive to conservative therapeutic interventions. Absolute contraindications to TKA include knee sepsis or other source of ongoing infection, extensor mechanism dysfunction, severe vascular disease, recurvatum deformity due to muscle weakness, and presence of a well-functioning knee arthrodesis. Relative contraindications may include neuropathic joint, morbid obesity, past history of osteomyelitis around the knee, and skin conditions such as psoriasis within the field of surgery [8].

Symptoms

Refractory knee pain is the most common symptom among patients who undergo TKA. Stiffness, deformity, and instability are symptoms also commonly seen in advanced osteoarthrosis or inflammatory polyarthropathy. In the postoperative period, acute surgical pain is most intense during the first 2 weeks. Disruption and inflammation of the periarticular soft tissues are manifested as a soft tissue stiffness pattern that differs in the severity of limitation of range of motion from the preoperative rigid stiffness of advanced arthrosis. Joint proprioception impairment may give rise to a sense of mild knee instability in the postoperative period. Uncommonly, debris may generate a sense of cracking, popping, or locking.

Physical Examination

Physical examination should include palpation of the knee to evaluate for effusion and joint line tenderness, which may indicate meniscal disease. Gait pattern should be documented with attention to the possible presence of knee thrust (abnormal medial or lateral movement of the knee), which may indicate ligamentous instability. Preoperative knee range of motion should be recorded to assess the extensor mechanism. Because of the importance of preserving the medial and lateral collateral ligaments during a total knee replacement, preoperative assessment of the stability of these ligaments is indicated. The skin over both legs should be assessed for signs of vascular disease or infection. The lower back and hip should be examined to rule out referred pain to the knee [9].

Functional Limitations

Osteoarthritis of the knee can result in pain or stiffness that can affect a person's functional ability to rise from a chair, to walk, or to use stairs. Table 80.1 depicts the required knee range of motion for specific functional mobility tasks. In an otherwise healthy patient population, osteoarthritis may impede participation in recreational or sporting activities, such as golf or tennis. The preoperative profile of a patient at risk for poor postoperative locomotor recovery is a woman with a high body mass index, many comorbidities, high intensity of knee pain, restriction in flexion amplitude, deficits in knee strength, and poor preoperative locomotor ability as measured by the 6-minute gait test. In addition, the preoperative gait power profiles, on the nonsurgical side, are characterized by low concentric push-off work by the plantar flexors and low concentric action of the hip flexors during early swing [10]. Postoperative pain scores and their associated psychological profiles ostensibly affect functional outcomes also [11].

Subsequent studies have further identified factors associated with a suboptimal postoperative functional outcome. Patients who have marked functional limitation, severe pain, low mental health score, and other comorbid conditions before TKA are more likely to have a worse outcome at 1 year and 2 years postoperatively [12]. One consistent finding is that preoperative joint function is a predictor of function at 6 months after TKA. Those patients who had lower preoperative functional status related to knee arthritis functioned at a lower level at 6 months than did patients with a higher preoperative functional status [13]. Studies have focused on quadriceps strength as a significant contributing factor. Functional measures underwent an expected decline early after TKA, but recovery was more rapid than anticipated and long-term outcomes were better than previously reported in

Table 80.1 Required Knee Range of Motion

Activity of Daily Living	Extension-Flexion
Walking in stance phase	15-40 degrees
Walking in swing phase	15-70 degrees
Stair climbing step over step	0-83 degrees
Standing up from a chair	0-93 degrees
Standing up from a toilet	0-105 degrees
Stooping to lift an object	0-117 degrees
Tying a shoelace	0-106 degrees

Modified from Kaplan RJ. Total knee replacement. In Frontera WR, ed. Essentials of Physical Medicine and Rehabilitation, 2nd ed. Philadelphia, WB Saunders, 2008.

the literature in patients with higher baseline quadriceps strength. The high correlation between quadriceps strength and functional performance suggests that emphasis on postoperative quadriceps strengthening is important to enhance the potential benefits of TKA [14]. However, preoperative quadriceps strength training has not been proved to enhance long-term functional outcome after TKA [15,16].

Diagnostic Studies

Plain radiographs of the knee remain the mainstay of diagnosis and preoperative planning. Three basic views include standing anteroposterior view (assesses medial and lateral joint space narrowing during normal leading of the joint), lateral view (assesses the patellofemoral joint and the position of the patella), and tangential patella or sunrise view (assesses the patellofemoral joint space) [9]. Magnetic resonance imaging is more sensitive than plain radiography in assessing cartilage but still may underestimate the amount of damage. Magnetic resonance imaging may also be used to evaluate meniscal or ligament disease [17].

In addition to the standard preoperative screening for surgical clearance, consideration should be given to radiographic evaluation of the cervical spine in rheumatoid arthritis patients. Rheumatoid arthritis patients are at increased risk for atlantodental instability and therefore may be at increased risk for spinal cord impingement as a result of perioperative manipulations with surgery and general anesthesia [18].

Rheumatoid arthritis patients are thought to be at 2.6-fold greater risk of infections than osteoarthritis patients are. Therefore, rheumatoid arthritis patients should be screened for potential sources of infections, including urinary tract infections, skin infections, and dental infections, before TKA. [19]

Differential Diagnosis of the Symptomatic Total Knee Arthroplasty

- Prosthetic loosening
- Infection
- Periprosthetic fracture
- Component failure

Treatment

Initial

Medical therapeutic interventions address the following.

Prophylaxis for Deep Venous Thrombosis and Pulmonary Embolism

Warfarin, a vitamin K antagonist, can be started preoperatively or postoperatively to prevent deep venous thrombosis (DVT) and pulmonary embolism (PE). The anticoagulant effects of vitamin K antagonists are not achieved until the third or fourth day of treatment. Thus, postoperative initiation of warfarin may not prevent small thrombi from forming. Nevertheless, warfarin does appear to effectively inhibit the extension of small thrombi, thereby preventing clinically significant DVT or PE. Because of its delayed reaction and its similar bleeding rates to low-molecular-weight heparin, warfarin tends to be the preferred thromboprophylactic medication by United States orthopedic surgeons [20].

New oral antithrombotic agents that inhibit either activated factor X or activated factor XI (thrombin) are now approved for use in the United States. Rivaroxaban inhibits activated factor X. The RECORD3 study demonstrated the superiority of a 10-mg once-daily oral dose of rivaroxaban over 40-mg subcutaneous daily dosing of enoxaparin in reducing the incidence of symptomatic venous thromboembolism (VTE) after total knee replacement [21]. The RECORD4 study compared rivaroxaban 10 mg orally daily with enoxaparin 30 mg subcutaneously twice daily. No statistically significant difference was shown in the incidence of major or symptomatic VTE [22].

Dabigatran etexilate is a direct thrombin inhibitor. It is active against both free and clot-bound thrombi. The RE-MOBILIZE trial compared dabigatran with enoxaparin (30 mg subcutaneously twice daily). Data for major VTE or death and major bleeding events were comparable [23]. Low-molecular-weight heparins are used in VTE prophylaxis after TKA. They have an advantage in that they can be given subcutaneously once or twice daily with constant dosing without the need for daily laboratory monitoring. They also carry a significantly reduced risk for heparin-induced thrombocytopenia compared with unfractionated heparin.

Intermittent pneumatic compression prevents venous thrombosis by increasing venous blood flow in the deep veins of the legs and by reducing plasminogen activator inhibitor [24]. Intermittent pneumatic compression is contraindicated in patients with evidence of leg ischemia due to peripheral vascular disease. The optimal use of intermittent pneumatic compression, which includes initiation in the operating room or recovery room, is an alternative option for VTE prophylaxis for patients at a high risk for bleeding. Aspirin is thought to be highly effective in reducing major arterial thrombotic events, but the benefit in reducing VTE is less clear. The 2008 American College of Chest Physicians anticoagulation guidelines recommended against use of aspirin alone as prophylaxis for VTE for any medical or surgical patient group [25]. The 2012 American College of Chest Physicians guidelines, however, have included aspirin as a recommended agent for thrombosis prophylaxis in patients undergoing TKA. This recommendation was not unanimously supported by the entire panel [26].

For patients undergoing total knee replacement, UpToDate recommends extending thrombosis prophylaxis beyond 10 days and up to 35 days after surgery [20].

Postoperative Care

During the first 48 to 72 hours, patients often receive controlled analgesia therapy administered through the intravenous or epidural route. Some anesthesiologists use a perioperative femoral nerve block. Subsequently, patients are given oral opioids. Controlled-release and short-acting opioids may be used. Depending on the clinician's and patient's preferences, fixed or rescue dose opioid medications are selected. The opioids can be titrated to achieve balance of analgesia versus emerging side effects [27–30].

Dry, sterile gauze dressings are applied as long as drainage is present. Staples and sutures can safely be removed 10 to 14 days after surgery [31,32]. Knee immobilizers may be used postoperatively to maintain knee extension and to avoid flexion contracture. Range of motion exercises supervised by a physical therapist should be initiated as soon as possible. Properly fitting, thigh-high elastic compression stockings, a continuous passive motion (CPM) machine, and possibly local cryotherapy are used to manage swelling [33–36].

The overall blood lost after unilateral TKA has been estimated at 2.2 units. Blood loss is greater for uncemented than for cemented prostheses. Patients are often advised before surgery to donate 1 to 3 units of packed red blood cells for autotransfusion, although this practice has recently been questioned [37]. In addition, postoperative blood collection and reinfusion through the surgical drain have been shown to be effective in reducing the need for bank blood and have a low morbidity rate with current techniques. Some patients are advised to commence a course of recombinant erythropoietin in conjunction with iron supplementation before surgery [38]. If the patient is receiving oral anticoagulation therapy, bridging therapy with a low-molecular-weight heparin compound may be considered by the patient's primary care physician or medical consultant [39]. If the perioperative red blood cell count reveals a macrocytic anemia, vitamin B_{12} and folic acid levels should be obtained. If the anemia is microcytic, serum iron level, total iron-binding capacity, or transferrin concentration should be determined along with a reticulocyte count.

Rehabilitation

Because preoperative function is a strong overall predictor of postoperative function for patients undergoing TKA, researchers are examining the potential role of prehabilitation (presurgical rehabilitation) in improving patient outcomes. Programs may include strength and flexibility training as well as nutritional counseling and education. Outcomes being studied include mobility, pain, self-care function, health-related quality of life, and self-efficacy (defined as the perception of one's ability to perform a task successfully). Although prehabilitation programs can have a positive effect on strength, function, and psychological health before surgery, it remains to be determined whether there is any significant long-term postoperative benefit [16,40].

The focus of postoperative rehabilitation should be joint range of motion, quadriceps strengthening, and training in gait and activities of daily living.

Rehabilitation programs that use clinical pathways enhance the efficiency of postoperative rehabilitation for the patient with TKA. The rehabilitation program can be conceptualized as occurring in stages or phases. The first stage commences in the immediate postoperative period. The final stage concludes when the patient returns to the community and pursues optimal independent functional living. See Table 80.2 for an example of a clinical pathway that addresses the schedule of progression during the first phase.

CPM devices may be used, but there is uncertainty whether the cost and inconvenience justify any significant clinical benefits. A 2010 meta-analysis review of 20 random trials comparing routine postoperative physical therapy and care with CPM to routine postoperative physical therapy and care without CPM showed only a small increase in range of motion (2-3 degrees) in the CPM group [41]. There is no evidence that short-term CPM application versus long-term CPM application influences outcome. There is no substantial evidence that CPM influences the degree of swelling, risk of VTE, or incidence of wound infection or incision site complications [42]. In the immediate postoperative period, the inhibited quadriceps and hamstrings may not adequately stabilize the knee. The patient may require a knee immobilizer for transfers and walking. The patient will often require a two-handed assistive device (e.g., walker or axillary crutches) for gait training initially. Adaptive equipment for bathing and dressing (e.g., tub or shower seat, grab bars, dressing sticks, sock aid) is generally necessary. Some patients may not have sufficient range of motion during the first week postoperatively to negotiate stairs. The motor reactions normalize by the third week; therefore, patients may return to driving activities if they can perform car transfers independently and can tolerate sitting for prolonged periods [43].

During the second stage of TKA rehabilitation (weeks 1 to 4), the patient progresses to low-resistance dynamic exercise for the involved lower extremity. This can be carried out with a stationary bicycle. Some patients may prefer aquatic-based exercise regimens during this period. Patients should be independent in ambulating with a two-handed or single-handed device if they are fully weight bearing on level surfaces up to 500 feet. They should be supervised in negotiating stairs. Electrical stimulation of the quadriceps can be considered for patients who have inhibited recruitment [44]. Soft tissue mobilization can be introduced to facilitate patellar glide. During this period, the patient should be independent in all basic activities of daily living. During the last 10 years, there has been a significant temporal shift in expediting home and outpatient (clinic) TKA rehabilitation. In this regard, there are no reproducible and enforceable guidelines that may be uniformly applied [45–47].

During the third stage of TKA rehabilitation (weeks 4 to 8), the available range of motion should reach 0 to 115 degrees. Patients are able to advance their dynamic resistance exercise regimens and more freely pursue both open and closed kinetic chain and dynamic balance exercises. Patients advance to a single-handed device or no device for ambulation and at different speeds and on different terrain. They should be independent in negotiating stairs. Patients advance to independence in instrumental activities of daily living.

In the final stage (weeks 8 to 12), patients may return to their preoperative exercise regimens and recreation activities and kneeling. Most patients who participated in sports before surgery are able to return to low-impact sport activities and exercise regimens. Patients are able to return to sedentary, light, and medium work categories. Patients who are on sick leave for more than 6 months preoperatively are less likely to return to work. There is published evidence that the degree of physical activity does not contribute to premature revision TKA [48]. However, younger patients may be at risk for earlier revision TKA, depending on their degree of physical activity [49]. Contact sports are advised against, and caution should be exercised with high-impact aerobic activities [50–54].

Procedures

Manipulation

Some patients with unsatisfactory gains in knee range of motion may be candidates for manipulation. The role of manipulation for the patient with a TKA contracture remains

Table 80.2 Clinical Pathway for First-Phase Rehabilitation

Postoperative Day	Exercise	Mobility	Ambulation	Activities of Daily Living
0	Deep breathing Incentive spirometer Quadriceps and gluteal sets	Sits to chair transfer Education on continuous passive motion machine		
	Straight-leg raise Hip abduction Ankle pumps			
1	Deep breathing	Bed mobility		Assess adaptive equipment: reachers, long-handled sponges, and shoehorns
	Lower extremity static resistance exercises	Bed to chair transfers with knee immobilizer		
	Ankle pumps and circles Continuous passive motion			
2	Continue previously described exercises	Continue bed mobility and transfers	Assisted ambulation in room, partial weight bearing or weight bearing as tolerated with knee immobilizer	Raised toilet seat
	Short arc quads			Grooming and dressing well while seated
	Straight-leg raise with knee immobilizer Upper extremity strengthening	Begin toilet transfers		
3	Continue previously described exercises	Decreased assistance in basic transfers	Independent ambulation with walker or crutches in room, partial weight bearing or weight bearing as tolerated with knee immobilizer	Independent toileting and grooming
	Sitting full arc motion flexion and extension in conjunction with supine passive flexion and extension		Trial of ambulation in corridor, possibly practice negotiating 2-4 stairs	Education on joint protection and energy conservation techniques
Depending on community resources and home safety and support availability, the patient may be ready for hospital discharge and post–acute care rehabilitation at this time.				
4	Continue previously described exercises with increased intensity	Independent in basic transfers	Gait training to improve pattern and endurance Discontinue knee immobilizer (if quadriceps strength is greater than 3/5)	Continue previously described activities of daily living
	Initiate active assistive range of motion exercises and quadriceps and hamstrings self-stretch			
5-6	Continue previously described exercises		Independent ambulation with assistive device	Independent dressing with tapered use of adaptive equipment
	Transition from passive to active assistive range of motion exercises		Begin stairs with railing, cane as needed	

From Kaplan RJ. Total knee replacement. In Frontera WR, ed. Essentials of Physical Medicine and Rehabilitation, 2nd ed. Philadelphia, WB Saunders, 2008.

controversial. Outcome studies are divided as to whether functional outcomes and quality of life are enhanced as a result of manipulation. When an orthopedic surgeon performs the procedure, it is carried out in an operating room with the use of general or epidural anesthesia. The goal is to overcome articular lesions with minimal force after quadriceps resistance is eliminated. Manipulation is most commonly performed during the second or third postoperative week if the range of motion of the involved knee is less than 75 degrees [55,56].

Arthrocentesis

Aspiration of the knee for aerobic and anaerobic cultures and sensitivities is the most reliable method for diagnosis of infection. Strict sterile technique must be used throughout the aspiration procedure [57].

Surgery

The most common materials presently used in replacement joints are cobalt-chromium and titanium on ultrahigh-molecular-weight polyethylene. In total knee arthroplasties, cobalt-chromium is commonly used on femoral weight-bearing surfaces because of its superior strength. Total knee arthroplasties can be stabilized with or without cement. In some cases, hybrid total knee arthroplasties are used.

There are three major surgical approaches for the standard TKA: the medial parapatellar retinacular approach, the midvastus approach, and the subvastus approach [58]. The medial parapatellar retinacular approach compromises the quadriceps tendon in its medial third, and this gives rise to more postoperative patellofemoral complications. The midvastus approach does not compromise the extensor mechanism of the knee joint. The subvastus approach also preserves the integrity of the extensor mechanism but does not expose the knee as well as the other two approaches do. The type of arthrotomy used will influence postoperative management. After a standard anteromedial arthrotomy between the vastus medialis and rectus tendons with eversion of the patella, active and passive range of motion may begin immediately. Protected ambulation with crutches or a walker is recommended for 4 to 6 weeks to allow healing of the arthrotomy repair and recovery of quadriceps strength. Although recovery after the subvastus approach may be more rapid than after the standard anteromedial approach, protected weight bearing with ambulatory aids for 3 to 6 weeks is still recommended to allow soft tissue healing. In the patient with limited preoperative range of motion, either tibial tubercle osteotomy or a V-Y quadricepsplasty needs to be performed. After tibial tubercle osteotomy, early range of motion and full weight bearing within 1 week of surgery is recommended. Variations of the conventional surgical exposures are also used in the minimally invasive TKA operative approaches [59].

Weight-bearing status depends on the details of the surgical reconstruction and whether the components were inserted with or without cement. For the otherwise uncomplicated primary cemented TKA, the patient can tolerate weight bearing within the confines of safety. Protected weight bearing can be performed only after the patient demonstrates adequate control of the limb to prevent falling. The time to weight bearing after total arthroplasty depends on the use of cement or cementless fixation and whether large structural bone grafting was required. In cemented total knees, no differences in the incidence of radiolucent lines have been observed between immediate weight bearing and protected weight bearing for 12 weeks. Although weight bearing after cementless fixation might increase micromotion, many surgeons allow early weight bearing [60].

The tibial and femoral components presently in use have a life expectancy of 10 to 20 years. This life span depends on the surgical technique, the components used, the bone stock, and the level of physical activity after TKA. Revision TKA is a surgical procedure that the patient with TKA may encounter several years after the original surgery [61].

Potential Disease Complications

Potential disease complications of conditions involving the knee, such as osteoarthritis, rheumatoid arthritis, and osteonecrosis of the femoral epicondyle or tibial condyle, include intractable pain, swelling, stiffness, contracture, and valgus or varus deformity. It is recommended that TKA not be significantly delayed once it is clinically indicated. Otherwise, the delay may allow the development of soft tissue contractures and excessive muscle atrophy, which could reduce the chances of a good postoperative recovery [62].

Potential Treatment Complications

The development of DVT with the subsequent risk for fatal PE is understandably the most feared complication of TKA. Without prophylaxis, the incidence of DVT after TKA ranges from 40% to 88%, the incidence of asymptomatic PE ranges from 10% to 20%, and the incidence of symptomatic PE ranges from 0.5% to 3%, with mortality up to 2%. With prophylaxis, the incidence of symptomatic DVT and PE drops to less than 1% and 0.3%, respectively [63].

Patellofemoral complications are thought to be the most common reason for reoperation after TKA. Examples include patella instability, patella component loosening or failure, patella fracture, patella clunk syndrome, and rupture of the exterior mechanism. Patella clunk syndrome results from formation of fibrous tissue on the quadriceps tendon. The patient feels a clunk as the knee is actively extended from 60 to 30 degrees. This syndrome was more commonly seen with earlier designs of posterior cruciate substitution prostheses. With changes in component design, the incidence of patella clunk has decreased [64].

The most common neurologic complication is peroneal nerve palsy. Clinical presentation includes paresthesias and ankle dorsiflexion weakness. Incidence is less than 1%. Recovery is variable, with one study reporting up to 50% full recovery [8]. Arterial vascular injuries, the majority of which are thrombosis, are exceedingly rare.

Periprosthetic fractures may occur in the patella, around the femoral component and the tibial component. Osteoporosis and rheumatoid arthritis increase the risk for periprosthetic fractures. Femoral fractures are associated with notching of the anterior femur at time of surgery. Tibial fractures remain rare [64].

Arthrofibrosis (stiffness) is a postoperative limited range of motion that may result in decreased function. In general, 67 degrees of knee flexion is needed during the swing phase of gait, 83 degrees to ascend stairs, 100 degrees to descend stairs, 93 degrees to rise from a standard chair, and 105 degrees to rise from a low chair [65]. It remains unclear whether the use of continuous passive motion reduces the risk of arthrofibrosis.

Although infection is a serious complication, the overall infection rate for initial TKA is low at around 1% [66]. This is higher in patients with diabetes mellitus, advanced rheumatoid arthritis, revision TKA, or constrained prostheses. Deep infection can occur any time from days to months after surgery. Musculoskeletal infection usually is manifested as increase in pain with or without weight bearing, increase in swelling, and fever. Diagnosis is confirmed by joint fluid analysis, as described earlier. The patient typically requires at least a 6-week course of antibiotic treatment between the period of component removal and reimplantation. The most successful technique for treatment of the infected total knee replacement is a two-stage reimplantation of the TKA components. Infection must never be overlooked as a cause of implant loosening. Infection can occur early or late and can be manifested with or without signs of systemic toxicity. The symptoms are commonly the same as those seen with aseptic loosening. A progressive radiolucency between the prosthesis and its adjacent bone almost always is considered an infection until proved otherwise. Negative aspirate from the knee, normal sedimentation rate and C-reactive protein level, and normal gallium or indium scans cannot rule out infection of the prosthetic device. The patient should be advised that even in the presence of normal test results, infection of the prosthetic device may be discovered intraoperatively and necessitate the removal of the prosthetic device.

Metallosis is a rare but severe complication of knee replacement surgery. Metallic debris may be deposited in the periprosthetic soft tissues from abrasion of the metallic components. This metallic debris may induce a massive release of cytokines from inflammatory cells. This release may accelerate osteolysis and loosening of the prosthesis [67]. The inflammatory cells may also infiltrate the synovium, resulting in synovitis, which may be manifested as an acutely painful effusion [68]. In addition, the metallic debris may have a direct toxic effect on human marrow stroma–derived mesenchymal stem cells; it is hypothesized that decreased viability of these mesenchymal stem cells may reduce the amount of viable osteoprogenitor cells, which would be a factor in the development of poor periprosthetic bone quality. The reduction in bone quality increases the risk of implant stability, which eventually requires revision surgery [69]. Titanium components appear to have an increased association with metallosis in comparison to chromium-cobalt components [68].

The most common reason for total arthroplasty failure has been loosening of the implant. Factors associated with loosening include infection, implant constraint, failure to achieve neutral mechanical alignment, instability, and cement technique. The prodromal features of impending loosening and failure of the components are an increase in pain and swelling with or without angular deformity of the knee [70]. The radiographic features include a widening radiolucent zone between the implant and the adjacent bone and subsidence of the implant. Loosening may occur at the component-cement interface or bone-cement interface. Implant loosening can be attributed to mechanical and biologic factors. The mechanical factors include limb alignment, ligamentous balance, and preservation of a contracted posterior cruciate ligament. Implant loosening can occur early or late. Early implant loosening usually occurs within the first 2 years and represents a mechanical failure of the interlock of the implant and host to bone. This early implant loosening is more appropriately called fixation failure and is often secondary to errors in judgment at the time of surgery or to problems with the technical aspects of the surgical procedure. Extremity malalignment, soft tissue imbalance, and poor cement technique individually or in combination contribute to loosening. Biologic factors are largely responsible for the phenomenon of late loosening. Late loosening of total knee implants is often secondary to the host biologic response to the implant's debris that weakens the mechanical bond of implant to bone established during surgery. Mechanical factors may contribute to late loosening, but they do not alone explain the loss of a fixation device that has been stable for many years. The volume of particles generated from the articulation is influenced by the patient's weight and activity level, duration of implantation, polyethylene thickness, and contact stresses. Wear may be accelerated by malalignment, instability, and ligament imbalance, resulting in increased volume of particulate released into the joint [71]. Aseptic loosening that will lead to failure of the prosthesis occurs in 5% to 10% of patients at around 10 to 15 years after surgery. Once a component becomes loose, it becomes mechanically unstable. This can lead to increased osteolyses. If the osteolyses becomes severe, revision surgery will be difficult [8]. Thirty-day mortality for TKA is around 0.6%, with no significant differences based on race or ethnicity [9].

References

[1] American Academy of Orthopaedic Surgeons. Primary total hip and total knee arthroplasty projections to 2030 (Appendix C). http://www.aaos.org.ezproxy.galter.northwestern.edu/wordhtml/pdfs_r/tjr.pdf.

[2] Lavernia CJ, Guzman JF, Gachupin-Garcia A. Cost effectiveness and quality of life in knee arthroplasty. Clin Orthop 1997;345:134–9.

[3] Kurtz S, Ong K, Lau E, et al. Projections of primary and revision hip and knee arthroplasty in the United States from 2005 to 2030. J Bone Joint Surg Am 2007;89:780.

[4] Gee AO, Lee GC. Alternative bearings in total knee arthroplasty. Am J Orthop 2012;41:280–3.

[5] Dunlop DD, Song J, Manheim LM, Chang RW. Racial disparities in joint replacement use among older adults. Med Care 2003;41:288–98.

[6] Hervey SL, Purves HR, Guller U, et al. Provider volume of total knee arthroplasties and patient outcomes in the HCUP-nationwide inpatient sample. J Bone Joint Surg Am 2003;85:1775–83.

[7] Kane RL, Saleh KJ, Wilt TJ, et al. Total knee replacement. Evidence Report/Technology Assessment No. 86, Rockville, Md: U.S. Dept. of Health and Human Services, Public Health Service, Agency for Healthcare Research and Quality; 2003, AHRQ publication 04-E006-2.

[8] Palmer SH. Total knee arthroplasty; June 2012. emedicine.medscape.com/article/1750275-overview.

[9] Martin GM, Thornhill TS. Total knee arthroplasty; September 2010. www.uptodate.com.

[10] Parent E, Moffet H. Preoperative predictors of locomotor ability two months after total knee arthroplasty for severe osteoarthritis. Arthritis Rheum 2003;49:36–50.

[11] Brander VA, Stulberg SD, Adams AD, et al. Predicting total knee replacement pain: a prospective, observational study. Clin Orthop Relat Res 2003;416:27–36.

[12] Lingard EA, Katz JN, Wright EA, Sledge CB, Kinemax Outcomes Group. Predicting the outcome of total knee arthroplasty. J Bone Joint Surg Am 2004;86:2179–86.

[13] Jones CA, Voaklander DC, Suarez-Alma ME. Determinants of function after total knee arthroplasty. Phys Ther 2003;83:696–706.

[14] Mizner RL, Petterson SC, Stevens JE, et al. Preoperative quadriceps strength predicts functional ability one year after total knee arthroplasty. J Rheumatol 2005;32:1533–9.

[15] Beaupre LA, Lier D, Davies DM, Johnston DB. The effect of a preoperative exercise and education program on functional recovery, health related quality of life, and health service utilization following primary total knee arthroplasty. J Rheumatol 2004;31:1166–73.

[16] McKay C, Prapavessis H, Doherty T. The effect of a prehabilitation exercise program on quadriceps strength for patients undergoing total knee arthroplasty: a randomized controlled pilot study. PM R 2012;4:647–56.

[17] Blackburn Jr WD, Chivers S, Bernreuter W. Cartilage imaging in osteoarthritis. Semin Arthritis Rheum 1996;25:273.

[18] Grauer JN, Tingstad EM, Rand N, et al. Predictors of paralysis in the rheumatoid cervical spine in patients undergoing total joint arthroplasty. J Bone Joint Surg Am 2004;86:1420.

[19] Poss R, Thornhill TS, Ewald FC, et al. Factors influencing the incidence and outcome of infection following total joint arthroplasty. Clin Orthop Relat Res 1984;182:117.

[20] Pineo GF. Prevention of venous thromboembolic disease in surgical patients. UpToDate; September 2012. www.uptodate.com.

[21] Lassen MR, Ageno W, Borris LC, et al. Rivaroxaban versus enoxaparin for thromboprophylaxis after total knee arthroplasty. N Engl J Med 2008;358:2776.

[22] Turpie AG, Lassen MR, Davidson BL, et al. Rivaroxaban versus enoxaparin for thromboprophylaxis after total knee arthroplasty (RECORD4): a randomised trial. Lancet 2009;373:1673.

[23] RE-MOBILIZE Writing Committee, Ginsberg JS, Davidson BL, Comp PC, et al. Oral thrombin inhibitor dabigatran etexilate vs North American enoxaparin regimen for prevention of venous thromboembolism after knee arthroplasty surgery. J Arthroplasty 2009;24:1.

[24] Comerota AJ, Chouhan V, Harada RN, et al. The fibrinolytic effects of intermittent pneumatic compression: mechanism of enhanced fibrinolysis. Ann Surg 1997;226:306.

[25] Geerts WH, Bergqvist D, Pineo GF, et al. Prevention of venous thromboembolism: American College of Chest Physicians Evidence-Based Clinical Practice Guidelines (8th Edition). Chest 2008;133:381S.

[26] Falck-Ytter Y, Francis CW, Johanson NA, et al. Prevention of VTE in orthopedic surgery patients: Antithrombotic Therapy and Prevention of Thrombosis, 9th ed: American College of Chest Physicians Evidence-Based Clinical Practice Guidelines. Chest 2012;141:e278S.

[27] Farag E, Dilger J, Brooks P, Tetzlaff JE. Epidural analgesia improves early rehabilitation after total knee replacement. J Clin Anesth 2005;17:281–5.

[28] Bourne MH. Analgesics for orthopedic postoperative pain. Am J Orthop 2004;33:128–35.

[29] Cheville A, Chen A, Oster G, et al. A randomized trial of controlled-release oxycodone during inpatient rehabilitation following unilateral total knee arthroplasty. J Bone Joint Surg Am 2001;83:572–6.

[30] Huenger F, Schmachtenberg A, Haefner H, et al. Evaluation of post-discharge surveillance of surgical site infections after total hip and knee arthroplasty. Am J Infect Control 2005;33:455–62.

[31] Lucas B. Nursing management issues in hip and knee replacement surgery. Br J Nurs 2004;13:782–7.

[32] Engel C, Hamilton NA, Potter PT, Zautra AJ. Comparing compression bandaging and cold therapy in postoperative total knee replacement surgery. Perianesthes Ambul Surg Nurs Update 2002;10:51.

[33] Esler CAN, Blakeway C, Fiddian NJ. The use of a closed-suction drain in total knee arthroplasty: a prospective, randomised study. J Bone Joint Surg Br 2003;85:215–7.

[34] Smith J, Stevens J, Taylor M, Tibbey J. A randomized, controlled trial comparing compression bandaging and cold therapy in postoperative total knee replacement surgery. Orthop Nurs 2002;21:61–6.

[35] Lieberman JR. A closed-suction drain was not beneficial in knee arthroplasty with cement. J Bone Joint Surg Am 2003;85:2257.

[36] Brosseau L, Milne S, Wells G, et al. Efficacy of continuous passive motion following total knee arthroplasty: a metaanalysis. J Rheumatol 2004;31:2251–64.

[37] Muller U, Roder C, Pisan M, et al. Autologous blood donation in total knee arthroplasties is not necessary. Acta Orthop Scand 2004;75:66–70.

[38] Rauh MA, Bayers-Thering M, LaButti RS, Krackow KA. Preoperative administration of epoetin alfa to total joint arthroplasty patients. Orthopedics 2002;25:317–20.

[39] Dunn AS, Wisnivesky J, Ho W, et al. Perioperative management of patients on oral anticoagulants: a decision analysis. Med Decis Making 2005;25:387–97.

[40] Topp R, Swank AM, Quesada PM, et al. The effect of prehabilitation exercise on strength and functioning after total knee arthroplasty. PM R 2009;1:729–35.

[41] Harvey LA, Brosseau L, Herbert RD. Continuous passive motion following total knee arthroplasty in people with arthritis. Cochrane Database Syst Rev 2010;3, CD004260.

[42] Lenssen AF, de Bie RA, Bulstra SK, van Steyn MJA. Continuous passive motion (CPM) in rehabilitation following total knee arthroplasty: a randomised controlled trial. Phys Ther Rev 2003;8:123–9.

[43] Pierson JL, Earles DR, Wood K. Brake response time after total knee arthroplasty: when is it safe for patients to drive? J Arthroplasty 2003;18:840–3.

[44] Avramidis K, Strike PW, Taylor PN, Swain ID. Effectiveness of electric stimulation of the vastus medialis muscle in the rehabilitation of patients after total knee arthroplasty. Arch Phys Med Rehabil 2003;84:1850–3.

[45] Epps CD. Length of stay, discharge disposition, and hospital charge predictors. AORN J 2004;79:975–6, 979-981, 984-988 passim.

[46] Weaver FM, Hughes SL, Almagor O, et al. Comparison of two home care protocols for total joint replacement. J Am Geriatr Soc 2003;51:523–8.

[47] Kramer JF, Speechley M, Bourne R, et al. Comparison of clinic- and home-based rehabilitation programs after total knee arthroplasty. Clin Orthop Relat Res 2003;410:225–34.

[48] Jones DL, Cauley JA, Kriska AM, et al. Physical activity and risk of revision total knee arthroplasty in individuals with knee osteoarthritis: a matched case-control study. J Rheumatol 2004;31:1384–90.

[49] Harrysson OL, Robertsson O, Nayfeh JF. Higher cumulative revision rate of knee arthroplasties in younger patients with osteoarthritis. Clin Orthop Relat Res 2004;421:162–8.

[50] Chatterji U, Ashworth MJ, Lewis PL, Dobson PJ. Effect of total knee arthroplasty on recreational and sporting activity. ANZ J Surg 2005;75:405–8.

[51] Kuster MS. Exercise recommendations after total joint replacement: a review of the current literature and proposal of scientifically based guidelines. Sports Med 2002;32:433–45.

[52] Lamb SE, Frost H. Recovery of mobility after knee arthroplasty: expected rates and influencing factors. J Arthroplasty 2003;18:575–82.

[53] Hassaballa MA, Porteous AJ, Newman JH, Rogers CA. Can knees kneel? Kneeling ability after total, unicompartmental and patellofemoral knee arthroplasty. Knee 2003;10:155–60.

[54] Clifford PE, Mallon WJ. Sports after total joint replacement. Clin Sports Med 2005;24:175–86.

[55] Bong MR, Di Cesare PE. Stiffness after total knee arthroplasty. J Am Acad Orthop Surg 2004;12:164–71.

[56] Ellis TJ, Beshires E, Brindley GW, et al. Knee manipulation after total knee arthroplasty. J South Orthop Assoc 1999;8:73–9.

[57] Lonner JH, Siliski JM, Della Valle C, et al. Role of knee aspiration after resection of the infected total knee arthroplasty. Am J Orthop 2001;30:305–9.

[58] Younger AS, Duncan CP, Masri BA. Surgical exposures in revision total knee arthroplasty. J Am Acad Orthop Surg 1998;6:55–64.

[59] Scuderi GR, Tenholder M, Capeci C. Surgical approaches in mini-incision total knee arthroplasty. Clin Orthop Relat Res 2004;428:61–7.

[60] Youm T, Maurer SG, Stuchin SA. Postoperative management after total hip and knee arthroplasty. J Arthroplasty 2005;20:322–4.

[61] Mehrotra C, Remington PL, Naimi TS, et al. Trends in total knee replacement surgeries and implications for public health, 1990–2000. Public Health Rep 2005;120:278–82.

[62] Weisman MH. Total joint replacement for severe rheumatoid arthritis. UpToDate; August 2007. www.uptodate.com.

[63] Januel JM, Chen G, Ruffieux C, et al. Symptomatic in-hospital deep vein thrombosis and pulmonary embolism following hip and knee arthroplasty among patients receiving recommended prophylaxis: a systematic review. JAMA 2012;307:294.

[64] Martin GM, Thornhill TS. Complications of total knee arthroplasty. UpToDate; January 2012. www.uptodate.com.

[65] Laubenthal KN, Smidt GL, Kettelkamp DB. A quantitative analysis of knee motion during activities of daily living. Phys Ther 1972;52:34.

[66] Leone JM, Hanssen AD. Management of infection at the site of a total knee arthroplasty. J Bone Joint Surg Am 2005;87:2335–48.

[67] Schiavone PA, Vasso M, Cerciello S, et al. Metallosis following knee arthroplasty: a histological and immunohistochemical study. Int J Immunopathol Pharmacol 2011;24:711–9.

[68] Romesburg JW, Wasserman PL, Schoppe CH. Metallosis and metal-induced synovitis following total knee arthroplasty: review of radiological findings. J Radiol Case Rep 2010;4:7–17.

[69] Wang ML, Tuli R, Manner PA, et al. Direct and indirect induction of apoptosis in human mesenchymal stem cells in response to titanium particles. J Orthop Res 2003;21:697–707.

[70] Dennis DA. Evaluation of painful total knee arthroplasty. J Arthroplasty 2004;19(Suppl. 1):35–40.

[71] Callaghan JJ, O'Rourke MR, Saleh KJ. Why knees fail: lessons learned. J Arthroplasty 2004;19(Suppl. 1):31–4.

SECTION IX
Foot and Ankle

CHAPTER 81

Achilles Tendinopathy

Michael F. Stretanski, DO

Synonyms

Achilles tendinosis
Peritendinosis
Heel cord tendinitis

ICD-9 Codes

726.71 Achilles bursitis or tendinitis
845.09 Sprains and strains of ankle and foot, Achilles tendon

ICD-10 Codes

M76.60 Achilles tendinitis, unspecified leg
M76.61 Achilles tendinitis, right leg
M76.62 Achilles tendinitis, left leg
S96.811 Sprain of other specified muscles and tendons at ankle and foot level, right foot
S96.812 Sprain of other specified muscles and tendons at ankle and foot level, left foot
S96.819 Sprain of other specified muscles and tendons at ankle and foot level, unspecified foot
Add the appropriate seventh character for episode of care to S96

Definition

Achilles tendinopathy exists along a spectrum of peritendinitis to tendinosis or tendinopathy. The pathologic process involves a painful, swollen, and tender area of the Achilles tendon and peritenon. Athletes with particularly tight heel cords are predisposed to this injury. This condition commonly affects middle-aged men who play tennis, basketball, or other quick start-and-stop sports. Achilles tendon rupture carries a 200-fold risk of sustaining a contralateral rupture of the Achilles tendon [1], but atraumatic disease associations, such as periarticular manifestation of poststreptococcal reactive arthritis [2], should remain in the atraumatic differential. Collagen vascular disease, inflammatory disease, and diabetes may also be risk factors. The relative avascularity of the region 5 to 7 cm proximal to the calcaneus insertion has long been considered a pathoanatomic structural risk factor, as is the thinning and twisting of the tendon at this midsection [3]. However, morphologic and biochemical differences present within the tendon during Achilles tendinopathy provide a modern addendum to this dogma. Upregulation of collagen 1 and collagen 3 together with mRNA of fibronectin, tenascin C, and fibromodulin as well as degradation factors matrix metalloproteinases 2 and 9 and tissue inhibitor of matrix metalloproteinase 2 in Achilles tendinopathy [4] seem to add to the growing understanding of the cellular and molecular basis of the clinical presentation. The histopathologic feature is angiofibroblastic hyperplasia (tendinosis) of the body of the tendon (a degenerative process) with a concomitant and potentially secondary inflammatory response in the peritenon [5,6]. The maladies often occur simultaneously but may occur individually. An association with chronic quinolone exposure is well documented [7–9] and is worse in patients concomitantly taking prednisone long term.

Symptoms

Pain and tenderness in the Achilles tendon are predominant symptoms, usually in association with running, sports with quick "cutting," and other fitness activities [10]. Activities with rapid starting and stopping or rapid eccentric contraction, such as classical ballet [11], increase the symptoms and risk of complete tear. In some patients, the pain actually improves with lower extremity exercise. Typically, the pain occurs with a change in activity or training schedule. The most common location for tendinosis symptoms is at the apex of the Achilles tendon curvature. Different activities can lead to pathologic change in other regions of the tendon, namely, at the calcaneal insertion with or without a Haglund deformity or at the myotendinous junction. A history of an acute traumatic event in which the patient reports a "pop" should suggest an Achilles tendon tear, although a similar pop can occur with tear or rupture of the plantaris, peroneus, or posterior tibial tendon. History of quinolone exposure, diabetes, collagen vascular disease, anabolic steroid use, or smoking should be noted.

Physical Examination

The essential element in the physical examination is localization of swelling and tenderness in the critical zone of the Achilles tendon at the apex of the Achilles curve approximately 2 ½ inches proximal to the os calcis insertion. Exquisite tenderness to palpation is a classic examination finding. The degree of ankle plantar force generated has been shown to have a strong negative relationship with pain, and a standardized strength testing system has been suggested and shown to be reliable on a small sample of patients [12]. Palpable heat is usually not evident unless peritendinitis is a major component. The Achilles tendon is usually tight, with ankle dorsiflexion rarely extending beyond 90 degrees. Associated findings may include abnormal foot posture (pes planus or cavus), tight hamstrings, and muscle weakness of the entire hip and leg. Heels may not move into a normal varus position in standing on toes. Neurologic evaluation findings, including strength, sensation, and deep tendon reflexes, are normal.

The examination should also include observation for a palpable defect and the Thompson test (squeezing the calf, which should result in plantar flexion in an attached tendon) to rule out rupture of the Achilles tendon (Fig. 81.1).

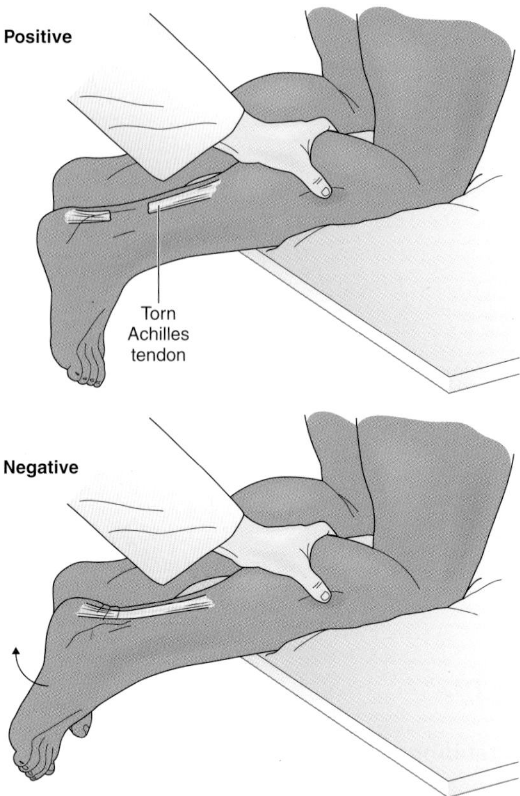

FIGURE 81.1 The Thompson test is a reliable clinical test to identify a complete tear in the Achilles tendon. When the Achilles tendon is torn, a positive test result is elicited by squeezing the calf and seeing no plantar flexion of the foot. The test result is negative when the calf is squeezed and plantar flexion occurs in the foot.

Functional Limitations

Impact weight-bearing activities, such as jogging and running, are usually limited. Dance or cutting "moves" typical of field sports are virtually impossible. Nonimpact fitness activities, such as cycling and using an elliptical trainer, may also result in symptoms. Patients may complain of pain with daily ambulatory activities, such as walking at work or climbing stairs. Whereas individual differences exist, early recovery of plantar flexion may be seen with little functional change, usually because of flexor hallucis longus compensation [13].

Diagnostic Studies

Unless a special form of calcified Achilles tendinosis occurs at the os calcis insertion, regular radiographs are usually normal. Diagnostic ultrasonography or magnetic resonance imaging is capable of defining the extent of both tendinosis and peritendinitis, but serial magnetic resonance examinations, especially postoperatively, are not indicated and do not correlate with functional outcome [14]. Partial rupture is a diagnostic dilemma for diagnostic ultrasonography [15], and if it is suspected, magnetic resonance imaging should still be considered the standard of care. Magnetic resonance imaging is also more useful in documenting a complete tear's distance and location as well as the existence of partial tear that may appear normal or questionable on diagnostic ultrasound examination. Electrodiagnostic studies, especially needle electromyography and H reflexes (the electrodiagnostic equivalent of an Achilles muscle stretch reflex), may help in defining S1 radicular features, but a normal electrodiagnostic study does not rule out sensory irritative radiculitis. These studies are generally recommended only to help define the prognosis or in patients who are unresponsive to rehabilitation and for whom surgery or other diagnoses are being considered. A slowly evolving role of positron emission tomography may exist [16], and blood work germane to systemic disease, sedimentation rate, antinuclear antibody, rheumatoid factor, and antistreptolysin antibody titer [2] may be appropriate.

Differential Diagnosis

Haglund deformity
Retrocalcaneal bursitis
Adventitial bursitis
Achilles tendon rupture
Tibial stress fracture
Medial gastrocnemius tear
S1 (L5) radiculopathy

Treatment

Initial

The initial treatment goal is to decrease pain and to reduce inflammation when it is present. Therefore rest from aggravating activities is critical. Icing (20 minutes, two or three times daily) and nonsteroidal anti-inflammatory drugs or analgesics can be used for pain and inflammation. A wide range of treatments from repetitive low-energy shock wave treatment [17], sclerosing agents [18], and topical nitroglycerin [19] to low-level laser therapy have been attempted with varying degrees of mixed results in small studies.

Counterforce bracing is often helpful, or a simple heel lift (⅛ to ½ inch) can decrease stress on the tendon. Warm-up before any weight-bearing activity and cooling with ice afterward are recommended. Good functional results can usually be achieved in about 75% of cases at 3 months with nonoperative treatment in compliant patients with a tendon separation distance of 10 mm or less apparent on diagnostic ultrasonography [20].

Rehabilitation

The rehabilitative process focuses on biologic improvement of the damaged tendon and peritenon and restoration of function, rather than the comfort efforts of the initial treatment phase. Rehabilitation is best initiated in a structured physical therapy program followed by home therapeutic exercise. Non–weight-bearing status and axillary crutches may have a role in the acute phase of treatment, with return to weight bearing as tolerated. A short leg cast or splint in 10 to 15 degrees of plantar flexion may also have a short-term role in acute phase treatment. Passive modalities including therapeutic ultrasound, iontophoresis, and phonophoresis often enhance compliance and enable the rehabilitation program. Electrical stimulation should be considered contraindicated in the face of the overuse etiology and counterphysiologic motor unit recruitment of muscle fibers.

Therapeutic exercise needs to be directed toward the complete kinetic chain because strength, endurance, and flexibility deficits are common, and most lower extremity sports activities occur as patterned motor engrams. Strength, proprioceptive, and endurance testing usually aids in uncovering relative weaknesses and monitoring the rehabilitation progress. Controlled eccentric exercise may be of benefit throughout the strength-building phase of rehabilitation and avoid additional tendon separation.

Control of abusive force loads can be accomplished by counterforce bracing of the Achilles tendon or orthotics to minimize abnormal foot posture. Gradual, controlled return to running may be initiated through running in water programs. As with any lower extremity injury, general fitness may be maintained by use of upper body land programs such as arm ergometry, resistance training, and water programs dedicated to the entire body. Return to sport or running is transitional, including plyometric and eccentric exercises. Full return generally requires normal strength, endurance, and flexibility. Repeated injury is not uncommon. Return to normal activity, generally in 6 to 12 weeks, depends on level of participation (professional athlete versus weekend warrior), severity of the injury, and general medical condition.

Procedures

Exogenous glucocorticoid injection is contraindicated as cellular death and tendon weakness with potential progression to tendon rupture are significant concerns. Although there may be a developing role for hylan G-F 20 [21], this has been studied, to date, only in corticosteroid-induced Achilles tendinopathy in an animal model. Likewise, pulsed ultrasound [22], indium-gallium-aluminum-phosphide diode laser irradiation [23], and substance P injection [24] in an animal tenotomy model have all shown potential results, and hyperbaric oxygen [25] may have a slightly more promising role.

Surgery

Rehabilitation failure may invite surgical intervention with a goal of problem resolution versus acceptance of the malady and alteration of activity level. Optimal surgical management strategy is controversial, but the relative avascularity of the region makes wound healing complications and deep infection ever-present threats. The concepts of surgery include removal of symptomatic peritendinitis tissue and resection of the abnormal tendinosis tissue in the body of the Achilles tendon with subsequent repair of the remaining adjacent normal tendon. This is usually accomplished with standard sutures or wires; however, fibrin sealant has been used [26], and at least on the surface, this may seem a more biologic approach. Surgical options consist of open, mini-open, or percutaneous repair. Surgery outcomes are better if all pathologic tissue is removed, reanastomosis is performed, and appropriate postoperative rehabilitation is implemented. The postoperative goals of neovascularization, reduction of atrophy, fibroblastic infiltration, and collagen production and the restoration of strength, endurance, and flexibility are best served by early mobilization [27].

In cases of suspected tendon rupture, a surgical consultation is warranted for consideration of other tendon ruptures. Endoscopic techniques have evolved alongside open and mini-open [28] approaches but with comparable rerupture rates. The percutaneous repair seems to be a better option for elite athletes with a greater likelihood of return to sport activities [29], but it has an increased complication rate. There are differences of opinion as to whether the percutaneous technique should be performed at all in lieu of a limited open technique [30].

Potential Disease Complications

Chronic symptoms can result in weakening and subsequent complete rupture of the Achilles tendon. Chronic intractable pain with other kinetic chain imbalances and secondary gait abnormality may develop. Significant alterations in gait can cause secondary knee, hip, forefoot, or low back pain. Consideration of undiagnosed systemic diseases that carry their own comorbidities should be entertained.

Potential Treatment Complications

Side effects of nonsteroidal anti-inflammatory drugs include gastric, renal, and hepatic complications. Bracing for prolonged periods may lead to pressure sores, disuse weakness, atrophy, poorly coordinated motor control when return to activity is attempted, and potential peroneal neuropathy. Sural nerve injury can occur with open or percutaneous repair [31]. Overly aggressive physical therapy or electrical stimulation of the gastrocnemius-soleus complex may cause increased pain and inflammation that can ultimately lead to tendon weakness and potential rupture. Surgical complications of bleeding, infection, and tibial, peroneal, or sural nerve injury are well known. Repeated tear may occur.

References

[1] Kongsgaard M, Aagaard P, Kjaer M, Magnusson SP. Structural Achilles tendon properties in athletes subjected to different exercise modes and in Achilles tendon rupture patients. J Appl Physiol 2005;99:1965–71.

[2] Sarakbi HA, Hammoudeh M, Kanjar I, et al. Poststreptococcal reactive arthritis and the association with tendonitis, tenosynovitis, and enthesitis. J Clin Rheumatol 2010;16:3–6.

[3] Theobald P, Benjamin M, Nokes L, Pugh N. Review of the vascularisation of the human Achilles tendon. Injury 2005;36:1267–72.

[4] Pingel J, Fredberg U, Qvortrup K, et al. Local biochemical and morphological differences in human Achilles tendinopathy. BMC Musculoskelet Disord 2012;13:53.

[5] Kraushaar B, Nirschl R. Tendinosis of the elbow (tennis elbow). Clinical features and findings of histological, immunohistochemical, and electron microscopy studies. J Bone Joint Surg Am 1999;81:259–78.

[6] Puddu G, Ippolito E, Postacchini F. A classification of Achilles tendon disease. Am J Sports Med 1976;4:145–50.

[7] Lado Lado FL, Rodriguez MC, Velasco GM, et al. Partial bilateral rupture of the Achilles tendon associated with levofloxacin. An Med Interna 2005;22:28–30.

[8] Chhajed PN, Plit ML, Hopkins PM, et al. Achilles tendon disease in lung transplant recipients: association with ciprofloxacin. Eur Respir J 2002;19:469–71.

[9] McGarvey WC, Singh D, Trevino SG. Partial Achilles tendon ruptures associated with fluoroquinolone antibiotics: a case report and literature review. Foot Ankle Int 1996;17:494–8.

[10] Nirschl R. Surgical considerations of ankle injuries. In: O'Connor F, Wilder R, editors. The complete book of running medicine. New York: McGraw-Hill; 2001.

[11] Stretanski MF, Weber GJ. Medical and rehabilitation issues in classical ballet. Am J Phys Med 2002;81:383–91.

[12] Paoloni JA, Appleyard RC, Murrell GA. The Orthopaedics Research Institute–Ankle Strength Testing System: inter-rater and intra-rater reliability testing. Foot Ankle Int 2002;23:112–7.

[13] Finni T, Hodgson JA, Lai AM, et al. Muscle synergism during isometric plantarflexion in Achilles tendon rupture patients and in normal subjects revealed by velocity-encoded cine phase-contrast MRI. Clin Biomech (Bristol, Avon) 2006;21:67–74.

[14] Wagnon R, Akayi M. Post-surgical Achilles tendon and correlation with functional outcome: a review of 40 cases. J Radiol 2005;86(Pt 1):1783–7.

[15] Kayser R, Mahlfeld K, Heyde CE. Partial rupture of the proximal Achilles tendon: a differential diagnostic problem in ultrasound imaging. Br J Sports Med 2005;39:838–42, discussion 838–842.

[16] Huang SS, Yu JQ, Chamroonrat W, et al. Achilles tendonitis detected by PDG-PET. Clin Nucl Med 2006;31:147–8.

[17] Rompe JD, Nafe B, Furia JP, Maffulli N. Eccentric loading, shockwave treatment, or a wait-and-see policy for tendinopathy of the main body of tendo Achillis: a randomized controlled trial. Am J Sports Med 2007;35:374–83.

[18] van Sterkenburg MN, de Jonge MC, Sierevelt IN, van Dijk CN. Less promising results with sclerosing ethoxysclerol injections for midportion Achilles tendinopathy: a retrospective study. Am J Sports Med 2010;38:2226–32.

[19] Paoloni JA, Appleyard RC, Nelson J, Murrell GA. Topical glyceryl trinitrate treatment of chronic noninsertional Achilles tendinopathy. A randomized, double-blind, placebo-controlled trial. J Bone Joint Surg Am 2004;86:916–22.

[20] Hufner TM, Brandes DB, Thermann H, et al. Long-term results after functional nonoperative treatment of Achilles tendon rupture. Foot Ankle Int 2006;27:167–71.

[21] Tatari H, Skiak E, Destan H, et al. Effect of hylan G-F 20 in Achilles' tendonitis: an experimental study in rats. Arch Phys Med Rehabil 2004;85:1470–4.

[22] Yeung CK, Guo X, Ng YF. Pulsed ultrasound treatment accelerates the repair of Achilles tendon rupture in rats. J Orthop Res 2006;24:193–201.

[23] Salate AC, Barbosa G, Gaspar P, et al. Effect of In-Ga-Al-P diode laser irradiation on angiogenesis in partial ruptures of Achilles tendon in rats. Photomed Laser Surg 2005;23:470–5.

[24] Steyaert AE, Burssens PJ, Vercruysse CW, et al. The effects of substance P on the biomechanic properties of ruptured rat Achilles' tendon. Arch Phys Med Rehabil 2006;87:254–8.

[25] Barata P, Cervaens M, Resende R, et al. Hyperbaric oxygen effects on sports injuries. Ther Adv Musculoskelet Dis 2011;3:111–21.

[26] Kuskucu M, Mahirogullari M, Solakoglu C, et al. Treatment of rupture of the Achilles tendon with fibrin sealant. Foot Ankle Int 2005;26:826–31.

[27] Sorrenti SJ. Achilles tendon rupture: effect of early mobilization in rehabilitation after surgical repair. Foot Ankle Int 2006;27:407–10.

[28] Rompe JD, Furia JP, Maffulli N. Mid-portion Achilles tendinopathy—current options for treatment. Disabil Rehabil 2008;30:1666–76.

[29] Maffulli N, Longo UG, Maffulli GD, et al. Achilles tendon ruptures in elite athletes. Foot Ankle Int 2011;32:9–15.

[30] Maes R, Copin G, Averous C. Is percutaneous repair of the Achilles tendon a safe technique? A study of 124 cases. Acta Orthop Belg 2006;72:179–83.

[31] Majewski M, Rohrbach M, Czaja S, Ochsner P. Avoiding sural nerve injuries during percutaneous Achilles tendon repair. Am J Sports Med 2006;34:793–8.

CHAPTER 82

Ankle Arthritis

David Wexler, MD, FRCS (Tr & Orth)
Dawn M. Grosser, MD
Todd A. Kile, MD

Synonym

Degenerative joint disease of the ankle

ICD-9 Codes

715.17 Osteoarthritis, localized, primary, ankle and foot
715.27 Osteoarthritis, localized, secondary, ankle and foot
716.17 Traumatic arthropathy, ankle and foot

ICD-10 Codes

M19.071 Primary osteoarthritis, right ankle and foot
M19.072 Primary osteoarthritis, left ankle and foot
M19.079 Primary osteoarthritis, unspecified ankle and foot
M19.271 Secondary osteoarthritis, right ankle and foot
M19.272 Secondary osteoarthritis, left ankle and foot
M19.279 Secondary osteoarthritis, unspecified ankle and foot
M12.571 Traumatic arthropathy, right ankle and foot
M12.572 Traumatic arthropathy, left ankle and foot
M12.579 Traumatic arthropathy, unspecified ankle and foot

Definition

Ankle arthritis is degeneration of the cartilage within the tibiotalar joint that can result from a wide range of causes, most commonly post-traumatic degenerative joint disease. An acute injury or trauma sustained a number of years before presentation or less severe, repetitive, minor injuries sustained during a longer period can lead to a slow but progressive destruction of the articular cartilage, resulting in degenerative joint disease [1]. Other common types are primary osteoarthritis, inflammatory arthritis (including rheumatoid, psoriatic, and gouty), and septic arthritis. Osteoarthritis is usually less inflammatory than rheumatoid arthritis but can also involve many joints simultaneously.

Symptoms

As with arthritis of any joint, the presenting symptoms are pain (which may be variable at different times of the day and exacerbated by activity), swelling, stiffness, and progressive deformity [1]. The ankle may be stiff on initial weight bearing; this improves after walking a while but then worsens with too much ambulatory activity. The pain is often relieved with rest. Pieces of the cartilage can break off, forming a loose body, and the joint can "lock" or "catch," sticking in one position and causing acute, excruciating pain until the loose body moves from between the two irregular joint surfaces. Another symptom is that of "giving way" or instability of the joint, which may be a result of surrounding muscle weakness or ligamentous laxity. With progression of the arthritis, night pain can become a major complaint.

Physical Examination

Swelling, pain, and possibly increased temperature on palpation may be present. The pain is usually maximal along the anterior talocrural joint line and typically chronic and progressive. If the patient's other ankle is normal, it is important to compare the two. Deformity and reduced range of motion in plantar flexion and dorsiflexion (normal: up to 20 degrees of dorsiflexion and 45 degrees of plantar flexion) may be seen. The patient may exhibit an antalgic gait or a limp. Acute arthritis is manifested very differently. Onset is rapid with associated warmth, erythema, swelling, and severe pain with passive range of motion and may be accompanied by constitutional symptoms such as fever and rigors.

It is appropriate to examine the other joints in the lower limb, particularly the knee. The findings on neurovascular examination are typically normal. Decreased sensation in the lower limb raises the possibility of a Charcot joint causing a destructive arthropathy (see Chapter 128).

Functional Limitations

Pain with walking distances and difficulty in negotiating stairs or inclines are particular functional disabilities. Even prolonged standing can become intolerable with advanced joint deterioration. Night pain can lead to disturbance of sleep. Patients will typically adjust their activities or eliminate many of them, particularly exercising, because of pain.

Diagnostic Studies

Plain anteroposterior and lateral standing radiographs provide sufficient information in the later stages of the disease (Figs. 82.1 and 82.2). Magnetic resonance imaging may show damage to articular cartilage and a joint effusion earlier in the course of the disease. In assessment of the radiographs, attention should also be paid to the other joints in the hindfoot because these will affect management options. Generalized bone density and alignment should also be noted.

In some cases, patients present with varying degrees of degeneration of other, adjacent joints, such as the subtalar joint or the knee. By performing differential blocks (i.e., isolated ankle block or subtalar block) with local anesthetic under radiographic control, the clinician may determine which of these joints are symptomatic. A bone scan might be of assistance. In acute presentations, complete blood cell count with a white blood cell count differential, serum urate concentration, and possible joint needle aspiration can help clarify the diagnosis.

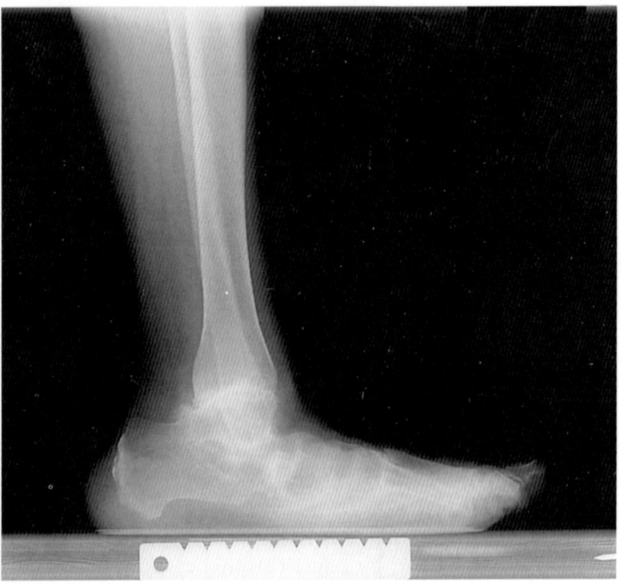

FIGURE 82.1 Lateral standing radiograph of the ankle in a patient with rheumatoid arthritis. This demonstrates loss of joint space and bone destruction of the ankle joint.

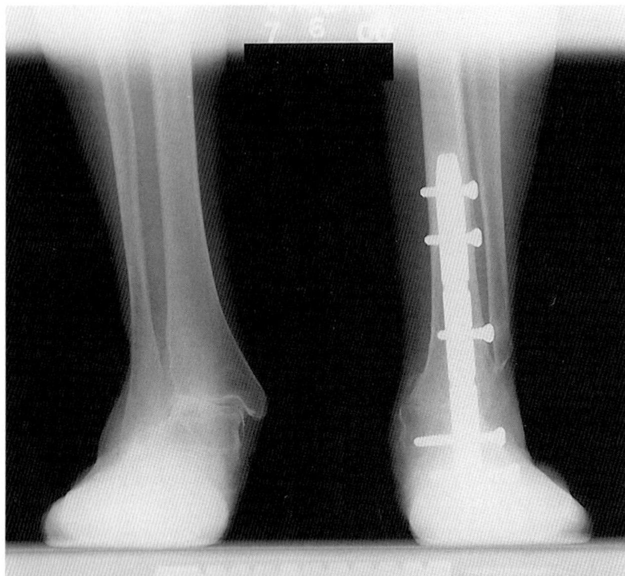

FIGURE 82.2 Anteroposterior standing radiograph of bilateral ankles in a patient with rheumatoid arthritis. This demonstrates the degenerative, destroyed joint on the left and one method of fusion with an intramedullary nail on the right.

Differential Diagnosis

Edema (e.g., edema secondary to congestive cardiac failure)
Subtalar joint degenerative disease
Posterior tibial tenosynovitis
Osteochondral defect
Fracture
Osteonecrosis

Treatment

Initial

Initial treatment focuses on pain relief and minimizing inflammation. Nonsteroidal anti-inflammatory drugs or simple analgesics are used to alleviate the pain. Prefabricated orthoses ranging from flexible neoprene braces and lace-up or wraparound ankle supports to more rigid braces or walking boots can be prescribed to enhance stability and to reduce movement in the ankle joint, thus reducing pain levels.

Rehabilitation

A custom-molded rigid ankle-foot orthosis fabricated by a skilled orthotist along with a rocker-bottom modification to the shoe (which can be accomplished by most cobblers) can provide dramatic pain relief for most patients with ankle arthritis. A physical therapist can instruct a patient in the proper technique for use of a walking stick or cane in the opposite hand. This is a simple but effective aid in reducing the forces across the ankle joint when the patient is ambulatory.

Mobilization, stretching techniques, and range of movement exercises may help alleviate pain and stiffness. Non–weight-bearing exercises are important, and if it is accessible, hydrotherapy has been shown to be an extremely useful and productive adjunct. Distraction and gliding mobilization techniques improve range of movement. Strengthening of surrounding muscle groups and proprioceptive rehabilitation will enhance stability.

Procedures

Other than the blocks that are performed to determine the location of the pathologic changes in confusing cases, injections are not typically done for ankle arthritis. Corticosteroid injection is generally of only limited duration, and steroids are chondrotoxic (cause cartilage damage). However, they can provide excellent temporary pain relief in patients with joints at end-stage disease. Viscosupplementation injections (as used in the management of knee arthritis) are still experimental and not recommended at this time.

Surgery

Surgery is indicated in patients who fail to respond to nonoperative management and especially in those with unremitting pain. In the earlier stages of arthritis, an arthroscopic washout and cartilage débridement of the ankle joint may provide significant improvement in pain levels.

As the disease progresses, more extensive surgery is required. Many different variations and techniques of fusion have been described, ranging from minimally invasive arthroscopic arthrodesis to open fusion with hardware [1–6]. Distraction arthroplasty (application of an external fixator for a period of time) has shown some promising results. Total ankle joint replacement (arthroplasty) has been an alternative to ankle fusion since the 1970s in certain select populations of patients. It has undergone a series of alterations because the earlier generation models were prone to failure and unpredictable results [7]. In recent times, there have been significant advances in and ongoing research comparing efficacy of arthrodesis and total joint arthroplasty [8,9]. Selection of patients is of paramount importance; those with high expectations and demands (hiking, tennis, running) may be better served with a more predictable, stable fusion than with a replacement that has a high likelihood of failure and need of revision.

Potential Disease Complications

Progressive immobility, permanent loss of motion of the ankle joint, bone collapse leading to leg length discrepancy, and chronic intractable pain can result from ankle arthritis.

Potential Treatment Complications

Analgesics and nonsteroidal anti-inflammatory drugs have well-known side effects that most commonly affect the gastric, hepatic, and renal systems. Arthroscopy can be complicated by nerve damage or, rarely, septic arthritis. On occasion, with arthrodesis, fusion can fail to occur [10]. An alteration in gait is common [11]. Arthroplasty complications include infection, thromboembolism, bone collapse, and implant migration.

References

[1] Richardson EG. Arthrodesis of ankle, knee and hip. In: Canale ST, editor. Campbell's operative orthopaedics. 9th ed. St. Louis: Mosby; 1988. p. 165–82.

[2] Thordarson DB. Ankle and hindfoot arthritis: fusion techniques. In: Craig EV, editor. Clinical orthopaedics. Philadelphia: Lippincott Williams & Wilkins; 1999. p. 883–90.

[3] Mann RA, Van Manen JW, Wapner K, Martin J. Ankle fusion. Clin Orthop 1991;268:49–55.

[4] Morgan CD, Henke JA, Bailey RW, Kaufer H. Long-term results of tibiotalar arthrodesis. J Bone Joint Surg Am 1985;67:546–50.

[5] Kile TA. Ankle arthrodesis. In: Morrey B, editor. Reconstructive surgery of the joints. 2nd ed. New York: Churchill Livingstone; 1996. p. 1771–87.

[6] Kile TA, Donnelly RE, Gehrke JC, et al. Tibiotalocalcaneal arthrodesis with an intramedullary device. Foot Ankle 1994;15:669–73.

[7] McGuire MR, Kyle RF, Gustilo RB, Premer RF. Comparative analysis of ankle arthroplasty versus ankle arthrodesis. Clin Orthop Relat Res 1988;226:174–81.

[8] Haddad SL, Coetzee JC, Estok R, et al. Intermediate and long-term outcomes of total ankle arthroplasty and ankle arthrodesis: a systematic review of the literature. J Bone Joint Surg Am 2007;89:1899–905.

[9] Cracchiolo III A, DeOrio JK. Design features of current total ankle replacements: implants and instrumentation. J Am Acad Orthop Surg 2008;16:530–40.

[10] Smith RW. Ankle arthrodesis. In: Thompson RC, Johnson KA, editors. Master techniques in orthopaedic surgery. The foot and ankle. Philadelphia: Raven Press; 1994. p. 467–82.

[11] Mazur JM, Schwartz E, Simon SR. Ankle arthrodesis: long term follow-up with gait analysis. J Bone Joint Surg Am 1979;61:964–75.

CHAPTER 83

Ankle Sprain

Brian J. Krabak, MD, MBA, FACSM

Synonym

Inversion sprain

ICD-9 Code

845.00 Sprains and strains of the ankle and foot

ICD-10 Codes

S93.401 Sprain of unspecified ligament of right ankle
S93.402 Sprain of unspecified ligament of left ankle
S93.409 Sprain of unspecified ligament of unspecified ankle
S93.601 Unspecified sprain of right foot
S93.602 Unspecified sprain of left foot
S93.609 Unspecified sprain of unspecified foot

Definition

Ankle sprain involves stretching or tearing of the ligaments of the ankle. Ankle injuries are a common cause of morbidity in the general and athletic population, with an estimated 25,000 ankle sprains requiring medical care in the United States per day [1]. Overall, ankle sprains are slightly more likely to occur in males (50.3%) than in females (49.7%) and nine times more likely to occur in younger than in older individuals [2]. In the high-school athlete, there are an average of 5.23 ankle injuries per 10,000 athlete-exposures, most often due to traumatic ligament injuries involving boys' basketball, girls' basketball, and boys' football [3]. In the collegiate athlete, ankle sprains represent 15% of all athletic injuries and account for almost 25% of injuries of men's and women's collegiate basketball and women's volleyball athletes [4,5].

Eighty-five percent of all ankle sprains occur on the lateral aspect of the ankle, involving the anterior talofibular ligament and calcaneofibular ligament (Fig. 83.1) [6]. Another 5% to 10% are syndesmotic injuries or high ankle sprains, which involve a partial tear of the distal anterior tibiofibular ligament. Identification of syndesmotic sprains is important; they may have a prolonged recovery compared with milder lateral ankle sprains and are more likely to require surgery. Only 5% of all ankle sprains involve the medial aspect of the ankle as the strong medial deltoid ligament is resistant to tearing. Most ankle sprains will recover during several weeks to months, depending on the grade of injury. It is estimated that 20% to 40% of ankle sprains result in chronic sequelae [7]. An ankle sprain that does not heal may be caused by injuries to other structures and will necessitate further investigation for other causes.

The exact structure torn will depend on the mechanism of injury. The most common mechanism of injury involves foot supination and inversion, resulting in a tear of the lateral ankle structures (primarily the anterotalofibular ligament). An eversion stress to the foot or ankle will tear the medial structures (deltoid ligament), and ankle dorsiflexion with external rotation will lead to a syndesmotic injury [6,8].

Ligamentous injuries are categorized into three gradations:

Grade I is a partial tear without laxity and only mild edema.

Grade II is a partial tear with mild laxity and moderate pain, swelling, tenderness, and instability.

Grade III is a complete rupture resulting in considerable swelling, increased pain, significant laxity, and often an unstable joint (Fig. 83.2).

Symptoms

Acutely, the injured patient will report pain, swelling, and tenderness over the injured ligaments. Some patients report a "pop" at the time of injury. Initially, they may have difficulty with weight bearing on the injured ankle and with subsequent ambulation. They may report some ecchymosis during the first 24 to 48 hours. There may be sensory symptoms in the sural, superficial peroneal, or deep peroneal nerve's distribution. Decreased function and range of motion along with instability are reported more often in grade II and grade III injuries.

Physical Examination

Inspection of the ankle will reveal edema and sometimes ecchymosis around the area of injury, depending on the extent of injury. Range of motion of the ankle joint may be limited by associated swelling and pain. Reduced

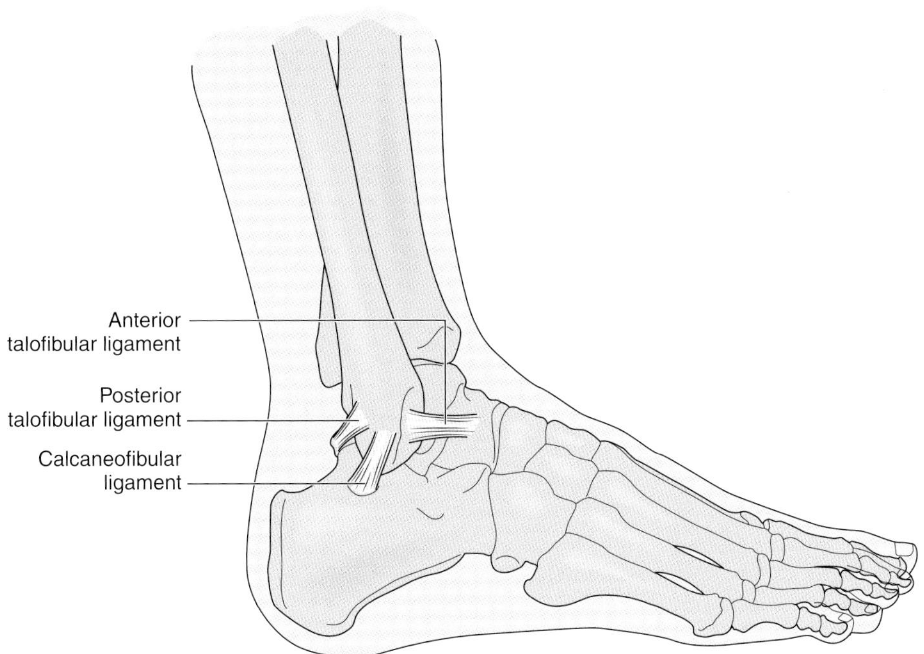

FIGURE 83.1 Ligaments of the lateral ankle.

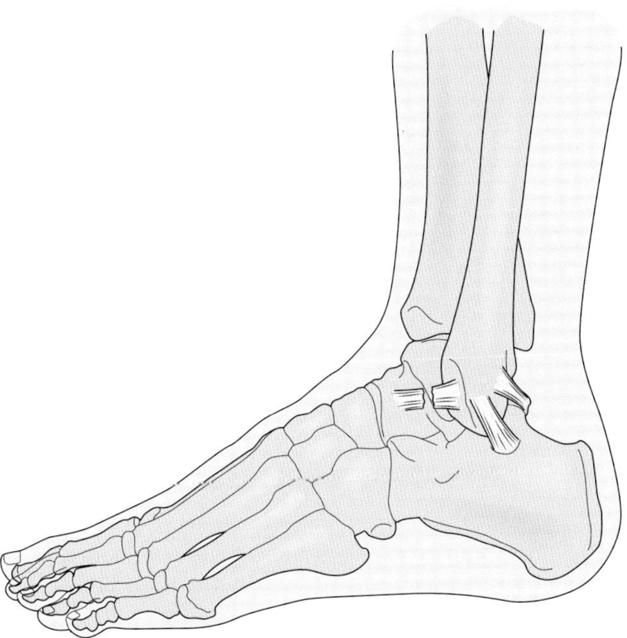

FIGURE 83.2 Grade III ankle sprain with a complete tear of the anterior talofibular ligament.

dorsiflexion may predispose the joint to an ankle sprain [9]. Palpation should include the anterior talofibular and calcaneofibular ligaments, syndesmotic area, and medial deltoid ligament. In addition, the examiner should palpate the distal fibula, medial malleolus, base of the fifth metatarsal, cuboid, lateral process of the talus (to assess for a possible snowboarder's fracture), and epiphyseal areas to assess for any potential fractures [10,11]. The patient should be examined for strength deficits, or reflex abnormalities, which could reveal concurrent injury. Although it is uncommon, ankle inversion injuries are sometimes associated with peroneal nerve injury and may result in sensory changes on the dorsum of the foot (superficial peroneal nerve) or the first web space (deep peroneal nerve). Deep peroneal nerve injury could result in decreased strength in dorsiflexion and eversion. If a fracture is not suspected, single-leg balance could be tested to assess the extent of proprioceptive compromise.

Ankle stability should be examined through a variety of tests and compared with the noninjured side to assess the amount of abnormal translation in the joint. The anterior drawer test of the ankle will assess the integrity of the anterior talofibular ligament. It is performed by plantar flexing the ankle to approximately 30 degrees and applying an anterior force to the calcaneus while stabilizing the tibia with the other hand. Increased translation compared with the other side implies injury to the anterior talofibular ligament. Studies in cadavers suggest that the test is accurate in detecting abnormal lateral ankle motion, with 100% sensitivity and 75% specificity [12,13]. The talar tilt test (Fig. 83.3) is performed with the ankle in a neutral position and assesses the integrity of the calcaneofibular ligament [13]. The squeeze test (Fig. 83.4) is used to diagnose a syndesmotic injury. It is performed by squeezing the proximal fibula and tibia at the midcalf and causes pain over the syndesmotic area. Similarly, the external rotation stress test is performed by placing the ankle in a neutral position and externally rotating the tibia, leading to pain in the syndesmotic region [14]. Unfortunately, several studies have demonstrated poor correlation between clinical stress test results and the degree of ligamentous disruption [15].

Functional Limitations

The patient may have difficulty in walking secondary to pain and swelling. Proprioception and balance on the injured ankle will be abnormal as noted by greater

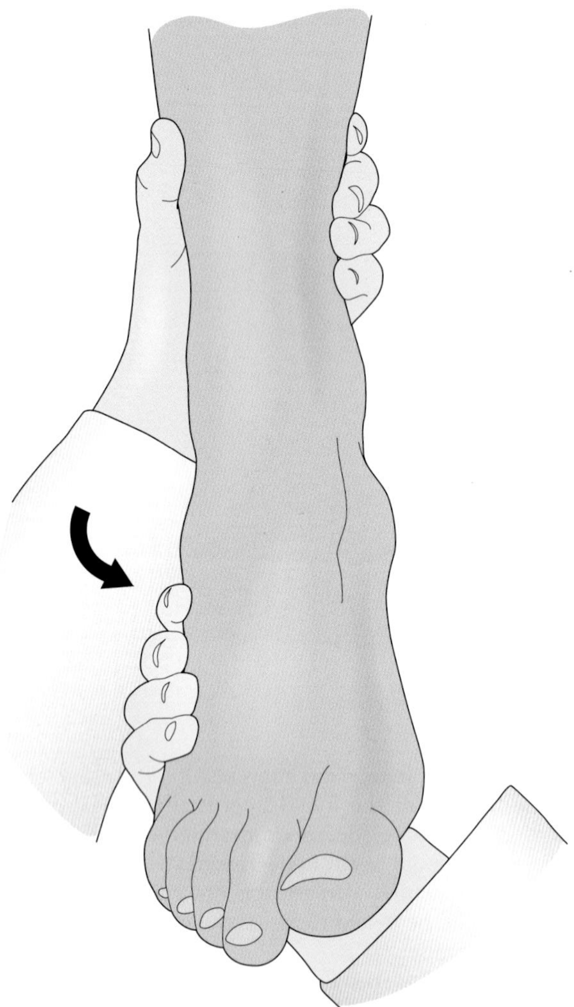

FIGURE 83.3 The talar tilt (inversion stress) test of the ankle.

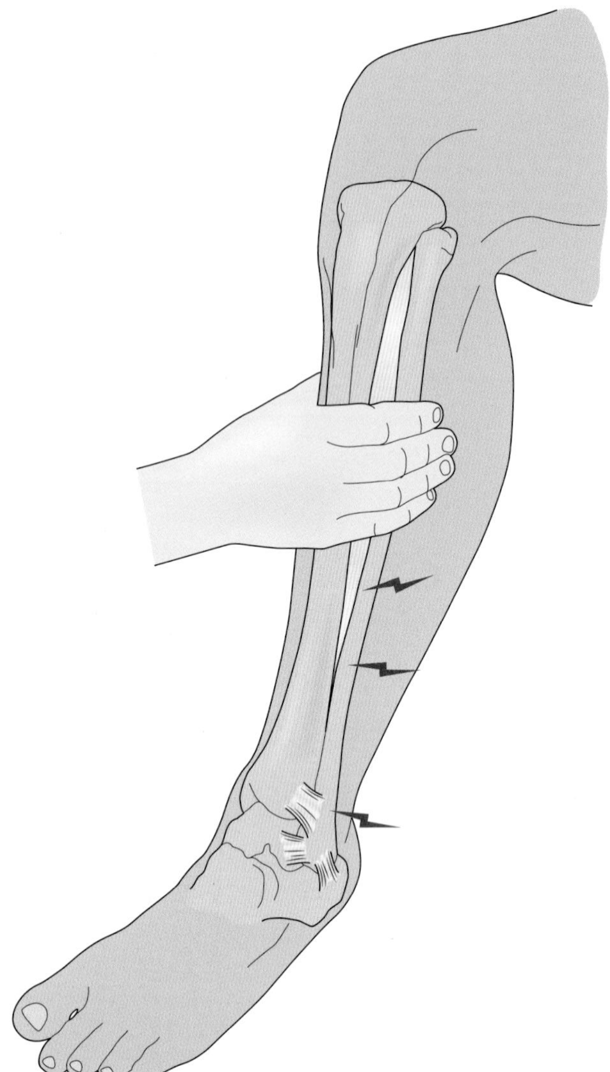

FIGURE 83.4 The squeeze test detects tears of the syndesmosis. The test result is positive when squeezing of the midcalf produces pain in the distal interosseous membrane and syndesmosis.

difficulty with single-leg standing on the injured leg [16]. The athlete will have difficulty with return to play until swelling and pain have diminished and rehabilitation is nearly completed. Incomplete recovery or inadequate rehabilitation may predispose the patient to reinjury [17]. Of note, the single-leg balance test can be helpful in predicting which athletes may sustain an ankle injury during the course of the upcoming season [18]. Chronic ankle sprains can result in mechanical instability, with objective instability or laxity noted on examination in all patients [19].

Diagnostic Studies

Standard anteroposterior, mortise, and lateral radiographs should be considered in cases in which there is tenderness over the lateral malleolus, ankle joint, syndesmosis, or other bony structure to rule out an underlying fracture [6,10]. The Ottawa ankle rules were developed and validated to clarify the indications for these ankle radiographs. The rules recommend imaging when there is tenderness along the lower 6 cm of the tibia or fibula, the navicular, or the fifth metatarsal head and an inability to bear weight immediately after injury and in the emergency department. Adherence to these rules has shown a 30% reduction in radiography use while missing no major fractures [10,11]. At 4 to 6 weeks, a slowly healing lateral ankle injury without significant pain resolution or improvement should be evaluated radiographically, especially if an initial radiograph was not obtained.

A magnetic resonance imaging scan can help identify the soft tissue disease as well as evaluate the osteochondral joint surface when the ankle does not heal despite adequate rehabilitation. Osteochondral injuries may not be seen immediately but occur later, especially in cases with chronic instability. Stress radiographs are optional and have questionable reliability because of the great range of normal joint movement [20]. Ultrasonography may be used to further evaluate the soft tissue structures of the ankle, including ligament injury and associated tendon subluxation. Advantages of ultrasonography include the lack of radiation and relatively low cost [21].

Differential Diagnosis

High ankle sprain, syndesmotic sprain
Osteochondral fracture of the talar dome
Neurapraxia of the common, superficial, or deep peroneal nerve
Fracture of the lateral process of the talus (snowboarder's fracture)
Avulsion or fracture of the tip of the fibula
Fracture of the base of the fifth metatarsal
Peroneal tendon injury
Subtalar joint instability
Posterior impingement or fracture of the os trigonum

Treatment

Initial

Protection, relative *rest*, *ice*, *compression*, and *elevation* (PRICE) are the proposed mainstay of initial treatment and are introduced immediately [22]. However, there appears to be insufficient evidence to determine the true effectiveness of RICE for acute ankle sprains [23]. It intuitively makes sense to use crutches if weight bearing causes pain. The crutches can be discontinued as ambulatory pain declines (usually in 2 to 3 days). Grade II and grade III sprains may require longer use of assistive devices. Patients should be cautioned to avoid hanging the ankle in a plantar flexed position because it may stretch the injured anterior talofibular ligament. Positioning in maximum dorsiflexion also minimizes resultant joint effusion. Plastic removable walking cast boots or air splints are occasionally used in higher grade injuries until pain-free weight bearing is achieved. These may be used for weeks to months, depending on the extent of injury. Caution should be taken with prolonged immobilization as a systematic review of randomized controlled trials suggests that prolonged immobilization (more than 4 weeks) is less effective than early functional treatment [24]. Local ice applications for 20 to 30 minutes three or four times daily combined with compression immediately after injury is effective in decreasing edema, pain, and dysfunction. Nonsteroidal anti-inflammatory drugs may be employed to decrease pain and inflammation. Other therapeutic modalities, including diathermy, electrotherapy, and therapeutic ultrasound, have not been shown to be effective.

Rehabilitation

The rehabilitation of ankle sprains has moved toward earlier mobilization in hopes of minimizing swelling, decreasing pain, and preventing chronic ankle problems [25,26]. Active range of motion in all planes is initially performed without resistance as soon as tolerated. Dorsiflexion and eversion strengthening can be started with static exercises and progress to concentric and eccentric exercises with tubing when the patient tolerates pain-free weight bearing. Double-leg toe raises should progress to single-leg toe raises and can be done in water if they are not tolerated on land. Endurance and lower extremity muscle strengthening exercises are incorporated and increased as tolerated by the patient. Proprioception training can start in a seated position and then advance to standing balance exercises. Standing exercises begin with single-leg stance while swinging the raised leg. Then, single-leg squats are required. Finally, exercises progress to single-leg stance and functional or sport-specific activity, such as dribbling, catching, or kicking. A more recent randomized study comparing PRICE therapy with early mobilization in patients with grade I or grade II ankle sprains reported better functional recovery in the first 2 weeks after injury in the early mobilization groups. There were no long-term differences at 16 weeks, and reinjury rate was the same for both groups [25]. A supervised program appeared to provide better results than a conventional home program [27].

Several studies have highlighted the importance of proprioceptive training in early recovery from ankle sprains and chronic functional instability. The study by Bahr and Bahr [28] of volleyball players demonstrated a 21% reduction in ankle sprains the first year and 49% reduction the second year in athletes who performed balance exercises. In addition, they reported fewer recurrent ankle sprains, and patients with more than one sprain benefited the most. A systematic review by McKeon and Hertel [29] showed that proprioceptive and balance training does in fact improve recovery acutely and can reduce recurrence rates of injury. Therefore, proprioceptive and balance exercises should be incorporated into the rehabilitation program as soon as possible.

The use of orthotic bracing is somewhat controversial. Earlier studies have suggested that bracing and taping may decrease recurrent injury rates in the previously injured ankle, but they have not been shown to be effective in athletes without a prior injury [30,31]. Beynnon and colleagues [30] studied 182 patients with first-time grade I and grade II ankle ligament sprains and showed that treatment with the air stirrup brace combined with an elastic wrap provided earlier return to preinjury function than with use of the air stirrup brace alone, an elastic wrap alone, or a walking cast for 10 days. Interestingly, a more recent meta-analysis suggests that the use of an ankle brace or ankle tape has no effect on enhancing proprioception in individuals with recurrent ankle sprains or who have functional ankle instability [32]. These studies suggest that the decrease in injury rates is due to something other than enhanced proprioception of the ankle.

Despite these findings, many athletes will consider using a brace to prevent a recurrent sprain. A study by Putnam and coworkers [33] suggested that use of ankle braces in healthy competitive recreational soccer players did not significantly affect performance in speed, agility, or kicking accuracy. The authors proposed the need for future studies to investigate the impact on athletes with ankle injuries.

Procedures

Procedures are generally not indicated for ankle sprains.

Surgery

Surgery is rare for ankle sprains. Most grade III ankle sprains with complete tears of the anterior talofibular ligament and instability are *not* treated surgically unless they result in chronic instability. If necessary, surgical repair may be completed after the sports season and is usually successful.

Reconstruction of the lateral ankle ligaments involves anatomic reconstruction of the ligament (modified Brostrom) and tendon weaving through the fibula (Watson-Jones, Chrisman-Snook) [34]. The direct repair of the ligament, even years after the injury, can be highly successful. Despite the various techniques, an extensive literature review recommended the need for randomized controlled studies to determine the relative effectiveness of surgical and conservative treatment for acute injuries of the lateral ligament complex of the ankle [35].

Potential Disease Complications

Recurrent sprains may lead to both mechanical (gross laxity) and functional (giving way) instability. The patient may present with undiagnosed secondary sources of pain, and these must be sought (see the section on differential diagnosis). Chronic intractable pain is another potential complication.

Potential Treatment Complications

Lack of recognition of and the prevalence of subacute sequelae in ankle sprains may lead to undertreatment and subsequent chronic pain or instability. Nonsteroidal anti-inflammatory drugs may cause gastric, hepatic, or renal complications. Prolonged immobilization can lead to inflexibility, muscle atrophy, and longer time loss from work or sport. Return to work, sport, or activity before adequate healing and rehabilitation may result in chronic pain and giving way (functional instability) and gross laxity (mechanical instability). As noted, heat and contrast baths should be avoided during the acute stage of injury as these modalities could promote swelling and bleeding. Finally, surgical complications could include joint injection, loss of range of motion, and compromised gait.

References

[1] Kerr ZY, Collins CL, Fields SK, Comstock RD. Epidemiology of player-player contact injuries among US high school athletes, 2005–2009. Clin Pediatr (Phila) 2011;50:594–603.

[2] Waterman BR, Owens BD, Davey S, et al. The epidemiology of ankle sprains in the United States. J Bone Joint Surg Am 2010;92:2279–84.

[3] Nelson AJ, Collins CL, Yard EE, et al. Ankle injuries among United States high school sports athletes, 2005-2006. J Athl Train 2007;42:381–7.

[4] Hootman JM, Dick R, Agel J. Epidemiology of collegiate injuries for 15 sports: summary and recommendations for injury prevention initiatives. J Athl Train 2007;42:311–9.

[5] Beynnon BD, Vacek PM, Murphy D, et al. First-time inversion ankle ligament trauma: the effects of sex, level of competition, and sport on incidence of injury. Am J Sports Med 2005;33:1485–91.

[6] Safran MR, Benedetti RS, Bartolozzi 3rd. AR, Mandelbaum BR. Lateral ankle sprains: a comprehensive review. Part 1: etiology, pathoanatomy, histopathogenesis, and diagnosis. Med Sci Sports Exerc 1999;31(Suppl. 7):S429–37.

[7] Rodriguez-Merchan EC. Chronic ankle instability: diagnosis and treatment. Arch Orthop Trauma Surg 2012;132:211–9.

[8] Tiemstra JD. Update on acute ankle sprains. Am Fam Physician 2012;85:1170–6.

[9] de Noronha M, Refshauge KM, Herbert RD, et al. Do voluntary strength, range of motion, or postural sway predict occurrence of lateral ankle sprain? Br J Sports Med 2006;40:824–8.

[10] Jenkin M, Sitler MR, Kelly JD. Clinical usefulness of the Ottawa ankle rules for detecting fractures of the ankle and midfoot. J Athl Train 2010;45:480–2.

[11] Bachmann LM, Kolb E, Koller MT, et al. Accuracy of Ottawa ankle rules to exclude fractures of the ankle and mid-foot: systematic review. BMJ 2003;326:417.

[12] Bahr R, Pena F, Shine J, et al. Mechanics of the anterior drawer and talar tilt tests. A cadaveric study of lateral ligament injuries of the ankle. Acta Orthop Scand 1997;68:435–41.

[13] Phisitkul P, Chaichankul C, Sripongsai R, et al. Accuracy of anterolateral drawer test in lateral ankle instability: a cadaveric study. Foot Ankle Int 2009;30:690–5.

[14] Hertel J, Denegar C, Monroe M, Stokes W. Talocrural and subtalar joint instability after lateral ankle sprain. Med Sci Sports Exerc 1999;31:1501–7.

[15] Fujii T, Luo ZP, Kitaoka HB, An KN. The manual stress test may not be sufficient to differentiate ankle ligament injuries. Clin Biomech (Bristol, Avon) 2000;15:619–23.

[16] Docherty CL, Valovich McLeod TC, Shultz SJ. Postural control deficits in participants with functional ankle instability as measured by the balance error scoring system. Clin J Sport Med 2006;16:203–8.

[17] Ross SE, Guskiewicz KM. Examination of static and dynamic postural stability in individuals with functionally stable and unstable ankles. Clin J Sport Med 2004;14:332–8.

[18] Trojian TH, McKeag DB. Single leg balance test to identify risk of ankle sprains. Br J Sports Med 2006;40:610–3.

[19] Hubbard TJ, Hertel J. Mechanical contributions to chronic lateral ankle instability. Sports Med 2006;36:263–77.

[20] Hubbard TJ, Kaminski TW, Vander Griend RA, Kovaleski JE. Quantitative assessment of mechanical laxity in the functionally unstable ankle. Med Sci Sports Exerc 2004;36:760–6.

[21] Guillodo Y, Varache S, Saraux A. Value of ultrasonography for detecting ligament damage in athletes with chronic ankle instability compared to computed arthrotomography. Foot Ankle Spec 2010;3:331–4.

[22] van den Bekerom MP, Kerkhoffs GM, McCollum GA, et al. Management of acute lateral ankle ligament injury in the athlete. Knee Surg Sports Traumatol Arthrosc 2013;21:390–5.

[23] van den Bekerom MP, Struijs PA, Blankevoort L, et al. What is the evidence for rest, ice, compression, and elevation therapy in the treatment of ankle sprains in adults? J Athl Train 2012;47:435–43.

[24] Kerkhoffs GM, Rowe BH, Assendelft WJ, et al. Immobilisation and functional treatment for acute lateral ankle ligament injuries in adults. Cochrane Database Syst Rev 2002;3, CD003762.

[25] Bleakley CM, O'Connor SR, Tully MA, et al. Effect of accelerated rehabilitation on function after ankle sprain: randomized controlled trial. BMJ 2010;340:c1964.

[26] Kerkhoffs GM, van den Bekerom M, Elders LA, et al. Diagnosis, treatment and prevention of ankle sprains: an evidence-based clinical guideline. Br J Sports Med 2012;46:854–60.

[27] van Rijn RM, van Ochten J, Luijsterburg PAJ, et al. Effectiveness of additional supervised exercises compared with conventional treatment alone in patients with acute lateral ankle sprains: systematic review. BMJ 2010;341:c5688.

[28] Bahr R, Bahr IA. Incidence of acute volleyball injuries: a prospective cohort study of injury mechanisms and risk factors. Scand J Med Sci Sports 1997;7:166–71.

[29] McKeon PO, Hertel J. Systematic review of postural control and lateral ankle instability, part II: is balance training clinically effective? J Athl Train 2008;43:305–15.

[30] Beynnon BD, Renstrom PA, Haugh L, et al. A prospective, randomized clinical investigation of the treatment of first-time ankle sprains. Am J Sports Med 2006;34:1401–12.

[31] Olmsted LC, Vela LI, Denegar CR, Hertel J. Prophylactic ankle taping and bracing: a numbers-needed-to-treat and cost-benefit analysis. J Athl Train 2004;39:95–100.

[32] Raymond J, Nicholson LL, Hiller CE, Refshauge KM. The effect of ankle taping or bracing on proprioception in functional ankle instability: a systematic review and meta-analysis. J Sci Med Sport 2012;15:386–92.

[33] Putnam AR, Bandolin SN, Krabak BJ. Impact of ankle bracing on skill performance in recreational soccer players. PM R 2012;4:574–9.

[34] Liu SH, Baker CL. Comparison of lateral ankle ligamentous reconstruction procedures. Am J Sports Med 1992;20:594–600.

[35] Kerkhoffs GM, Handoll HH, de Bie R, et al. Surgical versus conservative treatment for acute injuries of the lateral ligament complex of the ankle in adults. Cochrane Database Syst Rev 2007;2, CD000380.

CHAPTER 84

Bunion and Bunionette

David Wexler, MD, FRCS (Tr & Orth)
Dawn M. Grosser, MD
Todd A. Kile, MD

Synonyms

Hallux valgus
Lateral deviation of the great toe

ICD-9 Codes

727.1 Bunion
727.1 Bunionette
735.0 Hallux valgus (acquired)

ICD-10 Codes

M20.10 Hallux valgus (acquired), unspecified foot
M20.11 Hallux valgus (acquired), right foot
M20.12 Hallux valgus (acquired), left foot

Bunion

Definition

The term *bunion* stems from the Latin word *bunio*, which means "turnip," an image suggestive of an apparent growth or enlargement around the joint. The medical term for this is *hallux valgus*. There is no similar Latin term for the fifth toe, so a similar process involving the fifth metatarsophalangeal (MTP) joint is called a bunionette. Hallux valgus is a common deformity of the forefoot and the most common deformity of the first MTP, often causing pain (Figs. 84.1 and 84.2). The pathophysiologic process stems from both the proximal phalanx and the metatarsal bone. The proximal phalanx deviates laterally on the head of the first metatarsal, exacerbated by the pull of the adductor hallucis muscle. The lateral capsule becomes contracted, and the medial structures are attenuated. The metatarsal deviates medially, but the underlying sesamoids remain in their relationship to the second metatarsal, thus creating dissociation of the metatarsal-sesamoid complex. As these two processes occur together, the pull of the abductor hallucis moves more plantarward and the pull of the extensor tendon moves laterally, causing pronation and further lateral deviation of the great toe, respectively. As the metatarsal head becomes more uncovered, a prominent medial eminence, or bunion, is apparent. There is a bursa between the metatarsal head and the skin that may become inflamed and painful. Depending on the amount of axial rotation of the first metatarsal and pronation of the toe, the first ray becomes dysfunctional, leading to increased weight bearing on the more lateral metatarsal heads and "transfer metatarsalgia," causing pain under the plantar aspect of the forefoot [1].

The etiology of hallux valgus is multifactorial and can be either intrinsic or extrinsic [2]. The intrinsic causes are essentially genetic and are related to hypermobility of the first ray (hallux metatarsal) at its articulation with the medial cuneiform. Ligamentous laxity (e.g., Marfan syndrome, Ehlers-Danlos syndrome) can lead to this deformity as well as to variations in the shape of the metatarsal head (i.e., a rounder head is less stable than a flat one). Another contributing factor is metatarsus primus varus, or medial deviation of the first metatarsal, which is thought to be associated with a juvenile bunion [3]. Pes planus and first metatarsal length have also been evaluated for their contribution to hallux valgus, but findings are equivocal [4].

The principal extrinsic cause is inappropriate, nonconforming footwear, with abnormal valgus forces creating deformity [5]. This is particularly notable in women who wear high-heeled shoes with narrow toe boxes. The ratio of hallux valgus between women and men has been reported to be 15:1 [6].

Symptoms

Presenting symptoms can vary. The patient may complain only of a painless prominent medial eminence. However, more commonly, there will be pain that is worse when constrictive shoes are worn and relieved by walking barefoot or with open-toed shoes. If there is significant arthritis,

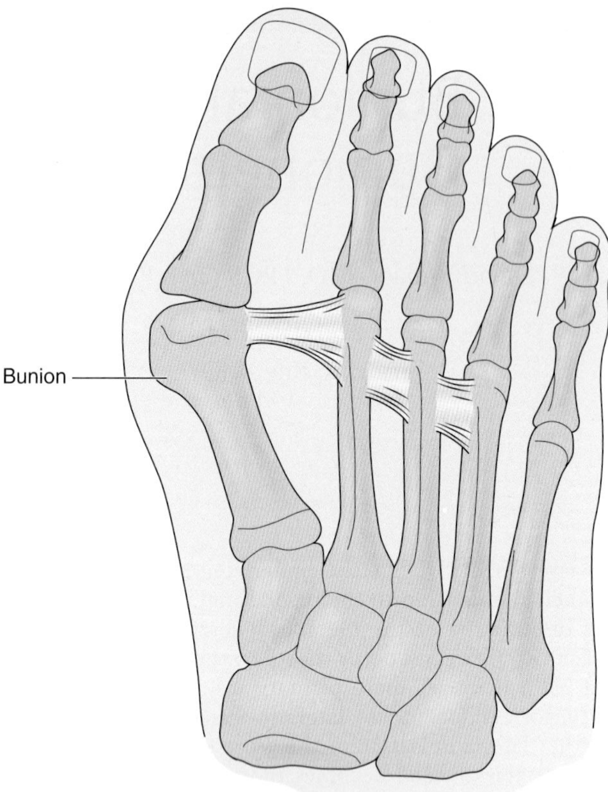

FIGURE 84.1 Anatomy of a bunion.

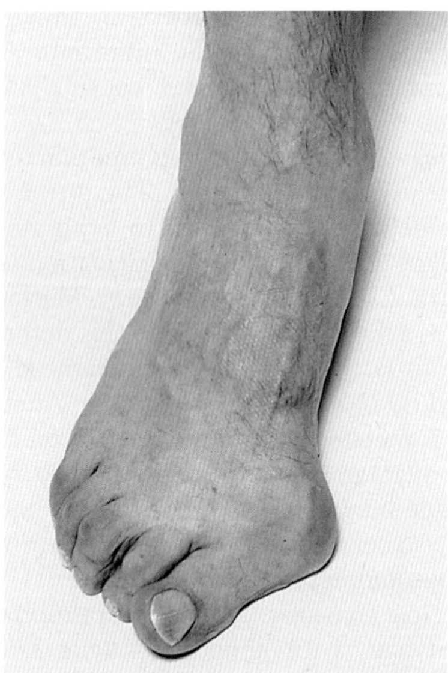

FIGURE 84.2 Clinical photograph demonstrating a bunion or hallux valgus deformity. Note also the pronation of the digit.

patients may have pain throughout range of motion of the MTP joint while walking. The bunion may become red and inflamed as the bursa enlarges and overlying skin becomes abraded by the shoe. The patient will have difficulty finding comfortable shoes. As the hallux deviates into increased valgus, it tends to impinge on the medial aspect of the pulp of the second toe, causing pressure and soreness [7].

Physical Examination

There is generally an obvious medial enlargement overlying the metatarsal head, with occasional signs of inflammation (bursitis). The great toe will be laterally deviated, and with progression of deformity, it will be pronated (axially rotated). There may be splaying of the forefoot and callosities visible under the metatarsal heads of the lesser toes. Metatarsalgia—tenderness under the metatarsal heads—may also be seen even without a callus. Passive extension of the hallux MTP joint will reveal possible limitation of range of motion (normally approximately 70 degrees). This may indicate concomitant degenerative joint disease of the MTP joint. Mobility of the hallux at the first metatarsal–medial cuneiform joint is assessed in relation to the second ray. Hammer toes are commonly noted as a consequence of the crowding in the shoe by the great toe. Depending on the patient's medical history (e.g., diabetes), the neuromuscular evaluation is important to assess for any vibratory loss, two-point discrimination loss, or other indications of neurologic compromise. Otherwise, the neurologic examination findings should be normal.

Functional Limitations

Limitations are principally in walking long distances and wearing shoes with a narrow toe box or high heels for prolonged periods. As hallux valgus progresses, arthritis may become a component and lead to stiffness and pain with any activity (biking, hiking, walking short distances, or even standing).

Diagnostic Studies

Weight-bearing plain radiographs will provide most of the necessary information. The anteroposterior view (Fig. 84.3) demonstrates the angle (Fig. 84.4) between the first and second metatarsals (intermetatarsal angle). The congruency of the first MTP joint can also be assessed for any evidence of arthritis. These all have a bearing on any proposed surgery [8,9].

Differential Diagnosis

Gout
Hallux rigidus
Rheumatoid arthritis
Infection

Treatment

Initial

Nonsteroidal anti-inflammatory medications and analgesics may be used to alleviate pain. However, key measures include education about footwear, namely, shoes with low heels, well-cushioned soles, extra depth, and broad toe boxes. Many orthoses are available and are of varying efficacy. These include sponge wedges to be placed in the first web space, more formal braces that attempt to pull the hallux into a more neutral position, and custom-molded orthotic appliances to resist foot pronation and to support the arch.

A study showed promising results of a total-contact insole with a fixed toe separator that improved pain, walking ability, and the radiographic hallux valgus angle in patients with painful hallux valgus treated nonoperatively [10].

Rehabilitation

Once the structural deformity has progressed, physical therapy has a limited role. This includes mobilization of the first MTP joint and strengthening of the intrinsic muscles of the foot, which may improve symptoms, as well as focus on gait training [11]. Distraction techniques like varus stretching or toe spacers may also be useful.

Procedures

Local anesthetic and steroid injection into the first MTP joint may provide short-term pain relief but is certainly not curative and generally not recommended because steroid injections may have a deleterious effect on the soft tissue and cartilage.

Surgery

After conservative management has failed, surgery is a consideration. Over the years, a vast array of different surgical procedures have been described [3,12]. Furthermore, no single procedure has provided sufficient evidence of being superior to any other. The complication and recurrence rates can be relatively high, and satisfaction of the patient is difficult to achieve. A study reported that the desired outcome of surgery for patients is threefold: a painless great toe that "when wearing conventional shoes, gives no problems," an improvement in the bursitis and appearance of the bunion, and the ability to walk as much as they wish [13]. These are not unreasonable goals, but it is very important to counsel patients preoperatively, explaining the complications and that there are no guarantees they will be able to return to wearing high-heeled fashionable footwear [14]. The principal goals of surgery are to relieve pain and to provide a foot capable of wearing a shoe.

The type of surgery, whether it is a distal soft tissue procedure [15] combined with a proximal metatarsal osteotomy, a distal osteotomy alone, or even an MTP arthrodesis, depends on the presenting anatomic deformity and its complexity.

Potential Disease Complications

Disease complications include ulceration of the medial eminence, metatarsalgia, callosities, hammer toe deformity, and stress fractures of the lesser toes.

Potential Treatment Complications

Analgesics and nonsteroidal anti-inflammatory drugs have well-known side effects that most commonly affect the gastric, hepatic, and renal systems. Treatment can result in recurrent hallux valgus deformity, hallux varus from surgical overcorrection [16], and hallux extensus (cock-up toe). Procedures in which the first metatarsal is excessively shortened may result in transfer metatarsalgia. Osteonecrosis of the first metatarsal head can occur if the blood supply is disrupted significantly. Nonunion can occur with the osteotomies and MTP arthrodesis.

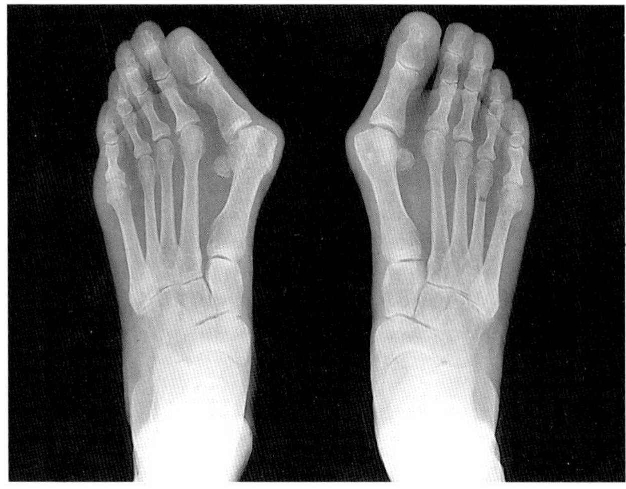

FIGURE 84.3 Standing anteroposterior radiograph of both feet in a patient with bilateral hallux valgus. This is more pronounced on the left. Note also the lateral deviation of the sesamoid bones.

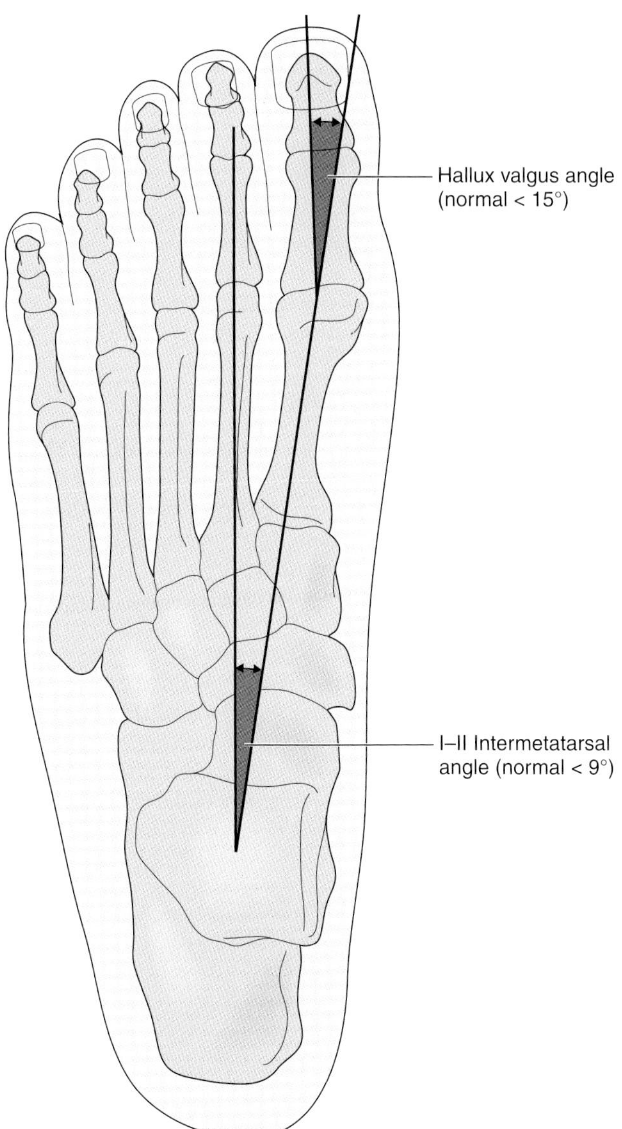

FIGURE 84.4 The hallux valgus angle and the intermetatarsal angle are measured from the patient's standing anteroposterior radiograph.

Bunionette

Definition

A bunionette is similar to a bunion as a painful bone prominence of a metatarsal head and overlying bursa, but it involves the fifth metatarsal. The fifth metatarsal deviates laterally and the fifth toe medially. It has also been called a tailor's bunion as a cross-legged sitting position, often associated with a tailor, can cause pressure over the fifth toe and potentially encourage this deformity. Like the bunion, a bunionette has a high association with constrictive shoes and is much more common in women than in men (4:1) [4].

Symptoms

Patients may be asymptomatic or complain of irritation over the lateral eminence with tight or stiff shoe wear. Typically, when they wear open shoes without pressure over the bunionette, they have no discomfort. However, they occasionally have an inflamed bursa that is acutely painful and red. If patients adjust their shoe wear, the pain can resolve.

Physical Examination

A prominent fifth metatarsal head with a widened appearance of the forefoot is often seen. Patients may develop lateral or plantar callosities over the bone prominence. Hallux valgus may be a concomitant finding, and the foot is considered a "splay foot" if both diagnoses are present [4].

Functional Limitations

Patients typically have pain with restrictive shoe wear that is improved or absent when they are barefoot or wearing open shoes, like flip-flops, that do not put pressure over the fifth metatarsal head. Their walking tolerance may be affected when inappropriate shoes are worn.

Diagnostic Studies

Three radiographic views of the foot are obtained: anteroposterior, lateral, and oblique. Anatomic differences that can be appreciated radiographically may influence the surgical approach. These are of three types: type I, an enlarged fifth metatarsal head; type II, an abnormal lateral bowing of the fifth metatarsal shaft; and type III, a wide intermetatarsal 4-5 angle.

Treatment

Initial

Addressing the constrictive shoe wear is the first approach. Wide, extra-depth shoes or tennis shoes may help decrease the irritation and bursitis. On occasion, pronation can exacerbate the pressure of the lateral eminence against the shoe, and an orthotic can unload or change the position enough to relieve this. Patients may also take their leather shoes to a shoemaker, who can create a focal stretch over the pressure area of the shoe.

Procedures

If a callus develops, it may be débrided, or patients can be advised to use a pumice stone after daily showers to gently buff the hypertrophic tissue that accumulates laterally or plantarly. Because the discomfort from the bunionette is a pressure phenomenon, injections are not helpful. The bursitis that occasionally accompanies this deformity will improve with appropriate shoe wear and keeping the callus thin.

Surgery

More than 20 different surgical procedures have been described for the correction of a bunionette deformity. These include lateral condylectomy or distal osteotomy for type I, midshaft or distal oblique osteotomy for type II, and proximal osteotomy for type III [4].

Potential Disease Complications

Ulcerations and callosities may develop if patients continue to wear restrictive shoes.

Potential Treatment Complications

Treatment can result in recurrence of deformity, particularly with an isolated lateral condylectomy; flail toe with metatarsal head resection; malunion or nonunion of osteotomies; and vascular compromise leading to osteonecrosis, particularly with proximal osteotomies.

References

[1] Richardson EG, Donley BG. Disorders of the hallux. In: Canale ST, editor. 9th ed. Campbell's operative orthopaedics, vol. 2. St. Louis: Mosby; 1998. p. 1621–711.
[2] Pedowitz W. Hallux valgus. In: Craig EV, editor. Clinical orthopaedics. Philadelphia: Lippincott Williams & Wilkins; 1999. p. 904–12.
[3] Austin D, Leventen E. A new osteotomy for hallux valgus: a horizontally directed V displacement osteotomy of the metatarsal head for hallux valgus and primus varus. Clin Orthop Relat Res 1981;157:25–30.
[4] Coughlin MJ, Mann RA. Surgery of the foot and ankle. 7th ed. St. Louis: Mosby; 1999, 150–178.
[5] Seale KS. Women and their shoes: unrealistic expectations? Instr Course Lect 1995;44:379–84.
[6] Hardy RH, Clapham JC. Observations on hallux valgus; based on a controlled series. J Bone Joint Surg Br 1951;33:376–91.
[7] Hertling D, Kessler RM. The leg, ankle and foot. In: Hertling D, Kessler RM, editors. Management of common musculoskeletal disorders. 3rd ed. Philadelphia: Lippincott Williams & Wilkins; 1996. p. 435–8.
[8] Mann RA. Decision making in bunion surgery. Instr Course Lect 1990;39:3–13.
[9] Bordelon RL. Evaluation and operative procedures for hallux valgus deformity. Orthopaedics 1987;10:38–44.
[10] Torkki M, Malmivaara A, Seitsalo S, et al. Hallux valgus: immediate operation versus 1 year of waiting with or without orthoses: a randomized controlled trial of 209 patients. Acta Orthop Scand 2003;74:209–15.
[11] Menz HB, Lord SR. Gait instability in older people with hallux valgus. Foot Ankle Int 2005;26:483–9.
[12] Donnelly RE, Saltzman CL, Kile TA, Johnson KA. Modified osteotomy for hallux valgus. Foot Ankle 1994;15:642–5.
[13] Schneider W, Knahr K. Surgery for hallux valgus. The expectations of patients and surgeons. Int Orthop 2001;25:382–5.
[14] Hattrup SJ, Johnson KA. Chevron osteotomy: analysis of factors in patients' dissatisfaction. Foot Ankle 1985;5:327–32.
[15] Mann RA, Rudicel S, Graves SC. Repair of hallux valgus with a distal soft-tissue procedure and proximal metatarsal osteotomy. J Bone Joint Surg Am 1992;74:124–9.
[16] Tourne Y, Saragaglia D, Picard F, et al. Iatrogenic hallux varus surgical procedure: a study of 14 cases. Foot Ankle Int 1995;16:457–63.

CHAPTER 85

Chronic Ankle Instability

Michael D. Osborne, MD
Stephan M. Esser, MD

Synonym

Weak ankle

ICD-9 Codes

718.87 Ankle-foot instability
719.47 Pain in joint, foot and ankle

ICD-10 Codes

M25.371 Other instability, right ankle
M25.372 Other instability, left ankle
M25.373 Other instability, unspecified ankle
M25.374 Other instability, right foot
M25.375 Other instability, left foot
M25.376 Other instability, unspecified foot
M25.571 Pain in right ankle and joints of right foot
M25.572 Pain in left ankle and joints of left foot
M25.579 Pain in unspecified ankle and joints of unspecified foot

Definition

Chronic ankle instability is a condition characterized by a constellation of symptoms, typically including pain, weakness, and a feeling that the ankle episodically gives way, that persist after an acute lateral ankle sprain. Although chronic ankle instability may occur after a single ankle sprain, it is more commonly a sequela of repeated sprains. It has been reported to occur in up to 40% of individuals with a history of ankle sprain and as late as 6½ years after an initial injury [1]. Anatomic lateral ankle ligament laxity and mechanical instability, peroneal muscle weakness, and ankle proprioceptive deficits are three primary factors thought to cause and to perpetuate symptoms. Arthrogenic muscle inhibition of the peroneal and soleus muscles has also been implicated as a possible contributing factor [2]. These causative factors may coexist with other pathologic processes of the ankle (such as those listed in the differential diagnosis section), which may serve to amplify and to perpetuate symptoms of functional instability. The establishment of additional diagnoses does not preclude a diagnosis of chronic ankle instability.

Symptoms

Usual symptoms are ankle pain, swelling around the lateral malleolus, weakness of the ankle evertors, and a feeling that the ankle is episodically unstable. The term *functional instability* describes the subjective sensation of "giving way" that often persists after ankle sprains [3]. Functional instability may occur in the absence of true mechanical ligament laxity and vice versa. Symptoms can continue for months or years after the original injury, range from mild to severe, and often are manifested as recurrent acute lateral ankle sprains.

Physical Examination

Objective findings are variable and can often be minimal. Potential examination findings in patients with chronic ankle instability may include reduced passive or active ankle range of motion, lateral ankle swelling, ecchymosis, lateral ankle tenderness (typically over the lateral ligament complex or peroneal tendons), weakness of the peroneal muscles, proprioceptive deficits (manifested by decreased ability to perform a single-leg stance), and mechanical laxity (demonstrated by increased motion on anterior drawer or talar tilt test compared with the contralateral ankle) [4]. Abnormal alignment, such as calcaneal varus, calcaneal valgus, or pes planus, may be evident. A limp may also be observed. Examination of the affected ankle should always be compared with the contralateral unaffected ankle.

Findings of the neurologic examination, including sensation and deep tendon reflexes, are commonly normal. Results of manual muscle testing should also be normal, with the exception of muscles surrounding the ankle that may exhibit weakness from disuse or because of pain. Balance testing commonly demonstrates deficits in the affected limb but may also reveal impairments in the contralateral ankle, making it unclear whether these findings represent a preexisting risk for injury or are the result of previous inversion injuries [5].

Functional Limitations

Affected persons may have difficulty participating in sports, particularly high-demand sports that require quick starts and stops, cutting, and jumping (such as soccer, football, and basketball) as well as sports that involve a lot of lateral movement (such as tennis). When symptoms are severe, limitations can include difficulty with climbing steps, ambulation, and activities that require prolonged standing. It is estimated that functional instability prevents 6% of patients from returning to their occupation; 5% to 15% remain occupationally disabled 9 months to 6½ years later, whereas 36% to 85% of patients report full recovery within a period of 3 years [1,2,6,7].

Diagnostic Studies

The diagnosis is made by confirming a history of prior sprain with subsequent development of typical symptoms of functional instability in conjunction with consistent examination findings. Adjunctive diagnostic testing can be helpful in establishing the diagnosis, particularly by identifying pathologic changes and conditions that may produce similar symptoms. Testing that may be useful when the diagnosis of chronic ankle instability is being considered includes routine radiography, stress radiography, computed tomography, bone scan, magnetic resonance imaging, ankle arthrography, and magnetic resonance arthrography.

Routine radiographs are useful to rule out old or chronic fractures (most commonly of the fibula, tibia, talus, and fifth metatarsal), to assess the integrity of the ankle mortise, and to assess for ankle arthritis. A routine radiographic series should include anteroposterior, lateral, and mortise views. Widening of the ankle mortise may indicate a syndesmotic disruption or significant deltoid ligament tear. Radiographs should be obtained in all cases with a history of significant trauma at initial injury.

Stress radiographs may be helpful in determining the presence of chronic mechanical instability. Although the routine use of stress radiographs remains controversial, a finding of more than 5 mm of anterior displacement of the talus during anterior drawer testing is considered to be abnormal [8]. Inversion stress radiographs are considered abnormal with a finding of more than 5 degrees of side-to-side difference in tibiotalar tilt [7]. However, a review found the published data regarding stress radiographs too variable to determine accepted normal values for acute and chronic sprains [9]. The sensitivity of stress radiographs in diagnosis of chronic lateral ligament tears (surgically confirmed) is low, although specificity is high [8].

Computed tomography can identify subtle talus fractures and other bone disease, such as tumors. Bone scans are particularly helpful in identifying stress fractures and can be a useful screening tool to evaluate for ongoing ankle disease, such as significant arthritis, infection, tumors, and reflex sympathetic dystrophy. Magnetic resonance imaging and magnetic resonance arthrography generally give the most information about soft tissue injury, although they also can be helpful in identifying fractures (such as osteochondral fractures), tumors, and chronic infections. Magnetic resonance imaging and magnetic resonance arthrography both have high specificity for identification of chronic ligament tears, but magnetic resonance arthrography has higher sensitivity [10]. The appropriate timing of advanced imaging is variable and governed by the clinical suspicion of further injury or pathologic change not evident on routine radiographs or persistent symptoms despite appropriate treatment. Figures 85.1 and 85.2 demonstrate anterior talofibular and calcaneofibular ligament tears as observed with ankle arthrography.

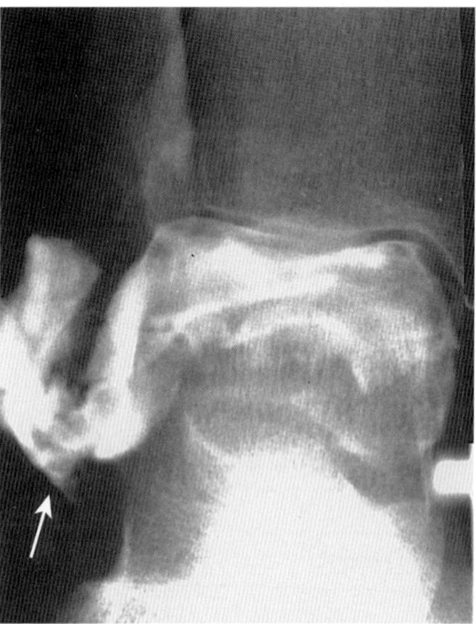

FIGURE 85.1 Ankle arthrogram. Anteroposterior view after ankle injection demonstrates extravasation laterally *(arrow)* resulting from anterior talofibular ligament tear. There is no filling of the peroneal tendon sheath. *(From Berquist TH. Radiology of the Foot and Ankle, 2nd ed. Philadelphia, Lippincott Williams & Wilkins, 2000. © Mayo Foundation, 2000.)*

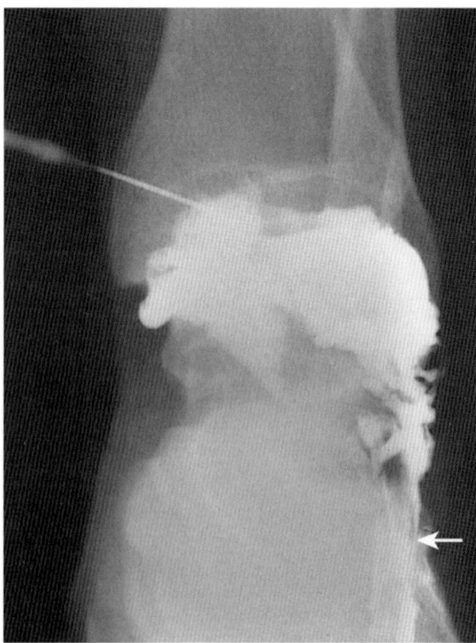

FIGURE 85.2 Ankle arthrogram. Anteroposterior view taken during ankle injection demonstrates filling of the peroneal tendon sheaths *(arrow)* resulting from calcaneofibular ligament disruption. *(From Berquist TH. Radiology of the Foot and Ankle, 2nd ed. Philadelphia, Lippincott Williams & Wilkins, 2000. © Mayo Foundation, 2000.)*

Differential Diagnosis

Peroneal tendinopathy: subluxation, tear, chronic tendinitis
Ankle impingement syndrome
Sinus tarsi syndrome
Subtalar instability
Sprain: midfoot, subtalar
Fracture: distal tibia-fibula, talar, osteochondral, stress fracture, fifth metatarsal, physeal
Arthropathy: degenerative, inflammatory, crystalline, infectious

Treatment

Initial

The initial treatment regimen depends, in part, on symptom acuity and whether a recent sprain has occurred. Initial treatment options include ice massage, compression, elevation, taping or bracing, and nonsteroidal anti-inflammatory drugs or analgesics. The goal with bracing at this juncture is to prevent recurrent sprains and further tissue trauma. Comprehensive literature reviews indeed validate the use of ankle supports to prevent reinjury [11–13]. Many patients can successfully be weaned from external supports after rehabilitation. However, high-demand athletes may choose to brace or to tape during athletic participation indefinitely. A thin lateral heel wedge will put the ankle in slight valgus alignment and potentially diminish symptoms of instability and the tendency for spontaneous ankle inversion with activity. This can be considered in patients with normal alignment for short-term symptom management. Eventually, restoration of neutral foot and ankle alignment should be pursued through orthotic prescription. A three-quarter-length rigid medial longitudinal arch support is recommended in patients with pes planus. In patients with varus or valgus alignment of the ankle, wearing of a shoe that has a firm heel counter is recommended.

Rehabilitation

Rehabilitation starts by normalizing ankle range of motion, with primary emphasis on restoring ankle dorsiflexion and eversion. This typically includes Achilles tendon stretching with the knee straight (to stretch the gastrocnemius) and flexed 30 degrees (to stretch the soleus) as well as eversion (posterior tibialis) stretching. Care must be taken to avoid recurrent inversion stress to the ankle, which can perpetuate lateral capsuloligamentous laxity.

As symptoms allow, the patient begins an ankle muscle group strengthening program with an emphasis on ankle evertor strengthening. Resistance exercises can begin when there is no pain through the available range of motion, with full weight bearing [14]. The rehabilitation program may start with low-level strengthening, such as submaximal static exercises, and progress in a pain-free fashion to dynamic and isokinetic strengthening. Typically, a combination of open and closed kinetic chain strengthening is employed in the rehabilitation process [15]. Open kinetic chain exercises include the use of ankle weights and resistance tubing. Closed kinetic chain exercises are more functionally based; the foot is planted on the ground, and the patient engages in an activity that requires the activation of antagonistic muscles that stabilize the ankle. Because eccentric muscle contractions place the greatest strain on the muscle, this mode of strengthening should be reserved for the final stages of the rehabilitation program.

Balance challenge and proprioceptive exercises are an important part of chronic ankle instability rehabilitation and have been found to decrease symptoms of functional instability as well as to reduce the rate of reinjury [16–18]. Ankle disks or wobble boards are devices that facilitate proprioceptive training. These exercises can be started without specialized equipment by having the patient perform a single-leg stance on the affected ankle; the skill level is then increased by having the patient close the eyes or stand on a pillow.

Functional exercises and sport-specific drills can begin when the patient has full range of motion, no pain, and at least 85% peroneal strength compared with the contralateral ankle [19]. These exercises add progressively difficult challenges and facilitate the attainment of dynamic strength and balance. Examples of these exercises are jogging, running, double-leg jumping, single-leg hopping, skipping rope, figure-eight drills, lateral cutting drills, and plyometrics. Patients should start at a low level of intensity and progress with increased intensity and difficulty only if they remain pain free while performing the exercise and have no pain or swelling after the training session.

Adjunctive modalities may be helpful throughout the rehabilitation process. These may include regular ice application (ice massage, ice pack, ankle Cryo/Cuff) after therapy sessions or heat application (superficial heat or ultrasound) to facilitate range of motion of a stiff joint. Electrical stimulation may be helpful for pain and edema control.

Procedures

Corticosteroid injections around the ankle ligaments are not advised and may further weaken the ligaments, accelerating mechanical instability. Prolotherapy, the injection of an irritant solution around the capsuloligamentous structures of the ankle, can be considered. The injectate (typically a low-concentration dextrose solution or a combination of phenol, glycerin, and glucose) acts as a local tissue irritant and activates the inflammatory cascade [20]. Given its mechanism of action, it can sometimes be a painful treatment. The purported result of this treatment is ligament and capsular hypertrophy causing reduction in laxity and thereby decreased pain [20]. At this time, no randomized controlled or large case series exists for the use of prolotherapy as a treatment of chronic ankle instability, but there is some suggestion of benefit in the treatment of knee laxity and pain due to osteoarthritis [21,22]. Further research is required.

Surgery

Surgery should be considered for patients who sustain recurrent lateral ankle sprains or exhibit significant symptoms of functional instability despite appropriate rehabilitation interventions. The goal of surgery is to restore mechanical stability to the ankle and thereby significantly reduce or eliminate chronic symptoms of instability. Late ankle reconstruction for chronic lateral instability is successful in approximately 85% of patients, regardless of the type of surgical procedure performed [23]. Intra-articular lesions (especially syndesmotic widening), osteochondral lesions of the talus, and ossicles are predictors of unsatisfactory results of ligament reconstruction [24]. Primary anatomic repair of the anterior talofibular and calcaneofibular ligaments is the preferred method of ankle ligament reconstruction [23]. However, in cases in which there is excessive joint laxity or insufficient capsular tissue is available, reconstructions such as the Chrisman-Snook procedure with use of the split peroneal brevis tendon, the semitendinosus, or an allograft may be preferred [25,26]. If the patient has significant varus predisposing to ankle instability, a Dwyer calcaneal closing wedge or lateral calcaneal slide may be appropriate.

Potential Disease Complications

Potential long-term sequelae of chronic ankle instability include the development of ankle impingement syndrome; chronic peroneal tendinopathy or subluxation; tibiotalar osteochondral injury; degenerative arthritis; superficial peroneal neuropathy; and chronic pain syndromes, such as complex regional pain syndrome type I (reflex sympathetic dystrophy).

Potential Treatment Complications

Potential treatment complications include frostbite from overly aggressive use of ice; exacerbation of edema from inappropriate ankle taping, wrapping, or bracing; and pain exacerbation or reinjury during physical therapy. Analgesics and nonsteroidal anti-inflammatory drugs have well-known side effects that most commonly affect the gastric, hepatic, and renal systems. Surgical complications include failed repair, wound or bone infection, loss of ankle range of motion from an aggressive reconstruction, and persistent ankle pain despite appropriate rehabilitation or surgical repair or reconstruction.

References

[1] Verhagen R, de Keizer G, van Dijk CN. Long term follow-up of inversion trauma of the ankle. Arch Orthop Trauma Surg 1995;114:92–6.

[2] McVey ED, Palmieri RM, Docherty CL, et al. Arthrogenic muscle inhibition in the leg muscles of subjects exhibiting functional ankle instability. Foot Ankle Int 2005;26:1055–61.

[3] Freeman M. Instability of the foot after injuries to the lateral ligaments of the foot. J Bone Joint Surg Br 1965;47:669–77.

[4] Hoch MC, Staton GS, Medina McKeon M, et al. Dorsiflexion and dynamic postural control deficits are present in those with chronic ankle instability. J Sci Med Sport 2012;15:574–9.

[5] Arnold BL, De La Motte S, Linens S, Ross S. Ankle instability is associated with balance impairments: a meta-analysis. Med Sci Sports Exerc 2009;41:1048–62.

[6] Schaap G, Keizer G, Marti K. Inversion of the ankle. Arch Orthop Trauma Surg 1989;108:272–5.

[7] van Rijn RM, van Os AG, Bernsen RM, et al. What is the clinical course of acute ankle sprains? A systematic literature review. Am J Med 2008;12:324–31.

[8] Miller MD, Cooper DE, Warner JP. Review of sports medicine and arthroscopy. Philadelphia: WB Saunders; 1995, 90.

[9] Frost SC, Amendola A. Is stress radiography necessary in the diagnosis of acute or chronic ankle instability? Clin J Sport Med 1999;9:40–5.

[10] Chandnani VP, Harper MT, Ficke JR, et al. Chronic ankle instability: evaluation with MR arthrography, MR imaging, and stress radiography. Radiology 1994;192:189–94.

[11] Handoll HH, Rowe BH, Quinn KM, de Bie R. Interventions for preventing ankle ligament injuries. Cochrane Database Syst Rev 2001;3, CD000018.

[12] Hume PA, Gerrard DF. Effectiveness of external ankle support: bracing and taping in rugby union. Sports Med 1998;25:285–312.

[13] Dizon J, Reyes J. A systematic review on the effectiveness of external ankle supports in the prevention of inversion ankle sprains among elite and recreational players. J Sci Med Sport 2010;13:309–17.

[14] Demaio M, Paine R, Drez D. Chronic lateral ankle instability-inversion sprains: part I. Orthopedics 1992;15:87–96.

[15] Osborne MD, Rizzo TD. Prevention and treatment of ankle sprain in athletes. Sports Med 2003;33:1145–50.

[16] Gauffin H, Tropp H, Odenrick P. Effect of ankle disk training on postural control in patients with functional instability of the ankle joint. Int J Sports Med 1988;9:141–8.

[17] Tropp H, Askling C, Gillquist J. Prevention of ankle sprains. Am J Sports Med 1985;13:259–62.

[18] Wortmann MA, Docherty CL. Effect of balance training on postural stability in subjects with chronic ankle instability. J Sport Rehabil 2013;22:143–9.

[19] Demaio M, Paine R, Drez D. Chronic lateral ankle instability-inversion sprains: part II. Orthopedics 1992;15:241–8.

[20] Rabago D, Best TM, Beamsley M, Patterson J. A systematic review of prolotherapy for chronic musculoskeletal pain. Clin J Sport Med 2005;15:376.

[21] Reeves KD, Hassanein KM. Long-term effects of dextrose prolotherapy for anterior cruciate ligament therapy. Altern Ther Health Med 2003;9:58–62.

[22] Rabago D, Zgierska A, Fortney L, et al. Hypertonic dextrose injections (prolotherapy) for knee osteoarthritis: results of a single-arm uncontrolled study with 1-year follow up. J Altern Complement Med 2012;18:408–14.

[23] Colville MR. Surgical treatment of the unstable ankle. J Am Acad Orthop Surg 1998;6:368–77.

[24] Choi WJ, Lee JW, Han SH, et al. Chronic lateral ankle instability: the effect of intra-articular lesions on clinical outcome. Am J Sports Med 2008;36:2167–72.

[25] Peters JW, Trevio SG, Renstrom PA. Chronic lateral ankle instability. Foot Ankle 1991;12:182–91.

[26] Marsh JS, Daigneault JP, Polzhofer GK. Treatment of ankle instability in children and adolescents with a modified Chrisman-Snook repair: a clinical and patient-based outcome study. J Pediatr Orthop 2006;26:94–9.

CHAPTER 86

Foot and Ankle Bursitis

Rathi L. Joseph, DO
Thomas H. Hudgins, MD

Synonyms

Fluid-filled sac of fibrous tissue
Glandular sac (a pouch at a joint to lessen friction)
Haglund deformity
Albert disease
Calcaneus altus
Cucumber heel
High-prow heel
Knobby heel
Prow beak deformity
Pump bump
Retrocalcaneal bursitis
Tendo Achilles bursitis
Winter heel
Hatchet-shaped heel
Achillodynia

ICD-9 Codes

726.71 **Achilles bursitis or tendinitis**
726.79 **Retrocalcaneal bursitis**
727.2 **Specific bursitis often of occupational origin**
727.3 **Other bursitis disorders**

ICD-10 Codes

M76.60 **Achilles tendinitis, unspecified leg**
M76.61 **Achilles tendinitis, right leg**
M76.62 **Achilles tendinitis, left leg**
M70.90 **Unspecified soft tissue disorder related to use, overuse and pressure of unspecified site**
M71.9 **Bursopathy, unspecified**

Definition

Bursae are closed sacs lined by a synovium-like membrane; they contain synovial fluid and are usually located in areas that are subject to friction. Their purpose is to mitigate friction and thus to facilitate the motion that occurs between bones and tendons, bones and skin, or tendons and ligaments [1].

Bursae are classified according to their location, as shown in Table 86.1 [1,2].

Symptomatic malleolar bursae most likely result from abnormal contact pressures. They may also be secondary to shear forces that arise between the bony malleoli and the patient s footwear, particularly boots or athletic shoes that surround the ankle. These may occur either medially or laterally. However, medial bursae are more common [1]. The bone prominences of the malleoli have little inherent soft tissue to protect them from these excessive pressures. The body responds to this abnormal stress by developing an adventitious bursa at this site. The skin and subcutaneous tissues are then able to glide over the bone prominences and thus dissipate these excessive forces. Sometimes, these bursae may become inflamed, resulting in bursitis.

The posterior heel includes the retrocalcaneal bursa, which is located between the calcaneus and the Achilles tendon insertion site, and the retroachilles bursa, which is located between the Achilles tendon and the skin. Each bursa is a potential site of inflammation. The most common cause of posterior heel bursitis is ill-fitting footwear with a stiff posterior edge that abrades the area of the Achilles tendon insertion. Retrocalcaneal inflammation may also be associated with a prominence of the posterosuperior lateral aspect of the calcaneus, causing irritation of the bursa, called a Haglund deformity or pump bump. This entity often goes hand-in-hand with retrocalcaneal bursitis, and frequently there is an element of insertional tendinitis as well.

Although Haglund deformity is more commonly found in women who wear high-heeled shoes, it is sometimes found in hockey players who wear a rigid heel counter that causes irritation. The population of patients that has this superolateral bone prominence tends to be younger than the patients with retrocalcaneal bursitis [3]. Numerous biomechanical risk factors have been associated with Haglund deformity. These include a high-arch cavus foot, rearfoot varus, rearfoot equinus, and trauma to the apophysis in childhood [4–6] (Fig. 86.1).

Table 86.1 Classification of Bursae According to Location

Bursal Type	Examples	Description
Deep	Retrocalcaneal	Found beneath the fibrous investing fascia Develop in utero Often communicate with joints
Subcutaneous	Olecranon, prepatellar	Develop during childhood Do not normally communicate with the adjacent joint
Adventitious	Malleolar, metatarsal head	Often have a thick, fibrous wall Are susceptible to inflammatory changes

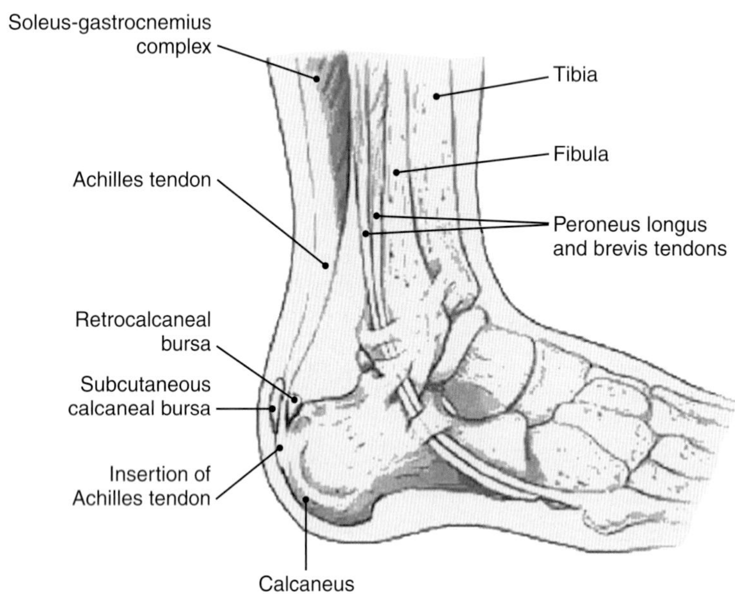

FIGURE 86.1 The anatomy of the structures around the ankle joint. *(From Morelli V, James E. Achilles tendonopathy and tendon rupture: conservative versus surgical management. Prim Care 2004;31:1039-1054.)*

Table 86.2 Risk Factors for Foot and Ankle Bursitis

Type of Bursitis	Risk Factors
Malleolar	Commonly found in repetitive overactivity in boot-wearing athletes, such as ice skaters
Retrocalcaneal	Athletic overactivity associated with repetitive trauma Most common in long-distance runners who run uphill as a training method Hindfoot varus Rigid plantar-flexed first ray
Retroachilles	Commonly found in women who wear high-heeled shoes In the athletic population, it is often found in hockey players who wear a rigid heel counter that causes irritation Retrocalcaneal bursitis Achilles tendinitis High-arch cavus foot Hindfoot varus Hindfoot equinus Trauma to the apophysis in childhood
Metatarsal	First metatarsal: dancers, squash players, or skiers Second to fourth metatarsals: chronic inflammatory arthritis

Bursitis can also occur in the forefoot and may involve the intermetatarsal bursae or the adventitial bursae beneath the metatarsal heads [2].

Risk factors for foot and ankle bursitis are outlined in Table 86.2. Runners, especially those who train uphill, sustain repeated ankle dorsiflexion. Repetitive stress through this motion can lead to bursitis. Also, runners and recreational walkers with sudden increase in mileage are at risk for acquiring symptoms of tenderness, swelling, redness, and pain near the insertion of the Achilles tendon. The most common cause of ankle bursitis is tight-fitting shoes with a firm heel counter. Women wearing high-heeled shoes, runners with improper shoe fit or overworn footwear, skaters, and patients with lower extremity edema are susceptible to development of ankle bursitis. Other important causes of bursitis, in general, are trauma, infection, rheumatoid arthritis, and gout.

Symptoms

With malleolar bursitis, there may be exquisite tenderness surrounding the inflamed bursa, a fluctuant mass over the medial malleolus, and decreased range of motion of the ankle.

Retrocalcaneal bursitis is hallmarked by pain that is anterior to the Achilles tendon and just superior to its insertion on the os calcis. Compression of the bursa between the calcaneus and the Achilles tendon occurs every time the ankle is dorsiflexed; in a runner, the repetitions are countless, particularly with uphill running, when ankle dorsiflexion is increased. Patients often develop a limp, and wearing of shoes may eventually become increasingly painful. Thus, it is not surprising that long-distance runners who use uphill running as a training method frequently develop retrocalcaneal bursitis.

Patients with retroachilles bursitis are often asymptomatic. However, when symptoms occur, the patient usually presents with a painful, tender subcutaneous swelling overlying the Achilles tendon, usually at the level of the shoe counter. The overlying skin may be hyperkeratotic or reddened.

Patients with metatarsal bursitis usually have exquisite tenderness surrounding the inflamed bursa, swelling over the metatarsal head, and decreased range of motion of the metatarsophalangeal joint.

Physical Examination

The physical examination findings in bursitis are described in Table 86.3.

The physical examination includes inspection of the patient's foot at rest and in a weight-bearing position. A visual survey of the foot may reveal swelling, bone deformities, bruising, or skin breaks. The physician should palpate bone prominences and tendinous insertions near the heel and midfoot, noting any tenderness or palpable defects. Passive range of motion of the foot and ankle joints is assessed for indications of restricted movement. Foot posture and arch formation are visually examined while the patient is bearing weight; the physician is looking for abnormal pronation or other biomechanical irregularities. The wear pattern on the posterior interior wall of the shoe should also be examined.

In general, the site of the inflamed bursa is fluctuant and may have some mild associated tenderness and warmth. The patient should be examined closely for any erythema, edema, hypersensitivity, fever, or swollen lymph nodes to rule out septic bursitis.

Insertional tendinosis involves degeneration, not inflammation, of the most distal portion of the Achilles tendon and its attachment on the calcaneal tuberosity. Distinguishing insertional Achilles tendinosis from retrocalcaneal bursitis or osseous impingement, although desirable, is difficult because both may be a continuum of the same disease process or can coexist.

Functional Limitations

Adhesions of the surface of a bursa limit the degree of movement of the associated joint. Pain is a common cause of decreased function. The patient may be limited in ambulation, climbing stairs, and sports activity. The patient also may be limited in footwear, such as protective boots for work.

Diagnostic Studies

Careful physical examination will often yield the cause of most heel pain. Nonetheless, physicians often order radiographs to aid in the diagnostic workup and to exclude osseous causes of the pain. The radiographic findings of bursitis are listed in Table 86.4.

Table 86.3 Bursitis—Physical Findings

Type of Bursitis	Physical Findings
Malleolar	Painful, tender subcutaneous swelling overlying the malleolus Overlying skin may be hyperkeratotic or reddened.
Retrocalcaneal	Tenderness and bogginess along the medial and lateral aspects of the Achilles tendon at its insertion Posterior heel pain with passive ankle dorsiflexion Posterior heel pain with active-resisted plantar flexion A positive two-finger squeeze test result: pain elicited by application of pressure both medially and laterally with two fingers just superior and anterior to the Achilles insertion
Retroachilles	Painful, tender subcutaneous swelling overlying the Achilles tendon, usually at the level of the shoe counter, and on lateral side of Achilles tendon Overlying skin may be hyperkeratotic or reddened.
Metatarsal	If a superficial bursa is affected, there will be signs of acute inflammation, with fluctuant swelling and warmth. If a deep bursa is affected, tissues are tight and congested. Pain with direct pressure, compression, or dorsiflexion of the associated digit An overlying callus may suggest that this is a high-pressure site during normal gait.

Table 86.4 Bursitis—Radiographic Findings

Type of Bursitis	Radiographic Findings
Malleolar	Diagnosis is essentially clinical, and further evaluation is not required.
Retrocalcaneal	Magnetic resonance imaging shows a bursal fluid collection with low signal intensity on T1-weighted images and high signal intensity on T2-weighted and STIR images. A bursa larger than 1 mm anteroposteriorly, 7 mm craniocaudally, or 11 mm transversely is considered abnormal [7].
Retroachilles	Diagnosis is essentially clinical, and further evaluation is not required. It may be discovered incidentally at magnetic resonance imaging performed to evaluate other heel injuries. Its appearance is similar to that of retrocalcaneal bursitis and consists of a bursal fluid collection just posterior to the distal Achilles tendon.
Metatarsal	Magnetic resonance imaging shows a well-defined fluid collection at a pressure point and demonstrates low signal intensity on T1-weighted images and high signal intensity on T2-weighted and STIR images. Small fluid collections with a transverse diameter of 3 mm or less in the first three intermetatarsal bursae may be physiologic. Peripheral enhancement is with gadopentetate dimeglumine [8].

Levy and colleagues [9] demonstrated that routine radiographs are of limited value in the initial evaluation of nontraumatic plantar heel pain in adults and are not necessary in the initial evaluation. They suggested that radiographs should be reserved for patients who do not improve as expected or present with an unusual history or confounding physical findings.

Multiple studies have attempted to delineate Haglund deformity radiographically by looking at the height, length, and angular relationships of the calcaneus. Most authors cannot recommend one particular radiographic view as being consistently helpful in demonstrating this bone prominence or in making a diagnosis or planning treatment. Ultrasonography can be used to visualize an anechoic area of fluid and can be helpful in medication placement [10].

Differential Diagnosis

METATARSAL BURSITIS

Trauma
Freiberg infraction
Infection
Arthritis
Tendon disorders
Non-neoplastic masses
Neoplasms

ANKLE OR HEEL BURSITIS

Achilles tendinitis
Calcaneus stress fracture
Rheumatoid arthritis
Gout
Seronegative spondyloarthropathies
Sural neuritis

Treatment

The treatment of bursitis is summarized in Table 86.5.

Initial

In general, nonoperative treatment of foot and ankle bursitis is always recommended first. Conservative treatment of heel pain, in general, includes use of nonsteroidal anti-inflammatory agents, physical therapy, and avoidance of repetitive high-impact activities [11]. If there is some associated Achilles tendon or plantar fascia disease present, a night splint may help relieve the acute pain many patients experience when they first get up in the morning.

Conservative treatment of general heel pain also includes use of heel lifts and open-back shoes. A portion of the heel counter can be cut away and replaced with a soft leather insert to cause less friction at the site where the heel counter meets the skin. Shoes without laces are to be avoided because they inherently fit close to the heel. Insertion of a heel cup in the shoe may help raise the inflamed region slightly above the restricting heel counter of the shoe. A heel cup also should be placed in the other shoe to avoid introducing leg length discrepancy. Pressure-off silicone sheet pads can be used long term when shoes with counters are worn. Custom orthoses are prescribed for those who have underlying structural abnormalities causing the symptoms.

Table 86.5 Bursitis—Treatment

Type of Bursitis	Treatment
Malleolar	Boot modification or change of footwear Doughnut-shaped cushion made to fit over malleoli Rest and activity modification
Retrocalcaneal	Rest and activity modification (e.g., avoidance of running and walking up hills and stairs) Encourage athletes to change running shoes on a regular basis Biomechanical control in the form of temporary heel lifts, tape immobilization, and, if abnormal pronation is present, custom foot orthotics Slight heel elevation with a felt heel pad A night splint to help keep the Achilles tendon and plantar fascia stretched to relieve acute morning pain and stiffness
Retroachilles	Rest and activity modification Heat application Padding Wearing a soft, nonrestrictive shoe without a counter (e.g., clogs, sandals)
Metatarsal	Rest and activity modification Protective padding Assess for any underlying deformity or foot type with abnormal function

Table 86.6 Bursitis—Rehabilitation

Type of Bursitis	Rehabilitation
Malleolar	Physical therapy is usually not necessary unless joint range of motion is affected. Physical therapy is then necessary to maintain ankle range of motion.
Retrocalcaneal	Physical therapy to teach stretching exercises of the Achilles tendon and plantar fascia Ice can be applied for 15 to 20 minutes, several times a day, during the acute period. Some clinicians also advocate use of contrast baths. Alternative means of maintaining strength and cardiovascular fitness include swimming, water aerobics, and other aquatic exercises.
Retroachilles	Physical therapy to teach stretching exercises of the Achilles tendon

Rehabilitation

The rehabilitation of bursitis is described in Table 86.6.

The patient is allowed weight bearing as tolerated and should be instructed to elevate the foot when not walking. If the patient has had surgery, the dressing is removed 3 days postoperatively, and the patient is allowed to shower. The patient is encouraged to perform active range of motion exercises at least three times a day for 10 minutes each time. The patient is allowed to wear regular shoes as soon as this is tolerated.

Physical therapy is used to teach stretching exercises of the Achilles tendon and plantar fascia to preserve range of motion. This gradual progressive stretching of the Achilles tendon may help relieve impingement on the subtendinous bursa.

Stretching of the Achilles tendon can be performed in the following manner: place the affected foot flat on the floor and lean forward toward the wall until a gentle stretch is felt within the ipsilateral Achilles tendon; maintain the stretch for 20 to 60 seconds and then relax. These stretches should be performed with the knee extended and repeated with the knee flexed, as seen in Figure 86.2. For the benefit of the stretching program to be maximized, repeat for several stretches per set, several times per day. Avoid ballistic (abrupt, jerking) stretches. Progress to calf dips on a stair for functional stretching and eccentric strengthening. Contrast baths and ice massage are also used in the acute management. Icing can be performed for 15 to 20 minutes, several times a day, during the acute period.

The athlete may be expected to return to play without restrictions after demonstrating resolution of symptoms, resolution of physical examination findings (e.g., limping, tenderness on palpation), and adequate performance of sports-specific practice drills without recurrence of symptoms or physical examination findings.

Procedures

If the patient remains symptomatic or finds the bursa to be aesthetically displeasing, the bursa can be aspirated and injected with a 1- to 2-mL solution of a corticosteroid. Many clinicians prefer not to repeat this injection more than once because the risk of tendon rupture is not worth the limited benefits offered by corticosteroid injection. However, tendon rupture is a known complication when corticosteroids are injected directly into the tendon substance [12,13]. There is no available evidence suggesting an association between corticosteroid injections of ankle bursae and Achilles tendon rupture, although most practitioners believe that ultrasound guidance can decrease the possibility of injection within the tendon itself.

Surgery

About 10% of patients with retrocalcaneal or supracalcaneal bursitis do not respond to conservative treatment and seek a surgical solution [14]. Open surgical techniques focus on resection of the posterosuperior portion of the calcaneus or performance of a calcaneal wedge osteotomy with or without débridement of diseased Achilles tendon. Endoscopic techniques provide visualization of the tendon-bone relationship with endoscopic inspection and allow precise débridement and evaluation for residual impingement. The smaller access allows easier closure and less extensive postoperative care. The small incision minimizes the potential for wound dehiscence, a painful scar, and nerve entrapment in scar tissue, and it provides a cosmetically superior result. Endoscopic techniques have had higher patient satisfaction and lower complication rates than open surgical treatment [15].

Potential Disease Complications

The primary disease complication is chronic bursitis with intractable pain that may limit footwear and joint mobility. Adhesive bursitis is another potential disease complication that may occur with chronic bursitis. In adhesive bursitis,

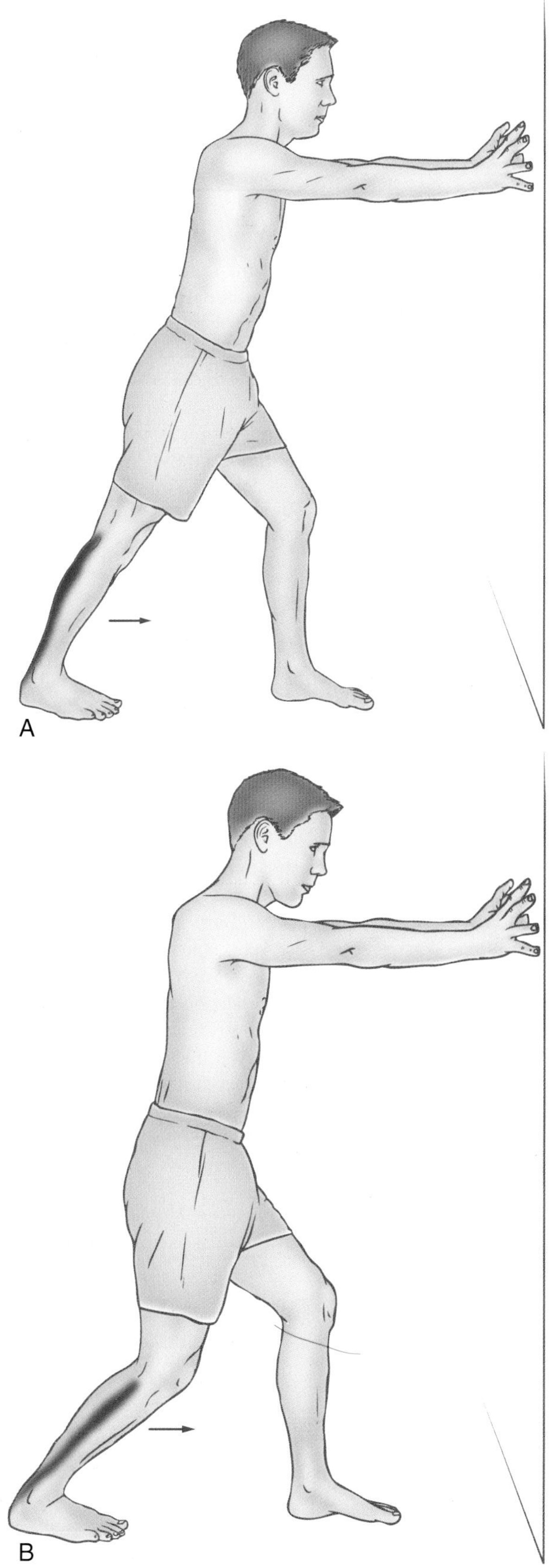

FIGURE 86.2 Stretching of the ankle plantar flexors. **A,** Gastrocnemius muscle. **B,** Soleus muscle. *(From Muscolino JE. The Muscle and Bone Palpation Manual with Trigger Points, Referral Patterns, and Stretching. St. Louis, Mosby, 2009.)*

two adjacent layers of the bursa may adhere and significantly decrease joint range of motion.

The course of bursitis may also be complicated by infection causing a septic bursitis. In this case, immediate surgical débridement and intravenous antibiotics are indicated. A *Staphylococcus aureus* organism is most often responsible and should be treated with appropriate antibiotics.

Potential Treatment Complications

Risks of chronic nonsteroidal anti-inflammatory drug use include gastrointestinal bleeding, renal toxicity, hypertension, and other cardiovascular complications; thus, duration should be kept to a minimum. Systemic complications may be lessened by use of topical nonsteroidal anti-inflammatory drugs to the affected area only.

Complications of open, endoscopic, and fluoroscopic surgical procedures include skin breakdown, avulsion of the Achilles tendon, inadequate decompression with recurrent pain, sensitive and disfiguring scars, altered sensation, and stiffness. In one series, open treatment was associated with a 14% rate of infection, a 17% rate of wound breakdown, a 23% rate of scar tenderness, and a 38% rate of altered sensation [16].

The role of corticosteroid injections in the treatment of retrocalcaneal bursitis is controversial. There have been numerous case reports of patients who have sustained a tendon rupture after peritendinous injections of corticosteroids for the treatment of tendinitis or tendinosis; however, little has been reported on retrocalcaneal intrabursal injections for the treatment of bursitis. Martin and associates [17] investigated the mechanical properties of and histologic changes in rabbit Achilles tendons after peritendinous steroid injection. They found that local injections of corticosteroid, both within the tendon substance and into the retrocalcaneal bursa, adversely affected the biomechanical properties of rabbit Achilles tendons. Another animal study also showed adverse effects of local injections of corticosteroid (within the tendon substance and into the retrocalcaneal bursa) on the biomechanical properties of Achilles tendons [18].

Prolonged immobilization may result in adhesions and subsequent joint stiffening. Thus, patients should have early mobilization after low-grade ankle sprains to prevent increased risk of ankle bursitis.

Patients with ankle bursitis may benefit from accelerated rehabilitation within 7 days of injury to improve muscle strength, sensorimotor control, and range of motion, much like patients after ankle sprains [19], but this has not yet been studied.

References

[1] Brown TD, Varney TE, Micheli LJ. Malleolar bursitis in figure skaters: indications for operative and nonoperative treatment. Am J Sports Med 2000;28:109–11.

[2] Ashman CJ, Klecker RJ, Yu JS. Forefoot pain involving the metatarsal region: differential diagnosis with MR imaging. Radiographics 2001;21:1425–40.

[3] Schepsis AA, Jones H, Hass AL. Achilles tendon disorders in athletes. Am J Sports Med 2002;30:287–305.

[4] Clement DB, Taunton JE, Smart GW, et al. A survey of overuse running injuries. Phys Sportsmed 1981;9:47–58.

[5] James SL, Bates BT, Osternig LR. Injuries to runners. Am J Sports Med 1978;6:40–50.

[6] Krissoff WB, Ferris WD. Runners' injuries. Phys Sportsmed 1979; 7:54–64.

[7] Narváez JA, Narváez J, Ortega R, et al. Painful heel: MR imaging findings. Radiographics 2000;20:333–52.

[8] West SG, Woodburn J. ABC of rheumatology: pain in the foot. BMJ 1995;310:860–4.

[9] Levy JC, Mizel MS, Clifford PD, Temple HT. Value of radiographs in the initial evaluation of nontraumatic adult heel pain. Foot Ankle Int 2006;27:427–30.

[10] Checa A, Chun W, Pappu R. Ultrasound-guided diagnostic and therapeutic approach to retrocalcaneal bursitis. J Rheumatol 2011;38:391–2.

[11] Mazzone MF, McCue T. Common conditions of the Achilles tendon. Am Fam Physician 2002;65:1805–10.

[12] Morelli V, James E. Achilles tendonopathy and tendon rupture: conservative versus surgical management. Prim Care 2004;31:1039–54.

[13] Wilson JJ, Best TM. Common overuse tendon problems: a review and recommendations for treatment. Am Fam Physician 2005;72:811–8.

[14] McGarvey WC, Palumbo RC, Baxter DE, Leibman BD. Insertional Achilles tendinosis: surgical treatment through a central tendon splitting approach. Foot Ankle Int 2002;23:19–25.

[15] Wiegerinck JI, Kok AC, van Dijk CN. Surgical treatment of chronic retrocalcaneal bursitis. Arthroscopy 2012;28:283–93.

[16] Taylor GJ. Prominence of the calcaneus: is operation justified? J Bone Joint Surg Br 1986;68:467–70.

[17] Martin DF, Carlson CS, Berry J, et al. Effect of injected versus iontophoretic corticosteroid on the rabbit tendon. South Med J 1999;92:600–8.

[18] Hugate R, Pennypacker J, Saunders M, Juliano P. The effects of corticosteroids on biomechanical properties of rabbit Achilles tendons. J Bone Joint Surg Am 2004;86:794–801.

[19] Bleakley CM, O'Connor SR, Tully MA, et al. Effect of accelerated rehabilitation on function after ankle sprain: randomised controlled trial. BMJ 2010;340:c1964.

CHAPTER 87

Hallux Rigidus

David Wexler, MD, FRCS (Tr & Orth)
Dawn M. Grosser, MD
Todd A. Kile, MD

Synonyms

Osteoarthritis or degenerative joint disease of the first metatarsophalangeal joint
Osteoarthritis of the great toe [1]

ICD-9 Code

735.2 Hallux rigidus

ICD-10 Codes

M20.20 Hallux rigidus, unspecified foot
M20.21 Hallux rigidus, right foot
M20.22 Hallux rigidus, left foot

Definition

Degenerative joint disease or loss of articular cartilage from the first metatarsophalangeal (MTP) joint leading to painful restriction of motion is called hallux rigidus. The normal range of motion of the first MTP joint is 30 to 45 degrees of plantar flexion to almost 90 degrees of dorsiflexion. The limited range of motion and pain with hallux rigidus are exacerbated by overgrowth of bone (osteophytes or "bone spurs") on the dorsal aspects of the base of the proximal phalanx and the head of the metatarsal, which impinge on one another as the great toe dorsiflexes [2]. Hallux rigidus is the second most common problem in the first MTP joint, after hallux valgus; 1 in 40 people older than 50 years will develop hallux rigidus [3].

In general, the cause is unknown, although it is associated with generalized osteoarthritis of other joints and repeated microtrauma (e.g., in soccer players). Sustaining repetitive turf toe–type injuries may lead to this form of early joint degeneration [4]. As the plantar capsuloligamentous complex of the first MTP joint is injured by hyperflexion of the great toe, it may acutely compress the articular surfaces of the joint, causing articular damage, or become chronically unstable, predisposing the MTP joint to degeneration and hallux rigidus [5].

Symptoms

Patients typically report pain, either intermittent or constant, that occurs with walking and is relieved by rest. It is insidious in onset and may be associated with stiffness, swelling, and sometimes inflammation. On occasion, there can be locking due to a cartilaginous loose body. Patients may notice that they are walking on the outside of the foot to avoid pushing off with the great toe during the terminal stance and toe-off phases of the gait cycle. As degeneration increases, the pain may intensify and result in an alteration of gait.

Physical Examination

On inspection, there will usually be swelling around the MTP joint with tenderness of the joint line. Dorsal osteophytes may be palpable and may cause irritation of overlying skin with shoe wear abrasion. Pain is reproduced with forcible dorsiflexion of the great toe, which is also restricted in range of movement. Plantar flexion may also be affected. Patients may have an antalgic (painful) gait, and single-stance heel raise may be difficult secondary to a painful MTP joint, as opposed to posterior tibial tendon deficiency. Findings of the neurologic examination, including strength, sensation, and reflexes, are typically normal.

Functional Limitations

Functional limitations include walking long distances, running any distance, and ascending stairs. As the severity increases, walking even short distances, daily errands, and standing for long periods may be difficult. Flexible shoes as well as shoes with a tight toe box may prove to be uncomfortable. This may lead to pressure areas dorsally over the osteophytes.

Diagnostic Studies

Plain anteroposterior and lateral standing radiographs will usually suffice in confirming the diagnosis (Fig. 87.1).

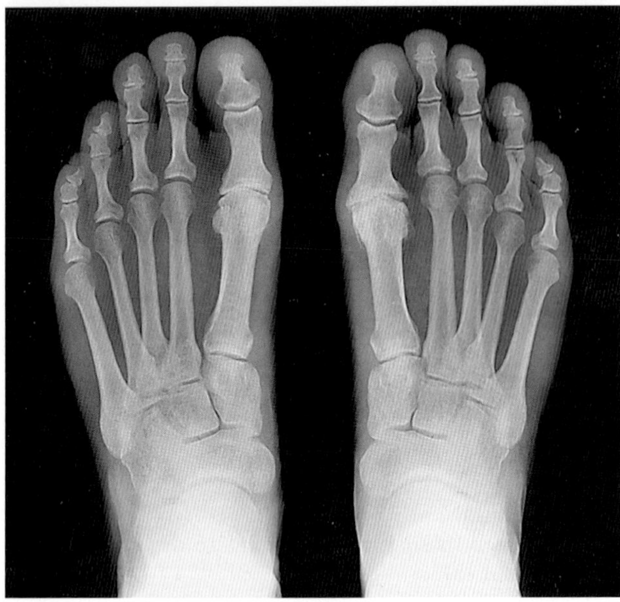

FIGURE 87.1 Standing anteroposterior radiograph of both feet. This demonstrates bilateral hallux rigidus or degenerative joint disease of the hallux MTP joints. The signs are narrowing of the joint space, osteophyte formation, and sclerosis. This is more pronounced on the right.

The signs are consistent with degenerative joint disease, namely, loss of joint space and congruency, large dorsal osteophytes (bone spurs), sclerosis (increased density of bone), and subchondral cysts. There may be evidence of a loose body. This disease process has been divided into three grades on the basis of the severity of radiographic and clinical findings, which help guide surgical treatment.

Grade I demonstrates small dorsal osteophytes with preservation of the MTP joint space on radiographic examination and typically intermittent pain with ambulation. Grade II demonstrates moderate dorsal osteophyte formation and asymmetric joint space narrowing radiographically and often constant pain with ambulation. Grade III has extensive osteophytes and severe dorsal and plantar joint space narrowing, often with noticeable loose bodies; clinically, patients will have constant pain with ambulation and significant limitation of motion [6].

Differential Diagnosis

Gout
Hallux valgus
Turf toe
Fracture

Treatment

Initial

Nonsteroidal anti-inflammatory drugs may provide symptomatic relief. Footwear modifications and orthoses to limit stresses at the MTP joint (carbon fiber inserts or Morton's extension orthotic devices) as well as avoidance of high heels or shoes with very flexible soles may be useful conservative treatment options [7].

Rehabilitation

More advanced shoe modifications can be made by a certified pedorthist. These include a steel shank and possibly a rocker-bottom. These may be applied to the soles of many different types of shoes, including athletic shoes. Anecdotally, many patients prefer first to try a steel shank because there is no cosmetic change to the shoe. With a rocker-bottom, the sole is altered, and this is sometimes less cosmetically acceptable to patients.

If there is evidence of other foot deformities, such as pes planus (flatfoot), orthotic inserts may provide correction and help with gait biomechanics.

Physical therapy is not generally necessary but may include basic mobilization and distraction techniques as well as strengthening exercises of the flexor and extensor hallucis muscles to enhance joint stability. Modalities such as contrast baths and ice may help with pain control.

Procedures

Intra-articular x-ray–guided or ultrasound-guided injection of the MTP joint with local anesthetic and steroid may provide short-term relief.

Surgery

The principal indications for surgery are continuing pain and failed nonoperative management. Depending on the severity of the degeneration, there are two broad approaches to surgery. For grade I and grade II, the appropriate treatment is joint preserving; the impinging dorsal osteophytes are excised and the joint is debulked, thus improving dorsiflexion [8–10]. A phalangeal osteotomy (i.e., Moberg procedure) may also be used to improve dorsiflexion. The second approach is joint sacrificing for grade III disease. These procedures range from resection arthroplasty, resulting in a floppy or flail shortened toe, to arthrodesis (Fig. 87.2), resulting in a stiff, rigidly fixed toe [6,11,12]. A number of manufacturers have tried to produce artificial great toe joints, made of Silastic, metal, and polyethylene or ceramic [13,14], but the long-term results of these have not lived up to expectations. A randomized controlled trial comparing arthrodesis to arthroplasty found better improvement in pain, satisfaction of patients, and cost ratio with arthrodesis. Patients receiving arthroplasty had minimal improvement in range of motion, had continued altered gait mechanics, and required removal secondary to loosening in a significant number [15]. Interposition arthroplasty (with use of autologous tissue attached between the two joint surfaces) has also been advocated as a reasonable option instead of fusing the joint for grade III disease [16]. Arthroscopic surgery has also been attempted.

Potential Disease Complications

Hallux rigidus may produce intractable pain and reduced mobility.

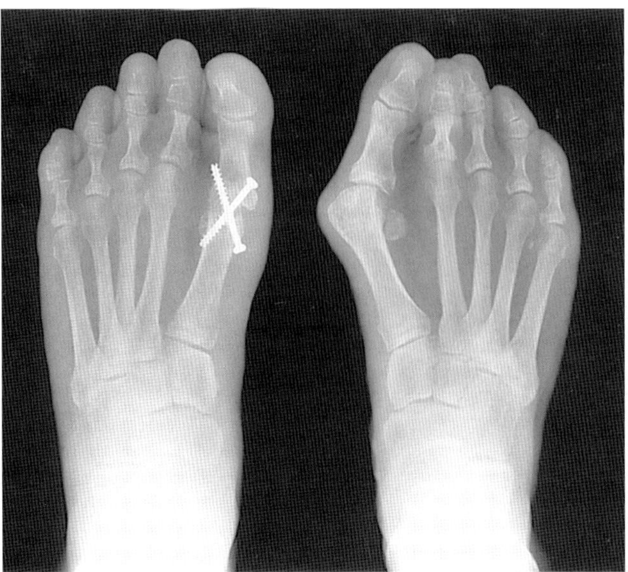

FIGURE 87.2 Standing anteroposterior radiograph of both feet. This demonstrates, on the left foot, one of the techniques for fusing the MTP joint, with crossed cannulated screws. The right foot shows a hallux valgus deformity.

Potential Treatment Complications

Analgesics and nonsteroidal anti-inflammatory drugs have well-known side effects that most commonly affect the gastric, hepatic, and renal systems. Steroid injection can rarely introduce infection.

Complications of surgery can range from failure of improvement with insufficient osteophyte resection to toe shortening with subsequent transfer metatarsalgia (pain under the metatarsal heads of the lesser toes). Arthroplasty complications include implant failure, silicone wear and subsequent debris production, foreign body reaction, and osteolysis. Arthrodesis complications include malunion and nonunion.

References

[1] O'Malley MJ. Hallux rigidus. In: Craig EV, editor. Clinical orthopaedics. Philadelphia: Lippincott Williams & Wilkins; 1999. p. 913–9.

[2] Richardson EG, Donley BG. Disorders of hallux. In: Canale ST, editor. 9th ed. Campbell's operative orthopaedics, vol. 2. St. Louis: Mosby; 1998. p. 1621–711.

[3] Coughlin MJ, Mann RA. Surgery of the foot and ankle. 7th ed. St. Louis: Mosby; 1999, 605–632.

[4] Mann RA. Disorders of the first metatarsophalangeal joint. J Am Acad Orthop Surg 1995;3:34–40.

[5] Sammarco GJ. Biomechanics of the foot. In: Frankel VH, Nordin M, editors. Biomechanics of the skeletal system. Philadelphia: Lea & Febiger; 1980. p. 193–219.

[6] Alexander IA. Hallux metatarsophalangeal arthrodesis. In: Thompson RC, Johnson KA, editors. Master techniques in orthopaedic surgery. The foot and ankle. Philadelphia: Raven Press; 1994. p. 49–64.

[7] Hertling D, Kessler RM. The leg, ankle and foot. In: Hertling D, Kessler RM, editors. Management of common musculoskeletal disorders. 3rd ed. Philadelphia: Lippincott Williams & Wilkins; 1996. p. 435–8.

[8] Geldwert JJ, Rock GD, McGrath MP, Mancuso JE. Cheilectomy: still a useful technique for grade I and grade II hallux limitus/rigidus. J Foot Surg 1992;31:154–9.

[9] Hattrup SJ, Johnson KA. Subjective results of hallux rigidus following treatment with cheilectomy. Clin Orthop 1988;226:182–9.

[10] Pfeffer GB. Cheilectomy. In: Thompson RC, Johnson KA, editors. Master techniques in orthopaedic surgery. The foot and ankle. Philadelphia: Raven Press; 1994. p. 119–33.

[11] Coughlin MJ. Arthrodesis of first metatarsophalangeal joint. Orthop Rev 1990;19:177–86.

[12] Curtis MJ, Myerson M, Jinnah RH, et al. Arthrodesis of the first metatarsophalangeal joint: a biomechanical study of internal fixation techniques. Foot Ankle 1993;14:395–9.

[13] Wenger RJ, Whalley RC. Total replacement of the first MTP joint. J Bone Joint Surg Br 1978;60:88–92.

[14] Townley CO, Taranow WS. A metallic hemiarthroplasty resurfacing prosthesis for the hallux metatarsophalangeal joint. Foot Ankle Int 1994;15:575–80.

[15] Gibson JN, Thomson CE. Arthrodesis or total replacement arthroplasty for hallux rigidus: a randomized controlled trial. Foot Ankle Int 2005;26:680–90.

[16] Kennedy JG, Chow FY, Dines J, et al. Outcomes after interposition arthroplasty for treatment of hallux rigidus. Clin Orthop Relat Res 2006;445:210–5.

CHAPTER 88

Hammer Toe

Daniel P. Montero, MD

Synonyms

Flexion contracture of the proximal interphalangeal joint
Lesser toe deformity
Hammer toe syndrome

ICD-9 Codes

735.4 Hammer toe (acquired)
735.8 Other acquired deformities of toe

ICD-10 Codes

M20.40 Hammer toe(s) (acquired), unspecified foot
M20.41 Hammer toe(s) (acquired), right foot
M20.42 Hammer toe(s) (acquired), left foot
M20.5X1 Other deformities of toe(s) (acquired), right foot
M20.5X2 Other deformities of toe(s) (acquired), left foot
M20.5X9 Other deformities of toe(s) (acquired), unspecified foot

Definition

Hammer toe refers to an abnormal flexion posture at the proximal interphalangeal (PIP) joint of one or more of the lesser four toes [1]. If the flexion contracture is severe and of long duration, concomitant hyperextension of the metatarsophalangeal (MTP) joint and extension of the distal interphalangeal (DIP) joint may occur (Fig. 88.1). In contrast to clawing, which tends to involve all toes, hammer toe deformity usually affects only one or two toes [2]. Hammer toes are classified as either flexible (passively correctable) or rigid (not passively correctable to the neutral position). The most commonly affected toe is the second, although multiple digits can be involved [3].

Hammer toe is the most common of the lesser toe deformities and occurs primarily in the sagittal plane. It is arguably the most common toe disorder that presents to the foot and ankle surgeon's office. Women are more commonly affected, and the incidence of hammer toe increases with age [4–6].

Contributing factors include long-term wear of poorly fitting shoes, especially those with tight, narrow toe boxes. Crowding and overlapping from hallux valgus are other causes. A long second ray with subsequent buckling of the toe may also lead to the deformity. Other predisposing factors are diabetes, connective tissue disease, and trauma [5].

Symptoms

Patients commonly complain of pain or tenderness in the area of the PIP joint, especially when wearing shoes or during weight-bearing activities. Patients also commonly present with cosmetic complaints. Pain may be the result of corn or callus formation over the dorsal aspect of the PIP joint from shoe compression. In cases in which hyperextension of the MTP joint has occurred, there is also increased pressure under the metatarsal heads. Metatarsalgia with subsequent callus formation underneath the metatarsal heads may occur secondary to their plantar displacement [2], with distal displacement of the plantar fat pad.

Physical Examination

The diagnosis is confirmed by the presence of MTP joint hyperextension, PIP joint flexion, and DIP joint extension in the affected toe. Palpation of the PIP joint usually causes tenderness, with the plantar aspect more commonly affected.

On inspection, determine the degree of PIP flexion. Also note accompanying foot deformities, such as ulcerations and callus formation over the PIP joint and tip of the toe. Hammer toe deformities become more prominent in stance phase. Examination of the joint range of motion of the affected toe will differentiate a fixed deformity from the one that is flexible. The presence or absence of crepitus should be noted. Flexor digitorum longus contracture is assessed with the ankle in dorsiflexion and plantar flexion. Correction of the deformity on plantar flexion signifies a flexible hammer toe. Dorsiflexion, in turn, accentuates the deformity [7].

The Kelikian push-up test is used to assess the degree of flexibility. Press upward on the plantar aspect of the

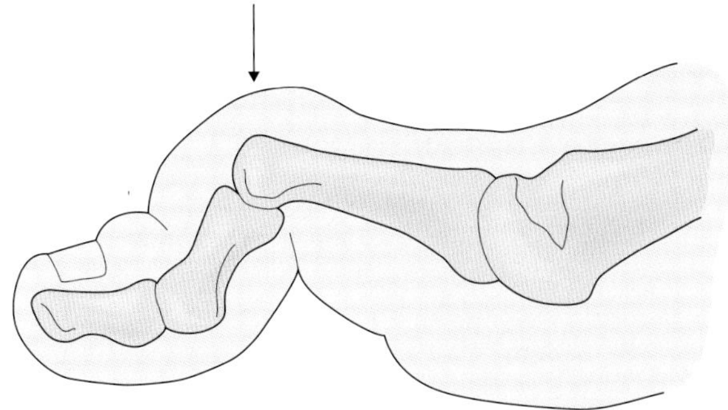

FIGURE 88.1 Diagrammatic representation of hammer toe. *(From Krug RJ, Lee EH, Dugan S, Mashey K. Hammer toe. In Frontera WR, Silver JK, Rizzo TD Jr, eds. Essentials of Physical Medicine and Rehabilitation, 2nd ed. Philadelphia, WB Saunders, 2008.)*

metatarsal head; in flexible deformities, the MTP joint will align and the proximal phalanx will assume a more normal position.

A mild deformity hammer toe implies no fixed contracture at the MTP or PIP joint, but the deformity increases with weight bearing. A moderate deformity hammer toe has a fixed or partially fixed contracture at the PIP joint and zero to mild extension contracture at the MTP joint. A severe deformity hammer toe involves fixed flexion contracture at the PIP joint with a fixed extension contracture of the MTP joint. Subluxation or dislocation of the proximal phalanx on the metatarsal head may also be present [7].

Also assess for signs of swelling, temperature change, or erythema that might indicate the presence of an infectious or rheumatic process responsible for the deformity.

Inspection of the patient's footwear is necessary to determine the ability of the toe box to accommodate the forefoot. The presence of corns or callus over the PIP joint, which may ulcerate, is often indicative of poorly fitting footwear.

Standard neurologic and vascular examinations will reveal no abnormal findings in uncomplicated hammer toe deformities. If there is a superficial peroneal nerve injury causing a dropfoot deformity, hammer toes will result because of extensor substitution. Likewise, a weakness of the gastrocnemius can lead to flexor substitution, causing a hammer toe.

If the patient has peripheral vascular disease or atherosclerosis, ulceration over a PIP joint may lead to toe loss unless the toe is revascularized.

Functional Limitations

Functional limitations mostly result from pain incurred by corn and callus formation. Walking and other weight-bearing activities can be painful. The ability to tolerate footwear with a narrow toe box is also impaired.

Diagnostic Studies

The diagnosis is primarily a clinical one. However, radiographs can be useful in the assessment of a rigid hammer toe, with weight-bearing views preferred. An apparent joint space narrowing on the anteroposterior view corresponds to subluxation of the proximal phalanx on the metatarsal head at the MTP joint [5,7].

Differential Diagnosis

Claw toes
Mallet toes
Interdigital neuroma
Nonspecific synovitis of the metatarsophalangeal joint
Triggering of the lesser toes (lower limb analogue of trigger finger) [8]
Rheumatoid or psoriatic arthritis
Plantar plate rupture

Treatment

Initial

Patient education is critical. The first step involves fitting for shoes with an adequate toe box to accommodate the dorsiflexed position of the proximal phalanx. High heels should be avoided as much as possible. A soft insole can also be used, which is useful for pressure relief [8]. Oral or topical nonsteroidal anti-inflammatory drugs (NSAIDs) can help with pain and inflammation. Analgesic medications may be taken for pain relief. Ulcer and callus management may be necessary, and patients should be educated about monitoring their skin for breakdown, especially in the setting of peripheral neuropathy.

Local icing may also help with acute pain (10 minutes, two or three times a day). However, ice should be avoided in patients with significant peripheral vascular disease because of its vasoconstrictive properties and in individuals with impaired sensation, such as peripheral neuropathy, because of the risk of frostbite.

Initial treatment is palliative rather than corrective and predominantly consists of attempts to accommodate the toe deformity by changing the patient's footwear and débridement of calluses if they are present. This may include stretching the shoes or switching to shoes with a deeper toe box or to extra-depth shoes. Padding, such as toe crest pads or custom or premade hammer toe regulators, may relieve pressure over the involved joints. Patients with calluses on the PIP joint may benefit from digital caps or silicone cushions.

Rehabilitation

Formal physical therapy is usually not required, although some patients might benefit from a supervised paraffin treatment, which should be followed by stretching exercises. Paraffin baths are contraindicated if ulcers or sensory deficits are present [9].

Stretching exercises can relieve the "tight" sensation in patients with a flexible or semiflexible deformity. Exercises such as picking up a towel with the toes are recommended for both stretching and strengthening of the intrinsic foot muscles.

Functional orthotics will provide flexor stabilization and, in some instances, symptomatic relief to overpronators with a flexible hammer toe deformity. Orthotics may slow the progression of the deformity by improving the biomechanics of the feet.

The clinician may prescribe shoes with deep, wide toe boxes. Alternatively, extra depth can be achieved in a standard shoe by trimming the existing shoe insert just distal to the metatarsal heads [10]. Lambswool or felt around the toes provides extra padding. An external metatarsal bar and rocker-bottom shoes may provide additional comfort-enhancing options. Specific strapping devices and hammer toe straightening orthoses are available. Again, patients with peripheral vascular disease or neuropathy should be cautious or avoid these.

Procedures

Steroid injections may be indicated for patients with painful PIP joint capsulitis or arthritic flare secondary to a hammer toe deformity. Combine steroid injections with padding or splinting for optimal relief. By use of a 27-gauge needle and corticosteroid with local anesthetic mixture, introduce the solution into the joint capsule through the dorsomedial or dorsolateral aspect of the joint. Always perform a surgical preparation before injecting the joint. The patient should be advised about the possibility of a steroid flare.

Surgery

Operative treatment should be pursued when conservative treatment fails. Cosmesis alone is not a good indication for surgery. Associated deformities must also be corrected for optimal surgical outcome (e.g., hallux valgus) [7].

Multiple procedures have been described for the surgical management of hammer toes. The procedures used are based on the degree of hammer toe deformity. A stepwise approach involving several procedures may be needed to accomplish correction on the basis of severity. Outcomes are varied by the specific procedures chosen. The following procedures are most commonly recommended and data supported [2]:

Mild deformity/flexible hammer toe (no fixed contracture at the MTP or PIP joint): flexor to extensor transfer using flexor digitorum longus.

Moderate deformity/rigid hammer toe with MTP subluxation (fixed flexion contracture at the PIP; MTP subluxation in extension): resection of the condyles of the proximal phalanx, dermodesis (removal of an ellipse of skin on the volar aspect of the joint); lengthening of extensor digitorum longus, tenotomy of extensor digitorum brevis; MTP capsulotomy, collateral ligament sectioning.

Moderate to severe deformity/rigid hammer toe with MTP dislocation: similar to subluxation treatment with addition of MTP arthroplasty or Weil osteotomy.

Severe deformity/crossover toe (fixed flexion contracture at the PIP joint; MTP subluxation in varus or valgus): resection of the condyles of the proximal phalanx, dermodesis; collateral ligament/capsular repair; extensor digitorum brevis transfer [2,11].

Replacement of the PIP or MTP joint with toe deformity is another option, as are implants that have been developed for intramedullary placement to stabilize the PIP joint, promoting fusion. Such implants are not universally accepted and are exceedingly difficult to remove should the surgery fail. Their removal could lead to substantial bone loss, making subsequent revision procedures challenging. Kirschner wires are usually used to stabilize the hammer toes for several weeks and are most accepted at this time.

Postoperative Rehabilitation

After 2 or 3 days of elevation of the foot, patients can bear weight as tolerated. Surgical shoes with limited activity and use of crutches are recommended for approximately 4 weeks postoperatively. If Kirschner wires are used, they are typically removed between 3 and 6 weeks after operation. This varies by the surgeon's preference [12]. Patients can start to gradually increase activities at approximately 8 weeks after surgery. More weight-bearing activities, such as running, are best started after 12 weeks of recovery. Such recommendations vary according to the severity of the deformity and complexity of the surgery.

Potential Disease Complications

Potential disease complications include chronic intractable pain that limits all mobility. Other complications may include metatarsalgia, plantar and point of contact ulcerations in the insensate foot, arthralgia and joint stiffness if subluxation has occurred, toenail deformities, and bursitis or synovitis [5]. Gait abnormalities may contribute to more proximal pain symptoms (e.g., low back and hip pain).

Diabetic neuropathy and advanced peripheral vascular disease are relative contraindications to splinting [13] when correction is nonsurgical.

Common potential complications include PIP joint ulceration due to excessive pressure, fixed foot deformity, and postural changes resulting from pain-induced gait deviations.

Potential Treatment Complications

Local icing can cause vasoconstriction and frostbite. Analgesics, NSAIDs, and cyclooxygenase 2 inhibitors have well-known side effects that most commonly affect the gastric, hepatic, and renal systems. Newer topical NSAIDs may have fewer side effects because of less systemic absorption. Postsurgical complications include toe ischemia, digital nerve palsy, nonunion, malalignment, reduced toe range of motion, rigid and excessively straight toe, persistent edema, flail toe, and osseous regrowth. Potential complications of surgical correction include flail or "floppy" toes, which can be repaired by collateral ligament repair or arthrodesis. Infection and, in severe cases, osteomyelitis can occur either before or as a complication of surgery. If intravenous antibiotic treatment is unsuccessful, partial or total toe amputation may be required. Because of the morbidity associated with surgical complications, appropriate patient selection is imperative in recommending operative correction of hammer toe deformities.

References

[1] Schrier JC, Verheyen CC, Louwerens JW. Definitions of hammer toe and claw toe: an evaluation of the literature. J Am Podiatr Med Assoc 2009;99:194–7.

[2] Canale ST, editor. 11th ed. Campbell's operative orthopedics, vol. 4. St. Louis: Mosby; 2007. p. 4630–40.

[3] Myerson MS, Shereff MJ. The pathological anatomy of claw and hammer toes. J Bone Joint Surg Am 1989;71:45–9.

[4] Preferred practice guidelines: hammertoe syndrome. J Foot Ankle Surg 1999;38:1067–2516.
[5] Hammer toe syndrome. American College of Foot and Ankle Surgeons. J Foot Ankle Surg 1999;38:166–78.
[6] Golightly YM, Hannan MT, Dufour AB, Jordan JM. Racial differences in foot disorders and foot type. Arthritis Care Res (Hoboken) 2012;64:1756–9.
[7] Wheeless CR. Hammer toes. Wheeless' textbook of orthopaedics. http://www.wheelessonline.com/ortho/hammer_toes; [accessed October 2012].
[8] Martin MG, Masear VR. Triggering of the lesser toes at a previously undescribed distal pulley system. Foot Ankle Int 1998;19:113–7.
[9] Hunt GC, McPoil TG, editors. Physical therapy of the foot and ankle. 2nd ed. New York: Churchill Livingstone; 1995.
[10] Kaye RA. The extra-depth toe box: a rational approach. Foot Ankle Int 1994;15:146–50.
[11] Shirzad K, Kiesau CD, DeOrio JK, Parekh SG. Lesser toe deformities. J Am Acad Orthop Surg 2011;19:505–14.
[12] Klammer G, Baumann G, Moor BK, et al. Early complications and recurrence rates after Kirschner wire transfixation in lesser toe surgery: a prospective randomized study. Foot Ankle Int 2012;33:105–12.
[13] McGlamry ED, Banks AS, Downey MS, editors. Comprehensive textbook of foot surgery. Baltimore: Williams & Wilkins; 1992. p. 341.

CHAPTER 89

Mallet Toe

Vasilios A. Lirofonis, DPM
Robert J. Scardina, DPM

Synonyms

Lesser toe deformity
Mallet toe syndrome
Claw toe
Claw toe syndrome
Hammer toe
Hammer toe syndrome
Contracted toe

ICD-9 Codes

735.8	**Other acquired deformities of the toe**
755.66	**Other anomalies of toes**

ICD-10 Codes

M20.5X1	**Other acquired deformities of the toe, right foot**
M20.5X2	**Other acquired deformities of the toe, left foot**
M20.5X9	**Other acquired deformities of the toe, unspecified foot**
M20.60	**Acquired anomalies of toe(s), unspecified, unspecified foot**
M20.61	**Acquired anomalies of toe(s), unspecified, right foot**
M20.62	**Acquired anomalies of toe(s), unspecified, left foot**

Definition

Mallet toe refers to an abnormal flexion deformity at the distal interphalangeal (DIP) joint (Fig. 89.1). Typically, the metatarsophalangeal and proximal interphalangeal joints are aligned in neutral position without extension or flexion. The most commonly affected toe is the longest toe, usually the second. The deformity may be fixed (rigid), semirigid, or flexible; it may occur unilaterally or bilaterally, and it may be acquired or congenital. High-heeled shoes and shoes with a narrow toe box may aggravate the deformity; it is present symptomatically more in women [1,2]. There is some observational evidence to suggest that a toe longer than adjacent toes is at increased risk for development of lesser toe deformities [3]. The incidence of a mallet toe deformity is much less common than that of a hammer toe deformity at almost 1:10 [4]. This is likely to be related to presentation rates as hammer toes are typically more problematic compared with mallet toe deformity.

Symptoms

Patients typically complain of pain or tenderness in the area of the dorsal DIP joint or distal aspect of the toe, most commonly when wearing shoes, particularly with a narrow toe box. The symptoms are also worse during weight-bearing activities, such as running. Patients may also have complaints of toenail deformities, which eventually may become painful. A painful corn or clavus may develop on either the dorsal aspect of the DIP joint (as a result of shoe irritation) or the distal aspect of the toe.

Physical Examination

The degree of DIP joint flexion should be evaluated, both weight bearing and non–weight bearing. Passive range of motion should be determined to evaluate whether the deformity is flexible, rigid, or semirigid, which will influence treatment options. One should inspect for cutaneous lesions (corns) on both the dorsal and distal aspects of the toe. Corns may progress to ulcers with subsequent superficial or deep infection, especially in the diabetic population with neuropathy. If the patient has peripheral arterial disease, ulceration may lead to necrosis and possible toe loss.

Swelling, increased temperature, or erythema might indicate inflammatory arthritis or joint infection. The patient's footwear should be examined to determine sufficient or insufficient toe box height to accommodate the deformity. Traditional neurologic and vascular examinations generally reveal no abnormal findings in uncomplicated mallet toe conditions.

Functional Limitations

Functional limitation in ambulation occurs most often as the result of pain, particularly with wearing of closed shoes and with weight-bearing activities. Walking may be limited, and

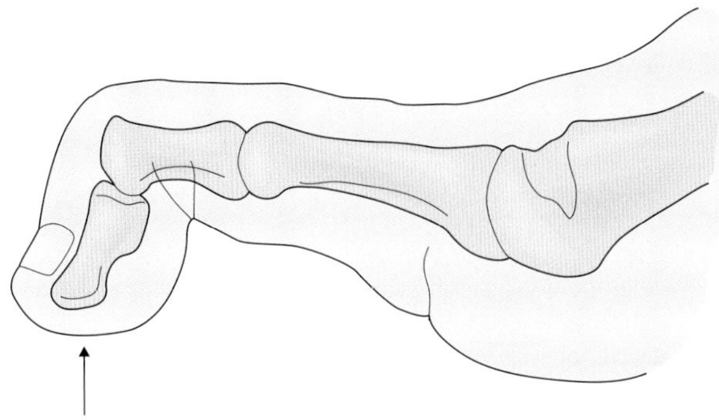

FIGURE 89.1 Mallet toe (arrow indicates usual area of hyperkeratosis or ulcer formation). *(From Maguire S. Mallet toe. In Frontera WR, Silver JK, Rizzo TD Jr, eds. Essentials of Physical Medicine and Rehabilitation, 2nd ed. Philadelphia, WB Saunders, 2008.)*

high-impact activities such as running may be altogether too painful. Women may complain that they are unable to wear shoes (dress and high heeled) required for their work environment. Painless deformity generally neither causes functional limitations nor requires treatment [5].

Diagnostic Studies

The diagnosis of a mallet toe is primarily clinical. However, foot radiographs can be useful in assessing the DIP joint with fixed deformity resulting from traumatic, degenerative, or inflammatory arthritis. Weight-bearing views are preferred in assessing for functional or dynamic (versus fixed) deformity. Non–weight-bearing isolated or magnification toe views also may be helpful. Noninvasive arterial studies (toe-brachial index) are used to assess perfusion in cases in which ischemia is suspected before initiation of conservative and especially surgical treatment.

Differential Diagnosis

Claw toe
Hammer toe
Cock-up toe
Triggering of the lesser toes (lower limb analogue of trigger finger) [6]
Rheumatoid arthritis
Psoriatic arthritis

Treatment

Initial

Patient education to provide an understanding of the deformity and proper footwear are essential. Shoes fabricated with soft upper material and having (or modified to achieve) adequate toe box depth to accommodate the deformity should be recommended (e.g., extra-depth shoes). Shoes incompatible with the deformity, especially high heels, should be avoided as much as possible. A soft shoe insole may be helpful in relieving pressure at the distal aspect of the toe [7,8]. Moleskin or adhesive felt padding may be applied to painful corns, but the use of medicated (salicylic acid) plasters should be avoided, especially in patients with diabetes or peripheral vascular disease. Oral nonsteroidal anti-inflammatory drugs and analgesics can help reduce pain but should be used only as a short-term measure. Initial care should be palliative and not directed toward deformity correction. Orthodigital devices (custom, premade, or hand fashioned), such as crest pads or mallet toe regulators, may relieve pressure over the involved joint or distal aspect of the toe, resulting in passive realignment of flexible deformities. Painful corns may be treated with digital cps, sleeves, or silicone cushions. Superficial ulcers developing from a corn or clavus are treated with off-loading measures and local wound care. Patients with "high-risk" neuropathic or dysvascular feet should be educated to perform diligent daily inspection for skin breakdown.

Rehabilitation

Formal physical therapy is usually not required unless the toe deformity is accompanied by more global foot deformity due to a neuromuscular disorder. Although toe and foot flexor tendon stretching exercises are generally of little or no benefit, they may relieve the "tight" sensation in patients with a flexible or semirigid deformity. Functional foot orthoses can provide flexor tendon stabilization and, in some instances, symptomatic relief in patients with subtalar joint hyperpronation and flexible mallet toe deformity. In occasional cases, when extra-depth shoes provide insufficient toe box room to accommodate the deformity, custom shoes may be prescribed. Physical therapy after surgical correction is usually indicated for reduction of edema.

Procedures

Steroid injections may be indicated for patients with a painful mallet toe deformity in the presence of inflammatory joint disease (Fig. 89.2). An intra-articular injection of a soluble corticosteroid with local anesthetic mixture, performed in sterile technique with a 27- or 30-gauge needle, may provide temporary relief. The patient should be advised about the possibility of a postinjection flare.

Surgery

Operative treatment should be considered when conservative treatments fail, painful cutaneous lesions persist, and especially if ulceration or infection develops. Cosmesis alone is a poor indication for surgical correction. Surgical treatment depends on the etiology, extent, and severity of the deformity. Contributory or associated digital or forefoot deformities

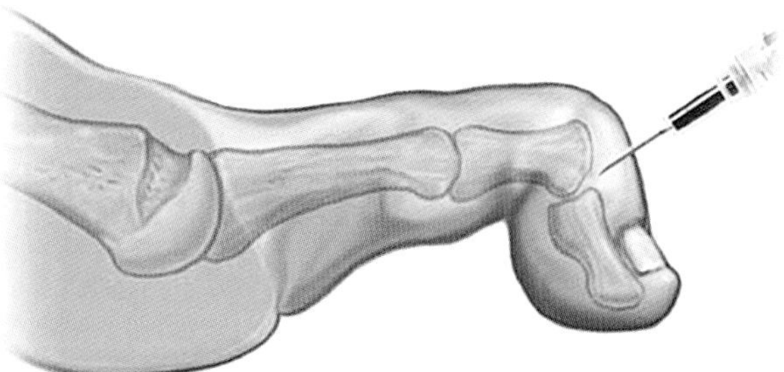

FIGURE 89.2 Injections are directed inside the distal interphalangeal joint, as indicated in the illustration.

(e.g., hallux valgus, hammer toe, neighboring underriding or overlapping toe deformities) may also require correction for optimal surgical outcome, including surgery for proximal interphalangeal joint flexion or metatarsophalangeal joint deformity of the same toe. For mild, flexible, manually reducible deformity, soft tissue procedures, such as long flexor tenotomy with or without plantar DIP joint capsulotomy, are indicated. For more severe and rigid deformity, DIP joint osseous and articular procedures (e.g., resection arthroplasty, arthrodesis, extension block method [9]) are required. Lesser toe mallet deformity does not absolutely require fusion [10]. Severe deformity, with the presence or threat of ulceration, may require partial digital amputation [11–13]. Cases involving osteomyelitis of the distal phalanx almost always require amputation at some level of the toe. In severe deformities, retrospective studies have shown that DIP joint resection arthroplasty combined with flexor tenotomy increases the likelihood of a good outcome [11,13]. Digital interphalangeal joint arthrodesis procedures may be performed in end-to-end or peg-in-hole fashion. The peg-in-hole technique has the advantage of shortening, which can reduce long flexor tendon tension. Temporary percutaneous 0.045-inch K-wire fixation of an end-to-end arthrodesis may result in better outcome.

Potential Disease Complications

Potential disease complications include mobility-limiting, chronic, intractable pain; metatarsalgia; dorsal or distal hyperkeratotic lesions or ulcerations, most commonly in the insensate foot; joint pain and stiffness; toenail deformities; bursitis; and synovitis. Gait abnormalities (antalgic) may contribute to more proximal pain of the low back, hip, and knee. A potential complication of nonsurgical treatment is deviation of the toes, especially overlapping second toes.

Potential Treatment Complications

Analgesics and nonsteroidal anti-inflammatory drugs have well-known side effects that most commonly affect the gastric, hepatic, and renal systems. Potential complications after corticosteroid injections include skin hypopigmentation at the injection site, infection, transient elevated blood glucose concentration, and postinjection flare (pain). Postsurgical complications include toe ischemia, digital nerve palsy, arthrodesis nonunion, joint malalignment, rigid or excessively straight toe, flail DIP joint, persistent or chronic toe edema, infection, flail toe, and periarticular osseous proliferation.

References

[1] Birrer RB, DellaCorte MP, Grisafi PJ, editors. Common foot problems in primary care. Philadelphia: Hanley & Belfus; 1992.
[2] Goud A, Khurana B, Chiodo C, Weissman BN. Woman's musculoskeletal foot conditions exacerbated by footwear: an imaging perspective. Am J Orthop 2011;40:183–91.
[3] Coughlin MJ, Mann RA. Lesser toe deformities. In: Coughlin MJ, Mann RA, editors. Surgery of the foot. 6th ed. St. Louis: Mosby; 1993. p. 341–412.
[4] Caselli MA, George DH. Foot deformities: biomechanical and pathomechanical changes associated with aging, part I. Clin Podiatr Med Surg 2003;20:487–509.
[5] Badlissi F, Dunn JE, Link CL, et al. Foot musculoskeletal disorders, pain, and foot-related functional limitation in older persons. J Am Geriatr Soc 2005;53:1029–33.
[6] Martin MG, Masear VR. Triggering of the lesser toes at a previously undescribed distal pulley system. Foot Ankle Int 1998;19:113–7.
[7] Hunt GC, McPoil TG, editors. Physical therapy of the foot and ankle. 2nd ed. New York: Churchill Livingstone; 1995.
[8] Guldemond NA, Leffers P, Schaper NC, et al. Comparison of foot orthoses made by podiatrists, pedorthists and orthotists regarding plantar pressure reduction in The Netherlands. BMC Musculoskelet Disord 2005;6:61–7.
[9] Wada K, Yui M. Surgical treatment of mallet toe of the hallux with the extension block method: a case report. Foot Ankle Int 2011;32:1086–8.
[10] Nakamura S. Temporary Kirschner wire fixation for a mallet toe deformity of the hallux. J Orthop Sci 2007;12:190–2.
[11] Coughlin MJ. Operative repair of the mallet toe deformity. Foot Ankle Int 1995;16:109–16.
[12] Molloy A, Shariff R. Mallet toe deformity. Foot Ankle Clin 2011;16: 537–46.
[13] Shirzad K, Kiesau CD, DeOrio JK, Parekh SG. Lesser toe deformities. J Am Acad Orthop Surg 2011;19:505–14.

CHAPTER 90

Metatarsalgia

Stuart Kigner, DPM
Robert J. Scardina, DPM

Synonyms

Ball of foot pain
Pain around the metatarsal heads
Plantar forefoot pain
Anterior metatarsalgia
Lesser metatarsalgia

ICD-9 Code

726.70 Enthesopathy of ankle and tarsus

ICD-10 Code

M77.9 Enthesopathy, unspecified

Definition

Metatarsalgia refers to pain in the forefoot under the metatarsal head region. Primary metatarsalgia is generally considered the result of mechanical overload of the metatarsal heads, whereas secondary metatarsalgia often has a rheumatic etiology. Primary metatarsalgia may be caused by hallux valgus, hallux rigidus, or sagittal plane first ray hypermobility, which causes a transfer of load to the lateral forefoot and lesser metatarsal heads (Fig. 90.1). A hammer toe with an associated dorsal contracture of a metatarsophalangeal (MTP) joint will cause a retrograde plantar flexion force on the metatarsal head (Fig. 90.2). Bunion surgery, with first metatarsal osteotomy resulting in excessive shortening or elevation of the first metatarsal and with resection of the base of the proximal phalanx of the hallux, is an iatrogenic cause of metatarsalgia [1]. Ankle equinus, leg length discrepancy, scoliosis, kyphosis, neuromuscular disorders, lower extremity trauma, or other foot surgery (elective or post-traumatic) may also result in increased forefoot pressures. Wearing of thin-soled high-heeled shoes may increase the risk for development of metatarsalgia. Although the relative risk of running barefoot or in "minimalist" shoes (compared with traditional running shoes) and developing metatarsalgia is not known, a case series of experienced runners who developed metatarsal stress fractures after transitioning to minimalist running footwear was recently reported [2]. Lieberman [3] has pointed out that runners who transition to barefoot or minimalist shoes may not have strong enough extensor muscles or metatarsal bones, which could lead to an increased risk of metatarsalgia or metatarsal stress fractures.

Secondary metatarsalgia has been associated with rheumatoid arthritis, psoriatic arthritis, reactive arthritis, and systemic lupus erythematosus. MTP joint synovitis may lead to weakening or rupture of the stabilizing structures around the joint, leading to dorsal subluxation of the toes on the lesser metatarsal heads [4]. Degenerative arthritis of the lesser MTP joint may be caused by Freiberg infraction (metatarsal head avascular necrosis).

Symptoms

Plantar forefoot pain is generally aggravated by weight bearing, is often worse during the propulsive phase of gait, and is often localized beneath the second metatarsal head or second MTP joint. Lesser MTP joint morning stiffness may be present. Neuritic radiating pain may occur from irritation, inflammation, or tethering of neighboring plantar intermetatarsal nerves.

Poorly defined pain in the forefoot is a common early symptom in patients with rheumatoid arthritis. Other symptoms include MTP joint symmetric swelling and stiffness after rest.

Physical Examination

The forefoot examination attempts to elicit pain on palpation directly beneath the metatarsal heads or MTP joints, commonly the result of mechanical overload from an unstable first ray or medial column. Pain elicited with lateral compression of neighboring metatarsal heads also suggests a plantar intermetatarsal neuroma. Stress fractures are commonly identified at the metatarsal neck, demonstrated by swelling, palpable pain, or bone fixation callus. Evaluate the excursion and pain of MTP joint passive range of motion and note the presence of swelling. Assess for first metatarsal hypermobility by applying a dorsiflexion force under the first metatarsal head. If hypermobility is present, the first metatarsal head will rise well above the second metatarsal head [5]. Examine for dorsal translation of the proximal phalangeal base on the

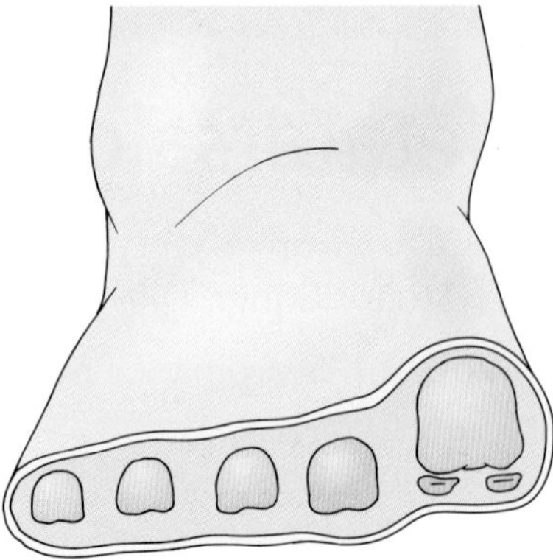

FIGURE 90.1 Cross-sectional view of metatarsal heads. Elevated first metatarsal head results in mechanical overload of lesser metatarsal heads.

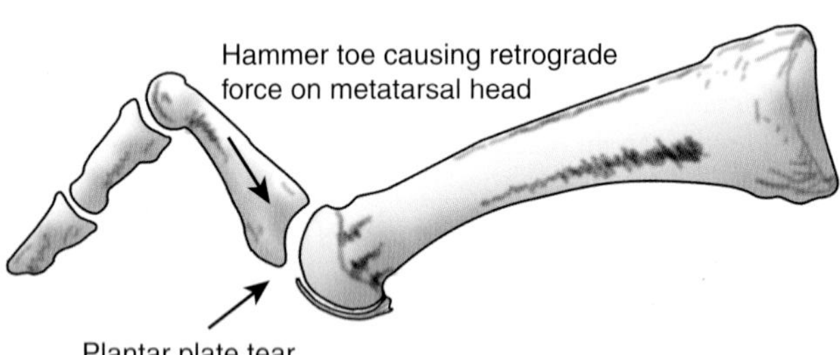

FIGURE 90.2 Hammer toe with associated plantar plate tear. The hammer toe causes a retrograde plantar flexion force on the metatarsal head.

metatarsal head (drawer test) to identify plantar plate or capsule disruption. Also check for Mulder sign, which may suggest a plantar intermetatarsal neuroma.

While the patient is standing, note the presence of forefoot deformities including hallux valgus, hammer toes, MTP joint dorsal contractures, and medial or lateral subluxation of the toes. The "paper pull-out test" to evaluate toe purchase is performed by asking the patient to flex the toe against a piece of paper placed on the floor under the toe. The test result is positive if the paper cannot be pulled out from under the toe. If there is a V-shaped alignment of adjacent toes noted while the patient is standing, indicative of web space widening, early synovitis [6], plantar intermetatarsal neuroma, or other space-occupying mass may be present. Weight-bearing bilateral or unilateral heel raise while standing barefoot often aggravates metatarsalgia pain. During gait examination, observe for early heel-off, antalgic gait, excessive or insufficient subtalar joint pronation, asymmetry, and lack of toe purchase. Inspect the skin for plantar calluses and their locations. Examine the shoe outsoles and insoles for signs of excessive or uneven wear indicative of areas of elevated pressure or abnormal foot mechanics.

Functional Limitations

Forefoot pain may limit standing, walking, and participation in high-impact activities, such as running or jumping. There will be a limitation to shoe style able to be worn comfortably. Metatarsalgia has its greatest impact on activities requiring prolonged standing or walking on hard floors (e.g., cashier, food preparation, or housekeeping jobs). Sales jobs requiring use of a dress shoe may be difficult. Walking speed may decrease while shopping or accessing public transportation. Recreational activities, such as walking, tennis, basketball, or running on a treadmill on an incline, may be particularly painful.

Diagnostic Studies

Weight-bearing foot radiographs will demonstrate the relative lengths of the metatarsals and transverse plane splaying, if it is present. A forefoot axial view may reveal a structural abnormality of the metatarsal head condyles or relative prolapse of a metatarsal head due to plantar flexion. Metatarsal stress fractures may be identified, but less so on initial radiographs, which may appear unremarkable. Radiographs may also reveal a displaced fracture, foreign body, and stigmata of tumor, osteomyelitis, and noninflammatory or inflammatory arthritis. Ultrasonography and magnetic resonance imaging may be used to evaluate inflammatory arthritis, MTP joint plantar plate disruption, early stress fracture, ligament or tendon tear, abscess, and plantar intermetatarsal neuroma. Laboratory tests may be ordered if inflammatory arthritis or infection is suspected. Although it is not widely used in the office setting, dynamic pedobarography including in-shoe pressure distribution measurement systems may reveal subtle regions of excessive plantar pressure and be used to monitor treatment results.

Differential Diagnosis

Bursitis (intermetatarsal or plantar metatarsal head)
MTP joint synovitis
Flexor tendon sheath synovitis
MTP joint capsulitis
MTP joint plantar plate rupture
Inflammatory and noninflammatory arthritis
Freiberg infraction
Intermetatarsal plantar neuroma
Metatarsal stress fracture
Infection (abscess or osteomyelitis)
Plantar callus
Intractable plantar keratoma
Plantar wart (verruca plantaris)
Foreign body
Neoplasm (soft tissue or bone)
Radiculopathy (lumbosacral)
Tarsal tunnel syndrome
Peripheral neuropathy or neuritis
Claudication

Treatment

Initial

Focal plantar pressure can be reduced by applying a felt or foam rubber aperture pad to off-load a single metatarsal head, or a foam rubber or felt metatarsal pad or bar may be applied just proximal to a single metatarsal head or multiple neighboring metatarsal heads. Prefabricated pads are commercially available. The pads may be applied directly to the foot or to the shoe insole (Fig. 90.3). Cushioned shoe insoles composed of materials such as Plastazote, Poron, and Spenco may be used to replace the entire existing shoe

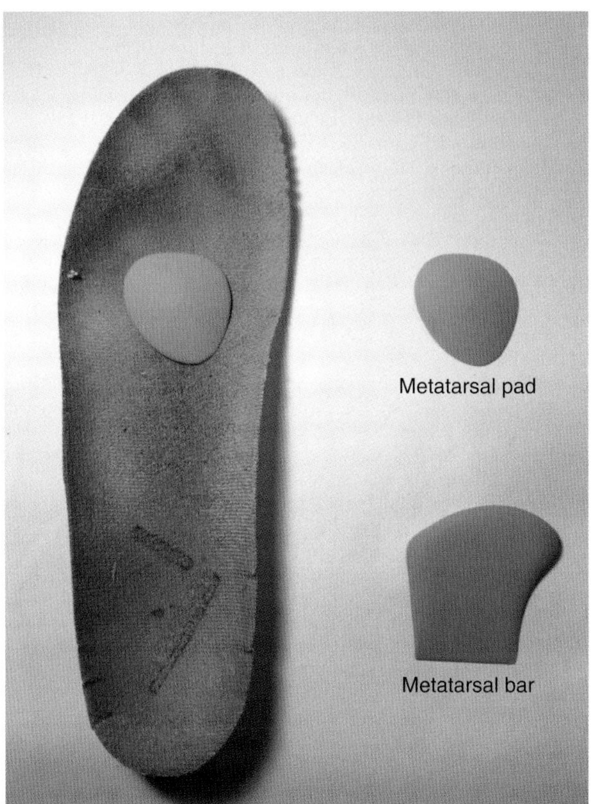

FIGURE 90.3 Metatarsal pad attached to shoe insole. The metatarsal pad and bar are designed to redistribute pressure away from metatarsal heads.

insole. Prefabricated insoles with an incorporated metatarsal pad or bar are also available. Custom fabricated foot orthoses may be designed with a depression under the painful metatarsal head areas or with an incorporated metatarsal pad or bar. Although there is limited scientific evidence to support their use, foot orthoses and running shoes with antitorsional features may address abnormal biomechanical forces causing elevated pressure and shearing under the metatarsal heads. Wearing of a shoe with a full-length stiff outsole or "rocker" outsole under the forefoot is advisable [7]. Shoes should have a low heel height, soft insole, and extra depth to accommodate a custom or commercial cushion insole. For patients who stand most of the day because of their occupation, a cushion floor mat can be used. If a capsule or plantar plate tear is suspected (Fig. 90.2), initial immobilization with a prefabricated walking boot may be indicated. Manually reducible dorsal MTP joint contractures may be addressed by applying tape around the base of the toe and securing it to the bottom of the foot [8]. A prefabricated removable toe splint may also be effective for this condition. Mechanically induced metatarsalgia may be treated with oral nonsteroidal anti-inflammatory drugs or a short tapered course of oral glucocorticoids. Metatarsalgia secondary to rheumatoid or other inflammatory arthritis may be addressed by early use of oral disease-modifying antirheumatic drugs [9].

Rehabilitation

If there is posterior lower leg muscle tightness, gastrocnemius or soleus stretching exercises are recommended [10]. Aquatic exercises and bicycle riding are preferable to exercises involving running and jumping. Decreasing stride length while running or fitness walking may also be helpful. Manipulation may be used to stretch out dorsal MTP joint contractures [8]. After the Weil surgical procedure on a lesser metatarsal, vigorous physical therapy to strengthen the toe flexors and to maintain plantar flexion range of motion soon after surgery has been recommended [11,12]. Rehabilitation after hallux valgus surgery, in an effort to avoid "transfer" metatarsalgia, may include strengthening of the peroneus longus muscle, manipulation to improve hallux plantar flexion, plantar and dorsal sliding of the hallux proximal phalanx, oscillating traction of the first MTP joint, and concentric strengthening of the hallux flexor and extensor muscles [13].

Procedures

A diagnostic local anesthetic block of a plantar intermetatarsal nerve may be performed to differentiate between pain originating from an intermetatarsal neuroma and metatarsalgia pain originating from the metatarsal head or MTP joint.

Surgery

Compared with more traditional elevating or shortening distal lesser metatarsal osteotomies, the Weil osteotomy, involving metatarsal head translation with or without elevation, has been reported to achieve good to excellent results [14]. Metatarsalgia in patients with rheumatoid arthritis has traditionally been addressed by excision of the lesser metatarsal heads combined with fusion of the first MTP joint. Recently, with early institution of disease-modifying antirheumatic drugs resulting in sustained low disease activity and remission, MTP joint–sparing surgery has been recommended. However, at this time, there is limited evidence to support this approach [15]. A rupture of the MTP joint plantar plate may be repaired primarily. Hammer toe surgery involving arthrodesis of the proximal interphalangeal joint combined with surgical capsular release and lengthening of the extensor tendons will decrease retrograde plantar pressure on the metatarsal head. A decrease in metatarsalgia has been reported after isolated gastrocnemius recession [16]. Bunionectomy with first metatarsal osteotomy, designed to decrease the angle between the first and second metatarsals, has been shown to decrease painful calluses under the second metatarsal head [17], and a lengthening osteotomy for an iatrogenic short first metatarsal has resulted in decreased metatarsalgia symptoms [18].

Potential Disease Complications

Metatarsalgia pain may result in functional limitation, including antalgic gait, and may lead to falls in the elderly patient population. Rupture of the plantar plate and collateral ligaments may result in MTP joint instability, dorsal toe subluxation, and transverse plane positional toe deformity, including overlapping toes.

Potential Treatment Complications

Intra-articular corticosteroid injections, especially acetate steroids, are generally not recommended in the presence of lesser MTP joint predislocation syndrome [8]. After corticosteroid injection, MTP joint dislocation [19] and plantar fat pad atrophy have been reported [20]. Other adverse reactions after injection of corticosteroids include skin hypopigmentation at injection site, infection, transient elevated blood glucose concentration, and postinjection flare (pain). Neuroma excision surgery was found to be more technically demanding because of the degree of fibrosis after a series of 20% ethyl alcohol (sclerosing) injections [21], which may also result in adhesive neuritis or "stump" neuroma formation. Topical salicylic acid used to treat painful plantar calluses may injure the skin and lead to open wounds and infection, especially in patients with diabetes. Adverse reactions associated with oral nonsteroidal anti-inflammatory drugs and disease-modifying antirheumatic drugs are listed elsewhere in the text. Shoes with stiff rocker outsoles may cause gait instability and possibly lead to falls, especially in the elderly patient population.

Because of the difficulty in precisely determining the optimal length of a metatarsal when a shortening osteotomy is performed to address metatarsalgia, excessive shortening may result in metatarsalgia of an adjacent metatarsal head and insufficient shortening may lead to some degree of persistent pain [10]. A not uncommon complication of the Weil lesser metatarsal osteotomy is a "floating toe" that does not purchase the floor while standing and walking [10]. Complications of foot orthotic therapy may include mild strain of ligaments, tendons, or muscles; orthotic edge irritation of the skin; and shoe fit difficulty. Improper positioning of a metatarsal pad may result in elevated pressure under the metatarsal head.

References

[1] Zembsch A, Trnka H, Ritschl P. Correction of hallux valgus metatarsal osteotomy versus excision arthroplasty. Clin Orthop Relat Res 2000;376:183–94.

[2] Salzler MJ, Bluman EM, Noonan S, et al. Injuries observed in minimalist runners. Foot Ankle Int 2012;33:262–6.

[3] Lieberman DE. What we can learn about running from barefoot running: an evolutionary medical perspective. Exerc Sport Sci Rev 2012;40:63–72.

[4] Loveday DT, Jackson GE, Geary NP. The rheumatoid foot and ankle: current evidence. Foot Ankle Surg 2012;18:94–102.

[5] Roberts MM, Greisberg J. Examination of the foot and ankle. In: DiGiovanni CW, Greisberg J, editors. Foot and ankle: core knowledge in orthopaedics. Philadelphia: Elsevier Mosby; 2007. p. 10–5.

[6] Panchbhavi VK, Trevino S. Clinical tip: a new clinical sign associated with metatarsophalangeal joint synovitis of the lesser toes. Foot Ankle Int 2007;28:640–1.

[7] Jeng CL, Logue J. Shoes and orthotics. In: Pinzur MS, editor. Orthopaedic knowledge update: foot and ankle. 4th ed. Rosemont, Ill: American Academy of Orthopaedic Surgeons; 2008. p. 15–24.

[8] Yu GV, Judge MS, Hudson JR, et al. Predislocation syndrome. Progressive subluxation/dislocation of the lesser metatarsophalangeal joint. J Am Podiatr Med Assoc 2002;92:182–99.

[9] Saag KG, Teng GG, Patkar NM, et al. American College of Rheumatology 2008 recommendations for the use of nonbiologic and biologic disease-modifying antirheumatic drugs in rheumatoid arthritis. Arthritis Rheum 2008;59:762–84.

[10] Espinosa N, Maceira E, Myerson MS. Current concept review: metatarsalgia. Foot Ankle Int 2008;29:871–9.

[11] Barouk P, Bohay DR, Trnka HJ, et al. Lesser metatarsal surgery. Foot Ankle Spec 2010;3:356–60.

[12] Myerson MS. Reconstructive foot and ankle surgery. 2nd ed. Philadelphia: WB Saunders; 2010.

[13] Schuh R, Hofstaetter SG, Adams SB, et al. Rehabilitation after hallux valgus surgery: importance of physical therapy to restore weight bearing of the first ray during the stance phase. Phys Ther 2009;89:934–45.

[14] Hofstaetter SG, Hofstaetter JG, Petroutsas JA, et al. The Weil osteotomy: a seven year follow-up. J Bone Joint Surg Br 2005;87:1507–11.

[15] Jeng C, Campbell J. Current concept review: the rheumatoid forefoot. Foot Ankle Int 2008;29:959–68.

[16] Maskill JD, Bohay DR, Anderson JG. Gastrocnemius recession to treat isolated foot pain. Foot Ankle Int 2010;31:19–23.

[17] Mann RA, Rudicel S, Graves S. Repair of hallux valgus with a distal soft-tissue procedure and proximal metatarsal osteotomy. J Bone Joint Surg Am 1992;74:124–9.

[18] Singh D, Dudkiewicz I. Lengthening of the shortened first metatarsal after Wilson's osteotomy for hallux valgus. J Bone Joint Surg Br 2009;91:1583–6.

[19] Reis ND, Karkabi S, Zinman C. Metatarsophalangeal joint dislocation after steroid injection. J Bone Joint Surg Br 1989;71:864.

[20] Basadonna P, Rucco V, Gasparini D, et al. Plantar fat pad atrophy after corticosteroid injection for an interdigital neuroma: a case report. Am J Phys Med Rehabil 1999;78:283–5.

[21] Hughes RJ, Ali K, Jones H, et al. Treatment of Morton's neuroma with alcohol injection under sonographic guidance: follow-up of 101 cases. AJR Am J Roentgenol 2007;188:1535–9.

CHAPTER 91

Morton Neuroma

Sammy M. Lee, DPM
Robert J. Scardina, DPM

Synonyms

Metatarsal neuralgia
Perineural fibroma
Plantar neuralgia
Morton neuralgia
Intermetatarsal neuroma
Pseudoneuroma
Metatarsal neuroma
Interdigital neuroma
Morton toe syndrome
Morton entrapment

ICD-9 Code

355.6 Mononeuritis of lower limb, lesion of plantar nerve

ICD-10 Codes

G57.90 Mononeuropathy of unspecified lower limb
G57.91 Mononeuropathy of right lower limb
G57.92 Mononeuropathy of left lower limb
G57.60 Lesion of plantar nerve, unspecified lower limb
G57.61 Lesion of plantar nerve, right lower limb
G57.62 Lesion of plantar nerve, left lower limb

Definition

Morton neuroma is not a neoplasm; rather, it is a local, mechanically induced, degenerative enlargement of the third plantar intermetatarsal nerve with associated perineural fibrosis [1] caused by an accumulation of collagenous material within the sheath of Schwann and usually the result of repetitive trauma (Fig. 91.1). As such, it is more accurately defined as an intermetatarsal compression or entrapment neuropathy [2]. The exact etiology has not been clearly identified or proved conclusively, but the following have been postulated as contributing factors: flatfoot (pes planus); anterior splay foot; high-arch foot (pes cavus); equinus deformity [3]; ill-fitting (tight or high-heeled) shoes; abnormal proximity of neighboring metatarsal heads [4]; and associated forefoot deformities, including hallux abductus, bunion, and lesser hammer toes. Plantar intermetatarsal nerves of the foot are purely sensory at and distal to the level of the metatarsophalangeal (MTP) joints, as they course through a fibro-osseous canal composed of neighboring metatarsal heads and the overlying deep transverse intermetatarsal ligament [5]. Anatomic (cadaver) studies have identified the third intermetatarsal nerve as most commonly receiving proximal branches from both the medial plantar and lateral plantar nerves, each arising from the common posterior tibial nerve. Therefore, anatomically, the third intermetatarsal nerve is usually enlarged to some degree as it develops from proximal trunks of two separate nerve branches. This anatomic configuration may or may not be a causative factor. The classic Morton neuroma occurs in the third intermetatarsal space. Similar nerve compression neuropathies occur, but less commonly, in the second plantar intermetatarsal space (Hauser neuroma) and rarely in the first (Heuter neuroma) and fourth (Iselin neuroma) plantar intermetatarsal spaces [2]. Symptomatic plantar neuromas in neighboring intermetatarsal spaces may occur in the same foot, but uncommonly. They are all treated in a similar fashion.

Symptoms

Morton neuroma may be manifested symptomatically in a variety of ways: localized sharp, lancinating, or burning pain; paresthesias and dysesthesias; numbness and tingling; and toe cramping. Symptoms typically radiate distally, involving the opposing plantar sides of the third and fourth toes, but pain exclusively in the fourth toe is not uncommon. Unilateral presentation is most common, whereas bilateral is less so. Symptoms occur predominantly during weight-bearing activities, but residual non–weight-bearing or nocturnal pain is sometimes present. Not uncommonly, patients may experience symptoms while driving an automobile with the foot held in a slightly dorsiflexed position. A characteristic patient maneuver is to remove the shoe and massage or manipulate the plantar forefoot and MTP joints, producing transient relief of symptoms [6].

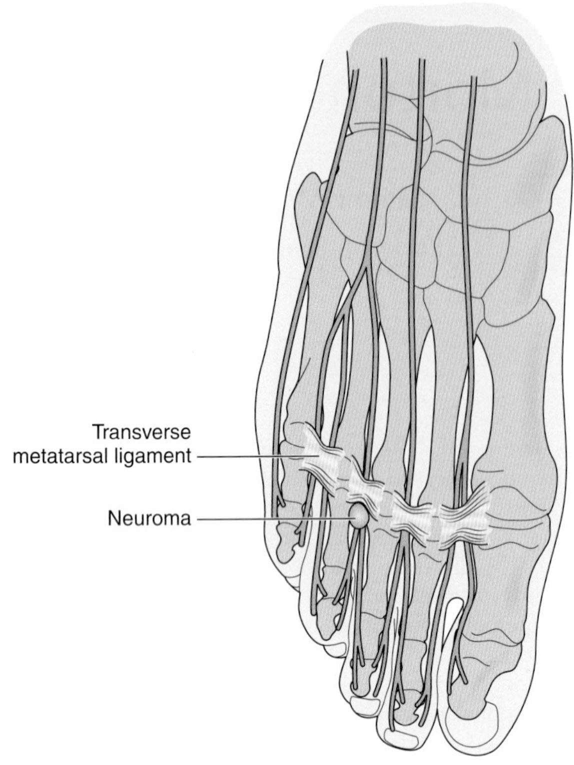

FIGURE 91.1 Morton neuroma.

Physical Examination

On inspection, the foot may appear normal or may demonstrate a subtle divergence of the third and fourth toes, usually more pronounced with weight bearing. When it is present, the regional palpable pain is typically plantar. The lateral forefoot squeeze test may mimic a tight shoe, thereby reproducing symptoms. In long-standing cases, hypoesthesia or anesthesia may be noted in the third interdigital web space, distally on the opposing plantar sides of the involved toes (toe tip sensation deficit [7]) or plantar, distal to the third and fourth metatarsal heads. The most diagnostic and reliable clinical maneuver is the Mulder test [8], performed by alternating lateral compression of the forefoot with one hand and dorsal-plantar compression of the involved distal intermetatarsal space with the opposite forefinger and thumb (Fig. 91.2) [6]. A Mulder sign is considered present when symptoms are reproduced and a palpable and sometimes audible click is detected. In general, there are no signs of proximal nerve involvement (e.g., tarsal tunnel syndrome), vasomotor instability, or arterial insufficiency. Predisposing foot types (pes planus or pes cavus) or a tight Achilles tendon (equinus) [3] may be evident on clinical examination. Passive range of motion of the neighboring MTP joints is usually pain free without crepitus. Unilateral antalgic (pain-avoidance) gait may also be observed.

Functional Limitations

Functional limitations include difficulty with walking or running any significant distance and in performing other weight-bearing physical activities as well as the inability to wear dress shoes comfortably (particularly women's high heels).

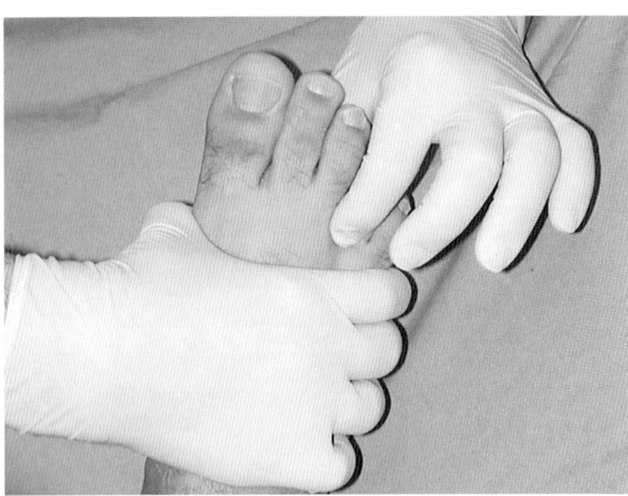

FIGURE 91.2 Technique to elicit Mulder sign.

Diagnostic Studies

The diagnosis of Morton neuroma is generally made from history and clinical examination. However, other supportive diagnostic studies may be helpful in establishing a diagnosis, especially when surgical intervention is being considered or in the event of failed conservative measures. Ultrasonography is a relatively simple, inexpensive, and helpful diagnostic tool [9,10]. In the evaluation of a primary neuroma, a 5-mm or greater hypoechoic mass, visualized in the coronal (frontal) plane projection between the neighboring metatarsal heads, is considered a positive finding [11,12]. Magnetic resonance imaging, although generally not recommended in the initial evaluation, may also be used, particularly in the presence of equivocal or normal ultrasonographic findings (e.g., small lesions) and when surgical excision is being considered [13–15]. Ultrasonography has a slightly higher sensitivity than magnetic resonance imaging, particularly for neuromas smaller than 5 mm in diameter [16]. Both ultrasonography and magnetic resonance imaging are used in the diagnosis of postsurgical recurrent or "stump" neuroma [17–19]. Performance of the Mulder test during sonography is a recently described real-time imaging method, helpful in assessing the dimensions of the nerve as well as the local "dynamics" of the pathologic process (Fig. 91.3) [11]. New high-resolution, high-frequency ultrasound scanning may provide a means of differentiating a neuroma from disease of neighboring soft tissue structures, including the plantar plate and flexor tendons [12]. The neuroma itself is not visible by plain radiographic imaging, but radiographs may be obtained to rule out metatarsal stress fracture, MTP joint disease (degenerative or inflammatory), or contributing neighboring metatarsal head abnormality. Sensory nerve conduction studies can be used, but because of the difficulty in isolating individual nerve trunks or branches, results are not consistently accurate or helpful. Differential latency testing is a new electrodiagnostic approach that is more sensitive, simpler to use, and less painful than conventional electrodiagnostic studies, and it requires no extra equipment. Values above 0.17 millisecond between branches of the common plantar interdigital nerves are consistent with Morton neuroma [20]. Last, a local anesthetic plantar intermetatarsal space injection can be a useful minimally invasive diagnostic maneuver to support the diagnosis.

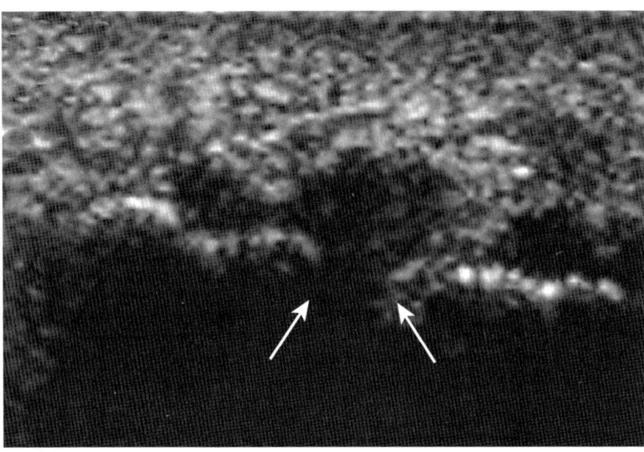

FIGURE 91.3 Dynamic frontal plane ultrasound image demonstrating plantar displacement of neuroma. The arrows indicate plantar displacement of neuroma beneath metatarsal heads. *(From Torriani M, Kattapuram S. Dynamic sonography of the forefoot: the sonographic Mulder sign. AJR Am J Roentgenol 2003;180:1121-1123.)*

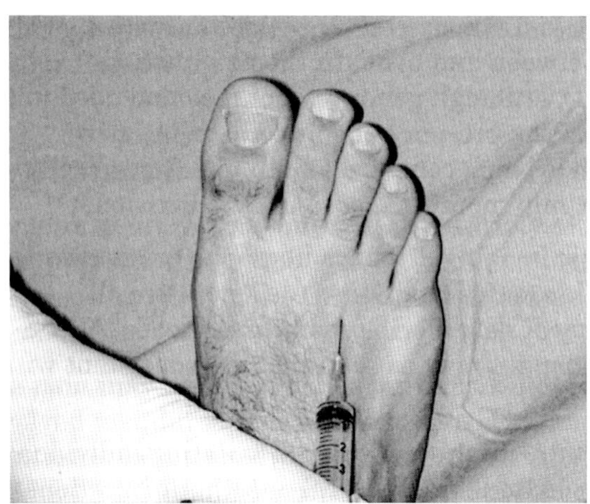

FIGURE 91.4 Technique of injection of a Morton neuroma.

Differential Diagnosis

Metatarsal stress fracture
Metatarsal head avascular necrosis (Freiberg infraction)
Metatarsal head osseous neoplasm
MTP joint soft tissue neoplasm
MTP joint synovitis
MTP joint plantar capsulitis
MTP joint plantar plate rupture or tear
MTP joint flexor tendinopathy
Oligoarticular systemic synovitis (e.g., rheumatoid)
MTP joint arthritis (e.g., degenerative, rheumatoid, post-traumatic)
Submetatarsal head bursitis
Localized forefoot ischemia
Tarsal tunnel syndrome
Proximal nerve root syndrome (e.g., lumbosacral radiculopathy)
Peripheral neuritis
Peripheral neuropathy (e.g., diabetic, alcoholic)
Rheumatoid nodule

Treatment

Initial

Conservative treatment modalities include shoe gear modifications (e.g., wider toe box), adhesive tape strapping or padding of the foot, and use of foot orthoses. Oral nonsteroidal anti-inflammatory drugs and analgesics may provide some relief from acute symptoms but are not recommended for long-term treatment. Posterior lower leg stretching exercises may be helpful in the presence of gastrocnemius equinus.

Rehabilitation

Physiotherapy modalities, including both iontophoresis and phonophoresis, may help manage acute pain. If symptoms respond to initial conservative "mechanical" measures, such as off-the-shelf arch supports, more individualized therapies such as custom foot orthoses may provide additional symptomatic relief; these usually require referral to a podiatrist or pedorthist for fabrication.

Procedures

Injections with sclerosing agents, such as absolute alcohol [21,22], phenol, and vitamin B_{12}, may be used if initial conservative noninvasive treatments fail. Local anesthetic-corticosteroid injections [15,23], however, are more commonly used and may provide transient (but rarely long-term) relief of symptoms (Fig. 91.4). These injections are limited to no more than three within a 3- to 6-month period because of the potential for plantar fat pad atrophy and MTP joint tendon or ligament rupture. Cryoablation and radiofrequency ablation have been used with mixed results and with a potential for iatrogenic injury to neighboring soft tissue structures.

Surgery

Conservative measures do not always result in symptomatic improvement [24]. The neuroma as well as the distal digital branches and proximal nerve trunk may be too large for their confined anatomic space. In these cases, surgical excision may be necessary [25]. The success rate of surgical excision is approximately 85% to 90%, and surgical revision or reexploration generally carries a poor prognosis [26]. Less traditional surgical techniques include neurolysis, decompression with dorsal nerve transposition [27], transection of the deep transverse intermetatarsal ligament (open or endoscopic), laser treatment (vaporization), distal lesser metatarsal osteotomies, and gastrocnemius recession (in the presence of soft tissue equinus deformity) [28–31].

Potential Disease Complications

Potential disease complications include persistent refractory or intractable nerve pain, reduced mobility, functional limitation, and shoe gear restrictions.

Potential Treatment Complications

Few complications may arise from conservative measures, such as padding, strapping, foot orthoses, and shoe modifications. On occasion, ipsilateral or contralateral knee, ankle, hip, or even low back pain may occur, but these respond rapidly after discontinuation of treatment. Likewise, there are no significant treatment complications from physiotherapy measures when they are used and applied properly. Long-term use of nonsteroidal anti-inflammatory drugs may lead to gastrointestinal irritation.

Injection therapy with corticosteroids may result in plantar fat pad atrophy and secondary metatarsalgia or MTP joint plantar plate or collateral ligament rupture and subsequent digital deformity. Injection therapy with sclerosing agents may result in perineural irritation, inflammation, and pain. Postsurgical complications include infection, hematoma, vascular compromise, dorsal cutaneous nerve injury, incomplete resection, recurrence [32,33], stump neuroma [34], plantar fat pad atrophy, painful hypertrophic scar formation (especially with plantar incision approach), and reflex sympathetic dystrophy [32,33].

References

[1] Addante JB, Peicott PS, Wong KY, Brooks DL. Interdigital neuromas: results of surgical excision of 152 neuromas. J Am Podiatr Med Assoc 1986;76:493–5.

[2] Larson EE, Barrett SL, Battiston B, et al. Accurate nomenclature for forefoot nerve entrapment: a historical perspective. J Am Podiatr Med Assoc 2005;95:298–306.

[3] Barrett SL, Jarvis J. Equinus deformity as a factor in forefoot nerve entrapment: treatment with endoscopic gastrocnemius recession. J Am Podiatr Med Assoc 2005;95:464–8.

[4] Levitsky KA, Alman BA, Jevsevar DS, Morehead J. Digital nerves of the foot: anatomic variations and implications regarding the pathogenesis of interdigital neuroma. Foot Ankle 1993;14:208–14.

[5] McMinn RM, Hutchings RT, Logan BM. Foot and ankle anatomy. London: Mosby-Wolfe; 1996, 71.

[6] Wu KK. Morton's interdigital neuroma. A clinical review of its etiology, treatment, and results. J Foot Ankle Surg 1996;35:112–9.

[7] Owens R, Gougoulias N, Guthrie H, Sakellariou A. Morton's neuroma: clinical testing and imaging in 76 feet, compared to a control group. Foot Ankle Surg 2011;17:197–200.

[8] Mulder JD. The causative mechanism in Morton's metatarsalgia. J Bone Joint Surg Br 1951;33:94–5.

[9] Pollak RA, Bellacosa RA, Dornbluth NC, et al. Sonographic analysis of Morton's neuroma. J Foot Surg 1992;31:534–7.

[10] Read JW, Noakes JB, Kerr D, et al. Morton's metatarsalgia: sonographic findings and correlated histopathology. Foot Ankle Int 1999;20:153–61.

[11] Torriani M, Kattapuram S. Dynamic sonography of the forefoot: the sonographic Mulder sign. AJR Am J Roentgenol 2003;180:1121–3.

[12] Kincaid BR, Barrett SL. Use of high-resolution ultrasound in evaluation of the forefoot to differentiate forefoot nerve entrapments. J Am Podiatr Med Assoc 2005;95:429–32.

[13] Biasca N, Zanetti M, Zollinger H. Outcomes after partial neurectomy of Morton's neuroma related to preoperative case histories, clinical findings, and findings on magnetic resonance imaging scans. Foot Ankle Int 1999;20:568–75.

[14] Waldt S, Rechl H, Rummeny EJ, Woertler K. Imaging of benign and malignant soft tissue masses of the foot. Eur Radiol 2003;13:1125–36.

[15] Tallia AF, Cardone DA. Diagnostic and therapeutic injection of the ankle and foot. Am Fam Physician 2003;68:1356–62.

[16] Fazal MA, Khan I, Thomas C. Ultrasonography and magnetic resonance imaging in the diagnosis of Morton's neuroma. J Am Podiatr Med Assoc 2012;102:184–6.

[17] Levine SE, Myerson MS, Shapiro PP, Shapiro SL. Ultrasonographic diagnosis of recurrence after excision of an interdigital neuroma. Foot Ankle Int 1998;19:79–84.

[18] Resch S, Stentstrom A, Jonnsson K. The diagnostic efficacy of magnetic resonance imaging and ultrasonography in Morton's neuroma: a radiological-surgical correlation. Foot Ankle Int 1994;15:88–92.

[19] Terk MR, Kwong PK, Suthar M, et al. Morton's neuroma: evaluation with MR imaging performed with contrast enhancement and fat suppression. Radiology 1993;189:239–41.

[20] Uludag B, Tataroglu C, Bademkiran F, et al. Sensory nerve conduction in branches of common interdigital nerves: a new technique for normal controls and patients with Morton's neuroma. J Clin Neurophysiol 2010;27:219–23.

[21] Dockery GL. The treatment of intermetatarsal neuromas with 4% alcohol sclerosing injections. J Foot Ankle Surg 1999;38:403–8.

[22] Fanucci E, Masala S, Fabiano S, et al. Treatment of intermetatarsal Morton's neuroma with alcohol injection under US guide: 10-month follow-up. Eur Radiol 2004;14:514–8.

[23] Greenfield J, Read J, Lifeld FW. Morton's interdigital neuroma: indication for treatment by local injections versus surgery. Clin Orthop 1984;185:142–4.

[24] Bennett GL, Graham CE, Mauldin DM. Morton's interdigital neuroma: a comprehensive treatment protocol. Foot Ankle Int 1995;16:760–3.

[25] Miller SJ. Intermetatarsal neuromas and associated nerve problems. In: Butterworth R, Dockery GL, editors. Color atlas and text of forefoot surgery. London: Mosby-Wolfe; 1996. p. 159–82.

[26] Mann RA, editor. Surgery of the foot. St. Louis: Mosby; 1986, 204.

[27] Vito GR, Talarico LM. A modified technique for Morton's neuroma. Decompression with relocation. J Am Podiatr Med Assoc 2003;93:190–4.

[28] Delon AL. Treatment of Morton's neuroma as a nerve compression. The role for neurolysis. J Am Podiatr Med Assoc 1992;82:389–402.

[29] Diebold PF, Daum B, Dang-Vu V, Litchinko M. True epineural neurolysis in Morton's neuroma: a 5-year follow up. Orthopedics 1996;19:397–400.

[30] Gauthier G. Thomas Morton's disease: a nerve entrapment syndrome. A new surgical technique. Clin Orthop 1979;142:90–2.

[31] Sharp RJ, Wade CM, Hennessy MS, Saxby TS. The role of MRI and ultrasound imaging in Morton's neuroma and the effect of size of lesion on symptoms. J Bone Joint Surg Br 2003;85:999–1005.

[32] Amis JA, Siverhus SW, Liwnicz BH. An anatomic basis for recurrence after Morton's neuroma excision. Foot Ankle 1992;12:153–6.

[33] Banks AS, Vito GR, Giorgini TL. Recurrent intermetatarsal neuroma. A follow-up study. J Am Podiatr Med Assoc 1996;86:299–306.

[34] Ernberg LA, Adler RS, Lane J. Ultrasound in the detection and treatment of a painful stump neuroma. Skeletal Radiol 2003;32:306–9.

CHAPTER 92

Plantar Fasciitis

Paul F. Pasquina, MD

Leslie S. Foster, DO

Matthew E. Miller, MD

Synonyms

Plantar tendinitis
Plantar tendinosis
Plantar fasciosis
Plantar fibromatosis

ICD-9 Code

728.71 Plantar fasciitis

ICD-10 Code

M72.2 Plantar fasciitis

Definition

The plantar fascia is a multilayered fibrous aponeurosis that originates from the medial calcaneal tuberosity and extends distally, becoming wider and thinner and splitting into five bands. Each band then divides into a superficial and deep layer to insert onto the transverse tarsal ligament, flexor sheath, volar plate, and periosteum of the base of the proximal phalanges of the toes [1] (Fig. 92.1). Plantar fasciitis is an overuse injury resulting from repetitive microtears of the plantar fascia at its origin at the tuberosity of the os calcis deep to the distal medial heel pad [2]. It is classically described as a local inflammatory reaction, although recent research has demonstrated the relative absence of inflammatory cells in the injured tissue, suggesting more of a degenerative process; therefore, the terms *tendinosis* and *fasciosis* are advocated [3].

Plantar fasciitis is one of the most common injuries of runners. This condition occurs equally in both sexes in young people; some studies show that a peak incidence may occur in women 40 to 60 years of age [4]. The condition is typically precipitated by a change in the athlete's training program. Such changes may include an increase in intensity or frequency, a decrease in recovery time, or a change in terrain or running surface. In the nonathlete, an increase in the amount of walking, standing, or stair climbing may also precipitate symptoms. There is a correlation of plantar fasciitis with professions requiring prolonged standing (e.g., police officers and hairdressers).

Risk factors such as pes planus (flat feet), pes cavus with rigid high arches, excessive pronation, obesity, Achilles tendon contracture, and poor footwear (usually a loose heel counter and inadequate arch support) may contribute to the development of this condition. Multiple authors have demonstrated that the successful treatment of plantar fasciitis is not contingent on the surgical removal of a heel spur (calcaneal enthesophyte). Studies have shown that only 50% of patients with plantar heel pain had a heel spur and that only 10% of patients with a heel spur were symptomatic [5].

Symptoms

Patients typically complain of sharp, knife-like pain in the plantar aspect of the heel at the base of the fascial insertion to the calcaneus. Pain is generally worse with standing or during the initial steps on awakening or after prolonged sitting. Patients will often complain of the classic "pain with the first steps in the morning" that eases after being up and about for a while. Pain also typically worsens at the beginning of an exercise session but decreases during exercise. The athlete may describe being able to "run through" the pain. Complaints of numbness, paresthesias, or weakness are atypical for plantar fasciitis; therefore, if these complaints are present, the clinician should suspect an underlying nerve injury.

Physical Examination

Palpation reveals tenderness at the origin of the fascia of the medial calcaneal tubercle, but there may be tenderness along the majority of the fascia. Range of motion often reveals limited great toe dorsiflexion from a tight plantar fascia as well as decreased ankle dorsiflexion from a tight Achilles tendon. Dorsiflexion should be tested with the knee straight (gastrocnemius on stretch) and with the knee bent (gastrocnemius relaxed, soleus on stretch) to better

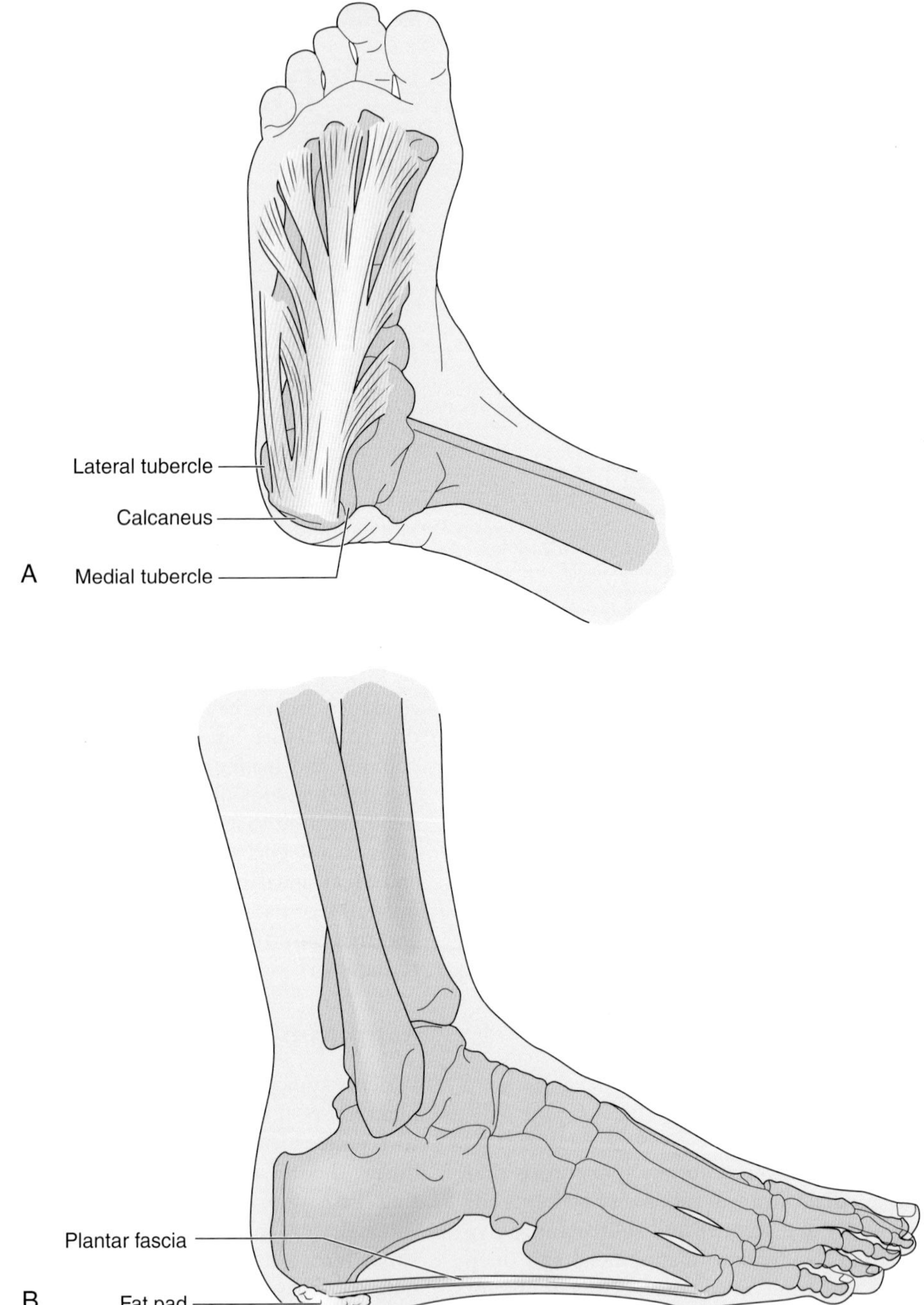

FIGURE 92.1 **A,** Plantar view of origin and insertion of plantar fascia. **B,** Bowstring effect of plantar fascia.

differentiate tightness of the gastrocnemius and soleus muscles. The neurologic examination should reveal normal muscle strength, sensation, and deep tendon reflexes, unless a concomitant neuropathy is present.

Functional Limitations

Depending on the severity of disease, patients may complain of symptoms only when they try to increase running intensity or distance. More severe cases may significantly limit a patient's ability to ambulate during daily activities or climbing stairs. Professions requiring extensive walking or standing (e.g., postal workers, nurses, or waitresses) may require job modification as well as more aggressive splinting or even casting during the initial phase of treatment.

Diagnostic Testing

Plantar fasciitis is usually a clinical diagnosis. However, radiographs of the foot may be helpful in ruling out other potential causes of heel or foot pain. It is a common misconception that the pain of plantar fasciitis is the direct result of the often (50%) associated anterior calcaneal enthesophyte (heel spur). In fact, a study of 461 asymptomatic patients showed radiographic evidence of heel spurs in 27% of those studied [5].

Electrodiagnostic testing (electromyography) may be helpful in ruling out the possibility of a nerve entrapment.

Ultrasound and magnetic resonance imaging studies may be helpful before surgical intervention is considered; these studies may demonstrate signal changes or swelling within the fascia. Magnetic resonance imaging usually demonstrates edematous involvement of the calcaneal insertion of the plantar aponeurosis, with marked thickening of the central cord of the plantar fascia.

Differential Diagnosis

The differential diagnosis of heel pain [6] includes the following inflammatory, metabolic, degenerative, nerve entrapment, and other conditions.

INFLAMMATORY
Juvenile rheumatoid arthritis
Rheumatoid arthritis
Ankylosing spondylitis
Reiter syndrome
Gout
Diffuse idiopathic skeletal hyperostosis
Psoriatic arthritis

METABOLIC
Migratory osteoporosis
Osteomalacia

DEGENERATIVE
Osteoarthritis
Atrophy of the heel fat pad

NERVE ENTRAPMENT
Tarsal tunnel syndrome
Entrapment of the medial calcaneal branch of the posterior tibial nerve

OTHER
Tumors
Vascular compromise
Infection

Treatment

Initial

As with most overuse injuries, initial treatment should follow the PRICEMM principles: *p*rotection, *r*est, *i*ce, *c*ompression, *e*levation, *m*edications, and *m*odalities. Protection and rest usually involve "relative rest"; the patient avoids aggravating activities while maintaining cardiovascular and muscle fitness by participating in low-impact activities such as swimming, bicycling, and weightlifting. Ice massage to the plantar fascia can easily be performed by the patient at home. Have the patient put a Styrofoam or paper cup full of water into the freezer. Once the water becomes ice, the patient may massage the block of ice along the origin of the plantar fascia for approximately 10 to 15 minutes. Icing is most helpful after activities or at the end of the day. Compression by way of taping the sole of the foot or applying an elastic wrap around the foot may offer comfort to the patient, as may soft gel heel cups, which may be placed in the patient's shoes. Casting in a neutral position helps in difficult cases. Keeping the foot elevated while sitting or lying down may also help reduce any local inflammation and swelling. Nonsteroidal anti-inflammatory drugs are often used to treat pain and any inflammatory component to the disease process. No studies have specifically examined the effectiveness of nonsteroidal anti-inflammatory drugs alone. More than 90% of patients with plantar fasciitis are cured with conservative measures [6]. Patients are often advised to obtain "stress mats" for prolonged standing on hard floors. Modalities are addressed in the following section.

Rehabilitation

The key elements of rehabilitation include stretching and strength training of not only the lower leg and foot but also the thigh, hip, and back. These include the plantar fascia, gastrocnemius-soleus complex, quadriceps, hamstrings, and hip flexors and extensors [7].

Increased flexibility is achieved through frequent stretching during the day. Each stretch should be held for 30 seconds. It is beneficial to tell patients that muscles need to be reminded to stay elongated; therefore it is better to stretch for 30 seconds 10 times per day than to dedicate an hour once a day to perform stretches. This also helps achieve the patient's compliance.

Strengthening of the foot intrinsic muscles may be achieved by placing a towel on the floor and having the patient crunch up the towel into a ball and then spread it back out by flexing and extending the toes. Alternative aerobic exercises or "cross-training" should be prescribed to minimize the effects of deconditioning. This can generally be achieved with running or swimming in the pool as well as by low-resistance cycling.

Therapeutic modalities include local ultrasound, iontophoresis, and phonophoresis. Although there is little evidence in the literature to suggest that these modalities hasten the resolution of the underlying problem, they may be helpful in controlling the patient's pain symptoms, thus allowing better participation in a rehabilitation exercise program. As symptoms resolve and the patient has achieved good flexibility as well as normal peroneal and posterior tibial muscle strength, a gradual return to sport is attempted. An appropriate return to running program should be established by the provider together with the patient. This can generally be achieved by having the patient start at half of the time or distance and intensity that he or she was running before the injury, divided into equal walk and jog intervals. For example, if a patient was running up to 30 minutes before the injury, an appropriate return to running schedule might be as follows: Alternate 4 minutes of walking with 1 minute of jogging for a total of 15 minutes. Increase by 5 minutes every week until 30 minutes is reached. Next, decrease the walk time intervals to 3 minutes each and increase the jog time intervals to 2 minutes. Each week, diminish walk time intervals by 1 minute and add 1 minute to the jog interval. Walk-jog sessions should be performed three times per week, allowing 24 hours of rest between workouts. If at any time the symptoms begin to reappear, return to the walk-jog intensity of the previous week for another week until advancing again. It is generally recommended to start on level surfaces before introducing hills. Patients must be cautioned to not "overdo it" and to stay within a structured rehabilitation program because reinjury is common.

Management of excessive foot pronation is essential to correction of a common contributing biomechanical factor [8]. This may be achieved simply by stretching the Achilles tendon; however, a change in footwear is often indicated. Numerous running shoes are on the market, and a good running shoe store with a knowledgeable staff may be helpful in finding the appropriate shoe for a particular type of foot. Essential components include a good heel counter and reasonable midfoot flexibility. Patients who demonstrate excessive hindfoot valgus and forefoot varus deformities typically benefit from custom-made orthotic devices that incorporate medial-side wedging. Patients should be cautioned about wearing high-heeled shoes, especially those with hard soles, as this will increase the forces across the plantar fascia as well as promote Achilles tendon shortening.

Procedures

Posterior night splinting may prove effective in resistant cases. Off-the-shelf devices are available, or fabrication of a posterior splint is simple with use of fiberglass casting tape. The patient's foot should be splinted in maximum dorsiflexion to allow maximum lengthening of the plantar fascia and to prevent the stiffening and contraction that normally occur during sleep. The splint should be applied every evening and worn throughout the night for 2 to 3 weeks. If the patient finds wearing the splints uncomfortable at first, a gradual "break-in" period may be necessary, with the goal of wearing the splints throughout the night in 1 to 2 weeks. A study demonstrated that about 90% of patients with refractory symptoms improved after only 1 month of treatment [9].

Corticosteroid injections can often be avoided if an effective treatment plan is adhered to. In refractory cases, however, a local steroid injection may allow the patient to be more compliant with the established rehabilitation program [10]. We prefer to inject a combination of 10 to 20 mg of triamcinolone (Kenalog) and 4 mL of 1% lidocaine with a 25-gauge, 1½-inch needle. A medial approach is used as it is generally better tolerated by the patient. The needle is aimed toward the medial tubercle of the calcaneus or most tender point, ensuring that the injection is above the fat pad to avoid potential fat pad atrophy (Fig. 92.2). Ultrasound guidance is now often used for more accurate injection with hopes of minimizing this complication (Fig. 92.3). Ultrasound-guided injection of dexamethasone sodium phosphate was shown to be safe and to provide some short-term benefit at 4 weeks [11].

Extracorporeal shock wave therapy is a treatment that generates shock waves by electrohydraulic, piezoelectric, or electromagnetic methods. A meta-analysis evaluated 20 published studies that clinically supported this treatment method as effective for plantar fasciitis. Two mechanisms are hypothesized for this treatment's efficacy. First, it is thought that the transmitted waves have an effect on pain receptor physiology. Second, the transmitted waves initiate fascial tissue healing through microtrauma and a subsequent healing response by the release of molecular agents and growth factors. An advantage to this treatment method is immediate weight bearing and return to most activities in 1 to 2 weeks [12].

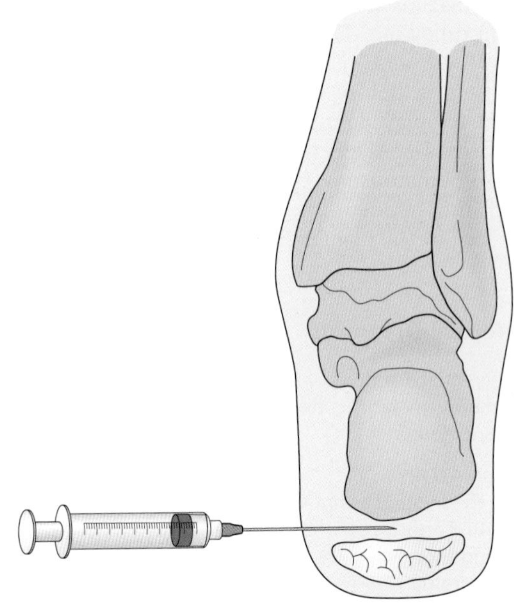

FIGURE 92.2 Proper approach for injection of plantar fascia.

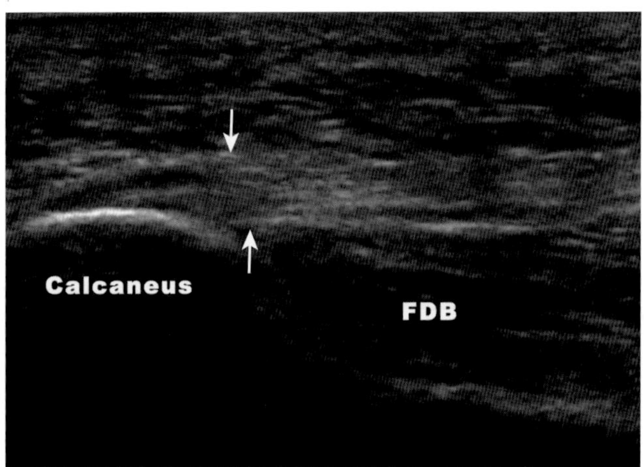

FIGURE 92.3 Ultrasound image (long-axis view) of the plantar fascia (*arrows*). *From superior to inferior: subcutaneous fat, plantar fascia, flexor digitorum brevis (FDB) muscle.*

Autologous blood injections have shown promise for recalcitrant plantar fasciitis. Martin [13] injected 1 mL of lidocaine and 2 mL of autologous blood where the plantar fascia was most tender. This treatment has been shown to decrease pain severity and to increase functional activity.

Babcock and Foster [14] investigated the effect of botulinum toxin in refractory plantar fasciitis. This randomized, double-blind, placebo-controlled study yielded significant improvements in pain relief and overall foot function at both 3 and 8 weeks after treatment.

Surgery

Surgery may be indicated in patients with significant disability and persistent pain when conservative measures have failed. The two most common surgical options are open and endoscopic release. Overall successful outcomes range from

48% to 90% [15]. A successful outcome could be expected for most patients who are treated for recalcitrant plantar fasciitis.

Potential Disease Complications

Patients who continue untreated and run through their pain typically have progressive symptoms, which begin to interfere with their activities of daily living and may lead to irreversible fascial degeneration and damage.

Potential Treatment Complications

Although corticosteroid injections may help selected patients to participate in a more effective rehabilitation program, this procedure should be performed with reservation because it may lead to heel fat pad atrophy or even plantar fascia rupture [16]. For this reason, it may be helpful to apply a walking splint or cast for several days after an injection.

Because of the risk of gastrointestinal bleeding, long-term use of nonsteroidal anti-inflammatory drugs should be avoided, and they should be used with caution in elderly patients or those with a history of gastrointestinal or bleeding disorders. The use of nonsteroidal anti-inflammatory drugs is contraindicated in patients with a known hypersensitivity to them.

Surgery, whether endoscopic or open, is associated with several risks (infection, complete rupture). Postoperative rehabilitation may require several weeks of limited or no weight bearing on the affected extremity.

References

[1] Karr SD. Subcalcaneal heel pain. Orthop Clin North Am 1994; 25:161–74.
[2] McBryde AM, Hoffman JL. Injuries to the foot and ankle in athletes. South Med J 2004;97:738–41.
[3] Dyck DD, Boyajian-O'Neill LA. Plantar fasciitis. Clin J Sport Med 2004;14:305–9.
[4] Gill LH, Kiebzak GM. Outcome of nonsurgical treatment for plantar fasciitis. Foot Ankle Int 1996;17:527–32.
[5] Rubin G, Witten M. Plantar calcaneal spurs. Am J Orthop 1963;5:38–41.
[6] Chacko K. Heel pain: diagnosis and treatment. Prim Care Case Rev 2003;6:50–6.
[7] DiGiovanni BF, Nawoczenski DA. Plantar fascia–specific stretching exercise improves outcomes in patients with chronic plantar fasciitis: a prospective clinical trial with two-year follow-up. J Bone Joint Surg Am 2006;88:1775–81.
[8] Riddle DL, Pulisic M. Risk factors for plantar fasciitis: a matched case-control study. J Bone Joint Surg Am 2003;85:872–7.
[9] Powell M, Post WR. Effective treatment of plantar fasciitis with dorsiflexion night splints. Foot Ankle Int 1998;19:10–8.
[10] Borchers JR, Best TM. Corticosteroid injection compared with extracorporeal shockwave therapy for plantar fasciopathy. Clin J Sport Med 2006;16:452–3.
[11] McMillan AM, Landorf KB, Gilheany MF, et al. Ultrasound guided corticosteroid injection for plantar fasciitis: randomised controlled trial. BMJ 2012;344:e3260.
[12] Ogden JA, Alvarez R. Shock wave therapy for chronic proximal plantar fasciitis. Clin Orthop Relat Res 2001;387:47–59.
[13] Kline A. Autologous blood injection in the treatment of plantar fasciitis. The Foot Health Blog; November 29, 2006. http://thefootblog.org.
[14] Babcock MS, Foster LS. Treatment of pain attributed to plantar fasciitis with botulinum toxin A: a short-term, randomized, placebo-controlled, double-blind study. Am J Phys Med Rehabil 2005;84:649–54.
[15] Davies MS, Weiss GA. Plantar fasciitis: how successful is surgical intervention? Foot Ankle Int 1999;20:803–7.
[16] Dimeff RJ. Complications of corticosteroid therapy in athletic injuries: a review. Clin J Sport Med 2006;16:279–80.

CHAPTER 93

Posterior Tibial Tendon Dysfunction

David Wexler, MD, FRCS (Tr & Orth)
Todd A. Kile, MD
Dawn M. Grosser, MD

Synonyms

Chronic tenosynovitis
Tibialis posterior tendon insufficiency
Asymmetric pes planus
Adult acquired flatfoot deformity [1]

ICD-9 Code

726.72 Tibialis tendinitis (posterior)

ICD-10 Codes

M76.821 Posterior tibial tendinitis, right leg
M76.822 Posterior tibial tendinitis, left leg
M76.829 Posterior tibial tendinitis, unspecified leg

Definition

The tibialis posterior muscle, originating from the proximal tibia and fibula, passes distally with a broad insertion on the plantar aspect of the navicular, cuneiform, cuboid, and metatarsal bases and normally functions to invert the subtalar joint and to adduct the forefoot. Its principal antagonist is the peroneus brevis, which normally everts the subtalar joint and abducts the forefoot. Posterior tibial tendon dysfunction is a condition, as its name suggests, that is characterized by the loss of function of the posterior tibial tendon. This disabling problem may be caused by trauma, degeneration, or inflammatory arthritides and is most commonly seen in the sixth to seventh decades of life [2]. These pathologic processes can lead to reduction of effective excursion of the tendon or even rupture, resulting in progressive loss of the medial arch, midfoot abduction, and forefoot pronation. Posterior tibial tendon dysfunction is the most common cause of acquired flatfoot in the adult. Usually, posterior tibial tendon dysfunction is a chronic, progressive process, but spontaneous rupture can occur in patients receiving long-term steroid therapy or after trauma.

In regard to pathophysiology, the posterior tibial tendon functions in concert with the gastrocnemius-soleus complex to stabilize the hindfoot. The longitudinal arch is stabilized primarily by bone articulations and ligamentous structures (spring ligament, talocalcaneal interosseous ligament, superficial deltoid) and only secondarily supported by the posterior tibial tendon. The initial pathologic change is typically tendinosis of the posterior tibial tendon with maintenance of the longitudinal arch. As the tendon becomes less efficient, more stress is placed on the medial ligamentous structures, which attenuate, leading to progressive loss of the arch and abduction of the midfoot [3]. The posterior tibial tendon begins to atrophy while the flexor digitorum longus hypertrophies in an attempt to compensate [4]. Next, the calcaneus will drift into a valgus malalignment, changing the lever arm of the Achilles and causing a heel cord contracture. Finally, the peroneus brevis becomes an unopposed antagonist and exacerbates the deformity.

Symptoms

Patients, most commonly middle-aged women, primarily complain of pain on the inner or medial aspect of the ankle and the hindfoot. As the insufficiency progresses, pronation increases, leading to pain over the dorsolateral aspect of the midfoot [5,6]. Typically, this results in a gradual loss of the arch associated with a corresponding increase in pain.

Rarely, there is a history of a rapid collapse from rupture after an acute injury [7,8]. There have been only six reported cases in the literature of athletes (basketball players and runners) younger than 30 years with acute posterior tibial tendon ruptures [9–12].

Physical Examination

The physical examination reveals swelling confined to the area around the medial malleolus. In general, there is tenderness along the course of the tendon, and there may be exquisite tenderness just distal to the medial malleolus where the tendon most commonly tears [13,14].

Assessment of the lower extremity in the weight-bearing position best demonstrates the essential elements of the deformity: valgus hindfoot (calcaneovalgus), midfoot abduction, and forefoot pronation. This complex deformity clinically demonstrates a "too many toes" sign, that is, when the feet are viewed from behind, there appear to be more toes on the affected side than on the unaffected side. The severity of the patient's presentation depends on the chronicity of the insufficiency and the magnitude of the tendon dysfunction. The medial longitudinal arch of the foot may be entirely lost.

The anterior tibial tendon may become more visible than on the normal side as the patient, subconsciously, tries to regain the arch. Patients may have difficulty walking on their tiptoes or have difficulty performing a one-sided toe-stand while holding on to the clinician's hands. The heel fails to invert into a varus position. Asking the patient to invert the plantar-flexed foot against resistance can be overcome by the clinician's hand. Assessment of the patient on the couch reveals altered posture of the foot due to the unopposed action of the peroneus brevis. A callosity can be seen in the region of the medial plantar aspect of the midfoot.

Posterior tibial tendon dysfunction can be classified in three stages that are correlated to the treatment. Stage I is a tenosynovitis, normal tendon function, and no deformity. Stage II is a spectrum of disease that includes tendinosis but also posterior tibial tendon dysfunction and weakness. Loss of the medial arch and progressive valgus of the heel with mild lateral impingement can be seen. Early in stage II, the patient may be able to perform a single heel raise, but as this stage progresses, this function is lost. Most important, the flexibility of the foot is maintained with nearly normal subtalar, midtarsal, and forefoot motion. This continuum of disease may progress to stage III as the deformity becomes more rigid and subtalar degeneration occurs with subsequent decreased motion. Lateral tenderness is present because of impingement of the distal fibula on the calcaneus. A heel cord contracture is also apparent in most cases.

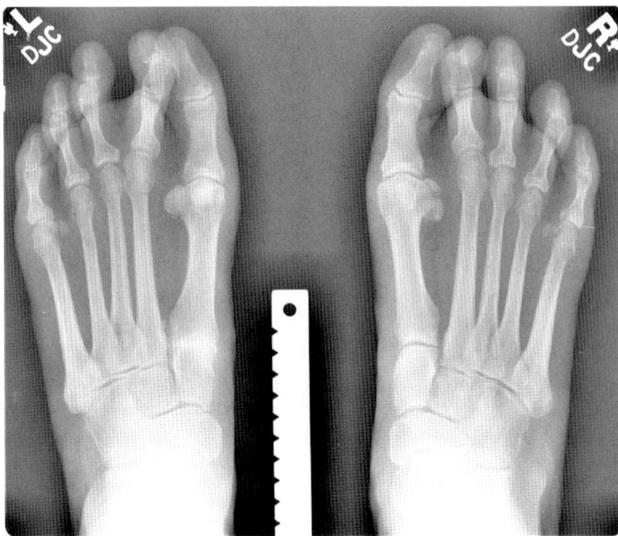

FIGURE 93.1 Anteroposterior view of the foot. Stage II with uncovering of the talar head.

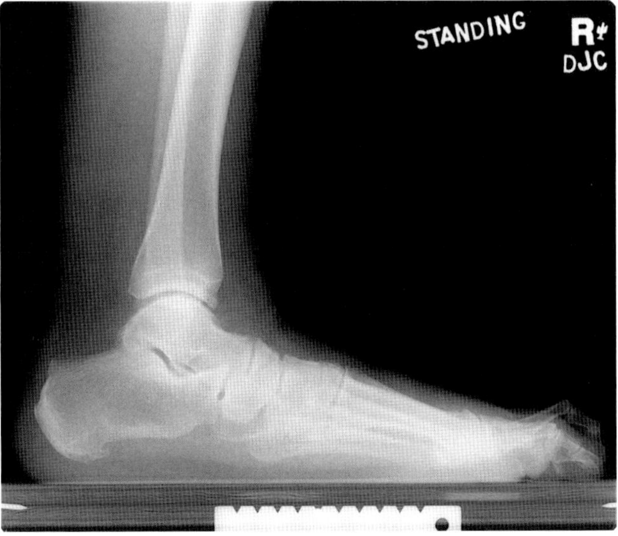

FIGURE 93.2 Lateral view of the foot. Stage II with decreased calcaneal height and talar–first metatarsal angle.

Functional Limitations

Patients may experience fatigue after only limited activity as their gait mechanics change with progressive pronation. They may have difficulty finding well-fitting footwear. Pain is usually the greatest complaint and also limits walking and sports-related activities [15].

Diagnostic Studies

Weight-bearing foot and ankle radiographs are usually helpful, depending on the severity of the clinical findings. In the earlier stages of tenosynovitis, the radiographs are usually normal, even if there is some mild clinical flattening of the medial longitudinal arch. As the problem progresses, radiographic changes occur (Figs. 93.1 and 93.2). These include, on the anteroposterior view, uncovering of the head of the talus (as the navicular moves laterally) and increase of the angle between the bodies of the talus and the calcaneus; on the lateral view, plantar flexion of the talus, collapse of the navicular-cuneiform joint, and overlapping of the four medial metatarsals are noted.

Ultrasonography has been used in the past to visualize the posterior tibial tendon both statically and dynamically and to demonstrate the tendon's excursion. Currently, the "gold standard" is magnetic resonance imaging to evaluate the continuity of the tendon. This provides a reasonably accurate view of the degree of inflammation and synovial fluid present within the tendon sheath as well as determines whether a tear of the tendon is present.

Differential Diagnosis

Tarsal coalition–spastic flatfoot
Degenerative arthritic deformity
Idiopathic flexible pes planus
Neuropathic arthropathy (e.g., secondary to diabetes mellitus)
Midtarsal collapse
Congenital pes planus
Lisfranc dislocation
Generalized dysplasia (ligamentous laxity)

Treatment

Initial

The first line of management, in stage I of posterior tibial tendon insufficiency, is with orthoses. Custom orthotic devices with longitudinal arch support and medial heel lift shoe inserts, University of California Biomechanics Laboratory (UCBL) inserts, rigid ankle-foot orthoses, and even double upright braces may be necessary. Unfortunately, there is no proof that any orthotic device can halt progression of the disorder, and if the deformity is less flexible, orthoses may be poorly tolerated. On occasion, a short leg cast is applied for 4 to 6 weeks for rest. Patients who have enough pain to require a boot or cast are also given a prescription for a wheelchair and walker. They are advised to be minimally weight bearing for at least 2 weeks. If the pain improves, they may gradually progress weight bearing in the boot. When they are pain free with weight bearing in the boot, they progress to a cushioned lace-up shoe and arch support. Pain should be the guide as to how fast patients may progress weight bearing. Anti-inflammatory medication may help alleviate some of the pain from the tenosynovitis. In obese individuals, weight loss can be critical.

Rehabilitation

Once the acute inflammation has settled, an exercise program may be started to strengthen the posterior tibial tendon. This can include active-resisted exercises with elastic materials (such as Cliniband or Thera-Band) and an exercise akin to trying to "pick up carpet with the sole of the foot" or "grasping a towel." Further methods include muscle stretching and strengthening techniques, particularly aimed at the Achilles tendon. Proprioceptive drills to improve balance on the wobble board and gait reeducation are also important.

Postoperative rehabilitation can include therapy for range of motion exercises after tenosynovectomy and most certainly after tendon transfer surgery to strengthen the muscle-tendon complex. After a subtalar or triple arthrodesis, the patient will have had a lengthy period of cast immobilization, and therefore gait reeducation can be beneficial.

Procedures

Injection of local anesthetic and steroid into the tendon sheath is a contentious subject and is not recommended because of the possibility of tendon rupture.

Surgery

Different surgical procedures are recommended, depending on the stage of the disease. Continuing pain and failure of nonoperative management of tenosynovitis (stage I) are the main indications for tenosynovectomy to remove all the inflamed synovium. This is followed by a period of cast immobilization. Repair of incomplete tears of the tendon may also be indicated and can be augmented by tendon transfers.

Complete tendon disruption, in the absence of bone collapse (stage II), can be treated with tendon transfers, combining a flexor digitorum longus transfer with a medial sliding calcaneal osteotomy. Subtalar or triple arthrodesis may be indicated for patients with progressively worsening deformity and lateral hindfoot pain (stage III) [16,17].

Postoperative gait analysis of patients after tendon transfer and osteotomy shows improvements compared with the preoperative analysis in ankle push-off power, step length, velocity, and cadence [18]. Long-term satisfaction with this procedure is high: 97% improvement in pain, 94% improvement in function, and 84% ability to wear shoes without modification or orthotic device [19].

Potential Disease Complications

Posterior tibial dysfunction can result in progressive pain and deformity, restriction of mobility, valgus deformity of the knee, and medial longitudinal arch ulceration as the medial midfoot collapses, causing increased pressure with weight bearing in this region.

Potential Treatment Complications

Analgesics and nonsteroidal anti-inflammatory drugs have well-known side effects that most commonly affect the gastric, hepatic, and renal systems. Steroid injection can cause tendon rupture. Complications of surgery include wound infection (in an area that can be notoriously slow to heal) and nonunion or failure of fusion in attempted arthrodesis.

References

[1] Deland JT. Posterior tibial tendon dysfunction. In: Craig EV, editor. Clinical orthopaedics. Philadelphia: Lippincott Williams & Wilkins; 1999. p. 883–90.

[2] Richardson EG. Disorders of tendons and fascia. In: Canale ST, editor. 9th ed. Campbell's operative orthopaedics, vol. 2. St. Louis: Mosby; 1998. p. 1889–923.

[3] Mann RA. Surgery of the foot and ankle. 7th ed. St. Louis: Mosby; 1999, 745–767.

[4] Wacker J, Calder JD, Engstrom CM, Saxby TS. MR morphometry of posterior tibial muscle in adult acquired flatfoot. Foot Ankle Int 2003;24:354–7.

[5] Hertling D, Kessler RM. The leg, ankle and foot. In: Hertling D, Kessler RM, editors. Management of common musculoskeletal disorders. 3rd ed. Philadelphia: Lippincott Williams & Wilkins; 1996. p. 435–8.

[6] Mann RA. Biomechanics of the foot and ankle. In: Mann RA, Coughlin MJ, editors. Surgery of the foot and ankle. 6th ed. St. Louis: Mosby; 1993. p. 3–44.

[7] Myerson MS. Adult acquired flatfoot deformity. J Bone Joint Surg Am 1996;78:780–92.

[8] Mann RA, Thompson FM. Rupture of the posterior tibial tendon causing flat foot. Surgical treatment. J Bone Joint Surg Am 1985;67:556–61.

[9] Henceroth 2nd WD, Deyerle WM. The acquired unilateral flatfoot in the adult: some causative factors. Foot Ankle 1982;2:304–8.

[10] Woods L, Leach RE. Posterior tibial tendon rupture in athletic people. Am J Sports Med 1991;19:495–8.

[11] Trevino S, Gould N, Korson R. Surgical treatment of stenosing tenosynovitis at the ankle. Foot Ankle 1981;2:37–45.

[12] Kettelkamp DB, Alexander HH. Spontaneous rupture of the posterior tibial tendon. J Bone Joint Surg Am 1969;51:759–64.

[13] Johnson KA, Strom DE. Tibialis posterior tendon dysfunction. Clin Orthop Relat Res 1989;239:196–206.

[14] Johnson KA. Tibialis posterior tendon rupture. Clin Orthop 1983;177:140–7.

[15] Pedowitz WJ, Jovatis P. Flatfoot in the adult. J Am Acad Orthop Surg 1995;3:293–302.

[16] Myerson MS, Corrigan J. Treatment of posterior tibial tendon dysfunction with flexor digitorum longus tendon transfer and calcaneal osteotomy. Orthopaedics 1996;19:383–8.

[17] Johnson KA. Tibialis posterior tendon release-substitution. In: Thompson RC, Johnson KA, editors. Master techniques in orthopaedic surgery. The foot and ankle. Philadelphia: Raven Press; 1994. p. 271–83.

[18] Brodsky JW. Preliminary gait analysis results after posterior tibial tendon reconstruction—a prospective study. Foot Ankle Int 2004;25:96–100.

[19] Myerson MS, Badekas A, Schon LC. Treatment of stage II posterior tibial tendon deficiency with FDL transfer and calcaneal osteotomy. Foot Ankle Int 2004;25:445–50.

CHAPTER 94

Tibial Neuropathy (Tarsal Tunnel Syndrome)

David R. Del Toro, MD

Synonyms

Tibial mononeuropathy at the ankle
Compression or entrapment neuropathy of the tibial nerve
Posterior tarsal tunnel syndrome
Posterior tibial nerve entrapment

ICD-9 Code

355.5 Tarsal tunnel syndrome

ICD-10 Codes

G57.50 Tarsal tunnel syndrome, unspecified lower limb
G57.51 Tarsal tunnel syndrome, right lower limb
G57.52 Tarsal tunnel syndrome, left lower limb

Definition

Tarsal tunnel syndrome can be described as a constellation of signs and symptoms caused by entrapment or compression of the tibial nerve or any of its branches within the tarsal tunnel, the region beneath the flexor retinaculum on the medial aspect of the ankle (Fig. 94.1). The tibial nerve branches that may be involved deep to the tarsal tunnel include the medial plantar nerve, lateral plantar nerve, Baxter nerve (also known as the first branch of the lateral plantar nerve or inferior calcaneal nerve), and medial calcaneal nerve [1]. Anatomically, the tarsal tunnel is a fibro-osseous structure that begins just posterior to the medial malleolus; the roof is the flexor retinaculum (also called the laciniate ligament), and the floor is formed by the tendons of the posterior tibialis, flexor digitorum longus, and flexor hallucis longus muscles. The tibial nerve usually divides into three branches at the level of the ankle: the medial plantar nerve, the lateral plantar nerve, and the medial calcaneal nerve. However, Baxter nerve (i.e., first branch of the lateral plantar nerve) usually branches from the lateral plantar nerve (but can branch off the tibial nerve) just distal to the origin of the medial calcaneal nerve at the level of the tarsal tunnel [2,3]. Baxter nerve then traverses laterally across the anterior aspect of the heel and terminates with motor branches to the abductor digiti quinti (or minimi) pedis muscle [2]. It is likely that tarsal tunnel syndrome occurs infrequently compared with other well-known focal entrapment neuropathies, such as carpal tunnel syndrome, ulnar neuropathy at the elbow, and peroneal (fibular) neuropathy at the knee. In fact, in a retrospective review of isolated tibial neuropathies in the foot, the incidence of Baxter neuropathy (17%) was much greater than that of tarsal tunnel syndrome (5%) [4].

There are generally considered to be five basic categories that account for the etiology of tarsal tunnel syndrome: trauma and post-traumatic changes, mass or space-occupying lesions causing compression, systemic diseases, biomechanical causes related to joint structure or deformity, and idiopathic causes. In addition, the underlying pathophysiologic mechanism of tarsal tunnel syndrome remains elusive; a portion of the literature supports the process of demyelination, whereas other sources implicate axonal degeneration as the primary process [5,6]. It is thought that the tibial nerve may be entrapped proximally within the tarsal tunnel, or one of its branches (e.g., the medial plantar nerve) may be entrapped distally in its own calcaneal chamber [1]. Entrapment of the first branch of the lateral plantar nerve (i.e., Baxter nerve) has also been described as a cause of heel pain [7–10]. Therefore in a case of clinically suspected tarsal tunnel syndrome, the tibial nerve and its major terminal branches (including the medial plantar nerve, lateral plantar nerve, and Baxter nerve) should be thoroughly evaluated [4].

In the current literature, there is no mention of an age or gender preference in patients with tarsal tunnel syndrome. One possible explanation for this is the relatively low incidence and various causes of tarsal tunnel syndrome.

Symptoms

The patient usually presents with pain or paresthesias along with numbness over the sole of the foot [1,11]. Pain is

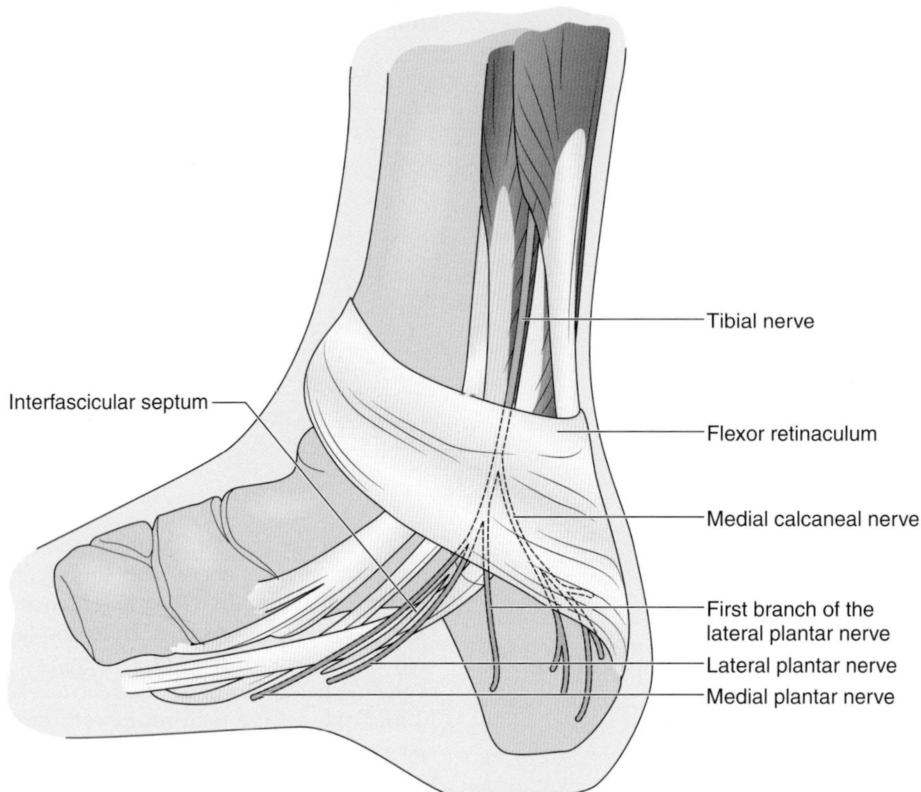

FIGURE 94.1 Medial aspect of the right foot. The tibial nerve traverses through the tarsal tunnel and then branches into the medial calcaneal nerve, medial plantar and lateral plantar nerves, and first branch of the lateral plantar nerve (i.e., Baxter nerve). Note that the medial calcaneal nerve branches may pierce the flexor retinaculum as they course toward the medial plantar aspect of the heel.

typically described as burning or a dull ache, but it may also be expressed as throbbing, cramping, or even tightness, and pain may extend proximally to the medial calf. Symptoms are often exacerbated by prolonged standing or walking and may be worse at night but may not be well localized. However, if the distribution of sensory disturbance is limited to a particular region of the foot, these symptoms could correspond to a specific tibial nerve branch that is involved (e.g., medial sole of foot due to medial plantar nerve involvement). Obvious weakness of the intrinsic foot muscles is an uncommon patient complaint and may be manifested only if the resulting foot deformity is grossly noticeable or so severe that it causes an unstable gait pattern. Patients with tarsal tunnel syndrome generally present with unilateral symptoms.

Physical Examination

Sensory examination of a patient with tarsal tunnel syndrome should reveal decreased light touch or pinprick over the plantar aspect of the foot corresponding to the distribution of one or all of the tibial nerve branches involved (Fig. 94.2). Motor examination of the intrinsic foot muscles is challenging because it is often difficult for patients to selectively activate these muscles. However, one may be able to appreciate muscle atrophy of the involved foot because its appearance may be asymmetric compared with the other foot [1]. A patient with tarsal tunnel syndrome often has a Tinel sign over the tibial nerve or one of its branches in the tarsal tunnel (Fig. 94.3). On occasion, percussion over the tibial nerve at the ankle will elicit pain extending proximally along the course of the tibial nerve; this sign is called the Valleix phenomenon. There may also be palpable tenderness over the tibial nerve in the tarsal tunnel. Two other provocative maneuvers that may reproduce symptoms in the foot or ankle are extension of the great toe and sustained

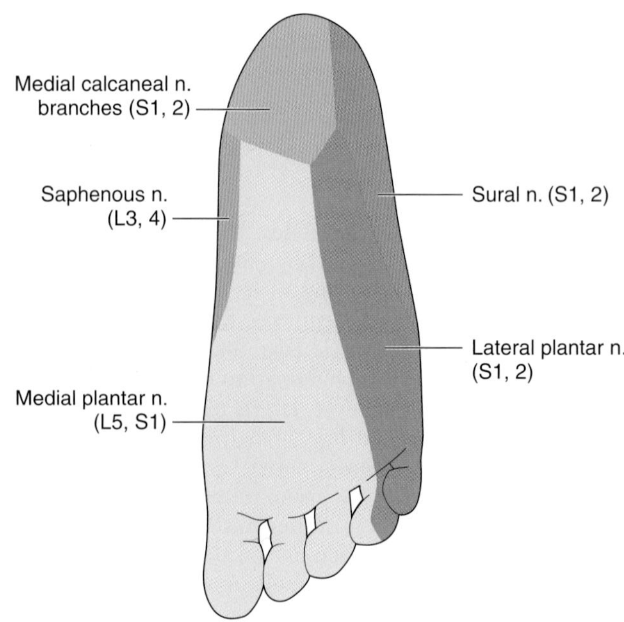

FIGURE 94.2 Cutaneous innervation of the sole of the foot.

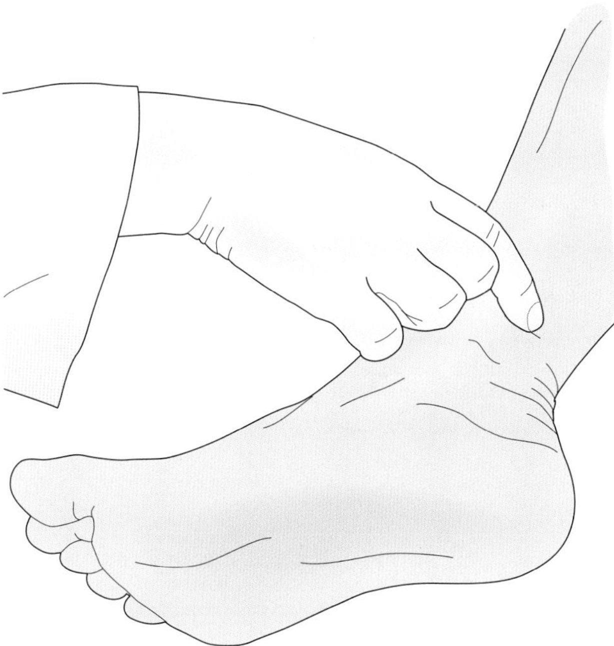

FIGURE 94.3 Tinel sign over the tibial nerve posterior to the medial malleolus.

passive eversion of the ankle [1]. Muscle stretch reflexes in the lower extremity (including patellar, medial hamstring, and Achilles) should be normal and symmetric compared with the unaffected side. Peripheral pulses (posterior tibial and dorsalis pedis) are usually palpable and unremarkable. If the biomechanical configuration of the foot is altered severely enough, gait deviations can be observed.

Functional Limitations

Impaired balance or a perception of instability due to diminished sensation or pain on the sole of the foot may be the only functional impairment that is reported by the patient. As a consequence, limited walking tolerance, reduced walking distance, stumbling, or falls may be reported by the patient.

Diagnostic Studies

Electrodiagnostic testing should be performed for any patient with clinically suspected tarsal tunnel syndrome; this is the only diagnostic study that evaluates the electrophysiologic function of the tibial nerve and its major terminal branches. Both needle electromyography and nerve conduction studies (i.e., motor, sensory, or mixed nerve studies) should be done. Furthermore, it is imperative that the tibial nerve be thoroughly evaluated from an electrophysiologic standpoint because either the tibial nerve or one or more of its terminal branches may be involved in clinically suspected tarsal tunnel syndrome [4,10]. A magnetic resonance imaging study may be useful in detecting a space-occupying mass that is impinging on or compressing the tibial nerve within the tarsal tunnel [12]. The magnetic resonance imaging study can also provide a "road map" for surgical exploration of the tarsal tunnel and then direct the procedure toward suitable anatomic decompression of the nerve [13]. The literature indicates that ultrasonography can be a complementary diagnostic imaging technique for cases of suspected tarsal tunnel syndrome by identifying space-occupying masses such as ganglia [14]. Plain radiographs and a bone scan may be needed to rule out a possible fracture or other bone lesion.

Differential Diagnosis

Plantar fasciitis
Peripheral neuropathy
Sciatic neuropathy
Lumbosacral plexopathy
Posterior tibialis dysfunction
Lumbosacral radiculopathy

Treatment

Initial

Conservative measures can be effective in the majority of tarsal tunnel syndrome cases, and therefore most patients should be given an adequate trial, which is generally at least 3 to 6 months. Initial management usually includes nonsteroidal anti-inflammatory drugs and possibly a neuropathic pain medication (such as gabapentin). If there is a biomechanical foot condition that can be corrected or supported, the patient could benefit from a medial arch support (for a pronated foot) or a foot orthosis (for hindfoot valgus) [7]. In some patients, a short leg walking cast or boot brace can provide symptomatic relief [15].

Rehabilitation

Physical therapy can be useful in certain cases, most typically with modalities such as iontophoresis to reduce symptoms of inflammation, deep massage to mobilize scar tissue, desensitization, and various exercises—such as stretching exercises of the toe flexors, both active and passive, and of the ankle muscle groups (i.e., dorsiflexors, plantar flexors, invertors and evertors) along with specific nerve mobilization exercises [16]. Strengthening exercises for the toe flexors and extensors and for the ankle muscle groups may also be prescribed for distinct motor deficits with a goal of equalizing any muscle imbalance. In addition, gait training along with balance training, both static and dynamic, may be necessary. The patient may require extra-depth shoes to accommodate a medial arch support or a custom-made foot orthosis. Therefore an orthotist or pedorthist may need to manufacture these custom-made orthotics or footwear.

Procedures

For diagnostic and therapeutic purposes, a local anesthetic-steroid injection into the tarsal tunnel can give relatively immediate relief of local swelling and inflammation surrounding the tibial nerve.

Surgery

Surgical management consists of release of the flexor retinaculum and possibly exploration for a mass or space-occupying lesion and neurolysis of the tibial nerve, depending on the surgeon [1]. In addition, some surgeons advocate release of the superficial and deep fascia of the abductor hallucis to more completely decompress the tibial nerve and its terminal branches. The success rate (good to excellent outcome) for tarsal tunnel release is variable and reported to be 44% to 78%, depending on the study [13]. Endoscopic release of the tarsal tunnel may be a potential surgical option in some cases [13,17].

Potential Disease Complications

Several potential disease complications may be a consequence of tarsal tunnel syndrome. Skin breakdown, including ulcerations, can occur over the plantar aspect of the foot as a result of impaired sensation. An altered gait pattern may develop with decreased balance or a "feeling of unsteadiness" because of impaired sensation, particularly with respect to proprioception and light touch or pressure in the foot, or because the biomechanical configuration of the foot is distorted. Low back pain or lower extremity joint pain (probably hip or knee) may arise as a consequence of the gait deviation.

Potential Treatment Complications

Nonsteroidal anti-inflammatory drugs may cause, most commonly, gastric or renal complications. Skin breakdown can develop over the foot or ankle from a poorly fitting foot orthosis. Tendon rupture may occur after steroid injection into the incorrect location (e.g., flexor tendon sheath). In addition, the symptoms of pain, numbness, and paresthesias in the foot can be exacerbated after a local anesthetic-steroid injection or after surgical decompression of the tarsal tunnel.

References

[1] Park TA, Del Toro DR. Electrodiagnostic evaluation of the foot. Phys Med Rehabil Clin N Am 1998;9:871–96.

[2] Sarrafian SK. Anatomy of the foot and ankle. Philadelphia: JB Lippincott; 1983, 356–390.

[3] Govsa F, Bilge O, Ozer MA. Variations in the origin of the medial and inferior calcaneal nerves. Arch Orthop Trauma Surg 2006;126:6–14.

[4] Zaza DI, Del Toro DR, White KT. A retrospective review of isolated tibial neuropathies in the foot. Muscle Nerve 2006;34:517.

[5] Kraft GH. Tarsal tunnel entrapment. Course E: entrapment neuropathies. Boston: AAEE Ninth Annual Continuing Education Course; 1986, 13–18.

[6] Spindler HA, Reischer MA, Felsenthal G. Electrodiagnostic assessment in suspected tarsal tunnel syndrome. Phys Med Rehabil Clin N Am 1994;5:595–612.

[7] Przylucki H, Jones CL. Entrapment neuropathy of muscle branch of lateral plantar nerve. J Am Podiatr Med Assoc 1981;71:119–24.

[8] Schon LC, Baxter DE. Heel pain syndrome and entrapment neuropathies about the foot and ankle. In: Gould JS, editor. Operative foot surgery. Philadelphia: WB Saunders; 1994. p. 192–208.

[9] Park TA, Del Toro DR. Isolated inferior calcaneal neuropathy. Muscle Nerve 1996;19:106–8.

[10] Ngo KT, Del Toro DR. Electrodiagnostic findings and surgical outcome in isolated first branch lateral plantar neuropathy: a case series with literature review. Arch Phys Med Rehabil 2010;91:1948–51.

[11] Patel AT, Gaines K, Malamut R, et al, American Association of Neuromuscular and Electrodiagnostic Medicine. Usefulness of electrodiagnostic techniques in the evaluation of suspected tarsal tunnel syndrome: an evidence-based review. Muscle Nerve 2005;32:236–40.

[12] Duran-Stanton AM, Bui-Mansfield LT. Magnetic resonance diagnosis of tarsal tunnel syndrome due to flexor digitorum accessorius longus and peroneocalcaneus internus muscles. J Comput Assist Tomogr 2010;34:270–2.

[13] Haddad SL. Compressive neuropathies of the foot and ankle. In: Myerson MS, editor. Foot and ankle disorders. Philadelphia: WB Saunders; 2000. p. 808–33.

[14] Nagaoka M, Matsuzaki H. Ultrasonography in tarsal tunnel syndrome. J Ultrasound Med 2005;24:1035–40.

[15] Mann RA. Diseases of the nerves. In: Coughlin MJ, Mann RA, editors. Surgery of the foot and ankle. St. Louis: Mosby; 1999. p. 502–24.

[16] Kavlak Y, Uygur F. Effects of nerve mobilization exercise as an adjunct to the conservative treatment for patients with tarsal tunnel syndrome. J Manipulative Physiol Ther 2011;34:441–8.

[17] Krishnan KG, Pinzer T, Schackert G. A novel endoscopic technique in treating single nerve entrapment syndromes with special attention to ulnar nerve transposition and tarsal tunnel release: clinical application. Neurosurgery 2006;59(Suppl. 1):ONS89–ONS100.

PART 2

PAIN

CHAPTER 95

Arachnoiditis

Michael D. Osborne, MD
Adam Wallace, MD

Synonyms

Spinal adhesive arachnoiditis
Lumbosacral spinal fibrosis
Chronic leptomeningitis

ICD-9 Code

322.9 Arachnoiditis

ICD-10 Code

G03.9 Arachnoiditis (spinal) NOS

Definition

The meninges are a system of three protective membranes that surround the central nervous system and consist of the pia mater, arachnoid mater, and dura mater layers. Arachnoiditis is the development of chronic inflammation and progressive fibrosis of the arachnoid and pia layers of the meninges. It can occur subsequent to a variety of conditions, although it is most commonly a sequela of spinal surgery or the result of intrathecal injection of radiographic dyes and chemicals with neurotoxic preservatives [1]. Some of the etiologic factors linked to the development of arachnoiditis are listed in Table 95.1. Because arachnoiditis is rare, specific incidence and prevalence are uncertain.

When microtrauma to the vasculature of the arachnoid membrane and pia mater occurs, it can impair the normal mechanisms for control of excessive meningeal fibrosis [1]. This may result in the deposition of fibrous collagen bands in the arachnoid-pia membranes and cause the nerve roots to adhere to each other as well as to the dural sac. The pathophysiologic mechanism of arachnoiditis involves a progression from root inflammation (radiculitis) to root adherence (fibrosis). In severe cases, the arachnoid fibrosis can cause compressive root ischemia, and progressive neurologic deficits may ensue [2]. When this condition occurs in the meninges of the cervical and thoracic regions, the spinal cord can become enmeshed and constricted as well. Pain is the result of dural adherence with nerve root traction and nerve ischemia. Typically, arachnoiditis develops slowly during the period of months after the initial insult, although it may continue to develop for years, resulting in worsening pain and paresthesias or progressive neurologic injury [1].

Symptoms

The symptoms associated with arachnoiditis are heterogeneous and often difficult to distinguish from other disease processes, such as radiculopathy, spinal stenosis, cauda equina syndrome, and neuropathies. Also, because arachnoiditis is often acquired iatrogenically during the course of evaluation and treatment of spinal disorders, patients often have concomitant symptoms of mechanical back pain or myofascial pain in addition to the arachnoiditis symptom complex.

Patients with arachnoiditis principally report burning pain or paresthesias. However, these symptoms often do not follow typical radicular patterns. Pain is usually constant but exacerbated by movement. Some patients experience secondary muscle spasms. Weakness and muscle atrophy may also occur, and bowel or bladder sphincter dysfunction is not uncommon. Onset is insidious, and symptoms may first be manifested years after the inciting event [3]. Symptoms can range from mild (such as slight tingling of the extremities) to severe (such as excruciating pain with progressive neurologic deterioration). The condition may also be asymptomatic and discovered only incidentally on magnetic resonance imaging (MRI).

Physical Examination

Neurologic examination typically reveals a patchy distribution of lower motor neuron deficits. Examination findings may include loss of reflexes, muscle weakness, muscle atrophy, anesthesia, gait instability, and reduced rectal tone [2]. Less commonly, arachnoiditis may involve the spinal cord; in these instances, upper motor neuron findings (hyperreflexia, spasticity, presence of Babinski response) can be found on examination.

A complete neurologic examination should be performed at the time of initial diagnosis. In the event that symptoms worsen, this examination may then be used as a benchmark to ascertain whether neurologic deterioration is occurring. In the setting of progressive neurologic decline, it is incumbent on the treating physician to rule out other pathologic processes (such as a new disc herniation) before neurologic

Table 95.1 Some Etiologic Factors Linked to the Development of Arachnoiditis

Agents Injected Into the Subarachnoid Space
Contrast media (especially Pantopaque)
Intrathecal chemotherapies (amphotericin B, methotrexate)
Local anesthetics with vasoconstrictors
Corticosteroids with polyethylene glycol or benzyl alcohol preservative
Spinal Surgery or Trauma
Extradural surgeries, such as laminectomy, discectomy, and fusion
Intradural Surgeries
Spinal fractures
Intrathecal blood
Subarachnoid hemorrhage
Bloody spinal tap
Blood patch with inadvertent intrathecal injection
Infection
Discitis, vertebral body osteomyelitis
Spinal tuberculosis
Other
Spinal stenosis
Idiopathic

Modified from Bourne IH. Lumbo-sacral adhesive arachnoiditis: a review. J R Soc Med 1990;83:262-265.

deterioration is attributed solely to progressive arachnoid fibrosis.

Functional Limitations

Patients with arachnoiditis may exhibit a variety of functional limitations, the degree of which corresponds to the extent of the neurologic impairments and the severity of the pain. Gait instability, reduced ambulatory capacity, and impairment in activities of daily living are not uncommon. As time goes by, patients tend to suffer secondary effects of immobilization and deconditioning, causing further functional impairment. The severe pain and impaired mobility tend to isolate patients socially and to limit their ability to work. Because the pain associated with arachnoiditis is usually present even at rest, sedentary work or light duty does not always improve a patient's symptoms enough to facilitate employment despite activity restrictions.

Diagnostic Studies

Presently, the diagnosis of arachnoiditis is most often made through the use of MRI. Historically, myelography was used routinely for diagnosis of arachnoiditis; characteristic findings included the observance of prominent nerve roots as well as various patterns of filling defects. The advent of computed tomography and MRI has made diagnosis easier.

MRI is preferred to computed tomographic myelography because of its noninvasive nature. Typical findings include adherent roots located centrally in the thecal sac (considered mild arachnoiditis), an "empty sac" (where roots are adherent to the wall of the thecal sac), and a mass of soft tissue replacing the subarachnoid space (severe disease) [4]. These findings are well seen on T2-weighted axial images (Figs. 95.1 and 95.2). Although the administration of contrast material

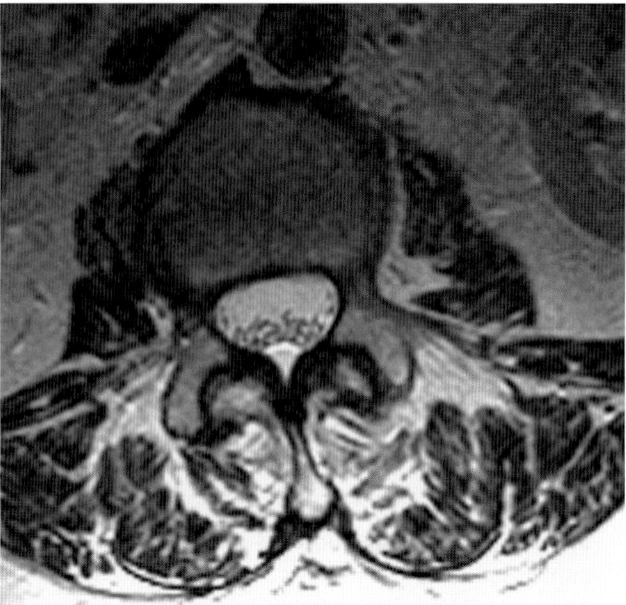

FIGURE 95.1 Normal MRI appearance of lumbar nerve roots on T2-weighted axial sequences.

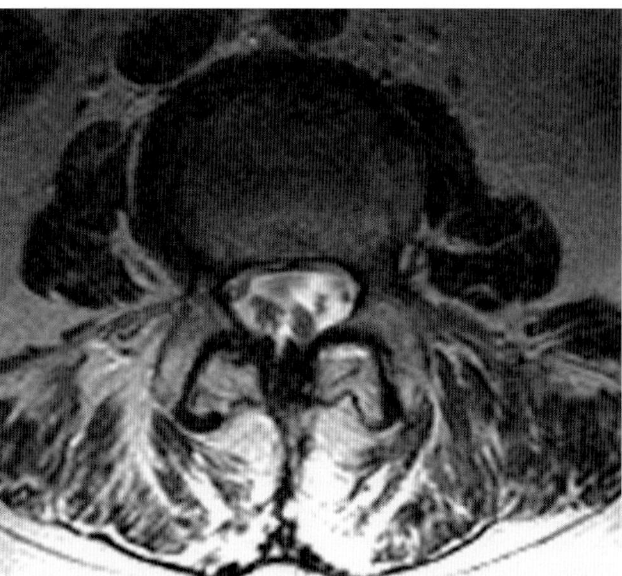

FIGURE 95.2 Lumbar MRI demonstrating the characteristic nerve root clumping indicative of arachnoiditis.

with MRI may help rule out other diseases in the differential diagnosis, such as tumors and infection, contrast enhancement is not necessary to visualize the characteristic appearance of arachnoiditis [5].

The diagnosis can also be made by computed tomographic myelography; even myelography with conventional radiography may be used if spinal instrumentation from prior fusion surgery creates too much artifact on MRI and computed tomography. The water-soluble myelographic contrast media used today (such as iohexol) are much safer than the prior oil-based media (Pantopaque), and serious adverse reactions involving the central nervous system are extremely rare (<0.1%) [6]. There have not been any documented cases of adhesive arachnoiditis with the use of iohexol myelography [6].

Differential Diagnosis

Spondylosis
Radiculopathy
Cauda equina syndrome
Neuropathy, plexopathy
Neurogenic claudication
Spinal tumors
Spinal infections
Postsurgical epidural fibrosis
Epidural hematoma
Meningitis

Treatment

Initial

The treatment of arachnoiditis is palliative, and medications are often used for this purpose. Antidepressant or anticonvulsant analgesics are considered the mainstay of medical management, although other classes of medications may provide benefit as well. Many antidepressants and anticonvulsants have been used for years off-label for the treatment of neuropathic pain with reasonable efficacy. The tricyclic antidepressants (such as amitriptyline) are the most common. The U.S. Food and Drug Administration has more recently approved several newer medications for use in specific neuropathic pain syndromes: duloxetine and pregabalin for diabetic neuropathy, and gabapentin and pregabalin for postherpetic neuralgia. These medications are often tried in patients with arachnoiditis with varying efficacy. Antidepressant and anticonvulsant analgesics are typically started at relatively low doses and titrated upward as tolerated. The precise starting dose and eventual maximal dose usually depend on how well the medication's side effects are tolerated. Some examples of dosing regimens are listed in Table 95.2. For most of these medications, it often takes a few weeks at any given dose for optimal analgesic effect to be reached.

Anti-inflammatory medications (nonsteroidal anti-inflammatory drugs) are commonly used as well with modest efficacy. This is probably because of the frequent occurrence of back pain in these patients. Often, patients with arachnoiditis have concomitant lumbar disc degeneration or osteoarthritis of the facet joints that may respond in part to anti-inflammatory medications. Likewise, patients with back pain may benefit from trials of muscle relaxants or more potent inhibitors of muscle contractions (antispasticity agents), such as baclofen and tizanidine. Baclofen has also been used off-label for treatment of neuropathic pain.

Opiates are often prescribed with varying degrees of success. In general, neuropathic pain seems to be less responsive to opiates. Some advocate the use of methadone because of its *N*-methyl-D-aspartate (NMDA) receptor antagonist activity, which may make it more effective for neuropathic pain syndromes. One of the chief limitations of opiates is the tendency for development of tolerance, requiring dose escalation.

Table 95.2 Examples of Dosing Regimens for Anticonvulsant and Antidepressant Analgesics

Medication	Starting Dose	Dose Increase and Interval	Maximal Dose
Tricyclic antidepressants	10-25 mg at night	10-25 mg per week	150 mg/day
Duloxetine	20-30 mg/day	20-30 mg per week	60 mg/day
Gabapentin	100-300 mg bid-tid	100-300 mg per week	1800-3600 mg/day
Pregabalin	50-75 mg bid-tid	50-75 mg per week	600 mg/day

Rehabilitation

Rehabilitation interventions can be divided into modalities for pain management and therapeutic exercise to improve pain as well as to aid function. Modalities such as heat application (superficial and deep) and ice application are most effective for treatment of the associated mechanical back pain and myofascial pain that often accompany arachnoiditis. Contrast baths can be used for distal extremity pain and can be helpful when the patient exhibits signs of peripheral sympathetic dysfunction. Electrical stimulation is primarily used to treat neuropathic pain, but it may also improve associated musculoskeletal and myofascial pain. Transcutaneous electrical nerve stimulation and percutaneous electrical nerve stimulation can be applied at the paraspinal level or along the course of a peripheral nerve to help attenuate neuropathic pain.

Unfortunately, exercise typically offers the patient very little as a direct means of symptom improvement for severe neuropathic pain; yet exercise is still an important part of treatment. As previously mentioned, patients with arachnoiditis may suffer from other musculoskeletal pain, and therapeutic exercise (such as stretching, strength training, and aerobic exercise) often improves these associated disorders in this subset of patients as well as in those with chronic pain [7,8]. Patients with intractable pain often avoid activity because of increased pain or fear of pain provocation. As such, they often become deconditioned and benefit from gentle progressive exercise regimens. Aquatic therapy is generally well tolerated and can be used as a method to improve many of the manifestations of deconditioning and prolonged immobility, such as to improve joint motion, flexibility, aerobic capacity, and muscle strength.

Procedures

There are few data to support the role of neuraxial corticosteroid injections, such as epidural steroids and nerve root blocks, in arachnoiditis treatment. Anecdotally, short-duration improvement may be observed, and any such procedures are usually performed as a "do and see" proposition.

The most promising intervention for the intractable pain associated with arachnoiditis is spinal cord stimulation. Spinal cord stimulation, also known as dorsal column stimulation, involves the placement of a stimulating electrode (either percutaneously or through a laminotomy)

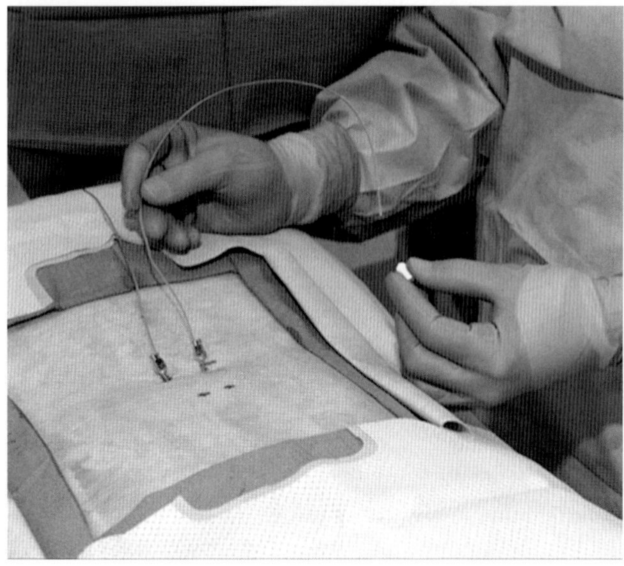

FIGURE 95.3 Intraoperative placement of spinal cord stimulator leads.

over the dorsal aspect of the spinal cord (Figs. 95.3 and 95.4). Exact level and location of electrode placement depend on the location of the patient's pain. Typically, patients undergo a percutaneous trial to test the stimulator's efficacy before permanent implantation. The goal is to stimulate the spinal cord with low levels of electrical impulses that produce a nonpainful paresthesia that modulates (masks) the patient's pain.

The largest studies investigating spinal cord stimulation have included patients with varied diagnoses, the most abundant of which is failed back surgery syndrome. It has been estimated that 11% of patients with failed back surgery syndrome have arachnoiditis. Approximately 50% to 60% of patients with failed back surgery syndrome treated with spinal cord stimulation receive more than 50% relief of their symptoms [9,10]. Studies investigating spinal cord stimulation efficacy in patients with a more specific diagnosis of epidural fibrosis or intradural fibrosis (arachnoiditis) have also found improvement in pain (60%), reduction of pain medication requirements (40%), and increased work capacity (25%) [11,12]. Spinal cord stimulation seems to be more effective for pain of neuropathic character than for pain of mechanical or musculoskeletal character. In addition, extremity pain is generally more easily treated compared with back pain–predominant symptoms [12].

Another option that could be considered is an intrathecal drug delivery system, which has been shown to be beneficial for those with chronic pain, whether it is neuropathic, nociceptive, or visceral in nature [13]. Medications such as opioids, local anesthetics, α-adrenergic receptor agonists, and NMDA receptor antagonists have all been successfully used. Recent use of intrathecal ziconotide has gained popularity for chronic neuropathic pain conditions. With all these interventions, one must consider the safety of the proposed treatment, taking special consideration of the risk of placing any intrathecal medication into an already pathologic spinal canal [13].

Surgery

There is very little role for surgical intervention in the treatment of arachnoiditis. There is no method of successfully surgically untangling the adherent nerve roots, although

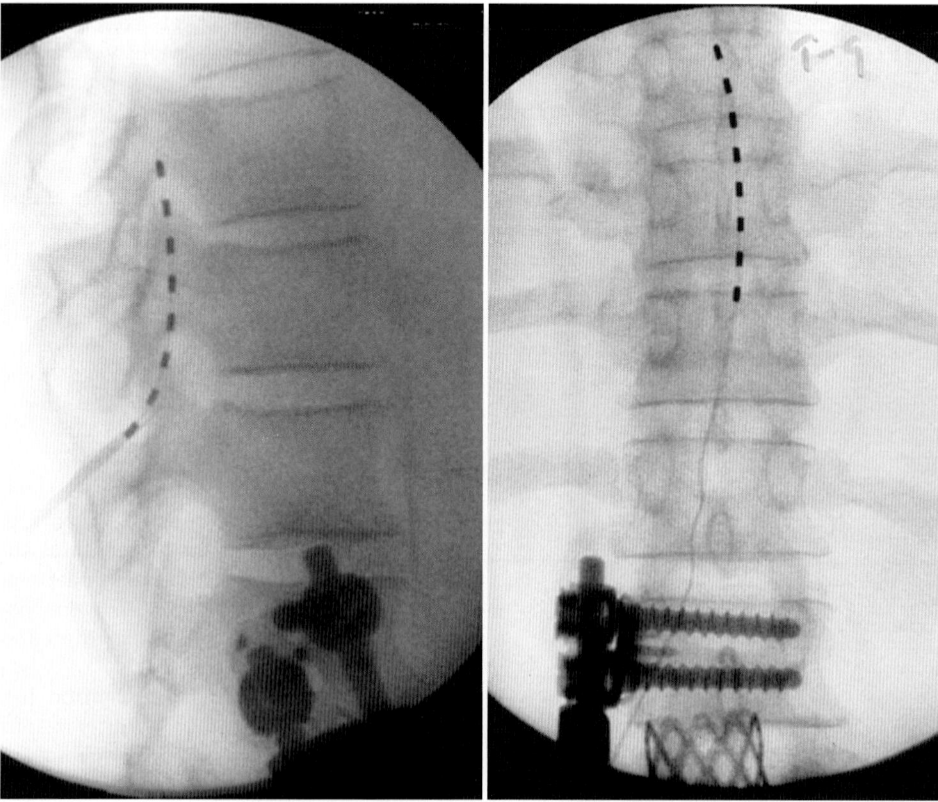

FIGURE 95.4 Fluoroscopic lateral and anteroposterior images of a percutaneous spinal cord stimulator lead in the dorsal thoracic spine.

attempts have been made [14]. Indications for surgery include rapidly progressive neurologic deterioration, such as myelopathy due to progressive syringomyelia or cauda equina syndrome from arachnoiditis ossificans. In these instances, surgical intervention (shunt placement or removal of the calcific mass) could be contemplated. The emphasis on such interventions is to halt or to retard further neurologic deterioration. The prospect that such procedures will improve pain remains speculative at best. There has been some documentation of subarachnoidal endoscopy (thecaloscopy) to perform adhesiolysis, but long-term benefit has not been established [15].

Potential Disease Complications

In severe cases of arachnoiditis, the fibrous bands that cause adherence of the nerve roots may become so prolific that progressive nerve root injury (radiculopathy, polyradiculopathy) or spinal cord injury (cauda equina syndrome, myelopathy) can ensue. Constriction of the spinal cord vasculature causes ischemia and focal areas of spinal cord demyelination. This vascular ischemia and associated alterations of normal cerebrospinal fluid flow have been observed to result in the formation of arachnoid cysts, syringomyelia, and even communicating hydrocephalus [16,17]. Calcification of the fibrotic milieu results in a condition termed arachnoiditis ossificans, which may result in progressive nerve root or spinal cord compression [18].

Potential Treatment Complications

Medication side effects are common. Anticonvulsant and antidepressant analgesics often produce sedation or alteration of mental status. Opiates, too, can produce sedation as well as severe constipation. Opiate dependence is generally anticipated as a ramification of use of this class of medication long term. Although true psychological addiction to opiates can occur, it is much less common than one might expect. The propensity for nonsteroidal anti-inflammatory drugs to cause gastrointestinal side effects is well known, as is their potential to adversely affect the kidneys and liver as well as to exacerbate hypertension and asthma.

Rehabilitation interventions are generally safe, although patients can suffer thermal injury from inappropriate application of superficial modalities. Transcutaneous electrical nerve stimulation and percutaneous electrical nerve stimulation are generally considered contraindicated in patients with pacemakers. Therapeutic exercise may potentially exacerbate pain symptoms.

Spinal cord stimulation poses some risk; however, complications are usually minor, and the incidence of new neurologic injury from something such as bleeding, infection, or neural trauma is quite small [10]. The most frequent complication usually entails electromechanical failure, such as percutaneous lead migration, when the stimulation no longer covers the symptomatic body region. The majority of electromechanical complications can be remedied with revision of the system.

References

[1] Bourne IH. Lumbo-sacral adhesive arachnoiditis: a review. J R Soc Med 1990;83:262–5.

[2] Rice I, Wee MY, Thomson K. Obstetric epidurals and chronic adhesive arachnoiditis. Br J Anaesth 2004;92:109–20.

[3] Wright MH, Denney LC. A comprehensive review of spinal arachnoiditis. Orthop Nurs 2003;22:215–9.

[4] Delamarter RB, Ross JS, Masaryk TJ, et al. Diagnosis of lumbar arachnoiditis by magnetic resonance imaging. Spine 1990;15:304–10.

[5] Johnson CE, Sze G. Benign lumbar arachnoiditis: MR imaging with gadopentetate dimeglumine. AJR Am J Roentgenol 1990;155:873–80.

[6] RxMed, Inc. Comprehensive resource for physicians, drug and illness information: omnipaque, http://www.rxmed.com/b.main/b2.pharmaceutical/b2.prescribe.html; [accessed 25.07.06].

[7] Demirbag C, Oguzoncul F. Effects of education and exercise on pain, depression and quality of life in patients diagnosed with fibromyalgia. HealthMed 2012;6:962–70.

[8] Verhagen AP, Cardoso JR, Bierma-Zeinstra SM. Aquatic exercise and balneotherapy in musculoskeletal conditions. Best Pract Res Clin Rheumatol 2012;26:335–43.

[9] Burchiel KJ, Anderson VC, Brown FD, et al. Prospective, multicenter study of spinal cord stimulation for relief of chronic back and extremity pain. Spine 1996;21:2786–94.

[10] Turner JA, Loeser JD, Bell KG. Spinal cord stimulation for chronic low back pain: a systematic literature synthesis. Neurosurgery 1995;37:1088–96.

[11] de la Porte C, Siegfried J. Lumbosacral spinal fibrosis (spinal arachnoiditis). Its diagnosis and treatment by spinal cord stimulation. Spine 1983;8:593–603.

[12] Probst C. Spinal cord stimulation in 112 patients with epi-/intradural fibrosis following operation for lumbar disc herniation. Acta Neurochir (Wien) 1990;107:147–51.

[13] Buvandendran A, Diwan S. Intrathecal drug delivery for pain and spasticity. Interventional and neuromodulatory techniques for pain management. vol. 2. Philadelphia: Elsevier Saunders; 2012.

[14] Mitsuyama T, Asamoto S, Kawamata T. Novel surgical management of spinal adhesive arachnoiditis by arachnoid microdissection and ventriculo-subarachnoid shunting. J Clin Neurosci 2011;18:1702–4.

[15] Warnke JP, Mourgela S. Endoscopic treatment of lumbar arachnoiditis. Minim Invasive Neurosurg 2007;50:1–6.

[16] Tumialan LM, Cawley CM, Barrow DL. Arachnoid cyst with associated arachnoiditis developing after subarachnoid hemorrhage. J Neurosurg 2005;103:1088–91.

[17] Koyanagi I, Iwasaki Y, Hida K, Houkin K. Clinical features and pathomechanisms of syringomyelia associated with spinal arachnoiditis. Surg Neurol 2005;63:350–5.

[18] Domenicucci M, Ramieri A, Passacantilli E, et al. Spinal arachnoiditis ossificans: report of three cases. Neurosurgery 2004;55:985–91.

CHAPTER 96

Chemotherapy-Induced Peripheral Neuropathy

Maryam R. Aghalar, DO
Christian M. Custodio, MD

Synonyms

Neuropathy
Peripheral neuropathy
Neurotoxicity

ICD-9 Codes

357.6 Polyneuropathy, drug related
357.4 Polyneuropathy, NOS
357.3 Polyneuropathy, cancer related

ICD-10 Codes

G62.0 Drug-induced polyneuropathy
G62.9 Polyneuropathy, unspecified
D49.9 and G63 Polyneuropathy, cancer related

Definition

Chemotherapy-induced peripheral neuropathy (CIPN) is damage and dysfunction of the peripheral nervous system secondary to chemotherapeutic agents, including platinum agents, taxanes, vinca alkaloids, thalidomide, bortezomib, and ixabepilone (Table 96.1). CIPN commonly occurs in 30% to 40% of patients, but its incidence can vary from 0% to 70% [1]. The degree of neuronal damage is dependent on many factors, such as the chemotherapeutic agent, the frequency and duration of therapy, the cumulative dose, the use of other neurotoxic agents, and the presence of preexisting neuropathies, most commonly from diabetes [1]. The severity of neuropathy generally increases until cessation of treatment. However, symptoms associated with platinum drugs may progress for weeks to months after treatment completion, a phenomenon called the "coasting" effect [2]. Many scales have been proposed to assess CIPN but lack standardization and reproducibility. The most widely used tool is the National Cancer Institute Common Terminology Criteria for Adverse Events (v4.03) (Table 96.2) [3]. Another scale is called the Total Neuropathy Score, which appears to be more sensitive in detecting changes in CIPN [4].

Symptoms

The onset of symptoms can be sudden or slowly progress over time. Symptoms can vary by what types of nerve fibers are affected. Sensory nerves are more commonly affected first because they have small fibers, they have little capacity for regeneration, and their cell bodies are located in dorsal root ganglion, where they are outside the protective blood-brain barrier. The dorsal root ganglion has a high supply of capillaries that are highly permeable to toxic compounds in the blood [5]. Patients can present with symmetric, distal, length-dependent, "stocking-glove" distribution of painful paresthesia, dysesthesia, cold sensitivity, allodynia, tingling, and numbness. The patients also may report muscle cramps and pain described as burning, lancinating, shock-like, or electric. Motor nerve fiber cell bodies located in the spinal cord are less affected as they are protected within the blood-brain barrier and they also have the capacity for distal sprouting and regeneration. Patients usually present with muscle weakness, myalgias, and difficulty in walking. If autonomic nerves are affected, patients can present with orthostatic hypotension, constipation, urinary retention, irregular heart rate, and sexual dysfunction [6].

Physical Examination

Physical examination should assess for impairments with any sensory modalities, including light touch, pinprick, proprioception, and temperature. Deep tendon reflexes may be absent. Motor strength, gait, and balance deficits should also be evaluated in detail. Lhermitte sign, which is defined as eliciting an electric sensation running down the spine with neck flexion, may be present, especially after platinum compounds secondary to demyelination in the spinal cord [7].

Table 96.1 Most Common Chemotherapeutic Agents Known to Induce Neuropathy

Drug	Mechanism of Action
Platinum compounds (cisplatin, carboplatin, oxaliplatin)	Damages DNA in dorsal root ganglion, causing neuronopathy or ganglionopathy with sensory axonal neuropathy
Vinca alkaloids (vincristine, vinblastine, vinorelbine, vindesine)	Antimicrotubule agents that inhibit axonal transport, causing sensorimotor axonal neuropathy
Taxanes (paclitaxel, paclitaxel albumin-stabilized nanoparticle formulation [Abraxane], docetaxel)	

Table 96.2 National Cancer Institute Common Terminology Criteria for Adverse Events (v4.03), Motor and Sensory Combined

Grade	Description	Action
0	Normal	No intervention
1	Asymptomatic, clinical or diagnostic observations only, weakness on examination only, loss of deep tendon reflexes or paresthesia	No intervention
2	Moderate symptoms, limiting instrumental activities of daily living	Decrease dosage
3	Severe symptoms, limiting self-care activities of daily living, assistive devices indicated	Decrease dosage or discontinue treatment
4	Life-threatening consequences, disabling	Discontinue treatment, urgent intervention indicated
5	Death	

Functional Limitations

The severity of the symptoms can range from mild discomfort and pain to severe disability and paralysis, with reduced functional independence and reduced quality of life. Weakness and proprioceptive impairments in the lower extremities may cause difficulty with mobility, balance, and gait, resulting in an increased risk of falls and injury. Weakness and sensory impairments in the upper extremities may cause difficulties with fine motor activities such as buttoning, tying shoelaces, cutting food, opening medication containers, typing on a computer keyboard, or operating a cell phone.

Diagnostic Studies

There is no standardized or "gold standard" diagnostic study to evaluate CIPN. Objective assessment such as nerve conduction studies, electromyography, and quantitative sensory testing can assess function and type of nerve damage (axonal vs demyelinating). These findings correlate poorly with the patient's report of symptoms, and changes in these tests can lag behind the onset of symptoms [7]. Other diagnostic tests should be used to screen for other causes of neuropathy (complete blood count; erythrocyte sedimentation rate; C-reactive protein level; vitamin B_{12}, methylmalonic acid, homocysteine, and folate concentrations; comprehensive metabolic panel to evaluate fasting blood glucose concentration; renal function and liver function tests; thyroid function tests; serum protein immunofixation electrophoresis; urinalysis and urine protein electrophoresis with immunofixation; drugs and toxin screen; paraneoplastic panel) [8]. Magnetic resonance imaging can also be done to rule out compression neuropathies and radiculopathy.

Differential Diagnosis

Myelopathy
Radiculopathy or polyradiculopathy
Polyradiculoneuropathy
Plexopathy
Mononeuropathy (e.g., carpal tunnel syndrome)
Peripheral neuropathy due to nonchemotherapy causes

Treatment

Initial

The main treatment of CIPN is to discontinue the offending agent or to reduce the dosage or frequency of administration. However, altering the treatment regimen needs to be weighed against the overall efficacy in treating the underlying disease. Many agents have been studied for prevention of CIPN (such as vitamin E and glutamine) but need larger randomized placebo-controlled trials to be scientifically proven to be effective. Other agents, such as calcium and magnesium infusions, glutathione, and α-lipoic acid, are currently under clinical trial investigation. Aside from stopping or decreasing the dose of the chemotherapeutic agent, there are no agents specifically approved for treatment of CIPN. Many drugs are being used on the basis of their efficacy in reducing pain intensity for other types of neuropathic pain, such as diabetic neuropathy [9]. In particular, pregabalin [10] and duloxetine [11] have been shown in clinical trials to be efficacious in reducing the symptoms of CIPN. Other agents commonly used for neuropathy, which have not been scientifically proven to be efficacious for CIPN, include gabapentin, venlafaxine, tricyclic antidepressants (amitriptyline and nortriptyline), and opioids. Topical agents such as capsaicin and lidocaine patches have also been found to be effective in certain forms of peripheral neuropathy [12]. A more recent topical gel formula, BAK-PLO (baclofen, amitriptyline, and ketamine in pluronic lecithin organogel), has shown moderate improvement in CIPN pain symptoms [13]. Medications are usually helpful in relieving the positive symptoms of CIPN (pain, paresthesia, dysesthesia, allodynia) but not effective for the treatment of negative neuropathic symptoms (weakness, numbness, or proprioceptive loss). Although rare, autonomic symptoms such as hypotension can be treated with getting up slowly, maintaining adequate salt and water intake, and using abdominal binders and compression stockings to decrease venous pooling. Resistant cases can be treated with midodrine or fludrocortisones.

Rehabilitation

Rehabilitation is successful when it is focused on specific individual impairments and subsequent disability, which could include imbalance, weakness, gait abnormality, and loss of proprioception. There should be a detailed evaluation for need of assistive devices or orthotics to prevent falls and to improve ambulation. Environmental and home modifications (removing throw rugs, installing adequate lighting) should be implemented as well. Aside from improving hand dexterity, occupational therapists can help with adaptive equipment (enlarged handles on eating utensils, buttonhooks) and increasing proprioceptive input, such as putting weights on the patient's arm.

Procedures

Neurostimulation with a transcutaneous nerve stimulation unit has been found to be helpful in some peripheral neuropathies but lacks sufficient evidence for treatment of CIPN. It can be used as an adjuvant therapy for patients with contraindications to pain medication or for whom it is ineffective, considering its ease of application and reversibility [6]. One small study suggested that acupuncture as a treatment of CIPN is effective in improving sensation, gait, and balance and that patients are able to reduce their use of pain medications [14]. There are no studies to date looking at the effectiveness of intrathecal medication delivery for the management of CIPN.

Surgery

Spinal cord stimulation has been reported to be successful in the treatment of many neuropathic pain syndromes [15] and should be reserved for patients with refractory pain. Spinal cord stimulation is a surgical procedure that involves placement of electrodes into the epidural space that send non-noxious electrical stimulation across the spine to displace painful sensations. This is used in refractory cases secondary to the risks and costs involved with the procedure.

Potential Disease Complications

Severe symptoms of CIPN can decrease a person's quality of life and impair activities of daily living. Also, CIPN can be a dose-limiting side effect that can interfere with the patient's ability to receive the full dose of cancer treatment or at a frequency required for optimal outcomes, which can eventually compromise survival.

Potential Treatment Complications

The main potential complication from the treatments or prevention of CIPN is the interference with the antineoplastic efficacy of chemotherapy. Other treatment complications arise from the different medications and their respective side effects. Gabapentin may cause somnolence, dizziness, gastrointestinal symptoms, mild edema, and cognitive impairment. Pregabalin has side effects similar to those of gabapentin but milder. Its faster onset of action, better absorption, and less need for titration make it a more preferred drug of choice. Duloxetine can cause nausea, xerostomia, constipation, or diarrhea. Duloxetine should be avoided with other serotonin reuptake inhibitors to prevent serotonin syndrome and also should be avoided with tamoxifen as it can decrease tamoxifen's active metabolite. Tricyclic antidepressants are usually less tolerated secondary to side effects of dry mouth, drowsiness, weight gain, and orthostasis.

References

[1] Windebank AJ, Grisold W. Chemotherapy-induced neuropathy. J Peripher Nerv Syst 2008;13:27–46.

[2] Siegal T, Haim N. Cisplatin-induced peripheral neuropathy: frequent off-therapy deterioration, demyelinating syndromes, and muscle cramps. Cancer 1990;66:1117–23.

[3] National Cancer Institute. Cancer therapy evaluation program. Common terminology criteria for adverse events (v4.03); December 2010. http://ctep.cancer.gov/protocolDevelopment/electronic_applications/ctc.htm.

[4] Cavaletti G, Frigeni B, Lanzani F, et al. The total neuropathy score as an assessment tool for grading the course of chemotherapy-induced peripheral neurotoxicity: comparison with the National Cancer Institute–Common Toxicity Scale. J Peripheral Nerv Syst 2007;12:210–5.

[5] Screnci D, McKeage MJ, Galettis P, et al. Relationships between hydrophobicity, reactivity, accumulation and peripheral nerve toxicity of a series of platinum drugs. Br J Cancer 2000;82:966–72.

[6] Stubblefield MD, Burstein HJ, Burton AW, et al. NCCN task force report: management of neuropathy in cancer. J Natl Compr Canc Netw 2009;7:S1–S26.

[7] Cavaletti G, Alberti P, Frigeni B, et al. Chemotherapy-induced neuropathy. Curr Treat Options Neurol 2011;13:180–90.

[8] England JD, Gronseth GS, Franklin G, et al. Evaluation of distal symmetric polyneuropathy: the role of laboratory and genetic testing (an evidence-based review). Muscle Nerve 2009;39:119.

[9] Bril V, England J, Franklin GM, et al. Evidence based guideline: treatment of painful diabetic neuropathy. PM R 2011;3:345–52.

[10] Saif MW, Syrigos K, Kaley K, et al. Role of pregabalin in treatment of oxaliplatin-induced sensory neuropathy. Anticancer Res 2010;30: 2927–33.

[11] Smith EML, Pang H, Cirrincione C, et al. A phase III double blind trial of duloxetine to treat painful chemotherapy-induced peripheral neuropathy. J Clin Oncol 2012;30(Suppl.).

[12] Attal N, Cruccu G, Baron R, et al. European Federation of Neurological Societies. EFNS guidelines on the pharmacological treatment of neuropathic pain; 2010 revision. Eur J Neurol 2010;17:1113–23.

[13] Barton D, Wos E, Qin R, et al. A double blind, placebo controlled trial of a topical treatment for chemotherapy induced peripheral neuropathy: NCCTG trial N06CA. Support Care Cancer 2011;19:833–41.

[14] Wong R, Sagar S. Acupuncture treatment for chemotherapy-induced peripheral neuropathy—a case series. Acupunct Med 2006;24:87–91.

[15] de Leon-Casasola OA. Spinal cord and peripheral nerve stimulation techniques for neuropathic pain. J Pain Symptom Manage 2009;38:S28–38.

CHAPTER 97

Chronic Pain Syndrome

Ali Mostoufi, MD, FAAPMR, FAAPM

Synonyms

Chronic pain disorder
Chronic intractable pain

ICD-9 Codes

338.4 Chronic pain syndrome
338.29 Chronic pain

ICD-10 Codes

G89.4 Chronic pain syndrome
G89.29 Chronic pain

Definition

Pain is an unpleasant sensory and emotional experience associated with actual or potential tissue damage [1]. Chronic pain is a pain status that persists beyond a reasonable expected healing period for the involved tissue. It is chronic if it persists for 6 months or more despite active treatment. It is called a syndrome because a constellation of symptoms develops in those patients facing chronic pain. The most common conditions leading to chronic pain syndrome (CPS) include headaches, repetitive stress injuries, back pain, whiplash injury, degenerative joint disorders, cancer, complex regional pain syndrome, shingles, fibromyalgia, neuropathy, central pain, and multiple surgeries [2]. In excess of 50 million Americans suffer from CPS and have a degree of impairment or disability from this condition [2]. Pain disorders cost $100 billion annually in lost work days, medical expenses, and other benefit costs [2]. Chronic pain is often a hidden problem and may be an issue that individuals are reluctant to share with family or friends. This may have an impact on the awareness of CPS in the community at large.

Chronic pain is prevalent in both adults and the pediatric population. Children suffering from chronic pain frequently continue to suffer from chronic pain as adolescents and young adults [3]. Some authors have reported a higher prevalence of CPS in individuals with a history of childhood abuse and personality disorder (borderline, narcissistic) [4]. CPS is more prevalent in women and by up to twofold in some diagnoses (e.g., fibromyalgia) [5,6]. Studies suggest a relationship between chronic pain and race as well as socioeconomic status. In a study of 3730 adults between ages 18 and 49, African Americans appear to have significantly more pain and disability and live in lower socioeconomic neighborhoods [7]. Living in a lower socioeconomic status neighborhood was associated with increased sensory, affective, pain-related disability and mood disorders [7].

Given its unclear pathophysiology and the lack of a definitive diagnostic test or successful treatment, CPS imposes a challenge to health care providers. Most patients are often unsatisfied with the treatment outcomes, leading to psychosocial stress, chronic pain behaviors, medication seeking, impairment, activity restriction, limited participation, and disability.

Symptoms

The primary symptom is a protracted pain that is out of proportion to the objective pathophysiologic process. Table 97.1 shows a list of common associated symptoms. Pain may be localized to a body segment, or it could be widespread. The measurement of pain severity is subjective and typically relies on the patient's report as well as on functional ability (work, activities of daily living, hobbies). The numeric (0-10) or the visual analogue scale that is used to assess pain often does not properly reflect the pain intensity, and despite adjustments to medical management, the reported pain level is unchanged. Because of this, clinicians may focus on functional gains as a measure of treatment success rather than on the patient's report of a decreased numeric or visual analogue scale score.

In CPS, there are often associated *pain behaviors* that help establish the diagnosis. Pain behaviors include assuming poor posture, abnormal gait (limping), facial grimacing, stiff movements, and use of assistive devices that have not been medically prescribed (canes, wheelchairs, and electric scooters). Decreasing pain behavior decreases the experience of pain. Behavioral treatments are a key component of multidisciplinary pain programs and can be effective for the relief of pain.

Mood and affect disorders including depression, anxiety, emotional instability, and anger are commonly associated

Table 97.1 Common Associated Symptoms and Signs in Chronic Pain Syndrome

Depression	Sleep disorders
Anxiety	Irritable bowel
Emotional lability	Cognitive difficulty (memory, concentration)
Chronic fatigue	Pain behaviors
Medication seeking	Dramatization of symptoms
Doctor shopping	Legal action—secondary gain

symptoms in patients with CPS [8]. Some studies have reported up to fourfold increased depression in patients with chronic back pain [9]. Chronicity of the pain, lack of clear etiology, and poor treatment outcomes contribute to the emotional aspect of this disorder. Just treating pain with medications without addressing the psychosocial component will lead to poor outcomes and further suffering. Part of the reasonable success associated with the multidisciplinary pain programs is related to management of the psychosocial component of the chronic pain.

Sleep disorders are prevalent in patients with CPS. Studies have shown that severity of insomnia contributes to the prediction of pain severity [10]. The insomnia associated with chronic pain needs to be anticipated and treated. Sleep-inducing medications often combined with cognitive-behavioral therapy can help improve insomnia. Sleep education, cognitive control and psychotherapy, sleep restriction, remaining passively awake, stimulus control therapy, sleep hygiene, relaxation training, and biofeedback are part of the cognitive-behavioral approach to treatment of insomnia [11]. Clinicians should be aware of increased cognitive impairment in elderly patients treated with medications for insomnia. This may lead to falls, injury, and increased pain [12].

Physical Examination

Physical examination is directed toward finding treatable causes of CPS. One of the most important parts of the physical examination is to observe the patient's gait, body motion, posture, and facial expression as well as abnormal pain behaviors. A systematic and detailed musculoskeletal and neurologic examination needs to be conducted. If the CPS follows an injury, focused examination of the injured body part is needed. Give-away weakness, nonmyotomal weakness, and nondermatomal numbness are often encountered on physical examination. If it is done repeatedly, there are likely to be inconsistencies in physical examination findings of a patient with CPS. Redirecting the patient's attention while repeating the examination may alter the findings and can point to pain behaviors. For example, diffuse tender points may not be tender if the patient's focus is diverted. Another example is a negative result of the seated straight-leg test (patients are less knowledgeable about it) versus a positive result of the supine straight-leg test in the same patient.

There are diagnosis-specific examination findings that may be noted, such as allodynia and trophic changes. These may be found in the area of the initial injury or in a different body part. Depending on the complaint, examination of other systems, including gastrointestinal, urologic, and pelvic girdle, may be indicated.

Functional Limitations

Typically, there is a disproportionate loss of function in patients with CPS when it is matched to the injury and the stated age. Fear-avoidance behavior will result in deconditioning and decline in function with activities of daily living [13]. Deconditioning leads to increased perception of pain, reduced quality of life, and further psychosocial stress and disability. If such abnormal pain behavior is reinforced by health care providers or the patient's family, it will result in chronicity of the pain and further decline in function.

Diagnostic Studies

In CPS, diagnostic studies are performed to find treatable causes that can lead to lingering pain. The results of such studies are often inconclusive or normal. Diagnostic testing may include laboratory work, electrodiagnostics, and imaging. Unless the presenting symptoms have changed, repeating costly diagnostic tests is of no value. Equally important is psychological testing. The Minnesota Multiphasic Personality Inventory is the most common psychological test used in patients with chronic pain and has been shown to help understand pain behaviors and the psychological impact on individuals with chronic pain [14] (Table 97.2).

Table 97.2 Differential Diagnosis of Chronic Pain Syndrome

Disorder	Description
Somatoform disorder	Group of psychiatric disorders, including somatization disorder, conversion disorder, hypochondriasis, and factitious disorder, that cause unexplained physical symptoms
Somatization disorder	Chronic physical symptoms that involve more than one part of the body, but no physical cause can be found Pain complaint is often associated with gastrointestinal, pseudoneurologic, and sexual complaints Symptoms are not intentionally fabricated
Conversion disorder	Dramatic loss of voluntary motor or sensory function (e.g., inability to walk, sudden blindness, paralysis) No evidence that the symptom is feigned or intentionally produced; loss of function is not due to medical illness
Hypochondriasis	Excessive preoccupation or worry about having a serious illness in absence of an actual medical condition
Factitious disorder	Deliberately produces or falsifies symptoms of illness for the sole purpose of assuming the sick role
Malingering	Fabricating or exaggerating the symptoms of mental or physical disorders for a variety of secondary gain motives

Differential Diagnosis

Somatoform disorder
Somatization disorder
Conversion disorder
Hypochondriasis
Factitious disorder
Malingering

Treatment

Initial

The initial treatment focuses on management of the pain and improvement in function. Numerous studies suggest a multidisciplinary approach for management of CPS [15]. These studies show that multidisciplinary treatments of chronic pain are superior to single-discipline treatments, such as medications or physical therapy. A team approach focuses on supporting patients in reaching individual goals. Goals should be improving pain and a better quality of life by means of enhancing physical and psychosocial function. The beneficial effect of multidisciplinary treatment is not limited to improvements in pain but also extend to variables such as return to work and use of the health care resources. An anesthesiologist, John J. Bonica, was the first to appreciate the need for a multidisciplinary approach to chronic pain [16]. Members of a multidisciplinary pain management team include a pain medicine specialist, mental health specialists, a physical therapist, an occupational therapist, the primary care provider, and the patient. Ideally, the rehabilitation component is 2 to 3 hours per day, 3 days per week, for several weeks [17]. In addition, patients will see mental health counselors weekly and are monitored by the pain specialist who is overseeing the entire care.

Education of the Patient

It is crucial for the patients dealing with CPS to be educated in the complexity of the disorder and possible factors affecting its management. Patients should be knowledgeable about their participation in the treatment plan. Both patient and family should have a good understanding of the multifactorial nature of chronic pain and the benefits of multidisciplinary management. Education of the patient should be done by all members of the treatment team.

Mental Health Treatment

Psychological interventions help patients find ways to accept the condition and to adjust to it. The focus of mental health counseling is to work on pain behaviors and to educate patients about the adverse consequences of this atypical behavior. Patients need to understand that negative thoughts stemming from pain will influence mood, behavior, sleep, and chronicity of the pain. Individual or group treatment may include biofeedback, relaxation training, coping mechanisms, clinical hypnosis, and cognitive therapy techniques [18]. These options may result in improved ability to manage pain. Advanced psychological or psychiatric treatments may include pharmacologic interventions to address emotional problems, affect disorders, anxiety disorders, sleep disturbances, and panic attacks. Common medications to treat psychological disorders in CPS are listed in Table 97.3. If opioid medications are being considered for treatment of CPS, a consultation with a pain psychologist is indicated to determine risk of future abuse.

Table 97.3 Common Medications Used to Address Psychological Issues in Chronic Pain Syndrome

Class	Examples
Antidepressants	Amitriptyline, nortriptyline, clonazepam, venlafaxine, citalopram, fluoxetine, bupropion, escitalopram, sertraline
Anxiolytics	Lorazepam, clonazepam, oxazepam, diazepam, alprazolam, buspirone
Mood stabilizers	Divalproex, lithium, gabapentin

Medications

In CPS, pain medications and adjunct medication are often not able to eliminate pain, but the analgesic effect may lead to increased function, improved rehabilitation outcomes, restored sleep, and enhanced mood. Commonly used pain medications and adjunct pharmaceutical substances in CPS are listed in Table 97.4. Pain medicine specialists should evaluate the patient, prescribe appropriate medications, monitor use and effect, and make adjustments when necessary. Short-term use of medications for pain is rarely worrisome, but prolonged use may increase the possibility of adverse reactions, including gastrointestinal side effects, cognitive and memory deficits, and gait instability. Use of opioid analgesics for chronic pain, although controversial, is fairly common. Opioid analgesics must be used with utmost caution and with understanding of the challenges related to chronic opioid management as well as the social stigma attached to them. The author recommends an opioid contract

Table 97.4 Analgesics and Adjunct Medications Prescribed for Chronic Pain

Class	Medication
Nonsteroidal analgesics	Salicylates: aspirin Arylalkanoic acids: diclofenac, etodolac, indomethacin, nabumetone Arylpropionic acids: ketoprofen, ibuprofen, naproxen Oxicams: piroxicam, meloxicam Coxibs: celecoxib
Opioid analgesics	Codeine, meperidine, hydrocodone, hydromorphone, morphine (short and long acting), oxycodone (short and long acting), methadone, fentanyl, tramadol, tapentadol
Partial μ opioid agonist and κ opioid receptor antagonist	Buprenorphine
Adjunct medications	Antiseizure medications: pregabalin, gabapentin, lamotrigine, topiramate, clonazepam Antidepressants (see Table 97.3)
Sedatives	Benzodiazepines: temazepam, diazepam, lorazepam Nonbenzodiazepines: eszopiclone, zaleplon, zolpidem

and involvement of the primary care physician in decision-making. Frequent and random blood or urine drug testing (for narcotic and illicit drugs), pill counts, opioid rotation, and routine reevaluation are needed to ensure safe use and effective treatment. Currently available evidence suggests that cannabis treatment is moderately efficacious for certain types of chronic pain (e.g., neuropathic, multiple sclerosis), but beneficial effects may be offset by potentially serious harms [19,20]. Smoked cannabis reduces pain, improves mood, and helps sleep in such patients [20]. More evidence from larger, well-designed trials is needed to clarify the true balance of benefits and harms.

Rehabilitation

Both outpatient and inpatient models of care are available to manage chronic pain, although it is difficult to obtain insurance coverage for inpatient care. This population of patients starts from a lower functional level, so the duration of treatment could be longer than the average for musculoskeletal pain issues. The rehabilitation team (physical therapist, occupational therapist, recreation therapist) will work with the patient to establish a structured day including supervised exercises. The basic exercise structure will include conditioning, stretching activities, progressive core and generalized strengthening, and aerobic exercise training. Aerobic exercise can be performed in an aquatic environment. The focus will also be on correction of body mechanics, proper posture, restoration of function, modification of maladaptive behaviors, and provision of pain relief by incorporation of modalities (heat, ice, and ultrasound) and relaxation techniques [21]. Deep tissue massage, myofascial release, transcutaneous electrical nerve stimulation, Pilates, Tai Chi, and yoga are additional treatments offered to patients with chronic pain. The accumulating evidence from recent reviews suggests that acupuncture is more than a placebo for commonly occurring chronic pain conditions [22]. Manipulative therapy, within the context of interdisciplinary treatment, has been shown to be an efficient and effective treatment to improve pain and function in patients with mechanical or compressive pain [23]. Transcutaneous electrical nerve stimulation units help relieve pain and foster independence in patients with chronic pain [21].

A recreational therapist examines previous interests of the patient and barriers to return to leisure activities. Within a formal program, recreational therapists evaluate and plan leisure activities that serve to promote mental and physical health. The challenge for the rehabilitation team remains the fear-avoidance behavior.

Procedures

Depending on the pain generator, specific procedures may help patients with CPS. This is especially true if previous medical care has insufficiently addressed the symptoms. Procedures that may be effective include neuraxial blocks, facet injections, radiofrequency neurotomy, sacroiliac injection, peripheral joint injections, peripheral nerve blocks, acupuncture, trigger point injections, and infiltration of inflamed bursa or tendons. Image guidance will enhance the accuracy of spine injections and will lead to improved outcome [24,25]. Chronic pain of complex regional pain syndrome (see Chapter 99) may be addressed with neuromodulation by spinal or peripheral nerve stimulator implantation. Implantable pain pumps are indicated in pain associated with terminal cancer but may also have limited indication in difficult to control pain of noncancer origin. When relative pain relief is achieved with procedures, tapering pain medications as well as increasing intensity of the rehabilitation program is encouraged.

Surgery

There is a limited indication for surgery in chronic pain. If the pain generator is identifiable and modern surgical methods are available to treat it, surgery may be considered. Patients suffering from chronic discogenic low back pain may benefit from interbody fusion or disc arthroplasty. Patients with end-stage degenerative joint disease suffering from chronic pain would likely benefit from arthroplasty. When it is clinically indicated and other noninvasive treatments have failed to help, an intrathecal drug delivery system and spinal or peripheral nerve stimulators could be considered, both of which require surgical implantation. It is possible that despite a surgical solution, the patient will continue to suffer from chronic pain.

Potential Disease Complications

Significant disability secondary to pain as well as suicidal ideation or attempt (secondary to psychosocial comorbidities) may complicate the clinical picture.

Potential Treatment Complications

Medications used to treat chronic pain can result in class-specific side effects. Nonsteroidal anti-inflammatory drugs commonly have gastrointestinal and renal side effects. Muscle relaxants, serotonin-norepinephrine reuptake inhibitors, anxiolytics, and tricyclics can cause central nervous system suppression. Narcotics can result in nausea, constipation, respiratory suppression, mental status changes, and suppressed endogenous opioids; dependency, tolerance, and abuse may also develop. Rehabilitation program intensity that is disproportionate to the functional status of the patient may lead to dissatisfaction and poor compliance and can worsen fear-avoidance behavior. Interventions and surgical care have their specific potential complications.

Acknowledgment

The author would like to thank resident physician Tony George for his valuable time and assistance in gathering updated literature on chronic pain syndrome.

References

[1] LaRocca H. A taxonomy of chronic pain syndromes. Spine 1992;17(Suppl.):S344–55.
[2] American Chronic Pain Association. Pain fact sheets. www.theacpa.org.
[3] Knook LM. The course of chronic pain with and without psychiatric disorders: a 6-year follow-up study from childhood to adolescence and young adulthood. J Clin Psychiatry 2012;73:e134–9.
[4] Craig TK, Drake H. The South London somatisation study II. Br J Psychiatry 1994;165:248–58.

[5] Unruh AM. Gender variations in clinical pain experience. Pain 1996;65:123–67.
[6] Wolfe F, Ross K, Anderson J, et al. The prevalence and characteristics of fibromyalgia in the general population. Arthritis Rheum 1995;38:19–28.
[7] Green CR. The association between race and neighborhood socioeconomic status in younger black and white adults with chronic pain. J Pain 2012;13:176–86.
[8] Currie SR, Wang J. Chronic back pain and major depression in the general Canadian population. Pain 2004;107:54–60.
[9] Sullivan MJ, Reesor K, Mikail S, Fisher R. The treatment of depression in chronic low back pain: review and recommendations. Pain 1992;50:5–13.
[10] Wilson KG, Eriksson MY, D'Eon JL, et al. Major depression and insomnia in chronic pain. Clin J Pain 2002;18:77–83.
[11] Pigeon WR. Treatment of adult insomnia with cognitive-behavioral therapy. J Clin Psychol 2010;66:1148–60.
[12] Jennifer G, Krista L, Nathan H. Sedative hypnotics in older people with insomnia: meta-analysis of risks and benefits. BMJ 2005;331:1169–73.
[13] Pfingsten M, Leibing E, Harter W, et al. Fear-avoidance behavior and anticipation of pain in patients with chronic low back pain: a randomized controlled study. Pain Med 2001;2:259–66.
[14] McGill JC, Lawlis GF, Selby D, et al. The relationship of Minnesota Multiphasic Personality Inventory (MMPI) profile clusters to pain behaviors. J Behav Med 1983;6:77–92.
[15] Scascighini L. Multidisciplinary treatment for chronic pain: a systematic review of interventions and outcomes. Rheumatology (Oxford) 2008;47:670–8.
[16] Schatman ME. Interdisciplinary chronic pain management: perspectives on history, current status and future viability. In: Fishman S, Ballantyne J, Rathmell J, editors. Bonica's management of pain. 4th ed. Philadelphia: Wolters Kluwer/Lippincott Williams & Wilkins; 2010. p. 1523–5.
[17] Gatchel R, Okifuji A. Evidence-based scientific data documenting the treatment and cost-effectiveness of pain programs for chronic nonmalignant pain. J Pain 2006;7:779–93.
[18] Weitz SE, Witt PH, Greenfield DP. Treatment of chronic pain syndrome. N J Med 2000;97:63–7.
[19] Martín-Sánchez E, Furukawa TA, Taylor J, Martin JL. Systematic review and meta-analysis of cannabis treatment for chronic pain. Pain Med 2009;10:1353–68.
[20] Ware M, Wang T, Shapiro S. Smoked cannabis for chronic neuropathic pain: a randomized controlled trial. CMAJ 2010;182:E694–701.
[21] Stanos SP, McLean J, Rader L. Physical medicine rehabilitation approach to pain. Med Clin North Am 2007;91:57–95.
[22] Hopton A. Acupuncture for chronic pain: is acupuncture more than an effective placebo? A systematic review of pooled data from meta-analyses. Pain Pract 2010;10:94–102.
[23] Lambert M. ICSI releases guideline on chronic pain assessment and management. Am Fam Physician 2010;82:434–9.
[24] Sehgal N, Shah RV, McKenzie-Brown AM, Everett CR. Diagnostic utility of facet (zygapophysial) joint injections in chronic spinal pain: a systematic review of evidence. Pain Physician 2005;8:211–24.
[25] Levin J, Wetzel R, Smuck M. The importance of image guidance during epidural injections: rates of incorrect needle placement during non–image guided epidural injections. J Spine 2012;1:2.

CHAPTER 98

Coccydynia

Ariana Vora, MD
Amy X. Yin, MD

Synonyms

Coccygodynia
Coccygalgia
Levator ani syndrome
Proctalgia fugax
Pelvic tension myalgia
Puborectalis syndrome

ICD-9 Codes

564.6 Proctalgia fugax
724.79 Coccydynia, coccygodynia

ICD-10 Codes

K59.4 Proctalgia fugax
M53.3 Coccydynia

Definition

Coccydynia is pain in the vicinity of the coccygeal bone at the base of the spine. It may be localized to the lower sacrum, the coccyx, or the adjacent muscles or soft tissues. Pain can be insidious or sudden in onset. Symptoms are usually triggered by sitting or rising from a sitting position.

The mean age at onset of coccydynia is 40 years, but it can occur over a wide range of ages [1]. The most common inciting factor is trauma to the coccyx or surrounding soft tissue from a vertical axial blow or cumulative trauma from a difficult vaginal delivery. Pathologic features may range from dislocated sacrococcygeal fracture to ligamentous damage of the caudal coccygeal segments. In most cases, the tip of the coccyx is subluxated or hypermobile [1] (Figs. 98.1 and 98.2).

The coccyx consists of three to five rudimentary vertebrae. The first coccygeal segment has transverse processes that articulate and occasionally fuse with the sacrum. This vertebra is usually separate from the remaining coccygeal vertebrae, which may partially or completely fuse, leading to anatomic variation of one to four total bony coccygeal segments [2].

The fibrous sacrococcygeal symphysis connects the sacrum to these segments of the coccyx. This joint is reinforced by sacrococcygeal ligaments, which enclose the final intervertebral foramen through which the S5 roots exit. The S4, S5, and coccygeal roots contribute to the coccygeal plexus, which provides rich somatic and autonomic innervation to the anus, perineum, and genitals [3]. The levator ani (innervated by S3-S5 nerve root branches through perineal and inferior rectal nerve branches of the pudendal nerve [4]) and coccygeal muscles (innervated by S3-S5 nerve root branches [5]) attach to and support the coccyx during defecation and childbirth. The gluteus maximus also attaches to the lateral coccyx and can contribute to a sensation of pressure while sitting.

Morphology of the coccyx may have a role in coccydynia. The coccyx that is markedly curved or angled forward, is anteriorly subluxed [2], or contains a bone spicule [6] is more prone to pain. Degeneration of disc structures [7] and referred pain from lumbar disc disease [2] have been implicated. There are also reported cases of rare coccydynia pathologic processes, including tuberculosis, tumors, and calcification of the joints or tendons. Prevalence of coccydynia is four to five times higher in women than in men [8,9]. In addition to obstetric trauma [10], the increased susceptibility to injury in women is attributed to anatomy as the female coccyx is more posterior in location and larger than the male coccyx [11]. Coccydynia is three times more frequent in obese women than in nonobese women [6], and this may be related to decreased pelvic rotation while sitting.

Symptoms

Coccygeal pain is located at the tip or sides of the coccyx. The quality of pain is usually dull and achy at baseline and intermittently sharp during activities that aggravate the symptoms. A sensation of pressure or an urge to defecate is also commonly described. Coccydynia has been associated with dyspareunia, dyschezia, dysmenorrhea, and piriformis syndrome. Symptoms are usually exacerbated by sitting on hard surfaces, prolonged sitting, and moving from the sitting to the standing position. Symptoms are generally relieved by taking weight off the coccyx.

Levator ani syndrome and proctalgia fugax are variants of coccydynia.

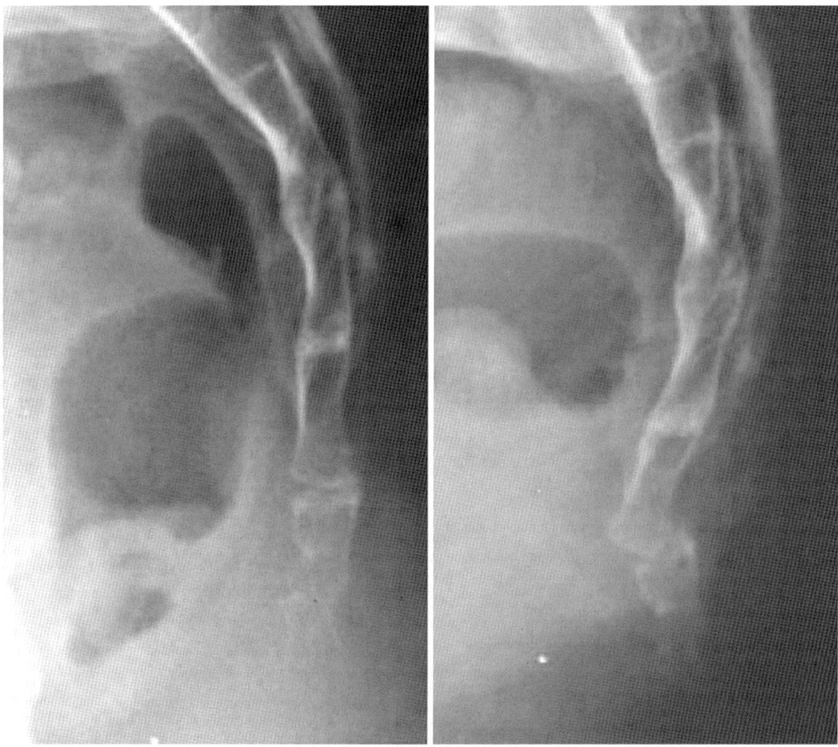

FIGURE 98.1 Lateral radiographs of coccygeal subluxation. *(From Doursounian L, Maigne JY, Faure F, et al. Coccygectomy for instability of the coccyx. Int Orthop 2004;28:176-179.)*

Levator ani syndrome is a dull ache or pressure sensation in the rectum, with pain episodes lasting more than 20 minutes at a time. Symptoms tend to be more severe during the day than at night. Symptoms may result from a hypertonic levator ani or puborectalis muscle or from inflammation of the arcus tendon of the levator ani [12,13]. This syndrome is associated with posterior traction of the puborectalis muscle and levator ani muscle tenderness on rectal examination.

Proctalgia fugax is the sudden onset of excruciating anal pain lasting a few seconds or minutes, then disappearing completely. Proctalgia fugax is characterized by spastic muscle contractions of the pelvic floor [14]. Episodes usually occur fewer than five times a year [15]. Symptoms are not typically related to defecation but are associated with sexual intercourse. Symptoms are usually nocturnal and awaken the patient from sleep. Unlike coccydynia, which is more common in women, proctalgia fugax occurs equally in men and women.

Physical Examination

- Inspect the sacrococcygeal region including the anus, surrounding skin, and soft tissue for cysts, fistulas, external hemorrhoids, and fissures.
- Palpate the pelvic area for evidence of lymphadenopathy or pelvic masses to rule out neoplastic or infectious disease (see the section on differential diagnosis).

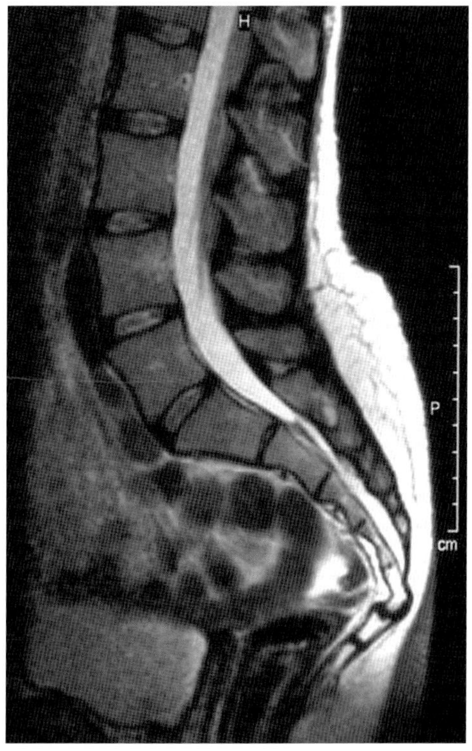

FIGURE 98.2 Sagittal magnetic resonance image of misaligned coccygeal fracture. *(From Pennicamp PH, Kraft CN, Stuetz A, et al. Coccygectomy for coccygodynia: does pathogenesis matter? J Trauma 2005;59:1414-1419.)*

- Assess for point tenderness or palpable abnormalities along the pelvic girdle, including the tip of the coccyx where a spicule would be located. It is also important to palpate surrounding joints. Classic findings in coccydynia are exquisite tenderness to direct palpation of the coccyx, sacrococcygeal ligaments, and pubococcygeal ligaments.
- Evaluate leg lengths, pelvic obliquity, sacroiliac motion, and sacroiliac joint tenderness because correction of these problems may be part of the treatment.

Lower extremity strength, reflexes, and sensation should be assessed for focal neurologic deficits and should be normal in coccydynia.

Digital rectal examination should include testing for occult blood, palpation for internal masses, and palpation of the levator ani muscles for tenderness. Manipulation of the coccygeal tip, the pubococcygeal ligament, and the sacrococcygeal joint should be performed to assess for tenderness and hypermobility [16].

Functional Limitations

Because coccydynia is often worsened by sitting, driving can become very painful. Sedentary work involving prolonged sitting may exacerbate symptoms; frequent breaks may be required. It is common to avoid social situations because of pain when sitting. Because of pressure to the coccyx and muscle contractions in the perineum during orgasm, sexual intimacy can worsen symptoms and is often avoided. Equestrian activities, cycling, and contact sports can also be particularly painful.

Diagnostic Studies

Coccydynia is often associated with subluxation or hypermobility of the tip of the coccyx (Fig. 98.3), which is usually seen on dynamic radiographs [1,17]. Single-position radiographs are seldom helpful in differentiating morphologic differences. Dynamic lateral radiographs are obtained in lateral and oblique views while the patient is sitting and standing. These demonstrate pelvis rotation and coccygeal mobility and may show fusion of the sacrococcygeal joint and superior intercoccygeal joints [1,17].

Bone scans and magnetic resonance imaging may show inflammation, fracture, or bone fragments. Because they are static tests, they are no more useful than dynamic radiographs in the diagnosis of hypermobility or subluxation [1]. However, advanced imaging modalities such as magnetic resonance imaging may be useful as second-line imaging to detect pericoccygeal inflammatory reactions, bone signal changes and edema, disc changes, or coccygeal tumors [18]. This may be clinically informative and guide treatment when dynamic radiographs are unremarkable.

Anal manometry testing has been described in the literature, with conflicting reports on its utility. The basis for manometry testing is the theory that prolonged sphincter contraction or dystonia may contribute to coccygeal pain. Abnormal anal manometric pressures support a diagnosis of proctalgia fugax, but the test is unlikely to diagnose proctalgia fugax because episodes are so infrequent. Anal manometry is not routinely recommended in the evaluation of coccydynia.

Differential Diagnosis

Coccygeal fracture, ligamentous strain, or dislocation
Bursitis at the coccygeal tip
Post-traumatic sacrococcygeal osteoarthritis
Coccygeal or lumbar disc degeneration
Internal pudendal nerve entrapment (Alcock canal syndrome)
Lower sacral nerve arachnoiditis
Rectal fissure
Pelvic or perirectal abscess
Pilonidal cyst or sinus
Thrombosed external hemorrhoid
Prostatitis
Pelvic organ prolapse
Tumors of the colorectum, sacrum, prostate, or ovaries
Postsurgical adhesion

Treatment

Initial

Conservative treatment is the "gold standard" for coccydynia as the natural history does not usually lead to deterioration. Medication management includes topical perianal

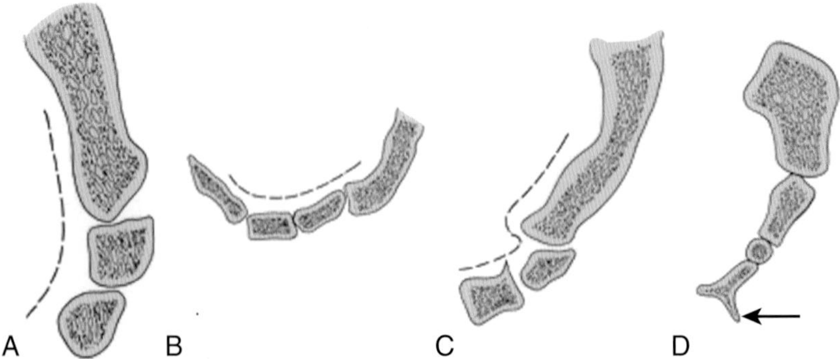

FIGURE 98.3 Schematic drawing of flexion mobility of the coccyx. **A,** Normal standing appearance of the coccyx. **B,** Increased flexion mobility of the coccyx when the patient is seated. **C,** Posterior subluxation of the coccyx when the patient is seated. **D,** Coccygeal spicule *(arrow)* arising from the dorsal surface of coccygeal segment. *(From Fogel GR, Cunningham PY, Esses DI. Coccygodynia: evaluation and management. J Am Acad Orthop Surg 2004;12:49-54.)*

lidocaine cream or gel, a bowel regimen or laxatives, acetaminophen, and nonsteroidal anti-inflammatory drugs.

Although they are relatively safe interventions, the efficacy of sitz baths, muscle relaxants, anticonvulsants, tricyclic antidepressants, acupuncture, iontophoresis, biofeedback, and electrogalvanic stimulation has not been established in the literature.

Rehabilitation

Ergonomic adaptation is commonly recommended. A trial of a doughnut-shaped pillow is always worthwhile to offload weight on the coccyx while sitting. Lifestyle recommendations, such as refraining from cycling, equestrian sports, or contact sports, may be beneficial.

Physical therapy should include pelvic massage and manipulation, pelvic relaxation techniques, pelvic floor strengthening exercises, pelvic joint mobilization, and postural correction. In patients with proctalgia fugax and levator ani symptoms, emphasis is placed on pelvic floor relaxation techniques. Correction of leg length discrepancy can help with referred sacroiliac pain. Psychological support is also crucial.

Procedures

Injection of the sacrococcygeal ligament and coccyx tip with 1% lidocaine can be diagnostic. A mixture of steroid (40mg methylprednisone) and a long-acting anesthetic (0.25% bupivacaine) may be used for therapeutic purposes [19]. This procedure can be done with use of physical landmarks. Ultrasound-guided injection can be considered but has not been well documented. Fluoroscopic guidance has been used, but utility may be limited as visualization of ligaments is not possible.

If there is dislocation of the coccyx, manipulation under anesthesia may be helpful, but there are no conclusive data on the efficacy of this approach.

Botulinum toxin injection of the puborectalis and pubococcygeus muscles may relieve pain associated with muscle hypertonicity [20,21].

Prolotherapy is an injection of proliferant solution that may relieve the pain of enthesopathy and facilitate regeneration of torn or painful sacrococcygeal and pubococcygeal ligaments. Its safety is well established. Although there are no randomized studies, a prospective observational study using dextrose prolotherapy for recalcitrant coccydynia indicated relief in 30 of 37 patients [22].

More recently, there has been some reported success with interventional procedures, such as ganglion impar nerve block or radiofrequency ablation. The ganglion impar (also known as ganglion of Walther) is a solitary structure in the precoccygeal space at the caudal end of the sympathetic chain implicated in nociceptive and sympathetic supply to the perineum. Various techniques including transcoccygeal and extracoccygeal approaches under fluoroscopy, ultrasonography, or computed tomography guidance have demonstrated pain relief in small prospective studies of patients with chronic perineal pain or coccydynia [23,24].

Pulsed radiofrequency has also been investigated for coccydynia. A prospective trial of 21 patients with coccydynia refractory to conservative management showed excellent to good results in 81% of patients [25].

These procedures may be considered possible alternatives to surgery.

Surgery

Most people recover with conservative treatment alone within weeks to months. A number of uncontrolled studies of patients with refractory coccydynia report pain relief with partial and total coccygectomy [1,26–30]. Successful treatment is usually associated with abnormal coccygeal motion.

Potential Disease Complications

Coccydynia is a symptom and not a disease. The primary complication is functional decline secondary to local pain, generally limiting sitting tolerance, sexual intercourse, and exercise tolerance.

Potential Treatment Complications

Gastrointestinal, hepatic, and renal complications may arise from prolonged use of acetaminophen or nonsteroidal anti-inflammatory drugs. Steroid injections may also be complicated by skin depigmentation and transient elevation in blood glucose level. Repeated steroid injections may result in ligamentous breakdown and altered mobility in the sacrococcygeal ligament. All procedures, including injections, nerve blocks, pulsed radiofrequency, and surgery, may result in infections. Coccygectomy complications also include bleeding or hematoma, delayed wound healing, and wound dehiscence [9].

References

[1] Fogel GR, Cunningham PY, Esses SI. Coccygodynia: evaluation and management. J Am Acad Orthop Surg 2004;12:49–54.

[2] Postacchini F, Massobrio M. Idiopathic coccygodynia. Analysis of fifty-one operative cases and a radiographic study of the normal coccyx. J Bone Joint Surg Am 1983;65:1116–24.

[3] DeAndres J, Chaves S. Coccygodynia: a proposal for an algorithm for treatment. J Pain 2003;4:257–66.

[4] Grigorescu BA, Lazarou G, Olson TR, et al. Innervation of the levator ani muscles: description of the nerve branches to the pubococcygeus, iliococcygeus, and puborectalis muscles. Int Urogynecol J Pelvic Floor Dysfunct 2008;19:107–16.

[5] Roshanravan SM, Wieslander CK, Schaffer JI, Corton MM. Neurovascular anatomy of the sacrospinous ligament region in female cadavers: implications in sacrospinous ligament fixation. Am J Obstet Gynecol 2007;197:660.e1–6.

[6] Maigne JY, Doursounian L, Chatellier G. Causes and mechanisms of common coccydynia: role of body mass index and coccygeal trauma. Spine (Phila Pa 1976) 2000;25:3072–9.

[7] Maigne JY, Guedj S, Straus C. Idiopathic coccygodynia: lateral roentgenograms in the sitting position and coccygeal discography. Spine (Phila Pa 1976) 1994;19:930–4.

[8] Ryder I, Alexander J. Coccydynia: a woman's tail. Midwifery 2000;16:155–60.

[9] Karadimas EJ, Trypsiannis G, Giannoudis PV. Surgical treatment of coccygodynia: an analytic review of the literature. Eur Spine J 2011;20:698–705.

[10] Kaushal R, Bhanot A, Luthra S, et al. Intrapartum coccygeal fracture, a cause for postpartum coccydynia: a case report. J Surg Orthop Adv 2005;14:136–7.

[11] Yamashita K. Radiological study of 1500 coccyces. Nippon Seikeigeka Gakkai Zasshi 1988;62:23–36.

[12] Park DH, Yoon SG, Kim KU, et al. Comparison study between local electrogalvanic stimulation and local injection therapy in levator ani syndrome. Int J Colorectal Dis 2005;20:272–6.

[13] Mazza L, Formento E, Fronda G. Anorectal and perineal pain: new pathophysiological hypothesis. Tech Coloproctol 2004;8:77–83.
[14] Pfenninger JL, Zainea GG. Common anorectal conditions: part I, symptoms and complaints. Am Fam Physician 2001;63:2391–8.
[15] Whitehead WE, Wald A, Diamant NE, et al. Functional disorders of the anus and rectum. Gut 1999;45(Suppl. 2):II55–9.
[16] Wald A. Functional anorectal and pelvic pain. Gastroenterol Clin North Am 2001;30:243–51.
[17] Hodges SD, Eck JC, Humphreys SC. A treatment and outcomes analysis of patients with coccydynia. Spine J 2002;4:138–40.
[18] Maigne JY, Pigeau I, Roger B. Magnetic resonance imaging findings in the painful adult coccyx. Eur Spine J 2012;21:2097–104.
[19] Wray CC, Easom S, Hoskinson J. Coccydynia. Aetiology and treatment. J Bone Joint Surg Br 1991;73:335–8.
[20] Jarvis SK, Abbott JA, Lenart MG, et al. Pilot study of botulinum toxin type A in the treatment of chronic pelvic pain associated with spasm of the levator ani muscles. Aust N Z J Obstet Gynaecol 2004;44:46–50.
[21] Katsinelos P, Kalomenopoulou M, Christodoulou K, et al. Treatment of proctalgia fugax with botulinum A toxin. Eur J Gastroenterol Hepatol 2001;13:1371–3.
[22] Khan SA, Kumar A, Varshney MK, et al. Dextrose prolotherapy for recalcitrant coccygodynia. J Orthop Surg (Hong Kong) 2008;16:27–9.
[23] Datir A, Connell D. CT-guided injection for ganglion impar blockade: a radiological approach to the management of coccydynia. Clin Radiol 2010;65:21–5.
[24] Gupta D, Jain R, Mishra S, et al. Ultrasonography reinvents the originally described technique for ganglion impar neurolysis in perianal cancer pain. Anesth Analg 2008;107:1390–2.
[25] Atim A, Ergin A, Bilgiç S, et al. Pulsed radiofrequency in the treatment of coccygodynia. Agri 2011;23:1–6.
[26] Karalezli K, Iltar S, Irgit K, et al. Coccygectomy in the treatment of coccygodynia. Acta Orthop Belg 2004;70:583–5.
[27] Perkins R, Schofferman J, Reynolds J. Coccygectomy for severe refractory sacrococcygeal joint pain. J Spinal Disord Tech 2003;16:100–3.
[28] Doursounian L, Maigne JY, Faure F, Chatellier G. Coccygectomy for instability of the coccyx. Int Orthop 2004;28:176–9.
[29] Pennicamp PH, Kraft CN, Stuetz A, et al. Coccygectomy for coccygodynia: does pathogenesis matter? J Trauma 2005;59:1414–9.
[30] Wood KB, Mehbod AA. Operative treatment for coccygodynia. J Spinal Disord Tech 2004;17:511–5.

CHAPTER 99

Complex Regional Pain Syndrome

Jiaxin Tran, MD

V.S. Ramachandran, MD, PhD

Eric L. Altschuler, MD, PhD

Synonyms

Reflex sympathetic dystrophy
Post-traumatic dystrophy
Sudeck atrophy
Sudeck syndrome
Causalgia
Osteodystrophy
Neuroalgodystrophy
Post-traumatic osteoporosis
Shoulder-hand syndrome
Sympathetically maintained pain

ICD-9 Codes

337.21 Reflex sympathetic dystrophy of the upper limb
337.22 Reflex sympathetic dystrophy of the lower limb
337.29 Reflex sympathetic dystrophy of other specified site
354.4 Causalgia of upper limb
355.71 Causalgia of lower limb
355.9 Mononeuritis of unspecified site, causalgia NOS

ICD-10 Codes

G90.511 Complex regional pain syndrome I of right upper limb
G90.512 Complex regional pain syndrome I of left upper limb
G90.519 Complex regional pain syndrome I of unspecified upper limb
G90.521 Complex regional pain syndrome I of right lower limb
G90.522 Complex regional pain syndrome I of left lower limb
G90.529 Complex regional pain syndrome I of unspecified lower limb
G90.59 Complex regional pain syndrome I of other specified site
G56.40 Causalgia of unspecified upper limb
G56.41 Causalgia of right upper limb
G56.42 Causalgia of left upper limb
G57.70 Causalgia of unspecified lower limb
G57.71 Causalgia of right lower limb
G57.72 Causalgia of left lower limb
G58.9 Mononeuropathy, unspecified

Definition

Complex regional pain syndrome (CRPS) is a perplexing medical condition. CRPS begins when a patient has an injury—to a nerve, bone, soft tissue, or connective tissue. The injury heals as assessed by both clinical examination and imaging, yet the patient still has pain significantly out of proportion not only to the healed injury but at times even to the injury itself. In addition to pain, the patient can have hyperesthesia or allodynia at the site of the injury. Curiously, the temperature of the affected limb can be different from that of the other side, and there can be hair, nail, and skin changes. In some cases, these changes can spread beyond the injury site to the entire limb, and in the worst case, in addition to excruciating pain and hyperesthesia, the skin becomes pachydermic.

Before 1994, this bizarre disease and constellation of symptoms was known, among other names, as reflex sympathetic dystrophy. Despite this moniker, it was never proved that the sympathetic nervous system mediates all the components of the disease, nor was a peripheral reflex or feedback loop causing the disease found. In 1994, a conference was held to clarify the classification of the disease [1]. It was renamed CRPS with two classifications, CRPS II for apparent major nerve injury and CRPS I for no major nerve injury. The disease is complex, and it can often be regional rather than confined to a dermatome, myotome, or territory of a single peripheral nerve. Pain is the hallmark of the disease and, for a patient with history of an injury, the sine qua non of diagnosis. It is multifaceted.

The new name, interestingly, is less specific than the former name, expressing the current lack of a full understanding of the disease. More than a decade ago, one of us (V.S.R.) suggested that central remapping of sensory neurons in the cerebral cortex in response to a peripheral injury to the corresponding body area might be a root cause of pain and ultimately other problems in this condition [2]. This hypothesis has not only collected evidence since but led to new and potentially most useful treatments [3].

CRPS is relatively rare. Even with fracture, the most common inciting event, only 1% of patients develop CRPS [4]. The incidence has been estimated to be up to 26 per 100,000 person-years [5]. The incidence of CRPS type I is generally higher than that of CRPS type II. The lower extremity is more often affected than the upper extremity. Female sex, adult age, postmenopausal status, and smoking are all risk factors for its development [6]. In the pediatric population, the incidence of CRPS increases just before puberty [7].

The pathophysiologic mechanism of the disease is, again, poorly understood. There is emerging evidence that CRPS does not only affect the peripheral nervous system. Functional and structural reorganization [8] of the central nervous system has been demonstrated with functional magnetic resonance imaging [9], single-photon emission computed tomography, electroencephalography, and transcranial magnetic stimulation mapping. Neuroplasticity of both the cortical somatosensory [10] and motor [11] systems is implicated. Distorted sensory and motor mapping is hypothesized to promote spontaneous pain and neglect symptoms in CRPS.

Symptoms

CRPS is a clinical diagnosis. The diagnosis can be suggested by the history of present illness alone. An individual experiences an injury. The injury can come in a variety of forms, whether traumatic (e.g., crush injury, gunshot wound, burn, or protracted labor [12]) or nontraumatic (e.g., leprosy [13]). The "injury" can also be an otherwise uncomplicated surgery. While healing takes place, the individual develops pain variably progressive in intensity, area involvement, and duration. Patients with both CRPS type I and type II may report neuropathic pain that is often intense, constant, burning, and present even without stimulation or movement. Symptoms are not confined to a particular nerve or anatomic territory; CRPS can spread [14] to the contralateral limb and even progress to all four limbs. In addition to pain, motor complaints are common and include weakness, cramps, and stiffness. There may also be signs of neglect [15], or more subtly, some patients may refer to the affected limb in the third person (e.g., "*it* is not moving"). It is important to ask about abnormal sweating patterns, localized edema, and skin flushing as clues of autonomic dysfunction in the history.

Symptoms and signs of CRPS are historically grouped into three stages. Stage 1 consists of severe pain and inflammatory signs (e.g., pitting edema, rubor, increased hair and nail growth). Stage 2 is marked by more intense pain, brawny edema, pallor, ridged nails, and osteoporosis. Unyielding pain and irreversible skin and bone changes (e.g., dystrophy, contracture, and extensive osteoporosis) are the primary features of stage 3. Although CRPS does not always follow a stepwise progression, these stages are useful descriptively. Classifying the syndrome solely on the basis of the severity of pain (i.e., mild, moderate, and severe) may be appropriate to follow its clinical course over time. We also classify CRPS as irreversible (i.e., presence of pachydermic skin changes) or potentially fully reversible (i.e., absence of pachydermic skin changes).

Mood disturbance is common in the chronic stages of the illness. Patients often report anxiety as the disease progresses beyond the second month; and by the sixth month, all patients will exhibit varying degrees of depression, sleep disturbance, and anxiety [16].

Physical Examination

Begin the examination by inspecting for signs of injury at or near the affected site. The injury may have been long ago and only a scar remains. If possible, compare all findings with the contralateral side to identify subtle asymmetry. Look for evidence of autonomic disturbances that are manifested as localized edema, skin color changes, and abnormal sweating pattern; note that skin color is best observed under natural light. Late-stage CRPS is characterized by trophic changes, such as abnormal hair and nail growth, thin and shiny skin, and fibrosis. At rest, disuse atrophy is the most apparent motor disturbance, but spontaneous muscle fasciculation, tremor, and cramp in the supporting muscles of the limb may also be observed.

Proceed to gentle palpation of the affected area. Make note of marked temperature asymmetry. Studies have shown that a clinician can adequately identify temperature and limb circumference asymmetry without special instruments [17]. Nonetheless, an infrared thermometer or a surface-probe thermometer can give more precise measurements. A temperature difference of more than 1.1° C between the affected area and a nonaffected, homologous body part is significant [1], but clinicians should have a low index of suspicion for CRPS such that even a small temperature change may be clinically relevant. Next, estimate the extent of involvement by sensory disturbances, such as increased sensitivity (hyperesthesia), exaggerated pain response to a painful stimulus (hyperalgesia), pain to an innocuous stimulus (allodynia), and paradoxically in some patients, hypoesthesia [18]. Ascertain abnormal findings with repeated testing. The sensory examination includes tests for light touch, pinprick, temperature, vibration, and proprioception. Consider testing the forehead because sensory disturbances on the ipsilateral side have been described [19].

Have the patient actively range the affected joints. Make note of difficulty with initiation of motion and range of motion deficits, which in turn require passive range to assess for contracture. The clinician can then perform a thorough musculoskeletal and neurologic examination including strength, stability, and reflexes to assess for deficits, be they related or unrelated to the CRPS.

Functional Limitations

The most immediate effects are dysfunction in activities of daily living from disuse of the affected limb. Lower limb involvement results in gait impairment. Even properly treated patients may continue to experience disability and decreased quality of life in the long term [20]. Permanent disability may ensue if contracture develops over time. Chronic pain also leads to the well-known syndrome of deconditioning, sleep disturbance, anxiety, and depression. With inadequate treatment, quality of life can be severely affected, often with devastating social, recreational, financial, and vocational consequences.

Diagnostic Studies

Several sets of diagnostic criteria (e.g., Bruehl and Veldman) exist, and none has been shown to be superior [21]. The International Association for the Study of Pain (IASP) criteria are most widely referenced in the literature and made up of the following four components: (1) presence of an identifiable noxious event or cause of immobilization; (2) persistent pain, allodynia, or hyperalgesia, disproportionate to any inciting event; (3) edema, changes in skin blood flow, or abnormal sudomotor activity; and (4) exclusion of other diagnoses as the cause of these symptoms [1]. IASP criteria are notably limited by poor inter-rater reliability and a specificity of only 36% [22]. They were subsequently revised in 2003 and published in 2007 as the Budapest criteria, which boast an increased specificity [23]. The Budapest criteria replace the second and third components of IASP criteria with at least one symptom and one sign in three of the following four categories: sensory, vasomotor, sudomotor or edema, and motor or trophic changes.

There is no "gold standard" for diagnosis of CRPS. It is a diagnosis of exclusion. Electromyography and nerve conduction studies can help identify nerve injury, if there is clinical suspicion. Doppler flowmeter, vascular scintigraphy, and vital capillaroscopy evaluate for vasomotor changes. Quantitative sudomotor axon reflex testing measures sweat output after mild electrical stimulation.

Plain films are often normal early in the course. Demineralization may become evident by the second month. Magnetic resonance imaging demonstrates nonspecific marrow edema, soft tissue swelling, and joint effusion. Even bone scintigraphy, in which the most suggestive finding is increased periarticular activity in the affected limb, has variable sensitivity and specificity [24]. A recent meta-analysis supports the use of triple-phase bone scan for assessment owing to its high sensitivity and negative predictive value [25].

Workup should focus on excluding other diagnoses. Frequently ordered tests include routine blood tests to screen for infection and acute inflammation, plain radiographs to screen for fracture, and electrodiagnostics to screen for coexisting nerve injury and muscle fiber loss.

Differential Diagnosis

Cellulitis
Lymphedema
Occult or stress fracture
Acute synovitis
Septic arthritis
Septic tenosynovitis
Scleroderma
Plexitis, peripheral neuropathy
Postherpetic neuralgia
Peripheral vascular disease, arterial insufficiency
Deep venous thrombosis, phlebitis
Vasculitis

Treatment

The old saying that prevention is the best treatment may hold true for CRPS. Since 1999 [26], a series of studies have suggested that a 50-day regimen of daily vitamin C of at least 500 mg, started immediately after upper extremity trauma [27] or extremity surgery [28]—including foot, ankle, distal radius, hand, and wrist—may prevent the development of CRPS. This recommendation has been adopted into the 2010 American Academy of Orthopaedic Surgeons clinical guideline [29].

When prevention is ineffective, aggressive management of CRPS early in the course of disease may minimize long-term impairment. Pharmacotherapy, physical therapy, interventional pain procedures, and neuromodulation are common management options. The treatment of CRPS, in reality, is highly controversial because quality evidence is lacking.

Anti-inflammatory Medications

Inflammation is implicated at least in the early development of CRPS; nonsteroidal anti-inflammatory drugs are thus often employed as first-line agents. There is no definitive evidence supporting this practice. Topical formulations of dimethyl sulfoxide and *N*-acetylcysteine, both free radical scavengers thought to buffer the excess byproducts from inflammatory processes, are viable options to consider. Three randomized controlled studies (RCTs) found topical dimethyl sulfoxide 50% and *N*-acetylcysteine formulations somewhat effective at reducing pain and improving function in CRPS type I [30]. Corticosteroids have also been used to manage inflammation with mixed success. Two RCTs showed that oral prednisone may improve inflammatory symptoms [31]. Conversely, an RCT of intrathecal methylprednisolone was stopped prematurely because there was no benefit at midpoint analysis [32].

Neuropathic Medications

Antidepressants and anticonvulsants have been extensively studied, and there is strong evidence demonstrating their effectiveness in treating neuropathic pain. There is, however, not yet a clinical study of antidepressants specifically on the treatment of CRPS. One RCT [33] demonstrated some efficacy of gabapentin, yet no statistical significance was found in another study [34]. The sedating side effects of both classes of medication can provide the added benefit of treating sleep disturbance.

Opioids and NMDA Receptor Antagonists

Opioids may be useful in the acute stages of CRPS for control of pain. Still, their use in chronic pain conditions remains controversial. Methadone may be considered for opioid-tolerant patients with severe neuropathic pain because of its *N*-methyl-D-aspartate (NMDA) receptor antagonist activity, which attenuates pain transmission through dorsal horn cells to the central nervous system.

Intravenous and 10% topical formulations of ketamine, a noncompetitive NMDA receptor antagonist, have been shown to significantly improve pain [35]. However, intravenous administration of ketamine warrants close monitoring, given a risk of psychedelic crisis, and repeated administrations have been associated with acute transaminitis [36]. Memantine is another noncompetitive NMDA receptor antagonist; its effectiveness when it is used alone has to be validated [37].

Bisphosphonates

Focal demineralization is a notable radiographic feature of CRPS, with a small contribution from disuse. Bisphosphonates are used to treat pathologic bone metabolism. Four RCTs have suggested that both oral and intravenous bisphosphonate formulations can improve pain in the acute inflammatory phase [32]. More research is necessary to determine the optimum formulation, dosage, and duration.

Novel Medications

A handful of novel medications were studied in the past decade. These studies are small and report only short-term outcomes, but they represent the continued effort of the medical community to find a better pharmacologic agent to treat CRPS. Tadalafil, a phosphodiesterase inhibitor aimed at reversal of the vasoconstrictive effect of CRPS, is one such medication under investigation and may provide pain reduction for patients with cold CRPS in the lower limbs [38]. Another promising RCT finds intravenous magnesium to improve pain and quality of life at 12 weeks after administration [39]. Last but not least is intravenous immune globulin [40], which significantly improved pain for three patients in an RCT with a sample size of 13.

Despite the early success described, many pharmacologic agents have proved ineffective. For more details on various medications that have been examined—including baclofen, lidocaine, and intranasal calcitonin—refer to a most comprehensive systematic review by Van Zundert et al [41].

Rehabilitation

Physical and Occupational Therapy

Existing RCTs find both physical and occupational therapies effective at improving pain and functional level. Relative to occupational therapy, physical therapy may provide quicker pain reduction at a lower cost [42]. Studies are unable to detect greater benefit with varying of the frequency of physical therapy or use of specific aspects of therapy.

Complementary Therapies

Three large RCTs suggest that acupuncture, opposing needling, and electroacupuncture for post-stroke CRPS may improve pain, edema, and function [43]. Similar benefits were not apparent in a separate RCT studying post-traumatic CRPS [44]. Hyperbaric oxygen therapy may improve pain and edema on the basis of the result of one medium-sized RCT [45]. Last but not least, Qigong may provide long-term anxiety relief for chronic, refractory CRPS [46].

Mirror Therapy

Mirror therapy was first devised as a therapeutic tool to relieve pain in amputees from a poorly mobile or spasmodic phantom limb [47]. In mirror therapy, a patient moves both limbs—the affected limb as best as possible—while watching the reflection of the good limb (Fig. 99.1). Visual feedback from the reflection of the good limb—which looks like the affected limb moving normally—feeds into and improves the motor control loop of the affected limb, ideally improving movement of the affected limb [3]. One of us (V.S.R.) was the first to suggest that mirror therapy might be helpful in reflex sympathetic dystrophy/CRPS [2]. RCTs [48,49] and case reports [3,50,51] have since affirmed the benefit of mirror therapy in CRPS.

Mirror therapy can be useful by visual feedback, providing an "active assist" to promote and to improve movement. It can also reduce hyperesthesia and allodynia through progressive contact exercises of both limbs while the reflection of the unaffected limb is watched in the mirror.

In general, we urge patients to use the limb as much as is safely possible and to take back "ownership" of the limb (e.g., not to speak of the limb in the third person). The hope is that with early intervention for CRPS with mirror therapy and rehabilitation, pharmacologic, and other methods, it may be possible to prevent patients from progressing to the pachydermic, irreversible stage of CRPS.

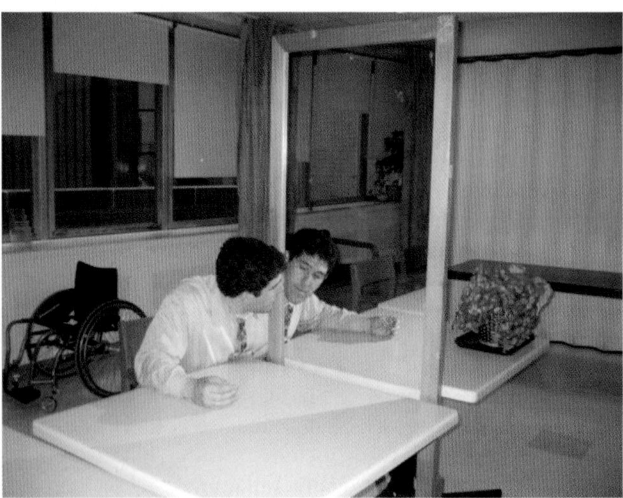

FIGURE 99.1 The affected limb (left upper in this picture) is hidden behind the mirror in mirror therapy. The subject then follows the reflection of the healthy limb to mobilize both limbs simultaneously.

Procedures

Neuromodulation

Repetitive transcranial magnetic stimulation, in contrast to spinal cord stimulation, is approved by the Food and Drug Administration only for resistant major depressive disorder. It employs electromagnetic currents to stimulate cortical targets, which has previously been shown effective in chronic pain management. Two RTCs [52,53] for CRPS found repetitive transcranial magnetic stimulation to improve pain, possibly in the sensory discrimination and emotional dimensions of pain. An early attempt to use direct motor cortex electrical stimulation has had some success, but further study is needed [54].

Regional Procedures

Two types of regional sympathetic blocks are commonly used for CRPS: stellate ganglion block and lumbar sympathetic block. Stellate ganglion block, also known as cervicothoracic ganglion block, targets ganglion cells along the pharynx. It theoretically interrupts afferent painful signals from the upper limbs. Lumbar sympathetic block targets ganglion cells along the spine at L2-L4 levels and attempts to interrupt afferent painful signals from the lower limbs. The effectiveness of stellate ganglion and lumbar sympathetic blocks is variable in existing RCTs and on average shows only transient analgesic benefits [55]. Of note, compared with lumbar sympathetic block using bupivacaine alone, one small RCT found that the addition of botulinum toxin A may prolong the effects [56]. Longer lasting effects from stellate ganglion and lumbar sympathetic blocks may be achieved with radiofrequency lumbar sympathectomy and phenol neurolysis, but no further studies have been published [57].

Bier block can be used in the upper or lower limbs, and it involves use of a tourniquet to restrain blood flow into the affected limb while intravenous local anesthetic is administered. A small RCT in the 1980s found serial Bier blocks with guanethidine to be as effective as serial Bier block with lidocaine in management of upper limb reflex sympathetic dystrophy pain. However, recent RCTs did not find intravenous guanethidine, bupivacaine, or methylprednisolone effective for most patients [58].

Surgery

Spinal cord stimulation is approved by the Food and Drug Administration for treatment of refractory CRPS and neuropathic pain. Its action is attributed to central excitability suppression. Three medium-sized RCTs found the combination of spinal cord stimulation with physical therapy to be more effective than physical therapy alone for pain control in the short term, but this result does not appear to carry over in the long term [59]. Percutaneous cervicothoracic or lumbar sympathectomy is reserved for patients with severe CRPS, but effectiveness is questionable [60].

Potential Disease Complications

Functional disability from pain and hyperesthesia of CRPS is a significant concern. The most feared complication is progression of an affected limb to pachydermia, an irreversible condition. Patients will then face severe, chronic pain. Limb contracture and muscle atrophy can result in loss of extremity function and potentially permanent disability.

Potential Treatment Complications

Adverse effects of pharmacotherapy vary according to the medication selected. For example, long courses of corticosteroids can produce significant endocrinologic disturbances and should be avoided; and nonsteroidal anti-inflammatory drugs have well-known adverse effects on the gastric, hepatic, and renal systems. Because polypharmacy may be necessary, care should be used in selection of interacting drugs that do not result in untoward side effects. Potential complications of stellate ganglion block are inadvertent arterial injection and seizures or recurrent laryngeal nerve injury. Perforation of the aorta, vena cava, or kidney can occur during lumbar sympathetic block. The most common complications of spinal cord stimulation include hardware failure, lead migration, infection, and failure to provide pain relief. Even for seemingly benign rehabilitation such as mirror therapy, one should be aware that patients can be at an increased risk for fall when they have increased mobility.

References

[1] Merskey H, Bogduk N. Classification of chronic pain: descriptions of chronic pain syndromes and definitions of pain terms. Seattle, Wash: IASP Press; 1994.

[2] Ramachandran VS. Decade of the brain symposium. University of California at San Diego; 1998.

[3] Ramachandran VS, Altschuler EL. The use of visual feedback, in particular mirror visual feedback, in restoring brain function. Brain 2009;132(Pt 7):1693–710.

[4] Baron R, Binder A, Pappagallo M. Complex regional pain syndromes. In: Pappagallo M, editor. The neurological basis of pain. New York: McGraw-Hill; 2005. p. 359–78.

[5] de Mos M, de Bruijn AG, Huygen FJ, et al. The incidence of complex regional pain syndrome: a population-based study. Pain 2007;129:12–20.

[6] An HS, Hawthorne KB, Jackson WT. Reflex sympathetic dystrophy and cigarette smoking. J Hand Surg Am 1988;13:458–60.

[7] Wilder RT. Management of pediatric patients with complex regional pain syndrome. Clin J Pain 2006;22:443–8.

[8] Schwenkreis P, Maier C, Tegenthoff M. Functional imaging of central nervous system involvement in complex regional pain syndrome. AJNR Am J Neuroradiol 2009;30:1279–84.

[9] Freund W, Wunderlich AP, Stuber G, et al. Different activation of opercular and posterior cingulate cortex (PCC) in patients with complex regional pain syndrome (CRPS I) compared with healthy controls during perception of electrically induced pain: a functional MRI study. Clin J Pain 2010;26:339–47.

[10] Maihöfner C, Handwerker HO, Neundörfer B, Birklein F. Cortical reorganization during recovery from complex regional pain syndrome. Neurology 2004;63:693–701.

[11] Maihöfner C, Baron R, DeCol R, et al. The motor system shows adaptive changes in complex regional pain syndrome. Brain 2007;130:2671–87.

[12] Butchart AG, Mathews M, Surendran A. Complex regional pain syndrome following protracted labour. Anaesthesia 2012;67:1272–4.

[13] Garg R, Dehran M. Leprosy: a precipitating factor for complex regional pain syndrome. Minerva Anestesiol 2010 Sep;76(9):758–60.

[14] van Rijn MA, Marinus J, Putter H, et al. Spreading of complex regional pain syndrome: not a random process. J Neural Transm 2011;118:1301–9.

[15] Kolb L, Lang C, Seifert F, Maihöfner C. Cognitive correlates of "neglect-like syndrome" in patients with complex regional pain syndrome. Pain 2012;153:1063–73.

[16] Brown GK. A causal analysis of chronic pain and depression. J Abnorm Psychol 1990;99:127–37.

[17] Perez RS, Burm PE, Zuurmond WW, et al. Physicians' assessments versus measured symptoms of complex regional pain syndrome type 1: presence and severity. Clin J Pain 2005;21:272–6.

[18] Rommel O, Malin JP, Zenz M, et al. Quantitative sensory testing, neurophysiological and psychological examination in patients with complex regional pain syndrome and hemisensory deficits. Pain 2001;93:279–93.

[19] Drummond PD, Finch PM. Sensory changes in the forehead of patients with complex regional pain syndrome. Pain 2006;123:83–9.

[20] Savaş S, Baloğlu HH, Ay G, et al. The effect of sequel symptoms and signs of complex regional pain syndrome type 1 on upper extremity disability and quality of life. Rheumatol Int 2009;29:545–50.

[21] Perez RS, Collins S, Marinus J, et al. Diagnostic criteria for CRPS I: differences between patient profiles using three different diagnostic sets. Eur J Pain 2007;11:895–902.

[22] Bruehl S, Harden RN, Galer BS, et al. External validation of IASP diagnostic criteria for complex regional pain syndrome and proposed research diagnostic criteria. Pain 1999;81:147–54.

[23] Harden RN, Bruehl S, Perez RS, et al. Validation of proposed diagnostic criteria (the "Budapest criteria") for complex regional pain syndrome. Pain 2010;150:268–74.

[24] Todorovic-Tirnanic M, Obradovic V, Han R, et al. Diagnostic approach to reflex sympathetic dystrophy after fracture: radiology or bone scintigraphy? Eur J Nucl Med 1999;22:1187–93.

[25] Cappello ZJ, Kasdan ML, Louis DS. Meta-analysis of imaging techniques for the diagnosis of complex regional pain syndrome type I. J Hand Surg Am 2012;37:288–96.

[26] Zollinger PE, Tuinebreijer WE, Kreis RW, Breederveld RS. Effect of vitamin C on frequency of reflex sympathetic dystrophy in wrist fractures: a randomised trial. Lancet 1999;354:2025–8.

[27] Zollinger PE, Tuinebreijer WE, Breederveld RS, Kreis RW. Can vitamin C prevent complex regional pain syndrome in patients with wrist fractures? A randomized, controlled, multicenter dose-response study. J Bone Joint Surg Am 2007;89:1424–31.

[28] Shibuya N, Humphers JM, Agarwal MR, et al. Efficacy and safety of high-dose vitamin C on complex regional pain syndrome in extremity trauma and surgery—systematic review and meta-analysis. J Foot Ankle Surg 2013;52:62–6.

[29] Lichtman DM, Bindra RR, Boyer MI, et al. Treatment of distal radius fractures. J Am Acad Orthop Surg 2010;18:180–9.

[30] Perez RS, Zollinger PE, Dijkstra PU, et al. Evidence based guidelines for complex regional pain syndrome type 1. BMC Neurol 2010;10:20.

[31] Kalita J, Vajpayee A, Misra UK. Comparison of prednisolone with piroxicam in complex regional pain syndrome following stroke: a randomized controlled trial. QJM 2006;99:89–95.

[32] Munts AG, van der Plas AA, Ferrari MD, et al. Efficacy and safety of a single intrathecal methylprednisolone bolus in chronic complex regional pain syndrome. Eur J Pain 2010;14:523–8.

[33] van de Vusse AC, Stomp-van den Berg SG, Kessels AH, et al. Randomised controlled trial of gabapentin in complex regional pain syndrome type 1. BMC Neurol 2004;4:13.

[34] Tan AK, Duman I, Taskaynatan MA, et al. The effect of gabapentin in earlier stage of reflex sympathetic dystrophy. Clin Rheumatol 2007;26:561–5.

[35] Azari P, Lindsay DR, Briones D, et al. Efficacy and safety of ketamine in patients with complex regional pain syndrome: a systematic review. CNS Drugs 2012;26:215–28.

[36] Noppers IM, Niesters M, Aarts LP, Bauer MC. Drug-induced liver injury following a repeated course of ketamine treatment for chronic pain in CRPS type 1 patients: a report of 3 cases. Pain 2011;152:2173–8.

[37] Gustin SM, Schwarz A, Birbaumer N, et al. NMDA-receptor antagonist and morphine decrease CRPS-pain and cerebral pain representation. Pain 2010;151:69–76.

[38] Groeneweg G, Huygen FJ, Niehof SP, et al. Effect of tadalafil on blood flow, pain, and function in chronic cold complex regional pain syndrome: a randomized controlled trial. BMC Musculoskelet Disord 2008;9:143.

[39] Collins S, Zuurmond WW, de Lange JJ, et al. Intravenous magnesium for complex regional pain syndrome type 1 (CRPS 1) patients: a pilot study. Pain Med 2009;10:930–40.

[40] Goebel A, Baranowski A, Maurer K, et al. Intravenous immunoglobulin treatment of the complex regional pain syndrome: a randomized trial. Ann Intern Med 2010;152:152–8.

[41] Van Zundert J, Hartrick C, Patijn J, et al. Evidence-based interventional pain medicine according to clinical diagnoses. Pain Pract 2011;11:423–9.

[42] Oerlemans HM, Oostendorp RA, de Boo T, et al. Adjuvant physical therapy versus occupational therapy in patients with reflex sympathetic dystrophy/complex regional pain syndrome type I. Arch Phys Med Rehabil 2000;81:49–56.

[43] Albazaz R, Wong YT, Homer-Vanniasinkam S. Complex regional pain syndrome: a review. Ann Vasc Surg 2008;22:297–306.

[44] Korpan MI, Dezu Y, Schneider B, et al. Acupuncture in the treatment of posttraumatic pain syndrome. Acta Orthop Belg 1999;65: 197–201.

[45] Kiralp MZ, Yildiz S, Vural D, et al. Effectiveness of hyperbaric oxygen therapy in the treatment of complex regional pain syndrome. J Int Med Res 2004;32:258–62.

[46] Wu WH, Bandilla E, Ciccone DS, et al. Effects of qigong on late-stage complex regional pain syndrome. Altern Ther Health Med 1999;5:45–54.

[47] Ramachandran VS, Rogers-Ramachandran D, Cobb S. Touching the phantom limb. Nature 1995;377:489–90.

[48] McCabe CS, Haigh RC, Halligan PW, Blake DR. Simulating sensory-motor incongruence in healthy volunteers: implications for a cortical model of pain. Rheumatology 2005;44:509–16.

[49] Cacchio A, De Blasis E, Necozione S, et al. Mirror therapy for chronic complex regional pain syndrome type 1 and stroke. N Engl J Med 2009;361:634–6.

[50] Vladimir Tichelaar YI, Geertzen JH, Keizer D, Paul van Wilgen C. Mirror box therapy added to cognitive behavioural therapy in three chronic complex regional pain syndrome type I patients: a pilot study. Int J Rehabil Res 2007;30:181–8.

[51] Bultitude JH, Rafal RD. Derangement of body representation in complex regional pain syndrome: report of a case treated with mirror and prisms. Exp Brain Res 2010;204:409–18.

[52] Picarelli H, Teixeira MJ, de Andrade DC, et al. Repetitive transcranial magnetic stimulation is efficacious as an add-on to pharmacological therapy in complex regional pain syndrome (CRPS) type I. J Pain 2010;11:1203–10.

[53] Pleger B, Janssen F, Schwenkreis P, et al. Repetitive transcranial magnetic stimulation of the motor cortex attenuates pain perception in complex regional pain syndrome type I. Neurosci Lett 2004;356:87–90.

[54] Velasco F, Carrillo-Ruiz JD, Castro G, et al. Motor cortex electrical stimulation applied to patients with complex regional pain syndrome. Pain 2009;147:91–8.

[55] Van Zundert J, Hartrick C, Patijn J, et al. Evidence-based interventional pain medicine according to clinical diagnoses. Pain Pract 2011;11:423–9.

[56] Carroll I, Clark JD, Mackey S. Sympathetic block with botulinum toxin to treat complex regional pain syndrome. Ann Neurol 2009;65:348–51.

[57] Manjunath PS, Jayalakshmi TS, Dureja GP, Prevost AT. Management of lower limb complex regional pain syndrome type 1: an evaluation of percutaneous radiofrequency thermal lumbar sympathectomy versus phenol lumbar sympathetic neurolysis—a pilot study. Anesth Analg 2008;106:647–9.

[58] van Eijs F, Stanton-Hicks M, Van Zundert J, et al. Evidence-based interventional pain medicine according to clinical diagnoses. 16. Complex regional pain syndrome. Pain Pract 2011;11:70–87.

[59] Kemler MA, de Vet HC, Barendse GA, et al. Effect of spinal cord stimulation for chronic complex regional pain syndrome type I: five-year final follow-up of patients in a randomized controlled trial. J Neurosurg 2008;108:292–8.

[60] Straube S, Derry S, Moore RA, McQuay HJ. Cervico-thoracic or lumbar sympathectomy for neuropathic pain and complex regional pain syndrome. Cochrane Database Syst Rev 2010;7, CD002918.

CHAPTER 100

Costosternal Syndrome

Marta Imamura, MD
David A. Cassius, MD

Synonyms

Anterior chest wall syndrome
Costochondritis
Costosternal chondrodynia
Atypical chest pain

ICD-9 Code

733.6 Tietze disease; costochondral junction syndrome and costochondritis

ICD-Code

M94.0 Chondrocostal junction syndrome [Tietze], costochondritis

Definition

Costosternal syndrome is a frequent cause of anterior chest wall pain that affects the costosternal [1–6] or costochondral [2,4–7] joints. The pathogenesis of costosternal syndrome is still unknown [2,8]. Costosternal syndrome is considered an entity distinct from the rarely occurring Tietze syndrome [1–7,9] because it is a frequent cause of benign anterior chest wall pain. Also, as opposed to Tietze syndrome, it is not associated with local swelling of the involved costosternal or costochondral joints [1–7,9], and it usually occurs at multiple sites. The onset is usually after 40 years of age instead of at a young age as in Tietze syndrome, and it affects more women than men. A traumatic cause has been proposed [8], and currently it is suspected that repetitive overuse lesions of the costosternal joint and anterior chest [6,10] may be involved in the development of the degenerative changes found at the costosternal joint [11,12]. The costosternal joints may also be inflamed by osteoarthritis, rheumatoid arthritis, ankylosing spondylitis, Reiter syndrome, psoriatic arthritis, and the SAPHO (*s*ynovitis, *a*cne, *p*ustulosis, *h*yperostosis, and *o*steitis) syndrome [3,7,12]. Infections of the costosternal joints are associated with tuberculosis, fungus (mycetoma, pulmonary aspergilloma, candidal costochondritis [13]), and syphilis as well as with viruses. The costosternal joints may also be the site of tumor invasion either from a primary malignant neoplasm, such as a chondrosarcoma or thymoma, or from a metastatic carcinoma, most commonly from the breast, kidney, thyroid, bronchus, lung, or prostate [12,14]. Chondromas and multiple exostoses are the most common benign tumors.

Costosternal syndromes may be a primary condition or secondary to these diseases. The condition occurs more frequently in women (a ratio of 2 to 3:1) and at an older age; two thirds of the patients are older than 40 years [1–4, 7,8]. The left side is more often involved. Costosternal joint disease is 1.69 times more frequent in patients who undergo median sternotomy than in normal controls of the same age [15].

Symptoms

The most common symptom in costosternal syndrome is pain of the anterior chest wall, usually localized at the precordium or at the left parasternal region [8,16]. Pain can radiate superiorly toward the left shoulder and left arm [8,16] and also to the neck, scapula, and anterior chest. Pain mainly develops after postural changes and maneuvers that place stress over the chest wall structures [16] rather than with physical efforts, such as those related to pain of cardiac origin [16]. Cardiac etiology for chest wall pain should be considered and ruled out [17]. Cough, deep breathing, and chest and scapular movements usually aggravate pain [5,11]. In contrast to Tietze syndrome, in which only one costal cartilage is involved in the majority of the patients, multiple sites are present in 90% of patients with costosternal syndromes [1,2,7–9]. The second to the fifth costal cartilages are most commonly affected [1–3,5,8,9]. Pain intensity may vary; it usually occurs at rest [12] and lasts for several weeks or months [8,16].

Physical Examination

Inspection of the patient suffering from costosternal syndrome reveals that the patient vigorously attempts to splint the joints by keeping the shoulders stiffly in neutral position [12]. Differing from the Tietze syndrome, the costosternal syndrome has no visible spherical local swelling or any inflammatory signs at the costal cartilages [1,4,5,7,9]. Pain is reproduced by active protraction or retraction of the shoulder, deep inspiration, and elevation of the arm [12]. Palpation of the affected portions of the thoracic cage elicits local tenderness at multiple sites [9]. It may reproduce the patient's spontaneous pain complaint, including its radiation [9,18,19]. Some authors, however, have not found pain reproduction on palpation [4,5,16–19].

Several maneuvers have been found to be helpful in establishing the diagnosis [8,16]. Application of firm steady pressure to the following chest wall structures elicits the patient's pain complaint: the sternum, the left and right parasternal junctions, the intercostal spaces, the ribs, the inframammary area, and the pectoralis major and left upper trapezius muscles [8,16,18]. All of these can precipitate pain similar in quality and location to the spontaneous pain [16]. Another maneuver, called the horizontal flexion test (Fig. 100.1), consists of having the arm flexed across the anterior chest with the application of steady prolonged traction in a horizontal direction while, at the same time, the patient's head is rotated as far as possible toward the ipsilateral shoulder [2,6,8,10,16,18]. Another test, called the crowing rooster maneuver, consists of having the patient extend the neck as much as possible by looking toward the ceiling while the examiner, standing behind the patient, exerts traction on the posteriorly extended arms [2,8,16,18]. Associated myofascial pain syndrome of the intercostal, pectoralis major, pectoralis minor, and sternal muscles is a common feature of the syndrome. These muscles may be tender on palpation. Because this syndrome is usually confused with pain of cardiac [1,2,11,20,21], abdominal [2,9,16,22], or pulmonary [20] origin, a comprehensive history and physical examination are essential in all patients [8,18,19], including athletes [6,10].

Functional Limitations

Functional limitations may be due to the severe incapacitating chest pain [16]. Activities such as lifting, bathing, ironing, combing and brushing hair, and other activities of daily living can be very problematic. Patients will need to be at light duty for weeks and to avoid physical efforts of the upper limbs and trunk [14]. Even after a cardiac origin is ruled out for the chest discomfort, many patients do not return to full employment, recreation, or daily activities [23,24] and remain functionally impaired for years [24]. This functional impairment may occur even in patients with chest pain and normal angiographic studies [23,24] without a proven myocardial infarction. Many of these patients may have a costosternal syndrome. However, the continuing regular physician visits, medication consumption, emergency department visits, repeated hospitalizations, and repeated arteriographies may be contributing to the functional impairment.

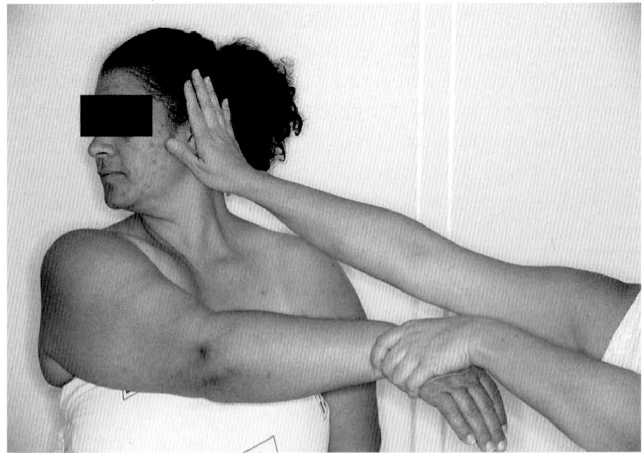

FIGURE 100.1 Horizontal flexion test for the diagnosis of costosternal syndrome.

Diagnostic Studies

The diagnosis of costosternal syndrome is usually a clinical diagnosis based on the detection of chest wall tenderness [11,16] that reproduces the spontaneous pain on physical examination [8,11,16,18,20,21]. Coronary heart disease [2,4,11,16,20,21], breast conditions [25], and pulmonary conditions [20,21] may be misdiagnosed as costosternal syndrome because of the anatomic proximity of the involved structures. Costosternal syndrome may also coexist with coronary artery disease [2,4,7,11,16,18] and other types of heart diseases [16]. The differentiation from anginal pain due to coronary heart disease may be judged by the pain characteristics. Typical anginal pain is substernal, provoked by exertion, and relieved by rest or nitroglycerin [20]. Atypical anginal pain has two of these symptoms, and nonanginal chest pain has only one of these symptoms [20]. Swap and Nagurney [21] described a low risk for acute coronary syndrome or acute myocardial infarction, with a likelihood ratio of 0.2 to 0.3, when chest pain is described as stabbing, pleuritic, or positional or is reproducible by palpation. The same authors also described a likelihood ratio of 2.3 to 4.7 for acute coronary syndrome when the chest pain radiates to one or both shoulders or arms or is precipitated by exertion [21]. In most patients with costosternal syndromes, the pain is usually localized in the anterior chest or parasternally at the level of the third or fourth intercostal space. As previously mentioned, it can also radiate superiorly toward the left shoulder and down the left arm. Patients experience pain at rest, and the pain can awaken them from sleep [8,16]. Chest pain characteristics, electrocardiographic abnormalities, or cardiac risk factors should be further evaluated by a cardiologist. Radionuclide cineangiographic testing is a sensitive method to differentiate between costosternal syndromes and cardiac diseases [16].

Laboratory and imaging procedures are helpful in the diagnosis of the possible secondary causes of the costosternal syndromes and to rule out other causes of anterior chest pain [11,14].

Plain radiographs are indicated for patients who present with pain possibly emanating from the costosternal joints to rule out occult bone tumors, infections, and congenital defects. If trauma has occurred, costosternal syndrome may coexist with occult rib fractures or fractures of the sternum. These fractures may be missed on plain radiographs and can require radionuclide bone scanning for proper diagnosis. Increased uptake of radioactivity on bone scans is seen in most patients; however, it is not a specific test for making the diagnosis of costosternal syndrome [26].

Additional testing, including complete blood count, prostate-specific antigen level, sedimentation rate, and antinuclear antibody titer, may be indicated to rule out other diseases that may cause a costosternal syndrome, such as rheumatoid arthritis, ankylosing spondylitis, Reiter syndrome, and psoriatic arthritis. Magnetic resonance imaging of the joints is indicated if joint instability or occult mass is suspected. Diagnostic ultrasonography may also be indicated to investigate the presence of an occult mass.

Neuropathic pain caused by diabetic polyneuropathies and acute herpes zoster involving the chest wall may also be confused or coexist with costosternal syndrome [12].

A highly reliable test (and an effective differential diagnostic procedure that can confirm the diagnosis of costosternal syndrome) is the complete pain relief noted after an intercostal block at the posterior axillary line [8]. Patients with cardiac disease will have little or no effect on their pain because the nociceptive pathways from the heart are in the sympathetic afferents located in the paravertebral region. This test is both diagnostic and therapeutic.

In the secondary forms of costosternal syndromes, the underlying conditions should be addressed for good results [16].

Differential Diagnosis

Angina pectoris
Acute myocardial infarction
Tietze syndrome
Dislocation and fracture of the ribs, sternum, and clavicle
Congenital sternoclavicular malformations
Myofascial pain syndrome at the anterior chest wall: sternal, pectoralis major, pectoralis minor, scalene, sternocleidomastoid (sternal head), subclavius, and cervical iliocostal muscles
Tumors of the costal cartilages
Costochondral dislocations
Trauma and arthritis of the sternoclavicular joint
Sternoclavicular hyperostosis
Manubriosternal arthritis
Trauma to the sternum
Xiphoidalgia syndrome
Diseases of the lung (pneumonia, lung abscess, atelectasis)
Spontaneous pneumothorax
Mediastinal emphysema
Mediastinitis
T1-12 radiculopathy (herpes zoster, postherpetic neuralgia)

Treatment

Initial

Initial treatment of the pain and functional disability associated with costosternal syndromes should include simple oral analgesics [2,18], such as acetaminophen and nonsteroidal anti-inflammatory drugs [12,27], alone or in combination with codeine [8] or tramadol. The use of an elastic rib belt may also provide symptomatic relief and help protect the costosternal joints from additional trauma [12]. Reassurance that the diagnosis is a non–life-threatening musculoskeletal pain syndrome can often by itself reduce the anxiety and fears and lead to symptomatic pain relief [2,6–9,11,16,27].

Rehabilitation

Physical modalities, such as local superficial heat for 20 minutes, two or three times a day, or ice for 10 to 15 minutes, three or four times a day, can be performed while symptoms are present [11,18]. Transcutaneous electrical nerve stimulation and electroacupuncture may be applied over the painful area. Gentle, pain-free range of motion exercises should be introduced as soon as tolerated. There is limited evidence to suggest that stretching exercises help for costochondritis pain [28]. Vigorous exercises should be avoided because they exacerbate the patient's symptoms. Perpetuating and aggravating factors [27], such as chronic coughing and bronchospasm, among others, should always be removed.

Procedures

For patients who do not respond to the initial or rehabilitation treatment modalities, a local anesthetic and steroid injection [5,6,9,11,12,25] can be performed as the next symptom control maneuver. Even in patients with coexisting true anginal pain, the relief of local chest pain is evident. Intra-articular injection of the costosternal joint (Fig. 100.2) is performed with the patient in the supine position [12]. The area of maximum tenderness can be infiltrated with a local anesthetic (2% lidocaine [7,25] or 0.25% preservative-free bupivacaine [12]) and methylprednisolone acetate [7,11,12,25] at the dosage of 10 mg per costosternal joint [25] by use of a 1½-inch, 25-gauge needle with strict aseptic technique [12]. The costosternal joints should be easily palpable as a slight bulging at the point where the rib attaches to the sternum [12]. An intercostal block at the posterior axillary line provides complete relief for 6 to 10 hours [8].

Surgery

Surgical procedures are rarely necessary [9]. Costosternal or sternoclavicular arthrodesis may be performed if conservative measures fail to provide satisfactory results.

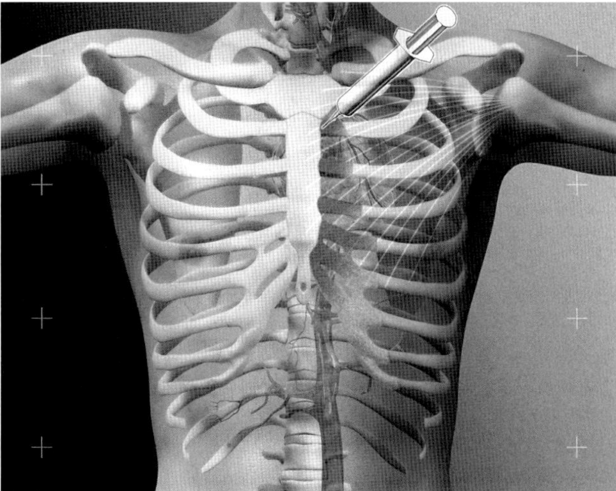

FIGURE 100.2 Schematic representation of the injection site at the second costosternal junction.

Potential Disease Complications

Costosternal syndromes are of benign origin, and complications rarely develop. They are self-limited [9], and spontaneous recovery usually occurs after 1 year in the majority of the cases [4]. Pain exacerbation due to physical activities and overload is usually followed by spontaneous recovery. However, as mentioned earlier, because of the many pathologic processes that may mimic the pain of costosternal syndrome, the clinician should always be careful to rule out underlying cardiac, lung, breast, and mediastinum diseases.

Potential Treatment Complications

The systemic complications of analgesics such as nonsteroidal anti-inflammatory drugs are well known and most commonly affect the gastric, hepatic, and renal systems. Local steroid combined with local anesthetic injections may cause pneumothorax if the needle is placed too laterally or deeply and invades the pleural space [12]. Cardiac tamponade as well as trauma to the contents of the mediastinum, although rare, can occur. This complication can be greatly decreased if the clinician pays close attention to accurate needle placement [12] or performs the injection with ultrasonographic guidance. Transient marked hypophosphatemia has been documented 8 hours after an intra-articular glucocorticoid injection in a patient with chronic costochondritis [29]. In this patient, hypophosphatemia was clinically characterized by limb paresthesia and weakness, followed by dysarthria [29]. All of these symptoms resolved within hours, even before the hypophosphatemia resolved [29]. Iatrogenic infections can also occur if strict aseptic techniques are not followed [12].

References

[1] Carabasi RJ, Christian JJ, Brindley HH. Costosternal chondrodynia: a variant of Tietze's syndrome? Dis Chest 1962;41:559–62.

[2] Fam AG, Smythe HA. Musculoskeletal chest wall pain. CMAJ 1985;133:379–89.

[3] Aeschlimann A, Kahn MF. Tietze's syndrome: a critical review. Clin Exp Rheumatol 1990;8:407–12.

[4] Disla E, Rhim HR, Reddy A, et al. Costochondritis. A prospective analysis in an emergency department setting. Arch Intern Med 1994;154:2466–9.

[5] Mukerji B, Mukerji V, Alpert MA, et al. The prevalence of rheumatologic disorders in patients with chest pain and angiographically normal coronary arteries. Angiology 1995;46:425–30.

[6] Gregory PL, Biswas AC, Batt ME. Musculoskeletal problems of the chest wall in athletes. Sports Med 2002;32:235–50.

[7] Freeston J, Karim Z, Lindsay K, et al. Can early diagnosis and management of costochondritis reduce acute chest pain admissions? J Rheumatol 2004;31:2269–71.

[8] Bonica JJ, Sola AF. Chest pain caused by other disorders. In: Bonica JJ, editor. The management of pain, vol II. Philadelphia: Lea & Febiger; 1990. p. 1114–45.

[9] Calabro JJ, Jeghers H, Miller KA, Gordon RD. Classification of anterior chest wall syndromes. JAMA 1980;243:1420–1.

[10] Rumball JS, Lebrun CM, Di Ciacca SR, et al. Rowing injuries. Sports Med 2005;35:537–55.

[11] Wolf E, Stern S. Costosternal syndrome: its frequency and importance in differential diagnosis of coronary heart disease. Arch Intern Med 1976;136:189–91.

[12] Waldman SD. Tietze's syndrome. In: Waldman SD, editor. Atlas of common pain syndromes. Philadelphia: WB Saunders; 2002. p. 158–60.

[13] Yang S-C, Shao P-L, Hsueh P-R, et al. Successful treatment of *Candida tropicalis* arthritis, osteomyelitis and costochondritis with caspofungin and fluconazole in a recipient of bone marrow transplantation. Acta Paediatr 2006;95:629–30.

[14] Wehrmacher WH. The painful anterior chest wall syndromes. Med Clin North Am 1958;38:111–8.

[15] Szántó D, Szücs G, Bíró BP, Priska M. Degenerative chondroarthropathy of the sternocostal joint following heart surgery. Orv Hetil 1994;135:2639–42.

[16] Epstein SE, Gerber LH, Borer JS. Chest wall syndrome: a common cause of unexplained cardiac pain. JAMA 1979;241:2793–7.

[17] McConaghy JR, Oza RS. Outpatient diagnosis of acute chest pain in adults. Am Fam Physician 2013;87:177–82.

[18] Levine PR, Mascette AM. Musculoskeletal chest pain in patients with "angina": a prospective study. South Med J 1989;82:580–91.

[19] Wise CM, Semble EL, Dalton CB. Musculoskeletal chest wall syndromes in patients with noncardiac chest pain: a study of 100 patients. Arch Phys Med Rehabil 1992;73:147–9.

[20] Cayley Jr WE. Diagnosing the cause of chest pain. Am Fam Physician 2005;72:2012–21.

[21] Swap CJ, Nagurney JT. Value and limitations of chest pain history in the evaluation of patients with suspected acute coronary syndromes. JAMA 2005;294:2623–9.

[22] Scobie BA. Costochondral pain in gastroenterologic practice. N Engl J Med 1976;295:1261.

[23] Lavey EB, Winkle RA. Continuing disability of patients with chest pain and normal coronary arteriograms. J Chron Dis 1979;32:191–6.

[24] Papanicolau MN, Calif RM, Hlatky MA, et al. Prognostic implications of angiographically normal and insignificant narrowed coronary arteries. Am J Cardiol 1986;58:1181–7.

[25] van Schalkwyk AJ, van Wingerden JJ. A variant of Tietze's syndrome occurring after reconstructive breast surgery. Aesthetic Plast Surg 1998;22:430–2.

[26] Mendelson G, Mendelson H, Horowitz SF, et al. Can ^{99m}technetium methylene diphosphonate bone scans objectively document costochondritis? Chest 1997;111:1600–2.

[27] Semble EL, Wise CM. Chest pain: a rheumatologist's perspective. South Med J 1988;81:64–8.

[28] Roberts-Thomson KC, Iyngkaran G, Fraser RJ. Intra-articular glucocorticoid injection: an unusual cause of transient hypophosphatemia. Rheumatol Int 2006;27:95–6.

[29] Rovetta G, Sessarego P, Monteforte P. Stretching exercises for costochondritis pain. G Ital Med Lav Ergon 2009;31:169–71.

CHAPTER 101

Fibromyalgia

Melissa Colbert, MD
Joanne Borg-Stein, MD

Synonym

Fibrositis

ICD-9 Code

729.1 Myalgia and myositis, unspecified

ICD-10 Codes

M79.1 Myalgia
M60.9 Myositis, unspecified

Definition

Fibromyalgia is a syndrome defined by chronic widespread pain of at least 3 months' duration. It is a multisystem illness associated with neuropsychological symptoms including fatigue, stiffness, unrefreshing sleep, cognitive dysfunction, anxiety, and depression. The majority of patients are women, for whom fibromyalgia is six times more common than in men [1]. The prevalence of the condition increases with age and is greater than 7% in women older than 60 years [2].

A discrete etiology of fibromyalgia has not been identified. Available evidence implicates sensitization of the central and peripheral nervous systems as key in maintaining pain and other core symptoms of fibromyalgia [3–6]. There may be a role for genetics, as individuals with certain genotypes are more likely to develop chronic pain and an overall increased sensitivity to pain during their lifetimes. These genes include catecholamine methyltransferase, sodium and potassium channels, and a number of others. Environmental factors, such as physical or emotional trauma, and infection (e.g., Epstein-Barr virus, Lyme disease, parvovirus), may interact with genetic factors to facilitate the development of fibromyalgia [6].

According to the 2010 American College of Rheumatology preliminary diagnostic criteria for fibromyalgia and measurement of symptom severity, a patient must have a widespread pain index score of at least 7 and a symptom severity scale score of at least 5 or a widespread pain index score of at least 3 and a symptom severity scale score of at least 9. The scoring is based on number and severity of somatic symptoms. In addition, symptoms must be present at a similar level for at least 3 months, and the patient must not have another disorder that would otherwise explain the pain (Table 101.1). These criteria do not include a tender point examination, as previously described by the 1990 American College of Rheumatology diagnostic criteria [7].

Symptoms

Fibromyalgia is characterized by widespread and long-lasting pain (>3 months) located above and below the waist, on both sides of the body. A series of other symptoms are frequently reported by patients. These include marked fatigue, stiffness, sleep disorders, cognitive disturbances (e.g., decreased comprehension, memory problems), anxiety, depression, temporomandibular joint syndrome, paresthesias, headache, genitourinary manifestations (e.g., pelvic or bladder pain), irritable bowel syndrome, and orthostatic intolerance [4].

Physical Examination

The findings of the general medical examination, including thorough joint inspection, should be normal. Blood pressure recording for orthostatic hypotension is performed. Mood and affect are noted.

The neurologic examination findings should also be largely normal but may demonstrate slight sensory or motor abnormalities [8]. By conducting a comprehensive neurologic and musculoskeletal examination, one may rule out superimposed pain generators, such as bursitis, tendinitis, radiculopathy, and myofascial trigger points.

Functional Limitations

Patients are limited in their daily activities and exercise tolerance by both pain and fatigue. Patients also report cognitive dysfunction with difficulty in concentration, organization, and motivation. This has been termed "fibro fog." Approximately 25% of patients with fibromyalgia report themselves disabled and are collecting some form of disability payment. Individuals are more likely to become disabled if they report higher pain scores, work at a job that requires

Table 101.1 Widespread Pain Index and Symptom Severity Scale Scores

Widespread Pain Index (score 0-19, 1 point for each location)				
Has the patient had pain in any of the following areas in the last week?				
Shoulder girdle (left)	Neck	Upper arm (left)	Upper leg (left)	Hip (left)
Shoulder girdle (right)	Upper back	Upper arm (right)	Upper leg (right)	Hip (right)
Jaw (left)	Chest	Lower arm (left)	Lower leg (left)	Lower back
Jaw (right)	Abdomen	Lower arm (right)	Lower leg (right)	
Symptom Severity Scale (score 0-12, total of specific symptoms plus general severity)				
Specific symptoms: How severe have the following symptoms been during the last week?				
(0 = no problem, 1 = slight/mild/intermittent, 2 = moderate/frequent, 3 = severe/pervasive/continuous)				
• Fatigue				
• Waking unrefreshed				
• Cognitive symptoms				
Number of general somatic symptoms (0 = none, 1 = few, 2 = moderate, 3 = many)				

A patient must have a widespread pain index score of at least 7 and a symptom severity scale score of at least 5 *or* a widespread pain index score of at least 3 and a symptom severity scale score of at least 9.

Data from Wolfe F, Clauw DJ, Fitzcharles M, et al. The American College of Rheumatology preliminary diagnostic criteria for fibromyalgia and measurement of symptom severity. Arthritis Care Res 2010;62:600-610.

heavy physical labor, have poor coping strategies and feel helpless, or are involved in litigation [9–11].

Diagnostic Studies

Fibromyalgia is a clinical diagnosis. For other conditions to be excluded, basic laboratory tests may be appropriate, such as complete blood count, erythrocyte sedimentation rate, thyroid-stimulating hormone concentration, liver transaminases, and creatine kinase activity. Primary sleep disorders may need to be identified by sleep studies. Radiography or magnetic resonance imaging may be indicated if osteoarthritis, radiculopathy, spinal stenosis, or intrinsic joint disease is suspected.

Electrodiagnostic studies may be useful to rule out an entrapment neuropathy or radiculopathy. The results of these studies will be normal in a patient with fibromyalgia but may be abnormal in the setting of a neuropathy.

Differential Diagnosis

Thyroid myopathy
Metabolic myopathy
Mood disturbances
Somatoform pain disorders
Rheumatic disease
Neuropathies

Treatment

Initial

Initial treatment includes education of the patient, pharmacologic treatment, gentle exercise, and relaxation training. A stepwise, multidisciplinary approach to fibromyalgia management is recommended. The first step is to confirm the diagnosis, to explain the condition, and to treat any comorbid illness, such as mood or sleep disturbance (see later). Education of the patient, which itself has been shown to have a therapeutic effect, includes individual and group classes that review the symptoms of fibromyalgia and emphasize the importance of adhering to a treatment program. It reassures the patient as to the generally benign course and outlines the treatment path [12–16].

The second step is to use pharmacologic and nonpharmacologic therapy, with emphasis on an individualized treatment plan. Trials with selective serotonin reuptake inhibitors, serotonin and norepinephrine reuptake inhibitors, or low-dose tricyclic antidepressants should be considered. One may use a combination medication trial or anticonvulsant [15]. The patient should begin a cardiovascular exercise program and be referred for cognitive-behavioral therapy or combine that with exercise.

The third step is specialty referral to rheumatology, physiatry, psychiatry, or pain management.

Pharmacologic management aims to normalize sleep patterns, to reduce fatigue, and to diminish pain. A low-dose tricyclic antidepressant at bedtime (e.g., amitriptyline, 10 to 25 mg) with a low-dose selective serotonin reuptake inhibitor (e.g., fluoxetine, 20 mg every morning) is an excellent and cost-effective combination. The combination works better than either medication alone. Cyclobenzaprine, which relies on a mechanism of action similar to that of tricyclic antidepressants, may also be used [17]. Studies demonstrate that the serotonin-norepinephrine reuptake inhibitors duloxetine and milnacipran are beneficial for patients with fibromyalgia, having the greatest impact on important symptoms such as pain and sleep [6,15,18].

Pain may be relieved with nonsteroidal anti-inflammatory drugs in combination with antidepressants or anticonvulsants, such as gabapentin or pregabalin. Pregabalin reduces pain in patients with fibromyalgia at doses of 300 to 450 mg/day in three divided doses, starting with 50 mg at bedtime and titrating up as tolerated. Opioids are rarely necessary. Tramadol, a μ opiate agonist with serotonergic and noradrenergic effects, may be used alone or in combination with acetaminophen [6,16]. Adjunctive nonpharmacologic pain control methods include acupuncture, massage, aqua therapy, yoga, Thai Chi, and biofeedback [6,19,20].

Rehabilitation

Physical therapy is used to educate the patient in a stretching, gentle strengthening, and cardiovascular fitness program. The aerobic exercise prescription includes low-impact interventions, such as walking and swimming, and should recommend low-intensity exercise that gradually increases to moderate intensity [1]. This can improve fitness and function and decrease pain. Occupational therapy is incorporated to review ergonomics of daily activities, and activities of daily living are reviewed at the work site. Task simplification, pacing, and maximization of function are emphasized [12,21–24].

Mental health professionals can be helpful in the rehabilitative phase to educate the patients in a mind-body stress reduction program, which may include cognitive-behavioral therapy, relaxation, and biofeedback. This provides the patient with positive coping strategies for living with chronic pain [15,25,26]. Associated depression and anxiety often need psychopharmacologic treatment as well.

Procedures

Trigger Point Injections

Myofascial trigger points may be injected with 1% lidocaine to decrease local pain and to increase pain thresholds [27]. Patients with recalcitrant chronic myofascial pain may respond to injections with botulinum toxin [28].

If patients have concurrent bursitis, tendinitis, or nerve entrapment, therapeutic injections may be performed to treat these specific diagnoses.

Acupuncture

Acupuncture can be used for treatment of pain and fatigue. Preliminary studies suggest that the benefit may last up to several months. Treatment two times per week for at least six visits appears necessary. Improvement lasts at least 1 month but is likely to wane over time. The optimal number and frequency of acupuncture treatments have not been determined [2,29–31].

Surgery

There is no surgery indicated for fibromyalgia.

Potential Disease Complications

Failure to make the diagnosis early may lead to delay in treatment, deconditioning, and expensive unnecessary medical testing and procedures. Chronic, intractable pain may occur despite treatment.

Potential Treatment Complications

Tricyclic antidepressant medications can be associated with anticholinergic side effects, such as urinary retention, sedation, constipation, and weight gain. Pregabalin may lead to dizziness, peripheral edema, and weight gain. Selective serotonin reuptake inhibitor medications may be associated with sexual dysfunction, gastrointestinal intolerance, and anorexia. Overly aggressive exercise programs may transiently increase pain in some patients. Injections may result in local pain, ecchymosis, intravascular injection, or pneumothorax if they are improperly executed. There is an increased risk of bleeding with use of nonsteroidal anti-inflammatory drugs and selective serotonin reuptake inhibitors. For patients taking high-dose serotonin reuptake inhibitors, consider avoidance or minimal use of nonsteroidal anti-inflammatory drugs [32]. There is also emerging concern for cardiovascular risks associated with nonsteroidal anti-inflammatory drugs [33]. The threshold for seizures is lowered by tramadol. In addition, the risk for seizure is enhanced by the concomitant use of tramadol with selective serotonin reuptake inhibitors [34].

References

[1] Wilson B, Spencer H, Kortebein P. Exercise recommendations in patients with newly diagnosed fibromyalgia. PM R 2012;4:252–5.

[2] Martin DP, Sletten CD, Williams BA, Berger IH. Improvement in fibromyalgia symptoms with acupuncture: results of a randomized controlled trial. Mayo Clin Proc 2006;81:749–57.

[3] Bennett R. Fibromyalgia: present to future. Curr Rheumatol Rep 2005;7:371–6.

[4] Goldenberg DL. Diagnosis and differential diagnosis of fibromyalgia. Am J Med 2009;122:S14–21.

[5] Staud R. Abnormal pain modulation in patients with spatially distributed chronic pain: fibromyalgia. Rheum Dis Clin North Am 2009;35:263–74.

[6] Goldenberg DL, Clauw DJ, Fitzcharles MA. New concepts in pain research and pain management of the rheumatic diseases. Semin Arthritis Rheum 2011;41:319–34.

[7] Wolfe F, Clauw DJ, Fitzcharles M, et al. The American College of Rheumatology preliminary diagnostic criteria for fibromyalgia and measurement of symptom severity. Arthritis Care Res 2010;62:600–10.

[8] Watson NF, Buchwald D, Goldberg J, et al. Neurologic signs and symptoms in fibromyalgia. Arthritis Rheum 2009;60:2839–44.

[9] Bennett RM. Fibromyalgia and the disability dilemma. Arthritis Rheum 1996;19:1627–33.

[10] Kurtze N, Gundersen KT, Svebak S. The impact of perceived physical dysfunction, health-related habits, and affective symptoms on employment status among fibromyalgia support group members. J Musculoskel Pain 2001;9:39–53.

[11] Henriksson CM, Liedberg GM, Gerdle B. Women with fibromyalgia: work and rehabilitation. Disabil Rehabil 2005;27:685–95.

[12] Adams N, Sim J. Rehabilitation approaches in fibromyalgia. Disabil Rehabil 2005;27:711–23.

[13] Dadabhoy D, Clauw DJ. Fibromyalgia: progress in diagnosis and treatment. Curr Pain Headache Rep 2005;9:399–404.

[14] Borg-Stein J. Treatment of fibromyalgia, myofascial pain and related disorders. Phys Med Rehabil Clin N Am 2006;17:491–510.

[15] Goldenberg DL, Burckhardt C, Crofford L. Management of fibromyalgia syndrome. JAMA 2004;292:2388–95.

[16] Arnold LM, Clauw DJ, Dunegan LJ, Turk DC. A framework for fibromyalgia management for primary care providers. Mayo Clin Proc 2012;87:488–96.

[17] Moldofsky H, Harris HW, Archambault WT, et al. Effects of bedtime very low dose cyclobenzaprine on symptoms and sleep physiology in patients with fibromyalgia syndrome: a double-blind randomized placebo-controlled study. J Rheumatol 2011;38:2653–63.

[18] Häuser W, Bernardy K, Üçeyler N, Sommer C. Treatment of fibromyalgia syndrome with antidepressants: a meta-analysis. JAMA 2009;301:198–209.

[19] Wang C, Schmid CH, Rones R, et al. A randomized trial of tai chi for fibromyalgia. N Engl J Med 2010;363:743–54.

[20] Carson JW, Carson KM, Jones KD, et al. A pilot randomized controlled trial of the yoga of awareness program in the management of fibromyalgia. Pain 2010;151:530–9.

[21] Gowans SE, deHueck A, Voss S, Richardson M. A randomized, controlled trial of exercise and education for individuals with fibromyalgia. Arthritis Care Res 1999;12:120–8.

[22] Rosen NB. Physical medicine and rehabilitation approaches to the management of myofascial pain and fibromyalgia syndromes. Baillieres Clin Rheumatol 1994;8:881–916.

[23] Kingsley JD, Panton LB, Toole T, et al. The effects of a 12-week strength-training program on strength and functionality in women with fibromyalgia. Arch Phys Med Rehabil 2005;86:1713–21.

[24] Tomas-Carus P, Gusi N, Häkkinen A, et al. Eight months of physical training in warm water improves physical and mental health in women with fibromyalgia: a randomized controlled trial. J Rehabil Med 2008;40:248–52.
[25] Kaplan KH, Goldenberg DL, Galvin-Nadeau M. The impact of a meditation-based stress reduction program on fibromyalgia. Gen Hosp Psychiatry 1993;15:284–9.
[26] Glombiewski JA, Sawyer AT, Gutermann J, et al. Psychological treatments for fibromyalgia: a meta-analysis. Pain 2010;151:280–95.
[27] Affaitati G, Costantini R, Fabrizio A, et al. Effects of treatment of peripheral pain generators in fibromyalgia patients. Eur J Pain 2011;15:61–9.
[28] Göbel H, Heinze A, Reichel G, et al,Dysport myofascial pain study group. Efficacy and safety of a single botulinum type A toxin complex treatment for the relief of upper back myofascial pain syndrome: results from a randomized double-blind placebo-controlled multicentre study. Pain 2006;125:82–8.
[29] Mayhew E, Ernst E. Acupuncture for fibromyalgia—a systematic review of randomized clinical trials. Rheumatology (Oxford) 2007;46:801–4.
[30] Targino RA, Imamura M, Kaziyama HHS, et al. A randomized controlled trial of acupuncture added to usual treatment for fibromyalgia. J Rehabil Med 2008;40:582–8.
[31] Amezaga Urruela M, Suarez-Almazor ME. Acupuncture in the treatment of rheumatic diseases. Curr Rheumatol Rep 2012;14:589–97.
[32] Mansour A, Perace M, Johnson B, et al. Which patients taking SSRIs are at greatest risk of bleeding? J Fam Pract 2006;55:206–8.
[33] Trelle S, Reichenbach S, Wandel S, et al. Cardiovascular safety of non-steroidal anti-inflammatory drugs: network meta-analysis. BMJ 2011;342:c7086.
[34] Gardner JS, Blough D, Drinkard CR, et al. Tramadol and seizures: a surveillance study in a managed care population. Pharmacotherapy 2000;20:1423–31.

CHAPTER 102

Headaches

Huma Sheikh, MD
Shivang Joshi, MD, MPH, BPharm
Elizabeth Loder, MD

Synonyms

General
- **Benign headaches**
- **Nonmalignant headache disorder**

Migraine
- **Sick headache**
- **Vascular headache**

Cluster
- **Suicide headache**
- **Alarm clock headache**
- **Histamine cephalgia**
- **Migrainous neuralgia**
- **Autonomic cephalgia**

Tension type
- **Ordinary headache**
- **Muscle contraction headache**
- **Tension headache**

ICD-9 Codes

307.81 **Tension headache**
346.9 **Migraine, unspecified**
784.0 **Headache**
339.0 **Cluster headache**

ICD-10 Codes

G44.209 **Tension-type headache, unspecified, not tractable**
G43.909 **Migraine, unspecified, not intractable, without status migrainosus**
R51 **Headache**
G44.029 **Chronic cluster headache, not intractable**

Definition

The three major primary headache disorders are migraine, cluster, and tension-type headache [1]. Although all three syndromes are characterized by chronic, recurrent, and potentially disabling headaches, specific diagnosis is important because of differing natural history and treatment.

Headache disorders are classified according to criteria outlined in the International Classification of Headache Disorders, originally developed by the International Headache Society in 1988 and revised in 2004 [1]. The criteria are available online (www.ihs-headache.org) and are due to be revised soon [2]. However, changes to criteria for the three primary headache disorders are expected to be minor. Diagnosis of all but a few rare migraine subtypes remains clinical, based on the patient's history and an examination that rules out secondary causes of headache (not covered in this chapter). The International Classification of Headache Disorders criteria were developed for research purposes and lack sensitivity when they are used in the clinical setting. Both migraine and tension-type headaches are more common in women than in men; cluster headache is generally a male disorder. Peak prevalence of migraine occurs during midlife, when it affects almost a quarter of all women and roughly 10% of men [3]. Recurrent headaches are not rare in children, but accurate diagnosis can be difficult because headache presentation in children varies from that in adults, and children may have difficulty describing the headache characteristics needed for a diagnosis to be made [4].

Migraine

Migraine is subclassified as migraine without aura (Table 102.1) and migraine with aura (Table 102.2). About 20% of patients have aura, usually preceding the headache, which consists of focal neurologic signs or symptoms that begin gradually and fade away within 30 to 60 minutes as the headache begins. The most common type of aura involves visual disturbances, typically an enlarging scotoma, but patients can also see shapes such as stars, zigzag lines, or other visual distortions, including field cuts and photopsias. Sensory or motor problems occur far less frequently. Blurry vision is usually not considered a part of aura. Migraine can also be classified as episodic or chronic (15 or more migraine headache days per month). Three gene mutations have been

Table 102.1 Diagnostic Criteria for Migraine without Aura

A. At least five attacks fulfilling B-D.
B. Headache attacks lasting 4-72 hours (untreated or unsuccessfully treated).
C. Headache has at least two of the following characteristics:
   1. Unilateral location
   2. Pulsating quality
   3. Moderate or severe intensity (inhibits or prohibits daily activities)
   4. Aggravated by or causes avoidance of routine physical activity
D. During headache at least one of the following:
   1. Nausea and/or vomiting
   2. Photophobia and phonophobia
E. At least one of the following:
   1. History, physical, and neurologic examinations do not suggest one of the disorders listed in groups 5-11.
   2. History and/or physical and/or neurologic examinations do suggest such disorder, but it is ruled out by appropriate investigations.
   3. Such disorder is present, but migraine attacks do not occur for the first time in close temporal relation to the disorder.

From Headache Classification Subcommittee of the International Headache Society. The International Classification of Headache Disorders: 2nd edition. Cephalalgia 2004;24(Suppl 1):1-160.

Table 102.2 Diagnostic Criteria for Migraine with Aura

A. At least two attacks fulfilling B.
B. At least three of the following four characteristics:
   1. One or more fully reversible aura symptoms indicating focal cerebral cortical and/or brainstem dysfunction.
   2. At least one aura symptom develops gradually over more than 4 minutes, or two or more symptoms occur in succession.
   3. No aura symptom lasts more than 60 minutes. If more than one aura symptom is present, accepted duration is proportionally increased.
   4. Headache follows aura with a free interval of less than 60 minutes. (It may also begin before or simultaneously with the aura.)
C. At least one of the following:
   1. History, physical, and neurologic examinations do not suggest one of the disorders listed in groups 5-11.
   2. History and/or physical and/or neurologic examinations do suggest such disorder, but it is ruled out by appropriate investigations.
   3. Such disorder is present, but migraine attacks do not occur for the first time in close temporal relation to the disorder.

From Headache Classification Subcommittee of the International Headache Society. The International Classification of Headache Disorders: 2nd edition. Cephalalgia 2004;24(Suppl 1):1-160.

identified that are associated with a particular subtype of migraine with aura known as familial hemiplegic migraine. These genes influence the stability of neuronal cell membranes [5,6]. Some patients are able to identify triggers for their headache, including exertion, certain foods, and hormonal influences.

Cluster

Cluster headaches are strictly unilateral headaches that are far more common in men than in women, but the prevalence in the general population overall is approximately 0.1% [7]. The pain is sharp and steady, in contrast to the throbbing pain of migraine, and localized to the orbital area. Diagnostic criteria require the presence of at least one autonomic sign or symptom during the headache, such as ipsilateral conjunctival injection, lacrimation, rhinorrhea, ptosis, or miosis.

Cluster headache is so called because the headaches occur regularly in most cases, from one to eight times a day, during a period of 2 weeks to 3 months that is referred to as a cluster episode. The headaches then completely remit for months or years. In chronic cluster headache, there are no headache-free periods or remissions, or they are less than 2 weeks in duration [8]. Patients with cluster headache usually describe alcohol intolerance during the cluster episode and generally note intense restlessness during the headache.

Tension Type

Tension-type headaches can vary in length from 30 minutes to 7 days. They are typically bilateral, moderate in intensity, and described as a pressing, squeezing sensation that is not affected by physical activity. Associated symptoms, such as nausea, vomiting, photophobia, and phonophobia, are generally not present or are mild. Tension-type headache is subclassified as infrequent episodic if it occurs less than 1 day per month, frequent episodic if it occurs from 1 day to 14 days per month, and chronic with attacks occurring 15 days or more per month for at least 6 months [1]. Patients with tension-type headache typically do not spontaneously report symptoms other than headache. A diagnosis of migraine should be reexamined if multiple associated symptoms are reported, like nausea and photophobia, which are thought to be a part of the sympathetic activation that occurs with migraines.

Symptoms

In addition to the aforementioned symptoms that are required for diagnosis, many patients with migraine report prodromal symptoms: yawning; neck and shoulder muscle discomfort; excessive salivation; and changes in appetite, mood, sleep, gastrointestinal function, and urination. Some of these can start days before the actual headache. Postdromal symptoms in migraine include fatigue, exercise intolerance, and neck and shoulder muscle discomfort. If headaches progress untreated, 80% of patients eventually develop allodynia, defined as pain in response to stimuli that normally are nonpainful. Once allodynia develops, treatment may be less successful [9].

Physical Examination

The primary headache disorders are diagnosed by history. The major purpose of physical and neurologic examination is to rule out the presence of secondary headache disorders. Accordingly, the most important parts of the physical examination are funduscopic examination to exclude papilledema and neurologic examination to exclude focal deficits that might suggest a malignant neoplasm, vascular causes like stroke or hemorrhage, collagen vascular disease, or infectious cause of headaches, among others.

Interictally, the physical and neurologic examination findings will be normal in primary headache disorders, or if another disorder is identified, it must not be causally related to the primary headache. Subtle cerebellar signs, such as dysmetria and balance abnormalities, have been detected in migraineurs compared with normal controls, but these are generally not detectable in a typical examination [10].

If the patient is examined during a headache attack, the following points should be specifically noted.

- Patients experiencing migraine lie quietly, avoid movement, and may appear pale and diaphoretic. They typically display marked photophobia and phonophobia and may be vomiting.
- Patients experiencing cluster headache are physically restless, in contrast to migraine sufferers.
- Head banging and agitation are common [11]. Autonomic signs should be documented to confirm the diagnosis. Between attacks, persistent ptosis and conjunctival injection may occasionally be seen.
- Patients experiencing tension-type headache may appear uncomfortable but generally are not incapacitated.
- Neck, shoulder, and jaw tightness is common in patients with prolonged episodes of all primary headache types and does not necessarily represent the underlying cause of the headache. In most cases, these complaints will improve with appropriate treatment of the headache and do not need to be treated separately. There is no evidence that patients with tension-type headache have abnormally elevated muscle tension. In fact, electromyographic findings do not have diagnostic or treatment implications in migraine or tension-type headache [12]. Although biofeedback-assisted muscle relaxation is clearly of benefit in migraine and tension-type headache, it may exert its effect through mechanisms other than muscle relaxation.

Functional Limitations

Quality of life surveys and other data suggest that patients with primary headache disorders are more functionally impaired than is commonly appreciated [13]. Obviously, acute attacks of migraine and cluster headache prohibit function and generally require bed rest if untreated. Visual aura can render driving or other hazardous activities dangerous or even impossible. Tension-type headache does not generally prohibit activities but may inhibit them. Patients commonly report feeling that they are not functioning at "full capacity." In many cases, severely affected patients report that fear and anxiety about possible attacks lead them to avoid, to cancel, or to decline work, social, and academic opportunities. Depression is a common comorbidity with poorly controlled headaches and also may lead to impaired function. The functional limitations imposed on many patients by nonspecific sedative treatments for migraine or by prophylactic treatments, which can cause fatigue, exercise intolerance, weight gain, and depression, are also underappreciated.

Diagnostic Studies

The primary headache disorders are clinical diagnoses, with the exception of the rare hemiplegic migraine syndromes. In general, imaging studies or laboratory tests are done to rule out secondary headache disorders, not to rule in primary disorders. With the exception of genetic testing for genes associated with familial hemiplegic migraine, there are currently no laboratory, genetic, or imaging markers that confirm a diagnosis of ordinary migraine with or without aura in individual patients. Biomarkers do exist that can distinguish subgroups of migraineurs, like those with hemiplegic migraine, from one another or from normal controls [14]. Some of the red flags to look out for that signal a secondary headache include change in pattern of headaches, headaches on awakening, any associated neurologic deficits, and headaches with onset in older age.

Differential Diagnosis

MIGRAINE
Seizure disorder
Sinus infection
Early subarachnoid hemorrhage
Collagen vascular disorders
Meningitis
Space-occupying central nervous system lesion
Post-traumatic headache

CLUSTER
Trigeminal neuralgia
Cavernous sinus thrombosis
Central nervous system or ear, nose, or throat tumor
Orbital cellulitis or fracture
Subarachnoid hemorrhage
Dental abscess

TENSION TYPE
Mild or forme fruste migraine attack
Temporomandibular disorder
Space-occupying central nervous system lesion

Treatment

Initial

Headache treatment consists of nonpharmacologic measures, lifestyle changes, and abortive treatment of acute attacks [15]. Another option, prophylactic treatment, in which daily medication is given to decrease the frequency and severity of headache episodes, is reserved for patients who do not obtain acceptable relief from abortive therapy or have more than two headache attacks a week. Although there is some overlap in treatment options among the various headache disorders, there are also important differences. In particular, cluster headache is often erroneously treated for years with migraine medication, to little or no avail [16].

Migraine

Lifestyle modification includes regular and adequate sleep and hydration, avoidance of excess caffeine, avoidance of missed meals, avoidance of alcohol (not a trigger for all migraine patients), and regular aerobic exercise. Although it is commonly advised, there is no scientific evidence that avoidance of chocolate, dairy products, or the myriad other dietary factors anecdotally implicated in migraine is helpful for the majority of patients with migraine. In the absence of good scientific evidence, it does not seem wise to promote food anxieties.

Nonpharmacologic treatment includes therapies such as cognitive-behavioral therapy, biofeedback-assisted relaxation, physical therapy, and acupuncture (although there is weak evidence of acupuncture's benefit). Physical therapy has *not* been shown to be useful in a trial that compared physical therapy and medication for migraine with medication alone [17]. If physical therapy is used, it should be short term and focus on development of an aerobic or other exercise program rather than on passive therapeutic modalities. One study did suggest that aerobic exercise 40 minutes three times a week is as effective as topiramate and relaxation training [18]. Biofeedback can also provide long-term benefits for patients with migraine.

Abortive therapy consists of nonsteroidal anti-inflammatory drugs, with or without caffeine; isometheptene compounds; opioids, with or without aspirin or acetaminophen; barbiturate-containing compounds (e.g., Fiorinal, Fioricet, Esgic, Phrenilin); ergots (e.g., Cafergot, Wigraine, D.H.E. 45); and triptans (sumatriptan, rizatriptan, zolmitriptan, naratriptan, frovatriptan, eletriptan, almotriptan). Keeping headache diaries should be emphasized for better monitoring.

Prophylactic therapy consists of nonsteroidal anti-inflammatory drugs; topiramate; beta blockers, especially propranolol (except those with sympathomimetic activity); calcium channel antagonists; tricyclic antidepressants, especially amitriptyline; riboflavin (vitamin B_2); sodium valproate; and selective serotonin reuptake inhibitors (weak evidence of benefit). Recently released preventive migraine treatment guidelines from the American Academy of Neurology and the American Headache Society assign sodium valproate, propranolol, metoprolol, and topiramate to the top level of treatment choices on the basis of an assessment of efficacy alone [19].

Cluster

Lifestyle modification includes alcohol avoidance and stress reduction.

Nonpharmacologic therapy employs 100% oxygen; 10 to 12 liters at headache onset by non-rebreather mask for 10 to 15 minutes aborts headache in 80% of patients.

Abortive therapy generally must be parenteral because headaches are short and onset is sudden. Options include oxygen, as previously described; dihydroergotamine, 1 mg subcutaneously; sumatriptan, 6 mg subcutaneously; and parenteral opioids.

Prophylactic therapy includes lithium carbonate, steroids (duration and dose must be limited to avoid side effects; principally used while results are awaited from other prophylactic medications), verapamil (high doses required), sodium valproate (benefit unclear), and topiramate (benefit unclear).

Tension Type

Lifestyle modification includes regular and adequate sleep and aerobic exercise.

Nonpharmacologic therapy includes biofeedback (thermal or electromyographic). Physical therapy focuses on stretching and strengthening exercise rather than on passive modalities.

Acute therapy consists of nonsteroidal anti-inflammatory drugs and isometheptene combinations. Potentially sedative or habit-forming opioid or barbiturate-containing compounds should generally be avoided.

Prophylactic therapy consists of nonsteroidal anti-inflammatory drugs, tricyclic antidepressants, and sodium valproate.

Rehabilitation

Patients whose headaches are refractory to currently available treatments suffer significant disability. Secondary depression and medication overuse may develop, along with family dysfunction and poor work performance. The development of chronic pain syndrome (in which patients develop disability out of proportion to the underlying disease, with associated behavioral abnormalities) requires interdisciplinary treatment for best results. The treatment philosophy, which must be accepted by the patient and family, shifts from cure to management. Medication reduction, increased "up" time and regular physical exercise, involvement in hobbies or return to work, and psychological intervention all help return the patient to some semblance of normal living, despite the persistence of headache [20]. Inpatient rehabilitation may be necessary for patients with severe medication overuse, who require special tapering from narcotic or barbiturate drugs, or who have associated medical or psychiatric morbidity that precludes outpatient treatment. Only a handful of such programs exist in the United States because of the reluctance of insurance companies to compensate for them.

Procedures

Onabotulinum toxin type A injections into the pericranial musculature received approval by the Food and Drug Administration for treatment of chronic migraines in 2010. Pooled data from two randomized controlled trials showed that it was useful in patients with chronic migraine (15 or more headache days per month), although its use is limited by cost and insurance coverage problems [21,22]. Episodic or chronic headaches associated with significant pericranial muscle spasm or pain may benefit from localized trigger point injections or occipital nerve blocks [23,24]. Trigger point injections for headache are small-volume injections into one or more tender or painful muscles in the head or neck. The injection may be of a local anesthetic alone, such as 0.5 to 1.5 mL of 0.25% or 0.5% bupivacaine, or in combination with a steroid, such as 1.5 mL of 0.5% bupivacaine and 0.25 mL of methylprednisolone sodium succinate (Solu-Medrol) 20 mg/mL. Trigger point injections may be repeated at 2-month intervals as needed [23]. Greater occipital nerve block is performed by injection of a combination of local anesthetic and steroid 2 cm lateral to the occipital protuberance; a common dose is 2 mL of 2% lidocaine with 5 mg of triamcinolone [24].

Surgery

Ablative surgical procedures on the fifth cranial nerve (radiofrequency, cryotherapy, and alcohol techniques) are employed in cases of refractory cluster headache. Implanted sphenopalatine ganglion stimulators are a promising but investigational approach for some patients. Some women with migraine contemplate oophorectomy, in the belief that elimination of hormonal cycling may eliminate migraine. In fact, abrupt surgical menopause seems to worsen, not improve, migraine, and this procedure should be discouraged. There is no clear evidence on whether closure of patent foramen ovale is helpful in the treatment of migraine with aura. Occipital nerve stimulators are under investigation for treatment of refractory migraine. Other surgical approaches, such as operations to release peripheral "trigger sites," have scanty evidence of benefit and in the absence of larger trials should not be recommended.

Potential Disease Complications

Inadequately managed headaches can directly or indirectly lead to depression, suicide, addiction and dependence syndromes, unemployment, divorce, and poor progress in school and the workplace. Emerging evidence indicates structural brain changes in some patients with long-duration, poorly controlled migraine attacks [25]. These include iron deposition in areas of the brainstem, white matter lesions, and reduction in gray matter volume. Migraine is a risk factor for ischemic stroke and may also increase the risk of coronary heart disease. Women with migraine are more likely to develop preeclampsia and to suffer postpartum stroke [26].

Potential Treatment Complications

Possible complications from injections include an allergic reaction to the medication and infection. Potential complications from cluster headache surgery include anesthesia dolorosa, dry eye, and facial anesthesia or weakness. Multiple reactions to oral medications are possible, and the clinician should be aware of the side effect profile for any medications prescribed. A 2006 Food and Drug Administration advisory warns about possible serotonin syndrome with concomitant use of selective serotonin reuptake inhibitors or serotonin-norepinephrine reuptake inhibitors and triptans. From a clinical perspective, the risk appears very low, but it is worth considering in patients using both medications who have unusual side effects. Most experts do not think, however, that the combination is absolutely contraindicated. Overuse of symptomatic medications for headache may lead to medication overuse headache syndromes that can be difficult to treat.

References

[1] Headache Classification Subcommittee of the International Headache Society. The international classification of headache disorders: 2nd edition. Cephalalgia 2004;24(Suppl. 1):1–160.

[2] International Headache Society. IHS classification ICHD-II. http://ihs-classification.org/en/; [accessed September 2012].

[3] Lipton RB, Stewart WF, Diamond S, et al. Prevalence and burden of migraine in the United States: data from the American Migraine Study II. Headache 2001;41:646–57.

[4] Laurell K, Larsson B, Mattsson P, Eeg-Olofsson O. A 3-year follow-up of headache diagnoses and symptoms in Swedish schoolchildren. Cephalalgia 2006;26:809–15.

[5] Vanmolkot KR, Kors EE, Turk U, et al. Two de novo mutations in the Na, K-ATPase gene ATP1A2 associated with pure familial hemiplegic migraine. Eur J Hum Genet 2006;14:555–60.

[6] Kors EE, Melberg A, Vanmolkot KR, et al. Childhood epilepsy, familial hemiplegic migraine, cerebellar ataxia and a new CACNA1A mutation. Neurology 2004;63:1136–7.

[7] Fischera M, Marziniak M, Gralow I, Evers S. The incidence and prevalence of cluster headache: a meta-analysis of population-based studies. Cephalalgia 2008;28:614.

[8] Sandrini G, Tassorelli C, Ghiotto N, Nappi G. Uncommon primary headaches. Curr Opin Neurol 2006;19:299–304.

[9] Burstein R, Yarnitsky D, Goor-Aryeh I, et al. An association between migraine and cutaneous allodynia. Ann Neurol 2000;47:614–24.

[10] Sándor PS, Mascia A, Seidel L, et al. Subclinical cerebellar impairment in the common types of migraine: a three-dimensional analysis of reaching movements. Ann Neurol 2001;49:668–72.

[11] Blau JN. Behavior during a cluster headache. Lancet 1993;342:723–5.

[12] Jensen R, Fuglsang-Frederiksen A, Olesen J. Quantitative surface EMG of pericranial muscles in headache. A population study. Electroencephalogr Clin Neurophysiol 1994;93:335–44.

[13] Lipton R, Stewart W, Sawyer J, et al. Clinical utility of an instrument assessing migraine disability: the Migraine Disability Assessment (MIDAS) questionnaire. Headache 2001;41:854–61.

[14] Loder E, Harrington MG, Cutrer M, et al. Selected confirmed, probable and exploratory migraine biomarkers. Headache 2006;46:1108–27.

[15] Silberstein SD, US Headache Consortium. Practice parameter: evidence-based guidelines for migraine headache (an evidence-based review): report of the Quality Standards Subcommittee of the American Academy of Neurology. Neurology 2000;55:754–62.

[16] van Vliet JA, Eekers PJ, Haan J, Ferrari MD. Features involved in the diagnostic delay of cluster headache. J Neurol Neurosurg Psychiatry 2003;74:1123–5.

[17] Biondi DM. Physical treatments for headache: a structured review. Headache 2005;45:738–46.

[18] Varkey E, Cider A, Carlsson J, Linde M. Exercise as migraine prophylaxis: a randomized study using relaxation and topiramate as controls. Cephalalgia 2011;31:1428–38.

[19] Loder E, Rizzoli P, Burch R. The 2012 AHS/AAN guidelines for prevention of episodic migraine: a summary and comparison with other recent clinical practice guidelines. Headache 2012;52:930–45.

[20] McAllister MJ, McKenzie KE, Schultz DM, Epshteyn MG. Effectiveness of a multidisciplinary chronic pain program for treatment of refractory patients with complicated chronic pain syndromes. Pain Physician 2005;8:369–73.

[21] Evers S, Olesen J. Botulinum toxin in headache treatment: the end of the road? Cephalalgia 2006;26:769–71.

[22] Aurora SK, Dodick DW, Turkel CC, et al. Onabotulinumtoxin A for treatment of chronic migraine: results from the double-blind, randomized, placebo-controlled phase of the PREEMPT 1 trial. Cephalalgia 2010;30:793–803.

[23] Mellick GA, Mellick LB. Regional head and face pain relief following lower cervical intramuscular anesthetic injection. Headache 2003;43:1109–11.

[24] Ashkenazi A, Young WB. The effects of greater occipital nerve block and trigger point injection on brush allodynia and pain in migraine. Headache 2005;45:350–4.

[25] Kruit MC, van Buchem MA, Hofman PAM, et al. Migraine as a risk factor for subclinical brain lesions. JAMA 2004;291:427–34.

[26] James AH, Bushnell CD, Jamison MG, Myers ER. Incidence and risk factors for stroke in pregnancy and the puerperium. Obstet Gynecol 2005;106:509–16.

CHAPTER 103

Intercostal Neuralgia

Susan J. Dreyer, MD

William J. Beckworth, MD

Synonyms

Intercostal neuralgia
Intercostal neuroma
Intercostal nerve pain

ICD-9 Codes

353.8 Intercostal neuralgia
954.8 Intercostal nerve injury

ICD-10 Codes

G58.0 Intercostal neuralgia
G58.0 Intercostal neuropathy

Definition

Intercostal neuralgia is pain in the thoracic region emanating from an intercostal nerve. The pain is typically a sharp, shooting, or burning pain radiating around the chest wall. It can be accompanied by altered sensitivity to touch, such as allodynia or an area of hyperalgesia. Intercostal neuralgia occurs commonly after thoracotomy [1–4]. It can also be seen in elderly debilitated patients without a known precipitating event [5]. Other causes include rib trauma, very rarely benign periosteal lipoma [6], and pregnancy [7].

Intercostal nerves are peripheral nerves that run along with the vascular bundle on the inferior surface of each rib (Fig. 103.1). Intercostal nerves are derived from the ventral rami of the first through twelfth thoracic nerves (Fig. 103.2), with the first, second, third, and twelfth being atypical on the basis of anatomic differences. Only 17% of intercostal nerves were found in the classic subcostal position in one study [8]. In Hardy's study, a midcostal location was the most prevalent at 73%; an additional 10% were supracostal. The intercostal nerve gives off four main branches as it travels anteriorly: gray rami communicantes, posterior cutaneous branch, lateral cutaneous division, and anterior cutaneous division.

Symptoms

Chest pain is the cardinal symptom. Because intercostal neuralgia involves a peripheral nerve, the pain is neuropathic rather than nociceptive. Neuropathic pain is often unrelenting, shooting, burning, and deep. The International Association for the Study of Pain defines neuropathic pain as "pain initiated or caused by a primary lesion or dysfunction in the nervous system." [9] Neuropathic pain is characterized by three symptoms: dysesthesia, paroxysmal pain, and allodynia [10]. Dysesthetic pain is an abnormal sensation described as unpleasant. Patients commonly use terms such as aching, cramping, pressure, and heat to describe a dysesthetic pain [11]. Paroxysmal pain is pain that comes in waves and is often described as lancinating or electric. Allodynia is the abnormal perception of pain after a normally nonpainful mechanical or thermal stimulus [11]. Patients with allodynia may respond to light touch with an exaggerated pain response or report a sensation of heat when a cold stimulus is applied. Intercostal neuralgia pain is unilateral. It is common (up to 81% of patients) after thoracotomy for coronary artery bypass grafting to the internal thoracic artery and after thoracotomy for tumor excision [3,4]. During thoracotomy (either open or video-assisted thoracoscopic surgery), the intercostal nerve may be directly injured during rib resection, compressed by a retractor, or later entrapped by a healing rib fracture. Intercostal neuralgia may follow other forms of chest trauma. It may mimic the pain of shingles (herpes zoster) but without the rash and can occur without significant trauma in the elderly.

The mechanism of neuropathic pain may be due to ectopic signals from neural "sprouts" after axonal injury. This new nerve growth may become a pain generator, especially if it becomes entrapped in scar tissue, forming a neuroma. Another mechanism may be compression or disruption of the nervi nervorum afferents in the connective tissue covering, producing a peripheral neuropathic pain.

Physical Examination

Much of the physical examination in intercostal neuralgia is done to exclude other sources of pain. First, it is

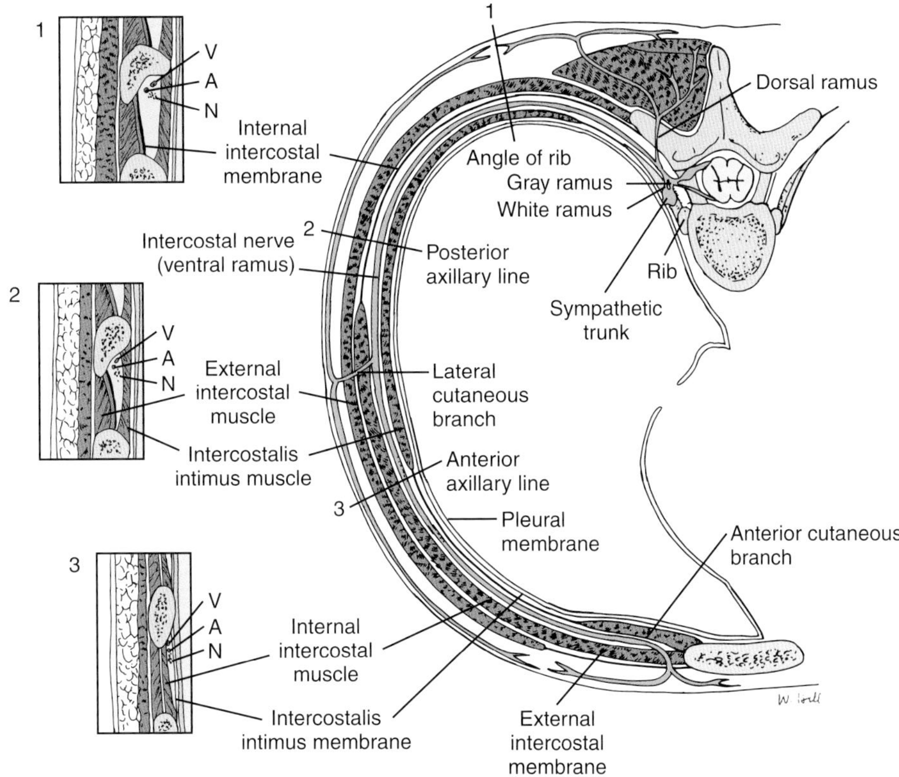

FIGURE 103.1 Intercostal nerve location. The intercostal nerve (N) runs along the inferior rib with the artery (A) and vein (V). *(From Chung J. Thoracic pain. In Sinatra RS, Hord A, Ginsberg C, Preble L, eds. Acute Pain. St. Louis, Mosby, 1992.)*

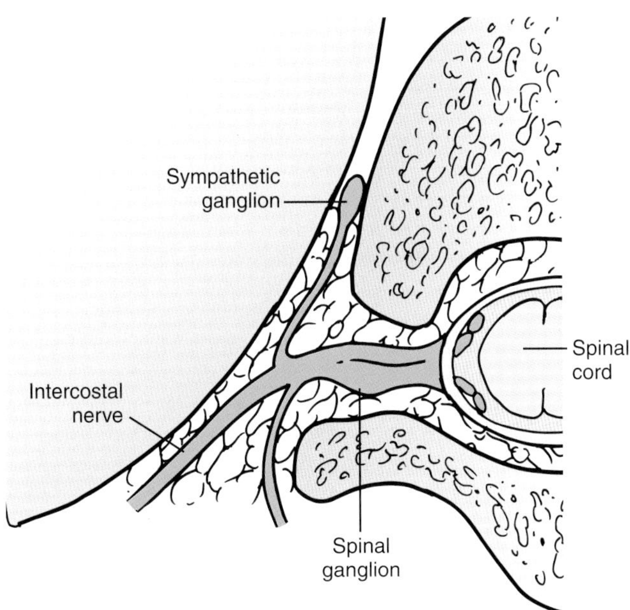

FIGURE 103.2 Intercostal nerves are derived from the ventral rami of the first through twelfth thoracic nerves. *(From Saberski LR. Cryoneurolysis in clinical practice. In Waldman S, ed. Interventional Pain Management, 2nd ed. Philadelphia, WB Saunders, 2001.)*

important to exclude cardiac and other visceral sources of chest pain (Table 103.1). Although point tenderness is uncommon during myocardial infarction, the presence of point tenderness does not exclude significant cardiac disease. In intercostal neuralgia, there are no constitutional signs, such as fever, dyspnea, diaphoresis, or shortness of breath. Cardiopulmonary examination findings should be normal or stable if prior cardiovascular or pulmonary disease exists.

Intercostal neuralgia is common after thoracotomy [1–3]. However, chest pain that recurs after a pain-free period following a thoracotomy for tumor resection is likely (90%) to be due to tumor recurrence. On the other hand, pain that persists for months or years after thoracotomy is most likely (70%) intercostal neuralgia [12].

Once the chest pain has been determined to be neuromusculoskeletal and nonvisceral, the task becomes one of differentiation of intercostal neuralgia from thoracic radiculopathy, herpes zoster, rib fracture, costochondritis, and local contusion. History of trauma, ecchymosis, crepitus, and point tenderness over a rib suggests rib fracture. If the trauma was minor, a contusion or intercostal neuralgia may be the source of discomfort. Contusions typically improve quickly during a period of weeks and are responsive to simple analgesics, such as acetaminophen and nonsteroidal anti-inflammatory medications. In contrast, pain from intercostal neuralgia persists and can be refractory to acetaminophen, nonsteroidal anti-inflammatory drugs, and even low-dose narcotics.

Careful palpation along the thoracotomy scar or rib may reveal a neuroma with the presence of a Tinel sign. Larger neuromas can often be visualized on magnetic resonance imaging. Sensory examination often reveals a small (1 to 2 cm) band of dermatomal sensory loss.

Table 103.1 Other Causes of Chest Pain

Cardiovascular
Myocardial ischemia
Pericarditis
Aortic dissection
Pulmonary
Pneumonia
Pneumothorax
Pleurisy
Pulmonary embolus
Tumor
Gastrointestinal
Esophageal
Esophagitis
Reflux
Perforation
Spasm
Cancer
Biliary
Cholelithiasis
Cholecystitis
Cholangitis
Colic
Pancreatic
Pancreatitis
Cancer
Intestinal
Peptic ulcer
Gastritis
Cancer
Musculoskeletal
Vertebral compression fracture
Tietze syndrome
Thoracic radiculopathy
Thoracic disc herniation
Cervical disc herniation
Costochondritis
Rib fracture
Costovertebral pain
Chest contusion
Spondylitis
Infective
Herpes zoster
Psychiatric
Depression
Anxiety
Hyperventilation
Renal
Nephrolithiasis
Pyelonephritis
Tumor

Examination of the thoracic spine in patients with intercostal neuralgia reveals full active range of motion without tenderness. In contrast, thoracic radiculopathy may be accompanied by pain with range of motion and at times thoracic spinal tenderness. Still, pain from thoracic radiculopathy is similar in quality and distribution to intercostal neuralgia.

Intercostal neuralgia is distinct from postherpetic neuralgia (shingles), and no herpes zoster virus can be identified in cases of intercostal neuralgia. Furthermore, in most cases of shingles, the chest pain is followed within a matter of days to weeks by a vesicular, linear eruption. The more debilitating pain of postherpetic neuralgia follows the skin lesions of shingles.

Functional Limitations

The pain of intercostal neuralgia is commonly mild to moderate but can be debilitating because it may interfere with one's ability to comfortably wear clothes. In one study, nearly 10% of post-thoracotomy patients observed for a mean of 19.5 months had moderate to severe pain that required daily analgesics, nerve blocks, relaxation therapy, acupuncture, or referral to a pain clinic [4]. The pain may also interfere with sleep. Trunk motion may stimulate the intercostal nerve, especially if a neuroma has formed. As a result, patients may begin restricting their activities.

Diagnostic Studies

Final diagnosis of intercostal neuralgia is often one of exclusion. Depending on which intercostal nerve is involved, chest pain from intercostal neuralgia may require an initial workup such as electrocardiography, cardiac enzyme analysis, cardiac computed tomography or magnetic resonance imaging, and other testing to exclude a cardiac source. Electromyographic recording of the paraspinal muscles is normal in intercostal neuralgia, whereas thoracic radiculopathy from thoracic disc herniation or foraminal stenosis may reveal active denervation potentials in the paraspinal muscles. Advanced imaging (thoracic magnetic resonance imaging, computed tomography, or computed tomographic myelography) also aids in demonstrating thoracic disc herniations or spinal stenosis as the source of the neural compression and confirms a diagnosis of thoracic radiculopathy. Larger intercostal neuromas may be visualized on magnetic resonance imaging of the ribs.

In the case of pain with a history of malignant disease, chest radiography, computed tomography, and bronchoscopy may be necessary to exclude recurrence of tumor. In patients whose history includes chest trauma, rib radiographs and at times bone scans help identify rib fractures.

Thoracic magnetic resonance imaging can exclude a disc herniation in an anatomically related area. Recall that it is not uncommon to identify asymptomatic disc herniations. In cases in which the disc protrusion does not cause clear compression but is abutting a thoracic nerve in the painful distribution, electrodiagnostic testing can exclude thoracic radiculopathy. Lesions of the intercostal nerve do not cause denervation in the thoracic paraspinal muscles.

When a postoperative neuroma is suspected, careful palpation often reveals a Tinel sign. Magnetic resonance imaging of the suspected area may reveal the neuroma. Small neuromas may be missed on magnetic resonance examination only to be identified later at the time of surgical resection.

Historical red flags including history of malignant disease, unexplained weight loss, malaise, and severe night pain raise the index of suspicion for rib metastases rather than intercostal neuralgia as the cause of the patient's chest pain. Appropriate oncologic workup, such as bone scans, laboratory investigation, and at times positron emission tomographic scans, should be performed.

Differential Diagnosis

Thoracic radiculopathy
Malignant neoplasm (primary or metastatic)
Rib fracture
Vertebral compression fracture
Chest wall contusion
Postherpetic neuralgia
Shingles
Referred pain from cardiac, pulmonary, vascular, or gastrointestinal disease
- Angina
- Aortic dissection
- Myocardial infarction
- Esophageal disorders
- Cholecystitis
- Peptic ulcer disease
- Pancreatitis
- Biliary colic
- Pleurisy
- Pulmonary embolism
- Pneumothorax

Costochondritis
Tietze syndrome
Nephrolithiasis
Pyelonephritis
Costovertebral or costochondral arthritis
Spondylitis

Treatment

Initial

Thoracic radiculopathy, postherpetic neuralgia, and intercostal neuralgia are all forms of neuropathic pain, and they share many initial conservative treatment options. Principles of treatment of neuropathic pain in general, rather than of a specific disease state, are employed [13,14]. Typically, drugs have not been specifically tested on populations of patients with intercostal neuralgia. Instead, physicians are left to extrapolate the data from treatment of other sources of neuropathic pain and to apply those principles in choosing medication to be used for this population. Often, neuropathic pain responds poorly to acetaminophen, nonsteroidal anti-inflammatory drugs, and low-dose narcotics, in contrast to nociceptive pain [15,16]. However, if the pain is mild to moderate, these agents are often tried first. Topical agents may be effective when there is significant allodynia or dysesthesia. The patient may need a family member to help apply the topical agent because it may be difficult to reach the involved area. Capsaicin creams are available over-the-counter, and a newer capsaicin patch (Qutenza) is available by prescription (the actual indication is for postherpetic neuralgia). The cream requires frequent application three or four times a day and may initially cause an exacerbation of pain as substance P is depleted. Topical lidocaine applied as a gel, eutectic mixture of local anesthetics (EMLA), or patch (Lidoderm) is another alternative [17].

Tricyclic antidepressants (e.g., amitriptyline, nortriptyline, desipramine) have been used for neuropathic pain for decades [18]. The dosage for analgesia is typically lower than that required to treat depression. Onset of action may be in days to weeks. The mechanism of action in neuropathic pain is believed to be modulation of descending inhibitory pathways by selective inhibition of norepinephrine or serotonin reuptake. Tricyclic antidepressants have anticholinergic effects and may cause confusion, increase the risk of falls and injury, and result in urinary retention. For these reasons, it is recommended that amitriptyline be avoided in persons older than 65 years. Despite this, amitriptyline (Elavil) is still a widely prescribed tricyclic antidepressant for neuropathic pain. It is usually started at 10 mg at bedtime and titrated upward as tolerated at 2- to 3-day intervals. Serotonin and norepinephrine reuptake inhibitors (SNRIs) such as duloxetine (Cymbalta), milnacipran (Savella), and venlafaxine (Effexor) are commonly used for neuropathic pain conditions, although only duloxetine is approved for a neuropathic diagnosis (painful diabetic neuropathy). Nausea can be seen with SNRIs. Milnacipran has a preference for norepinephrine reuptake inhibition and may lead to an increase in blood pressure. The SNRIs may be a better choice than the tricyclic antidepressants for elderly or debilitated patients with neuropathic pain.

Anticonvulsants are another mainstay for treatment of neuropathic pain. Anticonvulsants may work in several ways, including suppression of paroxysmal discharges and overall neuronal hyperexcitability [19]. Older agents such as carbamazepine and phenytoin have a narrow therapeutic window and risks of serious adverse drug reactions. These agents require careful monitoring if they are used. Bone marrow suppression occurs in up to 1% of patients, and severe dermatologic reactions such as Stevens-Johnson syndrome and epidermal necrolysis have also been reported with carbamazepine. Newer anticonvulsants, such as gabapentin (Neurontin) and pregabalin (Lyrica), are often chosen for their more favorable side effect profiles, efficacy, and limited interaction with other drugs. Gabapentin and pregabalin commonly cause sedation and may cause edema; both are indicated for neuropathic pain of diabetic peripheral neuropathy. These agents do not require blood samples for drug levels to be monitored. Dosing typically begins low and at night. For example, many practitioners start with gabapentin 300 mg at bedtime and titrate to 600 to 800 mg two or three times daily. At times, even higher doses are prescribed. Dosages are reduced in patients with renal insufficiency. Pregabalin can also be started at a low 50-mg bedtime dose and titrated to 300 mg twice daily, although it is uncommon to exceed 150 mg twice daily. Gabapentin and other anticonvulsants should be tapered before discontinuance. Like gabapentin and pregabalin, topiramate has also been used off-label for intercostal neuralgia [20].

Narcotics are often required for intercostal neuralgia. Adequate analgesia is needed to promote continued activity levels and to prevent deconditioning from disuse. Initial treatment should be with short-acting agents such as hydrocodone 5 mg with acetaminophen 325 mg every 4 hours as needed. Treatment of intercostal neuralgia can be protracted, and patients are often switched to long-acting agents for maintenance. If the pain is progressive, one should reevaluate the diagnosis and reconsider the possibility of occult tumor.

In refractory cases of neuropathic pain, clonidine, an adrenergic agonist, and ketamine, an *N*-methyl-D-aspartate

(NMDA) receptor antagonist, may be prescribed by pain specialists [10].

Rehabilitation

Physical and occupational therapy can be instrumental in combating disuse deconditioning. Also, desensitization techniques may be employed. Psychological consultation in patients who exhibit signs of anxiety, depression, or panic disorder may be beneficial to address the negative impact of these psychological stressors on the pain or the patient's behavior in response to the pain. Relaxation therapy and acupuncture have also been employed with anecdotal success [4].

If pain is severe, intercostal neuralgia may lead to avoidance of activity and deconditioning. It is important to keep patients physically active early in the rehabilitation process. The muscles of persons on strict bed rest lose 1.0% to 1.5% of their strength per day during a 2-week period. The loss is greatest during the first week of inactivity. Thus, if the patient is physically limited by pain, early prescription of a structured therapy program focusing on pain modulation helps prevent deconditioning. Desensitization techniques, heat, cold, and transcutaneous electrical nerve stimulation are all ways by which the therapist may assist in pain control while encouraging activity.

Psychological consultation in patients who exhibit signs of fear-avoidance, anxiety, and depression related to the pain may be beneficial later in the rehabilitation process. Biofeedback and relaxation therapy techniques are sometimes used. Biofeedback uses instrumentation to provide feedback on a variety of physiologic responses, such as muscle tension. It is typically used to facilitate relaxation and to enhance self-regulation. Two common relaxation therapies are autogenic training and progressive muscle relaxation. Relaxation training and biofeedback are thought to be equally effective in pain modulation.

Procedures

Local infiltration of a neuroma with corticosteroids and local anesthetics, intercostal nerve blocks, indwelling epidural catheters, and spinal nerve injections have all been used to control the pain associated with intercostal neuralgia when adequate relief is not achieved with oral and topical medications [2].

If a focal neuroma is identified, infiltration with several milliliters of local anesthetic with 40 mg of a long-acting corticosteroid, such as methylprednisolone (Depo-Medrol) or triamcinolone (Kenalog), often results in significant analgesia. In addition to its potent anti-inflammatory effect, the corticosteroid may also reduce neural discharges. Care must be taken during the injection to avoid pneumothorax.

Intercostal nerve blocks should be performed with appropriate monitoring. There are several techniques well described in interventional pain management books [21]. One common technique is to position the patient prone and to identify the angle of the rib just lateral to the sacrospinalis muscles (Fig. 103.3). The skin is moved up over the rib, and the needle is introduced down onto the posterior periosteum of the rib and then walked inferior. The advantage of moving the skin cephalad over the rib before needle insertion is that it allows the needle to be easily

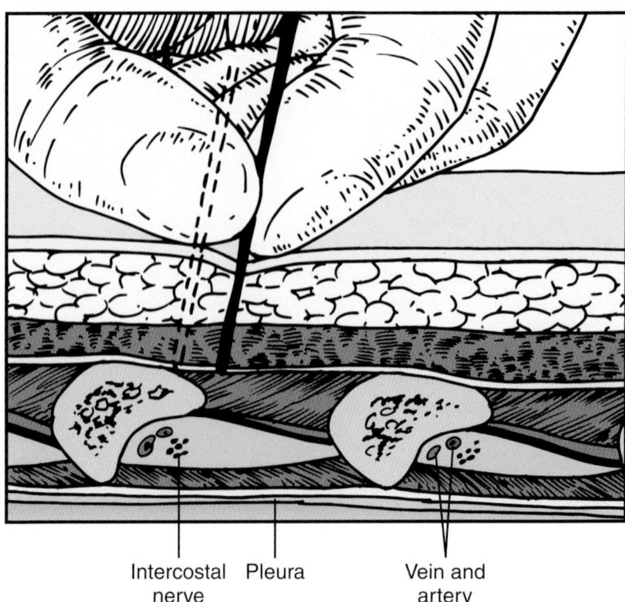

FIGURE 103.3 Intercostal nerve injection technique. The needle is advanced over the rib. Initial contact indicates posterior depth of the nerve. The skin and needle are then moved inferiorly off the rib, with care taken to avoid advancement of the needle too far, causing a pneumothorax. *(From Chung J. Thoracic pain. In Sinatra RS, Hord A, Ginsberg C, Preble L, eds. Acute Pain. St. Louis, Mosby, 1992.)*

moved inferior after the needle contacts bone. At the angle of the rib, the rib is typically 8 mm thick. Great care must be taken not to overpenetrate and cause a pneumothorax; 3 to 5 mL of local anesthetic is instilled along with a long-acting corticosteroid, such as triamcinolone, methylprednisolone, betamethasone, or dexamethasone. The needle is then withdrawn slightly and moved back over the rib before safe removal. Another approach is midaxillary and may be preferred in postoperative and acutely ill patients who cannot be easily positioned prone.

If symptoms are well controlled with intercostal nerve blocks but recur, neurolytic injection of phenol or alcohol has been used to denervate the peripheral nerve [21]. Indwelling epidural catheters have been used to provide regional anesthesia with minimal drug use. A report of pregnant patients who developed intercostal neuralgias found this technique safe and effective [7].

Cryotherapy involves another way of interrupting the peripheral nerve's ability to transmit pain by freezing it. Cryotherapy has been used on neuromas and the involved intercostal nerve [22].

Spinal cord stimulators have been implanted for intercostal neuralgia but with less success than in neuropathic pain due to diabetic peripheral neuropathy and causalgia [23]. Chronic post-thoracotomy pain and intercostal neuralgia can be difficult to control. In one study, up to 40% of post-thoracotomy patients required pain procedures including trigger point injections, intercostal nerve blocks, epidural steroid injections, and stellate ganglion blocks [2].

Surgery

Surgical resection of a neuroma can be effective but should be reserved for cases that have failed more conservative care and have demonstrated a temporary response to intercostal blocks. Dorsal root entry zone ablation involves surgical destruction of nociceptive secondary neurons in the spinal cord when pain is not adequately controlled with medical therapy [24,25]. The technique involves laminectomy with intradural exposure of the spinal cord. With an operating microscope, a radiofrequency probe is used to heat the dorsal horn of the affected side with a series of lesions.

Potential Disease Complications

Untreated upper intercostal neuralgia can potentially lead to a frozen shoulder as patients limit their use of the arm in response to the pain. Intercostal neuralgia can also cause a chronic pain syndrome with its comorbidities. Psychosocial dysfunction associated with chronic neuropathic pain includes impaired sleep, decreased appetite, and diminished libido.

Potential Treatment Complications

All medications carry risks. Many of the medications used for neuropathic pain (anticonvulsants, tricyclic antidepressants, narcotics) cause sedation. Injections in the area carry the risk of pneumothorax, bleeding, and infection. Surgical techniques may result in further nerve damage and pain, infection, bleeding, and pneumothorax.

References

[1] Landreneau RJ, Mack MJ, Hazelrigg SR, et al. Prevalence of chronic pain after pulmonary resection by thoracotomy or video-assisted thoracic surgery. J Thorac Cardiovasc Surg 1994;107:1079–85.
[2] Keller SM, Carp NZ, Levy MN, et al. Chronic post thoracotomy pain. J Cardiovasc Surg (Torino) 1994;35(Suppl. 1):161–4.
[3] Mailis A, Umana M, Feindel CM. Anterior intercostal nerve damage after coronary artery bypass graft surgery with the use of internal thoracic artery graft. Ann Thorac Surg 2000;69:1455–8.
[4] Dajczman E, Gordan A, Kreisman H, et al. Long-term postthoracotomy pain. Chest 1991;99:270–4.
[5] Jubelt B. Viral infections. In: Rowland P, editor. Merritt's neurology. 11th ed Philadelphia: JB Lippincott; 2005, Chapter 24.
[6] Kim HK. Intercostal neuralgia caused by a periosteal lipoma of the rib. Ann Thorac Surg 2006;85:1901–3.
[7] Sax TW, Rosenbaum RB. Neuromuscular disorders in pregnancy. Muscle Nerve 2006;34:559–71.
[8] Hardy PA. Anatomical variation in the position of the proximal intercostal nerve. Br J Anaesth 1988;61:338–9.
[9] International Association for the Study of Pain. IASP pain terminology. http://www.iasp-pain.org; [accessed 24.02.07].
[10] Milch RA. Neuropathic pain: implications for the surgeon. Surg Clin North Am 2005;85:1–10.
[11] Ropper AH, Brown RH. Pain. In: Victor M, Ropper AH, editors. Adams and Victor's principles of neurology. 8th ed. New York: McGraw-Hill; 2005, Chapter 8.
[12] McGarvey ML, Cheung AT, Stecker MM. Neurologic complications of cardiac surgery. UpToDate April 28, 2006.
[13] Woolf CJ. Pain: moving from symptom control toward mechanism-specific pharmacologic management. Ann Intern Med 2004;140:441–51.
[14] Smith HS, Sang CN. The evolving nature of neuropathic pain: individualizing treatment. Eur J Pain 2002;6(Suppl. B):13–8.
[15] Beydoun A. Neuropathic pain: from mechanisms to treatment strategies. J Pain Symptom Manage 2003;25(Suppl.):S1–3.
[16] Portenoy RK, Forbes K, Lussier D. Difficult pain problems: an integrated approach. In: Doyle D, Hanks G, MacDonald N, editors. Oxford textbook of palliative medicine. 2nd ed. New York: Oxford University Press; 1998. p. 438–58.
[17] Devers A, Galer BS. Topical lidocaine patch relieves a variety of neuropathic pain conditions: an open label study. Clin J Pain 2000;16:205–8.
[18] Onghena P, Van Houdenhove B. Antidepressant induced analgesia in chronic non-malignant pain: a meta-analysis of 39 placebo controlled studies. Pain 1992;49:205–19.
[19] Tremon-Lukats IW, Megeff C, Backonja MM. Anticonvulsants for neuropathic pain syndromes: mechanisms of action and place in therapy. Drugs 2000;60:1029–52.
[20] Bajwa ZH, Cami N, Warfield CA, et al. Topiramate relieves refractory intercostal neuralgia. Neurology 1999;52:1917–21.
[21] Kopacz DJ, Thompson GE. Intercostal nerve block. In: Waldman S, editor. Interventional pain management. 2nd ed. Philadelphia: WB Saunders; 2001. p. 401–8.
[22] Saberski LR. Cryoneurolysis in clinical practice. In: Waldman S, editor. Interventional pain management. 2nd ed. Philadelphia: WB Saunders; 2001. p. 226–42.
[23] Kumar K, Toth C, Nath RK. Spinal cord stimulation for chronic pain in peripheral neuropathy. Surg Neurol 1996;46:363–9.
[24] Brewer R, Bedlack R, Massey E. Diabetic thoracic radiculopathy: an unusual cause of post-thoracotomy pain. Pain 2003;103:221–3.
[25] Spaić M, Ivanović S, Slavik E, Antić B. DREZ (dorsal root entry zone) surgery for the treatment of the postherpetic intercostal neuralgia. Acta Chir Iugosl 2004;51:53–7.

CHAPTER 104

Myofascial Pain Syndrome

Martin K. Childers, DO, PhD
Jeffery B. Feldman, PhD
H. Michael Guo, MD, PhD

Synonyms

Myogelosis
Fibrositis
Fibromyalgia

ICD-9 Code

729.1 Myofascial pain syndrome

ICD-10 Code

M79.1 Myofascial pain syndrome

Definition

Myofascial pain syndrome (MPS) is a painful disorder characterized by the presence of myofascial trigger points (MTrPs), distinct sensitive spots in a palpable taut band of skeletal muscle fibers [1] that produce local and referred pain. Thus, MPS is characterized by both a motor abnormality (a taut or hard band within the muscle) and a sensory abnormality (tenderness and referred pain) [2] (Fig. 104.1). In addition to pain, the disorder is accompanied by referred autonomic phenomena as well as by anxiety and depression. The pathophysiologic mechanism of MPS is not clearly understood in part because of the scarcity of reliable valid studies. Moreover, concomitant disorders and frequent behavioral and psychosocial contributing factors in patients with MPS contribute to the complexity of human studies. Symptoms of MPS are generally associated with physical activities that are thought to contribute to "muscle overload," either acutely by sudden overload or gradually with prolonged repetitive activity [3]. MPS is reported to be prevalent in regional musculoskeletal pain syndromes; however, the syndrome can be classified as regional or generalized. Some authors broaden the definition of myofascial pain to include a regional pain syndrome of any soft tissue origin. Thus, MPS may be considered either a primary disorder causing local or regional pain syndromes or a secondary disorder that occurs as a consequence of some other condition, such as a radiculopathy.

The MTrP is generally considered the hallmark of MPS; therefore, much attention has been given to characteristic features of MTrPs in skeletal muscle [4,5]. One such feature of the MTrP is the so-called twitch response. This local response is considered a characteristic finding of the MTrP. Mechanical stimulation ("snapping" palpation, pressure, or needle insertion) can elicit a local twitch response that frequently is accompanied by referred pain [6]. The twitch response is accompanied by a burst of electrical activity ("end-plate noise") within the muscle band that contains the activated trigger point, whereas no activity is seen at other muscle bands. End-plate noise is significantly more prevalent in MTrPs than in sites that lie outside of the MTrP but still within the end-plate zone [7]. This observation has been attributed to a spinal reflex [4,6], as the response is abolished by motor nerve ablation or infusion of local anesthetic. Moreover, spinal cord transection above the neurologic level of the MTrP fails to permanently alter the characteristic response.

A number of hypotheses [8,9] have been put forward to explain the findings observed in MTrPs. One theory proposes that MTrPs are found only at the muscle spindle in an attempt to explain beneficial effects of α-adrenergic antagonists. However, this idea does not fully explain the electromyographic findings recorded at the MTrP. Further, there appears to be little evidence that painful muscle areas, such as MTrPs, are associated with any structural changes, such as an alteration in the appearance of the muscle spindle. Another theory is related to excessive release of acetylcholine in abnormal end plates [4], as the electromyographic activity recorded at trigger points resembles findings described at the end-plate region [7]. This idea has led some clinicians to study effects of botulinum toxin injection into MTrPs in an attempt to reduce release of excessive acetylcholine. To date, results of small cohort studies [10] examining effects of botulinum toxin on MTrPs have yielded inconsistent findings.

Central neurologic processes are increasingly viewed as essential factors in chronic pain syndromes. The medial

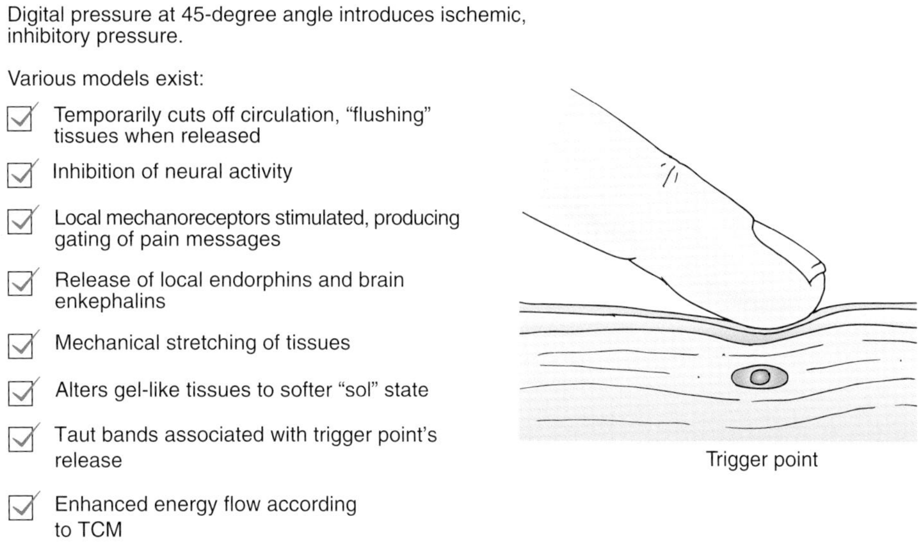

FIGURE 104.1 Schematic representation of myofascial trigger point. *TCM,* traditional Chinese medicine. *(From Chaitow L. Modern Neuromuscular Techniques, 3rd ed. New York, Churchill Livingstone, 2011.)*

thalamus is the principal relay of nociceptive input to the anterior cingulate cortex, and persistent stimulation of this pathway by pain in peripheral tissues has been demonstrated to change neurons in the cingulate cortex [11]. Thus, persistent pain is associated with long-term changes in the morphology, neurochemistry, and gene expression of the anterior cingulate cortex, which has the most direct connection with autonomic arousal, thereby contributing to the maintenance and exacerbation of pain [12].

Such central sensitization is characterized by an enhanced pain response to normally painful stimuli (hyperalgesia), a decrease in pain threshold to normally nonpainful stimuli (allodynia), and an increase in spontaneous activity (spontaneous pain). This process is clinically seen in MPS as the pain–muscle tension (in response to autonomic arousal and affective distress)–increased pain–increased tension and distress cycle.

Fibromyalgia (see Chapter 101), a chronic musculoskeletal pain condition that predominantly affects women, is characterized by diffuse muscle pain, fatigue, sleep disturbance, depression, and skin sensitivity [13]. Fibromyalgia may fit the classification of MPS as the diagnosis includes the presence of 11 of 18 tender points [14]. Furthermore, treatment of MPS and fibromyalgia is similar as evidence supports the role of exercise, cognitive-behavioral therapy, education, and social support in the management of both fibromyalgia and chronic MPS. However, there is controversy as to whether fibromyalgia and MPS represent specific pathologic processes or are descriptive terms of clinical conditions. Objective evidence of muscle abnormalities in fibromyalgia has been demonstrated by histologic studies showing disorganization of Z bands and abnormalities in the number and shape of muscle mitochondria. Biochemical studies and magnetic resonance spectroscopy have also shown inconstant abnormalities of adenosine triphosphate and phosphocreatine levels. It is unclear whether these abnormalities are a result of physical deconditioning or if abnormalities are due to problems in energy metabolism. There are no clear biochemical markers that distinguish patients with fibromyalgia. Thus, whereas the pathogenesis is still unknown, there has been evidence of increased corticotropin-releasing hormone and substance P in the cerebrospinal fluid of fibromyalgia patients as well as increased substance P and interleukins 6 and 8 in their serum [14]. One hypothesis supports the idea that fibromyalgia is an immunoendocrine disorder in which increased release of corticotropin-releasing hormone and substance P from neurons triggers local mast cells to release proinflammatory and neurosensitizing molecules. This hypothesis fits well with recent discoveries of neuropeptides found in the muscles of patients with active MTrPs [15].

Symptoms

The patient with MPS generally complains about dull or achy pain, sometimes poorly localized, particularly occurring during repetitive activities or during activities requiring sustained postures. Symptoms are exacerbated with digital pressure over tender areas of muscle with reproduction of the patient's usual pain. Symptoms are relieved with rest or cessation of repetitive activities. In contrast, the patient with fibromyalgia typically presents with sleep disturbances, depressed mood, and fatigue.

Physical Examination

The most important part of the physical examination is generally considered to be finding and localizing MTrPs to provide an accurate diagnosis of MPS. *Travell & Simons' Myofascial Pain and Dysfunction: The Trigger Point Manual* [16] is considered the criterion standard reference on locating and treating MTrPs. Active MTrPs, attributed to cause pain, exhibit marked localized tenderness and may refer pain to distant sites, disturb motor function, or produce autonomic changes. Specific clinical training is required to become adept at identifying MTrPs as evidence suggests that "non-trained" clinicians do not reliably detect the taut band and local twitch response [17].

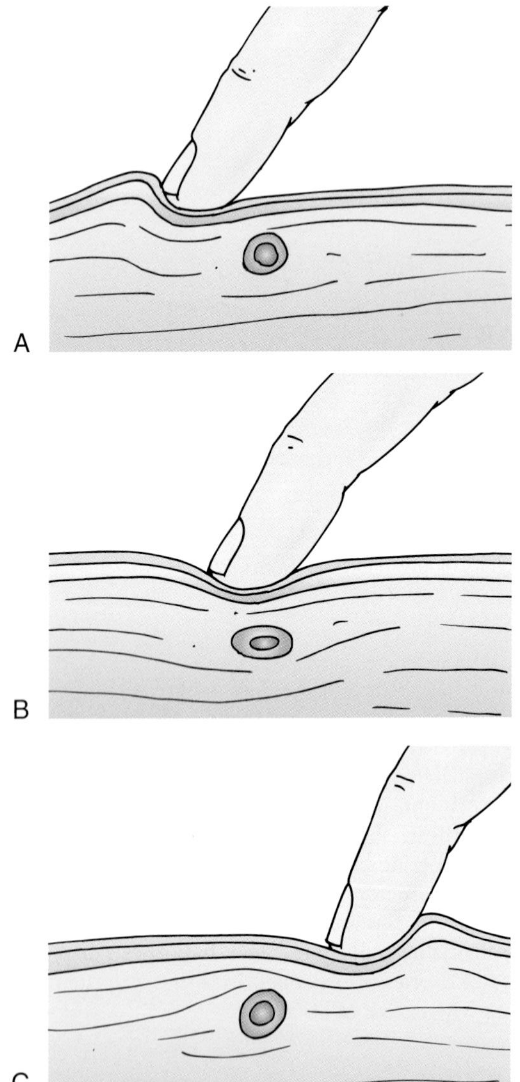

FIGURE 104.2 Flat palpation technique useful in examining muscles that are accessible only from one side. **A,** Index finger pushes skin to one side. **B,** Fingertip sweeps across the muscle to feel the taut band rolling beneath. **C,** Skin is pushed to the other side, completing the movement. When it is done vigorously, this technique is called snapping palpation. *(From Simons DG, Travell JG, Simons LS. Travell & Simons' Myofascial Pain and Dysfunction: The Trigger Point Manual, 2nd ed. Baltimore, Williams & Wilkins, 1999.)*

To clinically identify MTrPs, the clinician palpates a localized tender spot in a nodular portion of a taut, rope-like band of muscle fibers. Manual pressure over a trigger point should elicit pain at that area and may also elicit pain at a distant site (referred pain) from the point under the fingertip (Fig. 104.2). MTrPs, when palpated, should also elicit pain that mirrors the patient's experience. Applied pressure often reproduces the pain. Insertion of a needle, abrupt palpation, or even a brisk tap with the fingertip directly over the trigger point may induce a brief muscle contraction detectable by the examiner. This rapid contraction of muscle fibers of the ropy taut band is termed a local twitch response [3]. In muscles that move a relatively small mass or are large and superficial (such as the finger extensors or the gluteus maximus), the response is easily seen and may cause the limb to visibly move when the examiner introduces a needle into the trigger point. Localized abnormal response from the autonomic nervous system may cause piloerection, localized sweating, or even regional temperature changes in the skin attributed to altered blood flow [8,18,19].

Regional Examination of the Lower Extremity for Piriformis Syndrome

To evaluate individuals for piriformis syndrome [20], their usual buttock, hip, and lower limb pain may be reproduced during the following maneuvers: palpation over a point midway between the sacrum and greater trochanter of the femur, active hip abduction in the lateral recumbent position, and rectal palpation of the ipsilateral side of the involved limb [21,22]. Beatty described a maneuver [23,24] performed with the patient's lying with the painful side up, the painful leg flexed, and the knee resting on the table. Buttock pain is produced when the patient lifts and holds the knee several inches off the table. A positive finding in at least two of the preceding maneuvers is sufficient to confirm a diagnosis of piriformis syndrome, provided other potential causes have been eliminated from the differential diagnosis.

Diagnostic Studies

No definitive laboratory test or imaging method is diagnostic of MPS. Thus, diagnosis is made primarily by history and physical examination. Whereas no specific laboratory tests confirm (or refute) a diagnosis of MPS [25,26], some tests can be helpful in looking for predisposing conditions, such as hypothyroidism, hypoglycemia, and vitamin deficiencies. Specific tests that may be helpful include complete blood count, chemistry profile, erythrocyte sedimentation rate, and levels of vitamins C, B_1, B_6, B_{12}, and folic acid. If clinical features of thyroid disease are present, an assay for thyrotropin may be indicated [27].

Differential Diagnosis

Fibromyalgia
Trochanteric bursitis
Neuropathic pain
Postexercise muscle soreness
Articular dysfunction
Referred pain

Treatment

Initial

Therapeutic modalities such as biofeedback, ultrasound, lasers, and massage may be useful adjuncts in relieving initial pain to allow participation in an active exercise program [28]. Data suggest that addition of therapeutic physical modalities [1,3,25,29], such as heat, and various forms of muscle and nerve stimulation are beneficial in the initial treatment of MPS.

Nonsteroidal anti-inflammatory drugs (NSAIDs) may be a useful adjunct to active exercise-based treatment of MPS, but NSAIDs are generally considered beneficial when they are used in conjunction with an active treatment program. However, no randomized placebo-controlled clinical trials exist to support efficacy of NSAIDs in this condition. Interestingly, the NSAID diclofenac, when it is injected into the MTrP, was shown to be superior to lidocaine in one small clinical trial [30]. Low-dose amitriptyline is widely used in patients with fibromyalgia and is thought to help improve the patient's sleep cycle [31]. Muscle relaxants may also provide benefit to patients with MPS. For example, cyclobenzaprine hydrochloride, a commonly prescribed muscle relaxant, is indicated as an adjunct to rest and physical therapy for the relief of muscle spasm associated with acute, painful musculoskeletal conditions. In contrast to low-dose (5 mg three times daily) cyclobenzaprine, a higher dose (10 mg three times daily) is associated with more somnolence and dry mouth. Importantly, there does not appear to be a relationship between somnolence and pain relief. A large, multicenter, community-based trial of patients with acute pain and muscle spasm evaluated low-dose cyclobenzaprine (5 mg three times daily) alone compared with combination therapy with two doses of ibuprofen. It is possible that low-dose cyclobenzaprine or high-dose ibuprofen alone may be sufficient to relieve acute musculoskeletal pain and that no additional benefit is incurred by adding another medication. Future trials comparing various doses of muscle relaxants and NSAIDs alone or in combination will be required to address these questions in the treatment of patients with MPS.

Rehabilitation

Physical therapy techniques that focus on correction of muscle shortening by targeted stretching, strengthening of affected muscles, and correction of aggravating postural and biomechanical factors are generally considered to be the most effective treatment of MPS [32–34]. This idea is supported by a line of evidence examining the relationship between muscle overload and MTrPs [33,35], suggesting a direct relationship between exercise and MPS.

The goal for the treatment of MPS is to engage patients in active therapy to prevent the development of chronic pain syndrome or to rehabilitate patients from its disabling interacting symptoms if it has developed. Chronic MPS is not a diagnosis but a descriptive term for individuals who not only report persistent pain but also evidence poor coping, self-limitations in functional activities, significant life disruption, and dysfunctional pain behavior [36]. Other common symptoms of chronic pain syndrome related to an accompanying disuse syndrome include the multiple physical systems effects of deconditioning as well as insomnia, fatigue, anxiety, and depression [37]. A central feature of chronic MPS is a disability conviction and resulting avoidance of activity based on the fear that engaging in functional activity will increase pain (fear-avoidance) [37]. The critical importance of addressing such a belief is underlined by prior studies indicating that patients' beliefs about their pain are the best predictors of task performance [38], medical utilization [39], and long-term rehabilitation [40].

Preventing the development of such a disability conviction begins by assisting patients to shift from a biomedical perspective, in which there is an ongoing search for the cause of an illness to be "cured" or "fixed," to a biopsychosocial rehabilitation perspective [37,40]. This perspective views MPS as a multifactorial condition that need not be disabling if it is actively managed by the patient. Cognitive-behavioral therapy is the psychological approach that focuses on changing dysfunctional beliefs or "schemas" by which individuals process, store, and act on information [41]. For individuals with chronic pain to successfully participate in a functionally oriented rehabilitation approach, they need to understand or to believe the following:

1. The nature of the pain has been thoroughly evaluated, and there is no cure (i.e., surgery or another procedure) for the pain.
2. The rehabilitation approach involving physical activity and conditioning will increase functional capabilities and eventually reduce suffering.
3. The hurt engendered through physical conditioning will not cause harm.
4. Reinjury or worsening of the painful condition is unlikely, and it is in the individual's best interest to become more functional.

The first point most often can be addressed by the physician in the office, but the critical shift in belief that hurt will not cause harm generally requires the patient to have repeated experiences that contradict the prior life experience that if something hurts, you should stop doing it. For a patient with MPS to exercise consistently and sufficiently to contradict the common sense to avoid pain, an interdisciplinary team approach is often required. In such an approach, the physical therapist educates and guides the patient through a progressive physical reconditioning regimen. The physician periodically reevaluates the patient, reassuring and encouraging the patient that there is no problematic change in condition while adjusting medications to facilitate involvement in the program. Concurrently the psychologist provides training in stress management, pacing, and pain coping strategies. This is often best done in a group setting that normalizes the reactions and experience of the patient and where the social support and encouragement of the patient's peers is of significant benefit. Ultimately, though, it is the patient's repeated mild increases in pain without harm, as functioning improves, that change beliefs about pain and fear-avoidance of activity. It is largely for this reason that multidisciplinary pain programs that include a cognitive-behavioral approach have been found to be most effective for individuals with chronic pain on a range of key outcomes [42]. A cognitive-behavioral, functional restoration approach is particularly effective for chronic MPS because unlike in many other chronic pain conditions, one can be fairly certain that the hurt experienced through increased activity will not only not cause harm but will lead to long-term benefit.

Hypnosis

In addition to the cognitive changes noted, patients should be educated on the interacting effects of pain leading to increased sympathetic arousal ("stress response") that leads to increased muscle tension and increased pain. They therefore can reduce pain by reducing their reactivity to pain as well as other stressors in their life. Techniques for doing so include relaxation training, progressive muscle relaxation, mindfulness meditation, and hypnosis. Hypnosis is increasingly being integrated into multidisciplinary treatment approaches because it enables one to train patients to develop a relaxation response while also interspersing suggestions to encourage the changes in thinking noted before [43–51]. In other words, hypnosis is a tool that can be used not only to assist patients in reducing their attention to the sensation of pain but, more important, to reduce their affective distress and autonomic reactivity.

Mindfulness Meditation

Another approach to reducing affective distress and autonomic reactivity in response to pain that has received increasing attention is mindfulness meditation. Mindfulness has been defined as "paying attention in a particular way: on purpose, in the present moment, and nonjudgmentally." [52] Zeidan and colleagues [53] expanded on this description to operationally define mindfulness as involving "(a) regulated, sustained attention to the moment-to-moment quality and character of sensory, emotional and cognitive events, (b) the recognition of such events as momentary, fleeting and changeable (past and future representations of those events being considered cognitive abstractions), and (c) a consequent lack of emotional or cognitive appraisal and/or reactions to these events." Pragmatically, this tends to involve training in focused attention (Samatha meditation) and open awareness (Vipassana meditation). One is taught that such thoughts are momentary and fleeting and that one need not react to them. Whereas mindfulness-based stress reduction has been viewed as the "gold standard," there have been variations including mindfulness-based cognitive therapy [54]. For example, brief mindfulness training can have a significant impact on experimentally induced pain and cognition [53]. Although the specific mechanisms remain unclear, accruing evidence indicates that through processes of neuroplasticity, significant changes can occur in brain structures associated with the processing of pain, especially the prefrontal and anterior cingulate cortices [55]. In this way, one can therapeutically use the neuroplasticity of the brain to enhance pain control, in a manner that is the reverse of central sensitization described before.

Procedures

In combination with other therapies, interventional techniques can be an effective adjunct in the multidisciplinary management of patients with MPS [56]. In the treatment of MPS, other than trigger point injections, interventional procedures (e.g., epidural steroid injections, sacroiliac joint injections, and medial branch blocks) are usually not employed. However, at times, myofascial pain is associated with or caused by other underlying conditions. For instance, lumbar myofascial pain may also have some component of lumbar facet arthropathy. Lumbar medial branch blocks and radiofrequency denervation, alone or in combination with the other therapies (e.g., muscle relaxants), may work together to relieve myofascial pain. Similarly, epidural steroid injection may provide lumbar pain relief in a patient with spondylosis. It has been suggested that epidural steroid injections may be used to treat cervical MPS if conservative treatments fail [57]. Therefore, underlying disease may respond to more aggressive interventional methods and in turn synergistically provide pain relief to the patient with MPS.

MTrP injections should be individualized for both the patient and the clinician. Alcohol, if it is used to clean the skin, should be allowed to dry completely to prevent additional pain. Use of operating rooms or special procedure (sterile) rooms equipped with monitoring devices for the purpose of intramuscular injections with small-caliber needles is not necessary. Most patients can be treated safely in an office setting by experienced clinicians. The diagnostic skill required to find active MTrPs depends on considerable innate palpation ability, authoritative training, and extensive clinical experience [3]. Application of trigger point injection begins by determining the equipment needs according to the needs of the patient, the clinician's training, and the anatomic target for injection. Typically, a 1.0-mL tuberculin-type syringe with $\frac{5}{8}$-inch 25-gauge needle is adequate for superficial muscles. For small muscles (e.g., facial muscles), a 1-inch 30-gauge needle is sufficient. For larger muscles, a 1-inch or 1½-inch 25-gauge needle is adequate. After the patient is placed in a position in which the desired muscle can be relaxed, the MTrP is located. In the prone position, the MTrP is ascertained by gentle pressure from the end of a fingertip or a ballpoint pen applied at regular 1-cm intervals. The patient is observed closely during the palpation because pressure on the markedly tender MTrP usually causes the patient to jump, to wince, or to cry out. Each muscle has a characteristic elicited referred pain pattern that, for active MTrPs, is familiar to the patient. Thus, the patient will respond that this pressure reproduces the usual pain and, when questioned, will describe painful sensations at a site slightly distant to the point under the examiner's finger. Once the MTrP has been located, the skin is marked, and the site is injected with saline, anesthetic agent, or corticosteroid solution. Once the MTrP has been located, the skin is marked and prepared. The site is injected with no more than 1 mL injectate per site after negative aspiration for blood. When the needle is advanced to the MTrP, it may elicit a local twitch response, although a local twitch response is not observed all the time despite significant improvement of myofascial pain with trigger point injection. Other findings that may help determine the needle entrance to the MTrP are the patient's confirmation of reproduction of the usual pain pattern and the clinician's sensation of increased resistance as the needle is advanced from normal muscle tissue to the taut band.

Surgery

Surgery is not indicated in the treatment of patients with MPS.

Potential Disease Complications

Patients with MPS may go on to develop chronic pain syndrome. Treatment of individuals with chronic MPS is described earlier. Perhaps the biggest complication of untreated and progressive MPS is development of a syndrome of physical inactivity that may lead to cardiovascular disease. Evidence of a dose-response relation between physical activity and cardiovascular disease endpoints has been proposed [58], although the majority of the literature in this area has relied on prospective observational studies, and few randomized trials of physical activity and cardiovascular disease as a clinical outcome have been reported. This notwithstanding, evidence indicates that cardiovascular disease incidence and mortality are causally related to physical activity in an inverse, dose-response fashion. Thus, left untreated, patients with MPS who go on to develop chronic pain and lack physical activity are at high risk for cardiovascular disease and early death.

Potential Treatment Complications

The greatest risk of treatment of the patent with MPS is related to MTrP injections in the thoracic area. Because of the anatomic location of the apex of the lung to the proximity of the upper trapezius muscle or the scalene muscles, the clinician must be aware of the potential for pneumothorax as a result of MTrP injection in this area. The use of long (>1 inch) small-gauge needles should be avoided because long, thin needles can easily bend once they are inserted into the muscle, and the tip can inadvertently puncture the pleura. Rather, short (<1 inch) needles should be used for MTrP injections anywhere near the apex of the lung. In addition, the needle should be directed away from structures at risk of inadvertent puncture. To provide additional proprioceptive feedback during injection, grasping the muscle between the thumb and forefinger will allow the clinician to palpate the thickness of the tissue to be injected. Thin patients or those with reduced lung capacity from underlying diseases are particularly at risk, and thus the clinician should use extra precautions when performing MTrP injections in these patients.

References

[1] Borg-Stein J, Simons DG. Focused review: myofascial pain. Arch Phys Med Rehabil 2002;83:S40–7, S48–S49.

[2] Gerwin RD. Classification, epidemiology, and natural history of myofascial pain syndrome. Curr Pain Headache Rep 2001;5:412–20.

[3] Simons DG, Mense S. Diagnosis and therapy of myofascial trigger points. Schmerz 2003;17:419–24.

[4] Hong CZ, Simons DG. Pathophysiologic and electrophysiologic mechanisms of myofascial trigger points. Arch Phys Med Rehabil 1998;79:863–72.

[5] Macgregor J, Graf von Schweinitz D. Needle electromyographic activity of myofascial trigger points and control sites in equine cleidobrachialis muscle—an observational study. Acupunct Med 2006;24:61–70.

[6] Hong CZ. Pathophysiology of myofascial trigger point. J Formos Med Assoc 1996;95:93–104.

[7] Simons DG, Hong CZ, Simons LS. Endplate potentials are common to midfiber myofascial trigger points. Am J Phys Med Rehabil 2002;81:212–22.

[8] Rivner MH. The neurophysiology of myofascial pain syndrome. Curr Pain Headache Rep 2001;5:432–40.

[9] Simons DG. Myofascial pain syndromes: where are we? Where are we going? Arch Phys Med Rehabil 1988;69:207–12.

[10] Ho KY, Tan KH. Botulinum toxin A for myofascial trigger point injection: a qualitative systematic review. Eur J Pain 2007;11:519–27.

[11] Shyu BC, Vogt BA. Short-term synaptic plasticity in the nociceptive thalamic-anterior cingulate pathway. Mol Pain 2009;5:51.

[12] Cao H, Gao YJ, Ren WH, et al. Activation of extracellular signal-regulated kinase in the anterior cingulate cortex contributes to the induction and expression of affective pain. J Neurosci 2009;29:3307–21.

[13] Arnold LM. Biology and therapy of fibromyalgia. New therapies in fibromyalgia. Arthritis Res Ther 2006;8:212.

[14] Lucas HJ, Brauch CM, Settas L, Theoharides TC. Fibromyalgia—new concepts of pathogenesis and treatment. Int J Immunopathol Pharmacol 2006;19:5–10.

[15] Shah JP, Phillips TM, Danoff JV, Gerber LH. An in vivo microanalytical technique for measuring the local biochemical milieu of human skeletal muscle. J Appl Physiol 2005;99:1977–84.

[16] Simons DG, Travell JG, Simons LS. Travell & Simons' myofascial pain and dysfunction: the trigger point manual. Baltimore: Williams & Wilkins; 1999.

[17] Hsieh CY, Hong CZ, Adams AH, et al. Interexaminer reliability of the palpation of trigger points in the trunk and lower limb muscles. Arch Phys Med Rehabil 2000;81:258–64.

[18] McPartland JM. Travell trigger points—molecular and osteopathic perspectives. J Am Osteopath Assoc 2004;104:244–9.

[19] Mense S, Simons DG, Hoheisel U, Quenzer B. Lesions of rat skeletal muscle after local block of acetylcholinesterase and neuromuscular stimulation. J Appl Physiol 2003;94:2494–501.

[20] Burton DJ, Enion D, Shaw DL. Pyomyositis of the piriformis muscle in a juvenile. Ann R Coll Surg Engl 2005;87:W9–12.

[21] Childers MK, Wilson DJ, Gnatz SM, et al. Botulinum toxin type A use in piriformis muscle syndrome: a pilot study. Am J Phys Med Rehabil 2002;81:751–9.

[22] Nakamura H, Seki M, Konishi S, et al. Piriformis syndrome diagnosed by cauda equina action potentials: report of two cases. Spine (Phila Pa 1976) 2003;28:E37–40.

[23] Beatty RA. The piriformis muscle syndrome: a simple diagnostic maneuver. Neurosurgery 1994;34:512–4, discussion 514.

[24] Beatty RA. Piriformis syndrome. J Neurosurg Spine 2006;5:101, author reply 101–102.

[25] Auleciems LM. Myofascial pain syndrome: a multidisciplinary approach. Nurse Pract 1995;20:18, 21–22, 24–28, passim.

[26] Escobar PL, Ballesteros J. Myofascial pain syndrome. Orthop Rev 1987;16:708–13.

[27] Saravanan P, Dayan CM. Thyroid autoantibodies. Endocrinol Metab Clin North Am 2001;30:315–37, viii.

[28] Hou CR, Tsai LC, Cheng KF, et al. Immediate effects of various physical therapeutic modalities on cervical myofascial pain and trigger-point sensitivity. Arch Phys Med Rehabil 2002;83:1406–14.

[29] Fricton JR. Myofascial pain syndrome. Neurol Clin 1989;7:413–27.

[30] Frost A. Diclofenac versus lidocaine as injection therapy in myofascial pain. Scand J Rheumatol 1986;15:153–6.

[31] Borg-Stein J. Treatment of fibromyalgia, myofascial pain, and related disorders. Phys Med Rehabil Clin N Am 2006;17:491–510, viii.

[32] McClaflin RR. Myofascial pain syndrome. Primary care strategies for early intervention. Postgrad Med 1994;96:56–9, 63–66, 69–70, passim.

[33] Nicolakis P, Erdogmus B, Kopf A, et al. Effectiveness of exercise therapy in patients with myofascial pain dysfunction syndrome. J Oral Rehabil 2002;29:362–8.

[34] Rosen NB. Physical medicine and rehabilitation approaches to the management of myofascial pain and fibromyalgia syndromes. Baillieres Clin Rheumatol 1994;8:881–916.

[35] Itoh K, Okada K, Kawakita K. A proposed experimental model of myofascial trigger points in human muscle after slow eccentric exercise. Acupunct Med 2004;22:2–12, discussion 12–13.

[36] Feldman JB. The neurobiology of pain, affect and hypnosis. Am J Clin Hypn 2004;46:187–200.

[37] Aronoff GM, Feldman JB, Campion TS. Management of chronic pain and control of long-term disability. Occup Med 2000;15:755–70, iv.

[38] Lackner JM, Carosella AM. The relative influence of perceived pain control, anxiety, and functional self efficacy on spinal function among patients with chronic low back pain. Spine (Phila Pa 1976) 1999;24:2254–60, discussion 2260–2261.

[39] Reitsma B, Meijler WJ. Pain and patienthood. Clin J Pain 1997;13:9–21.

[40] Jensen MP, Turner JA, Romano JM. Changes in beliefs, catastrophizing, and coping are associated with improvement in multidisciplinary pain treatment. J Consult Clin Psychol 2001;69:655–62.

[41] Butler AC, Chapman JE, Forman EM, Beck AT. The empirical status of cognitive-behavioral therapy: a review of meta-analyses. Clin Psychol Rev 2006;26:17–31.

[42] Flor H, Fydrich T, Turk DC. Efficacy of multidisciplinary pain treatment centers: a meta-analytic review. Pain 1992;49:221–30.

[43] Rainville P, Carrier B, Hofbauer RK, et al. Dissociation of sensory and affective dimensions of pain using hypnotic modulation. Pain 1999;82:159–71.

[44] Malone MD, Strube MJ, Scogin FR. Meta-analysis of non-medical treatments for chronic pain. Pain 1988;34:231–44.

[45] Nielson WR, Weir R. Biopsychosocial approaches to the treatment of chronic pain. Clin J Pain 2001;17:S114–27.

[46] Osborne TL, Raichle KA, Jensen MP. Psychologic interventions for chronic pain. Phys Med Rehabil Clin N Am 2006;17:415–33.

[47] Turner JA, Chapman CR. Psychological interventions for chronic pain: a critical review. II. Operant conditioning, hypnosis, and cognitive-behavioral therapy. Pain 1982;12:23–46.
[48] Hofbauer RK, Rainville P, Duncan GH, Bushnell MC. Cortical representation of the sensory dimension of pain. J Neurophysiol 2001;86:402–11.
[49] Rainville P, Bao QV, Chretien P. Pain-related emotions modulate experimental pain perception and autonomic responses. Pain 2005;118:306–18.
[50] Rainville P, Duncan GH, Price DD, et al. Pain affect encoded in human anterior cingulate but not somatosensory cortex. Science 1997;277:968–71.
[51] Rainville P, Hofbauer RK, Bushnell MC, et al. Hypnosis modulates activity in brain structures involved in the regulation of consciousness. J Cogn Neurosci 2002;14:887–901.
[52] Kabat-Zinn J, Lipworth L, Burney R. The clinical use of mindfulness meditation for the self-regulation of chronic pain. J Behav Med 1985;8:163–90.
[53] Zeidan F, Gordon NS, Merchant J, Goolkasian P. The effects of brief mindfulness meditation training on experimentally induced pain. J Pain 2010;11:199–209.
[54] Ma SH, Teasdale JD. Mindfulness-based cognitive therapy for depression: replication and exploration of differential relapse prevention effects. J Consult Clin Psychol 2004;72:31–40.
[55] Zeidan F, Martucci KT, Kraft RA, et al. Brain mechanisms supporting the modulation of pain by mindfulness meditation. J Neurosci 2011;31:5540–8.
[56] Criscuolo CM. Interventional approaches to the management of myofascial pain syndrome. Curr Pain Headache Rep 2001;5:407–11.
[57] Murphy DR, Hurwitz EL. A theoretical model for the development of a diagnosis-based clinical decision rule for the management of patients with spinal pain. BMC Musculoskelet Disord 2007;8:75.
[58] Kohl 3rd HW. Physical activity and cardiovascular disease: evidence for a dose response. Med Sci Sports Exerc 2001;33:S472–83, discussion S493–S494.

CHAPTER 105

Occipital Neuralgia

Mark Young, MD

Aneesh Singla, MD, MPH

Synonyms

Cervicogenic headache
Occipital myalgia-neuralgia syndrome
Occipital headache
Occipital neuropathy
Occipital neuritis
Arnold neuralgia
Third occipital headache
Cervical migraine

ICD-9 Code

723.8 Other syndromes affecting cervical region; occipital neuralgia

ICD-10 Codes

G44.89 Other specified headache syndromes
M54.81 Occipital neuralgia

Definition

The International Headache Society categorizes occipital neuralgia as a cranial neuralgia and defines it with three diagnostic features: paroxysmal stabbing pain in the distribution of the occipital nerves with tenderness over the affected nerves temporarily relieved by local anesthetic block [1]. Occipital neuralgia can occur in the distribution of the greater and lesser occipital nerves (Fig. 105.1). However, the greater occipital nerve is more commonly involved (90%); in addition, unilateral symptoms are more common (85%) [2]. The condition appears to be more common in women [3].

The pain is described as lancinating, sharp, throbbing, electric shock–like, and often associated with posterior scalp dysesthesia or hyperalgesia [4–6]. Two broad categories of patients with occipital neuralgia are those with structural pathologic changes and those without an apparent cause [7]. Proposed causes include myofascial tightening, trauma of C2 nerve root (whiplash injury), prior skull or suboccipital surgery, other type of nerve entrapment, hypertrophied atlantoepistrophic (C1-C2) ligament, sustained neck muscle contractions, and spondylosis of the cervical facet joints [2,4,6,8–10]. Most patients with occipital neuropathy do not have discernible lesions [11].

Anatomy

The greater occipital nerve innervates the posterior skull from the suboccipital area to the vertex. It is formed from the medial (sensory) branch of the posterior division of the second cervical nerve [8]. It emerges between the atlas and lamina of the axis below the oblique inferior muscle and then ascends obliquely on this muscle between it and the semispinalis muscle [8]. The course of the greater occipital nerve does not appear to differ in men and women [12]. The lesser occipital nerve forms from the medial (sensory) branch of the posterior division of the third cervical nerve, ascends like the greater occipital nerve, and pierces the splenius capitis and trapezius muscles just medial to the greater occipital nerve [8]. It ascends along the scalp to reach the vertex, where it provides sensory fibers to the area of the scalp lateral to the greater occipital nerve.

The roots of the first two cervical nerves are not protected posteriorly by pedicles and facets because of the unique articulation of the atlas and axis relative to the rest of the spinal column. Thus, the first two cervical nerves are relatively vulnerable to injury. The joint between the atlas and occiput, between which the first cervical nerve emerges, is relatively immobile compared with the lower C1-C2 articulation. Thus the C2 nerve root emerges unprotected through a highly mobile joint, and this may explain the predominance of greater occipital nerve involvement in occipital neuralgia [13].

Symptoms

Although occipital neuralgia is defined by the International Headache Society as a paroxysmal headache, some patients complain of continuous pain [2]. In continuous occipital neuralgia, the headaches may be further classified as acute or chronic.

Paroxysmal occipital neuralgia describes pain occurring only in the distribution of the occipital nerve. The attacks are generally unilateral, and the pain is sudden and severe.

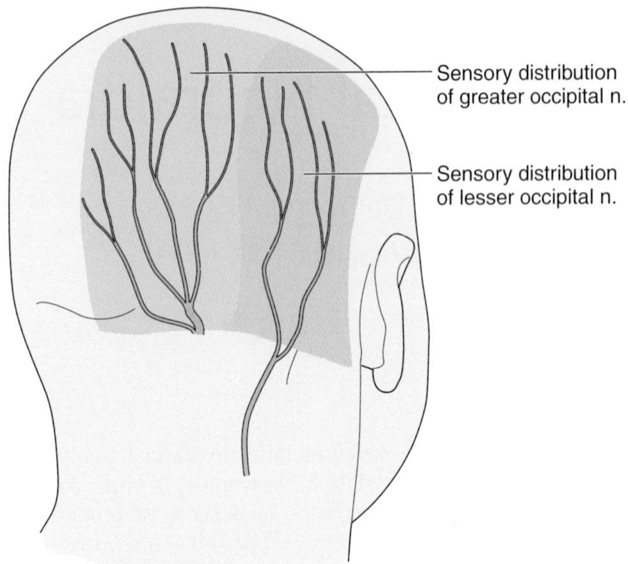

FIGURE 105.1 Occipital nerve anatomy. The greater occipital nerve pierces the fascia just below the superior nuchal ridge along with the artery. It supplies the medial portion of the posterior scalp. The lesser occipital nerve passes superiorly along the posterior border of the sternocleidomastoid muscle, dividing into the cutaneous branches that innervate the lateral portion of the posterior scalp and the cranial surface of the pinna. *(From Waldman SD. Greater and lesser occipital nerve block. In Waldman SD, ed. Atlas of Interventional Pain Management, 2nd ed. Philadelphia, WB Saunders, 2004.)*

The patient may describe the pain as sharp, twisting, a dagger thrust, or an electric shock. The pain rarely demonstrates a burning characteristic. Although single flashes of pain may occur, multiple attacks are more frequent. The attacks may occur spontaneously or be provoked by specific maneuvers applied to the back of the scalp or neck regions, such as brushing the hair or moving the neck [11].

Acute continuous occipital neuralgia often has an underlying cause. Exposure to cold is a common trigger [14]. The attacks last for many hours and are typically devoid of radiating symptoms (e.g., trigger zones to the face). The entire episode of neuralgia can continue up to 2 weeks before remission.

In chronic continuous occipital neuralgia, the patient may experience painful attacks that last for days to weeks. These attacks are generally accompanied by localized spasm of the cervical or occipital muscles. The reported pain originates in the suboccipital region up to the vertex and radiates to the frontotemporal region. Radiation to the orbital region is also common. Sensory triggers to the face or skull can initiate a painful episode. Similarly, pain may increase with pressure of the head on a pillow. Prolonged abnormal fixed postures that occur in reading or sleeping positions and hyperextension or rotation of the head to the involved side may provoke the pain. The pain may be bilateral, although the unilateral pattern is more common. Often, a previous history of cervical or occipital trauma or arthritic disease of the cervical spine is obtained. On occasion, patients may report other autonomic symptoms concurrently, such as nausea, vomiting, photophobia, diplopia, ocular and nasal congestion, tinnitus, and vertigo [11]. Severe ocular pain has also been described, as have symptoms in other distributions of the trigeminal nerve [9,10,12,13]. Convergence of sensory input from the upper cervical nerve roots into the trigeminal nucleus may explain this phenomenon [13]. Occipital neuralgia may occur in combination with other types of headaches. For example, one study found concurrent migraine in 20 of 35 consecutive patients presenting with occipital neuralgia [14].

Physical Examination

On examination, pain is generally reproduced by palpation of the greater and lesser occipital nerves. Allodynia or hyperalgesia may be present in the nerve distribution. Myofascial pain may be present in the neck or shoulders. Pain may limit cervical range of motion. Neurologic examination findings of the head, neck, and upper extremities are generally normal.

Entrapment of the nerve near the cervical spine may result in increased symptoms during flexion, extension, or rotation of the head and neck. Compression of the skull on the neck (Spurling maneuver), especially with extension and rotation of the neck to the affected side, may reproduce or increase the patient's pain if cervical degenerative disease is the cause of the neuralgia [11]. Pressure over both the occipital nerves along their course in the neck and occiput or pressure on the C2-C3 facet joints should cause an exacerbation of pain in such patients, at least when the headache is present. Even if the actual pathologic process is in the cervical spine, tenderness over the occipital nerve at the superior nuchal line is usually present.

Functional Limitations

In general, there are no neurologic deficits from occipital neuralgia. However, the pain from this entity may result in significant limitations in activities of daily living. During exacerbations, patients may have significant functional limitations, including insomnia, loss of work time, and inability to perform physical activity or to drive a vehicle. Tasks that involve the cervical spine or upper extremities, such as talking on the telephone, working at the computer, reading a book, cooking, gardening, and driving, may be painful and limited.

Diagnostic Studies

The diagnosis of occipital neuralgia is generally made clinically on the basis of history and physical examination. Imaging may help confirm the diagnosis when there is an anatomic cause. Diagnostic local anesthetic nerve blocks may be required for a definitive diagnosis to be obtained; these blocks are done with or without the addition of corticosteroid [5,8,11]. The relief of pain after a diagnostic local anesthetic block of the greater and lesser occipital nerves is generally confirmatory of the diagnosis of occipital neuralgia.

In addition, magnetic resonance imaging or computed tomography of the cervical spine should be performed to rule out an anatomic cause, such as tumor, vascular malformation, infection, or spondylotic arthritis, that may be compressing the medial (sensory) branches of C2-C3 [15]. Radiographs may be obtained to rule out gross abnormalities as an initial screening test but will not generally provide the level of detail needed for diagnostic purposes. Single-photon emission computed tomography and positron emission tomography are being increasingly used for diagnosis and treatment of certain headache syndromes and may be useful in occipital neuralgia if there is functional pathologic change involved or in trying to distinguish between occipital neuralgia and cluster or migraine headache [13]. Radiologic degenerative changes of the cervical spine do not necessarily correlate with the patient's symptoms and examination findings, but C2-C3 arthritic changes in the absence of other gross or radiographic abnormalities may explain the etiology. Other rare causes of occipital neuralgia reported in the literature include upper respiratory tract infection [16], herpes zoster infection or postherpetic neuralgia [17], myelitis [18], hypermobile C1 vertebra [19], and giant cell arteritis [20,21]. In patients with unilateral headaches in the distribution of the greater occipital nerve, ultrasonography can show enlargement of the ipsilateral nerve compared with the uninvolved contralateral nerve and thus lend further evidence to the diagnosis of occipital neuralgia [22].

Differential Diagnosis

C2-C3 subluxation or arthropathy
C2-C3 radiculopathy
Migraine headache
Cluster headache
Tension-type headache
Tumor (e.g., posterior fossa)
Congenital or acquired abnormalities at the craniocervical junction (e.g., Arnold-Chiari malformation or basilar invagination)
Rheumatoid arthritis
Atlantoaxial subluxation
Cervical myelopathy
Pott disease–osteomyelitis
Paget disease
Vascular abnormalities
Herpes zoster or postherpetic neuralgia
Giant cell arteritis
Trauma
Whiplash injury

Treatment

Initial

Treatments that may help with pain from occipital neuralgia include heat or cold therapy, massage, avoidance of excessive cervical spine flexion-extension or rotation, acupuncture, and application of transcutaneous electrical nerve stimulation.

Pharmacologic therapy with nonsteroidal anti-inflammatory drugs or acetaminophen as well as other analgesics may be used. Tricyclic antidepressants, anticonvulsants, and muscle relaxants may also prove useful. Anticonvulsants such as carbamazepine, gabapentin, and pregabalin have been used for neuropathic pain with good results. Certain patients with comorbid psychological stressors may have pain complaints out of proportion to physical examination findings and should have their psychological symptoms treated with appropriate medications and psychological or cognitive-behavioral therapy.

Patients will often benefit from adaptive equipment at home and work, such as a telephone earset or bookstand. It is also important to determine whether patients are using bifocal glasses and whether adjusting the neck to use these glasses is contributing to the condition.

Rehabilitation

The incorporation of stretching and strengthening exercises for the paracervical and periscapular muscles may be appropriate for the patient with subacute or chronic occipital neuralgia, particularly if the condition is provoked by cervical spine or trunk movement. Postural training and relaxation exercises should be incorporated into the exercise regimen. Principles of ergonomics should be addressed if work site activity is limited by pain exacerbations (e.g., use of a telephone headset, document holder) [11]. An ergonomic workstation evaluation may be beneficial.

Manual therapy, including spinal manipulation and spinal mobilization, has been used to treat patients with cervicogenic headaches. A review of trials done with spinal manipulation for cervicogenic headache revealed two with positive results regarding headache intensity, headache duration, and medication intake [23]. Only one trial showed a decrease in headache frequency. There is clearly a need for more well designed randomized controlled trials to evaluate these therapies [24]. Any spinal manipulation should be done with caution because there are serious risks if it is improperly performed [25]. Anecdotal reports support a trial of cervical traction in some cases [11].

Procedures

Blockade of the greater or lesser occipital nerve with a local anesthetic is diagnostic and therapeutic (Fig. 105.2). Pain relief can vary from hours to months. In general, at least 50% of patients will experience more than 1 week of relief after one injection. Isolated pain relief for more than 17 months has been reported after a series of five blocks [7]. The addition of a cortisone preparation is controversial, but it may provide additional benefit [3]. Botulinum toxin A injection into the greater occipital nerve has also been described [3], but the evidence is limited. Its use is currently ranked as grade C, the weakest strength recommendation [26]. Classically, landmark techniques have been used in occipital nerve blockade. Ward [27] described one such blind technique wherein the greater occipital nerve is found medial to the occipital artery along the superior nuchal line. Nerve stimulator–guided blocks [28] and computed tomography–guided blocks [6] have also been described. An ultrasound-guided technique was recently demonstrated [29] and postulated as superior to traditional landmark techniques in light of known variation of the greater occipital nerve [30], but clinical studies have not confirmed this presumption.

Dorsal rhizotomy of C1, C2, C3, and C4 has been described; about 71% to 77% of patients report significant benefit [7,25–27]. Before dorsal rhizotomy, local anesthetic blockade of the suspected medial (sensory) branches should be performed for diagnostic purposes.

Pulsed radiofrequency to the culprit occipital nerve was shown to improve symptoms for 6 months or more [31].

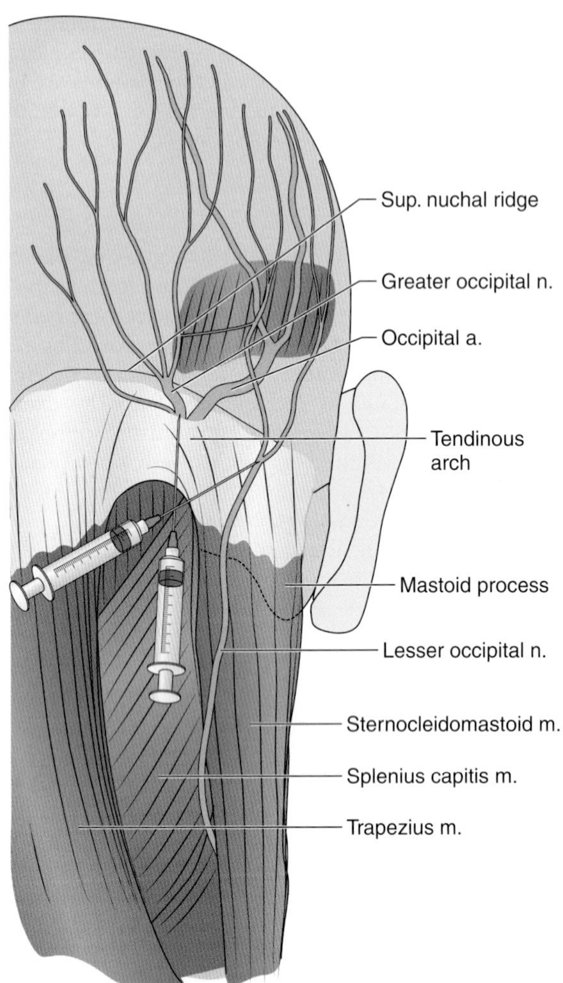

FIGURE 105.2 Occipital nerve block. The patient is placed in a sitting position with the cervical spine flexed and the forehead on a padded bedside table. A total of 8 mL of local anesthetic is drawn up in a 12-mL sterile syringe. A total of 80 mg of depot steroid is added to the local anesthetic with the first block and 40 mg with subsequent blocks. The occipital artery is palpated at the level of the superior nuchal ridge. After preparation of the skin with antiseptic solution, a 22- or 25-gauge, 1½-inch needle is inserted just medial to the artery and advanced perpendicularly until the needle approaches the periosteum of the underlying occipital bone. A paresthesia may be encountered. The needle is then redirected superiorly, and after gentle aspiration, 5 mL of solution is injected in a fan-like distribution, with care being taken to avoid the foramen magnum. *(From Waldman SD. Greater and lesser occipital nerve block. In Waldman SD, ed. Atlas of Interventional Pain Management, 2nd ed. Philadelphia, WB Saunders, 2004.)*

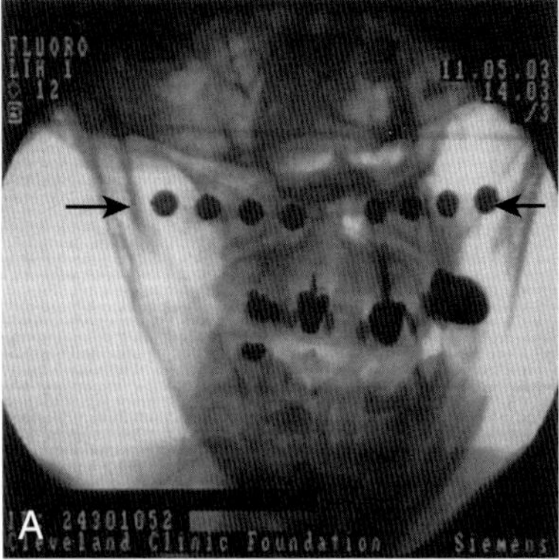

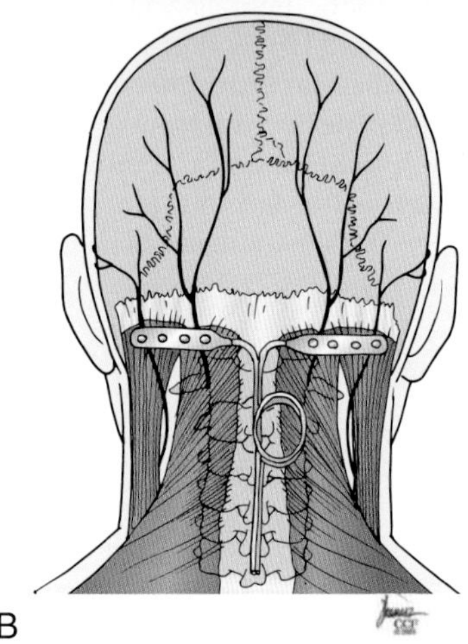

FIGURE 105-3 Occipital nerve stimulation. Radiograph (**A**) and schematic (**B**) of the midline subcutaneous approach in surgical lead positioning for electrical stimulation of the occipital nerve. **A,** Bilateral position of subcutaneous leads *(arrows)* after initial adjustment and just before intraoperative stimulation testing. Note that both leads are at the level of C1-C2 dens and aimed laterally. **B,** Schematic of the lead positioning in the subcutaneous occipital area. Note that the lead cable extensions form the loop just below the implant's position and through the same midline incision. *(From Kapural L, Mekhail N, Hayek SM, et al. Occipital nerve electrical stimulation via the midline approach and subcutaneous surgical leads for treatment of severe occipital neuralgia: a pilot study. Anesth Analg 2005;101:171-174.)*

A more recent report demonstrated benefit from pulsed radiofrequency in a significant portion of patients with treatment-refractory occipital neuralgia [32].

Surgery

One should consider surgical treatment after conservative therapy has failed, including but not limited to membrane stabilizers, tricyclic antidepressants, opioids, spinal manipulation, occipital nerve or cervical medial branch blocks, and partial posterior rhizotomy of C1-C3 [6]. Reversible interventions may be considered before destructive, irreversible surgical procedures [33]. In 1999, Weiner and Reed described successful treatment of occipital neuralgia with neurostimulation, whereby subcutaneous implantation of electrical leads in the suboccipital region modulates afferent pain nociceptive fibers to decrease the transmission of painful impulses. This is thought to occur through the gate control theory of pain or possibly through modulation of neurotransmitters in the central nervous system [34] (Fig. 105.3). A variety of surgical procedures for occipital neuralgia have been proposed, such as neurectomy, C1-C2 decompression, C2 ganglionectomy, and occipital nerve stimulation. The rate of meaningful pain relief from ganglionectomy has been reported to be 60% to 67% [35,36].

Surgical release of the inferior oblique muscles has been described as a potential treatment of occipital neuralgia, particularly when compression of the nerve by this muscle is suspected. In a small, retrospective study of 10 patients, the average visual analog score for pain decreased from 8 of 10 to 2 of 10 after the procedure [37]. Dorsal root entry zone lesioning has also been reported for occipital neuralgia [38].

Table 105.1 Pharmacologic Treatment of Occipital Neuralgia

Medication	Dosage	Common Side Effects
Nonsteroidal anti-inflammatory drugs	Variable	Gastrointestinal bleed, dyspepsia, nausea, headache, dizziness, rash, fluid retention, urticaria, hepatotoxicity, acute renal failure
Cyclooxygenase 2 inhibitors Celecoxib (Celebrex)	Celecoxib: 100 mg bid or 200 mg qd	Dyspepsia, nausea, abdominal pain, constipation, anorexia, elevated liver enzymes, acute renal failure, anaphylaxis, agranulocytosis
Tricyclic antidepressants Amitriptyline Nortriptyline Imipramine	Start at 10 mg qhs and titrate to 75 mg qhs or until clinical response	Dry mouth, constipation, urinary obstruction, sedation, postural hypertension, decreased seizure threshold
Carbamazepine (Tegretol)	Start at 100 mg bid; titrate to 400 mg bid	Sedation, unsteadiness, nausea, blurred vision, seizures, hepatitis, aplastic anemia
Gabapentin (Neurontin)	Start at 300 mg qd; titrate to 1200 mg tid	Dyspepsia, dizziness, tremor, coordination problems, insomnia, diarrhea, palpitations, nervousness, headache, tinnitus, depression, rash, dry mouth, anorexia, fatigue, arrhythmia
Mexiletine	Start at 150 mg qd × 3 d, then 300 mg qd × 3 d, then 10 mg/kg qd	Somnolence, dizziness, ataxia, fatigue, nystagmus, tremor, blurred vision, myalgia, weight gain, nausea, amnesia, leukopenia

Potential Disease Complications

Occipital neuralgia is generally a self-limited disease, but it may progress in some cases to a chronic intractable pain syndrome. In refractory cases, it is critical to rule out more ominous conditions. Patients involved in litigation or who have psychosocial stresses or vocational disputes may have a poorer outcome.

Potential Treatment Complications

Nonsteroidal anti-inflammatory drugs have a number of well-established side effects, as do tricyclic antidepressants (Table 105.1). The anesthetic block of the greater or lesser occipital nerve is considered relatively safe [39]. Contraindications to this block include coagulopathy and current infection. Potential complications include bleeding, infection, nerve injury, seizure from intravascular injection of local anesthetic, and headache exacerbation. Care must be taken not to puncture the posterior occipital artery. If the artery is punctured, pressure should be applied vigorously.

References

[1] Headache Classification Subcommittee of the International Headache Society. The international classification of headache disorders: 2nd edition. Cephalalgia 2004;24(Suppl. 1):9–160.

[2] Hammond SR, Danta G. Occipital neuralgia. Clin Exp Neurol 1978;15:258–70.

[3] Volcy M, Tepper SJ, Rapoport AM, et al. Botulinum toxin A for the treatment of greater occipital neuralgia and trigeminal neuralgia: a case report with pathophysiological considerations. Cephalalgia 2006;26:336–40.

[4] Slavin KV, Nersesyan H, Wess C. Peripheral neurostimulation for treatment of intractable occipital neuralgia. Neurosurgery 2006;58:112–9.

[5] Kapural L, Mekhail N, Hayek SM, et al. Occipital nerve electrical stimulation via the midline approach and subcutaneous surgical leads for treatment of severe occipital neuralgia: a pilot study. Anesth Analg 2005;101:171–4.

[6] Kapoor V, Rothfus WE, Grahovac SZ, et al. Refractory occipital neuralgia: preoperative assessment with CT-guided nerve block prior to dorsal cervical rhizotomy. AJNR Am J Neuroradiol 2003;24:2105–10.

[7] Loeser JD, editor. Bonica's management of pain. 3rd ed. Philadelphia: Lippincott Williams & Wilkins; 2001. p. 979.

[8] Star MJ, Curd JG, Thorne RP. Atlantoaxial lateral mass osteoarthritis. A frequently overlooked cause of severe occipitocervical pain. Spine 1992;17(Suppl.):S71–6.

[9] Kuhn WF, Kuhn SC, Gilberstadt H. Occipital neuralgias: clinical recognition of a complicated headache. A case series and literature review. J Orofac Pain 1997;11:158–65.

[10] Hecht JS. Occipital nerve blocks in postconcussive headaches: a retrospective review and report of ten patients. J Head Trauma Rehabil 2004;19:58–71.

[11] Handel TE, Kaplan RJ. Occipital neuralgia. In: Frontera WR, Silver JK, editors. Essentials of physical medicine and rehabilitation. Philadelphia: Hanley & Belfus; 2001. p. 38–43.

[12] Natsis K, Baraliakos X, Appell HJ, et al. The course of the greater occipital nerve in the suboccipital region: a proposal for setting landmarks for local anesthesia in patients with occipital neuralgia. Clin Anat 2006;19:332–6.

[13] Hunter CR, Mayfield FH. Role of the upper cervical roots in the production of pain in the head. Am J Surg 1949;78:743–51.

[14] Sahai-Srivastava S, Zheng L. Occipital neuralgia with and without migraine: difference in pain characteristics and risk factors. Headache 2010;51:124–8.

[15] Cerrato P, Bergui M, Imperiale D, et al. Occipital neuralgia as isolated symptom of an upper cervical cavernous angioma. J Neurol 2002;249:1464–5.

[16] Mourouzis C, Saranteas T, Rallis G, et al. Occipital neuralgia secondary to respiratory tract infection. J Orofac Pain 2005;19:261–4.

[17] Hardy D. Relief of pain in acute herpes zoster by nerve blocks and possible prevention of post-herpetic neuralgia. Can J Anaesth 2005;52:186–90.

[18] Boes CJ. C2 myelitis presenting with neuralgiform occipital pain. Neurology 2005;64:1093–4.

[19] Post AF, Narayan P, Haid Jr RW. Occipital neuralgia secondary to hypermobile posterior arch of atlas. Case report. J Neurosurg 2001;94(Suppl.):276–8.

[20] Gonzalez-Gay MA, Garcia-Porrua C, Branas F, Alba-Losada J. Giant cell arteritis presenting as occipital neuralgia. Clin Exp Rheumatol 2001;19:479.

[21] Jundt JW, Mock D. Temporal arteritis with normal erythrocyte sedimentation rates presenting as occipital neuralgia. Arthritis Rheum 1991;34:217–9.

[22] Cho JC, Haun DW, Kettner NW. Sonographic evaluation of the greater occipital nerve in unilateral occipital neuralgia. J Ultrasound Med 2012;31:37–42.

[23] Fernandez-de-las-Penas C, Alonso-Blanco C, Cuadrado ML, Pareja JA. Spinal manipulative therapy in the management of cervicogenic headache. Headache 2005;45:1260–3.

[24] Fernandez-de-las-Penas C, Alonso-Blanco C, San-Roman J, Miangolarra-Page JC. Methodological quality of randomized controlled trials of spinal manipulation and mobilization in tension-type headache, migraine, and cervicogenic headache. J Orthop Sports Phys Ther 2006;36:160–9.

[25] Oppenheim JS, Spitzer DE, Segal DH. Nonvascular complications following spinal manipulation. Spine J 2005;5:660–6, discussion 666–667.
[26] Linde M, Hagen K, Stovner LJ. Botulinum toxin treatment of secondary headaches and cranial neuralgias: a review of evidence. Acta Neurol Scand Suppl 2011;191:50–5.
[27] Ward JB. Greater occipital nerve block. Semin Neurol 2003;23:59–62.
[28] Naja ZM, El-Rajab M, Al-Tannir MA, et al. Occipital nerve blockade for cervicogenic headache: a double-blind randomized controlled clinical trial. Pain Pract 2006;6:89–95.
[29] Greher M, Moriggl B, Curatolo M, et al. Sonographic visualization and ultrasound-guided blockade of the greater occipital nerve: a comparison of two selective techniques confirmed by anatomical dissection. Br J Anaesth 2010;104:637–42.
[30] Cho JC. Benefits of sonographic examination for diagnosis and treatment of occipital neuralgia. OMICS J Radiol 2010;1:3.
[31] Vanelderen P, Rouwette T, De Vooght P, et al. Pulsed radiofrequency for the treatment of occipital neuralgia. Reg Anesth Pain Med 2010;35:148–51.
[32] Huang JHY, Galvagno SM, Hameed M, et al. Occipital nerve pulsed radiofrequency treatment: a multi-center study evaluating predictors of outcome. Pain Med 2012;13:489–97.
[33] Khan FR, Henderson JM. Does ganglionectomy still have a role in the era of neuromodulation? World Neurosurg 2012;77:280–2.
[34] Stojanovic MP. Stimulation methods for neuropathic pain control. Curr Pain Headache Rep 2001;5:130–7.
[35] Acar F, Miller J, Golshani KJ, et al. Pain relief after cervical ganglionectomy (C2 and C3) for the treatment of medically intractable occipital neuralgia. Stereotact Funct Neurosurg 2008;86:16–112.
[36] Lozano AM, Vanderlinden G, Bachoo R, Rothbart P. Microsurgical C-2 ganglionectomy for chronic intractable occipital pain. J Neurosurg 1998;89:359–65.
[37] Gille O, Lavignolle B, Vital JM. Surgical treatment of greater occipital neuralgia by neurolysis of the greater occipital nerve and sectioning of the inferior oblique muscle. Spine 2004;29:828–32.
[38] Rasskazoff S, Kaufmann AM. Ventrolateral partial dorsal root entry zone rhizotomy for occipital neuralgia. Pain Res Manag 2005;10:43–5.
[39] Waldman SD. Greater and lesser occipital nerve block. In: Waldman SD, editor. Atlas of interventional pain management. 2nd ed. Philadelphia: WB Saunders; 2004. p. 23–6.

CHAPTER 106

Pelvic Pain

Rebecca Posthuma, MD
Allison Bailey, MD

Synonyms

Pain in pelvic region
Chronic pelvic pain

ICD-9 Code

625.9 Pelvic pain

ICD-10 Code

R10.2 Pelvic and perineal pain

Definition

Chronic pelvic pain (CPP), a common condition among women, affects up to one in four women of reproductive age at some point in their lifetime [1,2]. It can be an elusive disorder to diagnose and to treat, challenging even the most experienced clinicians. Despite variable opinions as to what constitutes this disorder, a widely accepted definition of CPP is noncyclic pain localized primarily in the anatomic pelvis, the anterior abdominal wall at or below the umbilicus, the lumbosacral spine, or the buttocks [3]. Traditionally, CPP must be of 6 months' duration and severe enough to cause functional disability or to require treatment. It can be of gynecologic, urologic, gastrointestinal, musculoskeletal, or neurologic etiology. The pain that arises from CPP can be categorized into somatic, visceral, neuropathic, or referred pain.

The prevalence of CPP is estimated to be 3.8% in women aged 15 to 73 years, similar to that of asthma, back pain, and migraine headaches. In primary care practices, it is estimated that 39% of women have complained of pelvic pain [1,2,4]. There are no known demographic factors—age, race, ethnicity, education, or socioeconomic status—that put women at risk for development of CPP, although women with CPP tend to be of reproductive age.

Discovering the etiology of CPP (and therefore appropriate treatment) can be difficult because of the broad differential diagnoses and their many overlapping symptoms (see Table 106.1 for a complete list by organ system). In addition, these diagnoses are not mutually exclusive but in many cases may coexist. For example, endometriosis and myofascial pain are often known to overlap. Because of the diagnostic complexity of CPP, an accurate diagnostic approach cannot always be assumed. This is especially true if medical or surgical therapies for discrete diagnoses have failed to provide relief.

The initial diagnostic approach should begin with a thorough history to narrow the differential diagnosis. The pain history should include pain characteristics such as first occurrence, location, duration, temporal pattern, precipitating and alleviating factors, relationship to urination and defecation, patterns of radiation, intensity, and effect of pain on life activities (such as activities of daily living, sleep, work, sexual intercourse, and social or recreational activities). A monthly pain calendar, which records episodes, location, severity, and associated factors, is useful to obtain accurate and detailed information. The history should also include prior treatments; history of substance abuse; history of sexual, physical, and psychological abuse; and thorough review of systems. A pain map of the body is a useful tool to help the physician and patient specify pain patterns. The usual components of a patient history, such as medical problems, previous surgeries, and reproductive history, should be included as well. To streamline the process of obtaining a history for patients with CPP, the International Pelvic Pain Society has created the Pelvic Pain Assessment Form, which is an excellent and freely reproducible tool that can be found on its website [5].

The most common causes of CPP are of gynecologic, gastrointestinal, urologic, and musculoskeletal origin and include specific diagnoses, such as endometriosis, chronic pelvic inflammatory disease (PID), irritable bowel syndrome, bladder pain syndrome, and myofascial pelvic pain [6].

Gynecologic

Endometriosis

Endometriosis is a common gynecologic condition affecting women of reproductive age. It is characterized by the presence of endometrial tissue (the inner layer of the uterus) outside of the uterus. The extrauterine endometrial implants respond to the hormonal stimuli in the same way as intrauterine endometrium does, causing cyclic bleeding in the sensitive tissues of the peritoneum, ovaries, fallopian tubes, and elsewhere. This process can lead to formation of pelvic adhesions, scar tissue, and endometriomas.

Table 106.1 Conditions Associated with Pelvic Pain in Women

Gynecologic
Endometriosis*
Chronic pelvic inflammatory disease*
Pelvic adhesions
Pelvic congestion (pelvic varicosities)
Adenomyosis
Ovarian remnant syndrome
Residual ovary syndrome
Leiomyoma
Endosalpingiosis
Neoplasia
Fallopian tube prolapse (after hysterectomy)
Tuberculous salpingitis
Benign cystic mesothelioma
Postoperative peritoneal cysts
Mental Health Issues
Somatization
Substance abuse
Physical and sexual abuse
Depression
Sleep disorders
Urinary Tract
Interstitial cystitis/painful bladder syndrome*
Recurrent urinary tract infection
Urethral diverticulum
Chronic urethral syndrome
Neoplasia
Radiation cystitis
Gastrointestinal Tract
Irritable bowel syndrome*
Inflammatory bowel disease and other causes of colitis
Diverticular colitis
Chronic intermittent bowel obstruction
Neoplasia
Chronic constipation
Celiac disease (sprue)
Chronic appendicitis
Musculoskeletal
Pelvic floor myalgia*
Myofascial pain (trigger points)*
Coccygodynia
Piriformis syndrome
Hernia
Abnormal posture
Fibromyalgia
Peripartum pelvic pain syndrome
Neurologic Disorders
Neuralgia, especially of the iliohypogastric, ilioinguinal, genitofemoral, or pudendal nerves*
Herniated nucleus pulposus
Neoplasia
Neuropathic pain
Abdominal epilepsy
Abdominal migraine

*These diagnoses are the most common causes of chronic pelvic pain and are backed by substantial evidence.

This disorder is found in 10% to 15% of women of reproductive age, in 25% to 40% of women undergoing treatment for infertility, and in 33% of women who have laparoscopy for CPP. Risk factors include early menarche, short menstrual cycles (less than 27 days), and müllerian anomalies that involve vaginal or uterine obstruction of blood flow. Symptoms include long-standing cyclic pelvic pain, dysmenorrhea, menorrhagia, and deep dyspareunia. Severity of symptoms does not necessarily correlate with visual disease burden at time of surgery.

Uterine Leiomyomas

Leiomyomas (uterine fibroids, myomas) are benign smooth muscle tumors of the uterus and the most common neoplasm in women of reproductive age, with the highest prevalence in the fifth decade of life. The lifetime incidence of leiomyoma is 50% and up to 60% in women of African descent. Fibroids are thought to grow from estrogen stimulation. The most common symptoms are pressure from an enlarging pelvic mass, pain and dysmenorrhea, and abnormal uterine bleeding. The severity of symptoms is related to the size, number, and location of the tumors, although many women with fibroids are asymptomatic. In general, fibroids shrink after menopause. A myoma that grows rapidly after menopause is concerning for leiomyosarcoma, which occurs in 0.5% of fibroids.

Adenomyosis

Similar to endometriosis, adenomyosis is the presence of ectopic endometrial tissue in the myometrium (muscle layer) of the uterus. Adenomyosis develops from aberrant glands of the basalis layer of the endometrium and causes pain, dysmenorrhea, and menorrhagia. Some women experience intense pelvic cramping and pressure that radiates to the lower back, groin, rectum, and anterior thighs. Symptomatic adenomyosis usually is manifested in women aged 35 to 50 years, although adenomyosis can be found in asymptomatic women. The incidence of this disorder is unknown. As the ectopic endometrial tissue proliferates, the uterus takes on an enlarged, globular shape, which can sometimes be appreciated on examination.

Adhesive Disease

The correlation between abdominal adhesions and CPP is poorly understood, and studies of these are limited. It is thought that certain types of adhesions, particularly densely vascular adhesions to the bowel and peritoneum, cause CPP. Diagnosis can be made only at the time of laparoscopy as there are no examination findings, laboratory tests, or imaging studies that are reliably useful. Risk factors include a history of prior pelvic surgery, PID, endometriosis, inflammatory bowel disease, radiation therapy, and peritoneal dialysis.

Pelvic Congestion Syndrome

Pelvic congestion syndrome is a condition of vascular engorgement of the ovarian veins or internal iliac veins that leads to pelvic pain. Characteristic findings of gross dilation, incompetence, and reflux of the ovarian veins are seen on venography, sometimes forming parovarian pelvic varicosities. Dysfunction in the one-way valves of the ovarian veins is postulated as the underlying etiology. There is limited understanding of the prevalence of this condition as there are no definitive diagnostic criteria. As with most causes of pelvic pain, anatomic anomalies are not necessarily indicative of the presence or severity of pain. Pelvic congestion syndrome has been described only in premenopausal women. Typically, pain is worse after prolonged standing and improves in the morning after rest. Associated symptoms include marked ovarian tenderness, shifting location of pain, and deep dyspareunia or postcoital pain.

Chronic Pelvic Inflammatory Disease

PID starts as an acute condition and can become a chronic condition causing CPP. The transition from acute PID to chronic PID is incompletely understood and occurs in about 18% to 35% of women with acute PID. Women at risk for development of chronic PID include those who are not initially treated for the acute phase or are treated incompletely. In addition, the development of more severe adhesions or tubal damage and persistent pelvic tenderness 30 days after diagnosis and treatment increase the likelihood for development of CPP. Whether a woman is treated with an inpatient or outpatient regimen for acute PID does not have any bearing on the risk for later development of chronic PID or CPP [7]. Most PID is caused by *Chlamydia trachomatis* and *Neisseria gonorrhoeae*. Other implicated pathogens are *Gardnerella vaginalis, Haemophilus influenzae,* enteric gram-negative rods, and *Streptococcus agalactiae*. Diagnostic criteria and treatment of acute PID are published and maintained by the Centers for Disease Control and Prevention [8].

Gastrointestinal

Irritable bowel syndrome is a common functional bowel disorder of uncertain etiology characterized by a chronic, relapsing pattern of abdominopelvic pain and altered bowel habits in the absence of an organic cause. Although not all patients with this disorder seek treatment, the estimated prevalence is 10% to 15% in North America. The abdominal and pelvic pain is usually crampy in nature and varies in location, often exacerbated by emotional stress and eating habits and relieved by defecation. Patients also often complain of nongastrointestinal symptoms, such as altered sexual function, dysmenorrhea, urinary frequency, or dyspareunia.

The Rome III criteria are used to diagnose irritable bowel syndrome, and patients must have two of the following: pain relieved with defecation; onset of pain associated with a change in frequency of stool; or onset associated with a change in form (appearance) of stool [9].

Urologic

Chronic bladder pain in the absence of other identifiable etiology has been termed bladder pain syndrome (BPS). Previously called interstitial cystitis (IC), this is actually a misnomer as there is no evidence of underlying evidence of inflammation. For historical reasons, the nomenclature has changed to IC/BPS. IC/BPS is characterized by suprapubic or urethral pain, pressure, or discomfort that is worse with bladder filling and relieved with voiding. The severity of symptoms ranges greatly and may vary from day to day. Other urinary symptoms, such as frequency, urgency, and nocturia, accompany the pain [10]. IC/BPS often coexists with other chronic pain syndromes, such as fibromyalgia, irritable bowel syndrome, or myofascial pelvic pain syndrome [11]. The underlying etiology has not been exactly elucidated but may be related to altered integrity of the glycosaminoglycan layer of the bladder.

Because IC/BPS is a clinical diagnosis, there are no characteristic laboratory or imaging findings. A voiding diary that logs fluid intake, voiding volume, and frequency demonstrates the characteristic frequent, low-volume voiding pattern.

Musculoskeletal

Myofascial pelvic pain is pain attributed to short, tight, and tender pelvic floor muscles scattered with characteristic trigger points, small hypersensitive areas within a tight band of muscle (Fig. 106.1). A trigger point can cause local pain and over time lead to regional and diffuse pelvic pain as well as visceral dysfunction, such as constipation or irritative voiding. The exact prevalence of myofascial pelvic pain syndrome is unknown. Determining if CPP is due to a myofascial etiology or caused by another disorder can be challenging. In fact, overlap between pelvic pain disorders is common. For instance, studies have shown that 70% of women with bladder pain syndrome also have myofascial pain, most often involving the levator ani muscles of the pelvic floor [12]. Myofascial pelvic pain is thought to originate from an abnormal response to muscle fiber trauma, causing peripheral and then central sensitization. Inflammatory mediators are released locally when a muscle is injured. Over time, the muscle nociceptors become conditioned to the stimulus and a lower response threshold to inflammatory mediators and mechanical stimulation ensues, leading to muscle hyperalgesia. Continued input from the injured or painful muscle leads to neuroplastic changes in the dorsal spinal cord, resulting in amplified pain to both noxious and non-noxious stimuli. Furthermore, secondary hyperalgesia develops such that pain is perceived outside of the original area of injury [12].

Physical, mechanical, systemic, and psychological factors have been associated with the development of trigger points. Physical factors include injury to the nerves and muscles at the time of childbirth or surgery. Mechanical factors that contribute to myofascial pelvic pain include abnormal posture, leg length discrepancy, gait disturbances, sacroiliac joint dysfunction, and diastasis recti, all of which can trigger asymmetric use of the levator muscles. Systemic factors such as subclinical hypothyroidism, nutritional inadequacies, chronic allergies, and impaired sleep have also been linked to the development and activation of trigger points.

With myofascial pelvic pain, patients often have difficulty in localizing pain. The pain is characterized as achy, throbbing, or pressure-like in quality. Myofascial pelvic pain can radiate to the hip or back and commonly worsens throughout the day, with bowel or bladder function, or after intercourse. During the examination, attention should be paid to the pelvic floor examination. Patients with myofascial pelvic pain will complain of pain when pressure is placed on myofascial trigger points, which are often found in the pubococcygeus and ileococcygeus muscles of the pelvic floor.

Symptoms

The specific symptoms of CPP vary greatly but are important to elicit because they can give diagnostic clues. Pain caused by endometriosis typically worsens premenstrually and throughout menses. Pain accompanied by symptoms of poor urinary flow, urinary hesitancy, or constipation suggests myofascial pelvic pain, pelvic floor muscle dysfunction, or an anatomic defect such as pelvic organ prolapse. Pain with radiation to the lower extremities may indicate myofascial pelvic pain, sacroiliac joint dysfunction, or spinal disease,

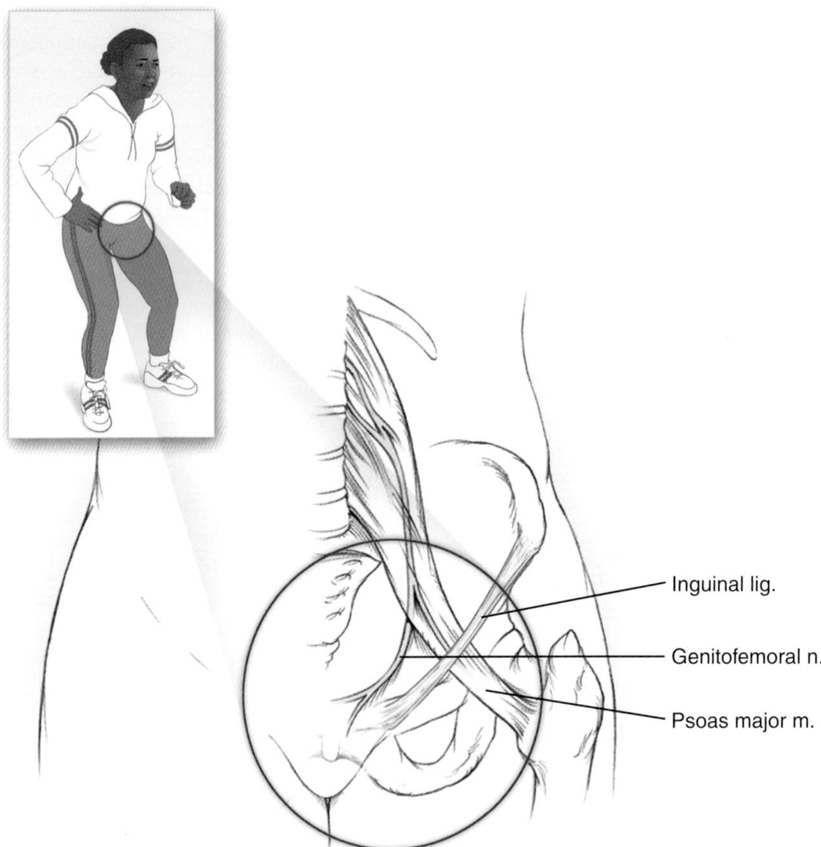

FIGURE 106.1 Myofascial pain involving the levator ani muscle of the pelvic floor. *(From Waldman SD. Atlas of Common Pain Syndromes, 3rd ed. Philadelphia, WB Saunders, 2012.)*

such as radiculopathy or cord compression. Improvement of pain while supine and aggravation of pain while upright suggest pelvic congestion syndrome. Lateralizing pain accompanied by hematuria may be indicative of urolithiasis or urinary tract obstruction. Crampy abdominal pain with diarrhea or constipation suggests irritable bowel syndrome or diverticular disease. Entry dyspareunia may be a symptom of lichen sclerosus, atrophic vaginitis, or vulvodynia; deep dyspareunia may be a symptom of endometriosis, myofascial pelvic pain syndrome, or chronic PID. Pain that increases with bladder filling and is associated with urinary frequency, nocturia, and painful voiding suggests IC/BPS.

Physical Examination

After a thorough history and review of systems, the clinician narrows the differential diagnosis. The goal of the physical examination is to reproduce, whenever possible, the patient's pain. Therefore it is important for the clinician to remember that this process can be a stressful and unpleasant experience for the patient. The physical examination—indeed, the entire evaluation—should be systematic and methodical. In the case of CPP, a multispecialty approach to both diagnosis and treatment is now considered standard of care. Therefore clinicians commonly treating patients with CPP should be familiar with the basic physical examination of the multiple organ systems around the pelvis that may give rise to pain symptoms. These clinicians ideally function within a team of experts from various specialties to ensure a complete diagnostic approach.

After a screening examination of the lumbosacral spine is performed, the examination of the pelvis continues with the patient supine. The patient should be asked to identify the areas of most pain. A four-quadrant abdominal examination is then performed with superficial and deep palpation (ideally with the patient's abdomen relaxed), leaving the area of most pain until last, and taking note of discomfort, hernia, masses, and surgical scars. If hypersensitivity is found on the superficial examination, this can suggest myofascial trigger points. A simple maneuver, the Carnett test, can be used to differentiate myofascial pain from visceral abdominal pain. For the Carnett test to be performed, the area of pain on the abdomen is palpated with one or two digits, and then the patient voluntarily contracts the abdomen by raising legs and head off the table. If pain at the palpation site increases, this is likely a myofascial trigger point, and if pain decreases, it is likely visceral in origin.

The examination continues in the dorsal lithotomy position. The patient should again show the clinician where the area of most pain is. First, begin with examination of the external pelvis, looking at the groin, external genitalia, and perineum for asymmetry or dermatologic abnormality. The soft end of a cotton swab can be used to assess pain in the vestibule, posterior fourchette, and labia; if pain is present, it can be indicative of vulvodynia or vulvar skin disorders.

A lubricated single-digit examination of the pelvic floor is performed next, before placing a speculum or performing a bimanual examination, which can aggravate the muscles of the pelvic floor. The base of the pelvic floor is palpated and the vagina should feel like a soft cylinder. In patients with hypertonic disorders, a shelf of contracted musculature can usually be felt in addition to myofascial trigger points. Myofascial trigger points are small areas of contracted tissue that are exquisitely tender on palpation and produce either direct or referred pain. The bladder base, cul-de-sacs, cervix, uterus, and adnexa should then be palpated, again noting tenderness, symmetry, and fullness, which can be indicative of endometriosis or pelvic masses.

The final part of the genitourinary examination is the speculum examination. A small speculum is suggested as a larger one can be difficult to pass into the vagina if there is pain and discomfort. The clinician should again note symmetry of the position of the cervix; shortening of the uterosacral ligaments causes lateral displacement of the cervix and is a classic finding of endometriosis. Vaginal and cervical culture specimens are obtained as indicated, particularly if chronic PID is suspected. Vaginal atrophy, seen in postmenopausal women with loss of vaginal rugae and lightening of the normal lush pink hue of the vaginal walls, can cause discomfort and is easily treated with vaginal estrogen.

Functional Limitations

CPP frequently results in significant functional limitations. In general, patients with chronic pain syndromes may have psychological distress because of delayed diagnosis and treatment. Chronic unrelieved pain is known to contribute to anxiety, depression, sleep disturbance, and altered family and social roles that may have an impact on all areas of function. Pelvic floor muscle myofascial pain may increase with prolonged sitting or standing, which may limit the patient's ability to participate in work, social, and recreational activities. In addition, bowel and bladder function may be affected, and in some cases incontinence may result. Many patients with CPP also complain of dyspareunia interfering with normal sexual function.

Diagnostic Studies

In the evaluation of CPP, history and physical examination are the mainstays of diagnosis, although several studies may help narrow the differential or confirm or exclude a specific diagnosis. In general, the most useful imaging modality for pelvic organs is ultrasonography, which can detect uterine fibroids, intrauterine disease, adnexal disease (e.g., endometrioma, ovarian neoplasm), and adenomyosis. Magnetic resonance imaging is preferable to assess adenomyosis. If there is a high suspicion for pelvic congestion syndrome, pelvic venography can be performed. Although there are no imaging studies that are useful in the diagnosis of myofascial pelvic pain syndrome, surface electromyography can provide objective evidence of muscle dysfunction.

Laboratory evaluation can include urine analysis and culture, sexually transmitted infection testing, complete blood count, erythrocyte sedimentation rate, or thyroid assay as indicated by the patient's risk factors and comorbid conditions. Results of laboratory tests, such as CA-125, can be elevated in the presence of endometriosis, but the sensitivity and specificity are too low to be of clinical value. When urinary symptoms are present, a urine analysis should be performed to rule out underlying infection, and patients with hematuria should be evaluated with cystoscopy.

Laparoscopy can be used as an extension of the diagnostic regimen. In fact, 40% of all laparoscopies are performed for CPP. When laparoscopy is performed for CPP, 33% of women are found to have endometriosis, 24% are found to have adhesive disease, and 35% have no visible disease [13]. Biopsy of any pathologic process found on laparoscopy is important because visual diagnosis of endometriosis is often unreliable. Diagnostic laparoscopy has the benefit of offering simultaneous treatment; if endometriosis or pelvic adhesions are found during the operation, ablation or resection can be performed. Patients who present with gastrointestinal symptoms should be referred to a gastroenterologist and will likely undergo colonoscopy as part of the evaluation.

Differential Diagnosis

Endometriosis
Pelvic inflammatory disease
Pelvic adhesions
Pelvic varicosities
Adenomyosis
Ovarian remnant syndrome
Leiomyoma
Endosalpingiosis
Neoplasia
Fallopian tube prolapse
Tuberculous salpingitis
Recurrent urinary tract infection
Urethral diverticulum
Inflammatory bowel disease
Diverticulitis
Bowel obstruction
Chronic constipation
Celiac disease
Chronic appendicitis
Coccygodynia
Piriformis syndrome
Hernia
Fibromyalgia
Iliohypogastric, ilioinguinal, genitofemoral, or pudendal neuralgia
Herniated nucleus pulposus

Treatment

Initial

Establishing a patient-physician relationship based on trust and confidence is important in treating CPP. During the arduous diagnostic process, concern for the patient should be expressed and her symptoms validated. As with any chronic pain condition, it is important to discuss expectations of symptom improvement and management. Treatment of CPP is a process that often requires time and a multimodality approach to treatment involving primary care providers, physicians from an array of specialties, and physical therapy.

While the patient is going through the diagnostic process, it is reasonable to start empirical treatment based on diagnostic probability. When a specific diagnosis is made, targeted therapy should be initiated. A 4- to 6-week trial of maximum-strength nonsteroidal anti-inflammatory drugs (NSAIDs) is an appropriate first-line therapy. If this is ineffective, a second NSAID may be tried because of variable responses of patients to individual drugs.

In addition to NSAIDs, when a gynecologic etiology is likely, hormonal therapy may be started either sequentially or simultaneously. Oral contraceptive pills should be attempted for two or three cycles, prescribed either in the standard manner or continuously. If the combination of NSAIDs and continuous oral contraceptive pills is unsuccessful after 2 to 3 months, second-line agents may be tried; these include progestins and gonadotropin-releasing hormone (GnRH) agonists.

Initial treatment of mild irritable bowel syndrome involves patient education, dietary modification, and behavioral changes. If patients have moderate or severe symptoms, pharmacologic agents may be added.

With IC/BPS, a stepwise approach should be taken for treatment; it may begin with simple measures such as heat or cold to the suprapubic area, avoidance of food or activities that exacerbate pain, and fluid management. Bladder analgesics, such as phenazopyridine or methenamine, may be used initially. For longer term management, non-narcotic and narcotic pain medications can be used, guided by principles used to manage other chronic pain conditions. Intravesical instillation of lidocaine with heparin or sodium bicarbonate may be used to manage pain exacerbations.

Some women find relief of CPP symptoms from complementary and alternative medical treatments, such as acupuncture, acupressure, and nutritional supplements. The decision to pursue these modalities should be individualized as there is a paucity of high-quality studies in the medical literature.

Endometriosis

Treatment of women with presumed or proven endometriosis usually begins with NSAIDs for pain management and combined oral contraceptive pills to induce a relative hypoestrogenic state, thereby decreasing the proliferation of extrauterine endometrial tissue. Long-acting progesterones, such as intramuscular medroxyprogesterone, etonogestrel subdermal implant, or levonorgestrel intrauterine device, are also useful in achieving a hypoestrogenic state. If these first-line therapies fail, GnRH agonists or aromatase inhibitors can be used [6]. If medical therapy fails, laparoscopy can be used to reduce disease burden, or the uterus and ovaries can be removed [13].

Uterine Leiomyomas

In women with fibroids, treatment should be guided by severity of symptoms, nearness to menopause, and desire for childbearing potential. A GnRH agonist, such as intramuscular leuprolide, can be used to help shrink the fibroid burden, although its side effect profile is onerous for some women. Uterine artery embolization, myomectomy (either hysteroscopically or abdominally), and hysterectomy are other treatments. Pregnancy should be avoided after uterine artery embolization, and a cesarean section is usually recommended in the case of pregnancy after myomectomy. If a woman is near menopause and has mild or moderate symptoms, it is reasonable to treat with NSAIDs and to reevaluate after menopause.

Myofascial Pelvic Pain Syndrome

Treatment of myofascial pelvic pain is best done with a multidisciplinary approach. Myofascial pelvic pain is often associated with other diagnoses, such as irritable bowel syndrome, endometriosis, depression, constipation, painful bladder syndrome, and chronic urinary tract infections. It is critical to treat a concomitant diagnosis if one is found because that may be the very thing that incites or exacerbates the myofascial pain. Neurogenic pain may be treated with tricyclic antidepressants or γ-aminobutyric acid analogues (such as gabapentin or pregabalin). However, the mainstay for treatment of myofascial pelvic pain is pelvic floor physical therapy, and specific techniques for physical therapists have been well described.

Rehabilitation

A comprehensive, multidisciplinary approach in managing CPP is of the utmost importance, and physical therapy plays an integral role in this. Physical therapists evaluate the structural, biomechanical, postural, functional, musculoskeletal, and neurologic dysfunctions that may cause, perpetuate, or result from pelvic pain. Involving the physical therapist in the early stage of pelvic pain is highly recommended. Rehabilitative interventions include connective tissue manipulation; behavioral retraining and education for posture, activity, and bowel and bladder habits; therapeutic exercise; neuromuscular reeducation; and manual therapy techniques for joints, soft tissue, and fascia [14]. Physical therapy appears to be most successful when all of these elements are considered and positive findings are addressed through a progressive and individualized treatment program.

Procedures

In the case of myofascial pelvic pain syndrome, patients who improve incompletely with physical therapy may benefit from trigger point injections into the pelvic floor muscles. Trigger point injections are most often performed with local anesthetic, such as lidocaine or bupivacaine [15]. Botulinum toxin A injections have also been used to reduce CPP and pelvic floor muscle spasm [16]. Sacral neuromodulation is an additional treatment option for women with myofascial pelvic pain and has been used in the treatment of refractory, nonobstructive urinary retention, urinary frequency or urgency, and urge incontinence. Although it is not approved by the Food and Drug Administration for the treatment of IC/BPS or pelvic pain, some studies suggest a benefit for these conditions [17].

Surgery

If medical therapy fails to bring improvement, diagnostic and potentially therapeutic laparoscopy should be pursued. Laparoscopic adhesiolysis can temporarily alleviate symptoms due to pelvic adhesions; however, adhesions often tend to recur rapidly. The role of hysterectomy in idiopathic CPP is controversial as there is a failure rate of pain resolution of 40%. In addition, there is an unclear understanding of which patients benefit from hysterectomy and which do not [18]. In the case of adenomyosis, hysterectomy is considered the definitive treatment for those who fail to respond to medical management. Other surgical procedures for CPP, such as presacral neurectomy and uterosacral nerve ablation, offer limited improvement in symptoms and are usually no longer performed.

Potential Disease Complications

If it is left untreated, CPP has the potential to cause severe debilitation, both from a personal standpoint and from a societal standpoint. Lessening of quality of life, depression, lost wages, and lack of participation in society can have long-reaching consequences.

Potential Treatment Complications

Potential adverse effects of NSAIDs are well publicized and include gastritis, gastrointestinal ulcers, renal impairment, and cardiac morbidity. GnRH agonists carry risk of early osteoporosis. Complications due to invasive procedures include bleeding and infection.

References

[1] Howard FM. Chronic pelvic pain. Obstet Gynecol 2003;101:594–611.

[2] Grace VM, Zondervan KT. Chronic pelvic pain in New Zealand: prevalence, pain severity, diagnoses and use of the health services. Aust N Z J Public Health 2004;28:369–75.

[3] ACOG Committee on Practice Bulletins—Gynecology. ACOG practice bulletin No. 51. Chronic pelvic pain. Obstet Gynecol 2004;103:589–605.

[4] Mathias SD, Kuppermann M, Liberman RF, et al. Chronic pelvic pain: prevalence, health-related quality of life, and economic correlates. Obstet Gynecol 1996;87:321–7.

[5] International Pelvic Pain Society, http://www.pelvicpain.org/resources/handpform.aspx; [accessed 02.01.13].

[6] ACOG Committee on Practice Bulletins—Gynecology. ACOG practice bulletin. Medical management of endometriosis. Number 11, December 1999 (replaces Technical Bulletin Number 184, September 1993). Clinical management guidelines for obstetrician-gynecologists. Int J Gynaecol Obstet 2000;71:183–96.

[7] Ness RB, Soper DE, Holley RL, et al. Effectiveness of inpatient and outpatient treatment strategies for women with pelvic inflammatory disease: results from the Pelvic Inflammatory Disease Evaluation and Clinical Health (PEACH) randomized trial. Am J Obstet Gynecol 2002;186:929–37.

[8] Centers for Disease Control and Prevention. Pelvic inflammatory disease, http://www.cdc.gov/std/treatment/2010/pid.htm; [accessed 02.01.13].

[9] Longstreth GF, Thompson WG, Chey WD, et al. Functional bowel disorders. Gastroenterology 2006;130:1480–91.

[10] Stanford EJ, Dell JR, Parsons CL. The emerging presence of interstitial cystitis in gynecologic patients with chronic pelvic pain. Urology 2007;69(4 Suppl.):53–9.

[11] Bogart LM, Berry SH, Clemens JQ. Symptoms of interstitial cystitis, painful bladder syndrome and similar diseases in women: a systematic review. J Urol 2007;177:450–6.

[12] Pulliam S, Silveira S. Pelvic floor muscle pain and dysfunction. In: Bailey A, Bernstein C, editors. Pain in women: a clinical guide. New York: Springer Science; 2012.

[13] Howard FM. The role of laparoscopy in the chronic pelvic pain patient. Clin Obstet Gynecol 2003;46:749–66.

[14] McKinney J. Pelvic floor muscle pain and dysfunction. In: Bailey A, Bernstein C, editors. Pain in women: a clinical guide. New York: Springer Science; 2012.

[15] FitzGerald MP, Kotarinos R. Rehabilitation of the short pelvic floor. I: background and patient evaluation. Int Urogynecol J Pelvic Floor Dysfunct 2003;14:261–8.

[16] Jarvis SK, Abbott JA, Lenart MB, et al. Pilot study of botulinum toxin type A in the treatment of chronic pelvic pain associated with spasm of the levator ani muscles. Aust N Z J Obstet Gynaecol 2004;44:46–50.

[17] Peters KM. Neuromodulation for the treatment of refractory interstitial cystitis. Rev Urol 2002;4(Suppl. 1):S36–43.

[18] ACOG criteria set. Hysterectomy, abdominal or vaginal for chronic pelvic pain. Number 29, November 1997. Committee on Quality Assessment. American College of Obstetricians and Gynecologists. Int J Gynaecol Obstet 1998;60:316–7.

CHAPTER 107

Phantom Limb Pain

Moon Suk Bang, MD, PhD
Se Hee Jung, MD, PhD

Synonyms

Painful phantom sensation
Phantom pain
Phantom limb syndrome

ICD-9 Codes

353.6 Phantom limb (syndrome)
729.2 Neuralgia, neuritis, and radiculitis, unspecified
905.9 Late effect of traumatic amputation (injury classifiable to 885-887 and 895-897)
997.60 Stump (surgical) (post-traumatic), abnormal, painful, or with complication (late)

ICD-10 Code

G54.6 Phantom limb syndrome with pain

Definition

Phantom pain refers to a painful sensation perceived in a body part that is no longer present subsequent to surgical or traumatic removal. It is most common after the amputation of a limb (i.e., phantom limb pain), but it has also been reported after the surgical removal of other body parts, such as breast, rectum, penis, testicles, eye, tooth, tongue, or lesion of peripheral or central nervous system [1]. Phantom limb pain is distinguished from stump pain, which is pain in the residual limb or stump, and phantom limb sensation, which is a nonpainful sensation of the absent part. Peripheral, spinal segmental, central, and psychological mechanisms are considered factors in the development of phantom limb pain, and an increasing number of studies with functional neuroimaging have suggested a central mechanism for phantom limb pain [2–5].

Although phantom limb pain is generally present within the first few days after an amputation, it can take several months or years to emerge. The reported prevalence of phantom limb pain differs considerably, ranging from about 40% to 90% [1,6]. However, phantom limb pain is less frequent in congenital amputation and loss of a limb early in childhood. The occurrence of phantom limb pain is independent of gender, age (in adults), level or side of amputation, dominance, and etiology of amputation.

In several reports, the intensity of pain remained constant but both the frequency and duration of pain attacks decreased significantly over time [7,8]. A small percentage of patients experienced a reduction in intensity of pain over time. Phantom limb pain leads to permanent disability in more than 40% of amputees, and pain persisting for more than 6 months is exceedingly difficult to treat.

Phantom limb pain has been reported to be significantly related to residual limb pain, physical activity, severity and duration of preamputation pain, noxious intraoperative inputs (such as pain brought about by cutting of tissues), acute postoperative pain, bilateral amputation, and lower limb amputation.

Symptoms

Pain is most prominent immediately after the operation; it is not static in nature and changes in quality over the years. Phantom limb pain is usually intermittent, but some patients report constant pain with superimposed exacerbations. The duration of an attack ranges from seconds or minutes to hours or days. Phantom limb pain is usually localized in distal parts of the absent limb, usually in the foot or hand.

The pain can be described as tingling, throbbing, aching, pins and needles, squeezing, stabbing, shooting, pinching, or cramping. Sometimes, the patients report that the amputated limb is positioned in a painful posture or that they sense spasms in the limb. The intensity as well as the quality of the pain varies greatly among patients from mild to severe. Phantom limb pain is triggered or worsened by physical (e.g., rainy weather, low temperature, prosthetic use, urination, defecation, reduced blood flow, and muscle tension), psychosocial (e.g., attention), and emotional (e.g., anxiety and stress) stimuli. Phantom limb pain is not relieved with position.

Physical Examination

Physical examination is generally unrevealing. However, patients can sometimes identify specific points on the residual limb that trigger phantom limb pain. Therefore the residual limb should be assessed for any sources of pain or trigger areas. The residual limb is examined for neuromas, cysts, bursae, bone spurs, or sites of excessive pressure. Other precipitating factors should be searched for, such as an ill-fitting prosthesis or mechanical stimulation.

Local problems, such as a herniated disc or spinal disease emitting sensations into the phantom limb or neuroma, can cause neuropathic pain. A comprehensive physical evaluation with particular attention to the neurologic examination, including strength, range of motion, muscle stretch reflexes, and muscle tone, should be done to rule out any concomitant central or peripheral neuropathic pain.

Functional Limitations

Functional complications of phantom limb pain include sleep disorders, interference with prosthesis training and use, reduction in walking ability, inability to return to work, change in employment status, and limitation of participation in social activities. Patients with phantom limb pain experience a greater degree of despair, more symptoms of depression, less satisfaction with social relations, poorer psychosocial adjustment, and poorer quality of life than amputees who are unaffected [9].

Diagnostic Studies

The diagnosis of phantom limb pain is generally made clinically on the basis of history and physical examination. Plain radiography and ultrasonography are performed for the diagnosis of underlying conditions, such as neuroma, abscess, bursitis, bone spur or fragment, or nerve entrapment. Magnetic resonance imaging, electrophysiologic tests, or laboratory tests may be indicated if other diagnoses are suspected.

Nerve block may be attempted as a diagnostic tool to identify candidates for specific procedures. Various pain scales and psychometric questionnaires are used to assess severity, treatment effect, and disability.

Differential Diagnosis

Nonpainful phantom sensation
Stump pain (residual limb pain)
Chronic postsurgical pain
Radicular pain
Neuralgia
Anginal pain

Table 107.1 Treatments Commonly Used for Phantom Limb Pain

Pharmacologic

Conventional analgesics
Opioids
Anticonvulsants
Antidepressants
NMDA receptor antagonists
Neuroleptics

Rehabilitation

Mirror therapy
Motor imagery
Biofeedback
Sensory discrimination training
Physiotherapy
Prosthesis training
Transcutaneous electrical nerve stimulation
Ultrasound
Manipulation

Psychological

Cognitive-behavioral pain management
Relaxation technique
Stress management
Distraction
Hypnosis

Anesthetic

Local anesthetics
Nerve blocks
Sympathetic block
Epidural blockade

Surgical

Stump revision
Neurectomy
Sympathectomy
Dorsal root entry zone ablation
Dorsal rhizotomy
Cordotomy
Thalamotomy
Spinal cord stimulation
Deep brain stimulation
Cortical resection of brain

Other

Acupuncture

Treatment

The treatments commonly used for phantom limb pain are listed in Table 107.1.

Initial

Patients should be taught before amputation that phantom limb pain is not a complication but a normal side effect of some amputations. Education about phantom limb pain reduces anxiety and distress in patients. The expected course of symptoms after amputation and during the prosthetic fitting process should be carefully reviewed with the patient. Preemptive analgesia in an attempt to prevent phantom limb pain by epidural or general routes during the preoperative and initial postoperative period has not been shown to be effective. Compression stockings or stump shrinkers during the early postoperative period can also be helpful.

Tricyclic antidepressants and anticonvulsants have long been considered to be the drugs of choice [1]. Controlled studies, however, showed conflicting data on the effect of tricyclic antidepressants in phantom limb pain [10,11]. Anticonvulsants such as carbamazepine, gabapentin, topiramate, and lamotrigine are effective.

Randomized controlled studies have demonstrated that opioids have analgesic efficacy in phantom limb pain and suggest an effect on cortical reorganization [12–14]. Morphine is effective in decreasing pain intensity in the short term [15]. Tramadol is an analgesic with both monoaminergic and opioid activity that is effective in long-standing phantom limb pain.

N-Methyl-D-aspartate (NMDA) receptor antagonists, such as ketamine and dextromethorphan, showed efficacy in controlling phantom limb pain [15,16].

Other pharmacologic interventions, such as beta blockers, topical capsaicin, nonsteroidal anti-inflammatory drugs, nonopioid analgesics, and botulinum toxin, have been suggested, but well-controlled trials have not been published.

Rehabilitation

Transcutaneous electrical nerve stimulation has long been considered an effective treatment modality; it can begin early in the postoperative period without significant side effects. However, a recent Cochrane review failed to find sufficient evidence to support the effectiveness of transcutaneous electrical nerve stimulation for phantom limb pain [17]. Heat and cold, manipulation, vibration, massage, and acupuncture can all be tried, but there is no evidence of their efficacy.

Several studies have reported positive results of biofeedback, including electromyographic biofeedback, thermal biofeedback, and muscle relaxation procedures [1,18]. Use of a prosthesis that provides sensory, visual, and motor feedback reportedly reduces phantom limb pain [19,20]. Sensory discrimination training or tactile stimulation has also been reported to reduce phantom limb pain with a reversal of cortical reorganization. Mirror therapy and motor imagery have been shown to decrease phantom limb pain, supporting a central mechanism for the presence of pain [2,4,21–23].

Psychological interventions such as relaxation technique, stress management, distraction, and hypnosis can also provide relief, although very few specific studies of patients with phantom limb pain were conducted.

Procedures

Regional anesthesia with local anesthetics, including plexus or nerve block, sympathetic block, and epidural block, can be applied to intractable phantom limb pain. A continuous perineural infusion of a local anesthetic was reported to be effective in preventing and decreasing phantom limb pain [24].

Surgery

Surgery is generally not indicated for phantom limb pain. Stump revision, such as neuroma resection, is indicated in selected patients with stump pain due to neuroma. The purpose of neuroma resection is relief of stump pain, not of phantom limb pain.

Spinal cord stimulation, dorsal root entry zone ablation, neurectomy, sympathectomy, dorsal rhizotomy, cordotomy, thalamotomy, and cortical resection of brain have been used in a few cases of intractable pain [25,26].

Potential Disease Complications

Phantom limb pain may cause significant disability. It keeps amputees from their usual activities and causes considerable interference with their daily, social, recreational, and work activities. The health-related quality of life of amputees with phantom limb pain is poorer than that of amputees without phantom limb pain.

Potential Treatment Complications

Side effects of pharmacologic treatment are well documented. Complications of regional anesthesia are systemic effects of local anesthetics, physiologic effects of the procedure (e.g., hypotension, inadvertent injection or block), and damage to adjacent structures. Spinal cord stimulation has few serious complications. Complications of surgical ablation techniques include Horner syndrome, dysesthesia, sudomotor paralysis, weakness, urinary complications, and respiratory problems. Selection of appropriate patients is important to successful surgical ablation.

References

[1] Flor H. Phantom-limb pain: characteristics, causes, and treatment. Lancet Neurol 2002;1:182–9.

[2] Raffin E, Mattout J, Reilly KT, et al. Disentangling motor execution from motor imagery with the phantom limb. Brain 2012;135:582–95.

[3] Vase L, Nikolajsen L, Christensen B, et al. Cognitive-emotional sensitization contributes to wind-up-like pain in phantom limb pain patients. Pain 2011;152:157–62.

[4] Diers M, Christmann C, Koeppe C, et al. Mirrored, imagined and executed movements differentially activate sensorimotor cortex in amputees with and without phantom limb pain. Pain 2010;149:296–304.

[5] Saitoh Y, Yoshimine T. Stimulation of primary motor cortex for intractable deafferentation pain. Acta Neurochir Suppl 2007;97(Pt 2):51–6.

[6] Kooijman CM, Dijkstra PU, Geertzen J, et al. Phantom pain and phantom sensations in upper limb amputees: an epidemiological study. Pain 2000;87:33–41.

[7] Nikolajsen L, Ilkjær S, Krøner K, et al. The influence of preamputation pain on postamputation stump and phantom pain. Pain 1997;72:393–405.

[8] Houghton A, Nicholls G, Houghton A, et al. Phantom pain: natural history and association with rehabilitation. Ann R Coll Surg Engl 1994;76:22–5.

[9] van der Schans CP, Geertzen JHB, Schoppen T, et al. Phantom pain and health-related quality of life in lower limb amputees. J Pain Symptom Manage 2002;24:429–36.

[10] Robinson LR, Czerniecki JM, Ehde DM, et al. Trial of amitriptyline for relief of pain in amputees: results of a randomized controlled study. Arch Phys Med Rehabil 2004;85:1–6.

[11] Wilder-Smith CH, Hill LT, Laurent S. Postamputation pain and sensory changes in treatment-naive patients: characteristics and responses to treatment with tramadol, amitriptyline, and placebo. Anesthesiology 2005;103:619–28.

[12] Huse E, Larbig W, Flor H, et al. The effect of opioids on phantom limb pain and cortical reorganization. Pain 2001;90:47–55.

[13] Wu CL, Tella P, Staats PS, et al. Analgesic effects of intravenous lidocaine and morphine on postamputation pain: a randomized double-blind, active placebo-controlled, crossover trial. Anesthesiology 2002;96:841–8.

[14] Bergmans L, Snijdelaar DG, Katz J, et al. Methadone for phantom limb pain. Clin J Pain 2002;18:203–5.

[15] Alviar M, Hale T, Dungca M. Pharmacologic interventions for treating phantom limb pain. Cochrane Database Syst Rev 2011;12, CD006380.

[16] Eichenberger U, Neff F, Sveticic G, et al. Chronic phantom limb pain: the effects of calcitonin, ketamine, and their combination on pain and sensory thresholds. Anesth Analg 2008;106:1265–73.

[17] de Roos C, Veenstra A, de Jongh A, et al. Treatment of chronic phantom limb pain using a trauma-focused psychological approach. Pain Res Manage 2010;15:65–71.

[18] Halbert J, Crotty M, Cameron ID. Evidence for the optimal management of acute and chronic phantom pain: a systematic review. Clin J Pain 2002;18:84–92.

[19] Lotze M, Grodd W, Birbaumer N, et al. Does use of a myoelectric prosthesis prevent cortical reorganization and phantom limb pain? Nat Neurosci 1999;2:501–2.

[20] Dietrich C, Walter-Walsh K, Preissler S, et al. Sensory feedback prosthesis reduces phantom limb pain: proof of a principle. Neurosci Lett 2012;507:97–100.
[21] Moseley GL, Gallace A, Spence C. Is mirror therapy all it is cracked up to be? Current evidence and future directions. Pain 2008;138:7–10.
[22] Chan BL, Witt R, Charrow AP, et al. Mirror therapy for phantom limb pain. N Engl J Med 2007;357:2206–7.
[23] Moseley GL. Graded motor imagery for pathologic pain: a randomized controlled trial. Neurology 2006;67:2129–34.
[24] Borghi B, D'Addabbo M, White PF, et al. The use of prolonged peripheral neural blockade after lower extremity amputation: the effect on symptoms associated with phantom limb syndrome. Anesth Analg 2010;111:1308–15.
[25] Mailis-Gagnon A, Furlan A, Sandoval J, et al. Spinal cord stimulation for chronic pain. Cochrane Database Syst Rev 2004;3, CD003783.
[26] Mailis-Gagnon A, Furlan A. Sympathectomy for neuropathic pain. Cochrane Database Syst Rev 2003;2, CD002918.

CHAPTER 108

Postherpetic Neuralgia

Ariana Vora, MD

Amy X. Yin, MD

Synonyms

Shingles
Herpes zoster
Varicella-zoster

ICD-9 Codes

053.12 Postherpetic trigeminal neuralgia
053.19 Postherpetic neuralgia (intercostal or ophthalmic)

ICD-10 Codes

B02.22 Postherpetic trigeminal neuralgia
B02.29 Postherpetic nervous system involvement

Definition

Varicella-zoster virus is a lipid-enveloped, double-stranded DNA herpesvirus that coevolved with ancestral primates for more than 70 million years [1]. It expresses its genes sequentially, leading to expression of nonstructural proteins, nonstructural protein enzymes, and late structural proteins [2]. Late structural proteins encapsulate the DNA core, infect host cells, and replicate in host cell nuclei.

Acute varicella-zoster infection is the initial activation of the virus manifested with a diffuse pruritic, vesicular rash. This is commonly known as chickenpox. Two viremic phases are thought to occur in acute zoster infection. Animal studies suggest that the first viremia occurs in regional lymph nodes and viscera, approximately 5 days after exposure [3]. The second viremia, approximately 14 days after exposure, promotes viral spread to the nasopharynx and the skin, causing the hallmark rash [4]. The virus usually infects children and spreads by aerosol droplets and skin-to-skin exposure to the vesicles, which contain large amounts of virus.

Herpes zoster, or shingles, is the reactivation of latent varicella-zoster virus. After acute herpes zoster infection, the virus remains dormant and resides in sensory ganglia, including the dorsal roots and cranial nerves [5]. Reactivation generally results from immunocompromised states such as stress, disease, or advanced age. The virus typically migrates along dermatomes, manifesting as a painful rash. The virus may spread to the spinal sensory nerves, dorsal horn, or cranial nerves. It is a painful condition with a highly age-related incidence, affecting about 50% of individuals who survive to the age of 85 years [6]. It affects men and women equally. Involvement of motor nerves is extremely rare.

Postherpetic neuralgia is pain persisting in affected dermatomes despite resolution of the rash. Although the timeline may be variable, many define postherpetic neuralgia as persistent pain 4 months or more after resolution of acute herpes zoster [7]. The likelihood for development of postherpetic neuralgia increases with older age, female sex, presence of a prodrome, greater rash severity, and greater acute pain severity [8]. It is the most common complication after an acute episode of shingles.

Symptoms

Prodromal symptoms may precede varicella-zoster reactivation by a few days up to 1 week. These include low-grade fever and malaise with hyperesthesia, dysesthesia, paresthesia, or pruritus along the distribution of affected dermatomes.

Fulminant shingles is marked by the emergence of erythematous macules accompanied by severe burning, stinging pain in a single sensory or cranial nerve distribution. This is followed by the eruption of fluid-filled papules, clusters, and vesicles. New skin eruptions generally continue to appear for 3 to 5 days. Thoracic dermatomes are most frequently affected. During this period, prodromal low-grade fever and malaise may continue to persist, and lymphadenopathy may also be present.

Zoster affecting exposed areas may result in sun or wind sensitivity. Sensitivity to light touch, intolerance to wearing of clothes over the erupted area, and brief jolts of shooting pain are also common.

Of the cranial nerves, the ophthalmic branch of the trigeminal nerve is the most often affected. If there is ophthalmic involvement, photophobia may be present. This is known as herpes zoster ophthalmicus and can result in monocular blindness. It has an incidence of 1% in the general population [9].

In very rare cases, zoster of the geniculate ganglion occurs, affecting the seventh and eighth cranial nerves. Symptoms include otalgia, vertigo, tinnitus, ataxia, loss of hearing, loss of taste, and even ipsilateral facial paralysis. This is known as Ramsay Hunt syndrome (herpes zoster oticus).

In most cases, symptoms tend to resolve shortly after healing of the rash. However, in more than 25% of patients, neuralgia persists for longer than 1 month after resolution of the rash [10]. This pain is commonly described as sharp, burning, aching, or shooting and may be accompanied by allodynia and hyperalgesia.

Physical Examination

In shingles, typical skin eruptions follow a dermatomal distribution, appearing as raised, fluid-filled vesicles. Once the vesicles burst and release fluid that contains live virus, they crust. Once the vesicles have crusted, the patient is no longer infectious. Lesions are often exquisitely tender to light touch. If deeper dermal involvement is present, scarring and discoloration may be seen.

Ophthalmic zoster is usually accompanied by a rash in the dermatomal distribution of the nasociliary nerve, along the side of the nose (Hutchinson sign). Periorbital edema, petechial hemorrhages, conjunctivitis, scleritis, and corneal sensitivity are also commonly associated with ophthalmic zoster [9]. Hutchinson sign and an unexplained red eye are indications for ophthalmologic consultation.

Ramsay Hunt syndrome is manifested as a rash on the auricle and external ear accompanied by exquisite otalgia, vestibulocochlear dysfunction, and facial nerve palsy. Any suspicion for Ramsay Hunt syndrome should lead to an urgent otolaryngology consultation.

With postherpetic neuralgia, there are no visible skin abnormalities on inspection. However, the patient may describe allodynia or hyperalgesia on even very gentle palpation.

Functional Limitations

Functional limitations due to herpes zoster include difficulty with activities involving pressure or heat exposure to the affected area. If the facial divisions of the trigeminal nerve or areas by the ear are affected, individuals may not tolerate wearing of protective headgear or facemasks and facial exposure to sun or wind. If the thoracic dermatomes are affected, clothing or even touching of the back against an office chair may increase pain. Both sex and contact sports may be intolerable. Difficulty in sleeping may arise from discomfort from sheets touching the skin. Bathing and toweling often exacerbate pain along the affected dermatome.

If the optic nerve or the ophthalmic branch to the trigeminal nerve is affected by shingles, monocular low vision may result in impaired depth perception and decreased field of view. If the patient has herpes zoster oticus, hearing, balance, tasting, and facial muscle movements are impaired. Thus, driving may be affected by zoster involvement of the trigeminal nerve or the geniculate ganglion.

Diagnostic Studies

Zoster is usually easy to diagnose on the basis of history and physical examination. In general, laboratory tests for diagnosis of reactivation of herpes zoster virus are not clinically useful [11]. For atypical cases, the Centers for Disease Control and Prevention guidelines suggest direct fluorescent antibody testing for rapid diagnosis [10]. To obtain a specimen, apply a sterile cotton swab to the base of an open lesion or, less preferably, a lesion crust.

Differential Diagnosis

Complex regional pain syndrome
Contact dermatitis
Drug-related allergic infection
Eczema
Other herpetic neuralgias
Nonherpetic viral infection
Radiculitis
Tertiary syphilis

Treatment

Initial

Prevention is important in this condition. Varicella vaccination in childhood is primary prevention for chickenpox. Zoster vaccination, recommended by the Centers for Disease Control and Prevention and the Advisory Committee on Immunization Practices for people 60 years of age or older [12], prevents herpes zoster reactivation as shingles. In a randomized double-blind placebo-controlled trial of the zoster vaccine, there was reduction of herpes zoster incidence by 51.3% and postherpetic neuralgia incidence by 66.5% [13]. However, there is still insufficient evidence for vaccination in the long-term prevention of postherpetic neuralgia [14].

If given within 72 hours of symptom onset, antiviral medication with oral acyclovir, valacyclovir, or famciclovir has been shown to relieve acute zoster pain and shorten rash duration, although there is no consistent evidence that it reduces the incidence of postherpetic neuralgia [15].

For patients with immunocompromise or malabsorption, the intravenous route of antiviral medication delivery is preferred to the oral route. There is limited evidence that a course of intravenous followed by oral antiviral treatment reduces pain in patients with postherpetic neuralgia of more than 3 months' duration [19].

Topical therapies that are approved by the Food and Drug Administration for postherpetic neuralgia include lidocaine and capsaicin. Lidocaine is available both as a 5% patch and in a gel cream form. A double-blind placebo-controlled efficacy and safety study with lidocaine patch has shown improvements in pain, allodynia, quality of life, and sleep measures [20,21].

Topical capsaicin is an extract of hot chili peppers that works as an agonist of the vanilloid receptor TRPV1. Capsaicin is available as an 8% patch and as different cream formulations. A small randomized double-blind controlled study with capsaicin showed a decrease in the numerical pain rating scale scores of patients by 33.8% compared with a 4.9% increase in controls [22]. Application of capsaicin should lead to desensitization of the unmyelinated epidermal nerve fibers and reduced hyperalgesia with repeated applications.

Other topical treatments that have been studied include topical aspirin, indomethacin, and diclofenac [23]. These have not been well studied and are not widely used in clinical practice.

Oral medications effective in treating postherpetic neuralgia include antiepileptic drugs, antidepressants, and opioid analgesics. The anticonvulsants gabapentin and pregabalin are approved by the Food and Drug Administration for treatment of postherpetic neuralgia. Both gabapentin and pregabalin are calcium channel ligands. Gabapentin can provide statistically significant improvement in daily pain rating, sleep, mood, and quality of life for patients with postherpetic neuralgia [24,25]. Pregabalin acts like gabapentin and is similarly useful in postherpetic neuralgia [26–28].

Whereas amitriptyline has been most studied, secondary amine tricyclics such as nortriptyline are usually preferred because of the side effect profile [28–30].

Use of opioids and opioid-like analgesics including tramadol, oxycodone, morphine, and methadone can also reduce severe pain in postherpetic neuralgia [31–33]. Use of opioids and opioid-like analgesics requires caution and close monitoring for side effects and medication abuse.

There are a number of guidelines for treatment of postherpetic neuralgia, with slight variations in recommended protocols [10,34,35]. Most would consider topical lidocaine, tricyclic antidepressants, and gabapentin or pregabalin first-line agents. Topical capsaicin, tramadol, and opioid analgesics are second- or third-line therapies [34,35]. Combination therapy may provide superior pain management while minimizing medication side effects [36,37].

Rehabilitation

Ultrasound may be effective in relieving acute zoster pain. In a clinical trial of acute zoster pain, more than 80% of participants receiving ultrasound were pain free at the end of the treatment compared with 46% in the placebo group [38]. The treatment parameters used in areas adjacent to the vertebral column were 1 MHz frequency, 25% pulsed cycle, applied for 1 minute per effective radiating area of the transducer at 0.8% W/cm^2 intensity and around the periphery of the vesicles at 0.5 W/cm^2.

Transcutaneous electrical nerve stimulation (TENS) is a widely used nonpharmacologic treatment thought to reduce nociception from small delta fibers and nonmyelinated fibers by stimulating larger, myelinated afferent nerve fibers, although its exact mechanism of action is still not well understood [39]. When TENS was applied to the second digit compared with the third and fifth digits in patients with carpal tunnel syndrome, fMRI showed temporarily decreased pain-related cortical activation [40]. When applied to the superficial radial nerve in healthy volunteers, TENS was found to increase the heat pain threshold [40a]. In a small RCT, patients with postherpetic neuralgia receiving a combination of TENS and oral pregabalin reported superior pain relief compared with those receiving a combination of sham TENS and pregabalin [40b]. In another combination therapy RCT, patients with postherpetic neuralgia reported significant pain reduction from baseline after receiving 8 weeks of TENS combined with local cobalamin injection [40c]. In summary, although there is theoretical support for TENS as a treatment for neuropathic pain and it has been recently studied in combination with other drugs, there is a need for studies comparing TENS alone against placebo in patients with postherpetic neuralgia. Although there is no consensus about voltage, pulse duration, or pulse frequency, TENS is thought to be most effective when applied at the maximum setting that is not uncomfortable.

Desensitizing treatments, such as alternating exposure to heat and cold, vibration, and repeated light tapping of the affected area, may be helpful but are not well studied.

In cases of ophthalmic involvement, occupational therapists can instruct in scanning techniques for low vision and decreased peripheral vision. If the geniculate ganglion is affected, occupational therapists may work on techniques for hearing impairment or vestibulocochlear dysfunction. Occupational therapists can also assist with fall risk reduction, such as by removal of loose rugs, improvement in lighting, and decrease of clutter in the home and work environment.

Other practical measures to improve function include rearrangement of workstations to reduce contact of sensitive areas with seat backs and armrests, use of low-friction fabrics such as silk, use of a hand-held showerhead to direct water flow away from painful dermatomes, and modification of sexual positions.

Procedures

Subcutaneous botulinum toxin injection has been successful in relieving postherpetic neuralgia pain in two small randomized, double-blind, placebo-controlled studies [41,42]. One study not only showed decreased pain, but patients who received botulinum toxin also had improved sleep and reduced opioid use compared with subcutaneous 0.5% lidocaine and placebo with 0.9% saline [42].

Retrospective studies on the effect of sympathetic nerve blocks have reported reduced duration of acute herpes zoster pain as well as short-term improvement with postherpetic neuralgia. However, the long-term effect of sympathetic nerve block in postherpetic neuralgia has not been established [43, 43a].

Paravertebral injection of bupivacaine and methylprednisolone may be helpful as adjuvant therapy to conservative management. A randomized study of 132 herpes zoster patients compared standard therapy of oral antivirals and analgesics or standard therapy with adjuvant paravertebral injections. The incidence of postherpetic neuralgia was 2% in the intervention group compared with 16% with standard treatment [44].

Epidural injection of steroids may provide modest, short-term pain relief in postherpetic neuralgia. In a randomized, controlled trial of 598 patients receiving standard oral antiviral and analgesic therapy with and without epidural steroid injection, the injection of bupivacaine and methylprednisolone was found to have a modest effect in reducing the pain of postherpetic neuralgia for 1 month but did not prevent long-term postherpetic neuralgia [45].

Intrathecal administration of methylprednisolone and lidocaine has led to significant decrease in pain intensity and area in a randomized trial of 277 patients with intractable postherpetic neuralgia. Patients in the intrathecal steroid group also had decrease in nonsteroidal anti-inflammatory drug use [46].

Other interventions, such as greater occipital nerve block, deep cervical nerve blocks, stellate ganglion blocks, and Jaipur block with subcutaneous lidocaine, bupivacaine, and methylprednisolone, have occasionally improved symptoms in case reports and observational studies [47–50]. The effects of cryotherapy, percutaneous nerve stimulation, and radiofrequency have not been well established. Spinal cord stimulation may be of benefit in medically complicated patients with multiple drug sensitivities, polypharmacy, and serious comorbid conditions [51]. Although these interventions have not been adequately studied, they may have some efficacy in treatment of recalcitrant postherpetic neuralgia symptoms.

Surgery

Surgery is not indicated for postherpetic neuralgia.

Potential Disease Complications

Acute optic neuritis from ophthalmic zoster may lead to permanent loss of vision, usually due to virus-induced impairment in retinal perfusion, leading to retinal necrosis. Retinal necrosis generally occurs in severely immunocompromised patients [52].

Herpes zoster ophthalmicus has also been associated with orbital apex syndrome, an inflammation of the oculomotor nerve thought to be related to secondary vasculitis within the orbital apex. This syndrome can cause impaired eye motility and often is manifested as dysconjugate gaze and diplopia.

Similarly, Ramsay Hunt syndrome may lead to permanent facial nerve paralysis and vestibulocochlear dysfunction.

Potential Treatment Complications

Topical lidocaine is generally well tolerated with only mild to moderate localized skin reactions reported [21]. However, topical capsaicin may cause greater local skin reaction including redness, burning pain, and itching [22].

The most common side effects of gabapentin and pregabalin are dizziness and somnolence. All tricyclic antidepressants may cause fatigue or sedation, dizziness, dry mouth, blurry vision, constipation, urinary retention, orthostatic hypotension, and QT prolongation or cardiac arrhythmias. Side effects of opioids and opioid-like analgesics include typical narcotic medication adverse effects of nausea, diarrhea, and constipation.

Gastrointestinal, hepatic, and renal complications may arise from prolonged use of acetaminophen, antiviral medications, or nonsteroidal anti-inflammatory drugs.

All interventional procedures carry a risk of pain, infection, and bleeding. Sympathetic nerve blocks may also cause hypotension, bradycardia, unintentional motor blockade, and neuropathic deafferentation pain. Epidural injections and paravertebral injection may result in hematoma or abscess formation. Complications of intrathecal methylprednisolone include hypotension, nerve root irritation, arachnoiditis, transverse myelitis, and chemical meningitis.

Spinal cord stimulation adverse effects include infection, dural puncture, pain from stimulator component, equipment failure, and dislocation. These may require reoperation or removal procedures.

References

[1] Grose D. Varicella zoster virus: out of Africa and into the research laboratory. Herpes 2006;13:32–5.
[2] Cohrs RJ, Hurley MP, Gilden DH. Array analysis of viral gene transcription during lytic infection of cells in tissue culture with varicella-zoster virus. J Virol 2003;77:11718–32.
[3] Dueland AN, Martin JR, Devlin ME, et al. Acute simian varicella infection: clinical, laboratory, pathologic, and virologic features. Lab Invest 1992;66:762–73.
[4] Tsolia M, Gershon AA, Steinberg SP, Gelb L. Live attenuated varicella vaccine: evidence that the virus is attenuated and the importance of skin lesions in transmission of varicella-zoster virus. National Institute of Allergy and Infectious Diseases Varicella Vaccine Collaborative Study Group. J Pediatr 1990;116:184–9.
[5] Cohrs R, Laguardia J, Gilden D. Distribution of latent herpes simplex virus type-1 and varicella zoster virus DNA in human trigeminal ganglia. Virus Genes 2005;31:223–7.
[6] Weiner DK, Schmader K. Postherpetic pain: more than sensory neuralgia? Pain Med 2006;7:243–9.
[7] Dworkin RH, Portenoy RK. Pain and its persistence in herpes zoster. Pain 1996;67:241–51.
[8] Jung BF, Johnson RW, Griffin DR, Dworkin RH. Risk factors for postherpetic neuralgia in patients with herpes zoster. Neurology 2004;62:1545–51.
[9] Opstelten W, Zaal MJ. Managing acute herpes zoster in primary care. BMJ 2005;331:147–51.
[10] Dubinsky RM, Kabbani H, El-Chami Z, et al. Practice parameter: treatment of postherpetic neuralgia: an evidence-based report of the Quality Standards Subcommittee of the American Academy of Neurology. Neurology 2004;63:959–65.
[11] Nicholson B. Differential diagnosis: nociceptive and neuropathic pain. Am J Manag Care 2006;12:S256–62.
[12] National Center for Immunization and Respiratory Diseases. General recommendations on immunization: recommendations of the Advisory Committee on Immunization Practices (ACIP). MMWR Recomm Rep 2011;60:1–64.
[13] Oxman MN, Levin MJ, Johnson GR, et al. A vaccine to prevent herpes zoster and postherpetic neuralgia in older adults. N Engl J Med 2005;352:2271–84.
[14] Chen N, Li Q, Zhang Y, et al. Vaccination for preventing postherpetic neuralgia. Cochrane Database Syst Rev 2011;3, CD007795.
[15] Watson P. Postherpetic neuralgia (updated). Clinical Evidence (BMJ online) 8 October 2010. Available at http://clinicalevidence.bmj.com/ceweb/conditions/ind/0905/0905.jsp.
[16] Deleted in proofs.
[17] Deleted in proofs.
[18] Deleted in proofs.
[19] Quan K, Hammack B, Kittelson J, Gilden D. Improvement of postherpetic neuralgia after treatment with intravenous acyclovir followed by oral valacyclovir. Arch Neurol 2006;63:940–2.
[20] Binder A, Bruxelle J, Rogers P, et al. Topical 5% lidocaine (lignocaine) medicated plaster treatment for post-herpetic neuralgia: results of a double-blind, placebo-controlled, multinational efficacy and safety trial. Clin Drug Investig 2009;29:393–408.
[21] Hans G, Sabatowski R, Binder A, et al. Efficacy and tolerability of a 5% lidocaine medicated plaster for the topical treatment of postherpetic neuralgia: results of a long-term study. Curr Med Res Opin 2009;25:1295–305.
[22] Backonja MM, Malan TP, Vanhove GF, et al. NGX-4010, a high concentration capsaicin patch, for the treatment of postherpetic neuralgia: a randomized, double-blind, controlled study with an open label extension. Pain Med 2010;11:600–8.
[23] De Benedittis G, Lorenzetti A. Topical aspirin/diethyl ether mixture versus indomethacin and diclofenac/diethyl ether mixtures for acute herpetic neuralgia and postherpetic neuralgia: a double-blind crossover placebo-controlled study. Pain 1996;65:45–51.
[24] Rice AS, Maton S, Postherpetic Neuralgia Study Group. Gabapentin in postherpetic neuralgia: a randomized, double blind, placebo-controlled study. Pain 2001;94:215–24.

[25] Moore RA, Wiffen PJ, Derry S, McQuay HJ. Gabapentin for chronic neuropathic pain and fibromyalgia in adults. Cochrane Database Syst Rev 2011;3, CD007938.

[26] Frampton JE, Foster RH. Pregabalin: in the treatment of postherpetic neuralgia. Drugs 2005;65:111–8, discussion 119–120.

[27] Moore RA, Straube S, Wiffen PJ, et al. Pregabalin for acute and chronic pain in adults. Cochrane Database Syst Rev 2009;3, CD007076.

[28] Collins SL, Moore RA, McQuay HJ, Wiffen P. Antidepressant and anticonvulsants for diabetic neuropathy and postherpetic neuralgia: a quantitative systematic review. J Pain Symptom Manage 2000;20:449–58.

[29] Watson CP, Evans RJ, Reed K, et al. Amitriptyline versus placebo in postherpetic neuralgia. Neurology 1982;32:671–3.

[30] Watson CP, Vernich L, Chipman M, Reed K. Nortriptyline versus amitriptyline in postherpetic neuralgia: a randomized trial. Neurology 1998;51:1166–71.

[31] Watson CP, Babul N. Efficacy of oxycodone in neuropathic pain: a randomized trial in postherpetic neuralgia. Neurology 1998;50:1837–41.

[32] Raja SN, Haythornthwaite JA, Pappagallo M, et al. Opioids versus antidepressants in postherpetic neuralgia: a randomized, placebo-controlled trial. Neurology 2002;59:1015–21.

[33] Boureau F, Legallicier P, Kabir-Ahmadi M. Tramadol in post-herpetic neuralgia: a randomized, double-blind, placebo-controlled trial. Pain 2003;104:323–31.

[34] Dworkin RH, O'Connor AB, Backonja M, et al. Pharmacologic management of neuropathic pain: evidence-based recommendations. Pain 2007;132:237–51.

[35] Attal N, Cruccu G, Baron R, et al. EFNS guidelines on the pharmacological treatment of neuropathic pain: 2010 revision. Eur J Neurol 2010;17:1113–e88.

[36] Rehm S, Binder A, Baron R. Post-herpetic neuralgia: 5% lidocaine medicated plaster, pregabalin, or a combination of both? A randomized, open, clinical effectiveness study. Curr Med Res Opin 2010;26:1607–19.

[37] Gilron I, Bailey JM, Tu D, et al. Nortriptyline and gabapentin, alone and in combination for neuropathic pain: a double-blind, randomized controlled crossover trial. Lancet 2009;374:1252–61.

[38] Cameron M, editor. Physical agents in rehabilitation: from research to practice. Philadelphia: WB Saunders; 2003. p. 289.

[39] Nathan PW, Hall PD. Treatment of postherpetic neuralgia by prolonged electric stimulation. BMJ 1974;3:645–7.

[40] Kara MK, Ozcakar L, Gokcay D, et al. Quantification of the effects of transcutaneous electrical nerve stimulation with functional magnetic resonance imaging: a double-blind randomized placebo-controlled study. Arch Phys Med Rehabil 2010;91:1160–5.

[40a] Buonocore M, Camuzzini N. Increase of the heat pain threshold during and after high-frequency transcutaneous peripheral nerve stimulation in a group of normal subjects. Eura Medicophys 2007;43:155–60.

[40b] Barbarisi M, Pace MC, Passavanti MB, et al. Pregabalin and transcutaneous electrical nerve stimulation for postherpetic neuralgia treatment. Clin J Pain 2010;26:567–72.

[40c] Xu G, Xú G, Feng Y, Tang WZ, et al. Transcutaneous electrical nerve stimulation in combination with cobalamin injection for postherpetic neuralgia: a single-center randomized controlled trial. Am J Phys Med Rehabil 2014;93:287–98.

[41] Ranoux D, Attal N, Morain F, Bouhassira D. Botulinum toxin type A induces direct analgesic effects in chronic neuropathic pain. Ann Neurol 2008;64:274–83.

[42] Xiao L, Mackey S, Hui H, et al. Subcutaneous injection of botulinum toxin A is beneficial in postherpetic neuralgia. Pain Med 2010;11:1827–33.

[43] Wu CL, Marsh A, Dworkin RH. The role of sympathetic nerve blocks in herpes zoster and postherpetic neuralgia. Pain 2000;87:121–9.

[43a] Kumar V, Krone K, Mathieu A. Neuraxial and sympathetic blocks in herpes zoster and postherpetic neuralgia: an appraisal of current evidence. Reg Anesth Pain Med 2004;29:454–61.

[44] Ji G, Niu J, Shi Y, et al. The effectiveness of repetitive paravertebral injections with local anesthetics and steroids for the prevention of postherpetic neuralgia in patients with acute herpes zoster. Anesth Analg 2009;109:1651–5.

[45] van Wijck AJ, Opstelten W, Moons KG, et al. The PINE study of epidural steroids and local anaesthetics to prevent postherpetic neuralgia: a randomized controlled trial. Lancet 2006;367:219–24.

[46] Kotani N, Kushikata T, Hashimoto H, et al. Intrathecal methylprednisolone for intractable postherpetic neuralgia. N Engl J Med 2000;343:1514–9.

[47] Naja ZM, Maaliki H, Al-Tannir MA, et al. Repetitive paravertebral nerve block using a catheter technique for pain relief in post-herpetic neuralgia. Br J Anaesth 2006;96:381–3.

[48] Hardy D. Relief of pain in acute herpes zoster by nerve blocks and possible prevention of post-herpetic neuralgia. Can J Anaesth 2005;52:186–90.

[49] Liu HT, Tsai SK, Kao MC, Hu JS. Botulinum toxin A relieved neuropathic pain in a case of post-herpetic neuralgia. Pain Med 2006;7:89–91.

[50] Puri N. Modified Jaipur block for the treatment of post-herpetic neuralgia. Int J Dermatol 2011;50:1417–20.

[51] Harke H, Gretenkort P, Ladleif HU, et al. Spinal cord stimulation in postherpetic neuralgia and in acute herpes zoster pain. Anesth Analg 2002;94:694–700.

[52] Zaal MJ, Volker-Dieben HJ, D'Amaro J. Visual prognosis in immunocompetent patients with herpes zoster ophthalmicus. Acta Ophthalmol Scand 2003;81:216–20.

CHAPTER 109

Post-Mastectomy Pain Syndrome

Justin Riutta, MD, FAAPMR

Synonyms

Post–axillary dissection pain
Mastodynia

ICD-9 Codes

457.1	**Lymphedema**
338.28	**Chronic postoperative pain**

ICD-10 Codes

I89.0	**Lymphedema, not elsewhere classified**
G89.28	**Chronic postoperative pain**

Definition

Post-mastectomy pain syndrome (PMPS) is a chronic pain condition, typically neuropathic in nature, that can follow surgery to the breast [1]. PMPS can occur with any surgery to the breast including mastectomy, lumpectomy, reconstruction, and augmentation, although symptoms of post-mastectomy pain are reduced with sentinel lymph node procedures [2,3]. PMPS affects approximately 40% to 52% of patients after breast surgery [3–5]. The risk factors for development of PMPS include younger age, more extensive surgery, more than 15 lymph nodes removed, more immediate postoperative pain, and anxiety [2,4,6]. Within the first 24 hours of surgery, 60% of patients have severe pain [7]. PMPS typically is manifested as phantom breast pain, intercostobrachial neuropathy, or incisional pain. Early management includes pain control, desensitization techniques, and shoulder range of motion. Chronic management includes neuropathic pain agents, interventional procedures, and rehabilitation. Primary objectives of management include sleep preservation, maintenance of shoulder function, and vocational rehabilitation.

Classification of PMPS can be divided into four categories: phantom breast pain, intercostobrachial neuralgia, myogenic pain, and neuroma pain [8]. Phantom pain is identified in 23% of post-mastectomy patients and consists of painful sensations in the area of the removed breast [9]. The intercostobrachial nerve is the lateral cutaneous nerve of the second thoracic root. It courses along the axillary vein and then provides sensation to the axilla and breast (Fig. 109.1). The intercostobrachial nerve is frequently stretched or sacrificed during axillary lymph node dissections and is a common cause of PMPS [8,10,11]. Myogenic pain is common after mastectomy and is associated with surgical irritation and immobilization. The scar from breast surgery can be a generator of pain. The pain has been attributed to underlying neuroma formation, axon impingement, and scar retraction [8,12].

Symptoms

The symptoms associated with PMPS include shooting, stabbing, burning, and pins and needles sensations in the breast, axilla, or medial arm [1,3,8,13–15]. In addition, patients complain of symptoms of tightness and fullness in the axilla. Pain is aggravated by shoulder movement, stretching, straining, and direct contact with clothes [3,13]. The symptoms of PMPS are usually nonprogressive and have been found to persist in half of patients observed for 9 years [1,13]. PMPS results in functional loss and sleep disruption, and these may be common presenting complaints [1,12].

Physical Examination

The primary aspects of the physical examination include exclusion of other causes of the identified pain and classification of PMPS. General inspection should be performed to evaluate for muscle wasting, asymmetry, and gross masses. The musculoskeletal examination should focus on shoulder range and function; muscle restriction in the pectoralis major and minor; and costovertebral, costochondral, and rib integrity. A careful skin examination should be performed to assess for scar adherence, fibrosis, scar tenderness, neuromas, infection, and recurrence of malignant disease. The lymphatic examination should be performed to assess for lymphadenopathy in lymphatic distributions not already dissected. The neurologic examination includes motor testing of the shoulder girdle, focusing on motor nerves potentially affected by breast surgery (thoracodorsal, long thoracic, medial and lateral pectoral). Sensory testing should include all breast dermatomes T1-T5. Particular attention should

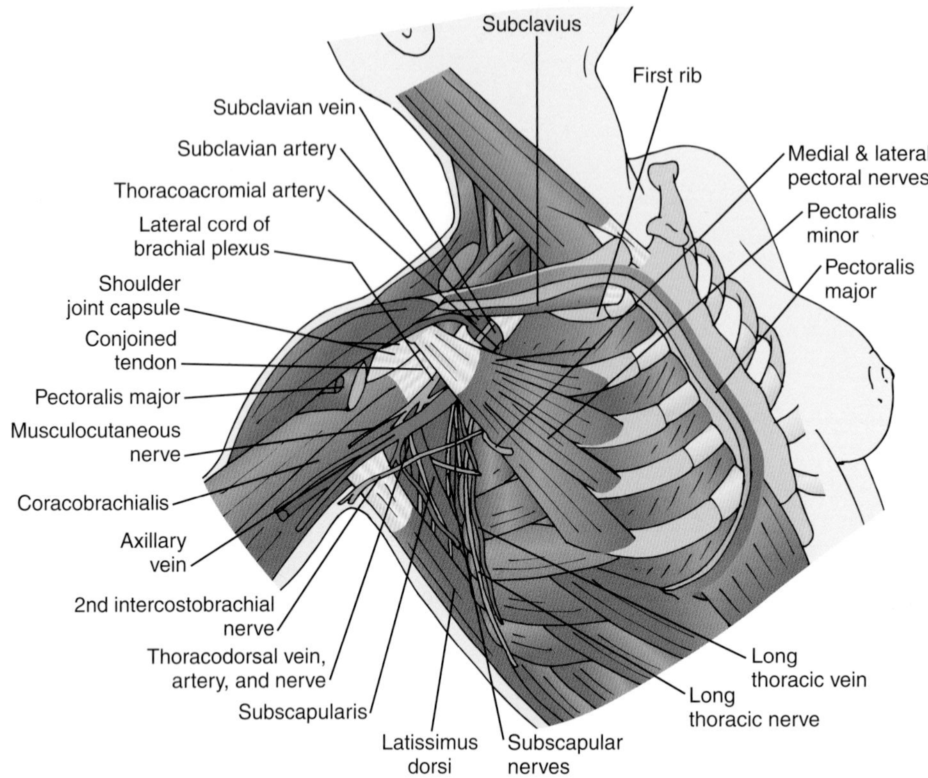

FIGURE 109.1 Regional anatomy relevant to post-mastectomy pain.

be paid to the posterior thorax dermatome as this can be a clue to spinal disease. The sensory examination of the axilla should identify the distribution, severity, and type of sensory abnormality. The complete neurologic examination should include a full assessment of ipsilateral upper extremity motor, reflex, and sensory function.

Functional Limitations

The major functional limitations with PMPS include loss of shoulder range of motion, lifting restrictions, and sleep disruption. Loss of shoulder range of motion is attributed to maintenance of the more comfortable adducted position, resulting in restricted abduction and external rotation [13]. Concurrently, restriction in the pectoralis minor and major results in decreased forward flexion and extension. Limitations with lifting result in diminished capacity to perform household duties (vacuuming, laundry), occupational duties (stocking shelves), and vocational pursuits [1,12,13]. Sleep disruption affects 50% of patients with PMPS and can lead to global daytime dysfunction [13].

Diagnostic Studies

Diagnostic studies are used primarily to exclude other causes of pain. Recurrent malignant neoplasms can be excluded by mammography, magnetic resonance imaging, or positron emission tomography scans. Dedicated imaging of the thoracic spine is warranted to exclude other suspected causes of neuropathic pain in the breast dermatomes, such as radiculopathy. Electrodiagnosis can be useful to exclude motor nerve abnormalities and plexopathy.

Differential Diagnosis

Tumor recurrence
Rib fracture
Paraneoplastic neuropathy
Intraparenchymal lung disease
Chemotherapy neuropathy
Thoracic nerve root impingement
Radiation plexopathy
Intercostal neuralgia

Treatment

Initial

The initial management of PMPS commences perioperatively. This includes minimizing dissection, nerve-sparing procedures, and early pain control. Early pain control is imperative because severe early postoperative pain is one of the most consistent factors in PMPS [5,7]. Early postoperative pain control is typically accomplished with judicious use of opiates and nonsteroidal anti-inflammatory drugs. A study found pregabalin in a single 75-mg dose preoperatively and 12 hours postoperatively to reduce pain [16]. Early desensitization techniques can help limit neuropathic symptoms and can be initiated once the incision is healed. For those with uncontrolled pain that limits sleep and daily function, neuropathic pain medications can be initiated. Some pharmaceuticals, such as capsaicin, amitriptyline, nortriptyline, gabapentin, pregabalin, and lidocaine patches, have been studied and found to be effective [8,14,16,17]. Long-acting opiates can be used when these agents fail to control symptoms [14].

Rehabilitation

From a rehabilitation perspective, PMPS management begins immediately postoperatively. The primary factor for rehabilitation management is to identify functional limits. Clearly, shoulder restriction is a major factor in the functional limitations from PMPS. Shoulder rehabilitation begins with stretching of the pectoralis complex and latissimus dorsi followed by glenohumeral range of motion and finally scapulohumeral retraining. Upper extremity strengthening commences once full shoulder range of motion is obtained. Targeted muscle groups for weight training include the latissimus dorsi, trapezius, scapular stabilizers, rotator cuff, and deltoid. Weight training should be performed with low weights and high repetitions. The final phase of rehabilitation is task-specific training, progressing from basic activities of daily living to household tasks, work-related duties, and recreational pursuits. It is important to guide the breast cancer survivor through resumption of full activity to avoid unnecessary injury.

Procedures

Procedural management of PMPS is typically limited to regional nerve blocks for pain control [14]. For those with progressive shoulder dysfunction and painful range of motion, local injections in the subacromial space may be beneficial. In addition, myofascial injections with anesthetic preparations or botulinum toxin can be beneficial for myogenic pain.

Surgery

Surgical management of PMPS typically relates to chest wall pain or shoulder dysfunction. Chest wall pain with scar retraction can be managed with scar removal. In addition, soft tissue adherence to chest wall structures may require surgical repair. Adhesive capsulitis as a result of progressive loss of shoulder range of motion may require manipulation under anesthesia for full shoulder range of motion to be obtained.

Potential Disease Complications

The primary potential disease complications from PMPS include adhesive capsulitis, loss of shoulder function, and diminished carrying capacity of the affected extremity. Resultant to this lack of function, patients can lose employment and vocational and recreational capacity. An insidious and life-altering complication of PMPS is sleep disruption. Sleep disruption can result in global dysfunction and health-related complications.

Potential Treatment Complications

Treatment complications are primarily related to side effects from medications. Capsaicin is known to cause painful skin reactions by its mechanism of action. Tricyclic antidepressants have anticholinergic side effects and must be used with caution in patients with cardiac arrhythmias. The main side effects of gabapentin include sedation, tremors, and dizziness. Topical lidocaine patches can result in skin excoriation. Bleeding, infection, and nerve irritation can complicate interventional procedures. Surgical procedures including manipulation under anesthesia and scar removal can result in increased pain and secondary soft tissue restriction.

References

[1] Macdonald L, Bruce J, Scott NW, et al. Long-term follow-up of breast cancer survivors with post-mastectomy pain syndrome. Br J Cancer 2005;92:225–30.
[2] Schulze T, Mucke J, Markwardt J, et al. Long-term morbidity of patients with early breast cancer after sentinel lymph node biopsy compared to axillary lymph node dissection. J Surg Oncol 2006;93:109–19.
[3] Smith WC, Bourne D, Squair J, et al. A retrospective cohort study of post mastectomy pain syndrome. Pain 1999;83:91–5.
[4] Alves Nogueira Fabro E, Bergmann A, do Amaral E Silva B, et al. Post-mastectomy pain syndrome: incidence and risks. Breast 2012;21:321–5.
[5] Tasmuth T, von Smitten K, Hietanen P, et al. Pain and other symptoms after different treatment modalities of breast cancer. Ann Oncol 1995;6:453–9.
[6] Katz J, Poleshuck EL, Andrus CH, et al. Risk factors for acute pain and its persistence following breast cancer surgery. Pain 2005;119:16–25.
[7] Fecho K, Miller NR, Merritt SA, et al. Acute and persistent postoperative pain after breast surgery. Pain Med 2009;10:708–15.
[8] Jung BF, Ahrendt GM, Oaklander AL, Dworkin RH. Neuropathic pain following breast cancer surgery: proposed classification and research update. Pain 2003;104:1–13.
[9] Rothemund Y, Grüsser SM, Liebeskind U, et al. Phantom phenomena in mastectomized patients and their relation to chronic and acute pre-mastectomy pain. Pain 2004;107:140–6.
[10] Vecht CJ. Arm pain in the patient with breast cancer. J Pain Symptom Manage 1990;5:109–17.
[11] Foley KM. Pain syndromes in patients with cancer. Med Clin North Am 1987;71:169–84.
[12] Kärki A, Simonen R, Mälkiä E, Selfe J. Impairments, activity limitations and participation restrictions 6 and 12 months after breast cancer operation. J Rehabil Med 2005;37:180–8.
[13] Stevens PE, Dibble SL, Miaskowski C. Prevalence, characteristics, and impact of postmastectomy pain syndrome: an investigation of women's experiences. Pain 1995;61:61–8.
[14] Kwekkeboom K. Postmastectomy pain syndromes. Cancer Nurs 1996;19:37–43.
[15] Wallace MS, Wallace AM, Lee J, Dobke MK. Pain after breast surgery: a survey of 282 women. Pain 1996;66:195–205.
[16] Kim SY, Song JW, Park B, et al. Pregabalin reduces post-operative pain after mastectomy: a double blinded, randomized, placebo-controlled study. Acta Anaesthesiol Scand 2011;55:290–6.
[17] Devers A, Galer B. Topical lidocaine patch relieves a variety of neuropathic pain conditions: an open-label study. Clin J Pain 2000;16:205–8.

CHAPTER 110

Post-Thoracotomy Pain Syndrome

Justin Riutta, MD, FAAPMR

Synonym

None

ICD-9 Code

338.22 Chronic post-thoracotomy pain

ICD-10 Code

G89.22 Chronic post-thoracotomy pain

Definition

Post-thoracotomy pain syndrome (PTPS) is pain that recurs or persists at the incision site or in the dermatomal distribution of the intercostal nerves for longer than 2 months after thoracotomy [1–3]. Thoracotomies are used to access intrathoracic contents, such as the lung, esophagus, and heart. The most common indication for a thoracotomy is tumor resection. The classic thoracotomy consists of a posterolateral incision of the thorax, bisection of the latissimus dorsi and serratus anterior, separation of the ribs, disruption of the intercostal nerves, and pleural incision. The thoracotomy is regarded as one of the most painful surgical procedures performed [1–10]. The incidence of PTPS has a wide range (2% to 90%), but on average, approximately 40% of patients will have chronic postoperative pain [2,4]. PTPS is mild to moderate in 92% of cases; 50% of patients will have disruption in the capacity to perform daily activities. Sleep disruption occurs in 25% to 30%. Fortunately, severe disabling pain occurs in only 3% to 5% of patients with PTPS [5,6]. Predictive factors for development of PTPS include increased pain 24 hours postoperatively, female gender, preoperative opiate use, and radiation therapy [4,8].

Intercostal neuralgia is the most commonly implicated cause of chronic PTPS [1]. Other factors contributing to pain are outlined in Table 110.1. Recognizing that local muscle disruption of the serratus anterior and latissimus dorsi results in abnormal scapulohumeral mechanics, shoulder abnormalities are one of the common causes of functional loss after thoracotomy [7].

Symptoms

PTPS generally is manifested with symptoms of allodynia, dysesthesias, and lancinating pain typically attributed to intercostal neuralgia [4]. In addition, patients will have symptoms of achiness, pleuritic pain, and focal tenderness over the incision site [1,4]. Shoulder movement, deep breathing, and lying directly on the affected side can aggravate these symptoms [4]. Pain is frequently encountered with shoulder maneuvers and direct contact with the incision site and can be manifested as shoulder dysfunction and sleep disruption.

Physical Examination

The examination of the patient with PTPS includes inspection of the incision site and chest wall movement with respiratory excursion. Deep breathing maneuvers to elicit pleuritic pain are another component of the examination. Palpation over the incision site to evaluate for scar adherence, hypersensitivity, or intercostal nerve pain is the next component of the examination. The rib cage is disrupted with surgery and must be assessed for persistent fractures, costochondral avulsions, and costochondritis. Assessment of regional musculature for postoperative disruption, atrophy, and myofascial pain is important. Adhesive capsulitis and shoulder girdle dysfunction are factors in PTPS; therefore active and passive range of motion of the shoulder and scapulohumeral mechanics should be evaluated. Neurologic examination includes motor testing of the affected extremity compared with the unaffected side, evaluation for scapular winging, and assessment of the dermatomal distribution of the transected intercostal nerves.

Functional Limitations

PTPS results in daily activity limitations in 50% of those affected [5]. Ochroch and associates [9] identified functional decrement using the 36-item short form health survey (SF-36) in most patients at 4 to 48 weeks postoperatively. Shoulder restriction secondary to chest wall pain, adhesive capsulitis, and disruption of the serratus anterior and latissimus dorsi has been identified in 15% to 33% of post-thoracotomy patients

Table 110.1 Factors Associated with Post-Thoracotomy Pain [1,4]
Intercostal neuroma
Rib fracture
Adhesive capsulitis
Infection
Pleurisy
Costochondral dislocation
Costochondritis
Local tumor recurrence
Myofascial pain
Vertebral collapse

at 1 year [7]. Shoulder restriction leads to limitations in sleep function, lifting capacity, and full range of motion activities of the shoulder girdle. In addition, functional limitations can be attributed to respiratory compromise related to surgery or underlying pulmonary disease.

Diagnostic Studies

The relevant diagnostic studies include baseline radiographs of the rib cage to evaluate for bone disruption. In addition, chest radiographs and computed tomography scans can be used to screen for intrathoracic processes, such as pleura-based dysfunction, pneumonia, and recurrence of primary malignant disease. A diagnostic intercostal nerve block can be performed to identify intercostal neuralgia.

Differential Diagnosis

Rib fracture
Costochondral dislocation
Vertebral collapse
Adhesive capsulitis
Costochondritis
Pleurisy
Myofascial pain
Muscle disruption pain
Tumor recurrence
Thoracic radiculopathy
Intercostal neuroma
Cardiac ischemia
Aortic dissection
Infection of incision, pleura, pleural space, and lung parenchyma

TREATMENT

Initial

The initial treatment of PTPS includes early aggressive management of pain. Preemptive analgesia is the concept of diminishing postoperative pain by disrupting pain pathways preoperatively [1]. Aspects of preemptive analgesia include thoracic epidural anesthesia, intercostal nerve blockade, opiates, and nonsteroidal anti-inflammatory drugs (NSAIDs) [1]. Thoracic epidural anesthesia has been shown to diminish acute postoperative pain in thoracotomy [10]. Balanced anesthesia with preoperative regional anesthesia, opiates, and NSAIDs diminishes the incidence of PTPS from 50% to 9.9% [2,4]. The surgical approach does have a bearing on postoperative pain. Smaller surgical incisions and muscle-sparing thoracotomies diminish postoperative pain [1]. In addition, early removal of chest tubes has been associated with diminished pain and improved pulmonary function [11].

Acute postoperative pain management includes thoracic epidural administration of opiates in combination with regional anesthesia and NSAIDs. Opiates alone decrease the incidence of PTPS to 23.4% [12]. In addition, opiates plus regional anesthesia decrease the incidence of PTPS to 14.8%. The opiates, anesthesia, and NSAIDs combine to diminish PTPS rates to 9.9% [12]. Further, early scar management, once healing is complete, can diminish long-term pain by reducing adhesions to chest wall structures and diminishing hypersensitivity. The primary technique to do this is gentle massage and repetitive stimulation of the incision site. Transcutaneous electrical nerve stimulation units have also been found to be effective in reducing PTPS [13,14].

Pharmacologic management of PTPS includes early postoperative use of opiates and NSAIDs in combination [2]. Delivery of topical anesthetics by patches (lidocaine) also can be used for pain control [2]. Management of chronic PTPS is usually through use of neuropathic pain medications. The only study specifically for PTPS used gabapentin and found that this was well tolerated and decreased pain in 73% of those studied; 42% of those studied had more than 50% pain relief [15]. Neuropathic pain medications used in other conditions that have not been studied in PTPS include amitriptyline and nortriptyline. If oral routes of pain control fail, intrathecal administration of opiates is an option.

Rehabilitation

The preoperative management of PTPS begins with nutritional assessment and augmentation. Patients with intrathoracic disease can frequently encounter nutritional issues as a result of their primary disease; it can be beneficial for postoperative recovery to maximize nutritional status. The second factor in preoperative management is to maintain or to obtain normal shoulder range of motion. As mentioned, shoulder dysfunction and muscle dysfunction occur in up to 33% of thoracotomy patients. Maximization of range, function, and muscle strength before surgery can reduce functional loss secondary to postoperative restriction.

Pulmonary rehabilitation is important in thoracotomy patients primarily because many have underlying pulmonary disease. Pulmonary rehabilitation preoperatively includes breathing techniques, energy conservation, instruction in medication use, secretion management, and aerobic endurance training. The objective is to reduce frequently encountered postoperative complications secondary to decreased depth of breathing, retention of secretions, atelectasis, and pneumonia [10]. Pulmonary rehabilitation begins postoperatively with breathing techniques, secretion management, and assisted coughing with stabilization of the disrupted thorax.

Scar mobilization is an important aspect of early pain relief. Scars can increase pain secondary to adherence to chest wall structures, underlying nerve entrapment, and restriction of range of motion of the shoulder. Early scar mobilization consists of gentle massage to maintain mobility of the incision and the soft tissue structures adjacent to the incision. Soft tissue massage techniques are not initiated until adequate wound healing has occurred.

Shoulder dysfunction is a common sequela of PTPS. The shoulder dysfunction has multiple factors, including muscle disruption, chest wall pain with shoulder movement, and myofascial pain. Surgical disruption of the latissimus dorsi and serratus anterior can lead directly to shoulder dysfunction. The serratus anterior stabilizes the scapula against the chest wall and aids in protraction. Normal shoulder abduction is limited without serratus anterior function. The latissimus dorsi is a powerful adductor of the arm. Latissimus dorsi restriction can lead to lack of forward flexion and abduction at the glenohumeral joint. The disruption of these two muscle groups is less of an issue with muscle-sparing procedures. The rehabilitation process is delayed primarily because of time for muscle continuity to return after disruption. The initial management includes gentle massage of the affected muscle group and pendulum exercises. This is followed by gentle active range of motion exercises that progress to passive range of motion exercises once full muscle continuity has been regained. Strengthening is the next process and can take up to a full year. Weakness in the latissimus muscle group may persist and requires attention and appropriate restrictions. The primary issue with the serratus anterior is obtaining normal scapular mechanics and normalizing scapulohumeral rhythm. This may require dedicated physical therapy by a therapist who understands shoulder mechanics. Shoulder rehabilitation may be delayed by postoperative restrictions. The standard restrictions are active range of motion only and no lifting of more than 10 pounds. These restrictions as standard practice are in place for 6 weeks after surgery. Full lifting as tolerated is typically not recommended until 12 weeks after surgery.

The next step in rehabilitation is regaining and perhaps surpassing of presurgical function with endurance training. Endurance training can include low-impact lower extremity exercise, such as walking and stationary biking once pain allows. The patient can progress to high-load activities (e.g., running, swimming, climbing) after full healing of the chest wall, typically at 12 weeks. The final step is return to work and vocational rehabilitation. It is important to address goals of the rehabilitation process early in management; this helps both physiatrist and patient to set goals that will maximize quality of life.

Procedures

Management of PTPS with interventional procedures consists of perioperative and chronic pain management. As mentioned, the perioperative management involves preemptive analgesia with regional anesthesia preoperatively [2,4]. Thoracic epidural anesthesia is the primary means of early postoperative management, and this typically consists of infusion of an opiate and an anesthetic [1]. Chronic PTPS management usually starts with intercostal nerve blockade [2]. Thoracic nerve root block and radiofrequency ablation of intercostal nerves are other procedures used for PTPS [2]. Long-term maintenance pain management can be accomplished with intrathecal opiate delivery and spinal cord stimulators [2].

Surgery

There are no surgical treatments for post-thoracotomy pain.

Potential Disease Complications

The potential complications of PTPS include postoperative respiratory dysfunction secondary to decreased depth of breathing, retention of secretions, and atelectasis [10]. In addition, persistent chest wall pain can result in decreased shoulder movement and adhesive capsulitis. Shoulder function also may be affected by the disruption of the serratus anterior and the latissimus dorsi, resulting in scapular dysfunction and glenohumeral dysfunction, respectively. In addition, sleep disruption, depression, loss of employment, and diminished functional and vocational capacities can be seen in PTPS.

Potential Treatment Complications

Complications of PTPS treatment include local complications from interventional procedures, including hematomas, infections, and nerve disruption. In addition, the use of opiates and NSAIDs postoperatively can lead to gastrointestinal dysfunction. The most common side effects identified with the use of gabapentin in this population are sedation (24%) and dizziness (6%) [13].

References

[1] Hazelrigg SR, Cetindag IB, Fullerton J. Acute and chronic pain syndromes after thoracic surgery. Surg Clin North Am 2002;82:849–65.

[2] Erdek M, Staats PS. Chronic pain after thoracic surgery. Thorac Surg Clin 2005;15:123–30.

[3] Merskey H. Classification of chronic pain: description of chronic pain syndromes and definitions of pain terms. Pain 1986;3:S138–9.

[4] Karmakar M, Ho A. Postthoracotomy pain syndrome. Thorac Surg Clin 2004;14:345–52.

[5] Maguire MF, Ravenscroft A, Beggs D, Duffy JP. A questionnaire study investigating the prevalence of the neuropathic component of chronic pain after thoracic surgery. Eur J Cardiothorac Surg 2006;29:800–5.

[6] Perttunen K, Tasmuth T, Kalso E. Chronic pain after thoracic surgery: a follow up study. Acta Anaesthesiol Scand 1999;43:563–7.

[7] Li W, Lee T, Yim A. Shoulder function after thoracic surgery. Thorac Surg Clin 2004;14:331–43.

[8] Gotoda Y, Kambara N, Sakai T, et al. The morbidity, time course and predictive factors for persistent post-thoracotomy pain. Eur J Pain 2001;5:89–96.

[9] Ochroch EA, Gottschalk A, Augostides J, et al. Long-term pain and activity during recovery from major thoracotomy using thoracic epidural analgesia. Anesthesiology 2002;97:1234–44.

[10] Yegin A, Erdogan A, Kayacan N, Karsli B. Early postoperative pain management after thoracic surgery; pre- and postoperative versus postoperative epidural analgesia: a randomised study. Eur J Cardiothorac Surg 2003;24:420–4.

[11] Refai M, Brunelli, Salati M, et al. The impact of chest tube removal on pain and pulmonary function after pulmonary resection. Eur J Cardiothorac Surg 2012;41:820–2.

[12] Richardson J, Sabanathan S, Mearns AJ, et al. Post-thoracotomy neuralgia. Pain Clin 1994;7:87–97.

[13] Erdogan M, Erdogan A, Erbil N, et al. Prospective, randomized, placebo-controlled study of the effects of TENS on postthoracotomy pain and pulmonary function. World J Surg 2005;29:1563–70.

[14] Fiorelli A, Morgillo F, Milione R, et al. Control of post-thoracotomy pain by transcutaneous electrical nerve stimulation: effect on serum cytokine levels, visual analogue scale, pulmonary function and medication. Eur J Cardiothorac Surg 2012;41:861–8.

[15] Sihoe AD, Lee TW, Wan IY, et al. The use of gabapentin for postoperative and post-traumatic pain in thoracic surgery patients. Eur J Cardiothorac Surg 2006;29:795–9.

CHAPTER 111

Radiation Fibrosis Syndrome

Katarzyna Ibanez, MD
Michael D. Stubblefield, MD

Synonyms

Late effects of radiation
Myelo-radiculo-plexo-neuro-myopathy
Dropped head syndrome
Radiation-induced cervical dystonia

ICD-9 Codes

909.2 Late effect of radiation
333.79 Cervical dystonia, acquired
781.0 Trismus

ICD-10 Codes

T66 Radiation sickness, unspecified
Add seventh character for episode of care
G24.8 Acquired torsion dystonia NOS
R25.2 Cramp and spasm

Definition

Radiation-induced toxicity after cancer treatment may result in significant long-term disability. Radiation fibrosis describes the insidious pathologic fibrotic tissue sclerosis that occurs in response to radiation exposure. Radiation fibrosis syndrome (RFS) is the term used to describe the myriad clinical manifestations of progressive fibrotic tissue sclerosis that can result from radiation treatment. It is estimated that about half of the approximately 14 million cancer survivors in the United States will receive radiation treatment during the course of their disease [1]. The incidence of RFS is unknown, and its severity is affected by multiple factors (see later). Radiotherapy is typically combined with surgery or chemotherapy; therefore the toxicities of these modalities may be cumulative and difficult to separate clinically.

The therapeutic goal of radiation therapy is to kill rapidly proliferating tumor cells by inducing apoptosis or mitotic cell death through free radical–mediated DNA damage [2]. Various dose-sculpting techniques have been developed to minimize exposure to normal tissues; however, radiation exposure to normal body cells cannot be completely eliminated [3]. The effects of radiation can be acute (occurring during or immediately after treatment), early-delayed (up to 3 months after completion of treatment), or late-delayed (occurring more than 3 months after completion of treatment) [4]. Radiation fibrosis is generally a late complication of radiation therapy and may become clinically apparent many years after treatment. Its progression can be insidious or rapid, but it is invariably irreversible [5,6]. It can damage any tissue type, including skin, muscle, ligament, tendon, nerve, viscera, and bone [7]. The underlying mechanism of radiation fibrosis is complex and not completely understood. It has been postulated that radiation-induced vascular endothelial injury causes thrombomodulin deficiency, resulting in its inability to scavenge locally formed thrombin, which in turn leads to abnormal accumulation of proliferative fibrin in the intravascular, perivascular, and extravascular compartments [2].

The long-term morbidity due to RFS is largely determined by the size of the radiation field, the type and susceptibility of underlying tissues to radiation, and the patient's individual resistance to the effects of radiation. Other factors include the patient's age, overall health, and medical and degenerative disorders, particularly degenerative spine disease; cancer status; exposure to neurotoxic, cardiotoxic, and other chemotherapy types; and time since radiation was administered [8]. For signs or symptoms to be considered referable to RFS, either the structures generating them must be within the radiation field or the neural, vascular, lymphatic, muscular, tendinous, or other structures important in their genesis must traverse the field. It is therefore necessary to understand which type of radiation field was used to treat a given patient to determine whether the signs, symptoms, or functional deficits can be attributable to RFS. The common radiation fields used in Hodgkin lymphoma (HL) are depicted in Figure 111.1. Extensive radiation fields, such as mantle field used to treat HL, can result in widespread sequelae of RFS. Patients with head and neck cancer (HNC) treated with radiation are also likely to develop RFS because of the high dose of radiation required for tumor control as well as the proximity of many vital tissues to the radiation field [9].

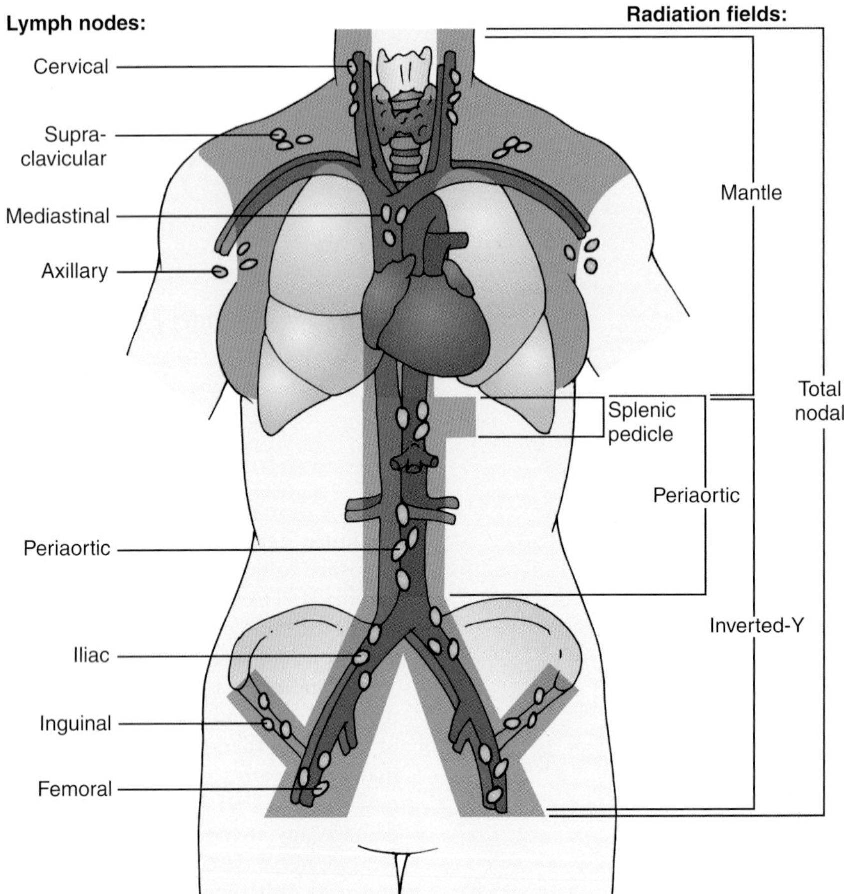

FIGURE 111.1 Radiation fields used to treat Hodgkin lymphoma. These fields encompass a vast amount of normal tissue and are well known to cause marked adverse late effects, particularly in patients treated with high doses in the mid-1980s.

Symptoms

Patients with RFS can present with a variety of symptoms as virtually every organ system can be affected. Symptoms should be anatomically congruent to the radiation field and involved tissues. HL survivors frequently present with neck extensor weakness (dropped head syndrome), pain and limited range of motion of the neck and shoulders, weakness, fatigue, gait and dexterity problems, neuropathic symptoms, and difficulty in performing activities of daily living. Spasms are frequently described as tight, pulling, or cramping sensations. Neuropathic pain is usually described as burning, stabbing, or searing. HNC patients commonly have trismus, cervical dystonia, facial lymphedema, dysphagia, and dysarthria. Radiation-induced trigeminal neuralgia (commonly in the V2-V3 distribution on the affected side, but bilateral involvement is possible) and anterior cervical neuralgia are also common complications. Neuropathic pain in patients with RFS can be severe and markedly out of proportion to the perceived pathologic process. If the spinal cord was in the radiation field, patients may present with spastic paraparesis or quadriparesis, depending on the level of the spinal cord affected by radiation. Early-delayed radiation-induced myelopathy is almost always reversible, whereas late-delayed is almost always progressive and permanent [10]. If autonomic nerves are affected, patients can present with orthostatic hypotension, baroreceptor failure, bowel and bladder dysfunction, and sexual dysfunction. Shortness of breath in HL patients treated with mantle field radiation may be due to pulmonary insufficiency from bilateral phrenic nerve dysfunction [11].

Physical Examination

Comprehensive examination, including detailed neuromuscular and musculoskeletal evaluation, is of paramount importance. Physical examination findings will vary greatly from patient to patient; however, a full account of physical examination findings is beyond the scope of this chapter.

Examination of patients treated for HL commonly demonstrates cervicothoracic paraspinal, shoulder girdle, and rhomboid muscle atrophy and often a C-shaped posture due to forwardly positioned neck and shoulders secondary to relatively strong pectoral muscles (Fig. 111.2). HNC patients commonly present with asymmetric positioning of the head and neck due to severe neck tightness, pain, and spasms of trapezius, sternocleidomastoid, and scalene muscles, among others. This radiation-induced cervical dystonia may progress to fixed contracture of the anterior cervical musculature [12]. Trismus seen in HNC patients is commonly associated with spasms in the masseter and pterygoid muscles (Fig. 111.3). Marked loss of range of motion and function may be seen if joints were involved in the radiation field. Rotator cuff tendinitis

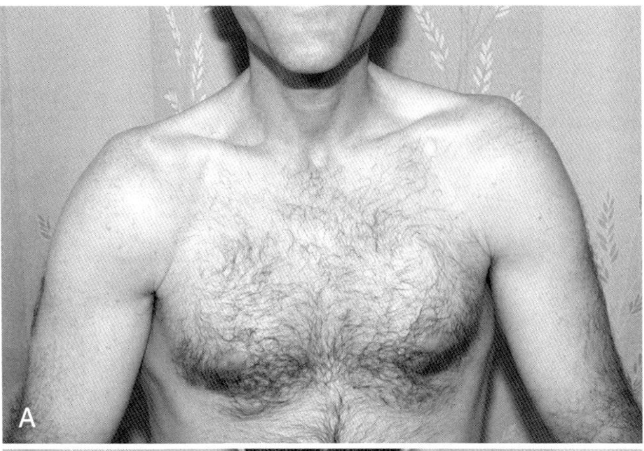

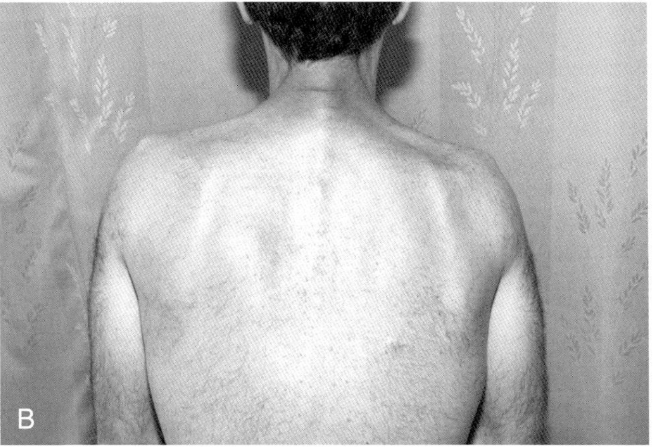

FIGURE 111.2 Typical pattern of C-shaped posture (**A**) and cervicothoracic muscle atrophy (**B**) in a Hodgkin lymphoma patient previously treated with mantle field radiation.

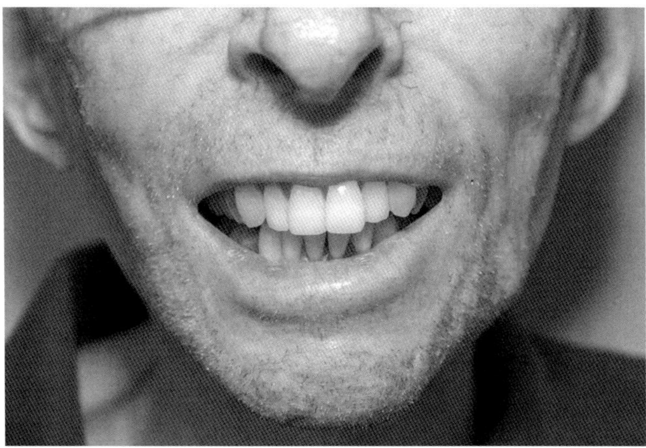

FIGURE 111.3 Severe trismus in a patient with tonsillar cancer treated with high-dose radiation. The patient is actively trying to open his mouth but has no clearance between his front teeth. He must ingest predominantly liquid nutrition between his back teeth. Oral hygiene and surveillance for recurrent cancer, among other functions, are severely compromised by his limited mouth opening.

and adhesive capsulitis may develop because of perturbation of normal shoulder motion secondary to C5 and C6 radiculopathy or upper brachial plexopathy [13]. Neurologic testing may reveal sensory loss, including light touch, pain, temperature, vibration, and proprioception. Weakness and gait dysfunction may be secondary to damage of neural tissue (spinal cord, plexus, cauda equina, peripheral nerves) or muscle itself. Not infrequently, the clinical picture fits that of myelo-radiculo-plexo-neuro-myopathy, with some or all components of the neuromuscular axis affected to varying degrees. The upper brachial plexus, frequently included in the radiation field of head and neck radiation ports, may be more susceptible to radiation injury because of its apical location in the neck and the long course traversed by its fibers relative to the middle and lower trunk. The pyramidal shape of the thorax and the clavicle may provide less protective tissue around the upper plexus, but the clinical validity of this phenomenon is unclear [14].

Functional Limitations

Sensory loss, pain, and weakness may have profound effects on gait and ability to perform activities of daily living. Loss of sensation also renders the patient more susceptible to secondary musculoskeletal injuries. Patients with severe trismus may have deficits including but not limited to difficulty in speaking, eating, drinking, and performing oral hygiene. Inability to position the head due to progressive fibrosis and contracture of the anterior cervical musculature can also affect swallowing, phonation, and work-related tasks. Patients with neck extensor weakness frequently have to stop driving and limit their work and leisure activities. Disability may also be related to bowel, bladder, and sexual dysfunction.

Diagnostic Studies

Imaging is often useful in the evaluation of RFS. A baseline magnetic resonance imaging (MRI) study of the entire spine for HL patients with RFS and of the cervical spine for HNC patients is often indicated to exclude degenerative processes of the spine or secondary malignant neoplasms. The addition of gadolinium contrast is required to exclude brain metastasis, intramedullary spinal tumor, or leptomeningeal disease and to differentiate tumor from scarring or fibrotic tissue in patients with a history of prior surgery. In addition, MRI of the spine may demonstrate overt demyelinating lesions or nodular enhancement of the cauda equina mimicking leptomeningeal disease in some patients treated for HL with high-dose radiation (Fig. 111.4). Computed tomography (CT) with contrast enhancement is used to evaluate the viscera of the chest, abdomen, and pelvis for metastatic or progressive disease. CT may also be used if MRI is contraindicated (because of a pacemaker, aneurysm clips, or breast tissue expanders, for example). CT myelography is indicated when metallic hardware causes excessive artifact, precluding adequate visualization of the spinal canal. Radiography is useful to evaluate suspected loosening or failure of spinal stabilization hardware or joint replacement prostheses.

Electrodiagnostic evaluation may provide invaluable information by identifying, localizing, confirming, or differentiating radiculopathy, plexopathy, neuropathy, or myopathy in patients with RFS. Needle electromyography can confirm muscle denervation and may identify myokymia, fasciculations, and muscle spasms. Given the

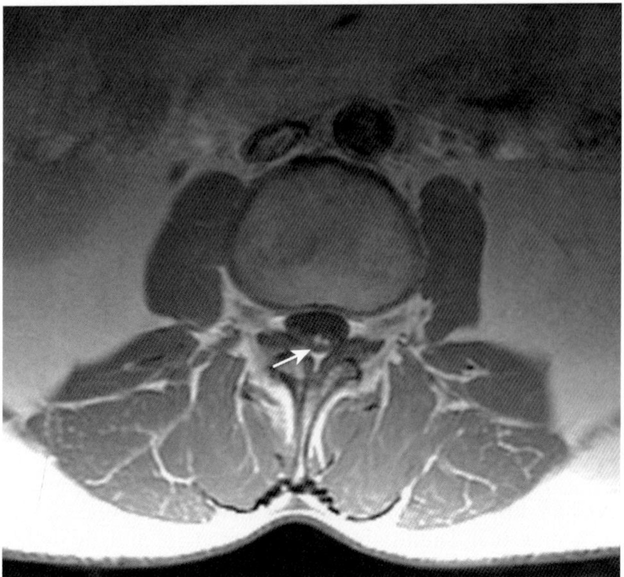

FIGURE 111.4 Gadolinium-enhanced T1-weighted magnetic resonance image depicting cauda equina enhancement (*arrow*) in a Hodgkin lymphoma patient who previously received periaortic radiation therapy.

high likelihood of multiple overlapping disorders present on electrodiagnostic testing, these studies should be interpreted by electromyographers with considerable experience in the evaluation of complex neuromuscular disorders.

Differential Diagnosis

FACIAL PAIN

Trigeminal neuralgia
Temporomandibular joint disorder
Trismus

NECK PAIN

Cervical dystonia
Spinal accessory mononeuropathy
Anterior cervical plexus neuralgia
Dropped head syndrome
Myofascial pain

SHOULDER PAIN

Rotator cuff tendinitis
Adhesive capsulitis
C5 or C6 cervical radiculopathy
Upper trunk brachial plexopathy

EXTREMITY PAIN AND WEAKNESS

Myelopathy
Radiculopathy
Plexopathy
Neuropathy
- Mononeuropathy
- Polyneuropathy

Myopathy
Tumor or neoplasm
- Primary
- Recurrent

Funicular pain
Musculoskeletal disorders
Fibromyalgia
Aromatase inhibitor–induced arthralgia or myalgia

Treatment

Initial

Whereas there is no cure for or way to stop progression of fibrotic tissue sclerosis leading to RFS, the patient's symptoms and function are likely to improve with appropriate treatment. Treatment is geared specifically toward the patient's complaints and functional deficits. Specialized care and a multidisciplinary approach are critical to successful rehabilitation. Patient education with an emphasis on the benefits of a lifelong home exercise program is of paramount importance. Many patients, especially HL survivors, require physical, occupational, and lymphedema therapy. The goals of physical therapy are to restore muscle balance and to correct the posture and body mechanics by stretching tight structures, strengthening weak musculature (core and neck extensors), and improving proprioception and endurance. Physical and occupational therapy are critical elements to rehabilitation of HNC patients with trismus and cervical dystonia. Patients with trismus also benefit from speech and swallowing therapy.

Rehabilitation

Orthotic devices are prescribed according to the principles used in other neuromuscular and musculoskeletal disorders, regardless of the underlying cause. Patients with weak neck extensors may benefit from a cervical collar, such as the Headmaster Collar (Symmetric Designs, Salt Spring Island, British Columbia, Canada). It is intended only for intermittent use and serves as an energy conservation device. Upper extremity orthotic devices may be appropriate in select patients with severe radiculopathy or plexopathy but are infrequently used. Lower extremity orthotic devices, such as ankle-foot orthoses, may be used for patients with a footdrop from any cause, including myelopathy, radiculopathy (usually L4-L5), plexopathy (lumbosacral trunk), and neuropathy (sciatic, common peroneal [fibular], deep peroneal [fibular] nerves). A posterior leaf spring ankle-foot orthosis is the most commonly used as it is lighter and less bulky than the alternatives. Patients with excessive spasticity (rarely seen in RFS unless myelopathy predominates) or significant mediolateral ankle instability require a custom molded ankle-foot orthosis. Control of the knee to prevent buckling is sometimes indicated. Patients with weak quadriceps may develop compensatory genu recurvatum, which may result in knee pain and degeneration. Older patients and those with weakness affecting multiple joints may benefit from a knee immobilizer. If weakness of both knee extension and ankle dorsiflexion is present, a knee immobilizer can often be fabricated to fit in a modular fashion over an ankle-foot orthosis and tends to be easier to manipulate than a knee-ankle-foot-orthosis.

Medications are often needed to control pain and muscle spasms in RFS. For the pain to be effectively managed, one must determine whether the pain is neuropathic or musculoskeletal (somatic) in nature. In many patients, both neuropathic and somatic pain may coexist. Neuropathic pain and, to some extent, muscle spasms associated with RFS may respond to nerve stabilizing agents. Pregabalin (Lyrica) is preferred to gabapentin (Neurontin), given its favorable pharmacokinetics, efficacy, and low potential for drug-drug interaction [15]. Duloxetine (Cymbalta) is also a suitable agent for neuropathic pain in RFS and can be used in conjunction with pregabalin. Duloxetine, as a serotonin and norepinephrine reuptake inhibitor, may adversely interact with other serotonin reuptake inhibitors and should generally be avoided with tricyclic antidepressants, tramadol, and triptans. Opioids are often added to pregabalin or duloxetine when needed but should be considered second-line agents. Tricyclic antidepressants might be helpful in neuropathic pain, but their unfavorable side effect profile (anticholinergic effects resulting in dry mouth, blurred vision, constipation, urinary retention, arrhythmia, drowsiness, orthostatic hypotension, sexual dysfunction) limits their use. A short course of a nonsteroidal anti-inflammatory drug (NSAID), especially during acute exacerbation of symptoms, may be used to control somatic pain from inflammation of the rotator cuff, adhesive capsulitis, and other underlying degenerative changes. Long-term use of NSAIDs is relatively contraindicated, given their known gastrointestinal and cardiovascular side effects, particularly in the HL survivor population, who are at increased risk. Opioids are often used to control somatic pain when NSAIDs are ineffective or contraindicated. Muscle relaxants, including baclofen, tizanidine (Zanaflex), and benzodiazepines, may help relieve pain associated with muscle spasms but should be discontinued if deemed ineffective after a short trial.

Patients with trismus should be evaluated for a jaw stretching device. In the first 6 months of treatment, the TheraBite Jaw Motion Rehabilitation System (Atos Medical Inc., West Allis, Wisconsin) may be used. The Dynasplint Trismus System (Dynasplint, Severna Park, Maryland) is generally preferred in patients with chronic trismus because it is customizable and uses the principle of low-torque, prolonged duration stretch, which may be more effective at improving range of motion in an experimental model [16].

Procedures

Trigger point injections and botulinum toxin injections are of particular benefit in specific conditions associated with RFS [17]. Trigger point injections may provide significant pain relief for up to 1 month and should be offered to patients with painful muscle spasms in the trapezius, levator scapulae, rhomboids, cervical paraspinal, and other muscles. Usually, 2 to 5 mL of 0.25% bupivacaine or a similar anesthetic is used per location, up to a maximum of 20 mL divided between one and ten sites. Botulinum toxin injections may be used as both primary and adjunctive treatment for musculoskeletal pain, muscle spasms, spasticity, migraines, neuropathic pain, and a variety of other disorders [18]. Some studied cancer-related indications for botulinum toxin injections include chronic and neuropathic pain after neck dissection, muscle spasms after radiation therapy to the head and neck, and radiation-induced trismus [12,19,20].

Patients with RFS-related neuromuscular and musculoskeletal pain who fail to respond to conservative management may also benefit from interventional procedures, including epidural steroid injections, peripheral nerve blocks, and intra-articular joint injections. Placement of implantable epidural drug pumps is usually discouraged because it would preclude patients from undergoing MRI in the future, which might be needed for disease surveillance.

Surgery

In general, conservative measures are the mainstay of treatment because surgery is unlikely to improve the marked and progressive neuromuscular disorders due to RFS. Severe dysfunction and atrophy of the underlying neuromuscular structures confer poor surgical outcomes. Coronoidectomy may be considered in a patient with severe trismus for whom conservative management failed, although clinical evidence for its efficacy is limited [21].

Potential Disease Complications

The clinical complications of RFS vary greatly and depend on multiple factors, as discussed earlier. Multiple non-neuromuscular complications (e.g., fatigue, alopecia, lymphedema, esophagitis, pericarditis, volvulus) as well as neuromuscular and musculoskeletal complications of RFS (e.g., myelo-radiculo-plexo-neuro-myopathy, osteoporosis, osteoradionecrosis, adhesive capsulitis) are well recognized. Patients with a history of HL treated with mantle or other types of radiation are at a greatly increased risk for development of secondary cancers (including thyroid, breast, lung, and sarcoma) and accelerated cardiovascular disease (including atherosclerosis, valvular heart disease, pericardial disease, cardiomyopathy, arrhythmias, and subclavian and carotid artery stenosis) [22]. Childhood cancer survivors are at the greatest risk for complications, including radiation-induced neoplasms, osteonecrosis, and abnormal bone growth either from cranial radiation affecting the endocrine system or from abnormal maturation of growth plates affected by radiation.

Potential Treatment Complications

Medications used to treat muscle spasms as well as neuropathic and musculoskeletal pain can result in significant side effects, in some cases leading to medication discontinuation by the patient. This can frequently be avoided by slow dose titration with the goal of finding the lowest effective dose of medications. Trigger point and botulinum toxin injections carry a low risk of adverse effects if they are given by an experienced practitioner. Altered anatomy from radiation and surgery should be taken into consideration. Some of the possible side effects include pneumothorax, bleeding, and infection. Botulinum toxin injections can cause focal muscle weakness ranging from a droopy eyelid or neck extension weakness to a severe dysphagia necessitating feeding tube placement; fortunately, these effects are transient. Starting doses of botulinum toxin should be low, and only relatively strong muscles should be targeted for injections.

References

[1] Mariotto AB, Yabroff KR, Shao Y, et al. Projections of the cost of cancer care in the United States: 2010–2020. J Natl Cancer Inst 2011;103:117–28.

[2] Hauer-Jensen M, Fink LM, Wang J. Radiation injury and the protein C pathway. Crit Care Med 2004;32(Suppl.):S325–30.

[3] Bhide SA, Nutting CM. Recent advances in radiotherapy. BMC Med 2010;8:25.

[4] New P. Radiation injury to the nervous system. Curr Opin Neurol 2001;14:725–34.

[5] Johansson S, Svensson H, Denekamp J. Dose response and latency for radiation-induced fibrosis, edema, and neuropathy in breast cancer patients. Int J Radiat Oncol Biol Phys 2002;52:1207–19.

[6] Johansson S, Svensson H, Denekamp J. Timescale of evolution of late radiation injury after postoperative radiotherapy of breast cancer patients. Int J Radiat Oncol Biol Phys 2000;48:745–50.

[7] Libshitz HI, DuBrow RA, Loyer EM, Charnsangavej C. Radiation change in normal organs: an overview of body imaging. Eur Radiol 1996;6:786–95.

[8] Zackrisson B, Mercke C, Strander H, et al. A systematic overview of radiation therapy effects in head and neck cancer. Acta Oncol 2003;42:443–61.

[9] Marcus KJ, Tishler RB. Head and neck carcinomas across the age spectrum: epidemiology, therapy, and late effects. Semin Radiat Oncol 2010;20:52–7.

[10] Giglio P, Gilbert MR. Neurologic complications of cancer and its treatment. Curr Oncol Rep 2010;12:50–9.

[11] Avila EK, Goenka A, Fontenla S. Bilateral phrenic nerve dysfunction: a late complication of mantle radiation. J Neurooncol 2011;103:393–5.

[12] Stubblefield MD, Levine A, Custodio CM, Fitzpatrick T. The role of botulinum toxin type A in the radiation fibrosis syndrome: a preliminary report. Arch Phys Med Rehabil 2008;89:417–21.

[13] Tytherleigh-Strong G, Hirahara A, Miniaci A. Rotator cuff disease. Curr Opin Rheumatol 2001;13:135–45.

[14] Jaeckle KA. Neurological manifestations of neoplastic and radiation-induced plexopathies. Semin Neurol 2004;24:385–93.

[15] Stubblefield MD, Burstein HJ, Burton AW, et al. NCCN task force report: management of neuropathy in cancer. J Natl Compr Canc Netw 2009;7(Suppl. 5):S1–26, quiz S27–S28.

[16] Usuba M, Akai M, Shirasaki Y, Miyakawa S. Experimental joint contracture correction with low torque–long duration repeated stretching. Clin Orthop Relat Res 2007;456:70–8.

[17] Stubblefield MD. Radiation fibrosis syndrome: neuromuscular and musculoskeletal complications in cancer survivors. PM R 2011;3:1041–54.

[18] Royal MA. Botulinum toxins in pain management. Phys Med Rehabil Clin N Am 2003;14:805–20.

[19] Lou JS, Pleninger P, Kurlan R. Botulinum toxin A is effective in treating trismus associated with postradiation myokymia and muscle spasm. Mov Disord 1995;10:680–1.

[20] Van Daele DJ, Finnegan EM, Rodnitzky RL, et al. Head and neck muscle spasm after radiotherapy: management with botulinum toxin A injection. Arch Otolaryngol Head Neck Surg 2002;128:956–9.

[21] Bhrany AD, Izzard M, Wood AJ, Futran ND. Coronoidectomy for the treatment of trismus in head and neck cancer patients. Laryngoscope 2007;117:1952–6.

[22] Ng AK, Mauch PM. Late effects of Hodgkin's disease and its treatment. Cancer J 2009;15:164–8.

CHAPTER 112

Repetitive Strain Injuries

Kelly C. McInnis, DO

Synonyms

Cumulative trauma disorders
Occupational overuse syndromes
Upper extremity musculoskeletal disorders
Nonspecific work-related upper limb disorders
Repetitive overuse disorders

ICD-9 Codes

719.44	**Hand pain**
729.5	**Limb pain**
729.1	**Myalgia and myositis, unspecified**

ICD-10 Codes

M79.641	**Pain in right hand**
M79.642	**Pain in left hand**
M79.643	**Pain in unspecified hand**
M79.609	**Pain in unspecified limb**
G70.9	**Myoneural disorder, unspecified (myalgia)**
M60.9	**Myositis, unspecified**

Definition

Repetitive strain injury (RSI) describes nonspecific upper extremity pain that often develops in occupational settings. RSIs are thought to result from the performance of repetitive and forceful hand-intensive tasks. These conditions are also referred to as cumulative trauma disorders, occupational overuse syndromes, and nonspecific work-related upper limb disorders. The varying nomenclature is controversial because it provides little insight into anatomy affected, disease severity, appropriate treatment, or expected prognosis. Classification systems of work-related musculoskeletal disorders often include specific diagnoses, such as carpal tunnel syndrome and de Quervain tenosynovitis, as RSIs, but the consensus in recent years has been to consider RSI an entirely separate category of occupational disorder [1]. RSIs have symptom complexes that do not fit neatly into another diagnostic classification, such as specific tendinopathy or nerve entrapment. RSIs typically have few objective physical findings and little in the way of demonstrable pathologic change.

RSI is a significant medical concern; approximately 65% of reported cases of occupational illness are attributed to repeated trauma annually [2,3]. In fact, occupational musculoskeletal disorders of the hand and wrist are associated with the longest absences from work and have greater lost productivity and wages than those of other anatomic regions [2]. There is evidence that this condition is actually underreported [4]. Important risk factors appear to be repetitive motion of the arm or wrist, movements that require extremes of hand or arm position, prolonged static postures, and vibration. Other risk factors may be poor ergonomic work environment, task invariability, lack of autonomy, and high levels of psychological distress in the workplace. In addition, the female gender appears to be more susceptible to development of RSI [5]. RSIs can develop outside of the workplace in individuals who participate in hobbies or activities that expose them to repetitive motion and prolonged postures on a consistent basis. A study demonstrated that the adult acquired upper limb amputee population is at increased risk of musculoskeletal pain in the neck/upper back and residual limb as well as in the contralateral remaining arm [6].

According to the U.S. Department of Labor, Bureau of Labor Statistics, occupations that appear to be at greatest risk for RSIs are those in the service and manufacturing industries, including any job involving computer processing and keyboard use [2]. These occupations have the most demand for upper extremity intensive tasks. Because of limitations in the assessment of risk factors, quantitative levels of exposure that are "acceptable" in each occupation are not available [7]. Clinically, it appears that the onset and perpetuation of RSIs are multifactorial. There is no proven etiology of RSI, but it is thought to develop from repetitive microtrauma to muscle, tendon, nerve, loose connective tissue, or bone that exceeds the ability of the tissue to heal itself. In animal models, when chronic repetitive motion is induced, an acute inflammatory response is stimulated in the tissue. This initial response eventually subsides and is followed by a fibrotic response that may lead to complete tissue repair if loads and repetition are sufficiently low [8]. However, in the presence of high repetition or high force, the acute inflammatory response is followed by tissue degeneration and fibrosis that leads to scarring. It is this tissue reorganization that may lead to a nonspecific pattern of pain in RSI.

Abnormal muscle fatigability may also contribute to pain [9]. Reduction in muscle blood flow and localized tissue hypoxia have been demonstrated in trapezius muscle biopsy specimens taken from assembly-line workers with prolonged, static shoulder postures who developed chronic trapezius myalgia [10]. In addition, diminished local muscle oxygenation and blood flow has been demonstrated in the forearms of individuals with RSI during static contraction, compared with controls at similar working intensities [11]. The same investigators later demonstrated that patients with RSI have an attenuated exercise-induced brachial artery blood flow and an impaired vascular endothelial function in the affected arm [12]. A subsequent study found that blood flow and oxygen consumption after exercise are similarly attenuated in both the affected and contralateral unaffected arms of patients with unilateral RSI, indicating that systemic vascular adaptations may occur [13]. These findings indicate that the underlying vasculature may be impaired in this condition. It is unclear whether these data can be extrapolated to explain the pathophysiologic mechanism of all RSIs in the upper extremity.

There may also be a neurogenic origin for RSI. There is evidence of neural reorganization at multiple levels of the central nervous system after the performance of repetitive tasks [2]. The repeated stimulation of nociceptive afferent nerve fibers may cause the receptors to become hypersensitive, to expand their receptive fields, and to increase the excitability of secondary neurons in the spinal cord. These changes may contribute to the hyperalgesia associated with chronic pain in RSIs. Moreover, there may also be an element of central nervous system reorganization at the level of the somatosensory cortex with repetitive tasks [2]. Figure 112.1 illustrates the distribution of somatosensory pathways in the central nervous system.

Regardless of the factors that contribute to the development of RSI, there is often a complex dynamic in managing patients with work-related musculoskeletal disorders. They are often involved in compensation claims. When the injured patient takes on the additional role of claimant, the perception of both patient and caregiver can change in many aspects of the healing and rehabilitation process. It is paramount for the physician treating RSI to take the medicolegal implications into account. Indeed, the workers' compensation system has a great impact on the reporting and control of work-related disorders [14].

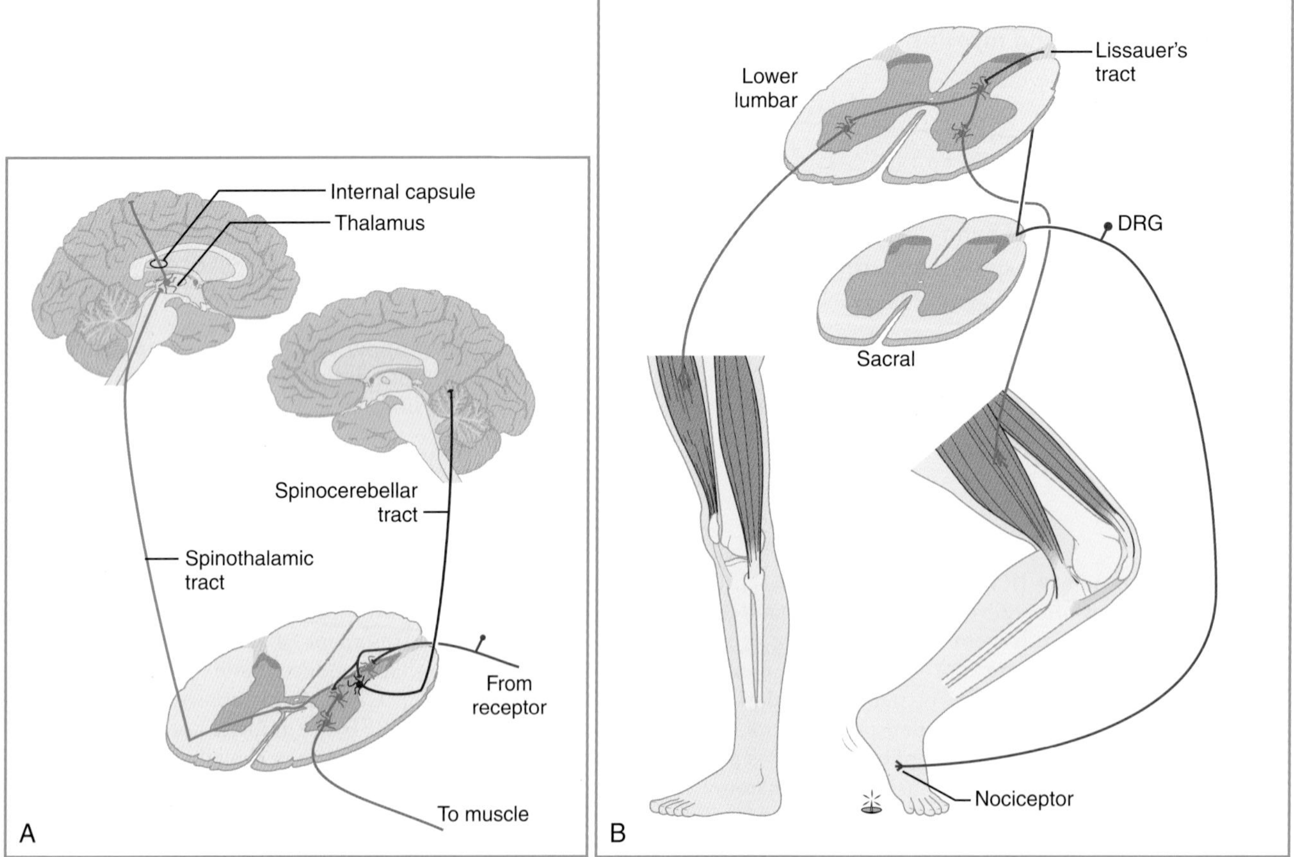

FIGURE 112.1 **A,** Spinothalamic and spinocerebellar tracts to muscle (*blue*) and from nociceptive receptor (*red*). **B,** Afferent sensory pathways from peripheral receptors to lumbosacral spine. *DRG,* dorsal root ganglion. *(From Nolte J. Elsevier's Integrated Neuroscience. St. Louis, Mosby, 2008.)*

Symptoms

The predominant symptom in RSI is upper extremity pain. The discomfort often begins as a dull ache in the forearm or hand after the performance of tasks of repetitive motion. Initially, it may be intermittent and alleviated with rest. As the offending activity is repeated with regularity, the pain may increase in intensity and be triggered by minimal exertion in the workplace and even while performing simple activities of daily living, such as dressing or grooming. The symptoms usually begin in one region of the limb in a fairly localized area (e.g., wrist, elbow, or forearm) but may quickly spread to involve the entire arm and at times the contralateral arm. Pain tends to gradually increase during the workday, with peak intensity during the last hours of work. It appears to get better over the weekends and during vacations from work.

Other symptoms may include paresthesias, numbness, and weakness. If these symptoms are present, they may not follow dermatomal or peripheral nerve distributions. Patients may also complain of arm or hand muscle cramping, allodynia, stiffness, and slowing or incoordination of fine motor movements of the hand.

Patients often complain of night pain, resulting in poor sleep. A detailed investigation of sleep habits is important because sleep disruption is common in RSI. Psychological distress and depression may result if pain and sleeplessness persist. In fact, self-reported upper extremity–specific health status measured by the Disabilities of the Arm, Shoulder, and Hand (DASH) questionnaire appears to correlate with depression and pain anxiety in these patients [15]. Some patients may also exhibit maladaptive illness beliefs, such as catastrophizing and fear-avoidance.

In taking a patient's history, the clinician should attain an accurate understanding of the patient's job description and daily workstation. It is important to thoroughly evaluate the biomechanics of body position and posture as well as the physical layout of the work site. Special attention should be given to the details of specific job duties, including the frequency, duration, and conditions under which they are performed. For example, if the patient works a desk job and spends each day on a computer, it is important to inquire about desk and chair setup and placement of the computer monitor and keyboard. The clinician should also take note of the patient's perception and satisfaction with the workplace. This information can give the clinician valuable insight as dissatisfied workers are notorious for work-related medical claims.

Physical Examination

RSI is a diagnosis of exclusion. Typically, there are no objective physical findings. Hence, the physical examination should be comprehensive and focus on ruling out alternative diagnoses. It should include a thorough musculoskeletal examination with inspection, palpation, and testing of passive and active range of motion of the cervical spine, shoulder, elbow, wrist, and fingers. There is typically no evidence of muscle atrophy or other deformity. There may be pain on active and passive range of motion, but there is generally no restriction of motion when the examiner takes the joint through a full arc. There may be diffuse myofascial pain with palpation over the symptomatic region. In addition, there may be evidence of one or more focal fibromyalgia tender points on the symptomatic as well as on the asymptomatic side [16] (Fig. 112.2).

Neurologic assessment can rule out localized nerve disease by investigating for dermatomal, myotomal, or peripheral nerve abnormalities. In RSI, deep tendon reflexes are normal and symmetric. Manual muscle strength testing should be performed but is generally inconsistent, depending on the patient's effort and pain level with exertion. Objective and reproducible strength tests can be performed with a hand or pinch dynamometer if level of strength is uncertain with examiner resistance. Computer-driven isokinetic dynamometers can also be used for more reliable measures of strength across uniaxial joints, such as the elbow. Sensory testing should be done by light touch as well as by pinprick. This portion of the neurologic examination is often difficult as subjective abnormalities are common. The reported impairments in sensation do not typically follow dermatomal distributions.

Provocative tests that reproduce specific pain patterns can help rule out alternative diagnoses. Examples include the Spurling test for cervical radiculopathy, Neer and Hawkins maneuvers for rotator cuff impingement, resisted wrist or finger extension for lateral epicondylitis, Tinel sign at the ulnar groove for ulnar neuritis, and Finkelstein test for de Quervain tenosynovitis. Provocative maneuvers that can rule out carpal tunnel syndrome include Tinel sign at the wrist, Phalen test, reverse Phalen test, and carpal tunnel compression. It is important to keep in mind that percussion over the median nerve at the wrist, the ulnar nerve at the cubital tunnel, or the radial nerve at the elbow may elicit pain or paresthesias in RSI, but this is not necessarily indicative of nerve injury.

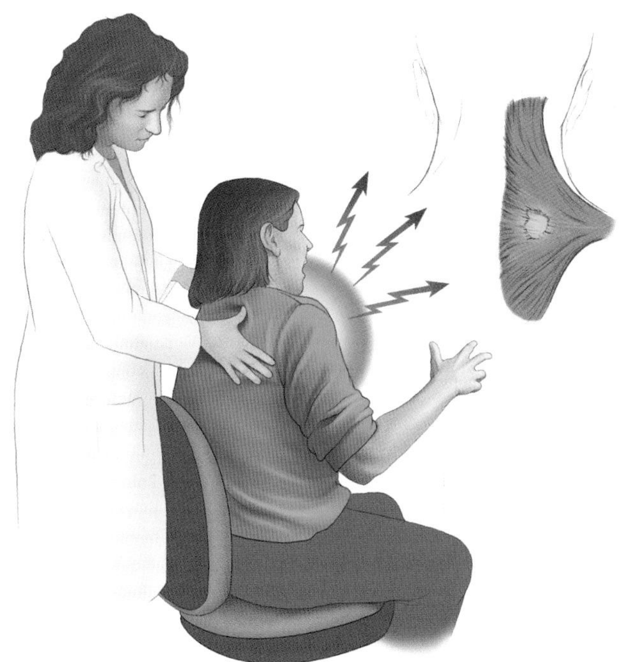

FIGURE 112.2 Fibromyalgia of the cervical musculature. *(From Waldman S. Atlas of Common Pain Syndromes, 3rd ed. Philadelphia, WB Saunders, 2012.)*

Functional Limitations

RSI can limit upper extremity function to highly variable degrees [17]. Patients may have difficulty in performing activities of daily living at home, such as dressing, grooming, or preparing a meal. The pain impairment may prevent them from participating in recreational activities that they formerly enjoyed. They can also be quite limited in terms of their work-related activity. For example, pain may prevent a patient from being productive at work because he or she finds it difficult to use a keyboard and computer to do different tasks. Employers often advocate functional capacity evaluations to define more objectively the amount of physical labor that the patient can perform safely.

Diagnostic Studies

Diagnostic tests are ordered if the diagnosis is not clear after the history and physical examination, if the results of the testing will change management, or if the testing is needed for medicolegal reasons. The tests are used to exclude other definitive conditions that may remain in the differential diagnosis after examination. Needle electromyography and nerve conduction studies are often necessary to rule out a peripheral nerve lesion, such as median nerve entrapment at the wrist. Electrodiagnostic studies provide the distinct advantage of offering objective data by quantifying the degree of nerve impairment in a manner that is independent of the patient's pain behaviors [18]. This can be important when injured workers have interest in substantial secondary gain and may not be reliable in their effort or honesty when motor and sensory nerve function is tested on physical examination.

Imaging is likely to be normal in RSI. Plain radiographs of the suspected site of disease will generally not reveal a fracture in the absence of blunt trauma but may reveal underlying degenerative changes that may or may not account for the patient's symptoms. Magnetic resonance imaging of the cervical spine and shoulder is often ordered to rule out disc herniation, neuroforaminal stenosis, and rotator cuff disease. This study may be useful only if there is concern for one of these diagnoses on the basis of the physical examination [19]. Magnetic resonance imaging is expensive, and abnormalities such as disc bulging and degenerative spondylosis are often found in asymptomatic individuals and may not explain the current symptom complex.

Laboratory work is seldom necessary at the time of initial evaluation unless an underlying systemic illness is suspected.

Differential Diagnosis

Cervical radiculopathy
Myofascial pain syndrome
Thoracic outlet syndrome
Rotator cuff or biceps tendinopathy
Lateral or medial epicondylitis
Compressive neuropathies (e.g., carpal tunnel syndrome)
de Quervain tenosynovitis
Osteoarthritis
Fractures

Treatment

Initial

Treatment of RSIs should focus on conservative measures. The first step is to limit exposure, if possible, to the particular repetitive activities that may have contributed to the development of the RSI and that continue to induce pain. Whenever possible, accommodations at the workplace should be optimized to allow the patient to continue to perform the duties that are required by the employer. Several strategies for computer-based occupations are discussed later in this chapter. Early return to work with transitional arrangements should be facilitated when necessary. Sick leave should be avoided because it may develop into chronic disability. A substantial proportion of workers experience additional injury-related absences even after their first return to work. Time off work has proved to be a powerful predictor of disability pension; fully following work-related restrictions can ensure that the patient remains a productive employee by going to work [20].

Unfortunately, there is little evidence for the effectiveness of any specific medical intervention for RSI. Clinical treatment is usually targeted at relief of pain and acute inflammation as well as restoration of range of motion. Inflammatory conditions are often treated with the PRICE regimen: protection (preventing further injury, perhaps by bracing), rest or activity modification (as mentioned before), ice, compression, and elevation to minimize swelling.

Icing of the limb for about 20 minutes three times daily in conjunction with wrist or elbow splinting can decrease symptoms. Other modalities that may be helpful in controlling pain symptoms in the acute phase of treatment include ultrasound, iontophoresis, and transcutaneous electrical nerve stimulation applied to the region of soft tissue pain. Manual therapy, spray and stretch techniques with a vapocoolant spray, and paraffin baths may also alleviate pain in some patients, although evidence for efficacy is lacking.

Medications may also be used to control pain and inflammation. Nonsteroidal anti-inflammatory drugs (NSAIDs) are usually the first-line pharmaceuticals for acute inflammation. There are many NSAIDs on the market from which to choose, and some can easily be purchased over-the-counter. It is often useful to try several different types of NSAIDs because patient responses can be idiosyncratic. Anticonvulsant medications, such as gabapentin, pregabalin, and carbamazepine, are also often used for pain. They are generally most effective for neuropathic pain. There is currently no evidence suggesting that they are specifically indicated in treatment of RSI. Local anesthetic patches (e.g., lidocaine) may be helpful if they are placed over a localized area of arm pain. Trigger point injections with local anesthetic or dry needling can also be considered to relieve myofascial pain. Oral narcotics are generally avoided.

Restoration of sleep can be helpful in reducing pain perception as well as in decreasing the risk for development of depression. The use of low-dose tricyclic antidepressants (e.g., nortriptyline or amitriptyline) can be effective. A randomized controlled trial found that low-dose amitriptyline did not significantly decrease arm pain compared with placebo among participants with RSI. However, low-dose amitriptyline did significantly improve arm function and well-being [21]. In addition, the antidepressant duloxetine that is indicated for treatment of fibromyalgia pain may be also be considered for treatment of pain associated with RSI. If signs of depression are present, appropriate comprehensive treatment and referral to a psychiatrist or psychologist may be indicated.

Rehabilitation

The rehabilitation of a patient with RSI is best achieved by a multidisciplinary approach with the physician overseeing the treatment plan and following the progress of the patient. A review of evidence-based management strategies suggests that biomedical treatment should not be ignored, but the psychosocial management approach appears to be more influential for occupational outcomes [22]. A referral to skilled physical and occupational therapy is essential [23]. Therapists may provide several therapeutic modalities (mentioned previously) to decrease pain and to facilitate an active stretching and strengthening program. The focus is not only on the affected limb but also on total body biomechanics and postural control at the workstation and at home. Progressive resistive exercise programs can be used, but worsening of pain symptoms with increasing exertion is often an issue. Progressive resistive exercises may have more benefit if they are introduced with small increments in resistance, allowing the patient to slowly adjust. This approach can improve participation of the patient and thus increase strength gains. Further physical conditioning with regimented aerobic training, catered to the patient's personal interests, and institution of a home exercise program may reduce pain, improve stress management, and increase work capacity. It is important to encourage physical activity as much as possible. General aerobic conditioning can be effective in encouraging a positive health perception.

Relaxation training may also be helpful for chronic, nonspecific regional arm pain [24]. Continued surveillance and treatment of mental health problems can be imperative in recovery. Cognitive-behavioral therapy techniques can be used to treat the maladaptive beliefs and misconceptions that may accompany upper extremity dysfunction [25]. Moreover, weight reduction, if needed, and smoking cessation should also be included in any plan to improve overall health.

Other rehabilitative measures for RSI include the fabrication of splints and the introduction of adaptive equipment that may assist in functional activities at home and in the workplace. Some therapists are specially trained to perform work site analysis and to suggest ergonomic modifications. Modifications can range from adjustment in chair height and computer mouse position to the substitution of large-handled tools, depending on the occupation. For computer users, it is generally recommended that chair height be such that the forearms are relatively horizontal to the floor and the wrists are in a neutral position. The volar aspect of the wrist can be supported during typing by a wrist support placed on the desktop or support tray in front of the keyboard. The keyboard should be located in a position directly in front of the typist, minimizing ulnar deviation of either wrist. The mouse should be placed close to midline. Split keyboards and those that provide a trackball can help with forearm and hand positioning. Voice-activated software is also available for those patients whose symptoms are refractory to these modifications [18]. Ergonomically designed computer touch pads, a foot-controlled mouse, and document holders are other tools that can help decrease symptoms in RSI.

There is limited evidence in published literature to confirm the usefulness of ergonomic interventions [26]. A systematic review by Goodman and colleagues [27] investigated the most effective interventions for upper extremity cumulative trauma disorders in computer users. The highest levels of evidence were found for education and training in ergonomics, forearm supports, ergonomic keyboards, ergonomic mice, and exercise and rest breaks. Most clinicians agree that such interventions are a worthwhile component of a comprehensive rehabilitation plan. Ergonomic interventions *may* make the workplace more comfortable, encouraging the patient to return to work and possibly preventing work disability [28]. Education about proper ergonomics should empower patients to make low-cost changes on their own at work and at home.

Many factors can limit the effectiveness of work hardening and work conditioning programs. Individuals who are having difficulty in returning to their previous level of work activity should be evaluated for alternative jobs. This can involve consideration of a new position with the current employer, if it is mutually agreed on. Job redesign that enriches career development opportunities may be effective. In fact, studies suggest that interventions aimed at altering workers' perceptions of monotonous or tedious work, through better job development opportunities, an increase of latitude over working patterns, and the improvement of communication between employers and employees, may be beneficial and cost-effective to the employer [29-31]. However, in some instances, an entirely different vocation must be pursued. If this is the case, a consultation with a vocational rehabilitation specialist is advised.

Procedures

Procedures are rarely indicated in RSI. In a population of patients with such a nondefinitive diagnosis, treatment failures are frequent. Therefore, trigger point injections, lateral epicondylar injections, carpal tunnel injections, and the like can be attempted to see if symptoms improve. The risk and benefits of each procedure should be explained in detail, including the risk of no relief of pain.

Surgery

Surgery is not indicated for RSI.

Potential Disease Complications

The most feared complication of RSI is increasing functional impairment and disability in all aspects of life. Negative outcomes can occur if the patient feels incapable of using his or her arms and hands. This may result in the inability to participate in home, work, and recreational activities. Depression and social isolation may accompany prolonged periods of absence from work.

Potential Treatment Complications

Treatment complications are rare. Most complications are associated with pain medication side effects. Analgesics and NSAIDs have well-known adverse reactions that most commonly affect the gastric, hepatic, and renal systems. Anticonvulsants can cause fatigue, ataxia, edema, or nausea. Tricyclic antidepressants have a high profile of fatigue, dizziness, dry mouth, and constipation. Patients should be informed of the side effect profile of each medication before administration. The patient's complete medication list should be reviewed to address potential adverse reactions between medications taken concurrently.

References

[1] Walker-Bone K, Cooper C. Hard work never hurt anyone—or did it? A review of occupational associations with soft tissue musculoskeletal disorders of the neck and upper limb. Ann Rheum Dis 2005;64:1112–7.

[2] Barr A, Barbe M, Clark B. Work-related musculoskeletal disorders of the hand and wrist: epidemiology, pathophysiology, and sensorimotor changes. J Orthop Sports Phys Ther 2004;34:610–27.

[3] Giang GM. Epidemiology of work-related upper extremity disorders: understanding prevalence and outcomes to impact provider performances using a practice management reporting tool. Clin Occup Environ Med 2006;5:267–83.

[4] Morse T, Dillon C, Kenta-Bibi E, et al. Trends in work-related musculoskeletal disorder reports by year, type, and industrial sector: a capture-recapture analysis. Am J Ind Med 2005;48:40–9.

[5] Lacerda E, Nacul L, Augusto L, et al. Prevalence and associations of symptoms of upper extremities, repetitive strain injuries (RSI) and "RSI-like condition." A cross-sectional study of bank workers in Northeast Brazil. BMC Public Health 2005;5:107–16.

[6] Ostlie K, Franklin R, Skjeldal O, et al. Musculoskeletal pain and overuse syndromes in adult acquired major upper-limb amputees. Arch Phys Med Rehabil 2011;92:1967–73.

[7] Mani L, Gerr F. Work-related upper extremity musculoskeletal disorders. Prim Care 2000;27:845–64.

[8] Barr A, Barbe M. Pathophysiological tissue changes associated with repetitive movement: a review of the evidence. Phys Ther 2002;82:173–87.

[9] Helliwell P, Taylor W. Repetitive strain injury. Postgrad Med J 2004;80:438–43.

[10] Larsson S, Bodegard L, Henriksson K, et al. Chronic trapezius myalgia: morphology and blood flow studied in 17 patients. Acta Orthop Scand 1990;61:394–8.

[11] Brunnekreef J, Oosterhof J, Thijssen D, et al. Forearm blood flow and oxygen consumption in patients with bilateral repetitive strain injury measured by near-infrared spectroscopy. Clin Physiol Funct Imaging 2006;26:178–84.

[12] Brunnekreef J, Benda N, Schreuder T, et al. Impaired endothelial function and blood flow in repetitive strain injury. Int J Sports Med 2012;33:835–41.

[13] Brunnekreef J, Thijssen D, Oosterhof J, et al. Bilateral changes in forearm oxygen consumption at rest and after exercise in patients with unilateral repetitive strain injury: a case-control study. J Orthop Sports Phys Ther 2012;42:371–8.

[14] Harding W. Worker's compensation litigation of the upper extremity claim. Clin Occup Environ Med 2006;5:483–90.

[15] Ring D, Kadzielski J, Fabian L, et al. Self-reported upper extremity health status correlates with depression. J Bone Joint Surg Am 2006;88:1983–8.

[16] Helliwell P, Bennett R, Littlejohn G, et al. Towards epidemiological criteria for soft-tissue disorders of the arm. Occup Med 2003;53:313–9.

[17] Ring D, Guss D, Malhotra L, et al. Idiopathic arm pain. J Bone Joint Surg Am 2004;86:1387–91.

[18] Foye P, Cianca J, Prathers H. Cumulative trauma disorders of the upper limb in computer users. Arch Phys Med Rehabil 2002;83:S12–5.

[19] Hassett R. The role of imaging of work-related upper extremity disorders. Clin Occup Environ Med 2006;5:285–98, vii.

[20] Baldwin M, Butler R. Upper extremity disorders in the workplace: costs and outcomes beyond the first return to work. J Occup Rehabil 2006;16:303–23.

[21] Goldman R, Stason W, Park S, et al. Low-dose amitriptyline for treatment of persistent arm pain due to repetitive use. Pain 2010;149:117–23.

[22] Burton A, Kendall N, Pearce B, et al. Management of work-relevant upper limb disorders: a review. Occup Med (Lond) 2009;59:44–52.

[23] Driver D. Occupational and physical therapy for work-related upper extremity disorders: how we can influence outcomes. Clin Occup Environ Med 2006;5:471–82, xi.

[24] Spence S, Sharpe L, Newton-John T, et al. Effect of EMG biofeedback compared to applied relaxation training with chronic, upper extremity cumulative trauma disorders. Pain 1995;63:199–206.

[25] Derebery J, Tullis W. Prevention of delayed recovery and disability of work-related upper extremity disorders. Clin Occup Environ Med 2006;5:235–47, vi.

[26] Verhagen A, Karels C, Bierma-Zeinstra S, et al. Ergonomic and physiotherapeutic interventions for treating work-related complaints of the arm, neck or shoulder in adults. Cochrane Database Syst Rev 2006;3: CD003471.

[27] Goodman G, Kovach L, Fisher A, et al. Effective interventions for cumulative trauma disorders of the upper extremity in computer users: practice models based on systematic review. Work 2012;42:153–72.

[28] Pearce B. Ergonomic considerations in work-related upper extremity disorders. Clin Occup Environ Med 2006;5:249–66, vi.

[29] Silverstein B, Clark R. Interventions to reduce work-related musculoskeletal disorders. J Electromyogr Kinesiol 2004;14:135–52.

[30] Colombini D, Occhipinti E. Preventing upper limb work-related musculoskeletal disorders (UL-WMSDs): new approaches in job (re)design and current trends in standardization. Appl Ergon 2006;37:441–50.

[31] Juul-Kristensen B, Jensen C. Self-reported workplace related ergonomic conditions as prognostic factors for musculoskeletal symptoms: the "BIT" follow up study on office workers. Occup Environ Med 2005;62:188–94.

CHAPTER 113

Temporomandibular Joint Dysfunction

Steven Scott, DO
Robert Kent, DO, MHA, MPH
Julie Martin, PT
Marissa McCarthy, MD
Jill Massengale, MS, ARNP
Tony Urbisci, BS

Synonyms

Temporomandibular joint dysfunction
Temporomandibular joint dysfunction syndrome
Temporomandibular disorder

ICD-9 Code

524.60 Unspecified temporomandibular joint disorder

ICD-10 Codes

M26.60 Temporomandibular joint disorder, unspecified
M26.29 Other specified disorders of temporomandibular joint

Definition

The temporomandibular joint (TMJ) is the synovial articulation between the mandible and the cranium. The TMJ is unusual in that the articular surfaces are covered by fibrous tissue rather than hyaline cartilage, as in most joints, and that it is divided into two joint spaces by an intra-articular disc. TMJ dysfunction (TMD) includes a collection of symptoms that refer to intrinsic and extrinsic TMJ conditions. These conditions are commonly referred to as TMJ, although they should more accurately be referred to as TMD to specify a difference between the joint itself and a true dysfunction. These symptoms include issues that cause pain or dysfunction relating to the TMJ itself as well as to the muscles of mastication. Because of the high number of issues that can be manifested in the facial and temporal area, a thorough history and physical examination are necessary to identify the true cause of pain in this area.

Studies report that approximately 28% of the population exhibits signs of TMD. Of those people suffering from symptoms, 14% had actual restricted range of motion of the mandible [1]. There is historically a predominance in women (5:1 versus men), and it occurs most often in patients between the ages of 15 and 45 years [2–4]. The most common cause of TMD is myofascial pain dysfunction of the muscles of mastication, and stress is often associated with this dysfunction [5–7]. This dysfunction can also be associated with macrotrauma, such as a motor vehicle accident, or microtrauma, such as teeth grinding and clenching at night. Identification of specific mechanical causes is important as well to correct issues that may be lending themselves to TMD. Examples of mechanical causes can be prolonged mouth or upper respiratory breathing, postural abnormalities, and sleeping prone with increased pressure on the TMJ. A third major cause of TMD is dental malalignment. No matter the physical cause, stress and psychosocial impact should always be considerations [5–7].

Within the TMJ, there is a biconcave cartilage disc that normally moves with the mandibular condyle in the fossa (Fig. 113.1). The TMJ is a modified hinge joint that has two separate periods and types of motion. In the initial third of opening, the joint moves in a rotational manner. In the latter two thirds of opening, the joint moves in both a rotational and translational motion, allowing increased range of motion. Muscles commonly involved with TMD are the temporalis, masseter, and internal and external pterygoids. The TMJ is innervated by branches of the mandibular nerve. Irritation to these nerves, muscle spasms, intra-articular disease, and myofascial irritation can cause symptoms related to TMD [8].

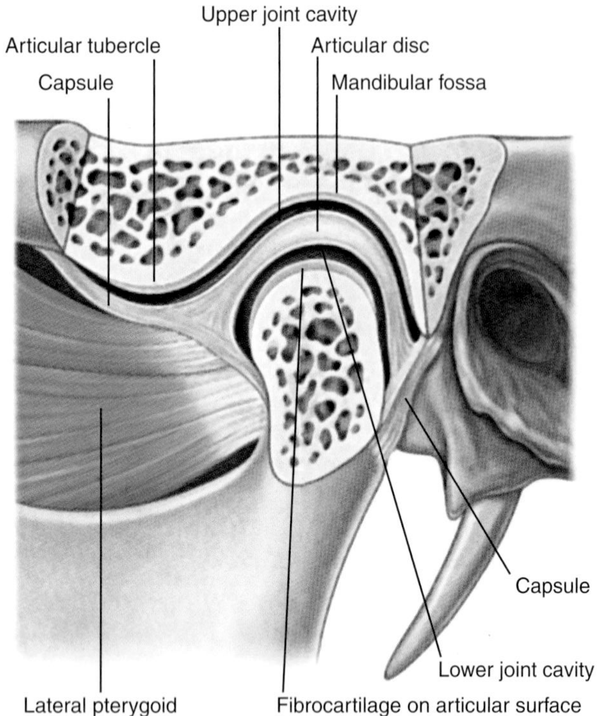

FIGURE 113.1 Anatomy of the temporomandibular joint. *(Image from http://www.usa.gov/Topics/Graphics.shtml.)*

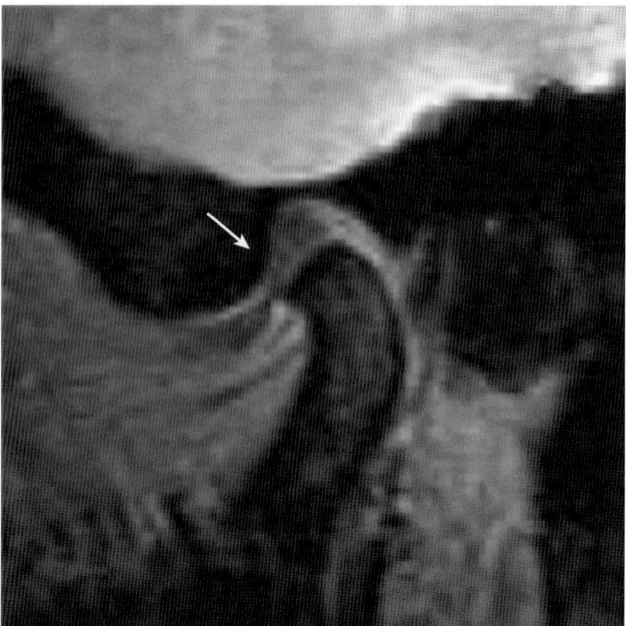

FIGURE 113.2 Magnetic resonance image of normal temporomandibular joint in closed position. The intra-articular disc is marked by the arrow. *(Image from http://www.usa.gov/Topics/Graphics.shtml.)*

Symptoms

Symptoms of TMD are varied and may at first seem unrelated. A common complaint with which patients may present is noise stemming from the TMJ, including crepitus, clicking, grinding, and popping. Pain at the level of the TMJ or surrounding areas also is a common complaint that may lead a patient to seek care from a health care provider. Whereas pain directly over the TMJ or mandible may lead patients to believe that they have a problem with the jaw, TMD can often be manifested as nontraditional headaches or upper cervical pain as well and is often made worse with chewing. Another common complaint in TMD is decreased range of motion of the jaw with "locking" of the joint in severe cases. Other symptoms, such as generalized facial pain, earaches, tinnitus, dysphagia, and even photosensitivity, have been reported with TMD [7,9].

Physical Examination

The diagnosis of TMD is made by observation of the range of motion of the mandible and palpation of the musculoskeletal structures of the face and head. It is essential to determine whether the patient has an intrinsic or extrinsic dysfunction of the TMJ. The translation can be felt by placing a finger over the TMJ just anterior to the tragus of the ear and asking the patient to open the mouth wide and repeat this motion. With palpation, the provider should identify whether the movement is smooth or if crepitus or joint dysfunction is noted. At maximal mouth opening, measure the opening in millimeters between the upper and lower incisal edges; the normal range is between 38 and 45 mm [10,11]. The average individual should have roughly three fingerbreadths between the teeth without any discomfort or pain. Monitoring of mandible opening for lateralization during opening can also suggest pathologic change. Have the patient also move the mandible left and right, noting restriction on one side versus the other or pain with this motion.

If the disc in the TMJ is displaced (Fig. 113.2) or if there are arthritic changes, clicking and crepitus can be heard or palpated as the disc clicks into its normal position with jaw opening. There will also be a click as the disc slips out of its normal position on closing. If the disc is fully displaced (anterior disc displacement with no reduction), there is no clicking and limited opening with an opening shift toward the locked side and no lateral movement toward the contralateral side. Full lateral and protrusive movements with limited openings might suggest muscle spasm versus disc displacement.

The provider gently palpates both masseters and temporalis muscles, insertion of the sternocleidomastoid muscle, and suboccipital area; any sensitivity should be noted. If the TMD symptoms are of new onset after trauma, a thorough cervical spine examination should be completed as well.

Functional Limitations

Pain may limit speaking and mastication. In patients with chronic pain, sleep and mood disorders may persist as well. Underlying psychosocial stress or depression that may be leading to TMD must also be identified as a possible hindrance of function [6].

Diagnostic Studies

Radiography can identify major arthritic changes, malalignments, or fractures but is not diagnostic if there are no abnormal findings. If it is available, panoramic oral radiography

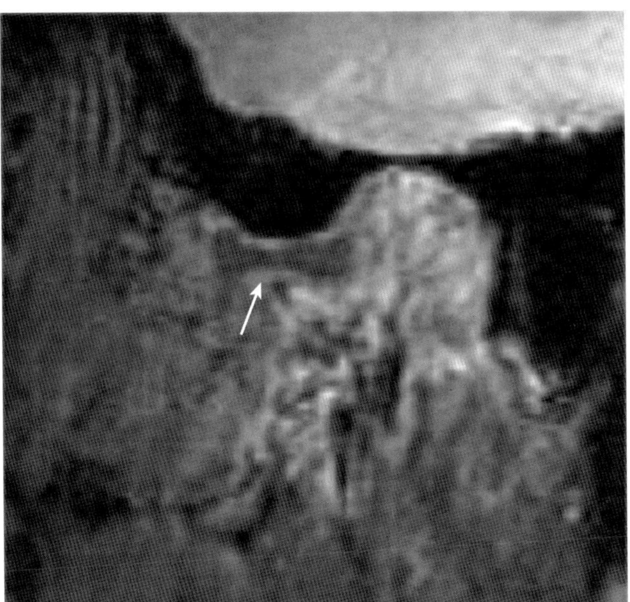

FIGURE 113.3 Medial displacement of the temporomandibular joint disc (*arrow*). *(Image from http://www.usa.gov/Topics/Graphics.shtml.)*

may be beneficial to visualize bilateral TMJs and alignment. Magnetic resonance imaging is necessary to visualize the disc and to provide definitive diagnosis of the disc position (Fig. 113.3), but it is not generally required for nonlocking joints that click [5,8].

Differential Diagnosis

Trauma to surrounding structures
Fractures
Tumors
Infected teeth or gums
Acute trismus or muscle spasm
Facial nerve injuries
Upper cervical whiplash injuries
Headaches
Parotid gland disease
Trigeminal neuralgia

Treatment

Initial

There are different philosophical approaches of dental clinicians managing TMD. Some dentists attempt to calm symptoms with oral appliances and have the patient discontinue the daytime appliance after the first few months. Others believe that permanent bite changes are necessary for long-term relief and will grind the bite surfaces of teeth to balance the irregular bite. If there is dental malalignment, an occlusal stabilizing appliance may prove beneficial.

Acute pain with full lateral mandibular excursive and protrusive movement is treated as an acute muscle spasm. Nonsteroidal anti-inflammatory medications, moist heat, and ice massage as well as eating of softer food during the acute period may decrease pain and ease the burden on the musculature [10]. If the pain does become chronic in nature, lasting more than 3 months, more attention should be paid to stress as a common cause, and medications that treat both pain and emotional stress, such as tricyclic antidepressants, should be considered [7].

Rehabilitation

Manual manipulation can be beneficial in treatment of TMD when the underlying dysfunction is myofascial or muscle spasm. For a unilateral muscle spasm causing TMD, the muscle energy technique takes the patient's mandible away from the restriction and into the barrier away from the direction of chin deviation, and the patient pushes back three times. After the third activation is completed by the patient, the provider should take the jaw laterally to the physiologic barrier. If a patient has bilateral muscle spasms, have the patient open the mouth against resistance and close the mouth against resistance, repeating each three times to attempt to release the TMJ complex. For more complex TMD cases in which there is some locking, an intraoral technique may be used. In this technique, the provider should put on gloves (with cotton or gauze wrapped around the thumbs). Start by placing the thumbs on the patient's lower molars and wrap the remaining fingers around the ramus of the mandible, pushing inferiorly and anteriorly until release is felt. This technique stretches bilateral muscle groups at the same time as well as allows myofascial release [11].

Jaw exercises and stretching of the muscles of mastication are paramount to treatment of acute TMD as well as to prevention of progression or recurrences. Following Rocabado's original research, main goals should focus on joint distraction, elimination of compression, restoration of physiologic articular rest, mobilization of soft tissues, and improvement in the condyle-disc-glenoid fossa relationship. A working example of this exercise is the placement of hands under the chin and opening downward with pressure against the hand for a few seconds at a time for six times, six times a day (classic six by six exercises), which may benefit the patient [12].

Stress reduction and biofeedback to decrease teeth grinding or clenching can be beneficial to help break acute spasms and to avoid progressive weakness or dysfunction.

Correction of posture also may be beneficial to patients suffering from TMD. Holding a posture with increased thoracic kyphosis and decreased cervical lordosis (forward leaning) can increase stress on the TMJ as well as lead to myofascial dysfunction. Other postural issues, such as postures or chronic dysfunction of the subcranial spine, most notably the occipitoatlantal joint, can contribute to TMJ pain. Correction of this posture with exercise and active therapy, such as chin tucks and scapular retraction, is recommended. Also, for patients who tend to sit in this head forward position, a lumbar roll or support while sitting may also be beneficial.

Along with the multiple modalities discussed, the patient should be counseled on avoidance of specific tasks that may exacerbate the symptoms or stress the jaw, such as yawning, singing, chewing gum, or resting the chin on a hard surface.

Procedures

For patients diagnosed with a myofascial cause of TMD, trigger point injections are a viable option to aid in release of the taut bands within these muscles. For recurrent myofascial cases, trigger point injections should be considered an adjunct to continuing therapy to correct the mechanical issues leading to repeated episodes. Intra-articular injections may be beneficial for patients with TMD that has not responded to more conservative treatments. Multiple injectants have been used in TMJ dysfunctions, including local anesthetic, steroids, and viscosupplementation [8,13]. Botulinum toxin has also demonstrated some efficacy in refractory cases and may be considered before surgical intervention [14].

Complementary medicine techniques can also be considered in approaching the treatment of a patient with TMD. For example, Chinese scalp acupuncture can play a role in management. This technique addresses the sensory area of the scalp for abnormal sensations of the face that are hypersensitive, including pain, tingling, and numbness. Treatment by scalp acupuncture has shown positive results in disorders with TMJ pain. Treatment of the lower two fifths of the sensory area focuses on the face, head, and TMJ pain, and it has proved to be a useful adjunct to current treatments [15].

Surgery

Although surgery is rarely needed, there are surgical procedures that may benefit patients with refractory TMD. If imaging demonstrates intra-articular bone or disc fragments, surgical removal is an option. For patients with refractory TMD not responding to less invasive treatment, shaving of the condyle has also been shown to be beneficial. A joint replacement is possible for the TMJ, allowing return to function (Fig. 113.4). This is more often used when there is significant ankylosis of the joint, which may be seen in patients with severe cases or with a neurogenic cause due to paralysis of the muscles of mastication.

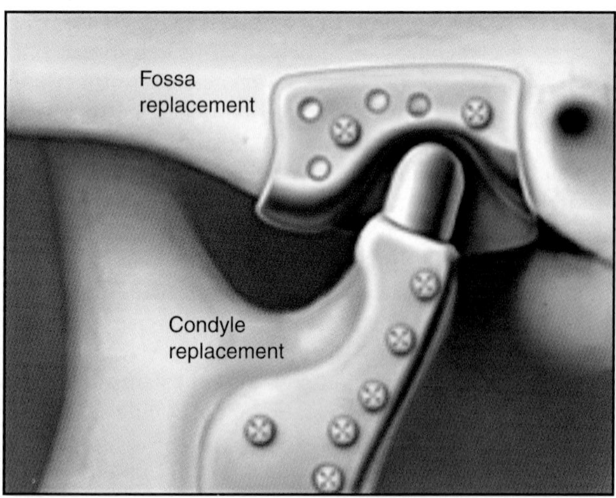

FIGURE 113.4 Temporomandibular joint replacement. *(Image from http://www.usa.gov/Topics/Graphics.shtml.)*

If the problem persists for several weeks or remains refractory to initial treatments and therapies, referral to a provider specializing in TMD may be warranted. When there is unilateral restricted translation of the TMJ and limited opening with a deviation or acute inability to close the mouth, called an open lock or subluxation, consultation with a TMD specialist with experience in unlocking these subluxations is recommended.

Potential Disease Complications

A potential complication is bruxism or rhythmic grinding of the teeth from other conditions, such as traumatic brain injury, especially at night. Trismus, or overactivity of the muscles of mastication, can restrict jaw mobility and be a severe functional problem. If there is anterior disc displacement without reduction, it can limit mouth opening on that side and cause significant pain if there is forced opening. Degenerative joint disease in the older population can affect the TMJ with increased symptoms of pain, tenderness, crepitus, and limitations of jaw movement. TMJ ankylosis may occur from rheumatoid arthritis or trauma, and surgery is often needed. Infections of the TMJ are rare, and there are usually local or systemic signs of inflammation. Finally, local TMD pain during several months can become a widespread chronic pain disorder affecting sleep and causing mood swings, depression, and anxiety.

Potential Treatment Complications

Oral appliances used 24 hours a day for many months may create a permanent bite change. When this occurs, the patient cannot bring his or her teeth fully together when clenching. If it is not properly managed, this may increase symptoms. Athletic mouth guards bought in stores and heated to conform to bite may aggravate TMD symptoms. Inherent risks in injection techniques include ecchymosis, bleeding, infection, and vascular or nerve damage. Medications used to treat TMD carry the same risk as they would for treatment of any pain condition as defined by each individual medication. Surgical interventions have risks similar to those of any open surgical procedure, and these should be discussed between the surgeon and the patient.

References

[1] Okeson J. Bell's orofacial pains. Chicago: Quintessence Publishing; 1995.
[2] Okeson J. Orofacial pain: guidelines for assessment, classification, and management. Carol Stream, Ill: Quintessence Publishing; 1996.
[3] Köhler AA. On temporomandibular disorders. Time trends, associated factors, treatment need and treatment outcome. Swed Dent J 2013;227:111–9.
[4] Schmid-Schwap M, Bristela M, Kundi M, Piehslinger E. Sex-specific differences in patients with temporomandibular disorders. J Orofac Pain 2013;27:42–50.
[5] Sharma S, Gupta DS, Pal US, Jurel SK. Etiological factors of temporomandibular joint disorders. Natl J Maxillofac Surg 2011;2:116–9.
[6] Resende CM, Alves AC, Coehlo LT, et al. Quality of life and general health in patients with temporomandibular disorders. Braz Oral Res March 2013;27:116–21.
[7] Pimentel MJ, Gui MS, Martins de Aquino LM, Rizzatti-Barbosa CM. Features of temporomandibular disorders in fibromyalgia syndrome. Cranio 2013;31:40–5.
[8] Warfield CA, Bajwa ZH. Principles and practice of pain medicine. 2nd ed. New York: McGraw-Hill; 2004.

[9] Kino K, Sugisaki M, Haketa T, et al. The comparison between pains, difficulties in function, and associating factors of patients in subtypes of temporomandibular disorders. J Oral Rehabil 2005;32:315–25.

[10] Travell JG, Simons DG. Myofascial pain and dysfunction: the trigger point manual. Baltimore: Williams & Wilkins; 1983.

[11] Nicholas AS, Nicholas EA. Atlas of osteopathic techniques. Philadelphia: Wolters Kluwer Health/Lippincott Williams & Wilkins; 2008.

[12] Deodato F, Christiano S, Truscendi R, Giorgetti R. A functional approach to TMJ disorders. Prog Orthod 2003;4:20–37.

[13] Waldman SD. Atlas of pain management injection techniques. 3rd ed. Philadelphia: Elsevier/Saunders; 2013.

[14] Persaud R, Garas G, Silva S, et al. An evidence-based review of botulinum toxin (Botox) applications in non-cosmetic head and neck conditions. JRSM Short Rep 2013;4:10.

[15] La Touche R, Goddard G, De-la-Hoz J, et al. Acupuncture in the treatment of pain in temporomandibular disorders: a systematic review and meta-analysis of randomized controlled trials. Clin J Pain 2010;26:541–50.

CHAPTER 114

Central Post-Stroke Pain (Thalamic Pain Syndrome)

Alice J. Hon, MD
Eric L. Altschuler, MD, PhD

Synonyms

Central post-stroke pain
Thalamic pain syndrome
Thalamic pain syndrome of Dejerine-Roussy
Central pain

ICD-9 Code

338.0 Central pain syndrome

ICD-10 Code

G89.0 Central pain syndrome

Definition

Central post-stroke pain (CPSP), formerly known as thalamic pain syndrome, is a chronic complex disabling pain syndrome characterized by pain and temperature sensation abnormalities after a cerebrovascular accident, infarct, or hemorrhage. It was first described, with pathophysiologic correlation to a lesion in the thalamus, in 1906 by Dejerine and Roussy as a "severe persistent, paroxysmal, often intolerant pain on the hemiplegic side, not yielding to analgesic treatment" [1]. There were previous descriptions of pain after a central lesion by Edinger [2] and others earlier in the 19th century.

The disease affects up to 8% of patients with stroke and, in one study, 9% of hemorrhagic stroke patients with thalamic lesions [3–5]. Pain onset in stroke patients occurs weeks to months after a cerebrovascular accident [5]. CPSP is considered a persistent central neuropathic pain that follows an ischemic or hemorrhagic stroke without a peripheral cause. Although the pathogenesis remains unclear, there appears to be involvement not only of the thalamus as initially studied by Dejerine but of the spinothalamic pathway because of the pain and temperature sensitivity [6,7]. Interestingly, not all patients with lesions along the spinothalamic pathway have CPSP [8,9]. Many CPSP patients have many lesions noted on magnetic resonance imaging that are unrelated to the pain [10].

Predictors as to those at risk are unclear, but in one study controls with thalamic stroke without thalamic pain had lesions mainly in the more anterolateral nuclei. Thalamic pain patients were noted to have lesions mainly in lateral and posterior thalamic nuclei on magnetic resonance imaging [11]. In one study at 16 months, patients with higher pain intensity were female [12].

Symptoms

CPSP is characterized by mild hemiplegia, hemihypoesthesia, hyperpathia with burning sensation, hemiataxia, astereognosis, dyskinesias (especially choreoathetosis), and positive or negative pain sensations that occur for hours to continuously in the entire half the body, arm, leg, foot, or hand [13,14]. Patients describe pain sensations as burning, cold, stabbing, sharp, aching, pricking, squeezing, shooting, tingling, or heavy when they are exposed to changes in temperature measured by a thermal probe, monofilament for tactile stimuli, and brushing with a stiff brush typically used for oil painting [15]. Particularly excruciating are the sensory abnormalities, especially the thermal sensations that can include burning, scalding, or burning and freezing in addition to other vague descriptions of positive and negative sensory abnormalities. Symptoms can be constant or intermittent, described as burning by some CPSP patients, and triggered by touching of an item, being touched, or changes in temperature [14]. Because of the variable onset and symptom constellation, patients are often misdiagnosed [16].

Physical Examination

It is important in considering the diagnosis of CPSP to perform a thorough musculoskeletal and neurologic physical examination to rule out other causes of pain. Physical findings in patients with CPSP may include mild or more severe hemiplegia, hyperesthesia, or hypoesthesia. Patients may have impaired pinprick, temperature, and touch sensation, whereas vibration and joint proprioception are less commonly affected [10].

In a prospective study of 207 stroke patients, 87 subjects (16 with CPSP and 71 with no pain) with abnormal sensation were observed. The CPSP group was noted to have more abnormal sensibility to cold and warm stimuli compared with nonpain subjects with abnormal sensation. The 16 CPSP patients had evoked dysesthesia or allodynia (sensation of pain by stimuli that are usually nonpainful) [5].

Functional Limitations

Strokes that cause CPSP are typically associated with only mild hemiplegia, though some patients can have moderate or severe hemiplegia and the functional limitations that accompany these. The pain of CPSP can often be a much more severe cause of functional limitation, at times to the point of being incapacitating.

Diagnostic Studies

Brain imaging of patients with CPSP will typically show a lesion in the spinothalamic pathway, but not all patients with such lesions will have CPSP [8,9].

Differential Diagnosis

Peripheral neuropathy
Traumatic brain injury
Syringomyelia
Multiple sclerosis
Complex regional pain syndrome
Shoulder disease (frozen shoulder, rotator cuff disease)
Deep venous thrombosis

Treatment

Initial

Historically, CPSP has been resistant to both medical and surgical management. Despite the severe impact on quality of life for patients with CPSP, there is limited scientific evidence of its treatment [17].

The only medications that have shown pain reduction in a randomized controlled trial are amitriptyline (at least 75 mg daily) [18], lamotrigine (at least 200 mg daily) [19], and gabapentin [20]. Thus, these medicines are considered first-line management for CPSP. Unfortunately, even with these medicines, only mild pain relief was achieved, and many patients did not respond at all. Other medicines that have been found to have some benefit in open trials, such as nortriptyline, desipramine, imipramine, doxepin, venlafaxine, maprotiline, gabapentin, pregabalin, carbamazepine, mexiletine, fluvoxamine, and phenytoin, are considered second-line treatment [10,17–19,21–28].

For patients resistant to treatment, opioids (such as levorphanol, studied in a double-blind randomized controlled study) have been used, resulting in some pain reduction in a small group but not in a large population [29]. In one study, intravenous morphine showed a modest short-term benefit in some patients [30]. Long-term benzodiazepines are not recommended because of potentiation of inhibitory effects of γ-aminobutyric acid, but there is a possible role of short-term use in CPSP patients with anxiety [13]. Intravenous administration of the γ-aminobutyric acid agonist thiopental, intravenous propofol, and intrathecal baclofen alleviated some pain in patients with CPSP [31–33], but oral doses of baclofen and amobarbital were ineffective [33,34].

Rehabilitation

Rehabilitation begins with management of the various deficits resulting from the stroke. Barriers to treatment include cogitative and communication limitations due to the cerebrovascular event [16].

To date, CPSP has been difficult to treat with medical or surgical interventions [16]. The pain in CPSP is a "false" signal being generated by the brain. Pain can be a useful symptom indicating an injury, but in CPSP there is no corporeal injury. It would be ideal if some method could be found to "connect to" and retrain the thalamus or other brain areas to the fact that there is no injury, so there should be no pain. For movement problems after stroke, mirror therapy [35], in which visual feedback from the reflection of the good limb helps regularize the motor control loop, can be beneficial [36]. This approach does not work for CPSP (even in patients with CPSP and hemiparesis after stroke for whom mirror therapy helped the hemiparesis), nor should one expect it to because the problem is sensory pain, not a movement difficulty.

Procedures

There has been one case report finding acupuncture helpful in CPSP [37]. Acupuncture, perhaps by sensory stimulation, may be a way to "reconnect" with and retrain the thalamus or associated structures. Further studies of acupuncture for CPSP are warranted.

Surgery

When all other modalities have failed, deep brain stimulation has been tried in a couple of cases. For example, one male patient had some improvement in pain at 6-month follow-up [38]; another male patient with deep brain stimulation by an electrode implanted in his periventricular gray region had pain relief lasting 4 months [39].

Neurosurgical destructive options include medial thalamotomy and mesencephalic tractotomy, which in limited cases of patients with central and deafferentation pain improved the allodynia and hyperpathia, but with less promising outcome for the burning or dysesthetic pain [40]. As ablation is considered the final resort, more conservative measures, including deep brain stimulation, should be tried.

Potential Disease Complications

Disease complications include severe pain and its typical sequelae that affect the quality of life of the individual with CPSP. Because of the physical and psychological effects of central pain, work and social life are often affected, requiring different cognitive and behavioral techniques to cope [41]. In one study, 27 patients with CPSP reported pain to be a great burden, and most rated the intensity as high, interfering more with leisure activities compared with brainstem lesions [42]. Problem-centered coping with focus on external or environmental etiology is used more often by men, whereas emotion-centered coping is more often used by women. For example, women in one group were noted to use spiritual and religious activities as coping strategies more often than men did [41].

Potential Treatment Complications

Treatment complications include adverse effects of the medications or surgical procedure and vary by the medication or surgery implemented. It is important to consider and to minimize drug interactions in patients, especially those who are taking multiple medications as these patients often are.

References

[1] Dejerine J, Roussy G. Le syndrome thalamique. Rev Neurol (Paris) 1906;14:521–32.
[2] Edinger L. Giebt es central antstehender schmerzen? Dtsch Z Nervenheilkd 1891;1:262–82.
[3] Schott GD. From thalamic syndrome to central poststroke pain. J Neurol Neurosurg Psychiatry 1996;61:560–4.
[4] Kumral E, Kocaer T, Ertubey NO, Kumral K. Thalamic hemorrhage. A prospective study of 100 patients. Stroke 1995;26:964–70.
[5] Andersen G, Vestergaard K, Ingeman-Nielsen M, Jensen TS. Incidence of central post-stroke pain. Pain 1995;61:187–93.
[6] Bowsher D, Leijon G, Thuomas KA. Central poststroke pain: correlation of MRI with clinical pain characteristics and sensory abnormalities. Neurology 1998;51:1352–8.
[7] Boivie J, Leijon G, Johansson I. Central post-stroke pain—a study of the mechanisms through analyses of the sensory abnormalities. Pain 1989;37:173–85.
[8] Vestergaard K, Nielsen J, Andersen G, et al. Sensory abnormalities in consecutive, unselected patients with central post-stroke pain. Pain 1995;61:177–86.
[9] Bogousslavsky J, Regli F, Uske A. Thalamic infarcts: clinical syndromes, etiology, and prognosis. Neurology 1988;38:837–48.
[10] Kumar B, Kalita J, Kumar G, Misra UK. Central poststroke pain: a review of pathophysiology and treatment. Anesth Analg 2009;108:1645–57.
[11] Sprenger T, Seifert CL, Valet M, et al. Assessing the risk of central post-stroke pain of thalamic origin by lesion mapping. Brain 2012;135(Pt 8):2536–45.
[12] Jonsson AC, Lindgren I, Hallstrom B, et al. Prevalence and intensity of pain after stroke: a population based study focusing on patients' perspectives. J Neurol Neurosurg Psychiatry 2006;77:590–5.
[13] Segatore M. Understanding central post-stroke pain. J Neurosci Nurs 1996;28:28–35.
[14] Widar M, Ek AC, Ahlstrom G. Coping with long-term pain after a stroke. J Pain Symptom Manage 2004;27:215–25.
[15] Greenspan JD, Ohara S, Sarlani E, Lenz FA. Allodynia in patients with post-stroke central pain (CPSP) studied by statistical quantitative sensory testing within individuals. Pain 2004;109:357–66.
[16] Henry JL, Lalloo C, Yashpal K. Central poststroke pain: an abstruse outcome. Pain Res Manag 2008;13:41–9.
[17] Frese A, Husstedt IW, Ringelstein EB, Evers S. Pharmacologic treatment of central post-stroke pain. Clin J Pain 2006;22:252–60.
[18] Leijon G, Boivie J. Central post-stroke pain—a controlled trial of amitriptyline and carbamazepine. Pain 1989;36:27–36.
[19] Vestergaard K, Andersen G, Gottrup H, et al. Lamotrigine for central poststroke pain: a randomized controlled trial. Neurology 2001;56:184–90.
[20] Serpell MG. Gabapentin in neuropathic pain syndromes: a randomised, double-blind, placebo-controlled trial. Pain 2002;99:557–66.
[21] Lampl C, Yazdi K, Roper C. Amitriptyline in the prophylaxis of central poststroke pain. Preliminary results of 39 patients in a placebo-controlled, long-term study. Stroke 2002;33:3030–2.
[22] McQuay HJ, Tramer M, Nye BA, et al. A systematic review of antidepressants in neuropathic pain. Pain 1996;68:217–27.
[23] Bowsher D. The management of central post-stroke pain. Postgrad Med J 1995;71:598–604.
[24] Gonzales GR. Central pain: diagnosis and treatment strategies. Neurology 1995;45(Suppl. 9):S11–6, discussion S35–S36.
[25] Sumpton JE, Moulin DE. Treatment of neuropathic pain with venlafaxine. Ann Pharmacother 2001;35:557–9.
[26] Canavero S, Bonicalzi V. Lamotrigine control of central pain. Pain 1996;68:179–81.
[27] Awerbuch GI, Sandyk R. Mexiletine for thalamic pain syndrome. Int J Neurosci 1990;55:129–33.
[28] Agnew DC, Goldberg VD. A brief trial of phenytoin therapy for thalamic pain. Bull Los Angeles Neurol Soc 1976;41:9–12.
[29] Rowbotham MC, Twilling L, Davies PS, et al. Oral opioid therapy for chronic peripheral and central neuropathic pain. N Engl J Med 2003;348:1223–32.
[30] Attal N, Guirimand F, Brasseur L, et al. Effects of IV morphine in central pain: a randomized placebo-controlled study. Neurology 2002;58:554–63.
[31] Yamamoto T, Katayama Y, Hirayama T, Tsubokawa T. Pharmacological classification of central post-stroke pain: comparison with the results of chronic motor cortex stimulation therapy. Pain 1997;72:5–12.
[32] Canavero S, Bonicalzi V, Pagni CA, et al. Propofol analgesia in central pain: preliminary clinical observations. J Neurol 1995;242:561–7.
[33] Taira T, Tanikawa T, Kawamura H, et al. Spinal intrathecal baclofen suppresses central pain after a stroke. J Neurol Neurosurg Psychiatry 1994;57:381–2.
[34] Koyama T, Arakawa Y, Shibata M, et al. Effect of barbiturate on central pain: difference between intravenous administration and oral administration. Clin J Pain 1998;14:86–8.
[35] Ramachandran VS, Rogers-Ramachandran D, Cobb S. Touching the phantom limb. Nature 1995;377:489–90.
[36] Ramachandran VS, Altschuler EL. The use of visual feedback, in particular mirror visual feedback, in restoring brain function. Brain 2009;132(Pt 7):1693–710.
[37] Yen HL, Chan W. An East-West approach to the management of central post-stroke pain. Cerebrovasc Dis 2003;16:27–30.
[38] Alves RV, Asfora WT. Deep brain stimulation for Dejerine-Roussy syndrome: case report. Minim Invasive Neurosurg 2011;54:183–6.
[39] Pickering AE, Thornton SR, Love-Jones SJ, et al. Analgesia in conjunction with normalisation of thermal sensation following deep brain stimulation for central post-stroke pain. Pain 2009;147:299–304.
[40] Tasker RR. Thalamotomy. Neurosurg Clin N Am 1990;1:841–64.
[41] Nogueira M, Teixeira MJ. Central pain due to stroke: cognitive representation and coping according to gender. Arq Neuropsiquiatr 2012;70:125–8.
[42] Leijon G, Boivie J, Johansson I. Central post-stroke pain—neurological symptoms and pain characteristics. Pain 1989;36:13–25.

CHAPTER 115

Thoracic Outlet Syndrome

Karl-August Lindgren, MD, PhD

Synonyms

Cervical rib syndrome
Costoclavicular syndrome
Scalenus anticus syndrome

ICD-9 Code

353.0 Thoracic outlet syndrome

ICD-10 Code

G54.0 Thoracic outlet syndrome

Definition

Thoracic outlet syndrome is a symptom complex caused by compression or irritation of the neurovascular structures as they leave the thoracic cage through its narrow outlet. The thoracic outlet contains many structures in a confined space. The base of the thoracic outlet is formed by the first rib and the fascia of Sibson, which is attached to the transverse process of the seventh cervical vertebra, the pleura, and the first rib. The outlet is bounded superiorly by the subclavius muscle and the clavicle, anteriorly by the anterior scalene muscle, and posteriorly by the middle scalene muscle. The brachial plexus and the subclavian artery pass over the first rib between the anterior and middle scalene muscles (Fig. 115.1).

Neurovascular compression occurs most frequently at three levels:

- in the superior thoracic outlet, bordered posteriorly by the spine, anteriorly by the manubrium, and laterally by the first rib;
- in the costoscalene hiatus, bordered anteriorly by the anterior scalene muscle, posteriorly by the middle scalene muscle, and caudally by the first rib; and
- in the costoclavicular passage, bordered laterally by the clavicle, posteriorly by the scapula, and medially by the first rib.

The clinical symptoms of thoracic outlet syndrome are divided into categories according to the structures under pressure. True neurologic thoracic outlet syndrome is often caused by the distal C8-T1 roots or proximal fibers of the lower trunk of the plexus being stretched over a taut congenital band extending from the tip of a rudimentary cervical rib to the first rib. The most common form of thoracic outlet syndrome is the disputed neurologic thoracic outlet syndrome. The term *disputed* has been chosen because so many of the basic tenets of this syndrome are in dispute. Symptoms caused by pure venous compression (venous thoracic outlet syndrome) occur in 1.5% of patients and are manifested as axillary-subclavian vein thrombosis, usually in young patients engaged in vigorous physical activity that emphasizes upper limb and shoulder motion (such as cricket, tennis, and baseball). Arterial thoracic outlet syndrome is very rare and may be suspected if the patient presents with claudication of the arm, coldness, and ischemia of a finger or a hand. Individuals who have congenital bone or fibromuscular variations at these spaces and experience trauma are at risk for development of thoracic outlet syndrome. Anatomic variations and anomalies probably play a secondary role in the etiology. Congenital bands and ligaments are observed in a large majority of patients with thoracic outlet syndrome, and nine different types have been recognized [1]. In a human cadaver study, only 10% had a bilaterally normal anatomy. Anatomic anomalies of the thoracic-cervical-axillary region were found in 60% of human fetuses [2]. It is suggested that anatomic abnormalities confer a predisposition to symptoms of thoracic outlet syndrome after stress or injury [3]. Variation in the course of the brachial plexus that may predispose to symptoms of thoracic outlet syndrome has also been presented. Cervical ribs are regarded as predisposing factors, and a prevalence of cervical ribs was found to be 2.21% in a London population [4]. However, cervical ribs are present since birth. In 80% of patients with cervical ribs, symptoms did not develop until after a neck injury. Post-traumatic thoracic outlet syndrome has been presented in several articles [5–7].

According to Roos [1], anomalies are always the reason behind symptoms of thoracic outlet syndrome. However, only a few other surgeons have observed such anomalies. In the case of the first rib, the costovertebral and costotransverse joints allow a fair amount of rotation to take place along the long axis of the rib. Moreover, this rib has attached to it the anterior and middle scalene muscles, which act either

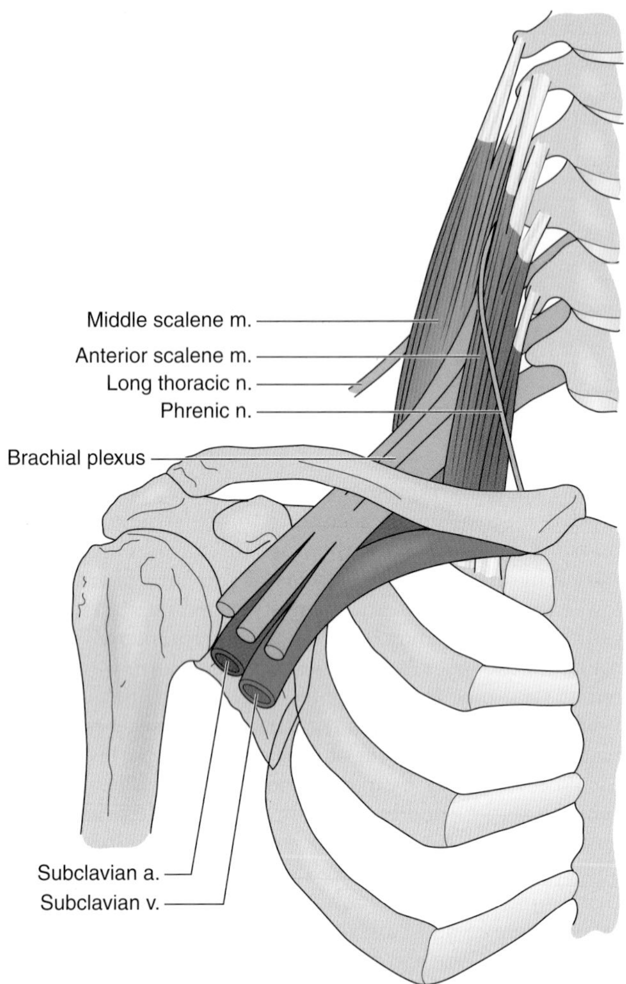

FIGURE 115.1 Anatomy of the thoracic outlet area. *(Reprinted from the Christine M. Kleinert Institute for Hand and Microsurgery, Inc.)*

by raising the thorax or by flexing and rotating the cervical part of the spine. In consequence, this first rib bears more stresses and strains than any of the other ribs, and these are greatest at the costotransverse joint [8]. Osteoarthritic changes are found more frequently in the costotransverse joint of the first rib. The lack of a superior supporting ligament may explain why this joint of the first rib is relatively weaker than those of the other ribs [8].

The elevation of the ribs during inspiration increases the anteroposterior diameter of the upper thorax. The range of this motion is reduced in older people. A disturbance of the function of the upper thoracic aperture will predispose to thoracic outlet syndrome symptoms. A dysfunction of the first rib at the costotransverse joint causes a restricted movement of the first rib [9]. In patients with thoracic outlet syndrome, the C8 and T1 nerve roots are most commonly affected. These roots constitute the part of the brachial plexus closest to the costotransverse joint. The stellate ganglion is located in the immediate vicinity of the first costotransverse joint and has numerous connections to the C8 and T1 roots. Minimal trauma associated with static, repetitive work, especially in young women, can cause abnormal stress on the upper aperture, and the poorly stabilized first rib can subluxate at the costotransverse joint. A subluxation at the first costotransverse joint could irritate

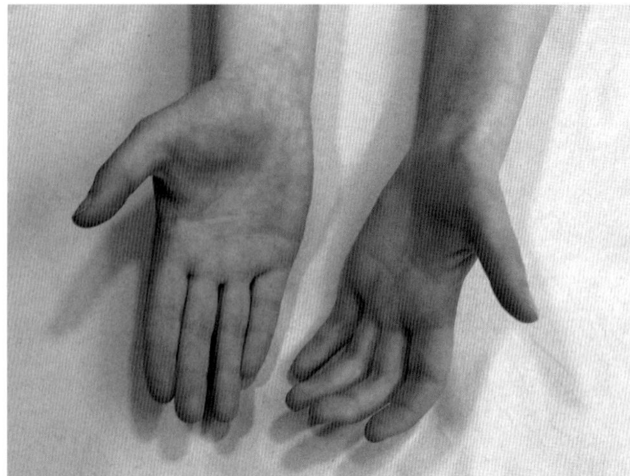

FIGURE 115.2 The hands of a patient with true neurologic thoracic outlet syndrome. Wasting of the muscles is clearly shown in the left hand.

the nerve roots C8 and T1 emerging in front of this joint. This irritation could explain the predominantly subjective pain and sensory loss in the ulnar distribution. The weakness of the hand and the various symptoms resembling complex regional pain syndrome may be explained by the irritation of the stellate ganglion.

Symptoms

True neurologic thoracic outlet syndrome is manifested with a long history of sensory symptoms, mainly along the medial forearm, associated with hand weakness and wasting, particularly of the thenar muscles (Fig. 115.2). In the upper plexus type presented by Roos [1], pain is felt over the brachial plexus radiating from the ear, through the anterior cervical region, over the clavicle into the upper part of the chest, posteriorly into the rhomboid and scapular areas, across the trapezius, and down the outer arm into the radial aspect of the forearm in a C5-C6 distribution. In the lower plexus type, pain is felt in the supraclavicular and infraclavicular fossae, radiating into the upper part of the back and from the axilla down the inner arm along the ulnar nerve distribution.

In contrast, disputed neurologic thoracic outlet syndrome possesses none of these characteristics. The most common symptoms are pain and paresthesias in an ulnar distribution and numbness, tingling, weakness, or dysfunction of the hand. The list of symptoms attributed to disputed neurologic thoracic outlet syndrome is long. These patients are often told by their physicians that their symptoms are exaggerated or that their complaints are not real. Coldness, easy fatigability, ischemia of a finger or a hand, and pallor on elevation are considered to be symptoms of arterial origin. Swelling, discoloration, and a heavy feeling in the hand are considered to be symptoms of venous origin. Swelling, hyperesthesia, discoloration, and a feeling of alternate cold and warm could also be signs of complex regional pain syndrome. Traction on the stellate ganglion has also been considered a possible cause of pain in these patients [8]. In general, in the absence of peripheral emboli, most "vascular symptoms" or "Raynaud phenomena" probably result from irritation of the sympathetic nerves rather than from compression of the subclavian artery in the thoracic outlet. A common feature of the symptoms is their intermittence and provocation by use of the arm above shoulder level. Aggravation of the symptoms often occurs after rather than during exercise.

Physical Examination

The diagnosis of thoracic outlet syndrome is a clinical one based on a detailed history and physical examination. This takes time and effort. Years of inappropriate diagnosis and ineffective therapy take a heavy toll on these patients. In the physical examination, the individual as a whole must be taken into consideration. One must remember that many of these patients have some psychological complaints. A thorough clinical examination including a logical explanation for the symptoms will often relieve the psychic burden.

The physical examination starts with an inspection of the neck, shoulders, and upper extremities. Color, muscle atrophy, edema, temperature, and nails are examined. This examination requires the patient to be examined with the shirt off. The cervical spine is then examined to exclude symptoms of cervical origin caused by a cervical disc or spondylarthrotic intervertebral foramen. A typical pain radiculation in C5 to C8 distribution indicates that a nerve root irritation is present. A local distribution of pain with neck extension indicates a facet joint problem.

A neurologic examination is performed to include sensory testing, muscle strength testing (C5-C8), and reflexes. Tinel sign is tested to exclude carpal tunnel syndrome. Palpation of the median, ulnar, and radial nerves from the axilla to the hand may reveal tenderness. This tenderness will vanish if a successful therapy is administered [10].

Almost all clinical tests used in the examination of the patient with thoracic outlet syndrome aim to provoke the symptoms felt by the patient, presuming that the compressing structure may be provoked to irritate the neurovascular bundle in the area of the thoracic outlet during the test. These maneuvers are unreliable in general [11]. A clinical test in extensive use is the Adson test [12]. With the patient sitting, hands resting on the thighs, both radial pulses are simultaneously palpated. During forced inspiration, hyperextension of the neck, and turning of the head to the affected side, the radial pulse is palpated for obliteration, and auscultation is done for supraclavicular bruit. The test has changed during the years. In 1927, when Adson described his test, the vascular changes were considered to be pathognomonic of thoracic outlet syndrome. Later, neurologic changes occurred more frequently than vascular ones, and these can be detected better when the head is rotated to the contralateral rather than the ipsilateral side, as initially described.

Radial pulse obliteration or subclavian bruit is found in 69% of normal patients [13]. All studies clearly indicate that pulse obliteration with the arm and head in various positions is a normal finding and has no relation to thoracic outlet syndrome.

In the hyperabduction test, symptoms are reproduced by hyperabduction of the arm. However, more than 80% of normal individuals experience obliteration of the radial pulse during this test [14]. In the exaggerated military maneuver, also called Eden test, symptoms are reproduced by pulling back the acromioclavicular joint in an exaggerated military "attention" position. The neurovascular structures could be compressed between the first rib and the clavicle, without any anatomic predisposing factors. This maneuver is also referred to as the costoclavicular test. Arterial compression is found in 60% of asymptomatic individuals by this test.

In the abduction–external rotation test, also called Roos test or elevated arm stress test (EAST), the hands are in the "stick up" position and are then repeatedly opened and closed for 3 minutes. Roos [1] considered the symptoms to be due to both arterial and brachial plexus compression and referred to this procedure as a claudication test; he was later convinced that thoracic outlet syndrome was neurologic rather than vascular in origin but claimed that the EAST procedure was the most reliable procedure. Roos has also claimed that the EAST procedure has great specificity, with a positive result in thoracic outlet syndrome but generally negative results in carpal tunnel syndrome and cervical radiculopathy. However, in a controlled study, it was found that the EAST procedure is an excellent test for carpal tunnel syndrome; the result is positive in 92% of patients with carpal tunnel syndrome and in 74% of normal controls [15]. Positional compression during all of these tests is a common phenomenon in normal subjects, and diminishing of the pulse in Adson test, the costoclavicular maneuver, and the hyperabduction test is considered to be a normal finding rather than a pathologic one. None of these tests unequivocally establishes the presence or absence of thoracic outlet syndrome. Ribbe and colleagues [16] used a "thoracic outlet syndrome index" to establish the diagnosis of thoracic outlet syndrome. According to these authors, a patient with thoracic outlet syndrome should have at least three of the following four symptoms or signs:

1. A history of aggravation of symptoms with the arm in the elevated position
2. A history of paresthesia in the segments C8-T1
3. Tenderness over the brachial plexus supraclavicularly
4. A positive "hands-up" (abduction–external rotation) test result

Because all of these provocative maneuvers are unreliable, one should examine the function of the thoracic upper aperture. The function of the upper thoracic aperture should be analyzed with the cervical rotation–lateral flexion test [17]. The test is carried out as follows. The neutrally positioned cervical spine is first passively and maximally rotated away from the side being examined and then, in this position, gently flexed as far as possible, moving the ear toward the chest. This is done in both directions. A restriction blocking the lateral flexion part of the movement indicates a positive test result; a free movement indicates a negative test result (Fig. 115.3). This test indicates an abnormal function of the upper thoracic aperture. The test is indicative of a subluxation of the first rib at the costotransverse joint. The test has been used to identify patients who did not gain from surgery [18] as well as in a 2-year follow-up study after conservative treatment [10].

In the surgery series [18], it was hypothesized that the remaining stump of the first rib was subluxated and that is why the symptoms persisted after surgery. The importance of the length of the remaining stump has also been stressed

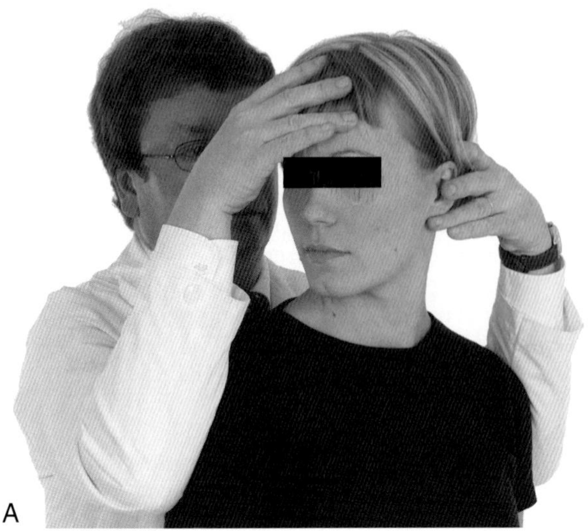

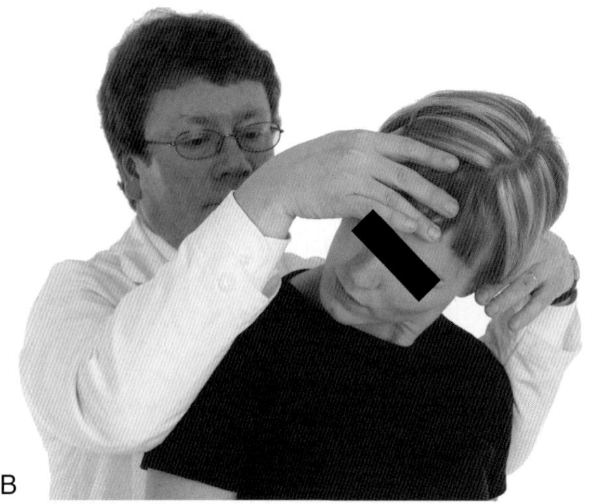

FIGURE 115.3 The performance of the cervical rotation–lateral flexion test. **A,** The head is rotated away from the side to be examined. **B,** In this position, the neck is tilted forward, bringing the ear toward the chest. If this movement is restricted, the test result is considered positive and is indicative of a malfunction of the first rib. A normal free movement indicates a negative test result. *(Reproduced with permission of Kustannus Oy Duodecim.)*

by other authors [19,20]. It is mandatory to analyze the function of the upper thoracic aperture and not rely only on provocative maneuvers that may lead to unnecessary surgical interventions.

Functional Limitations

The patients with symptoms of thoracic outlet syndrome have difficulty in working over the horizontal level, such as cleaning windows and putting up draperies. Static work, such as working with a keyboard, may be difficult because of paresthesias and difficulty in controlling the movements of the arm. Many patients cannot "rely" on the hand. Sleep is disturbed because of pain and tingling after exertion during the day.

Diagnostic Studies

Radiologic examination in the thoracic outlet syndrome can detect cervical ribs, bone anomalies of the first or second ribs, tumors, or the "droopy shoulder" syndrome. The incidence of arterial compression of clinical significance is extremely low, and arteriography should not be used in the diagnosis of thoracic outlet syndrome, except in patients with signs of pronounced compression or ischemia. Arterial compression inside the thoracic outlet can be detected with Doppler ultrasonography.

Magnetic resonance imaging has been used to detect anomalies, but these may not correlate with symptoms [21]. Functional magnetic resonance imaging may show a smaller distance between the first rib and the clavicle, but the significance remains to be shown. A cineradiographic study can detect abnormal movement of the structures of the upper aperture, but this can be detected with clinical tests [17].

Somatosensory evoked potentials can document the neurocompressive component of thoracic outlet syndrome and provide an objective assessment. The theory of the "double crush" syndrome suggests that nerve compression at one level makes the whole nerve more vulnerable to compression injury at another level. Symptoms after an unsuccessful carpal tunnel operation disappeared after a first rib excision [22]. The double crush phenomenon should be taken into account and neurophysiologic examination should be performed to exclude more distal sites of nerve compression than the thoracic outlet, such as nerve entrapment in the carpal tunnel.

Differential Diagnosis

Radiculopathy
Multiple sclerosis
Syringomyelia
Glenohumeral instability
Tumors of the cervical spine
Pancoast tumor
Myofascial pain syndrome in the cervical region
Trapezius strain

Treatment

Initial

After the thorough clinical examination and detailed history (including the question, "Have you had a trauma to your neck region?") [5,6,23], what the examining physician suspects to be the origin of the symptoms must be explained to the patient. Good pain management, not only using pain medications but also taking into account sleeping hygiene, is important. A multiprofessional team [24] should be consulted so that all therapy modalities are taken into account. This includes physiatrists, physiotherapists, occupational therapists, social workers, and psychologists; also, there must be a possibility to consult specialists in neurology and psychiatry, thoracic surgeons, and neurosurgeons.

Rehabilitation

The outcome of conservative therapy varies among different studies. Sällström and Celegin's program [25] brought relief to 83% of patients with mild symptoms but only 9% of those with severe symptoms. Even a success rate of 100% has been reported (a supervised physiotherapy program of graduated resisted shoulder elevation exercises in eight patients). Almost all authors have emphasized exercises to improve patients' posture as well as strengthening exercises of the shoulder girdle. However, it is difficult to compare the different studies because the diagnostic criteria are seldom mentioned, the severity of the symptoms varies, and rarely is the type of therapy described.

Procedures

During the last 25 years, I have recommended and used a multidisciplinary approach [10]. The therapy itself starts with shoulder exercises, the purpose of which is to restore the movement of the whole shoulder girdle and to provide more space for the neurovascular structures. Restoration of the movement and function of the cervical spine follows. The exercises that aim to activate the anterior, middle, and posterior scalene muscles are the most important part (Fig. 115.4). These exercises have been shown to correct any malfunction of the first ribs, thus normalizing the function of the upper thoracic aperture [26] and enabling normal movement of the first ribs. Stretching of the muscles of the shoulder girdle involves the upper part of the trapezius muscles, the sternocleidomastoid muscles, the levator scapulae, and the small pectoral muscle. The role of the small pectoral muscle has been emphasized elsewhere [27]. Further stretching exercises should be administered as needed, depending on the clinical findings in the individual case. Strengthening exercises for the anterior serratus muscle should be included, thus enhancing the stability of the scapula. Nerve gliding exercises are used to restore the mobility of the nerves. It is mandatory that physiotherapists, psychologists, occupational therapists, and social workers be consulted during the whole process. The patients should be observed for a long time because relapses are common. With use of this program, I found that 88.1% of the patients were satisfied with the outcome, that is, their symptoms had either disappeared or were much abated or the real cause of the symptoms had been diagnosed.

Recommendations were carried through during a 2-year follow-up period in 87.9% of cases. Of the patients who were advised to retire because of symptoms, the primary problem was found to be other than thoracic outlet syndrome (psychiatric causes, complex regional pain syndrome, polyneuropathy, multiple sclerosis, other) [10]. Conservative therapy is the treatment of choice in thoracic outlet syndrome because it is safe and can be implemented as a self-treatment program.

If symptoms are not abated despite restored function, the differential diagnosis should be reviewed. The fact that conservative treatment is tedious and relapses are common should not be considered a reason for surgical intervention. Surgery is a viable option only if there are signs of significant

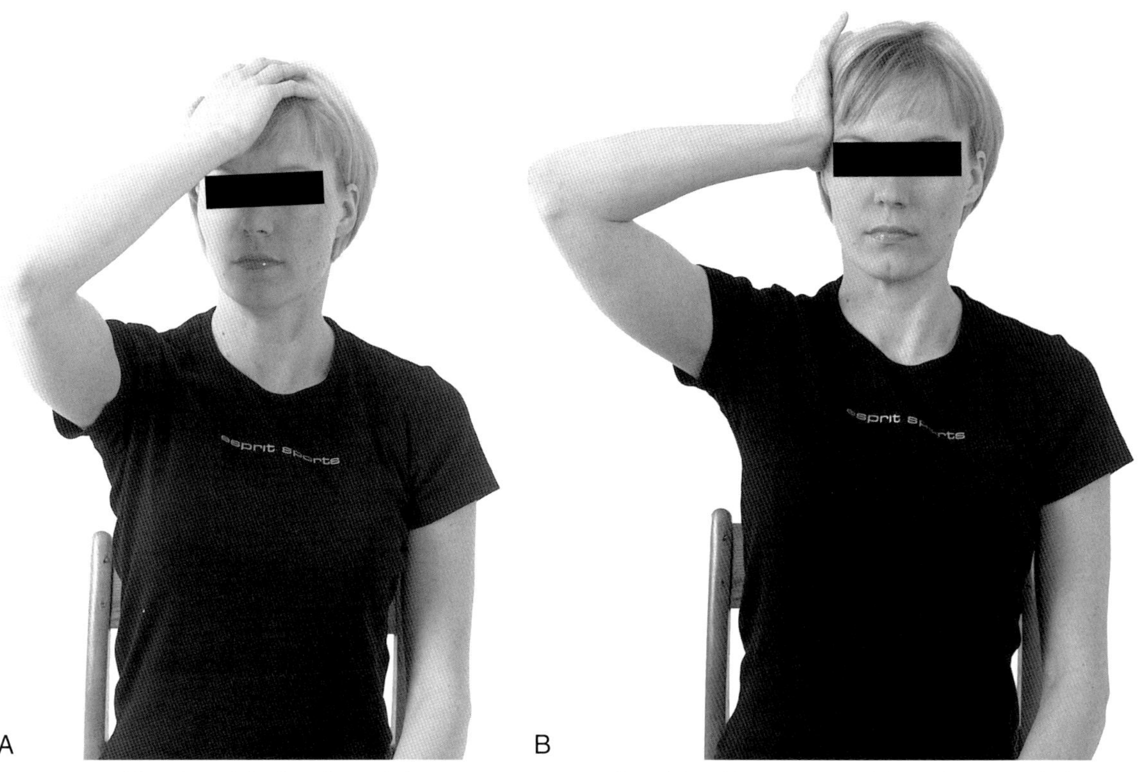

FIGURE 115.4 Normal function of the first ribs and the upper aperture can be achieved by activation of the scalene muscles by the patient. **A,** The patient first activates the anterior scalene muscles by pressing the forehead against the palm, with the cervical spine being all the time in a neutral position. **B,** The middle scalene muscles are activated by pressing sidewards against the palm. The exercises are done five or six times for a duration of 5 seconds each and with about 15 seconds between the exercises. The exercises are done on both sides. *(Reproduced with permission of Kustannus Oy Duodecim.)*

motor loss, atrophy, or vascular thrombosis. Psychosocial aspects should always be taken into account. It is extremely important to evaluate the degree of disability that thoracic outlet syndrome symptoms cause in relation to the patient's life situation and psychosocial abilities.

There is a link between the workplace and the individual in the pathogenesis and course of thoracic outlet syndrome. The role of occupational factors must be considered, and one has to go back to "the scene of the crime."

Surgery

Cherington [28] stated already in 1991, "It is important for surgeons and primary care physicians to be aware of the rising tide of skepticism surrounding the diagnosis and treatment of the thoracic outlet syndrome." Skepticism is indeed justified for several reasons. The most often diagnosed and surgically treated form of thoracic outlet syndrome in the United States, disputed neurologic thoracic outlet syndrome, has no objective clinical, radiologic, or electrodiagnostic criteria. In 1927, Adson [12] introduced scalenotomy as an approach to relieve structures from compression. Roos [1] presented a transaxillary resection of the first rib, and this operation has perhaps been the most used approach. Supraclavicular approaches have also been presented. Some authors claim the results of surgical management to be good, excellent, or favorable in more than 90% of patients [29]. Different studies, however, are difficult to compare because of the various criteria used to assess the outcome. In addition, the numbers of patients have ranged from 26 to 1336 and the follow-up times from 1 month to 15 years. Some authors do not state the follow-up time at all. A combined surgical treatment using transaxillary first rib resection and transcervical scalenotomy is said to be more effective than either of these alone [30]. There have been only a couple of studies in which the follow-up examination was done by independent examiners not involved in the surgical procedure or selection of the patients. This seems to affect the results after surgery. Among the different operative procedures, scalenotomy seems to speed up patients' retirement [31]. Cuetter and Bartoszek [32] and Lindgren [18] have reevaluated patients treated unsuccessfully with surgery for thoracic outlet syndrome; they found that in each case, another disease or functional disturbance explained the patient's complaints.

Recurrence after unsuccessful procedures may be a disabling and difficult problem for patients. This is extremely tragic in patients who have been found to have pulse changes in provocative positions in the absence of any other symptoms. Even abnormal electrodiagnostic findings before an operation do not predict the outcome of surgery [33]. Clinical tests show a good sensitivity but a poor specificity and cannot be used as the predictors for the outcome after surgery [34]. Long-term results of operation for thoracic outlet syndrome may be much worse than those initially achieved. Patients who present with poorly systematized neurologic symptoms have poor results after surgery and should be denied surgery or at least informed that postoperative results may be disappointing [35].

Botulinum chemodenervation of the scalene muscles has been found useful in alleviating symptoms in patients with thoracic outlet syndrome, especially if they are waiting for definitive surgical decompression. However, a randomized trial showed that chemodenervation did not result in clinically or statistically significant improvement in pain, paresthesias, or function in a population with thoracic outlet syndrome [36].

Potential Disease Complications

It is very important to detect those patients with post-traumatic thoracic outlet syndrome. These may present with worsening of the symptoms, such as a decrease in muscle strength, increase of pain, and tingling in the radicular territory, as well as unspecific disturbances, such as dizziness and face pain. In the case of these patients, one must consider surgical options [23]. It has been said that true neurogenic thoracic outlet syndrome is rare. Overdiagnosis of this syndrome results from a failure to realize that a wide range of symptoms occur regularly in patients with carpal tunnel syndrome and that these are commonly outside the anatomic distribution of the median nerve. The failure to recognize this can reinforce abnormal behavior in patients, particularly when they are subjected to unnecessary brachial plexus or ulnar nerve surgery, undertaken without neurophysiologic identification of an appropriate neurogenic abnormality [37]. If they are not dealt with correctly, these patients will suffer for long periods with more than one symptom. These may include muscle atrophy, swelling in the supraclavicular fossa, abnormal posture, and tendency to faint with certain movements. The leading symptom is numbness and clumsiness of the hand, but pain in the occiput-shoulder area is an important symptom too [38]. These may worsen without proper therapy.

Potential Treatment Complications

Surgery for thoracic outlet syndrome is not as innocuous as it was once thought. Dale [39] found that more than half of those who reported performing the surgery had encountered brachial plexus injuries severe enough to produce clinical weakness, nearly one fifth of which were permanent. Large numbers of failed thoracic outlet syndrome surgery have been reported during the last decades. Brachial plexus lesions, infections, and cases of life-threatening hemorrhage have been published. Even deaths have been reported. Franklin and colleagues [40] reported that 60% of workers were still work disabled 1 year after thoracic outlet syndrome decompression surgery.

References

[1] Roos DB. Thoracic outlet and carpal tunnel syndromes. In: Rutherford RB, editor. Vascular surgery. Philadelphia: WB Saunders; 1984. p. 708–24.
[2] Fodor M, Fodor L, Ciuce C. Anomalies of thoracic outlet in human fetuses: anatomical study. Ann Vasc Surg 2011;25:961–8.
[3] Juvonen T, Satta J, Laitala P, et al. Anomalies at the thoracic outlet are frequent in the general population. Am J Surg 1995;170:33–7.
[4] Brewin J, Hill M, Ellis H. The prevalence of cervical ribs in a London population. Clin Anat 2009;22:331–6.
[5] Casbas L, Chauffour X, Cau J, et al. Post-traumatic thoracic outlet syndromes. Ann Vasc Surg 2005;19:25–8.
[6] Crotti FM, Carai A, Carai M, et al. Post-traumatic thoracic outlet syndrome (TOS). Acta Neurochir Suppl 2005;92:13–5.
[7] Sanders R, Hammond SL. The significance and management of cervical ribs and anomalous first ribs. J Vasc Surg 2002;36:51–6.
[8] Schulman J. Brachial neuralgia. Arch Phys Med Rehabil 1949;30:150–3.

[9] Lindgren KA, Leino E. Subluxation of the first rib: a possible thoracic outlet syndrome mechanism. Arch Phys Med Rehabil 1988;69:692–5.
[10] Lindgren KA. Conservative treatment of thoracic outlet syndrome: a 2-year follow-up. Arch Phys Med Rehabil 1997;78:373–8.
[11] Nord KM, Kapoor P, Fisher J, et al. False positive rate of thoracic outlet syndrome diagnostic maneuvers. Electromyogr Clin Neurophysiol 2008;48:67–74.
[12] Adson AW, Coffey JR. Cervical rib: a method of anterior approach for relief of symptoms by division of the scalenus anticus. Ann Surg 1927;85:839–57.
[13] Gilroy J, Meyer JS. Compression of the subclavian artery as a cause of ischaemic brachial neuropathy. Brain 1963;86:733–46.
[14] Wright IS. The neurovascular syndrome produced by hyperabduction of the arms. Am Heart J 1945;29:1–29.
[15] Costigan DA, Wilbourn AJ. The elevated arm stress test: specificity in the diagnosis of the thoracic outlet syndrome. Neurology 1985;35(Suppl. 1):74–5.
[16] Ribbe E, Lindgren S, Norgren L. Clinical diagnosis of thoracic outlet syndrome—evaluation of patients with cervicobrachial symptoms. Man Med 1986;2:82–5.
[17] Lindgren KA, Leino E, Manninen H. Cervical rotation lateral flexion test in brachialgia. Arch Phys Med Rehabil 1992;73:735–7.
[18] Lindgren KA. Reasons for failures in the surgical treatment of thoracic outlet syndrome. Muscle Nerve 1995;18:1484–6.
[19] Geven LI, Smit AJ, Ebels T. Vascular thoracic outlet syndrome. Longer posterior rib stump causes poor outcome. Eur J Cardiothorac Surg 2006;30:232–6.
[20] Mingoli A, Sapienza P, di Marzo L, et al. Role of first rib stump length in recurrent neurogenic thoracic outlet syndrome. Am J Surg 2005;190:156.
[21] Cherington M, Wilbourn AJ, Schils J, et al. Thoracic outlet syndromes and MRI. Brain 1995;118:819–21.
[22] Wilhelm A, Wilhelm F. Thoracic outlet syndrome and its significance for surgery of the hand (on the etiology and pathogenesis of epicondylitis, tendovaginitis, median nerve compression and trophic disorders of the hand). Handchir Mikrochir Plast Chir 1985;17:173–87.
[23] Alexandre A, Coro L, Azuelos A, et al. Thoracic outlet syndrome due to hyperextension-hyperflexion cervical injury. Acta Neurochir Suppl 2005;92:21–4.
[24] Brooke BS, Freischlag JA. Contemporary management of thoracic outlet syndrome. Curr Opin Cardiol 2010;25:535–40.
[25] Sällström J, Celegin Z. Physiotherapy in patients with thoracic outlet syndrome. Vasa 1983;12:257–61.
[26] Lindgren KA, Manninen H, Rytkonen H. Thoracic outlet syndrome—a functional disturbance of the thoracic upper aperture? Muscle Nerve 1995;18:526–30.
[27] Sanders RJ. Recurrent neurogenic thoracic outlet syndrome stressing the importance of pectoralis minor syndrome. Vasc Endovascular Surg 2011;45:33–8.
[28] Cherington M. Thoracic outlet syndrome: rise of the conservative viewpoint. Am Fam Physician 1991;43:1998.
[29] Karamustafaoglu YA, Yoruk Y, Tarladacalisir T, et al. Transaxillary approach for thoracic outlet syndrome: results of surgery. Thorac Cardiovasc Surg 2011;59:349–52.
[30] Atasoy E. Combined surgical treatment of thoracic outlet syndrome: transaxillary first rib resection and transcervical scalenectomy. Handchir Mikrochir Plast Chir 2006;38:20–8.
[31] Gockel M, Vastamaki M, Alaranta H. Long-term results of primary scalenotomy in the treatment of thoracic outlet syndrome. J Hand Surg [Br] 1994;19:229–33.
[32] Cuetter AC, Bartoszek DM. The thoracic outlet syndrome: controversies, overdiagnosis, overtreatment, and recommendations for management. Muscle Nerve 1989;12:410–9.
[33] Lepantalo M, Lindgren KA, Leino E, et al. Long term outcome after resection of the first rib for thoracic outlet syndrome. Br J Surg 1989;76:1255–6.
[34] Sadeghi-Azandaryani M, Burklein D, Ozimek A, et al. Thoracic outlet syndrome: do we have clinical tests as predictors for the outcome after surgery? Eur J Med Res 2009;14:443–6.
[35] Degeorges R, Reynaud C, Becquemin JP. Thoracic outlet syndrome surgery: long-term functional results. Ann Vasc Surg 2004;18:558–65.
[36] Finlayson HC, O'Connor RJ, Brasher PM, et al. Botulinum toxin injection for management of thoracic outlet syndrome: a double-blind, randomized, controlled trial. Pain 2011;152:2023–8.
[37] Burke D. Symptoms of thoracic outlet syndrome in women with carpal tunnel syndrome. Clin Neurophysiol 2006;117:930–1.
[38] Muizelaar JP, Zwienenberg-Lee M. When it is not cervical radiculopathy: thoracic outlet syndrome—a prospective study on diagnosis and treatment. Clin Neurosurg 2005;52:243–9.
[39] Dale WA. Thoracic outlet compression syndrome. Critique in 1982. Arch Surg 1982;117:1437–45.
[40] Franklin GM, Fulton-Kehoe D, Bradley C, et al. Outcome of surgery for thoracic outlet syndrome in Washington state workers' compensation. Neurology 2000;54:1252–7.

CHAPTER 116

Tietze Syndrome

Marta Imamura, MD
Satiko T. Imamura, MD

Synonyms

Parasternal chondrodynia
Costochondral junction syndrome
Thoracochondralgia
Chondropathia tuberosa
Costal chondritis

ICD-9 Code

733.6 Tietze's disease; costochondral junction syndrome and costochondritis

ICD-10 Code

M94.0 Chondrocostal junction syndrome (Tietze)

Definition

Tietze syndrome is a benign, self-limited, nonsuppurative localized painful swelling of the upper costal cartilages of unknown etiology [1–10]. It affects the costochondral, costosternal, or sternoclavicular joints [2,5–7,9]. The manubriosternal and xiphisternal joints are less frequently affected [5,10]. First described in 1921 by a German surgeon in Breslau, Alexander Tietze, it is different from the costosternal syndrome [5–12]. Tietze syndrome is a rare cause of benign anterior chest wall pain associated with local swelling of the involved costal cartilages (Fig. 116.1) [5,6,12]. It is typically described in young adults and is a disease of the second and third decades of life [10,12]. Although it is not common, Tietze syndrome may also appear in children, infants [10,13], and elderly people [14]. It affects both men and women in a 1:1 ratio [4–6,9,10,15]. Lesions are unilateral and single in more than 80% of patients [4,10], and the second and third costal cartilages are most commonly involved [1,4,6,9–12]. Costosternal syndrome, a frequent cause of benign anterior chest wall pain, is not associated with a local swelling of the involved costal cartilages [5–12]. Costosternal syndrome usually occurs during and after the fourth decade of life, more frequently in women in a rate of 2 to 3:1 [9,10]. Multiple costal cartilages are involved in 90% of patients with costosternal syndrome [5,9,10].

The pathogenesis of Tietze syndrome is unknown [1–4,6, 8–10]. Recurrent functional overloading or microtrauma to the costal cartilages from severe coughing, heavy manual work, and sudden movement of the rib cage as well as malnutrition, sprain of the intra-articular sternocostal ligament, and respiratory tract infections may influence the development of Tietze syndrome [2,5,6,8–10,12,15]. Costal swelling may be due to focal enlargement [4,7], ventral angulation or irregular calcification of the affected costal cartilage [4,16], and thickening of overlying muscle [16,17]. Tietze syndrome may mimic a variety of life-threatening clinical entities [4,6,15] and must be considered in the differential diagnosis of any painful mass in the peristernal area. Clinical awareness of this syndrome and of its benign course may minimize performance of invasive diagnostic procedures [13].

Symptoms

Clinical manifestations include the sudden or gradual onset of pain of variable intensity [3,4,10,15] in the upper anterior chest wall in association with a fusiform and tender swelling of the involved costal cartilage [4,15]. Despite descriptions that pain may radiate to the shoulder, arm, and neck [3,4,12], its distribution usually occurs within the segment innervated by the afferent fibers carrying the painful impulse [2]. It is often aggravated by motion of the thoracic wall, sneezing, coughing, deep breathing, bending, exertion [1–8,15], and lying prone or over the affected side [10]. Some patients report inability to find a comfortable position in bed and have pain on turning over in the bed [1]. Weather change, anxiety, worry, and fatigue may exacerbate the pain [4]. Symptoms are usually unilateral, with no preferential side [3]. There is no reported association with sternotomy.

Physical Examination

On physical examination, a slight firm swelling is noted at the involved site [1–4,15]. Systemic manifestations [4,6,10,13,15] and inflammation are usually absent [1,4,5,7,10,15], but

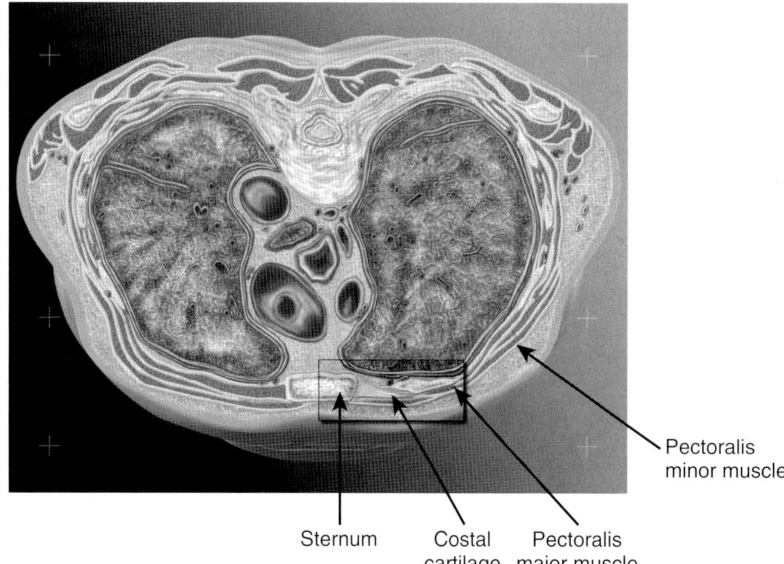

FIGURE 116.1 Schematic representation of the area of Tietze syndrome (costal cartilage, costosternal and costochondral joints) and anatomic relations with the mediastinal structures and other anterior chest wall structures.

there may be local heat [15]. Pain is reproduced with active protraction or retraction of the shoulder, deep inspiration, and elevation of the arm [12] (Fig. 116.2). A unique visible, spherical, nonsuppurative, tender tumor of elastic-hard and pasty consistency can be palpated, usually over the second and third costochondral joints. Local palpation with firm pressure over the localized tender swelling reproduces the spontaneous pain complaint [12] (Fig. 116.3). Physical examination findings of the musculoskeletal and neurologic systems of reported cases from the literature are usually normal except for the local findings [4–6,13,15,17]. Muscle strength and upper limb range of motion may be decreased because of pain. Dermatomal and subcutaneous hyperalgesia (Fig. 116.4) and hyperemia (Fig. 116.5) may be present in the involved thoracic spinal segments. The adjacent intercostal [12], sternal, and pectoralis major and minor muscles may be tender to palpation [14].

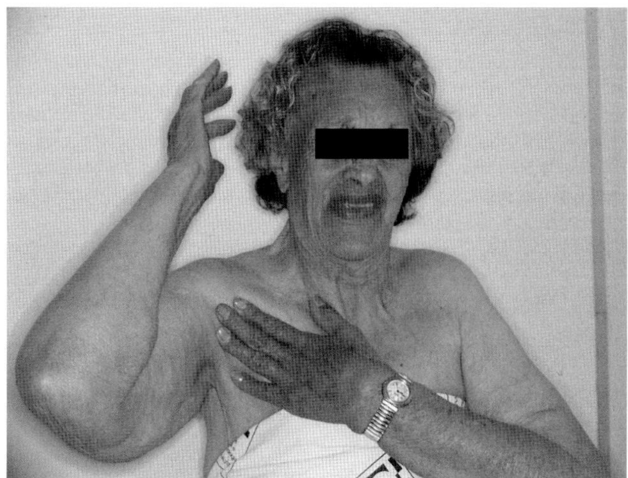

FIGURE 116.2 Reproduction of the spontaneous pain complaint during arm elevation in a patient diagnosed with Tietze syndrome.

Functional Limitations

The disability produced by Tietze syndrome is usually minor, although it can be severe with activity restriction involving the trunk and upper limbs. Activities such as lifting, bathing, ironing, combing and brushing hair, and other activities of daily living can be problematic. Patients who have physically vigorous jobs may need to be put on light duty for weeks and avoid physical efforts of the upper limbs and trunk [1]. Functional limitations may also be due to chronic pain [18]; however, even of those patients who continue to have pain after 1 year, most lead a life without disability.

Diagnostic Studies

Diagnosis of Tietze syndrome is essentially made on a clinical basis: anterior chest wall pain confirmed by palpation of a tender swelling at the second or third costochondral junction that reproduces the patient's complaint in the absence of another definite diagnosis [3–5,7–9,11,15]. Results of laboratory analysis including inflammatory and immunologic parameters are usually normal [4–9,15]. Some cases may show a slight increase in the erythrocyte sedimentation rate [7,13,15].

Chest, rib, and sternum plain films and conventional tomograms of the costochondral junction are generally normal [6,17,19]. Plain radiographs may show cartilage enlargement on tangential views, chondral calcification, irregularities at the joint surface, osteosclerosis, and presence of osteophytes at the costal joint. However, these radiographic changes may also be found in physiologic costochondral calcifications [20]. Plain radiographs are therefore mainly indicated to rule out occult bone diseases including tumors, low-grade infections, tender fat or lipomas, chest wall contusion, and congenital deformity [4,12,16]. Tuberculosis, chondroma, and chondrosarcoma are mostly located at the costochondral junction [16].

Ultrasonographic findings of the affected costochondral joints are characterized by an increase of the size of the

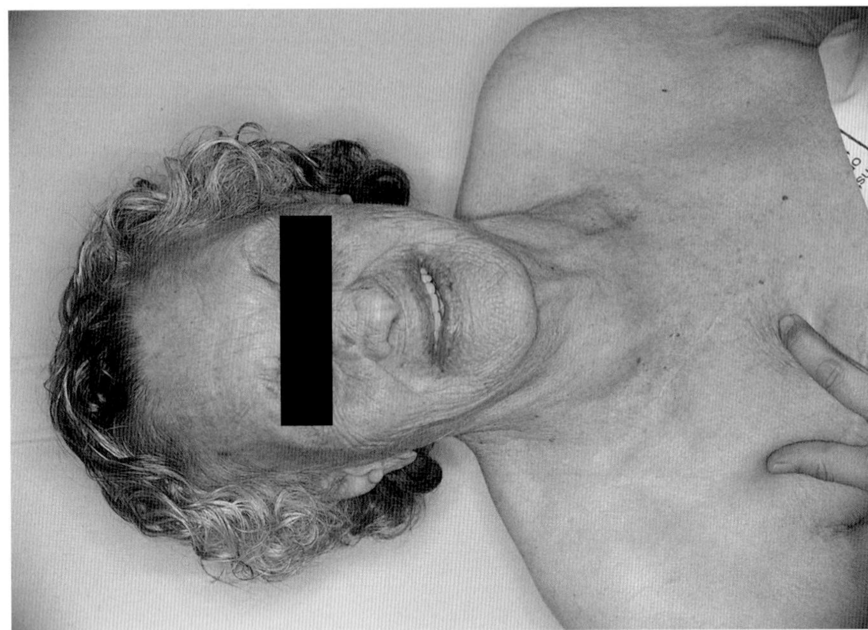

FIGURE 116.3 Local palpation with firm pressure over the localized tender swelling reproduces the spontaneous pain complaint.

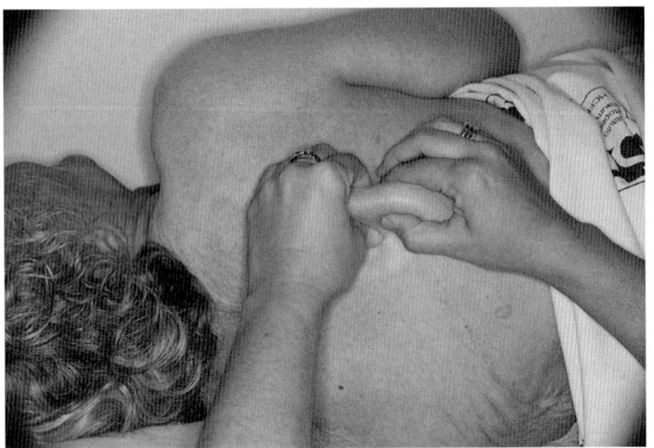

FIGURE 116.4 Subcutaneous hyperalgesia during the pinch and roll maneuver at the thoracic level.

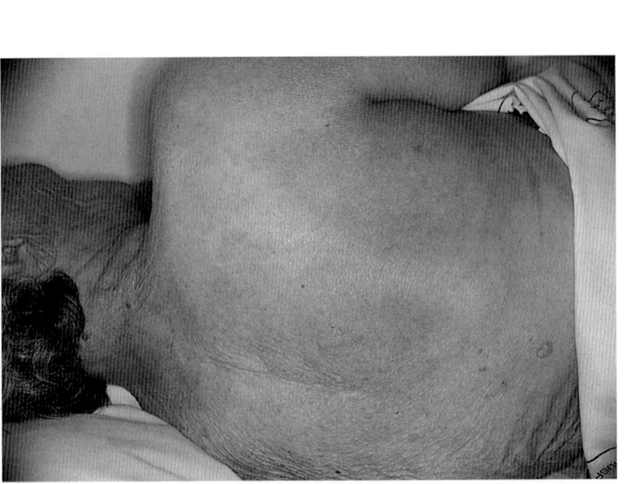

FIGURE 116.5 Hyperemia localized at the involved thoracic spinal segments after the pinch and roll maneuver.

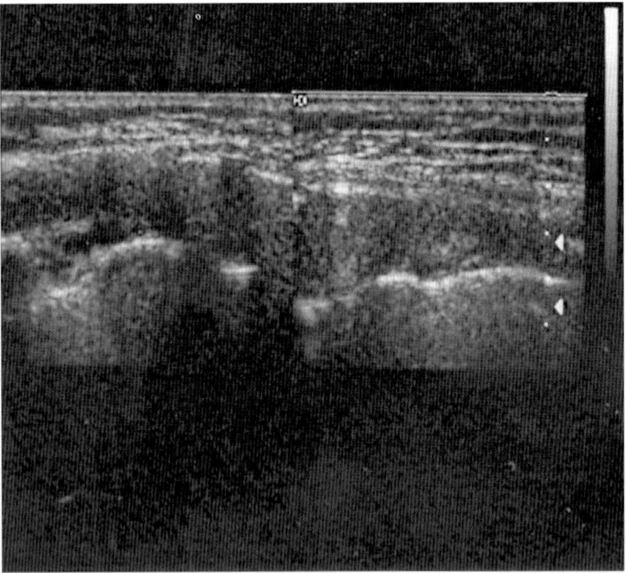

FIGURE 116.6 Comparison of the ultrasonographic findings of the affected costochondral joint *(left)* and the nonaffected contralateral joint *(right)* in an 82-year-old woman diagnosed with Tietze syndrome. The affected costochondral joint appears with a discrete increased size and as a nonhomogeneous hyperechoic cartilage with dotty, hyperreflective echoes and broad posterior acoustic shadows. *(Courtesy Marcelo Bordalo Rodrigues.)*

affected costal cartilage compared with the contralateral symmetric joint and normal age- and gender-matched controls (Fig. 116.6) [21]. There is also a nonhomogeneous increase in the echogenicity in the diseased cartilage, with dotty, hyperreflective echoes and intense broad posterior acoustic shadow [21]. The normal ultrasonographic picture of the costal cartilage (Fig. 116.7) is manifested as a hypoechoic oval area with the absence of posterior acoustic

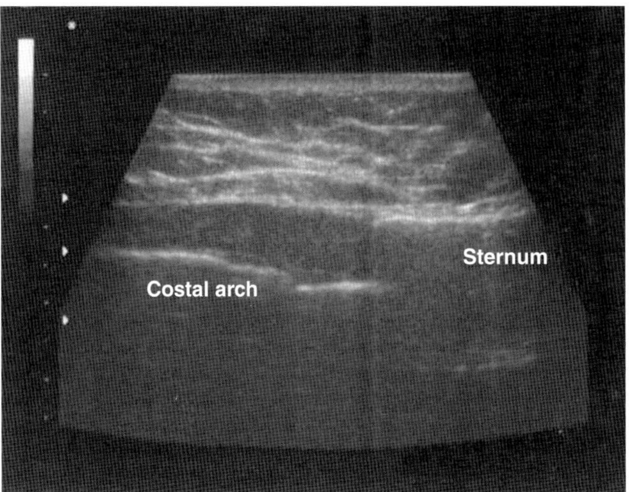

FIGURE 116.7 Normal ultrasonographic appearance of the costal cartilage. The normal costal cartilage appears as the homogeneous hypoechoic oval area between the sternum and the costal arch. *(Courtesy Marcelo Bordalo Rodrigues.)*

shadows in the longitudinal scans [21], and it appears as a ribbon-shaped homogeneous hypoechogenicity in the transverse scan with no posterior acoustic shadowing [21].

Computed tomography of the chest is an effective noninvasive means of imaging costal cartilage and adjacent structures in patients with Tietze syndrome [17,19,21]. Costal cartilage is normally symmetric in size and orientation at any level and is normally oriented along the horizontal axis [17]. Cartilage density is uniform and greater than that of the overlying muscle but less than calcium density [17]. Reported computed tomographic abnormalities of patients with Tietze syndrome include focal enlargement of the involved costal cartilage [6,17,19], ventral angulations [6,15,17,19], swelling or irregular calcification of the affected costal cartilage [17,19], perichondral soft tissue swelling, and periarticular bone sclerosis [5,22]. Computed tomography scan is useful to exclude other possible causes of chest wall or thoracic mass [6], such as malignant lymphoma [17,23] and mediastinal carcinoma [24]. Fluorodeoxyglucose–positron emission tomography can also be used in the differential diagnosis with malignant neoplasms [25].

Asymmetric thickening of the pectoralis major muscle simulating a chest wall mass can also be excluded [17]. Planar bone scanning with technetium Tc 99 usually reveals intense tracer uptake, but the findings are not specific [4,6,15,20,22]. Bone scintigraphy allows the precise localization of the involved joint [6] and the delineation of the number of involved joints; it should be considered to rule out occult fractures of the ribs and sternum in cases of local trauma [12].

Pinhole skeletal scintigraphy seems to enhance diagnostic specificity [20]. It is able to show a characteristic appearance of a drumstick-like pattern in acute cases and a C- or inverted C–shaped uptake in the chronically affected costal cartilage [20].

Magnetic resonance imaging of the costosternal and sternoclavicular joints usually shows thickening at the site of complaint; focal or widespread increased signal intensities of affected cartilage on both T2-weighted and short T1 inversion recovery or fat-saturated images; bone marrow edema in the subchondral bone; and intense gadolinium uptake in the areas of thickened cartilage, in the subchondral bone marrow, or in capsule and ligaments [26]. Magnetic resonance imaging is also indicated if an occult mass is suspected [9,12]. Magnetic resonance imaging allows differentiation of cartilage and bone abnormalities [26].

The histopathologic characteristics of costal cartilage in Tietze syndrome are usually normal [15] or nonspecific [3,6,7,15]. These characteristics include increased vascularity and degenerative changes with patchy loss of ground substance leading to a fibrillar appearance [6,22,27]. Degenerative changes occur with the formation of clefts, which may undergo calcification [1,22,27].

Differential Diagnosis

ANTERIOR CHEST WALL PAIN OF LOCAL ORIGIN

Costosternal syndrome
Trauma: dislocation and fractures of the ribs, sternum, clavicle, costal cartilage, costochondral or sternoclavicular joint
Arthritis: osteoarthritis, rheumatoid arthritis, ankylosing spondylitis, Reiter syndrome, psoriatic arthritis, SAPHO syndrome (synovitis, acne, pustulosis, hyperostosis, osteitis), gout
Infection: osteomyelitis, low-grade infection of the costal cartilage (tuberculosis, syphilis, typhoid and paratyphoid infections, blastomycosis, actinomycosis, brucellosis)
Tumors of the costochondral cartilages
- Benign: chondroma, multiple exostosis, lipomas
- Malignant neoplasms: Hodgkin and non-Hodgkin lymphoma [28], metastatic bone diseases (carcinoma of breast, lung, thyroid, kidney, or prostate), multiple myeloma, plasmacytoma, thymoma, chondrosarcoma

Myofascial pain syndrome at the anterior chest wall: sternal, pectoralis major, pectoralis minor, scalene, sternocleidomastoid (sternal head), subclavius, iliocostalis cervicis muscles
Other: slipping rib syndrome, condensing osteitis of the clavicle, congenital sternoclavicular malformations, xiphoidalgia syndrome, T1-T12 radiculopathy, intercostal neuritis (postherpetic neuralgia)

ANTERIOR CHEST WALL PAIN OF VISCERAL ORIGIN

Cardiac: myocardial infarction, angina pectoris, stenocardia
Pulmonary: pneumonia, pulmonary embolism, pleurisy, lung abscess, atelectasis, spontaneous pneumothorax
Breast: cyclic breast pain, duct ectasia, breast carcinoma
Abdominal: peptic duodenal ulcer, epigastric hernia, gastritis or pancreatitis, acute cholecystitis, diffuse peritonitis

Treatment

Initial

Treatment is symptomatic because the pathogenesis of the disease is still unclear [3,4,6,14,15]. The natural history of patients diagnosed with true Tietze syndrome is, in general, good and benign because of the self-limited characteristic of the condition. In the majority of cases, pain disappears spontaneously within a few weeks and swelling in a few months [15] without treatment [9]. Symptoms may be exacerbated after manual work and severe cough. During this period, the use of an elastic rib belt may also provide symptomatic relief and help protect the costosternal joints from additional trauma [9,12]. Initial treatment of the pain and functional disability associated with Tietze syndrome should include simple oral analgesics such as acetaminophen, oral or topical nonsteroidal anti-inflammatory drugs (NSAIDs) alone [6,9,11,14] or in combination with codeine [5,8,9,15], or tramadol. Reassurance about the benign nature of the disorder and the diagnosis of a non–life-threatening but real and well-recognized musculoskeletal pain disease can often by itself reduce the anxiety and fears and lead to symptomatic pain relief [2–5,8–11,15,29]. Avoidance of iatrogenic worries is usually helpful [29]. Removal of aggravating and perpetuating factors (including physical efforts of the upper limbs and trunk, chronic cough, and bronchospasm) and improved nutrition are also important [1,5,8,9,14]. Human calcitonin at the dosage of 0.25 mg/day was given for a course of 1 month to five women diagnosed with Tietze syndrome who had intense pain not relieved by conventional treatment [30]. Three patients reported complete remission of symptoms and imaging findings, and symptoms improved in two patients with disappearance of pain [30].

Rehabilitation

Physical modalities including local superficial heat for 20 minutes, two or three times a day, and ice for 10 to 15 minutes, three or four times a day, can be performed until symptoms are improved [3,12,14]. Heat and cold are equally effective, and the choice of modality relies on the patient's preference and tolerance. Transcutaneous electrical nerve stimulation and electroacupuncture may be applied over the painful area [14]. Electroacupuncture is applied by introducing the acupuncture disposable needle over the skin points of lower electrical skin resistance [14] that are located within the involved spinal segments. Galvanic or faradic low-frequency electrical currents are applied at the inserted needle [14]. Administration of corticosteroids by iontophoresis may provide more prolonged pain relief [11]. Gentle, pain-free range of motion exercises should be introduced as soon as tolerated [12]. Vigorous exercises should be avoided if they exacerbate the patient's symptoms [12]. Proper posture during sitting or working activities should be restored [5,8,9]. Inactivation of associated pectoralis major trigger points followed by relaxation and stretching exercises with relaxation of the involved muscles may also be helpful. Stretching exercises of the pectoralis major muscle, such as the standing pushup in the corner for 10 seconds, repeated for 1 or 2 minutes several times a day, may be helpful [8,31]. Vapocoolant spray applied to the involved areas may also relieve chest wall pain [8]. Patients should be instructed to avoid improper posture or repetitive misuse of chest wall muscles [8].

Psychological and psychopharmacologic treatment should be considered for patients with continuing symptoms and disability, especially if these are associated with abnormal health beliefs, depressed mood, panic attacks, or other symptoms such as fatigue or palpitations [29]. Both cognitive-behavioral therapy and selective reuptake inhibitors have been shown to be effective [29]. Tricyclic antidepressants are helpful in reducing reports of pain in patients with chest pain and normal coronary arteries [29].

Procedures

Most patients respond to NSAIDs, heat, and activity modification. For patients who do not respond to the initial and rehabilitation treatment modalities, however, a local anesthetic [2,4,6] and steroid injection can be performed as the next symptom control maneuver [2,5,6,8,9,11,12,15,21]. Injection of the costal cartilage is performed by placing the patient in the supine position [12,21]. Proper preparation with antiseptic solution of the skin overlying the affected costal cartilage is carried out with isopropyl alcohol and soluble iodine solution to swab the injection site [21]. The exact position for injection is identified by clinical and ultrasonographic examination [21]. The injection site is the point of maximum tenderness by palpation or the point of maximum cartilaginous hypertrophy by ultrasonographic examination [21]. A refrigerant spray may be used to anesthetize the overlying skin before the needle is inserted [21]. There should be limited resistance to injection [12]. If significant resistance is found, the needle should be withdrawn slightly and repositioned until the injection proceeds with only limited resistance [12]. This procedure should be repeated for each affected joint [12]. After the needle is removed, a sterile pressure dressing and ice pack are placed at the injection site [12]. Local steroid injections associated with local anesthetics have shown good therapeutic results [21]. There is an average of 82% decrease in the size of the affected costal cartilage 1 week after the local anesthetic and steroid injection, and the posterior acoustic shadowing is absent [21]. Clinical examination of the injected patients detected complete resolution and substantial improvement of signs and symptoms of pain and swelling. This shows a strong correlation between clinical changes and ultrasonographic findings in patients with Tietze syndrome. An intercostal nerve block performed 1.5 to 2 inches proximal to the costochondral joint of the affected level provides even longer lasting pain relief and is indicated if other measures are not effective [11].

Surgery

Surgical procedures are rarely necessary and indicated only if the symptomatic conservative measures failed to alleviate symptoms [9]. Surgical excision of the localized involved cartilage can be performed in severe and refractory cases [9]. Costosternal or sternoclavicular arthrodesis may be performed if conservative measures fail to provide satisfactory results.

Potential Disease Complications

Tietze syndrome is a benign condition and rarely presents complications. It is self-limited with spontaneous recovery of the pain after a few weeks or several months [1,3,4,15] to 1 year in the majority of cases. Swelling may persist for months [15] to years [4]. The course of this condition is characterized by periods of recurrence and improvement [1,3,4,14].

Potential Treatment Complications

The systemic complications of NSAIDs are well known and most commonly affect the gastric, hepatic, and renal systems. The major complication of the local steroid combined with local anesthetic injections is pneumothorax if the needle is placed too laterally or deeply and invades the pleural space [12]. Cardiac tamponade as well as an iatrogenic infection, although rare, can occur if, respectively, the needle is placed in the direction of the heart and strict aseptic techniques are not performed [12]. The possibility of trauma to the contents of the mediastinum remains another possibility [12]. This complication can be greatly decreased if the clinician pays close attention to accurate needle placement [12] or performs the injection with ultrasound guidance [21].

References

[1] Geddes AK. Tietze's syndrome. Can Med Assoc J 1945;53:571–3.

[2] Wehrmacher WH. The painful anterior chest wall syndromes. Med Clin North Am 1958;38:111–8.

[3] Kayser HL. Tietze's syndrome: a review of the literature. Am J Med 1956;21:982–9.

[4] Levey GS, Calabro JJ. Tietze's syndrome: report of two cases and review of the literature. Arthritis Rheum 1962;5:261–9.

[5] Fam AG, Smythe HA. Musculoskeletal chest wall pain. CMAJ 1985;133:379–89.

[6] Boehme MW, Scherbaum WA, Pfeiffer EF. Tietze's syndrome—a chameleon under the thoracic abdominal pain syndrome. Klin Wochenschr 1988;66:1142–5.

[7] Jurik AG, Graudal H. Sternocostal joint swelling—clinical Tietze's syndrome. Report of sixteen cases and review of the literature. Scand J Rheumatol 1988;17:33–42.

[8] Semble EL, Wise CM. Chest pain: a rheumatologists perspective. South Med J 1988;81:64–8.

[9] Aeschlimann A, Kahn MF. Tietze's syndrome: a critical review. Clin Exp Rheumatol 1990;8:407–12.

[10] Bonica JJ, Sola AF. Chest pain caused by other disorders. In: Bonica JJ, editor. The management of pain, II. Philadelphia: Lea & Febiger; 1990. p. 1114–45.

[11] Jensen S. Musculoskeletal causes of chest pain. Austral Fam Physician 2001;30:834–9.

[12] Waldman SD. Tietze's syndrome. In: Waldman SD, editor. Atlas of common pain syndromes. Philadelphia: WB Saunders; 2002. p. 158–60.

[13] Mukamel M, Kornreich L, Horev G, et al. Tietze's syndrome in children and infants (clinical and laboratory observations). J Pediatr 1997;131:774–5.

[14] Imamura ST, Imamura M. Síndrome de Tietze. In: Cossermelli W, editor. Terapêutica em Reumatologia. São Paulo: Lemos Editorial; 2000. p. 773–7.

[15] Hiramuro-Shoji F, Wirth MA, Rockwood CA. Atraumatic conditions of the sternoclavicular joint. J Shoulder Elbow Surg 2003;12:79–88.

[16] Jurik AG, Justesen T, Graudal H. Radiographic findings in patients with clinical Tietze syndrome. Skeletal Radiol 1987;16:517–23.

[17] Edelstein G, Levitt RG, Slaker DP, et al. Computed tomography of Tietze syndrome. J Comput Assist Tomogr 1984;8:20–3.

[18] Mayou RA, Bass C, Hart G, et al. Can clinical assessment of chest pain be made more therapeutic? Q J Med 2000;93:805–11.

[19] Edelstein G, Levitt RG, Slaker DP, et al. CT observation of rib anomalies: spectrum of findings. J Comput Assist Tomogr 1985;9:65–72.

[20] Yang W, Bahk YW, Chung SK, et al. Pinhole skeletal scintigraphic manifestations of Tietze's disease. Eur J Nucl Med 1994;21:947–52.

[21] Kamel M, Kotob H. Ultrasonographic assessment of local steroid injection in Tietze's syndrome. Br J Rheumatol 1997;36:547–50.

[22] Honda N, Machida K, Mamiya T, et al. Scintigraphic and CT findings of Tietze's syndrome: report of a case and review of the literature. Clin Nucl Med 1989;14:606–9.

[23] Fioravanti A, Tofi C, Volterrani L, et al. Malignant lymphoma mimicking Tietze's syndrome. Arthritis Rheum 2002;47:229–30.

[24] Thongngarm T, Lemos LB, Lawhon N, et al. Malignant tumor with chest wall pain mimicking Tietze's syndrome. Clin Rheumatol 2001;20:276–8.

[25] Mathew AS, El-Haddad G, Lilien DL, Takalkar AM. Costosternal chondrodynia simulating recurrent breast cancer unveiled by FDG PET. Clin Nucl Med 2008;33:330–2.

[26] Volterrani L, Mazzei MA, Giordano N, et al. Magnetic resonance imaging in Tietze's syndrome. Clin Exp Rheumatol 2008;26:848–53.

[27] Cameron HU, Fornasier VL. Tietze's syndrome. J Clin Pathol 1974;27:960–2.

[28] Jeon IH, Jeong WJ, Yi JH, et al. Non-Hodgkin's lymphoma at the medial clavicular head mimicking Tietze syndrome. Rheumatol Int 2012;32:2531–4.

[29] Bass C, Mayou R. ABC of psychological medicine. Chest pain. BMJ 2002;325:588–91.

[30] Ricevuti G. Effects of human calcitonin on pain in the treatment of Tietze's syndrome. Clin Ther 1985;7:669–73.

[31] Rovetta G, Sessarego P, Monteforte P. Stretching exercises for costochondritis pain. G Ital Med Lav Ergon 2009;31:169–71.

CHAPTER 117

Trigeminal Neuralgia

Josemaria Paterno, MD

Aneesh Singla, MD, MPH

Synonyms

Tic douloureux
Cranial neuralgia
Facial pain
Facial neuralgia
Trifacial neuralgia

ICD-9 Code

350.1 Trigeminal neuralgia: tic douloureux, trifacial neuralgia, trigeminal neuralgia NOS

ICD-10 Code

G50.0 Trigeminal neuralgia, tic douloureux, trifacial neuralgia, syndrome of paroxysmal facial pain

Definition

Trigeminal neuralgia is pain in the distribution of the trigeminal dermatomes. The pain is described as an electric shock–like, stabbing, unilateral pain having abrupt onset and termination. Intervals between attacks are pain free. Non-noxious triggers occur in the same or different sensory areas of the face, and there is minimal or no sensory loss in the region of pain [1–7]. Trigeminal neuralgia has an incidence of 4 or 5 per 100,000 people up to 20 per 100,000 per year after the age of 60 years [7–9] and a prevalence of 0.1 to 0.2 per 1000. The female-to-male ratio is about 3:2 [8].

The trigeminal nerve (cranial nerve V) is the largest of the cranial nerves. It begins in the brainstem at the trigeminal nucleus and travels along the ventrolateral surface of the pons and through the subarachnoid space until it enters the temporal bone, where it forms into the gasserian ganglion located in the Meckel cave [10]. The divisions are the ophthalmic or V1 branch, the maxillary or V2 branch, and the mandibular or V3 branch (Figs. 117.1 and 117.2). The relative distribution of pain in trigeminal neuralgia is as follows: V1, 20%; V2, 44%; V3, 36% [10].

Most patients with classic symptoms have mechanical compression of the trigeminal nerve as it leaves the pons and travels in the subarachnoid space toward the Meckel cave [10–12]. Most commonly, there is cross-compression by a major vessel. Other proposed causes include demyelinating plaques from multiple sclerosis, neoplastic disease, and abscess formation with bone resorption and irritation of the trigeminal nerve in the maxilla or mandible. Trigeminal neuralgia occurs in about 1% of patients with multiple sclerosis, and approximately 2% to 8% of patients with trigeminal neuralgia have multiple sclerosis [7,8,13].

Regardless of the etiology, it is likely that both peripheral and central mechanisms play a role in the pathogenesis of this syndrome.

Symptoms

Typical trigeminal neuralgia symptoms involve electric shock–like pain in the distribution of one or more branches of the trigeminal nerve. Pain is often intermittent, with pain-free intervals of months or even years [10]. The pain may last a few seconds to less than 2 minutes. The pain has at least four of the following five characteristics: distribution along one or more divisions of the trigeminal nerve; sudden intense, sharp, superficial, stabbing, or burning quality; severe intensity; precipitation from trigger areas or by certain daily activities, such as eating, talking, washing the face, or cleaning the teeth; and between paroxysms, the patient is completely asymptomatic [6,14]. In general, patients do not report any other neurologic deficit.

Physical Examination

The diagnosis of trigeminal neuralgia is made primarily by history. The Sweet criteria for this diagnosis are five pain descriptors. The diagnosis must be questioned if these criteria are not met [5], as follows: the pain is paroxysmal; the pain may be provoked by light touch to the face (trigger zones); the pain is confined to the trigeminal distribution; the pain is unilateral; and the findings on clinical sensory examination are normal [5,15]. When possible, physical examination of the oral cavity, dentition, and trigeminal nerve distribution should be performed to rule out other diseases. A complete cranial nerve examination should be performed. In general, no sensory or motor deficits are present, but serial examinations may detect a change and identify a secondary cause of trigeminal neuralgia [6].

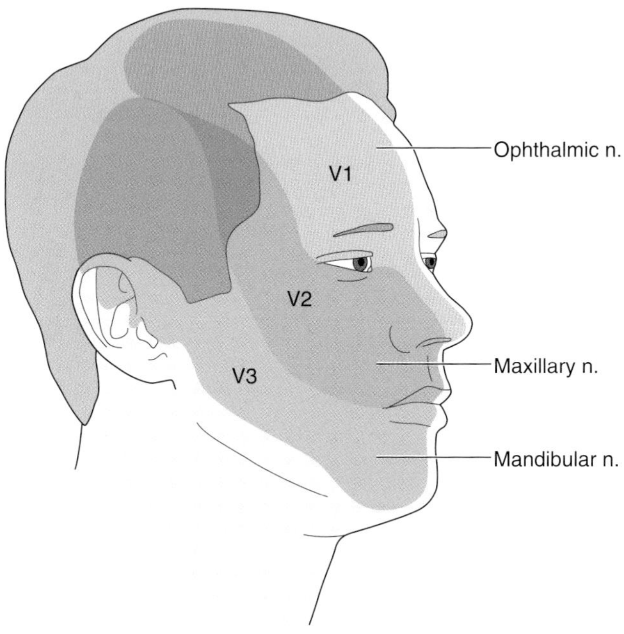

FIGURE 117.1 Dermatomes for trigeminal nerve. V1, ophthalmic nerve. V2, maxillary nerve. V3, mandibular nerve. *(From Waldman SD. Trigeminal nerve block: coronoid approach. In Waldman SD, ed. Atlas of Interventional Pain Management, 2nd ed. Philadelphia, WB Saunders, 2004.)*

Functional Limitations

In general, there are no impairments associated with trigeminal neuralgia. However, the pain from this entity may result in significant limitation in several activities of daily living. During exacerbations, patients may be functionally incapacitated because of pain and may be unable to perform activities such as comb hair, chew food, or shave. Talking on the telephone may be painful. Wearing glasses or makeup may not be possible. The pain from trigeminal neuralgia is not continuous but paroxysmal, suggesting spontaneous discharges from specific neurons, and it frequently occurs by innocuous tactile stimuli [4]. Therefore any activity that involves contact with the face may become difficult or impossible.

Diagnostic Studies

When a diagnosis of trigeminal neuralgia is suspected, patients should have diagnostic brain imaging with magnetic resonance imaging. Magnetic resonance imaging with gadolinium contrast can aid in diagnosis of multiple sclerosis plaques, neoplasm, and any neurovascular compressive relationship to the trigeminal root [5]. Electromyography, nerve conduction studies, and quantitative sensory testing may provide sensitive, quantitative, and objective results for the diagnosis, localization, and accuracy of damage to the trigeminal nerve [16]. Other studies that may have a role in diagnosis include intraoral, skull, and sinus radiographs and daily diaries of pain.

Differential Diagnosis

See Table 117.1.

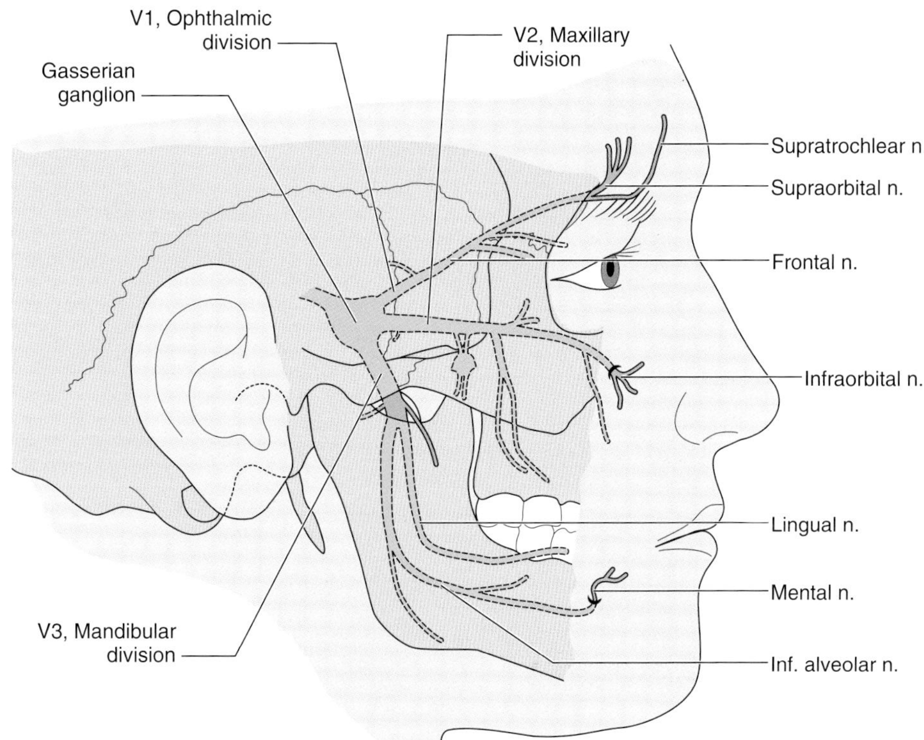

FIGURE 117.2 Anatomy of trigeminal nerve. The gasserian ganglion is formed from two roots that exit the ventral surface of the brainstem at the midpontine level. These roots pass in a forward and lateral direction in the posterior cranial fossa across the border of the petrous bone. They then enter the Meckel cave. The gasserian ganglion has three sensory divisions, the ophthalmic (V1), the maxillary (V2), and the mandibular (V3). *(From Waldman SD. Gasserian ganglion block. In Waldman SD, ed. Atlas of Interventional Pain Management, 2nd ed. Philadelphia, WB Saunders, 2004.)*

Table 117.1 Differential Diagnosis of Trigeminal Neuralgia or Facial Pain

Condition	Prevalence	Major Location and Radiation	Timing	Character and Severity	Provoking Factors	Associated Factors
Dental						
Pulpal	Very common	Well localized to a tooth	Can last 10-20 minutes after sugary stimulus	Sharp, stabbing, throbbing, dull, moderate to severe	Hot, cold, or sweet foods provoke it, rarely spontaneous	Immediate relief on removal of stimulus
Fractured or cracked tooth	Fairly common	Localized to one or two teeth, but may be poorly localized, difficult to visualize	Very short lasting, seconds, intermittent	Sharp, moderate	Biting, never spontaneous, may be sensitive to heat	Rebound pain, worse after force removed, opposing natural tooth normally present
Pulpal—chronic pulpitis	Common	Poorly localized intraorally	Intermittent, hours	Mild, dull, throbbing	Occasionally heat	Often large restoration
Periodontal—chronic apical periodontitis	Common	Poorly localized, intraoral	Intermittent, minutes to hours	Mild, dull, throbbing	Large restoration	Sinus may be visible, bad taste
Bone pain–osteomyelitis	Rare	Most often mandible, widespread	Continuous	Throbbing, severe	Biting on mobile teeth	Pyrexia, malaise, trismus, swelling, may be paresthesia, pus, mobile teeth, sequestra
Denture pain, pressure on mental nerve, secondary trigeminal neuralgia	Rare	Localized intraoral	Intermittent, daily	Aching, may be sharp if over mental nerve	Eating with denture	Often redness, ulceration in area of pressure
Neurologic Trigeminal Neuralgia						
Classic, typical [14]	Rare	Intraoral or extraoral in trigeminal region	Each episode of pain lasts for seconds to minutes; refractory periods and long periods of no pain	Sharp, shooting, moderate to very severe	Light touch provoked (e.g., eating, washing, talking)	Discrete trigger zones
Atypical trigeminal neuralgia [17]	Rare	Intraoral or extraoral in trigeminal region	Sharp attacks lasting seconds to minutes, more continuous-type background pain, less likely to have complete pain remission	Sharp, shooting, moderate to severe but also dull, burning, continuous mild background pain	Light touch provoked, but continuous-type pain not so clearly provoked	May have small trigger areas, variable pattern
Trigeminal neuropathy [18]	Very rare	Trigeminal area, but may radiate beyond	Continuous	Dull with sharp exacerbation	Areas of allodynia, light touch	Sensory loss, subjective-objective, progressive, vasodilation and swelling may occur

Glossopharyngeal neuralgia	Very rare	Intraoral in distribution of glossopharyngeal	Each episode lasts for seconds up to 2 minutes	Sharp, stabbing, burning, severe	Swallowing, chewing, talking	No neurologic deficit
Postherpetic neuralgia [19]	Rare	Most commonly first division of trigeminal	Continuous pain	Tingling, severity varies	Tactile allodynia	More than 6-12 months after acute herpes zoster
Vascular						
Cluster headache, episodic pain-free periods, chronic, no remissions [14]	Rare	Orbital, supraorbital, temporal	15-180 minutes to several hours, from 1 every other day to 8 per day	Hot, searing, punctuate, severe	Vasodilators (e.g., alcohol)	Conjunctival injection, lacrimation, nasal congestion, rhinorrhea, sweating, miosis, ptosis, eyelid edema, restlessness
SUNCT [20]	Very rare	Ocular, periocular, but may radiate to frontotemporal area, upper jaw, and palate	Each episode last up to 2 minutes; intermittent, several attacks per day and then may remit	Burning, electrical, stabbing, severe	Neck movements	Conjunctival injection, lacrimation, nasal stuffiness, rhinorrhea
Chronic paroxysmal hemicrania [20]	Very rare	Eye, forehead	Pain lasts 2-45 minutes, 5-10 times daily	Stabbing, throbbing, boring	Head movements, responds to indomethacin	Autonomic symptoms as for SUNCT
Giant cell arteritis [20]	Rare	May be bilateral, mostly over temporal artery	Continuous	Aching, throbbing, boring, sharp	Chewing	Jaw claudication, neck pain, anorexia, visual symptoms; temporal artery biopsy is "gold standard"
Temporomandibular disorders, idiopathic orofacial pain, facial arthromyalgia [19]	Relatively common	May be bilateral, periauricular, radiate to neck, temples	Intermittent, may last for hours, may have severe exacerbations	Throbbing, sharp, or dull aching	Clenching and grinding, opening wide, psychosocial factors, trauma	May be limitation in opening, tenderness of muscles of mastication, altered occlusion, responds to relaxation
Atypical facial pain [21]	Relatively common	May be bilateral or unilateral, can radiate widely beyond trigeminal area, variable location	Intermittent or continuous, often long history of pain	Nagging, throbbing, aching, sharp (wide range of words used), and severity mild to moderate	Life events, stress, weather changes, movements	Dysesthesia, facial edema, headaches, depression
Atypical odontalgia, phantom tooth [19]	Rare	Intraoral in a tooth or teeth, gingival, moves to another area	Continuous, few minutes to hours	Dull, throbbing, may be sharp, mild to moderate	Life events, emotional, teeth hypersensitive to temperature and pressure	Often history of tooth extraction

Reprinted with permission from Zakrzewska JM. Diagnosis and differential diagnosis of trigeminal neuralgia. Clin J Pain 2002;18:14-21.

Treatment

Initial

Treatments that may help with trigeminal neuralgia include heat or cold therapy, massage, avoidance of triggers, and application of transcutaneous electrical nerve stimulation [8,9]. Topical ointments such as lidocaine, ketamine, and ketoprofen may help as well [8,9]. Pharmacologic options are listed in Table 117.2. The anticonvulsant carbamazepine is considered a first-line therapy and has been efficacious in several controlled trials [22–25]. Carbamazepine can be associated with systemic issues affecting the hematologic and endocrine system (see "Potential Treatment Complications"). The carbamazepine derivative oxcarbazepine is associated with fewer side effects and often better tolerated. Baclofen and lamotrigine have also been helpful in controlled trials [22,26,27]. Uncontrolled observations, clinical practice, and the authors' experience also suggest that phenytoin, clonazepam, topiramate, sodium valproate, gabapentin, pregabalin, zonisamide, levetiracetam, mexiletine, and lidocaine may be useful [22]. Pharmacologic therapy with nonsteroidal anti-inflammatory agents, acetaminophen, tricyclic antidepressants, serotonin-norepinephrine reuptake inhibitors, and muscle relaxants may be useful. One study showed that intranasal lidocaine 8% administered by a metered-dose spray produced prompt but temporary analgesia without serious adverse reactions in patients with second-division trigeminal neuralgia [28]. In general, 80% of patients will respond to medical therapy [7].

Rehabilitation

Modalities for pain control, such as electrical stimulation, ice massage, and hot packs, can play a role in rehabilitation and recovery from trigeminal neuralgia. Speech therapy may be indicated to help with oral motor deficits that affect speech or swallowing.

Adaptive equipment, such as a telephone earset, may be recommended. Some general chronic pain rehabilitation approaches may also be useful, such as improved sleep hygiene, low-intensity aerobic exercise, biofeedback, cognitive-behavioral therapy, and relaxation techniques. Acupuncture may also have a role in the management of trigeminal neuralgia [29]. After surgical intervention with microvascular decompression, the rehabilitation process is often brief. Trigeminal neuralgia pain relief is usually immediate, and neuropathic medications are gradually discontinued in the weeks after surgery. If pain does recur, medications may be restarted, or if necessary, a second interventional procedure may eventually be needed.

Trigeminal neuralgia patients with underlying multiple sclerosis face many therapeutic challenges. Rehabilitation exercises that improve multiple sclerosis symptoms and quality of life can help modulate the impact of trigeminal neuralgia. Aerobic exercise has been shown to improve quality of life, pain, fitness, and function in multiple sclerosis patients with moderate to severe disability [30].

Table 117.2 Pharmacologic Options for Trigeminal Neuralgia Reported in the Literature

Drug	Daily Dose	NNT
*Carbamazepine	300-2400 mg	1.4-2.1 (1.1-3.9)
*Baclofen	60-80 mg	1.4 (1.0-2.6)
*Lamotrigine	400 mg	2.1 (1.3-6.1)
Phenytoin	300-400 mg	
Clonazepam	6-8 mg	
Valproate	1200 mg	
Oxcarbazepine	1200-1400 mg	
Gabapentin	600-2000 mg	
Intravenous lidocaine	2-5 mg/kg	
Mexiletine	10 mg/kg	

*Indicates data from placebo-controlled trials.
NNT is number needed to treat to obtain 1 patient with at least 50% pain relief.
From Sindrup SH, Jensen TS. Pharmacotherapy of trigeminal neuralgia. Clin J Pain 2002;18:22-27.

Procedures

With medically refractory trigeminal neuralgia, physicians and patients can choose among several interventions, such as transient nerve blocks, rhizotomy by radiofrequency (RF) ablation, stereotactic radiosurgery, and surgical microvascular decompression. Local anesthetic trigeminal nerve blocks may reduce the intensity or the episodes of pain (Fig. 117.3), but the pain often outlasts the duration of the local anesthetic. Nerve blocks can be repeated at intervals but are more useful as a diagnostic test to judge candidacy for percutaneous RF ablation [3]. RF ablation is the most common nonsurgical intervention performed for trigeminal neuralgia, with a reported initial success rate of more than 90% [31–33]. However long-term efficacy of RF ablation is lower than that of microvascular decompression, with approximately 20% reporting recurrence of pain within 12 months [31,32,34]. In a review of 1600 RF ablations of the trigeminal nerve, Kanopolat reported the most common side effects to be weakened corneal reflex (5.7%), masseter weakness (4.1%), and dysesthesia (1%) [31]. Regarding specific RF technique, conventional RF was clearly more efficacious than pulsed RF in a double-blind randomized trial of 40 patients with idiopathic trigeminal neuralgia [34].

Stereotactic radiosurgery is another option for trigeminal neuralgia. A focused beam of radiation is used to target the trigeminal nerve root. Success rates of 80% have been reported, but microvascular decompression still offers superior long-term outcomes [33,35,36]. However, both RF ablation and stereotactic radiosurgery are viable alternatives to microvascular decompression, especially for high-risk elderly patients, the patient's preference to avoid surgery, or prior failed microvascular decompression.

Other forms of rhizotomy have reported good short-term results with neurolytic agents such as alcohol and glycerol. The consensus among most physicians is that these particular techniques have lower success rates and higher morbidity [3].

Surgery

Overall nonsurgical interventions are effective but lack robust long-term efficacy, leading to repeated interventions. Definitive surgical therapy is microvascular decompression, which entails a craniotomy to insert a felt barrier or inert

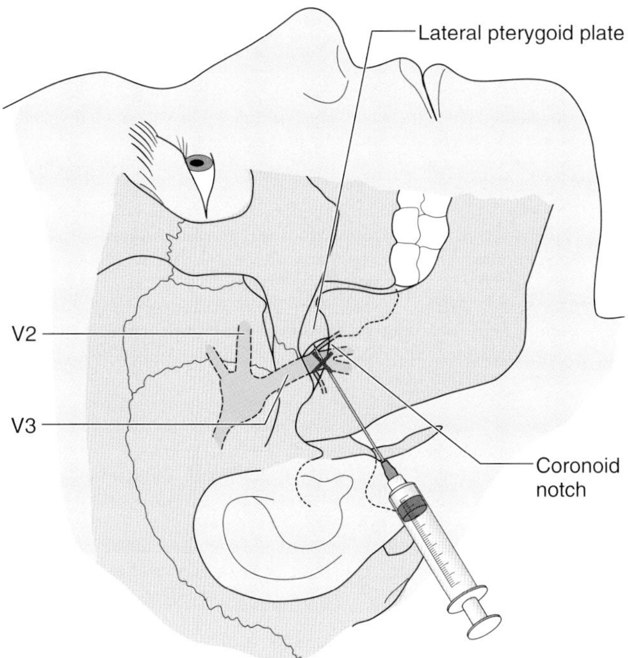

FIGURE 117.3 Technique of trigeminal nerve block. The patient is placed in the supine position with the cervical spine in the neutral position. The coronoid notch is identified by asking the patient to open and close the mouth several times and palpating the area just anterior and slightly inferior to the acoustic auditory meatus. After the notch is identified, the patient is asked to hold the mouth in neutral position. A total of 4 mL of local anesthetic is drawn up in a 12-mL sterile syringe. In treatment of trigeminal neuralgia, atypical facial pain, or other painful conditions involving the maxillary and mandibular nerves, a total of 80 mg of depot steroid is added to the local anesthetic. After the skin overlying the coronoid notch is prepared with antiseptic solution, a 22-gauge, 3½-inch styleted needle is inserted just below the zygomatic arch directly in the middle of the coronoid notch. The needle is advanced approximately 1½ to 2 inches in a plane perpendicular to the skull until the lateral pterygoid plate is encountered. At this point, if blockade of both the maxillary and mandibular nerves is desired, the needle is withdrawn slightly. After careful aspiration, 6 mL of solution is injected in incremental doses. During the injection procedure, the patient must be observed carefully for signs of local anesthetic toxicity. *(From Waldman SD. Trigeminal nerve block: coronoid approach. In Waldman SD, ed. Atlas of Interventional Pain Management, 2nd ed. Philadelphia, WB Saunders, 2004.)*

sponge between the compressing vessel and trigeminal nerve origin in the cerebellopontine angle cistern. Overall long-term outcomes are excellent, with complete pain relief as high as 70% to 86% several years after surgery [37–39]. Although the elderly have traditionally been considered a higher risk group for microvascular decompression, more recent data from small prospective studies indicate that some older patients can safely undergo microvascular decompression [38,39].

Furthermore, although it is still experimental, intracranial neurostimulation provides an alternative means for trigeminal neuralgia pain relief in surgically and medically refractory cases. By implantation of electrodes to the facial motor cortex, motor cortex stimulation has shown efficacy for neuropathic facial pain. Motor cortex stimulation has shown particular promise in the treatment of trigeminal neuropathic pain and central pain syndromes, such as thalamic pain syndrome [40].

Potential Disease Complications

Trigeminal neuralgia is generally amenable to surgical treatment or pharmacotherapy. However, it can progress to become a chronic intractable pain syndrome. In refractory cases, it is important to consider other diagnoses or facial pain syndromes.

Potential Treatment Complications

Carbamazepine can be associated with numerous side effects, including aplastic anemia and the syndrome of inappropriate diuretic hormone secretion; hence, frequent monitoring is necessary. Our practice is to check a CBC and chemistry panel 2 weeks after starting the medication, monthly for 3 months, and then every 6 to 9 months thereafter. If the patient is on a stable dose and a dose adjustment is made, we recheck the labs within 1 month after the dose change. For Gamma Knife radiosurgery, post-treatment facial numbness was reported as bothersome in 5%, commonly in patients who underwent another invasive treatment [36]. Although microvascular decompression has the best efficacy and durability of all treatments, known complications can be serious and include up to a 4% risk of cerebellar hematoma, cranial nerve injury, cerebrospinal fluid leak, stroke, and death—complications not seen with the less invasive ablative procedures [41]. In addition, in a case series of 67 elderly patients undergoing posterior fossa exploration for trigeminal neuralgia, complications occurred in 10 patients (15%) and included ataxia (10%), hearing loss (5%), trigeminal dysesthesias (5%), facial weakness (3%), aseptic meningitis (2%), and pulmonary embolus (2%) [39].

References

[1] Kitt CA, Gruber K, Davis M, et al. Trigeminal neuralgia: opportunities for research and treatment. Pain 2000;85:3–7.
[2] Devor M, Amir R, Rappaport ZH. Pathophysiology of trigeminal neuralgia: the ignition hypothesis. Clin J Pain 2002;18:4–13.
[3] Fishman SM, Ballantyne JC, Rathmell JP, editors. Bonica's management of pain. 4th ed. Philadelphia: Lippincott Williams & Wilkins; 2009. p. 865–6.
[4] Nurmikko TJ, Eldridge PR. Trigeminal neuralgia—pathophysiology, diagnosis and current treatment. Br J Anaesth 2001;87:117–32.
[5] Scrivani SJ, Mathews ES, Maciewicz RJ. Trigeminal neuralgia. Oral Surg Oral Med Oral Pathol Oral Radiol Endod 2005;100:527–38.
[6] Zakrzewska JM. Diagnosis and differential diagnosis of trigeminal neuralgia. Clin J Pain 2002;18:14–21.
[7] Kapur N, Kamel IR, Herlich A. Oral and craniofacial pain: diagnosis, pathophysiology, and treatment. Int Anesthesiol Clin 2003;41:115–50.
[8] Larsen A, Piepgras D, Chyatte D, Rizzolo D. Trigeminal neuralgia: diagnosis and medical and surgical management. JAAPA 2011;24:20–5.
[9] Baron R, Binder A, Wasner G. Neuropathic pain: diagnosis, pathophysiological mechanisms, and treatment. Lancet Neurol 2010;9:807–19.
[10] Fishman SM, Ballantyne JC, Rathmell JP, editors. Bonica's management of pain. 4th ed. Philadelphia: Lippincott Williams & Wilkins; 2009. p. 833–66.
[11] Dandy W. Concerning the cause of trigeminal neuralgia. Am J Surg 1934;204:447–55.
[12] Zakrzewska JM, Coakham HB. Microvascular decompression for trigeminal neuralgia: update. Curr Opin Neurol 2012;25:296–301.
[13] Silberstein SD, Young WB. Headaches and facial pain. In: Goetz CG, editor. Textbook of clinical neurology. Philadelphia: WB Saunders; 1999. p. 1089–105.

[14] Classification and diagnostic criteria for headache disorders, cranial neuralgias and facial pain. Headache Classification Committee of the International Headache Society. Cephalalgia 1988;8(Suppl. 7):1–96.
[15] White J, Sweet WH. Pain and the neurosurgeon. Springfield, Ill: Charles C Thomas; 1969.
[16] Jaaskelainen SK. The utility of clinical neurophysiological and quantitative sensory testing for trigeminal neuropathy. J Orofac Pain 2004;18:355–9.
[17] Zakrzewska JM, Jassim S, Bulman JS. A prospective, longitudinal study on patients with trigeminal neuralgia who underwent radiofrequency thermocoagulation of the Gasserian ganglion. Pain 1999;79:51–8.
[18] Goadsby PJ, Lipton RB. A review of the paroxysmal hemicranias, SUNCT syndrome and other short-lasting headaches with autonomic feature, including new cases. Brain 1997;120:193–209.
[19] Merskey H, Bogduk N. Classification of chronic pain. Descriptors of chronic pain syndromes and definitions of pain terms. Seattle: IASP Press; 1994, 1.
[20] Hayreh SS, Podhajsky PA, Raman R, Zimmerman B. Giant cell arteritis: validity and reliability of various diagnostic criteria. Am J Ophthalmol 1997;123:285–96.
[21] Pfaffenrath V, Rath M, Pollmann W, Keeser W. Atypical facial pain: application of the IHS criteria in a clinical sample. Cephalalgia 1993;13(Suppl. 12):84–8.
[22] Sindrup SH, Jensen TS. Pharmacotherapy of trigeminal neuralgia. Clin J Pain 2002;18:22–7.
[23] Campbell FG, Graham JG, Zilkha KJ. Clinical trial of carbamazepine (Tegretol) in trigeminal neuralgia. J Neurol Neurosurg Psychiatry 1966;29:265–7.
[24] Killian JM, Fromm GH. Carbamazepine in the treatment of neuralgia. Use of side effects. Arch Neurol 1968;19:129–36.
[25] Nicol CF. A four year double-blind study of tegretol in facial pain. Headache 1969;9:54–7.
[26] Fromm GH, Terrence CF, Chattha AS. Baclofen in the treatment of trigeminal neuralgia: double-blind study and long-term follow-up. Ann Neurol 1984;15:240–4.
[27] Zakrzewska JM, Chaudhry Z, Nurmikko TJ, et al. Lamotrigine (Lamictal) in refractory trigeminal neuralgia: results from a double-blind placebo controlled crossover trial. Pain 1997;73:223–30.
[28] Kanai A, Suzuki A, Kobayashi M, Hoka S. Intranasal lidocaine 8% spray for second-division trigeminal neuralgia. Br J Anaesth 2006;97:559–63.
[29] Millan-Guerrero RO, Isais-Millan S. Acupuncture in trigeminal neuralgia management. Headache 2006;46:532.
[30] Brown TR, Kraft GH. Exercise and rehabilitation for individuals with multiple sclerosis. Phys Med Rehabil Clin N Am 2005;16:513–55.
[31] Kanpolat Y, Avman N, Gokalp HZ, et al. Effectiveness of radiofrequency thermocoagulation in recurrent trigeminal neuralgia after previous retrogasserian rhizotomy. Appl Neurophysiol 1985;48:258–61.
[32] Kanpolat Y, Savas A, Bekar A, Berk C. Percutaneous controlled radiofrequency trigeminal rhizotomy for the treatment of idiopathic trigeminal neuralgia: 25-year experience with 1,600 patients. Neurosurgery 2001;48:524–32, discussion 532–534.
[33] Dhople AA, Adams JR, Maggio WW, et al. Long-term outcomes of gamma knife radiosurgery for classic trigeminal neuralgia: implications of treatment and critical review of the literature. Clinical article. J Neurosurg 2009;111:351–8.
[34] Erdine S, Ozyalcin NS, Cimen A, et al. Comparison of pulsed radiofrequency with conventional radiofrequency in the treatment of idiopathic trigeminal neuralgia. Eur J Pain 2007;11:309–13.
[35] Elaimy AL, Hanson PW, Lamoreaux WT, et al. Clinical outcomes of gamma knife radiosurgery in the treatment of patients with trigeminal neuralgia. Int J Otolaryngol 2012;2012:919186.
[36] Lopez BC, Hamlyn PJ, Zakrzewska JM. Stereotactic radiosurgery for primary trigeminal neuralgia: state of the evidence and recommendations for future reports. J Neurol Neurosurg Psychiatry 2004;75:1019–24.
[37] Barker 2nd. FG, Jannetta PJ, Babu RP, et al. Long-term outcome after operation for trigeminal neuralgia in patients with posterior fossa tumors. J Neurosurg 1996;84:818–25.
[38] Sekula Jr RF, Frederickson AM, Jannetta PJ, et al. Microvascular decompression for elderly patients with trigeminal neuralgia: a prospective study and systematic review with meta-analysis. J Neurosurg 2011;114:172–9.
[39] Sekula RF, Marchan EM, Fletcher LH, et al. Microvascular decompression for trigeminal neuralgia in elderly patients. J Neurosurg 2008;108:689–91.
[40] Levy R, Deer TR, Henderson J. Intracranial neurostimulation for pain control: a review. Pain Physician 2010;13:157–65.
[41] Lopez BC, Hamlyn PJ, Zakrzewska JM. Systematic review of ablative neurosurgical techniques for the treatment of trigeminal neuralgia. Neurosurgery 2004;54:973–82, discussion 982–983.

PART 3

REHABILITATION

CHAPTER 118

Upper Limb Amputations

Timothy R. Dillingham, MD, MS
Diane W. Braza, MD

Synonyms

Hand amputations
Below-elbow amputations
Above-elbow amputations

ICD-9 Codes

886 Traumatic amputation of other finger(s) (complete) (partial)
886.0 Without mention of complication
886.1 Amputated finger, complicated
887 Traumatic amputation of arm and hand (complete) (partial)
887.0 Unilateral, below elbow, without mention of complication
887.1 Unilateral, below elbow, complicated
887.2 Unilateral, at or above elbow, without mention of complication
887.3 Unilateral, at or above elbow, complicated
887.4 Unilateral, level not specified, without mention of complication
887.5 Unilateral, level not specified, complicated
887.6 Bilateral (any level), without mention of complication
887.7 Bilateral (any level), complicated
905.9 Late effect of traumatic amputation
997.60 Amputation stump complication, unspecified
997.61 Neuroma of amputation stump
997.62 Infection (chronic) of amputated stump
V52 Fitting and adjustment of prosthetic device and implant
V52.0 Artificial arm (complete) (partial)

ICD-10 Codes

S68.110 Complete traumatic metacarpophalangeal amputation of right index finger
S68.111 Complete traumatic metacarpophalangeal amputation of left index finger
S68.112 Complete traumatic metacarpophalangeal amputation of right middle finger
S68.113 Complete traumatic metacarpophalangeal amputation of left middle finger
S68.114 Complete traumatic metacarpophalangeal amputation of right ring finger
S68.115 Complete traumatic metacarpophalangeal amputation of left ring finger
S68.116 Complete traumatic metacarpophalangeal amputation of right little finger
S68.117 Complete traumatic metacarpophalangeal amputation of left little finger
S68.118 Complete traumatic metacarpophalangeal amputation of other finger
S68.119 Complete traumatic metacarpophalangeal amputation of unspecified finger
S68.120 Partial traumatic metacarpophalangeal amputation of right index finger
S68.121 Partial traumatic metacarpophalangeal amputation of left index finger
S68.122 Partial traumatic metacarpophalangeal amputation of right middle finger

S68.123 **Partial traumatic metacarpophalangeal amputation of left middle finger**
S68.124 **Partial traumatic metacarpophalangeal amputation of right ring finger**
S68.125 **Partial traumatic metacarpophalangeal amputation of left ring finger**
S68.126 **Partial traumatic metacarpophalangeal amputation of right little finger**
S68.127 **Partial traumatic metacarpophalangeal amputation of left little finger**
S68.128 **Partial traumatic metacarpophalangeal amputation of other finger**
S68.129 **Partial traumatic metacarpophalangeal amputation of unspecified finger**
S48.911 **Complete traumatic amputation of right shoulder and upper arm, level unspecified**
S48.912 **Complete traumatic amputation of left shoulder and upper arm, level unspecified**
S48.919 **Complete traumatic amputation of unspecified shoulder and upper arm, level unspecified**
S48.921 **Partial traumatic amputation of right shoulder and upper arm, level unspecified**
S48.922 **Partial traumatic amputation of left shoulder and upper arm, level unspecified**
S48.929 **Partial traumatic amputation of unspecified shoulder and upper arm, level unspecified**
S58.011 **Complete traumatic amputation at elbow level, right arm**
S58.012 **Complete traumatic amputation at elbow level, left arm**
S58.019 **Complete traumatic amputation at elbow level, unspecified arm**
S58.021 **Partial traumatic amputation at elbow level, right arm**
S58.022 **Partial traumatic amputation at elbow level, left arm**
S58.029 **Partial traumatic amputation at elbow level, unspecified arm**
S58.111 **Complete traumatic amputation at level between elbow and wrist, right arm**
S58.122 **Complete traumatic amputation at level between elbow and wrist, left arm**
S58.119 **Complete traumatic amputation at level between elbow and wrist, unspecified arm**
T87.9 **Unspecified complication of amputation stump**
T14.8 **Other injury of unspecified body region**
T87.30 **Neuroma of amputation stump, unspecified extremity**
T87.31 **Neuroma of amputation stump, right upper extremity**
T87.32 **Neuroma of amputation stump, left upper extremity**
T87.33 **Neuroma of amputation stump, right lower extremity**
T87.34 **Neuroma of amputation stump, left lower extremity**
T87.40 **Infection of amputation stump, unspecified extremity**
Z44.9 **Encounter for fitting and adjustment of unspecified external prosthetic device**
Z44.011 **Encounter for fitting and adjustment of complete right artificial arm**
Z44.012 **Encounter for fitting and adjustment of complete left artificial arm**
Z44.019 **Encounter for fitting and adjustment of complete artificial unspecified arm**
Z44.021 **Encounter for fitting and adjustment of partial artificial right arm**
Z44.022 **Encounter for fitting and adjustment of partial artificial left arm**
Z44.029 **Encounter for fitting and adjustment of partial artificial unspecified arm**

Definition

Upper limb amputations are devastating occurrences for individuals, with profound functional and vocational consequences. In the United States, overall, there are approximately 1.7 million people living with a limb loss, or approximately 1 of every 200 people [1]. In contrast to lower limb loss, upper extremity amputation is much less frequent, affecting approximately 41,000 persons, or about 3% of the U.S. amputee population [2]. The primary reason for upper limb loss is trauma; cancer is the next most common reason [2–4]. The rates for traumatic amputations declined by 50% during the period 1988 to 1996 [3], probably because of changing work force patterns and greater concerns for industrial safety. However, as a result of the recent wars in Afghanistan and Iraq, the number of catastrophic injuries due to explosive devices has increased [5]. Traumatic amputation is the major reason for upper extremity loss in the military [5]. As of September 2010, 21% of major limb loss sustained in Operation New Dawn, Operation Iraqi Freedom, and Operation Enduring Freedom involved the upper extremity [5,6]. As of September 2010, there were 1219 major limb and 399 partial limb amputations [6].

Upper limb amputations from trauma occur at a rate of 3.8 individuals per 100,000; finger amputations are the most common (2.8 per 100,000). Hand amputations from trauma occur at a rate of 0.02 per 100,000 [3]. Traumatic transradial amputations occur at a rate of 0.16 per 100,000 persons, and transhumeral limb loss from trauma occurs at a rate of 0.1 per 100,000 [3].

Limb amputations that result from malignant neoplasms have declined approximately 42% from 1988 to 1996 [3]. Their rates of occurrence are lower than for trauma, with an upper limb loss rate in 1996 of 0.09 per 100,000 [3]. These rates of upper limb amputations are lower than the incidence rates of lower limb dysvascular amputations due to diabetes and peripheral arterial diseases, which occur in 45 per 100,000 individuals and disproportionately affect minority individuals [3,7].

In an analysis of the National Trauma database between the years 2000 and 2004, upper limb amputations were more likely to be seen than lower limb amputations in motor vehicle crashes. Motorcyclists and pedestrians were more likely to sustain a lower limb amputation [8]. Machinery, power tools, explosions, self-inflicted injury and assaults, and power tools are among the most common reasons for traumatic upper limb amputations [8]. Electrical burn is an uncommon cause of upper extremity amputation. Heating causes coagulative necrosis, and the passage of the electrical current through the tissues causes disruption of cell membranes [9]. Men are at far greater risk for traumatic amputation than women are, demonstrating about 6.6 times the female rate for minor amputations of the finger and hand [4].

Traumatic amputations often result in irregularly shaped residual limbs and frequently require skin grafts. Efforts to reduce edema and to promote proper limb shaping should be instituted as soon as possible [10]. The level of amputation is the single most important determinant of function after amputation. The primary surgical principle is to save as much limb as possible while ensuring removal of devitalized tissues and residual limb wound healing. Saving of the most distal joint possible dramatically improves the amputee's function. The elbow joint, for instance, when it is preserved, allows the arm to function in carrying and supporting activities. For the mangled hand, saving of any fingers or remnants provides reconstructive hand surgeons the possibility of constructing a hand that can perform grasping activities.

Rates of prosthetic rejection are high among upper limb amputees [5]. Persons sustaining upper limb amputations present complex rehabilitative needs that are ideally best managed by a rehabilitation center with therapists, prosthetists, and physicians possessing specialized knowledge and experience. Proper rehabilitation and a comfortable and functional prosthesis will facilitate functional restoration. Vocational counseling and vocational retraining are vital aspects of any program as this condition often afflicts young, vocationally productive persons, primarily men. A continuum of care is vital to successful rehabilitation. Patients must be transitioned effectively from the inpatient postsurgical unit, sometimes to an inpatient rehabilitation unit and always to a long-term outpatient rehabilitation and prosthetic program.

Symptoms

Congenital upper limb amputees may report no specific symptoms except the lack of full upper extremity function. In contrast, traumatic upper limb amputees may describe phantom pain (pain perceived in the missing part of the limb) or phantom sensation (nonpainful perceptions of the missing part of the limb). Discomfort with prosthetic fit or skin breakdown on the residual limb may be reported in prosthetic users.

Physical Examination

Upper limb amputees require a thorough musculoskeletal examination that includes muscle strength testing, sensory testing, and examination of the contralateral limb. Examination of the residual limb should assess for areas of skin breakdown, redness, painful neuroma, and volume changes that could affect prosthetic fit. Persons with traumatic amputations of the upper limb can have brachial plexus injuries or rotator cuff tears that weaken the residual upper limb muscles. Insensate skin can predispose a patient to breakdown at the site of contact with a prosthesis. Joint range of motion should be assessed. In particular, the scapulothoracic motion is important as protraction of the scapulae provides the force for a dual-control cable system for body-powered prostheses. Reduced elbow or shoulder range of motion from heterotopic ossification, joint capsule contracture, or muscle contracture can impede maximum recovery of function or use of a prosthesis.

Functional Limitations

An upper limb amputee's functional status depends on the level of amputation. Persons with finger loss (not including the thumb) are quite functional without a prosthesis. Persons with thumb amputations lose the ability to grip large objects as well as fine motor skills that require opposition with another finger. Reconstructive surgery by pollicization with another remaining finger dramatically improves hand function.

Transradial and transhumeral amputees lose hand function and have limitations in basic and higher level activities of daily living, such as dressing. Jang and colleagues [11] surveyed upper extremity amputees regarding the impact on activities of daily living. Subjects reported difficulty with complex tasks and either changed jobs or became unemployed. The most common difficulties in daily living were lacing shoes, using scissors, and removing bottle tops [11]. Upper limb amputees frequently sustain new vocational limitations that can preclude return to their previous work activities. Most persons can adapt to almost all basic daily activities with use of the intact contralateral hand and upper limb.

Prosthetic devices may or may not improve function. Some amputees find upper limb prosthetic devices cumbersome, discarding their use altogether. Datta and colleagues [12] found a 73.2% return to work rate after upper limb amputation, although 66.6% had to change jobs. The overall rejection rate of the prosthesis in this study population of predominantly traumatic upper limb amputees was about 34%. The vast majority used the prosthesis primarily for cosmesis; 25% of patients reported that the prosthesis was beneficial for driving, and a small proportion used it for employment and recreational activities. Some amputees require a specialized prosthesis to continue their specific work-related activities. Recreational activities such as golf, tennis, and other sports can often be accomplished with the use of adaptive prosthetic devices designed for these specific purposes. Return after amputation to such enjoyable pursuits can be quite therapeutic.

Diagnostic Testing

No special diagnostic testing is generally required beyond a careful physical examination. If there is weakness of the limb, electrodiagnostic testing may clarify whether a plexopathy is also present. Radiographs may be necessary to evaluate for osteomyelitis, heterotopic ossification, or a bone spur in the distal limb causing poor prosthetic fit. If myoelectric prostheses are considered, electromyographic signals and voluntary control of key muscles can be tested by a specialized therapist to determine if such control is possible and to train the amputee to independently use these potential control muscles.

Treatment

Initial

Management of persons with upper limb amputations involves a continuum of care [3,10,13–16]. This begins with provision of preoperative information when the amputation is elective, as in the case of cancer. The overriding concern in planning the amputation is to save all possible length, particularly the elbow joint. This preserves elbow flexion and prevents the need for a dual-control cable system. The early input of a physiatrist, nurse, and physical or occupational therapist with expertise in this area is highly advantageous. Early involvement of the rehabilitation team can provide helpful information about prosthetic options, the rehabilitation continuum, and what can be expected after amputation (such as phantom sensations).

Rehabilitation

Initial Rehabilitation Care

Immediately after amputation, the primary goals are wound healing, edema control, and prevention of contractures and deconditioning. Persons sustaining upper limb amputations due to trauma or cancer generally have normal underlying blood supply, and most surgical sites can readily heal. Edema is prevented by use of a shrinker sock, elastic bandage wrapping with a figure-of-eight technique that provides pressure distally without choking the limb, or a rigid dressing system. In sophisticated centers, immediate postoperative prosthesis fitting in the operating room is implemented. The immediate postoperative prosthesis is placed over the limb after padding of the skin with soft dressings. The immediate postoperative prosthesis accommodates surgical drains yet prevents the formation of edema. Prosthetic components can be attached to the immediate postoperative prosthesis and early training implemented.

Postoperative early identification and treatment of adherent scar tissue are important. Scar can form between skin, muscle, and bone. These adherences can cause pain when muscles are contracted or a joint is moved during operation of the prosthesis [17].

Residual limb pain and phantom pain are two conditions that can affect patients with upper limb amputations [14]. Phantom sensations are common; yet fortunately, disabling phantom pain occurs in only about 5% of amputees [13]. Despite the many interventions used for phantom pain, there are no uniformly effective treatments [13,15]. Medication and physical modalities must be tried in a rational fashion to determine the most effective intervention. Physical modalities include a transcutaneous electrical nerve stimulation unit, physical manipulation, and massage of the residual limb [13]. Fitting of a comfortable prosthesis can often help reduce these painful sensations.

Neuromodulating medications, such as tricyclic antidepressants and antiepileptics (gabapentin and pregabalin), are frequently used with variable results [13,15]. Beta blockers (propranolol and atenolol) have been found to be somewhat effective in treating phantom pain [13]. If patients require cardiac or hypertension medications, the choice of a beta blocker may serve two purposes for these amputees with phantom pain.

Opiates may be effective for these problems when other methods fail to relieve phantom pain [15]. If it is anticipated that the person with phantom pain will need analgesia for a long period, long-acting opiates should be used. Longer acting opiates have less habituation and addiction potential. Most amputees with phantom pain have intermittent severe pain that can be treated with small doses on an as-needed basis of a short-acting opiate, such as oxycodone. For the few patients with severe, unremitting, phantom and residual limb pain, referral to a specialized pain center is suggested.

Rehabilitative and Prosthetic Management

Prevention of contractures in the residual limb and prevention of generalized deconditioning are important goals of early rehabilitation. Any other injuries, as are common in persons sustaining severe trauma, should be identified and rehabilitation efforts directed at their remediation. For body-powered prostheses, scapulothoracic motion provides power through a cable system to operate the prosthesis. Therefore, to optimize function, therapeutic exercise to optimize shoulder range of motion and scapular stabilization is important. Likewise, elbow contractures or shoulder contractures or capsulitis will severely impede maximal prosthetic use, and these problems should be aggressively addressed. Early training in activity of daily living skills should be pursued as well. Therapies should be directed toward amelioration of weakness through exercises or of contractures through active-assisted range of motion exercises and prolonged stretching.

A detailed discussion of prosthetic devices is beyond the scope of this chapter, and consultation with a skilled prosthetist and physiatrist is desirable. Prostheses can serve a cosmetic (passive) role or a functional role, or both [18]. In general, there are two types, body-powered and myoelectric devices [3,16,18]. Body-powered prostheses enable an amputee to harness residual body movements to generate controlled movement and force of a terminal device [18]. Body-powered devices are usually less cosmetic and associated with limited range of motion and limited prehensile strength, yet they are less expensive and much more durable [18]. Myoelectric prostheses are controlled by electrical signals generated in muscles from the remaining residual limb or shoulder girdle. Myoelectric prosthetic devices extract signals from remaining muscles under voluntary control to activate and to control drive motors in the prosthesis [19]. These devices are expensive, and special prosthetic skills are required to fabricate and to maintain them, but they are generally more cosmetic in appearance and well suited for selected patients. Prosthetic functional outcomes depend on an individual's goals related to cosmesis, function, and psychological factors [17]. Prosthetic prescription should also consider an individual's level of cognitive functioning and ability to learn to operate a device. Skin breakdown can occur over bone prominences, where there are skin grafts, or where skin is adherent to underlying bone. Alteration of the prosthetic socket and suspension systems or temporary discontinuation of prosthetic use until the skin has healed may be necessary.

To meet the needs of military amputees, the Defense Advanced Research Projects Agency (DARPA) has funded development of two advanced upper limb prosthetic solutions. One of the technologies uses neural control; the other, DEKA arm, uses a "strap and go" system that can be controlled by noninvasive means [5]. Implementation of advanced technology requires a coordinated approach using multiple members of the rehabilitation team. Success is largely contingent on the availability of highly trained and specialized personnel to fit and train amputees and resources to pay for these services [5]. Telemedicine may help overcome some of these barriers. The field of upper extremity prosthetics is changing with the development of implantable neurologic sensing devices and targeted muscle innervation. Targeted motor reinnervation incorporates the transfer of residual peripheral nerves into muscles in or near the residual limb, with subsequent reinnervation of those muscles. By use of these surface electromyographic signals that relate directly to the original function of the limb, control of the externally powered prosthesis occurs [20]. Multidextrous terminal devices may soon be available [17].

Procedures

Most procedures related to the care of upper extremity amputees focus on pain management techniques, such as injection of local anesthetic around a painful neuroma, nerve blocks, massage, or chiropractic manipulation. Acupuncture, hypnosis, and biofeedback have also been used in the management of phantom limb pain with variable success [15].

Surgery

Revision surgeries are sometimes necessary to remove bone spurs that interfere with prosthetic fitting. The initial surgery should spare all length possible, particularly the elbow joint. A well-healed surgical site with good distal soft tissue coverage of the bone end is an optimal result that facilitates prosthetic use. In addition, surgical treatment of adherent scar tissue may be necessary to improve function of a prosthesis. In a study of combat-related upper extremity amputations, 42% underwent revision surgery. The most common indications for revision surgery, in order of decreasing frequency, are heterotopic ossification excision, wound infection, neuroma excision, wound dehiscence, scar revision, and contracture release. In the group that underwent revision surgery, regular prosthesis use increased from 19% before the revision to 87% after it [21].

Potential Disease Complications

As a result of the upper limb amputation, residual limb pain, including severe phantom pain, can occur. Joint contractures can develop in the remaining part of the limb, as can frozen shoulder and adhesive capsulitis. This is a particular concern with coexistent peripheral nerve or brachial plexus injury. Self-reported musculoskeletal pain is more frequent in upper limb amputees than in controls, frequently located in the neck, upper back, and shoulder region [22].

Depression brought on by the difficulties of adjusting to limb loss is reported. Psychological counseling and support groups incorporating peer support are valuable resources.

Potential Treatment Complications

Surgical complications include postoperative wound infections and postoperative failure of the surgical wounds to heal. Neuroma formation can occur after transection of a nerve. Burying the nerve ending under large soft tissue masses may reduce the likelihood of neuroma irritation.

Many medications used in the treatment of phantom pain associated with amputations have potential side effects, including dry mouth, constipation, weight gain, mental cloudiness, cardiovascular effects, and addiction. The side effect profiles vary by the medication class and dosage.

Skin breakdown from a poorly fitting prosthesis can occur. This can be aggravated by hyperhidrosis, folliculitis, or poor hygiene.

Overuse injuries in the nonamputated limb reportedly are higher than expected in the normal population [12]. These include repetitive strain-type injuries due to the individual's performing certain tasks with poor body posture and ergonomics [23].

References

[1] National Limb Loss Information Center. Amputation statistics by cause. Limb loss in the United States. NLLIC fact sheet; 2008. http://www.amputee-coalition.org/fact_sheets/amp_stats_cause.pdf [accessed 07.10.12].

[2] Ziegler-Graham K, MacKenzie EJ, Ephraim PL, et al. Estimating the prevalence of limb loss in the United States: 2005–2050. Arch Phys Med Rehabil 2008;89:422–9.

[3] Dillingham TR, Pezzin LE, MacKenzie EJ. Limb amputation and limb deficiency: epidemiology and recent trends in the United States. South Med J 2002;95:875–83.

[4] Dillingham TR, Pezzin LE, MacKenzie EJ. Incidence, acute care length of stay, and discharge to rehabilitation of traumatic amputee patients: an epidemiologic study. Arch Phys Med Rehabil 1998;79:279–87.

[5] Resnik L, Meucci MR, Lieberman-Klinger S, et al. Advanced upper limb prosthetic devices: implications for upper limb prosthetic rehabilitation. Arch Phys Med Rehabil 2012;93:710–7.

[6] Fischer H. CRS report to Congress. U.S. military casualty statistics: Operation New Dawn, Operation Iraqi Freedom, and Operation Enduring Freedom. http://www.fas.org/sgp/crs/natsec/RS22452.pdf [accessed 07.10.12].

[7] Dillingham TR, Pezzin LE, MacKenzie EJ. Racial differences in the incidence of limb loss secondary to peripheral vascular disease: a population-based study. Arch Phys Med Rehabil 2002;83:1252–7.

[8] Barmparas G, Inaba K, Teixeira P, et al. Epidemiology of post-traumatic limb amputation: a national trauma databank analysis. Am Surg 2010;76:1214–22.

[9] Tarim A, Ezer A. Electrical burn is still a major risk factor for amputations. Burns 2013;39:354–7. http://dx.doi.org/10.1016/j.burns.2012.06.012, Published online August 1, 2012. Accessed October 3, 2012.

[10] Nelson VS, Flood KM, Bryant PR, et al. Limb deficiency and prosthetic management. 1. Decision making in prosthetic prescription and management. Arch Phys Med Rehabil 2006;87:S3–9.

[11] Jang CH, Yang HE, Yang HE, et al. A survey on activities of daily living and occupations of upper extremity amputees. Ann Rehabil Med 2011;35:907–21.

[12] Datta D, Selvarajah K, Davey N. Functional outcome of patients with proximal upper limb deficiency—acquired and congenital. Clin Rehabil 2004;18:172–7.

[13] Vaida G, Friedmann LW. Postamputation phantoms: a review. Phys Med Rehabil Clin N Am 1991;2:325–53.

[14] Roberts TL, Pasquina PF, Nelson VS, et al. Limb deficiency and prosthetic management. 4. Comorbidities associated with limb loss. Arch Phys Med Rehabil 2006;87:S21–7.

[15] Hanley MA, Ehde DM, Campbell KM, et al. Self-reported treatments used for lower-limb phantom pain: descriptive findings. Arch Phys Med Rehabil 2006;87:270–7.

[16] Dillingham TR. Rehabilitation of the upper limb amputee. In: Dillingham TR, Belandres P, editors. Rehabilitation of the injured combatant. Washington, DC: Office of the Surgeon General; 1998. p. 33–77.

[17] Lake C, Dodson R. Progressive upper limb prosthetics. Phys Med Rehabil Clin N Am 2006;17:49–72.

[18] Behrend C, Reizner W, Marchessault J, Hammert W. Update on advances in upper extremity prosthetics. J Hand Surg [Am] 2011;36:1711–7.

[19] Dawson M, Carey J, Fahimi F. Myoelectric training systems. Expert Rev Med Devices 2011;8:581–9.

[20] Kuiken T. Targeted reinnervation for improved prosthetic function. Phys Med Rehabil Clin N Am 2006;17:1–13.

[21] Tintle S, Baechler M, Nanos G, et al. Reoperations following combat-related upper-extremity amputations. J Bone Joint Surg Am 2012;94:e1191–6.

[22] Ostlie K, Franklin RJ, Skjeldal OH, et al. Musculoskeletal pain and overuse syndromes in adult acquired major upper-limb amputees. Arch Phys Med Rehabil 2011;92:1967–73.

[23] Jones LE, Davidson JH. Save the arm: a study of problems in the remaining arm of unilateral upper limb amputees. Prosthet Orthot Int 1999;23:55–8.

CHAPTER 119

Lower Limb Amputations

Michelle Gittler, MD

Synonyms

Below-knee amputation—transtibial amputation
Above-knee amputation—transfemoral amputation
Syme amputation (foot disarticulation)
Neuropathic pain—dysesthetic pain
Residual limb—stump

ICD-9 Codes

353.6 Phantom limb (syndrome)
718.45 Joint contracture (hip), pelvis and thigh
718.46 Joint contracture (knee), lower leg
719.7 Difficulty walking (ankle and foot)
Note: all 89_ codes are for traumatic amputations
895 Traumatic amputation of toe(s) (complete) (partial)
895.0 Without mention of complication
895.1 Complicated
896 Traumatic amputation of foot (complete) (partial)
896.0 Unilateral, without mention of complication
896.1 Unilateral, complicated
896.2 Bilateral, without mention of complication
896.3 Bilateral, complicated
897 Traumatic amputation of leg(s) (complete) (partial)
897.0 Unilateral, below knee, without mention of complication
897.1 Unilateral, below knee, complicated
897.2 Unilateral, at or above knee, without mention of complication
897.3 Unilateral, at or above knee, complicated
897.4 Unilateral, level not specified, without mention of complication
897.5 Unilateral, level not specified, complicated
897.6 Bilateral (any level), without mention of complication
897.7 Bilateral (any level), complicated
905.9 Late effect of traumatic amputation
997.60 Amputation stump complication, unspecified
997.61 Neuroma of amputation stump
997.62 Infection (chronic)
V52 Fitting and adjustment of prosthetic device and implant
V52.1 Artificial leg (complete) (partial)
V49.70 Unspecified level lower limb amputation
V49.75 Below knee amputation status
V49.76 Above knee amputation status

ICD-10 Codes

G54.7 Phantom limb syndrome with pain
G54.6 Phantom limb syndrome without pain
M24.551 Contracture, right hip
M24.552 Contracture, left hip
M24.559 Contracture, unspecified hip
M24.561 Contracture, right knee
M24.562 Contracture, left knee
M24.569 Contracture, unspecified knee
R26.2 Difficulty walking
S98.131 Complete traumatic amputation of one right lesser toe
S98.132 Complete traumatic amputation of one left lesser toe
S98.139 Complete traumatic amputation of one unspecified lesser toe
S98.141 Partial traumatic amputation of one right lesser toe

S98.142 Partial traumatic amputation of one left lesser toe
S98.149 Partial traumatic amputation of one unspecified lesser toe
S98.911 Unspecified injury of right ankle
S98.912 Unspecified injury of left ankle
S98.919 Unspecified injury of unspecified ankle
S98.921 Unspecified injury of right foot
S98.922 Unspecified injury of left foot
S98.929 Unspecified injury of unspecified foot
S88.911 Complete traumatic amputation of right lower leg, level unspecified
S88.912 Complete traumatic amputation of left lower leg, level unspecified
S88.919 Complete traumatic amputation of unspecified lower leg, level unspecified
S88.921 Partial traumatic amputation of right lower leg, level unspecified
S88.922 Partial traumatic amputation of left lower leg, level unspecified
S88.929 Partial traumatic amputation of unspecified leg, level unspecified
S88.111 Complete traumatic amputation at level between knee and ankle, right lower leg
S88.112 Complete traumatic amputation at level between knee and ankle, left lower leg
S88.119 Complete traumatic amputation at level between knee and ankle, unspecified lower leg
S88.121 Partial traumatic amputation at level between knee and ankle, right lower leg
S88.122 Partial traumatic amputation at level between knee and ankle, left lower leg
S88.129 Partial traumatic amputation at level between knee and ankle, unspecified lower leg
S88.011 Complete traumatic amputation at knee level, right lower leg
S88.012 Complete traumatic amputation at knee level, left lower leg
S88.019 Complete traumatic amputation at knee level, unspecified leg
S88.021 Partial traumatic amputation at knee level, right lower leg
S88.022 Partial traumatic amputation at knee level, left lower leg
S88.029 Partial traumatic amputation at knee level, unspecified lower leg
T87.40 Infection of amputation stump, unspecified extremity
T87.30 Neuroma of amputation stump, unspecified extremity
T87.31 Neuroma of amputation stump, right upper extremity
T87.32 Neuroma of amputation stump, left upper extremity
T87.33 Neuroma of amputation stump, right lower extremity
T87.34 Neuroma of amputation stump, left lower extremity
Z44.9 Encounter for fitting and adjustment of unspecified external prosthetic device
Z89.511 Acquired absence of right leg below knee
Z89.512 Acquired absence of left leg below knee
Z89.519 Acquired absence of unspecified leg below knee
Z89.611 Acquired absence of right leg above knee
Z89.612 Acquired absence of left leg above knee
Z89.619 Acquired absence of unspecified leg above knee

Definition

In 2005, an estimated 1.6 million persons in the United States were living with loss of a limb, of whom 65% have had a lower limb amputation [1]. Vascular conditions account for most cases of amputation (54%), with two thirds of these having a secondary diagnosis of diabetes [2]. Lower limb amputations account for 97% of all dysvascular amputations. More than half of dysvascular amputations are major lower limb amputations (transfemoral, 25.8%; transtibial, 27.6%) [2,3]; 42.8% involve other levels (ray, toes). Most of these amputations occur in people aged 60 years and older. There are approximately 82,000 nontraumatic diabetes-related lower extremity amputations each year [3]. Trauma is the next most common cause of lower extremity amputation (22%), followed by tumors (5%). However, in children aged 10 to 20 years, tumor is the most common cause of both upper and lower extremity amputations. Male amputees outnumber female amputees 2.1:1 in disease and 7.2:1 in trauma [4]. Across all causes, 42% of the persons living with the loss of a limb are 65 years or older; 65% are men, and 42% are nonwhite [2].

Symptoms

The postoperative or post-traumatic sequela of an amputation is that the patient is missing all or part of a limb. In addition, there may be associated symptoms, such as phantom limb sensation, phantom pain, stump pain, and pain from the surgery itself.

Phantom limb sensation is the perception that the extremity is still present and occasionally distorted in position. Phantom limb sensation typically fades away within the first year after amputation, usually in a "telescoping" phenomenon. This includes the perception that the distal aspect of the limb (that is, the foot) is moving closer and closer to the site of amputation.

Phantom limb pain is differentiated as a painful perception within the absent body part. The incidence of phantom limb pain is variable and has been reported from 0.5% to virtually 100% of persons with amputations. This variability is due to differences in study methods and population. The most recent studies suggest that up to 85% of people with amputations will experience phantom pain [5]. Patients may describe the pain in the absent foot or the absent limb as cramping, stabbing, burning, or icy cold.

Pain at the surgical site is common and should resolve within a few weeks of surgery. Residual limb pain is perceived in the residual limb in the region of the amputation. The incidence of residual limb pain has been reported between 10% and 25%; it may be diffuse or focal and is commonly associated with neuroma, which is palpable around the amputation site.

Physical Examination

Wound healing, range of motion, muscle strength, and incisional integrity must be evaluated in the residual limb. Upper extremity strength should be assessed to determine capability for use of assistive devices.

Visualization of the contralateral foot is a mandatory component of the examination. The unaffected foot is assessed for areas of potential breakdown. These include the plantar surface of the foot, web spaces, and areas of bone prominence.

Skin breakdown in the residual limb is typically a result of pressure or shear forces in the healed limb. Skin necrosis may be evidence of ischemia with need for surgical revision. Skin breakdown can be manifested as abrasions from tape or the unraveling of an elastic wrap or be true partial- or full-thickness (pressure) sores. Pressure sore phenomenon typically occurs at bone prominences. The fibular head, hamstring tendons, patellar tendon, medial and lateral femoral condyles, and anterior distal tibia should routinely be examined for skin breakdown.

Joint contractures are a loss of full range of motion at a joint. They may be conceptualized as functional or mechanical. Functional contractures are the result of (inappropriate) positioning. A transtibial amputee may develop knee or hip flexion contractures merely by sitting with the hip flexed and the knee flexed at 90 degrees (the knee and hip extensors remain intact but are not being used). A mechanical contracture may result from unopposed muscle action. In the transfemoral amputee, the insertion of the hip adductors is sacrificed and the unopposed (and firmly attached) hip abductors may result in an abduction contracture.

The transtibial and Syme amputee requires evaluation of range of motion of the knee in flexion and extension. Medial and lateral knee stability must also be assessed. For successful ambulation with a prosthesis, knee extension muscle strength should be graded at least higher than 4/5. A knee flexion contracture of 10 degrees up to 18 degrees can usually be accommodated in a transtibial prosthesis; however, the absence of limb contractures is related to better success in prosthetic ambulation [6]. A contracture of more than 20 degrees requires that the individual ambulate with a bent socket, weight bearing through the knee.

In the transfemoral (above-knee) amputee, the range of motion evaluation should include hip flexion, hip extension, hip adduction, and hip abduction. A transfemoral prosthesis can functionally accommodate up to a 20-degree hip flexion contracture; a contracture of more than this makes prosthetic fitting and successful ambulation less likely. Strength should also be assessed, and grades of 4/5 or higher in muscles responsible for hip flexion-extension and abduction are required for ambulation.

Stump or residual limb pain is assessed first by inspection. Areas of obvious necrosis indicating poor blood flow may require surgical débridement. Nonhealing incisions are manifestations of ischemia, underlying hematoma, or abscess. The surrounding area should be palpated and assessed for induration and discharge. An attempt should be made to "milk" fluctuance, and drainage should be sent for Gram stain and culture. Sutures (if present) may need to be removed to facilitate evacuation of the abscess or hematoma. In some instances, the incision may need to be reopened for drainage and healing to take place.

Stump pain without signs or symptoms of infection should be evaluated for neuroma (palpation along the anatomic course of the sciatic nerve). Stump pain with or without skin breakdown may also be due to poor prosthetic fit, so the fit of the prosthesis ought to be evaluated, preferably with a prosthetist present. Nonblanchable erythema is a pressure sore until proved otherwise, and the prosthesis should not be worn until appropriate adjustments are made. Bruising at the distal aspect of the stump in the prosthetic wearer is indicative of a poor prosthetic fit. That is, the residual limb may be falling too deeply into the socket. Similarly, a choke phenomenon occurs with lack of total contact or inability to get the residual limb all the way into the socket. This can progress to verrucous hyperplasia, which predisposes the individual to fissuring and infection.

Gait evaluation with the prosthesis should be performed with an appropriate assistive device. Observed gait deviations should be communicated to the prosthetist for prosthesis modifications and to the therapist for focused gait training.

Functional Limitations

Functional limitations are largely dependent on the premorbid status of the individual. Ambulation with one limb or hopping (with a walker or crutches) requires approximately 60% increased energy over normal human locomotion. The energy cost of ambulation with a prosthesis varies. In the diabetic or dysvascular amputee, it approaches 38% to 60% increased energy for a below-knee amputee and 52% to 116% higher for an above-knee amputee [2,6]. An otherwise healthy person who has sustained a traumatic limb amputation or an individual who had been ambulating with crutches or another assistive device before having an amputation (often because of non–weight-bearing status on the affected limb) will probably be discharged from the acute care setting to home with outpatient services, at an "ambulatory" level with the appropriate assistive device; the energy expenditure will be less than that of a dysvascular amputee.

An older individual or person with multiple comorbidities should be encouraged to pursue functional independence by optimizing wheelchair mobility and transfers when there is inadequate cardiopulmonary reserve to ambulate with an assistive device [7]. This person may have had an acute or subacute rehabilitation hospital stay after the acute care hospitalization.

Functional limitations due to pain are associated with an inability to participate in ongoing activities of daily living. In general, symptoms of phantom sensation tend not to be an issue, whereas phantom pain can be severely limiting, preventing a person from participating in pre-prosthetic and prosthetic rehabilitation. Functional limitations related to stump or residual limb pain include the inability to tolerate stump shrinkage by appropriate modalities and an inability to tolerate gait training with a prosthesis. To accommodate stump pain, the patient may develop gait deviations to decrease pressure under the residual limb.

Individuals with significantly impaired cardiac output may not be able to perform pre-prosthetic training with a walker (or crutches). These patients may not be prosthetic candidates at all because of the increased energy demands of prosthetic ambulation [6]. Coronary artery calcification scores were very high in amputees compared with Framingham Risk Score–matched control groups. This suggested moderate to extensive coronary artery disease in more than two thirds of amputees studied. It may be relevant to carefully evaluate amputees for asymptomatic coronary artery disease and to consider prophylactic revascularization [8]. Keep in mind that individuals with preexisting amputations who undergo coronary artery bypass grafting will not be able to use an assistive device postoperatively (maintenance of sternal precautions), and alternative mobility options (e.g., power wheelchair) should be considered.

Rates of clinical depression range from 18% to 35% among amputees. Those with amputation-related pain are more prone to depression. Depression should be differentiated from the grief response and postoperative adjustment period [9].

Diagnostic Studies

The individual with phantom limb pain may benefit from diagnostic as well as therapeutic sympathetic nerve block. On occasion, electrodiagnostic tests (electromyography and nerve conduction studies) are helpful to differentiate symptoms of radiculopathy or other disease in the phantom limb.

In the younger amputee, it is occasionally necessary to obtain plain radiographs of the residual limb to assess the bone overgrowth. This is typically visually evident on inspection; the radiograph confirms the extent of overgrowth.

The individual with new amputation secondary to peripheral vascular disease may require cardiac evaluation to establish parameters for an exercise prescription.

Differential Diagnosis

Secondary conditions related to residual limb
Edema
Neuroma
Incision
  Postsurgical
  Infection
Bone overgrowth
Ischemia
Phantom pain
Sympathetic pain
Radiculopathy
Ischemia

Treatment

Initial

Initial treatment focuses on edema control and shaping of the residual limb as well as wound healing, prevention of contractures, and pain management. Options for edema control are listed in Table 119.1 [10,11].

Patients with a transtibial amputation have the potential for knee flexion and hip flexion contractures as a result of positioning (usually, sitting in a wheelchair or in bed). Therefore, avoidance of pillows under the knee and promotion of lying prone in bed can be helpful.

Persons with a transfemoral amputation may also develop hip flexion contractures as a result of sitting. In addition, there is the tendency for development of hip abduction contractures, so positioning of the hip in relative adduction, avoidance of pillows under the residual limb, and promotion of the prone position are essential.

Phantom sensation is not typically painful, although it can be frightening or disorienting for the patient. The best treatment is to reassure the patient that this is a normal reaction after amputation. Education and reassurance of the patient as well as ongoing tactile input (i.e., massaging the distal residual limb and using the limb) will enhance the accommodation to phantom sensation. There are many proposed treatments of phantom pain; however, there is no one definitive treatment that seems to work best. Initial pharmacologic intervention includes non-narcotic and narcotic analgesics; nonsteroidal anti-inflammatory drugs; anticonvulsants and membrane stabilizers, particularly gabapentin, duloxetine, and pregabalin; and tricyclic antidepressants [9].

Rehabilitation

Pre-prosthetic training focuses on functional independence in mobility and self-care from the ambulatory (single limb) or wheelchair level, avoidance of hip and knee contractures, and residual limb management. Prosthetic training is initiated once the residual limb is ready—the edema is resolved and the incision has healed; the prosthesis is then fabricated. A description of prostheses is beyond the scope of this chapter; however, the reader is referred to one of several texts on prosthetic components and prescription [12,13]. K levels are used by Medicare to determine an individual's functional potential and thus to justify prosthetic

Table 119.1 Treatment Options for Edema Control

Treatment Options	Advantages	Disadvantages
In a Below-Knee Amputee		
Above-knee cast	Prevents knee flexion contracture Provides protection No patient "skill" or management necessary to remove Very low cost	Bulky, awkward, heavy to move Unable to visualize wound Unable to remove Potential for skin breakdown
"Stump shrinker"	Easy to don and doff Enables visualization of wound Accustoms individual to use of a sock Provides shaping of residual limb	Cost—may need to be replaced after stump has begun to shrink
Rigid removable dressing (Fig. 119.1)	Excellent for preparing residual limb for eventual prosthesis Fosters patient's independence in assessing need for stump socks Good edema management Provides some soft tissue protection Able to view wound	Therapist, physician, and prosthetist must be skilled in fabrication Potential for skin breakdown if applied incorrectly
Elastic bandage (ACE wrap)	Easily available Able to visualize wound Accommodates all shapes and sizes Good edema control	Requires excellent dexterity for patient to don and doff Potential for shear injury if wrap unravels Must be reapplied multiple times a day secondary to potential loosening
In an Above-Knee Amputee		
Stump shrinker, elastic bandage	Same advantages and disadvantages as described for below-knee amputee	

Table 119.2 K Levels

K0 (level 0)	Does not have the ability or potential to ambulate or to transfer safely with or without assistance, and a prosthesis does not enhance the quality of life or mobility
K1 (level 1)	Has the ability or potential to use a prosthesis for transfers or ambulation on level surfaces at fixed cadence—typical of the limited and unlimited household walker
K2 (level 2)	Has the ability or potential for ambulation with the ability to traverse low-level environmental barriers, such as curbs, stairs, or uneven surfaces—typical of the limited community walker
K3 (level 3)	Has the ability or potential for walking with variable cadence—typical of the community walker who is able to traverse most environmental barriers and may have vocational, therapeutic, or exercise activity that demands prosthetic use beyond simple walking
K4 (level 4)	Has the ability or potential for prosthetic use that exceeds basic walking skills, exhibiting high impact, stress, or energy levels—typical of the prosthetic demands of the child, active adult, or athlete

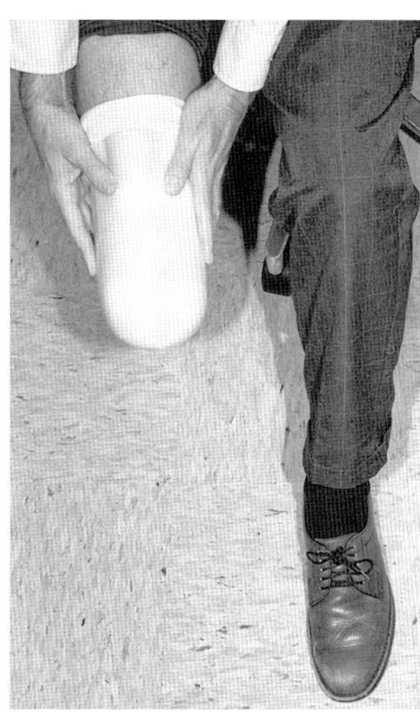

FIGURE 119.1 Application of the removable rigid dressing. *(From Lennard TA. Pain Procedures in Clinical Practice, 2nd ed. Philadelphia, Hanley & Belfus, 2000.)*

components (Table 119.2). When the prosthesis has been fabricated, an outpatient appointment with the ordering physician is scheduled that is attended by the patient and the prosthetist. A basic evaluation of the fit of the prosthesis is conducted, and referral for physical therapy that focuses on prosthetic training is made at that time, or adjustments to the prosthesis are made. The patient must be taught how to put on (don) and take off (doff) the prosthesis as well as when to add socks for a better fit. The patient should also be encouraged to routinely inspect the skin on the residual limb (often done best with a long-handled mirror).

Occupational therapy consists of identifying necessary equipment (e.g., toilet safety frame, tub transfer bench) and establishing independence in self-care from the wheelchair or ambulatory level with use of just the unaffected limb (single-limb stance). Occupational therapy should also be ordered when the patient receives the prosthesis to establish independence in self-care, particularly with lower extremity dressing, toileting, and homemaking while the prosthesis is worn.

Return to driving is an important aspect of functional independence. The majority (80.5%) of prosthetic users with major lower extremity amputations are able to return to automobile driving 3.8 months after amputation. People with left-sided amputations have significantly fewer concerns about driving; those with right-sided amputations may need vehicle modifications (40%) or may need to switch to left-foot driving style [14].

Procedures

Treatment of postamputation phantom pain includes sympathetic blocks, which are typically performed under fluoroscopic guidance. Neuromas, which typically form 1 to 12 months after amputation, may be manifested as a focal soft tissue mass with reproducible pain on palpation. Local anesthetic injection may provide pain relief. Surgical resection is an option but can result in a new (painful) neuroma [15].

Surgery

Surgery is indicated when a residual limb requires wound revision or higher level of amputation. Hamstring releases have a limited role or no role because they would inhibit the ability to walk. There does not appear to be any role for surgical stump revision for treatment of phantom pain.

There are few data to promote dorsal root entry zone ablation, dorsal rhizotomy, dorsal column tractotomy, thalamotomy, or cortical resection in the treatment of phantom pain. A small trial to surgically treat phantom pain locally was performed. The sciatic nerve was split proximal to the popliteal fossa, and the two parts were reconnected in a sling fashion. Of 15 patients, 14 reported that the procedure was "very helpful." [15]

Bone overgrowth develops in 10% to 30% of children with congenital amputations, and this must be addressed surgically. This is much less common in the adult with an acquired amputation.

Potential Disease Complications

The most common complications are dehiscence or breakdown of the incision and nonhealing wounds. Infection or ischemia is the most likely cause of dehiscence or a nonhealing incision. A trial of conservative management including antibiotics (after a culture specimen is obtained) and appropriate local wound care is reasonable. Increasing wound necrosis, foul drainage, and fever or chills warrant reevaluation by the surgeon.

Other potential complications may involve cardiac ischemia as a heretofore inactive (i.e., energy conservative) individual begins using up to 100% more energy for gait training [6]. A reasonable guideline for gait training is assessment of an individual's ability to ambulate with the intact lower extremity with crutches or another assistive device. This consumes approximately 60% more energy than bipedal human locomotion. A person who is not able to gait train (hop on one foot short distances) with use of an assistive device is probably not a potential prosthetic ambulator. Major limb amputation continues to result in significant morbidity and mortality. One-year survival for dysvascular and diabetic individuals is 50.6% for transfemoral amputees and 74.5% for transtibial amputees. Five-year survival is 22.5% and 37.8% (survival in end-stage renal disease is as low as 14% at 5 years after amputation) [2,3].

Potential Treatment Complications

Once the prosthesis has been fabricated, skin breakdown is the most common complication. Breakdown commonly occurs at the distal anterior tibia (clapper-in-bell phenomenon, a result of continued forward motion of the distal residual limb in the socket during swing phase), the hamstring tendons (tight brim), and the patellar tendon.

Patients should be instructed to inspect these areas and immediately report to the prosthetist signs of persistent, nonblanchable erythema. The prosthesis should not be worn until modifications are made.

Medication side effects depend on the particular medication being used as well as potential for drug interactions when multiple medications are being used.

References

[1] Esquenazi A, Yoo SK. Epidemiology and assessment lower limb amputations. Knowledgenow.com. Published November 7, 2012. Accessed Feb. 19, 2014.

[2] Ziegler-Graham K, MacKenzie EJ, Ephraim PL, et al. Estimating the prevalence of limb loss in the United States: 2005-2050. Arch Phys Med Rehabil 2008;89:422–9.

[3] Dillingham TR, Pezzin LE, MacKenzie EJ. Limb amputation and limb deficiency: epidemiology and recent trends in the United States. South Med J 2002;95:875–83.

[4] Leonard EI, McAnelly RD, Lomba M, Faulker VW. Lower limb prosthesis in physical medicine and rehabilitation. In: Braddom RL, editor. Physical medicine and rehabilitation. 2nd ed. Philadelphia: WB Saunders; 2000. p. 279–310.

[5] Ehde DM, Czerniecki JM, Smith DG, et al. Chronic phantom sensations, phantom pain, residual limb pain, and other regional pain after lower limb amputation. Arch Phys Med Rehabil 2000;81:1039–44.

[6] Friedan RA, Brar AK, Esquinazi A. Fitting an older patient with medical comorbidities with a lower limb prosthesis. PM R 2012;4:59–64.

[7] Morgenroth DC, Czerniecki JM. The complexities surrounding decisions related to prosthetic fitting in elderly dysvascular amputees [letter]. PM R 2012;4:540–2.

[8] Nallegowda M, Lee E, Brandstater M, et al. Amputation and cardiac comorbidity: analysis of severity of cardiac risk. PM R 2012;4:657–66.

[9] Roberts TL, Pasquina PF, Nelson VS, et al. Limb deficiency and prosthetic management. 4. Comorbidities associated with limb loss. Arch Phys Med Rehabil 2006;87:S21–7.

[10] Mueller MS. Comparison of rigid removable dressings and elastic bandages in preprosthetic management of patients with below-knee amputations. Phys Ther 1982;62:1438–41.

[11] Wu Y, Krick H. Rigid removable dressings for below knee amputees. Clin Prosthet Orthot 1987;11:33–44.

[12] Nelson VS, Flood KM, Bryant PR, et al. Limb deficiency and prosthetic management. 1. Decision making in prosthetic prescription and management. Arch Phys Med Rehabil 2006;87:S3–9.

[13] Walsh NE, Bosker G, Santa Maria D. Upper and lower extremity prosthetics. In: Frontera WR, editor. DeLisa's physical medicine and rehabilitation: principles and practice. 5th ed. Philadelphia: Lippincott Williams & Wilkins; 2010. p. 2017–49.

[14] Boulias C, Meikle B, Pauley T, Devlin M. Return to driving after lower extremity amputation. Arch Phys Med Rehabil 2006;87:1183–8.

[15] Prantl L, Schreml S, Heine N, et al. Surgical treatment of chronic phantom limb sensation and limb pain after lower limb amputation. Plast Reconstr Surg 2006;118:1562–72.

CHAPTER 120

Ankylosing Spondylitis

George W. Deimel IV, MD
Steven E. Braverman, MD

Synonyms

Seronegative spondyloarthropathy
Seronegative arthritis
Seronegative spondylarthritides

ICD-9 Code

720.0 Ankylosing spondylitis

ICD-10 Codes

M45.0 Ankylosing spondylitis of multiple sites in spine
M45.1 Ankylosing spondylitis of occipito-atlanto-axial region
M45.2 Ankylosing spondylitis of cervical region
M45.3 Ankylosing spondylitis of cervicothoracic region
M45.4 Ankylosing spondylitis of thoracic region
M45.5 Ankylosing spondylitis of thoracolumbar region
M45.6 Ankylosing spondylitis of lumbar region
M45.7 Ankylosing spondylitis of lumbosacral region
M45.8 Ankylosing spondylitis of sacral and sacrococcygeal region
M45.9 Ankylosing spondylitis of unspecified sites in spine

Definition

Ankylosing spondylitis is a chronic, inflammatory, rheumatologic disorder that primarily affects the spinal column and sacroiliac joints. It is classified as a seronegative spondyloarthropathy. Enthesitis (inflammation of the soft tissues attaching tendons, ligaments, and joint capsules to bone), synovitis, and inflammation of the synovial capsule are characteristic of its involvement. The most common sites include sacroiliac, apophyseal, and discovertebral joints of the spine; costochondral and manubriosternal joints; paravertebral ligaments; and attachments of the Achilles tendon and plantar fascia. Peripheral joint involvement is less common but occurs in the more severe forms of the disease or with younger age at onset [1].

The onset of symptoms is usually in late adolescence or early adulthood, and there is a 3:1 male predilection. It is not associated with the presence of rheumatoid factor or antinuclear antibodies. Although there is a genetic association with the HLA-B27 histocompatibility antigen (approximately 90% of ankylosing spondylitis patients express the HLA-B27 genotype), this antigen has not proved to be an adequate screening marker as only 5% of individuals with the HLA-B27 genotype contract the disease. Thus, HLA-B27 is not necessary to confirm the diagnosis [2].

Symptoms

Inflammatory spondyloarthropathies should be considered in any young adult patient who complains of insidious onset, progressively worsening, dull, thoracolumbar or lumbosacral back pain. Other characteristics that should raise suspicion for inflammatory-mediated axial disease include back pain that improves with exercise, shows no improvement with rest, and is responsive to nonsteroidal anti-inflammatory medications and pain at night [3].

Ankylosing spondylitis can have a variable presentation, but sacroiliac pain is a common complaint along with progressive morning stiffness and prolonged stiffness after inactivity. Tendon and ligament attachment sites may become painful and swollen, and one third of patients may have hip or shoulder pain. Chest pain with deep breathing and eye pain with blurred vision, floaters, and photophobia are late symptoms of more severe disease [4]. Neurologic symptoms, such as paresthesias and motor weakness, are usually absent.

Physical Examination

The most typical findings on physical examination are signs of decreased spine mobility and pain at sites of ligament

Note: The opinions in this article are those of the author and not necessarily those of the U.S. Army or Department of Defense.

and tendon attachments. Tests of spinal mobility include the modified Schober test, finger to floor distance, cervical rotation, occiput to wall distance, and chest expansion. The modified Schober test is performed with the patient initially standing in erect position. The examiner identifies the posterosuperior iliac crest line (i.e., lumbosacral junction) and makes two midline marks, one 10 cm above the iliac crest line and one 5 cm below the iliac crest line. The patient is then instructed to perform forward trunk flexion while the examiner measures the distance between the two marks. Normal spinal mobility is indicated by an increase of more than 5 cm or a total distance of more than 20 cm; an increase of less than this would suggest limited lumbar spine mobility. The inability to touch the occiput to the wall while standing against it and the inability to expand the chest by more than 3 cm in full inhalation are late findings in the disease [5].

On palpation of the spine, the lower paraspinal muscles and sacroiliac joints may be tender. A Gaenslen test result may also be positive (Fig. 120.1). Palpation of extremities demonstrates pain at attachment sites of ligaments and tendon (enthesitis), particularly around the heel (e.g., calcaneal enthesitis) and knee (i.e., tibial tuberosity). Peripheral joint swelling and pain with decreased range of motion can be seen in 25% to 30% of patients. A discolored and edematous iris with circumferential corneal congestion occurs in iritis and anterior uveitis. The neurologic evaluation is typically normal with regard to motor, sensory, and reflex examination findings. Weakness may be noted, but it is usually associated with pain, loss of mobility, or disuse.

Functional Limitations

The functional limitations of the patient with ankylosing spondylitis are typically related to spine pain and immobility. The three best predictors of decreased spinal mobility are cervical rotation, modified Schober test, and finger to floor distance, although these measurements have not correlated

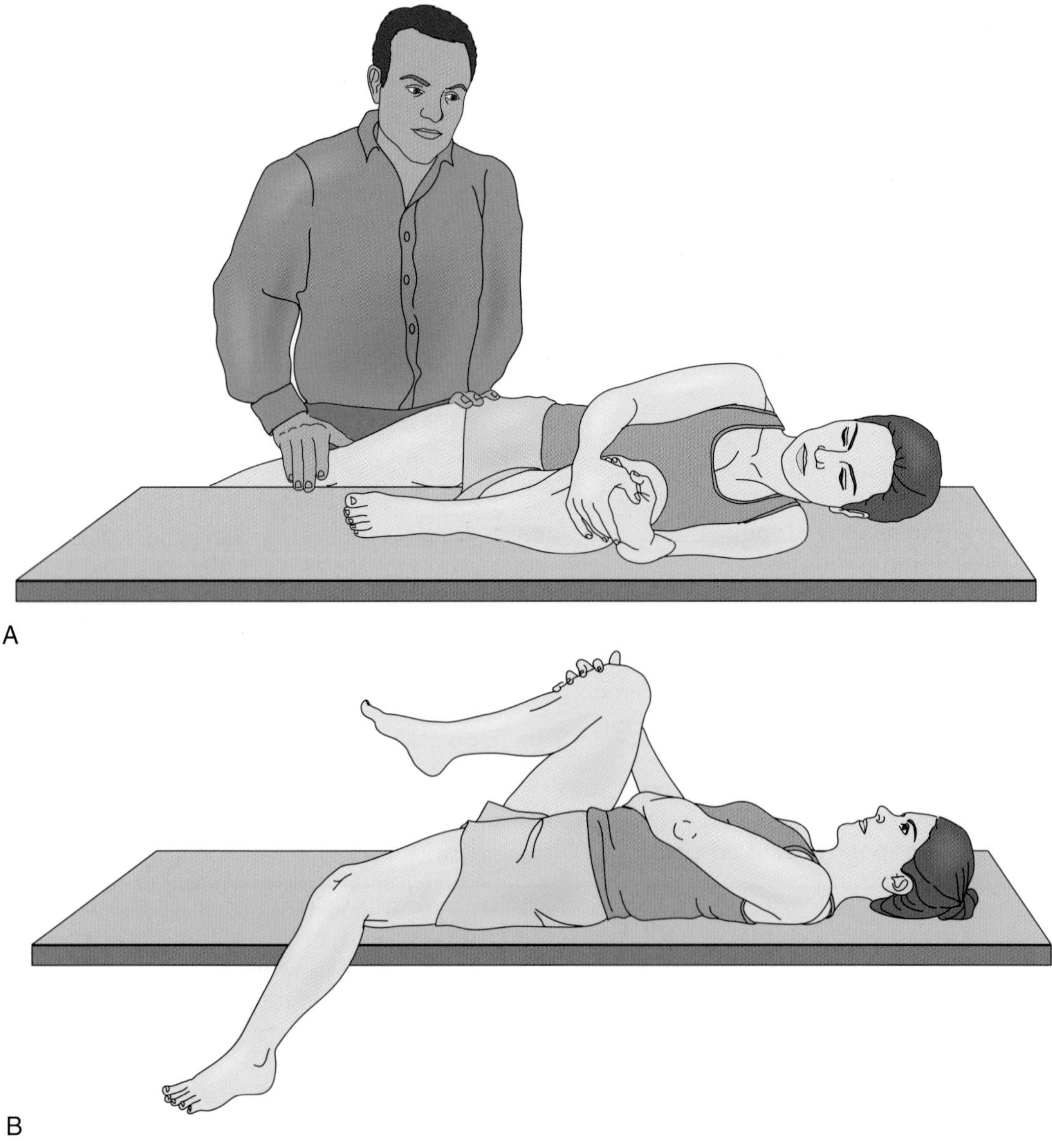

FIGURE 120.1 Gaenslen test. **A,** With the patient in side-lying position, the clinician extends the test leg. **B,** With the patient supine, the test leg is extended over the edge of the table. Pain in the sacroiliac joints indicates a positive test result.

with the patient's assessment of disease activity [5,6]. Early in the disease process, decreased spine range of motion is secondary to back pain and muscle spasms. Most dysfunction is mild and self-limited, typically improving with treatment. In severe disease, positioning from hip flexion contractures, thoracic kyphosis, and loss of cervical rotation decrease patients' ability to view activities in front of them and side to side. The most commonly reported activity limitations are interrupted sleeping, turning the head while driving, carrying groceries, and having energy for social activities [7]. Limitations in chest wall motion lead to a reliance on diaphragmatic breathing and a secondary drop in aerobic capacity. Pain, posture, and functional impairments can also significantly affect sexual relationships [8].

The Bath Ankylosing Spondylitis Functional Index and the Dougados Functional Index are functional assessment tools used by clinicians specializing in the care of patients with ankylosing spondylitis that provide a measure of daily function [9–11]. Past studies have shown that approximately 90% of patients with ankylosing spondylitis remain employed, although recent evidence suggests that up to one third of patients experience some form of employment disruption because of pain and physical limitations [4,6,12].

Diagnostic Studies

There is a well-documented lag time between initial onset of symptoms and diagnosis that ranges from 7 to 11 years [13]. Given the lack of specific signs and symptoms for early ankylosing spondylitis, a high level of suspicion is required in young patients presenting with back pain. Laboratory investigation should include inflammatory markers: erythrocyte sedimentation rate and C-reactive protein [11]. Although neither is required for diagnosis and approximately 40% of patients will have normal values, the elevation of acute phase reactants can indicate severity, responsiveness to treatment, peripheral joint involvement, or extra-articular disease. HLA-B27 is present in 90% of patients with ankylosing spondylitis. A negative test result suggests milder disease with a better prognosis. Rheumatoid factor and antinuclear antibodies are absent.

Radiography of the spine and pelvis is the standard imaging modality in diagnosis and assessment of disease, although computed tomography and magnetic resonance imaging are more sensitive for detection of bone changes, especially early in the disease course and particularly in the assessment of the sacroiliac joints [14]. Spine radiographs show ossification of spinal ligaments and apophyseal joints, sclerosis, and syndesmophytes with eventual ankylosis that leads to the classic bamboo spine appearance. Pelvic (sacroiliac and hip) radiographs demonstrate symmetric involvement of the sacroiliac joints with bone erosions, sclerosis, and blurring of the subchondral bone plate eventually progressing to complete ankylosis. On the basis of the modified New York criteria for ankylosing spondylitis, radiographic features of moderate bilateral sacroiliitis or moderate to severe unilateral sacroiliitis plus one clinical feature are required for definite diagnosis of ankylosing spondylitis. Additional radiographic findings include bone erosions at entheses, symmetric and concentric joint narrowing, and subchondral sclerosis of the hip joints with ankylosis in severe disease. Once initial radiographs are abnormal, further radiographic progression correlates with worsening results of the modified Schober test, although it is recommended that assessment of spinal mobility be used as a proxy for radiographic evaluation [15].

Early computed tomography imaging findings demonstrate pseudowidening of the sacroiliac joints followed by sclerosis, narrowing, and ankylosis. Magnetic resonance imaging can show similar findings but also provides the additional benefit of revealing active inflammation. Sonography can be used to diagnose enthesitis and can also be particularly useful to guide therapeutic interventions and to follow disease progression [16,17].

Differential Diagnosis

Rheumatoid arthritis
Other seronegative spondyloarthropathies
Reiter syndrome
Psoriatic arthritis
Enteropathic spondylitis
Behçet syndrome

Treatment

Initial

Evidence-based treatment guidelines must be tailored to the disease progression and functional impact on the individual with ankylosing spondylitis. The goals of management have been outlined by the European League Against Rheumatism (EULAR) and the Assessment of Spondyloarthritis International Society (ASAS) and should include concurrent medical, rehabilitation, and surgical treatment with the goals of optimizing pain control, maintaining maximal functional capacity with emphasis on spinal range of motion, reducing fatigue, and minimizing impact of extra-axial manifestations [18–20]. Given the variable presentation and progression of symptoms in each patient, an individualized program tailored to the patient's specific needs is necessary.

From a medical standpoint, nonsteroidal anti-inflammatory drugs (NSAIDs) are considered the first-line treatment of patients with ankylosing spondylitis. NSAIDs provide symptomatic relief and have been shown to slow radiographic progression [21–23]. The choice of NSAID is based on individual therapeutic response, compliance, and side effects. Continuous dosing (as opposed to intermittent administration of NSAIDs during periods of exacerbation) is the favored dosing regimen based on the most recent 2010 ASAS/EULAR recommendations; this dosing regimen has been shown to slow structural damage with only marginal increase in side effects [19,22,24].

The recent discovery of biologics has revolutionized the treatment of rheumatologic diseases [25]. Specifically, tumor necrosis factor-α antagonists (infliximab, etanercept, adalimumab, and golimumab) have demonstrated clinical effectiveness in the treatment of ankylosing spondylitis [20]. The choice of tumor necrosis factor-α blocker is based on individual therapeutic response and other factors, such as the presence of extra-axial manifestations or concomitant inflammatory bowel disease. Other disease-modifying agents have shown limited efficacy and are not generally recommended in the treatment of ankylosing spondylitis with the exception of sulfasalazine, which can be used in cases with a predominance of peripheral disease, inflammatory bowel disease, or psoriasis [20,26]. Pulsed methylprednisolone may be effective for NSAID-resistant flares, although long-term use is not generally recommended because of concern for osteoporosis [19,27]. Pamidronate, when it is used to treat associated osteoporosis, may also decrease ankylosing spondylitis disease progression [28].

Rehabilitation

The benefits of exercise for patients with ankylosing spondylitis are well documented [29]. Individualized programs should include activities to optimize aerobic capacity, flexibility, and pulmonary function [30–32]. Hip range of motion increases with regular stretching with use of the contraction-relaxation-stretching technique. Strengthening of back and hip extensors should follow the flexibility exercises. Aerobic activities may maintain chest expansion. However, an exercise stress test should be considered before an aerobic program if aortic insufficiency is suspected [31].

Despite the well-documented benefits of exercise programs, patients with ankylosing spondylitis are poorly compliant, and not surprisingly, the benefits of these programs are lost once the exercise is discontinued. There is no evidence that a particular type of exercise is superior to another, although specific exercise programs that target strengthening and flexibility of shortened muscle chains show promise [33]. One particular area that has clearly shown benefit is the setting in which the program is performed [19]. A physical therapy supervised group was superior to a home exercise program and both were superior to no intervention for improvements in pain, function, mobility, and patient global assessment. Group exercise also demonstrated improved compliance [29,34,35].

Spa therapy and balneotherapy can be safely recommended and have shown moderate benefit for treatment of pain and improving the patient's assessment of disease activity [36]. Splinting and spinal orthoses are generally not effective. Foot orthotics can help with calcaneal enthesopathies. A firm mattress may help with sleep, along with a small cervical pillow that will help maintain cervical lordosis. Wide mirrors assist drivers with limited cervical mobility [32]. There are no data to support or to refute the use of diet, education, or self-help groups [19].

Procedures

Periarticular corticosteroid injections and fluoroscopically guided sacroiliac joint injections may help during NSAID-resistant flares or when NSAIDs are contraindicated [37]. Local injections for enthesopathies may be effective, but injections in and around the Achilles tendon insertion should be avoided.

Surgery

Hip and knee arthroplasties are effective for patients with intractable pain, limitations in mobility, and poor quality of life. Early referral to an orthopedic surgeon should be considered as joint replacement is optimal before progression to ankylosis. Age is not considered a limiting factor as young patients have fared well, and long-term studies have demonstrated that more than 50% of patients exceed a 20+-year life span of their prosthesis [38,39]. Spinal osteotomy is an option for patients with severe kyphosis to improve horizontal vision and balance, although there is considerable risk [19,40].

Potential Disease Complications

Potential complications include iritis or uveitis, inflammatory bowel disease, aortic insufficiency, and aortic root dilation [41]. Osteoporosis (best evaluated with bone densitometry of the femur) is common, which increases risk of spine fracture and associated neurologic injury due to relatively minor trauma [42,43]. Recent evidence suggests an increased morbidity and mortality due to cardiovascular disease in patients with ankylosing spondylitis [44].

Potential Treatment Complications

NSAIDs may produce gastrointestinal and renal toxic effects [45]. Corticosteroids increase risk of osteoporosis. Tumor necrosis factor-α antagonists increase the risk of infection, including reactivation of latent tuberculosis. Total hip arthroplasty increases the risk of anterior dislocations. Spinal osteotomy carries the risk of paralysis and a mortality rate of up to 4% [40].

References

[1] Sieper J, Braun J, Rudwaleit M, et al. Ankylosing spondylitis: an overview. Ann Rheum Dis 2002;61(Suppl. 3):iii8–iii18.

[2] Reveille JD. Major histocompatibility genes and ankylosing spondylitis. Best Pract Res Clin Rheumatol 2006;20:601–9.

[3] Sieper J, van der Heijde D, Landewé R, et al. New criteria for inflammatory back pain in patients with chronic back pain: a real patient exercise by experts from the Assessment of SpondyloArthritis international Society (ASAS). Ann Rheum Dis 2009;68:784–8.

[4] Ozgul A, Peker F, Taskaynatan MA, et al. Effect of ankylosing spondylitis on health-related quality of life and different aspects of social life in young patients. Clin Rheumatol 2006;25:168–74.

[5] Haywood KL, Garratt AM, Jordan K, et al. Spinal mobility in ankylosing spondylitis: reliability, validity and responsiveness. Rheumatology (Oxford) 2004;43:750–7.

[6] Dalyan M, Güner A, Tuncer S, et al. Disability in ankylosing spondylitis. Disabil Rehabil 1999;21:74–9.

[7] Dagfinrud H, Kjeken I, Mowinckel P, et al. Impact of functional impairment in ankylosing spondylitis: impairment, activity limitation, and participation restrictions. J Rheumatol 2005;32:516–23.

[8] Healey EL, Haywood KL, Jordan KP, et al. Ankylosing spondylitis and its impact on sexual relationships. Rheumatology (Oxford) 2009;48:1378–81.

[9] Calin A, Garrett S, Whitelock H, et al. A new approach to defining functional ability in ankylosing spondylitis: the development of the Bath Ankylosing Spondylitis Functional Index. J Rheumatol 1994;21:2281–5.

[10] Dougados M, Gueguen A, Nakache JP, et al. Evaluation of a functional index and an articular index in ankylosing spondylitis. J Rheumatol 1988;15:302–7.

[11] Zochling J, Braun J, van der Heijde D. Assessments in ankylosing spondylitis. Best Pract Res Clin Rheumatol 2006;20:521–37.

[12] Fabreguet I, Koumakis E, Burki V, et al. Assessment of work instability in spondyloarthritis: a cross-sectional study using the ankylosing spondylitis work instability scale. Rheumatology (Oxford) 2012;51:333–7.

[13] Feldtkeller E, Khan MA, van der Heijde D, et al. Age at disease onset and diagnosis delay in HLA-B27 negative vs. positive patients with ankylosing spondylitis. Rheumatol Int 2003;23:61–6.

[14] Braun J, van der Heijde D. Imaging and scoring in ankylosing spondylitis. Best Pract Res Clin Rheumatol 2002;16:573–604.
[15] Wanders A, Landewé R, Dougados M, et al. Association between radiographic damage of the spine and spinal mobility for individual patients with ankylosing spondylitis: can assessment of spinal mobility be a proxy for radiographic evaluation? Ann Rheum Dis 2005;64:988–94.
[16] Aydin SZ, Karadag O, Filippucci E, et al. Monitoring Achilles enthesitis in ankylosing spondylitis during TNF-alpha antagonist therapy: an ultrasound study. Rheumatology (Oxford) 2010;49:578–82.
[17] Spadaro A, Iagnocco A, Perrotta FM, et al. Clinical and ultrasonography assessment of peripheral enthesitis in ankylosing spondylitis. Rheumatology (Oxford) 2011;50:2080–6.
[18] Zochling J, van der Heijde D, Burgos-Vargas R, et al. ASAS/EULAR recommendations for the management of ankylosing spondylitis. Ann Rheum Dis 2006;65:442–52.
[19] van den Berg R, Baraliakos X, Braun J, van der Heijde D. First update of the current evidence for the management of ankylosing spondylitis with non-pharmacological treatment and non-biologic drugs: a systematic literature review for the ASAS/EULAR management recommendations in ankylosing spondylitis. Rheumatology (Oxford) 2012;51:1388–96.
[20] Baraliakos X, van den Berg R, Braun J, van der Heijde D. Update of the literature review on treatment with biologics as a basis for the first update of the ASAS/EULAR management recommendations of ankylosing spondylitis. Rheumatology (Oxford) 2012;51:1378–87.
[21] Zochling J, van der Heijde D, Dougados M, Braun J. Current evidence for the management of ankylosing spondylitis: a systematic literature review for the ASAS/EULAR management recommendations in ankylosing spondylitis. Ann Rheum Dis 2006;65:423–32.
[22] Wanders A, Heijde Dv, Landewé R, et al. Nonsteroidal antiinflammatory drugs reduce radiographic progression in patients with ankylosing spondylitis: a randomized clinical trial. Arthritis Rheum 2005;52:1756–65.
[23] Kroon F, Landewé R, Dougados M, van der Heijde D. Continuous NSAID use reverts the effects of inflammation on radiographic progression in patients with ankylosing spondylitis. Ann Rheum Dis 2012;71:1623–9.
[24] Koehler L, Kuipers JG, Zeidler H. Managing seronegative spondarthritides. Rheumatology (Oxford) 2000;39:360–8.
[25] Khan MA. Ankylosing spondylitis and related spondyloarthropathies: the dramatic advances in the past decade. Rheumatology (Oxford) 2011;50:637–9.
[26] Clegg DO, Reda DJ, Abdellatif M. Comparison of sulfasalazine and placebo for the treatment of axial and peripheral articular manifestations of the seronegative spondylarthropathies: a Department of Veterans Affairs cooperative study. Arthritis Rheum 1999;42:2325–9.
[27] Peters ND, Ejstrup L. Intravenous methylprednisolone pulse therapy in ankylosing spondylitis. Scand J Rheumatol 1992;21:134–8.
[28] Haibel H, Brandt J, Rudwaleit M, et al. Treatment of active ankylosing spondylitis with pamidronate. Rheumatology (Oxford) 2003;42:1018–20.
[29] Dagfinrud H, Kvien TK, Hagen KB. Physiotherapy interventions for ankylosing spondylitis. Cochrane Database Syst Rev 2008;1; CD002822.
[30] Sweeney S, Taylor G, Calin A. The effect of a home based exercise intervention package on outcome in ankylosing spondylitis: a randomized controlled trial. J Rheumatol 2002;29:763–6.
[31] Ince G, Sarpel T, Durgun B, Erdogan S. Effects of a multimodal exercise program for people with ankylosing spondylitis. Phys Ther 2006;86:924–35.
[32] Gall V. Exercise in the spondyloarthropathies. Arthritis Care Res 1994;7:215–20.
[33] Fernandez-de-Las-Penas C, Alonso-Blanco C, Alguacil-Diego IM, Miangolarra-Page JC. One-year follow-up of two exercise interventions for the management of patients with ankylosing spondylitis: a randomized controlled trial. Am J Phys Med Rehabil 2006;85:559–67.
[34] Passalent LA. Physiotherapy for ankylosing spondylitis: evidence and application. Curr Opin Rheumatol 2011;23:142–7.
[35] Passalent LA, Soever LJ, O'Shea FD, Inman RD. Exercise in ankylosing spondylitis: discrepancies between recommendations and reality. J Rheumatol 2010;37:835–41.
[36] Aydemir K, Tok F, Peker F, et al. The effects of balneotherapy on disease activity, functional status, pulmonary function and quality of life in patients with ankylosing spondylitis. Acta Reumatol Port 2010;35:441–6.
[37] Luukkainen R, et al. Periarticular corticosteroid treatment of the sacroiliac joint in patients with seronegative spondylarthropathy. Clin Exp Rheumatol 1999;17:88–90.
[38] Sweeney S, Gupta R, Taylor G, Calin A. Total hip arthroplasty in ankylosing spondylitis: outcome in 340 patients. J Rheumatol 2001;28:1862–66.
[39] Joshi AB, Markovic L, Hardinge K, Murphy JC. Total hip arthroplasty in ankylosing spondylitis: an analysis of 181 hips. J Arthroplasty 2002;17:427–33.
[40] Van Royen BJ, De Gast A. Lumbar osteotomy for correction of thoracolumbar kyphotic deformity in ankylosing spondylitis. A structured review of three methods of treatment. Ann Rheum Dis 1999;58:399–406.
[41] Lautermann D, Braun J. Ankylosing spondylitis—cardiac manifestations. Clin Exp Rheumatol 2002;20(Suppl. 28):S11–5.
[42] Waldman SK, Brown C, Lopez de Heredia L, Hughes RJ. Diagnosing and managing spinal injury in patients with spondylitis. J Emerg Med 2013;44:e315–9.
[43] Robinson Y, Sanden B, Olerud C. Increased occurrence of spinal fractures related to ankylosing spondylitis: a prospective 22-year cohort study in 17,764 patients from a national registry in Sweden. Patient Saf Surg 2013;7:2.
[44] Papagoras C, Voulgari PV, Drosos AA. Atherosclerosis and cardiovascular disease in the spondyloarthritides, particularly ankylosing spondylitis and psoriatic arthritis. Clin Exp Rheumatol 2013;31:612–20.
[45] Zochling J, Bohl-Bühler MH, Baraliakos X, et al. Nonsteroidal anti-inflammatory drug use in ankylosing spondylitis—a population-based survey. Clin Rheumatol 2006;25:794–800.

CHAPTER 121

Burns

Jeffrey C. Schneider, MD
Amy X. Yin, MD

Synonyms

Thermal injury
Late effects of burn injury
Burn contracture
Hypertrophic scarring from burns

ICD-9 Codes

906.5 Late effect of burn of eye, face, head, and neck
906.6 Late effect of burn of wrist and hand
906.7 Late effect of burn of other extremities
906.8 Late effect of burns of other specified sites
906.9 Late effect of burn of unspecified site
949 Burn, unspecified
949.1 Erythema (first degree)
949.2 Blisters, epidermal loss (second degree)
949.3 Full-thickness skin loss (third-degree NOS)
949.4 Deep necrosis of underlying tissues (deep third degree) without mention of loss of a body part
949.5 Deep necrosis of underlying tissues (deep third degree) with loss of a body part

ICD-10 Codes

T20.00XS Late effect of burn of unspecified degree of head, face, and neck, unspecified site
T20.07XS Late effect of burn of unspecified degree of neck
T26.40XS Late effect of burn of unspecified eye and adnexa, part unspecified
T26.41XS Late effect of burn of right eye and adnexa, part unspecified
T26.42XS Late effect of burn of left eye and adnexa, part unspecified
T30.0 Burn of unspecified body region, unspecified degree (Note: This code is not for inpatient use.)
Burns have to be coded by location and then degree (see section T20-T25)
I96 Gangrene, not elsewhere classified

Definition

There are approximately 450,000 burn injuries requiring medical treatment and 45,000 burn hospitalizations, including 25,000 at burn centers, in the United States each year [1]. Adult burn injury patients are most likely to be young (average age at injury for adults is 42 years) and male (70%-75%) [1,2]. Most burns in adults result from fire or flame injuries (44%-61%) [1,2]. Other causes of burns that are also commonly reported include scald, contact, grease, electrical, and chemical injuries [1,2]. Burns usually happen in the home (68%) but also occur in the workplace (10%) or as a result of motor vehicle accidents (7%) [1]. For children, scald injuries are the most common cause and occur more frequently in children younger than 5 years. However, there are disproportionally more scald and inhalation injuries in minority populations [3].

Although there are 3500 estimated deaths from fire and burns annually in the United States [1], the incidence of burns has decreased dramatically in the past 50 years as a result of public education as well as home and work safety efforts. In addition, mortality from burn injury has declined by approximately 50% during the same period [4]. Advances in medical care and the development of comprehensive burn centers (Table 121.1) have contributed to this improved mortality rate. Survival of patients admitted to burn centers is estimated to be 96% [1]. Currently, once survival is ensured, medical management and treatment of burn injury are focused on wound healing, management of complications, and rehabilitation.

Symptoms

The symptoms of burn injury are directly related to the depth, size, and location of the injury. As expected,

Table 121.1 Criteria for Referral to a Burn Center

Burn Injuries that Should be Referred to a Burn Center
Partial-thickness burns greater than 10% of the total body surface area
Burns that involve the face, hands, feet, genitalia, perineum, or major joints
Third-degree burns in any age group
Electrical burns, including lightning injury
Chemical burns
Inhalation injury
Burn injury in patients with preexisting medical disorders that could complicate management, prolong recovery, or affect mortality
Any patient with burns and concomitant trauma (such as fractures) in which the burn injury poses the greatest risk of morbidity or mortality
Burned children in hospitals without qualified personnel or equipment for the care of children
Burn injury in patients who will require special social, emotional, or rehabilitative intervention

From American College of Surgeons, Committee on Trauma. Guidelines for the operation of burn centers. Resources for Optimal Care of the Injured Patient. Chicago, Ill, American College of Surgeons, 2006.

nociceptive pain is a major symptom of burn injury. Involvement of nerve endings in the dermal layer may also result in impaired or altered sensations causing neuropathic pain. Pruritus is common in the acute period and is linked to both the chronic inflammatory state and altered pain pathways of burns. Furthermore, postburn pain and pruritus may persist for years after injury, and regular monitoring with use of standardized measures is recommended. The visual analog scale, numeric pain rating scale, and 5-D scale for itching [5] are useful in assessing symptoms and treatment response.

Deep partial-thickness and full-thickness burns interrupt the function of skin appendages. Damaged skin appendages may include the apocrine sweat glands, resulting in dry, friable skin that does not heal well and is susceptible to infection. In larger burns, the loss of sweat glands may also impair body temperature regulation. The overall poor skin condition after burn injury may lead to chronic wounds.

Scar tissue develops weeks to months after closure of deep partial-thickness and full-thickness burns. Hypertrophic scars and contractures may result. This can be painful, cause deformity, and interfere with joint function. Contractures may lead to subluxation of hand or feet joints and dislocation of hips or shoulders. Scoliosis and kyphosis can result from burn scar contracture and postural changes.

Other symptoms are related to the multitude of other burn complications (see section on potential disease complications), some of which arise from the complex and prolonged intensive care and hospital course. Severe deep injury of extremities can require amputations of nonviable limbs. Formation of osteophytes and heterotopic ossification occur in burns and are associated with long-term immobilization [6]. Chronic infections from skin wounds and immune compromise are significant concerns. Other issues include complications from inhalation injury resulting in chronic pulmonary symptoms, hormone imbalances, deconditioning and malnutrition, and loss of bone and muscle mass [7]. Last, premorbid psychiatric disorders and psychiatric complications from the burn itself are prevalent and include sleep disturbances, depression, anxiety, substance abuse, and post-traumatic stress.

Physical Examination

A thorough physical examination is necessary to assess the burn itself as well as resulting complications. The evaluation should begin with an examination of the skin for burn location and depth, sensation, and signs of infection. Determination of burn depth allows categorization of wound severity.

The current burn classification system groups burns into four categories of varying depth: superficial, superficial and deep partial thickness, and full thickness. Superficial injuries, traditionally known as first-degree burns, solely affect the epidermal layer. The category of second-degree burns is divided into superficial and deep partial-thickness burns. Superficial partial-thickness burns interrupt the epidermis and superficial (papillary) dermis. These often have good vascular supply and are painful with a pink or red and sometimes blistered appearance [8]. Deep partial-thickness burns extend into the deep (reticular) dermis and damage skin appendages, which affects some degree of sensory and apocrine function. Full-thickness burns, also called third-degree burns, affect the entire epidermal and dermal layers and result in complete loss of skin appendages. Deep partial-thickness and full-thickness burns usually have poor blood flow and can be painless and appear less red [8]. Severe injuries also may penetrate to the muscle, tendon, and bone. Such deep injuries, classified as fourth-degree burns, are not part of the newer anatomic classification system (Fig. 121.1 and Table 121.2).

The depth of burn is an important factor in determining acute management of wounds. Burn surgeons often classify burns as superficial wounds, which heal by conservative management, or deep wounds, which require surgical intervention. Clinical assessment is the most widely used

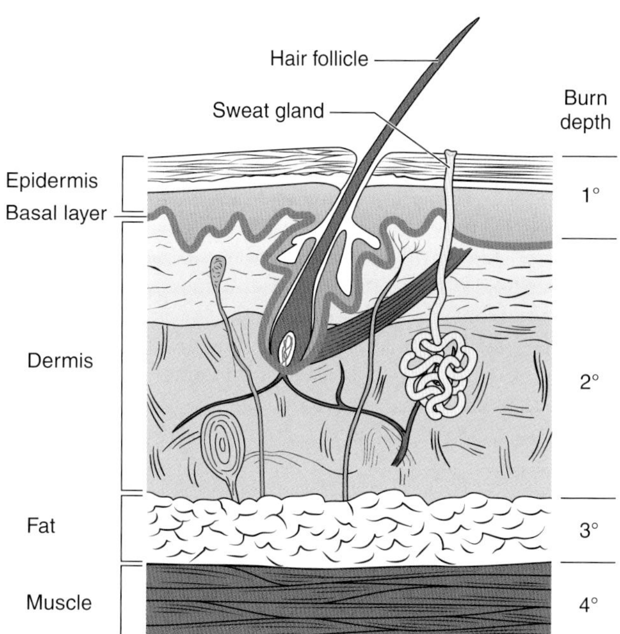

FIGURE 121.1 Diagram of skin anatomy with subdivisions by degree of burn.

Table 121.2 Burn Severity Classifications

Classic Classification	New Classification	Appearance and Symptoms	Course and Treatment
First degree (epidermis)	Superficial thickness	Erythematous; dry, mildly swollen; blanches with pressure; painful	Exfoliation; heals spontaneously in 1 week; no scarring
Second degree (dermis)	Superficial partial thickness	Blistering; moist, weeping; blanches with pressure; painful	Reepithelialization in 7-20 days
	Deep partial thickness	No blisters; wet or waxy dry; variable color; less painful; at risk for conversion to full thickness because of marginal blood supply	Reepithelialization in weeks to months; skin grafting may speed recovery; associated with scarring
Third degree (all of dermis and epidermis)	Full thickness	White waxy to leathery gray to charred black; insensate to pain; does not blanch to pressure	Reepithelialization does not occur; requires skin grafting; associated with scarring
Fourth degree (extends to muscle, bone, tendon)	—	Black (eschar); exposed bones, ligaments, tendons	May require amputation or extensive deep débridement

technique to evaluate burn wound depth and severity. Unfortunately, the clinical evaluation is accurate only about 64% to 76% of the time, and other techniques, briefly discussed in diagnostic studies, may also be used to evaluate wound depth [9,10]. Because of the evolving nature of burn wounds in the first few days after injury, monitoring the progression of the wound over time allows one to best assess its ultimate anatomic classification and management plan.

Postoperative burn wounds should also be closely watched in the rehabilitation setting. Postoperative wound evaluation includes inspection of grafts for hematoma, seroma, infections, and areas of graft loss [8]. After skin grafting, and as the skin matures, one should monitor for signs of hypertrophic scarring, which initially appears as erythematous, raised, and hardened skin.

A complete neurologic examination including an assessment of motor and sensory function, reflexes, and cognition should also be performed. Immediately after injury or surgery, the sensory examination is primarily limited to light touch modality because of pain. However, after wound closure, the sensory examination enables one to evaluate for small- and large-fiber neuropathies. Deep burn wounds may involve the vascular supply and affect wound healing. A pertinent vascular examination includes assessment of peripheral pulses of the involved extremities. The musculoskeletal examination should assess not only strength but also joint range of motion and deformities. The motor examination of joints crossed by a deep partial-thickness or full-thickness burn should not be performed until after skin graft "take" is ensured, usually within a week after grafting. Note that burn patients may have significant weakness from deconditioning and lean muscle loss. A complete cardiac and pulmonary examination should be performed with particular attention to signs of respiratory complications and hypermetabolic state. Psychiatric examination should include a thorough screening for signs of sleep disturbance, depression, anxiety, substance abuse, and post-traumatic stress. Patients who exhibit symptoms of a major psychiatric disorder should receive a complete psychiatric evaluation.

Functional Limitations

Functional limitations are directly related to the severity and location of the burn and related complications. Those with burns to the upper extremities may experience impairments in activities of daily living, fine motor tasks, and occupational activities. Burns to the lower extremities may result in impairments in mobility and higher level exercise and sport activities. Small burns to sensitive areas such as the face, including the eyes, ears, nose, or mouth, and genitals may result in significant impairments in specific functions.

Another effect is impaired psychological function. Psychological impairments are common and significant, leading to difficulty with community and social integration [11,12]. Factors associated with delayed return to work include increased hospital length of stay, electrical etiology, injury at work, and the need for inpatient rehabilitation. After hospitalization, barriers for returning to work include pain, neurologic issues, and impaired mobility [13].

Diagnostic Studies

Many different diagnostic tests are useful in the initial assessment of the burn patient. These may include tests to assess wound depth. The "gold standard" of burn depth analysis is biopsy with histologic assessment, but this is not standard practice [14]. Techniques using laser Doppler imaging, thermography, vital dyes, ultrasonography, and confocal laser scanning microscopes have been suggested for wound depth assessment, but these methods are not routinely used clinically. Bronchoscopic evaluation of the airway is performed for inhalation injury along with serum carboxyhemoglobin level.

In the rehabilitation setting, diagnostic tests are targeted toward short- and long-term sequelae of burns. Plain radiographs are used to evaluate for abnormal bone and joint changes, such as bone growth deformity in children, osteophytes, or joint subluxation and dislocation. Plain films are also used to evaluate heterotopic ossification but may not demonstrate findings until 3 weeks (see Chapter 130) [15]. Heterotopic ossification is diagnosed as early as 7 days after formation with a triple-phase bone scan. The aberrant ossification is visualized by increased uptake in the third phase of the scan. For patients with signs or symptoms of peripheral nerve injury, nerve conduction study and electromyography are used for the diagnosis of neuropathy.

Differential Diagnosis

Thermal injury
Electrical burns
Chemical burns
Radiation burns
Scalding

Treatment

Initial

The initial management of the severely burned patient focuses on the ABCs: airway, breathing, and circulation. Aggressive fluid resuscitation to compensate for insensible fluid losses is a mainstay of acute management [16], but recent literature has shown overresuscitation to be a possible complicating issue [17]. Other principles of initial management include maintenance of clean and protected wounds, use of antimicrobial agents and infection prevention, emergent relief of ischemic compression by fasciotomy or escharotomy, and early excision and grafting of open wounds. A detailed review of the rapid advances in acute management of burn injuries is beyond the scope of this chapter.

Rehabilitation

Rehabilitation of burn patients is a complex issue. The most common and significant issues are discussed in this section.

Pain

Pain management after burn injury is an integral part of rehabilitation. Background nociceptive pain from the injury itself and exacerbations of pain from therapy, dressing changes, débridement, and other procedures can cause significant discomfort. Long-acting opioid pain medications are commonly used to treat background pain [18]. Premedication with short-acting opioid analgesics before dressing changes or procedures and for breakthrough pain is standard of care [18,19]. Because of the development of drug tolerance or a history of recreational opioid use, both common in burn patients, selection of opioids and doses has to be individualized to patients and may exceed standard dosing guidelines for appropriate symptom control. As the wounds heal, a slow and careful opioid taper is needed to prevent withdrawal. Although there is limited evidence for sole use of nonopioids in severe burn pain, nonsteroidal anti-inflammatory drugs and acetaminophen can be valuable in combination with opioids [18]. Other nonopioid pain medications, like muscle relaxants and antiepileptics, may also be used but have not been well studied.

Strong consideration should also be given to nonpharmacologic pain treatment options. Techniques that demonstrate reduction of pain scores include massage, hypnosis, multimodal distraction techniques, cognitive-behavioral techniques, and music therapy [18,20,21]. Off-the-shelf virtual reality has been shown to reduce acute pain intensity during wound care procedures [22].

Clinicians should note that pain is often a multifactorial experience and therefore should make extended efforts to treat all possible contributing factors, including pruritus, neuropathy, anxiety, sleep disturbance, depression, and post-traumatic stress.

Pruritus

Moisturizing is encouraged for treatment of pruritus; not only do emollients such as aloe vera and lanolin help improve skin quality, but massaging may provide itch relief by the gate theory and desensitization of the skin [23]. Studies have also shown that topical treatments with colloidal oatmeal, liquid paraffin, EMLA (eutectic mixture of local anesthetics) application, and doxepin cream can be effective for symptom management.

A mainstay of treatment is antihistamines. Histamine is found in abundance in burn wounds and is implicated as a primary mediator of pruritus. Selective H_1 and H_2 antihistamines are generally preferred to nonspecific antihistamines for their limited side effect profile. The use of cetirizine and cimetidine was also shown to be more effective than diphenhydramine and placebo in treatment of postburn pruritus [23]. However, the effect of any antihistamine is often limited. A study of 35 adult patients using diphenhydramine, hydroxyzine, and chlorpheniramine showed similar effect with complete relief in only 20%, partial relief in 60%, and no relief in 20% of patients [24].

Gabapentin has been shown in recent studies to relieve pruritus both as monotherapy and in combination with antihistamines. Some consider postburn pruritus to be a neuropathic process, and the effect of gabapentin may be due to the similar nerve pathways for pain and pruritus. A comparative study of gabapentin, cetirizine, and the combination of the two in 60 patients showed significantly better results in the gabapentin group and the combination group compared with the cetirizine-only group [25]. Pregabalin may be similarly effective but has not been studied in postburn pruritus. Other agents including ondansetron, paroxetine, and naltrexone have shown potential usefulness as adjunctive treatments.

Biofeedback therapy and psychological support may attenuate symptoms. Modalities including laser treatment, massage, and transcutaneous electrical nerve stimulation have also demonstrated positive results and may be useful [26–28]. The use of botulinum toxin injection is under investigation [29].

Wounds

The goal of wound care is to provide a moist, clean environment for reduced bacterial colonization and reepithelialization. Silver-based dressings are the cornerstone of wound management because silver ions have broad antimicroorganism activity. Silver sulfadiazine is the best known and most widely used silver-based agent for burns. More recent research suggests that new dressings that elute nanocrystalline silver have better antimicrobial activity, including against methicillin-resistant *Staphylococcus aureus* [30]. These dressings allow longer intervals between dressing changes and increase the patient's comfort. Hydrofiber dressings are another new dressing type that may be less painful and are commonly used for exudative burns [31]. There has also been increasing interest in honey. Several trials comparing honey with traditional dressing in minor burns showed shorter healing times [30]. In general, there are many dressing options, and dressing selection should take into account knowledge and familiarity of the health care providers.

Hypertrophic Scarring

Compression garments are considered standard of care for treatment of hypertrophic scars. Such garments are initiated with closure of wounds. Initially, pressure wrappings are applied around the affected areas with plastic elastic (ACE), cotton elastic (Tubigrip), or adhesive elastic (Coban) bandages. As edema resolves, the scarred area assumes a more stable shape, and custom-made pressure garments are then fitted. These garments are usually recommended to be worn 23 hours per day for up to 1 to 2 years after a burn. Compliance with this schedule is difficult for many patients. The efficacy of this treatment has not been established in the literature [32], but a number of studies show some improvement in clinical appearance in moderate or severe scarring [33].

Silicone gel sheeting is also considered first-line treatment, but the use of silicone gel sheeting or silicone spray does not demonstrate greater effect compared with pressure garment use alone [34].

Contractures

Positioning and splinting are used to prevent development of contractures and to maximize joint function. Preventive treatment ideally begins on admission to the intensive care unit. The optimal position to minimize contracture development is depicted in Figure 121.2. Particular attention is given to burns that cross joints and exposed tendons. Such joints are at high risk for contracture development and should receive empirical splinting and exercises to maintain range of motion.

Positioning should always be paired with passive or active range of motion exercises to prevent the development of contractures. Range of motion exercises can begin immediately if the patient has not undergone skin grafting and usually within 1 week after grafting so as not to interfere with graft take. Once a contracture develops, rehabilitation interventions such as splinting, positioning, range of motion exercises, and serial casting have been shown to prevent worsening of the contracture and to improve joint motion [35–38].

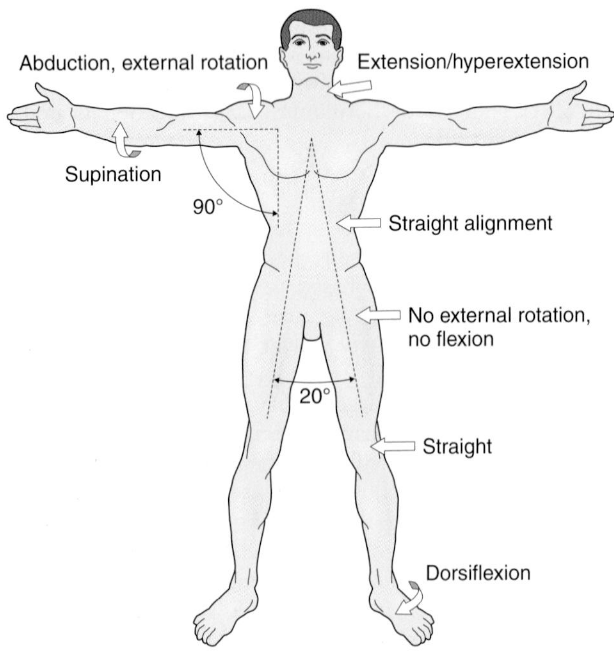

FIGURE 121.2 Optimal positioning to prevent burn contractures.

Heterotopic Ossification (see Chapter 130)

Conservative treatments include positioning and range of motion exercises. Medications such as nonsteroidal anti-inflammatory drugs or bisphosphonates and radiation therapy are efficacious in the prevention of heterotopic ossification in other disease populations (e.g., spinal cord injury and hip arthroplasty). Their use can be considered, but studies have not examined their effect in burn patients [15].

Hypermetabolism and Deconditioning

After severe burns, survivors often experience a hypermetabolic state with increased catabolism and loss of lean body and bone mass. Meeting nutritional needs, often under the guidance of a dietitian, is an important part of burn care. Enteral feeding may be needed in the acute setting for effective nutrition. Consideration should also be given to nutritional supplementation including vitamins C and D, zinc, and thiamine. Oxandrolone, an anabolic steroid, has been shown in multiple randomized controlled trials, with up to 1 year of use, to increase muscle protein synthesis and weight gain and to decrease hospital length of stay [39]. Because of prolonged hospitalization and the loss of muscle, burn survivors are often severely deconditioned. Long-term exercise training programs are needed for return to premorbid functional level. Aerobic and progressive resistance training programs have been shown to be efficacious in improving strength, peak oxygen consumption, lean body mass, and pulmonary function in burn survivors [40].

Psychological Comorbidity

There is limited literature validating treatment of depression, acute stress disorder, post-traumatic stress disorder, and sleep disorders specifically in the burn population [41]. One small study suggests that sertraline may be useful in preventing post-traumatic stress disorder in burned children [42]. Regardless, a large body of evidence documents the efficacy of both pharmacologic and nonpharmacologic treatments of these disorders in other populations [43–45], and psychological conditions in burn patients should be addressed on the basis of these guidelines. Treatment of the burn-injured patient ideally involves collaboration with a mental health team to assist in the diagnosis and treatment of these problems.

Procedures

Botulinum toxin injection is under study as a treatment for postburn pruritus. Another procedure being evaluated is extracorporeal shock wave therapy, which may promote perfusion, increase angiogenesis, and accelerate burn wound healing [46]. Extracorporeal shock wave therapy may also have a role in improving pliability and appearance of postburn scarring [47]. However, both these procedures are investigational at this time.

Surgery

Excision and grafting of open wounds are ideally performed within 1 week of injury in clinically stable patients. The goal is to remove necrotic and inflamed tissue for promotion of physiologic wound closure. Studies have shown that early excision and grafting minimizes fluid loss, reduces metabolic demand, and decreases the risk of infection and sepsis [48].

There are many techniques for grafting. Most commonly, partial-thickness burns are treated with split- and full-thickness grafts of epidermis and superficial (papillary) dermis harvested from a nonaffected area (autograft). For larger wounds, mesh grafts or tissue expanders may be used [8]. Allograft, dermal substitutes, cultured epithelial autograft, and Meek technique for micrografts can be used for extensive burns with minimal viable tissue. Deeper burns may require excision and coverage with skin, muscle, or myocutaneous flaps, but these may lead to great deformity [8].

Bone marrow mesenchymal stem cells are under investigation for the possible regeneration of sweat gland–like structures. A few centers have performed face transplants for severe burn patients [49].

In spite of aggressive rehabilitation after a burn injury, significant contractures may still develop. Surgical release of the contracted joint is indicated when there are significant functional impairments despite appropriate conservative treatment.

Surgical resection of heterotopic bone is indicated if it results in significant joint impairment despite a course of conservative treatment or nerve entrapment.

Scarring, disfigurement, and other cosmetic concerns are addressed with reconstructive surgical efforts. Severely burned patients may undergo multiple surgeries during the span of years after their injury. Planning of the myriad possible procedures is a task that should involve multiple members of the burn team, including the patient and his or her family, physiatrist, surgeon, therapists, and mental health professionals.

Potential Disease Complications

Long-term Pain and Pruritus

Pain and pruritus after burn injury are difficult to manage and may become chronic and include physical impairments. Hypersensitivity can be a chronic consequence of burn injury regardless of the severity of the burn [50]. Patients with long-term severe pain and depression are associated with lower physical function at 2 years after injury [51]. This should be taken into account for rehabilitation, return to work, and community integration.

Hypertrophic Scarring

Hypertrophic scarring is common (32%-67%) among those severely burned and is more prevalent among darker pigmented individuals [52]. When it crosses a joint, it may result in deformities and contractures, leading to psychological, functional, and cosmetic impact [15].

Contractures

Contractures are a common and significant complication of burn injury. They result in cosmetic deformity as well as decreased joint range of motion and function. Contractures are most common at the shoulder, elbow, and knee. Length of stay, inhalation injury, and extent of burn are associated with increased incidence and severity of contracture [53]. Contractures of the hand most commonly occur at the wrist but may involve the metacarpophalangeal, proximal interphalangeal, and distal interphalangeal joints of all digits. Predictors of hand contracture development include concomitant medical problems, total body surface area grafted, and presence of hand burn and hand grafting [54].

Amputation

Amputations may complicate burn injuries and are most commonly associated with electrical injury. Low-voltage (<1000 V) injuries most commonly result in amputation of the digits. High-voltage injuries frequently result in major amputation (10%-50%).

Osteophytes and Heterotopic Ossification

Osteophytes are the most frequently observed skeletal alteration in adult burn patients and are most often seen at the elbow.

Heterotopic ossification occurs in approximately 1% of burn injuries and also is most frequently located at the elbow. It commonly is manifested with a decrease in range of motion and may cause impairments in joint function and activities of daily living.

Neuropathy

Mononeuropathies, mononeuropathy multiplex, and peripheral neuropathy have all been documented after burn injury. Risk factors for the development of mononeuropathy include electrical injury, intensive care, and history of alcohol abuse. Compression neuropathy can also result from bulky dressing and improper and prolonged positioning. Mononeuropathy multiplex and peripheral neuropathy in burn patients may be due to a combination of direct thermal injury and the body's systemic response to injury. Risk factors for the development of a generalized peripheral neuropathy include intensive care stay, age, and diabetes [55].

Thermoregulation

Full-thickness burns damage the sweat glands present in the dermal layer. After skin grafting, these glands do not regenerate, leading to impaired sweating in involved areas. For those with larger burns, this may affect thermoregulation, particularly with physical activity in warm climates.

Psychological and Cognitive Complications

Psychological complications are some of the most significant sequelae of burn injury. Acute stress disorder, post-traumatic stress (11%-45%), depression (16%-53%), and sleep disturbances (13%-73%) are common after burn injuries. Preexisting psychiatric disorders are associated with longer hospital stays and require more surgical interventions. Burn patients, regardless of premorbid psychiatric history, often require long-term psychiatric follow-up.

Cognitive impairments may result from anoxia associated with inhalation injury or hypoperfusion associated with shock. A high index of suspicion is needed for diagnosis and treatment of patients with mild cognitive impairments. Neuropsychological evaluation may assist in diagnosis.

Potential Treatment Complications

Medications used to treat pruritus and pain have diverse side effects. The most common adverse effects of opioids and opioid-like pain medications are nausea, diarrhea, and constipation. Gastrointestinal, hepatic, and renal complications may arise from prolonged use of acetaminophen or nonsteroidal anti-inflammatory drugs. Antihistamines used for pruritus have sedating effects. The most common side effects of gabapentin and pregabalin are dizziness and somnolence. Topical treatments, such as silicone gel sheets for hypertrophic scarring, may result in skin maceration or contact dermatitis and rash. Splinting and casting for contractures may cause skin abrasions or pressure sores. Improper positioning and splinting may also lead to compression neuropathies, most commonly seen at the peroneal nerve. Surgical interventions always carry a risk of bleeding, infection, and poor wound healing. This is especially true for burn patients with immune compromise and poor skin integrity.

References

[1] Burn incidence and treatment in the United States: 2011 fact sheet. http://www.ameriburn.org/resources_factsheet.php.

[2] 2012 Burn injury model systems national database update: adults. http://bms-dcc.ucdenver.edu/images/docs/2012BMS_Database_Update_adults.pdf.

[3] Kramer CB, Rivara FP, Klein MB. Variations in US pediatric burn injury hospitalizations using the National Burn Repository data. J Burn Care Res 2010;31:734–9.

[4] Ryan CM, Schoenfeld DA, Thorpe WP, et al. Objective estimates of the probability of death from burn injuries. N Engl J Med 1998;338:362–6.

[5] Elman S, Hynan LS, Gabriel V, Mayo MJ. The 5-D itch scale: a new measure of pruritus. Br J Dermatol 2010;162:587–93.

[6] Chen HC, Yang JY, Chuang SS, et al. Heterotopic ossification in burns: our experience and literature reviews. Burns 2009;35:857–62.

[7] Jeschke MG, Chinkes DL, Finnerty CC, et al. Pathophysiologic response to severe burn injury. Ann Surg 2008;248:387–401.

[8] Orgill DP. Excision and skin grafting of thermal burns. N Engl J Med 2009;360:893–901.

[9] Brown RF, Rice P, Bennet NJ. The use of laser Doppler imaging as an aid in clinical management decision making in the treatment of vesicant burns. Burns 1998;24:692–8.

[10] Heimbach D, Afromowitz M, Engrav L, et al. Burn depth estimation—man or machine. J Trauma 1984;24:373–8.

[11] Fauerbach JA, Heinberg LJ, Lawrence JS, et al. Coping with body image changes following a disfiguring burn injury. Health Psychol 2002;21:115–21.

[12] Lawrence JW, Fauerbach JA, Heinberg L, et al. Visible vs hidden scars and their relation to body esteem. J Burn Care Rehabil 2004;25:25–32.

[13] Schneider JC, Bassi S, Ryan CM. Barriers impacting employment after burn injury. J Burn Care Res 2009;30:294–300.

[14] Heimbach D, Engrav L, Grube B, et al. Burn depth: a review. World J Surg 1992;16:10–5.

[15] Hunt JL, Arnoldo BD, Kowalske K, et al. Heterotopic ossification revisited: a 21-year surgical experience. J Burn Care Res 2006;27:535–40.

[16] Davies J. The fluid therapy given to 1027 patients during the first 24 hours after burning. 1. Total fluid and colloid input. Burns 1975;1(4):319.

[17] Cartotto R, Zhou A. Fluid creep: the pendulum hasn't swung back yet! J Burn Care Res 2010;31:551–8.

[18] Patterson DR, Hofland HW, Espey K, et al. Pain management. Burns 2004;30:A10–5.

[19] Finn J, Wright J, Fong J, et al. A randomised crossover trial of patient controlled intranasal fentanyl and oral morphine for procedural wound care in adult patients with burns. Burns 2004;30:262–8.

[20] Frenay MC, Faymonville ME, Devlieger S, et al. Psychological approaches during dressing changes of burned patients: a prospective randomised study comparing hypnosis against stress reducing strategy. Burns 2001;27:793–9.

[21] Sen S, Greenhalgh D, Palmieri T. Review of burn research for the year 2010. J Burn Care Res 2012;33:577–86.

[22] Kipping B, Rodger S, Miller K, et al. Virtual reality for acute pain reduction in adolescents undergoing burn wound care: a prospective randomized controlled trial. Burns 2012;38:650–7.

[23] Baker RA, Zeller RA, Klein RL, et al. Burn wound itch control using H1 and H2 antagonists. J Burn Care Rehabil 2001;22:263–8.

[24] Vitale M, Fields-Blache C, Luterman A. Severe itching in the patient with burns. J Burn Care Rehabil 1991;12:330–3.

[25] Ahuja RB, Gupta R, Gupta G, et al. A comparative analysis of cetirizine, gabapentin and their combination in the relief of post-burn pruritus. Burns 2011;37:203–7.

[26] Allison KP, Kiernan MN, Waters RA, et al. Pulsed dye laser treatment of burn scars. Alleviation or irritation? Burns 2003;29:207–13.

[27] Field T, Peck M, Hernandez-Reif M, et al. Postburn itching, pain, and psychological symptoms are reduced with massage therapy. J Burn Care Rehabil 2000;21:189–93.

[28] Hettrick HH, O'Brien K, Laznick H, et al. Effect of transcutaneous electrical nerve stimulation of the management of burn pruritus: a pilot study. J Burn Care Rehabil 2004;25:236–40.

[29] Akhtar N, Brooks P. The use of botulinum toxin in the management of burns itching: preliminary results. Burns 2012;38:1119–23.

[30] Bezuhly M, Fish JS. Acute burn care. Plast Reconstr Surg 2012;130:349e–58e.

[31] Dokter J, Boxma H, Oen IM, et al. Reduction in skin grafting after the introduction of hydrofiber dressings in partial thickness burns: a comparison between a hydrofiber and silver sulphadiazine. Burns 2013;39:130–5.

[32] Kealey GP, Jensen KL, Laubenthal KN, et al. Prospective randomized comparison of two types of pressure therapy garments. J Burn Care Rehabil 1990;11:334–6.

[33] Engrav LH, Heimbach DM, Rivara FP, et al. 12-Year within-wound study of the effectiveness of custom pressure garment therapy. Burns 2010;36:975–83.

[34] Steinstraesser L, Flak E, Witte B, et al. Pressure garment therapy alone and in combination with silicone for the prevention of hypertrophic scarring: randomized controlled trial with intraindividual comparison. Plast Reconstr Surg 2011;128:306e–13e.

[35] Richard R, Staley M, Miller S, et al. To splint or not to splint: past philosophy and present practice. Part I. J Burn Care Rehabil 1996;17:444–53.

[36] Richard R, Staley M, Miller S, et al. To splint or not to splint: past philosophy and current practice. Part II. J Burn Care Rehabil 1997;18:64–71.

[37] Richard R, Staley M, Miller S, et al. To splint or not to splint: past philosophy and present practice. Part III. J Burn Care Rehabil 1997;18:251–5.

[38] Schneider JC, Qu HD. Efficacy of inpatient burn rehabilitation: a prospective pilot study examining range of motion, hand function and balance. Burns 2012;38:164–71.

[39] Wolf SE, Edelman LS, Kemalyan N, et al. Effects of oxandrolone on outcome measures in the severely burned: a multicenter prospective randomized double-blind trial. J Burn Care Res 2006;27:131–9.

[40] Cucuzzo NA, Ferrando A, Herndon DN. The effects of exercise programming vs traditional outpatient therapy in the rehabilitation of severely burned children. J Burn Care Rehabil 2001;22:214–20.

[41] Esselman PC, Thombs BD, Magyar-Russell G, et al. Burn rehabilitation: state of the science. Am J Phys Med Rehabil 2006;85:383–414.
[42] Stoddard Jr FJ, Luthra R, Sorrentino EA, et al. A randomized controlled trial of sertraline to prevent posttraumatic stress disorder in burned children. J Child Adolesc Psychopharmacol 2011;21:469–77.
[43] Vieweg WV, Julius DA, Fernandez A, et al. Posttraumatic stress disorder: clinical features, pathophysiology, and treatment. Am J Med 2006;119:383–90.
[44] Pagel JF, Parnes BL. Medications for the treatment of sleep disorders: an overview. Prim Care Companion J Clin Psychiatry 2001;3:118–25.
[45] Arroll B, Macgillivray S, Ogston S, et al. Efficacy and tolerability of tricyclic antidepressants and SSRIs compared with placebo for treatment of depression in primary care: a meta-analysis. Ann Fam Med 2005;3:449–56.
[46] Arno A, Garcia O, Hernan I, et al. Extracorporeal shock waves, a new non-surgical method to treat severe burns. Burns 2010;36:477–82.
[47] Fioramonti P, Cigna E, Onesti MG, et al. Extracorporeal shock wave therapy for the management of burn scars. Dermatol Surg 2010;38:778–82.
[48] Ong YS, Samuel M, Song C. Meta-analysis of early excision of burns. Burns 2006;32:145–50.
[49] Pomahac B, Pribaz J, Eriksson E, et al. Restoration of facial form and function after severe disfigurement from burn injury by a composite facial allograft. Am J Transplant 2011;11:386–93.
[50] Wollgarten-Hadamek I, Hohmeister J, Demirakca S, et al. Do burn injuries during infancy affect pain and sensory sensitivity in later childhood? Pain 2009;141:165–72.
[51] Ullrich PM, Askay SW, Patterson DR. Pain, depression, and physical functioning following burn injury. Rehabil Psychol 2009;54:211–6.
[52] Bambaro KM, Egrav LH, Carrougher GJ, et al. What is the prevalence of hypertrophic scarring following burns? Burns 2003;29:299–302.
[53] Schneider JC, Holavanahalli R, Goldstein R, et al. A prospective study of contractures in burn injury: defining the problem. J Burn Care Res 2006;27:508–14.
[54] Schneider JC, Holavanahalli R, Helm P, et al. Contractures in burn injury part II: investigating joints of the hand. J Burn Care Res 2008;29:606–13.
[55] Kowalske K, Holavanahalli R, Helm P. Neuropathy after burn injury. J Burn Care Rehabil 2001;22:353–7.

CHAPTER 122

Cardiac Rehabilitation

Alan M. Davis, MD, PhD

Synonyms

None

ICD-9 Codes

410.00–410.92	Acute myocardial infarction
411.0–411.89	Other acute and subacute forms of ischemic heart disease
412	Old myocardial infarction
413.0–413.9	Angina pectoris
414.0–414.9	Other forms of chronic ischemic heart disease
428.0-428.9	Congestive heart failure
429.2	Cardiovascular disease, unspecified
V42	Cardiac valve replacement status
V42.1	Cardiac transplant status
V43.2	Implantable heart assist system insertion status
V45.81	Aortocoronary bypass status

ICD-10 Codes

I21.3	ST elevation (STEMI) myocardial infarction of unspecified site
I25.2	Old myocardial infarction
I25.9	Chronic ischemic heart disease, unspecified
I20.9	Angina pectoris, unspecified
I50.9	Heart failure, unspecified
I25.10	Atherosclerotic heart disease of native coronary artery without angina pectoris
Z95.2	Presence of prosthetic heart valve
Z95.812	Presence of fully implantable artificial heart
Z95.811	Presence of heart assist device
Z95.1	Presence of aortocoronary bypass graft

Definition

Cardiac rehabilitation is the integrated treatment of individuals after cardiac events or procedures with the goals of maximizing physical function, promoting emotional adjustment, modifying cardiac risk factors, and addressing return to previous social roles and responsibilities. The American Heart Association 2012 update estimates cardiovascular disease prevalence to be 86,200,000 people in the United States; coronary heart disease affects 16,300,000. Of those with coronary heart disease, 7,900,000 have had myocardial infarction, 9,000,000 have angina pectoris, 5,700,000 have heart failure, and 650,000 to 1,300,000 have congenital cardiovascular defects.

Cardiovascular diseases have continued to be the leading cause of mortality in both men and women for more than a century and accounted for 32.8% of all deaths in 2008 [1]. Cardiac rehabilitation supports those who survive to change their lifestyle, to maximize their functional capacity and quality of life, and to decrease their risk for future cardiac events. Cardiac rehabilitation may benefit individuals after acute coronary syndrome, cardiac surgery (coronary artery bypass graft, valve replacement, transplantation, ventricular reduction surgery, correction of congenital heart defect), and compensated congestive heart failure. Cardiac rehabilitation comprehensively addresses risk factor modification and secondary prevention through exercise training, smoking cessation, diet modification, evaluation and treatment of psychosocial stressors, education about the disease process, return to work, and maximizing the medical treatment of comorbidities (such as diabetes mellitus, hypertension, and obesity). In a meta-analysis of exercise-based cardiac rehabilitation programs, cardiovascular mortality was decreased 26%, overall mortality was decreased 13%, and hospital readmissions were reduced 31% compared with usual care in patients with myocardial infarction, percutaneous interventions, coronary artery bypass graft, or known cardiac disease [2].

Symptoms

The individual with a recent cardiac event or procedure frequently complains of decreased endurance for walking or climbing stairs, increased dyspnea during physical activity, and fatigue. If arrhythmia is present, the patient may feel palpitations. Chest pain may accompany physical exertion or emotional stress. Pain due to surgical incisions of the extremities or chest wall may also be present. Symptoms of heart failure, such as orthopnea and paroxysmal nocturnal dyspnea, may also be present. The person may feel anxious about any type of physical exercise, resumption of sexual activities, and return to work. In many cases, the patient may have symptoms suggesting depression, such as emotional lability, listlessness, poor sleep with frequent or early morning awakenings, and lack of interest in previously enjoyed activities.

Physical Examination

Observation of the patient should look for signs of depression and anxiety. During the examination of the cardiac patient, the clinician will search for signs of complications after the cardiac event or cardiac procedure. Findings of congestive heart failure or fluid overload, such as dyspnea at rest, rales, decreased basilar lung sounds, pleural or pericardial rub, dependent edema, elevated jugular venous distention, or S_3 gallop, should be evaluated. Palpation of decreased or absent pulses in the extremities may suggest the common comorbidity of peripheral vascular disease. Wounds such as sternotomies, vascular harvest sites, chest tube insertion sites, pacemaker insertion sites, and arterial puncture sites should be carefully examined for appropriate healing or signs of infection before exercise programs are prescribed. Manual muscle testing of the extremities provides an indication of the degree of skeletal muscle atrophy due to decreased physical activity. Observation of the patient should look for signs of undue dyspnea during standing and ambulation. The patient should be able to comfortably walk at a slow cadence unless there is marked congestive heart failure or lung disease.

Functional Limitations

Functional limitations due to cardiac disease alone are related to the workload the myocardium can sustain before signs of cardiac dysfunction result. Overall endurance is decreased. The degree and severity of cardiac impairment may limit a patient's physical progress and ultimate maximum level of function. The patient may later return to physically demanding activity, such as heavy labor or competitive tennis (both 8 metabolic equivalents or METs), after rehabilitation that follows uncomplicated coronary angioplasty or stenting without myocardial infarction. However, for the patient who experienced myocardial infarction complicated by congestive heart failure and arrhythmia, the 3 to 5 METs required for walking to a neighbor's home or performing the household chores may be limited by dyspnea. Further compromise of progress is related to the common comorbidities of obesity, cerebrovascular disease, intrinsic lung disease, diabetes mellitus, and peripheral vascular disease. Impairment due to neurologic, rheumatologic, or orthopedic disease may require specific adaptations to allow conditioning and strengthening exercise.

Most patients with uncomplicated cardiac disease are able to ambulate and perform their self-care on discharge from the hospital. A slow stroll and being able to perform basic activities of daily living are not adequate for most individuals and do not predict excellent quality of life for the individual not referred to rehabilitation. Cardiac rehabilitation maximizes the person's functional restoration, allowing return to work, social roles, and recreational activity. Despite the known benefits of cardiac rehabilitation, the majority of eligible individuals are not enrolled [3].

Emotional stress and an individual's response to it may also produce functional limitations when return to social roles and responsibilities is considered. This may range from anxiety about physical exertion to major reactive depression. Dysfunction such as ischemia, arrhythmia, or even sudden death may be produced by emotional demands such as anxiety [4–6]. This is likely to be due to increased sympathetic drive in the autonomic nervous system, which predisposes the individual to more endothelial damage and cardiac arrhythmias mediated by catecholamines. Depression accounts for approximately the same (35%) risk for myocardial infarction as smoking does [7]. This argues strongly for a clear psychological screening of patients with cardiac events. Patients whose depression was diagnosed and treated by selective serotonin reuptake inhibitors (SSRIs) at the time of their initial myocardial infarction had 43% less new myocardial infarction and cardiac death compared with treatment with non-SSRIs [8]. This is due to an antiplatelet aggregation effect unrelated to aspirin or clopidogrel bisulfate (Plavix).

Diagnostic Studies

The clinician should evaluate the patient's lipid profile to guide pharmacologic and dietary management of hyperlipidemia and hypercholesterolemia. Tight diabetes control may decrease the rate of atheroma formation, and glycosylated hemoglobin (HbA_{1c}) level is used to ascertain the recent success of blood glucose control [9]. Calculation of body mass index assists in targeting ideal body weight.

For the individual with dyspnea on exertion and the comorbidity of lung disease, pulmonary function testing will clarify the contribution of obstructive or restrictive lung disease to the symptoms. Treatable conditions, such as reactive airways and hypoxia during exercise, should be addressed before beginning of cardiac rehabilitation for maximal benefit. Combined ventilatory gas analysis by use of a metabolic cart and electrocardiographic monitoring may differentiate cardiac versus pulmonary exercise-induced dyspnea, chest pain, or fatigue. This may be especially useful in patients with congestive heart failure [10].

A symptom-limited functional exercise test with a metabolic cart is administered 2 to 6 weeks after adequate time for healing and provides the best guide to exercise prescription. The specific timing of exercise testing depends on the amount of myocardium damage, the amount of time needed for healing of surgical sites, the need for return to work, and the practice pattern of the clinician administering the test. As opposed to commonly performed *diagnostic* exercise test protocols, such as the Bruce protocol, that seek to elicit cardiac symptoms, *functional* exercise testing documents work capacity and cardiopulmonary function. Functional exercise testing protocols start at a lower exercise intensity level than common diagnostic protocols do and increase fewer METs per stage. Treadmill testing following a ramp, modified Naughton, or Naughton-Balke protocol is especially well suited to guide cardiac rehabilitation exercise training because these protocols use smaller increments of intensity that more accurately portray functional capacity. Alternatively, bicycle ergometer protocols may also use smaller gradations of exercise intensity. Bicycle ergometry protocols should be considered for individuals with balance deficits, mild neurologic impairment, or orthopedic limitations.

Echocardiographic, pharmacologic, or nuclear medicine exercise stress testing should be considered for patients with marked lower extremity limitations, severe debility, or electrocardiograms that are difficult to interpret. Most patients have had many electrocardiograms during their hospital stay or evaluation. In the outpatient setting, electrocardiograms should be ordered if there is a change in clinical status, such as new symptoms (e.g., the resumption of angina). For the most part, patients are also monitored by telemetry during at least the initial part of their cardiac rehabilitation.

Patients should be screened for psychosocial stressors, such as anxiety and depression. Besides asking the patient about the symptoms of anxiety, anger, persistent sadness, excessive fatigue, and abnormal sleep architecture, commonly used questionnaires that are easy to administer in an office setting are the Beck Depression Inventory and the State-Trait Anxiety Inventory. Both take only a few minutes to complete and can be used to monitor the effectiveness of treatment.

Treatment

Initial

Cardiac rehabilitation begins with risk factor reduction. Fully integrated cardiac rehabilitation programs enroll the individual into exercise training, dietary interventions, and psychosocial interventions. The referring physician then becomes the supporter of the patient, shifting the patient's lifestyle to making responsible health choices. Consider a discussion of the cardiac rehabilitation experience. The initial medical management focuses on optimizing the cardiac medication regimen to control or to prevent hypertension, ischemia, arrhythmia, hyperlipidemia, fluid overload, or other complications that follow the patient's cardiac event. Diabetes management is also critical to secondary prevention of cardiovascular disease. Concurrent with medical management, the clinician prescribing cardiac rehabilitation must promote choices for healthy living. Each cardiac patient has choices about smoking, diet, exercise, and stress management. Smoking cessation has the highest rates of success by combining participation in a smoking cessation support group with pharmacologic management of the craving due to nicotine addiction. Bupropion combined with a nicotine patch, gum, or lozenges works well. Have the patient begin taking the bupropion hydrochloride (150 mg every day for the first 3 days, then 150 mg twice daily) 1 to 2 weeks before the chosen date to quit smoking and begin using the nicotine supplement at the time of smoking cessation. This should coincide with the first smoking cessation support group meeting.

Dietary modification has been documented to improve the lipid profile [11]. Ask the patient to keep a food diary for at least 3 days to bring to the cardiac rehabilitation program or refer the patient to a registered dietitian for evaluation and education on appropriate heart healthy dietary choices. The American Heart Association revised cardiac diet recommendations of 2006 are substantially more stringent on the saturated fat intake (Table 122.1) [11]. The dietitian may recommend the American Heart Association diet, but other choices could be the Mediterranean diet or the lacto-ovovegetarian diet. None of these three diets has been shown to be superior, and the choice of diet is based primarily on the patient's ability to follow the diet.

Table 122.1 American Heart Association 2006 Diet and Lifestyle Recommendations for Cardiovascular Disease Risk Reduction

Balance calorie intake and physical activity to achieve or maintain a healthy body weight.
Consume a diet rich in vegetables and fruits.
Choose whole-grain, high-fiber foods.
Consume fish, especially oily fish, at least twice a week.
Limit your intake of saturated fat to <7% of energy, *trans* fat to <1% of energy, and cholesterol to <300 mg per day by choosing lean meats and vegetable alternatives; selecting fat-free (skim), 1%-fat, and low-fat dairy products; and minimizing intake of partially hydrogenated fats.
Minimize your intake of beverages and foods with added sugars.
Choose and prepare foods with little or no salt.
If you consume alcohol, do so in moderation.
When you eat food that is prepared outside of the home, follow the American Heart Association Diet and Lifestyle Recommendations.

The individual with cardiac disease often needs to learn strategies to decrease the emotional stress of anxiety and depression. Patients with either of these based on the original screening should be treated. SSRIs treat both components fairly well with few side effects. A referral for counseling with a mental health professional can provide patients with an assortment of tools to learn relaxation and provides a forum for the discussion of emotional symptoms surrounding cardiac events in their life. Women have a higher rate of anxiety and psychosomatic complaints than do men beginning cardiac rehabilitation and can benefit from greater attention to psychosocial interventions [12,13]. In the busy clinic, the clinician can teach the individual a simple stress reduction technique. A relaxation response documented by augmented parasympathetic activity has been noted during the simple exercise of paced breathing. Ask the patient to pace his or her breathing, using a clock, for 5 to 10 minutes twice daily. The patient should time inhalation and exhalation equally for 3 to 5 seconds each while avoiding air hunger or hyperventilation. Once he or she performs this exercise with facility, additional relaxation can be achieved from further slowing of the breathing rate or prolonging the period of exhalation [14].

Return to sexual activity should be frankly discussed with patients and their sexual partners to decrease their anxiety about sexual activity after a cardiac event [15]. Sexual activity between couples with a long-standing relationship requires 3 to 5 METs. Extramarital sex causes higher energy demands. In a statement from the American Heart Association, sexual activity is safe to be resumed, although erectile dysfunction medications should be avoided in patients using nitrates for angina due to coronary artery disease [16].

Return to work and recreational activities should be based on patients' clinical status and their previous work. In a meta-analysis of European cohort studies, significant job-related emotional stress also increased the risk for cardiac events [17]. The exercise test performance predicts the level of vocational work capacity. If the patient's work capacity is only 3 to 4 METs or less, return to work may be unrealistic. Even self-care activities are likely to produce symptoms at this low level. With a capacity of 5 to 7 METs, the person should be able to perform sedentary work and most domestic roles. If the person can exercise beyond 7 METs, most types of work can be performed without restriction, except those involving heavy physical labor. For recreational activity, the MET level required should be evaluated before return to play is recommended. The *Compendium of Physical Activities* can be used to guide return to work and recreation activities and can also be accessed online (https://sites.google.com/site/compendiumofphysicalactivities/) [18]. The following are some common recreational activities and their MET requirements: walking at a moderate pace, 3.5; tennis, 4.5 to 8; golf, 4 to 5; downhill skiing, 4 to 8; bowling, 3 to 5; and volleyball, 3 to 4.

Rehabilitation

Cardiac rehabilitation begins in the hospital with early mobilization, dietary instruction, and medication and disease process education. Many patients have relatively minimally invasive procedures without the loss of heart muscle function, such as coronary stent placement during acute angina. The following recommendations assume some kind of cardiac debility.

Consider a short stay in acute inpatient rehabilitation if the person is stable but unable to perform basic mobility and self-care tasks at a household level. Recommend a self-directed walking program if the patient is unable to begin a supervised exercise training program on discharge from the hospital. This should be reserved for individuals with an uncomplicated hospital course and for whom exercise is not contraindicated (Table 122.2). The patient should walk primarily on level surfaces at a slower pace with the goal of 10 to 30 minutes of walking at least three to five times per week at an intensity that will allow talking. Ask patients to keep a walking journal and review it with them.

Table 122.2 Possible Contraindications for Entry into Inpatient or Outpatient Exercise Programs

Unstable angina
Resting systolic blood pressure > 200 mm Hg
Resting diastolic blood pressure > 100 mm Hg
Orthostatic blood pressure drop or drop during exercise training of 20 mm Hg
Moderate to severe aortic stenosis
Acute systemic illness or fever
Uncontrolled atrial or ventricular dysrhythmias
Uncontrolled sinus tachycardia (120 beats per minute)
Uncontrolled congestive heart failure
Third-degree atrioventricular block
Active pericarditis or myocarditis
Recent embolism
Thrombophlebitis
Resting ST displacement (>3 mm)
Uncontrolled diabetes
Orthopedic problems that prohibit exercise

From American College of Sports Medicine. Guidelines for Exercise Testing and Prescription, 4th ed. Philadelphia, Lea & Febiger, 1991.

If no significant cardiac damage has occurred, such as after angioplasty, the period of convalescence may be shortened on the basis of the clinician's judgment and considerations such as the individual's need to return to previous pursuits.

Physical training with referral to cardiac rehabilitation begins at the end of the convalescence period. Ideally, this is based on functional exercise testing described in the preceding section on diagnostic studies. Arguments have been made that exercise testing at this stage does not improve the outcome or safety of a supervised cardiac rehabilitation therapy program, but functional exercise testing is still the "gold standard." [19] Exercise prescription includes type, target intensity, frequency, and duration of exercise. Aerobic exercises, such as walking and bicycling, are the mainstay of most programs. Prescribe aerobic exercise intensity on the basis of heart rate, exercise intensity (METs), or perceived exertion (Table 122.3). The visual analog Borg scale rates perceived exertion (Fig. 122.1) and has been shown to correlate linearly with heart rate and oxygen consumption [20]. For the patient taking beta blockers, perceived exertion is a good guideline as the heart rate response is somewhat blunted. The frequency of exercise sessions is usually three to five times per week.

Aerobic exercise sessions begin with a warm-up phase of 2 to 5 minutes at a lower intensity of exercise to limber the joints, to open collateral circulation, and to decrease peripheral vascular resistance. The stimulus or conditioning phase may be continuous or discontinuous, with the 3- to 12-month goal of at least 20 to 30 minutes of aerobic exercise. This may be broken down as a discontinuous exercise with rest breaks between periods of conditioning exercise. A cool-down phase at a lower intensity of exercise will prevent hypotension and, later, joint pain. Duration of aerobic exercise sessions depends on the individual's level of fitness. For the markedly debilitated patient, 3 to 5 minutes in the target range will provide benefit initially. The deconditioned individual should be progressed during 4 to 12 weeks to this 20- to 30-minute stimulus phase. Electrocardiographic monitoring during aerobic exercise is recommended for patients with low ejection fraction, abnormal blood pressure response to exercise, ST-segment depression during low-level exercise testing, or serious ventricular arrhythmia [21].

Strength training or circuit training with resistance exercises adds skeletal muscle strength and facilitates building of local muscle endurance for those with good left ventricular function. This should especially be considered for the cardiac patient who may be returning to a physically demanding job. Patients who use free weights should begin with the lowest weight that produces a perceived exertion of 11 to 13 after 10 to 15 repetitions (see Fig. 122.1). One to three sets will build strength. This should involve enough different exercises to include all major muscle groups of the upper and lower extremities.

The clinic-based supervised exercise program typically lasts 1 to 3 months, with the exercise prescription upgraded monthly. Monthly reevaluation should include consideration of increasing the stimulus-phase intensity or duration of aerobic exercise. After 2 to 3 months of a conditioning

Table 122.3 Cardiac Rehabilitation Exercise Prescription

Type	Aerobic	Treadmill Bicycle (circle one)
Include	Strength training?	Yes No (circle one)
Intensity: Based on heart rate		
Target heart range		
70% to 85% of maximum heart rate if the patient is not taking β-adrenergic blockade		
85% maximum completed on treadmill if the patient is taking β-adrenergic blockade		
High resting heart rate (HR), by exercise testing results (Karvonen formula):		
Target HR = resting HR + $[(HR_{max} - HR_{rest}) \times (60 + MT_{max}/100)]$		
Intensity: Based on workload		
Target 66% MET level completed on treadmill testing		
Target 25 watts or 150 kpm less than completed stage on bicycle ergometer testing		
Intensity: Based on perceived exertion		
Borg scale target 11 to 15		
Warm-up phase		
Treadmill ambulation at _____ speed _____grade for _____ minutes.		
Bicycle ergometry at _____ kpm/watts for _____ minutes.		
Check blood pressure, pulse rate, and perceived exertion.		
Advance to stimulus phase.		
Stimulus phase		
Treadmill ambulation at _____ speed _____ grade _____ minutes with/without rest. Repeat _____ sets.		
Bicycle ergometry at _____ kpm/watts for _____ minutes with/without rest. Repeat _____ sets.		
Check blood pressure, pulse rate, and perceived exertion.		
Advance to cool-down phase.		
Cool-down phase		
Treadmill ambulation at _____ speed _____ grade for _____ minutes.		
Bicycle ergometry at _____ kpm/watts for _____ minutes.		
Check blood pressure, pulse rate.		
Frequency	3 times per week	
Duration	1 hour per visit for 12 weeks	

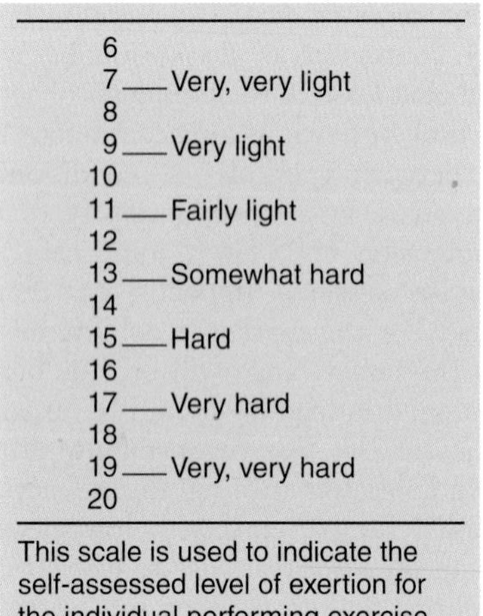

FIGURE 122.1 Borg scale of perceived exertion. *(From Borg G. Perceived exertion as an indicator of somatic stress. Scand J Rehabil Med 1970;2:92-98.)*

exercise program, the individual should have the ability to achieve 7 to 8 METs of sustained exercise. Once the patient has achieved this goal, repeat of the exercise test will show the level of improvement and guide the transition to a self-directed maintenance program. The patient may choose to follow his or her target heart rate or exertion level during exercise.

The benefits of exercise training include increased maximum oxygen uptake, increased endurance for activities of daily living, increased functional capacity, decreased heart rate during exercise, decreased rate-pressure product, decreased fatigue, decreased dyspnea, and decreased symptoms of heart failure. Exercise training reduces atherogenic and thrombotic risk factors by managing or preventing excess body weight, increasing high-density lipoprotein cholesterol concentration, decreasing plasma triglyceride levels, decreasing platelet aggregation, and improving glucose levels. Myocardial perfusion may be improved by increased coronary blood flow. The progress of coronary atherosclerosis may be slowed or possibly reversed.

Home-based cardiac rehabilitation programs should be considered for less medically complex patients unable to attend outpatient programs. A review comparing home-based versus center-based rehabilitation for low-risk cardiac patients after uncomplicated myocardial infarction or coronary artery bypass graft showed no difference in morbidity and mortality, health-related quality of life, or modifiable risk factor reduction [22].

Psychosocial interventions provide specific tools to live with emotional stress, depression, anxiety, and returning to work. Adjunct treatment with medication may be necessary if counseling and lifestyle management are inadequate alone.

Procedures

Medically stabilized cardiac patients need few procedures. Large pulmonary effusions may decrease exercise capacity, requiring the need for thoracentesis. Interventional cardiology procedures may be needed for acutely occluded stents, angioplasty, or grafts. For the patient with significant arrhythmias, pacemaker or defibrillator placement or adjustment may be necessary. The patient with worsening cardiac symptoms may need to repeat coronary angiography or other diagnostic testing if medication adjustment is unsuccessful.

Surgery

Surgical interventions may be needed for failed coronary bypass vascular grafts, infected wounds, or pseudoaneurysms at arterial puncture sites. Permanent pacemaker or implantable defibrillators may be necessary for individuals with arrhythmias not controlled with medications.

Potential Disease Complications

The most common cause of mortality in the United States is cardiac disease. Decreased exercise tolerance and decreased work capacity are the most common functional impairments. Medical complications include congestive heart failure, arrhythmia, repeated infarction, and possible closure of coronary artery grafts and stents or angioplasties. Sternotomies may not heal or become infected, requiring surgical débridement or revision. Because coronary artery disease is associated with generalized atherosclerotic vascular disease, one should be aware of possible stroke, peripheral vascular insufficiency, and other end-organ manifestations of compromised vascular supply. Even with referral to cardiac rehabilitation, individuals may still experience loss of social roles, vocational barriers, and difficulty with emotional adjustment despite excellent physical improvement and appropriate psychosocial interventions.

Potential Treatment Complications

There is a slight risk of precipitation of a cardiac event during cardiac rehabilitation. In one study, the risk of a significant cardiac event during exercise training, such as new infarct or death, occurred at a rate of 1/50,000 to 1/120,000 person-hours of exercise [23]. Preventing the enrollment into cardiac rehabilitation of patients who are not medically stabilized can minimize the risk. Exercise testing has relative and absolute contraindications that should be followed. These contraindications have been elucidated in great detail elsewhere [10]. In general, however, do not test patients with unstable angina, malignant cardiac arrhythmia, pericarditis, endocarditis, severe left ventricular dysfunction, severe aortic stenosis, or any other acute noncardiac disease. Common adverse treatment events are postexercise hypotension or arrhythmia and muscle or joint pain. These are minimized if exercise testing guides the cardiac rehabilitation prescription.

References

[1] Roger VL, Go AS, Lloyd-Jones DM, et al. Heart disease and stroke statistics—2012 update: a report from the American. Circulation 2012;125:e2–e220.
[2] Heran BS, Chen JM, Ebrahim S, et al. Exercise-based cardiac rehabilitation for coronary heart disease. Cochrane Database Syst Rev 2011;7, CD001800.
[3] Arena R, Williams M, Forman DE, et al. Increasing referral and participation rates to outpatient cardiac rehabilitation. Circulation 2012;125:1321–9.
[4] Davis A, Natelson B. Brain-heart interactions. The neurocardiology of arrhythmia and sudden cardiac death. Tex Heart Inst J 1993;20:158–69.
[5] Roest AM, Zuidersma M, de Jonge P. Myocardial infarction and generalised anxiety disorder: 10-year follow-up. Br J Psychiatry 2012;200:324–9.
[6] Watkins L, Blumenthal J, Davidson J, et al. Phobic anxiety, depression, and risk of ventricular arrhythmias in patients with coronary heart disease. Psychosom Med 2006;68:651–6.
[7] Yusuf S, Hawken S, Ounpuu S, et al. Effect of potentially modifiable risk factors associated with myocardial infarction in 52 countries (the INTERHEART study): case-control study. Lancet 2004;364:937–52.
[8] Berkman LF, Blumenthal J, Burg M, et al. Effects of treating depression and low perceived social support on clinical events after myocardial infarction: the Enhancing Recovery in Coronary Heart Disease Patients (ENRICHD) randomized trial. JAMA 2003;289:3106–16.
[9] Reusch JE, Wang CC. Cardiovascular disease in diabetes: where does glucose fit in? J Clin Endocrinol Metab 2011;96:2367–76.
[10] Arena R, Myers J, Guazzi M. Cardiopulmonary exercise testing is a coreassessment for patients with heart failure. Congest Heart Fail 2011;17:115–9.
[11] Lichtenstein AH, Appel LJ, Brands M, et al. Diet and lifestyle recommendations revision 2006: a scientific statement from the American Heart Association. Circulation 2006;114:82–96.
[12] Brezinka V, Kittel F. Psychosocial factors of coronary heart disease in women: a review. Soc Sci Med 1996;42:1351–65.
[13] Davidson P, Digiacomo M, Zecchin R, et al. A cardiac rehabilitation program to improve psychosocial outcomes of women with heart disease. J Womens Health (Larchmt) 2008;17:123–34.
[14] Davis A. Respiratory modulation of heart rate variability and parasympathetic influence on the heart [doctoral dissertation]. Newark, NJ: University of Medicine and Dentistry of New Jersey–New Jersey Medical School; 1997.
[15] Friedman S. Cardiac disease, anxiety, and sexual functioning. Am J Cardiol 2000;86:46f–50f.
[16] Levine GN, Steinke EE, Bakaeen FG, et al. Sexual activity and cardiovascular disease: a scientific statement from the American Heart Association. Circulation 2012;125:1058–72.
[17] Kivimaki M, Nyberg ST, Batty GD, et al. Job strain as a risk factor for coronary heart disease: a collaborative meta-analysis of individual participant data. Lancet 2012;380:1491–7.
[18] Ainsworth BE, Haskell WL, Herrmann SD, et al. 2011 Compendium of Physical Activities: a second update of codes and MET values. Med Sci Sports Exerc 2011;43:1575–81.
[19] Mezzani A, Hamm LF, Jones AM, et al. Aerobic exercise intensity assessment and prescription in cardiac rehabilitation. J Cardiopulm Rehabil Prev 2012;32:327–50.
[20] Borg G. Subjective effort and physical abilities. Scand J Rehabil Med Suppl 1978;6:105–13.
[21] American Association for Cardiopulmonary Rehabilitation. Guidelines for cardiac rehabilitation and secondary prevention programs. 4th ed. Champaign, Ill: Human Kinetics; 2004.
[22] Taylor RS, Dalal H, Jolly K, et al. Home-based versus centre-based cardiac rehabilitation. Cochrane Database Syst Rev 2010;1, CD007130.
[23] Franklin BA, Bonzheim K, Gordon S, Timmis GC. Safety of medically supervised outpatient cardiac rehabilitation exercise. Chest 1998;114:902–6.

CHAPTER 123

Cancer-Related Fatigue

Andrea Cheville, MD, MSCE

Synonyms

Cancer-related fatigue syndrome
Paraneoplastic dysfunction

ICD-9 Codes

357.6 Polyneuropathy due to drugs
780.79 Other malaise and fatigue
781.2 Abnormality of gait

ICD-10 Codes

G62.0 Drug-induced polyneuropathy
R53.81 Other malaise
R26.9 Abnormalities of gait and mobility

Definition

Cancer causes one in four deaths in the United States and is a major public health problem worldwide. Projections for 2013 were that more than 1,660,290 new cancer cases would be diagnosed and that more than 580,305 patients would die of cancer [1]. Cancers vary widely in prognosis, natural history, management, treatment responsiveness, adverse sequelae, and associated physical impairments. As a consequence, cancer rehabilitation is not amenable to one-size-fits-all treatment approaches. Physical impairments vary with the location and stage of cancer as well as by the type of treatment. For example, cancers of the head and neck may require neck dissection and irradiation. Common sequelae include shoulder dysfunction and fibrosis of cervical soft tissue. In contrast, primary breast cancer treatment may cause myofascial pain and upper extremity swelling. The reader is referred to chapters specific to these conditions and anatomic locations (e.g., scapular winging, lymphedema).

A more uniform approach can be applied to the management of cancer-related fatigue (CRF). The National Comprehensive Cancer Network defines CRF as a distressing, persistent, subjective sense of physical, emotional, or cognitive tiredness or exhaustion related to cancer or cancer treatment that is not proportional to recent activity and interferes with usual functioning [2]. CRF is the most common cancer-associated symptom among the more than 12 million cancer survivors in the United States [3]. Its effects can be overwhelming and, depending on the nature and treatment of the cancer, can limit the lives of as many as 70% of disease-free survivors [4–7]. Whereas severe post-treatment CRF is particularly common among lung cancer survivors [8,9], high levels of persistent CRF are also reported among the survivors of most malignant neoplasms, including but not limited to those of the breast, brain, head, and neck and childhood malignant neoplasms [7–21]. CRF, even at it mildest levels, affects all health-related quality of life domains [4,22–24]. On a vocational level, CRF intensity predicts failure to return to work [4,25–27], and it is estimated that 1 million cancer survivors may be receiving disability payments as a consequence of its persistence [28]. On a general level, multiple investigators have found that increased CRF is considered an important unmet care need by patients [29–31] and explains a significant proportion of performance and mobility degradations [32–38] across a wide range of cancers [39–42]. Not surprisingly, the indirect costs associated with patients with CRF are increased, with research showing that patients with CRF visit general practitioners 50%, specialists 350%, physical therapists 130%, and complementary caregivers 520% more often than those without the condition do [4,43,44]. Fortunately, effective CRF treatment has been shown to improve vocational productivity and performance of activities of daily living while reducing family stress and caregiver burden [45].

Symptoms

Before formal evaluation is undertaken, it is important to establish the patient's current place on the cancer trajectory, which influences all elements of the history and physical examination. Three important distinctions must be made:

1. Is the patient receiving active treatment?
2. Does the patient have residual cancer?
3. Is the patient deemed curable?

The willingness and capacity of patients to engage in the rehabilitation process will be reflected in the answers to these questions.

A characteristic constellation of symptoms should not be anticipated in patients' reporting of CRF. As emphasized before, patients' neoplasms, treatment regimens, and disease trajectories are variable. CRF may therefore be manifested differently, contingent on the particulars of each case. Patients' descriptions of their fatigue may be inconsistent and, at times, puzzling to clinicians. Any of the following subjective complaints should raise concern about possible CRF: weakness (generalized or proximal), dyspnea on exertion, orthostatic hypotension, sedation, hypersomnolence, exertional intolerance, or cognitive compromise (e.g., attention or concentration deficits, short-term memory dysfunction). Patients may report the sensation that their legs are leaden or that they are walking through water. Validated self-report fatigue scales (e.g., Brief Fatigue Inventory, Functional Assessment of Cancer Treatment—Fatigue, Profile of Mood States) can be exceedingly useful to quantify severity of symptoms and to monitor treatment response [46]. A brief screen for depression or other mood disorders is essential, and validated screening tools are widely available.

Patients' cancer histories warrant attention, including prior and ongoing radiation therapy and chemotherapy as well as any surgical procedures. Awareness of a patient's primary cancer will shift the focus toward particular causes of symptoms. Information comparable with that solicited through a good pain history should be elicited for fatigue: acuity of fatigue onset, activity- or treatment-related precipitants, diurnal fluctuation, associated symptoms (e.g., pain, nausea), progressive worsening or improvement, exacerbating and alleviating factors, and prior treatments and degree of response. Questions about sleep patterns, sleep hygiene, and daytime napping are useful. Reports suggest that frequent daytime napping may actually worsen fatigue [47].

The extent to which fatigue limits vocational, avocational, and familial pursuits as well as autonomous mobility and self-care should be comprehensively reviewed. Because fatigue most commonly interferes with activities requiring stamina and exertional tolerance, changes in a patient's comfortable walking distance, duration of physical activity, and willingness to climb stairs will help characterize the impact of fatigue.

Physical Examination

Special tests are rarely indicated on physical examination. Rather, clinicians should perform a comprehensive evaluation with emphasis on musculoskeletal and neurologic elements. Assessment of range of motion, gait (including tandem), static and dynamic balance, and ability to squat repetitively may identify potential contributing factors amenable to therapeutic exercise. Examination may reveal evidence of congestive heart failure or pulmonary compromise. Signs of hypothyroidism should be sought, particularly in patients irradiated for head and neck cancers. For patients without evidence of cancer, the neurologic examination findings should be normal beyond chemotherapy-related peripheral neuropathy. Weakness in proximal hip and shoulder musculature suggests steroid myopathy. Identification of new neurologic deficits should trigger evaluation for malignant progression or emerging treatment toxicity. The mental status examination may reveal evidence of compromised arousal, attention, memory, or concentration, particularly in patients who have received whole-brain radiation therapy or intrathecal chemotherapy.

Functional Limitations

Although fatigue is rarely so severe that it undermines basic mobility or performance of activities of daily living apart from the palliative context [48], evaluation of these functional domains is integral to comprehensive evaluation. Severe functional compromise may be a red flag, contingent on the clinical context that triggers evaluation for significant comorbidity or recurrent cancer. Ambulation for moderate distances may produce limiting dyspnea in patients with cancer-related cardiac or pulmonary dysfunction. Patients with steroid myopathy or generalized muscle weakness may have difficulty in rising from low surfaces, such as a toilet, soft chair, or car seat. These patients may also demonstrate decreased ability to independently complete their activities of daily living in a reasonable time frame. As suggested previously, many patients describe generalized heaviness of the limbs and global decrements in activity level without precise functional limitations.

Dysfunction in social, vocational, psychological, and sexual domains may be present. Patients should be questioned about compromised social interactions, sleep, and intimacy as well as work-related and leisure pursuits. Many patients abandon their avocational activities as a consequence of fatigue, with the potential for isolation and secondary depression. Patients with cognitive deficits related to radiation therapy or chemotherapy may experience difficulty in maintaining their vocational productivity. Financial and domestic management skills may be compromised as well.

Diagnostic Studies

Diagnostic tests should be informed by patients' symptoms and findings on clinical examination. Dyspnea should be assessed with pulse oximetry during activity, chest radiography, and electrocardiography. Patients who exhibit severe dyspnea with minimal activity may have pulmonary fibrosis. Definitive diagnosis may require computed tomographic scanning. Positron emission tomography may help distinguish fibrosis from cancer involving the lung parenchyma. Patients with cancer are at an elevated risk for venous thrombosis; therefore, a venous duplex study and possibly a ventilation-perfusion scan should be considered for persistent shortness of breath. Patients who have received doxorubicin (Adriamycin) or trastuzumab (Herceptin) should be evaluated with a multigated acquisition scan to rule out possible chemotherapy-related cardiac toxicity. Most patients will have undergone multigated acquisition screening before the administration of chemotherapy. The results of baseline tests can be compared with new evaluations for evidence of deterioration. Pericardial effusions may be a consequence of malignant spread or radiation-induced irritation or occur as a paraneoplastic phenomenon. An echocardiogram should be obtained for patients with a suggestive history and physical examination. Patients reporting insomnia or a failure to feel rested after a night's sleep may benefit from a sleep study to rule out sleep apnea or related disorders.

Serologic evaluation may include thyroid-stimulating hormone concentration (to screen for thyroid myopathy in patients who have received irradiation to the anterior neck), calcium concentration, electrolyte values (Addison disease may occur with adrenal metastases or irradiation), hemoglobin concentration, and hematocrit. Hypercalcemia or persistent mechanical pain should be evaluated with a bone scan or plain films. *Multiple myeloma and malignant neoplasms producing lytic metastases may fail to generate an abnormal bone scan despite diffuse skeletal involvement.* Blood levels of centrally acting medications (e.g., tricyclic antidepressants, anticonvulsants) may warrant assessment in patients who describe fatigue with a significant cognitive dimension.

For patients with focal neurologic deficits, imaging of those portions of the neural axis implicated on physical examination should be performed. Magnetic resonance images should be obtained with gadolinium. Steroids administered in conjunction with chemotherapy may be of sufficient doses to cause myopathy. Electrodiagnostic studies can rule out alternative, treatable sources of neurologic compromise.

Patients complaining of generalized cognitive dysfunction may benefit from neuropsychological evaluation. Cognitive deficits have been detected after chemotherapy [49]. Multifocal brain metastases may be manifested with a global decrement in mental acuity and capacity to attend. Enhanced computed tomographic scanning of the head may be warranted when there is a high clinical probability of brain metastases (e.g., patients with melanoma, breast or lung cancers).

Screening for depression, anxiety, and other psychological distress is integral to the CRF evaluation. The Patient Health Questionnaire (PHQ-9) is a brief and valid screen for use in cancer populations. The PHQ-9 distinguishes both the presence and severity of depression [50]. The Generalized Anxiety Disorder (GAD-7) screen is another valid measure with low respondent burden that can be facilely integrated into routine history taking [51].

Differential Diagnosis

- Depression
- Nutritional insufficiency
- Anemia
- Infection
- Metabolic or endocrine abnormality (e.g., hypercalcemia, hypothyroidism, adrenal insufficiency)
- Steroid myopathy
- Medication side effects
- Chemotherapy- or radiation therapy–induced cognitive dysfunction
- Cachexia
- Pulmonary parenchymal disease, bleomycin toxicity, radiation therapy–induced fibrosis
- Pleural or pericardial effusion
- Doxorubicin- or trastuzumab-related cardiotoxicity
- Disturbed disorder
- Neural axis compromise (e.g., brain metastasis, epidural metastasis, brachial or lumbosacral plexopathy)

Treatment

Initial

It is important to address any remediable endocrine, hematologic, metabolic, or physical abnormalities before initiation of treatment (e.g., exercise that targets fatigue). Uncontrolled pain mandates the initiation or modification of analgesics. Opioid-based pharmacotherapy has emerged as the cornerstone of cancer pain management [52]. Secondary infections related to cancer therapy–induced neutropenia must be treated before aerobic conditioning can begin. The discovery of disease progression may warrant initiation or alteration of an antineoplastic regimen or the administration of radiation therapy. Cardiac toxicity may improve after the initiation of digoxin or medications to reduce afterload. Anemia generally responds to therapy with recombinant erythropoietin with associated improvements in the patient's function and quality of life [53]. Patients with pulmonary fibrosis induced by radiation therapy or chemotherapy and those who have undergone lobectomy or pneumonectomy may require supplemental oxygen during rehabilitative efforts. Nutritional evaluation may be needed for cachectic or hypoproteinemic patients.

Rehabilitation

Well-powered, randomized, controlled trials have established that both strengthening and aerobic exercise can, regardless of the phase of the disease, effectively reduce the effects of CRF [54–63]. Modest exercise intensity levels (e.g., 60% of maximum oxygen consumption up to 5 days per week) suffice and are well tolerated by patients irrespective of treatment phase. A significant proportion of positive studies have used home-based exercise approaches [57–61], which work in noncancer populations suggests may be particularly effective in enhancing long-term adherence [64–66]. It is significant that whereas structured programs, particularly when they are augmented with supportive counseling [60,61], have proved highly efficacious, a more flexible program lacking specific exercise recommendations has not [67].

Exercise is not the only beneficial approach. Psychoeducational interventions emphasizing activity and stress management [68–71], mindfulness training [72], coping skills and problem-solving training [68,73], and cognitive-behavioral therapy [74] have also been shown to be capable of significantly reducing CRF. Although randomized, controlled trials of supportive and exercise therapies in isolation have yielded mixed results [75–79], supportive therapy alone may be effective when CRF is the principal therapeutic focus [79]. To date, no trial that has combined aerobic exercise with structured psychological support has failed to note significant improvements in fatigue [58,60,61]. However, treatments may be less effective in the advanced stages of cancer [80].

Unfortunately, the patient volumes, staff expertise, and infrastructure necessary to support these group and 1:1 interventions are available only at large tertiary medical centers. According to the National Cancer Institute estimates, only about 15% of U.S. cancer patients are diagnosed and treated at these centers, suggesting that the remaining 85% are being treated at facilities incapable of providing effective CRF management programs.

The literature supports interval training at 50% to 70% of the heart rate reserve or while working at an exertion of 11 to 14 (moderate intensity) on the 6 to 20 perceived rate of exertion scale. The intensity of the exercise program depends on baseline fitness levels, intensity of cancer treatment, and stage of cancer treatment. While the patient is undergoing treatment, most studies recommend decreasing the intensity to the lower end of the heart rate range. Once active chemotherapy or radiation therapy has been completed, the program may be progressed toward the higher end of the range. The intensity must also take into account daily laboratory values and patterns of fatigue associated with treatment. For example, fatigue peaks within the middle and end of the radiation therapy cycle, and the program should account for this pattern. Finally, duration and frequency should closely match the American College of Sports Medicine guidelines, which recommend that patients with cancer exercise for a total of 20 to 30 minutes three to five times per week [81].

Exercise precautions for cancer patients are seldom evidence based. They vary significantly between institutions and clinicians. The following limitations are conservative suggestions and should not be interpreted as absolute exercise contraindications. Aerobic and resistive exercise should be carefully reviewed if not discontinued when platelet levels fall below 10,000/μL. Contact and high-impact sports should be avoided when platelet levels fall below 50,000/μL or in patients with primary or metastatic bone disease. Light exercise is allowed when hemoglobin concentration is less than 8g/dL, with patients closely monitored for symptoms. Therapeutic activities should be restricted to indoor exercise for patients at nadir with an absolute neutrophil count below 500/μL. Exercise should be deferred for febrile patients with temperatures above 101.5°F.

In addition to aerobic conditioning, referral to occupational and physical therapy for training in energy conservation strategies, use of adaptive equipment, and progressive resistive exercise will benefit appropriate patients. Instruction in compensatory strategies for mobility and performance of activities of daily living can optimize autonomy within the constraints imposed by CRF. Adaptive equipment, such as canes, crutches, and walkers, may improve mobility; provision with adaptive devices, such as long-handled shoehorns and reachers, may facilitate independent self-care activities. Interventions for mobility and performance of activities of daily living benefit even end-stage cancer patients. For these patients, education and empowerment of caretakers may emerge as the primary therapeutic focus.

A psychiatric consultation may be indicated if depression emerges during evaluation. All nonessential centrally acting drugs should be eliminated. Pain medications should be chosen to minimize neuropsychological toxicity. Among the opioids, hydromorphone, fentanyl, and oxycodone have fewer active metabolites than morphine sulfate [82]. Their use may be associated with a more tolerable side effect profile in the elderly and patients with renal impairment. Pharmacologic approaches for cancer fatigue center predominantly around the administration of psychostimulants. The utility of these agents is equivocal since controlled trials of methylphenidate and pemoline have produced mixed results [83].

Procedures

Patients with pleural or pericardial effusions will benefit from percutaneous drainage of the fluid. Pleurocentesis or pericardiocentesis may be required to prevent the reaccumulation of effusions. Percutaneous stenting procedures have become commonplace when tumor compression narrows the lumen of ureters, bile ducts, bronchi, or blood vessels with adverse physiologic sequelae. When cancer pain cannot be adequately managed with systemic therapy or if side effects become untenable, neuraxial analgesic delivery may restore normal arousal, energy, and cognition [33]. Radiation therapy may be used palliatively to treat pain or to reduce tumor bulk that is compressing neurologic structures.

Surgery

Cancer patients with deconditioning and fatigue may benefit from surgical debulking of tumor or resection of isolated lung, liver, bone, or brain metastases. Fatigue, however, is not an independent indication for surgery. If focal sensory or motor deficits result from tumor compression of neural pathways, emergent resection may be required.

Potential Disease Complications

Patients commonly deteriorate functionally because of incremental tumor burden and morbidities as their cancers advance. Consequences of malignant progression may include new or worsening neurologic deficits, dyspnea, cognitive deterioration from intracranial metastases or radiation therapy–induced changes, pathologic fractures, visceral obstruction, and somatic pain syndromes.

Potential Treatment Complications

Potential complications of anticancer modalities are extensive. Radiation therapy can cause fibrosis, neurologic compromise, and worsening of CRF. Chemotherapy can similarly exacerbate CRF. Various chemotherapeutic agents have the capacity to impair cognitive, renal, pulmonary, cardiac, and neurologic function. The pharmacologic agents used to manage cancer-associated symptoms and pain can adversely affect neurologic, gastrointestinal, and urinary function as well as exacerbate peripheral edema and CRF.

Complications associated with rehabilitative interventions are few when strategies are used appropriately. Patients with bone-avid cancers (e.g., lung, prostate, breast, thyroid, multiple myeloma, and renal) are at risk for pathologic fractures, particularly those with lytic metastases. A recent bone scan or skeletal survey should be reviewed before initiating an exercise program.

Cancer patients should generally be considered more susceptible to common exercise-induced complications. Overly aggressive aerobic conditioning or strengthening programs may worsen CRF. Uncustomary exertion may aggravate chemotherapeutically induced electrolyte and fluid imbalances. Therapeutic regimens for cancer patients should be adapted and scrutinized accordingly.

References

[1] Siegel R, Naishadham D, Jemal A. Cancer statistics, 2013. CA Cancer J Clin 2013;63:11–30.

[2] National Comprehensive Cancer, Network. Cancer-related fatigue, http://www.nccn.org/professionals/physician_gls/pdf/fatigue.pdf; [accessed 16.04.13].

[3] Horner M, Ries L, Krapcho M, et al. SEER cancer statistics review, 1975–2006. National Cancer Institute. http://seer.cancer.gov/csr/1975_2006/.

[4] Curt GA, Breitbart W, Cella D, et al. Impact of cancer-related fatigue on the lives of patients: new findings from the Fatigue Coalition. Oncologist 2000;5:353–60.

[5] Cella D, Davis K, Breitbart W, Curt G. Cancer-related fatigue: prevalence of proposed diagnostic criteria in a United States sample of cancer survivors. J Clin Oncol 2001;19:3385–91.

[6] Fobair P, Hoppe RT, Bloom J, et al. Psychosocial problems among survivors of Hodgkin's disease. J Clin Oncol 1986;4:805–14.

[7] Andrykowski MA, Greiner CB, Altmaier EM, et al. Quality of life following bone marrow transplantation: findings from a multicentre study. Br J Cancer 1995;71:1322–9.

[8] Hjermstad MJ, Fossa SD, Oldervoll L, et al. Fatigue in long-term Hodgkin's disease survivors: a follow-up study. J Clin Oncol 2005;23:6587–95.

[9] Fox SW, Lyon DE. Symptom clusters and quality of life in survivors of lung cancer. Oncol Nurs Forum 2006;33:931–6.

[10] Zeltzer LK, Recklitis C, Buchbinder D, et al. Psychological status in childhood cancer survivors: a report from the childhood cancer survivor study. J Clin Oncol 2009;27:2396–404.

[11] Andrykowski MA, Curran SL, Lightner R. Off-treatment fatigue in breast cancer survivors: a controlled comparison. J Behav Med 1998;21:1–18.

[12] Bower JE, Ganz PA, Desmond KA, et al. Fatigue in long-term breast carcinoma survivors: a longitudinal investigation. Cancer 2006;106:751–8.

[13] Bower JE, Ganz PA, Desmond KA, et al. Fatigue in breast cancer survivors: occurrence, correlates, and impact on quality of life. J Clin Oncol 2000;18:743–53.

[14] Servaes P, Verhagen S, Bleijenberg G. Determinants of chronic fatigue in disease-free breast cancer patients: a cross-sectional study. Ann Oncol 2002;13:589–98.

[15] Crom DB, Hinds PS, Gattuso JS, et al. Creating the basis for a breast health program for female survivors of Hodgkin disease using a participatory research approach. Oncol Nurs Forum 2005;32:1131–41.

[16] Ruffer JU, Flechtner H, Tralls P, et al. Fatigue in long-term survivors of Hodgkin's lymphoma; a report from the German Hodgkin Lymphoma Study Group (GHSG). Eur J Cancer 2003;39:2179–86.

[17] Fossa SD, Dahl AA, Loge JH. Fatigue, anxiety, and depression in long-term survivors of testicular cancer. J Clin Oncol 2003;21:1249–54.

[18] Kyrdalen AE, Dahl AA, Hernes E, et al. Fatigue in hormone-naive prostate cancer patients treated with radical prostatectomy or definitive radiotherapy. Prostate Cancer Prostatic Dis 2010;13:144–50.

[19] Djarv T, Lagergren J, Blazeby JM, Lagergren P. Long-term health-related quality of life following surgery for oesophageal cancer. Br J Surg 2008;95:1121–6.

[20] Chaukar DA, Walvekar RR, Das AK, et al. Quality of life in head and neck cancer survivors: a cross-sectional survey. Am J Otolaryngol 2009;30:176–80.

[21] Pourel N, Peiffert D, Lartigau E, et al. Quality of life in long-term survivors of oropharynx carcinoma. Int J Radiat Oncol Biol Phys 2002;54:742–51.

[22] Shih YC, Wang XS, Cantor SB, Cleeland CS. The association between symptom burdens and utility in Chinese cancer patients. Qual Life Res 2006;15:1427–38.

[23] Ferreira KA, Kimura M, Teixeira MJ, et al. Impact of cancer-related symptom synergisms on health-related quality of life and performance status. J Pain Symptom Manage 2008;35:604–16.

[24] Brown DJ, McMillan DC, Milroy R. The correlation between fatigue, physical function, the systemic inflammatory response, and psychological distress in patients with advanced lung cancer. Cancer 2005;103:377–82.

[25] Spelten ER, Verbeek JH, Uitterhoeve AL, et al. Cancer, fatigue and the return of patients to work—a prospective cohort study. Eur J Cancer 2003;39:1562–7.

[26] Yabroff KR, Lawrence WF, Clauser S, et al. Burden of illness in cancer survivors: findings from a population-based national sample. J Natl Cancer Inst 2004;96:1322–30.

[27] Buckwalter AE, Karnell LH, Smith RB, et al. Patient-reported factors associated with discontinuing employment following head and neck cancer treatment. Arch Otolaryngol Head Neck Surg 2007;133:464–70.

[28] Horner MJ RL, Krapcho M, Neyman N, et al, eds. SEER cancer statistics review, 1975–2006. National Cancer Institute. http://seer.cancer.gov/csr/1975_2006/.

[29] Janda M, Steginga S, Dunn J, et al. Unmet supportive care needs and interest in services among patients with a brain tumour and their carers. Patient Educ Couns 2008;71:251–8.

[30] Hwang SS, Chang VT, Cogswell J, et al. Study of unmet needs in symptomatic veterans with advanced cancer: incidence, independent predictors and unmet needs outcome model. J Pain Symptom Manage 2004;28:421–32.

[31] Baker F, Denniston M, Smith T, West MM. Adult cancer survivors: how are they faring? Cancer 2005;104(Suppl.):2565–76.

[32] Dodd MJ, Miaskowski C, Paul SM. Symptom clusters and their effect on the functional status of patients with cancer. Oncol Nurs Forum 2001;28:465–70.

[33] Given CW, Given BA, Stommel M. The impact of age, treatment, and symptoms on the physical and mental health of cancer patients. A longitudinal perspective. Cancer 1994;74(Suppl.):2128–38.

[34] Cella D, Eton D, Hensing TA, et al. Relationship between symptom change, objective tumor measurements, and performance status during chemotherapy for advanced lung cancer. Clin Lung Cancer 2008;9:51–8.

[35] Kurtz ME, Given B, Kurtz JC, Given CW. The interaction of age, symptoms, and survival status on physical and mental health of patients with cancer and their families. Cancer 1994; 74(Suppl.):2071–8.

[36] Dahele M, Skipworth RJ, Wall L, et al. Objective physical activity and self-reported quality of life in patients receiving palliative chemotherapy. J Pain Symptom Manage 2007;33:676–85.

[37] Hansen JA, Feuerstein M, Calvio LC, Olsen CH. Breast cancer survivors at work. J Occup Environ Med 2008;50:777–84.

[38] Lavigne JE, Griggs JJ, Tu XM, Lerner DJ. Hot flashes, fatigue, treatment exposures and work productivity in breast cancer survivors. J Cancer Surviv 2008;2:296–302.

[39] Silver HJ, de Campos Graf Guimaraes C, Pedruzzi P, et al. Predictors of functional decline in locally advanced head and neck cancer patients from South Brazil. Head Neck 2010;32:1217–25.

[40] Given B, Given C, Azzouz F, Stommel M. Physical functioning of elderly cancer patients prior to diagnosis and following initial treatment. Nurs Res 2001;50:222–32.

[41] Kurtz ME, Kurtz JC, Given CW, Given B. Loss of physical functioning among patients with cancer: a longitudinal view. Cancer Pract 1993;1:275–81.

[42] Kurtz ME, Kurtz JC, Stommel M, et al. Loss of physical functioning among geriatric cancer patients: relationships to cancer site, treatment, comorbidity and age. Eur J Cancer 1997;33:2352–8.

[43] van de Poll-Franse LV, Mols F, Vingerhoets AJ, et al. Increased health care utilisation among 10-year breast cancer survivors. Support Care Cancer 2006;14:436–43.

[44] Passik SD, Kirsh KL. A pilot examination of the impact of cancer patients' fatigue on their spousal caregivers. Palliat Support Care 2005;3:273–9.

[45] Berndt E, Kallich J, McDermott A, et al. Reductions in anaemia and fatigue are associated with improvements in productivity in cancer patients receiving chemotherapy. Pharmacoeconomics 2005;23:505–14.

[46] Minton O, Stone P. A systematic review of the scales used for the measurement of cancer-related fatigue (CRF). Ann Oncol 2009;20:17–25.

[47] O'Donnell JF. Insomnia in cancer patients. Clin Cornerstone 2004;(Suppl. 1D)S6–14.

[48] Yennurajalingam S, Bruera E. Palliative management of fatigue at the close of life: "it feels like my body is just worn out." JAMA 2007;297:295–304.

[49] Jim HS, Phillips KM, Chait S, et al. Meta-analysis of cognitive functioning in breast cancer survivors previously treated with standard-dose chemotherapy. J Clin Oncol 2012;30:3578–87.

[50] Kroenke K, Spitzer RL, Williams JB. The PHQ-9: validity of a brief depression severity measure. J Gen Intern Med 2001;16:606–13.

[51] Spitzer RL, Kroenke K, Williams JB, Lowe B. A brief measure for assessing generalized anxiety disorder: the GAD-7. Arch Intern Med 2006;166:1092–7.
[52] Foley KM. Treatment of cancer-related pain. J Natl Cancer Inst Monogr 2004;32:103–4.
[53] Cortesi E, Gascon P, Henry D, et al. Standard of care for cancer-related anemia: improving hemoglobin levels and quality of life. Oncology 2005;68(Suppl. 1):22–32.
[54] Mock V, Frangakis C, Davidson NE, et al. Exercise manages fatigue during breast cancer treatment: a randomized controlled trial. Psychooncology 2005;14:464–77.
[55] Segal RJ, Reid RD, Courneya KS, et al. Randomized controlled trial of resistance or aerobic exercise in men receiving radiation therapy for prostate cancer. J Clin Oncol 2009;27:344–51.
[56] Segal RJ, Reid RD, Courneya KS, et al. Resistance exercise in men receiving androgen deprivation therapy for prostate cancer. J Clin Oncol 2003;21:1653–9.
[57] Mock V, Dow KH, Meares CJ, et al. Effects of exercise on fatigue, physical functioning, and emotional distress during radiation therapy for breast cancer. Oncol Nurs Forum 1997;24:991–1000.
[58] Mock V, Burke MB, Sheehan P, et al. A nursing rehabilitation program for women with breast cancer receiving adjuvant chemotherapy. Oncol Nurs Forum 1994;21:899–907, discussion 908.
[59] Headley JA, Ownby KK, John LD. The effect of seated exercise on fatigue and quality of life in women with advanced breast cancer. Oncol Nurs Forum 2004;31:977–83.
[60] Courneya KS, Friedenreich CM, Sela RA, et al. The group psychotherapy and home-based physical exercise (group-hope) trial in cancer survivors: physical fitness and quality of life outcomes. Psychooncology 2003;12:357–74.
[61] Pinto BM, Frierson GM, Rabin C, et al. Home-based physical activity intervention for breast cancer patients. J Clin Oncol 2005;23:3577–87.
[62] Courneya KS, Mackey JR, Bell GJ, et al. Randomized controlled trial of exercise training in postmenopausal breast cancer survivors: cardiopulmonary and quality of life outcomes. J Clin Oncol 2003;21:1660–8.
[63] Burnham TR, Wilcox A. Effects of exercise on physiological and psychological variables in cancer survivors. Med Sci Sports Exerc 2002;34:1863–7.
[64] Jones MI, Greenfield S, Jolly K. Patients' experience of home and hospital based cardiac rehabilitation: a focus group study. Eur J Cardiovasc Nurs 2009;8:9–17.
[65] Opdenacker J, Boen F, Coorevits N, Delecluse C. Effectiveness of a lifestyle intervention and a structured exercise intervention in older adults. Prev Med 2008;46:518–24.
[66] Ashworth NL, Chad KE, Harrison EL, et al. Home versus center based physical activity programs in older adults. Cochrane Database Syst Rev 2005;1, CD004017.
[67] Thorsen L, Skovlund E, Stromme SB, et al. Effectiveness of physical activity on cardiorespiratory fitness and health-related quality of life in young and middle-aged cancer patients shortly after chemotherapy. J Clin Oncol 2005;23:2378–88.
[68] Fawzy FI, Cousins N, Fawzy NW, et al. A structured psychiatric intervention for cancer patients. I. Changes over time in methods of coping and affective disturbance. Arch Gen Psychiatry 1990;47:720–5.
[69] Boesen EH, Ross L, Frederiksen K, et al. Psychoeducational intervention for patients with cutaneous malignant melanoma: a replication study. J Clin Oncol 2005;23:1270–7.
[70] Barsevick AM, Dudley W, Beck S, et al. A randomized clinical trial of energy conservation for patients with cancer-related fatigue. Cancer 2004;100:1302–10.
[71] Jacobsen PB, Meade CD, Stein KD, et al. Efficacy and costs of two forms of stress management training for cancer patients undergoing chemotherapy. J Clin Oncol 2002;20:2851–62.
[72] Speca M, Carlson LE, Goodey E, Angen M. A randomized, wait-list controlled clinical trial: the effect of a mindfulness meditation–based stress reduction program on mood and symptoms of stress in cancer outpatients. Psychosom Med 2000;62:613–22.
[73] Telch CF, Telch MJ. Group coping skills instruction and supportive group therapy for cancer patients: a comparison of strategies. J Consult Clin Psychol 1986;54:802–8.
[74] Gaston-Johansson F, Fall-Dickson JM, Nanda J, et al. The effectiveness of the comprehensive coping strategy program on clinical outcomes in breast cancer autologous bone marrow transplantation. Cancer Nurs 2000;23:277–85.
[75] Goodwin PJ, Leszcz M, Ennis M, et al. The effect of group psychosocial support on survival in metastatic breast cancer. N Engl J Med 2001;345:1719–26.
[76] Sandgren AK, McCaul KD. Short-term effects of telephone therapy for breast cancer patients. Health Psychol 2003;22:310–5.
[77] Bordeleau L, Szalai JP, Ennis M, et al. Quality of life in a randomized trial of group psychosocial support in metastatic breast cancer: overall effects of the intervention and an exploration of missing data. J Clin Oncol 2003;21:1944–51.
[78] Spiegel D, Bloom JR, Yalom I. Group support for patients with metastatic cancer. A randomized outcome study. Arch Gen Psychiatry 1981;38:527–33.
[79] Forester B, Kornfeld DS, Fleiss JL. Psychotherapy during radiotherapy: effects on emotional and physical distress. Am J Psychiatry 1985;142:22–7.
[80] Payne C, Wiffen PJ, Martin S. Interventions for fatigue and weight loss in adults with advanced progressive illness. Cochrane Database Syst Rev 2012;1, CD008427.
[81] Schmitz KH, Courneya KS, Matthews C, et al. American College of Sports Medicine roundtable on exercise guidelines for cancer survivors. Med Sci Sports Exerc 2011;42:1409–26.
[82] Coller JK, Christrup LL, Somogyi AA. Role of active metabolites in the use of opioids. Eur J Clin Pharmacol 2009;65:121–39.
[83] Minton O, Richardson A, Sharpe M, et al. Psychostimulants for the management of cancer-related fatigue: a systematic review and meta-analysis. J Pain Symptom Manage 2011;41:761–7.

CHAPTER 124

Cerebral Palsy

Sathya Vadivelu, DO
Marlís González-Fernández, MD, PhD

Synonym

Little disease

ICD-9 Codes

343	**Infantile cerebral palsy**
343.0	**Diplegic**
343.1	**Hemiplegic; congenital hemiplegia**
343.2	**Quadriplegic**
343.3	**Monoplegic**
343.4	**Infantile hemiplegia; infantile hemiplegia NOS**
343.8	**Other specified infantile cerebral palsy**
343.9	**Infantile cerebral palsy, unspecified**
V54.8	**Orthopedic aftercare: changes, check or removal of casts, splints (external)**

ICD-10 Codes

G80.0	**Spastic quadriplegic cerebral palsy (congenital)**
G80.1	**Spastic diplegic cerebral palsy**
G80.2	**Spastic hemiplegic cerebral palsy**
G80.3	**Athetoid cerebral palsy**
G80.4	**Ataxic cerebral palsy**
G80.8	**Other cerebral palsy (mixed cerebral palsy syndromes)**
G80.9	**Cerebral palsy, unspecified**
G83.0	**Diplegia of upper limbs**
G82.50	**Quadriplegia, unspecified**
G82.51	**Quadriplegia, C1-C4 complete**
G82.52	**Quadriplegia, C1-C4 incomplete**
G82.53	**Quadriplegia, C5-C7 complete**
G82.54	**Quadriplegia, C5-C7 incomplete**
G83.30	**Monoplegia, unspecified affecting unspecified side**
G83.31	**Monoplegia, unspecified affecting right dominant side**
G83.32	**Monoplegia, unspecified affecting left dominant side**
G83.33	**Monoplegia, unspecified affecting right nondominant side**
G83.34	**Monoplegia, unspecified affecting left nondominant side**
G81.90	**Hemiplegia, unspecified affecting unspecified side**
G81.91	**Hemiplegia, unspecified affecting right dominant side**
G81.92	**Hemiplegia, unspecified affecting left dominant side**
G81.93	**Hemiplegia, unspecified affecting right nondominant side**
G81.94	**Hemiplegia, unspecified affecting left nondominant side**
Z47.89	**Encounter for other orthopedic aftercare**

Definition

Cerebral palsy (CP) is a neurodevelopmental condition caused by a nonprogressive lesion of the brain. Whereas CP is typically diagnosed early in life and brain lesions are not progressive, it continues to bear effects that may worsen throughout the life span.

Many definitions of CP have been proposed. The most recent was agreed on in 2006 after review of the proposed definition by the International Workshop on Definition and Classification of CP. Through this review, it was decided that CP would be used as a clinically descriptive term instead of an etiologic diagnosis, defined as follows:

Cerebral palsy describes a group of permanent disorders of the development of movement and posture, causing activity limitation, that are attributed to nonprogressive disturbances that occurred in the developing fetal or infant brain. The motor disorders of cerebral palsy are often accompanied by disturbances of sensation, perception, cognition, communication, and behavior, by epilepsy, and by secondary musculoskeletal problems [1].

Prevalence

The prevalence of CP has been reported to range from 1 to 3 per 1000 live births [2–4]. Yeargin-Allsopp and coworkers [3] reported a higher incidence of CP in boys compared with girls, with a ratio of 1.4 to 1. The same study found a higher prevalence of CP in black compared with white children or those of Hispanic descent [3]. Subsequent studies confirmed this finding [5–8]. Maenner and colleagues [8] also evaluated mobility. In this study, the majority of children were ambulatory, followed by those who were nonambulatory or had limited mobility, with the smallest number walking with an assistive device.

Mobility difficulties have been associated with increased mortality of children with CP. In a study by Strauss and coworkers [9], those who were categorized as having poor mobility (defined by the inability to lift the head while in a prone position) had twice the mortality rate as those with high mobility (defined by the ability to roll or to sit). However, the same study found that the overall mortality rate of children with severe disabilities is declining by an estimated 3.4% per year.

Etiology

Risk factors for CP can be divided into pre-pregnancy risk factors, maternal disease, and pregnancy related. Pre-pregnancy risk factors, which have been associated with thrombosis and perinatal stroke, include advanced maternal age and primiparity, respectively. Maternal diseases such as diabetes, anemia, hypertension, epilepsy, thyroid dysfunction, and chronic renal disease have also been associated with CP. Associations have been found with multiple gestation (twins, triplets) and delivery factors such as assisted fertilization, plurality, placental disease, bleeding during pregnancy, preeclampsia or eclampsia, intrauterine exposure to infection (urinary tract infections, sexually transmitted diseases, and rubella, among others) or maternal fever in labor, restricted or excessive growth for gestational age, abnormal presentation at time of delivery, rupture of membranes longer than 24 hours before delivery, and induced labor [10,11]. Apgar score of less than 7 at 5 minutes, low birth weight, and gestational age of less than 37 weeks are also risk factors for CP.

Although many risk factors for CP exist, the actual cause is a cerebral abnormality. CP may be caused by neonatal encephalopathy from hypoxic-ischemic events, ischemic stroke, or congenital malformations [12].

Classification

CP has been classified on the basis of the dominant presentation of tone or movement into spastic, dyskinetic (dystonic or choreoathetotic), and ataxic [1]. It has been further divided on the basis of limb involvement into unilateral (or hemiplegia) or bilateral (either diplegia or quadriplegia) [1,13]. It is also recommended to account for accompanying impairments and anatomic findings in classifying CP [1].

Neuroimaging findings have been associated with specific CP subtypes. Bilateral spastic CP has most frequently been found to have periventricular white matter changes on imaging. On the other hand, unilateral spastic CP has been associated with periventricular white matter lesions, periventricular gliosis, focal cortical dysplasia, and unilateral schizencephaly. Athetoid CP has been associated with cortical or deep gray matter lesions. In ataxic CP, lesion patterns are less common, but imaging may demonstrate cerebellar malformations [14].

Symptoms

Whereas CP has a profound effect on the musculoskeletal system, it can be accompanied by myriad symptoms affecting other body systems. Symptoms vary by disease severity and may include intellectual disability, seizures, learning disorders, skeletal deformities, pain, abnormal tone, weakness, developmental delay, poor dental health, difficulties with bowel and bladder management, difficulties with oral-motor control, tremors, difficulties with sleep, and difficulties with mood. Here we discuss the body systems most commonly affected by CP.

Head, Eyes, Ears, Nose, and Throat

CP may be accompanied by visual deficits, sensorineural hearing loss, poor oral-motor control, and poor dentition. Vision may be hindered by strabismus (esotropia) or nystagmus. Depending on etiology, there may also be concern for retinopathy of prematurity. Difficulty with oral-motor control may lead to excessive drooling, dysphagia, dysarthria, or aphasia [15,16].

Cardiovascular

Cardiovascular disease may be of concern as those with CP age. Increased circulatory system disease in adult CP cases compared with age-matched peers has been reported [17].

Pulmonary

Many CP-associated symptoms can lead to deterioration of the pulmonary system. Dysphagia may lead to aspiration, which in turn can lead to pneumonia. Changes in tone and development of scoliosis can lead to decreased vital capacity and restricted airway disease. As patients age with CP, there may be an increase in respiratory illnesses, including pneumonia, influenza, and chronic obstructive pulmonary disease [16,17].

Gastrointestinal and Genitourinary

Along with oral-motor impairment, feeding may be affected by swallowing dysfunction. A high incidence of gastroesophageal reflux disease has also been reported [16]. This may be due to associated hiatal hernias, scoliosis, increased intra-abdominal pressure from spasticity, seizures, or neuromuscular incoordination. Regardless of cause, chronic gastroesophageal reflux may lead to esophagitis. This may be manifested with dystonic posturing of the head and neck, hematemesis or vomiting, anemia, or chronic irritability. Chronic peptic esophagitis may potentially cause esophageal mucosal ulceration and stricture formation. Constipation may also arise because of low-fiber or liquid diet, use of medications (including opioids, antispasmodics, antihistamines, and anticonvulsants), immobility, decreased bowel motility, hypotonia, or skeletal abnormalities. Chronic constipation may in turn lead to megarectum, anal fissures, or soiling [16,17].

Musculoskeletal

Musculoskeletal disease is the hallmark of CP. Its impact is lifelong and causes arthritic changes, deformity or contracture, and joint dislocation. This can lead to decreased mobility, osteoporosis, fracture, skin breakdown, and pain [15,17].

Pain is reported in both children and adults with CP and may be caused by muscle imbalance or spasticity. Back pain is commonly reported, followed by pain in weight-bearing joints. The presentation of CP can influence the location of pain. Foot pain is commonly reported in those with diplegic CP, whereas knee pain is more frequent in quadriplegic CP. Neck pain, shoulder pain, and headaches are reported in those with dyskinesia [17]. Pain can affect socialization and education as well as lead to fatigue and decreased mobility [18,19].

Pain affects not only mobility but also strength, endurance, balance, and spasticity. A study looking at aging with CP found that 39% of 20-year-old CP patients could ambulate 20 feet without an assistive device. This declined progressively to 37% by 40 years and 25% by 60 years of age. Subtype also played a role; spastic diplegic patients most commonly showed this progressive decline in mobility [17].

Decreased mobility can lead to osteoporosis. A study in 2008 reported that adults and children with spastic quadriplegia who are nonambulatory have decreased bone density of the lower spine across their life span [17]. Decreased mobility may also influence scoliosis progression over time. It was reported that curves of more than 4 degrees by the age of 15 years led to progressive worsening of spine curvature with age. Curvature of the spine, whether scoliosis, kyphosis, or lordosis, can affect sitting balance, increase pain, and cause difficulties with bowel and bladder management [17].

Sitting may also be influenced by hip subluxation due to muscle imbalance, especially in spastic CP [20]. Hip subluxation can lead to difficulties with wheelchair seating and fit, which may result in skin breakdown and pain, as persistent hip dislocations have been reported to increase pelvic obliquity [20].

Other joints commonly affected in CP include the knee, foot, and ankle. The most common disorders of the foot are equinus deformity, equinoplanovalgus deformity, and equinocavovarus deformity (Fig. 124.1). Equinus deformity is a disorder of the hindfoot characterized by excessive plantar flexion of the hindfoot in reference to the ankle. It is seen with hypertonicity of the gastrocnemius or soleus muscles. Equinoplanovalgus deformity is seen with pronation of the forefoot and midfoot and is typically accompanied by hallux valgus and valgus deformity at the ankle. This is commonly seen with increased tone to the gastrocnemius and the peroneals. Equinovarus deformity is seen with supination of the midfoot and involves the gastrocnemius and posterior tibialis muscles [21]. Increased tone at the gastrocnemius can also produce toe walking, which is a common occurrence in CP.

Excessive knee flexion due to increased tone in the hamstrings may be seen. However, increased tone alone does not lead to the crouched gait pattern commonly seen in CP. This pattern may be due to a combination of skeletal deformity, weakness, spasticity, and poor motor control [22,23]. It is characterized by flexion at the hips, due in part to increased tone of the iliopsoas, and flexion at the knees. Increased tone of the hip adductors may lead to further gait abnormality, producing a scissoring gait pattern.

Neurologic

Neurologic symptoms are manifested across a range of body systems. This may include impairments of oral-motor control, vision deficits, and sensorineural hearing loss [15,16]. Patients may have seizures, cognitive problems, sensory impairments, weakness, movement disorders, abnormal motor control, and muscle hypertonicity.

Seizures are most commonly seen in those with spastic quadriplegia. Their presentation can vary from generalized tonic-clonic to focal, complex partial, simple partial, myoclonic, typical absence, atypical absence, or atonic. Seizures may progress to epilepsy. A study by Humphreys and coworkers [24] found an association between the development of epilepsy and the presence of neonatal seizures in CP patients with periventricular leukomalacia.

Sensory impairments can also be seen in patients with CP. Difficulties with proprioception, two-point discrimination, and stereognosis may be present. This is most common in those with the spastic hemiplegic subtype [25]. Recent literature supports these findings and notes a correlation between sensory impairment and involvement of the thalamocortical pathways [26,27].

The predominant neurologic findings in those with CP are changes in tone or movement. This is evident by the way in which CP is classified: spastic, dyskinetic (dystonic or choreoathetotic), or ataxic [1]. Spastic CP is the most common, and spasticity is its predominant feature. Spasticity is defined as hypertonia that produces increased resistance in response to increased speed of stretch. The dystonic pattern seen in dyskinetic CP is characterized by involuntary muscle contractions that can be sustained or intermittent, leading to twisting or repetitive movements or abnormal postures [28]. The choreoathetotic pattern is characterized by the combination of athetoid (slow, writhing) and choreiform (abrupt, jerky) movements. The ataxic subtype is characterized by uncoordinated movements. Hypotonia may be seen early in infancy, although it may still be present intermittently with dyskinetic CP.

Other

Sleep may be affected in those with CP as a result of sleep anxiety, night wakings, parasomnias, sleep disordered breathing, intellectual impairment leading to difficulty in self-soothing to sleep, altered light perception, reduced melatonin secretion, epilepsy, or pain. Pain may be due to restricted movement, contracture, or spasms. Wayte and

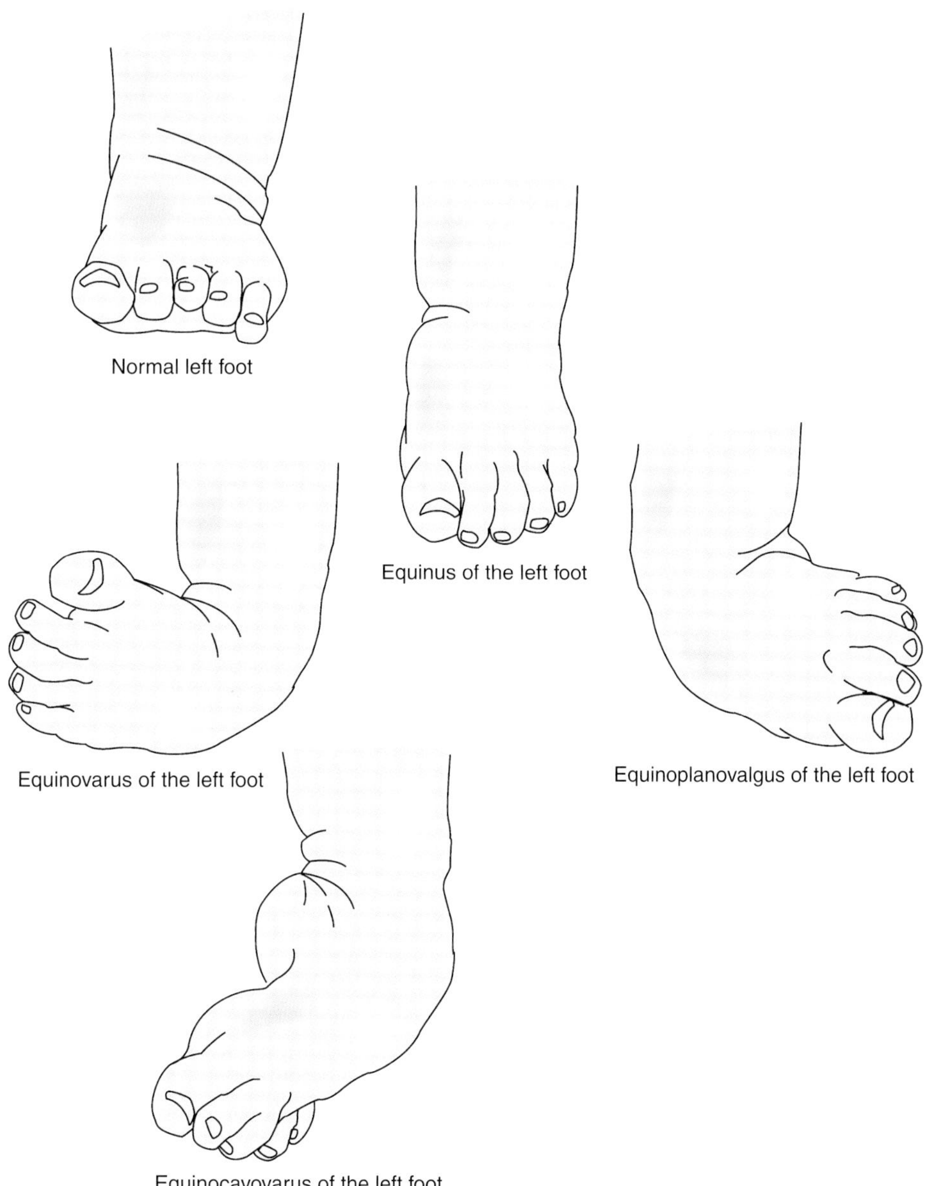

FIGURE 124.1 Common disorders of the foot.

coworkers [29] reported that persons with CP needed parental support at night most commonly for restless sleep and turning over in bed. This need for parental support led to increased caregiver burden and depression [30].

Depression has also been reported in patients with CP. It was found that adults older than 40 years with CP experienced greater levels of loneliness and depression than did 60-year-olds without a disability [17]. Depression has been associated with concern about lack of resources and expertise in care for adults with CP [31].

Physical Examination

As CP may bear influence on all body systems, it is necessary to obtain a complete history and to perform a thorough examination. It is important to consider the age of the patient and to modify the examination accordingly. Assessment should include an evaluation of function, a detailed musculoskeletal examination (to evaluate joint range of motion, deformity, or malalignment), and a thorough neurologic examination (including evaluation of strength, tone, and sensation). Psychological and cognitive assessment may also be performed.

Mobility is classified by the Gross Motor Functional Classification System, which is divided into five categories based on independence with mobility and use of assistive devices (Table 124.1) [1,13,32–34]. Upper extremity function is categorized by the Manual Ability Classification System. This system accounts for age and primarily assesses how patients handle objects in daily life. The classification system was originally designed for those between 8 and 12 years old. It is divided into five levels with progressive involvement from level I to level V (Table 124.2). In a study by Eliasson and colleagues [35], children with hemiplegia were primarily level II, those with diplegia were either level I or level IV, and those with quadriplegia were level IV or level V.

Table 124.1 Gross Motor Functional Classification System

Level	Abilities
Level I	Children are able to walk both indoors and outdoors and climb stairs without assistance.
Level II	Children have some difficulties with mobility on uneven surfaces and hold onto a railing while climbing stairs. They are able to walk indoors and outdoors.
Level III	Children require use of an assistive device for mobility on level surfaces. This may be by walking with an assistive device or propelling a manual wheelchair.
Level IV	Children require wheeled mobility as their primary means of mobility and may walk only short distances with use of an assistive device.
Level V	Children rely on caregivers for mobility.

Table 124.2 Manual Ability Classification System

Level	Abilities
Level I	Handles objects easily, but may have difficulty with speed or accuracy
Level II	Handles most objects, but may use compensatory means to complete task
Level III	Has difficulty handling objects and requires assistance to prepare or to modify task
Level IV	Handles limited objects and requires continuous support
Level V	Does not handle objects and requires total assistance

Table 124.3 Tests for Evaluation of Musculoskeletal Abnormalities

Maneuver	Purpose	Assessment
Barlow	Posterior hip dislocation	Femurs are pushed posteriorly while the hips and knees are in flexion and the thighs are in adduction. The result is positive if the maneuver produces dislocation.
Ortolani	Hip dislocation	Hips are abducted with the knees and hips flexed at 90 degrees. The result is positive if there is a palpable relocation of the hip.
Galeazzi	Hip dislocation or subluxation	Hips and knees are flexed to 90 degrees and the pelvis is in neutral position. The result is positive if there is an asymmetry.
Thomas	Hip flexion contracture	The unaffected hip and knee are passively flexed. The result is positive if this produces flexion of the affected hip.
Popliteal angle	Knee flexion contracture or tight hamstrings	Hips and knees are flexed to 90 degrees, then the knees are passively extended while the hips remain flexed.

Musculoskeletal abnormalities should be carefully evaluated as they have great impact on overall function. Signs of scoliosis should be observed. Passive and active range of motion should be assessed at all joints and may be measured with a goniometer. Specific tests can be used for the evaluation of common abnormalities (Table 124.3). Examination of the hips in infants should include assessment of hip dislocation with the Barlow and Ortolani tests. The Galeazzi or Allis sign may indicate hip dislocation or subluxation. It will be seen as an asymmetry when hips and knees are flexed to 90 degrees and the pelvis is in neutral position. It is important to assess hip abduction because increased tone to the hip adductors or hip deformity can lead to difficulties with perineal care. This is tested in the supine position, with knees flexed and hips flexed to 90 degrees, after which the hips are abducted. Internal and external rotation of the hips should be assessed. The Thomas test may be used evaluate for hip flexion contracture [36,37]. Popliteal angles should be measured with hips flexed to 90 degrees and knees initially in a flexed position, then passively extended. Ankle dorsiflexion should be measured with the knee flexed to assess tightness of the soleus and the knee extended to assess gastrocnemius tightness [37]. Deformity of the foot and ankle should also be documented. Analysis of gait in a formal gait laboratory may be useful in assessing the musculoskeletal system and mobility [34].

Neurologic examination should be appropriate for the patient's age. Primitive infantile reflexes, such as the Moro, palmar grasp, asymmetric tonic neck, plantar grasp, and Galant, should be provoked. The asymmetric tonic neck reflex should subside by 3 months. It is elicited by rotation of the patient's head, causing extension of extremities on the chin side and flexion on the occiput side. The Galant reflex is seen with curvature of the trunk toward the side of stimulation when the examiner scratches the skin of the patient down the back. This response should be extinguished by 4 months. The palmar grasp response, which is seen with finger flexion of the patient when the examiner's finger is placed in the palm, should disappear by 6 months. The Moro reflex, which is caused by sudden head extension and leads to upper extremity abduction, then adduction and flexion, should resolve by 6 months. The plantar grasp response is seen with flexion of the toes when the sole of the foot is touched. This should be extinguished by 15 months [38].

Muscle strength may be evaluated by observation or through formal manual muscle testing, depending on the patient's age. Developmental milestones should be discussed with parents or observed. Emergence of hand dominance at an early age should be discussed with parents as this may indicate weakness or difficulties with the nondominant hand. Variations in tone should be assessed. Spasticity may be classified by the Ashworth scale, the modified Ashworth scale, or the Tardieu rating scale. The Ashworth scale rates spasticity from 1 to 5 with increasing severity, and the modified Ashworth scale rates spasticity from 0 to 4 with increasing severity; the Tardieu rating scale measures spasticity at varying velocities [39]. Sensory examination may also be performed with assessment of proprioception, two-point discrimination, and stereognosis [25–27].

Muscle stretch reflexes should be obtained and may be increased. Formal vision and hearing assessment to ascertain visual impairment or hearing loss is often necessary. Mood should be discussed because depression is seen in those aging with CP [31]. Neuropsychological examination may be beneficial in assessment of cognitive concerns.

Functional Limitations

Functional limitations vary by subtype and comorbidities, many of which are described earlier and involve activities of daily living and mobility. It is reported that gross motor function may improve up to the age of 7 years, but musculoskeletal disease may worsen, potentially affecting mobility in children with CP [34]. Research by Palmer [40] suggests that the best predictor of functional limitation is the rate of motor development. This can be evaluated by use of the developmental quotient (chronologic age divided by developmental age) or through videotape assessment of spontaneous general movements during the first months of life [40].

Engel-Yeger and colleagues [41] reported that people with CP, compared with their typically developing peers, were more limited in their activities, were limited in the frequency of activity participation outside of school, and did not as frequently interact with peers during activities. This same article suggested that it may be the physical limitations that account for these differences.

Diagnostic Studies

Head, Eyes, Ears, Nose, and Throat

Audiometry may be obtained to assess hearing. Neuro-ophthalmology referral may be necessary for visual assessment.

Cardiovascular

With aging (if cardiac concerns arise), electrocardiography, thallium or exercise-induced stress testing, or echocardiography may be warranted.

Pulmonary

Chest radiographs may be obtained if pneumonia is suspected or there is a change in respiratory status.

Pulmonary function tests may be performed if there is concern for development of chronic obstructive pulmonary disease.

Gastrointestinal and Genitourinary

Abdominal plain films should be obtained if chronic constipation develops. Gastroenterology consultation and upper endoscopy may be necessary if there is concern for peptic esophagitis or hematemesis. If dysphagia is suspected, formal evaluation by a speech-language pathologist is warranted. This evaluation may include instrumental examination (modified barium swallow study or fiberoptic endoscopic evaluation of swallowing).

Musculoskeletal

Scoliosis films should be obtained to measure and to evaluate scoliotic curves. Hip radiographs should be ordered when concern for congenital dysplasia or dislocation exists. Radiographs may be obtained for any suspected fracture of the limbs or vertebral compression fracture. Radiographs may also be useful in assessing degenerative changes of the peripheral joints or spine. To assess bone density, a bone density study (DEXA scan) may be ordered.

Neurologic

Initial evaluation of suspected intracranial disease in infancy may begin with cranial ultrasonography [40]. This technique is useful before cranial suture and fontanelle closure and may reveal hemorrhage, ventricular enlargement, or cystic changes. In children and adults, computed tomography may assess for hemorrhagic changes, but its use should be carefully considered, given the amount of radiation exposure. Magnetic resonance imaging is used to assess the underlying pathologic brain changes associated with the development of CP. Common findings may include hypoxic-ischemic injuries, periventricular leukomalacia, schizencephaly, and cerebellar malformations. Krageloh-Mann and Horber [42] reported that 86% of magnetic resonance images obtained in children with CP were abnormal and 83% of those gave insight into the etiology of the child's CP. There is also evidence to suggest that diffusion magnetic resonance imaging to evaluate white matter lesions, specifically looking at the corticomotor and sensorimotor tracts, is useful [26,27].

Treatment

Treatment of CP should focus on management of symptoms, maximization of function, and prevention of complications. Currently there is no cure for CP.

Initial

When treatment of CP is initiated, existing symptoms and comorbidities as well as potential complications should be considered. One such symptom may be pain, which should be addressed on the basis of etiology. If pain is due to degenerative changes, nonsteroidal anti-inflammatories may be used. Pain may arise from a trigger point and may be treated with trigger point injection. Complications from immobility, such as skin breakdown, may arise. These can be treated by off-loading of pressure but may require further interventions, such as débridement or surgical closure. Immobility can lead to pain and fatigue, for which physical or occupational therapy can be implemented. Immobility may also lead to constipation, which may require dietary modifications (increasing fiber intake), stool softeners, enemas, or other laxatives [16]. Discomfort may also arise from gastroesophageal reflux disease, for which proton pump inhibitors have been shown to be effective [16]. Depression may also arise, which may be treated pharmacologically. Referral to a psychologist or psychiatrist may also be necessary.

Rehabilitation

In establishing a treatment program, it is important to take a multidisciplinary approach with focused and clear goals in mind. Physical therapists, occupational therapists, speech-language pathologists, and neuropsychologists may all be involved to varying degrees and at varying frequencies. Patients' goals will vary significantly and may range from independence in basic activities of daily living to assistance with management of tone, prevention of contracture, and maximizing independence with vocational or sports interests.

A wide range of interventions are available for management of abnormal tone. Assessment must be made as to whether a focal or generalized intervention is required. Physical therapy or occupational therapy may be started in either scenario to work toward implementing a home stretching program and providing education to the patient and the family on the importance of stretching. This is especially important during growth. A wide variety of orthotics may be used as well to help preserve range of motion and for functional tasks, such as providing support at the foot and ankle with mobility or support at the wrist while performing manual activities. Constraint-induced movement therapy may also be considered to promote functional use of the affected limb in those with unilateral involvement.

Generalized interventions for management of spasticity may include oral medications or intrathecal medications. Oral medications include baclofen, dantrolene, clonidine, tizanidine, and benzodiazepines. Most oral medications can have systemic effects that can affect cognition or lead to sedation. Intrathecal delivery of medication is known to have fewer systemic effects. Baclofen may be delivered through an intrathecal pump to manage spasticity [34].

Procedures

If focal intervention is needed, patients may benefit from localized procedures such as botulinum toxin or phenol injections. Botulinum toxin has been shown to be effective in reducing spasticity short term. Long-term efficacy of botulinum toxin is still unclear [34]. Botulinum toxin may be used in combination with serial casting; however, there is mixed evidence about the efficacy of this combined intervention [34].

Surgery

Surgery is an option for both focal and generalized interventions. Selective dorsal rhizotomy may be considered as a surgical treatment to help manage focal spasticity. Orthopedic surgeries to correct contracture or deformity may be necessary as well. This may include tendon lengthening (typically of the Achilles or adductors) and bone correction (such as derotational osteotomies). Generalized interventions for surgical management of spasticity may include placement of an intrathecal pump for delivery of intrathecal medications. Intrathecal delivery of medication is known to have fewer systemic effects. Baclofen may be delivered through an intrathecal pump to manage spasticity [34].

Potential Disease Complications

Because CP is a lifelong disorder, complications associated with aging are often seen. These complications may affect all body systems but predominantly include changes in tone, development of contracture, pain, weakness, decreased mobility, and depression. As described in previous sections of this chapter, there may be increased risk of circulatory system disease, respiratory illnesses, chronic obstructive pulmonary disease, gastroesophageal reflux disease, constipation, osteoporosis, and seizures. Early-onset arthritis may also be of concern [15].

Potential Treatment Complications

Complications associated with the treatment of CP vary on the basis of the intervention. All medications have potential side effects. Oral medications, such as baclofen, dantrolene, tizanidine, and benzodiazepines, may cause varying degrees of weakness and sedation. Baclofen and benzodiazepines may lead to cognitive changes. Use of clonidine may lead to hypotension and bradycardia. Intrathecal administration of baclofen has fewer systemic effects, but other potential risks are associated with the pump and catheter. Programming errors, kinked or broken catheter, or pump malfunctioning can lead to baclofen overdose (sedation, lethargy, respiratory failure, and urinary retention) or baclofen withdrawal (cognitive changes, increased spasticity, pruritus, and seizures). Use of focal injections to treat spasticity may lead to infection at the injection site, soreness, or bleeding. Phenol may lead to dysesthesias when it is injected at the site of a mixed sensory-motor nerve. Botulinum toxin may cause weakness and in rare cases botulism-like symptoms, including difficulty in breathing and dysphagia.

Serial casting may lead to skin irritation and potential skin breakdown. Range of motion and stretching can cause pain and have the potential to cause fracture if stretching is performed too aggressively in an osteoporotic patient. Surgery, including dorsal rhizotomy and orthopedic surgeries, may have complications of postoperative pain and constipation in addition to risks of the actual procedure. There are also increased risks associated with anesthesia use when respiratory muscle compromise is present.

References

[1] Rosenbaum P, Paneth N, Leviton A, et al. A report: the definition and classification of cerebral palsy. Dev Med Child Neurol Suppl 2007;109:8–14.

[2] Paneth N, Hong T, Korzeniewski S. The descriptive epidemiology of cerebral palsy. Clin Perinatol 2006;33:251–67.

[3] Yeargin-Allsopp M, Van Naarden Braun K, Doernberg NS, et al. Prevalence of cerebral palsy in 8-year-old children in three areas of the United States in 2002: a multisite collaboration. Pediatrics 2008;121:547–54.

[4] Bhasin TK, Brocksen S, Avchen R, Van Naarden K. Prevalence of four developmental disabilities among children aged 8 years: Metropolitan Atlanta Developmental Disabilities Surveillance Program, 1996 and 2000. MMWR Surveill Summ 2006;55:1–9.

[5] Arneson CL, Durkin MS, Benedict RE, et al. Prevalence of cerebral palsy: Autism and Developmental Disabilities Monitoring Network, three sites, United States, 2004. Disabil Health J 2009;2:45–8.

[6] Kirby RS, Wingate MS, Van Naarden Braun K, et al. Prevalence and functioning of children with cerebral palsy in four areas of the United States in 2006: a report from the Autism and Developmental Disabilities Monitoring Network. Res Dev Disabil 2011;32:462–9.

[7] Wu YW, Xing G, Fuentes-Afflick E, et al. Racial, ethnic, and socioeconomic disparities in the prevalence of cerebral palsy. Pediatrics 2011;127:e674–81.

[8] Maenner MJ, Benedict RE, Arneson CL, et al. Children with cerebral palsy: racial disparities in functional limitations. Epidemiology 2012;23:35–43.

[9] Strauss D, Shavelle R, Reynolds R, et al. Survival in cerebral palsy in the last 20 years: signs of improvement? Dev Med Child Neurol 2007;49:86–92.

[10] Nelson KB. Causative factors in cerebral palsy. Clin Obstet Gynecol 2008;51:749–62.
[11] Stoknes M, Andersen GL, Elkamil AI, et al. The effects of multiple pre- and perinatal risk factors on the occurrence of cerebral palsy. A Norwegian register based study. Eur J Paediatr Neurol 2012;16:56–63.
[12] Longo M, Hankins GD. Defining cerebral palsy: pathogenesis, pathophysiology and new intervention. Minerva Ginecol 2009;61:421–9.
[13] Andersen GL, Irgens LM, Haagaas I, et al. Cerebral palsy in Norway: prevalence, subtypes and severity. Eur J Paediatr Neurol 2008;12:4–13.
[14] Krägeloh-Mann I, Cans C. Cerebral palsy update. Brain Dev 2009;31:537–44.
[15] Young NL. The transition to adulthood for children with cerebral palsy: what do we know about their health care needs? J Pediatr Orthop 2007;27:476–9.
[16] Sullivan PB. Gastrointestinal disorders in children with neurodevelopmental disabilities. Dev Disabil Res Rev 2008;14:128–36.
[17] Svien LR, Berg P, Stephenson C. Issues in aging with cerebral palsy. Top Geriatr Rehabil 2008;24:26–40.
[18] Tervo RC, Symons F, Stout J, Novacheck T. Parental report of pain and associated limitations in ambulatory children with cerebral palsy. Arch Phys Med Rehabil 2006;87:928–34.
[19] Houlihan CM, O'Donnell M, Conaway M, Stevenson RD. Bodily pain and health-related quality of life in children with cerebral palsy. Dev Med Child Neurol 2004;46:305–10.
[20] Senaran H, Shah SA, Glutting JJ, et al. The associated effects of untreated unilateral hip dislocation in cerebral palsy scoliosis. J Pediatr Orthop 2006;26:769–72.
[21] Davids JR. The foot and ankle in cerebral palsy. Orthop Clin North Am 2010;41:579–93.
[22] Hoang HX, Reinbolt JA. Crouched posture maximizes ground reaction forces generated by muscles. Gait Posture 2012;36:405–8.
[23] Ross SA, Engsberg JR. Relationships between spasticity, strength, gait, and the GMFM-66 in persons with spastic diplegia cerebral palsy. Arch Phys Med Rehabil 2007;88:1114–20.
[24] Humphreys P, Deonandan R, Whiting S, et al. Factors associated with epilepsy in children with periventricular leukomalacia. J Child Neurol 2007;22:598–605.
[25] Sanger TD, Kukke SN. Abnormalities of tactile sensory function in children with dystonic and diplegic cerebral palsy. J Child Neurol 2007;22:289–93.
[26] Hoon Jr AH, Stashinko EE, Nagae LM, et al. Sensory and motor deficits in children with cerebral palsy born preterm correlate with diffusion tensor imaging abnormalities in thalamocortical pathways. Dev Med Child Neurol 2009;51:697–704.
[27] Scheck SM, Boyd RN, Rose SE. New insights into the pathology of white matter tracts in cerebral palsy from diffusion magnetic resonance imaging: a systematic review. Dev Med Child Neurol 2012;54:684–96.
[28] Sanger TD, Delgado MR, Gaebler-Spira D, et al. Task Force on Childhood Motor Disorders. Classification and definition of disorders causing hypertonia in childhood. Pediatrics 2003;111:e89–97.
[29] Wayte S, McCaughey E, Holley S, et al. Sleep problems in children with cerebral palsy and their relationship with maternal sleep and depression. Acta Paediatr 2012;101:618–23.
[30] Hemmingsson H, Stenhammer AM, Paulsson K. Sleep problems and the need for parental night-time attention in children with physical disabilities. Child Care Health Dev 2008;35:89–95.
[31] Horsman M, Suto M, Dudgeon B, Harris SR. Growing older with cerebral palsy: insiders' perspectives. Pediatr Phys Ther 2010;22:296–303.
[32] Westbom L, Hagglund G, Nordmark E. Cerebral palsy in a total population of 4-11 year olds in southern Sweden. Prevalence and distribution according to different CP classification systems. BMC Pediatr 2007;7:41.
[33] Sigurdardottir S, Thorkelsson T, Halldorsdottir M, et al. Trends in prevalence and characteristics of cerebral palsy among Icelandic children born 1990 to 2003. Dev Med Child Neurol 2009;51:356–63.
[34] Narayanan UG. Management of children with ambulatory cerebral palsy: an evidence-based review. J Pediatr Orthop 2012;32(Suppl. 2): S172–81.
[35] Eliasson AC, Krumlinde-Sundholm L, Rosblad B, et al. The Manual Ability Classification System (MACS) for children with cerebral palsy: scale development and evidence of validity and reliability. Dev Med Child Neurol 2006;48:549–54.
[36] O'Neil ME, Fragala-Pinkham MA, Westcott SL, et al. Physical therapy clinical management recommendations for children with cerebral palsy–spastic diplegia: achieving functional mobility outcomes. Pediatr Phys Ther 2006;18:49–72.
[37] McDowell BC, Salazar-Torres JJ, Kerr C, Cosgrove AP. Passive range of motion in a population-based sample of children with spastic cerebral palsy who walk. Phys Occup Ther Pediatr 2012;32:139–50.
[38] Zafeiriou DI. Primitive reflexes and postural reactions in the neurodevelopmental examination. Pediatr Neurol 2004;31:1–8.
[39] Haugh AB, Pandyan AD, Johnson GR. A systematic review of the Tardieu Scale for the measurement of spasticity. Disabil Rehabil 2006;28:899–907.
[40] Palmer FB. Strategies for the early diagnosis of cerebral palsy. J Pediatr 2004;145(Suppl.):S8–S11.
[41] Engel-Yeger B, Jarus T, Anaby D, Law M. Differences in patterns of participation between youths with cerebral palsy and typically developing peers. Am J Occup Ther 2009;63:96–104.
[42] Krageloh-Mann I, Horber V. The role of magnetic resonance imaging in elucidating the pathogenesis of cerebral palsy: a systematic review. Dev Med Child Neurol 2007;49:144–51.

CHAPTER 125

Chronic Fatigue Syndrome

Gerold R. Ebenbichler, MD

Synonyms

Chronic fatigue and immune dysfunction syndrome
Myalgic encephalomyelitis
Neurasthenia
Post-viral fatigue syndrome
Iceland disease
Royal Free disease
Yuppie flu

ICD-9 Code

780.71 Chronic fatigue syndrome

ICD-10 Code

R53.82 Chronic fatigue syndrome

Definition

Chronic fatigue syndrome (CFS) is a debilitating condition of unknown nature and cause, but most medical authorities now accept its existence. CFS is characterized by severe, disabling, medically unexplained fatigue for more than 6 months and prominently features subjective impairments in concentration, short-term memory, and sleep as well as musculoskeletal pain [1]. Sufferers experience significant disability and distress, which may be further exacerbated by a lack of understanding from others, including health professionals. CFS affects both adults and children.

Epidemiologic research in Western countries has demonstrated that among adults, between 230 and 500 of every 100,000 persons are affected with CFS [2–4]. Women have CFS more commonly [5], as do minority groups and people with lower educational status and educational attainment [2].

The causes of CFS remain uncertain. CFS may start either gradually or suddenly. In the latter case, it is often triggered by an influenza-like viral or similar illness. Some progress in the understanding of the disease has been made when causes were divided into predisposing, triggering or precipitating, and perpetuating factors [6,7]. Personality (neuroticism, introversion) and lifestyle factors, inactivity in childhood and inactivity after infectious mononucleosis, and genetic factors are presumed to influence vulnerability in CFS. Certain infectious illnesses (e.g., Epstein-Barr virus infection, Q fever, and Lyme disease), precipitating somatic events (e.g., serious injuries), and psychological distress (e.g., serious life events) may precipitate the disorder. The perceptions, illness attributions, and beliefs of patients may encourage avoidant coping and perpetuate the illness.

Among various pathophysiologic hypotheses tested, some evidence has emerged supporting subtle hypoactivity in the hypothalamic-pituitary-adrenal axis with lower than normal cortisol response to increased corticotropin levels [8] and a hyperserotonergic state or upregulated serotonin receptors in CFS [9,10]. Whether these alterations are a cause or a consequence of CFS, however, remains unclear. Dysfunction in the immune system in CFS is inconsistently evidenced by findings of abnormal cytokine production, mainly concentrating on proinflammatory ones that are known to be involved in the regulation of the hypothalamic-pituitary-adrenal axis and sympathetic nervous system, such as tumor necrosis factor, interleukin-1, and interleukin-6 [11]. On the tissue level, cytokines such as interleukin-6 are involved in the stress response and represent crucial inducers of sickness behavior [12], which is characterized by avoidance behavior, apathy, sleepiness, impaired memory and concentration, anorexia, mild fever, and increased sensitivity to pain. No convincing evidence exists to support CFS as a continuing viral infection [11]. Increasing evidence suggests that in a large subgroup of CFS patients, central sensitization with widespread hyperalgesia, delayed diffuse noxious inhibitory control, and dysfunction of endogenous inhibition during exercise seems to corroborate several psychological influences on the illness [13]. Functional magnetic resonance imaging studies in patients with CFS revealed findings indicative of increased neuronal resource allocation [14] or dysfunctional motor planning [15], which seems to be consistent with cognitive impairment in these patients.

Symptoms

Patients with CFS typically present with a variety of symptoms that may widely overlap with symptoms of functional somatic syndromes, including the irritable bowel syndrome, fibromyalgia, multiple chemical sensitivity, chronic pelvic pain, temporomandibular joint dysfunction, and Gulf War illness [11].

Patients experience profound, overwhelming exhaustion, both mentally and physically, which is worsened by exertion and is not completely relieved by rest [16]. Fatigue is highly subjective, multidimensional, and variable in nature, and it does not necessarily need to be the major and most debilitating symptom in this condition [1]. Patients may express their complaints of fatigue in different ways. Patients' expectations and causal attribution of symptoms to somatic factors, hidden agenda involving insurance issues, and invalidity of benefit claims have been related to an increase in symptoms and may contribute to a diversity of symptoms reported [7].

In addition to fatigue, patients with CFS usually complain about a wide variety of multisystem symptoms that are nonspecific and variable in both nature and severity over time. These may be just as prominent as fatigue and are best summarized in different categories [16,17].

- Complaints of cognitive dysfunction. CFS patients may experience forgetfulness, confusion, difficulties in thinking, and "mental fatigue" or "brain fog."
- Postexertional malaise. Patients report a period of deep fatigue and exhaustion that lasts for more than 24 hours after physical exertion.
- Complaints of pain. These include headaches of a new type, pattern, or severity; muscle pain; and multijoint pain. Patients may further report pain in bones, eyes, and testicles; abdominal and chest pain; chills; and painful skin sensitivity.
- Unrefreshing sleep and rest is a hallmark of CFS, and insomnia is also common. Patients report more difficulty in falling asleep, more interrupted sleep, and more daytime napping. It is extremely difficult for many patients to maintain a sleep schedule. Patients report that exercise, unlike in healthy persons, worsens the insomnia and unrefreshing sleep symptoms alike.
- Psychological complaints of emotional lability, anxiety, depressive mood, irritability, and sometimes a curious emotional "flattening" most likely due to exhaustion may be reported by CFS patients. CFS patients with preexisting psychiatric symptoms may report that these worsen with the onset of CFS. Treatment of psychiatric symptoms alone does not relieve the physical symptoms of CFS, indicating that the disease is not only psychological in nature.
- Other frequently reported complaints refer to general hypersensitivity and poor temperature control; these include low-grade fevers, photophobia, vertigo, nausea, allergies, hot flashes, and rashes [18,19].

Physical Examination

The physical examination is directed toward determination of whether symptoms are caused by any other disease or illness. The findings of the general medical and neurologic examinations should be normal. There may be low-grade fever with temperatures between 37.5° C and 38.5° C orally, nonexudative pharyngitis, and tender cervical or axillary lymph nodes up to 2 cm in diameter. A mild hypotension, elicited mainly with tilt-table testing and reversed by mineralocorticoids, may be observed. In some patients, orthostatic hypotension with wide swings in blood pressure resulting in syncope as well as intermittent hypertension may be found [20]. Complaints of paresthesias usually prove to be odd on sensory testing, particularly numbness in the bones or muscles or fluctuating patches of numbness or paresthesias on the chest, face, or nose. A few patients report blurred or "close to" double vision. In neither case are there physical findings to corroborate the sensory experiences [20]. Unsteadiness on standing with closed eyes may be found.

A thorough mental status examination is performed to rule out any exclusionary psychiatric disorders. The psychological examination may reveal abnormalities in mood, intellectual function, memory, concentration, and personality. Particular attention should be paid to anxiety, self-destructive thoughts, and observable signs such as psychomotor retardation [1].

The musculoskeletal examination findings should be normal. In CFS patients with arthralgia and myalgia, joint swelling and inflammation and other superimposed pain generators, such as bursitis, tendinitis, and radiculopathy, have to be ruled out. Palpatory examination of muscles may reveal tender muscles, tender points that are not numerous enough to be classified as fibromyalgia, and individual trigger points.

Functional Limitations

Disablement varies widely among patients with CFS. Whereas some are able to lead a relatively normal life, others are totally bed bound and unable to care for themselves. In a rehabilitative assessment, body functions that represent the patient's core subjective symptoms may reveal the most pronounced impairment; these are energy and drive functions, sensation of pain, sleep functions, attention function, emotional functions, memory functions, and exercise tolerance functions. Both muscle and cardiopulmonary function as demonstrated by cardiopulmonary stress testing may be reduced in these patients. Avoidance behavior as a consequence of patients' experiencing worsening of symptoms after previously well-tolerated levels of exercise and kinesiophobia—a specific kind of fear-avoidance behavior that is defined as an excessive, irrational, and debilitating fear of physical movement and activity resulting from a feeling of vulnerability to painful injury or reinjury—may increase sedentariness in CFS patients. However, kinesiophobia was not correlated with reduced exercise capacity by bicycle ergometer exercise stress testing [21].

CFS patients may be able to begin but not to complete mental or physical activities that were previously easily accomplished. Thus, tasks that predominantly challenge the cognitive performance, like focusing attention, solving problems, handling stress, making decisions, undertaking multiple tasks, or driving a car, may limit patients in carrying out their daily routine, especially at the workplace. Tasks that require predominantly physical performance, like walking or household tasks, may limit the patient's activities of daily life. Many patients have to modify or give up physical hobbies and exercise and find themselves

Table 125.1 Case Definition (1994) for Chronic Fatigue Syndrome from the U.S. Centers for Disease Control and Prevention

Characterized by Persistent or Relapsing Unexplained Chronic Fatigue
Fatigue lasts for at least 6 months
Fatigue is of new or definite onset
Fatigue is not the result of an organic disease or of continuing exertion
Fatigue is not alleviated by rest
Fatigue results in a substantial reduction in previous occupational, educational, social, and personal activities
Four or more of the following symptoms, concurrently present for ≥6 months: impaired memory or concentration, sore throat, tender cervical or axillary lymph nodes, muscle pain, pain in several joints, new headaches, unrefreshing sleep, or malaise after exertion
Exclusion Criteria
Medical condition explaining fatigue
Major depressive disorder (psychotic features) or bipolar disorder
Schizophrenia, dementia, or delusional disorder
Anorexia nervosa, bulimia nervosa
Alcohol or substance abuse
Severe obesity

Modified from Fukuda K, Straus SE, Hickie I, et al; International Chronic Fatigue Syndrome Study Group. The chronic fatigue syndrome: a comprehensive approach to its definition and study. Ann Intern Med 1994;121:953-959; and Prins JB, van der Meer JW, Bleijenberg G. Chronic fatigue syndrome. Lancet 2006;367:346-355.

Table 125.2 Laboratory Tests Recommended for the Exclusion of Diseases That May Cause Chronic Fatigue

Complete blood count with differential cell count
Blood and serum chemistries (serum electrolytes, blood urea nitrogen, glucose, creatinine, calcium)
Erythrocyte sedimentation rate
Urinalysis
Thyroid function studies
Antinuclear antibodies
Serum cortisol concentration
Immunoglobulin levels
Rheumatoid factor
Tuberculin skin test
Human immunodeficiency virus serology
Lyme serology (when endemic)
Magnetic resonance imaging of head (to rule out multiple sclerosis)
Polysomnography (to rule out sleep disorder)
Optional Tests to be Used When Clinically Indicated
Quantification of natural killer cells
Quantification of B- and T-cell subsets
Functional elevation of natural killer cells
T-cell response to mitogenic stimulation
Measurements of delayed hypersensitivity
Production of and response to cytokines
Enzyme-linked immunosorbent assay/activated cell test
Serologic tests for *Candida albicans*
RNase L enzymatic activity assay or RNase L protein quantification
Spinal tap for oligoclonal bands
Tilt table
Catecholamine testing
Nerve conduction studies including electromyography
Anti–acetylcholine receptor antibodies
Vitamin B_{12} deficiency
Circulating immune complexes including CD3 and CD4
Viral serologies

Modified from Craig T, Kakumanu S. Chronic fatigue syndrome: evaluation and treatment. Am Fam Physician 2002;65:1083-1090; and Wikipedia 2007/results from an NIH consensus conference.

unable to work full-time or at all [17]. Categories related to intimate relationships, family relationships, communication, and complex interpersonal relationships may be altered in CFS patients, thereby restricting them from participation in social and work life.

Cognitive avoidance coping as a major illness-perpetuating factor was found negatively related to social functioning [22], and a strong association seems to exist between kinesiophobia and self-reported activity limitations and participation restrictions in CFS patients [21]. In addition to environmental factors related to the immediate family and friends, health professionals may reinforce patients' symptom severity and illness behavior and facilitate further impaired functioning in these patients. Personal beliefs, practices, ideologies, spirituality, laws, and societal norms may also facilitate or hinder functioning in CFS patients. A considerable number of patients with CFS in many countries are receiving disability benefits or private insurance or have made claims and been denied [23].

Diagnostic Studies

There are no accepted diagnostic tests for CFS. Diagnosis of CFS is primarily based on the patient's symptoms that fit scientific case definitions of CFS, which aim to effectively distinguish CFS from other types of unexplained fatigue. Among numerous scientific case definitions available, the U.S. Centers for Disease Control and Prevention criteria are the most widely supported [1]. This case definition characterizes CFS by a grouping of nonspecific symptoms and a diagnosis of exclusion (Table 125.1). To receive a diagnosis of CFS, fatigue must have persisted or recurred during 6 or more consecutive months. Concomitant symptoms must have persisted or recurred during 6 or more consecutive months of illness and cannot have predated the fatigue [16]. Clinicians may have difficulties in diagnosis of CFS, especially by not acknowledging the diagnosis of fatigue when its onset is gradual or by the diversity of patients' fatigue reports. Instruments developed to assess fatigue, such as the Checklist Individual Strength, the Chalder Fatigue Scale, and the Krupp Fatigue Severity Scale, are widely used in research studies and may assist physicians with objectivation of fatigue and establishment of the medical diagnosis.

Fatigue and similar symptoms can be caused by a wide variety of conditions. Thus, diagnosis of CFS needs to include a diagnostic process that eliminates potential causes of the patient's symptoms (see the section on differential diagnosis). In addition to a thorough history and a meticulous physical examination, diagnostic studies include a mental status examination and a minimum array of laboratory tests.

A structural psychiatric interview is essential to identify permanent psychiatric exclusions (see Table 125.1 and the section on differential diagnosis). Reliable detection instruments may be helpful when physicians perform screening for psychiatric diagnoses, such as the Composite International Diagnostic Interview [24] and the Structured Clinical Interview for DSM-IV Axis I (SCID) [25].

Laboratory examination is intended to detect other disorders, not to find out whether a patient has CFS. Recommendations for laboratory testing have been provided (Table 125.2).

Questionnaires such as the Epworth Sleepiness Scale and the Centre for Sleep and Chronobiology Sleep Assessment Questionnaire are useful to screen for and to profile sleep abnormalities [26]. Polysomnography defines sleep architecture, duration and timing of sleep, respiratory obstruction, and abnormal limb movements and may be indicated when primary sleep disorders exclusionary to CFS, such as sleep apnea and narcolepsy, have to be ruled out.

Assessment of a patient's functioning and health according to the International Classification of Functioning, Disability, and Health (ICF) [27] would further complete the diagnostic studies in patients with CFS. The classification might be recommended, but compared with other chronic conditions like osteoarthritis and back pain, ICF core sets that best describe the prototypical spectrum of disability have not yet been developed for CFS [28,29]. Furthermore, ICF core sets have to be psychometrically validated after they have been developed. This can be best accomplished by item response theory–based computerized adaptive testing, a method selecting only those items out of the item pool that are most relevant for the individual patient [30,31]. For the time being, instruments that have been recommended in a consensus conference may be used to measure the symptom-specific disablement and quality of life of patients with CFS [16].

Differential Diagnosis [32,33]

- Blood
  - Anemia
  - Hemochromatosis
- Infections
  - Chronic Epstein-Barr virus infection
  - Influenza
  - Hepatitis
  - Human immunodeficiency virus infection
  - Lyme disease
  - Occult abscess
  - Poliomyelitis, postpoliomyelitis syndrome
  - Tuberculosis
  - Bacterial endocarditis
  - Chronic brucellosis
- Parasites
- Fungi
- Autoimmune disease
  - Behçet syndrome
  - Dermatomyositis
  - Lupus erythematosus
  - Polyarteritis
  - Polymyositis
  - Reiter syndrome
  - Rheumatoid arthritis
  - Sjögren syndrome
  - Vasculitis
- Liver disease
- Chronic heart disease
- Chronic lung disease
- Metabolic and toxic conditions
- Endocrine disease
  - Diabetes mellitus
  - Hyperthyroidism and hypothyroidism
  - Addison disease
  - Cushing syndrome
  - Panhypopituitarism
- Ovarian failure
- Malignant neoplasms
- Neuromuscular disorders
  - Fibromyalgia
  - Multiple sclerosis
  - Parkinson disease
  - Myasthenia gravis
  - Head injuries
- Sleep disorders
  - Obstructive sleep syndromes (sleep apnea, narcolepsy)
- Psychiatric
  - Bipolar affective disorders
  - Schizophrenia of any subtype
  - Delusional disorders of any subtype
  - Dementias of any subtype
  - Organic brain disorders and alcohol or substance abuse within 2 years before onset of the fatiguing illness
- Other
  - Pharmacologic side effects
  - Alcohol and substance abuse
- Body weight fluctuation (severe obesity or marked weight loss)

Treatment

Initial

Treatment of CFS is symptom based and aims to improve fatigue and comorbid conditions, such as sleep disturbances, depression, and painful symptoms.

Treatment of CFS with pharmacologic therapies has had disappointing results in most cases. So far, no pharmacologic treatments have been proved effective in the treatment of fatigue. The subtle changes found in the hypothalamic-pituitary-adrenal axis have led to a few randomized controlled trials that overall did not establish steroids as a treatment of choice [34]. For immunologic therapies like immunoglobulin G, staphylococcus toxoid, ribonucleic acid, and others, there is insufficient evidence about their effectiveness in CFS [34].

Anecdotal evidence suggests that low doses of antidepressant medication (e.g., 10 to 30 mg of nortriptyline) administered at bedtime improve sleep and diminish pain, although the benefit of these medications has not been demonstrated in CFS [34,35]. In addition, the use of acetaminophen, nonsteroidal anti-inflammatory drugs, and opioids may be worthwhile in patients with prominent musculoskeletal complaints or headaches.

Complementary medicine has gained increasing popularity among patients with chronic diseases. These treatments include homeopathy, herbal remedies, supplements, megavitamins, special diets, and energy healing. Although individual studies revealed beneficial effects for homeopathy and supplements in the treatment of CFS, there is insufficient evidence for the effectiveness of these interventions [34].

Rehabilitation

Management based on a rehabilitation model is now recommended for patients with CFS. The individual rehabilitative assessment is necessary to identify those treatment targets that are most likely to reach the rehabilitation aims of the patient with CFS. These rehabilitation programs may involve different professions and therapies, and increasing evidence for the effectiveness of individual rehabilitation interventions has emerged [34–37].

Cognitive-behavioral therapy for CFS addresses changing of condition-related cognitions and behaviors and incorporates two elements: (1) a cognitive element focusing on the modification of thoughts and beliefs thought relevant for the disease process and (2) a behavioral element consisting of a graded increase of activity. Several systematic reviews suggest that cognitive-behavioral therapy for adults with CFS is an effective treatment in improving both physical functioning and symptoms such as fatigue, anxiety, and mood compared with either routine care or relaxation therapy [34–36]. Furthermore, one study provided evidence supporting the effectiveness of cognitive-behavioral therapy in children and adolescents [38]. In this study, cognitive-behavioral therapy was associated with a significant positive effect on fatigue, symptoms, physical functioning, and school attendance.

Graded exercise is designed to overcome deconditioning and to increase strength and cardiovascular health. Cycle ergometer training, swimming, or walking may be combined according to the patient's preferences. Graded exercise has no intentions of explicitly treating cognition but should incorporate considerable education wherein the sufferer learns to start at an appropriate level of activity (based on intensity and duration) that is gradually increased, at a rate that does not substantially increase symptoms. If severe fatigue follows exercise, lasting more than 24 hours, the exercise prescription is adjusted so it is less demanding; there are no specific and firm guidelines because of the wide spectrum found in this syndrome. Overall results from systematic reviews suggest that graded aerobic exercise therapy, at intensities between 40% and 70% of the maximum oxygen consumption performed three to five times per week for 30 minutes, is a promising intervention with positive effects on CFS patients' symptoms and quality of life [34,37]. Compared with the symptom-oriented approach of exercise therapy, the time-contingent approach, which considers the duration and frequency of exercise therapy to reverse deconditioning (and in which exercise intensity is based on achievable exercise at baseline, followed by a negotiated gradual increase) [39], seems to clearly offer more advantages in symptom reduction and improving functioning [40]. A few patients may find health benefits and pain relief from other than aerobic exercises, like gentle stretching and gentle strengthening including yoga or Tai Chi.

Education of the individual as to what is known and not known about CFS, its impact on function at work and home, and its prognosis should be included in the rehabilitation programs. Education of patients in self-management strategies that consider when, how, and why people change their behavior over time (transtheoretical model) [41] is of utmost importance in modern rehabilitation. The transtheoretical model describes a "meta" model and critically incorporates aspects of other models into its theoretical framework. These are self-initiated and professionally facilitated changes in health beliefs, behavioral intentions, decision-making processes, self-efficacy, and coping to overcome the temptations component of the transtheoretical model. Patients are better prepared for coping on a daily basis, have more realistic expectations, and think that the physician is not ignoring their concerns. In addition, when appropriate, the individual should be informed that periodic reassessment for a possible treatable underlying process may ensue. This may help relieve anxiety about abandonment. Avoidance of heavy meals, alcohol, caffeine, and total rest can help, as can minimizing intake of substances that alter sleep patterns or alter one's self-image [42].

Procedures

Treatment is symptomatic; therefore, procedures may be chosen to help with trigger points, dizziness, headache, or other symptoms as they occur. If trigger points are noted, appropriate therapy may be initiated. Spray and stretch techniques, dry needling, and trigger point injection with a local anesthetic or small amount of steroid have all met with some success [43].

Acupuncture is an important constituent of traditional Chinese medicine. It is believed in traditional Chinese medicine that acupuncture can strengthen the vital essence of the human body and remove the blockage in energy channels. The application of acupuncture for CFS is mainly empirically based; a few clinical trials that included a control group suggest that this procedure may be effective in reducing symptoms [44].

Surgery

No specific surgery is performed for CFS.

Potential Disease Complications

Recovery without treatment is rare, with a median recovery rate of 5% and improvement rate of 39.5% [5]. Recovery episodes seem more likely in patients with less severe fatigue and if patients do not attribute the illness to physical causes [5]. The primary complication of the disease is continued fatigue and loss of function, which commonly occur despite treatment. Predictors of poor treatment outcome were membership in a self-help group, receipt of a sickness benefit, claiming of a disability-related benefit, low sense of control, strong focus on symptoms, and pervasively passive activity pattern [7].

Both reduced functioning and sedentariness may increase the progress or severity of chronic diseases of the cardiovascular and metabolic systems, thereby further increasing the disablement of patients with CFS.

Potential Treatment Complications

Physicians who convey understanding and compassion to patients, despite the lack of a known "cure," can alter a patient's quality of life; fear, or the perception of being abandoned, can markedly accentuate frustration and accelerate a decline in function. Medication side effects should be reviewed on an intermittent basis to be certain that the nonspecific symptoms found in CFS are not being accentuated. Care should be taken to avoid too strenuous an exercise program because the fatigue that may ensue can be both physically and mentally debilitating. Despite optimal care, depression, fatigue, and a loss of function may still occur. Physicians and patients should both be aware that symptoms found in CFS may persist for months or years but that remittance or recovery is still possible.

Acknowledgment

The author thanks Dr. Thomas Brockow, FBK German Institute for Health Care Research, for his valuable comments on the manuscript.

References

[1] Fukuda K, Straus SE, Hickie I, et al. The chronic fatigue syndrome: a comprehensive approach to its definition and study. International Chronic Fatigue Syndrome Study Group. Ann Intern Med 1994;121:953–9.

[2] Reyes M, Nisenbaum R, Hoaglin DC, et al. Prevalence and incidence of chronic fatigue syndrome in Wichita, Kansas. Arch Intern Med 2003;163:1530–6.

[3] Jason LA, Richman JA, Rademaker AW, et al. A community-based study of chronic fatigue syndrome. Arch Intern Med 1999;159:2129–37.

[4] Nacul LC, Lacerda EM, Pheby D, et al. Prevalence of myalgic encephalomyelitis/chronic fatigue syndrome (ME/CFS) in three regions of England: a repeated cross-sectional study in primary care. BMC Med 2011;9:91.

[5] Cairns R, Hotopf M. A systematic review describing the prognosis of chronic fatigue syndrome. Occup Med (Lond) 2005;55:20–31.

[6] White PD. What causes chronic fatigue syndrome? BMJ 2004; 329:928–9.

[7] Prins JB, van der Meer JW, Bleijenberg G. Chronic fatigue syndrome. Lancet 2006;367:346–55.

[8] Cleare AJ. The neuroendocrinology of chronic fatigue syndrome. Endocr Rev 2003;24:236–52.

[9] Cleare AJ, Messa C, Rabiner EA, Grasby PM. Brain 5-HT_{1A} receptor binding in chronic fatigue syndrome measured using positron emission tomography and [^{11}C]WAY-100635. Biol Psychiatry 2005;57:239–46.

[10] Yamamoto S, Ouchi Y, Onoe H, et al. Reduction of serotonin transporters of patients with chronic fatigue syndrome. Neuroreport 2004;15:2571–4.

[11] Cho HJ, Skowera A, Cleary A, Wessely S. Chronic fatigue syndrome: an update focusing on phenomenology and pathophysiology. Curr Opin Psychiatry 2006;19:67–73.

[12] Konsman JP, Parnet P, Dantzer R. Cytokine-induced sickness behaviour: mechanisms and implications. Trends Neurosci 2002;25:154–9.

[13] Nijs J, Meeus M, Van Oosterwijck J, et al. In the mind or in the brain? Scientific evidence for central sensitization and chronic fatigue syndrome. Eur J Clin Invest 2012;42:203–12.

[14] Lange G, Steffener J, Cook DB, et al. Objective evidence of cognitive complaints in chronic fatigue syndrome: a BOLD fMRI study of verbal working memory. Neuroimage 2005;26:513–24.

[15] de Lange FP, Kalkman JS, Bleijenberg G, et al. Neural correlates of the chronic fatigue syndrome—an fMRI study. Brain 2004; 127(Pt 9):1948–57.

[16] Reeves WC, Lloyd A, Vernon SD, et al. Identification of ambiguities in the 1994 chronic fatigue syndrome research case definition and recommendations for resolution. BMC Health Serv Res 2003;3:25.

[17] Afari N, Buchwald D. Chronic fatigue syndrome: a review. Am J Psychiatry 2003;160:221–36.

[18] CFIDS Association of America. http://www.cfids.org/; [accessed 01.11.07].

[19] Levine PH. Chronic fatigue syndrome comes of age. Am J Med 1998;105:2s–4s.

[20] Ropper AH, Brown RH. Fatigue, asthenia, anxiety, and depressive reactions. In: Ropper AH, Brown RH, editors. Adams and Victor's principles of neurology. 8th ed. New York: McGraw-Hill; 2005. p. 433–47.

[21] Nijs J, de Meirleir K, Duquet W. Kinesiophobia in chronic fatigue syndrome: assessment and associations with disability. Arch Phys Med Rehabil 2004;85:1586–92.

[22] Heijmans MJ. Coping and adaptive outcome in chronic fatigue syndrome: importance of illness cognitions. J Psychosom Res 1998;45(Spec No):39–51.

[23] Ross SD, Estok RP, Frame D, et al. Disability and chronic fatigue syndrome: a focus on function. Arch Intern Med 2004;164:1098–107.

[24] Andrews G, Peters L. The psychometric properties of the Composite International Diagnostic Interview. Soc Psychiatry Psychiatr Epidemiol 1998;33:80–8.

[25] Taylor RR, Friedberg F, Jason LA. A clinician's guide to controversial illnesses: chronic fatigue syndrome, fibromyalgia, and multiple chemical sensitivities. Sarasota, Fla: Professional Resource Press; 2001.

[26] Unger ER, Nisenbaum R, Moldofsky H, et al. Sleep assessment in a population based study of chronic fatigue syndrome. BMC Neurol 2004;4:6.

[27] World Health Organization. International classification of functioning, disability and health (ICF). Geneva: World Health Organization; 2001.

[28] Cieza A, Stucki G, Weigl M, et al. ICF core sets for low back pain. J Rehabil Med 2004;44(Suppl.):69–74.

[29] Dreinhöfer K, Stucki G, Ewert T, et al. ICF core sets for osteoarthritis. J Rehabil Med 2004;44(Suppl.):75–80.

[30] Weiss DJ. Adaptive testing by computer. J Consult Clin Psychol 1985;53:774–89.

[31] Ware Jr JE, Bjorner JB, Kosinski M. Practical implications of item response theory and computerized adaptive testing: a brief summary of ongoing studies of widely used headache impact scales. Med Care 2000;38(Suppl.):II73–82.

[32] Royal College of Paediatrics and Child Health. Evidence based guidelines for the management of CFS/ME (Chronic Fatigue Syndrome/ Myalgic Encephalopathy) in children and young people. London: RCPCH; December 2004. 1–22, www.rcpch.ac.uk/recent_publications.html.

[33] Reid S, Chalder T, Cleare A, et al. Chronic fatigue syndrome. Clin Evid (Online) 2011 May 26.

[34] Chambers D, Bagnall A, Hempel S, Forbes C. Interventions for the treatment, management and rehabilitation of patients with chronic fatigue syndrome/myalgic encephalomyelitis: an updated systematic review. J R Soc Med 2006;99:506–20.

[35] Whiting P, Bagnall A, Sowden A, et al. Interventions for the treatment and management of chronic fatigue syndrome: a systematic review. JAMA 2001;286:1360–8.

[36] Price JR, Mitchell E, Tidy E, Hunot V. Cognitive behaviour therapy for chronic fatigue syndrome in adults. Cochrane Database Syst Rev 2008;3, CD001027.

[37] Edmonds M, McGuire H, Price J. Exercise therapy for chronic fatigue syndrome. Cochrane Database Syst Rev 2004;3, CD003200.

[38] Stulemeijer M, de Jong LW, Fiselier TJ, et al. Cognitive behaviour therapy for adolescents with chronic fatigue syndrome: randomised controlled trial. BMJ 2005;330:14–7.

[39] White PD, Goldsmith KA, Johnson AL, et al. Comparison of adaptive pacing therapy, cognitive behaviour therapy, graded exercise therapy, and specialist medical care for chronic fatigue syndrome (PACE): a randomised trial. Lancet 2011;377:823–36.

[40] Van Cauwenbergh D, De Kooning M, Ickmans K, Nijs J. How to exercise people with chronic fatigue syndrome: evidence-based practice guidelines. Eur J Clin Invest 2012;42:1136–44.

[41] Prochaska J, DiClemente CC, Norcross JC. In search of how people change. Am Psychol 1992;47:1102–14.

[42] Manningham R. The symptoms, nature and causes, and cure of the febricula, or little fever. London: J. Robinson; 1750.

[43] Robinson J, Arendt Nielsen L. Muscle pain syndromes. In: Braddom RL, editor. Physical medicine and rehabilitation. Philadelphia: WB Saunders; 2006. p. 989–1020.

[44] Porter NS, Jason LA, Boulton A, et al. Alternative medical interventions used in the treatment and management of myalgic encephalomyelitis/chronic fatigue syndrome and fibromyalgia. J Altern Complement Med 2010;16:235–49.

CHAPTER 126

Joint Contractures

Mark Campbell, MD, MSc
Nancy Dudek, MD, MEd
Guy Trudel, MD, MSc, FRCPC, DABPMR

Synonyms

Arthrofibrosis
Capsulitis
Ankylosis

ICD-9 Codes

M24.5 Contracture of joint
M24.6 Ankylosis of joint
M96.0 Arthrodesis

ICD-10 Codes

M24.50 Contracture, unspecified joint
M24.60 Ankylosis, unspecified joint
Z98.1 Arthrodesis status

Definition

A joint contracture is a limitation in the passive range of motion of a joint. Changes in articular structures (bone, cartilage, capsule) or nonarticular structures (muscles, tendons, skin) can prevent a joint from moving passively through its full range. A classification according to the tissue limiting the range of motion is proposed in Table 126.1.

By this definition, regardless of the nature of the tissue alteration, if it results in joint motion limitation, the joint condition is called a joint contracture. For example, a muscle with adaptive shortening or fibrosis restricting joint motion is classified as joint contracture—myogenic type. It should not be referred to as a muscle contracture.

As such, joint motion limited by pain or spasticity qualifies as a joint contracture only if the limitation is demonstrated after the pain or the influence of the hyperactive upper motor neuron (increased tone, spasticity, co-contraction) has been removed. For example, when a person with a spinal cord injury is treated for spasticity, the tone in the lower extremities will be reduced and an apparent chronic ankle plantar flexion contracture may disappear.

Conventionally, a joint contracture is named according to the joint involved and the direction *opposite* the lack of range. Some examples: a knee flexion contracture lacks full extension; an elbow extension contracture lacks full flexion; and an ankle plantar flexion contracture lacks dorsiflexion.

A contracture is the final common path of numerous conditions preventing movement of a joint through its full range of motion. Pain, trauma, immobility, weakness, and edema commonly contribute to reduced joint range of motion. The body's natural reaction to a painful joint is to "splint" or immobilize it. Not moving the joint through its full range, with time, can cause structural changes to one or more articular or nonarticular tissues, and a joint contracture can ensue [1]. Joints traumatized by fracture or reconstructive surgery, such as anterior cruciate ligament repair or arthroplasty, are susceptible to contractures [2]. Joint contractures can happen as a consequence of the disease (prolonged immobility in bed in intensive care units; Fig. 126.1) or as part of the treatment (casting after fracture or prolonged use of a brace). Any joint can be affected. At the spine, affected vertebral amphiarthrodial and facet diarthrodial joints can limit the range at one or more segments.

Neurologic conditions that increase muscle tone or cause weakness contribute to contractures because of unequal forces generated by opposing muscle groups. In upper motor neuron conditions, such as after a stroke or traumatic brain injury, spasticity and excessive muscle tone prevent a joint from accessing portions of its normal range [3]. Similarly, in lower motor neuron injuries, such as a plexopathy or peripheral nerve injury, the unopposed muscle pull will limit joint motion toward the paralyzed muscle. The range of motion not accessed will eventually be lost, resulting in a joint contracture.

A number of other local conditions, such as arthritis, joint infections, and burns, will cause contractures [4]. In addition, conditions affecting multiple systems, such as muscular dystrophy, diabetes, and Parkinson and Alzheimer diseases, can limit mobility or initiation and put the patient at risk for contractures.

Data on incidence and prevalence of joint contractures are limited and often describe one specific joint [4]. Nevertheless, these studies indicate a common problem. At least one joint contracture was noted in 7% to 51% of

Table 126.1 Classification of Contractures According to the Tissue Restricting the Range of Motion of the Joint

Type	Condition*
Arthrogenic	
Bone	Intra-articular fracture, osteophyte
Cartilage	Osteochondritis dissecans
Synovium	Pigmented villonodular synovitis, synovial chondromatosis
Capsular	Secondary to immobility and capsular shortening, adhesive capsulitis, arthrofibrosis
Other	Meniscal tear, labrum tear, palmar or plantar fibromatosis
Myogenic	
Muscle	Muscle fibrosis, myositis ossificans, muscle adaptation to altered neurologic supply (spasticity, flaccidity)
Fascia	Eosinophilic fasciitis
Tendinous	Tendon transposition, shortening
Cutaneous	Burn, scleroderma
Mixed (any combination of the above types)	Burn and adhesive capsulitis

*One or more clinical conditions illustrate each type of joint contracture.

persons after a spinal cord injury [5–7]. Between 16% and 81% of persons with an acquired brain injury developed a joint contracture [3,8,9], and 51% of children who had an obstetric brachial plexus injury were found to have a shoulder contracture [10]. In institutionalized elderly, one study reported that 71% of those who were immobile had a joint contracture, whereas none of the mobile patients had a joint contracture [11].

Symptoms

Joint contractures develop insidiously and may progress asymptomatically. They are painful only with attempts to move the joint through its full range beyond the restriction. Many daily activities do not require a joint to move through its entire range. Therefore a contracture may develop unnoticed for extended periods until the joint restriction

Table 126.2 Range of Motion Required to Perform Select Activities of Daily Living

Activity	Joint	Required Range
Walking	Knee	60° of flexion [12]
	Ankle	15° of dorsiflexion [13]
		20° of plantar flexion [13]
Ascending stairs	Knee	94° of flexion [14]
	Hip	67° of flexion [14]
Eating (fork to mouth)	Elbow	128° of flexion [15]
Combing hair	Shoulder	105° of abduction [12]
		90° of external rotation [12]
Perineal hygiene	Shoulder	90° of internal rotation [12]
	Wrist	54° of flexion [16]
Open a door with doorknob	Elbow	35° of pronation [15]
		23° of supination [15]
	Wrist	32° of ulnar deviation [16]
Open and close jar lid	Wrist	10° of radial deviation [16]
		36° of ulnar deviation [16]

interferes with functional activity (Table 126.2). In the outpatient setting, patients with hand and finger joint contractures might present with complaints of a weak or ineffective grasp. A patient with a knee flexion contracture may complain of a limp [17] or of hip or low back pain. Nearly half of tetraplegic spinal cord injury patients with a shoulder contracture experienced shoulder pain [18]. Subjects with spinal muscular atrophy or congenital myopathy were more than eight times more likely to experience elbow pain if they had an elbow contracture [19].

Physical Examination

The patient must be relaxed, properly positioned, and in no pain. The clinician inspects the patient for abnormalities of limb shape, size, symmetry, and position. Edema, effusion, or deformity of the joints is noted. Skin is also assessed for any areas of breakdown or thickening complicating a contracture. Palpation of joints for swelling and tenderness must be completed. Passive range of motion is particularly important when weakness prevents normal active movement. The most precise tool for joint

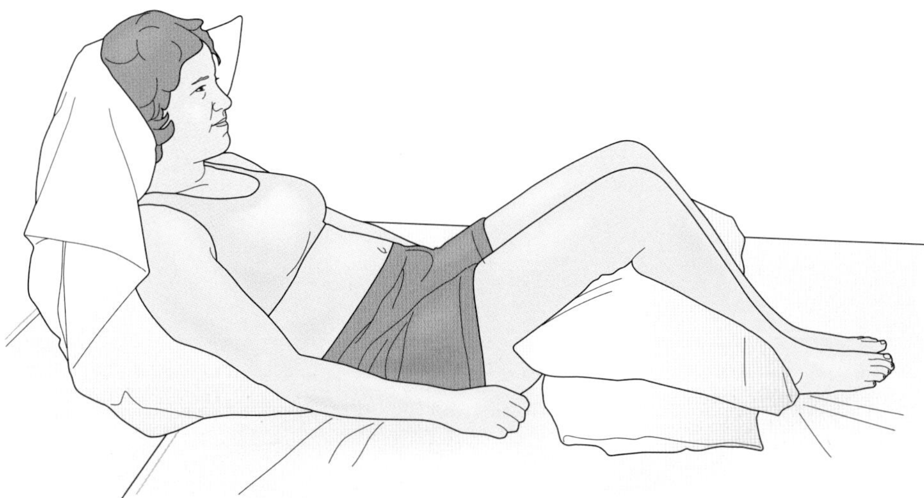

FIGURE 126.1 Prolonged bed rest is a risk factor for contractures in multiple joints.

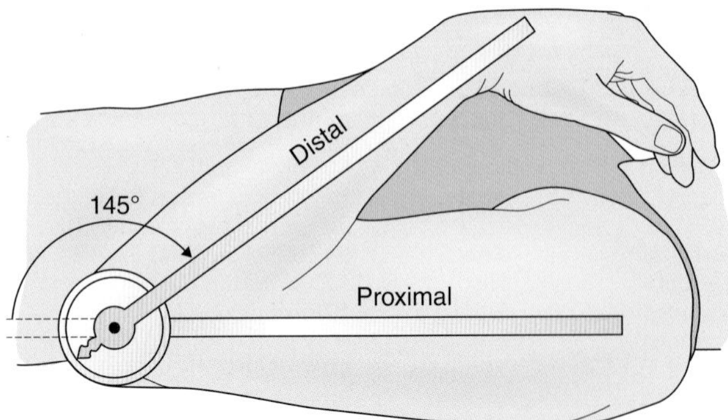

FIGURE 126.2 Example of how to measure a joint with a universal goniometer. *(Modified from Norkin CC, White DJ. Measurement of Joint Motion: A Guide to Goniometry, 3rd ed. Philadelphia, FA Davis, 2003.)*

measurement is a universal goniometer (Fig. 126.2). Spine combined movements can be assessed with an inclinometer. Comparison is made with the contralateral side or with normative values [20].

A complete neuromuscular examination can detect potential causes of contractures. Particular attention must be paid to strength and specifically to the presence of muscle imbalance in opposing muscle groups. Reflexes and tone are assessed. In the presence of spasticity, the clinician should first apply prolonged passive stretch to determine whether a full range of motion can be achieved. If it is not achieved, the clinician can use modalities (e.g., therapeutic heating), optimize medication, or use motor block injections to rule out that spasticity is masking normal passive range of the joint. Finally, a sensory examination detecting abnormal sensation will influence the choice of treatment modalities.

Functional Limitations

Joint contractures affect the performance of activities of daily living. Functional limitations depend on the underlying medical condition, the joints affected, and the severity of the joint contractures (Table 126.2). Upper extremity contractures of the elbow, wrist, and fingers impair the performance of all basic activities of daily living, such as dressing and grooming, as well as advanced skills requiring fine motor coordination, like writing. In a disabled elderly population, half as many subjects with an upper limb contracture fed themselves compared with those without a contracture [21]. Upper limb contractures can also limit mobility in patients using gait aids. Lower extremity contractures interfere mainly with mobility [21]. Hip and knee flexion contractures alter gait pattern, increase energy expenditure, and impair wheelchair mobility and car transfers. Fixed spinal deformity may limit many activities of daily living. Patients with transtibial amputations are at risk for development of a knee flexion contracture after their amputation (Fig. 126.3A). This may result in an inability to fit that patient with the most functional below-knee prosthesis. Instead, a bent-knee prosthesis, offering the patient less function and increased energy cost, must be used (Fig. 126.3B). Multiple upper and lower limb joint contractures exacerbate disability.

Diagnostic Studies

The diagnosis of a joint contracture is clinical. Radiographic evaluation can identify contributing conditions, such as osteophytes and heterotopic ossification. If a systemic cause is suspected, specific investigations are indicated.

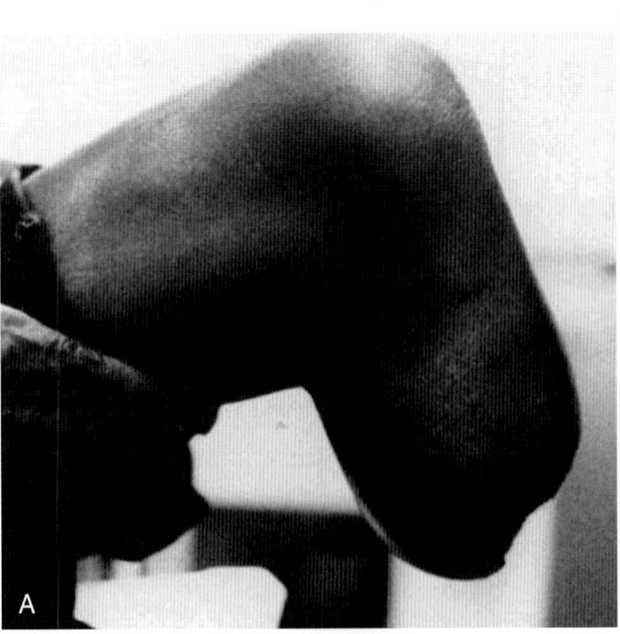

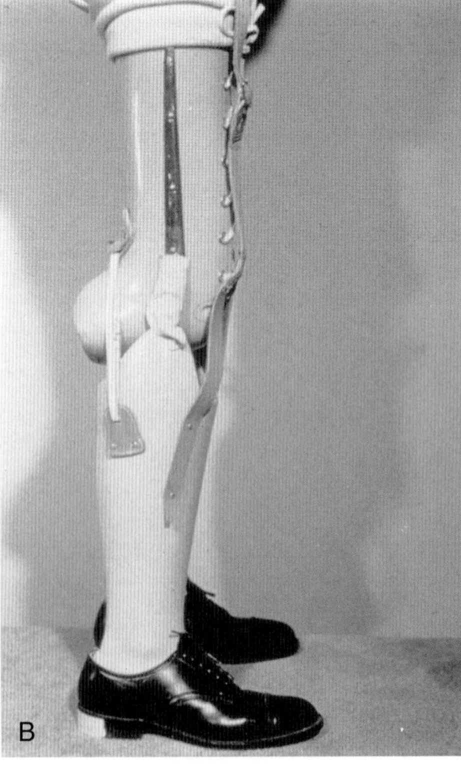

FIGURE 126.3 **A,** Knee flexion contracture in a below-knee (transtibial) amputee. **B,** Example of a bent-knee prosthesis.

Differential Diagnosis

Spasticity
Heterotopic ossification
Degenerative joint disease
Fracture
Dislocation
Loose body in a joint
Meniscal tears
Psychogenic

Treatment

Initial

Successfully treating a medical condition that limits the joint range of motion may resolve the contracture; however, such conditions can also produce an irreversible joint contracture. A stepwise assessment and treatment plan may therefore be needed.

Prevention is at the heart of joint contracture management. Moving joints actively or passively through their full range on a daily basis prevents contractures. Continuous passive motion devices, such as those used after total knee joint arthroplasty, can achieve this postoperatively [22].

Pain control is essential to the prevention and treatment of contractures, particularly after an acute injury or after a surgical procedure [23]. Rest, ice, compression, elevation, and joint protection can help reduce pain in the acute stage, allowing earlier initiation of range of motion. Appropriate use of analgesics will promote the patient's comfort and compliance with stretching sessions.

Therapeutic positioning and splinting prevent contractures in immobilized patients [23]. These measures maintain the correct length of connective tissue and alternate between different positions of the joint. An example of therapeutic positioning is lying prone to stretch the hip joints in extension. External rotation and abduction of the shoulders with an arm support attached to the bed of patients in the intensive care unit will maintain shoulder range. Standing upright or on an incline will help stretch the ankle joints. Hand and finger as well as ankle static orthoses are useful for preventing finger and ankle contractures.

Rehabilitation

Once contractures have developed, rehabilitation includes sustained stretching and exercises to increase range of motion. Again, analgesia and control of spasticity should be optimized to benefit the stretching sessions. A recent Cochrane review has questioned the effectiveness of up to 7 months of stretching in the treatment of contracture in both neurologic and non-neurologic conditions [24]; therefore, aggressive treatment may be required during a longer period.

Therapeutic modalities are commonly used to potentiate the effect of stretching sessions. The combination of modalities that heat soft tissues with stretching is an effective treatment [25]. Ultrasound, for example, heats soft tissues around large joints to a therapeutic temperature range of 40° C to 43° C, improving their elasticity [23]. Small joints can be heated by the use of paraffin bath dips or hydrotherapy (e.g., for hand and finger contractures in scleroderma or nerve injury).

Dynamic bracing can achieve prolonged, continuous stretching of joint contractures. Serial casting or serial splinting is also used with the same intent. After maximal stretching, a cast or orthosis is applied to preserve gains. The cast or orthosis is removed every 2 or 3 days, stretching is repeated, and the cast or orthosis is reapplied at an enhanced angle (Fig. 126.4). Joints casted or splinted at the end range of motion for longer periods led to improved benefit [26]. Serial casting or splinting should be carefully monitored on limbs with circulatory or sensory compromise because of increased risk of skin breakdown and ulcer formation.

Provision of assistive devices to lessen specific disability and of gait aids to try to normalize gait completes the rehabilitation process.

Procedures

If spasticity is thought to maintain contractures, despite optimized oral medication, treatments such as motor point blocks with phenol or botulinum toxin injections or intrathecal baclofen are considered. These procedures can be diagnostic as well as therapeutic because they can differentiate a joint contracture from spasticity. These procedures

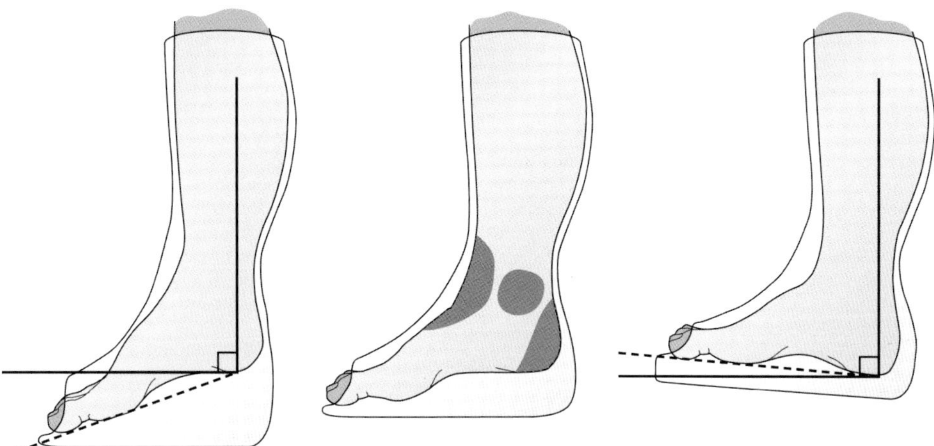

FIGURE 126.4 Serial short leg casts depicting a reduction of plantar flexion contracture of 20 degrees to a final holding cast at 5 degrees of dorsiflexion. Several intermediate casts between the initial and final holding casts may be required to achieve gradual dorsiflexion range.

can constitute an adjunct to dynamic bracing and serial casting or splinting.

Extracorporeal shock wave lithotripsy [27] and ablative laser therapy [28] are being evaluated for skin-related contractures.

Surgery

In fixed contractures, surgical treatments include tenotomy, tendon lengthening, joint capsule release, and joint reconstruction. In some cases, skin grafts or flaps may be necessary to close resulting large skin defects [29]. These procedures are reserved for patients in whom less aggressive methods of treatment have failed and the fixed contractures significantly affect function [23].

Potential Disease Complications

Joint contracture can lead to ankylosis of a joint with corresponding loss of function. Upper limb contractures, especially if they are affecting multiple joints, can lead to dependency for all aspects of care. Mobility can be decreased to a bedridden state. Pressure sores can develop because of the limited options for mobility and weight-bearing areas. Infection by bacterial and fungal agents can occur in the skinfolds if contractures prevent adequate access for hygiene.

Potential Treatment Complications

Aggressive stretching can inadvertently result in pain; tears in muscle, ligament, or capsule; and joint subluxation. These complications can lead to bleeding, especially in patients receiving anticoagulation or those with a bleeding diathesis or thrombopenia.

Splinting and casting can result in skin ulceration or limb ischemia if patients are inappropriately selected or not closely monitored. This risk is increased if the patient lacks protective sensation because of the underlying disease.

References

[1] Farmer SE, James M. Contractures in orthopaedic and neurological conditions: a review of causes and treatment. Disabil Rehabil 2001;23:549–58.

[2] Scuderi GR. The stiff total knee arthroplasty—causality and solution. J Arthroplasty 2005;20:23–6.

[3] Singer BJ, Jegasothy GM, Singer KP, et al. Incidence of ankle contracture after moderate to severe acquired brain injury. Arch Phys Med Rehabil 2004;85:1465–9.

[4] Fergusson D, Hutton B, Drodge A. The epidemiology of major joint contractures: a systematic review of the literature. Clin Orthop Relat Res 2007;456:22–9.

[5] Krause JS. Aging after spinal cord injury: an exploratory study. Spinal Cord 2000;38:77–83.

[6] Vogel LC, Krajci KA, Anderson CJ. Adults with pediatric-onset spinal cord injury: part 2: musculoskeletal and neurological complications. J Spinal Cord Med 2002;25:117–23.

[7] Bryden AM, Kilgore KL, Lind BB, Yu DT. Triceps denervation as a predictor of elbow flexion contractures in C5 and C6 tetraplegia. Arch Phys Med Rehabil 2004;85:1880–5.

[8] Pohl M, Mehrholz J. A new shoulder range of motion screening measurement: its reliability and application in the assessment of the prevalence of shoulder contractures in patients with impaired consciousness caused by severe brain damage. Arch Phys Med Rehabil 2005;86:98–104.

[9] Yarkony GM, Sahgal V. Contractures. A major complication of craniocerebral trauma. Clin Orthop Relat Res 1987;219:93–6.

[10] Hoeksma A, Ter Steeg AM, Dijkstra P, et al. Shoulder contracture and osseous deformity in obstetrical brachial plexus injuries. J Bone Joint Surg Am 2003;85:316–22.

[11] Selikson S, Damus K, Hamerman D. Risk factors associated with immobility. J Am Geriatr Soc 1988;36:707–12.

[12] Brinkmann JR, Perry J. Rate and range of knee motion during ambulation in healthy and arthritic subjects. Phys Ther 1985;65:1055–60.

[13] Magee DJ. Orthopedic physical assessment. 5th ed. St. Louis: Saunders Elsevier; 2008.

[14] Protopapadaki A, Drechsler WI, Cramp MC, et al. Hip, knee, ankle kinematics and kinetics during stair ascent and descent in healthy young individuals. Clin Biomech (Bristol, Avon) 2007;22:203–10.

[15] Morrey BF, Askew LJ, Chao EY. A biomechanical study of normal functional elbow motion. J Bone Joint Surg Am 1981;63:872–6.

[16] Ryu J, Cooney III. WP, Askew LJ, et al. Functional ranges of motion of the wrist joint. J Hand Surg [Am] 1991;16:409–19.

[17] Buschbacher RM, Porter CD. Deconditioning, conditioning, and the benefits of exercise. In: Braddom RL, editor. Physical medicine and rehabilitation. 2nd ed. Philadelphia: WB Saunders; 2000. p. 706–8.

[18] Dalyan M, Sherman A, Cardenas DD. Factors associated with contractures in acute spinal cord injury. Spinal Cord 1998;36:405–8.

[19] Willig TN, Bach JR, Rouffet MJ, et al. Correlation of flexion contractures with upper extremity function and pain for spinal muscular atrophy and congenital myopathy patients. Am J Phys Med Rehabil 1995;74:33–8.

[20] Norkin CC, White DJ. Measurement of joint motion: a guide to goniometry. 3rd ed. Philadelphia: FA Davis; 2003.

[21] Yip B, Stewart DA, Roberts MA. The prevalence of joint contractures in residents in NHS continuing care. Health Bull (Edinb) 1996;54:338–43.

[22] Salter RB. Continuous passive motion (CPM): a biological concept for the healing and regeneration of articular cartilage, ligaments, and tendons: from origination to research to clinical applications. Williams & Wilkins: Baltimore; 1993.

[23] Halar EM, Bell KR. Immobility and inactivity: physiological and functional changes, prevention, and treatment. In: DeLisa JA, editor. Physical medicine and rehabilitation: principles and practice. 4th ed. Philadelphia: Lippincott Williams & Wilkins; 2004. p. 1452–63.

[24] Katalinic OM, Harvey LA, Herbert RD, et al. Stretch for the treatment and prevention of contractures. Cochrane Database Syst Rev 2010;9: CD007455.

[25] Usuba M, Miyanaga Y, Miyakawa S, et al. Effect of heat in increasing the range of knee motion after the development of a joint contracture: an experiment with an animal model. Arch Phys Med Rehabil 2006;87:247–53.

[26] Flowers KR, LaStayo PC. Effect of total range time on improving passive range of motion. J Hand Ther 2012;25:48–54.

[27] Fioramonti P, Cigna E, Onesti MG, et al. Extracorporeal shock wave therapy for the management of burn scars. Dermatol Surg 2012;38:778–82.

[28] Kineston D, Kwan JM, Uebelhoer NS, et al. Use of a fractional ablative 10.6-μm carbon dioxide laser in the treatment of a morphea-related contracture. Arch Dermatol 2011;147:1148–50.

[29] Kim KS, Kim ES, Hwang JH, et al. Medial sural perforator plus island flap: a modification of the medial sural perforator island flap for the reconstruction of postburn knee flexion contractures using burned calf skin. J Plast Reconstr Aesthet Surg 2012;65:804–9.

CHAPTER 127

Deep Venous Thrombosis

Blessen C. Eapen, MD

Synonyms

Venous thromboembolism
Blood clot
Thrombophlebitis
Phlebothrombosis

ICD-9 Code

451.1 Phlebitis and thrombophlebitis, of deep vessels of lower extremities

ICD-10 Codes

I80.201 Phlebitis and thrombophlebitis of unspecified deep vessels of right lower extremity
I80.202 Phlebitis and thrombophlebitis of unspecified deep vessels of left lower extremity
I80.203 Phlebitis and thrombophlebitis of unspecified deep vessels of lower extremities, bilateral
I80.209 Phlebitis and thrombophlebitis of unspecified deep vessels of unspecified lower extremity

Definition

Venous thromboembolism is a major cause of mortality and morbidity and is manifested by deep venous thrombosis (DVT) and pulmonary embolism. This chapter is limited to the discussion of DVT. DVT occurs when a fibrin clot abnormally occludes a vein in the deep venous system, predominantly in the lower extremities. The prevailing theory explaining the development of DVT is known as Virchow triad, which includes alterations in blood flow (stasis), vascular endothelial injury, and hypercoagulation disorder. The risk for development of DVT varies according to specific characteristics of the patient, the medical condition, or the surgical procedure (Table 127.1). Conditions that may increase the risk for development of DVT are advanced age, morbid obesity, varicose veins, prolonged immobility, pregnancy, malignant disease, stroke, inflammatory bowel disease, congestive heart failure, and previous DVT. Certain hereditary conditions may also predispose to development of DVT, such as deficiencies in protein C and protein S and familial thrombophilia. Acquired deficiencies of the natural anticoagulant system include antibodies directed against antiphospholipid and heterozygous factor V Leiden mutations [1].

Patients can be categorized according to their risk for development of DVT [2] on the basis of the type of surgical procedure; orthopedic patients carry the highest risk [3] (Table 127.2). It is believed that orthopedic procedures carry such a high risk for DVT because the mechanical destruction of bone marrow during most orthopedic procedures causes intravasation of marrow cells and cell fragments and elevations of plasma tissue factor [4]. Plasma tissue factor is a potent trigger of blood clotting [5] and is found in high concentrations in bone marrow and the adventitia surrounding the major blood vessels and the brain, which places neurosurgical patients at great risk for development of DVT. After neurosurgery, the incidence of DVT has been reported to be as high as 50% [6]. Risk factors that increase the rates of DVT in neurosurgery patients include intracranial surgery, malignant tumors, duration of the surgery, and presence of paresis or paralysis of the lower limbs [7]. Patients can remain in a hypercoagulable state up to 5 weeks postoperatively [8]. In addition to surgical patients, victims of orthopedic and neurologic trauma are at great risk for development of DVT, especially if long bone fracture or paralysis is sustained. Patients who suffer injury to the spinal cord are at high risk for DVT because of stasis and hypercoagulability.

Symptoms

Venous thrombosis often occurs asymptomatically. Symptoms of DVT may include ipsilateral lower extremity edema, fever, extremity warmth, and pain. Symptoms do not rule in or rule out DVT but can serve only as a trigger for further diagnostic inquiry.

Table 127.1 Risk Factors for Deep Venous Thrombosis

Patient Factors	Diseases	Procedures
Age >40 years Obesity Varicose veins Prolonged immobilization Pregnancy High-dose estrogen therapy Tamoxifen Bevacizumab Previous deep venous thrombosis	Thrombophilia Antithrombin III, protein C, protein S deficiency Antiphospholipid antibody, lupus anticoagulant Malignant disease Major medical illness Trauma Spinal cord injury Paralysis	Pelvic surgery Lower limb orthopedic surgery Neurosurgery

Modified from Sokolof J, Knight R. Deep venous thrombosis. In Frontera WR, Silver JK, Rizzo TD Jr, eds. Essentials of Physical Medicine and Rehabilitation, 2nd ed. Philadelphia, WB Saunders, 2008.

Physical Examination

The classic signs of DVT are tenderness, ipsilateral swelling, and warmth. A palpable cord can sometimes be felt, which reflects a thrombosed vein. In the past, emphasis was placed on the presence of Homan sign and calf tenderness in making a clinical diagnosis of DVT; however, these physical examination findings have been found to be nonspecific with poor positive predictive values [9]. Significant asymmetric calf edema is an important sign and can be determined by taking the circumferential measurement of the calf 10 cm below the tibial tuberosity. A 3-cm difference in calf girth is considered a significant clinical difference. When it is massive, the swelling can obstruct not only venous outflow but arterial inflow, leading to phlegmasia cerulea dolens due to ischemia. Here, the leg is usually blue and painful.

Like symptoms, physical examination findings are not sensitive or specific. In more than 50% of the instances of DVT, physical examination findings are normal.

Functional Limitations

DVT rarely causes functional compromise, except calf pain during walking. Absolute bed rest is generally not indicated, and early walking is safe in patients with acute DVT and may help reduce acute symptoms [10]. However, patients should suspend their lower extremity exercise program until they are fully anticoagulated.

Diagnostic Studies

The Wells prediction rules (Table 127.3) are a group of clinical characteristics that are useful in estimating the pretest probability of DVT. High-quality evidence exists to support the validity of these rules, and their use is recommended as a practice guideline by the American Academy of Family Physicians and the American College of Physicians [11]. They are easily implemented before more definitive testing is performed on patients [12].

Invasive and noninvasive diagnostic tests are available to screen for DVT. These include contrast venography, compression ultrasonography, impedance plethysmography, D-dimer testing, and magnetic resonance venography.

Contrast venography is an invasive test that is considered the "gold standard" for the diagnosis of DVT and is the only test that can reliably detect DVT isolated to the calf veins, the iliac veins, and the inferior vena cava (Figs. 127.1 and 127.2). The drawbacks to venography are its technical complexity, the requirement for the use of contrast media, the risk of allergic reaction, and the patient's discomfort. Therefore it is not recommended as an initial screening test.

Compression ultrasonography (real-time, B-mode venous) is the procedure of choice for the investigation of patients with suspected DVT. Venous ultrasonography allows direct visualization of the vein lumen. The inability to compress the lumen of the vein is the main criterion for a positive test result. Other adjunctive findings include vein distention, absence of flow, echogenic signals within the vessel lumen, and visualization of filling defects by color Doppler studies. Systematic reviews have demonstrated

Table 127.2 Risk Categories of Venous Thromboembolism in Surgical Patients without Prophylaxis

Risk Category	Calf DVT	Proximal DVT	Fatal PE
High	40%-80%	10%-30%	1%-5%
Major orthopedic surgery of the lower limb Major general surgery in patients >40 years with cancer or recent DVT or PE Multiple trauma Thrombophilia			
Moderate	10%-40%	2%-10%	0.1%-0.8%
General surgery in patients >40 years that lasts 30 minutes or more without additional risk factors General surgery in patients <40 years receiving estrogen or with a history of DVT or PE Emergency cesarean section in women >35 years			
Low	<10%	<1%	<0.01%
Minor surgery (i.e., <30 minutes in patients >40 years without additional risk factors) Uncomplicated surgery in patients <40 years without additional risk factors			

DVT, deep venous thrombosis; *PE,* pulmonary embolism.
From Sokolof J, Knight R. Deep venous thrombosis. In Frontera WR, Silver JK, Rizzo TD Jr, eds. Essentials of Physical Medicine and Rehabilitation, 2nd ed. Philadelphia, WB Saunders, 2008. Modified from Bounameaux H. Integrating pharmacologic and mechanical prophylaxis of venous thromboembolism. Thromb Haemost 1999;82:931-939.

Table 127.3 Wells Prediction Rules: Clinical Evaluation Table for Predicting Pretest Probability of Deep Venous Thrombosis

Clinical Characteristic	Score
Active cancer (treatment ongoing, within previous 6 months, or palliative)	1
Paralysis, paresis, or recent plaster immobilization of the lower extremities	1
Recently bedridden >3 days or major surgery within 12 weeks requiring general or regional anesthesia	1
Localized tenderness along the distribution of the deep venous system	1
Entire leg swollen	1
Calf swelling 3 cm larger than asymptomatic side (measured 10 cm below tibial tuberosity)	1
Pitting edema confined to the symptomatic leg	1
Collateral superficial veins (nonvaricose)	1
Alternative diagnosis at least as likely as deep venous thrombosis	−2

Clinical probability: low, ≤0; intermediate, 1-2; high, ≥3. In patients with symptoms in both legs, the more symptomatic side is used.

From Wells PS, Anderson DR, Bormanis J, et al. Value of assessment of pretest probability of deep-vein thrombosis in clinical management. Lancet 1997;350:1795-1798.

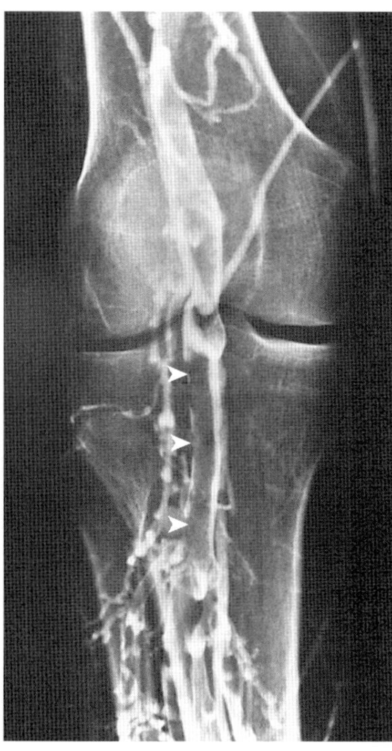

FIGURE 127.1 Acute deep venous thrombosis of popliteal vein. Note the intraluminal filling defect *(arrowheads)* and "tram-tracking" of contrast material around the thrombus. *(From Sokolof J, Knight R. Deep venous thrombosis. In Frontera WR, Silver JK, Rizzo TD Jr, eds. Essentials of Physical Medicine and Rehabilitation, 2nd ed. Philadelphia, WB Saunders, 2008.)*

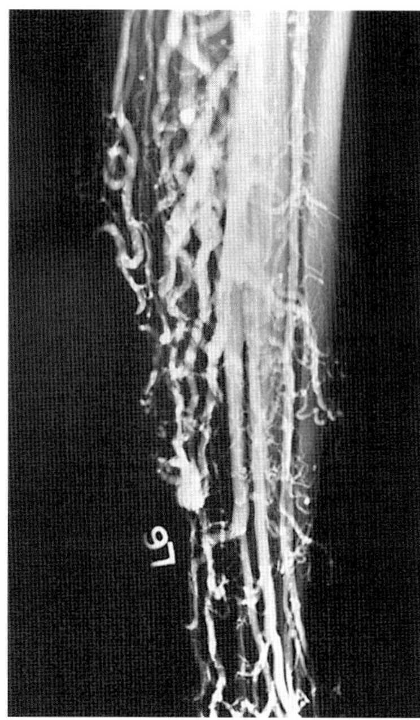

FIGURE 127.2 Chronic lower extremity deep venous thrombosis with abundant collaterals. *(From Katz DS, Math KR, Groskin SA. Radiology Secrets. Philadelphia, Hanley & Belfus, 1998.)*

high sensitivities and specificities for the diagnosis of DVT in the proximal lower extremity by ultrasonography. However, sensitivities are poor for determination of the presence of calf vein thrombosis. Visualization of calf veins by ultrasonography is technically more difficult and less reliable than diagnosis of venous thrombus in the area between the trifurcation of the popliteal vein and the femoral vein in the groin.

Impedance plethysmography, a noninvasive diagnostic test for detection of blood vessel occlusion, determines volumetric changes in the limb by measuring changes in its girth as indicated by changes in the electric impedance of mercury-containing polymeric silicone tubes in a pressure cuff. The method is based on the principle that any circumferential rate of change in a limb segment is directly proportional to the volumetric rate of change, which in turn reflects occlusion of venous and arterial blood flow. However, the technique does not accurately identify the presence or absence of partially obstructing thrombi in major vessels [13]. Impedance plethysmography has limitations including the possibility of false-positive results because of arterial insufficiency and muscle tension [14].

D-dimer assay has emerged as a method to help predict the presence of DVT. D-dimer is a degradation product of the cross-linked fibrin blood clot and is typically elevated in patients with DVT. However, D-dimer levels may also be elevated in a variety of nonthrombotic disorders, including recent major surgery, hemorrhage, trauma, malignant disease, and sepsis. Because of the high sensitivity and low specificity of the D-dimer assay, it is a good tool for exclusion of DVT if the test result is negative. However, a high level does not have as much clinical value.

The first step in the diagnostic approach is the determination of risk. Patients can be separated by clinical criteria into high-, moderate-, and low-risk categories. All symptomatic patients thought to have DVT should, at the very least, undergo venous ultrasound imaging of the proximal venous system. Patients at moderate or high risk should have the ultrasound study repeated in 1 week. DVT also may be ruled out on the basis of a negative result of the D-dimer assay. If the D-dimer assay result is positive, a follow-up ultrasound study in 1 week is indicated.

Magnetic resonance venography is as accurate as contrast venography for the diagnosis of DVT. This was illustrated in a study that evaluated 85 patients thought to have DVT, all of whom underwent both magnetic resonance and contrast venography [15]. Although the diagnostic accuracy of magnetic resonance venography is comparable to that of contrast venography, outcome data are lacking. In addition, the present high cost of magnetic resonance venography makes it unlikely that it will gain prominence as a noninvasive test for DVT. However, magnetic resonance venography is a useful approach when contrast venography is required but precluded because of allergy to contrast media.

Differential Diagnosis

Claudication
Ruptured popliteal (Baker) cysts
Cellulitis
Hematoma
Lymphedema
Superficial thrombophlebitis
Drug-induced edema
Calf muscle pull or tear

Treatment

Initial

The most appropriate choice of prophylaxis depends on the clinical scenario and the risk-benefit profile for a particular patient. The prophylactic options that are currently available for hospitalized medical patients include low-dose unfractionated heparin (UFH), low-molecular-weight heparin (LMWH), fondaparinux, aspirin, warfarin, intermittent pneumatic compression, and graduated compression stockings [16]. UFH and LMWH have been shown to reduce venous thromboembolic risk in hospitalized medical patients, but neither agent altered mortality [17]. On direct comparison, LMWH was more effective than UFH in preventing DVT [17]. Large meta-analyses comparing LMWH with UFH in general and orthopedic surgery have shown that LMWH is safer and more efficacious than UFH [18].

Fondaparinux has been approved by the Food and Drug Administration for the prophylaxis of DVT in patients undergoing surgery for hip fracture, hip replacement, or knee replacement; for extended DVT prophylaxis after hip fracture surgery; and for patients at risk for thromboembolic complications after abdominal surgery [19]. The approved dose for prevention of postoperative DVT is 2.5 mg subcutaneously once daily (in adults over 50 kg; prophylaxis is contraindicated in patients <50 kg), to be initiated 6 to 8 hours after completion of surgery.

Antiplatelet agents such as aspirin reduce the risk of DVT and pulmonary embolism in some patients; however, there is little evidence that antiplatelet agents have a significant effect on the prevention of venous thromboembolic events in medical patients. Also, low-dose aspirin did not significantly reduce the rate of recurrence of venous thromboembolism but resulted in a significant reduction in the rate of major vascular events, with improved net clinical benefit [19]. The 2012 American College of Chest Physicians guidelines did not recommend the use of aspirin, either alone or in combination, as prophylaxis against DVT in any medical patient group [20].

Low-dose warfarin is better than aspirin or placebo in patients with hip fractures but may not be satisfactory in preventing DVT after elective hip and knee surgery. The use of warfarin can be associated with a transient hypercoagulable state in the first 36 hours after administration because it causes a rapid decline in protein C levels before the anticoagulant effect, which does not occur until 36 to 72 hours after drug administration.

Mechanical DVT prophylaxis can be achieved with intermittent pneumatic leg compression, intermittent pneumatic foot compression, or graduated compression stockings. Intermittent pneumatic leg compression provides increases in peak velocity and flow in the common femoral vein and is better than placebo in preventing DVT. Intermittent pneumatic foot compression is a high-pressure system that exerts compression limited to the foot. These devices are best for patients who undergo lower extremity orthopedic surgery and cannot be fitted with the intermittent pneumatic leg compression devices. The intermittent pneumatic foot compression offers no advantage over LMWH in the prevention of DVTs, except for a lower rate of bleeding complications. Graded compression elastic stockings work by increasing venous blood flow velocity. Knee-length stockings are sized to fit, and they deliver graduated pressure of 40 mm Hg at the ankle, 36 mm Hg at the lower calf, and 21 mm Hg at the upper calf. Recent clinical practice guidelines from the American College of Chest Physicians recommend the use of either intermittent pneumatic compression or graduated compression stockings over no mechanical prophylaxis in acutely ill hospitalized medical patients at increased risk for thrombosis who are bleeding or are at high risk for major bleeding [20].

The optimal duration of pharmacologic prophylaxis varies with individual risk and clinical situation. Current standard of care is to stop prophylaxis 7 to 10 days after a surgical procedure or when medical patients are ambulating freely. After major orthopedic surgery, prolonged prophylaxis of 4 to 6 weeks is most advantageous. In patients with spinal cord injuries, prophylaxis is best maintained for 6 to 10 weeks.

In someone who presents with a DVT, the primary goal of treatment is to prevent extension of the clot, recurrence of the thrombosis, acute pulmonary embolism, and development of late complications of DVT (e.g., post-thrombotic syndrome, chronic thromboembolic pulmonary hypertension, and chronic venous insufficiency). The cornerstone of medical treatment of DVT is anticoagulation therapy. Anticoagulation therapy is indicated in patients with symptomatic proximal lower extremity DVT because pulmonary embolism may occur in up to 50% of untreated individuals [21]. One study showed death in 26% of patients who had clinically suspected pulmonary embolism and did not receive anticoagulation, compared with no deaths in the treatment group [22]. Current recommendations per the 2012 American College of Chest Physicians evidence-based clinical practice guidelines for antithrombotic and thrombolytic therapy are that patients with DVT or pulmonary embolism should be treated acutely with LMWH, fondaparinux, intravenous UFH, or dose-adjusted subcutaneous UFH [20]. An analysis of 16 systematic reviews of clinical trials revealed that there is high-quality evidence to support the use of

LMWH over UFH in the treatment of established DVT [23]. Furthermore, the risk of major bleeding during initial therapy appears to be reduced with these agents compared with UFH [23]. When UFH is used, the dose should be sufficient to prolong the activated partial thromboplastin time to 1.5 to 2.5 times the mean of the control value, or the upper limit of the normal activated partial thromboplastin time range [24].

Many medical centers have adopted weight-adjusted nomograms to increase the likelihood of obtaining a therapeutic anticoagulation effect early. The nomogram that has been found to achieve the most rapid acquisition of the target activated prothrombin time is an initial bolus of 80 units/kg of UFH followed by an infusion rate of 18 units/kg per hour. Activated prothrombin time should be checked every 4 to 6 hours until a therapeutic range of 1.5 is achieved. The duration of UFH treatment ranges between 4 and 10 days. Patients with a large iliofemoral vein thrombosis or major pulmonary embolism require a 7- to 10-day course of heparin, with a delay in the initiation of warfarin until the activated prothrombin time is in the therapeutic range. Studies demonstrate that a 4- to 5-day course of heparin with warfarin administered within 24 hours of heparin initiation in patients without major pulmonary embolism of large proximal clots was as effective as 9 to 10 days of UFH alone.

LMWHs are fragments of UFH produced by either chemical or enzymatic depolymerization. LMWHs display improved bioavailability, dose-independent clearance, and more predictable dose response compared with UFH. Therefore, these agents can usually be given once or twice daily subcutaneously in weight-adjusted doses without laboratory monitoring. The U.S. Food and Drug Administration has approved two LMWHs, dalteparin (Fragmin) and enoxaparin (Lovenox), for perioperative DVT prophylaxis (Table 127.4). There are two other LMWHs available for use in DVT treatment: tinzaparin (Innohep) and nadroparin.

Table 127.4 U.S. Food and Drug Administration–Approved Uses of Low-Molecular-Weight Heparins

Name	FDA-Approved Indications	Dosage
Dalteparin (Fragmin)	DVT prophylaxis after hip replacement	5000 units SC daily; start 2500 units SC ×1 dose 4-8h postop; allow >6h between first and second doses
Enoxaparin (Lovenox)	DVT prophylaxis after knee surgery	30 mg SC q12h
	DVT prophylaxis after hip surgery	30 mg SC q12h or 40 mg SC daily
	DVT prophylaxis after abdominal surgery	40 mg SC daily
	Inpatient treatment of acute DVT with or without PE	1 mg/kg SC q12h or 1.5 mg/kg SC daily
	Outpatient treatment of acute DVT without PE	1 mg/kg SC q12h

DVT, deep venous thrombosis; *PE,* pulmonary embolism; *SC,* subcutaneously.
From Sokolof J, Knight R. Deep venous thrombosis. In Frontera WR, Silver JK, Rizzo TD Jr, eds. Essentials of Physical Medicine and Rehabilitation, 2nd ed. Philadelphia, WB Saunders, 2008.

Enoxaparin and tinzaparin are approved for DVT treatment in the United States and Canada. Dalteparin and nadroparin are approved for this use only in Canada. Ardeparin (Normiflo) is another LMWH previously used for DVT treatment, but it was later withdrawn from the market. Enoxaparin can be used for hospitalized patients with DVT with or without pulmonary embolism and for outpatient treatment of DVT without pulmonary embolism.

Unmonitored outpatient therapy with LMWH is thought to be as safe and effective as in-hospital intravenous administration of UFH in patients with proximal DVT [25]. Like patients receiving UFH, those treated with LMWH should begin taking warfarin within 24 to 48 hours. LMWH can be discontinued after a minimum of 5 days, provided the international normalized ratio (INR) has been therapeutic for 2 consecutive days.

Thrombolytic therapy has a limited role in the treatment of DVT. It has been suggested that pharmacologic lysis of DVT could prevent post-thrombotic syndrome if complete lysis can be achieved before valve destruction occurs. However, thrombolysis, whether it is given systemically or by catheter, is expensive, the risk of bleeding complications is high, and the evidence of additional benefit is not convincing. Thrombolysis should be reserved for patients with massive iliofemoral thrombosis or unstable cardiac or pulmonary disease with no contraindications to thrombolytic therapy.

After initial treatment with LMWH, long-term anticoagulation therapy to prevent recurrent DVT is needed.

Oral anticoagulation with warfarin should prolong the INR to a target of 2.5 (range, 2-3), which generally is considered effective in preventing recurrent DVT, and risk of bleeding is lower than with higher INR levels. If oral anticoagulants are contraindicated or inconvenient, long-term therapy can be undertaken with adjusted-dose UFH, LMWH, or fondaparinux. Because of ease of use, especially in the outpatient setting, LMWH or fondaparinux is preferred to UFH [26].

Treatment duration ranges between 3 and 6 months; the short duration is reserved for those who had some risk factor (e.g., immobility) before surgery. Indefinite therapy is preferred in patients with a first unprovoked episode of proximal DVT, who have a greater relative risk of recurrent venous thromboembolism and a relatively lower concern about the burdens of long-term anticoagulant therapy [26].

The risk of recurrent DVT is serious on cessation of anticoagulation treatment. There is some evidence to suggest that post-treatment residual thrombus increases the risk of recurrent DVT and mortality [27]. The monitoring of serial D-dimer levels has been shown to be useful in determining the likelihood of DVT recurrence [28]. Treatment is indicated for at least 12 months in patients with recurrent DVT or for individuals with continuous risk factors for thromboembolic disease, such as malignant disease [25]. Untreated calf vein thrombosis does not commonly result in clinically significant pulmonary embolism unless the thrombus extends into the proximal venous segments, which occurs in about 25% of the cases. It is safe to monitor calf thrombi with serial venous ultrasound examinations or impedance plethysmography and to initiate therapy only if the thrombus extends into the popliteal or more proximal veins. Treatment of superficial venous thrombosis is usually not indicated. Pregnant women with DVT are classically treated with subcutaneous UFH or LMWH at full doses until delivery. Current recommendations indicate that the patient should be switched to UFH 2 weeks before the expected delivery, and a 4- to 6-week course of warfarin should be completed after delivery. Warfarin freely crosses the placental barrier, and therefore it is contraindicated during pregnancy but is safe for the mother and nursing child after delivery.

Rehabilitation

There is no strict contraindication to therapeutic exercises and ambulatory activities after DVT, but it is recommended that these activities be suspended until the patient is in the therapeutic range for heparin or has been receiving LMWH for 24 hours. On the other hand, physical and occupational therapy ordered immediately after high-risk surgical procedures can greatly improve a patient's postoperative mobility and lessen the chance for development of DVT.

Procedures

Inferior vena caval filters are indicated in patients with DVT who have an absolute contraindication to anticoagulation, high risk of bleeding, or recurrent DVT despite adequate anticoagulation. Caval interruption has been found to be effective in preventing subsequent pulmonary embolism; however, this is counterbalanced by the increased incidence of recurrent DVT. Patients who have significant but temporary contraindications to the use of anticoagulants who receive caval interruption devices should begin taking anticoagulation medication as soon as possible after placement.

Surgery

Surgical removal of acute DVT by thrombectomy or embolectomy is rarely used. It should be considered only in patients with massive thrombosis and compromised arterial circulation who do not respond to or who have an absolute contraindication to thrombolytic therapy.

Potential Disease Complications

If untreated, proximal DVT is linked with a 10% immediate risk of fatal pulmonary embolism and approximately 20% higher risk for development of a severe post-thrombotic syndrome 5 to 10 years later [29] (Fig. 127.3). There are two predominant patterns of DVT: an ascending pattern, with DVT arising in the calf veins; and a descending pattern, with DVT occurring initially in the iliac or common femoral vein. The descending pattern more commonly results in pulmonary embolus. Post-thrombotic syndrome is a condition characterized by chronic edema and debilitating pain and can lead to ulceration, infection, or, in rare cases, amputation. Heparin use and the wearing of graduated compression stockings have been associated with a lower risk for development of post-thrombotic syndrome.

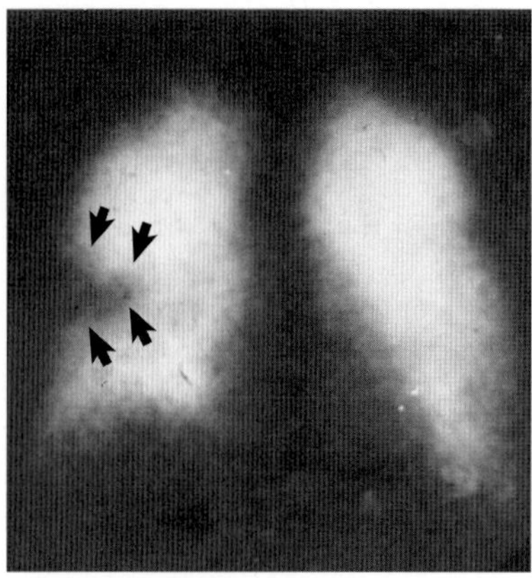

FIGURE 127.3 Frontal image from subsequent perfusion lung scan shows a corresponding peripheral, pleura-based area of absent perfusion in the right midlung *(arrowheads)*. The ventilation study showed diminished ventilation in this area, consistent with pulmonary embolus with infarction, and multiple unmatched perfusion defects were seen in the left lung, indicating that the probability of pulmonary embolism is high. *(From Katz DS, Math KR, Groskin SA. Radiology Secrets. Philadelphia, Hanley & Belfus, 1998.)*

Potential Treatment Complications

All pharmacologic anticoagulation agents alter the hemostatic mechanisms to some extent by decreasing blood coagulation or platelet function, and all carry a risk of bleeding. Both UFH and LMWH are associated with similar increased risk of bleeding complications. Heparin-induced thrombocytopenia is a potential complication of heparin use and can be seen slightly less commonly with LMWH compared with UFH because of the lower affinity of LMWH for platelet binding. A diagnosis of heparin-induced thrombocytopenia is made when there is a 50% reduction in platelet count or a presence of antiplatelet antibodies. Once the diagnosis is made, all heparin products are contraindicated. Skin necrosis is a rare complication of warfarin use, and it can be prevented if high-dose warfarin is delayed until the activated prothrombin time is therapeutic with heparin. Complications from caval interruption include problems related to the deployment of the device: hemorrhage, hematoma, femoral artery injury, femoral nerve injury, infection, and site pain. Another potential complication is pulmonary embolism from embolization of the device itself or from failure of the device to capture an embolus. A clot-laden caval interruption device can impede venous flow and lead to lower extremity venous stasis and edema. Osteoporosis and risk of bone fracture are associated with long-term use of UFH [30], but the risk may be less with LMWH [31]. Contraindications to the use of warfarin include advanced liver disease, alcoholism, poor compliance with follow-up, poorly controlled hypertension, major bleeding, and pregnancy [32].

References

[1] Ridker PM, Glynn RJ, Miletich JP, et al. Age-specific incidence rates of venous thromboembolism among heterozygous carriers of factor V Leiden mutation. Ann Intern Med 1997;126:528–31.
[2] Clagett GP, Anderson Jr FA, Geerts W, et al. Prevention of venous thromboembolism. Chest 1998;114:531s–60s.
[3] Pineo GF, Hull RD. Prophylaxis of venous thromboembolism following orthopedic surgery: mechanical and pharmacological approaches and the need for extended prophylaxis. Thromb Haemost 1999;82:918–24.
[4] Giercksky KE, Bjorklid E, Prydz H, Renck H. Circulating tissue thromboplastin during hip surgery. Eur Surg Res 1979;11:296–300.
[5] Camerer E, Kolsto AB, Prydz H. Cell biology of tissue factor, the principal initiator of blood coagulation. Thromb Res 1996;81:1–14.

[6] Hamilton MG, Yee WH, Hull RD, Ghali WA. Venous thromboembolism prophylaxis in patients undergoing cranial neurosurgery: a systematic review and meta-analysis. Neurosurgery 2011;68:571–81.

[7] Flinn W, Sandager G, Silva M. Prospective surveillance for perioperative venous thrombosis: experience in 2643 patients. Arch Surg 1996;131:472–80.

[8] Dahl OE, Aspelin T, Arnesen H, et al. Increased activation of coagulation and formation of late deep venous thrombosis following discontinuation of thromboprophylaxis after hip replacement surgery. Thromb Res 1995;80:299–306.

[9] Handler J, Hedderman M, Davodi D, et al. Implementing a diagnostic algorithm for deep venous thrombosis. Permanente J 2003;7:54–60.

[10] Kahn SR, Shrier I, Kearon C. Physical activity in patients with deep venous thrombosis: a systematic review. Thromb Res 2008;122:763–73.

[11] Qaseem A, Snow V, Barry P, et al. Joint American Academy of Family Physicians/American College of Physicians Panel on Deep Venous Thrombosis/Pulmonary Embolism. Current diagnosis of venous thromboembolism in primary care: a clinical practice guideline from the American Academy of Family Physicians and the American College of Physicians. Ann Fam Med 2007;5:57–62.

[12] Segal JB, Eng J, Tamariz LJ, Bass EB. Review of the evidence on diagnosis of deep venous thrombosis and pulmonary embolism. Ann Fam Med 2007;5:63–73.

[13] Hull R, Taylor DW, Hirsh J, et al. Impedance plethysmography: the relationship between venous filling and sensitivity and specificity for proximal vein thrombosis. Circulation 1978;58:898–902.

[14] Hull R, van Aken WG, Hirsh J, et al. Impedance plethysmography using the occlusive cuff technique in the diagnosis of venous thrombosis. Circulation 1976;53:696–700.

[15] Carpenter JP, Holland GA, Baum RA, et al. Magnetic resonance venography for the detection of deep venous thrombosis: comparison with contrast venography and duplex Doppler ultrasonography. J Vasc Surg 1993;18:734–41.

[16] Geerts WH, Bergqvist D, Pineo GF, et al. American College of Chest Physicians. Prevention of venous thromboembolism: American College of Chest Physicians evidence-based clinical practice guidelines (8th Edition). Chest 2008;133(Suppl.):381S–453S.

[17] Wein L, Wein S, Haas SJ, et al. Pharmacological venous thromboembolism prophylaxis in hospitalized medical patients: a meta-analysis of randomized controlled trials. Arch Intern Med 2007;167:1476–86.

[18] Nurmohamed MT, Rosendaal FR, Buller HR, et al. Low-molecular-weight heparin versus standard heparin in general and orthopaedic surgery: a meta-analysis. Lancet 1992;340:152–6.

[19] Brighton TA, Eikelboom JW, Mann K, et al. Low-dose aspirin for preventing recurrent venous thromboembolism. N Engl J Med 2012;367:1979–87.

[20] Kearon C, Akl EA, Comerota AJ, et al. Antithrombotic therapy for VTE disease: antithrombotic therapy and prevention of thrombosis, 9th ed: American College of Chest Physicians evidence-based clinical practice guidelines. Chest 2012;141:e419S.

[21] Mannucci PM, Poller L. Venous thrombosis and anticoagulant therapy. Br J Haematol 2001;114:258–70.

[22] Barritt DW, Johnson SC. Anticoagulation drugs in the treatment of pulmonary embolism trial. Lancet 1960;1:1309–12.

[23] Snow V, Qaseem A, Barry P, et al. Management of venous thromboembolism: a clinical practice guideline from the American College of Physicians and the American Academy of Family Physicians. Ann Fam Med 2007;5:74–8.

[24] Corbin SB, Clark NL, McClendon BJ, Snodgrass NK. Patterns of sealant delivery under variable third party requirements. J Public Health Dent 1990;50:311–8.

[25] Siragusa S, Cosmi B, Piovella F, et al. Low-molecular-weight heparins and unfractionated heparin in the treatment of patients with acute venous thromboembolism: results of a meta-analysis. Am J Med 1996;100:269–77.

[26] Guyatt GH, Akl EA, Crowther M, et al. American College of Chest Physicians Antithrombotic Therapy and Prevention of Thrombosis Panel. Executive summary: antithrombotic therapy and prevention of thrombosis, 9th ed: American College of Chest Physicians evidence-based clinical practice guidelines. Chest 2012;141(Suppl.):7S–47S.

[27] Young L, Ockelford P, Milne D, et al. Post-treatment residual thrombus increases the risk of recurrent deep vein thrombosis and mortality. J Thromb Haemost 2006;4:1919–24.

[28] Shrivastava S, Ridker PM, Glynn RJ, et al. D-dimer, factor VIII coagulant activity, low intensity warfarin and the risk of recurrent venous thromboembolism. J Thromb Haemost 2006;4:1208–14.

[29] Bounameaux H, Ehringer H, Gast A, et al. Differential inhibition of thrombin activity and thrombin generation by a synthetic direct thrombin inhibitor (napsagatran, Ro 46-6240) and unfractionated heparin in patients with deep vein thrombosis. ADVENT Investigators. Thromb Haemost 1999;81:498–501.

[30] Dahlman T. Osteoporotic fractures and the recurrence during pregnancy and puerperium in 94 women undergoing thromboprophylaxis with heparin. Am J Obstet Gynecol 1983;168:1265–70.

[31] Monreal M, Lafoz E, Olive A, et al. Comparison of subcutaneous unfractionated heparin with a low molecular weight heparin (Fragmin) in patients with thromboembolism and contraindications to coumadin. Thromb Haemost 1994;71:7–11.

[32] Schulman S, Kearon C, Kakkar AK, et al. Dabigatran versus warfarin in the treatment of acute venous thromboembolism. N Engl J Med 2009;361:2342–52.

CHAPTER 128

Diabetic Foot and Peripheral Arterial Disease

Timothy R. Dillingham, MD, MS
Diane W. Braza, MD

Synonyms

Vascular claudication
Poor circulation
Arterial insufficiency

ICD-9 Codes

250.00 Diabetes mellitus
250.60 Diabetic neuropathy
443.9 Peripheral arterial disease

ICD-10 Codes

E11.9 Type 2 diabetes without complications
E11.40 Type 2 diabetes with diabetic neuropathy, unspecified
I73.9 Peripheral vascular disease, unspecified

Definition

The incidence of lower limb amputations due to vascular disease has increased in the United States by approximately 20% during the last decade, disproportionately in minorities [1]. Persons with diabetes mellitus and peripheral vascular disease should be identified and prophylactic foot education and preventive care instituted to reduce the risk of limb loss [2].

Diabetes mellitus, a multisystem disease, causes two conditions that place the foot at high risk for amputation: polyneuropathy and peripheral arterial disease (PAD). Diabetes affects about 25.8 million Americans [3]. Diabetes is also on the rise in the United States, particularly in African American and Hispanic populations [4]. Data from the Framingham Heart Study [5] revealed that 20% of symptomatic patients with PAD had diabetes, but the true prevalence of PAD in patients with diabetes has been difficult to determine as most patients are asymptomatic, many do not report their symptoms, screening modalities have not uniformly been agreed on, and pain perception may be blunted by the presence of peripheral neuropathy [6].

Risk factors for diabetic ulcers include male sex, hyperglycemia, and diabetes duration. Foot ulcers often result from severe macrovascular disease, and diabetic neuropathy exacerbates the risk [7]. More than 60% of nontraumatic lower limb amputations occur in people with diabetes, underscoring the need to prevent foot ulcers and subsequent limb loss [8]. Multidisciplinary clinics that identify and manage patients with at-risk feet have demonstrated impressive reductions of 44% to 85% in the incidence of foot ulcers and lower limb amputations [9]. Minor foot trauma in a person with poor underlying circulation and reduced sensation can lead to skin ulceration. Skin ulcers, if they fail to heal, may lead to gangrene and progress to a point such that an amputation becomes necessary. This sequence of events can often be prevented before it starts.

Numerous studies have further shown that attention to lifestyle modification can dramatically reduce progression to type 2 diabetes [10]. The importance of identifying and treating a core set of risk factors (prediabetes, hypertension, smoking, dyslipidemia, and obesity) cannot be overstated [11].

Atherosclerosis is a vascular disease that can involve the peripheral arterial system. PAD is underdiagnosed, undertreated, and increasing in prevalence [12]. The American Heart Association estimates that 8 to 12 million Americans have PAD and that nearly 75% of them are asymptomatic. Annually, approximately 1 million Americans develop symptomatic PAD [13]. Despite its association with other cardiovascular risks including stroke and heart disease, only 25% of Americans with PAD are undergoing active treatment [14]. Major risk factors associated with the development of PAD or that accelerate its progression are high plasma cholesterol and lipoprotein levels, cigarette smoking, hypertension, diabetes, hyperhomocysteinemia, older age, positive family history, and chronic kidney disease [15–17]. African American ethnicity is a strong and independent risk factor for PAD [8]. Hypertension is an important risk factor for PAD, conferring a twofold to threefold increased risk for development of PAD [18]. The risk of PAD is increased two to four times by diabetes [19]. Given that men have more risk factors for PAD, they are more commonly affected than women are.

Symptoms

The patient with a diabetic foot may demonstrate no symptoms because peripheral neuropathy can result in a lack of sensation. Peripheral neuropathy can mask painful ulcers and ischemic skin. Foot collapse due to Charcot joints can progress asymptomatically. Alternatively, diabetic patients can have pain sensations in the feet from sensory polyneuropathy, including burning, tingling, and painful numbness. Because of impaired sensation, patients may report imbalance and falls.

Persons with PAD have claudication pain with walking because of insufficient arterial blood supply to meet the demand of exercising muscles. Pain with vascular claudication is typically in the calf, worsened with ambulation and relieved by resting [20]. Symptoms of pain, ache, or cramp with walking can also occur in the buttock, hip, thigh, or calf [20]. Patients with neurogenic claudication due to spinal stenosis can have similar leg or calf pain with walking but must bend at the waist or sit to relieve the symptoms. Persons may present with gangrene, ischemic ulcers on the distal foot, or, when PAD is severe, pain at rest.

Physical Examination

In addition to a standard physical examination, special neurovascular areas must be highlighted [21].

Inspect the skin for ulcerations, cracks, callus, or trophic changes (thin, shiny skin; distal hair loss).

Evaluate for any foot deformities that predispose it to abnormal stress distribution. These include hammer toes, collapsed foot arches due to Charcot joints, high-arch feet due to intrinsic muscle atrophy from polyneuropathy, and changes in stress distribution from previous toe or ray amputations.

Assess distal pulses, particularly dorsalis pedis and posterior tibial. If they are absent or weak, it suggests the need for further testing for vascular integrity.

Assess sensation because persons with loss of protective sensation are at risk for skin ulceration. The instrument most frequently used for detection of neuropathy is the nylon Semmes-Weinstein monofilament. Inability to perceive the 10-g force applied by a 5.07 monofilament is associated with clinically significant large-fiber neuropathy [22].

Evaluate gait and balance. Peripheral neuropathy predisposes to falls and skin trauma. Probe any ulcers with sterile cotton-tipped applicators or surgical instruments. If bone is reached, this identifies persons with osteomyelitis, and other special bone imaging is unnecessary [23]. Assess shoes for uneven wear patterns, areas of breakdown, and width of the toe box.

Assess skin for redness and pressure points.

Functional Limitations

Persons with diabetes can develop peripheral polyneuropathy with loss of position sense and weakness. These can lead to gait instability and falls. Persons with PAD are often limited in community ambulation and vocational activities because of pain from claudication.

Diagnostic Studies

There are many noninvasive and invasive tests for PAD that are beyond the scope of this discussion. Angiography can identify surgically remediable lesions.

In the outpatient setting, the ankle-brachial index, a ratio of Doppler-recorded systolic pressures in the lower and upper extremities, is a convenient, accurate, noninvasive test that provides objective assessment of lower limb vascular status for screening and diagnosis of PAD [24]. Based on the results of the Ankle Brachial Index Collaboration, values above 1.40 indicate noncompressible arteries. Normal values are 1.00 to 1.40; borderline, 0.91 to 0.99; and abnormal, 0.90 or less [25]. The American College of Cardiology Foundation and American Heart Association Task Force on Practice Guidelines recommend resting ankle-brachial index to establish the diagnosis of lower extremity PAD in patients with exertional leg symptoms, nonhealing wounds, and age 65 years and older or 50 years and older with a history of smoking or diabetes [25]. Measurement of systolic pressure in the foot also provides a measure of arterial integrity.

Transcutaneous oximetry is the best method for assessment of cutaneous ischemia [9]. Transcutaneous oximetry pressures of more than 40 mm Hg are normal; pressures of 20 to 40 mm Hg indicate moderate disease, and potential for healing of a skin ulcer is less likely. With pressures below 20 mm Hg, severe skin ischemia is present, and skin healing is poor.

Systolic blood pressures in the foot are also helpful in quantifying the severity of ischemia. Persons with ischemic ulcers and ankle systolic pressures of less than 40 to 60 mm Hg are considered to have severe ischemia. Persons with persistently recurring ischemic rest pain and ankle systolic pressures of 50 mm Hg or less are severely involved [9].

If a person complains of numbness in the legs or feet or has low back pain, electrodiagnostic testing should be conducted to identify whether peripheral polyneuropathy is present or whether lumbosacral radiculopathy is responsible for these symptoms. Nerve conduction study findings may include reduced sensory and motor amplitude, latencies, and slowed conduction velocity. Electromyographic findings in radiculopathy include increased insertional activity, abnormal spontaneous activity, and changes in motor unit morphology; when these electromyographic findings are seen in a myotomal pattern, this suggests radiculopathy.

Differential Diagnosis [15]

NONVASCULAR

Neurogenic claudication from lumbar spinal stenosis
Calf pain due to S1 radiculopathy
Foot pain due to plantar fasciitis
Pain in legs and feet due to polyneuropathy
Arthritis of the hips
Restless legs syndrome

VASCULAR

Arterial embolus
Deep venous thrombosis
Thromboangiitis obliterans (Buerger disease)

Treatment

Initial

Efforts to achieve smoking cessation are recommended for individuals with lower extremity PAD. Cigarette smoking is the most important risk factor for development of PAD [26]. Observational studies have demonstrated that the risk of death, myocardial infarction, and amputation is substantially greater in those individuals with PAD who continue to smoke [25]. The risk of smoking for vascular disease is even greater for women than for men [27].

For diabetes control, minimize hyperglycemia. The presence of PAD is 20% to 30% higher in diabetics than in the general population. According to recently published guidelines, patients with diabetes and PAD should have aggressive control of blood glucose levels with a hemoglobin A_{1c} level below 7.0% or as close to 6% as possible to reduce the risk of microvascular complications [25].

For hypertension control, management of blood pressure is required. The desired blood pressure range is less than 140/90 mm Hg or less than 130/80 mm Hg if diabetes or renal insufficiency is present [12]. Choice of antihypertensive medication is generally guided by the presence of underlying diseases, such as diabetes, chronic kidney disease, or proteinuria [12].

Elevated total and low-density lipoprotein cholesterol levels, reduced high-density lipoprotein level, and hypertriglyceridemia are associated with lower extremity PAD [20]. Several clinical trials have demonstrated the benefits of lipid-lowering therapy in patients with PAD and coexistent coronary and cerebral arterial disease [15].

High serum homocysteine levels are associated with a twofold to threefold increased risk for PAD [28]. Dietary supplementation with B vitamins and folate may lower homocysteine levels, but no controlled trials to date demonstrate this clinical benefit in PAD [15].

Aerobic exercise can improve lipid profiles and optimize weight, blood pressure, and glycemic control, thus playing a role in medical management of PAD.

The 2012 American College of Chest Physicians Evidence-Based Clinical Practice Guidelines for antithrombotic therapy and prevention of thrombosis recommend aspirin, 75 to 100 mg/day, for individuals with asymptomatic PAD for the primary prevention of cardiovascular events. For secondary prevention of cardiovascular disease in patients with symptomatic PAD, long-term aspirin, 75 to 100 mg/day, or clopidogrel, 75 mg/day, is recommended [29]. Warfarin is not recommended. For patients with refractory claudication despite exercise therapy and smoking cessation, cilostazol, 100 mg twice daily, is recommended in addition to aspirin, 75 to 100 mg/day, or clopidogrel, 75 mg/day [29] (Table 128.1).

Table 128.1 Medical Management of Peripheral Arterial Disease

Smoking cessation
Lipid modification: target low-density lipoprotein cholesterol level <100 mg/dL
Treatment of hypertension: target blood pressure <140/90 mm Hg
Control of hyperglycemia: target hemoglobin A_{1c} level <7%
Antiplatelet therapy: aspirin, 75-100 mg daily, or clopidogrel, 75 mg daily
Aerobic exercise

Rehabilitation

Exercise

Patients with symptomatic PAD have impaired walking tolerance. A program of supervised exercise is recommended for patients with intermittent claudication. A meta-analysis of training programs concluded that supervised exercise therapy showed statistically significant and clinically relevant differences in improvement of maximal treadmill walking distance compared with nonsupervised exercise therapy regimens of approximately 150 meters [30]. A study comparing the efficacy of cycle training versus treadmill exercise in the treatment of intermittent claudication concluded that cycle exercise is not effective in improving walking performance in all claudication patients [31]. A cross-transfer effect between training modes was noted for patients reporting common limiting symptoms at baseline for both cycling and walking. Therefore, the current recommendation for exercise in intermittent claudication is walking [31]. Exercise should be performed for a minimum of 30 to 45 minutes, at least three times per week. Supervised exercise can induce increases in maximal walking ability that exceed those attained with drug therapies alone and translate into improved functional ability [26,32]. Exercise is contraindicated in the presence of an ischemic ulcer or rest pain.

Foot Care

Meticulous attention to the feet by both patient and physician and detailed education of the patient are the mainstays of preventive foot care. Deformities should prompt the clinician to consider custom shoe inserts to distribute pressures evenly over the foot. Extra-depth shoes may be necessary to accommodate hammer toes. Extra-width shoes can accommodate bunions and other foot deformities. Sneakers may be another alternative for persons with or without mild foot deformities. However, if there are any aberrations in foot bone architecture, custom footwear with molded sole inserts is desirable. Gentle rocker-bottom modifications affect weight transfer from heel to toe during the gait cycle.

Skin Ulcers

Early treatment of skin infections with antibiotics is warranted along with minimization or elimination of weight bearing during healing. Achievement of a therapeutic antibiotic concentration at the site of infection is key. Intravenous antibiotics may therefore be necessary for patients with severe infection or systemic illness and for treatment of pathogens that are not susceptible to oral agents [33].

For more involved wounds, débridement with dressing changes or whirlpool is sometimes necessary. Deep infections into bone or infections that extend along fascial planes require débridement. If osteomyelitis is suspected, at least a 6-week course of parenteral or oral antibiotic therapy guided by culture samples obtained during débridement is an effective clinical approach. Other wound care measures, such as total contact casting, can assist with improved healing of plantar surface ulcers [34]. However, when both PAD and infection are present or the patient has a heel ulcer, outcome is poor and alternative strategies should be sought [34].

Hyperbaric oxygen therapy may improve wound healing and reduce the rate of amputation [35]. However, given its expense and limited resource, it is mostly limited to deep infections unresponsive to standard therapy.

Edema hinders wound healing. Measures to control edema, such as leg elevation, compression stockings, and pneumatic compression devices, are often used [36].

Procedures

An acute painful, pale, pulseless limb should be evaluated emergently as this indicates acute arterial compromise. Likewise, gangrene or an ulcer extending to bone should prompt surgical consultation. Sharp débridement for a necrotic wound is often necessary to remove devitalized tissue and to promote healing of ulcers.

Percutaneous endovascular interventions to treat peripheral arterial occlusion include transluminal angioplasty with balloon dilation, stents, atherectomy, laser, cutting balloons, thermal angioplasty, and fibrinolysis or fibrinectomy. This intervention may be necessary to provide enough oxygenated arterial blood to a limb to heal open sores, to improve symptoms of claudication, or to save an extremity at risk for amputation [22].

Endovascular procedures are indicated for individuals with severe vocational or lifestyle-limiting disability due to intermittent claudication for whom exercise and pharmacologic therapy have failed. Clinical features must suggest a reasonable likelihood of symptomatic improvement with endovascular intervention with a favorable risk-benefit ratio [25].

Outcomes of percutaneous transluminal angioplasty and stents depend on anatomic and clinical factors. Durability of patency after percutaneous transluminal angioplasty is greatest for lesions in the common iliac artery and decreases distally. Durability decreases with increasing length of the stenosis, multiple and diffuse lesions, poor-quality runoff, diabetes, renal failure, and smoking. Hormone replacement in women has been shown to decrease patency of iliac stents [25].

Surgery

Surgical treatment of intermittent claudication is indicated in individuals who do not derive adequate functional benefit from nonsurgical therapies, who have limb arterial anatomy favorable to a durable clinical result, and in whom the risk of cardiovascular complications is low.

The exact surgical procedure (aortobifemoral bypass, aortoiliac bypass, iliofemoral bypass, axillofemoral-femoral bypass) is determined by the site and severity of the occlusive lesion, prior revascularization attempts, general medical condition, and desired outcome [25].

Similar considerations are given in the management of limb-threatening ischemia. Surgical lower limb amputation may be necessary if revascularization attempts are unsuccessful in the management of limb-threatening ischemia or gangrene.

Potential Disease Complications

As a result of PAD, patients may develop ischemic pain from arterial insufficiency defined as claudication (pain with ambulation) or rest pain. Other potential complications include nonhealing or slow to heal foot ulcers, cellulitis, and deeper wound infections in the foot. If those complications cannot be treated medically, amputation of a portion of the lower limb may be necessary to save the remaining viable limb and to prevent disseminated infection. Charcot joints and bone fractures in the foot due to diabetic polyneuropathy can be seen, potentially leading to skin ulcer and breakdown.

Potential Treatment Complications

Potential treatment complications depend on the intervention implemented. For example, in surgical revascularization, infection of arterial bypass grafts, ischemic cardiac disease, and worsening of renal azotemia are potential complications. Patients undergoing wound débridement should be closely observed for possible infection of foot ulcers after débridement. For PAD patients initiating an exercise program, potential complications include cardiac ischemic events, given the strong correlation of arterial disease and cardiovascular disease. Therefore, in such patients, supervised exercise instruction after cardiac stress testing is initially recommended to stratify patients at potential risk.

References

[1] Dillingham T, Pezzin L, MacKenzie E. Limb amputation and limb deficiency: epidemiology and recent trends in the United States. South Med J 2002;95:875–83.

[2] Sanders L. Diabetes mellitus: prevention of amputation. J Am Podiatr Med Assoc 1994;84:322–8.

[3] National diabetes fact sheet. 2011. http://www.cdc.gov/diabetes/pubs/pdf/ndfs_2011.pdf [accessed 15.10.20].

[4] Harris MI. Diabetes in America: epidemiology and scope of the problem. Diabetes Care 1998;21(Suppl. 3):C11–4.

[5] Murabito JM, D'Agnostino RB, Silbershatz H, Wilson WF. Intermittent claudication: a risk profile from the Framingham Heart Study. Circulation 1997;96:44–9.

[6] American Diabetes Association. Peripheral arterial disease in people with diabetes. Diabetes Care 2003;26:12.

[7] Beckman JA, Creager MA, Libby P. Diabetes and atherosclerosis: epidemiology, pathophysiology, and management. JAMA 2002;287:2570–81.

[8] Criqui MH, Vargas V, Denenberg JO, et al. Ethnicity and peripheral arterial disease: the San Diego Population Study. Circulation 2005;112:2703–7.

[9] Pandian G, Hamid F, Hammond MC. Rehabilitation of the patient with PVD and diabetic foot problems. In: DeLisa J, Gans BM, editors. Rehabilitation medicine: principles and practice. Philadelphia: Lippincott-Raven; 1998. p. 1517–44.

[10] Tuomilehto J, Lindstrom J, Eriksson JG, et althe Finnish Diabetes Prevention Study Group. Prevention of type 2 diabetes mellitus by changes in lifestyle among subjects with impaired glucose tolerance. N Engl J Med 2001;344:1343–50.

[11] Eckel RH, Kahn R, Robertson RM, Rizza RA. Preventing cardiovascular disease and diabetes mellitus: a call to action from the ADA and AHA. Circulation 2006;113:2943–6.

[12] Simmons A, Steffen K, Sanders S. Medical therapy for peripheral arterial disease. Curr Opin Cardiol 2012;27:592–7.

[13] American Heart Association. Peripheral arterial disease, http://www.heart.org/HEARTORG/Conditions/More/PeripheralArteryDisease/Peripheral-Artery-Disease-PAD_UCM_002082_SubHomePage.jsp; [accessed 15.10.12].

[14] Becker GJ, McClenny TE, Kovacs ME, et al. The importance of increasing public and physician awareness of peripheral arterial disease. J Vasc Interv Radiol 2002;13:7–11.

[15] Sontheimer D. Peripheral vascular disease: diagnosis and treatment. Am Fam Physician 2006;73:1971–6. http://www.aafp.org/afp/2006/0601/p1971.html [accessed 15.10.12].

[16] Meijer WT, Grobbee DE, Hunink MG, et al. Determinants of peripheral arterial disease in the elderly: the Rotterdam study. Arch Intern Med 2000;160:2934–8.

[17] Chen J, Mohler ER, Xie D, et al. Risk factors for peripheral arterial disease among patients with chronic kidney disease. Am J Cardiol 2012;110:136–41.

[18] Lane DA, Lip GY. Treatment of hypertension in peripheral arterial disease. Cochrane Database Syst Rev 2009;4: CD003075.

[19] National Heart, Lung, and Blood Institute. NHLBI workshop on peripheral arterial disease (PAD): developing a public awareness campaign, http://www.nhlbi.nih.gov/health/prof/heart/other/pad_sum.pdf; [accessed 08.12.12].

[20] Peripheral arterial disease (PAD) fact sheet, http://www.cdc.gov/dhdsp/data_statistics/fact_sheets/docs/fs_PAD.pdf; [accessed 15.10.12].

[21] American Diabetes Association. Standards of medical care in diabetes—2006. Diabetes Care 2006;29:S4–42.

[22] Singh N, Armstrong DG, Lipsky BA. Preventing foot ulcers in patients with diabetes. JAMA 2005;293:217–28.

[23] Grayson M, Gibbons G, Balough K, et al. Probing to bone in infected pedal ulcers: a clinical sign of underlying osteomyelitis in diabetic patients. JAMA 1995;273:721–3.

[24] U.S. Preventive Services Task Force recommendation statement. Screening for peripheral arterial disease. Am Fam Physician 2006;73:1–8.

[25] Rooke TW, Hirsch AT, Misra S, et al. ACCF/AHA focused update of the guideline for the management of patients with peripheral artery disease (updating the 2005 guideline): a report of the American College of Cardiology Foundation/American Heart Association Task Force on practice guidelines. J Am Coll Cardiol 2011;58:2020–45.

[26] Regensteiner JG, Hiatt WR. Current medical therapies for patients with peripheral arterial disease: a critical review. Am J Med 2002;112:49–57.

[27] Huxley RR, Woodward M. Cigarette smoking as a risk factor for coronary heart disease in women compared to men: a systematic review and meta-analysis of prospective cohort studies. Lancet 2011;378:1297–305.

[28] Graham IM, Daly LE, Refsum HM, et al. Plasma homocysteine as a risk factor for vascular disease. JAMA 1997;277:1775–81.

[29] Alonso-Coella P, Bellmunt S, McGorrian C, et al. Antithrombotic therapy in peripheral artery disease: antithrombotic therapy and prevention of thrombosis, 9th ed: American College of Chest Physicians Evidence-Based Clinical Practice Guidelines. Chest 2012;141(Suppl.):e669S–90S.

[30] Bendermacher BLW, Willigendael EM, Teijink JAW, Prins MH. Supervised exercise therapy versus non-supervised exercise therapy for intermittent claudication. Cochrane Database Syst Rev 2009; http://onlinelibrary.wiley.com/doi/10.1002/14651858.CD005263.pub2/pdf [accessed 15.10.12].

[31] Sanderson B, Askew C, Stewart I, et al. Short-term effects of cycle and treadmill training of exercise tolerance in peripheral arterial disease. J Vasc Surg 2006;44:119–27.

[32] Watson L, Ellis B, Leng G. Exercise for intermittent claudication. Cochrane Database Syst Rev 2008; http://onlinelibrary.wiley.com/doi/10.1002/14651858.CD000990.pub2/abstract [accessed 15.10.12].

[33] Lipsky BA. Medical treatment of diabetic foot infections. Clin Infect Dis 2004;39:S104–14.

[34] Nabuurs-Franssen MH, Sleegers R, Huijberts M, et al. Total contact casting of the diabetic foot in daily practice. Diabetes Care 2005;28:243–7.

[35] Wunderlich RP, Peters EJD, Lavery L. Systemic hyperbaric oxygen therapy: lower-extremity wound healing and the diabetic foot. Diabetes Care 2000;23:1551–5.

[36] Armstrong DG, Nguyen HC. Improvement in healing with aggressive edema reduction after débridement of foot infection in persons with diabetes. Arch Surg 2000;135:1405–9.

CHAPTER 129

Dysphagia

Koichiro Matsuo, DDS, PhD
Jeffrey B. Palmer, MD

Synonyms

Swallowing disorder
Swallowing impairment
Deglutition disorder

ICD-9 Codes

438.82 Other late effects of cerebrovascular disease, dysphagia
787.2 Dysphagia, difficulty in swallowing

ICD-10 Codes

I69.891 Dysphagia following other cerebrovascular disease
R13.10 Dysphagia, difficulty in swallowing

Definition

Dysphagia generally refers to any difficulty with swallowing, including occult or asymptomatic impairments. It is a common problem, affecting one third to one half of all stroke patients [1] and about one sixth of elderly individuals [2]. It is frequent in head and neck cancer, traumatic brain injury, degenerative disorders of the nervous system, gastroesophageal reflux disease, and inflammatory muscle disease (Table 129.1). Dysphagia is classified according to the location of the problem as oropharyngeal (localized to the oral cavity or pharynx, not just the oropharynx) or esophageal. It may also be classified as mechanical (due to a structural lesion of the foodway) or functional (caused by a physiologic abnormality of foodway function) [3].

Sudden onset is suggestive of stroke. Concomitant limb weakness suggests a neurologic or neuromuscular disorder. Medication-induced dysphagia is commonly overlooked. Medications that impair level of consciousness (such as sedatives and tranquilizers), have anticholinergic effects (tricyclics, propantheline), or can damage mucous membranes (nonsteroidal anti-inflammatory drugs, aspirin, quinidine) may also cause dysphagia [4].

Symptoms

The most common symptoms of dysphagia are coughing or choking during eating [5] and the sensation of food sticking in the throat or chest. Some of the many symptoms and signs of dysphagia are listed in Table 129.2. A history of drooling, significant weight loss, or recurrent pneumonia suggests that the dysphagia is severe. The history is most useful for identification of esophageal dysphagia; the complaint of food sticking in the chest is usually associated with an esophageal disorder. In contrast, the complaint of food sticking in the throat has little localizing value and is often caused by an esophageal disorder. Coughing and choking during swallowing suggest an oropharyngeal origin and may be precipitated by aspiration (penetration of material through the vocal folds and into the trachea). However, some patients have impaired cough reflexes, resulting in silent aspiration (without cough) [5,6]. Silent aspiration occurs in 28% to 94% of people with dysphagia, depending on the population of patients [7,8]. Patients with neurologic disorder have a higher incidence of silent aspiration. Pain on swallowing (odynophagia) may occur transiently in pharyngitis, but persistent pain is unusual and is suggestive of neoplasia. Heartburn is a nonspecific complaint that is usually not associated with swallowing but occurs after meals. Heartburn may occur in gastroesophageal reflux disease, but a more specific symptom of gastroesophageal reflux disease is regurgitation of sour or bitter-tasting material into the throat after eating.

Physical Examination

An examination of the oral cavity and neck may identify structural abnormalities, weakness, or sensory deficits. The finding of dysarthria (abnormal articulation of speech) or dysphonia (abnormal voice quality) is often associated with oropharyngeal dysphagia. However, the examination is primarily useful for finding evidence of underlying neurologic, neuromuscular, or connective tissue disease. The examination should always include trial swallows of water [9–11]. During the swallow, there should be prompt elevation of the hyoid bone and larynx. Changes in voice quality and spontaneous coughing after swallowing suggest pharyngeal dysfunction. The history and physical examination are

Table 129.1 Selected Causes of Oral and Pharyngeal Dysphagia

Neurologic Disorders and Stroke	Structural Lesions	Connective Tissue Diseases
Cerebral infarction Brainstem infarction Intracranial hemorrhage Parkinson disease Multiple sclerosis Amyotrophic lateral sclerosis Poliomyelitis Myasthenia gravis Dementias	Thyromegaly Cervical hyperostosis Congenital web Zenker diverticulum Caustic ingestion Neoplasm Post–ablative surgery Radiation fibrosis	Polymyositis Muscular dystrophy Psychiatric disorders Psychogenic dysphagia

Table 129.2 Symptoms and Signs of Dysphagia

Oral or Pharyngeal Dysphagia

Coughing or choking with swallowing
Difficulty with initiation of swallowing
Food sticking in the throat
Drooling
Unexplained weight loss
Change in dietary habits
Recurrent pneumonia
Change in voice or speech
Nasal regurgitation
Dehydration

Esophageal Dysphagia

Sensation of food sticking in the chest or throat
Oral or pharyngeal regurgitation
Drooling
Unexplained weight loss
Change in dietary habits
Recurrent pneumonia
Dehydration

limited in their ability to detect and to characterize dysphagia, so instrumental studies are usually necessary [12].

Neurologic examination is important in the evaluation of dysphagic individuals because neurologic disorders commonly cause dysphagia. Disorders of either upper or lower motor neurons may produce dysphagia. The findings of atrophy or fasciculations of the tongue or palate suggest lower motor neuron dysfunction of the brainstem motor nuclei. In contrast to the prevailing wisdom, the gag reflex is not strongly predictive of the ability to swallow. It may be absent in normal individuals and normal in individuals with severe dysphagia and aspiration [13].

Functional Limitations

Functional limitations depend on the nature and severity of the dysphagia. Many individuals modify their diets to eliminate foods that are difficult to swallow; others require special postures or respiratory maneuvers. Some require inordinate amounts of time to consume a meal. In severe cases, tube feeding is necessary. These alterations in the ability to eat a meal can have a profound effect on psychological and social function [14]. Interaction with family and friends often centers on mealtime—family dinners, "going out" for a drink or for dinner, "coming over" for a snack or for dessert. Difficulty in eating a meal may disrupt relationships and result in social isolation. Some patients may require supervision during meals or feel unsafe when they eat alone, causing further disruption of social and vocational function.

Diagnostic Testing

Because the mechanics of swallowing are largely invisible to the naked eye, diagnostic studies are commonly needed. The sine qua non for diagnosis of oropharyngeal swallowing disorders is the videofluorographic swallowing study (VFSS) [15]. In this test, the patient eats and drinks a variety of solids and liquids combined with barium while images are recorded with videofluorography (x-ray videotaping). The VFSS is usually performed jointly by a physician (physiatrist or radiologist) and a speech-language pathologist. A unique benefit of the VFSS is that therapeutic techniques (such as modification of food consistency, body position, or respiration) can be tested and their effects on swallowing observed during the study. A routine barium swallow study is frequently sufficient if the problem is clearly esophageal.

If a VFSS cannot be performed because of the physical limitation of the patient, the fiberoptic endoscopic evaluation of swallowing is useful to visualize the anatomy of the pharynx and larynx and vocal fold function during eating with no x-ray exposure [16]. It is also highly sensitive for detection of aspiration [8]; but it does not visualize essential aspects of swallowing, such as the oral and esophageal stages of swallowing, or critical events of pharyngeal swallowing including opening of the upper esophageal sphincter, elevation of the larynx, and contraction of the pharynx.

In cases of esophageal dysphagia, esophagoscopy is frequently necessary to detect mucosal lesions or masses. Biopsy is indicated when mucosal abnormalities are detected. Manometry is useful for detection and characterization of motor disorders of the esophagus and is sometimes performed on the pharynx as well. Electromyography is indicated when neuromuscular disease is suspected and is useful for detection of lower motor neuron dysfunction of the larynx and pharynx.

Differential Diagnosis

Myocardial ischemia
Globus sensation
Heartburn due to gastroesophageal reflux disease
Indirect aspiration (aspiration of refluxed gastric contents)

Treatment

Initial

The treatment of dysphagia depends on its causes and mechanism. Common treatments are listed in Table 129.3. Whenever possible, initial treatment should be directed at the underlying disease process; for example, steroids for inflammatory muscle disease. Esophageal dysphagia necessitates evaluation and treatment by a gastroenterologist. When no therapy exists for the underlying disease or the

Table 129.3 Principal Treatments of Selected Disorders Affecting Swallowing

Problems	Principal Treatments
Amyotrophic lateral sclerosis	Dietary modification Compensatory maneuvers Counseling and advance directives
Carcinoma of esophagus	Esophagectomy and radiation therapy
Gastroesophageal reflux disease	Dietary modification No eating at bedtime Pharmacologic therapy Smoking cessation
Polymyositis, myasthenia gravis	Pharmacologic treatment of underlying disease (dietary modification, compensatory maneuvers, and dysphagia therapy only if necessary)
Esophageal stricture or web	Dilation
Stroke, multiple sclerosis	Dietary modification Compensatory maneuvers Dysphagia therapy

therapy is ineffective or contraindicated, rehabilitative strategies are appropriate. Patients and their family members are encouraged to learn the Heimlich maneuver; this is important because airway obstruction is potentially fatal.

Rehabilitation

Many patients benefit from a structured swallowing therapy provided by a speech-language pathologist, including instruction and supervision about diet, compensatory maneuvers, and exercise [17]. The goals of therapy are to reduce aspiration, to improve the ability to eat and drink, and to optimize nutritional status. Therapy is individualized according to the patient's specific anatomic and structural abnormalities and the initial responses to treatment trials observed at the bedside or during the VFSS [18]. A fundamental principle of rehabilitation is that the best therapy for any activity is the specific activity itself; swallowing is generally the best therapy for swallowing disorders, so the rehabilitation evaluation is directed at identifying the circumstances for safe and effective swallowing for each individual patient.

Diet modification is a common treatment of dysphagia [19]. Patients vary in ability to swallow thin and thick liquids, and that determination is usually best made by VFSS. A patient can usually receive adequate oral hydration with either thin (e.g., water or apple juice) or nectar-thick liquids (e.g., apricot nectar, tomato juice). Rarely, a patient may be limited to honey-thick or pudding consistency if thin and thick liquids are freely aspirated. Most patients with significant dysphagia are unable to safely eat meats or similarly tough-textured foods and require a mechanical soft diet. A pureed diet is recommended for patients who exhibit oral preparatory phase difficulties, pocket food in the buccal recesses (between the teeth and the cheek), or have significant pharyngeal retention after swallowing with chewed solid foods. Maintenance of oral feeding often requires compensatory techniques to reduce aspiration or to improve pharyngeal clearance. A variety of behavioral techniques are used, including modifications of posture, head position (Fig. 129.1), and respiration, as well as specific swallow maneuvers [20].

Exercise therapy for dysphagia is indicated when the problem is related to weakness of the muscles of swallowing [21]. The choice of exercises must be individualized according

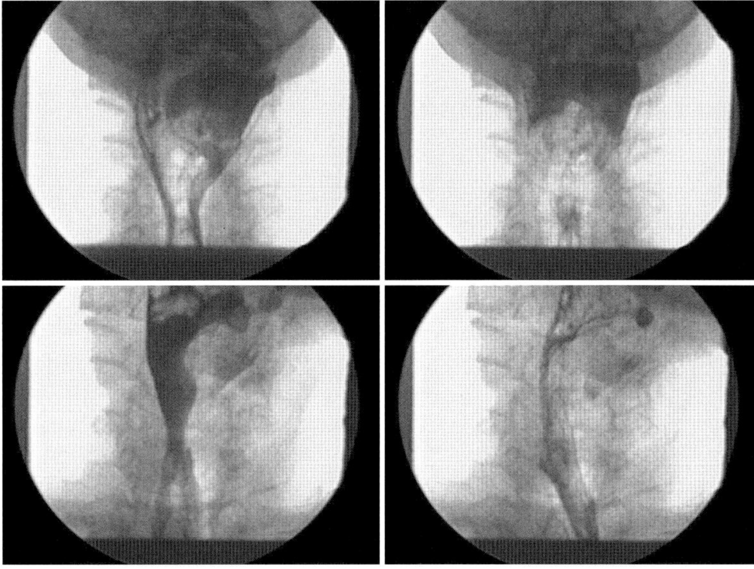

FIGURE 129.1 Turning the head toward the weak side improves pharyngeal emptying in some individuals with dysphagia due to lateral medullary infarction. This series of video prints is taken from a videofluorographic swallowing study of an individual with severe dysphagia due to lateral medullary infarction. The top images show an anteroposterior projection of swallowing with the head in anatomic position. The top left image was obtained in mid-swallow. There is stasis of barium in the left piriform recess, with only minimal flow of barium through the upper esophageal sphincter. The top right image shows the large amount of residual barium in the pharynx after swallowing. The bottom images show swallowing with the head turned toward the weak left side. The lower left image, in mid-swallow, shows enhanced flow of barium. The lower right image shows dramatically reduced retention of barium after the swallow.

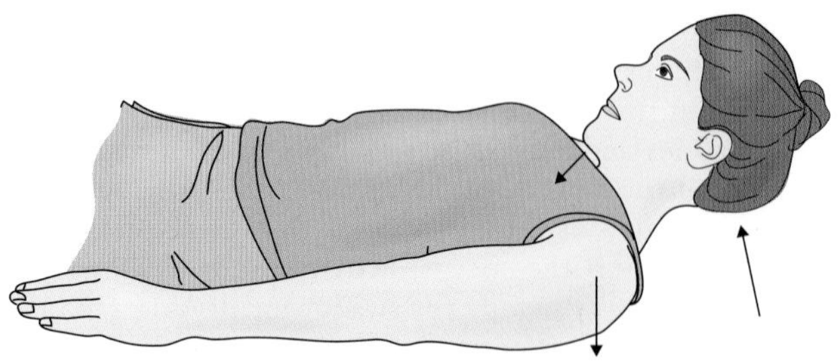

FIGURE 129.2 Shaker (pronounced "shock-air") exercise augments upper esophageal sphincter opening by strengthening the anterior suprahyoid muscles. The neck is actively flexed, raising the head so the patient can see the toes and touching the chin to the chest, without lifting the shoulders and with the mouth closed.

to the physiologic assessment. The full range of exercises is beyond the scope of this chapter, but several examples illustrate the principles.

- Tongue weakness can be treated with lingual resistance exercise [22].
- Strengthening of the anterior suprahyoid muscles is useful when the upper esophageal sphincter opens poorly. Flexing the neck against gravity while lying supine can strengthen these muscles (Fig. 129.2) [23,24].
- Vocal fold adduction exercises may be useful in cases of aspiration due to weakness of these muscles. These exercises are done several times a day whenever possible.

Procedures

VFSS functions as both a diagnostic and a therapeutic procedure for dysphagia, especially oropharyngeal dysphagia, because it can be used to test the effectiveness of modifying food consistency and other compensatory techniques [25]. Endoscopy with dilation of the esophagus is often indicated in cases of partial esophageal obstruction due to stricture or web. Dilation is also appropriate in stenosis of the upper esophageal sphincter. Endoscopy can be used for biofeedback, especially to demonstrate movements of the larynx during swallowing maneuvers. Electromyography is also used for biofeedback. Activities of the infrahyoid and suprahyoid muscles are recorded with surface electrodes during swallowing therapy. Biofeedback itself is not a dysphagia therapy but can be a useful adjunct to therapy. Surface electrical stimulation on the submental or anterior cervical muscles is a new treatment of dysphagia, but the evidence for its efficacy is weak [26].

Surgery

Surgery is rarely indicated in the care of patients with oral or pharyngeal dysphagia. The most common procedure for pharyngeal dysphagia is cricopharyngeal myotomy, during which the upper esophageal sphincter is disrupted to reduce the resistance of the pharyngeal outflow tract. However, the effectiveness of myotomy is highly controversial [27]. Esophagectomy may be necessary in case of esophageal cancer or obstructive strictures. Feeding gastrostomy (usually percutaneous endoscopic gastrostomy) is indicated when the severity of the dysphagia makes it impossible for adequate alimentation or hydration to be obtained orally, although intravenous hydration or nasogastric tube feedings may be sufficient on a time-limited basis [28]. Orogastric tube feedings have been used successfully by patients who have absent gag reflexes and can tolerate intermittent oral catheterization. Laryngectomy or surgical closure of the larynx is rarely performed in cases of recurrent, intractable aspiration pneumonia.

Potential Disease Complications

Severe dysphagia may result in aspiration pneumonia [29], airway obstruction, bronchiectasis, dehydration, or starvation and is potentially fatal. Severe dysphagia often causes social isolation because of the inability to consume a meal in the usual manner. This can lead to clinical depression. Suicide has been reported.

Potential Treatment Complications

The VFSS is safe and well tolerated. Prescription of a modified diet often means the substitution of thick for thin liquids. Some patients find these unpalatable and reduce fluid intake to the point of dehydration and malnutrition. Failure to reevaluate patients in a timely manner can lead to unnecessary prolongation of dietary restrictions, increasing the risk of malnutrition and adverse psychological effects of dysphagia. Dilation of the esophagus or sphincters can result in perforation, but this complication is uncommon. Percutaneous endoscopic gastrostomy can have direct or indirect sequelae. Direct sequelae, such as pain, infection, and obstruction of the feeding tube, are common. Percutaneous endoscopic gastrostomy tube feeding can promote aspiration pneumonia in individuals with severe gastroesophageal reflux disease.

References

[1] Martino R, Foley N, Bhogal S, et al. Dysphagia after stroke: incidence, diagnosis, and pulmonary complications. Stroke 2005;36:2756–63.
[2] Achem SR, Devault KR. Dysphagia in aging. J Clin Gastroenterol 2005;39:357–71.
[3] Palmer JB, Drennan JC, Baba M. Evaluation and treatment of swallowing impairments. Am Fam Physician 2000;61:2453–62.
[4] Buchholz DW. Oropharyngeal dysphagia due to iatrogenic neurological dysfunction. Dysphagia 1995;10:248–54.
[5] Smith Hammond CA, Goldstein LB. Cough and aspiration of food and liquids due to oral-pharyngeal dysphagia: ACCP evidence-based clinical practice guidelines. Chest 2006;129:154S–68S.
[6] Smith CH, Logemann JA, Colangelo LA, et al. Incidence and patient characteristics associated with silent aspiration in the acute care setting. Dysphagia 1999;14:1–7.
[7] Weir KA, McMahon S, Taylor S, Chang AB. Oropharyngeal aspiration and silent aspiration in children. Chest 2011;140:589–97.
[8] Rodrigues B, Nobrega AC, Sampaio M, et al. Silent saliva aspiration in Parkinson's disease. Mov Disord 2011;26:138–41.
[9] DePippo KL, Holas MA, Reding MJ. Validation of the 3-oz water swallow test for aspiration following stroke. Arch Neurol 1992;49:1259–61.
[10] Tohara H, Saitoh E, Mays KA, et al. Three tests for predicting aspiration without videofluorography. Dysphagia 2003;18:126–34.
[11] Wu MC, Chang YC, Wang TG, Lin LC. Evaluating swallowing dysfunction using a 100-ml water swallowing test. Dysphagia 2004;19:43–7.
[12] Palmer JB. Evaluation of swallowing disorders. In: Grabois M, Garrison SJ, Hart KA, Lehmkuhl DL, editors. Physical medicine and rehabilitation: the complete approach. Malden, Mass: Blackwell Science; 1999. p. 277–90.
[13] Leder SB. Gag reflex and dysphagia. Head Neck 1996;18:138–41.

[14] Kumlien S, Axelsson K. Stroke patients in nursing homes: eating, feeding, nutrition and related care. J Clin Nurs 2002;11:498–509.

[15] Palmer JB, Kuhlemeier KV, Tippett DC, Lynch C. A protocol for the videofluorographic swallowing study. Dysphagia 1993;8:209–14.

[16] Langmore SE. Endoscopic evaluation and treatment of swallowing disorders. New York: Thieme; 2001.

[17] Carnaby G, Hankey GJ, Pizzi J. Behavioural intervention for dysphagia in acute stroke: a randomised controlled trial. Lancet Neurol 2006;5:31–7.

[18] Ott DJ, Hodge RG, Pikna LA, et al. Modified barium swallow: clinical and radiographic correlation and relation to feeding recommendations. Dysphagia 1996;11:187–90.

[19] Robbins J, Gensler G, Hind J, et al. Comparison of 2 interventions for liquid aspiration on pneumonia incidence: a randomized trial. Ann Intern Med 2008;148:509–18.

[20] Ashford J, McCabe D, Wheeler-Hegland K, et al. Evidence-based systematic review: oropharyngeal dysphagia behavioral treatments. Part III—impact of dysphagia treatments on populations with neurological disorders. J Rehabil Res Dev 2009;46:195–204.

[21] Logemann JA. The role of exercise programs for dysphagia patients. Dysphagia 2005;20:139–40.

[22] Robbins J, Kays SA, Gangnon RE, et al. The effects of lingual exercise in stroke patients with dysphagia. Arch Phys Med Rehabil 2007;88:150–8.

[23] Shaker R, Easterling C, Kern M, et al. Rehabilitation of swallowing by exercise in tube-fed patients with pharyngeal dysphagia secondary to abnormal UES opening. Gastroenterology 2002;122:1314–21.

[24] Mepani R, Antonik S, Massey B, et al. Augmentation of deglutitive thyrohyoid muscle shortening by the Shaker Exercise. Dysphagia 2009;24:26–31.

[25] Palmer JB, Carden EA. The role of radiology in rehabilitation of swallowing. In: Jones B, editor. Normal and abnormal swallowing: imaging in diagnosis and therapy. 2nd ed. New York: Springer-Verlag; 2003. p. 261–73.

[26] Clark H, Lazarus C, Arvedson J, et al. Evidence-based systematic review: effects of neuromuscular electrical stimulation on swallowing and neural activation. Am J Speech Lang Pathol 2009;18:361–75.

[27] Tieu BH, Hunter JG. Management of cricopharyngeal dysphagia with and without Zenker's diverticulum. Thorac Surg Clin 2011;21:511–7.

[28] Dennis MS, Lewis SC, Warlow C. Effect of timing and method of enteral tube feeding for dysphagic stroke patients (FOOD): a multicentre randomised controlled trial. Lancet 2005;365:764–72.

[29] van der Maarel-Wierink CD, Vanobbergen JN, Bronkhorst EM, et al. Meta-analysis of dysphagia and aspiration pneumonia in frail elders. J Dent Res 2011;90:1398–404.

CHAPTER 130

Heterotopic Ossification

Amanda L. Harrington, MD
Jeffrey B. Eliason, MD
William L. Bockenek, MD

Synonyms

Myositis ossificans
Ossifying fibromyopathy
Neurogenic heterotopic ossification
Periarticular ossification
Heterotopic ossification in paraplegia
Neurogenic ossifying fibromyositis
Neurogenic osteoma
Paraosteoarthropathy

ICD-9 Codes

728.1 **Muscular calcification and ossification**
728.10 **Calcification and ossification, unspecified**
Massive calcification (paraplegic)
728.11 **Progressive myositis ossificans**
728.12 **Traumatic myositis ossificans**
Myositis ossificans (circumscripta)
728.13 **Postoperative heterotopic calcification**
733.99 **Other and unspecified disorders of bone and cartilage**
Hypertrophy of bone

ICD-10 Codes

M61.9 **Calcification and ossification of muscle, unspecified**
M61.20 **Paralytic calcification and ossification of muscle, unspecified site**
M61.10 **Myositis ossificans progressiva, unspecified site**
M61.00 **Myositis ossificans traumatica, unspecified site**
M61.40 **Other calcification of muscle, unspecified site**
M89.30 **Hypertrophy of bone, unspecified site**

Definition

Heterotopic ossification is the formation of mature, lamellar bone in nonskeletal tissue, usually in soft tissue surrounding joints [1,2]. Its exact etiology is unknown. Heterotopic ossification is commonly seen in patients with traumatic brain injury, spinal cord injury, cerebrovascular accident, burns, fractures, trauma, or muscle injuries and after total joint arthroplasty. Heterotopic ossification has also been described in medically complex patients after prolonged sedation, ventilation, critical illness, and immobilization [3,4]. In addition, heterotopic ossification has been found to be a complication after both cervical and lumbar disc replacement [5,6]. Riedel first described heterotopic ossification after trauma to the spinal cord in 1883 [7]. The term *neurogenic heterotopic ossification* has been commonly used for heterotopic ossification in patients with traumatic brain injury, spinal cord injury, and cerebrovascular accident [2,8]. The bone formation in heterotopic ossification differs from that in other disorders of calcium deposition in that heterotopic ossification results in encapsulated bone between muscle planes, which is not intra-articular or connected to periosteum [9].

The incidence rate reported in the literature varies from 11% to 75% in patients with severe traumatic brain injury and spinal cord injury [10,11]. Approximately 33% of patients with traumatic brain injury and spinal cord injury diagnosed with heterotopic ossification show a loss of joint range of motion; 10% to 16% progress to complete joint ankylosis [2,10]. The incidence of heterotopic bone formation after total hip arthroplasty and acetabular fracture is estimated at 16% to 53% and 18% to 90%, respectively [12].

Heterotopic ossification is both more common and more extensive in patients with severe spasticity. Increased spasticity and lower level of limb function increase the risk for development of heterotopic ossification and the rate of recurrence after surgical resection [8]. In addition, when other factors are controlled for, the incidence of heterotopic ossification increases with body mass index in patients with acetabular fracture [13]. In patients with spinal cord injury, the number of pressure ulcers and duration of time since injury are also associated with the development of heterotopic ossification [14]. When ectopic bone is discovered in patients with paraplegia, it is never found above the level of injury. Heterotopic ossification is rarely seen in flaccid limbs [8]. Interestingly, heterotopic ossification is infrequently reported in cerebral palsy or in children with anoxic brain injury [2].

The pathogenic mechanisms of heterotopic ossification are still being investigated. Whether genetic factors or local phenomena (trauma, tissue hypoxia, venous insufficiency, edema) are triggering factors, the final common pathway is inflammation and increased blood flow in the tissues [1,8,15]. Undifferentiated mesenchymal cells in connective tissue surrounding muscle or vasculature are transformed by bone morphogenetic proteins into osteoblasts, which lay down new bone matrix [4,12,13,15–17]. The scientific literature suggests that overactive bone morphogenetic protein signaling is involved in the development of both acquired heterotopic ossification and congenital heterotopic ossification, which is seen in fibrodysplasia ossificans progressiva.

The temporal relationship between injury and initiation of ossification is not clear. However, clinical signs, symptoms, and positive diagnostic test results may appear as early as 2 weeks after injury [12]. Mineralization and true bone formation are usually completed by 6 to 18 months [8]. The extent of bone formation has been described in the Brooker classification [2,11,17–19] for heterotopic ossification of the hip (Fig. 130.1). Only class III and class IV are clinically significant. Although modifications to the Brooker classification have been suggested, many clinicians continue to use this system to describe the extent of heterotopic bone formation (Table 130.1).

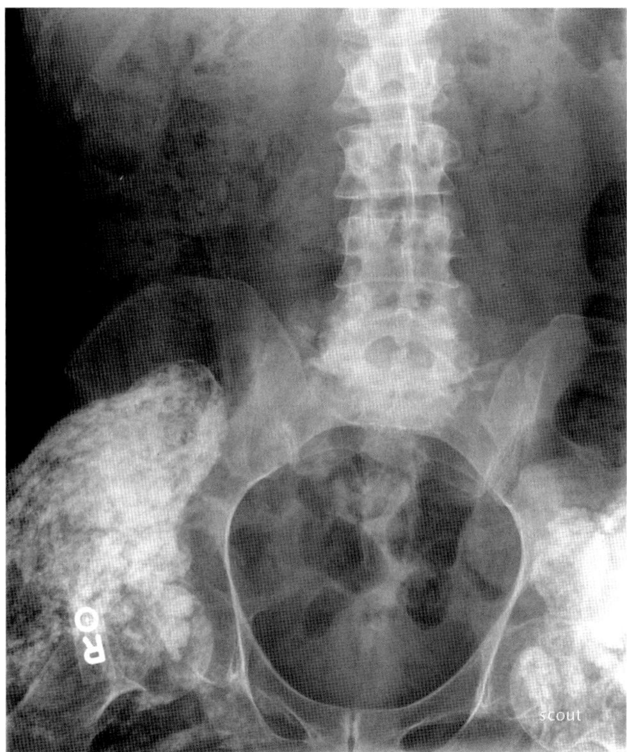

FIGURE 130.1 Radiograph of Brooker class IV heterotopic ossification of the right hip.

Table 130.1 Brooker Classification for Heterotopic Ossification of the Hip

Class	Description
I	Islands of bone within soft tissue
II	Bone spurs from pelvis or proximal femur, at least 1 cm between bone surfaces
III	Bone spurs from pelvis or proximal femur with space between bone surfaces of less than 1 cm
IV	Apparent bone ankylosis of the hip (Fig. 130.1)

Symptoms

Individuals demonstrate great variability in the initial symptoms and degree of heterotopic bone involvement. Patients are often asymptomatic [1,20]. In neurogenic heterotopic ossification, the most common symptom is pain (although this is often absent in spinal cord injury because of sensory deficits). Limitation to joint range of motion is commonly reported [8,12]. Symptoms range in onset from 2 weeks to 12 months after the inciting event, and patients may report warmth, swelling, and tenderness [2,11,21,22]. Heterotopic ossification may trigger autonomic dysreflexia in patients with spinal cord injury at or above the T6 level [23].

Physical Examination

Time at onset, location, and degree of heterotopic bone formation vary between individuals. Therefore, joints should be examined frequently in those at risk to assess range of motion and to assist in early diagnosis. The clinician should also inspect each joint for erythema and palpate for point tenderness or masses. The most common physical finding is decreased range of motion of the joint.

Distal joints of the hands and feet are almost never involved. Heterotopic ossification is typically limited to hips, knees, shoulders, and elbows [8]. In neurogenic heterotopic ossification secondary to traumatic brain injury or spinal cord injury, the hip is the most common joint affected [15]. Ossification is usually found inferomedial to the joint and is typically associated with adductor spasticity [2].

Functional Limitations

The loss of range of motion secondary to heterotopic ossification interferes with hygiene, transfers, and daily activities [22]. Pain from heterotopic ossification can be a significant cause of functional limitation.

Diagnostic Studies

The three-phase bone scan is the current "gold standard" for early detection of heterotopic ossification. It is possible to discover increased metabolic activity as early as 2 to 4 weeks after injury. This procedure involves intravenous injection of technetium Tc 99m–labeled polyphosphate, which is

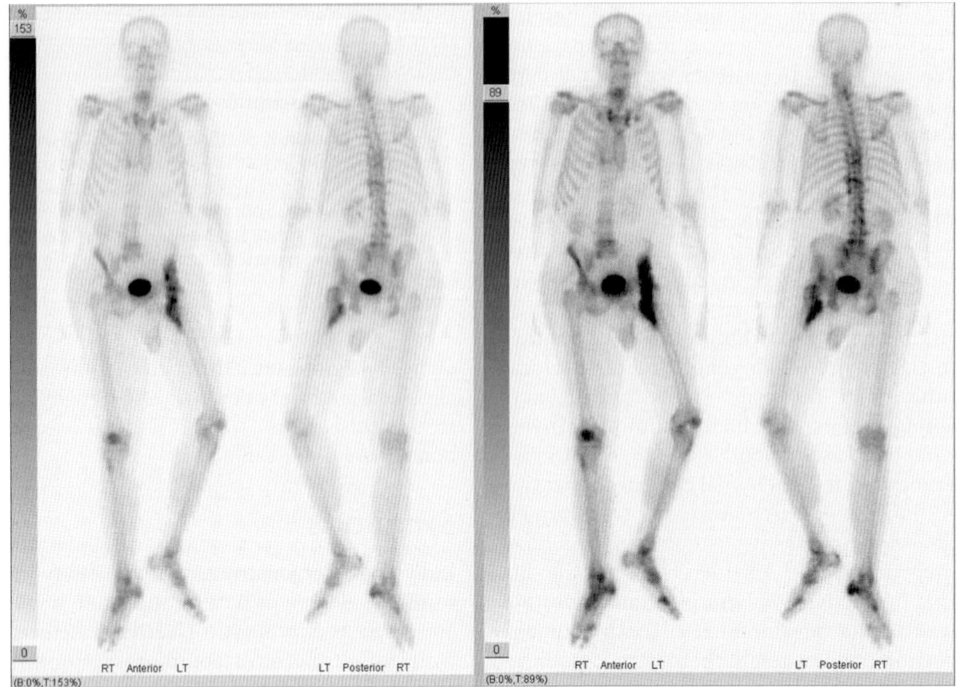

FIGURE 130.2 Three-phase bone scan showing increased activity at the left hip juxta-articular ossification site.

known to accumulate in areas of active bone growth. The three phases are as follows [8,22] (Fig. 130.2):

Phase 1: Dynamic blood flow occurs immediately after injection.

Phase 2: Immediate static scan detects areas of blood flow after injection.

Phase 3: Static phase involves a repeated bone scan after several hours.

A disadvantage of the three-phase bone scan is its lack of specificity. It therefore may be difficult to differentiate bone tumor, metastasis, or osteomyelitis from heterotopic ossification [8]. In addition, false-negative bone scans have been described after spinal cord injury [24].

Radiographs are readily available and economical but may not show calcification until after clinical signs and symptoms have developed or until 4 to 6 weeks after an abnormality is detected on the bone scan [11]. Heterotopic ossification has been described in three radiologic stages with variable time frames [2,25]:

1. early: increased activity on bone scan, no radiologic evidence;
2. intermediate: radiographically appearing immature bone; and
3. mature: well-developed, mature-appearing bone.

Both mature and immature bone can coexist. It is not uncommon for mature ossification to radiographically obscure immature bone [2]. Therefore, radiographic determination of the maturity of heterotopic bone is often unreliable [2,8].

Computed tomographic scanning is rarely used in detection of heterotopic ossification. There has been some evidence to suggest that magnetic resonance imaging of the knee may help to confirm an early diagnosis of heterotopic ossification [26]. Both computed tomography and magnetic resonance imaging have proved especially helpful in preoperative planning for resection to establish relationships of bone to muscle and neurovascular bundles [8,11].

Ultrasonography and angiography are not often used for the diagnosis of heterotopic ossification. However, cases have been reported in which ultrasound examination has been used to help differentiate heterotopic ossification from primary bone tumor, hematoma, or abscess. Similarly, angiography has been used to differentiate traumatic myositis ossificans from tumor and to define anatomy before surgical resection [8,12].

Many laboratory tests have been investigated for use in the diagnosis of heterotopic ossification. No one test has been found to be completely reliable with high sensitivity and specificity for heterotopic ossification. Although it is nonspecific, a widely used laboratory test for monitoring of heterotopic bone formation is the alkaline phosphatase (ALP) level. ALP has been shown to be elevated during the active bone formation of heterotopic ossification (normal range is 38 to 126 U/L). ALP levels rise as early as 2 weeks after injury, reaching a peak around 10 weeks [8]. ALP is helpful for diagnosis because it may be elevated up to 7 weeks before development of clinical symptoms [4]. Because the specificity of ALP elevation is low, it is recommended that three-phase bone scan be used to confirm suspected cases of heterotopic ossification [27].

Serum and urinary calcium concentrations, frequently nonspecific responses to trauma, do not provide any information about the ongoing ossification process and are therefore not used for diagnosis and monitoring of heterotopic ossification [15]. Other urinary markers, including hydroxyproline, deoxypyridinoline, and prostaglandin E_2, have been suggested for use in detection of heterotopic ossification [3,4,8,12]. Serum intact osteocalcin, C-reactive protein, erythrocyte sedimentation rate, and creatine kinase have been used as markers for heterotopic bone formation in some studies. In patients with spinal cord injury, the inflammatory phase of heterotopic bone formation can be monitored by C-reactive protein levels, and creatine kinase can be used to estimate the severity of ossification [3,16]. Both C-reactive protein and creatine kinase levels may be used to assist in therapeutic and treatment decisions. When markers suggest active formation of heterotopic ossification, medical and rehabilitation treatments may be indicated; however, if markers suggest ongoing inflammation, surgical resection for definitive treatment may be delayed [16].

Differential Diagnosis

Deep venous thrombosis
Cellulitis or infection
Acute arthritis
Superficial thrombophlebitis
Contracture
Complex regional pain syndrome
Spasticity
Tumoral calcinosis
Secondary hyperparathyroidism
Hypervitaminosis D
Fracture
Gout
Pseudogout
Para-articular chondroma
Calcinosis circumscripta
Hematoma or hemorrhage

Treatment

Initial

Nonsurgical strategies for treatment of heterotopic ossification include mobilization of the joint, medications to decrease inflammation or bone formation, and prophylactic low-dose radiation therapy. These therapies and preventive strategies may be combined to improve outcome [2,20]. Spasticity and pain can be barriers to providing proper range of motion. Both should be managed appropriately to ensure that mobilization can occur.

Nonsteroidal anti-inflammatory drugs (NSAIDs) can be used not only for analgesia of the patient but also to reduce bone formation by the inhibition of prostaglandin synthetase. NSAIDs inhibit arachidonic acid metabolism, thereby inhibiting prostaglandin production, reducing inflammation, and slowing bone metabolism.

Studies have shown that indomethacin, ibuprofen, and other NSAIDs have been effective for the prevention of heterotopic ossification in total hip arthroplasty and in high-risk spinal cord–injured patients [2,8,12,16,21,28]. A recent review suggested that NSAIDs have the greatest efficacy in preventing heterotopic ossification when they are given early after a spinal cord injury [29,30]. Indomethacin has been the most widely used NSAID in prophylaxis for heterotopic ossification and is commonly used after surgical resection to prevent recurrence. Traditionally, indomethacin is started on postoperative day 1 at a dose of 25 mg three times a day for 3 weeks and is continued for up to 2 months [2,8,17]. Shorter treatment durations have been found effective for prophylaxis [31].

Etidronate disodium (EHDP), a bisphosphonate, has been shown to delay the aggregation of apatite crystals into large, calcified clusters in patients with traumatic brain injury and spinal cord injury [2,8,10]. Although EHDP does not eradicate bone that has already formed, it reduces further progression of ossification [16]. EHDP is not routinely used for prophylaxis, but some clinicians advocate prophylactic use in high-risk spinal cord–injured patients. Bisphosphonates are thought to be most effective for treatment once the diagnosis of heterotopic ossification is established, particularly if they are given early in the disease course before there is radiographic evidence of bone formation [29,30]. The treatment recommendation for established heterotopic ossification in spinal cord injury is 20 mg/kg daily orally for 6 months [32]. For patients with traumatic brain injury, it has been suggested that oral treatment be initiated at 20 mg/kg per day for 3 months, then reduced to 10 mg/kg per day for 3 months [10].

Observational evidence suggests that warfarin is associated with a reduced incidence of heterotopic ossification in patients with spinal cord injury; however, it is not used solely for prevention of heterotopic ossification, in part because of the side effect profile [30]. After elective total hip arthroplasty, aspirin thromboprophylaxis has been shown to reduce prevalence of heterotopic ossification [33]. At the molecular level, treatments aimed at the reduction of bone morphogenetic protein signaling may help reduce formation of heterotopic bone. Although not used in clinical treatment at this time, bone morphogenetic protein receptor antagonists, retinoic acid receptor agonists, and free radical scavengers are current research targets [34].

Rehabilitation

Comprehensive physical and occupational therapy can be considered both preventive and a first-line treatment modality. Several studies have shown that early range of motion exercises are beneficial in the prevention and treatment of heterotopic ossification [9]. Some have suggested that joint manipulation may increase the inflammatory response, thereby increasing production of heterotopic bone, but there is no objective evidence to show this to be true [2]. Joint manipulation may not alter bone formation, but it can prevent soft tissue contractures and maintain functional range of motion. Because physical therapy is often difficult secondary to pain or spasticity, forceful manipulation under anesthesia has been tried but is not a standard treatment modality. Exercises to maintain joint range of motion are still considered the mainstay for prevention of heterotopic ossification [2,21]. Continuous passive motion machines are beneficial in increasing range of motion after surgical resection of heterotopic bone [4,12].

Procedures

Radiation therapy has been shown to help prevent heterotopic ossification after total hip arthroplasty and after resection of mature heterotopic bone [1,27]. It is the only therapy for heterotopic ossification that acts locally [8]. Although opinions differ as to the most effective treatment method, single doses of 5 to 8 Gy are more frequently used than fractionated doses, and similar results are found when preoperative and postoperative treatments are compared [1]. Radiation therapy has been used successfully after heterotopic bone resection in patients with traumatic brain injury and spinal cord injury to help prevent recurrence and for local treatment of heterotopic ossification in spinal cord injury [2,16,17,35]. Pulse low-intensity electromagnetic therapy uses magnetic fields to improve blood flow to the target area and has been shown in one study to prevent the formation of heterotopic ossification after spinal cord injury [30,36].

Surgery

Although heterotopic ossification may recur after surgical resection, it remains the only definitive treatment for mature heterotopic bone. In fact, surgical excision is the most common treatment of heterotopic ossification after traumatic brain injury [29]. Surgical indications include joint immobility causing difficulty in activities of daily living, ankylosed joints leading to pressure ulcers or skin breakdown, and conditions in which heterotopic ossification contributes to focal peripheral neuropathy [2]. Preoperative planning often requires three-dimensional computed tomography and magnetic resonance imaging to assess the relationship between heterotopic bone and neurovascular structures at risk. Careful dissection with isolation of neurovascular bundles reduces risk of morbidity associated with hemorrhage, sepsis, or repeated ankylosis [2]. Functional range of motion can typically be reached with a wedge resection of the ectopic bone [2].

Controversy exists as to the timing of the procedure because bone maturity is difficult to assess. It has been shown that immature heterotopic bone has a greater incidence of recurrence [16,27]. Traditionally, three-phase bone scan and ALP levels have been used to monitor bone maturity. However, because both may remain abnormal indefinitely, many clinicians no longer wait for normalization of bone scans and ALP levels to proceed with resection [16]. Still, it is not uncommon for surgery to be delayed for up to 2 to 2.5 years in patients with traumatic brain injury or spinal cord injury; however, the suggested optimal timing is 12 to 18 months [29,37]. After heterotopic bone resection, radiation therapy and NSAIDs are often used to prevent recurrence [2,8].

Potential Disease Complications

Heterotopic bone deposition impairs normal joint range of motion and causes secondary soft tissue contractures, which involve surrounding skin, muscles, ligaments, and neurovascular bundles [2]. The resulting restrictive position predisposes the patient to the development of pressure ulcers and subsequent infections. Direct pressure or chronic spasticity can cause nerve ischemia and compression, resulting in focal peripheral neuropathy [2]. Vascular compression, deep venous thrombosis, and lymphedema may also result. Decreased range of motion predisposes to osteoporosis and subsequent pathologic fracture during transfer or lifting of the patient [2].

Potential Treatment Complications

NSAIDs have well-known side effects that most commonly affect the gastric, hepatic, and renal systems. There is also a risk of defective bone-prosthesis union and poor bone healing in orthopedic populations when NSAIDs are used for the prevention of heterotopic ossification [8,31].

EHDP is generally a safe method for treatment of heterotopic ossification. The most common side effects are nausea and diarrhea. Twice-daily divided dosing of EHDP helps alleviate these symptoms. EHDP also carries a potential risk of bone fracture secondary to osteomalacia; if it is withdrawn after a short treatment duration, a rebound ossification secondary to prolonged osteoclast inhibition may result [10,32].

Radiation therapy is rarely associated with malignant neoplasia and does not disrupt wound healing, provided wounds are not in the field of irradiation [8,38]. In orthopedic populations after total hip arthroplasty, increased rates of trochanteric nonunion have been described with both high-dose fractionated and single-dose protocols [31,38].

Surgical complications, which carry a high morbidity and are not uncommon, include hemorrhage, sepsis, wound infection, repeated ankylosis, and heterotopic bone recurrence [8,27]. Chronic pain and recurrent contracture may also result. The distorted anatomy in heterotopic ossification makes dissection visibility difficult, endangering neurovascular structures [2]. Postoperative blood loss requiring transfusion is not uncommon despite good surgical hemostasis [2].

References

[1] Balboni TA, Gobezie R, Mamon HJ. Heterotopic ossification: pathophysiology, clinical features, and the role of radiotherapy for prophylaxis. Int J Radiat Oncol Biol Phys 2006;65:1289–99.
[2] Botte MJ, Keenan ME, Abrams RA, et al. Heterotopic ossification in neuromuscular disorders. Orthopedics 1997;20:335–41.
[3] Sugita A, Hashimoto J, Maeda A, et al. Heterotopic ossification in bilateral knee and hip joints after long-term sedation. J Bone Miner Metab 2005;23:329–32.
[4] Pape HC, Marsh S, Morley JR, et al. Current concepts in the development of heterotopic ossification. J Bone Joint Surg Br 2004;86:783–7.
[5] Park SJ, Kang KJ, Shin SK, et al. Heterotopic ossification following lumbar total disc replacement. Int Orthop 2011;35:1197–201.
[6] Suchomel P, Jurák L, Benes 3rd V, et al. Clinical results and development of heterotopic ossification in total cervical disc replacement during a 4-year follow-up. Eur Spine J 2010;19:307–15.
[7] Riedel B. Demonstration eine durch achttägiges Umhergehen total destruirten Kniegelenkes von einem Patienten mit Stichverletzung des Rückens. Verh Dtsch Ges Chir 1883;12:93.
[8] Buschbacher R. Heterotopic ossification: a review. Crit Rev Phys Med Rehabil 1992;4:199–213.
[9] Venier LH, Ditunno JF. Heterotopic ossification in the paraplegic patient. Arch Phys Med Rehabil 1971;52:475–9.
[10] Spielman G, Gennarelli TA, Rogers CR. Disodium etidronate: its role in preventing heterotopic ossification in severe head injury. Arch Phys Med Rehabil 1983;64:539–42.
[11] Garland DE. Clinical observations on fractures and heterotopic ossification in the spinal cord and traumatic brain injured populations. Clin Orthop Relat Res 1988;233:86–101.
[12] Bossche LV, Vanderstraeten G. Heterotopic ossification: a review. J Rehabil Med 2005;37:129–36.
[13] Mourad WF, Packianathan S, Shourbaji RA, et al. The impact of body mass index on heterotopic ossification. Int J Radiat Oncol Biol Phys 2012;82:831–6.
[14] Coelho CV, Beraldo PS. Risk factors of heterotopic ossification in traumatic spinal cord injury. Arq Neuropsiquiatr 2009;67:382–7.
[15] McCarthy EF, Sundaram M. Heterotopic ossification: a review. Skeletal Radiol 2005;34:609–19.
[16] Banovac K, Sherman AL, Estores IM, et al. Advanced clinical solutions: prevention and treatment of heterotopic ossification after spinal cord injury. J Spinal Cord Med 2004;27:376–82.

[17] Puzas JE, Miller MD, Rosier RN. Pathologic bone formation. Clin Orthop Relat Res 1989;245:269–81.
[18] Shi S, de Gorter DJ, Hoogaars WM, et al. Overactive bone morphogenetic protein signaling in heterotopic ossification and Duchenne muscular dystrophy. Cell Mol Life Sci 2013;70:407–23.
[19] Brooker AF, Bowerman JW, Robinson RA, et al. Ectopic ossification following total hip replacement. Incidence and a method of classification. J Bone Joint Surg Am 1973;55:1629–32.
[20] Pakos EE, Pitouli EJ, Tsekeris PG, et al. Prevention of heterotopic ossification in high-risk patients with total hip arthroplasty: the experience of a combined therapeutic protocol. Int Orthop 2006;30:79–83.
[21] Stover SL, Hataway CJ, Zeiger HE. Heterotopic ossification in spinal cord–injured patients. Arch Phys Med Rehabil 1975;56:199–204.
[22] Johns JS, Cifu DX, Keyser-Marcus L, et al. Impact of clinically significant heterotopic ossification on functional outcome after traumatic brain injury. J Head Trauma Rehabil 1999;14:269–76.
[23] Blackmer J. Rehabilitation medicine: 1. Autonomic dysreflexia. CMAJ 2003;169:931–5.
[24] Svircev JN, Wallbom AS. False-negative triple-phase bone scans in spinal cord injury to detect clinically suspect heterotopic ossification: a case series. J Spinal Cord Med 2008;31:194–6.
[25] Haider T, Winter W, Eckholl D, et al. Primary calcification as a mechanism of heterotopic ossification. Orthop Trans 1990;14:309–10.
[26] Argyropoulou MI, Kostandi E, Kosta P, et al. Heterotopic ossification of the knee joint in intensive care unit patients: early diagnosis with magnetic resonance imaging. Crit Care 2006;10:R152.
[27] Garland DE. A clinical perspective on common forms of acquired heterotopic ossification. Clin Orthop Relat Res 1991;263:13–29.
[28] Moore KD, Goss K, Anglen JO. Indomethacin versus radiation therapy for prophylaxis against heterotopic ossification in acetabular fractures: a randomized, prospective study. J Bone Joint Surg Br 1998;80:259–63.
[29] Aubut JL, Mehta S, Cullen N, et al. A comparison of heterotopic ossification treatment within the traumatic brain and spinal cord injured population: an evidence based systemic review. NeuroRehabilitation 2011;28:151–60.
[30] Teasell RW, Mehta S, Aubut JL, et al. A systematic review of therapeutic interventions for heterotopic ossification following spinal cord injury. Spinal Cord 2010;48:512–21.
[31] Dahners LE, Mullis BH. Effects of nonsteroidal anti-inflammatory drugs on bone formation and soft-tissue healing. J Am Acad Orthop Surg 2004;12:139–43.
[32] Banovac K. The effect of etidronate on late development of heterotopic ossification after spinal cord injury. J Spinal Cord Med 2000;23:40–4.
[33] Cohn RM, Della Valle AG, Cornell CN. Heterotopic ossification is less after THA in patients who receive aspirin compared to coumadin. Bull NYU Hosp Jt Dis 2010;68:266–72.
[34] Pavlou G, Kyrkos M, Tsialogiannis E, et al. Pharmacological treatment of heterotopic ossification following hip surgery: an update. Expert Opin Pharmacother 2012;13:619–22.
[35] Sautter-Bihl ML, Hultenschmidt B, Liebermeister E, et al. Fractionated and single-dose radiotherapy for heterotopic bone formation in patients with spinal cord injury. Strahlenther Onkol 2001;177:200–5.
[36] Durović A, Miljković D, Brdareski Z, et al. Pulse low-intensity electromagnetic field as prophylaxis of heterotopic ossification in patients with traumatic spinal cord injury. Vojnosanit Pregl 2009;66:22–8.
[37] Mavrogenis AF, Soucacos PN, Papagelopoulos PJ. Heterotopic ossification revisited. Orthopedics 2011;34:177.
[38] Coventry MB, Scanlon PW. The use of radiation to discourage ectopic bone. A nine-year study in surgery about the hip. J Bone Joint Surg Am 1981;63:201–8.

CHAPTER 131

Lymphedema

Mabel Caban, MD, MS

Lori Hall, PT, MS, CLT-LANA

Synonyms

Primary lymphedema
Secondary lymphedema
Post-mastectomy lymphedema
Nonne-Milroy-Meige syndrome
Familial lymphedema

ICD-9 Codes

457.0	**Postmastectomy lymphedema syndrome**
457.1	**Lymphedema**
	Acquired
	Praecox
	Secondary
757.0	**Hereditary edema of legs**
	Chronic hereditary
	Congenital
997.99	**Surgical**

ICD-10 Codes

I97.2	**Postmastectomy lymphedema syndrome**
I89.0	**Lymphedema, not elsewhere classified, praecox and secondary**
Q82.0	**Hereditary lymphedema**

Definition

Between 3 and 5 million people in the United States suffer from lymphedema, which in a significant number develops from cancer and its treatment [1]. The incidence of post-mastectomy lymphedema ranges from 6% to 48%, depending on whether the patient received axillary radiation and surgery; if only lumpectomy is performed, the incidence drops to only 6%. This increases to 23% with use of sentinel node biopsy and radiation therapy; but if axillary lymph node dissection and radiation therapy are used, the incidence is even higher at about 35% to 48% [1].

About 80% of lymphedema cases involve the lower limbs and relate to peripheral vascular disease [1]. Cervical cancer, melanoma, and pelvic cancers increase the frequency of secondary lymphedema of the lower extremity. An incidence of 21% to 49% is reported after cervical cancer surgery and radiation therapy. In women with endometrial cancer, 11% developed lower limb lymphedema after surgery and radiation therapy. Around the world, infection in the form of filariasis is the most common cause of lymphedema. An estimated 15 million people present with lower extremity lymphedema in filariasis-endemic regions in the world [2].

Lymphedema is a condition of an abnormal enlargement of part of the body associated with lymphostasis from dysfunction of the lymphatic system (Fig. 131.1). The dysfunction is due to the abnormal morphology of the lymphatic system, high production of lymph, or blockage in drainage [3,4]. The lymphatic system consists of vessels with lymph traveling through lymph nodes. The lymphatic vessels transport fluid, plasma proteins, and other substances from the tissue back into the circulatory system. Lymphedema results from the inability to drain the lymphatic fluid and the accumulation of it in the limb. Chronic edema initiates a cascade of events that cause transformation of the tissue with skin thickening, fibrosis, deposition of fat, and unhealthy skin changes after months to years. A classification of lymphedema includes primary (heritable) and secondary (acquired) causes [5]. Phlebolymphedema pertains to dysfunction of the lymphatic system in association with chronic venous insufficiency [6]. Chronic venous insufficiency is a manifestation of deep venous thrombosis, angiodysplasia, lack of valves in the venous system, or varicosities.

The radical excision of lymph nodes for malignant disease does not always cause lymphedema [7]. Lymphedema could occur as a late complication of surgery for malignant disease because of gradual failure, making the distal lymphatics pump harder through the most proximal damaged ducts over time. The body compensates by regenerating the transected lymphatics to some extent. With irradiation, fibrous scarring forms, increasing the risk of lymphedema. The diagnosis depends on the history and characteristic changes of the skin on clinical examination (Fig. 131.1).

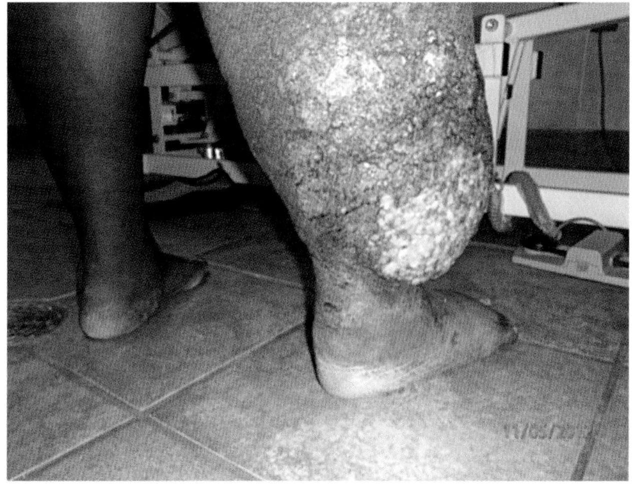
FIGURE 131.1 Abnormal skin changes in the patient with lymphedema.

Symptoms

The hallmark of lymphedema is painless swelling. Although many people believe that pain is a major component of lymphedema, this is not typically present, especially in the early stages. One of the first symptoms of lymphedema is tightness of the cutis and subcutis [8]. Chronic indolent swelling of a limb is the most common presentation of lymphedema. Patients may complain that the arm feels heavy or that rings feel tight. Hypertrophy of fatty tissue occurs and eventually fibrosis too. In true lower extremity lymphedema, the feet are involved. The skin condition changes from being soft initially to becoming harder over time. Early or postsurgical lymphedema can spread proximally, an unusual finding after the first year, and lasts about 3 months after surgery [7].

Physical Examination

The patient with limb edema requires a thorough physical examination before the initiation of therapy. Swelling of a limb with or without pain may be the presentation of an infection, deep venous thrombosis, or obstruction caused by a tumor at the level of the lymph nodes. Limb temperature and discoloration should be noted. In early stages, the edema is pitting, but as lymphedema progresses, the edema becomes nonpitting. In the absence of treatment, distal enlargement of the wrist or ankle occurs. A discrepancy of 2 cm in circumference or a difference of 200 mL in volume from side to side has been accepted for the diagnosis of lymphedema. A multitude of skin changes occur over time (Table 131.1) [9]. Signs of lymphedema progression include a cool limb, skin thickening, limited range of motion, increased presence of papillomas, mycosis, and bacterial infection. Infection, such as cellulitis, erysipelas, and lymphangitis, must be recognized to prevent systemic malaise and worsening of the swelling [3].

Staging of the condition helps assess progression and evaluate better treatment options. Stages of lymphedema are as follows:

Stage 0 Preclinical: there is no swelling, and it can lasts months or years.

Stage I Reversible stage: swelling is soft and pitting.

Stage II Spontaneously irreversible stage: increased swelling and change in tissues with fibrosis formed.

Stage III Lymphostatic elephantiasis: limb becomes extremely swollen with thickened skin.

Lymphedema does not cause neurologic deficits, but paresthesias and numbness may occur in the same distribution of the edema. Explanations include coexistence of neurologic damage from node dissection, peripheral nerve injury, plexopathy, and chemotherapy-induced polyneuropathy. The possibility of cancer recurrence must be ruled out with imaging, such as computed tomography or magnetic resonance imaging with contrast enhancement.

Lipedema can occur with lymphedema. This is an abnormality of the deposition of fat involving the lower body, most commonly in women, of symmetric appearance. Swelling starts at the waist and finishes at the ankles without inclusion of the feet as opposed to lymphedema, in which the feet are involved. Lipedema does not respond to dietary intervention or complete decongestive therapy. If underlying hormonal imbalance exists, correction will improve this condition, and although it is controversial, liposuction can improve it in some cases [10,11].

Unilateral or bilateral venous insufficiency may be manifested with varicosities, fibrosis, thickened cutis, and brownish skin discoloration. Superimposed venous ulcers may occur in advanced cases [3,7].

Functional Limitations

Impaired mobility due to the excessive weight of the limb may occur in severe cases (Table 131.2) [4]. Tight clothing, restriction of movement, and loss of body image and self-esteem are frequent complaints leading to psychosocial impairment. Women with breast cancer–related lymphedema report problems with their sexual well-being and social interaction [12]. In the past, avoidance of physical activity was the norm for fear of worsening the edema. This has changed with new evidence supporting the benefits of physical activity and exercise [12]. Wearing of a compression garment during exercise is advised (Fig. 131.2).

Table 131.1 Common Skin Changes Observed in Lymphedema
Hyperkeratosis: skin becomes thicker
Papillomatosis
Skin turgor increases
Skin breaks may allow lymph to seep
Peau d'orange
Dyschromia
Pachydermia

Table 131.2 Functional Deficits Arising in Chronic Lymphedema
Poor posture
Pain
Scar or tissue tension
Weakness
Gait impairment
Psychosocial impairment

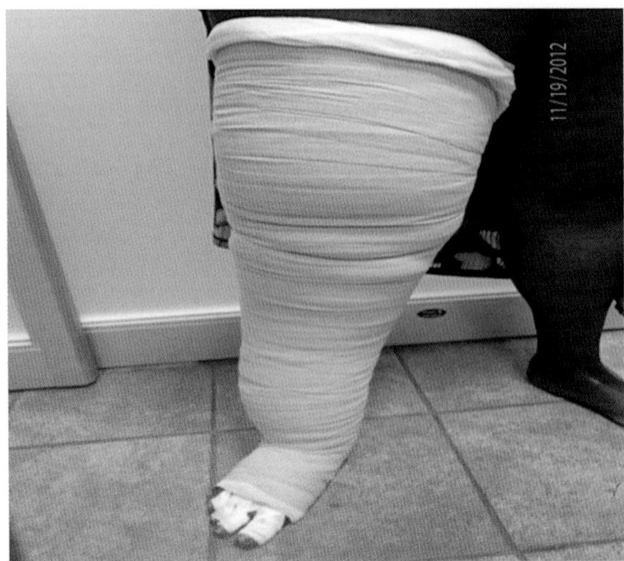

FIGURE 131.2 Short-stretch, multilayered compression bandaging.

Diagnostic Studies

The diagnosis of lymphedema is based on the history, physical examination, and noninvasive diagnostic procedures. New-onset lymphedema should be a diagnosis of exclusion after deep venous thrombosis and malignant disease (including cancer recurrence) are ruled out. Therefore, most patients with new-onset lymphedema will have a workup for malignant disease as well as a Doppler ultrasound examination to rule out deep venous thrombosis. The diagnosis can be confounded with conditions such as obesity, chronic venous insufficiency, occult trauma, fracture, and repeated infections. Genetic testing may be necessary if gene therapy becomes clinically viable in the future [13]. Currently, research with animal models is targeting the vascular endothelial growth factor receptor 3 (VEGFR-3) and its primary ligands (VEGF-C and VEGF-D), looking for potential molecular treatment strategies.

Differential Diagnosis of Chronic Edema [7]

SYSTEMIC ETIOLOGY
Congestive heart failure
Renal failure
Hypoalbuminemia
Protein-losing nephropathy
Myxedema

LOCAL ETIOLOGY
Primary or secondary lymphedema
Lipedema
Deep venous thrombosis
Chronic venous disease
Ipsilateral surgery
Cellulitis
Baker cyst
Cyclic or idiopathic edema
Tumor recurrence

Treatment

Initial

The risk of lymphedema can be reduced by use of sentinel node biopsy as part of the treatment for malignant neoplasms [14]. Early lymphedema may revert with appropriate compression of the limb and by maintaining an active lifestyle. The goals of the initial treatment include reduction of swelling, arrest of progression, improvement of other related symptoms, avoidance of infection, and optimization of function and quality of life. Treatment includes conservative, surgical, pharmacologic, and alternative methods.

The most commonly used drugs are the diuretics. However, diuretics are believed to worsen other types of lymphedema because they increase urination and produce hemoconcentration of tissue proteins. Because the edema is protein rich, the diuretic prompts protein to remain stagnant in the congested area, leading to fibrosclerosis. Diuretics may be used in the presence of ascites or hydrothorax. A short course of diuretics can help in the presence of malignant lymphedema [4].

Benzopyrones may increase the number of macrophages that hydrolyze tissue proteins to facilitate the removal of protein. Their exact mechanism of action is not well understood, the benefits remain unproven, and the use is limited because of the potential for liver toxicity [3]. Selenium, a free radical scavenger, reportedly has an antiedematous effect that potentiates the effect of complete decongestive therapy and reduces the risk of erysipelas infections in patients with lymphedema [15].

Antiseptic dressings for minor wounds and the early use of antibiotics for infections can prevent long-term complications. Prophylaxis with antibiotics such as phenoxymethylpenicillin (500 mg daily) is recommended for cases with recurrent cellulitis [3].

Rehabilitation

Treatment outcomes are most favorable with diagnosis and treatment early before fibrosis and hardening of the tissue occur. When pitting edema exists, the lymphedema is more responsive to treatment [16]. Complete decongestive therapy, the standard of care for lymphedema, is a multifaceted treatment approach performed by a certified lymphedema therapist that consists of two phases.

Phase one is the reductive phase. During this phase, manual lymphatic drainage, a technique similar to a gentle light touch massage that stimulates the lymphatics and facilitates drainage of congested areas, is used. Compression bandages employ multiple layers of short-stretch bandages and other materials, such as foam padding, to create a bandage with a low resting pressure and a high working pressure in the affected limb. Remedial exercises are movements with light exertion and stretches done while compression bandages or garments are worn. These exercises stimulate the lymph drainage into the thoracic duct [17]. Finally, meticulous skin and nail care requires moisturizing with a low-pH lotion; this prevents skin from drying and cracking and also discourages the growth of bacteria and fungus, which can cause infections and wounds. The initial phase of complete decongestive therapy ends when the maximum volume reduction is achieved and there is no further improvement. Relative contraindications to institution of complete decongestive therapy include acute infections, cardiac edema, peripheral arterial occlusive disease, renal dysfunction, and acute deep venous thrombosis. Recurrent tumor should be treated before the use of massage (manual lymphatic drainage).

During phase two, or the maintenance phase, the patient is fitted with a compression garment to wear during the day and taught how to continue bandaging at night or to apply a nighttime compression device [17]. The patient may also be taught self-drainage of lymph or the use of an intermittent pneumatic compression device. The use of the intermittent pneumatic compression device is controversial, and there are concerns that a high-pressure single chamber may cause damage to superficial structures, edema in the trunk or genitals, and development of a fibrosclerotic ring above the device sleeve. In response to some of the concerns, the latest models have multichambers, with sequential pressure delivery, programmable pressures, and truncal clearance [18]. In this phase, it is important that the patient continue to take care of the skin and perform the home exercise program. Weight reduction has been proved to have a positive impact by reducing limb volume [19].

Studies have shown some success when other modalities are included together with complete decongestive therapy. For example, low-level laser therapy was approved by the Food and Drug Administration in 2006 for professional treatment and self-treatment of lymphedema. Studies have shown moderate to strong evidence for the effectiveness of low-level laser therapy [20]. Kinesio tape is widely used to treat edema and may be an alternative to short-stretch bandaging for breast cancer–related lymphedema when compliance with short-stretch bandaging after 1 month of intervention is poor [21]. Kinesio tape in conjunction with compression may improve results but has yet to be sufficiently studied. Oscillation therapy involves the use of electrostatic impulses to create a kneading effect to promote lymphatic drainage [22].

Surgery

Surgical options can benefit a few patients when the size of the limb interferes with mobility. Surgical procedures are still controversial. These are debulking procedures to remove excess tissue overgrowth; microsurgery to restore lymphatic continuity by use of a lymphatic collector or vein segment, also known as lymphaticovenous anastomosis [23]; and liposuction when lymphedema is nonresponsive to conservative management from the excess fat overgrowth. Patients still need to wear compression garments long term [24].

The standard of care in the past was to excise all of the regional lymph nodes during cancer surgery, but this is no longer the case to prevent morbidity such as lymphedema. For example, in breast cancer patients, sentinel lymph node dissection is associated with lower incidence of lymphedema than axillary lymph node dissection is. Sentinel lymph node dissection facilitates the resection of the sentinel node that combined with frozen-section histologic examination prevents unnecessary secondary surgeries, prevents lymphedema, and improves disease-specific survival [25].

Potential Disease Complications

Recurrent cellulitis and infections with staphylococcal resistant bacteria may occur. Delay in treatment increases the risk of sepsis. If it is untreated, lymphedema may progress to fibrosclerosis of the tissue and elephantiasis. A rare complication is lymphangiosarcoma, a malignant neoplasm in a lymphedematous limb described in post-mastectomy lymphedema and congenital lymphedema [7]. Stewart-Treves syndrome was first described in women who had undergone a radical mastectomy with subsequent lymphedema and lymphangiosarcoma.

Potential Treatment Complications

Potential complications include disease progression, liver complications from the use of benzopyrones, and worsening of lymphedema after liposuction from disruption of the remaining lymphatics.

References

[1] Lawenda BD, Mondry TE, Johnstone PA. Lymphedema: a primer on the identification and management of a chronic condition in oncologic treatment. CA Cancer J Clin 2009;59:8–24.

[2] Dreyer G, Addiss D, Gadelha P, et al. Interdigital skin lesions of the lower limbs among patients with lymphoedema in an area endemic for bancroftian filariasis. Trop Med Int Health 2006;11:1475–81.

[3] Mortimer PS. Swollen lower limb-2: lymphoedema. BMJ 2000;320:1527–9.

[4] Foeldi M, Foeldi E. Textbook of lymphology. Munich, Germany: Elsevier; 2006.

[5] Lohrmann C, Foeldi E, Speck O, et al. High-resolution MR lymphangiography in patients with primary and secondary lymphedema. AJR Am J Roentgenol 2006;187:556–61.

[6] Piller N. Phlebolymphoedema/chronic venous lymphatic insufficiency: an introduction to strategies for detection, differentiation and treatment. Phlebology 2009;24:51–5.

[7] Tiwari A, Cheng KS, Button M, et al. Differential diagnosis, investigation, and current treatment of lower limb lymphedema. Arch Surg 2003;138:152–61.

[8] Johansson K, Branje E. Arm lymphoedema in a cohort of breast cancer survivors 10 years after diagnosis. Acta Oncol 2010;49:166–73.

[9] Rockson SG, Rivera KK. Estimating the population burden of lymphedema. Ann N Y Acad Sci 2008;1131:147–54.

[10] Fife CE, Maus EA, Carter MJ. Lipedema: a frequently misdiagnosed and misunderstood fatty deposition syndrome. Adv Skin Wound Care 2010;23:81–92.

[11] Aldrich MB, Guilliod R, Fife CE, et al. Lymphatic abnormalities in the normal contralateral arms of subjects with breast cancer–related lymphedema as assessed by near-infrared fluorescent imaging. Biomed Opt Express 2012;3:1256–65.

[12] Hayes SC, Janda M, Cornish B, et al. Lymphedema after breast cancer: incidence, risk factors, and effect on upper body function. J Clin Oncol 2008;26:3536–42.

[13] Rockson SG. Causes and consequences of lymphatic disease. Ann N Y Acad Sci 2010;1207(Suppl. 1):E2–6.

[14] Goldberg JI, Riedel ER, Morrow M, et al. Morbidity of sentinel node biopsy: relationship between number of excised lymph nodes and patient perceptions of lymphedema. Ann Surg Oncol 2011;18:2866–72.

[15] Micke O, Bruns F, Mucke R, et al. Selenium in the treatment of radiation-associated secondary lymphedema. Int J Radiat Oncol Biol Phys 2003;56:40–9.

[16] Silver JK, Gilchrist LS. Cancer rehabilitation with a focus on evidence-based outpatient physical and occupational therapy interventions. Am J Phys Med Rehabil 2011;90:S5–15.

[17] Korpan MI, Crevenna R, Fialka-Moser V. Lymphedema: a therapeutic approach in the treatment and rehabilitation of cancer patients. Am J Phys Med Rehabil 2011;90:S69–75.

[18] Mayrovitz HN. The standard of care for lymphedema: current concepts and physiological considerations. Lymphat Res Biol 2009;7:101–8.

[19] Shaw C, Mortimer P, Judd PA. A randomized controlled trial of weight reduction as a treatment for breast cancer–related lymphedema. Cancer 2007;110:1868–74.
[20] Omar MT, Shaheen AA, Zafar H. A systematic review of the effect of low-level laser therapy in the management of breast cancer–related lymphedema. Support Care Cancer 2012;20:2977–84.
[21] Tsai HJ, Hung HC, Yang JL, et al. Could Kinesio tape replace the bandage in decongestive lymphatic therapy for breast-cancer-related lymphedema? A pilot study. Support Care Cancer 2009;17:1353–60.
[22] Jones J. Case study: use of oscillation therapy and MLLB in cancer-related oedema. Br J Community Nurs 2012;(Suppl.)S17–21 April.
[23] Campisi C, Davini D, Bellini C, et al. Lymphatic microsurgery for the treatment of lymphedema. Microsurgery 2006;26:65–9.
[24] Brorson H. Liposuction of arm lymphoedema. Handchir Mikrochir Plast Chir 2003;35:225–32.
[25] Giuliano AE, Hunt KK, Ballman KV, et al. Axillary dissection vs no axillary dissection in women with invasive breast cancer and sentinel node metastasis: a randomized clinical trial. JAMA 2011;305:569–75.

CHAPTER 132

Motor Neuron Disease

Nanette C. Joyce, DO, MAS

Gregory T. Carter, MD, MS

Synonyms

Amyotrophic lateral sclerosis (Lou Gehrig's disease)
Progressive muscular atrophy
Primary lateral sclerosis
Progressive bulbar palsy
Adult spinal muscular atrophy
Spinobulbar muscular atrophy (Kennedy disease)

ICD-9 Codes

335.10	**Spinal muscular atrophy**
	Spinal muscular atrophy, unspecified
335.11	**Kugelberg-Welander disease**
335.19	**Other spinal muscular atrophy**
	Adult spinal muscular atrophy
335.20	**Amyotrophic lateral sclerosis**
	Motor neuron disease
335.21	**Progressive muscular atrophy**
	Duchenne-Aran muscular atrophy
	Progressive muscular atrophy (pure)
335.22	**Progressive bulbar palsy**
335.23	**Pseudobulbar palsy**
335.24	**Primary lateral sclerosis**
335.29	**Other motor neuron diseases**

ICD-10 Codes

G12.9	**Spinal muscular atrophy, unspecified**
G12.1	**Other inherited spinal muscular atrophy, including adult spinal muscular atrophy, Kugelberg-Welander disease**
G12.21	**Amyotrophic lateral sclerosis, progressive spinal muscle atrophy**
G12.20	**Motor neuron disease, unspecified**
G12.22	**Progressive bulbar palsy**
G12.29	**Other motor neuron disease, primary lateral sclerosis**

Definition

The term *motor neuron disease* encompasses a heterogeneous group of progressive neuromuscular disorders characterized by the selective loss of upper or lower motor neurons. However, motor neuron disease is also used interchangeably with *amyotrophic lateral sclerosis* (ALS), which can be confusing for the uninitiated. ALS is the most common adult motor neuron disease. For the diagnostic criteria for ALS to be met, both upper and lower motor neuron involvement is necessary [1,2]. In sporadic cases with only lower motor neuron dysfunction, the disease is called progressive muscular atrophy; if upper motor neuron dysfunction is singularly present, it is primary lateral sclerosis; and if dysfunction is localized to the bulbar region, the disease is called progressive bulbar palsy. Most patients initially diagnosed as having progressive muscular atrophy, primary lateral sclerosis, or progressive bulbar palsy eventually progress to meet diagnostic criteria for ALS [3]. Those who do not convert have a slower rate of disease progression. This chapter focuses on ALS as the management principles are similar for the entire class of motor neuron diseases.

The prevalence of ALS is about 6 to 8 per 100,000 people, with an annual incidence of approximately 2 cases per 100,000 people. Men are more commonly affected than women, with a ratio nearing 2:1. Most cases of ALS are sporadic, having unknown etiology. Only 5% to 10% of patients have familial ALS, which is most commonly transmitted in an autosomal dominant fashion. Approximately 30% to 40% of familial cases in the United States and Europe are caused by mutations in the *C9orf72* gene; 20% worldwide are caused by mutations in the *SOD1* (superoxide dismutase) gene; and rarer forms of familial ALS have been linked to mutations in the *TARDBP, FUS, ANG, ALS2, SETX,* and *VAPB* genes [4,5]. Other inherited adult motor neuron diseases are Kennedy disease (X-linked recessive) and adult spinal muscular atrophy (autosomal recessive), which are purely lower motor neuron disorders with greatly increased life span compared with ALS.

ALS causes rapid, progressive skeletal muscle weakness and atrophy, leading to premature death by respiratory failure. Weakness begins in a focal region, such as a single limb, the bulbar muscles, or the respiratory muscles, and spreads to affect other regions. Extraocular muscles and bowel and bladder sphincter function are often spared until late in the disease course. Mean age at onset is the mid-50s, but ALS may develop in adults of any age. Rare juvenile familial forms exist with onset before the age of 25 years. Mean survival, without tracheostomy, is 3 years from diagnosis but ranges from less than 1 year to more than 20 years. One explanation for this extreme variability is that ALS is multiple disorders without a single etiology but rather with multiple causes, sharing a common final step in the pathophysiologic pathway—motor neuron apoptosis. This is illustrated by the varying phenotypes associated with familial forms of ALS [3]. Theories about the pathogenesis of sporadic ALS have implicated RNA toxicity, glutamate excitotoxicity, oxidative stress, neuroinflammation, protein misfolding, glial cell activation, and mitochondrial dysfunction, to name a few [5].

Symptoms

Early symptoms of ALS can be subtle and include muscle twitching and cramping, weakness, and loss of coordination. Patients with a predominantly upper motor neuron syndrome often present with muscle stiffness, weakness, loss of dexterity, and loss of voluntary motor control from spasticity that may affect vocal quality or limb function. Patients with a predominantly lower motor neuron syndrome may present with weakness and muscle atrophy, fasciculations, muscle cramps, and flaccid dysarthria. Bulbar symptoms include dysarthria, dysphagia, sialorrhea (drooling), and pseudobulbar affect—laughing or crying in exaggeration of or incongruent with mood. Symptoms are initially painless and asymmetric across limbs. As the disease relentlessly progresses, weakness and atrophy spread to affect all skeletal muscles, causing significant impairment and disability. If patients do not succumb first to respiratory failure, they will ultimately transition from independent function to total dependence.

Respiratory failure is the presenting symptom in a rare few. Constitutional symptoms of weight loss and generalized fatigue are common. Cognitive symptoms including behavioral or executive dysfunction have been reported to occur in 33% to 51% of patients [6]. Most have milder symptoms; approximately 5% to 14% meet clinical criteria for a diagnosis of frontotemporal dementia [6].

Physical Examination

Physical examination of a patient with suspected motor neuron disease should be aimed at establishing the certainty of diagnosis. ALS is diagnosed clinically, and the patient with suspected motor neuron disease requires a thorough neurologic examination, assessing each of the four major body regions (bulbar, cervical, thoracic, and lumbar) for signs of upper and lower motor neuron involvement. The "gold standard" for the diagnosis of upper motor neuron disease is establishment of the presence of pathologic reflexes—a brisk jaw jerk, Hoffmann sign, abdominal skin reflex, and Babinski sign. Increased muscle stretch reflex responses as demonstrated by increased spread and amplitude or clonus are considered pathologic. Reflexes that would be graded normal but are elicited from atrophied and weak muscles should also be considered pathologic. Evidence of lower motor neuron disease includes muscle weakness, atrophy, hypotonia, hyporeflexia, and fasciculations. Patients with ALS may be hyperreflexic and hyporeflexic, depending on the stage at which they are in the disease process and whether they have a predominance of upper or lower motor neuron phenotype. For example, hyperreflexia occurs in the patient with upper motor neuron dysfunction, but this sign can be overcome and silenced by concomitant lower motor neuron loss causing muscle atrophy and hyporeflexia. Because ALS is an asymmetric and spreading process, the upper motor neuron signs may be more predominant than the lower motor neuron signs, or vice versa, within any single limb or between limbs and body regions. These examination findings will change over time as the disease progresses. The tongue should be examined for fasciculations, atrophy, strength, and range of motion. The patient's mental status, nonmotor cranial nerve function, sensory examination, and cerebellar examination findings are usually normal.

In patients with an established diagnosis, the physical examination documents disease progression and includes the musculoskeletal and cardiorespiratory systems in addition to the neurologic evaluation. The musculoskeletal examination focuses on assessment of range of motion and evaluation of painful joints or soft tissue structures. Because progressive respiratory failure is a ubiquitous manifestation of ALS, follow-up appointments should be scheduled regularly (i.e., every 3 months) and the cardiorespiratory system assessed at each visit. Forced vital capacity (FVC) and maximal inspiratory, maximal expiratory, and peak cough pressures can be measured with a spirometer in the office setting and should be considered part of the regular cardiorespiratory follow-up evaluation, providing relevant information for clinical decision-making and prognosis (Table 132.1).

Table 132.1 Pulmonary Function Testing in Amyotrophic Lateral Sclerosis

Measure	Key Values	Significance
Forced vital capacity	<75% of predicted at time of diagnosis [49]	Poor prognostic indicator
	Slower rate of monthly decline (<3.1%/month) [50]	Predicts slower disease progression
	50% of predicted [37]	Meets Medicare guidelines for initiation of noninvasive ventilation
Maximal inspiratory pressure	−60 cm H_2O [37]	Meets Medicare guidelines for initiation of noninvasive ventilation
Maximal expiratory pressure	Normal value [50]	Associated with 2-year survival
	Abnormal value	Associated with abnormal cough
Peak cough flow	270 L/min [37]	Initiate mechanical cough assistance
Sniff nasal inspiratory pressure	−40 cm H_2O [37]	Meets Medicare guidelines for initiation of noninvasive ventilation

Functional Limitations

The pattern of progressive functional limitation is directly related to the patient's motor neuron disease phenotype. Bulbar-onset ALS initially affects the patient's ability to speak and to swallow and typically spreads to involve the muscles of the upper extremities before the lower extremities [7]. These patients have a difficult time maintaining their weight both because of dysphagia and because of the loss of upper limb strength that impairs their ability to feed themselves. Eventually, bulbar-predominant patients become anarthric with accompanying severe dysphagia that limits their ability to control their secretions and to swallow their own saliva.

The functional limitations that develop in patients with spinal-onset ALS are the direct or indirect result of muscle weakness and atrophy. In lumbar spine onset, gait is abnormal early in the disease secondary to footdrop or hip flexion weakness. As the disease progresses, the patient's mobility worsens. Eventually, even the most basic activities of daily living become impossible to perform. Patients often transition quickly from independence to total dependence.

Reactive depression, generalized fatigue, and musculoskeletal pain may further limit function.

Diagnostic Studies

The diagnosis of ALS is based on the combined clinical and electrodiagnostic examinations. Neuroimaging and clinical laboratory studies are used to exclude other conditions that mimic ALS. All patients thought to have a motor neuron disease should undergo electrodiagnostic testing. The Awaji-shima revised El Escorial criteria (Table 132.2) are used to establish the certainty level of the diagnosis of ALS [1,2]. These criteria were developed as a tool for clinical trial enrollment but are commonly used in the clinic. The revised criteria classify the certainty level of diagnosis into one of three categories: definite, probable, and possible, which no longer includes the categories of Suspected ALS or Probable ALS Laboratory Supported that were part of the El Escorial criteria (Fig. 132.1). In addition to both upper and lower motor neuron findings, a diagnosis of ALS requires evidence of progressive spread of signs or symptoms within a single body region or from one of the four body regions to another. Certainty level of diagnosis depends on how many regions reveal upper motor neuron and lower mo-

Table 132.2 Awaji-shima Revised El Escorial Criteria: Clinical Certainty Levels for the Diagnosis of Amyotrophic Lateral Sclerosis [1]

Clinical Certainty	Clinical or Electrophysiologic Evidence
Clinically definite	UMN and LMN findings in at least three body regions
Clinically probable	UMN and LMN findings in at least two body regions with UMN findings rostral to LMN findings
Clinically possible	UMN and LMN findings in one body region, *or* UMN findings in at least two body regions without LMN findings, *or* LMN findings that are rostral to UMN findings

LMN, lower motor neuron; *UMN*, upper motor neuron. Four body regions: bulbar, cervical, thoracic, lumbar.

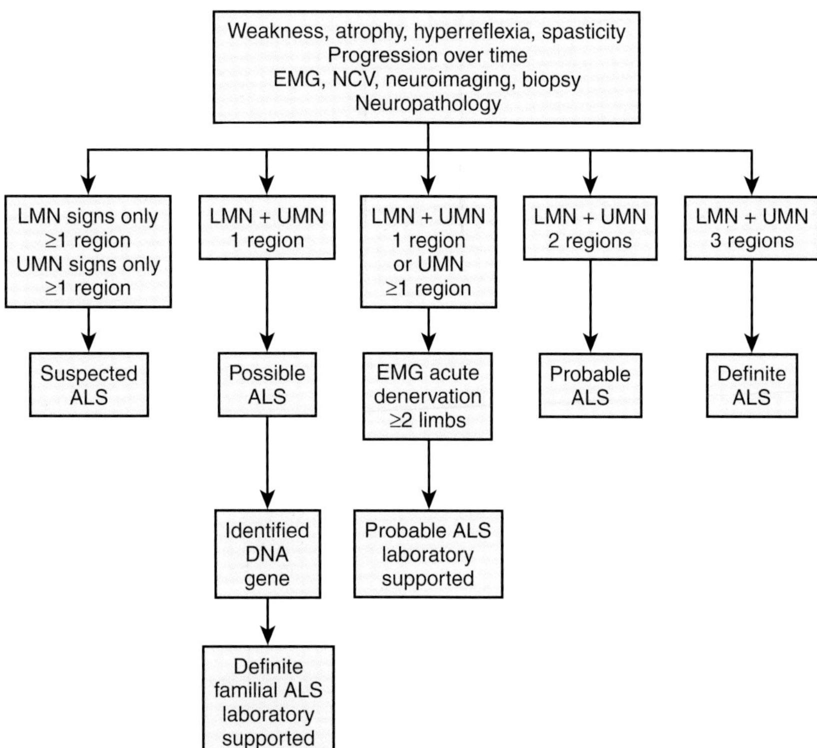

FIGURE 132.1 El Escorial criteria for the diagnosis of amyotrophic lateral sclerosis (ALS). *EMG*, electromyography; *LMN*, lower motor neuron; *NCV*, nerve conduction velocity; *UMN*, upper motor neuron. *(From Krivickas LS. Motor neuron disease. In Frontera WR, Silver JK, Rizzo TD Jr, eds. Essentials of Physical Medicine and Rehabilitation, 2nd ed. Philadelphia, WB Saunders, 2008.)*

tor neuron disease [1]. Electrophysiologic findings of denervation, including positive sharp waves, fibrillation potentials, and fasciculation potentials, are used to confirm lower motor neuron dysfunction in clinically affected regions and to detect subclinical lower motor neuron dysfunction, thereby extending the clinical examination. Signs of denervation observed during electromyography are now considered equivalent to lower motor neuron symptoms on clinical examination [1].

Imaging studies are used to exclude possibilities other than motor neuron disease from the differential diagnosis. Magnetic resonance imaging is the primary imaging modality in the evaluation of patients with suspected ALS. Almost all patients should have magnetic resonance imaging of the cervical spine to exclude cord compression, syrinx, or other spinal cord disease. The location of symptoms will dictate whether other regions of the spinal cord should be imaged. In those presenting with bulbar symptoms, brain magnetic resonance imaging should be performed to exclude stroke, tumor, syringobulbia, and other pathologic processes.

In most neuromuscular clinics, a routine panel of laboratory tests is performed for all patients thought to have ALS. A suggested set of such tests is provided in Table 132.3. The rationale behind the performance of this extensive battery of tests is to assess the general health of the patient and to exclude treatable conditions. The differential diagnosis, developed after the history and physical examination, may suggest that more specialized testing be performed. Table 132.4 suggests additional tests that may be warranted when the presentation is atypical with a progressive muscular atrophy, primary lateral sclerosis, or progressive bulbar palsy phenotype. When there is a family history of motor neuron disease, genetic testing may be considered.

Table 132.3 Suggested Laboratory Studies

Hematology

Complete blood count
Sedimentation rate

Chemistry

Electrolytes, blood urea nitrogen, creatinine
Glucose
Hemoglobin A_{1c}
Calcium
Phosphorus
Magnesium
Creatine kinase
Liver function tests
Serum lead level
Urine heavy metal screen
Vitamin B_{12}
Folate

Endocrine

Thyroxine
Thyroid-stimulating hormone
25-Hydroxyvitamin D
Intact parathyroid hormone

Immunology

Serum immunoelectrophoresis
Urine assay for Bence Jones proteins
Antinuclear antibody
Rheumatoid factor

Microbiology

Lyme titer
VDRL test

Optional

Human immunodeficiency virus test (if risk factors are present)
Anti-Hu antibody (if malignant disease is suspected)
DNA test for *SOD1* mutation (with family history)

Modified from Krivickas LS. Motor neuron disease. In Frontera WR, Silver JK, Rizzo TD Jr, eds. Essentials of Physical Medicine and Rehabilitation, 2nd ed. Philadelphia, WB Saunders, 2008.

Table 132.4 Specialized Laboratory Testing

Phenotype	Test	Diagnosis Excluded
Progressive muscular atrophy	DNA test: CAG repeat on X chromosome	Kennedy disease
	DNA test: *SMN* gene mutation	Spinal muscular atrophy
	Hexosaminidase A	Hexosaminidase A deficiency (heterozygous Tay-Sachs disease)
	Voltage-gated calcium channel antibody test	Lambert-Eaton myasthenic syndrome
	Cerebrospinal fluid examination	Polyradiculopathy, infectious or neoplastic
	GM_1 antibody panel	Multifocal motor neuropathy
Primary lateral sclerosis	Very long chain fatty acids	Adrenoleukodystrophy
	Human T-lymphotropic virus 1 (HTLV-1) antibodies	HTLV-1 myelopathy (tropical spastic paraparesis)
	Parathyroid hormone	Hyperparathyroid myelopathy
	Cerebrospinal fluid examination	Multiple sclerosis
Progressive bulbar palsy	Acetylcholine receptor antibodies	Myasthenia gravis
	DNA test: CAG repeat on X chromosome	Kennedy disease
	Cerebrospinal fluid examination	Multiple sclerosis

From Krivickas LS. Motor neuron disease. In Frontera WR, Silver JK, Rizzo TD Jr, eds. Essentials of Physical Medicine and Rehabilitation, 2nd ed. Philadelphia, WB Saunders, 2008.

Differential Diagnosis

The differential diagnosis varies on the basis of phenotype and is stratified by lower motor neuron, upper motor neuron, bulbar, or mixed lower and upper motor neuron involvement.

LOWER MOTOR NEURON ONLY

Progressive muscular atrophy
Spinal muscular atrophy
Kennedy disease
Poliomyelitis, postpoliomyelitis syndrome
Benign monomelic amyotrophy
Hexosaminidase A deficiency
Polyradiculopathy
Multifocal motor neuropathy with conduction block
Chronic inflammatory demyelinating polyneuropathy
Motor neuropathy or neuronopathy
Lambert-Eaton syndrome
Plexopathy
Benign fasciculations

UPPER MOTOR NEURON ONLY
Primary lateral sclerosis
Multiple sclerosis
Adrenoleukodystrophy
Subacute combined systems degeneration
Hereditary spastic paraparesis
Myelopathy
Syringomyelia

BULBAR
Progressive bulbar palsy
Myasthenia gravis
Multiple sclerosis
Foramen magnum tumor
Brainstem glioma
Stroke
Syringobulbia
Head and neck cancers
Polymyositis
Oculopharyngeal muscular dystrophy
Kennedy disease

UPPER AND LOWER MOTOR NEURONS
Familial or sporadic amyotrophic lateral sclerosis
Cervical myelopathy with radiculopathy
Syringomyelia
Spinal cord tumor or arteriovenous malformation
Lyme disease

Table 132.5 Pharmacologic Management of Amyotrophic Lateral Sclerosis–Related Symptoms

Symptom	Potential Therapy
Pseudobulbar affect	Amitriptyline, selective serotonin reuptake inhibitors, Nuedexta (dextromethorphan hydrobromide 20 mg/quinidine sulfate 10 mg)
Sialorrhea	Glycopyrrolate (Robinul), amitriptyline, atropine 0.5% sublingual drops, scopolamine transdermal patch, botulinum toxin, radiation therapy
Thick secretions	Guaifenesin, beta blocker
Spasticity	Oral or intrathecal baclofen, tizanidine, regional botulinum toxin injection
Laryngospasm	Treat underlying gastroesophageal reflux: proton pump inhibitors (omeprazole), H_2 receptor blockers (ranitidine)
Cramps	Mexiletine, stretching
Depression	Tricyclic antidepressants, selective serotonin reuptake inhibitors
Anxiety	Lorazepam, buspirone
Fatigue	Modafinil
Insomnia	Address nocturnal hypoventilation first; amitriptyline, zolpidem, trazodone
Urinary urgency	Oxybutynin, amitriptyline
Constipation	Increased hydration, fiber supplements (Metamucil), osmotics (MiraLax), saline laxatives (milk of magnesia), stool softeners (Colace), stimulants (Dulcolax), enemas

Treatment

Initial

Pharmacologic

There is no cure for ALS; however, ongoing research is focused on identifying disease mechanisms and finding drugs to slow disease progression. Riluzole (Rilutek) is the only medication approved by the Food and Drug Administration (FDA) specifically for treatment of ALS. It is an antiglutamate agent that was approved by the FDA for treatment of ALS in 1995 after two clinical trials showed that the drug slowed disease progression [8,9]. A Cochrane review reporting a meta-analysis of riluzole clinical trials showed a survival benefit of approximately 2 months [10]. Unfortunately, no functional benefit was derived as strength declined at a rate similar to that in those taking riluzole and placebo. The recommended dose of riluzole is 50 mg twice daily. The most common adverse side effects are fatigue, nausea, and elevation of hepatic enzymes. Riluzole is contraindicated in those with hepatic enzyme activity of more than five times the upper limit of normal.

Offering patients pharmacologic treatment of their disease and access to clinical trials has psychological benefits that may outweigh the actual slowing of disease progression currently able to be achieved. The following is an abbreviated list of compounds and biologics that are currently in clinical trial for ALS: arimoclomol, creatine combined with tamoxifen, edaravone, neural stem cells, and mesenchymal stem cells. Negative ALS clinical trials have tested many therapeutics and supplements, including multiple growth factors, dexpramipexole, creatine, lithium, ceftriaxone, glutamate antagonists, anti-inflammatory agents (celecoxib), calcium channel blockers, and amino acids [11]. Whereas many ALS patients take multiple supplements, no double-blind, placebo-controlled trials have proved their efficacy. In the future, a cocktail approach to slowing of disease progression may be the ideal treatment strategy [12].

Symptomatic

A number of drugs are useful for treatment of spasticity, sialorrhea, pseudobulbar affect, depression, and anxiety (Table 132.5).

Spasticity requires treatment only if it interferes with function. Nonpharmacologic management involves teaching patients stretching exercises and positioning techniques that decrease muscle tone. Baclofen (Lioresal) is the most effective pharmacologic agent, followed by tizanidine (Zanaflex). Diazepam (Valium) should be avoided because it may suppress respiration, and dantrolene (Dantrium) is not recommended because it causes excessive muscle weakness. In general, pharmacologic management of spasticity is less successful in ALS than in multiple sclerosis or spinal cord injury because the lower motor neuron component of ALS makes patients extremely susceptible to the development of excessive weakness.

Patients with bulbar dysfunction experience sialorrhea because they have difficulty swallowing and managing the oral secretions they normally produce. A variety of anticholinergic drugs may be used to dry the mouth. Tricyclic antidepressants are often tried first but may not be tolerated because of adverse side effects (excessive dry mouth, somnolence, urinary retention). One benefit of the tricyclic antidepressants is that they may treat other ALS-related symptoms, such as pseudobulbar affect, insomnia, and pain. Tricyclic antidepressants are contraindicated in patients with cardiac arrhythmia or conduction disorder. When tricyclic antidepressants are not tolerated, a scopolamine patch (Transderm Scōp) or glycopyrrolate (Robinul) may be helpful. If these treatments are inadequate, patients may benefit from salivary gland botulinum toxin injection [13–15].

Pseudobulbar affect, sometimes called emotional incontinence, may become distressing for both the patient and the family. Amitriptyline (Elavil) or fluvoxamine (Luvox) may help blunt the intensity of these inappropriate or exaggerated reactions. A combination preparation of dextromethorphan and quinidine (Nuedexta) was found to be effective in a large randomized clinical trial [16] and was granted FDA approval in late 2010 for the treatment of pseudobulbar affect. Nuedexta is contraindicated in patients with heart failure, long QT syndrome, and conduction block.

Reactive depression and anxiety are both normal responses to a diagnosis of ALS [17]. Patients and their families may benefit from individual counseling and participation in ALS support groups. Anxiety may be treated with benzodiazepines as long as the patient does not have significant reduction of vital capacity. Undetected hypoventilation may produce or contribute to preexisting feelings of anxiety. Depression should be treated pharmacologically because not treating it may have a significant negative impact on the quality of life remaining [18,19]. Selective serotonin reuptake inhibitors (SSRIs) are good first choices because of their minimal side effects. Tricyclic antidepressants may be preferred if they are also needed to treat other symptoms, such as sialorrhea or pseudobulbar affect. Caution should be taken in prescribing both an SSRI and a tricyclic antidepressant as SSRIs will increase the serum level of the tricyclic antidepressant and increase the potential for serious drug-related events.

Rehabilitation

Exercise

Skeletal muscle weakness is the primary impairment in ALS and causes the majority of the clinical problems. In the early stages of ALS, patients often inquire about the role of exercise in preventing or forestalling the development of weakness. There remains scarce evidence on which to base recommendations for exercise in ALS. Little research has been published since the 2008 Cochrane review of Dal Bello-Haas et al [20]. However, a search of www.clinicaltrials.gov identified two ongoing clinical trials, one studying the effects of resistance training in patients with ALS and the other studying aerobic exercise training [21]. Rehabilitation strategies later in the disease focus on augmenting function by compensating for muscle weakness to maintain independence.

Three forms of exercise training are most relevant to patients with ALS: flexibility, strengthening, and aerobic exercise. Flexibility training helps prevent the development of painful contractures, is considered first-line treatment of spasticity, and aborts painful muscle spasms. A home stretching program, designed by a knowledgeable therapist, is appropriate for the ALS patient throughout the course of the disease. The stretching routine initially may be created for independent performance but necessarily will be transitioned to caregiver-assisted exercises when the patient is no longer capable of performing them alone.

Physicians caring for ALS patients have traditionally been reluctant to recommend strengthening exercises. The reasons for this appear to be twofold; epidemiologic studies have inconsistently suggested a link between high-intensity physical exercise and disease onset, and reports of overuse weakness accelerating disease progression have appeared in the literature [22,23]. This philosophy promotes the development of disuse weakness, compounding the disability produced by ALS itself. The literature supporting the development of overwork weakness in neuromuscular patients is anecdotal and has not been demonstrated in controlled prospective studies. A single randomized trial of strength training in ALS has been published [24]. It demonstrated a slowing of decline in physical function as measured by the ALS Functional Rating Scale out to 6 months after exercise initiation compared with the control group. No adverse effects were observed. Studies of patients with more slowly progressive neuromuscular diseases and postpoliomyelitis syndrome suggest that only muscles mildly affected by the disease process can be strengthened by a moderate-intensity resistance program [25–27]. Interested ALS patients should be encouraged to begin or to continue a resistance program to maximize the strength of unaffected or mildly affected muscles with the goal of prolonging function. Until further studies have been completed examining the effects of high-intensity strength training in ALS, resistance exercise can safely be accomplished by instructing the patient to use a weight that can be lifted 20 times in submaximal sets of 10 to 15 repetitions. This ensures that the training is performed at a low to moderate level of resistance. Common sense would suggest that if an exercise regimen consistently produces immediate or severe delayed muscle soreness or fatigue lasting longer than a half-hour after exercise, it is too strenuous and is impairing function. If the patient chooses to exercise, the level of postexercise fatigue and recovery time should be ascertained during the regular follow-up appointments. Recommendations for modification of exercise intensity and duration should be provided on the basis of the patient's response.

Aerobic exercise helps maintain cardiorespiratory fitness. A study of moderate aerobic activity in patients with ALS demonstrated a short-term positive effect on disability up to 3 months after exercise initiation compared with controls [28]. Multiple studies in transgenic mouse models of ALS have shown that aerobic exercise prolongs survival [29–31]. Given the lack of any apparent contraindication, aerobic exercise training is recommended for patients with ALS as long as it can be performed safely without a risk of falling or injury. In addition to the physical benefits, strengthening and aerobic exercise may have a beneficial effect on mood, psychological well-being, bone health, appetite, and sleep. Further studies are needed to assess the impact of regular exercise and varying exercise intensities on the patient with ALS.

Assistive Technology for Mobility

As ALS progresses, the rehabilitation focus shifts from exercise to maintenance of independent mobility and function for as long as possible. Interventions include assistive devices such as canes, walkers, braces, hand splints, wheelchairs, and scooters; home equipment such as dressing aids, adapted utensils, grab bars, raised toilet seats, shower benches, and lifts; home modifications (ramps, wide doorways); and automobile adaptations, such as hand controls, environmental control units, and voice-activated software. These rehabilitation interventions are best provided by a multidisciplinary team that includes a physiatrist, physical therapist, occupational therapist, and orthotist.

Pain Management

Patients frequently have musculoskeletal pain syndromes, such as adhesive capsulitis (frozen shoulder), low back pain, and neck pain due to muscle weakness and inability to change positions. Measures to prevent adhesive capsulitis include range of motion exercises and adequate support for a hypotonic arm rather than allowing it to dangle at the patient's side. Low back pain can be triggered by an ill-fitting seating system. Preventive measures include a lumbar support for the wheelchair, a good cushion on a solid seat, the encouragement of frequent weight shifts, and a reclining back and tilt-in-space wheelchair. Neck pain associated with head drop is one of the most difficult musculoskeletal pain issues to remedy. A variety of cervical collars may be tried, but a head support on the wheelchair or a reclining lounge chair may be more comfortable than a collar. Nonpharmacologic measures such as massage and transcutaneous electrical nerve stimulation can also be used for pain control. Acetaminophen alone or combined with nonsteroidal anti-inflammatory drugs, lidocaine patches, or, if necessary, opioid medications can be used to alleviate musculoskeletal pain. The major concerns with opiate use are respiratory depression and constipation. The respiratory depression of opiates may be acceptable in the late and terminal stages of the disease when morphine is needed to relieve air hunger.

Dysphagia

Adequate swallowing function is necessary to maintain the nutritional status of the patient with ALS (unless a feeding tube is in place). If nutritional status is not properly maintained, patients tend to use muscle as fuel and thus lose muscle mass and strength earlier than they would otherwise [32]. Swallowing dysfunction may also precipitate aspiration pneumonia or respiratory failure. Early signs and symptoms of dysphagia are drooling, a wet voice, coughing during or after drinking thin liquids, nasal regurgitation, and requiring an excessive amount of time to complete meals. Patients should be referred to a speech pathologist when the first signs of dysphagia develop. Those with mild swallowing difficulties can be taught compensatory techniques to reduce the risk of aspiration and choking [33]. Recommendations may be given concerning modification of food consistencies. Feeding tube placement is indicated with the development of aspiration pneumonia, with loss of more than 10% of body weight, and when an excessive amount of time is required to eat such that quality of life is impaired.

Dysarthria

Early or mild dysarthria may be managed by having a speech therapist teach patients adaptive strategies, such as overarticulation and slowing of the speaking rate to avoid vocal fatigue. Speech therapy with the intent of improving speech quality has not been shown to be effective and is not indicated for ALS patients. In patients with hypernasal speech caused by palatal weakness and primarily lower motor neuron dysfunction, a palatal lift or augmentation prosthesis may improve speech clarity [34]. As dysarthria worsens, patients require alternative forms of communication. Low-technology interventions include letter and word boards for written communication in those with good hand function. Higher technology solutions include iPad (Apple, Inc., Cupertino, Calif) voice applications and more traditional augmentative communication devices with a voice synthesizer (i.e., DynaVox, Pittsburgh, Pa; Tobii Technology, Stockholm, Sweden). As long as one muscle, somewhere in the body, can be voluntarily activated (including the extraocular muscles), the patient should be able to operate a communication device. High-technology solutions to communication problems are not suitable for all patients. The most enduring systems are flexible so that the method of access can be modified as weakness progresses.

Pulmonary Rehabilitation (see also Chapter 150)

Respiratory failure is the primary cause of death in ALS. In the absence of underlying intrinsic pulmonary disease, the respiratory failure in ALS is purely mechanical. Because of muscle weakness, the lungs do not inflate fully on inspiration. Most patients with ALS remain asymptomatic until the FVC is less than 50% of predicted. Pulmonary function tests, particularly the FVC, should be monitored every few months, depending on rate of disease progression. Nocturnal hypoventilation is typically the earliest manifestation of respiratory insufficiency; symptoms include poor sleep with frequent awakening, nightmares, early morning headaches, and excessive daytime fatigue and sleepiness [35]. Another early sign of respiratory muscle weakness is a weak cough and difficulty in clearing secretions.

The management of respiratory failure in ALS involves prevention of infection and provision of noninvasive or invasive mechanical ventilatory assistance. All patients with ALS should receive a yearly influenza vaccination and a pneumococcal vaccination with boosters every 5 years. Patients with an inadequate cough, as determined by a peak cough flow measurement of 270 L/min or less, can be helped by manually assisted coughing or an in-exsufflator device that mechanically augments the cough [35]. Providing patients with supplemental oxygen should typically be avoided as it may suppress respiratory drive, exacerbate alveolar hypoventilation, and ultimately lead to carbon dioxide retention and respiratory arrest [36]. Supplemental oxygen is recommended only for patients with a concomitant pulmonary disease or as a comfort measure for those who decline assisted ventilation. Noninvasive positive pressure ventilation (NIPPV) is considered standard of care for patients with ALS. The American Academy of Neurology's practice parameter on ALS recommends that NIPPV be introduced when the FVC falls to 50% of predicted or earlier if the patient is symptomatic [37]. However, others have suggested that earlier introduction of NIPPV may further improve survival and quality of life [38,39]. With good patient acceptance, NIPPV can extend the life of an ALS patient well beyond that of available disease-modifying medications.

NIPPV can be delivered through a variety of oral or nasal mask interfaces with use of bilevel positive airway pressure machines or portable volume-cycled ventilators. Bilevel positive airway pressure is currently the most commonly used form of NIPPV. Gaining popularity are newer technologies that offer volume-assured pressure support and provide automatic inspiratory and expiratory pressure adjustments to meet the tidal volume or alveolar ventilation needs of patients with progressive restrictive lung disease. Initially, NIPPV is used at night. As FVC continues to decline, ventilator use can be extended into the day and eventually become continuous. Although studies have confirmed that use of NIPPV prolongs survival and may slow the decline of FVC [40,41], it is a temporary measure. Patients wishing to prolong their life to the fullest extent possible may consider invasive mechanical ventilation.

Discussion concerning respiratory failure should be initiated soon after the diagnosis of ALS is confirmed so that patients and their families can learn about their choices and, ideally, make a decision about invasive ventilator use in a noncrisis situation. These discussions should include both the benefits and limitations of invasive ventilation. An increasing number of patients are choosing tracheotomy and mechanical ventilation. In a recently published study, 31.3% of patients attending an ALS clinic chose mechanical ventilation with a median increase in survival of 16 months compared with nontracheostomized patients [42].

Before initiation of mechanical ventilation, patients should outline their wishes about withdrawal of treatment as part of an advance directive and inform their family and physicians; continued muscle atrophy and weakness may lead to a "locked-in" state in which patient communication is no longer possible. In one retrospective study, the most common reason for withdrawal of mechanical ventilation by ALS patients was a "loss of meaning in life." [43]

Procedures

Management of Sialorrhea

Botulinum toxin injection of the salivary glands is the preferred method for management of sialorrhea in patients who do not respond to pharmacologic therapy [13–15]. Botulinum toxins A and B have been found to be equally effective. The safety of injection is increased with ultrasound guidance. Another treatment option for the patient refractive to more conservative treatments is radiotherapy of the parotid glands [44].

Gastrostomy Tube

A gastrostomy tube is recommended in ALS patients when they show signs of nutritional deficiency (i.e., lose 10% of their weight). The American Academy of Neurology's practice parameter on ALS states that the morbidity and mortality of percutaneous endoscopic gastrostomy tube placement increase when the FVC falls below 50% of predicted [37] and recommends placement before that time. Some studies have shown that percutaneous endoscopic gastrostomy tubes can be safely placed with bilevel positive airway pressure assistance in patients with lower FVCs [45,46]. In addition, radiologically inserted gastrostomy tube placement appears to be safer, better tolerated in patients with ALS, and preferable in patients with low FVCs; less sedation is required, incidence of aspiration is lower, tube placement is more often successful, and acute respiratory decompensation observed with percutaneous endoscopic gastrostomy is avoided [47,48].

Tracheostomy

Every effort should be made to have a tracheotomy performed on a planned basis after a patient has chosen to use invasive ventilation. However, this is often not the case, and the procedure is commonly performed during a crisis situation. Patients should be given early access to unbiased literature describing the procedure and reviewing care and cost considerations to enable an informed decision. Once it is placed, a cuffless tracheostomy tube or a tube with a deflated cuff is preferred.

Potential Disease Complications

Disease complications include progressive weakness, joint contractures, musculoskeletal pain syndromes, osteoporosis, fractures due to falls, dysphagia, dehydration, impaired nutrition, aspiration, dysarthria, depression, progressive respiratory failure, pneumonia, pressure wounds, deep venous thrombosis, and death.

Potential Treatment Complications

The potential treatment complications include drug reactions (e.g., to riluzole, tricyclic antidepressants) and misplacement, malfunction, or infection of the percutaneous endoscopic gastrostomy tube or radiologically inserted gastrostomy tube.

Complications of long-term ventilation by tracheostomy are tracheomalacia, pneumonia, loss of all skeletal muscle function including extraocular movements causing a locked-in state, and dementia.

References

[1] de Carvalho M, Dengler R, Eisen A, et al. Electrodiagnostic criteria for diagnosis of ALS. Clin Neurophysiol 2008;119:497–503.

[2] Brooks BR, Miller RG, Swash M, Munsat TLWorld Federation of Neurology Research Group on Motor Neuron Diseases. El Escorial revisited: revised criteria for the diagnosis of amyotrophic lateral sclerosis. Amyotroph Lateral Scler Other Motor Neuron Disord 2000;1:293–9.

[3] Rosenfeld J, Swash M. What's in a name? Lumping or splitting ALS, PLS, PMA and other motor neuron diseases. Neurology 2006;66:624–5.

[4] Genetics home reference. Amyotrophic lateral sclerosis, http://ghr.nlm.nih.gov/condition/amyotrophic-lateral-sclerosis; [accessed December 2012].

[5] Paratore S, Pezzino S, Cavallaro S. Identification of pharmacological targets in amyotrophic lateral sclerosis through genomic analysis of deregulated genes and pathways. Curr Genomics 2012;13:321–33.

[6] Raaphorst J, de Visser M, Linssen WH, et al. The cognitive profile of amyotrophic lateral sclerosis: a meta-analysis. Amyotroph Lateral Scler 2010;11:27–37.

[7] Fujimura-Kiyono C, Kimura F, Ishida S, et al. Onset and spreading patterns of lower motor neuron involvements predict survival in sporadic amyotrophic lateral sclerosis. J Neurol Neurosurg Psychiatry 2011;82:1244–9.

[8] Bensimon G, Lacomblez L, Meininger V, et al. A controlled trial of riluzole in amyotrophic lateral sclerosis. N Engl J Med 1994;330:585–91.

[9] Lacomblez L, Bensimon G, Leigh PN, et al. Dose-ranging study of riluzole in amyotrophic lateral sclerosis. Lancet 1996;347:1425–31.

[10] Miller R, Mitchell J, Lyon M, Moore D. Riluzole for amyotrophic lateral sclerosis (ALS)/motor neuron disease (MND). Cochrane Database Syst Rev 2002;2, CD001447.

[11] de Carvalho M, Costa J, Swash M. Clinical trials in ALS: a review of the role of clinical and neurophysiological measurements. Amyotroph Lateral Scler Other Motor Neuron Disord 2005;6:202–12.

[12] Rosenfeld J. ALS combination treatment. Drug cocktails. Amyotroph Lateral Scler Other Motor Neuron Disord 2004;5:115–7.

[13] Guidubaldi A, Fasano A, Ialongo T, et al. Botulinum toxin A versus B in sialorrhea: a prospective, randomized, double-blind, crossover pilot study in patients with amyotrophic lateral sclerosis or Parkinson's disease. Mov Disord 2011;26:313–9.

[14] Gilio F, Iacovelli E, Frasca V, et al. Botulinum toxin type A for the treatment of sialorrhoea in amyotrophic lateral sclerosis: a clinical and neurophysiological study. Amyotroph Lateral Scler 2010;11:359–63.

[15] Costa J, Rocha ML, Ferreira J, et al. Botulinum toxin type-B improves sialorrhea and quality of life in bulbar onset amyotrophic lateral sclerosis. J Neurol 2008;255:545–50.

[16] Brooks B, Thisted R, Appel S, et al. Treatment of pseudobulbar affect in ALS with dextromethorphan/quinidine: a randomized trial. Neurology 2004;63:1364–70.

[17] Ganzini L, Johnston WS, Hoffman WF. Correlates of suffering in amyotrophic lateral sclerosis. Neurology 1999;52:1434–40.

[18] Lou J, Reeves A, Benice T, Sexton G. Fatigue and depression are associated with poor quality of life in ALS. Neurology 2003;60:122–3.

[19] Kubler A, Winter S, Ludolph A, et al. Severity of depressive symptoms and quality of life in patients with amyotrophic lateral sclerosis. Neurorehabil Neural Repair 2005;19:182–93.

[20] Dal Bello-Haas V, Florence JM, Krivickas LS. Therapeutic exercise for people with amyotrophic lateral sclerosis or motor neuron disease. Cochrane Database Syst Rev 2008;2:CD005229.

[21] ClinicalTrials.gov. ALS exercise. http://clinicaltrials.gov/ct2/results?term=ALS+exercise; [accessed December 2012].

[22] Beghi E, Logroscino G, Chiò A, et al. Amyotrophic lateral sclerosis, physical exercise, trauma and sports: results of a population-based pilot case-control study. Amyotroph Lateral Scler 2010;11:289–92.

[23] Francis K, Bach J, DeLisa J. Evaluation and rehabilitation of patients with adult motor neuron disease. Arch Phys Med Rehabil 1999;80:951–63.

[24] Dal Bello-Haas V, Florence JM, Kloos AD, et al. A randomized controlled trial of resistance exercise in individuals with ALS. Neurology 2007;68:2003–7.

[25] Lindeman E, Leffers P, Spaans F, et al. Strength training in patients with myotonic dystrophy and hereditary motor and sensory neuropathy: a randomized clinical trial. Arch Phys Med Rehabil 1995;76:612–20.

[26] Aitkens SG, McCrory MA, Kilmer DD, Bernauer EM. Moderate resistance exercise program: its effect in slowly progressive neuromuscular disease. Arch Phys Med Rehabil 1993;74:711–5.

[27] Agre JC, Rodriquez AA, Franke TM. Strength, endurance, and work capacity after muscle strengthening exercise in postpolio subjects. Arch Phys Med Rehabil 1997;78:681–6.

[28] Drory V, Goltsman E, Reznik J, et al. The value of muscle exercise in patients with amyotrophic lateral sclerosis. J Neurol Sci 2002;191:133–7.

[29] Kirkenezos I, Hernandez D, Bradley W, Moraes C. Regular exercise is beneficial to a mouse model of amyotrophic lateral sclerosis. Ann Neurol 2003;53:804–7.

[30] Veldink J, Bar P, Joosten E, et al. Sexual differences in onset of disease and response to exercise in a transgenic model of ALS. Neuromuscul Disord 2003;13:737–43.

[31] Kaspar B, Frost L, Christian L, et al. Synergy of insulin-like growth factor-1 and exercise in amyotrophic lateral sclerosis. Ann Neurol 2005;57:649–55.

[32] Braun MM, Osecheck M, Joyce NC. Nutrition assessment and management in amyotrophic lateral sclerosis. Phys Med Rehabil Clin N Am 2012;23:751–71.

[33] Strand EA, Miller RM, Yorkston KM, Hillel AD. Management of oral-pharyngeal dysphagia symptoms in amyotrophic lateral sclerosis. Dysphagia 1996;11:129–39.

[34] Esposito S, Mitsumoto H, Shanks M. Use of palatal lift and palatal augmentation prostheses to improve dysarthria in patients with amyotrophic lateral sclerosis: a case series. J Prosthet Dent 2000;83:90–8.

[35] Wolfe LF, Joyce NC, McDonald CM, et al. Management of pulmonary complications in neuromuscular disease. Phys Med Rehabil Clin N Am 2012;23:829–53.

[36] Gay P, Edmonds L. Severe hypercapnia after low flow oxygen therapy in patients with neuromuscular disease and diaphragmatic dysfunction. Mayo Clin Proc 1995;70:327–30.

[37] Miller RG, Jackson CE, Kasarskis EJ, et al. Practice parameter update: the care of the patient with amyotrophic lateral sclerosis: drug, nutritional, and respiratory therapies (an evidence-based review): report of the Quality Standards Subcommittee of the American Academy of Neurology. Neurology 2009;73:1218–26.

[38] Jackson C, Rosenfeld J, Moore D, et al. A preliminary evaluation of a prospective study of pulmonary function studies and symptoms of hypoventilation in ALS/MND patients. J Neurol Sci 2001;191:75–8.

[39] Bourke S, Tomlinson M, Williams T, et al. Effects of non-invasive ventilation on survival and quality of life in patients with amyotrophic lateral sclerosis: a randomised controlled trial. Lancet Neurol 2006;5:140–7.

[40] Kleopa KA, Sherman M, Neal B, et al. BiPAP improves survival and rate of pulmonary function decline in patients with ALS. J Neurol Sci 1999;164:82–8.

[41] Aboussouan L, Khan S, Banerjee M, et al. Objective measures of the efficacy of noninvasive positive-pressure ventilation in amyotrophic lateral sclerosis. Muscle Nerve 2001;24:403–9.

[42] Spataro R, Bono V, Marchese S, La Bella V. Tracheostomy mechanical ventilation in patients with amyotrophic lateral sclerosis: clinical features and survival analysis. J Neurol Sci 2012;323:66–70.

[43] Dreyer PS, Felding M, Klitnæs CS, Lorenzen CK. Withdrawal of invasive home mechanical ventilation in patients with advanced amyotrophic lateral sclerosis: ten years of Danish experience. J Palliat Med 2012;15:205–9.

[44] Kasarskis EJ, Hodskins J, St Clair WH. Unilateral parotid electron beam radiotherapy as palliative treatment for sialorrhea in amyotrophic lateral sclerosis. J Neurol Sci 2011;308:155–7.

[45] Gregory S, Siderowf A, Golaszewski A, et al. Gastrostomy insertion in ALS patients with low vital capacity: respiratory support and survival. Neurology 2002;58:485–7.

[46] Boitano L, Jordan T, Benditt J. Noninvasive ventilation allows gastrostomy tube placement in patients with advanced ALS. Neurology 2001;56:413–4.

[47] Blondet A, Lebigot J, Nicolas G, et al. Radiologic versus endoscopic placement of percutaneous gastrostomy in amyotrophic lateral sclerosis: multivariate analysis of tolerance, efficacy, and survival. J Vasc Interv Radiol 2010;21:527–33.

[48] Thornton F, Fotheringham T, Alexander M, et al. Amyotrophic lateral sclerosis: enteral nutrition provision—endoscopic or radiologic gastrostomy? Radiology 2002;224:713–7.

[49] Czaplinski A, Yen AA, Appel SH. Forced vital capacity (FVC) as an indicator of survival and disease progression in an ALS clinic population. J Neurol Neurosurg Psychiatry 2006;77:390–2.

[50] Baumann F, Henderson RD, Morrison SC, et al. Use of respiratory function tests to predict survival in amyotrophic lateral sclerosis. Amyotroph Lateral Scler 2010;11:194–202.

CHAPTER 133

Movement Disorders

Kenneth H. Silver, MD

Synonyms

Extrapyramidal disease
Hypokinesias
Hyperkinesias
Dyskinesias

ICD-9 Codes

307.2	**Tics**
307.20	**Tic disorder, unspecified**
307.22	**Chronic motor tic disorder**
307.23	**Gilles de la Tourette disorder**
332	**Parkinson disease**
332.0	**Parkinsonism or Parkinson disease: primary, idiopathic**
332.1	**Secondary parkinsonism**
	Parkinsonism due to drugs
333.0	**Other degenerative diseases of the basal ganglia**
	Progressive supranuclear ophthalmoplegia
	Shy-Drager syndrome
333.1	**Essential and other specified forms of tremor**
333.2	**Myoclonus**
333.4	**Huntington chorea**
333.5	**Other choreas**
333.6	**Idiopathic torsion dystonia**
333.84	**Organic writers' cramp**
781.0	**Abnormal involuntary movements: abnormal head movements, spasms, fasciculation, tremor**

ICD-10 Codes

F95.9	**Tic disorder, unspecified**
F95.1	**Chronic motor or vocal tic disorder**
F95.2	**Tourette's disorder**
G20	**Parkinson's disease**
G21.9	**Secondary parkinsonism, unspecified**
G21.19	**Other induced secondary parkinsonism**
G23.9	**Degenerative disease of basal ganglia, unspecified**
G23.1	**Progressive supranuclear ophthalmoplegia**
G90.3	**Multi-system degeneration of the autonomic nervous system**
G25.0	**Essential tremor, familial**
G25.3	**Myoclonus**
G10	**Huntington's disease**
G25.5	**Chorea NOS**
G24.1	**Genetic torsion dystonia**
G25.89	**Other specified extrapyramidal and movement disorders**
R25.1	**Tremor, unspecified**

Definition

Involuntary movement disorders can be characterized by either too little (hypokinetic) or too much (hyperkinetic) movement. Hypokinetic problems include Parkinson disease and Parkinson-like conditions, such as progressive supranuclear palsy, vascular or trauma-induced parkinsonism, and multisystem atrophy (which encompasses the related disorders of Shy-Drager syndrome, striatonigral degeneration, and olivopontocerebellar degeneration). Hyperkinetic disorders include parkinsonian and nonparkinsonian tremor, tics, Gilles de la Tourette syndrome, dystonia, dyskinesias (including tardive dyskinesias), hemifacial spasm, athetosis, chorea (including Huntington disease), hemiballismus, myoclonus, and asterixis [1].

Essential tremor, the most common movement disorder, is 5 to 10 times more prevalent than Parkinson disease in the general population. Parkinson disease affects 1 million Americans including 1% of those older than 60 years. Idiopathic Parkinson disease constitutes approximately 85% of all the Parkinson-like conditions; neuroleptic-induced Parkinson disease (7%-9%), vascular parkinsonism (3%), multisystem atrophy (2.5%), and progressive supranuclear palsy (1.5%) represent much smaller fractions. Relatively rare, Huntington disease occurs with a frequency in the population as low as 0.004% by some estimates [2,3].

Symptoms

Tremors, the most common form of involuntary movement disorders, are characterized by rhythmic oscillations of a body part. Tremors can be classified as to the situation in which they are most prominent, that is, most pronounced at rest or with movement. Tremors with movement are subdivided into those occurring with maintained posture (postural or static tremor, tested by holding the arms out in front), with movement from point to point (kinetic or intentional tremor, tested by finger to nose pointing), or with only a specific type of movement (task-specific tremor). Tremors that are at their worst at rest are exclusively associated with Parkinson disease or other parkinsonian states (such as those produced by neuroleptics) [2,4].

Parkinsonian patients commonly show a resting tremor, slowness of movement or bradykinesia, and a form of increased muscle tone called rigidity (see Chapter 141 for more details). Other common features are reduction in movements of facial expression resulting in "masked facies," stooped posture, and reduction of the amplitude of movements (hypometria). Also seen are changes in speech to a soft monotone (hypophonia) and small, less legible handwriting (micrographia). Walking becomes slower, stride length is reduced, and pivoting is replaced with a series of small steps (turning "en bloc") [5,6]. The nonmotor symptoms associated with Parkinson disease can be equally disabling: fatigue, pain, and neuropsychiatric disturbances, among others [3]. The following syndromes typically are manifested with the listed features in addition to the characteristic symptoms of Parkinson disease (tremor and rigidity) [7].

- Shy-Drager syndrome: autonomic failure with prominent postural hypotension
- Progressive supranuclear palsy: reduction in vertical gaze and slowing of eye movements
- Vascular parkinsonism: early dementia with brisk tendon reflexes
- Multiple head trauma, "parkinsonism pugilistica": early dementia with brisk tendon reflexes
- Olivopontocerebellar degeneration: prominent intention tremor, imbalance, and ataxia

Tics are sustained nonrhythmic muscle contractions that are rapid and stereotyped, often occurring in the same extremity or body part during times of stress. The muscles of the face and neck are usually involved, with movement of a rotational sort away from the body's midline. They are commonly familial and often seen in otherwise normal children between the ages of 5 and 10 years and usually disappear by the end of adolescence. Tourette syndrome is characterized by motor and vocal tics lasting for more than 1 year and may involve involuntary use of obscenities and obscene gestures, although such behavior may be mild and transient and occurs only in a minority of afflicted persons [6,8].

Dystonias are slow, sustained contractions of muscles that frequently cause twisting movements or abnormal postures. The disorder resembles athetosis but shows a more sustained static contraction. When rapid movements are involved, they are usually repetitive and continuous. Dystonia often increases with emotional or physical stress, anxiety, pain, or fatigue and disappears with sleep. The dystonias are further classified as focal, segmental, or multifocal on the basis of the distribution of muscles affected. Symptoms of hemifacial spasm usually begin in the orbicularis oculi and later involve other muscles innervated by cranial nerve VII [1,6,9].

Tardive dyskinesia is a condition characterized by involuntary, choreiform movements of the face and tongue associated with chronic neuroleptic medication use. Common movements include chewing, sucking, mouthing, licking, "fly-catching movements," puckering, and smacking (buccal-lingual-masticatory syndrome). Choreiform movements of the trunk and extremities can also occur along with dystonic movements of the neck and trunk.

Athetosis is characterized by involuntary, slow, writhing, and repetitious movements. They are slower than choreiform movements and less sustained than dystonia. Athetosis may be seen alone or in combination with other movement disorders and itself leads to bizarre but characteristic postures. Any part of the body can be affected, but it is usually the face and distal upper extremities that are involved. Chorea is manifested as nonstereotyped, unpredictable, and jerky movements that interfere with purposeful motion. The movements are rapid, erratic, and complex and can be seen in any or all body parts but usually involve the oral structures, causing abnormal speech and respiratory patterns. Hemiballismus is an uncommon disorder consisting of extremely violent flinging of the arms and legs on one side of the body.

Myoclonus is one of the most common involuntary movement disorders of central nervous system origin. It is characterized by sudden, jerky, irregular contractions of a muscle or groups of muscles. It can be subdivided into stimulus-sensitive myoclonus (reflex myoclonus), appearing with volitional movement, muscle stretch, or superficial stimuli such as touch, and non–stimulus- sensitive myoclonus, which occurs at rest (spontaneous myoclonus). Myoclonic movements can be either irregular or periodic [1,6].

Physical Examination

A complete physical examination is key to ruling out treatable causes of the presenting movement disorder, such as infectious (encephalitis), medication side effect (tardive dyskinesia), genetic (Tourette syndrome), or endocrinologic (tremor-associated thyrotoxicosis).

A good neurologic examination of patients thought to have a movement disorder helps identify an underlying causative condition, such as stroke (e.g., cerebrovascular-based Parkinson disease, hemiballismus, or ataxia), tumor, brain trauma, or even peripheral nerve injury–associated focal dystonias. Other aspects of physical examination focus on characterization of the type of abnormal movements by detailing of their body distribution (limb, trunk, head, face, or widespread), their quality (tremor, writhing, explosive, rigidity), their frequency (rapid and repetitive or slow and sustained), and their general quantity or lack thereof (hyperactive or hypoactive).

For instance, essential tremor (senile tremor) is usually rapid and fine and occurs when the patient is asked to hold the arms outstretched, whereas parkinsonian tremor decreases with voluntary movement. Intention (cerebellar) tremor is slow and broad, occurring at the end of a purposeful motion, as when the patient executes a finger to nose task. In addition to tests of cerebellar function, tests for upper motor neuron syndrome (hyperreflexia, spasticity, presence of Babinski sign) may assist the examiner in distinguishing movement disorders more commonly associated with stroke or brain injury.

Functional Limitations

Functional limitations depend on the severity of the movement disorder. Some tremors and tics may be more a cosmetic and psychological concern, whereas severe postural disturbance in Parkinson disease or stroke-induced ataxia can clearly impair ambulation or upper extremity control. In Parkinson disease, postural changes, such as stooping with the development of permanent kyphosis, can occur after years of disease. Many physical activities require additional effort to be performed. Manual dexterity is invariably impaired as Parkinson disease worsens, affecting many daily activities, such as dressing, cutting food, writing, and handling small objects such as coins [10]. Soft, monotone, hoarse voice quality and imprecise articulation, together with restricted facial expression (masked facies), contribute to limitations in communication in a large majority of individuals with Parkinson disease, with 30% reporting it the most debilitating deficit. These functional losses negatively affect quality of life, leading to declining efficiency at work and, in many cases, abandonment of many leisure activities. Depression and social isolation are commonly seen in patients with Parkinson disease.

In cervical dystonia (torticollis), social stigmatization is a major concern, as are functional impairments, which can include driving, reading, and activities that involve looking down and using the hands. In another focal dystonia, writer's or occupational cramp, the symptoms are manifested in a certain posture or position; for instance, a patient may be able to write at a blackboard but not seated at a desk. With lingual involvement in oromandibular dystonia, the tongue has abnormal movements during speaking or deglutition. The result of such dystonias is impairment of speech and eating [9]. In Huntington chorea, along with the choreiform movement, progressive dementia and emotional and behavioral abnormalities are seen. As the disease progresses, the presentation becomes less choreiform and more parkinsonian and dystonic (i.e., restricted motions, immobility, and unsteadiness of gait). Intellectual impairment and psychosis invariably occur and progress rapidly to become the most disabling features [6].

Diagnostic Studies

In most cases of movement disorders, such as Parkinson disease, tardive dyskinesia, essential tremor, and dystonia, the diagnosis is made on the grounds of clinical examination and history; no one specific test is pathognomonic for the disease [5–7]. Positron emission tomography and single-photon emission computed tomography scans are able to identify altered brain dopaminergic activity; however, their superiority over clinical diagnosis is unclear at this time [6]. Evaluation for potential causes of the other movement disorders, such as stroke, traumatic brain injury, normal-pressure hydrocephalus, tumor, infection, and metabolic or endocrinologic disease, should be performed with appropriate tests, including head and spinal magnetic resonance imaging and computed tomography, cerebrospinal fluid analysis, and blood serum analysis. Electrodiagnostic tests (electromyography and nerve conduction studies) may be useful in some cases, such as focal dystonias, to rule out coexisting or causative peripheral nerve entrapment. Electroencephalography is often helpful in distinguishing focal seizures from myoclonus or other repetitive movement presentations [11]. More tests may be necessary to confirm or to exclude other diagnoses, such as human immunodeficiency virus–related diseases, central nervous system infection, toxic exposures, Wilson disease, and psychiatric illnesses. Videofluoroscopy should be ordered to more accurately characterize swallow dysfunction and to assist with treatment planning when the clinical examination findings or symptoms suggest dysphagia.

Differential Diagnosis

Seizures
Psychiatric illness
Spasticity, spasms

Treatment

Initial

Treatment is highly dependent on which specific category of movement disorder is present. Typically, pharmacologic treatment is initiated when the symptoms become severe enough to cause discomfort or disability (Fig. 133.1).

Antiparkinson medications replace dopamine (levodopa), act as a postsynaptic (dopamine) agonist, increase the availability of levodopa or dopamine by preventing their metabolism (catechol-*O*-methyltransferase, monamine oxidase B inhibitors), or reestablish the dopamine-acetylcholine balance in the striatum (anticholinergics). Levodopa in combination with carbidopa (Sinemet) continues to be the most effective medication for treatment of Parkinson disease symptoms, but it is usually not the first medication given to those newly diagnosed, particularly in younger patients. The dopamine agonists bromocriptine (Parlodel), ropinirole (Requip), and pramipexole (Mirapex) or the recently approved rotigotine (Neupro) transdermal patch can be used as monotherapies in mild, early Parkinson disease, as can the monamine oxidase B inhibitors selegiline (Eldepryl, Zelapar) and rasagiline (Azilect). Loss of levodopa efficacy usually develops within 3 to 5 years after the medication is begun, so an effort is made to manage early Parkinson disease with other medications. A guiding principle is to start levodopa treatment in patients with symptoms that interfere with the performance of daily life functions despite other treatment. Its long-term use is associated with the development of motor fluctuations and dyskinesias. Over time, as the disease worsens, the patient's frequency of levodopa dosing and the total dose needed will increase, along with the need for other supplemental medications, such as the dopamine agonists and monamine oxidase B inhibitors, to help counter

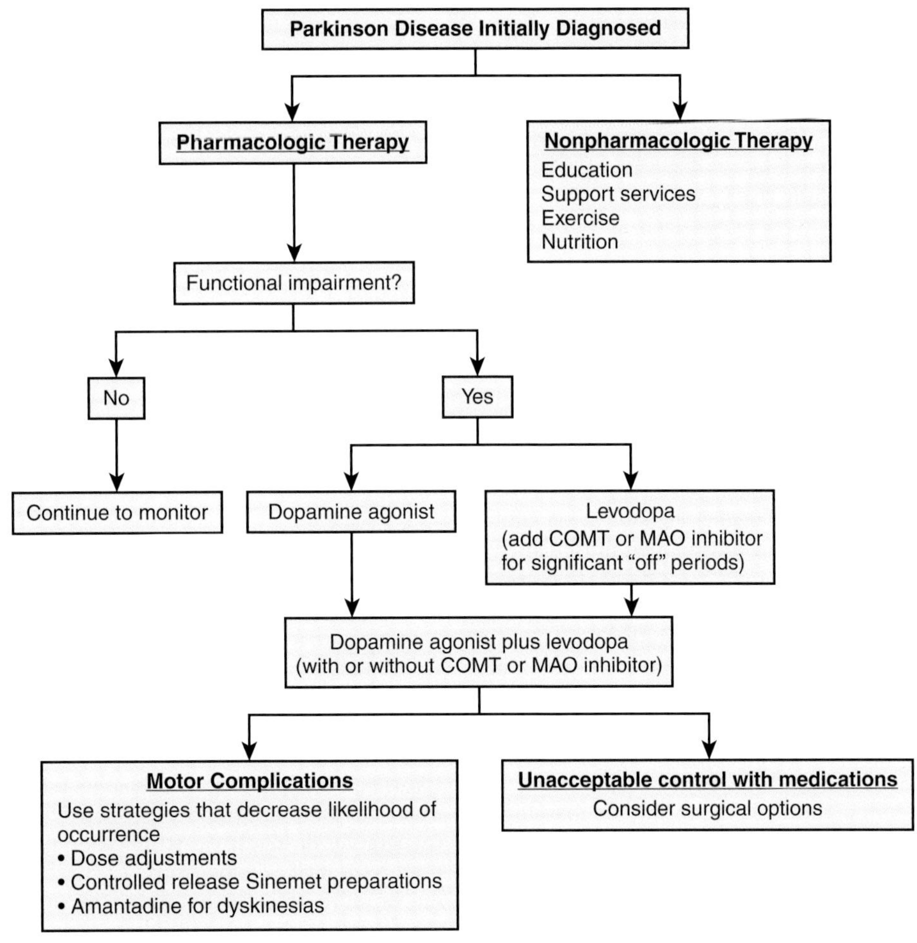

FIGURE 133.1 Algorithm for medication management of Parkinson disease. *COMT,* catechol-O-methyltransferase; *MAO,* monamine oxidase.

worsening motor fluctuations [12]. For patients with significant "off time," the catechol-*O*-methyltransferase inhibitors entacapone (Comtan) and tolcapone (Tasmar) are used in combination with levodopa/carbidopa, slowing its breakdown and augmenting its effectiveness. Because hepatic disease has been reported with tolcapone use, liver function test monitoring is required.

Anticholinergic drugs such as trihexyphenidyl (Artane) and benztropine (Cogentin) are used less widely today because of their side effect profile and limited efficacy for rigidity and bradykinesia. They are useful primarily for younger patients with tremor as their primary symptom [3,5,6,12,13].

A continuous pump-based infusion of levodopa/carbidopa directly into the small intestines through an implanted catheter has shown efficacy in Parkinson disease patients suffering motor fluctuations and is presently undergoing clinical trials the United States [14].

Propranolol is the most useful medication in treating essential tremor (the most common symptomatic tremor), task-specific tremor, and action tremor. Other beta blockers have fewer side effects but are less effective. The anticonvulsant primidone and the benzodiazepine clonazepam are also effective antitremor drugs. Gabapentin and botulinum toxin injections may be of some benefit in tremor management [1,2,6]. Tics can be managed with neuroleptics; pimozide and haloperidol are generally effective, but sedation limits their use. Newer atypical neuroleptics may have fewer side effects, including risperidone, quetiapine, olanzapine, and clozapine. Other medications shown to be of some benefit include clonazepam, clonidine, calcium channel blockers, and antidepressant agents [1,6]. Anticholinergic medications, such as trihexyphenidyl and benztropine, are the most effective oral agents for both generalized and focal dystonias in younger patients. Baclofen (either orally or by intrathecal pump), carbamazepine, and the benzodiazepines, such as diazepam and clonazepam, are sometimes helpful. Dopamine-blocking or dopamine-depleting agents may be used to treat some patients with dystonia. Focal dystonias are now commonly treated with botulinum toxin injections [6,9] (see the section on procedures).

Replacement of typical antipsychotic drugs with the atypical neuroleptics, such as clozapine and risperidone, is useful to control psychosis in patients with tardive dyskinesia without worsening of symptoms. Other drugs, such as benzodiazepines, adrenergic antagonists, and dopamine agonists, may also be beneficial for suppression of the movements. The most important step in the treatment of tardive dyskinesia is prevention by limiting the use of neuroleptic medications [15]. The response to drug therapy has been poor in patients with ataxia; many agents have been touted as useful (propranolol, isoniazid, carbamazepine, clonazepam, tryptophan, buspirone, thyroid-stimulating hormone), but none has demonstrated efficacy [16]. A number of drugs have been used to treat myoclonus and can be effective in some situations. These include diazepam, clonazepam, valproate, and levetiracetam (Keppra) as well as botulinum toxin injections [11].

Rehabilitation

In general, the patient with Parkinson disease needs to be counseled to maintain a reasonable level of activity at all costs as physical exertion becomes more difficult and the risk of deconditioning increases. Exercises focus on proper body alignment (upright posture) and postural reflexes (response to dynamic balance challenges) as well as on limb range of motion and strengthening of proximal musculature to assist in stair climbing and coming to a stand. Exercises are also aimed at the restoration of diminished reciprocal limb motions and an increase in step length and can include treadmill training. A number of randomized studies in Parkinson disease patients have demonstrated benefits such as improved walking speed and endurance, step length, and balance with several forms of exercise [17,18].

The tendency to freeze can be reduced with visual targets, such as markers on the floor, counting, or marching rhythmically. The difficulty in rising from sitting surfaces can be addressed with elevated sitting surfaces (chair, toilet) and strategically placed grab rails or bars (bed, bathtub). Although wheeled walkers are useful in assisting ambulation, particularly by preventing backward instability, patients with significant postural deficits may prefer more stable devices, such as a supermarket shopping cart or walking behind a wheelchair. Adaptive equipment is provided when deficits in upper extremity control limit efficient and safe function [19,20]. Speech therapy is useful in patients with Parkinson disease to improve articulation and loudness as well as to diagnose and to manage dysphagia [13,21].

In tremor, measures to reduce or to alleviate anxiety (e.g., biofeedback, relaxation exercises) are useful, as are strategies to control oscillation excursion with weights or other mechanical compensations [20]. Lifestyle changes may include restriction of caffeine intake or other stimulants that may temporarily augment symptoms. In addition, alcohol consumption may lead to transient improvement for many with essential tremor [2,6].

Stretching exercises may be important for maintenance or recovery of range of motion for affected joints in a dystonic limb. Certain types of occupation-based focal limb dystonias (e.g., writer's or musician's cramp) may be treated with muscle reeducation techniques, including biofeedback. A regular program of stretching exercises may assist affected individuals in regaining full range of motion after a botulinum toxin injection has weakened a dystonic muscle. Some patients use so-called sensory tricks to temporarily relieve their symptoms. These commonly involve touching or stroking a particular spot on the skin. In addition, in some patients, certain types of braces may provide the same stimulation and be equally effective [14,20].

Ataxic patients may benefit from rehabilitation to help them learn compensatory techniques for performance of basic self-care and occupational activities and to assess the benefits of weighted bracelets or similar devices to damp the oscillations. Gait training and education in the use of assistive devices for walking can prevent falls and enhance mobility in the ataxic individual. In disorders involving athetosis, ballismus, or Huntington disease, careful weighting of the extremities can help at times. Rehabilitation techniques involving improvement of coactivation and trunk stability, rhythmic stabilization, and traditional relaxation techniques including biofeedback have been mentioned as reasonable strategies. Some have suggested value in oral desensitization when hyperreactivity to sensory stimuli exists for reducing excessive facial movements in tardive dyskinesia, but other rehabilitation strategies are not of proven utility [20].

Procedures

Botulinum toxin injections are beneficial in numerous hyperkinetic movement disorders, including focal dystonias, tremor, and myoclonus. Trigger point injections may provide relief in painful muscles associated with focal dystonias (e.g., cervical torticollis).

The muscles selected for botulinum toxin injection are based on understanding of the primary clinical patterns of spasticity or dystonia. Direct injection by palpation technique may be appropriate for superficial muscles; electromyography or electrical stimulation guidance is commonly used to identify deeper muscles. Each muscle is injected in one or more sites, the number being a function of the size of the muscle. Dosage is variable but typically does not exceed 400 units total body dose for a 3-month period. Botulinum toxin A is reconstituted in the vial with preservative-free normal saline, at varying dilutions depending on the muscle size. For example, an average size muscle, such as flexor carpi radialis, could receive a concentration of 10 units per 0.1 mL.

The skin is cleaned with an alcohol or iodine swab and allowed to dry. When electromyography or electrical stimulation guidance is used, a specialized needle with an exposed tip connected by wire to the recording or stimulating device is needed. Needles are typically 37 mm in length and 27-gauge; larger or smaller needles are often needed, depending on muscle size and depth. In adults, preanesthetization of the skin is usually unnecessary; in children, local anesthetic creams are helpful. When botulinum toxin is injected, aspiration of the syringe to prevent injection into a blood vessel is standard technique. Before the injection, informed consent is obtained.

For Parkinson patients, cell transplants and gene therapies continue as experimental procedures still under investigation [13].

Surgery

Deep brain stimulation (subthalamic nuclei, globus pallidus) has been proven efficacious and has largely replaced neuroablative lesion procedures, such as thalamotomy and pallidotomy, for Parkinson disease [1,6,22]. Both deep brain stimulation and ablative surgery are also used for severe cases of other movement disorders, such as tremor or dystonia. In addition, peripheral destructive procedures, such as myectomy, rhizotomy, and peripheral nerve denervation, are occasionally performed on individuals with dystonic limbs who have proved refractory to more conventional management.

Potential Disease Complications

Many of the movement disorders, particularly Parkinson disease, are progressive and can result in muscle weakness and immobility, severe limb contractures, aspiration of food and respiratory compromise, social isolation and depression, and intellectual impairment and dementia.

Potential Treatment Complications

Antiparkinson medications may have numerous side effects, including nausea and other gastrointestinal symptoms, drowsiness, confusion, hallucinations, psychosis, and motor dyskinesia. Similar adverse medication effects are described with other agents used to suppress unwanted movements. Botulinum toxin is generally well tolerated but can cause transient unwanted weakness in target or adjacent muscles, including dysphagia. Risks associated with surgical approaches to central nervous system structures are considerable and need to be properly weighed before these options are selected [1,6,22].

References

[1] Fahn S, Jankovic J, Hallett M. Principles and practices of movement disorders. 2nd ed. Philadelphia: Saunders Elsevier; 2011.
[2] Aboud H, Ahmed A, Fernandez H. Essential tremor: choosing the right management plan for your patient. Cleve Clin J Med 2011;78:821–8.
[3] Fernandez H. Updates in the medical management of Parkinson disease. Cleve Clin J Med 2012;79:28–35.
[4] Chen JJ, Lee KC. Nonparkinsonism movement disorders in the elderly. Consult Pharm 2006;21:58–71.
[5] Nutt J, Wooten G. Diagnosis and initial management of Parkinson's disease. N Engl J Med 2005;353:1021–7.
[6] Jankovic J. Movement disorders. In: Daroff R, Fenichel G, Jankovic J, Mazziotta J, editors. Bradley's neurology in clinical practice. Philadelphia: WB Saunders; 2012. p. 1762–801.
[7] Weiner WJ. A differential diagnosis of parkinsonism. Rev Neurol Dis 2005;2:124–31.
[8] Scahill L, Sukhodolsky DG, Williams SK, Leckman JF. Public health significance of tic disorders in children and adolescents. Adv Neurol 2005;96:240–8.
[9] Tarsy D, Simon DK. Dystonia. N Engl J Med 2006;355:818–29.
[10] Chapuis S, Ouchchane L, Metz O, et al. Impact of the motor complications of Parkinson's disease on quality of life. Mov Disord 2005;20:224–30.
[11] Caviness JN, Truong DD. Myoclonus. Handb Clin Neurol 2011; 100:399–420.
[12] Pahwa R, Factor D, Lyons K, et al. Practice parameter: treatment of Parkinson disease with motor fluctuations and dyskinesia (an evidence-based review). Report of the Quality Standards Subcommittee of the American Academy of Neurology. Neurology 2006;66:983–95.
[13] Hauser R. Parkinson disease treatment and management. http://emedicine.medscape.com/article/1831191. Updated July 30, 2012. Accessed October 2012.
[14] Santos-Garcia D, Macias M, Llaneza M, et al. Experience with continuous levodopa enteral infusion (Duodopa) in patients with advanced Parkinson's disease in a secondary level hospital. Neurologia 2010;25:536–43.
[15] Margolese HC, Chouinard G, Kolivakis TT, et al. Tardive dyskinesia in the era of typical and atypical antipsychotics. Part 2: incidence and management strategies in patients with schizophrenia. Can J Psychiatry 2005;50:703–14.
[16] Ogawa M. Pharmacological treatments of cerebellar ataxia. Cerebellum 2004;3:107–11.
[17] De Goede C, Keus S, Kwakkel G, Wagenaar R. The effect of physical therapy in Parkinson's disease: a research synthesis. Arch Phys Med Rehabil 2001;82:509–15.
[18] Tomlinson CL, Patel S, Meek C, et al. Physiotherapy versus placebo or no intervention in Parkinson's disease. Cochrane Database Syst Rev 2012;7, CD002817.
[19] Suchowersky O, Gronseth G, Perlmutter J, et al. Practice parameter: neuroprotective strategies and alternative therapies for Parkinson disease (an evidence-based review). Report of the Quality Standards Subcommittee of the American Academy of Neurology. Neurology 2006;66:976–82.
[20] Francisco G, Kothari S, Schiess M, Kaldis T. Rehabilitation of persons with Parkinson's disease and other movement disorders. In: DeLisa JA, Gans BM, Walsh NE, editors. Physical medicine and rehabilitation: principles and practice. 4th ed. Philadelphia: Lippincott Williams & Wilkins; 2005. p. 809–28.
[21] Ramig L, Sapir S, Fox C, Countryman S. Changes in vocal loudness following intensive voice treatment (LSVT) in individuals with Parkinson's disease: a comparison with untreated patients and normal age-matched controls. Mov Disord 2001;16:79–83.
[22] Weaver FM, Follett K, Stern M, et al. Bilateral deep brain stimulation vs. best medical therapy for patients with advanced Parkinson disease: a randomized controlled trial. JAMA 2009;301:63–73.

CHAPTER 134

Multiple Sclerosis

Ann-Marie Thomas, MD, PT

Synonyms

Disseminated sclerosis
Focal sclerosis
Insular sclerosis

ICD-9 Code

340 Disseminated or multiple sclerosis
Brain stem
Cord
Generalized

ICD-10 Code

G35 Multiple sclerosis

Definition

Multiple sclerosis (MS) can be defined as an inflammatory disorder that results in damage, primarily to myelin sheaths and oligodendrocytes and less so to axons and nerve cells, in the central nervous system [1,2].

The prevalence of MS has been estimated at 300,000 to 400,000 in the United States and 2 million worldwide [3]. The disease usually becomes clinically apparent between the ages of 20 and 40 years, with a peak incidence at 24 to 30 years and onset as late as the seventh decade [3]. The disease appears twice as likely to develop in women as in men, and whites are more frequently diagnosed than are other races [3]. Although African Americans may experience greater MS-related disability than white individuals do, the disease progresses similarly for both races [3,4].

There are four common clinical courses in MS:

- Relapsing-remitting MS: Patients experience episodes of acute worsening of neurologic function followed by periods of remission. Patients may exhibit residual deficits after the episode of exacerbation. Most patients start with this course.
- Secondary progressive MS: Patients initially experience a relapsing-remitting course followed by progression of the disease with or without additional episodes of exacerbation and improvement. Most patients eventually transition to this disease course.
- Primary progressive MS: Patients experience a relentless progression of symptoms from the onset [5,6].
- Progressive relapsing MS: Patients experience a baseline progressive course with episodes of acute relapses followed by a return to the baseline progressive course.

MS can be diagnosed if there is evidence of two attacks disseminated in time and space with clinical, laboratory, or imaging evidence of at least two lesions in the brain or spinal cord [1–3,7]. Evidence may be obtained from clinical findings, magnetic resonance imaging, cerebrospinal fluid analysis, or visual evoked potentials [6,7]. Other diseases that could explain the symptoms must be excluded (see differential diagnosis) [8,9]. The most recent guidelines and revisions do not recommend the use of "clinically definite MS" or "probable MS"; the outcome of a diagnostic evaluation is MS, "possible MS," or "not MS" (Table 134.1) [2,6,7].

Symptoms

Symptoms of MS may involve multiple systems [10,11] (Table 134.2). Motor symptoms typically include weakness and spasticity [11]. Up to 85% of patients with MS may experience spasticity, and as many as a third may be affected by spasticity that is severe enough to diminish their quality of life [12]. Patients with MS may report paroxysmal spasms or nocturnal spasms.

MS may be the cause of decreased or even absent sensation in various body parts, including sensory levels that most often affect the trunk. Paresthesia (uncomfortable abnormal sensation that may be described by the patient as pain, pins and needles, or tingling) can occur in up to 50% of patients with MS and most commonly is neuropathic. Lhermitte sign is an electric shock–like sensation that radiates down the spine to the legs when the neck is flexed [10]. It may occur in up to 40% of patients with MS [7]. Multiple pain syndromes may occur in patients with MS [11,13] (Table 134.3). Visual symptoms may include optic neuritis that results from inflammation of the optic nerves and typically is manifested as retro-orbital pain or painful eye movements [14]. Visual deficits can range from mild distortions to complete visual loss [14]. Scotoma may be present as an area in the visual field with absent or impaired vision and dyschromatopsia as imperfect color vision [14]. Ocular motor deficits usually include internuclear ophthalmoplegia and nystagmus and are manifested as diplopia, blurry vision, and reading fatigue [14].

Table 134.1 The 2010 McDonald Criteria for Diagnosis of Multiple Sclerosis

Clinical Presentation	Additional Data Needed for MS Diagnosis
≥2 attacks*; objective clinical evidence of ≥2 lesions or objective clinical evidence of 1 lesion with reasonable historical evidence of a prior attack†	None‡
≥2 attacks*; objective clinical evidence of 1 lesion	Dissemination in space, demonstrated by: ≥1 T2 lesion in at least 2 of 4 MS-typical regions of the CNS (periventricular, juxtacortical, infratentorial, or spinal cord)§; or Await a further clinical attack* implicating a different CNS site
1 attack*; objective clinical evidence of ≥2 lesions	Dissemination in time, demonstrated by: Simultaneous presence of asymptomatic gadolinium-enhancing and nonenhancing lesions at any time; or A new T2 and/or gadolinium-enhancing lesion(s) on follow-up MRI, irrespective of its timing with reference to a baseline scan; or Await a second clinical attack*
1 attack*; objective clinical evidence of 1 lesion (clinically isolated syndrome)	Dissemination in space and time, demonstrated by: For DIS: ≥1 T2 lesion in at least 2 of 4 MS-typical regions of the CNS (periventricular, juxtacortical, infratentorial, or spinal cord)§; or Await a second clinical attack* implicating a different CNS site; and For DIT: Simultaneous presence of asymptomatic gadolinium-enhancing and nonenhancing lesions at any time; or A new T2 and/or gadolinium-enhancing lesion(s) on follow-up MRI, irrespective of its timing with reference to a baseline scan; or Await a second clinical attack*
Insidious neurological progression suggestive of MS (PPMS)	1 year of disease progression (retrospectively or prospectively determined) plus 2 of 3 of the following criteria§: 1. Evidence for DIS in the brain based on ≥1 T2 lesions in the MS-characteristic (periventricular, juxtacortical, or infratentorial) regions 2. Evidence for DIS in the spinal cord based on ≥2 T2 lesions in the cord 3. Positive CSF (isoelectric focusing evidence of oligoclonal bands and/or elevated IgG index)

If the criteria are fulfilled and there is no better explanation for the clinical presentation, the diagnosis is "MS"; if suspicious, but the criteria are not completely met, the diagnosis is "possible MS"; if another diagnosis arises during the evaluation that better explains the clinical presentation, then the diagnosis is "not MS."

MS, multiple sclerosis; *CNS,* central nervous system; *MRI,* magnetic resonance imaging; *DIS,* dissemination in space; *DIT,* dissemination in time; *PPMS,* primary progressive multiple sclerosis; *CSF,* cerebrospinal fluid; *IgG,* immunoglobulin G.

*An attack (relapse; exacerbation) is defined as patient-reported or objectively observed events typical of an acute inflammatory demyelinating event in the CNS, current or historical, with duration of at least 24 hours, in the absence of fever or infection. It should be documented by contemporaneous neurological examination, but some historical events with symptoms and evolution characteristic for MS, but for which no objective neurological findings are documented, can provide reasonable evidence of a prior demyelinating event. Reports of paroxysmal symptoms (historical or current) should, however, consist of multiple episodes occurring over not less than 24 hours. Before a definite diagnosis of MS can be made, at least 1 attack must be corroborated by findings on neurological examination, visual evoked potential response in patients reporting prior visual disturbance, or MRI consistent with demyelination in the area of the CNS implicated in the historical report of neurological symptoms.

†Clinical diagnosis based on objective clinical findings for 2 attacks is most secure. Reasonable historical evidence for 1 past attack, in the absence of documented objective neurological findings, can include historical events with symptoms and evolution characteristics for a prior inflammatory demyelinating event; at least 1 attack, however, must be supported by objective findings.

‡No additional tests are required. However, it is desirable that any diagnosis of MS be made with access to imaging based on these criteria. If imaging or other tests (for instance, CSF) are undertaken and are negative, extreme caution needs to be taken before making a diagnosis of MS, and alternative diagnoses must be considered. There must be no better explanation for the clinical presentation, and objective evidence must be present to support a diagnosis of MS.

§Gadolinium-enhancing lesions are not required; symptomatic lesions are excluded from consideration in subjects with brainstem or spinal cord syndromes.

From Polman CH, Reingold SC, Banwell B, et al. Diagnostic criteria for multiple sclerosis: 2010 revisions to the McDonald criteria. Ann Neurol 2011;69:292-302.

Cerebellar symptoms may include tremor, which can range from mildly annoying to disabling, be gross or fine, and occur at rest or with purposeful actions. Various parts of the body may be involved, including the head, the upper or lower limbs, and the trunk.

Constipation and bowel incontinence may occur in up to 73% of patients with MS [15]. More than 70% of patients with MS may suffer from bladder dysfunction [15]. MS lesions in the spinal cord can result in a small spastic bladder due to detrusor overactivity. This usually is manifested as urinary urgency, frequency, voiding of small amounts of urine, and eventually incontinence [15]. Bladder underactivity can result in retention and overflow incontinence. Bladder dysfunction is often associated with urinary tract infections that can worsen MS symptoms. Sexual dysfunction commonly includes erectile and ejaculatory dysfunction in men; vaginal dryness in women; and increased time to arousal, decreased genital sensation, and decreased libido in men and women [15]. Factors contributing to sexual dysfunction include disease progression, antidepressants, fatigue, and depression [15].

Involvement of cranial nerves VII, IX, X, and XII may result in dysphagia or swallowing difficulties. These are manifested as coughing, frequent throat clearing, complaints of

Table 134.2 Common Symptoms in Multiple Sclerosis

Bladder symptoms	Urgency, frequency, hesitancy, retention, incontinence
Bowel symptoms	Constipation, urgency, incontinence
Cerebellar symptoms	Incoordination, imbalance, tremor
Cognition	Concentration, memory, executive dysfunction
Fatigue	Lassitude, reduced endurance
Mood disorders	Depression, anxiety, emotional lability
Motor	Weakness, spasticity
Sensory symptoms	Loss of sensation, positive sensations
Sexual dysfunction	Decreased libido, erectile dysfunction
Vision	Visual loss and double vision

From Goldman MD, Cohen JA, Fox RJ, Bethoux FA. Multiple sclerosis: treating symptoms, and other general medical issues. Cleve Clin J Med 2006;73:178.

food "sticking" in the throat, weight loss, weak voice, choking, or even aspiration pneumonia [16].

Fatigue has been reported to occur in more than 90% of MS patients and is regarded as the most disabling symptom in as many as 60% of these patients [15,17]. MS-related fatigue has been described as an overwhelming feeling of tiredness, lack of energy, or exhaustion exceeding the expected [15,17].

As many as 50% of patients with MS may have cognitive deficits that are manifested as problems with memory, planning, concentration, judgment, problem solving, and processing speed [18–21]. MS patients frequently report heat intolerance with an exacerbation of symptoms in warm or humid environments [22].

Physical Examination

Inflammation of the optic nerve may result in optic or retrobulbar neuritis manifesting as acute vision loss. Even after treatment, vision deficits may persist in the form of poor vision, especially in dim light, or blind spots in the visual field known as scotomas. Demyelination in the medial longitudinal fasciculus may result in varying degrees of horizontal nystagmus; involvement of the third cranial nerve may be manifested as a persistently enlarged pupil. Double vision may be attributable to weakened strength and coordination in the eye muscles. Cataracts may develop at an earlier age in the MS population because of the use of steroids. Visual problems may worsen with stress, increased temperature, and infection [14].

Speech dysfunction may include dysarthria with diminished fluency, slurring, decreased speed, and eventually incomprehensibility.

Sensory testing may reveal deficits in pinprick, temperature, proprioception, or vibration. A sensory level may be evident.

Manual muscle testing can show varying degrees of muscle weakness. The patient may exhibit poor control of a limb or insufficient clearance of the foot during gait. Spastic gait may be another motor finding. Cerebellar involvement may be manifested as dysmetria with past pointing on finger to nose testing and uncoordinated heel to shin movements. The Ashworth Scale (or Modified Ashworth Scale) [23] is commonly used to measure the amount of spasticity, and the 88-item Multiple Sclerosis Spasticity Scale is a reliable and valid measure of the impact of spasticity in patients with MS [24].

Early in the course, deep tendon reflexes tend to be hyperactive. Decreased or absent reflexes can represent segmental levels of deficit. Corticospinal tract involvement may be evident with an asymmetric plantar response or loss of the abdominal reflex. Deep tendon reflexes can also be asymmetric; testing them in more than one position can determine the consistency of the findings.

Cognitive testing may reveal multiple deficits, including in memory, problem solving, judgment, and concentration.

Functional Limitations

The combinations of deficits in MS lead to difficulties with activities of daily living and mobility. Weakness, incoordination, spasticity, or sensory deficits may each or in combination contribute to falls. In addition to possible injuries, these falls may lead to decreased mobility because of fear of repeated falls. Decreased mobility itself leads to further weakness, decreased endurance, and less independence. Weakness or spasticity can also lead to difficulties with feeding and self-care, resulting in the need for personal care

Table 134.3 Multiple Sclerosis Pain Syndromes and Their Treatment

Pain Syndrome	Acute or Chronic	Clinical Example	Treatment Approaches
Neuralgia	Both	Trigeminal neuralgia	Gabapentin, 100-900 mg three or four times daily Carbamazepine, 200-400 mg three times daily (extended-release form also available) Dilantin, 300-600 mg daily Oxcarbazepine, 150-900 mg daily Amitriptyline, 10-100 mg daily at bedtime Other tricyclic antidepressants Baclofen (oral or intrathecal) as adjuvant therapy
Meningeal irritation	Acute	Optic neuritis	Intravenous corticosteroids directed at underlying inflammation
Sensory pain	Both	Paresthesias	Same as for neuralgia
Skeletal muscle pain	Chronic	With spasticity or limited mobility	Rehabilitation (physical and occupational therapy) Assistive devices Nonsteroidal anti-inflammatory drugs

From Goldman MD, Cohen JA, Fox RJ, Bethoux FA. Multiple sclerosis: treating symptoms, and other general medical issues. Cleve Clin J Med 2006; 73:182.

attendants. The Multiple Sclerosis Functional Composite is a clinical measure developed by a task force of the National Multiple Sclerosis Society [25,26] and is mostly used in clinical trials. It measures ambulation, arm and hand function, and cognition and has been found to have greater reliability, sensitivity, and validity than the Kurtzke Expanded Disability Status Scale [3].

Bowel and bladder dysfunction can contribute to many embarrassing moments in the community, causing patients with MS to fear leaving home or to become distracted by seeking out the locations of bathrooms in areas they plan to visit. Many resort to wearing diapers or catheters. Fear of bladder incontinence may also lead a patient to decrease fluid intake, resulting in dehydration.

Depression, insomnia, and fatigue can all contribute to activity intolerance.

Visual deficits may limit activities such as driving and reading, thus limiting participation in work and recreation.

Diagnostic Studies

Magnetic resonance imaging is the most important test in the diagnosis and management of MS [27]. The use of gadolinium allows enhancement of active inflammatory lesions that represent areas with blood-brain barrier breakdown. These hyperintense lesions on T2-weighted images are more specific for MS if they are located in the cerebral white matter, especially the corpus callosum, periventricular area, and brainstem [6].

Cerebrospinal fluid studies, visual evoked potentials, and brainstem auditory evoked potentials can assist in the diagnosis of MS when magnetic resonance imaging findings but not clinical findings support a diagnosis of MS [6,22].

Differential Diagnosis

Acute disseminated encephalomyelitis
Cerebrovascular disease
Primary cerebral vasculitis
Systemic lupus erythematosus
Polyarteritis nodosa
Familial cavernous hemangiomas
Eales disease with neurologic involvement
Sjögren syndrome
Inflammatory central nervous system disease
Migratory sensory neuritis
Behçet disease
Lyme disease
Chronic fatigue syndrome
Neurobrucellosis
Neurosarcoidosis
Metastatic and remote effects of cancer
Multiple metastases
Paraneoplastic syndromes
Vitamin B_{12} deficiency
Myasthenia gravis
Human T-lymphotropic virus 1–associated myelopathy
Acquired immunodeficiency syndrome myelopathy
Other human immunodeficiency virus syndromes
Adult-onset leukodystrophy
Herpes zoster myelitis
Arachnoiditis

Treatment

Initial

Treatment of patients with MS requires a multidisciplinary approach that should involve careful identification of the symptoms with consideration given to the consequences of these symptoms. Symptoms then need to be prioritized and a treatment plan formulated with use, where appropriate, of nonpharmacologic interventions first [28–33].

Education of the patient and family should be included in any initial treatment plan involving patients with MS. This provides information about a balanced diet [34], including adequate fluid intake, weight control, and appropriate exercise [35]. The patient is encouraged to continue working and participating in recreational activities for as long as possible. Modifications may be necessary to allow these activities to continue. The health care providers, the family, and the patient should closely monitor emotional stability, especially mood, because such conditions as depression can contribute to disability. Disabled parking placards can make the task of driving and parking more convenient for the disabled patient with MS.

High-dose methylprednisolone for 3 to 5 days has been established as effective treatment of acute relapses [36,37]. This can be given in a home or hospital setting with similar efficacy [38]. The medications approved by the U.S. Food and Drug Administration (FDA) that are available as first-line treatment to decrease the relapse rate in relapsing-remitting MS include interferon beta-1a (Avonex, Rebif), interferon beta-1b (Betaseron, Extavia), glatiramer acetate (Copaxone), mitoxantrone (Novantrone), natalizumab (Tysabri), and fingolimod (Gilenya) [39]. Fingolimod offers the advantage of oral administration and may be the most effective in decreasing relapse frequency in relapsing-remitting MS [40].

Spasticity management can be complex (see Chapter 153). Some patients use their spasticity to assist with transfers or gait; therefore, spasticity should be treated only if it interferes with mobility or activities of daily living. The first step is seeking and treatment of noxious stimuli, such as pain or infection, especially urinary tract infections, because such stimuli can exacerbate spasticity [41]. Treatment options include physical therapy (see the section on rehabilitation), oral or intrathecal medications, and nerve or muscle blocks [41].

Oral baclofen is the usual first-line treatment, starting with 5 mg two or three times per day and titrating up to the FDA-recommended maximum of 80 mg/day in divided doses. Patients with severe spasticity may require and have been shown to tolerate higher doses (up to 160 mg/day) [42]. Tizanidine, an α-adrenergic receptor antagonist, has been shown to be effective in reducing muscle tone in patients with MS [43]. Dosing should be started at 2 mg and slowly increased to the effective dose of 24 to 36 mg/day in three divided doses [41]. Side effects can include sedation, dry mouth, and weakness. Tizanidine may cause less weakness but more severe dry mouth compared with baclofen [44]. The GABAergic drugs gabapentin (Neurontin) and pregabalin (Lyrica) have been shown to have antispasticity properties [41] and can be used as monotherapy or in addition to baclofen or tizanidine. Sedation is the most common side effect. Benzodiazepines, such as diazepam (Valium) at

5 to 7.5 mg and clonazepam (Klonopin) at 0.5 to 1.5 mg, can be sedating and so are best used at bedtime for nocturnal spasms. They have addiction potential.

A third-line oral antispasticity option is dantrolene sodium, a direct-acting muscle relaxant [41]. It may be best for the nonambulatory patient with MS with severe spasticity who may be unaffected by the resultant weakness.

Back spasms in patients with MS may respond to cyclobenzaprine (Flexeril). Intractable spasticity may be managed with muscle or nerve blocks or intrathecal administration of baclofen (see the section on procedures).

Bladder dysfunction should be initially assessed with a urinalysis and urine culture to determine if a urinary tract infection is present. Appropriate antibiotics should be used for a urinary tract infection. If there is no infection or improvement after antibiotic treatment, a postvoid residual urine volume by ultrasound can help determine failure-to-empty (postvoid residual > 100 mL) or failure-to-store (postvoid residual < 100 mL) dysfunction [45]. A urodynamic study can help determine the presence (or absence) of detrusor hyperreflexia, detrusor-sphincter dyssynergia, or detrusor areflexia. Nonpharmacologic interventions for bladder dysfunction include timed voiding, minimizing the intake of bladder irritants such as caffeine, and regulation of fluid intake. Detrusor hyperactivity may respond to anticholinergic medications, such as the nonselective muscarinics oxybutynin (Ditropan), tolterodine (Detrol), trospium (Sanctura), and fesoterodine (Toviaz). Alternatively, the selective M_2 and M_3 antimuscarinics darifenacin (Enablex) and solifenacin (VESIcare) may be used [15]. The main side effects of the anticholinergics are dry mouth and constipation. Transdermal oxybutynin may offer even fewer side effects. Botulinum toxin type A injections into the detrusor muscle have shown efficacy in reducing symptoms in patients with detrusor hyperreflexia [46]. Detrusor underactivity is best managed with clean intermittent catheterization [45]. Cholinergic agents such as bethanechol (Urecholine) and tamsulosin may also reduce bladder urine volume [15]. Detrusor-sphincter dyssynergia may respond to a combination of clean intermittent catheterization and anticholinergic drugs [15]. Patients with MS and bladder dysfunction may eventually need continuous drainage by a suprapubic catheter. Urology consultation may be necessary for further workup and treatment in complicated cases that are not responding well to medications or for those patients requiring suprapubic catheterization. Surgical procedures may be necessary (see the section on surgery).

Sexual dysfunction in men with MS may be treated with oral medications such as sildenafil, vardenafil, and tadalafil if the problem is erectile dysfunction [47]. Intraurethral or penile injections of papaverine or alprostadil, mechanical vibrators, and vacuum devices can enhance arousal and orgasm [11,18]. Treatment of sexual dysfunction should include counseling and education [18,48]. Sildenafil may help improve lubrication in women with MS and sexual dysfunction [49].

Bowel dysfunction manifesting as constipation is best managed by establishment of a bowel program. This consists of adequate fluid intake, incorporation of fiber, adherence to a bowel elimination schedule, biofeedback, maintenance of physical activity, and judicious use of medications [15,18]. Fluid intake should be at least 8 cups each day. Fiber can be found in such foods as raw fruits and vegetables, whole grains, nuts, and seeds. Bowel elimination is most likely to occur shortly after a meal when the gastrocolic reflex results in an increase in the movement of intestinal contents; allow up to 30 minutes of uninterrupted time. Bulk formers, stool softeners, laxatives, rectal stimulants such as suppositories, or occasional use of enemas may be necessary. Diarrhea may be managed by bulk formers taken once per day without the extra fluid as in treatment of constipation. Medications such as loperamide, to slow bowel activity, may be necessary in patients with chronic diarrhea with fecal incontinence [18]. Workup should seek to eliminate other causes of diarrhea, such as *Clostridium difficile* infection or lactose intolerance.

Factors contributing to or mimicking fatigue should be ruled out or identified and addressed. Common factors are thyroid dysfunction, anemia, sleep disturbance, infections, and sedating medications [15,18]. Treatment should include nonpharmacologic [50] (Table 134.4) and, if necessary, pharmacologic interventions. First-line medications include amantadine [51,52] (Symmetrel), started at 100 mg in the morning and early afternoon, and modafinil [51] (Provigil), 100 to 400 mg in the morning. Pemoline (Cylert) and methylphenidate (Ritalin) are third-line medications [15]. Aspirin has been shown to improve fatigue in patients with MS [52].

The multiple pain syndromes in patients with MS are amenable to nonpharmacologic and pharmacologic interventions [11,53,54] (see Table 134.3).

Cognitive impairment can be detected during daily interactions with family, colleagues, and friends or during interactions with speech-language pathologists, physical therapists, and occupational therapists. Formal neuropsychological testing can determine the presence and severity of even subtle cognitive impairments [19]. Speech-language pathologists can teach compensatory techniques, such as repetition and maintaining a memory book. Donepezil was not shown

Table 134.4 Nonpharmacologic Interventions for Management of Fatigue in Patients with Multiple Sclerosis

Intervention	Method
Treat underlying factors that exacerbate fatigue	Correction of sleep disturbances Treatment of depression Reversal of thyroid abnormalities Management of medication adverse effects
Improve physical fitness	Aerobic exercise
Improve mobility	Physical and occupational therapy Instruction in proper use of mobility aids and techniques
Teach energy conservation	Timed rest periods Work simplification techniques
Teach cooling techniques	Avoidance of heat Use of cooling vests or other garments

From Crayton HJ, Rossman HS. Managing the symptoms of multiple sclerosis: a multimodal approach. Clin Ther 2006;28:449.

to improve MS-related cognitive dysfunctions [55,56]. Identifying and treating depression with antidepressant medication and counseling can be helpful [32].

Acute visual deficits attributable to inflammation may improve more rapidly after high-dose intravenous administration of methylprednisolone. Prism lenses may help compensate for double vision. Regular patching should be avoided because this may prevent the brain from learning to compensate for double vision; patching can be limited to specific activities, such as watching television or reading.

Rehabilitation

Physical therapy interventions to decrease spasticity include range of motion exercises, stretching, positioning, aerobic exercise, and relaxation techniques [32].

The physical therapist may also improve mobility by training the patient to use various assistive devices to compensate for weakness and fatigue. The physical therapist may also use transcutaneous electrical nerve stimulation to assist with pain management. Physical therapists can teach aerobic exercises to prevent deconditioning, to improve endurance, and thus to delay or to minimize the effects of fatigue [35]. Weakness due to the "short circuiting" in demyelinated nerves, as can occur in MS, may be made worse if the patient exercises to the point of fatigue. Exercise programs should be individualized and updated as the patient's condition changes [35]. Occupational therapists can help mitigate the effects of fatigue by teaching energy conservation and work simplification through the use of adaptive equipment and techniques.

Ataxia and tremor can be difficult symptoms to manage. Weighted utensils and weights on the distal limbs or assistive devices may lessen the effect of the tremor on a patient's function [15]. Compensatory techniques taught by occupational therapy may improve activities of daily living. Medications for tremor may include beta blockers, buspirone, and clonazepam [15].

A speech-language pathologist can teach the patient techniques to improve speech intelligibility. Various oromotor exercises can help maintain oral muscle coordination [57]. Swallowing dysfunction should be evaluated with a videofluoroscopy study. The speech-language pathologist can also help determine the safest food texture for a patient with dysphagia [57]. Severe dysphagia may require placement of a gastrostomy tube for nutrition to be maintained [57].

A vocational rehabilitation counselor can play an important role in integrating the disabled MS patient back into the workforce.

Procedures

Muscle or nerve blocks should be reserved for patients with focal spasticity or generalized spasticity with a focal target, such as hip adductor spasticity that interferes with toileting. The most commonly used agents are botulinum toxin and phenol [41]. Intramuscular injection of botulinum toxin to specific muscles usually takes effect within a week, peaks in 2 to 3 weeks, and lasts 3 to 4 months. Side effects may include muscle weakness, atrophy, and diffusion to other muscles. The maximum recommended dose of botulinum toxin is 400 units at a minimum interval of 3 months [41,58]. Resistance may occur from development of neutralizing antibodies. The neurolytic effect from phenol usually lasts 3 to 12 months, and the injection can be repeated. Side effects of the procedure include local soreness, edema, and fibrosis. Intrathecal administration of phenol has been used in selected patients whose spasticity was resistant to conventional treatment [41].

Surgery

Intrathecal administration of baclofen from a pump implanted in the abdomen is a reasonable option when oral antispasticity medications or muscle and nerve blocks are not tolerated or effective [59]. In rare cases, severe spasticity may need to be treated with stereotactic radiosurgery or deep brain stimulation [60] and refractory tremors with deep brain stimulation [61,62], thalamic stimulation, or thalamotomy [61–63]. Trigeminal neuralgia may be amenable to gamma knife radiosurgery [64]. Augmentation cystoplasty may be an option in patients with detrusor hyperreflexia that is refractory to conservative treatments [65].

Potential Disease Complications

MS has the potential to progress in such a way as to render the patient severely disabled both physically and cognitively. Dysphagia may lead to aspiration pneumonia that can cause death. Cervical myelopathy or severe demyelination in the brainstem may lead to respiratory failure. Complications related to the relative immobility include pneumonia, deep venous thrombosis, pulmonary embolism, and decubitus ulcers. Neurogenic bladder may contribute to urinary tract infections and even urosepsis. In a sample population of MS patients, half the deaths were due to pneumonia, pulmonary embolism, aspiration, urosepsis, and decubitus ulcers; respiratory complications accounted for most of the deaths [66]. The other deaths were similar to those in the general population. There may be a higher incidence of suicide in patients with MS [67]. If suicides are excluded, the life expectancy of patients with MS may be 6 to 7 years less than that of the general population [68].

Potential Treatment Complications

Corticosteroids may cause myriad adverse effects, including osteoporosis, immunosuppression, edema, cataracts, glaucoma, avascular necrosis, and myopathy. Interferon beta-1b and beta-1a may result in influenza-like symptoms and injection site reactions. Continued use of interferons may lead to the development of antibodies, rendering them less effective [69]. Baclofen and other antispasticity medications can lead to weakness, drowsiness, and dizziness [41]. If oral or intrathecal baclofen is abruptly withdrawn, hallucinations or seizures may occur [41]. Medications such as opiates for severe pain and benzodiazepines for tremor and spasticity have abuse potential. Dantrolene or tizanidine for spasticity may result in hepatitis, and liver enzymes should be monitored especially during the first 4 months [21]. Antidepressants may contribute to sexual dysfunction.

References

[1] Polman CH, Wolinsky JS, Reingold SC. Multiple sclerosis diagnostic criteria: three years later. Mult Scler 2005;11:5–12.

[2] McDonald WI, Compston A, Edan G, et al. Recommended diagnostic criteria for multiple sclerosis: guidelines from the International Panel on the diagnosis of multiple sclerosis. Ann Neurol 2001;50: 121–7.

[3] Fox RJ, Bethoux F, Goldman MD, Cohen JA. Multiple sclerosis: advances in understanding, diagnosing, and treating the underlying disease. Cleve Clin J Med 2006;73:91–102.

[4] Marrie RA, Cutter G, Tyry T, et al. Does multiple sclerosis–associated disability differ between races? Neurology 2006;66:1235–40.

[5] Montalban X, Sastre-Garriga J, Filippi M, et al. Primary progressive multiple sclerosis diagnostic criteria: a reappraisal. Mult Scler 2009;15:1459–65.

[6] Polman CH, Reingold SC, Banwell B, et al. Diagnostic criteria for multiple sclerosis: 2010 revisions to the McDonald criteria. Ann Neurol 2011;69:292–302.

[7] Al-Araji AH, Oger J. Reappraisal of Lhermitte's sign in multiple sclerosis. Mult Scler 2005;11:398–402.

[8] Bagnato F, Centonze D, Galgani S, et al. Painful and involuntary multiple sclerosis. Expert Opin Pharmacother 2011;12:763–77.

[9] Miller DH, Weinshenker BG, Filippi M, et al. Differential diagnosis of suspected multiple sclerosis: a consensus approach. Mult Scler 2008;14:1157–74.

[10] Ben-Zacharia AB. Therapeutics for multiple sclerosis symptoms. Mt Sinai J Med 2011;78:176–91.

[11] Goldman MD, Cohen JA, Fox RJ, Bethoux FA. Multiple sclerosis: treating symptoms, and other general medical issues. Cleve Clin J Med 2006;73:177–86.

[12] Rizzo MA, Hadjimichael OC, Preiningerova J, Vollmer TL. Prevalence and treatment of spasticity reported by multiple sclerosis patients. Mult Scler 2004;10:589–95.

[13] Martinelli Boneschi F, Colombo B, Annovazzi P, et al. Lifetime and actual prevalence of pain and headache in multiple sclerosis. Mult Scler 2008;14:514–21.

[14] Graves J, Balcer LJ. Eye disorders in patients with multiple sclerosis: natural history and management. Clin Ophthalmol 2010;4:1409–22.

[15] Samkoff LM, Goodman AD. Symptomatic management in multiple sclerosis. Neurol Clin 2011;29:449–63.

[16] Poorjavad M, Derakhshandeh F, Etemadifar M, et al. Oropharyngeal dysphagia in multiple sclerosis. Mult Scler 2010;16:362–5.

[17] Amato MP, Portaccio E. Management options in multiple sclerosis–associated fatigue. Expert Opin Pharmacother 2012;13:207–16.

[18] Frohman TC, Castro W, Shah A, et al. Symptomatic therapy in multiple sclerosis. Ther Adv Neurol Disord 2011;4:83–98.

[19] Chiaravalloti ND, DeLuca J. Cognitive impairment in multiple sclerosis. Lancet Neurol 2008;7:1139–51.

[20] Amato MP, Portaccio E, Goretti B, et al. Cognitive impairment in early stages of multiple sclerosis. Neurol Sci 2010;31(Suppl 2):S211–4.

[21] Goretti B, Portaccio E, Zipoli V, et al. Impact of cognitive impairment on coping strategies in multiple sclerosis. Clin Neurol Neurosurg 2010;112:127–30.

[22] Leavitt VM, Sumowski JF, Chiaravalloti N, Deluca J. Warmer outdoor temperature is associated with worse cognitive status in multiple sclerosis. Neurology 2012;78:964–8.

[23] Platz T, Eickhof C, Nuyens G, Vuadens P. Clinical scales for the assessment of spasticity, associated phenomena, and function: a systematic review of the literature. Disabil Rehabil 2005;27:7–18.

[24] Hobart JC, Riazi A, Thompson AJ, et al. Getting the measure of spasticity in multiple sclerosis: the Multiple Sclerosis Spasticity Scale (MSSS-88). Brain 2006;129(Pt 1):224–34.

[25] Ontaneda D, LaRocca N, Coetzee T, et al. Revisiting the multiple sclerosis functional composite: proceedings from the National Multiple Sclerosis Society (NMSS) Task Force on Clinical Disability Measures. Mult Scler 2012;18:1074–80.

[26] Rudick R, Antel J, Confavreux C, et al. Recommendations from the National Multiple Sclerosis Society Clinical Outcomes Assessment Task Force. Ann Neurol 1997;42:379–82.

[27] Ceccarelli A, Bakshi R, Neema M. MRI in multiple sclerosis: a review of the current literature. Curr Opin Neurol 2012;25:402–9.

[28] Duddy M, Haghikia A, Cocco E, et al. Managing MS in a changing treatment landscape. J Neurol 2011;258:728–39.

[29] Derwenskus J. Current disease-modifying treatment of multiple sclerosis. Mt Sinai J Med 2011;78:161–75.

[30] Filippi M. Multiple sclerosis in 2010: advances in monitoring and treatment of multiple sclerosis. Nat Rev Neurol 2011;7:74–5.

[31] Hartung HP, Montalban X, Sorensen PS, et al. Principles of a new treatment algorithm in multiple sclerosis. Expert Rev Neurother 2011;11:351–62.

[32] Schapiro RT. The symptomatic management of multiple sclerosis. Ann Indian Acad Neurol 2009;12:291–5.

[33] Schapiro RT. Managing symptoms of multiple sclerosis. Neurol Clin 2005;23:177–87, vii.

[34] Schapiro RT. Diet and nutrition. In: Schapiro RT, editor. Managing the symptoms of multiple sclerosis. New York: Demos; 2003.

[35] Doring A, Pfueller CF, Paul F, Dörr J. Exercise in multiple sclerosis—an integral component of disease management. EPMA J 2011;3:2.

[36] Sellebjerg F, Barnes D, Filippini G, et al. EFNS guideline on treatment of multiple sclerosis relapses: report of an EFNS task force on treatment of multiple sclerosis relapses. Eur J Neurol 2005;12:939–46.

[37] Nicholas R, Rashid W. Multiple sclerosis. Clin Evid (Online) 2012 Feb 10;2012.

[38] Chataway J, Porter B, Riazi A, et al. Home versus outpatient administration of intravenous steroids for multiple-sclerosis relapses: a randomised controlled trial. Lancet Neurol 2006;5:565–71.

[39] Loma I, Heyman R. Multiple sclerosis: pathogenesis and treatment. Curr Neuropharmacol 2011;9:409–16.

[40] Del Santo F, Maratea D, Fadda V, et al. Treatments for relapsing-remitting multiple sclerosis: summarising current information by network meta-analysis. Eur J Clin Pharmacol 2012;68:441–8.

[41] Kheder A, Nair KP. Spasticity: pathophysiology, evaluation and management. Pract Neurol 2012;12:289–98.

[42] Smith CR, LaRocca NG, Giesser BS, Scheinberg LC. High-dose oral baclofen: experience in patients with multiple sclerosis. Neurology 1991;41:1829–31.

[43] Malanga G, Reiter RD, Garay E. Update on tizanidine for muscle spasticity and emerging indications. Expert Opin Pharmacother 2008;9:2209–15.

[44] Chou R, Peterson K, Helfand M. Comparative efficacy and safety of skeletal muscle relaxants for spasticity and musculoskeletal conditions: a systematic review. J Pain Symptom Manage 2004;28:140–75.

[45] Fowler CJ, Panicker JN, Drake M, et al. A UK consensus on the management of the bladder in multiple sclerosis. Postgrad Med J 2009;85:552–9.

[46] Kalsi V, Gonzales G, Popat R, et al. Botulinum injections for the treatment of bladder symptoms of multiple sclerosis. Ann Neurol 2007;62:452–7.

[47] Fowler CJ, Miller JR, Sharief MK, et al. A double blind, randomised study of sildenafil citrate for erectile dysfunction in men with multiple sclerosis. J Neurol Neurosurg Psychiatry 2005;76:700–5.

[48] Bitzer J, Platano G, Tschudin S, Alder J. Sexual counseling for women in the context of physical diseases—a teaching model for physicians. J Sex Med 2007;4:29–37.

[49] Dasgupta R, Wiseman OJ, Kanabar G, et al. Efficacy of sildenafil in the treatment of female sexual dysfunction due to multiple sclerosis. J Urol 2004;171:1189–93, discussion 1193.

[50] Crayton HJ, Rossman HS. Managing the symptoms of multiple sclerosis: a multimodal approach. Clin Ther 2006;28:445–60.

[51] Lapierre Y, Hum S. Treating fatigue. Int MS J 2007;14:64–71.

[52] Shaygannejad V, Janghorbani M, Ashtari F, Zakeri H. Comparison of the effect of aspirin and amantadine for the treatment of fatigue in multiple sclerosis: a randomized, blinded, crossover study. Neurol Res 2012;34:854–8.

[53] O'Connor AB, Schwid SR, Herrmann DN, et al. Pain associated with multiple sclerosis: systematic review and proposed classification. Pain 2008;137:96–111.

[54] Nick ST, Roberts C, Billiodeaux S, et al. Multiple sclerosis and pain. Neurol Res 2012;34:829–41.

[55] O'Carroll CB, Woodruff BK, Locke DE, et al. Is donepezil effective for multiple sclerosis–related cognitive dysfunction? A critically appraised topic. Neurologist 2012;18:51–4.

[56] Krupp LB, Christodoulou C, Melville P, et al. Multicenter randomized clinical trial of donepezil for memory impairment in multiple sclerosis. Neurology 2011;76:1500–7.

[57] Giusti A, Giambuzzi M. Management of dysphagia in patients affected by multiple sclerosis: state of the art. Neurol Sci 2008;29(Suppl 4): S364–6.

[58] Francisco GE. Botulinum toxin: dosing and dilution. Am J Phys Med Rehabil 2004;83(Suppl):S30–7.

[59] Erwin A, Gudesblatt M, Bethoux F, et al. Intrathecal baclofen in multiple sclerosis: too little, too late? Mult Scler 2011;17:623–9.

[60] Patwardhan RV, et al. Neurosurgical treatment of multiple sclerosis. Neurol Res 2006;28:320–5.

[61] Schuurman PR, Bosch DA, Merkus MP, Speelman JD. Long-term follow-up of thalamic stimulation versus thalamotomy for tremor suppression. Mov Disord 2008;23:1146–53.

[62] Yap L, Kouyialis A, Varma TR. Stereotactic neurosurgery for disabling tremor in multiple sclerosis: thalamotomy or deep brain stimulation? Br J Neurosurg 2007;1:349–54.

[63] Hassan A, Ahlskog JE, Rodriguez M, Matsumoto JY. Surgical therapy for multiple sclerosis tremor: a 12-year follow-up study. Eur J Neurol 2012;19:764–8.

[64] Zorro O, Lobato-Polo J, Kano H, et al. Gamma knife radiosurgery for multiple sclerosis–related trigeminal neuralgia. Neurology 2009;73:1149–54.

[65] Zachoval R, Pitha J, Medova E, et al. Augmentation cystoplasty in patients with multiple sclerosis. Urol Int 2003;70:21–6, discussion 26.

[66] Cottrell DA, Kremenchutzky M, Rice GP, et al. The natural history of multiple sclerosis: a geographically based study. 5. The clinical features and natural history of primary progressive multiple sclerosis. Brain 1999;122(Pt 4):625–39.

[67] Sadovnick AD, Eisen K, Ebers GC, Paty DW. Cause of death in patients attending multiple sclerosis clinics. Neurology 1991;41:1193–6.

[68] Sadovnick AD, Ebers GC, Wilson RW, Paty DW. Life expectancy in patients attending multiple sclerosis clinics. Neurology 1992;42:991–4.

[69] Killestein J, Polman CH. Determinants of interferon beta efficacy in patients with multiple sclerosis. Nat Rev Neurol 2011;7:221–8.

CHAPTER 135

Myopathies

Kristian Borg, MD, PhD
Erik Ensrud, MD

Synonym

Muscular dystrophies

ICD-9 Codes

359.0 **Congenital hereditary muscular dystrophy**
359.1 **Hereditary progressive muscular dystrophy**
359.2 **Myotonic disorders**
359.4 **Toxic myopathy**
359.5 **Endocrine myopathy**
359.6 **Inflammatory myopathy in other diseases**
359.8 **Other myopathies**
359.9 **Myopathy, unspecified**
710.3 **Dermatomyositis**
710.4 **Polymyositis**

ICD-10 Codes

G71.0 **Muscular dystrophy, congenital**
G71.19 **Myotonic disorders**
G72.2 **Myopathy due to other toxic agents**
E34.9 **[G73.7] Endocrine myopathy**
G72.49 **Inflammatory myopathy, not elsewhere classified**
G72.9 **Myopathy, unspecified**
M33.90 **Dermatopolymyositis, unspecified, organ involvement unspecified**
M33.20 **Polymyositis, organ involvement unspecified**

Definition

Myopathy is the common name for diseases derived from the muscle. Myopathies have different causes and different courses, that is, they may have acute, subacute, or chronic presentations (Table 135.1). Myopathies affect proximal or distal muscle groups; some of them also affect heart muscle, leading to cardiomyopathy [1]. Many myopathies are inherited disorders (Table 135.2); in an increasing number of disorders, the genetic background and the abnormal or missing muscle protein have been revealed during the last decade. An updated gene table is published online [2]. There is also a gene table updated for 2012 and published in *Neuromuscular Disorders* [3]. Muscle diseases are rare, with a prevalence of approximately 50 per 100,000. Myopathy is more common in females than in males, although Duchenne muscular dystrophy is found only in males because of an X-linked inheritance.

Muscular Dystrophies

Muscular dystrophies are inherited disorders of muscle due to abnormal structural muscle proteins, for example, dystrophin in Duchenne muscular dystrophy and sarcoglycans, calpain, and dysferlin in different limb-girdle dystrophies [2,3]. They are characterized by progressive course and early onset.

Congenital Myopathies

Congenital myopathies form a clinically heterogeneous group characterized by findings on muscle biopsy. They are slowly progressive or nonprogressive and usually are manifested in the neonatal period.

Metabolic Myopathies Including Mitochondrial Myopathies

Metabolic myopathies form a clinically heterogeneous group of muscle disorders resulting from inherited defects in intracellular energy production. They may be manifested as cramps and myoglobinuria. Patients with cramps and myoglobinuria often have disorders in the glycogen or lipid metabolism pathways. They may be asymptomatic at rest, but symptoms develop after exercise. Mitochondrial myopathies may be a part of a neurologic syndrome often involving the central nervous system.

Inflammatory Myopathies

Inflammatory myopathies are characterized by inflammatory changes in the muscle and are associated with infections or an immunologic process. They are divided into polymyositis, dermatomyositis, and inclusion body myositis [4]. The course is acute or subacute and is almost always associated with an elevated serum creatine kinase (CK) level.

Drug-Induced and Endocrine Myopathies

Drug-induced myopathies are caused by different drugs, for example, colchicine, azidothymidine (AZT), chloroquine, hydroxychloroquine, and corticosteroids. Myopathy due to intake of statins, the cholesterol-lowering agents, has been reported [5]. Endocrine myopathies include both hyperthyroid and hypothyroid myopathies as well as myopathy due to hyperparathyroidism.

Myotonic Syndromes

A number of disorders are associated with clinical or electrical myotonia. The myotonic disorders are divided into myotonic dystrophies and "pure" myotonia [6]. The myotonias are inherited disorders due to alterations in ion channels in the muscle and seldom give rise to persistent muscle weakness. Myotonic dystrophy (MD 1) or Steinert disease exists in a congenital and an adult form. Individuals with myotonic dystrophy may not notice any problems until adolescence or early adult life [7]. The first symptom may be difficulty in releasing an object due to myotonia. Progressive weakness with onset in distal muscles follows. The genetic explanation to MD 1 is an expansion of a CTG repeat in chromosome 19 (*DMPK* gene). The gene encodes a protein kinase that occurs in different tissues, leading, for example, to cardiomyopathy. The clinical affection is correlated to the number of repeats, and the number of repeats increases between generations, leading to a clinical anticipation. There is also a more rare form with later onset, a slower course, and proximal muscle weakness (MD 2). The genetic background to MD 2 is a CCTG repeat in chromosome 3 (*ZNF9* gene) [8].

Symptoms

Muscle weakness, most often affecting proximal muscles, is the cardinal symptom. Almost all myopathies affect the proximal muscles to the greatest extent. Another prominent symptom is muscle fatigue. The earliest symptoms are often related to weakness of the hip and proximal leg muscles; patients experience difficulty in rising from a chair and often require support of their arms. Compensation for leg extensor weakness by bracing of the legs with the hands and climbing with the hands on the legs when rising to a standing position is known as the Gower maneuver. Walking up and down stairs may be difficult because of quadriceps and hip extensor weakness, respectively. Weakness of proximal muscles in the upper extremities can be manifested as fatigue or inability to perform overhead tasks, such as hair brushing, brushing teeth, and lifting objects to elevated shelves.

In hereditary distal myopathies [9] and inclusion body myositis, the distal muscle weakness leads to footdrop and ankle instability as well as difficulty with manual tasks, such as turning doorknobs and opening jars.

Pain is not a common symptom in myopathies. However, inflammatory and metabolic myopathies are associated with

Table 135.1 Myopathic Disorders

Muscular Dystrophies

X-linked (dystrophinopathy)
Limb-girdle
Congenital
Facioscapuloperoneal
Scapuloperoneal
Distal myopathy

Congenital Myopathies

Central core disease
Nemaline myopathy
Myotubular myopathy
Centronuclear myopathy
Desmin-related myopathy
Other

Metabolic Myopathies

Glycogenosis
Lipid storage myopathies
Mitochondrial myopathies
Periodic paralysis

Inflammatory Myopathies

Polymyositis
Dermatomyositis
Inclusion body myositis
Other (e.g., viral)

Endocrine Myopathies

Thyroid
Parathyroid
Adrenal, steroid
Pituitary

Drug-Induced/Toxic Myopathies
Myotonic Syndromes

Myotonic dystrophy (DM type 1)
Myotonic dystrophy, proximal type (DM type 2)
Chloride channel myotonia (myotonia congenita Thomsen)
Sodium channel myotonia (paramyotonia congenita Eulenburg, hyperkalemic periodic paralysis)
Calcium channel disorders (hypokalemic periodic paralysis)
Potassium channel disorders (hypokalemic periodic paralysis)
Schwartz-Jampel
Drug induced

Table 135.2 Myopathic Disorders: Major Forms of Inheritance

Disorder	Inheritance
Duchenne muscular dystrophy	X-linked recessive
Becker muscular dystrophy	X-linked recessive
Facioscapulohumeral dystrophy	Autosomal dominant
Scapuloperoneal dystrophy	X-linked dominant
Limb-girdle dystrophy	Autosomal recessive/dominant
Oculopharyngeal dystrophy	Autosomal dominant
Distal myopathy/muscular dystrophy	Autosomal dominant/recessive
Congenital muscular dystrophy	Autosomal recessive/dominant/sporadic
Congenital myopathies	Autosomal recessive
Myotonic syndromes	Autosomal dominant
Metabolic myopathies	Autosomal dominant/recessive, X-linked recessive

Modified from Dumitru D. Electrodiagnostic Medicine. Philadelphia, Hanley & Belfus, 1995:1067.

pain. Exercise-induced muscle pain suggests a metabolic myopathy. The pain has an aching, dull, and crampy quality and is usually poorly localized. An exercise-induced weakness suggests a neuromuscular junction disorder. Symptoms of hypoventilation and cardiac failure should be considered.

Physical Examination

A general examination is performed to assess for signs of cardiac failure and rashes found in dermatomyositis. Muscle atrophy assessment and testing of muscle strength are central and should involve examination of proximal and distal muscles in all extremities as well as facial muscles and neck flexors and extensors. Hip girdle muscles are best isolated for strength testing while the patient is in the supine and prone positions. The abilities of walking, rising from a chair (or floor in pediatric patients), and stepping onto a low chair are often helpful in evaluating leg weakness. Examination of the shoulder may reveal winging of the scapula, a characteristic finding in facioscapulohumeral muscular dystrophy. Facial weakness and temporalis muscle wasting are also present in facioscapulohumeral muscular dystrophy and in myotonic dystrophy.

Range of motion at joints should be examined because contractures may have marked functional effects. Reflexes should be normal or decreased proportional to muscle weakness in myopathies. Abnormalities on sensory testing suggest involvement of sensory nerves (i.e., a neuromuscular disorder).

Functional Limitations

The most common functional limitations are related to the prominent symptom of proximal weakness, which can have a marked effect on transfers, ascending and descending stairs, and ambulation. In severe myopathies, patients may be restricted to wheelchair mobility. Proximal upper extremity weakness can interfere with activities of daily living, such as dressing, grooming, and cooking. Fatigue is common secondary to the increased effort required with weakened muscles. Cardiac failure and respiratory insufficiency requiring ventilation can result in difficulty with daily activities and increased fatigue. The dysphagia involved in some myopathies may make eating time-consuming and difficult.

Diagnostic Studies

The serum CK concentration is the most important test in myopathies. Patients with Duchenne muscular dystrophy may have very high CK values. Serum CK concentration is usually elevated in inflammatory myopathies and metabolic myopathies. It is often normal or nearly normal in congenital myopathies.

Exercise, especially if it is strenuous or performed in a sedentary individual, can cause marked CK elevation. Thus, patients should be advised to abstain from strenuous exercise for 5 days before serum CK testing. CK concentration may also be elevated in neuromuscular disorders, such as motor neuron disease.

Nerve conduction studies are important in cases of suspected myopathy. Sensory and motor nerve conduction studies are usually normal. However, distal compound muscle action potentials may be reduced. Exceptions include patients with inclusion body myositis (30% have a sensory or sensorimotor polyneuropathy) [4]. In cases with abnormal nerve conduction velocities, coexisting neuropathies such as diabetic polyneuropathy should be considered.

The electromyographic examination is helpful in the evaluation of myopathies. Primarily, the size of motor units is decreased by the dysfunction or loss of individual muscle fibers, leading to motor unit action potentials that characteristically have decreased duration, decreased amplitude, and increased phases in contrast with the neuropathic motor unit action potential findings. In addition, denervating potentials (fibrillations and positive sharp waves) occur in many myopathic disorders.

Muscle biopsy is often useful in the diagnosis of myopathy. The selection of muscle for biopsy is important because a muscle that is end stage is likely to show only fibrotic replacement of muscle tissue, and an unaffected muscle may be normal. In an acute myopathy, it is best to select a muscle for biopsy that is clinically weak; in a chronic myopathy, it is preferable to select a muscle that is only mildly weak. The muscle selected should not have been sampled by needle electromyography, which may result in temporary inflammation. The pathologist, to investigate possible causes, performs specific histochemical and immunohistochemical stains and occasionally electron microscopy on the specimen.

Magnetic resonance imaging may be an additional diagnostic tool in clinical practice. The pattern of muscle involvement is often specific for the different entities [10].

Genetic testing is nowadays routine in the evaluation of many of the muscular dystrophies and is also useful in the evaluation of other chronic myopathies. With similar phenotypes, such as limb-girdle muscular dystrophy, the only way to accurately diagnose the condition is by genetic testing. A helpful resource is the gene table published online [2].

Differential Diagnosis

- Motor neuron disease
  - Amyotrophic lateral sclerosis
  - Late-onset spinal muscular atrophy
- Neuromuscular junction disorders
  - Myasthenia gravis
  - Lambert-Eaton myasthenic syndrome
- Motor neuropathies
  - Demyelinating motor neuropathies, such as multifocal motor neuropathy and diabetic amyotrophy
- Spinal stenosis or myelopathy
- Parkinson disease
- Poliomyelitis, postpoliomyelitis syndrome

Treatment

Initial

Of great importance is an initial detailed explanation to the patient and relatives. Patients are informed that they must not exert themselves to the point of exhaustion. Referral to the Muscular Dystrophy Association is helpful for education and support of the patient.

Steroids are often effective in the treatment of inflammatory myopathies (as are other immunosuppressants) and have been shown to slow progression in some muscular dystrophies. In a recent Cochrane report [11], corticosteroids were shown to improve muscle strength and function in Duchenne muscular dystrophy in the short term. Carnitine is used in lipid storage myopathies. Much work is now devoted to development of new therapeutic strategies, including gene [12] and stem cell [13] therapies. Otherwise, the only therapeutic option is symptomatic treatment (e.g., pain treatment with different analgesics).

Rehabilitation

Physical therapy and occupational therapy are often necessary for gait training and stretching. Assistive devices, such as canes, walkers, and wheelchairs, as indicated in a particular patient, can minimize disability. Assistive devices should be used, preferably after training with a physical therapist. Bracing may be helpful for footdrop.

Adaptive equipment may be prescribed to assist a patient to perform daily activities. Home adaptations, such as tub bars and entrance ramps, may be of great assistance to patients with proximal muscle weakness.

Exercise can help maintain joint range of motion. There has been debate about whether patients with muscle disorders benefit from exercise training. There is an increasing knowledge on the effect of exercise training in different muscle disorders [14,15]. High-resistance training at submaximal level seems to be beneficial in slowly progressive disorders in the short term. In rapidly progressive disorders, such as Duchenne muscular dystrophy, high-resistance training is questionable [14]. On the basis of this, moderate exercise, not to the point of exhaustion, is preferable. It is important to start exercise training early in the course of the disease so that there are still trainable muscle fibers left.

The common opinion on exercise training in inflammatory myopathies has changed during recent years. Patients with inflammatory myopathies have been strongly advised to avoid exercise. However, results from training studies have shown that exercise training has beneficial effects on muscle function [16].

Procedures

Assisted ventilation, including negative pressure ventilation, noninvasive positive pressure ventilation, and invasive positive pressure ventilation (i.e., endotracheal tube or tracheostomy), may be indicated for patients with insufficient ventilation [17]. Feeding tubes may be necessary for patients with dysphagia due to severe bulbar myopathy.

Surgery

Patients with muscular dystrophies may require contracture release and spine stabilization surgeries.

Potential Disease Complications

Severe myopathies, including muscular dystrophies, can cause restrictive pulmonary disease due to chest wall muscle weakness and scoliosis. Assisted ventilation, including negative pressure ventilation, noninvasive positive pressure ventilation, and invasive positive pressure ventilation (by endotracheal tube or tracheostomy), may be indicated. Decreased mobility can result from proximal lower and upper extremity weakness. Contractures can be caused by disuse and fibrosis as well as by scoliosis due to paraspinal muscle weakness. Cardiac involvement is present in some forms of muscle disorders [1]. Gastrointestinal symptoms due to smooth muscle involvement are common in patients with muscular dystrophies.

Potential Treatment Complications

Immunosuppression may have associated side effects. Steroid use and decreased mobility may lead to osteoporosis and the subsequent risk of pathologic fractures, and analgesics have well-known side effects. Special attention should be paid to patients undergoing general anesthesia because of the risk of malignant hyperthermia, which is a potentially lethal condition appearing in different myopathies, including a specific disorder with a mutation in the skeletal muscle ryanodine receptor.

References

[1] Goodwin FC, Muntoni F. Cardiac involvement in muscular dystrophies: molecular mechanisms. Muscle Nerve 2005;32:577–88.

[2] GeneTable of Neuromuscular Disorders. http://www.musclegenetable.org.

[3] Kaplan JC. The 2012 version of the gene table of monogenic neuromuscular disorders. Neuromuscul Disord 2011;21:833–61.

[4] Greenberg SA. Pathogenesis and therapy of inclusion body myositis. Curr Opin Neurol 2012;25:630–9.

[5] Miller JAL. Statins—challenges and provocations. Curr Opin Neurol 2005;18:494–6.

[6] Davies NP, Hanna MG. The skeletal muscle channelopathies: distinct entities and overlapping syndromes. Curr Opin Neurol 2003;16:559–68.

[7] Schara U, Schoser BG. Myotonic dystrophies type 1 and 2: summary on current aspects. Semin Pediatr Neurol 2006;13:71–9.

[8] Liquori CL, Ricker K, Moseley ML, et al. Myotonic dystrophy type 2 caused by a CCTG expansion in intron 1 of ZNF9. Science 2001;293:864–7.

[9] Mastaglia FL, Lamont PJ, Laing NL. Distal myopathies. Curr Opin Neurol 2005;18:504–10.

[10] Mercuri E, Jungbluth H, Muntoni F. Muscle imaging in clinical practice: diagnostic value of muscle magnetic resonance imaging in inherited neuromuscular disorders. Curr Opin Neurol 2005;18:526–37.

[11] Manzur AY, Kuntzer T, Pike M, Swan A. Glucocorticoid corticosteroids for Duchenne muscular dystrophy. Cochrane Database Syst Rev 2008;1, CD003725.

[12] Verhaart IEC, Aartsma-Rus A. Gene therapy for Duchenne muscular dystrophy. Curr Opin Neurol 2012;25:588–96.

[13] Tedesco FS, Cossu GA. Stem cell therapies for muscle disorders. Curr Opin Neurol 2012;25:597–603.

[14] Ansved T. Muscle training in muscular dystrophies. Acta Physiol Scand 2001;171:359–66.

[15] Voet NB, van der Kooi EL, Riphagen II, et al. Strength training and aerobic exercise training for muscle disease. Cochrane Database Syst Rev 2010;1, CD003907.

[16] Alexandersson H, Lundberg IE. Exercise as a therapeutic modality in patients with idiopathic inflammatory myopathies. Curr Opin Rheumatol 2012;24:201–7.

[17] Mellies U, Dohna-Schwake C, Voit T. Respiratory function assessment and intervention in neuromuscular disorders. Curr Opin Neurol 2005;18:543–7.

CHAPTER 136

Neural Tube Defects

Jess Nordin, DO
Glendaliz Bosques, MD

Synonyms

Craniorachischisis
Anencephaly
Encephalocele
Spinal dysraphism
Myelodysplasia
Hydrocele spinalis
Spina bifida (occulta, aperta, manifesta, cystica)
Myelomeningocele
Myelocele
Hemimyelomeningocele
Hemimyelocele
Lipoma with dural involvement
Lipomyelomeningocele
Lipomyeloschisis
Myelocystocele
Meningocele
Filum terminale lipoma
Tight filum terminale
Dorsal enteric fistula
Neurenteric cyst
Split notochord syndrome
Diastematomyelia
Diplomyelia
Dermal sinus
Caudal regression syndrome
Segmental spinal dysgenesis

ICD-9 Codes

655.0 Central nervous system malformation in fetus
740.0 Anencephalus
740.1 Craniorachischisis
740.2 Iniencephaly
741.0 Spina bifida with hydrocephalus
741.9 Spina bifida without mention of hydrocephalus
742.0 Encephalocele
742.51 Diastematomyelia
742.59 Other specified congenital anomalies of spinal cord
742.9 Unspecified anomaly of brain, spinal cord, and nervous system
756.17 Spina bifida occulta
781.2 Abnormality of gait

ICD-10 Codes

O35.0 Maternal care for (suspected) central nervous system malformation in fetus
Add seventh character for number of gestations
Q00.0 Anencephaly
Q00.1 Craniorachischisis
Q00.2 Iniencephaly
Q05.4 Unspecified spina bifida with hydrocephalus
Q05.9 Spina bifida, unspecified
Q01.9 Encephalocele, unspecified
Q06.2 Diastematomyelia
Q06.9 Congenital malformation of spinal cord, unspecified
Q04.9 Congenital malformation of brain, unspecified
Q07.9 Congenital malformation of nervous system, unspecified
Q76.0 Spina bifida occulta
R26.9 Unspecified abnormalities of gait and mobility

Definition

A neural tube defect occurs when the neural tube, the embryologic precursor to the brain and spinal cord, fails to close between the third and fourth weeks of embryogenesis. Neural tube defects are a subset of central nervous system congenital anomalies leading to varying degrees of neurologic impairment from complete failure of neurulation to spina bifida occulta, a posterior vertebral defect without protrusion of neural tissue. Myelomeningocele (MMC), a form of spina bifida cystica, is the most common spinal dysraphism. MMC occurs when the meninges and the spinal cord project through a vertebral defect, forming a sac most commonly located in the lumbosacral region.

The etiology of neural tube defects is multifactorial. Genetic factors have been implicated; there is a 4% risk of recurrence of MMC after having one affected child [1,2]. Associated environmental factors include low socioeconomic status, parental occupation, maternal diabetes mellitus, maternal hyperthermia, maternal obesity, and drug exposures, such as to valproic acid [1]. Since the mandatory fortification of grain products with folate in the United States in 1998, the prevalence rate of spina bifida declined 31% to a rate of 3.49 per 10,000 [1]. The highest prevalence, in the United States, is among women of Hispanic ethnicity [1].

Symptoms

Neurologic

Clinical presentation (Table 136.1) will vary by the extent of involvement of sensory, motor, and autonomic nerves. Dysphagia, aspiration, stridor, vocal cord paralysis, nystagmus, spasticity, bradycardia, and sleep apnea are all symptoms of *brainstem dysfunction*. A high index of suspicion is sometimes necessary for early assessment and management because severe apnea may lead to respiratory arrest, which could in turn result in death.

The symptoms of *hydrocephalus* will vary by age. In an infant, symptoms include lethargy, poor appetite, vomiting, accelerated head enlargement, bulging anterior fontanelle, dilated scalp veins, spasticity, and clonus. In an older child, headache is a prominent symptom. Mechanical obstruction of a ventriculoperitoneal shunt (VPS) is manifested acutely with signs of hydrocephalus. VPS infections are associated with fever, headache, and meningismus. Adults with VPS can develop chronic idiopathic headaches.

Tethered cord syndrome can result in progressive scoliosis, decline in lower extremity strength, development of lower extremity contractures, spasticity, change in gait or urinary symptoms, low back pain, and skin ulcers. Patients with spina bifida occulta may present to providers with tethered cord syndrome symptoms beginning during adulthood [3].

A noted increase in spasticity can be caused by hydrocephalus, syringomyelia, tethered cord, urinary tract infection, and decubitus ulcers. Seizures may be common in children with MMC.

Orthopedic

Symptoms from progressive scoliosis can include pain, cardiopulmonary dysfunction, and severe disability interfering

Table 136.1 Clinical Presentation and Functional Considerations of Myelomeningocele by Neurosegmental Level

	Neurosegmental Levels			
	T6-12	**L1-L3**	**L4-L5**	**S1-S4**
Muscles involved	Abdominal muscles, trunk flexors and extensors	Iliopsoas (L1-L3) Hip adductors (L2-L4) Quadriceps (L2-L4)	Hip adductors (L2-L4) Quadriceps (L2-L4) Gluteus medius (L4-S1) Gluteus maximus (L5-S1) Hamstring (L5-S2) Tibialis anterior (L4-L5) Peroneal (L5-S1) Tibialis posterior (L4-L5) Toe extensors (L5-S1) Toe flexors (L5-S3) Foot intrinsics (L5-S3)	Gluteus medius (L4-S1) Gluteus maximus (L5-S1) Hamstring (L5-S2) Peroneal (L5-S1) Gastrocnemius (S1-S2) Toe extensors (L5-S1) Toe flexors (L5-S3) Foot intrinsics (L5-S4)
Orthopedic complications				
Spine	Kyphosis Scoliosis	Scoliosis Lordosis	Scoliosis Lordosis	
Hips	Hip flexion contractures	Hip dislocation Hip flexion and adduction contractures	Hip dislocation Hip flexion contractures	
Legs	Knee flexion contractures	Knee flexion contractures		
Feet	Equinus	Equinus	Calcaneovarus Calcaneus	Cavus
Ambulatory potential	Can ambulate with equipment; however, poor long-term probability	Household ambulation (may cease ambulation during second decade of life)	Community ambulation	Community ambulation
Equipment needs	Wheelchair TLSO HKAFO KAFO RGO Standers	Wheelchair RGO KAFO Dynamic standers Hip abduction splint	Forearm crutches Walkers KAFO AFO	AFO SMO

AFO, ankle-foot orthosis; *HKAFO,* hip-knee-ankle-foot orthosis; *KAFO,* knee-ankle-foot orthosis; *RGO,* reciprocating gait orthosis; *SMO,* supramalleolar orthosis; *TLSO,* thoracolumbar-sacral orthosis.

with sitting balance and ambulation. Hip deformities, including contractures and dislocations, may result in popping sensation, leg length discrepancy, and pain. Pelvic obliquity can lead to progression of scoliotic curve and difficulties with sitting and positioning. Presence of knee flexion or extension contractures may interfere with functional tasks, such as transfers. Foot deformities are common and may depend on which spinal segments are affected. Pathologic fractures in the lower limbs may be manifested with localized erythema and swelling [4]. Musculoskeletal pain in the shoulder area may be extremely common in wheelchair users, especially in adult patients.

Urinary

Patients may present with urinary retention or incontinence from neurogenic bladder. Urinary tract infections can be associated with fever, changes in urinary control like new-onset leakage between catheterizations, and change in urine quality (color, foul odor, or sediment).

Gastrointestinal

Stool incontinence and constipation are symptoms of neurogenic bladder. Chronic constipation may lead to incontinence due to overflow.

Endocrine

Short stature due to growth hormone deficiency is the most common endocrine symptom [5].

Reproductive

Many men with MMC are infertile [6]. Fertility among women with MMC is thought to be normal [7]. Change in urologic status (i.e., new-onset incontinence) or back pain may be a presenting sign of pregnancy or labor.

Pulmonary

Brainstem dysfunction associated with Chiari II malformation can lead to hypoventilation, apnea, and respiratory failure. Restrictive lung disease can be seen with severe progression of neuromuscular scoliosis. In thoracic-level MMC, partial innervations of abdominal and intercostal musculature may result in respiratory insufficiency.

Cardiovascular

Lower extremity swelling may be due to positional edema or lymphedema. There is evidence showing increased prevalence of lymphedema [8]. Hypertension may be prevalent as well with associated metabolic syndrome and early-onset arteriosclerosis from sedentary lifestyle and obesity.

Allergy and Immunology

There is an increased prevalence of latex allergy. Careful precautions should be taken as a severe reaction can include angioedema and anaphylaxis. This can be life-threatening.

Dermatology

Patients with MMC are at risk for pressure ulcers because of insensate skin, incontinence, impaired mobility, orthopedic abnormalities, and orthoses.

Nutrition

Obesity is common, especially in older adolescents and adults. Significant dysphagia, on the other hand, may lead to failure to thrive and difficulty in gaining weight from brainstem dysfunction.

Psychosocial

Difficulties with motivation and academic performance may be reported by parents. Depression may be common in older adolescents and adults [9].

Physical Examination

A full physical examination should be performed and will vary on the basis of the level of the lesion. Particular focus for the physiatrist lies in the neurologic and musculoskeletal examination and its relation to functional status. Criteria for assessment of motor level in patients with MMC should be used (Table 136.2). Examination should include assessment of the cranial nerves, mental status, motor strength, sensation, reflexes, range of motion in joints, muscle tone, spinal alignment, and gait. Developmental screening includes assessment of gross and fine motor, language, and cognitive abilities. Anthropometric measurements should be monitored in the MMC population because of a high incidence of decreased height or linear length from associated musculoskeletal deformities [10]. Arm span measurements allow a more accurate assessment of body mass index [10]. The Centers for Disease Control and Prevention growth charts used for able-bodied children may not provide all the information necessary for assessment of appropriate growth and nutrition. Evaluation for skin breakdown and for cutaneous midline lesions of the spine, which may signal an underlying form of occult dysraphism, should be performed. The patient's equipment should be routinely evaluated.

Functional Limitations

Functional limitations vary by the degree of associated neurologic impairments and orthopedic abnormalities. Children with MMC generally have delay in ambulation [11]. The strength of the iliopsoas, quadriceps, and gluteus medius muscles is an important predictor of ambulatory potential. In general, patients with thoracic lesions are wheelchair dependent. Patients with upper lumbar lesions usually ambulate household distances with variable wheelchair dependency. Patients who have lower lumbar and sacral lesions ambulate longer community distances. These patients may still require some bracing or assistive devices.

Other factors, such as presence of hydrocephalus, seizures, muscle tone, contractures, fractures, weight, cognition, and motivation, among others, have been implicated with ambulation and mobility [11,12].

Table 136.2 International Myelodysplasia Study Group: Criteria for Assigning Motor Levels

Motor Level	Criteria for Assigning Motor Levels	Functional Movement Noted
T10 or above	Determined by sensory level and/or palpation of abdominal muscles	
T11	Trunk extensors (thoracic and lumbar)	
T12	Abdominal and paraspinal muscles provide some pelvic control. Hip hiking from the quadratus lumborum may also be present.	Hip hike
L1	Grade 2 **weak iliopsoas,** quadratus lumborum	Hip hike
L1-2	Exceeds criteria for L1 but does not meet L2 criteria	
L2	Meets or exceeds criteria for L1 +	
	Grade 3 iliopsoas	Hip flexion
	Grade 3 sartorius	
	Grade 3 hip adductors (adductor magnus, brevis, longus; pectineus; gracilis)	Hip adduction
L3	Meets or exceeds the criteria for L2 +	
	Grade 3 quadriceps	Knee extension
L3-4	Exceeds criteria for L3 but does not meet L4 criteria	
L4	Meets or exceeds the criteria for L3 +	
	Grade 3 medial hamstrings	Medial knee flexion
	Grade 3 tibialis anterior	Ankle dorsiflexion
	A weak peroneus tertius may also be seen.	
L4-5	Exceeds criteria for L4 but does not meet L5 criteria	
L5	Meets or exceeds the criteria for L4 +	
	Grade 2 **gluteus medius**	Hip abduction
	Grade 3 lateral hamstring (biceps femoris)	Knee flexion
	Grade 3 tibialis posterior	Ankle inversion
L5-S1	Exceeds criteria for L5 but does not meet S1 criteria	
S1	Meets or exceeds the criteria of L5 +	
	Grade 3 gluteus medius	Hip abduction
	Grade 2 **gastrocnemius/soleus complex**	Ankle plantar flexion
S1-2	Exceeds criteria for S1 but does not meet S2 criteria	
S2	Meets or exceeds the criteria for S1 +	
	Grade 4 gluteus maximus	Hip extension
	Grade 3 gastrocnemius/soleus complex	Ankle plantar flexion
S2-3	All of the lower limb muscle groups are of normal strength (grade 4 in 1-2 muscle groups)	
	Also includes normal-appearing infants who are too young to be bowel and bladder trained	
"No loss"	Meets all of the criteria for S2-3 + has no bowel or bladder dysfunction	

Bold text indicates main muscle tested.

From McDonald CM, Jaffe KM, Shurtleff DB, Menelaus MB. Modifications to the traditional description of neurosegmental innervation in myelomeningocele. Dev Med Child Neurol 1991;33:473-481.

Diagnostic Studies

Prenatal

Elevated serum levels of α-fetoprotein detected in the second trimester suggest a neural tube defect. Fetal ultrasonographic imaging and magnetic resonance imaging can aid in determining prognosis and parental decision-making [13]. Amniocentesis may show elevated levels of α-fetoprotein and acetylcholinesterase, also consistent with a neural tube defect.

Postnatal

At birth, the determination of neurologic status is clinical. A head ultrasound examination is performed to assess for ventricular size. Echocardiography can be performed before surgical repair to rule out congenital heart disease. Cranial or spinal ultrasound examination can be used for noninvasive assessment of neurologic status in an infant. Beyond infancy, magnetic resonance imaging is performed to assess the spinal cord, and computed tomography is used to assess for hydrocephalus. A shunt series can be performed if there is concern for shunt malfunction. A VPS tap may be performed to rule out infection. Plain film radiography or computed tomography is used when there is concern for a joint or spine deformity or pathologic fracture.

Urologic studies include renal and bladder ultrasonography, voiding cystourethrography, urodynamic studies, DMSA nuclear scan, and postvoid residual measurement [14]. Cystoscopy is performed for bladder cancer surveillance, especially if the patient has undergone bladder augmentation procedures [15]. Routine blood work may include a complete blood count, comprehensive metabolic profile, lipid panel [16], 25-hydroxyvitamin D level, and cystatin C level [14]. Depending on clinical presentation, other diagnostic studies may include determination of endocrine hormone levels and prealbumin concentration, electroencephalography, dual-energy x-ray absorptiometry scan, polysomnography, and latex allergy assay. Throughout childhood and adulthood, health care providers should continue to perform routine health maintenance. Neuropsychological testing should be performed before entrance into school.

Differential Diagnosis

Alternating hemiplegia of childhood
Arthrogryposis
Cerebral palsy
Charcot-Marie-Tooth disease
Congenital hypothyroidism
Congenital myopathies
Congenital neuropathies
Currarino syndrome
Hereditary spastic paraparesis
Inborn error of metabolism
Intracranial tumor
Ischemic or hemorrhagic stroke
Multiple vertebral segmentation defects
Myotonia congenita
OEIS complex (omphalocele, exstrophy of the cloaca, imperforate anus, and spinal defects)
Poliomyelitis
Sacrococcygeal teratoma
Spinal epidural abscess
Spinal cord hemorrhage
Spinal cord infarct
Spinal cord injury
Spinal muscle atrophy
Spinal tumor
VACTERL association (vertebral defects, anal atresia, cardiac defects, tracheoesophageal fistula, renal anomalies, and limb abnormalities)

Treatment

Initial

Surgical closure of MMC within 48 hours is customary. Fetal surgery can be performed before 26 weeks of gestational age. Lower incidences of hindbrain abnormalities and shunt-dependent hydrocephalus as well as improved motor outcomes have been reported for in utero compared with postnatal surgical closure [17]. However, fetal surgery has not shown improvement in lower urinary tract function [18].

First-line management of hydrocephalus is placement of a VPS. Endoscopic third ventriculostomy combined with choroid plexus cauterization represents an alternative technique by addressing both the communicating and noncommunicating mechanisms of hydrocephalus without introducing shunt dependency [19].

Infants who are unable to void or who have large postvoid residuals should begin clean intermittent catheterization programs. Children can be taught to perform clean intermittent catheterization as early as 5 years of age, although it may take longer because of the high executive function impairments related to hydrocephalus. Patients with detrusor-sphincter dyssynergia or hydronephrosis may be treated with anticholinergic medications. Children with vesicoureteral reflux are often prescribed prophylactic antibiotics. Various treatments exist for hyperactive sphincter function.

A bowel management program may consist of stool softeners, bulking agents, suppositories, digital stimulation, manual removal, or enemas. Clinicians often recommend performing bowel programs after a meal to take advantage of the gastrocolic reflex.

An acute change in the respiratory status of a patient may warrant posterior fossa decompression or treatment of hydrocephalus. If this is unsuccessful, tracheostomy and long-term mechanical ventilation may be considered.

Other treatment modalities may include antiepileptics, growth hormone or gonadotropin-releasing hormone analogue treatment, bisphosphonates, and calcium and vitamin D. Recommendations for daily physical activity and dietary management must be included. Genetic counseling and appropriate folic acid supplementation are advised for affected women considering pregnancy. Current guidelines for folic acid supplementation are 0.4 mg/day for any woman of childbearing age and 4 mg/day for women with a previous neural tube defect pregnancy or who are at high risk [20].

Rehabilitation

Rehabilitation and comprehensive medical care for patients with MMC involve a family-centered approach by a multidisciplinary team to include physiatrists, physical therapists, occupational therapists, speech-language pathologists, recreational therapists, behavioral psychologists, neuropsychologists, teachers, social workers, and child life specialists in collaboration with other physicians and surgeons. Educational needs should be assessed for implementation of an individualized education plan or 504 plans. Vocational rehabilitation should be considered as well. Educating the patient about the condition and promoting independence in self-care and maintenance of mobility status are essential to improve quality of life and to decrease preventable conditions [21]. Advancements in the medical and surgical management of children with MMC, especially after 1975, have resulted in increased life expectancy [22,23]. Survival to 16 years of age is estimated at 54% for those treated before 1975 and 85% for those treated after 1975 [22]. If a shunt is in place, there is a risk of decreased survival after 34 years of age [22]. Effective transition to adult health care providers remains an area of further research.

The general goals of the treatment plan include maintaining range of motion, strengthening, promoting functional independence through development, encouraging weight-bearing exercises, and maximizing mobility and cardiovascular fitness. It is important to establish a home exercise program. Equipment should be optimized for functional level and modified for proper fit. Wheelchair users may require pressure mapping. A reciprocating gait orthosis may be considered in higher level lesions and requires active hip flexion for use. Other equipment may include walkers, crutches, canes, standers, parapodiums, resting splints, adaptive equipment, and orthoses, depending on the functional level. Patients may cease ambulation during the second year of life as a result of weight gain and axial growth [11].

Procedures

Spasticity may be treated with onabotulinum toxin or phenol injections. Functional electrical stimulation may be beneficial. Nonoperative management of various orthopedic abnormalities may include bracing and casting. Management of neurogenic bladder may include intravesical onabotulinum toxin injections or anticholinergics.

Surgery

Children with a VPS may develop obstruction requiring shunt revision. Studies show that shunted patients, presenting with shunt malfunction, may be freed from shunt dependence by an endoscopic third ventriculostomy, instead of a shunt revision [19]. A symptomatic Chiari II malformation warrants craniovertebral decompression. Severe brainstem involvement may lead to placement of a gastrostomy tube and tracheostomy because of respiratory insufficiency and dysphagia. Tethered cord syndrome with neurologic decline may require surgical intervention for release. Surgical options for spasticity and contracture management include contracture release, tendon lengthening, joint capsule release, targeted rhizotomy, and intrathecal baclofen pump placement.

Patients who have progressive scoliosis should undergo a spinal arthrodesis or fusion. Surgical treatment of hip contractures and dislocations is controversial [24]. Surgery for hip dislocation may not improve walking ability and should mostly be considered in unilateral dislocation in lesions below L4 [24]. Surgical correction of various foot deformities is performed to allow a functional position for ambulation and to prevent pressure ulceration.

Surgical procedures for neurogenic bladder and bowel include an artificial urinary sphincter, bladder augmentation, bladder neck sling or closure, continent catheterizable stoma, vesicotomy, antegrade continence enema, and colostomy.

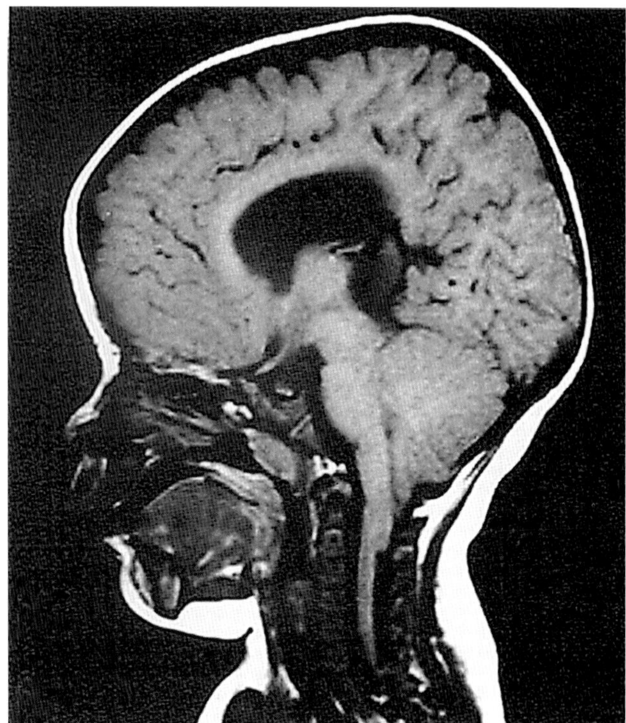

FIGURE 136.1 T1-weighted magnetic resonance image of the brain: Arnold-Chiari type II malformation with tonsillar displacement, of more than 3 mm, through the foramen magnum (hindbrain herniation), resulting in obstructive hydrocephalus.

Potential Disease Complications

MMC is associated with Arnold-Chiari type II malformation, a posterior fossa malformation in which the caudal vermis, cerebellar tonsils, and medulla can herniate through the foramen magnum, resulting in obstructive hydrocephalus (Fig. 136.1). As a result, brainstem dysfunction can occur. In spinal dysraphisms, the spinal cord is generally anatomically fixed at the site of the anomaly after neonatal repair. Neurologic decline can occur secondary to traction, or tethering, on the cord from aggravating factors such as growth spurts, trauma, and existing deformities. An increase in spasticity can be caused by hydrocephalus, syringomyelia, tethered cord, urinary tract infection, and decubitus ulcers. Seizures may be common in children with MMC. Other complications may include supratentorial cerebral malformations and visuospatial dysfunction.

Scoliosis, kyphosis, or lordosis may result from muscle imbalances and congenital spinal deformities. Vertebral congenital abnormalities are associated with MMC and can cause worsening of spinal deformities. Orthopedic deformities of hips, knees, and ankles, including contractures and dislocations, are related to positioning and muscle imbalance. Some orthopedic deformities, such as foot deformities and early hip dislocation, may be congenital. Others, such as late hip subluxation, contractures, osteoporosis, and fragility fractures, may be acquired. Foot deformities are common in all MMC levels. Charcot joints from poor sensation, pressure, weight bearing, and repetitive microtrauma can be seen.

Neurogenic bladder may lead to chronic kidney disease from vesicoureteral reflux, recurrent urinary tract infections, and urinary incontinence or retention. Patients with neurogenic bladder and chronic use of indwelling urinary catheters or bladder augmentation procedures may be at higher risk for development of bladder cancer. Early surveillance is recommended.

Neurogenic bowel may lead to fecal impaction or incontinence. Early-onset diverticulosis and complications with megacolon have been reported as well.

Hypothalamic-pituitary dysfunction may be present because of hydrocephalus or other central nervous system abnormalities. However, underdevelopment of the lower limbs, from neurogenic atrophy, and spinal deformities present in MMC also play a role in short stature. Other reported complications include precocious puberty, cryptorchidism, sexual dysfunction, and male infertility. Fertility in women is mostly normal; however, a higher risk of having a child with MMC has been reported. Instead of 400 μg of folic acid recommended for the general female population, these patients should supplement with 4 mg of folic acid during childbearing age.

Lack of sensation, orthopedic deformities, equipment or medical device malfunction (including poor fit), and obesity may lead to pressure ulcers. Wound healing may be impaired because of autonomic dysfunction. Chronic nonhealing ulcers may require specialized medical or surgical management. Chronic occult osteomyelitis may be seen.

Obesity rates are higher among adults with spina bifida compared with the general population, especially affecting adult women [25]. This can have an impact on mobility and equipment needs.

Patients with thoracic-level lesions and hydrocephalus are at greater risk for cognitive impairment [26]. Other factors implicated in intellectual outcome include incidence of shunt revision and infection, epilepsy, and associated cerebral malformations [27]. Common findings include neuropsychological deficits in visual perception, academic difficulties in mathematics, and better verbal skills than written skills [26]. Mood disorders, such as depression, may be common in older adolescents and adults [9].

Potential Treatment Complications

VPS complications can include obstruction, infection, and intellectual delay. Other treatment complications include deterioration in neurologic status, cerebrospinal fluid leak, surgical wound dehiscence or infection, spinal cord injury, pain, osteoporotic fractures during therapy, development of latex allergy, and death.

References

[1] Boulet SL, Yang Q, Mai C, et al. Trends in the postfortification prevalence of spina bifida and anencephaly in the United States. Birth Defects Res A Clin Mol Teratol 2008;82:527–32.
[2] Goodrich LV, Jung D, Higgins KM, Scott MP. Overexpression of ptc1 inhibits induction of Shh target genes and prevents normal patterning in the neural tube. Dev Biol 1999;211:323–34.
[3] Rajpal S, Tubbs RS, George T, et al. Tethered cord due to spina bifida occulta presenting in adulthood: a tricenter review of 61 patients. J Neurosurg Spine 2007;6:210–5.
[4] Dosa NP, Eckrich M, Katz DA, et al. Incidence, prevalence, and characteristics of fractures in children, adolescents, and adults with spina bifida. J Spinal Cord Med 2007;30(Suppl 1):S5–9.
[5] Trollmann R, Bakker B, Lundberg M, Doerr HG. Growth in pre-pubertal children with myelomeningocele (MMC) on growth hormone (GH): the KIGS experience. Pediatr Rehabil 2006;9:144–8.
[6] Bong GW, Rovner ES. Sexual health in adult men with spina bifida. ScientificWorldJournal 2007;7:1466–9.
[7] Visconti D, Noia G, Triarico S, et al. Sexuality, pre-conception counseling and urological management of pregnancy for young women with spina bifida. Eur J Obstet Gynecol Reprod Biol 2012;163:129–33.
[8] Garcia AM, Dicianno BE. The frequency of lymphedema in an adult spina bifida population. Am J Phys Med Rehabil 2011;90:89–96.
[9] Essner BS, Holmbeck GN. The impact of family, peer, and school contexts on depressive symptoms in adolescents with spina bifida. Rehabil Psychol 2010;55:340–50.
[10] Shurtleff DB, Walker WO, Duguay S, et al. Obesity and myelomeningocele: anthropometric measures. J Spinal Cord Med 2010;33:410–9.
[11] Williams EN, Broughton NS, Menelaus MB. Age-related walking in children with spina bifida. Dev Med Child Neurol 1999;41:446–9.
[12] Chang CK, Wong TT, Huang BS, et al. Spinal dysraphism: a cross-sectional and retrospective multidisciplinary clinic-based study. J Chin Med Assoc 2008;71:502–8.
[13] Van Der Vossen S, Pistorius LR, Mulder EJ, et al. Role of prenatal ultrasound in predicting survival and mental and motor functioning in children with spina bifida. Ultrasound Obstet Gynecol 2009;34:253–8.
[14] Filler G, Gharib M, Casier S, et al. Prevention of chronic kidney disease in spina bifida. Int Urol Nephrol 2012;44:817–27.
[15] Austin JC, Elliott S, Cooper CS. Patients with spina bifida and bladder cancer: atypical presentation, advanced stage and poor survival. J Urol 2007;178(Pt 1):798–801.
[16] Rendeli C, Castorina M, Ausili E, et al. Risk factors for atherogenesis in children with spina bifida. Childs Nerv Syst 2004;20:392–6.
[17] Adzick NS, Thom EA, Spong CY, et al. A randomized trial of prenatal versus postnatal repair of myelomeningocele. N Engl J Med 2011;364:993–1004.
[18] Lee NG, et al. In utero closure of myelomeningocele does not improve lower urinary tract function. J Urol 2012;188(Suppl):1567–71.
[19] Warf BC, Campbell JW. Combined endoscopic third ventriculostomy and choroid plexus cauterization as primary treatment of hydrocephalus for infants with myelomeningocele: long-term results of a prospective intent-to-treat study in 115 East African infants. J Neurosurg Pediatr 2008;2:310–6.
[20] ACOG Committee on Practice Bulletins. ACOG practice bulletin. Clinical management guidelines for obstetrician-gynecologists. Number 44, July 2003. (Replaces Committee Opinion Number 252, March 2001). Obstet Gynecol 2003;102:203–13.
[21] Mahmood D, Dicianno B, Bellin M. Self-management, preventable conditions and assessment of care among young adults with myelomeningocele. Child Care Health Dev 2011;37:861–5.
[22] Davis BE, Daley CM, Shurtleff DB, et al. Long term survival of individuals with myelomeningocele. Pediatr Neurosurg 2005;41:186–91.
[23] Bowman RM, McLone DG, Grant JA, et al. Spina bifida outcome: a 25-year prospective. Pediatr Neurosurg 2001;34:114–20.
[24] Wright JG. Hip and spine surgery is of questionable value in spina bifida: an evidence-based review. Clin Orthop Relat Res 2011;469:1258–64.
[25] Dosa NP, Foley JT, Eckrich M, et al. Obesity across the lifespan among persons with spina bifida. Disabil Rehabil 2009;31:914–20.
[26] Iddon JL, Morgan DJ, Loveday C, et al. Neuropsychological profile of young adults with spina bifida with or without hydrocephalus. J Neurol Neurosurg Psychiatry 2004;75:1112–8.
[27] Juranek J, Salman MS. Anomalous development of brain structure and function in spina bifida myelomeningocele. Dev Disabil Res Rev 2010;16:23–30.

CHAPTER 137

Neurogenic Bladder

Ayal M. Kaynan, MD, FACS
Meena Agarwal, MD, PhD, MS, Dip Urol, FRCS, FRCS(Urol)
Inder Perkash, MD, FRCS, FACS

Synonyms

None

ICD-9 Codes

344.61 **Cauda equina syndrome with neurogenic bladder**
596.4 **Atony of bladder**
596.51 **Hypertonicity of bladder**
596.52 **Low bladder compliance**
596.53 **Paralysis of bladder**
596.54 **Neurogenic bladder NOS**
596.55 **Detrusor-sphincter dyssynergia**
596.59 **Other functional disorder of bladder**
596.9 **Unspecified disorder of bladder**

ICD-10 Codes

G83.4 **Cauda equina syndrome with neurogenic bladder**
N31.2 **Flaccid neuropathic bladder, atonic neuropathic bladder**
N31.8 **Other neuromuscular dysfunction of bladder**
N31.9 **Neuromuscular dysfunction of bladder, unspecified**
N36.44 **Muscular disorders of urethra, bladder sphincter dyssynergy**
N32.9 **Bladder disorder, unspecified**
N32.89 **Other specified disorders of bladder**

Definition

The term *neurogenic bladder* describes a process of dysfunctional voiding as the result of neurologic impairment. This can interfere with urine storage at low bladder pressures, disrupt voluntary coordinated voiding, and lead to varying degrees of incontinence. Neurologic control of bladder function is at multiple levels throughout the central nervous system and subject to multiple pathophysiologic processes. Voiding dysfunction occurs in most of the neurologically impaired patients [1].

The micturition reflex center has been localized to the pontine mesencephalic reticular formation in the brainstem [2,3]. Efferent axons from the pontine micturition center travel down the spinal cord in the reticulospinal tract to the detrusor motor nuclei located in the S2, S3, and S4 segments in the sacral gray matter (vertebral levels T12 to L2). Parasympathetic nerves take their origin from nuclei at the intermediolateral gray column of the spinal cord at S2, S3, and S4 and travel by the pelvic nerve and pelvic plexus to ganglia in the bladder wall. The predominant parasympathetic nerve root supplying the bladder is usually S3. Acetylcholine is released from the postganglionic nerves, which in turn excites muscarinic receptors [4,5].

Preganglionic sympathetic neurons originate in the intermediolateral gray column of the spinal cord from spinal segments T10 to L2. These nerves course to the sympathetic chain ganglion and through the pelvic plexus to the bladder neck and fundus of the bladder. Receptors at the bladder neck are primarily α-adrenergic [6], stimulation of which results in closure of the internal sphincter during urinary storage and, in men, during ejaculation as well. In contrast to the bladder neck, the fundus of the bladder is populated with β-adrenergic receptors, which contribute to bladder relaxation (and therefore urinary storage) during sympathetic activation.

The external urethral sphincter (striated muscle, voluntary) surrounds the membranous urethra and extends up and around the distal part of the prostatic urethra. The pudendal nerves, which innervate the external sphincter, take their origin from the somatic motor nuclei in the anterior gray matter of the sacral cord (conus, S2-S4); however, it is the S2 spinal segment that provides the principal motor contribution. Toe plantar flexors also have S1 and S2 innervations. Thus, the preservation of toe plantar flexors after spinal cord injury suggests that the external urethral sphincter is intact.

The central control of the bladder is a complex multilevel process. Advances in functional brain imaging have allowed research into this control in humans. The regions of the brain that have been implicated in the central control of continence include the pontine micturition center, periaqueductal gray, thalamus, insula, anterior cingulate gyrus, and prefrontal cortices. The pontine micturition center and the periaqueductal gray are thought to be crucial in the supraspinal control of continence and micturition. Higher centers, such as the insula, anterior cingulate gyrus, and prefrontal regions, are probably involved in the modulation of this control and cognition of bladder sensation. Further work should aim to examine how the regions interact to achieve urinary continence [7].

Symptoms

The symptoms of neurogenic bladder have a wide spectrum of presentation and include urinary incontinence, urinary retention, suprapubic or pelvic pain, incomplete voiding, paroxysmal hypertension with diaphoresis (autonomic dysreflexia), recurrent urinary tract infections, and occult deterioration in renal function. The symptoms vary according to the level of spinal cord injury and pathophysiologic basis of the neurologic disorder.

Abnormalities in the midbrain (e.g., Parkinson disease) lead to detrusor hyperreflexia due to loss of dopamine. Lesions in segmental areas of the spinal cord lead to detrusor-sphincter dyssynergia (DSD). Cortical lesions (lesions above the pontine micturition center) usually result in loss of voluntary inhibition of the micturition reflex. Lesions in the forebrain, such as cerebrovascular accidents with change in blood flow to the cingulate gyrus, can lead to hyperreflexic bladder because of reduced dopamine D_1 with increased glutamate activity. Thus, the cingulate gyrus plays an important role in urine storage. Patients with Parkinson disease have less severe urinary dysfunction with little evidence of internal or external sphincter denervation. By contrast, in multiple system atrophy, patients have more symptoms and wide-open bladder neck. The result is a hyperreflexic bladder with coordinated (synergic) sphincter function [8,9]. In the absence of outflow obstruction (e.g., urethral stricture, benign prostatic hyperplasia, large uterine leiomyoma, fecal impaction), complete bladder evacuation with some incontinence is the outcome. The findings of postmicturition residuals of more than 100 mL, detrusor–external sphincter dyssynergia, and open bladder neck at the start of bladder filling, with significant postural hypotension and neurogenic sphincter motor unit potentials, are highly suggestive of multiple system atrophy [8,9]. It seems DSD reported in such patients may be a voluntary contraction of external sphincter to avoid leakage and is therefore not true DSD. The patient can have unstable blood pressure, which is aggravated with a postural change, indicating some degree of autonomic failure. Similarly, after a severe head injury, an autonomic failure can result in unstable postural hypotension and wide-open bladder neck. The insula and anterior cingulate seem to be responsible for the modulation of autonomic function [10].

All lesions from the pons to spinal cord level S2 result in a loss of cortical inhibition and loss of coordinated sphincter activity during reflex voiding. The micturition reflex is without an inhibitory or coordinated control from higher centers. This results in a hyperreflexic bladder with dyssynergic sphincter function, which often results in incomplete voiding and high bladder pressures; it can lead to vesicoureteral reflux. Urinary retention from functional obstruction occurs, and overflow incontinence may occur with an overdistended bladder.

Spinal cord lesions above T5-T6 result in autonomic dysreflexia above the key level (T5-T8) that innervates the splanchnic bed and regulates blood supply to control blood pressure. Accentuated visceral activity (e.g., full bladder, fecal impaction), which causes sympathetically mediated vasoconstriction, is normally inhibited by secondary output (a negative feedback) from the medulla and is countered by vasodilation in the splanchnic bed through the greater splanchnic nerve. Without the proper inhibitory reflexes or control of the splanchnic bed to redistribute circulating blood volume, blood pressure rises sharply. With the carotid bodies and vagal nerves intact, bradycardia results. The full syndrome is characterized by paroxysmal and extreme elevation in blood pressure, facial flushing, perspiration, goose pimples, headache, and some degree of bradycardia. This is virtually always seen in conjunction with detrusor-sphincter dyssynergia [11].

Spinal cord lesions in the conus at S2 or below result in lower motor neuron injury to the bladder and external sphincter. The effect on the bladder is predictable: areflexia. Because the parasympathetic ganglia reside in or near the bladder wall, bladder tone is generally maintained. Bladder compliance therefore tends to decrease with time as a result of neural decentralization (or infection-related fibrosis) [1,12]. The result on the bladder neck and external sphincter is not as intuitive. An atonic synergic sphincter system might be expected; the external sphincter usually retains some fixed tone, although not under voluntary control; and the bladder neck is often competent because of the intact sympathetic innervations (α-adrenergic activity) but is nonrelaxing. Even though bladder pressures are generally low during filling and storage, obstructive physiology is often the case during voiding [1,13]. Overflow incontinence is possible. A small, titrated dose of alpha blockers can maintain some continence and improve voiding.

In the acute phase of injury, most central nervous system lesions result in a temporarily areflexic bladder [14,15]. This phase, termed central nervous system shock, is variable and can last several weeks. Reappearance of knee jerks heralds recovery from the shock phase. The specific patterns of voiding dysfunction with the most common neurologic abnormalities in the chronic phase are detailed in Table 137.1 and Figure 137.1.

Confounding medical problems, such as diabetes and many cardiovascular drugs (Table 137.2), will profoundly affect bladder function. Patients who catheterize themselves intermittently should be asked about the size of catheter used and whether there is any resistance or trauma during catheterization—clues to the presence of a urethral stricture. Patterns of voiding should be elicited, and changes in voiding habits should be scrutinized. Patients with suprasacral spinal cord injury, for example, often give a history of intermittent stream coinciding with spasticity of their lower extremities, a strong clue to detrusor-sphincter dyssynergia. Spinal cord–injured patients with incomplete lesions can void with excessive Valsalva maneuver and can produce very high intra-abdominal pressures. This can lead to vesicoureteral reflux, upper tract changes, repeated pyelonephritis, and even bladder and kidney stone disease. They therefore need to be monitored frequently with urodynamics and managed

Table 137.1 Patterns of Voiding Dysfunction in Chronic Neurologic Disease

Neurologic Disorder	Detrusor Activity	Striated Sphincter	Comments
Suprapontine	***Hyperreflexic***	***Synergic***	
Brain tumor, cerebral palsy			Detrusor-sphincter dyssynergia may occur in those with spinal cord damage; voluntary control may be impaired
Cerebrovascular accident			Voluntary control may be impaired
Delayed central nervous system maturation			Persistence of uninhibited bladder beyond age 2-3 years; enuresis later
Dementia			Voluntary control is impaired
Parkinson disease			Detrusor contractility and voluntary control may be impaired
Pernicious anemia			Bladder compliance may be decreased
Shy-Drager syndrome			Bladder neck remains open; bladder compliance may be decreased; autonomic instability (low blood pressure)
Pons-S1	***Hyperreflexic***	***Dyssynergic***	
Anterior spinal cord ischemia			Bladder compliance may be decreased
Multiple sclerosis			Varies with lesions
Myelodysplasia, trauma			Variable
Below S1	***Areflexic***	***Fixed tone***	
Acute transverse myelitis			Bladder neck may be closed but nonrelaxing
Diabetes, Guillain-Barré syndrome, herniated intervertebral disc			Usually overdistended bladder
Myelodysplasia, poliomyelitis			Decreased bladder compliance may develop; bladder neck may be open (sympathetic denervation)
Radical pelvic surgery			Bladder neck is open
Tabes dorsalis, trauma			Bladder neck may be closed but nonrelaxing

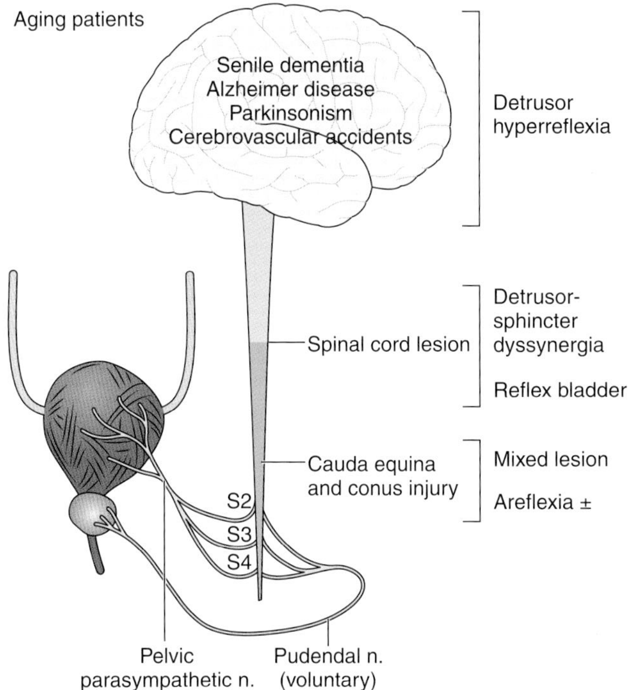

FIGURE 137.1 Diagrammatic illustration of central nervous system disorders leading to different neurologic manifestations. *(From Perkash I. Incontinence in patients with spinal cord injuries. In O'Donnell P, ed. Geriatric Urology. Boston, Little Brown, 1994.)*

appropriately to achieve low-pressure voiding. Approximately 50% of men ultimately have benign prostatic hyperplasia. Thus, even in the case of stable neurologic disease, these men may develop difficulty in voiding from progressive outflow obstruction. Typical symptoms include nocturia, decreased force of stream, hesitancy, and postvoid dribbling. However, patients with outflow obstruction frequently have irritative voiding symptoms as well. It is important to make sure that these symptoms are not due to symptomatic infection: back pain, suprapubic pain, fever, dysuria, urgency, frequency, or hematuria. These symptoms are not specific and can reflect many of the processes discussed. Their presence must therefore be interpreted according to context.

Physical Examination

General considerations include the level of disability and the capability to use upper and lower extremities. The neurologic examination focuses on the strength and dexterity of the upper extremities and the tone and reflexes of the lower extremities. Neurourologic examination includes perianal sensation for evidence of sacral sparing, anal sphincter voluntary contraction, and bulbocavernosus reflex.

The genitalia are examined for the condition of the penis: whether it is circumcised, its size, and adequacy of the meatus; attention is also paid to the presence of meatal erosion due to an indwelling catheter. In women, it is important to note the appearance of the urethral meatus; this structure erodes quite readily with long-standing catheterization. Pelvic examination will identify confounding factors to voiding dysfunction, such as uterine prolapse or leiomyoma. Rectal examination yields information on anal tone, size of prostate, and presence of fecal impaction. Voluntary contraction of the anal sphincter indicates control over the perineal muscles; in the presence of quadriplegia, it indicates an incomplete central cord–type lesion. To determine voluntary contraction, the clinician places a

Table 137.2 Pharmacologic Action on the Bladder

Drug	Indication	Mechanism	Side Effects and Cautions
Cholinergics Bethanechol	Areflexic bladder	Muscarinic receptor agonists Bladder has M_2 and M_3 receptors; M_3 receptors are responsible for normal detrusor contraction	Bronchospasm, miosis
Anticholinergics Hyoscyamine Oxybutynin Tolterodine Trospium chloride (quaternary amine) Darifenacin Solifenacin	Hyperreflexic bladder	Muscarinic receptor antagonists	Constipation, dry mouth, tachycardia
Sympathomimetics Norepinephrine Pseudoephedrine	Open bladder neck	α-Receptor antagonists	Arrhythmia, hypertension, coronary vasospasm, excitability, tremors
Antiadrenergics (alpha blockers) Phenoxybenzamine Phentolamine Terazosin Doxazosin Tamsulosin Alfuzosin	Smooth sphincter dyssynergia (competent, nonrelaxing bladder neck)	α-Receptor agonists	Orthostatic hypotension, dizziness, rhinitis, retrograde ejaculation
Tricyclic antidepressants Amitriptyline Imipramine	Hyperreflexic bladder with stress incontinence	Anticholinergic and sympathomimetic properties	Myocardial infarction, tachycardia, stroke, seizures, blood dyscrasias, dry mouth, drowsiness, constipation, blurred vision
Benzodiazepines Chlordiazepoxide	Extremity spasticity with detrusor-sphincter dyssynergia	γ-Aminobutyric acid (GABA) channel activator, centrally acting muscle relaxant	Dizziness, drowsiness, extrapyramidal effects, ataxia, agranulocytosis
Baclofen	Extremity spasticity with detrusor-sphincter dyssynergia	$GABA_B$ channel activator (?); exact mechanism unknown; centrally acting muscle relaxant	Central nervous system depression, cardiovascular collapse, respiratory failure, seizures, dizziness, weakness, hypotonia, constipation, blurred vision*
Dantrolene	Extremity spasticity with detrusor-sphincter dyssynergia	Direct muscle relaxant by calcium sequestration in the sarcoplasmic reticulum	Hepatic dysfunction, seizures, pleural effusion, incoordination, dizziness, nausea, vomiting, abdominal pain
Botulinum toxin	Detrusor-sphincter dyssynergia	Inhibits release of acetylcholine	Repeated injections necessary

*Note that baclofen is also administered intrathecally by an implanted pump in these patients, and adverse effects are primarily limited to the central nervous system. Bladder contractility may also be reduced. No significant change occurs in detrusor-sphincter dyssynergia.

finger in the patient's anal canal. The bulbocavernosus reflex should be tested. Because deep tendon reflexes at the patella reflect status of the spinal cord at L3-L4, hyperreflexia at the knee almost certainly indicates increased tone at the pelvic diaphragm and thus detrusor-sphincter dyssynergia. Absence of the toe plantar flexors reflects either damage to S2 or a supraconal lesion, and it therefore predicts damage to the external urinary sphincter and possible involvement of the bladder. For patients with spinal cord injury, the return of deep reflexes below the level of injury heralds the recovery from spinal cord shock. The first and most important determination with regard to bladder function is the establishment of good bladder evacuation. The abdomen must therefore be examined for bladder palpability after a trial of voiding. Either a bladder ultrasound scan or urinary catheterization should be performed to determine the postvoid residual.

Functional Limitations

Functional limitations are typically due to incontinence and include social rejection and isolation. Incontinence may also affect a patient's ability to work, to participate in recreational activities, and to sustain interpersonal relationships.

Diagnostic Studies

All patients with neural injury should have blood chemistries at baseline and periodically during follow-up for blood urea nitrogen and creatinine concentrations. Renal and bladder ultrasound examination should be performed to assess the status of the urinary tract: size, shape, and echogenicity of the kidneys; presence of hydronephrosis or hydroureter; presence of renal or bladder stones; change in hydronephrosis during and after voiding; and completeness of the void.

If vesicoureteral reflux or urethral strictures are suspected, voiding cystourethrography may be performed.

If renal stones are suspected, non–contrast-enhanced computed tomography (renal stone protocol) is an excellent tool for identification of the size and location of the stones. In dealing with renal stones, it is sometimes important to assess calyceal or ureteral anatomy or differential renal function, in which case intravenous urography may be performed. Finer qualitative assessment of differential renal function may be performed by technetium Tc 99m mertiatide (^{99m}Tc-MAG3) nuclear renal scan. When compromise of renal function is suspected, this test may be useful.

Transrectal linear array ultrasonography may be performed to assess prostate size, prominent median prostatic lobe, ledge at the bladder neck [16], or proximal urethral and bladder neck strictures. Voiding videofluoroscopy or ultrasonography can show abrupt cessation of urine flow.

Cystoscopy is an excellent tool for studying bladder and urethral anatomy; it quickly identifies the presence of a urethral stricture (although it may not determine its length or depth), provides an assessment of internal prostatic size, provides indirect evidence of high intravesical pressures (bladder trabeculation), and readily demonstrates bladder stones. Cystoscopy is essential in the assessment of hematuria (more than five red blood cells per high-power field on two or more urine specimens). Whereas hematuria in neurally injured patients is commonly related to infection or traumatic catheterization, the use of indwelling catheters for a long time places these patients at a significantly higher risk for bladder cancer [17]. It has been suggested, therefore, that these patients undergo surveillance cystoscopy annually, particularly if they have other risk factors for bladder cancer, such as smoking or a family history with bladder cancer. After bladder irrigation with normal saline, a urine specimen for malignant cell cytology may be helpful as a screening test. No test is as sensitive for the detection of bladder tumors as the cystoscopic examination and biopsy of a suspicious area.

Note that cystoscopy does not provide functional information. The best single test for bladder function is urodynamic testing. Formal urodynamic testing, including cystometrography and electromyography, is crucial to the proper documentation of bladder and outlet function. The test is subject to inherent errors in technique, interpretation, and cooperation of the patient; however, the astute clinician must interpret the results in light of the entire clinical scenario. Properly performed, it will elucidate and quantify postvoid residual of urine, bladder capacity, bladder compliance, bladder pressures during filling and voiding, and external sphincteric coordination. In conjunction with videofluoroscopic monitoring, ureteral reflux, bladder position, and internal and external sphincteric function may be visualized. Urodynamics should be performed at baseline for all patients with neurologic disease. Because of central nervous system shock in the acute phase of injury, it is best to perform urodynamics after the shock resolves—on return of distal reflexes. Figure 137.2 illustrates a normal voiding pattern. Figure 137.3 illustrates the urodynamic findings of an areflexic bladder. Figure 137.4A, B shows detrusor-sphincter dyssynergia. The sonographic correlate of detrusor-sphincter dyssynergia is shown in Figure 137.4C (nonrelaxation of the external urethral sphincter is demonstrated).

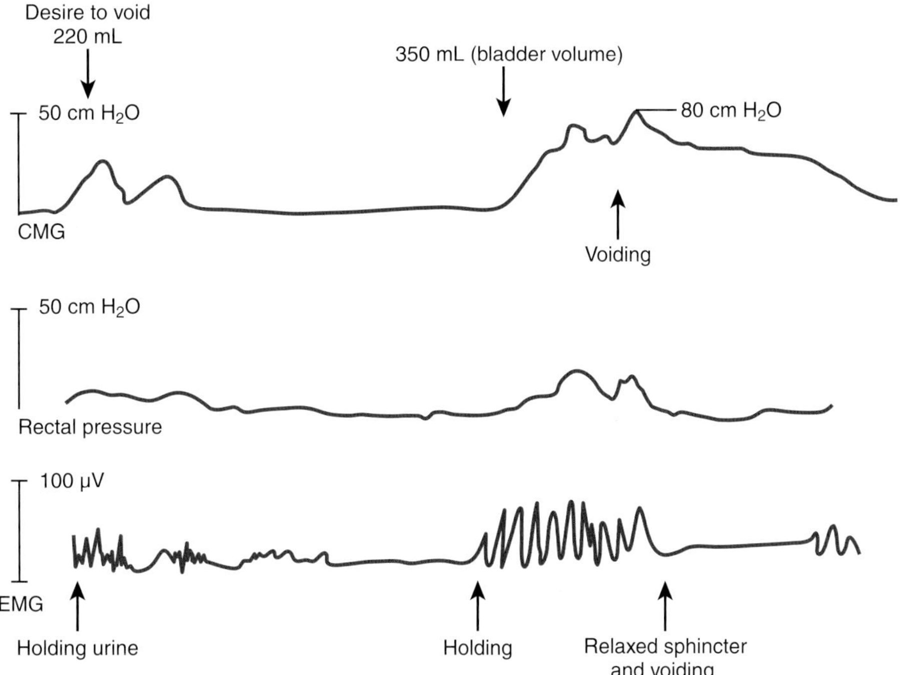

FIGURE 137.2 Urodynamic study consisting of simultaneous cystometrography (CMG), rectal pressure, and electromyography (EMG) of the external urethral sphincter. During bladder filling, the desire to void is usually expressed between 300 and 400 mL. When the normal person is asked to hold urine, the external urethral sphincter contracts and the bladder relaxes. When asked, this person voided voluntarily at a filling volume of approximately 350 mL; the external urethral sphincter relaxed just before voiding, indicating a normal study.

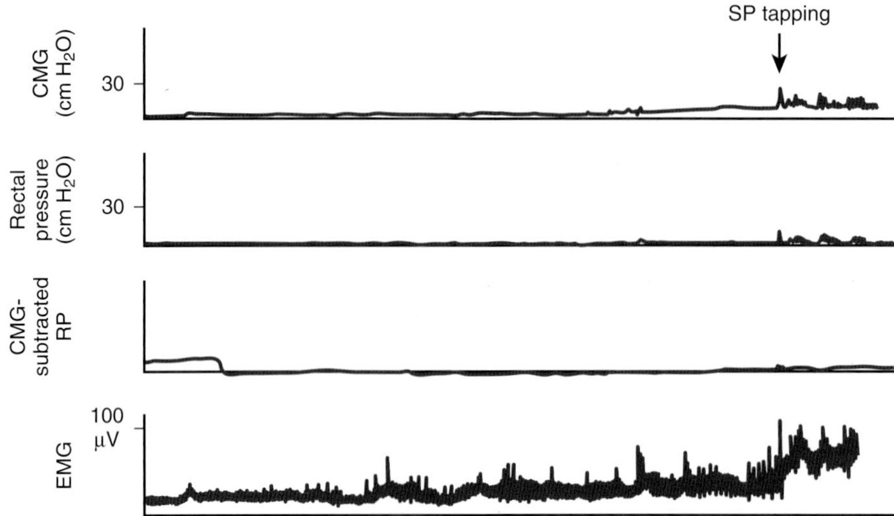

FIGURE 137.3 Urodynamic study demonstrating an areflexic bladder in a patient with spinal cord injury. There is minimal increase in electromyographic (EMG) activity during filling of the bladder. There is no bladder contraction, even after suprapubic (SP) tapping, indicating overdistention areflexia or a lower motor neuron lesion. *CMG*, cystometrography; *RP*, rectal pressure.

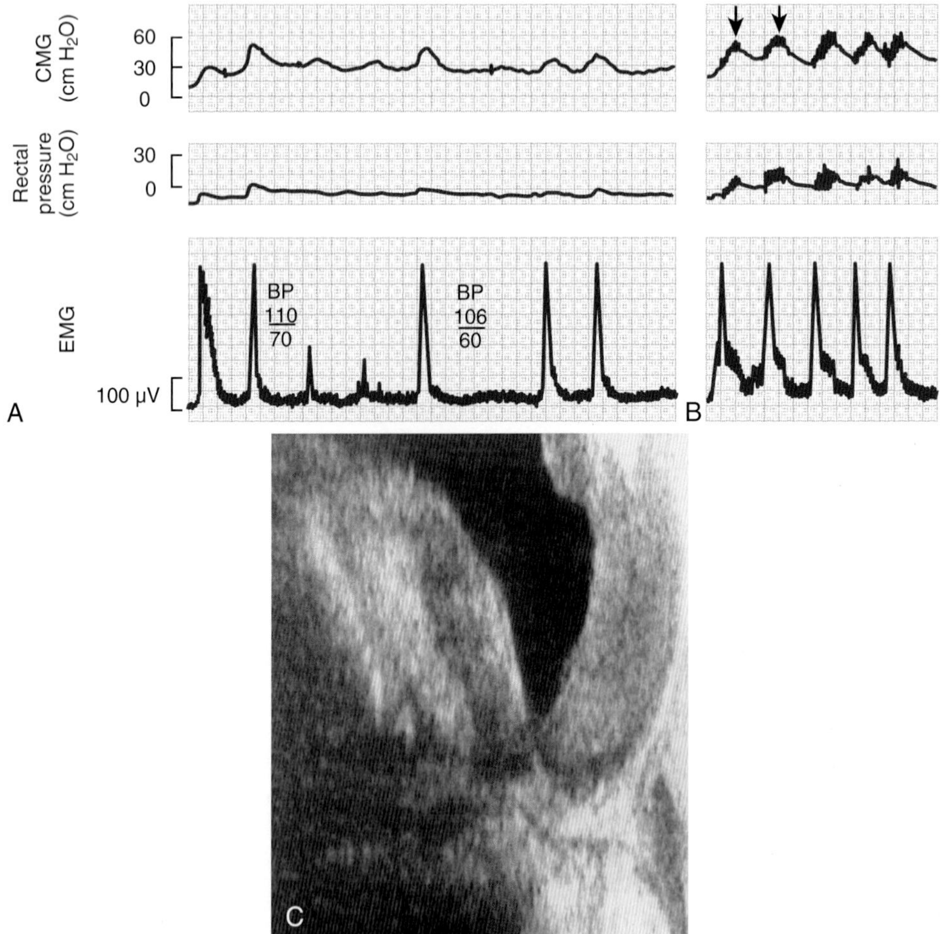

FIGURE 137.4 **A** and **B,** Detrusor-sphincter dyssynergia in a patient with spinal cord injury; each bladder contraction on the cystometrogram (CMG) is accompanied by a marked increase in electromyographic (EMG) activity of the external urethral sphincter. *BP,* blood pressure. **C,** Ultrasound cystourethrogram during an attempted void in a patient with spinal cord injury with detrusor-sphincter dyssynergia. The passage of urine is abruptly stopped by closure of the external urethral sphincter, and the posterior urethra is dilated.

Differential Diagnosis

The diseases listed in Table 137.1 are the most common causes of neurogenic bladder.

Treatment

Initial

The priorities of bladder management relate first to preservation of renal function and abolition of infection and second to social concerns. Overflow incontinence, ureteral reflux, or high bladder pressures in the presence of renal insufficiency or active infection must be managed aggressively by ensuring proper egress for urine. A source for persistent infection, such as urinary lithiasis, must be sought and, if found, eliminated. High bladder pressure, particularly if it is sustained (>40 cm H_2O), ultimately results in deterioration of renal function and should therefore be addressed actively, even if renal function is normal [18].

Rehabilitation

Patients at risk for degenerative neurogenic bladders, particularly those with (or at risk for) sensory neuropathies (e.g., diabetic patients, phenytoin users), should have a timed voiding schedule to prevent overdistention and progression to bladder areflexia. A 24-hour voiding diary, including fluid intake, time and quantity voided, and postvoid residual (by catheterization or ultrasound evaluation), should be recorded periodically. These patients should void every 6 hours, void again immediately after the first void, and adjust their fluid intake and voiding frequency according to the voiding diary. Patients with diabetes should be careful to maintain good glycemic control, not only for global prevention of related degenerative disease but also to prevent osmotic diuresis.

Most neurogenic bladder lesions are associated with impaired bowel function. Fecal impaction and obstructed constipation may also cause mechanical obstruction to the passage of urine. Further, many of the medications used to reduce bladder contractility, particularly the anticholinergics, exacerbate bowel motility dysfunction. It is therefore important that these patients be routinely prescribed high-fiber diets, stool softeners (e.g., docusate, 100 mg orally, three times daily), laxatives (e.g., psyllium, 1 packet [3.4 g] orally every day), and suppositories (e.g., bisacodyl, 10 mg per rectum every day) and undergo digital stimulation either daily or every other day. Digital stimulation is best performed after either a meal or coffee or tea to take advantage of the gastrocolic reflex.

The Credé method (suprapubic pressure) alone can lead to high intravesical pressures and even vesicoureteral reflux. Such pressure, or persistent tapping of the suprapubic region for 2 minutes at a time, should be performed only when methods to relieve bladder outlet obstruction have been ensured. This should not be performed in patients with active detrusor-sphincter dyssynergia and detrusor hyperreflexia because it will only exacerbate already high bladder pressures, and urine will not be completely evacuated.

Acute Phase and Central Nervous System Shock Phase

This phase usually lasts days to weeks. The bladder is areflexic during this period, and adequate bladder drainage should be secured to prevent the areflexic bladder from developing overdistention and myogenic failure. Indwelling continuous Foley catheterization (14 F) is the easiest way to ensure bladder drainage. Alternatively, intermittent catheterization may be performed (after the initial phase of diuresis) and, when it is used from the onset, reduces the incidence of infection and stone disease [19].

Patients do need training or assistance in self-catheterization. Rehabilitation nurses may also be involved in this educational process. Catheterization is performed every 4 to 6 hours and fluid is restricted to a maximum of 2 liters per day, if possible. The frequency of catheterization should be adjusted so that residuals are no more than 300 to 400 mL. For patients with a hyperreflexic bladder, long-term intermittent catheterization requires mitigation of the detrusor reflex with anticholinergics (Table 137.2).

Anticholinergic Drugs (Drugs to Increase Bladder Capacity)

In the human being, bladder (detrusor muscle) has muscarinic receptors (M_2 and M_3 receptors). M_3 receptors compared with M_2 receptors are small in number but are mainly responsible for bladder contraction. The antimuscarinic drugs oxybutynin, tolterodine, darifenacin, solifenacin, and trospium are the five major drugs (Table 137.3) currently available to modulate detrusor hyperreflexia, to increase bladder capacity, and to reduce bladder voiding pressures. Comparative clinical studies have shown that oxybutynin and solifenacin may be marginally more effective than tolterodine, although tolterodine seems to be better tolerated; but dry mouth and constipation are still major problems for compliance of patients with all of them because of the widespread existence of M_3 receptors, particularly in the salivary glands. Except for trospium chloride, most of the other drugs shown in Table 137.3 are tertiary amines and cross the blood-brain barrier, enhancing the anticholinergic factor. There is evidence that they may lead to some loss of memory, particularly in elderly patients [20].

Anticholinergic drugs have been, on the whole, a disappointment in the treatment of incontinence associated with neurogenic detrusor overactivity. Whereas urodynamic parameters often improve and the number of incontinence episodes is often reduced by anticholinergics, incontinence often remains a problem. Mirabegron (Myrbetriq; Astellas Pharma US, Inc), a selective β_3-receptor agonist that causes detrusor fundus relaxation, has emerged recently as a pharmaceutical alternative for patients failing to respond to anticholinergic therapy in the able-bodied idiopathic overactive bladder population [21]. It has not yet been studied in the neurogenic bladder population, although a trial is certain for this in the near future. According to the Food and Drug Administration, its most important side effect is significant hypertension, noted in 11.3% (compared with 7.6% in the placebo arm), which is reversible with discontinuation of the drug. It is dosed at 25 mg or 50 mg orally once daily. Botox injections are used in the bladder wall to reduce bladder

Table 137.3 Summary of Anticholinergic Agents

Anticholinergic*	$T_{1/2}$ (h)	Typical Side Effects	Comments
Oxybutynin Ditropan	2-3	Dry mouth, constipation, blurry vision, headaches Elderly: cognitive impairment, hallucinations	Typical dose is 5 mg orally tid
Ditropan XL	13	Same as oral oxybutynin	Slower absorption with more stable blood concentration Typical dose is 10 mg orally daily, but doses up to 40 mg daily are generally safe
Oxytrol (oxybutynin patch)	2-5	Same as oral oxybutynin, plus local skin irritation	Bypasses first pass of the liver, which reduces the concentrations of active metabolites that are thought to contribute to side effects Dosed at 3.9 mg/day, 1 patch 2 times/week, alternating skin sites
Tolterodine Detrol	2-10	Same as oral oxybutynin	Possibly more selective to urinary M receptors, resulting in fewer side effects Typical dose is 2 mg orally bid
Detrol LA	2-10	Same as oral oxybutynin	Slower absorption with more stable blood concentration Typical dose is 4 mg orally daily
Darifenacin (Enablex)	13-19	Same as oral oxybutynin	Typical dose is 7.5 mg or 15 mg orally daily
Trospium	20	Same as oral oxybutynin	Quaternary amine does not cross the blood-brain barrier well, resulting in minimal central nervous system anticholinergic effect, and it may limit cognitive side effects (particularly in the elderly) Typical dose is 20 mg orally bid
Sanctura XR	36	Same as oral oxybutynin	More stable blood concentration Typical dose is 60 mg orally daily
Solifenacin (VESIcare)	45-68	Same as oral oxybutynin	Typical dose is 5 mg or 10 mg orally daily

*Unless patients with urinary retention are managed with a catheter, anticholinergic therapy is contraindicated for them. Anticholinergics are also contraindicated in patients with gastric retention and patients with uncontrolled narrow-angle glaucoma.
$T_{1/2}$ (h), pharmacokinetic half-life (hours).

pressures to safe levels (<40 cm H_2O) and to achieve continence between catheterizations.

Procedures

Another alternative to long-term management of bladder drainage is placement of a suprapubic catheter. This is preferable to chronic transurethral catheterization because it eliminates the risk of urethral or meatal erosion and is less often the cause of epididymitis or orchitis. Urinary tract infections, however, are just as likely, and these catheters require changing once a month. They are best placed either in the operating room under cystoscopic guidance or, better, through suprapubic incision to ascertain that the catheter ultimately resides as superiorly as possible, far from the bladder neck. This helps prevent irritation at the bladder neck, which often causes reflex bladder contractions, particularly if the catheter balloon (also in an indwelling Foley catheter) drops down into the posterior urethra (Fig. 137.5).

Botulinum Toxin

Patients with neurogenic overactive bladder failing to respond to anticholinergic therapy may benefit from periodic administration of intravesical onabotulinumtoxinA, the leading manufactured agent being Botox. Its purported mechanism of action is the inhibition of release of acetylcholine at the presynaptic cholinergic junction [22], which effectively suppresses detrusor contraction [23]. Botox is typically administered by submucosal injection cystoscopically in 0.5-mL aliquots; the total dose ranges from 100 to 300 units through a rigid or flexible cystoscope.

Prospective randomized double-blind placebo-controlled trials showed that Botox is efficacious and safe in patients with neurogenic detrusor overactivity and incontinence, with clinical benefits seen up to 9 months after injection [24,25]. Botox reduced incontinence episodes and improved quality of life in patients with multiple sclerosis and in patients with spinal cord injury (T1 or lower). Median time to a request for re-treatment was 42 weeks [24]. In a 7-year retrospective review of 216 patients given Botox or Dysport in 365 sessions, significant improvement was seen in maximum detrusor pressure, detrusor compliance, and bladder capacity at 6 weeks and 6 months; a quarter of the patients never stopped anticholinergic therapy; half discontinued after 6 weeks; and after 6 months, 35% still had not resumed anticholinergic therapy [26]. In a randomized placebo-controlled study [27], similar improvement was demonstrated in urodynamic outcomes. Reitz and colleagues [28] showed that 73% of neurogenic detrusor overactivity incontinent patients achieved continence with Botox at 12 weeks.

After Botox injection, postvoid residuals may be significantly elevated in a dose-dependent fashion; a third of patients had urinary retention and required intermittent catheterization [24]. Another drawback of this agent is need for repeated treatment periodically. Rarely, generalized weakness, difficulty in swallowing, or dysarthria ensues, although these side effects reverse spontaneously in several weeks [26].

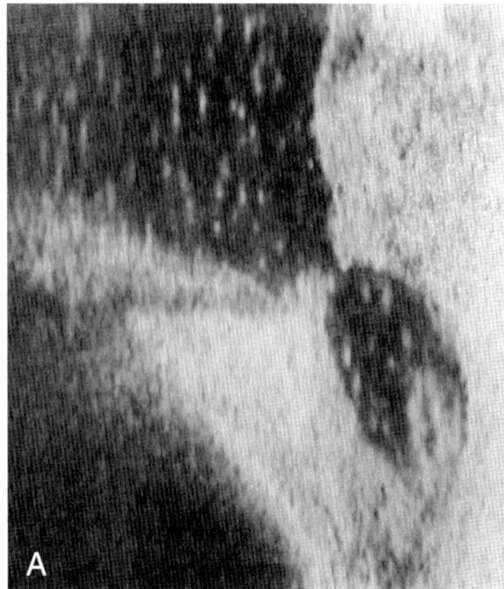

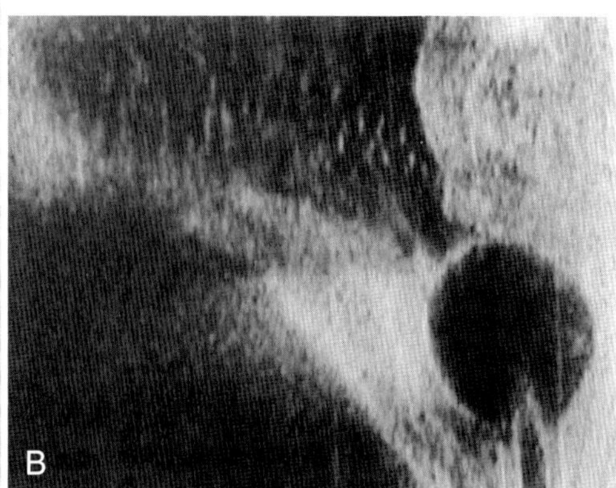

FIGURE 137-5 **A,** Linear array ultrasound–voiding cystourethrogram shows a contracted bladder neck and dilated prostatic urethra. **B,** The balloon of the urethral Foley catheter is lodged in the prostatic urethra. This occurs uncommonly; however, it may lead to inadequate bladder drainage and, in patients with lesions above T6, autonomic dysreflexia.

Sacral Nerve Stimulation

For patients with hyperreflexic bladders, electrical stimulation through peripheral patch electrodes or implantation of a sacral nerve root stimulator may be of some benefit [29–31]. The treatment is dependent on an intact sacral reflex and works by modulation of signaling from somatic and afferent nerves involved in the micturition reflex pathway. Patients must be able to empty the bladder voluntarily (or by Valsalva maneuver) when the device is turned off or be capable of performing intermittent self-catheterization.

Installation of a sacral nerve stimulator may be done in two stages: a test phase with temporary wires, typically lasting about 1 week; and pending a successful outcome with the test phase, installation of a permanent system. Correct placement of the lead is done under local anesthesia with the patient awake and conversant in the prone position. Its placement in the correct foramen level (typically S3) and depth of penetration to the anterior nerve root are confirmed by real-time fluoroscopic imaging, assessment for a tapping sensation in the vagina or perineum, dorsiflexion of the ipsilateral great toe, and bellowing contraction of the perineal area. For those having a permanent implant, the patient is then typically sedated for subcutaneous placement of the implantable pulse generator and tunneling of the wire.

The studies reported are primarily in able-bodied populations with idiopathic detrusor hyperreflexia. Limited evaluation thus far in the neurogenic population, however, has shown promise. In a review and meta-analysis of 26 studies, including 357 patients, and a mean follow-up of 26 months concerning the safety and efficacy of sacral nerve stimulation in neurogenic lower urinary tract dysfunction, the pooled success rate was 68% for the test phase and 92% for permanent sacral nerve stimulator implantation [32]. Adverse events were seen in none in the test placement group and 24% in the permanent placement group. Adverse effects include pain, infection, and lead migration. In one study, 33% required surgical revision [33]. The life span of these implantable pulse generators varies with intensity of use but averages about 5 years.

Sacral nerve stimulator implantation is relatively contraindicated in multiple sclerosis patients to the extent that these patients are frequently studied by magnetic resonance imaging over time. It is also not appropriate for patients with significant spinal and sacral bone abnormalities.

Surgery

Transurethral sphincterotomy has been used in suprasacral lesions in the past and has fallen into disfavor because of intraoperative and delayed bleeding potential. Use of a laser in a contact mode causes virtually no intraoperative bleeding [11,34]. This procedure results in incontinence postoperatively and requires the use of an external condom catheter.

There are rare circumstances in which bladder management has aggravated renal function, evidenced by recurrent ascending urinary tract infections or a bladder that is too contracted to store sufficient volumes. Some patients find it socially unacceptable to be incontinent and are willing to perform intermittent self-catheterization, but the body habitus precludes them from this. In such cases, there are certain reconstructive options that should be considered. An incontinent urinary diversion with a stoma in abdomen that drains urine in a bag may be performed [35,36]. Cystectomy may be combined with this procedure or the bladder may be left in situ with a small risk of pyocystis.

In patients willing and able to perform intermittent self-catheterization, the most common reconstructive alternative is an augmentation cystoplasty. The bladder is augmented by a segment of ileum, and the ureters remain in their native locations. Bladder pressure is reduced and capacity increased, thus protecting the upper tracts from side effects of high pressure bladder. The drainage of urine is performed by intermittent self-catheterization. This procedure may be combined with an artificial rrinary sphincter in patients with incompetent sphincter.

For bladders that have low pressures and good compliance but leak through fixed sphincters, the Mitrofanoff and bladder neck closure may be an excellent option. Spina bifida patients with conus lesions might be good candidates for this procedure. Egress through the bladder neck is eliminated, and the appendix is interposed between the bladder and the umbilicus where it is opened. In the common event that the bladder has poor compliance, an ileal bladder augmentation will raise bladder volume and lower bladder pressure. Patients would then catheterize their augmented bladders through the umbilicus.

Potential Disease Complications

Urinary tract infections, kidney stones, and autonomic dysreflexia are common disease complications associated with neurogenic bladder. Social isolation due to incontinence may lead to depression.

Patients with spinal cord injury who have a urinary tract infection commonly may not present with symptoms [4]. Fevers, chills, back pain, suprapubic pain, dysuria, frequency, and testicular swelling in the setting of positive urine cultures should be regarded as a urinary tract infection. Patients without overt symptoms of pyelonephritis, prostatitis, epididymitis-orchitis, or cystitis are more difficult to diagnose, particularly if they have an indwelling catheter or are being managed by intermittent catheterization. Those using catheters are virtually always colonized with bacteria, and the injudicious use of antibiotics will only select out resistant strains. Factors indicating a need for treatment include urinary lithiasis, as this is most often related to infection (struvite, magnesium ammonium phosphate), and pyuria (8 to 10 white blood cells per high-power field, or 100 white blood cells per milliliter) in the setting of bacteriuria (more than 10,000 colony-forming units per milliliter). Urine pH should be checked periodically; pH above 7 is invariably associated with infection from urea-splitting organisms, which may lead to struvite stone formation.

Patients with detrusor-sphincter dyssynergia or urinary retention of any kind should have the bladder drained expeditiously with a fresh Foley catheter during the course of their treatment to ascertain good egress of infected urine. If prostatitis is suspected, transurethral insertion of a Foley catheter is relatively contraindicated, and drainage should be ensured suprapubically. Fluoroquinolones are an excellent first choice for most urinary tract infections; therapy may then be tailored to culture and sensitivity results. Three to 5 days is sufficient for cystitis. Pyelonephritis requires 2 weeks of therapy. Epididymitis requires at least 3 weeks of therapy, and prostatitis often requires 6 weeks. A higher incidence of bladder cancer (squamous cell) has been reported in patients with long-term indwelling bladder drainage [37].

Autonomic Dysreflexia

The control of widespread sympathetic activity below the spinal lesion is the key factor in the management of autonomic dysreflexia, and prevention is the first concern. Noxious stimuli, such as overdistention of the bladder, should be reversed immediately by catheter drainage. Local instillation of 20 mL of lidocaine jelly of 0.3% tetracaine through the Foley catheter or suprapubic tube may provide topical anesthesia of the vesical mucosa and reduce triggering impulses to the spinal cord. Consideration of procedures for patients at risk (spinal lesions above T6) should include spinal anesthesia, use of ganglion blockers, and use of adrenergic blockers.

In the acute episode, if reversal of the noxious stimulus fails to control symptoms, administration of nifedipine (10-30 mg sublingually [38]) or nitropaste (about 1 inch applied on the body surface) is usually adequate to reduce blood pressure. Note that normal blood pressure for a patient with spinal cord injury is less than 100 mm Hg systolic. If nifedipine fails, hydralazine (10 to 20 mg intravenously or 10 to 50 mg intramuscularly) may be administered. Use lower doses initially and repeat every 20 to 30 minutes as necessary to maintain a low blood pressure. Other useful drugs include alpha blockers (such as prazosin, terazosin, guanethidine, and clonidine) and anticholinergics (such as oxybutynin and tolterodine). For long-term management of autonomic dysreflexia, clonidine (0.1 to 0.3 mg orally twice daily) is useful. Note that the chronic form of this syndrome is often related to active detrusor-sphincter dyssynergia, and methods aimed at control of this phenomenon, such as transurethral sphincterotomy, may alleviate the patient of autonomic dysreflexia [11].

Potential Treatment Complications

For those who have had indwelling Foley catheters for an extended period (more than several days) and require catheter removal or exchange, antibiotics should be administered prophylactically before, during, and after removal of the existing catheter. Gentamicin (80 mg intramuscularly once just before removal of the catheter) is appropriate for most patients with stable renal function, even if function is impaired, and has both gram-positive and gram-negative coverage. Those with prosthetics, aortic stenosis, or other risk factors for seeding should have coadministration of ampicillin (1 g intravenously) for enterococcus coverage. Alternatively, amoxicillin–clavulanic acid (750 mg) or ciprofloxacin (500 mg) may be given orally twice daily before and 24 hours after placement of the new catheter. In addition, the bladder should be irrigated gently through the catheter with 50 mL of Neosporin G.U. irrigant (DSM Pharmaceutical, Inc., Greenville, North Carolina) (at body temperature) containing 40 mg/L Neomycin and 200,000 units/L Polymixin B. Irrigation should be avoided in patients with a defect/ulceration in the bladder mucosa or in postoperative patients for the toxic absorption of these drugs; ideally, a new catheter is placed and urine for culture is obtained to avoid culturing bacteria in the biolayer around the catheter [32]. Bladder is irrigated with GU irrigant every 4 hours for at least 48 hours. Irrigation is continued while the catheter is being pulled through the urethra to remove urethral pathogens. This method has been shown to significantly reduce urinary tract infection related to catheter changes [33, 34].

Attention to hygiene is paramount in the prevention of urinary tract infections in the spinal cord–injured population. Those on condom catheter drainage should change it once a day. Leg bags should be routinely disinfected with 6% Clorox solution or bleach (most cost-efficient) and then washed well with running water. Wheelchair seat cushions should be changed and cleaned, and the patient should take a shower daily to reduce colony counts at the perineum. Suppressive treatment should be considered for patients who demonstrate recurrent infections. Nitrofurantoin, 100 mg orally daily, is sufficient. Methenamine hippurate

(1 g orally twice a day) and ascorbic acid (500 mg orally daily) acidify the urine and may be good for prophylaxis of urinary tract infection [40,41].

Stoma care after colostomy is a source of great consternation for many who have it because of frequent appliance leaks and skin irritation. Also, the stoma must be situated properly on the abdomen according to the patient's habitus and positioning in the wheelchair. Bladder augmentations of any kind are susceptible to perforations and life-threatening infections (as much as 10%). These patients have a 3% chance of small bowel obstruction from adhesions during their lifetime. Chronic indwelling Foley catheters carry the potential for urinary infection, meatal erosion, epididymitis-orchitis, stone disease, and urethral fistula. In women, the urethra becomes patulous in time and incontinence ensues with or without a catheter. Finally, with time and repeated infections, indwelling catheters put patients at risk for development of squamous cell cancer of the bladder [37]. Although the incidence is low, gross hematuria should be evaluated with great suspicion in these patients because this disease is often advanced at the time of discovery and is often fatal [39].

References

[1] Wein AJ, Dmochowski RR. Neuromuscular dysfunction of the lower urinary tract. In: Wein AJ, Kavoussi LR, Novick AC, et al., editors. Campbell-Walsh urology. 10th ed. Philadelphia: Saunders Elsevier; 2011. p. 351–8.

[2] Bradley WE, Timm GW, Scott FB. Innervation of the detrusor muscle and urethra. Urol Clin North Am 1974;1:3–27.

[3] Denny-Brown D, Robertson EG. On the physiology of micturition. Brain 1933;56:149.

[4] Perkash I. Long-term urologic management of the patient with spinal cord injury. Urol Clin North Am 1993;3:423–34.

[5] Igawa Y. Discussion: functional role of M_1, M_2, and M_3 muscarinic receptors in overactive bladder. Urology 2000;55(Suppl 5A):47–9.

[6] Gosling JA, Dixon JS. The structure and innervation of smooth muscle in the wall of the bladder neck and proximal urethra. Br J Urol 1975;47:549–58.

[7] Kavia RB, Dasgupta R, Fowler CJ. Functional imaging and the central control of the bladder [review]. J Comp Neurol 2005;493:27–32.

[8] Khan A, Hertanu J, Yang WC, et al. Predictive correlation of urodynamic dysfunction and brain injury after cerebrovascular accident. J Urol 1981;126:86–8.

[9] Sakakibara R, Hattori T, Uchiyama T, Yamanishi TJ. Videourodynamic and sphincter motor unit potential analyses in Parkinson's disease and multiple system atrophy. J Neurol Neurosurg Psychiatry 2001;71:600–6.

[10] deGroat WC, Steers WD. Autonomic regulation of the urinary bladder and sexual organs. In: Loewy AD, Spyer KM, editors. Central regulation of autonomic functions. Oxford: Oxford University Press; 1990. p. 313–4.

[11] Perkash I. Transrectal sphincterotomy provides significant relief in autonomic dysreflexia in spinal cord injured patients: long term follow up results. J Urol 2007;177:1026–9.

[12] Fam B, Yalla SV. Vesicourethral dysfunction in spinal cord injury and its management. Semin Neurol 1988;8:150–5.

[13] Wein AJ. Neuromuscular dysfunction of the lower urinary tract and its treatment. In: Walsh PC, Retik AB, Vaughan ED, et al., editors. Campbell's urology. 7th ed. Philadelphia: WB Saunders; 1998. p. 961.

[14] Burney TL, Senapti M, Desai S, et al. Acute cerebrovascular accident and lower urinary tract dysfunction: a prospective correlation of the site of brain injury with urodynamic findings. J Urol 1996;156:1748–50.

[15] Borrie MJ, Campbell A, Caradoc-Davies TH, et al. Urinary incontinence after stroke: a prospective study. Age Ageing 1986;15:177–81.

[16] Perkash I, Friedland GW. Posterior ledge at the bladder neck: crucial diagnostic role of ultrasonography. Urol Radiol 1986;8:175–83.

[17] West DA, Cummings JM, Longo WE. Role of chronic catheterization in the development of bladder cancer in patients with spinal cord injury. Urology 1999;53:292–7.

[18] Flood HD, Ritchey ML, Bloom DA, et al. Outcome of reflux in children with myelodysplasia managed by bladder pressure monitoring. J Urol 1994;152:1574–7.

[19] Guttman L, Frankel H. The value of intermittent catheterization in early management of traumatic paraplegia and tetraplegia. Paraplegia 1966;4:63–84.

[20] Katz IR, Prouty Sands L, Bilker W, et al. Identification of medications that cause cognitive impairment in older people: the case of oxybutynin chloride. J Am Geriatr Soc 1988;46:8–13.

[21] Otsuki H, Kosaka T, Nakamura K, et al. β_3-Adrenoceptor agonist mirabegron is effective for overactive bladder that is unresponsive to antimuscarinic treatment or is related to benign prostatic hyperplasia in men. Int Urol Nephrol 2013;45:53–60.

[22] Simpson LL. Molecular pharmacology of botulinum toxin and tetanus toxin. Annu Rev Pharmacol Toxicol 1986;26:427–53.

[23] Nitti VW. Botulinum toxin for the treatment of idiopathic and neurogenic overactive bladder: state of the art. Rev Urol 2006;8:198–208.

[24] Herschorn S, Gajewski J, Ethans K, et al. Efficacy of botulinum toxin A injection for neurogenic detrusor overactivity and urinary incontinence: a randomized, double-blind trial. J Urol 2011;185:2229–35.

[25] Cruz F, Herschorn S, Aliotta P, et al. Efficacy and safety of onabotulinumtoxinA in patients with urinary incontinence due to neurogenic detrusor overactivity: a randomised, double-blind, placebo-controlled trial. Eur Urol 2011;60:742–50.

[26] Stoehrer M, Wolff A, Kramer G, et al. Treatment of neurogenic detrusor overactivity with botulinum toxin A: the first seven years. Urol Int 2009;83:379–85.

[27] Schurch B, de Seze M, Denys P, et al. Botulinum toxin type A is a safe and effective treatment for neurogenic urinary incontinence: results of a single treatment, randomized, placebo controlled 6-month study. J Urol 2005;174:196–200.

[28] Reitz A, Stohrer M, Kramer G, et al. European experience of 200 cases treated with botulinum-A toxin injections into the detrusor muscle for urinary incontinence due to neurogenic detrusor overactivity. Eur Urol 2004;45:510–5.

[29] Gasparini ME, Schmidt RA, Tanagho EA. Selective sacral rhizotomy in the management of the reflex neuropathic bladder: a report on 17 patients with long-term followup. J Urol 1992;148:1207–10.

[30] Ohlsson BL, Fall M, Frankenberg-Sommars D. Effects of external and direct pudendal nerve maximal electrical stimulation in the treatment of the uninhibited overactive bladder. Br J Urol 1989;64:374–80.

[31] Jonas U, Fowler CJ, Chancellor MB, et al. Efficacy of sacral nerve stimulation for urinary retention: results 18 months after implantation. J Urol 2001;165:15–9.

[32] Kessler TM, La Framboise D, Trelle S, et al. Sacral neuromodulation for neurogenic lower urinary tract dysfunction: systematic review and meta-analysis. Eur Urol 2010;58:865–74.

[33] Vasdev N, Biles BD, Sandher R, Hasan TS. The surgical management of the refractory overactive bladder. Indian J Urol 2010;26:263–9.

[34] Perkash I. Contact laser sphincterotomy: further experience and longer follow-up. Spinal Cord 1996;34:227–33.

[35] McDougal WS. Use of intestinal segments and urinary diversion. In: Walsh PC, Retik AB, Vaughan ED, et al., editors. Campbell's urology. 7th ed Philadelphia: WB Saunders; 1998. p. 3146.

[36] Rink RC, Adams MCL. Augmentation cystoplasty. In: Walsh PC, Retik AB, Vaughan ED, et al., editors. Campbell's urology. 7th ed. Philadelphia: WB Saunders; 1998. p. 3167–89.

[37] Serretta V, Pomara G, Piazza F, Gange E. Pure squamous cell carcinoma of the bladder in western countries. Report on 19 consecutive cases. Eur Urol 2000;37:85–9.

[38] Messerli FH, Grossman E. The use of sublingual nifedipine: a continuing concern. Arch Intern Med 1999;159:2259–60.

[39] Banovac K, Wade N, Gonzalez F, et al. Decreased incidence of urinary tract infections in patients with spinal cord injury: effect of methenamine. J Am Paraplegia Soc 1991;14:52–4.

[40] Rhame FS, Perkash I. Urinary tract infections occurring in recent spinal cord injury patients on intermittent catheterization. J Urol 1979;122:669–73.

[41] Pearman JW. Prevention of urinary tract infections following spinal cord injury. Paraplegia 1971;9:95–104.

CHAPTER 138

Neurogenic Bowel

Inder Perkash, MD, FRCS, FACS
Meena Agarwal, MD, PhD, MS, Dip Urol, FRCS, FRCS(Urol)

Synonyms

None

ICD-9 Code

564.81 Neurogenic bowel

ICD-10 Code

K59.2 Neurogenic bowel

Definition

Within the nervous system, there are peripheral, somatic, and autonomic (sympathetic and parasympathetic) contributions to the various organ-based functions. Related to the gastrointestinal system, several end-organ problems resulting from neurologic dysfunction include prolonged colonic transit time, reduced anorectal sensibility, and lack of voluntary control of the external anal and urethral sphincters, often associated with a dyssynergic response. The severity of colorectal dysfunction depends on the degree of completeness and level of the spinal cord injury [1,2]. However, specific evaluation is required in individual cases. These problems have an extensive impact on quality of life. Our study based on interviews of 125 consecutive male patients and 2 female patients with spinal cord injury showed that 27% of patients had chronic disabling gastrointestinal problems requiring alteration of their lifestyle; symptoms usually appeared 5 to 10 years after injury ($P < .05$) [3]. Severity of bowel dysfunction correlated with high level of lesion, completeness of cord injury, and longer duration of injury (≥10 years) [4,5].

Bowel Innervations and Gastrointestinal Motility

Unlike in the bladder, small and large bowel movements are mainly autonomous and may be influenced with some spinal cord lesions. The vagus nerve, which arises intracranially and provides parasympathetic innervations from the esophagus to the splenic flexure of the colon, is spared in spinal cord lesions (Fig. 138.1). The pelvic nerve carries parasympathetic fibers from S2-S4 to the descending colon and rectum. Some pelvic nerve branches travel proximally and innervate the transverse and ascending colon [6]. Sympathetic innervations are supplied by the superior and inferior mesenteric (T9-T12) and hypogastric (T12-L2) nerves. The somatic pudendal nerve (S2-S4) innervates the pelvic floor.

The intrinsic nervous system of the gastrointestinal tract, which includes Auerbach plexus, is situated in the colonic wall between the longitudinal and circular muscle layers. This nerve supply helps coordinate colonic wall movement and the advancement of stool through the colon. The behavior of the bowel can be controlled by the intrinsic innervations of the gut independently of input from the central nervous system.

The extrinsic nervous system also innervates the colon and includes the parasympathetic, sympathetic, and somatic nerves [4,5]. Peristaltic waves travel both toward and away from the ileocecal valve in the ascending colon; but in the descending colon, the waves travel mainly to push the contents to the anus [4]. The motility of the colon is performed by three primary mechanisms: myogenic, chemical, and neurogenic. The myogenic transmission of signals occurs between enteric smooth muscle cells that are interconnected by gap junctions, which produces transmission from cell to cell. Most intestinal muscle displays autorhythmicity that causes colonic wall contractions [4].

Chemical control is through the activity of neurotransmitters and hormones. The chemicals influence the promotion or inhibition of contractions through the action of the central nervous system or autonomic nervous system or by direct action on muscle cells. This activity can be triggered by luminal stimuli that are detected by nerves through epithelial intermediation. Epithelial enterochromaffin cells act as sensory transducers that activate the mucosal processes of both intrinsic and extrinsic primary afferent neurons through their release of 5-hydroxytryptamine (5-HT). Intrinsic primary afferent neurons are present in both the submucosal and myenteric plexuses. Peristaltic and secretory reflexes are initiated by submucosal intrinsic primary afferent neurons, which are stimulated by 5-HT acting at 5-HT_{1P} receptors. Serotonergic transmission within the enteric nervous system and the activation of myenteric intrinsic primary afferent neurons are 5-HT_3 mediated [6]. Signaling to the central nervous system is also predominantly 5-HT_3

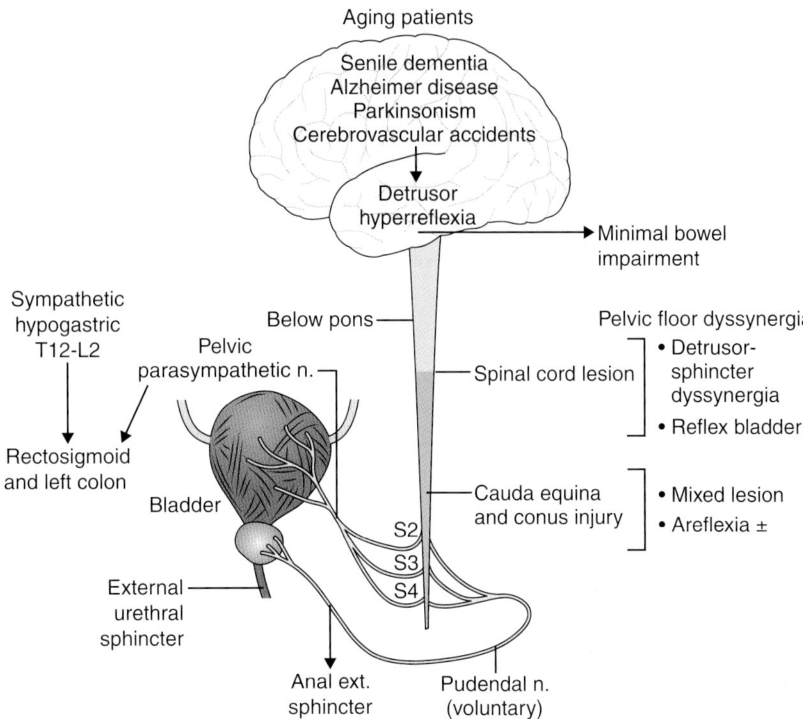

FIGURE 138-1 Important central neural control of the pelvic organs and resultant dysfunctions after denervation. *(Modified with permission from Zafar Khan.)*

mediated. The gut is thus the only organ that can display reflexes and integrate neuronal activity even when it is isolated from the central nervous system.

The neurogenic mechanism of colonic control is through the enteric nervous system, which coordinates all segmental motility and some propagated movement. The number of intrinsic neurons in the gut greatly exceeds the number of fibers in the vagus and splanchnic nerves. In humans, the enteric nervous system contains up to 100 million neurons, compared with only 2000 efferent fibers in the vagus nerve, suggesting that intrinsic nerves may direct most reflex and control activities and that the extrinsic innervations may serve only a modulatory function [7,8].

Normal defecation is the result of a complex interaction between muscles, nerves, and central nervous system. For a normal defecation, there needs to be a mass movement of colonic contents associated with relaxation of internal and external anal sphincters. Mass movement of colonic contents before defecation associated with internal sphincter relaxation has recently been shown to result from high-amplitude propagating contractions in children even with sigmoid dysmotility [9]. The colon absorbs fluids, electrolytes, and short-chain fatty acids; provides for growth of symbiotic bacteria; secretes mucus for lubrication of feces; and slowly propels stool toward the anus [10]. The contents in the distal colon are retained until bowel evacuation. Transport of contents may take 12 to 30 hours from the ileocecal valve to the rectum [2].

Neurogenic Bowel

A neurogenic bowel occurs when there is a dysfunction of the colon or rectosigmoid due to the lack of nervous control [11–13]. The enteric nervous system remains intact after spinal cord injury. However, depending on the level of the injury, different bowel problems and complications may arise. The lower motor neuron bowel syndrome or areflexic bowel results from a lesion affecting the parasympathetic cell bodies in the conus medullaris, cauda equina lesions, or damage to the pelvic nerves. No spinal cord–mediated peristalsis occurs, and there is slow stool propulsion. Only the myenteric plexus coordinates segmental colonic peristalsis, and a dryer, rounder stool shape occurs. Because of the denervated external anal sphincter, there is increased risk for incontinence. The levator ani muscles lack tone, and this reduces the rectal angle and causes the lumen of the rectum to open. The lower motor neuron bowel syndrome produces constipation and a significant risk of incontinence due to the lax external anal sphincter. A lesion above the conus medullaris causes an upper motor neuron bladder and bowel syndrome or hyperreflexic bladder and bowel. There is increased colonic wall and anal tone. The voluntary control of the external anal sphincter is lacking, and the sphincter remains tight, thereby retaining stool. The nerve connections between the spinal cord and the colon, however, remain intact; therefore, there is reflex coordination and stool propulsion. The upper motor neuron bowel syndrome with supraconal lesions in the spinal cord produces constipation and fecal retention at least in part owing to the hyperactivity of the external anal sphincter.

Pathophysiology of Constipation in Neurologically Impaired Patients

In neuropathic bowel, constipation is usually a major consequence [11–13]. The pathophysiologic mechanisms of constipation are obstructed defecation, weak abdominal muscles, impaired rectal sensation, and delayed colonic transit time. Both incomplete and complete lesions can have an obstructed defecation or fecal incontinence [14]. The mechanism for fecal incontinence is due to areflexic or atonic anal sphincter, uninhibited rectal contractions, poor rectal sensibility, and lack of anal sphincter tone and contraction (conus and cauda equina lesions).

During attempts to defecate, in some able-bodied persons with chronic constipation, there is also an inappropriate contraction (or failed relaxation) of the puborectalis and of the external anal sphincter muscles. This paradoxical contraction of the pelvic floor musculature during straining at defecation is also called pelvic floor dysfunction [14,15] or pelvic floor dyssynergic response. This is not a true dyssynergia because it can be relaxed with volitional control. The diagnostic criteria were elucidated in the Rome II report and include those for functional constipation plus at least two of three investigations among manometry, electromyography, and defecography showing inappropriate contraction of or failure to relax the pelvic floor muscles [14,15]. Patients can learn to relax the pelvic floor musculature with biofeedback to manage functional obstructed defecation. This dyssynergic response, therefore, needs to be distinguished from true detrusor anal sphincter dyssynergia due to neurologic impairment, in which biofeedback may not have any role for the functional improvement.

Symptoms

There is a high prevalence and wide spectrum of gastrointestinal symptoms after spinal cord injury. Abdominal bloating and constipation are usually related to specific spinal cord levels of injury [16]. The limited manner through which spinal cord–injured patients can manifest symptoms resulted in complaints that were characteristically vague [3]. The most common problems that impaired quality of life were poorly localized abdominal pain (14%) and difficulty with bowel evacuation (20%), hemorrhoids (74%), abdominal distention (43%), and autonomic dysreflexia. Twenty-three percent of our population required at least one admission to the hospital for a gastrointestinal complaint after their injury. The prevalence of chronic gastrointestinal symptoms increased with time after injury [3].

Physical Examination

For the rehabilitation of neurogenic bowel, an individual evaluation [17,18] is important with a careful rectal examination and anorectal neurologic testing to document degree of neurologic impairment. A neurologic examination can reveal the extent of the nerve damage and the completeness of the spinal cord injury. The abdomen should be inspected and palpated for distention, palpable fecal masses, increased abdominal muscle tone indicative of spasticity, and bowel sounds. The rectal examination can provide information about external anal sphincter tone, stool in the rectal vault, presence of hemorrhoids, cystocele in women, or masses, and it assesses the tone and ability to produce voluntary contraction of the puborectalis muscles.

The bulbocavernosus reflex assesses the integrity of the local spinal reflex arc; its absence along with poor anal tone indicates a conus or cauda equina lesion (lower motor neuron). It is also important to assess the patient's strength in the upper and lower extremities, hand function, sitting balance, and ability to transfer; the length of the patient's arms, legs, and trunk; and the patient's weight. These factors are helpful to determine whether the patient can perform his or her own bowel program or whether assistance will be needed. Berkowitz and colleagues [19] found that 37% of all patients with spinal cord injury need assistance with bowel care. People with tetraplegia are more likely to need assistance than are people with paraplegia.

Functional Limitations

There is some degree of loss of voluntary control for bowel evacuation, constipation, unpredicted incontinence, abdominal distention, and associated discomfort, depending on the degree and level of completeness of the neurologic lesion.

Diagnostic Studies

Colonic and anorectal dysfunctions are recognized as the principal pathophysiologic mechanism underpinning chronic constipation and particularly obstructed constipation in neurologically impaired patients [20].

Colonic motor activity comprises four main components: myoelectric activity [21], phasic contractile activity, tonic contractile activity, and intraluminal transit. Specific methods are available for the assessment of each separate component, but no single investigation gives information about all four types of activity. In current clinical practice, evaluation of colonic motor function is almost exclusively limited to assessment of intraluminal pressure and transit time [22,23]. Although the direct assessment of colonic contractile activity can be achieved through colonic manometry, this procedure is only slowly gaining clinical acceptance, notably in pediatrics. Other novel methods are also available; two techniques exist for the routine assessment of colonic (or whole gut) transit, both of which involve irradiation of the subjects: radiopaque markers [24] and radionuclide scintigraphy [25]. Wireless (telemetric) motility capsules [26] with magnetic markers to obviate irradiation are currently being tried, but they need further validation before being incorporated into general clinical practice. Together with assessment of rectal evacuation and rectal sensation, studies of colonic transit should form the cornerstone of investigation of chronic idiopathic constipation in patients with functional or partial neurologic impairment. These investigations have led to the conceptualization of constipation in three broad and overlapping categories: normal-transit constipation, slow-transit constipation, and evacuation disorders.

Anorectal Dyssynergia

For the precise diagnosis of anorectal dyssynergia, particularly in incomplete or functional lesions, anorectal manometry along with simultaneous electromyography of the external anal sphincter is important to distinguish between functional constipation [15,16] and obstructed constipation due to a neurologic lesion. It is also important to evaluate impairment due to an incomplete lesion (e.g., multiple sclerosis, pudendal nerve lesion after childbirth, lumber disc disease, back injury, or spinal tumor). Defecography, nerve stimulation and pudendal latency, ultrasonography, and magnetic resonance imaging may also be required for better understanding of gastrointestinal dysfunction. A rectal examination should be performed to look for a rectocele, voluntary anal contraction, and bulbocavernosus reflex to evaluate sacral nerve root lesions. Defecography detects structural abnormalities and assesses functional information on the movement of the pelvic floor and the organs that it supports; conversely, excessive descent (descending perineum syndrome) can also be a pathophysiologic mechanism of constipation. Defecography can also help complement anorectal manometry studies in ruling out slow transit and other causes of constipation. Magnetic resonance imaging or pelvic floor sonography can further complement the studies. This will help reduce morbidity rates and will improve the quality of life for the neurologically impaired patient.

Treatment

Initial

Unless there is an associated acute abdomen, the small bowel and the bulk of the colon are functional and are not paralyzed. Management of bowel evacuation will also depend on level of injury. In cauda equina lesions and also during the shock phase after spinal cord injury, there is a flaccid bowel; the management generally involves manual removal (disimpaction) of stool and use of a suppository. Digital stimulation may also be helpful with intact bulbocavernosus reflex. In patients with a supraconal lesion with spastic bowel, routine use of stool softeners, suppository insertion, and digital stimulation help evacuation of the fecal matter. Digital stimulation with and without suppository for about 20 to 30 minutes usually evokes bowel evacuation. Glycerin or Microlax suppository has been commonly used.

Rehabilitation

Bowel Management after Spinal Cord Injury

In the rehabilitation of the spinal cord–injured patient, adequate bowel evacuation in less than 60 minutes is an ideal goal; however, a large number of patients may require up to 180 minutes. It is therefore important to individualize the bowel program for adequate evacuation on the basis of the neurologic and physical status with a set time, diet control, and digital stimulation with or without a glycerin suppository [11]. Additional help to regulate the bowel with bulking agents by increasing water content (e.g., Metamucil) or stool softeners by increasing water penetration of stool (e.g., Coloxyl) has been useful in children. Iso-osmotic laxative (e.g., Movicol) and osmotic laxative (e.g., lactulose) are also widely used to help individualize the bowel program.

The addition of bisacodyl to aid myoelectric propagation activity, transit in the ascending colon, and rectal tone in humans has been reported. Internal anal sphincter relaxation associated with bisacodyl-induced colonic high-amplitude propagating contractions in children with constipation has also been reported: a coloanal reflex [27,28]. Bisacodyl has been widely prescribed for the management of neurogenic bowel [29]. The dosage is normally 5 or 10 mg, but up to 30 mg can be taken for complete cleansing of the bowel before a procedure. If it is taken at the maximum dosage, there will likely be a sudden, extremely powerful, uncontrollable bowel movement, and so precautions should be taken. When it is administered rectally in suppository form, it is usually effective in 15 to 60 minutes. Two suppositories can be inserted at once if a very strong, purgative, enema-like result is needed. A few hours after the initial evacuation, there can be a secondary action that will continue as long as there is unexpelled bisacodyl present in the rectum.

For design of the bowel program, a variety of factors need to be considered. Is this an upper motor neuron or lower motor neuron bowel dysfunction? Is it a complete or an incomplete lesion? Is this associated with anorectal dyssynergia? A detailed history is needed to find out any bowel problems antedating spinal cord injury, such as diabetes, irritable bowel syndrome, lactose intolerance, inflammatory bowel disease, or past rectal bleeding. These disorders may affect the management and choice of medications used in the bowel regimen. Other medications frequently used by patients with spinal cord injury for other problems, such as anticholinergics for treatment of neurogenic bladder, antidepressants, narcotics, and antispasticity medications, also affect the bowel.

In addition, the person's dietary habits and the amount of fluid intake need to be documented as part of bowel management. It is helpful to evaluate psychosocial and family circumstances to provide guidelines to modify convenient timing for the bowel program and to develop rehabilitation strategies through diet, pelvic floor exercises, and biofeedback (in partial lesions).

Patient Education and Awareness of Risk Factors

It is critical to develop a comprehensive, individualized, and structured education program for prevention of incontinence, bowel accidents, and skin breakdown during sitting on a toilet seat. It is also important to identify other risk factors for negative outcomes: colonic overdistention, irritable bowel syndrome, bladder dysfunction, or autonomic dysreflexia in high spinal cord lesions. Equipment essential during bowel care also has been studied, although new technology in bowel chair design and manufacture has been slow to evolve [30,31]. There are flaws in commode-shower chair design, as reported by consumers, which increase the risk of falls during transfers and risk of pressure ulcers due to inadequate padding as well as the long duration of the bowel care process.

The current and most frequently used neurogenic bowel management strategies in some persons with only digital stimulation or a suppository insertion may be associated with incomplete evacuation, some incontinence, increased risk of pressure-induced tissue damage resulting from longer duration of commode sitting, and more damage to the mucosal tissue than with other methods available to persons with spinal cord injury. The use of the docusate mini enema may be an option in neurogenic bowel management because it has been shown to reduce the occurrence of bowel incontinence; it reduces the duration of commode sitting and thus reduces the risk of pressure ulcers, and it does not cause inflammation or seepage of the mucosal lining of the lower bowel [32]. All of these may improve quality of life and social and community integration of persons with spinal cord injury.

Use of Prokinetic Drugs

When conservative management is not effective, prokinetic agents, such as cisapride, prucalopride, metoclopramide, neostigmine, and fampridine, have been used and are supported by strong evidence for the treatment of chronic constipation in spinal cord–injured patients. They need to be used carefully for their side effects. Serious cardiac arrhythmias including ventricular tachycardia, fibrillation, and QT prolongation have been reported in patients taking cisapride. Cisapride has therefore been removed from the U.S. market [33–35]. The gastroprokinetic effects make metoclopramide useful in the treatment of gastric stasis and in gastroesophageal reflux disease. Because of the risk of tardive dyskinesia with chronic or high-dose use of the drug, the U.S. Food and Drug Administration recommends that metoclopramide be used for short-term treatment, preferably less than 12 weeks [35]; in 2009, it required all manufacturers of metoclopramide to issue a black box warning [35].

Procedures

Botulinum Toxin in Gastrointestinal Disorders

Botulinum neurotoxin inhibits contraction of gastrointestinal smooth muscles and sphincters; it has also been shown that the neurotoxin blocks cholinergic nerve endings in the autonomic nervous system, but it seems not to block noradrenergic responses mediated by nitric oxide. This has attracted use of botulinum neurotoxin for overactive smooth muscles, such as the anal sphincters for treatment of anal fissure and the lower esophageal sphincter for treatment of esophageal achalasia [36]. It is critical to appreciate the anatomic and functional organization of the denervation of the gastrointestinal tract for neuropathic bowel dysfunctions, particularly in patients with long-term constipation and incomplete bowel evacuation for whom a bowel rehabilitation program has failed. An early resolution of obstruction may be with botulinum neurotoxin to control the pelvic floor dyssynergic response. It might thus prevent back pressure effects on the rectosigmoid and colon in a neuropathic bowel.

Despite uncontrolled data, botulinum toxin is now being used for a variety of spastic disorders of gastrointestinal smooth muscle. Its usefulness has been exploited in anismus patients with pelvic floor dyssynergia. This is one of the common causes of constipation, in which the pelvic floor muscles contract too much or do not relax enough during a bowel movement. In one study [37], either 100 units of botulinum toxin (Botox; Allergan, Irvine, Calif) or 500 units (equivalent dose) of Dysport (Ipsen Ltd; Slough, United Kingdom) was diluted in 2 mL of normal saline, and a 21-gauge needle was passed cranially through the external sphincter to the level of the puborectalis muscle. The needle was then gradually withdrawn, injecting small amounts of mixture along the length of the puborectalis–external sphincter muscle; 1 mL was given bilaterally at the 3- and 9-o'clock positions. In these patients, initially 39% (21 patients) benefited, but after the second injection, 95% had resolution of symptoms. At a median follow-up of 19.2 (7.0-30.4) months, 20 (95%) of 21 patients had a sustained response and required no further treatment [37]. One unit of Botox is equivalent to about 3 units of Dysport. Most others have used only about 50 mg of Botox for anorectal injections.

So far, few placebo-controlled trials have been performed despite widespread use of the toxin for the past 10 years. Botulinum toxin appears to be safe, and side effects are uncommon. The short-term efficacy of intrasphincteric injection of botulinum neurotoxin in achalasia is now well established. The U.S. Food and Drug Administration has not approved Botox for any of these conditions.

Surgery

In patients with severe bowel dysfunction and markedly prolonged colon transit time [24], we evaluated indications for transverse colostomy [38]. In a follow-up study [39], the effect on quality of life of this procedure was evaluated with 100% satisfaction and reduction of bowel care from 117 minutes to 12.8 minutes per day ($P<.00001$). Indications for and usefulness of intestinal diversion have also been reported with positive results in patients with severe bowel dysfunctions after spinal cord injury [40]. In an another study [41], the difference in the long-term outcome among left-sided colostomies, right-sided colostomies, and ileostomies was evaluated; The average daily time to bowel care was significantly shortened in all groups (right-sided colostomies, 102 to 11 minutes, $P<.05$; left-sided colostomies, 123 to 18 minutes, $P<.05$; and ileostomies, 73 to 13 minutes, $P<.05$). The successful outcome noted in all groups suggests that preoperative symptoms and colonic transit time studies may have been helpful in optimal choice of stoma site selection. However, the choice of colostomy in the descending colon was considered better because of the lesser fluid content in the fecal matter (more solid fecal matter) and the easy management of the collecting devices. In a systematic review of electronic databases (MEDLINE and CINAHL) from January 1960 to November 2007, colostomy in selected patients provided equivocal or superior quality of life outcomes compared with conservative bowel management strategies [11].

Surgical interventions, such as colostomy, Malone antegrade continence enema, and implanted stimulators [1,42], are not routinely used, although all are supported by lower levels of evidence (pre–post studies) in reducing bowel-related complications and improving quality of life. Overall, more intervention trials are needed to assess management programs for neurogenic bowel among individuals with spinal cord injury, especially trials involving multiple centers [1]. The use of common and validated scoring systems, such as the Neurogenic Bowel Dysfunction score and those found in the International Bowel Function data sets [43,44], will be helpful if they are implemented so that comparison of results and meta-analyses may be conducted to further our knowledge on the treatment and management of neurogenic bowel after spinal cord injury.

Potential Disease Complications

In spinal cord lesions above T6 level, one of the serious complications is autonomic dysreflexia. It usually accompanies poor bladder drainage and impacted fecal matter in the rectum. It needs immediate attention with gentle bowel evacuation after lidocaine jelly (4%) insertion in the rectum and use of alpha blockers to control blood pressure [11].

In a slow-transit bowel, marked abdominal distention with chronic constipation and dilated colon further aggravates bowel evacuation. A barium contrast enema will delineate an obstructing lesion, if it is present, or may reveal a huge colon with redundant bowel. Although this finding will not delineate the specific cause, it will indicate the magnitude of the anatomic abnormality. If the impaction is located more proximally in the bowel, oral stimulants, such as magnesium citrate solution or bisacodyl tablets, may be required. Caution in the use of oral medication is needed if a bowel obstruction is suspected. Intestinal perforation could result. In addition, oil retention enemas may be helpful in combination with oral agents to loosen the stool. The decision to proceed with colonoscopy depends on the individual's clinical history and findings as well as on whether the physician is satisfied with the results of the contrast enema. To clear the contrast material and to prevent constipation, oral laxatives and frequent bowel care should be used for a few days after studies that require barium [11].

Fecal incontinence can lead to overgrowth of microorganisms around the anus, which weakens the skin, and skin sores can develop. Also, sitting on an unpadded bowel care seat for a long time without frequent pressure relief could result in skin sores.

Hemorrhoids occur frequently [3] and may become more symptomatic as they increase in size; they may be exacerbated by physical interventions, such as suppositories, enemas, or digital stimulation, to regulate the bowels in individuals with spinal cord injury. When hemorrhoids become clinically significant, they may cause pain (if sensation is present), bleeding, mucus incontinence secondary to prolapsed mucosa, or symptoms of autonomic dysreflexia. Persistent bleeding and autonomic dysreflexia that are not responsive to changes in bowel care routine are indications for consideration of banding [45] or hemorrhoidectomy.

Potential Treatment Complications

In 27% of spinal cord–injured patients, chronic gastrointestinal problems appeared usually 5 to 10 years after the initial injury. This seems to be related mostly to anorectal dyssynergia with resultant obstructed constipation and incomplete evacuation with the back pressure effect on the colon [3], suggesting that these problems are acquired and may therefore be avoided by the adoption of certain chronic care routines to manage obstructed constipation with anal stretch, high-fiber diet, and adequate fluid intake. Chronic use of stimulant laxatives can lead to damage of the myenteric plexus with aggravated colonic dysmotility.

References

[1] Krassioukov A, Eng JJ, Claxton G, et al. SCIRE Research Team. Neurogenic bowel management after spinal cord injury: a systematic review of the evidence. Spinal Cord 2010;48:718–33.

[2] Menardo G, Bausano G, Corazziari E, et al. Large-bowel transit in paraplegic patients. Dis Colon Rectum 1987;30:924–8.

[3] Stone JM, Nino-Murcia M, Wolfe VA, Perkash I. Chronic gastrointestinal problems in spinal cord injury patients: a prospective analysis. Am J Gastroenterol 1990;85:1114–9.

[4] Bassotti G, Germani U, Morelli A. Human colonic motility: physiological aspects. Int J Colorectal Dis 1995;10:173–80.

[5] Linsenmeyer TA, Stone JM. Neurogenic bladder and bowel dysfunction. In: DeLisa JA, editor. Rehabilitation medicine: principles and practice. Philadelphia: Lippincott-Raven; 1998. p. 1073–106.

[6] Glatzle J, Sternini C, Robin C, et al. Expression of 5-HT_3 receptors in the rat gastrointestinal tract. Gastroenterology 2002;123:217–26.

[7] Kunze WA, Furness JB. The enteric nervous system and regulation of intestinal motility. Annu Rev Physiol 1999;61:117–42.

[8] Bornstein JC, Costa M, Grider JR. Enteric motor and interneuronal circuits controlling motility. Neurogastroenterol Motil 2004;16(Suppl. 1): 34–8.

[9] Zhang WQ, Yan GZ, Ye DD, Chen CW. Simultaneous assessment of the intraluminal pressure and transit time of the colon using a telemetry technique. Physiol Meas 2007;28:141–8.

[10] Stephen AM, Cummings JH. The microbial contribution to human faecal mass. J Med Microbiol 1980;13:45–56.

[11] Consortium for Spinal Cord Medicine. Neurogenic bowel management in adults with spinal cord injury. Washington, DC: Paralyzed Veterans of America; March 1998, 9.

[12] Staas Jr WE, Cioschi HS. Neurogenic bowel dysfunction: critical review. Phys Rehabil Med 1989;11–21.

[13] Benevento BT, Sipski ML. Neurogenic bladder, neurogenic bowel, and sexual dysfunction in people with spinal cord injury. Phys Ther 2002;82:601–12.

[14] Vallès M, Mearin F. Pathophysiology of bowel dysfunction in patients with motor incomplete spinal cord injury: comparison with patients with motor complete spinal cord injury. Dis Colon Rectum 2009;52:1589–97.

[15] Drossman DA, Corazziari E, Talley NJ, et al, editors. ROME II. The functional gastrointestinal disorders. Diagnosis, pathophysiology and treatment: a multinational consensus. 2nd ed. McLean, Va: Degnon Associates; 2000.

[16] Levi R, Hultling C, Nash MS, Seiger A. The Stockholm spinal cord injury study: 1. Medical problems in a regional SCI population. Paraplegia 1995;33:308–15.

[17] Stiens SA, Bergman SB, Goetz LL. Neurogenic bowel dysfunction after spinal cord injury: clinical evaluation and rehabilitative management. Arch Phys Med Rehabil 1997;78(Suppl.):S86–S102.

[18] Liu CW, Huang CC, Chen CH, et al. Prediction of severe neurogenic bowel dysfunction in persons with spinal cord injury. Spinal Cord 2010;48:554–9.

[19] Berkowitz M, Harvey C, Greene G, et al. The economic consequences of traumatic spinal cord injury. New York: Demos; 1992.

[20] Dinning PG, Smith TK, Scott SM. Pathophysiology of colonic causes of constipation. Neurogastroenterol Motil 2009;21(Suppl. 2): 20–30.

[21] Frexinos J, Bueno L, Fioramonti J. Diurnal changes in myoelectric spiking activity of the human colon. Gastroenterology 1985;88 (Pt 1):1104–10.

[22] Scott SM. Manometric techniques for the evaluation of colonic motor activity: current status. Neurogastroenterol Motil 2003;15:483–513.

[23] Camilleri M, Bharucha AE, di Lorenzo C, et al. American Neurogastroenterology and Motility Society consensus statement on intraluminal measurement of gastrointestinal and colonic motility in clinical practice. Dig Dis Sci 1985;30:289–94.

[24] Murcia MN, Stone JM, Chang PJ, Perkash I. Colonic transit time in spinal cord–injured patients. Invest Radiol 1990;25:109–12.

[25] Stivland T, Camilleri M, Vassallo M, et al. Scintigraphic measurement of regional gut transit in idiopathic constipation. Gastroenterology 1991;101:107–15.

[26] Rao SS, Kuo B, McCallum RW, et al. Investigation of colonic and whole-gut transit with wireless motility capsule and radiopaque markers in constipation. Clin Gastroenterol Hepatol 2009;7:537–44.

[27] Rodriguez L, Siddiqui A, Nurko S. Internal anal sphincter relaxation associated with bisacodyl-induced colonic high amplitude propagating contractions in children with constipation: a colo-anal reflex? Neurogastroenterol Motil 2012;24:1023–e545.

[28] Preston DM, Lennard-Jones JE. Pelvic motility and response to intraluminal bisacodyl in slow-transit constipation. Dig Dis Sci 1985;30:289–94.

[29] Stiens SA, Luttrel W, Binard JE. Polyethylene glycol versus vegetable oil based bisacodyl suppositories to initiate side-lying bowel care: a clinical trial in persons with spinal cord injury. Spinal Cord 1998;36:777–81.

[30] Nelson AL, Malassigne P, Murray J. Comparison of seat pressures on three bowel care/shower chairs in spinal cord injury. SCI Nurs 1994;11:105–7.

[31] Malassigne P, Nelson AL, Cors MW, Amerson TL. Design of the advanced commode-shower chair for spinal cord–injured individuals. J Rehabil Res Dev 2000;37:373–82.

[32] Amir I, Sharma R, Bauman WA, Korsten MA. Bowel care for individuals with spinal cord injury: comparison of four approaches. J Spinal Cord Med 1998;21:21–4.
[33] Walker AM, Szneke P, Weatherby LB, et al. The risk of serious cardiac arrhythmias among cisapride users in the United Kingdom and Canada. Am J Med 1999;107:356–62.
[34] Hennessy S, Leonard CE, Newcomb C, et al. Cisapride and ventricular arrhythmia. Br J Clin Pharmacol 2008;66:375–85.
[35] U.S. Food and Drug Administration. FDA requires boxed warning and risk mitigation strategy for metoclopramide-containing drugs [press release]. February 26, 2009.
[36] Vittal H, Pasricha PF. Botulinum toxin for gastrointestinal disorders: therapy and mechanisms. Neurotox Res 2006;9:149–59.
[37] Hompes R, Harmston C, Wijffels N, et al. Excellent response rate of anismus to botulinum toxin if rectal prolapse misdiagnosed as anismus ('pseudoanismus') is excluded. Colorectal Dis 2012;14:224–30.
[38] Stone JM, Wolfe VA, Nino-Murcia M, Perkash I. Colostomy as treatment for complications of spinal cord injury. Arch Phys Med Rehabil 1990;71:514–8.
[39] Rosito O, Murcia NM, Wolfe VA, et al. The effects of colostomy on the quality of life in patients with spinal cord injury: a retrospective analysis. J Spinal Cord Med 2002;25:174–83.
[40] Hocevar B, Gray M. Intestinal diversion (colostomy or ileostomy) in patients with severe bowel dysfunction following spinal cord injury. J Wound Ostomy Continence Nurs 2008;35:159–66.
[41] Safadi BY, Rosito O, Nino-Murcia M, et al. Which stoma works better for colonic dysmotility in the spinal cord injured patient? Am J Surg 2003;186:437–42.
[42] Valles M, Rodriguez A, Borau A, Mearin F. Effect of sacral anterior root stimulator on bowel dysfunction in patients with spinal cord injury. Dis Colon Rectum 2009;52:986–92.
[43] Krogh K, Perkash I, Stiens SA, Biering-Sørensen F. International bowel function basic spinal cord injury data set. Spinal Cord 2009;47:230–4.
[44] Krogh K, Perkash I, Stiens SA, Biering-Sørensen F. International bowel function extended spinal cord injury data set. Spinal Cord 2009;47:235–41.
[45] Cosman BC, Stone JM, Perkash I. Gastrointestinal complications of chronic spinal cord injury. J Am Paraplegia Soc 1991;14:175–81.

CHAPTER 139

Osteoarthritis

Amy X. Yin, MD
Allen N. Wilkins, MD
Edward M. Phillips, MD

Synonym

Degenerative joint disease

ICD-9 Codes

715.0 Osteoarthrosis, generalized
715.1 Osteoarthrosis, localized, primary
715.2 Osteoarthrosis, localized, secondary
715.3 Osteoarthrosis, localized, not specified whether primary or secondary
715.9 Osteoarthrosis, unspecified whether generalized or localized
716.1 Traumatic arthropathy
716.9 Arthropathy, unspecified

ICD-10 Codes

M15.9 Generalized osteoarthritis
M19.91 Primary osteoarthritis, unspecified site
M19.93 Secondary osteoarthritis, unspecified site
M19.90 Unspecified osteoarthritis, unspecified site
M12.50 Traumatic arthropathy, unspecified
M12.9 Arthropathy, unspecified

Definition

Osteoarthritis (OA) is generally considered a family of degenerative joint disorders characterized by specific clinical and radiographic findings. OA is the most prevalent chronic joint disease and has become the most common cause of walking disability in older adults in the United States [1–3]. It is estimated that 26.9 million adults have clinical OA, and the total cost for all arthritis, including OA, is more than 2% of the United States gross domestic product [4,5]. The disease burden of OA is likely to continue to increase with the aging population and higher incidence of obesity [2,5].

OA has traditionally been thought of as just a condition of cartilage degeneration [6]. It is actually a complex combination of genetic, metabolic, biomechanical, and biochemical joint changes that lead to failure of the normal cartilage remodeling process (Fig. 139.1). The joint then accumulates increasing cartilage degeneration changes in response to stress or injury [2,6]. More recent evidence implicates bone changes and synovial inflammation also as integral to the pathologic process of OA [2]. As a whole, OA is characterized by degradation and loss of articular cartilage, hypertrophic bone changes with osteophyte formation, subchondral bone remodeling appearing as sclerosis or cysts, and chronic synovitis or inflammation of the synovial membrane [1,6].

Joint involvement in OA is usually asymmetric, with a predilection for weight-bearing joints. Common sites of involvement are the hips, knees, hands, feet, and spine. Less common sites of involvement are the ankles, wrists, shoulders, and sacroiliac joints. Secondary arthritis may be manifested with an atypical pattern of joint involvement.

OA is classified into two groups: primary and secondary. Primary or idiopathic OA can be localized or generalized. Localized OA usually refers to a single joint; generalized OA describes involvement of three or more joints. Secondary OA is due to a specific condition known to cause or to worsen development of OA (Table 139.1).

Multiple risk factors have been linked to the development of OA (Table 139.2). Systemic factors include age, gender, genetics, bone mineral density, and body weight. Age is consistently one of the strongest if not the strongest risk factor for OA [3,5]. Female gender is associated with higher prevalence of symptomatic knee, hip, and hand OA [3,5]. Heritable genetic traits may play a role in OA, but identification of such traits has been challenging. Some genetic markers strongly implicated in OA include *GDF5*, *MCF2L*, and the genomic region 7q22 [7,8]. There is an inverse relationship between bone mineral density and OA [3,9]. Both overweight and obese people are shown to be at a greater risk for OA, especially in weight-bearing joints like the knee [3,10,11]. Low levels of factors like vitamin C, vitamin D, vitamin E, and vitamin K may have an effect on OA, but there is no consensus recommendation currently [3].

Local biomechanical factors implicated in OA include previous joint injury, joint malalignment, bone anatomic

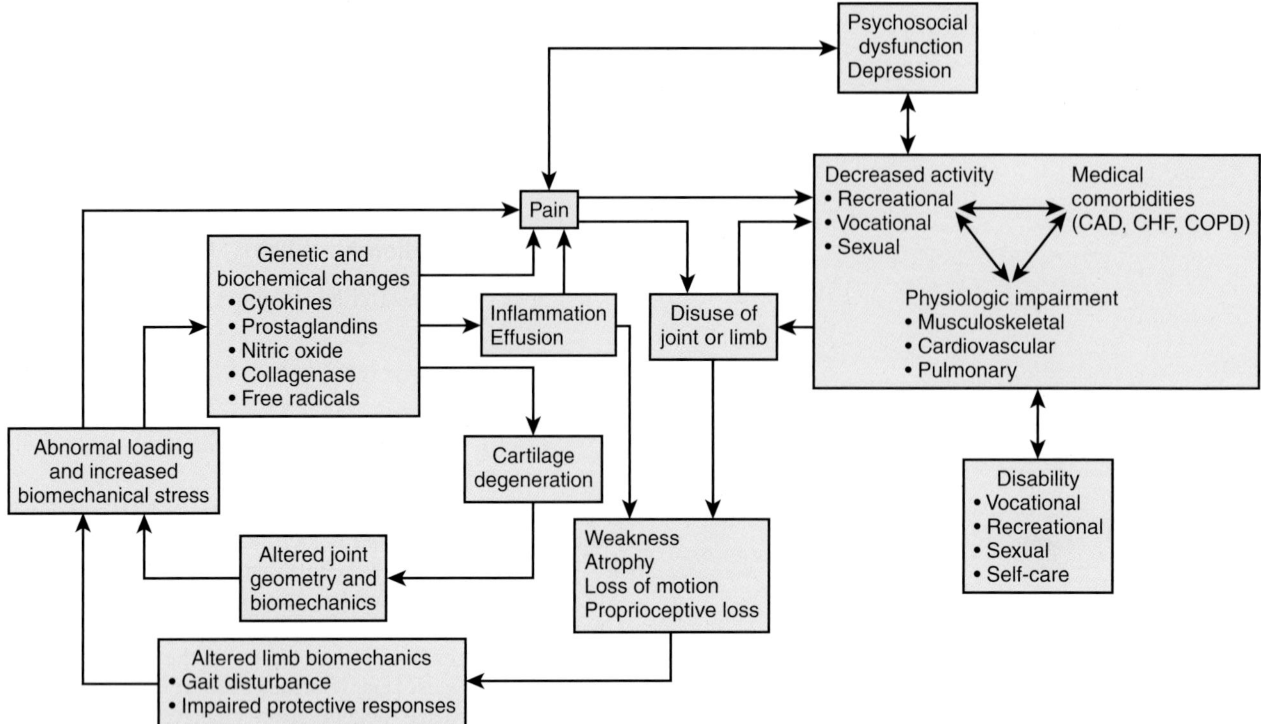

FIGURE 139.1 Model of multifactorial process of degeneration, pain, psychosocial and physiologic dysfunction, and disability that may occur in osteoarthritis. *CAD,* coronary artery disease; *CHF,* congestive heart failure; *COPD,* chronic obstructive pulmonary disease.

Table 139.1 Causes of Secondary Osteoarthritis

Bone and joint disorders, such as osteonecrosis and Paget disease
Calcium crystal deposition disorders
Congenital or developmental disorders
Endocrine disorders, such as acromegaly and hypothyroidism
Infectious diseases, such as septic arthritis
Inflammatory arthritis, such as rheumatoid arthritis
Metabolic disorders
Neuropathic disorders, such as diabetes mellitus and Charcot arthropathy
After trauma

Table 139.2 Major Risk Factors for Development of Osteoarthritis

Systemic Factors
Age
Bone mineral density
Gender
Genetics
Obesity
Biomechanical Factors
Joint injury
Joint malalignment
Bone variation or abnormality
Muscle weakness

variation or abnormality, and muscle weakness. Those with previous injury have a 15% greater lifetime risk of symptomatic knee OA [11]. Lower extremity malalignment may be associated with greater radiographic knee OA. Bone abnormality like acetabular dysplasia is associated with greater incidence of hip OA [12]. Muscle weakness, specifically of the knee extensor muscles, predicts knee OA in most cohorts of women [3,13].

In terms of physical loading, some suggest that there is greater risk of knee OA with work activities such as squatting, lifting, prolonged standing, or climbing stairs, but this is not seen consistently [11]. Currently, there is no strong evidence to show that sports or physical activity itself leads to an increased risk of symptomatic OA [3]. Historical data have correlated certain sports with OA of specific joints, but there are many confounders in these studies that make interpretation inconclusive [3].

Symptoms

Patients usually complain of pain, stiffness, reduced movement, and swelling in the affected joints that is exacerbated with activity and relieved by rest. Pain at rest or at night suggests severe disease or another diagnosis. Early morning stiffness, if it is present, is typically less than 30 minutes. Joint tenderness and crepitus on movement may also be present. Swelling may be due to bone deformity, such as osteophyte formation, or an effusion caused by synovial fluid accumulation. Systemic symptoms are absent.

In early disease, pain is usually gradual in onset and mild in intensity. Pain is typically self-limited or intermittent. Patients with advanced disease may describe a sense of grinding or locking with joint motion and buckling or instability of joints during demanding tasks. Periarticular muscle pain may be prominent. Patients may complain of fatigue if biomechanical changes lead to increased energy requirements for activities of daily living. Overuse of alternative muscle groups can lead to development of pain syndromes in other parts of the musculoskeletal system.

Physical Examination

Joint Examination

Diagnosis of OA involves assessment of the affected joints for common clinical features (Table 139.3). These usually include tenderness, bone enlargement, and malalignment. Osteophytes, joint surface irregularity, or chronic disuse may also result in decreased range of motion, pain, effusion, and crepitus. Locking during range of motion may suggest loose bodies or floating cartilage fragments in the joint. Joint contracture can result from holding a joint in slight flexion, which is less painful for inflamed or swollen joints. There may be secondary abnormalities in joints above or below the primarily involved joint. Remember to assess joints bilaterally because asymptomatic joints may also have abnormal findings.

Neuromuscular and General Examination

A thorough musculoskeletal examination should include inspection, palpation of soft tissues surrounding the joint of interest, assessment of muscle strength and flexibility, and joint-specific provocative maneuvers. First, gait should be observed. There may be an antalgic gait or a slow gait pattern because of pain in a specific joint. If the patient uses a cane, appropriate use of the cane should be assessed during gait.

Both functional strength and manual muscle testing should be performed. Periarticular muscle atrophy and weakness may be present in chronic OA. However, manual muscle testing is typically unreliable in the lower extremities because of the high baseline strength of these muscle groups. Function tests like sit-to-stand testing may be more informative. Palpation and dynamic testing of soft tissues may differentiate pain from tendinopathy or bursitis from OA. Joint-specific provocative maneuvers may help isolate the source in symptomatic patients with poorly localized pain. A careful neurologic examination should be performed to ensure that pain is not the result of nerve impingement or a neuropathic process.

Clinicians may also consider performing a general examination. Evaluation of other systems may also help differentiate primary OA from secondary OA due to a systemic process. Because obesity has been identified as a risk factor for OA, assessment of the patient's body mass index may also be useful.

Functional Limitations

Functional limitations will depend on the joints affected by OA. Patients with disease in the hips and knees will have impairments in mobility, locomotion, and activities of daily living involving the lower body. Patients may complain of increasing difficulty with climbing up and down stairs, walking, making chair or toileting transfers, and lower body dressing and grooming. Degeneration in the shoulders or hands limits vocational and recreational activities, self-care, and upper body activities of daily living. Patients may initially have trouble with using the computer or lifting boxes, which then progresses to difficulties with activities of daily living like feeding, grooming, bathing, and dressing. Spine OA can result in limitations with all mobility.

Table 139.3 Clinical Features of an Osteoarthritic Joint

Tenderness to palpation
Bone enlargement
Malalignment
Joint effusion or swelling
Crepitus
Periarticular muscle spasm, atrophy, or weakness
Decreased, painful range of motion

Diagnostic Studies

Although imaging studies are not needed to confirm the diagnosis, plain radiographs may help elucidate the severity of joint damage and progression of OA. The classic findings include asymmetric joint space narrowing, osteophytes at joint margins, subchondral sclerosis, and subchondral cyst formation. There is a well-demonstrated discordance between x-ray findings and symptoms in OA. Asymptomatic individuals may have significant radiographic disease, and severe pain and dysfunction can occur in the setting of limited radiologic changes. Computed tomography scans, ultrasonography, and magnetic resonance imaging are typically not needed for evaluation of OA but can be helpful in providing better visualization not only for OA severity evaluation but also for identification of other tissue pathologic processes and diagnosis [1].

Routine laboratory test results should be normal, and laboratory testing is usually not needed in uncomplicated cases of OA. If laboratory tests are available, clinicians should take care in interpreting the results. There is a high prevalence of laboratory abnormalities in elderly people, such as a raised erythrocyte sedimentation rate or anemia, because of comorbid conditions. Autoimmune markers may be useful to differentiate OA from other musculoskeletal disorders like inflammatory arthritides.

Joint aspiration should be pursued in patients with significant joint effusion or inflammation. Joint fluid analysis can be helpful in ruling out crystal deposition disease like gout or pseudogout, inflammatory arthritis, or infectious arthritis. In contrast to other arthritides, synovial fluid in OA is usually clear with normal viscosity and leukocyte counts typically less than 1500 to 2000 cells/mm^3.

Differential Diagnosis

Neoplasm
Deep venous thrombosis
Osteomyelitis
Occult fracture
Aseptic necrosis
Chondromalacia
Soft tissue infection
Bursitis
Tendinitis
Ligamentous injury
Overuse injury
Radiculopathy
Neuropathy
Polymyalgia rheumatica
Inflammatory arthritis
Crystal deposit arthritis

Treatment

Initial

The major principles of OA management involve relieving pain and other symptoms as well as maximizing joint function and quality of life. Initial treatment should include both pharmacologic and nonpharmacologic rehabilitation modalities. Here we provide a broad overview of major concepts. Site-specific management of OA is discussed in more detail in other chapters.

No pharmacologic intervention has been shown conclusively to alter disease progression in OA. A number of topical and oral medications have been used to alleviate symptoms and to improve functional status. Topical treatment of OA includes nonsteroidal anti-inflammatory drugs (NSAIDs), capsaicin, rubefacients, and opioids. Many treatment guidelines from 2008 or later recommend topical NSAIDs as first-line OA treatment, especially in elderly patients, in whom drug safety and tolerability are significant concerns [1,14,15]. In a meta-analysis of 7688 participants in 34 studies, topical NSAIDs were significantly more effective than placebo in treating chronic musculoskeletal conditions such as OA [16]. Topical diclofenac is the only NSAID approved for use by the U.S. Food and Drug Administration. Studies of topical diclofenac in OA indicate a number needed to treat of 6.4 to 11 for at least 50% pain relief during 8 to 12 weeks compared with placebo [16]. Topical NSAIDs are recommended over oral NSAIDs by the American College of Rheumatology (ACR) for treatment of hand OA in patients older than 75 years [15].

Topical capsaicin cream has also been shown to reduce pain in joints affected by OA. This derivative of cayenne pepper causes exuberant release and depletion of substance P, which diminishes pain transmission from C fibers. Limited data from controlled trials have shown improvements in OA pain with capsaicin, and its use is recommended by the ACR and Osteoarthritis Research Society International as an adjunct or additional treatment [14,15].

Topical rubefacients containing salicylate or nicotinate esters are available for treatment of musculoskeletal pain without a prescription. They are thought to produce counterirritation and vasodilation of the skin for pain relief. Although they may be efficacious in the treatment of acute musculoskeletal pain in the short term (1 week), research on effectiveness is limited [17]. The ACR conditionally recommends trolamine salicylate as treatment of hand OA [15].

One randomized placebo-controlled trial looked at the use of transdermal fentanyl in moderate to severe OA [18]. Although there may be some pain relief, use of transdermal opioids is not routinely recommended because of the potential negative effects of opioid use [18–20].

Oral agents often discussed in the treatment of OA include acetaminophen, NSAIDs, opioids and opioid-like medications, serotonin-norepinephrine reuptake inhibitors, and glucosamine and chondroitin. Acetaminophen and NSAIDs are typically considered first-line oral agents [1,14,15]. A meta-analysis of acetaminophen demonstrated a statistically significant reduction in pain compared with placebo in seven randomized controlled trials with a number needed to treat of 4 to 16 [21]. Although NSAIDs are more efficacious than acetaminophen, effects were modest and associated with greater rates of adverse gastrointestinal effects [21].

Tramadol acts not only as a weak opioid but through modulation of serotonin and norepinephrine levels. A meta-analysis of 11 randomized controlled trials with a total of 1019 patients showed less pain intensity, greater symptom relief, and improved function for those receiving some form of tramadol compared with placebo or control. However, adverse effects were often noted to cause patients to stop taking the medication [22]. Tramadol alone or in combination with acetaminophen is conditionally recommended by the ACR as initial treatment of OA in several joints [15].

The use of opioid medications in OA has risen. Although opioids can improve pain and function in patients with OA, there is a high rate of adverse events and withdrawal of patient treatment [1,20]. Opioids should be considered second-line treatment at best, even when OA pain is severe [20]. The ACR strongly recommends use of opioids only for patients who are either not willing to undergo or have contraindications to total knee arthroplasty after medical therapy has failed [15].

Duloxetine is a serotonin-norepinephrine reuptake inhibitor that is conditionally recommended by the ACR for treatment of knee OA [15]. In pooled data from two randomized controlled trials, patients with knee OA treated with duloxetine were more likely to experience an improvement in outcomes, pain, and function with a number needed to treat of 5 to 9 [23].

Significant attention has focused on the use of supplements such as chondroitin and glucosamine in OA. The Glucosamine/chondroitin Arthritis Intervention Trial (GAIT), a randomized controlled trial of 1583 patients with painful knee OA, demonstrated no clinically significant effective pain reduction [24]. Multiple other randomized controlled trials and meta-analyses of both chondroitin and glucosamine have had conflicting conclusions, and the topic is still hotly debated [1,25–27]. The ACR conditionally recommends against the use of chondroitin and glucosamine in knee OA and hip OA [15]. Patients considering the use of glucosamine or chondroitin should be cautioned that these products are not subject to regulation of purity or accuracy of labeling.

Other treatments of OA include avocado soybean unsaponifiables and diacerein, but these are not widely used [1].

Rehabilitation

A comprehensive rehabilitative approach is important and effective in promoting wellness and reducing disability in patients with OA.

Self-management interventions and programs foster active participation of patients and are thought to be a key element of chronic disease management [1]. These programs provide education and experiential skills in not only disease management but mental and social well-being. Studies have demonstrated that these interventions reduce pain, improve health behaviors, and reduce use of health care resources in patients with chronic pain and arthritis [28]. Group-based self-management programs are often available through a local chapter of the Arthritis Foundation and are conditionally recommended by the ACR for patients with hip and knee OA [15].

Lifestyle changes like exercise and weight loss are an integral part of rehabilitation of OA. There is significant evidence that physical activity is important in patients with OA. Both aerobic and muscle strengthening exercises seem to be beneficial in terms of improving pain, function, and quality of life [29–32]. A meta-analysis of 32 studies indicates platinum level [33] of evidence that land-based therapeutic exercises have at least short-term benefit for reduction of pain and improved physical function for knee OA [34]. There is silver level [33] of evidence for land-based therapeutic exercises for reduction of pain and improvement of physical function in symptomatic hip OA [35]. Therapeutic exercises should include joint protection techniques, stretching and range of motion exercises, muscle strengthening, and aerobic exercises.

Weight loss is important in overweight patients with OA. A meta-analysis of weight reduction in patients with knee OA showed diminished physical disability with a weight loss of more than 5% within a 20-week period [36].

The ACR strongly recommends land-based cardiovascular (aerobic) and resistance exercises, aquatic exercises, Tai Chi, and weight loss (in persons overweight) for patients with OA of hip and knee [15]. Physiatrists, occupational therapists, physical therapists, and other health care professionals can help make recommendations on appropriate exercise, weight loss techniques, and therapeutic modalities for individualized patient care.

Clinical experience suggests that cold, heat, and manual therapy can be helpful in decreasing pain and increasing mobility. Thermal agents and manual therapy in combination with supervised exercise are also recommended by the ACR [15].

Braces and splints may be helpful for symptomatic relief of certain joints. Knee bracing had additional benefit compared with medical treatment alone on the basis of limited evidence [37]. Splints may be useful for OA of the thumb [38]. The ACR recommends splinting for patients with hand OA, specifically of the trapeziometacarpal joint, but offers no recommendations on knee bracing [15].

Orthotic wedged insoles and medially directed patellar taping may be helpful for knee OA to off-load the joint or to improve biomechanics.

Adaptive equipment, such as a cane or walker, can be used if necessary for patients with impaired balance to prevent falls or for pain reduction by decreasing joint loading. In the setting of significant functional impairments, therapists can provide assistive devices that help with feeding, grooming, dressing, and other activities of daily living.

The use of transcutaneous electrical nerve stimulation is supported by a few small, short-term trials. Systematic review of the data has been inconclusive [39]. For most patients in these studies, pain relief was experienced only during active use of the device. Regardless, transcutaneous electrical nerve stimulation is conditionally recommended by the ACR in knee OA [15]. Ultrasound appears to have no proven benefit in the treatment of OA.

Acupuncture is also recommended for the treatment of chronic moderate to severe painful knee OA. A multicenter, 26-week National Institutes of Health–funded randomized controlled trial found acupuncture to be effective as adjunctive therapy for reducing pain and improving function in patients with knee OA [40]. A meta-analysis of acupuncture in the treatment of OA showed statistically significant benefits compared with sham or waiting list controls [41].

Procedures

Intra-articular corticosteroid injection is conditionally recommended by the ACR for patients with painful knee or hip OA who do not have a satisfactory clinical response to full-dose acetaminophen [15]. The short-term effect of intra-articular corticosteroid injection has been well demonstrated in meta-analysis, and it is routinely used in treatment of OA [42,43]. There is clinically significant improved pain relief and patient global assessment compared with placebo injections, although the effects typically last only 1 to 3 weeks [42,43].

Intra-articular hyaluronic acid injections (viscosupplementation) are conditionally recommended by the ACR for people 75 years of age or older with knee OA but are not routinely recommended for OA of other joints [15]. Although conflicting evidence exists, multiple meta-analyses of randomized controlled trials suggest that there may be a small benefit in comparison with intra-articular placebo injection or noninterventional control [43,44]. The clinical significance is difficult to determine and may be irrelevant. In comparison with glucocorticoid injections, hyaluronic acid injections had greater benefit between 5 and 13 weeks after injection, but this was not sustained [43].

Procedures such as botulinum toxin type A injection, intra-articular injection of platelet-rich plasma, and adipose stem cell injections are under investigation [42,45–48]. A few studies showed positive effect of platelet-rich plasma in patients with knee OA, but no standardized protocol has been established [47,48].

Surgery

In patients for whom pain and loss of mobility are disabling despite conservative management, orthopedic consultation should be obtained to assess risks and benefits of surgery.

Surgical interventions performed for OA include arthroscopic lavage and débridement, osteotomy, joint fusion, joint distraction, and arthroplasty. Joint replacement surgery or total joint arthroplasty is a mainstay of surgical OA treatment. Protocols for total joint arthroplasty include different approaches and minimally invasive techniques. A systematic review of hip replacement surgery trials concluded that in 70% of subjects, pain and function scores were rated good or excellent 10 years postoperatively [49]. Observational studies have suggested that better outcomes are associated with patients between the ages of 45 and 75 years; with weight less than 70 kg; and with a good social support, higher educational level, and lower preoperative morbidity [50]. Similar favorable results have been achieved in total knee replacement for OA. In both hip and knee joint replacements, early inpatient rehabilitation after arthroplasty has been shown to reduce hospital stays and cost of care in older patients with medical comorbidities [51].

Systematic review of arthroscopic lavage and débridement in OA showed no short- or long-term benefit compared with placebo, and it is not advised [52]. Osteotomy has been used to correct biomechanics and to unload areas of high stress with some success. Fusion may be helpful in situations in which joint replacement is not appropriate. Joint distraction or distraction arthroplasty is increasingly performed for ankle OA to avoid fusion and to maintain range of motion. Hip joint resurfacing is an effective alternative to total arthroplasty in severe hip OA [53], but patellar resurfacing is not recommended in knee pain, for which no benefit has been shown [54].

Potential Disease Complications

Potential complications of OA include chronic pain, muscle weakness, decreased range of motion, limited physical function, inability to participate in work or the community, and loss of self-care skills.

Potential Treatment Complications

The safety profile of topical OA medications is generally good. Topical NSAIDs may cause increased local adverse events (mostly mild skin reactions) compared with placebo or oral NSAIDs [16]. However, topical NSAIDs have decreased incidence of gastrointestinal, cardiovascular, and renal adverse events compared with traditional oral NSAIDs [15,16]. Topical capsaicin and rubefacients are known for local skin reactions like redness, burning pain, and itching. It is worthwhile to caution patients that they may experience increased pain when beginning therapy.

Oral analgesics including acetaminophen and NSAIDs have well-known side effects that most commonly affect the gastric, hepatic, and renal systems. Although use of acetaminophen is associated with only mild side effects for the most part, it does carry a significant risk of hepatic toxicity. NSAIDs are known to have both gastrointestinal toxicity and nephrotoxicity and are associated with increased risk of myocardial infarction, stroke, and erectile dysfunction. In patients with high gastrointestinal risk for ulceration and bleeding, a cyclooxygenase-2 inhibitor or NSAID with concurrent use of a proton pump inhibitor may be considered [1]. Selective cyclooxygenase-2 inhibitors carry greater cardiovascular risk and should be used only in patients with minimal cardiovascular risk factors and no history of cardiovascular disease. The most common adverse drug reactions of tramadol and opioids are nausea, vomiting, itching, sweating, constipation, and drowsiness. Drug addiction and dependence with both are widely reported.

All intra-articular injections usually have mild side effects but, like any procedure, may result in bleeding, infection, and local irritation and pain. Complications common to all surgical techniques include pain, bleeding, infection, and effects of anesthesia. Studies have well documented the adverse effects or events associated with total arthroplasty. Intraoperative complications include fracture, nerve injury, vascular injury, and cement-related hypotension. Postoperative complications of total joint arthroplasty include thromboembolism, dislocation, osteolysis, aseptic loosening, implant failure or fracture, and heterotopic ossification. Aseptic loosening, implant failure, and fractures are often painful and require surgical revision.

References

[1] Bijlsma JW, Berenbaum F, Lafeber FP. Osteoarthritis: an update with relevance for clinical practice. Lancet 2011;377:2115–26.

[2] Brashaw RT, Tingstad EM. Rehabilitation of the osteoarthritic patient: focus on the knee. Clin Sports Med 2005;24:101–31.

[3] Suri P, Morgenroth DC, Hunter DJ. Epidemiology of osteoarthritis and associated comorbidities. PM R 2012;4(Suppl.):S10–9.

[4] Felson DT, Niu J, Clancy M, et al. Effect of recreational physical activities on the development of knee osteoarthritis in older adults of different weights: the Framingham Study. Arthritis Rheum 2007;57:6–12.

[5] Lawrence RC, Felson DT, Helmick CG, et al. Estimates of the prevalence of arthritis and other rheumatic conditions in the United States. Part II. Arthritis Rheum 2008;58:26–35.

[6] Pearl AD, Warren RF, Rodeo SA. Basic science of articular cartilage and osteoarthritis. Clin Sports Med 2005;24:1–12.

[7] Chapman K, Valdes AM. Genetic factors in OA pathogenesis. Bone 2012;51:258–64.

[8] Loughlin J. Genetic indicators and susceptibility to osteoarthritis. Br J Sports Med 2011;45:278–82.

[9] Nevitt MC, Zhang Y, Javaid MK, et al. High systemic bone mineral density increases the risk of incident knee OA and joint space narrowing, but not radiographic progression of existing knee OA: the MOST study. Ann Rheum Dis 2010;69:163–8.

[10] Losina E, Walensky RP, Reichmann WM, et al. Impact of obesity and knee osteoarthritis on morbidity and mortality in older Americans. Ann Intern Med 2011;154:217–26.

[11] Blagojevic M, Jinks C, Jeffery A, et al. Risk factors for onset of osteoarthritis of the knee in older adults: a systematic review and meta-analysis. Osteoarthritis Cartilage 2010;18:24–33.

[12] Reijman M, Hazes JM, Pols HA, et al. Acetabular dysplasia predicts incident osteoarthritis of the hip: the Rotterdam study. Arthritis Rheum 2005;52:787–93.

[13] Segal NA, Glass NA, Torner J, et al. Quadriceps weakness predicts risk for knee joint space narrowing in women in the MOST cohort. Osteoarthritis Cartilage 2010;18:769–75.

[14] Arnstein PM. Evolution of topical NSAIDs in the guidelines for treatment of osteoarthritis in elderly patients. Drugs Aging 2012;29:523–31.

[15] Hochberg MC, Altman RD, April KT, et al. American College of Rheumatology 2012 recommendations for the use of nonpharmacologic and pharmacologic therapies in osteoarthritis of the hand, hip, and knee. Arthritis Care Res (Hoboken) 2012;64:465–74.

[16] Derry S, Moore RA, Rabbie R. Topical NSAIDs for chronic musculoskeletal pain in adults. Cochrane Database Syst Rev 2012;9, CD007400.

[17] Matthews P, Derry S, Moore RA, et al. Topical rubefacients for acute and chronic pain in adults. Cochrane Database Syst Rev 2009;3 CD007403.

[18] Langford R, McKenna F, Ratcliffe S, et al. Transdermal fentanyl for improvement of pain and functioning in osteoarthritis: a randomized, placebo-controlled trial. Arthritis Rheum 2006;54:1829–37.

[19] Bannwarth B. Transdermal fentanyl in patients with osteoarthritis: comment on the article by Langford et al. Arthritis Rheum 2007;56:697–8.

[20] Nüesch E, Rutjes AW, Husni E, et al. Oral or transdermal opioids for osteoarthritis of the knee or hip. Cochrane Database Syst Rev 2009;4, CD003115.

[21] Towheed TE, Maxwell L, Judd MG, et al. Acetaminophen for osteoarthritis. Cochrane Database Syst Rev 2006;1: CD004257.

[22] Cepeda MS, Camargo F, Zea C, et al. Tramadol for osteoarthritis. Cochrane Database Syst Rev 2006;3: CD005522.

[23] Hochberg MC, Wohlreich M, Gaynor P, et al. Clinically relevant outcomes based on analysis of pooled data from 2 trials of duloxetine in patients with knee osteoarthritis. J Rheumatol 2012;39:352–8.

[24] Clegg DO, Reda DJ, Harris CL, et al. Glucosamine, chondroitin sulfate, and the two in combination for painful knee osteoarthritis. N Engl J Med 2006;354:795–808.

[25] Lee YH, Woo JH, Choi SJ, et al. Effect of glucosamine or chondroitin sulfate on the osteoarthritis progression: a meta-analysis. Rheumatol Int 2010;30:357–63.

[26] Wandel S, Jüni P, Tendal B, et al. Effects of glucosamine, chondroitin, or placebo in patients with osteoarthritis of hip or knee: network meta-analysis. BMJ 2010;341:c4675.

[27] Reichenbach S, Sterchi R, Scherer M, et al. Meta-analysis: chondroitin for osteoarthritis of the knee or hip. Ann Intern Med 2007;146:580–90.

[28] Lorig KR, Sobel DS, Stewart AL, et al. Evidence suggesting that a chronic disease self-management program can improve health status while reducing hospitalization: a randomized trial. Med Care 1999;37:5–14.

[29] Pelland L, Brosseau L, Wells G, et al. Efficacy of strengthening exercises for osteoarthritis (Part I): a meta-analysis. Phys Ther Rev 2004;9:77–108.
[30] Brosseau L, Pelland L, Wells G, et al. Efficacy of aerobic exercises for osteoarthritis (Part II): a meta-analysis. Phys Ther Rev 2004;9:125–45.
[31] Loew L, Brosseau L, Wells GA, et al. Ottawa panel evidence-based clinical practice guidelines for aerobic walking programs in the management of osteoarthritis. Arch Phys Med Rehabil 2012;93:1269–85.
[32] Hernández-Molina G, Reichenbach S, Zhang B, et al. Effect of therapeutic exercise for hip osteoarthritis pain: results of a meta-analysis. Arthritis Rheum 2008;59:1221–8.
[33] Maxwell L, Santesso N, Tugwell P, et al. Method guidelines for Cochrane Musculoskeletal Group systematic reviews. J Rheumatol 2006;33:2304–11.
[34] Fransen M, McConnell S. Exercise for osteoarthritis of the knee. Cochrane Database Syst Rev 2008;4, CD004376.
[35] Fransen M, McConnell S, Hernandez-Molina G, Reichenbach S. Does land-based exercise reduce pain and disability associated with hip osteoarthritis? A meta-analysis of randomized controlled trials. Osteoarthritis Cartilage 2010;18:613–20.
[36] Christensen R, Bartels EM, Astrup A, Bliddal H. Effect of weight reduction in obese patients with knee osteoarthritis: a systematic review and meta-analysis. Ann Rheum Dis 2007;66:433–9.
[37] Brouwer RW, Jakma TS, Verhagen AP, et al. Braces and orthoses for treating osteoarthritis of the knee. Cochrane Database Syst Rev 2005;1, CD004020.
[38] Rannou F, Dimet J, Boutron I, et al. Splint for base-of-thumb osteoarthritis: a randomized trial. Ann Intern Med 2009;150:661–9.
[39] Rutjes AW, Nüesch E, Sterchi R, et al. Transcutaneous electrostimulation for osteoarthritis of the knee. Cochrane Database Syst Rev 2009;4, CD002823.
[40] Hochberg M, Lixing L, Bausell B, et al. Traditional Chinese acupuncture is effective as adjunctive therapy in patients with osteoarthritis of the knee [abstract]. Arthritis Rheum 2004;50:S644.
[41] Manheimer E, Cheng K, Linde K, et al. Acupuncture for peripheral joint osteoarthritis. Cochrane Database Syst Rev 2010;1, CD001977.
[42] Hameed F, Ihm J. Injectable medications for osteoarthritis. PM R 2012;4(Suppl.):S75–81.
[43] Bellamy N, Campbell J, Robinson V, et al. Viscosupplementation for the treatment of osteoarthritis of the knee. Cochrane Database Syst Rev 2006;2, CD005321.
[44] Rutjes AW, Jüni P, da Costa BR, et al. Viscosupplementation for osteoarthritis of the knee: a systematic review and meta-analysis. Ann Intern Med 2012;157:180–91.
[45] Kwon DR, Park GY, Lee SU. The effects of intra-articular platelet-rich plasma injection according to the severity of collagenase-induced knee osteoarthritis in a rabbit model. Ann Rehabil Med 2012;36:458–65.
[46] Ter Huurne M, Schelbergen R, Blattes R, et al. Antiinflammatory and chondroprotective effects of intraarticular injection of adipose-derived stem cells in experimental osteoarthritis. Arthritis Rheum 2012;64:3604–13.
[47] Gobbi A, Karnatzikos G, Mahajan V, et al. Platelet-rich plasma treatment in symptomatic patients with knee osteoarthritis: preliminary results in a group of active patients. Sport Health 2012;4:162–72.
[48] Spaková T, Rosocha J, Lacko M, et al. Treatment of knee joint osteoarthritis with autologous platelet-rich plasma in comparison with hyaluronic acid. Am J Phys Med Rehabil 2012;91:411–7.
[49] Faulkner A, Kennedy LG, Baxter K, et al. Effectiveness of hip prostheses in primary total hip replacement: a critical review of evidence and an economic model. Health Technol Assess 1998;2:1–33.
[50] Young NL, Cheah D, Waddell JP, et al. Patient characteristics that affect the outcome of total hip arthroplasty: a review. Can J Surg 1998;41:188–95.
[51] Munin MC, Rudy TE, Glynn NW, et al. Early inpatient rehabilitation after elective hip and knee arthroplasty. JAMA 1998;279:847–52.
[52] Laupattarakasem W, Laopaiboon M, Laupattarakasem P, et al. Arthroscopic debridement for knee osteoarthritis. Cochrane Database Syst Rev 2008;1, CD005118.
[53] Smith TO, Nichols R, Donell ST, et al. The clinical and radiological outcomes of hip resurfacing versus total hip arthroplasty: a meta-analysis and systematic review. Acta Orthop 2010;81:684–95.
[54] Pavlou G, Meyer C, Leonidou A, et al. Patellar resurfacing in total knee arthroplasty: does design matter? A meta-analysis of 7075 cases. J Bone Joint Surg Am 2011;93:1301–9.

CHAPTER 140

Osteoporosis

David M. Slovik, MD

Synonyms

Thin bones
Brittle bones

ICD-9 Code

733.00 Osteoporosis, unspecified

ICD-10 Code

M81.0 Age-related osteoporosis without current pathological fracture, osteoporosis NOS

Definition

Osteoporosis is a skeletal disorder characterized by compromised bone strength predisposing a person to an increased risk for fracture. Bone strength primarily reflects the integration of bone density and bone quality. Bone quality refers to factors such as microarchitectural changes, bone turnover, collagen structure, damage accumulation (e.g., microfractures), and degree of mineralization [1].

Osteoporosis can also be defined according to the World Health Organization criteria on the basis of bone mineral density and bone mineral content measurements (see section on diagnostic studies).

Osteoporosis is the most common metabolic bone disease. The National Osteoporosis Foundation estimates that at least 10 million Americans have osteoporosis and another 34 million have decreased bone mass, putting them at increased risk for osteoporosis and fractures. Of the 10 million, 8 million are women and 2 million are men. Annually in the United States, more than 1.5 million fractures attributable to osteoporosis occur, including approximately 750,000 vertebral, 300,000 hip, and 250,000 wrist fractures. The annual cost of caring for osteoporosis-related fractures in the United States is in excess of $16 billion. In addition, there is a 15% to 25% excess mortality within the first year after a hip fracture. In recent years, the hip fracture rate has been reported to be declining [2].

Symptoms

Osteoporosis is a silent disease until a fracture occurs. Pain and deformity are usually present at the site of fracture. Vertebral fractures often occur with little trauma, such as coughing, lifting, or bending over. Acute back pain may be related to a vertebral compression fracture, with pain localized to the fracture site or in a radicular distribution. New back pain or chronic back pain in a patient with osteoporosis and prior vertebral fractures may be related to new fractures, muscle spasm, or other causes.

With vertebral fractures, even if they are asymptomatic, there may be a gradual loss of height and the development of a kyphosis. Breathing may be difficult, and early satiety and bloating—a sensation of fullness and dyspepsia—may develop because of less room in the abdominal cavity.

Physical Examination

In evaluating patients with osteoporosis, it is important to diagnose treatable and reversible causes and to assess the risk factors for development of osteoporosis and osteoporotic fractures. Table 140.1 lists common causes of osteoporosis. Table 140.2 lists risk factors for osteoporosis.

The physical examination focuses on findings suggestive of secondary causes of osteoporosis (e.g., hyperthyroidism and Cushing syndrome). One should also examine areas previously involved with fractures (e.g., back, hip, and wrist) to assess for deformity and limitation of function. A baseline measurement of height should be obtained and reevaluated at subsequent visits. Localized vertebral tenderness may be present from fracture, paravertebral muscle spasm, or exaggerated thoracic kyphosis. The findings of the neurologic examination looking for any deficits due to vertebral fracture are usually normal.

Functional Limitations

Functional limitations are related to the type of fracture and its long-term consequences. With vertebral fractures, the functional limitation may initially be related to the acute pain and inability to move. The chronic limitations may be related to loss of height, chronic back pain, difficulty in moving, abdominal distention, and difficulty in breathing.

The functional limitations after a hip fracture are related to the decreased functional mobility, often the need for long-term use of assistive devices, the lack of independence, and the long-term need for assistive care. An assistive device will be needed permanently for ambulation by

Table 140.1 Common Causes of Osteoporosis

Age Related
Postmenopausal
Senile
Endocrine and Metabolic Related
Hypogonadism
Hyperthyroidism
Primary hyperparathyroidism
Adrenal-cortical hormone excess
Diabetes mellitus, type 1
Hypercalciuria
Genetics and Collagen Disorders
Osteogenesis imperfecta
Ehlers-Danlos syndrome
Homocystinuria
Marfan syndrome
Hematologic Disorders
Multiple myeloma
Systemic mastocytosis
Thalassemia
Drug Related
Glucocorticoids
Thyroid hormone excess
Chemotherapy, immunosuppressants
Anticonvulsant drugs
Aromatase inhibitors
Androgen deprivation therapy (men)
Proton pump inhibitors
Selective serotonin reuptake inhibitors
Thiazolidinediones
Miscellaneous
Rheumatoid arthritis
Immobilization
Organ transplantation

Table 140.2 Risk Factors for Osteoporosis

Advanced age
Female
Small-boned, thin women
White and Asian women
Estrogen deficiency
Personal history of fracture as adult
Fracture in first-degree family members
Inactivity
Low calcium intake
Cigarette smoking
Alcoholism
Medications such as glucocorticoids, excessive thyroid hormone, chemotherapy and immunosuppressants, antiseizure drugs, aromatase inhibitors; androgen deprivation therapy in men

50% of people with a hip fracture, and two thirds will lose some of their ability to perform ordinary daily activities.

Wrist fractures usually heal completely, but some people have chronic pain, deformity, and functional limitations.

Diagnostic Studies

Bone density measurements are the standard for assessment of risk, diagnosis, and long-term management of patients with osteoporosis. Bone density measurement is often essential to make management decisions. Available techniques include single-photon absorptiometry, dual-energy x-ray absorptiometry, quantitative computed tomography, and quantitative ultrasonography. Dual-energy x-ray absorptiometry, although it is not as sensitive as quantitative computed tomography for detection of early trabecular bone loss, is the method of choice for measurement of bone mineral density because of its good precision, low radiation dose, and fast examination time.

Bone mineral density testing should be based on an individual's fracture risk profile and skeletal health assessment. It should be performed only if the results will influence a treatment decision.

Bone mineral density testing should be considered on the basis of the National Osteoporosis Foundation guidelines, as follows [3]:

- Women age 65 and older and men age 70 and older, regardless of clinical risk factors
- Younger postmenopausal women and men age 50-69 about whom you have concern based on their clinical risk factor profile
- Adults who have a fracture after age 50
- Adults with a condition (e.g., rheumatoid arthritis) or taking a medication (e.g., glucocorticoids in a daily dose of 5 mg or more for >3 months) associated with low bone mass or bone loss
- Anyone being considered for pharmacologic therapy for osteoporosis
- Anyone being treated for osteoporosis, to monitor treatment effect
- Anyone not receiving therapy in whom evidence of bone loss would lead to treatment
- Postmenopausal women discontinuing estrogen

Bone mineral density is reported by T and Z scores (Table 140.3). The T score compares an individual's bone mineral density with the mean value for young normal individuals expressed as a standard deviation (SD); the Z score compares the values to age- and sex-matched adults.

- Normal: a T score value for bone mineral density or bone mineral content that is not more than 1 SD below the young adult mean value.
- Low bone mass (osteopenia): a T score value for bone mineral density or bone mineral content that lies between1.0 and 2.5 SDs below the young adult mean value.
- Osteoporosis: a T score value for bone mineral density or bone mineral content that is 2.5 SDs or more below the young adult mean value.

The lower the T score, the higher the risk for subsequent fractures. However, the score will not predict who will fracture because other factors come into play (e.g., fall velocity, type of fall, direction of fall, and protective padding). A low Z score may suggest excessive bone loss due to secondary causes of osteoporosis.

Specific laboratory tests are obtained to help in the differential diagnosis of osteoporosis and to rule out osteomalacia. The general laboratory tests include a complete blood count,

Table 140.3 Bone Mineral Density Reporting

T score	Standard deviations (SDs) above or below peak bone mass in young, normal, sex-matched adults
Z score	Standard deviations (SDs) above or below age- and sex-matched adults

chemistry profile including calcium and phosphorus, liver and kidney tests, serum and urine protein electrophoresis, and thyroid-stimulating hormone concentration. A 24-hour collection of urine for calcium and creatinine measurement is also helpful. Because of the high prevalence of vitamin D deficiency in the adult population, especially elderly individuals, a serum 25-hydroxyvitamin D level should be obtained. A parathyroid hormone level should be determined in suspected cases of primary or secondary hyperparathyroidism. Blood and urine test results are usually normal in uncomplicated cases of osteoporosis. After a fracture, the alkaline phosphatase activity may be elevated. Biochemical markers of bone turnover, including urine N-telopeptide and serum C-telopeptide, may be helpful in selective patients to assess for bone turnover and whether someone is responding to treatment.

Differential Diagnosis

Common causes of osteoporosis are listed in Table 140.1.

Treatment [4]

Initial

The initial approach to the prevention and treatment of osteoporosis involves nonpharmacologic interventions and, in appropriate patients, the use of various pharmacologic agents (Table 140.4). Prevention and treatment guidelines are presented in Tables 140.5 and 140.6.

Calcium

Adequate calcium is important for all age groups. Epidemiologic studies suggest that long-standing dietary calcium deficiency can result in lower bone mass. The average dietary calcium intake in postmenopausal women is less than 600 mg/day. Several studies have shown that calcium supplementation along with vitamin D, especially in the elderly, may slow bone loss and reduce vertebral and nonvertebral fracture rates [5]. A total calcium intake of 1200 to 1300 mg/day is recommended for postmenopausal women [6]. This can be achieved primarily by consumption of foods that have a high calcium content, such as milk and dairy products and calcium-fortified foods, especially yogurt. Calcium supplementation is often required, especially in elderly individuals. Calcium carbonate supplements have the highest calcium content but may cause abdominal discomfort with bloating and constipation and are better absorbed when they are taken with foods. Calcium citrate preparations are generally better absorbed and are not dependent on gastric acid.

Table 140.4 Treatment Options

Nonpharmacologic Intervention

Calcium
Vitamin D
Exercise
Smoking cessation
Fall prevention

Pharmacologic Agents

Hormone replacement therapy
Selective estrogen receptor modulators
  Raloxifene (Evista)
Bisphosphonates
  Alendronate (Fosamax)
  Risedronate (Actonel)
  Ibandronate (Boniva)
  Zoledronic acid (Reclast)
Calcitonin (Miacalcin and Fortical nasal sprays)
Teriparatide (Forteo)
Denosumab (Prolia)

Table 140.5 Osteoporosis Prevention Guidelines

Hormone replacement therapy for menopausal symptoms
Raloxifene, 60 mg/day
Alendronate, 5 mg/day or 35 mg once weekly by mouth (prevention dose)
Risedronate, 5 mg/day or 35 mg weekly or 150 mg monthly by mouth
Ibandronate, 2.5 mg daily or 150 mg monthly by mouth
Zoledronic acid, 5 mg intravenously every other year

Table 140.6 Osteoporosis Treatment Guidelines

Alendronate, 10 mg/day or 70 mg once weekly (treatment dose)
Risedronate, 5 mg/day or 35 mg weekly or 150 mg monthly by mouth
Ibandronate, 2.5 mg/day or 150 mg monthly orally; 3 mg intravenously every 3 months
Zoledronic acid, 5 mg intravenously yearly
Raloxifene, 60 mg/day
Calcitonin (nasal spray), 200 units once daily
Teriparatide, 20 μg subcutaneously daily for 2 years
Denosumab, 60 mg subcutaneously every 6 months

Vitamin D

Vitamin D insufficiency and deficiency are common in postmenopausal women, especially in those who have sustained a hip fracture and those who are chronically ill, housebound, institutionalized, and poorly nourished [6,7]. Vitamin D improves muscle strength and balance and reduces the risk of falling. There may also be other unproven nonskeletal beneficial effects. A dose of 800 to 1000 IU/day (from supplements, multivitamins, and other sources) should be administered to prevent vitamin D deficiency. Some need higher amounts. Many calcium supplements now contain vitamin D. Maintaining a serum 25-hydroxyvitamin D level of more than 30 ng/mL (70 nmol/L) is suggested by many experts, although the Institute of Medicine suggests levels above 20 ng/mL.

Exercise

There is increasing evidence that weight-bearing and strength training exercises are beneficial to bone in helping achieve peak bone mass and preserving bone later in life [8]. Bone adapts to physical and mechanical loads placed on it by altering its mass and strength. This occurs either by the direct impact from the weight-bearing activity or by the action of muscle attached to bone. Exercising can also help strengthen back muscles, improve balance, lessen the likelihood of falling, and give one a sense of well-being [9]. Back extension exercises and abdominal strengthening exercises are helpful. However, acute stresses to the back, such as trunk flexion, side-bending, high impact, and heavy weights, should be avoided to lessen the likelihood of injury and fracture. A proper exercise program should be established. Older postmenopausal women and even the frail elderly can tolerate and potentially show improvements in muscle strength and bone mineral density in response to strength training and resistive exercise programs.

Smoking Cessation

A 5% to 10% reduction in bone density has been seen in women who smoked one pack per day in adulthood. Therefore, it is recommended that physicians aggressively pursue smoking cessation in their treatment plans.

Fall Prevention

Many factors can lead to falls, including poor vision, frailty, medication (especially narcotic pain medications, hypotensive agents, and psychotropic drugs), and balance disturbances [10]. Each area needs to be assessed appropriately. Prevention measures include keeping rooms free from clutter and having good lighting. Advise patients to wear supportive shoes, to be aware of thresholds, and to avoid slippery floors; rugs should be tacked down. Grab bars are useful in the bathroom. A portable telephone and a personal alarm activator are helpful, and someone should check on the individual regularly.

Guidelines for Treatment

The guidelines for treatment of postmenopausal women based on National Osteoporosis Foundation recommendations are as follows:

- Hip or spine fracture
- T score −2.5 or below at the spine, femoral neck, or total hip
- T score between −1.0 and −2.5 and high 10-year fracture risk by the U.S.-adapted World Health Organization Fracture Risk Assessment Calculator (FRAX). Treat if 10-year risk is 3% or more for hip fractures or 20% or more for major osteoporosis-related fractures [11].

Hormone Replacement Therapy

Hormone replacement therapy can be used in the short-term management of postmenopausal women with symptoms of estrogen deficiency, including hot flashes, memory deficits, urinary frequency, and vaginal dryness. Long-term hormone replacement therapy can slow bone loss and lower the incidence of fractures [12]. In the Women's Health Initiative (WHI) study with estrogen and progestin, there was a 34% reduction in vertebral and hip fractures. However, there was an increase in breast cancer, coronary heart disease, stroke, and thromboembolic disease [13]. The mean age of patients in the WHI was 63 years. A recent reanalysis from the WHI showed no increase in coronary heart disease risk in women when hormone replacement therapy was started within 10 years of the onset of menopause [14]. Significant controversy still exists about the results of the WHI. Estrogen is approved for the prevention of osteoporosis but not for treatment. The major reason to use hormone replacement therapy is to treat menopausal symptoms. The lowest dose of estrogen and progesterone should be used to effectively relieve these symptoms. Women who have had a hysterectomy should be given estrogen alone. A progestin should be added to the estrogen regimen if the uterus is still present.

Selective Estrogen Receptor Modulators

Selective estrogen receptor modulators are synthetic compounds that have both estrogen-antagonistic and estrogen-agonistic properties. Raloxifene (Evista) is approved by the Food and Drug Administration (FDA) for the prevention and treatment of osteoporosis at an oral dose of 60 mg daily. Raloxifene is also approved for the reduction in risk of invasive breast cancer in postmenopausal women with osteoporosis and in postmenopausal women at high risk of invasive breast cancer. Raloxifene reduces new vertebral fractures by 40% to 50% but not the risk of nonspine fractures [15]. Raloxifene acts as an antiestrogen on breast tissue and reduces the risk of invasive breast cancer similar to the reduction by tamoxifen. It does not produce uterine hypertrophy and does not significantly affect the risk of coronary heart disease. Raloxifene has no beneficial effects on menopausal symptoms and may increase hot flashes and the risk of deep venous thrombosis.

Bisphosphonates

The bisphosphonates are a group of compounds related chemically to pyrophosphate. They are characterized by a P-C-P structure. Changes in the side chains affect the binding and potency of the bisphosphonates. They are potent inhibitors of osteoclastic bone resorption.

Alendronate (Fosamax) was the first approved by the FDA in 1995 for the prevention and treatment of postmenopausal osteoporosis. Alendronate is also approved for the treatment of glucocorticoid-induced osteoporosis [15] and osteoporosis in men. In postmenopausal women, the dose for prevention is 5 mg/day or 35 mg once weekly; the dose for treatment is 10 mg/day or 70 mg once weekly. Alendronate significantly increases bone mineral density at various sites. In addition, there is a significant decrease in the incidence of vertebral, hip, and wrist fractures as well as painful vertebral fractures, hospitalization days, and other measurements of functional impairment [16].

Risedronate (Actonel) is approved by the FDA for the prevention and treatment of postmenopausal osteoporosis with an oral dose of 5 mg daily, 35 mg weekly, or 150 mg monthly. Studies have shown an increase in bone mineral density at various sites along with a decrease in vertebral and nonvertebral fractures [17]. Risedronate is also approved for the prevention and treatment of glucocorticoid-induced osteoporosis and osteoporosis in men.

Ibandronate (Boniva) is approved by the FDA for the prevention and treatment of postmenopausal osteoporosis. The oral dose is either 2.5 mg daily or 150 mg monthly. An intravenous preparation is also available for the treatment of postmenopausal osteoporosis in a dose of 3 mg intravenously every 3 months. Studies have shown an increase in bone density and a reduction in vertebral fractures [18].

The bisphosphonates are poorly absorbed and must be given on an empty stomach to maximize their absorption. Alendronate and risedronate must be taken at least 30 minutes (ibandronate, 60 minutes) before the first food, beverage, or medication with a full glass of plain water, and patients should not lie down for at least 30 minutes (ibandronate, 60 minutes) to avoid the potential upper gastrointestinal side effects, especially of esophagitis. Patients with a history of reflux should not be given these medications.

Zoledronic acid (Reclast) is approved by the FDA for the treatment of postmenopausal osteoporosis, osteoporosis in men, and glucocorticoid-induced osteoporosis and after surgical repair of hip fracture,. It is administered as a once-yearly infusion of 5 mg, administered usually during 15 to 20 minutes. It significantly reduces spine, hip, and nonhip fractures and increases bone density [19].

The major side effects with the intravenous bisphosphonates are the acute phase symptoms, including fever, muscle and joint pains, influenza-like symptoms, and headache. These usually last for no more than 24 to 72 hours. These symptoms have been reported in 32% of patients with the first infusion, in 7% after the second yearly infusion, and in 3% after the third infusion of zoledronic acid. Very uncommon but serious adverse complications from long-term use of the bisphosphonates include osteonecrosis of the jaw [20] and atypical femur fractures [21]. Osteonecrosis of the jaw has been reported primarily in cancer patients who receive bisphosphonates for skeletal metastases at a dose much higher than the dose given for osteoporosis.

Calcitonin

Synthetic salmon calcitonin given parenterally by injection and nasal spray (Miacalcin, Fortical) is approved for the treatment of postmenopausal osteoporosis. The injectable calcitonin is given as 100 units daily subcutaneously or intramuscularly. The nasal spray of calcitonin is approved in a dose of 200 units (one spray) daily. A reduction in new vertebral fractures but not in hip or nonvertebral fractures has been reported [22]. Occasional nasal irritation or headache may be seen with the nasal spray.

Parathyroid Hormone

As long ago as the late 1920s, there was evidence that parathyroid extract, administered in an intermittent once-a-day injection, stimulated osteoblast activity in animal models. This is in contrast to bone loss seen with chronic elevations in parathyroid hormone in primary hyperparathyroidism. After human parathyroid hormone was sequenced in the early 1970s, clinical studies with use of the 1-34 amino-terminal fragment started. Early results in osteoporosis trials showed increases in bone accretion, calcium balance, and trabecular bone volume with normal skeletal architecture. In the multicenter trial of recombinant human parathyroid hormone 1-34 fragment (teriparatide), 20 μg administered subcutaneously daily produced an increase in vertebral and hip bone density and a 55% reduction in vertebral fracture risk [23]. Teriparatide (Forteo) is generally well tolerated and is self-administered for up to 2 years by use of a 31-gauge needle and a prefilled syringe with a 28-day supply of medication. It is currently the only anabolic agent available (in contrast to the antiresorptive agents) and is approved for the treatment of postmenopausal women with osteoporosis who are at high risk for fracture. It is also approved for treatment of osteoporosis in men and glucocorticoid-induced osteoporosis. In rats given teriparatide in doses up to 60 times the exposure in humans, there was an increase in osteosarcoma, which was dose and duration dependent. Thus, teriparatide should not be administered to patients who have an increased baseline risk for osteosarcoma, including patients with Paget disease of bone, those with unexplained elevated alkaline phosphatase, and those who have received prior external beam or implant radiation therapy involving the skeleton.

Denosumab

Denosumab (Prolia) is a human monoclonal antibody directed against RANKL, a cytokine mediator responsible for accelerating osteoclast formation. It is approved for the treatment of postmenopausal osteoporosis at high risk for fractures and osteoporosis in men. The dose is 60 mg subcutaneously every 6 months. Reductions in spine, hip, and nonspine fractures are seen, and there is an increase in bone density. Side effects include a small increase in serious infection, such as skin infections. It is not affected by renal function and can be given to patients with reduced renal function [24].

Rehabilitation

Rehabilitation efforts in osteoporosis should commence long before a fracture. Either a physical or occupational therapist can be involved in assessing the patient's home to make sure it is safe and to decrease the risk of falls. Specialized equipment, such as grab bars for the bathroom and hand-held reachers for high cupboards, can be very helpful. It is important to educate patients about keeping the floors clear of clutter and throw rugs. Small pets also can be a hazard underfoot.

Therapists can assess whether the patient would be safer ambulating with an assistive device (e.g., cane or walker) in the home and community. It is important for all assistive devices to be appropriately prescribed and fitted for the patient.

Finally, therapists can instruct patients about how to exercise to improve strength, flexibility, and balance. All of these activities can help prevent falls, and weight-bearing strengthening exercises may also improve bone density.

In patients with a hip fracture or other disabling fracture, a multidisciplinary coordinated team approach involving the physician, therapists, and other rehabilitation specialists (e.g., nurse, social worker) is necessary for the patient to regain maximal function and to lead a productive life. The initial rehabilitation program also involves pain control, bowel and bladder care, and maintenance of skin integrity. The therapists, in addition to working on a program involving bed mobility, transfers, gait activities, safety precautions, and activities of daily living, must be cognizant of the medical problems in each patient. After an acute rehabilitation stay, some patients may need an additional stay in a transitional setting on their way to eventually going home or else require long-term placement. For those able to go home, the team needs to teach the patient a home exercise program, to order appropriate equipment, and to arrange for continued therapy, either at home or in an outpatient setting.

Back Braces

Back braces may be helpful, especially in the short term, to get patients out of bed and ambulatory so they can participate in activities. Back braces, however, can be very uncomfortable and often are not tolerated. Long-term use should be discouraged unless it helps the patient in functional activities and with control of pain.

Procedures

Other than surgery for fracture repair, procedures are generally not needed in the management of osteoporosis. Two procedures—vertebroplasty and kyphoplasty—are available to stabilize vertebral fractures and to alleviate pain.

Surgery

The preferred treatment of hip fracture and some other fractures is surgical repair and stabilization.

Potential Disease Complications

As bone density decreases, the risk for sustaining a fracture increases. Osteoporosis is asymptomatic until a fracture occurs. Thereafter, all complications are related to the problems from these fractures, to the surgery (if it is required), and to the recuperative period and eventually to the loss of function and independence.

After vertebral fractures, acute pain may limit mobility. Bed rest and narcotic analgesics may be necessary. Severe constipation and urinary retention may ensue. Chronically, patients may suffer from severe back pain and have respiratory problems, abdominal distention, bloating, and constipation. Many patients who wear a back brace complain about the discomfort and difficulty in using it.

Potential Treatment Complications

The complications of treatment can be related either to the surgical repair of the fracture and the recuperative phase or to medications used to prevent or to treat osteoporosis.

Most osteoporotic fractures occur in older patients and result in loss of function and loss of independence and the need for long-term care. Because surgery is required to repair a hip fracture, complications from surgery, anesthesia, bed rest, and pain medications (often narcotics) are common. Pneumonia, phlebitis, urinary tract infection, constipation, and respiratory problems also are frequent.

Complications from drug therapy for osteoporosis include the following: potential increase in breast cancer (estrogen), heart disease (estrogen), clotting and thromboembolic problems (estrogen, raloxifene), and endometrial cancer (in those using only estrogen); hot flashes (raloxifene); upper gastrointestinal symptoms and esophagitis from oral alendronate, risedronate, and ibandronate; fever, muscle and joint aches, and influenza-like symptoms from intravenous ibandronate and zoledronic acid; osteonecrosis of the jaw and atypical femur fractures with long-term bisphosphonates; running nose and headache from calcitonin; and transient mild hypercalcemia with teriparatide and a small increase in infections with denosumab.

References

[1] NIH Consensus Development Panel on Osteoporosis Prevention, Diagnosis, and Therapy. Osteoporosis prevention, diagnosis, and therapy. JAMA 2001;285:785–95.

[2] Brauer CA, Coca-Perraillon M, Cutler DM, Rosen AB. Incidence and mortality of hip fractures in the United States. JAMA 2009;302:1573–9.

[3] National Osteoporosis Foundation. Clinician's guide to prevention and treatment of osteoporosis. Washington, DC: National Osteoporosis Foundation; 2010.

[4] Watts NB, Bilezikian JP, Camacho PM, et al. American Association of Clinical Endocrinologists medical guidelines for clinical practice for the diagnosis and treatment of postmenopausal osteoporosis. Endocr Pract 2010;16:1–37.

[5] Dawson-Hughes B, Harris SS, Krall EA, Dallal GE. Effect of calcium and vitamin D supplementation on bone density in men and women 65 years of age or older. N Engl J Med 1997;337:670–6.

[6] Ross AC, Manson JE, Abrams SA, et al. The 2011 report on dietary reference intakes for calcium and vitamin D from the Institute of Medicine: what clinicians need to know. J Clin Endocrinol Metab 2011;96:53–8.

[7] Rosen CJ. Vitamin D, insufficiency. N Engl J Med 2011;364:248–54.

[8] Slovik DM. Osteoporosis. In: Frontera WF, Slovik DM, Dawson DM, editors. Exercise in rehabilitation medicine. 2nd ed. Champaign, Ill: Human Kinetics; 2006. p. 221–48.

[9] Nelson ME, Wernick S. Strong women, strong bones. updated ed. New York: Putnam Penguin; 2006.

[10] Greenspan SL, Myers ER, Kiel DP, et al. Fall direction, bone mineral density, and function: risk factors for hip fracture in frail nursing home elderly. Am J Med 1998;104:539–45.

[11] FRAX algorithm. www.shef.ac.uk/FRAX. Also available at www.NOF.org.

[12] The North American Menopause Society. Management of osteoporosis in postmenopausal women: 2010 position statement of the North American Menopause Society. Menopause 2010;17:25–54.

[13] Writing Group for the Women's Health Initiative Investigation. Risks and benefits of estrogen plus progestin in healthy postmenopausal women: principal results from the Women's Health Initiative randomized controlled trial. JAMA 2002;288:321–33.

[14] Rossouw JE, Prentice RL, Manson JE, et al. Postmenopausal hormone therapy and risk of cardiovascular disease by age and years since menopause. JAMA 2007;297:1465–77.

[15] Ettinger B, Black DM, Mitlak BH, et al. Multiple Outcomes of Raloxifene Evaluation (MORE) Investigators. Reduction of vertebral fracture risk in postmenopausal women with osteoporosis treated with raloxifene: results from a 3-year randomized clinical trial. JAMA 1999;282:637–45.

[16] Black DM, Cummings SR, Karpf DB, et al. Randomized trial of effect of alendronate on risk of fracture in women with existing vertebral fractures. Lancet 1996;348:1535–41.

[17] Harris ST, Watts NB, Genant HK, et al. Vertebral Efficacy with Risedronate Therapy (VERT) Study Group. Effects of risedronate treatment on vertebral and nonvertebral fractures in women with postmenopausal osteoporosis: a randomized, controlled trial. JAMA 1999;282:1344–52.

[18] Chesnut CH, Skag A, Christiansen C, et al. Effects of oral ibandronate administered daily or intermittently on fracture risk in postmenopausal osteoporosis. J Bone Miner Res 2004;19:1241–9.

[19] Black DM, Delmas PD, Eastell R, et al. Once-yearly zoledronic acid for treatment of postmenopausal osteoporosis. N Engl J Med 2007;356:1809–22.

[20] Hellstein JW, Adler RA, Edwards B, et al. Managing the care of patients receiving antiresorptive therapy for prevention and treatment of osteoporosis. Recommendations from the American Dental Association Council on Scientific Affairs. J Am Dent Assoc 2011;142:1243–51.

[21] Shane E, Burr D, Eberling PR, et al. Atypical subtrochanteric and diaphyseal femoral fractures: report of a task force of the American Society for Bone and Mineral Research. J Bone Miner Res 2010;25:2267–94.

[22] Chesnut CH, Silverman S, Andriano K, et al. PROOF Study Group. A randomized trial of nasal spray salmon calcitonin in postmenopausal women with established osteoporosis: the prevent recurrence of osteoporotic fractures study. Am J Med 2000;109:267–76.

[23] Neer RM, Arnaud CD, Zanchetta JR, et al. Effect of parathyroid hormone$_{1\text{-}34}$ on fractures and bone mineral density in postmenopausal women with osteoporosis. N Engl J Med 2001;344:1434–41.

[24] Cummings SR, Marten JS, McClung MR, et al. Denosumab for prevention of fractures in postmenopausal women with osteoporosis. N Engl J Med 2009;361:756–65.

CHAPTER 141

Parkinson Disease

Nutan Sharma, MD, PhD

Synonyms

Shaking palsy
Paralysis agitans
Idiopathic parkinsonism

ICD-9 Codes

332.0 **Parkinson disease/parkinsonism**
333.1 **Essential tremor**
333.0 **Other degenerative diseases of the basal ganglia (This includes multiple system atrophy, progressive supranuclear palsy, and corticobasal degeneration.)**

ICD-10 Codes

G20 **Parkinson disease**
G25.0 **Essential tremor**
G23.9 **Degenerative disease of basal ganglia, unspecified**
G23.1 **Progressive supranuclear palsy**
G90.3 **Multi-system degeneration of the autonomic nervous system**
G31.85 **Corticobasal degeneration**

Definition

Parkinson disease (PD) is a chronic, progressive neurodegenerative disease. On pathologic examination, it is characterized by preferential degeneration of dopaminergic neurons in the substantia nigra pars compacta and the presence of cytoplasmic inclusions known as Lewy bodies. It is characterized clinically by a resting tremor, bradykinesia, and rigidity. It is important to distinguish PD from the disorders that are known collectively as the Parkinson-plus syndromes. These are relatively rare disorders that share some of the features of PD, such as rigidity and bradykinesia. However, the Parkinson-plus syndromes do not respond to medical treatment and have some unique clinical features as well.

The prevalence of PD has been estimated in more than 80 studies conducted around the world. The most consistent finding is that PD is an age-related disease. Between the ages of 50 and 59 years, the prevalence is estimated at 273 per 100,000, whereas between 70 and 79 years, the prevalence is estimated at 2700 per 100,000 [1]. Some studies have reported a higher prevalence of PD in men, whereas other studies have not.

The genetic contribution to the development of PD is an area of intense study. A variety of gene mutations that can cause PD have been identified in family studies [1]. However, their contribution to the development of PD in a larger population is not yet fully appreciated. Environmental risk factors are also thought to play a role in the pathogenesis of PD. Numerous studies have focused on the risk of pesticide and heavy metal exposure to the development of PD. Whereas the methodology varies in different studies, in those with an occupational exposure to pesticides or heavy metals, the data have been mixed, indicating either an increased risk for development of PD or no increased risk [1].

Symptoms

The most common initial manifestations of PD are rest tremor and bradykinesia. The resting tremor is suppressed by either purposeful movement or sleep and exacerbated by anxiety. The bradykinesia may produce a sensation of stiffness in the affected arm or leg. Pain is also a part of PD. An aching pain in the initially affected limb may first be attributed to bursitis or arthritis. Less common presenting complaints include gait difficulty and fatigue. It is not uncommon for one of these features to be present for months or even years before others develop.

As the disease progresses, there is marked difficulty in both initiating and terminating movement. There is difficulty in rising from a seated position, particularly when one is seated in a sofa or chair without armrests. Handwriting becomes smaller and more difficult to read. Friends and family members often complain that the patient's speech is more difficult to understand, particularly on the telephone. The symptom of a softer voice with a decline in enunciation is known as hypophonia.

Physical Examination

The most distinctive clinical feature is the rest tremor. It is typically present in a single upper extremity early in the course of the disease. As the disease progresses, the resting tremor may spread to both the ipsilateral lower limb and the contralateral limbs. Examination of motor tone reveals cogwheel rigidity in the affected limb. Motor strength, however, remains unaffected.

Additional features that must be evaluated in an examination include rapid, repetitive limb movements and gait. Examination of repetitive movements of the fingers or entire hand will reveal bradykinesia and decreased amplitude and accuracy of finger tapping or toe tapping movements in the affected limb. Examination of gait will reveal decreased arm swing on the affected side, smaller steps, and an inability to pivot turn. Typically, patients make several steps to complete a turn because of some degree of postural instability. Deep tendon reflexes and sensation are not affected in PD.

In advanced PD, loss of postural reflexes becomes evident. Individuals are unable to maintain balance when turning. Other manifestations of advanced PD include freezing episodes and dysphagia. There is also a spectrum of cognitive impairment in PD, extending from minimal cognitive impairment to PD with dementia. Minimal cognitive impairment is defined as a gradual decline in cognitive function, identified by the patient or caregiver, that does not interfere significantly with functional independence [2]. PD with dementia is dementia with a slowly progressive course of cognitive impairment that most prominently affects attention, executive, and visuospatial functions [3].

In examination of someone who is taking medication for PD, it is important to record the time at which the last dose of medication was taken relative to the time at which the examination occurs. Medications for PD are particularly good at ameliorating the rest tremor and bradykinesia, particularly in the early stages of the disease. Typically, the rest tremor will subside for 1 to 3 hours after the last dose of medication. Other features, such as reduced arm swing, hypophonia, and loss of postural reflexes, do not respond to oral medication.

Functional Limitations

Functional limitations depend on which symptoms are most prominent in a particular patient. Early in the course of PD, the sole limitation may be in one's ability to write legibly. Affected individuals are still able to perform activities of daily living, although they may prefer to use the unaffected limb for tasks such as shaving and dressing. Although the rest tremor may result in a feeling of self-consciousness or embarrassment, it does not affect one's independence as it is suppressed with purposeful movement.

As the disease progresses, the ability to perform fine motor skills declines, and difficulty with standing and gait develops. An individual will have difficulty in buttoning a shirt or tying shoelaces. More time will be required to stand and to initiate gait. Postural instability with a tendency to retropulse also develops. Thus patients have difficulty in climbing stairs and walking safely and quickly. Slowed reaction times may also affect one's ability to drive safely. Decisions about whether someone should drive are often difficult and must be made on an individual basis. Marked hypophonia may make speaking on the telephone difficult as well. As the voice becomes more affected, dysphagia is likely to develop.

One aspect of PD that has historically received little attention is the effect it has on sexual activity. Men may experience erectile dysfunction and difficulty with ejaculation as part of the autonomic dysfunction found in PD. Women may experience inadequate lubrication and a tendency to urinate during sex secondary to autonomic dysfunction. In both genders, hypersexuality may be seen as a side effect of treatment with dopamine agonists [4].

In end-stage PD, limitations include marked dysphagia and severe abnormalities of gait that require both devices and one or two persons for assistance. At this stage, help is necessary for all activities of daily living as well.

Diagnostic Studies

PD is a clinical diagnosis. Conventional laboratory investigations do not contribute to the diagnosis or management of PD. Computed tomography and magnetic resonance imaging scans of the brain do not reveal any consistent abnormalities. A dopamine transporter radioligand has recently become available for clinical use, in single-photon emission computed tomography scanning, to assist in the evaluation of those with suspected PD. The scan is known as a DaTscan, and a recent analysis demonstrates that it does not provide greater accuracy than a clinical diagnosis based on history and examination of a patient [5].

Differential Diagnosis

The differential diagnosis includes essential tremor and several diseases known collectively as the Parkinson-plus syndromes: Lewy body dementia, progressive supranuclear palsy, multiple system atrophy, and corticobasal degeneration.

Essential tremor	An involuntary, rhythmic tremor of a body part, most commonly affecting arms and hands but that can also involve head, voice, tongue, trunk, or legs
Lewy body dementia	Motor symptoms of Parkinson disease with rapidly progressive dementia within the first year; visual hallucinations are common
Progressive supranuclear palsy	Bradykinesia, rigidity, frequent falls early in disease course, rest tremor, and inability to voluntarily move the eyes upward
Multiple system atrophy	Bradykinesia, rigidity, ataxia, and autonomic dysfunction (flushing, palpitations, nausea, vomiting)
Corticobasal degeneration	Bradykinesia, rigidity, inability to coordinate purposeful movements (apraxia), and sense that limbs are not one's own (alien limb syndrome)

Treatment

Initial

The decision to initiate medical treatment is based on the degree of disability and discomfort that the patient is experiencing. Six classes of drugs are used to treat PD (summarized in Table 141.1). The selection of a particular drug

Table 141.1 Classes of Antiparkinson Medications, Mechanisms of Action, Beneficial Effects, and Side Effects

Drug Class	Specific Agents	Mechanism of Action	Effective for	Side Effects
Anticholinergic	Benztropine	Muscarinic receptor blocker	Tremor, rigidity	Dry mouth, blurred vision, constipation, urinary retention, confusion, hallucinations, impaired concentration
Antiviral	Amantadine	Promotes synthesis and release of dopamine	Tremor, rigidity, akinesia	Leg edema, livedo reticularis, confusion, hallucinations
Dopamine replacement	Levodopa	Converted to dopamine	Tremor, rigidity, akinesia, freezing	Nausea, diarrhea, confusion, hallucinations
Dopamine agonists (D_1 and D_2)	Bromocriptine, pergolide	Dopamine analogues that bind to D_1 and D_2 receptors	Rigidity, akinesia	Leg edema, nausea, confusion, hallucinations
Dopamine agonists (D_2)	Ropinirole, pramipexole	Dopamine analogues that bind to D_2 receptors	Rigidity, akinesia	Leg edema, sleep attacks, nausea, confusion, hallucinations
Monoamine oxidase B inhibitors	Selegiline, rasagiline	Inhibit the metabolism of dopamine	Mild reduction in "wearing off" from levodopa	Nausea, hallucinations, confusion
Catechol O-methyltransferase inhibitor	Entacapone	Inhibits the metabolism of dopamine	Mild reduction in "wearing off" from levodopa	Dyskinesia, nausea, diarrhea

depends on the patient's main complaint, which is usually either a rest tremor or bradykinesia. There is no evidence to suggest that expediting or delaying the onset of treatment for PD has any effect on the overall course of the disease. However, it is clear that those who do not receive treatment and are bradykinetic are at greater risk of falling and injuring themselves.

Anticholinergic agents are the oldest class of medications used in PD. They are most effective in reducing the rest tremor and rigidity associated with PD. However, the side effects associated with anticholinergic agents typically limit their usefulness. Amantadine is also used in the treatment of PD. Amantadine produces a limited improvement in akinesia, rigidity, and tremor.

Dopamine replacement remains the cornerstone of antiparkinson therapy. Levodopa is the natural precursor to dopamine and is converted to dopamine by the enzyme aromatic amino acid decarboxylase. To ensure that adequate levels of levodopa reach the central nervous system, levodopa is administered simultaneously with a peripheral decarboxylase inhibitor. In the United States, the most commonly used peripheral decarboxylase inhibitor is carbidopa. Levodopa is most effective in reducing tremor, rigidity, and akinesia. The most common side effects, seen with the onset of treatment, are nausea, abdominal cramping, and diarrhea. Long-term treatment with levodopa is associated with three types of complications: hourly fluctuations in motor state, dyskinesias, and a variety of psychiatric complaints including hallucinations and confusion. However, it is not clear whether the motor fluctuations are due to the levodopa treatment alone, the disease progression alone, or a complex interplay of imperfect dopamine replacement and the inexorable progression of disease. In summary, current evidence supports the use of dopamine replacement as soon as the symptoms of PD become troublesome to the individual patient. There is no evidence that supports withholding of treatment to minimize long-term motor complications.

Dopamine agonists, which directly stimulate dopamine receptors, are also used in the treatment of PD. These agents can be used either as an adjunct to levodopa therapy or as monotherapy. The older dopamine agonists, which are relatively nonspecific and exert their effects at both D_1 and D_2 receptors, are bromocriptine and pergolide. In comparison to the side effects seen with levodopa, there is a lower frequency of dyskinesias and a higher frequency of confusion and hallucinations. The newer dopamine agonists pramipexole and ropinirole are more specific for D_2 receptors. These newer agents have been reported to cause daytime somnolence, peripheral edema, and impulse control disorders [6]. All dopamine agonists can cause orthostatic hypotension, particularly when they are first introduced. It is best to start with a small dose of medication at bedtime and then slowly increase the total daily dose.

Inhibitors of dopamine metabolism are also used in the medical treatment of PD. Both selegiline and rasagiline inhibit monoamine oxidase B, which metabolizes dopamine in the central nervous system. Thus, inhibitors of monoamine oxidase B are thought to improve an individual's response to levodopa by alleviating the motor fluctuations that are seen with long-term levodopa treatment. Another agent that inhibits the metabolism of dopamine is entacapone. Entacapone inhibits catechol O-methyltransferase in the periphery. Entacapone is administered in conjunction with levodopa and, by inhibiting peripheral catechol O-methyltransferase activity, increases the amount of levodopa that reaches the central nervous system. The benefits of entacapone treatment include a reduction in total daily levodopa dose and an improvement in the length of time of maximum mobility [7].

Rehabilitation

The clinical pathologic process seen in PD reveals that patients tend to become more passive, less active, and less motivated as the disease progresses. The benefits to physical and occupational therapy are thus more far reaching than a simple improvement in motor function. The physical benefits include improvement in muscle strength and tone as well as maintenance of an adequate range of motion in the joints. The psychological benefits include enlistment of the patient as an active participant in treatment and provision of a sense of mastery over the effects of PD. Both physical therapy and occupational therapy focus on mobility, the use of adaptive equipment, and safety in both the home and community.

Because the symptoms of PD gradually worsen over time, individuals can benefit from periodic physical therapy training throughout the course of their illness. The training may take place through either community-based programs that are more readily accessible for those who live far from an academic center or home-based programs for those who cannot easily travel. An emphasis on gait training is particularly helpful to prevent falls and injury. Gait training typically involves training an individual to be conscious of taking a longer stride and putting the foot down with each step. Another method is to use visual cues to maintain a regular size for each step. For example, one can put strips of masking tape on the floor, at a regular interval that is comfortable for one's height, weight, and gender. As PD progresses, episodes of frozen gait, in which the feet seem to be stuck to the floor, occur. Freezing episodes can be broken by multiple techniques, such as visualizing that one is stepping over an imaginary line on the floor, counting in a rhythmic cadence, or marching in place.

Occupational therapy is particularly helpful in recommending adaptive devices or establishing new routines that allow people with PD to continue to live independently. For example, the use of a long-handled shoehorn eliminates the need to bend over and thus reduces the risk that a person with PD will fall while getting dressed. Other examples of adaptive equipment are a firmly secured grab bar in the bathtub and a relatively high toilet seat with armrests to minimize the risk of freezing while on the toilet.

Speech therapy plays a critical role for those PD patients who suffer from communication difficulties. Although dysarthria is difficult to treat, hypophonia can be overcome with training. Specifically, the Lee Silverman Voice Treatment program has been shown to be effective in improving both the volume and clarity of speech in those with PD [8]. Swallow evaluation and therapy are also helpful in the treatment of dysphagia, which occurs as PD progresses.

Procedures

Feeding tubes are sometimes used in individuals who have severe end-stage PD. Some patients choose hospice care, without artificial feeding at that point. Individuals who do get feeding tubes may need to have medication doses adjusted (e.g., carbidopa/levodopa will now bypass the esophagus and have a shortened time to onset of action).

Surgery

Although a large number of medications are available for the treatment of early and moderately advanced PD, they are of limited efficacy in those with advanced PD. Several surgical procedures are currently available for those with advanced PD. These procedures consist of either creation of a permanent lesion or insertion of an electrical stimulator in a specific nucleus of the brain.

Thalamotomy consists of introduction of a lesion in the ventral intermediate nucleus of the thalamus. Thalamotomy has been reported to produce a reduction in tremor of the contralateral limb in 85% of the patients who were treated. Thalamotomy is recommended in PD patients with an asymmetric, severe, medically intractable tremor.

Unilateral pallidotomy consists of introduction of a lesion in the globus pallidus. The most striking benefits are a reduction in contralateral drug-induced dyskinesias, contralateral tremor, bradykinesia, and rigidity. Unilateral pallidotomy is recommended in PD patients with bradykinesia, rigidity, and tremor who experience significant drug-induced dyskinesia despite optimal medical therapy. However, data regarding the long-term cognitive effects of unilateral pallidotomy are limited and varied in their findings [9,10]. Thus neuropsychological evaluation is recommended in all patients both before and after surgery.

Deep brain stimulation (DBS) for PD consists of high-frequency electrical stimulation in either the globus pallidus or the subthalamic nucleus. DBS requires surgery, in which the source of electrical stimulation is placed subcutaneously in the chest wall and the leads to which it is attached are placed in one of the locations listed. The advantage of DBS is that the degree of electrical stimulation can be easily adjusted, externally, once the DBS unit is in place. In contrast, both thalamotomy and pallidotomy result in permanent, fixed lesions in the brain. DBS of the ventral intermediate nucleus of the thalamus is effective in the treatment of a severe and disabling tremor that is unresponsive to medical therapy, with reports of approximately 80% improvement in tremor 5 years after DBS implantation [11]. DBS of the globus pallidus results in a marked reduction in dyskinesia. There are also improvements in bradykinesia, speech, gait, rigidity, and tremor. DBS of the subthalamic nucleus also results in marked improvement in tremor, akinesia, gait, and postural stability [12].

Potential Disease Complications

Depression is found in approximately 35% of those with PD [13]. It may be difficult to distinguish true depression from the apathy associated with PD. The crucial factor is to determine whether the patient has a true disturbance of mood, with loss of interest, sleep disturbance, and sometimes suicidal thoughts. The reasons for depression in PD are a subject of debate. There is a suspicion that the pathologic process of PD itself may predispose to depression. Regardless of the cause, recognition and treatment of depression may have a significant impact on the overall disability caused by the illness. Many PD patients have been treated safely and effectively with selective serotonin reuptake inhibitors, such as fluoxetine and paroxetine. Tricyclic antidepressants can be used, although their anticholinergic properties may limit their effectiveness.

Gastrointestinal complications also occur in PD. Dysphagia is typically due to poor control of the muscles of both mastication and the oropharynx. Soft food is easier to eat, and antiparkinson medication improves swallowing. Constipation is a frequent complaint in those with PD. Treatment includes increase in physical activity; discontinuation of anticholinergic drugs; and maintenance of a diet with intake of adequate fluids, fruit, vegetables, fiber, and lactulose (10 to 20 g daily).

Potential Treatment Complications

The motor complications seen with pharmacologic treatment are divided into two categories: fluctuations (off state) and levodopa-induced dyskinesias. The off state consists of a return of the signs and symptoms of PD: bradykinesia, tremor, and rigidity. Patients may also experience anxiety, dysphoria, or panic during an off state.

The development of levodopa-induced dyskinesias appears to be related to the degree of dopamine receptor supersensitivity. As PD progresses, there is an increasing loss of dopamine receptors. This results in an increased sensitivity of the remaining dopamine receptors to dopamine itself. Thus, there is a greater chance for development of dyskinesias at a given dose of levodopa. Treatment options are to lower each dose of levodopa but with an increase in the frequency with which it is taken; to add or to increase the dose of a dopamine agonist while the dose of levodopa is decreased; and to add amantadine, which has been shown to be an antidyskinetic agent in some patients [14]. There are potential complications to each of these solutions: reducing each dose of levodopa while increasing the frequency of doses (e.g., once every 2 hours) is a difficult schedule for a patient to maintain; adding or increasing the dose of dopamine agonist may result in compulsive behaviors (shopping, gambling, hypersexuality), excessive daytime sleepiness, and peripheral edema; and amantadine may cause confusion. An alternative is to treat those who continue to experience an improvement in their mobility with levodopa but develop dyskinesias that become more pronounced as the day progresses with DBS.

References

[1] Wirdefeldt K, Adami H, Cole P, et al. Epidemiology and etiology of Parkinson's disease: a review of the evidence. Eur J Epidemiol 2011;26:S1–58.

[2] Litvan I, Goldman JG, Troster AI, et al. Diagnostic criteria for mild cognitive impairment in Parkinson's disease: movement disorder society task force guidelines. Mov Disord 2012;27:349–56.

[3] Goetz CG, Emre M, Dubois B. Parkinson's disease dementia: definitions, guidelines and research perspectives in diagnosis. Ann Neurol 2008;64:S81–92.

[4] Bronner G, Vodusek DB. Management of sexual dysfunction in Parkinson's disease. Ther Adv Neurol Disord 2011;4:375–83.

[5] de la Fuente-Fernandez. Role of DaTSCAN and clinical diagnosis in Parkinson disease. Neurology 2012;78:696–701.

[6] Antonini A, Tolosa E, Mizuno Y, et al. A reassessment of risks and benefits of dopamine agonists in Parkinson's disease. Lancet Neurol 2009;8:929–37.

[7] Fox SH, Katzenschlager R, Lim SY, et al. The movement disorder society evidence-based medicine review update: treatments for the motor symptoms of Parkinson's disease. Mov Disord 2011;26(Suppl. 3):S2–41.

[8] Sapir S, Spielman JL, Ramig LO, et al. Effects of intensive voice treatment (the Lee Silverman Voice Treatment [LSVT]) on vowel articulation in dysarthric individuals with idiopathic Parkinson disease: acoustic and perceptual findings. J Speech Lang Hear Res 2007;50:899–912.

[9] Alegret M, Valldeoriola F, Tolosa E, et al. Cognitive effects of unilateral posteroventral pallidotomy: a 4-year follow-up study. Mov Disord 2003;18:323–8.

[10] Strutt AM, Lai EC, Jankovic J, et al. Five year follow-up of unilateral posteroventral pallidotomy in Parkinson's disease. Surg Neurol 2009;71:551–8.

[11] Pahwa R, Lyons KE, Wilkinson SB, et al. Long-term evaluation of deep brain stimulation of the thalamus. J Neurosurg 2006;104:506–12.

[12] Walter BL, Vitek JL. Surgical treatment for Parkinson's disease. Lancet Neurol 2004;3:719–28.

[13] Aarsland D, Pahlhagen S, Ballard CG, et al. Depression in Parkinson's disease—epidemiology, mechanisms and management. Nat Rev Neurol 2011;8:35–47.

[14] Hubsher G, Haider M, Okun MS. Amantadine: the journey from fighting flu to treating Parkinson disease. Neurology 2012;78:1096–9.

CHAPTER 142

Peripheral Neuropathies

Seward B. Rutkove, MD

Synonyms

Polyneuropathies
Neuropathies

ICD-9 Codes

356.2	**Hereditary sensory neuropathy**
356.4	**Idiopathic progressive polyneuropathy**
356.9	**Idiopathic neuropathy, unspecified**
357.1	**Polyneuropathy in collagen vascular disease**
357.2	**Polyneuropathy in diabetes**
357.3	**Polyneuropathy in malignant disease**
357.4	**Polyneuropathy in other diseases classified elsewhere**
357.5	**Alcoholic polyneuropathy**
357.6	**Polyneuropathy due to drugs**
357.7	**Polyneuropathy due to other toxic agents**
357.9	**Inflammatory and toxic neuropathy, unspecified**

ICD-10 Codes

G60.8	**Hereditary and idiopathic neuropathies**
G60.3	**Idiopathic progressive neuropathy**
M35.9 [G63]	**Polyneuropathy in collagen vascular disease**
E11.42	**Type 2 diabetes mellitus with diabetic polyneuropathy**
D49.9 [G63]	**Polyneuropathy in malignant disease**
G62.9	**Polyneuropathy, unspecified**
G62.1	**Alcoholic polyneuropathy**
G62.0	**Drug-induced polyneuropathy**
G62.2	**Polyneuropathy due to other toxic agents**

Definition

Peripheral neuropathies are a collection of disorders characterized by the generalized dysfunction of peripheral nerves. This group of diseases is heterogeneous, including those that predominantly affect the nerve axon, others that primarily affect the myelin sheath, and still others that involve both parts of the nerve simultaneously. In addition, some peripheral neuropathies affect only small, unmyelinated fibers, whereas others predominantly involve only large myelinated ones. Table 142.1 contains a list of the most frequently encountered forms of peripheral neuropathy.

Peripheral neuropathy is common; one Italian study suggested a prevalence of about 3.5% in the general population [1]. In diabetes, one study demonstrated clinical peripheral neuropathy affecting 8.3% of individuals compared with a control population, in whom 2.1% of individuals were affected [2]. After 10 years, 41.9% of the diabetic patients had peripheral neuropathy compared with 6% of the control subjects.

Defining peripheral neuropathy remains no simple task. Members of the American Academy of Neurology along with those of the American Association of Electrodiagnostic Medicine and the American Academy of Physical Medicine and Rehabilitation have developed a formal case definition for distal symmetric polyneuropathy (the most common form) [3]. The authors chose to use a combination of symptoms, signs, and electrodiagnostic testing results to formulate an ordinal ranking system to identify the likelihood of the disease in a given patient. Although it is a useful tool for future research studies, the necessity of applying such a complex approach underscores the difficulty in attempting to define peripheral neuropathy in any simple fashion.

Symptoms

Patients with peripheral neuropathy present with a number of specific sensory complaints, including decreased sensation often associated with pain, tingling (paresthesias), and burning. They may complain of a "sock-like" feeling in the feet or that the feet are persistently cold. Some patients, usually with more advanced disease, will note atrophy of the intrinsic foot muscles and some weakness, especially with the development of partial footdrop. Walking difficulties usually also develop once sensation is significantly

Table 142.1 Specific Disorders of Peripheral Nerves

Predominantly Axonal Disorders

Diabetic neuropathy
Alcoholic neuropathy
Medication-related neuropathy (e.g., metronidazole, colchicine, nitrofurantoin, isoniazid)
Systemic disease–related neuropathy (e.g., chronic renal failure, inflammatory bowel disease, connective tissue disease)
Thyroid neuropathy
Heavy metal toxic neuropathy (lead, arsenic, cadmium)
Porphyric neuropathy
Paraneoplastic neuropathy
Syphilitic, Lyme neuropathy
Sarcoid neuropathy
Human immunodeficiency virus–related neuropathy
Hereditary neuropathies (Charcot-Marie-Tooth, type 2; familial amyloid; mitochondrial)
Critical illness neuropathy

Predominantly Demyelinating Disorders

Idiopathic chronic inflammatory demyelinating polyradiculoneuropathy (CIDP)
CIDP associated with monoclonal proteins
Antimyelin-associated glycoprotein neuropathy (a form of CIDP)
Human immunodeficiency virus–associated CIDP
Guillain-Barré syndrome
Hereditary (Charcot-Marie-Tooth, types 1 and 3)

impaired. Sensory symptoms in the hand (paresthesias and reduced tactile sensation) usually develop once an axonal peripheral neuropathy has progressed up to about the level of the knees. In patients with generalized demyelinating peripheral neuropathies, more generalized symptoms of weakness and sensory loss are often present, although distally predominant paresthesias often occur. The history includes a detailed past medical history, review of systems, and any prior exposure to toxins (Table 142.2).

Table 142.2 Toxins Producing Peripheral Nerve Degeneration

Industrial Chemicals

Affect peripheral nervous system preferentially
- Lead
- Acrylamide
- Organophosphates
- Thallium

Some effects on central nervous system
- Carbon disulfide
- Methylmercury
- Methyl bromide

Large amounts required
- Arsenic
- Trichloroethylene
- Tetrachloroethane
- 2,4-Dichlorophenoxyacetic acid (2,4-D)
- Pentachlorophenol
- DDT

Some effects on other than nervous tissue
- Carbon tetrachloride
- Carbon monoxide

Pharmaceutical Substances

Arsenic
Arsenic-based chemicals
Clioquinol
Disulfiram
Gold
Hydralazine
Nitrofurantoin
Phenytoin
Sulfonamides
Thalidomide
Thallium
Vincristine

Modified from Gilliatt RW. Recent advances in the pathophysiology of nerve conduction. In Desmedt JE, ed. New Developments in Electromyography and Clinical Neurophysiology. Basel, Karger, 1973:2-18.

Physical Examination

The physical examination demonstrates distinct abnormalities that depend on the form of peripheral neuropathy present. Most commonly, patients present with a sensorimotor axonal peripheral neuropathy. In this condition, decreased sensation to pinprick, vibration, light touch, and temperature may be identified distally in the lower extremities with normal sensation more proximally. Of note, vibration sensation testing with a tuning fork has been shown to be reliable [4]. Some weakness of toe or foot extension and flexion may also be apparent. Deep tendon reflexes will be hypoactive distally (e.g., ankle jerks decreased relative to knee jerks).

In patients with acquired demyelinating peripheral neuropathy, the examination may demonstrate marked generalized weakness with some abnormal sensory findings, usually including decreased joint position sense. In this disorder, deep tendon reflexes may be reduced or diffusely absent. Patients with hereditary demyelinating polyneuropathies may demonstrate distal muscle atrophy in the feet and lower legs. Such patients may develop a pes cavus foot deformity, in which the foot is foreshortened and has a very high arch. A "champagne bottle" appearance to the legs (where muscle atrophy of the lower leg, especially of the calf, is prominent) may also be present. As any peripheral neuropathy progresses, lower extremity sensory loss may lead to gait unsteadiness, and upper extremity sensory loss may produce decreased hand dexterity.

Functional Limitations

Patients with peripheral neuropathy face a number of potential functional limitations. In those individuals with a distal axonal peripheral neuropathy, limitations usually include problems with gait and unsteadiness, especially as the neuropathy progresses. If pain is a prominent symptom, the activities of daily living may be compromised to some extent. Pain may also be prominent at night, interfering with sleep. In those patients with very advanced axonal peripheral neuropathy or demyelinating forms, such as hereditary Charcot-Marie-Tooth disease, weakness can produce major functional limitations, restricting the patient's walking ability and in some cases leading to dyspnea and nocturnal hypoventilation. In patients with some chronic forms of demyelinating polyneuropathy, weakness of both proximal and distal muscles can become severe, limiting the performance of many activities of daily living. Sensory deficits can limit one's ability to button shirts, to zip pants, to turn a key in a lock, to tie shoelaces, or to type on a computer.

Diagnostic Studies

Electrodiagnostic studies (including electromyography and nerve conduction studies) remain the most important first tests in the evaluation of polyneuropathy [5]. Nerve conduction studies assist in determination of whether the peripheral neuropathy is mainly demyelinating, axonal, or mixed (Figs. 142.1 and 142.2) by evaluation of the amplitude and conduction velocities of the motor and sensory responses obtained [6]. In axonal neuropathies, amplitudes are reduced and conduction velocities are relatively normal; in demyelinating neuropathies, amplitudes are generally preserved but conduction velocities are decreased; in mixed neuropathies, a combination of reduced amplitude and conduction velocities is present. In small-fiber neuropathies, nerve conduction studies are generally normal. Likewise, nerve conduction studies help determine the severity of the process as well. Although needle electromyography plays a more limited role in the diagnosis of peripheral neuropathy, a gradient of reinnervation, in which distal muscles are most abnormal and proximal muscles less affected, helps determine the degree of motor involvement. In addition, needle electromyography may assist in determining whether a superimposed problem, such as polyradiculopathy, is also contributing.

In general, a number of serologic tests are also performed to identify the cause of the peripheral neuropathy. These are outlined in Table 142.3.

Additional workup is occasionally necessary. Sural nerve biopsy can be useful for determining the cause of the polyneuropathy for some conditions that are difficult to diagnose, such as amyloid neuropathy, as well as some other unusual forms of peripheral neuropathy. The analysis of cutaneous sensory fibers through the use of skin biopsy to identify the presence of peripheral neuropathy involving only small, unmyelinated fibers is now also routinely performed to assist with the diagnosis of idiopathic small-fiber neuropathy or that associated with certain conditions, such as amyloid [7]. On occasion, muscle biopsy may be helpful in this regard as well because vasculitic abnormalities or amyloid can also be identified in skeletal muscle. Lumbar puncture may aid in the determination of whether an acquired demyelinating peripheral neuropathy is present by the identification of a very elevated cerebrospinal fluid protein concentration in the presence of a normal number of white cells (so-called albuminocytologic dissociation). Autonomic testing, such as quantitative sudomotor axon reflex texting, tilt-table testing, and heart rate variability to deep breathing, can also be helpful in delineating the involvement of the autonomic nervous system in the neuropathic process [8].

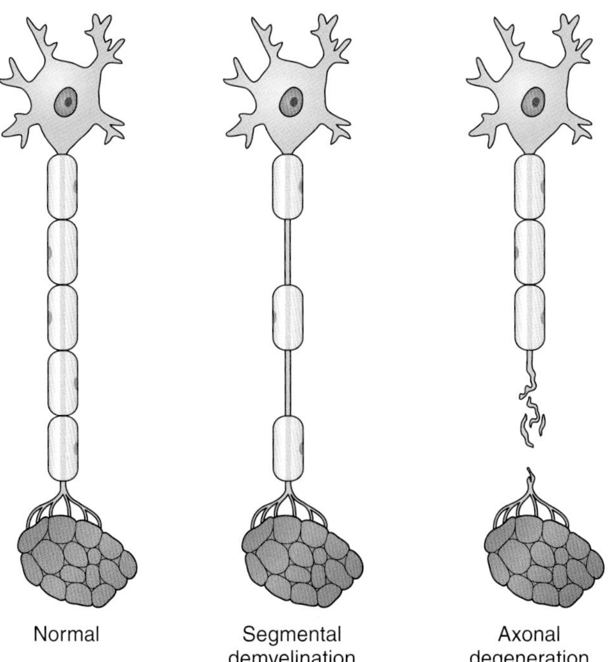

FIGURE 142.1 Types of peripheral nerve damage.

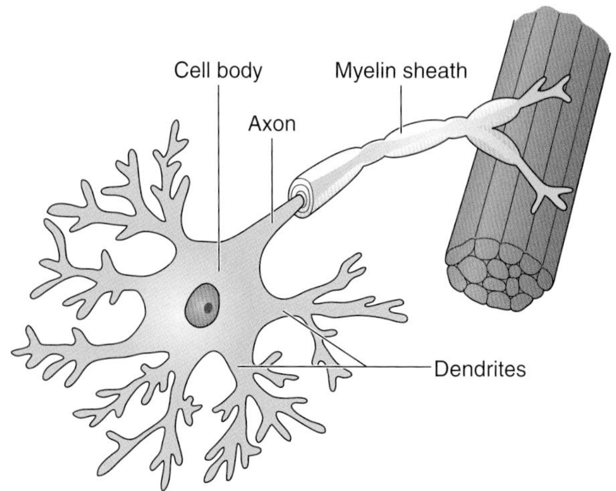

FIGURE 142.2 Schematic representation of a motor nerve extending from a cell body to the muscle it innervates.

Table 142.3 Serologic Testing in Peripheral Neuropathy

Baseline Testing
Vitamin B_{12}
Thyroid-stimulating hormone
Rapid plasma reagin (or VDRL test)
Serum glucose
Serum hemoglobin A_{1c}
Antinuclear antibody
Erythrocyte sedimentation rate
Serum protein electrophoresis
Urine protein electrophoresis
Some Additional Tests, Depending on Clinical Suspicion
Serum protein immunophoresis
24-Hour urine collection for heavy metals
24-Hour urine collection for porphyrins
Glucose tolerance testing
Human immunodeficiency virus infection testing
Anti-Ro, anti-La antibodies (Sjögren syndrome)
Anti-Hu antibody (paraneoplastic neuropathy)
Additional antibody testing in certain demyelinating disorders
Antimyelin-associated glycoprotein
Genetic testing (for disorders such as familial amyloidosis, Charcot-Marie-Tooth disease)

Differential Diagnosis

Myelopathy (spinal cord compression)
Lumbosacral polyradiculopathy (lumbar stenosis)
Mononeuropathy multiplex

Treatment

Initial

If a cause of the axonal peripheral neuropathy is known or identified (which generally is achieved about 80% of the time), treatment geared toward the underlying disorder itself might help slow progression of the polyneuropathy. For example, improved glucose control can help improve neuronal function in diabetic neuropathy [9]. Likewise, in those people with a neuropathy secondary to toxin exposure, such as alcoholic neuropathy, decreased exposure to the toxin may be helpful.

In patients with axonal peripheral neuropathies, treatment is usually symptom based, with efforts toward reducing pain and dysesthesias. A number of drugs have proved useful in this regard [10]. The tricyclic antidepressants remain most effective (generally nortriptyline or amitriptyline, starting with 10 mg at bedtime and increasing as needed until improvement occurs). Gabapentin (starting at a dose of 100 to 300 mg three times daily) has also gained wide acceptance in the treatment of this disorder during the past several years [11]. Two newer drugs specifically approved for use in diabetic polyneuropathy, duloxetine (Cymbalta), at 30 mg or 60 mg daily, and pregabalin (Lyrica) at a dose of 50 mg three times daily, increasing to 100 mg three times daily if needed, can be useful in a variety of peripheral neuropathies [12,13]. However, it is not clear that either of these is more efficacious than previously available and more inexpensive medications [14]. In patients in whom these measures prove of limited value, the use of long-acting narcotic agents may occasionally be necessary. In patients with certain forms of demyelinating peripheral neuropathy (such as chronic inflammatory demyelinating polyradiculoneuropathy), immunosuppressive or immunomodulating therapies can make a dramatic difference in the patient's symptoms and level of function. Drugs including corticosteroids, azathioprine, cyclosporine, and cyclophosphamide can be used [15]. Intravenous immune globulin and plasmapheresis are also widely used in this group of disorders [16,17]. Finally, in all patients with distal sensory loss due to peripheral neuropathy, and especially in those with diabetic peripheral neuropathy, regular podiatric care is extremely important in preventing the development of serious foot complications, such as ulcerations [18].

Rehabilitation

Physical therapy may be recommended to improve mobility, muscle strength, and balance. In patients with moderate to severe peripheral neuropathy, gait training may consist of balance exercise and use of an assistive device, such as a cane or walker. Either a physical or occupational therapist can review falls precautions (e.g., avoiding throw rugs in the home, using a chair in the bath or shower). Some patients may benefit from an ankle-foot orthosis. However, in patients with compromised sensation, monitoring of the skin to prevent breakdown when a brace is used is critical. Patients can be taught to self-monitor their skin with use of a long-handled mirror to check the bottom of their feet. Custom shoes (e.g., extra depth and width) may be beneficial, as can custom shoe orthoses.

In patients with more advanced peripheral neuropathy, evaluation by an occupational therapist may help maximize the function of the hands and arms. The occupational therapist can provide the patient with information about adaptive equipment, such as elastic shoelaces, wide grip handles for cookware and utensils, and shoehorns. An occupational or physical therapist experienced in assistive technology can also be helpful in specialized equipment, such as voice-activated computer software, driving adaptations, and environmental control units.

If pain is an issue, therapeutic modalities may be used to alleviate the pain. These may include instruction on use of transcutaneous electrical nerve stimulation, paraffin baths, and the like. It is important to caution the patient with impaired sensation not to use any heat or ice that may cause burns or frostbite. Individuals with impaired vascular status also should be advised not to use ice because of its vasoconstrictive effects.

Procedures

Patients with peripheral neuropathy are generally at increased risk for development of superimposed compressive neuropathies, such as carpal tunnel syndrome, that can be challenging to diagnose [19]. Treatment with local corticosteroid injections can be helpful for this problem (see Chapter 36).

Surgery

Surgery may be necessary for some associated conditions, including severe carpal tunnel syndrome, but it is usually more relevant to patients who develop infections of the distal lower extremities and require amputations. Other, less severe distal leg problems may also develop, requiring orthopedic or podiatric surgery. Although lower extremity nerve release surgeries are sometimes performed in the hope of treating neuropathic symptoms [20], there is little evidence to support the use of these procedures to treat peripheral neuropathy [21].

Potential Disease Complications

A number of potential foot complications can occur, including persistent, intractable pain, skin ulcerations, and foot trauma, possibly leading to amputations. Serious trauma secondary to increased gait unsteadiness is another potential problem. Finally, depression due to immobility and persistent pain also often plays a role in patients with more advanced peripheral neuropathy.

Potential Treatment Complications

The tricyclic antidepressants and other pain medications have the potential side effect of drowsiness. Dry mouth, constipation, and urinary retention also occur commonly with the tricyclic antidepressants. Side effects of duloxetine include dizziness, nausea, and constipation. Side effects of pregabalin include dizziness and somnolence. Addiction remains a major concern with narcotic use.

Treatment of the autoimmune peripheral neuropathies poses significant risk, given the inherent toxicity of the medications employed. Patients using immunosuppressive medications are at increased risk for infection, malignant neoplasia, anemia, and multiple other side effects (e.g., liver toxicity with azathioprine, renal failure with intravenous immune globulin, hemorrhagic cystitis with cyclophosphamide).

Skin breakdown can occur with improper bracing.

References

[1] Italian General Practitioner Study Group. Chronic symmetric symptomatic polyneuropathy in the elderly: a field screening investigation in two Italian regions. Neurology 1995;45:1832–6.

[2] Partanen J, Niskanen L, Lehtinen J, et al. Natural history of peripheral neuropathy in patients with non–insulin dependent diabetes mellitus. N Engl J Med 1995;333:89–94.

[3] England JD, Gronseth GS, Franklin G, et al. American Academy of Neurology, American Association of Electrodiagnostic Medicine, American Academy of Physical Medicine and Rehabilitation. Distal symmetric polyneuropathy: a definition for clinical research: report of the American Academy of Neurology, the American Association of Electrodiagnostic Medicine, and the American Academy of Physical Medicine and Rehabilitation. Neurology 2005;64:199–207.

[4] Botez SA, Liu G, Logigian E, Herrmann DN. Is the bedside timed vibration test reliable? Muscle Nerve 2009;39:221–3.

[5] Dyck P, Dyck P, Grant I, Fealey R. Ten steps in characterizing and diagnosing patients with peripheral neuropathy. Neurology 1996;47:10–7.

[6] Albers J. Clinical neurophysiology of generalized polyneuropathy. J Clin Neurophysiol 1993;10:149–66.

[7] Hermann D, Griffin F, Hauer P, et al. Epidermal nerve fiber density and sural nerve morphometry in peripheral neuropathies. Neurology 1999;53:1634–40.

[8] England JD, Gronseth GS, Franklin G, et al. American Academy of Neurology, American Association of Neuromuscular and Electrodiagnostic Medicine, American Academy of Physical Medicine and Rehabilitation. Practice parameter: the evaluation of distal symmetric polyneuropathy: the role of autonomic testing, nerve biopsy, and skin biopsy (an evidence-based review). Report of the American Academy of Neurology, the American Association of Neuromuscular and Electrodiagnostic Medicine, and the American Academy of Physical Medicine and Rehabilitation. PM R 2009;1:14–22.

[9] Tron W, Carta Q, Cantello R, et al. Peripheral nerve function and metabolic control in diabetes mellitus. Ann Neurol 1984;16:178–83.

[10] Sindrup S, Jensen T. Pharmacologic treatment of pain in polyneuropathy. Neurology 2000;55:915–20.

[11] Backonja M, Beydoun A, Edwards KR, et al. Gabapentin for the symptomatic treatment of painful neuropathy in patients with diabetes mellitus: a randomized controlled trial [see comments]. JAMA 1998;280:1831–6.

[12] Raskin J, Pritchett YL, Wang F, et al. A double-blind, randomized multicenter trial comparing duloxetine with placebo in the management of diabetic peripheral neuropathic pain. Pain Med 2005;6:346–56.

[13] Shneker BF, McAuley JW. Pregabalin: a new neuromodulator with broad therapeutic indications. Ann Pharmacother 2005;39:2029–37.

[14] Tesfaye S, Selvarajah D. Advances in the epidemiology, pathogenesis and management of diabetic peripheral neuropathy. Diabetes Metab Res Rev 2012;28(Suppl. 1):8–14.

[15] Barnett MH, Pollard JD, Davies L, McLeod JG. Cyclosporin A in resistant chronic inflammatory demyelinating polyradiculoneuropathy. Muscle Nerve 1998;21:454–60.

[16] Hahn A, Bolton C, Zochodne D, Feasby T. Intravenous immunoglobulin treatment in chronic inflammatory demyelinating polyneuropathy. Brain 1996;119:1067–77.

[17] Hahn A, Bolton C, Pillay N, et al. Plasma-exchange therapy in chronic inflammatory demyelinating polyneuropathy. Brain 1996;119:1055–66.

[18] Boulton AJ. What you can't feel can hurt you. J Vasc Surg 2010;52(Suppl.):28S–30S.

[19] Gazioglu S, Boz C, Cakmak VA. Electrodiagnosis of carpal tunnel syndrome in patients with diabetic polyneuropathy. Clin Neurophysiol 2011;122:1463–9.

[20] Aszmann OC, Kress KM, Dellon AL. Results of decompression of peripheral nerves in diabetics: a prospective, blinded study. Plast Reconstr Surg 2001;108:1452–3.

[21] Chaudhry V, Russell J, Belzberg A. Decompressive surgery of lower limbs for symmetrical diabetic peripheral neuropathy. Cochrane Database Syst Rev 2008;3, CD006152.

CHAPTER 143

Plexopathy—Brachial

Erik Ensrud, MD
John C. King, MD
John D. Alfonso, MD

Synonyms

Brachial plexopathy
Neuralgic amyotrophy
Parsonage-Turner syndrome
Brachial amyotrophy
Idiopathic shoulder girdle neuropathy
Brachial plexitis
Erb palsy
Klumpke palsy

ICD-9 Codes

353.0	Brachial plexus lesions
353.5	Neuralgic amyotrophy
723.4	Brachial neuritis or radiculitis NOS
767.6	Birth trauma

ICD-10 Codes

G54.0	Brachial plexus disorders
G54.5	Neuralgic amyotrophy
M54.10	Radiculopathy, site unspecified
M54.11	Radiculopathy, occipito-atlanto-axial region
M54.12	Radiculopathy, cervical region
M54.13	Radiculopathy, cervicothoracic region
M54.14	Radiculopathy, thoracic region
P14.0	Erb's paralysis due to birth injury
P14.1	Klumpke's paralysis due to birth injury
P14.3	Other brachial plexus birth injuries
P14.9	Birth injury to peripheral nervous system, unspecified
P15.9	Birth injury, unspecified

Definition

Brachial plexopathy is the pathologic dysfunction of the brachial plexus, a complex peripheral nerve structure in the proximal upper extremity. The brachial plexus starts just outside the spinal cord in the lower neck and extends to the axilla. The total average brachial plexus length is approximately 6 inches [1]. The plexus is divided into five sections: roots, trunks, divisions, cords, and branches or terminal nerves. The spinal nerves C5 through T1 classically supply anterior primary rami of the nerve roots, which then form the plexus. Variations in nerve root supply that involve other nerve roots are said to be expanded. When the C4 nerve root also supplies the brachial plexus and T1 contribution is minimal, the plexus is called prefixed. When the T2 nerve root supplies the brachial plexus and C5 contribution is minimal, the plexus is said to be postfixed [2]. The nerve roots combine to form the trunks behind the clavicle. There are three trunks, the upper, middle, and lower. The upper is formed from the C5 and C6 nerve roots, the middle is a continuation of C7, and the lower is formed from C8 and T1. The trunks then divide behind the clavicle into anterior and posterior divisions. Just inferior to the clavicle, the divisions coalesce into cords. The cords travel along the axillary artery, just inferior to the clavicle, and are named for their spatial relationship to the artery. The posterior cord is formed from the union of the three posterior divisions. The lateral cord is formed by the union of the anterior divisions of the upper and middle trunks. The medial cord is the continuation of the anterior division of the lower trunk. Nerve branches are the most distal elements of the brachial plexus and are the major nerves of the upper extremity. These branches begin in the distal axilla and other than the median nerve, which is formed by contributions from the medial and lateral cords, are continuations of the cords. There are also numerous peripheral nerves that arise directly from the roots, trunks, and cords (Fig. 143.1).

Brachial plexopathy can be due to wide-ranging causes, including idiopathic, iatrogenic, autoimmune, traumatic, neoplastic, and hereditary. It can occur in any age group; but other than when it is secondary to obstetric trauma, it usually occurs from the ages of 30 to 70 years. Men are affected two to three times as often as are women, and the reason is likely due to their more frequent participation in vigorous athletic activities that can lead to trauma. About half of the cases have no identified precipitating event; in others, brachial plexopathy follows an antecedent infection, trauma, surgery, or immunization.

Symptoms

Brachial plexopathy can result in symptoms of pain, weakness, and numbness, both at the level of the brachial plexus and distally in the supplied upper extremity. The area of pain and other symptoms correlates with the portion of the brachial plexus involved and the specific nerve elements from that area. Depending on the cause of the plexopathy, symptom onset can range from sudden to insidious. Because of the complex muscle suspension of the shoulder joint, chronic brachial plexopathy may result in glenohumeral subluxation and instability due to stretching of the shoulder capsule. Brachial plexopathy usually does not cause prominent neck pain. Some brachial plexopathies may occur bilaterally and therefore cause symptoms in both upper extremities.

Physical Examination

The physical examination of the brachial plexus for brachial plexopathy must be thorough because of the complexity of its structure and function. The shoulder girdle and

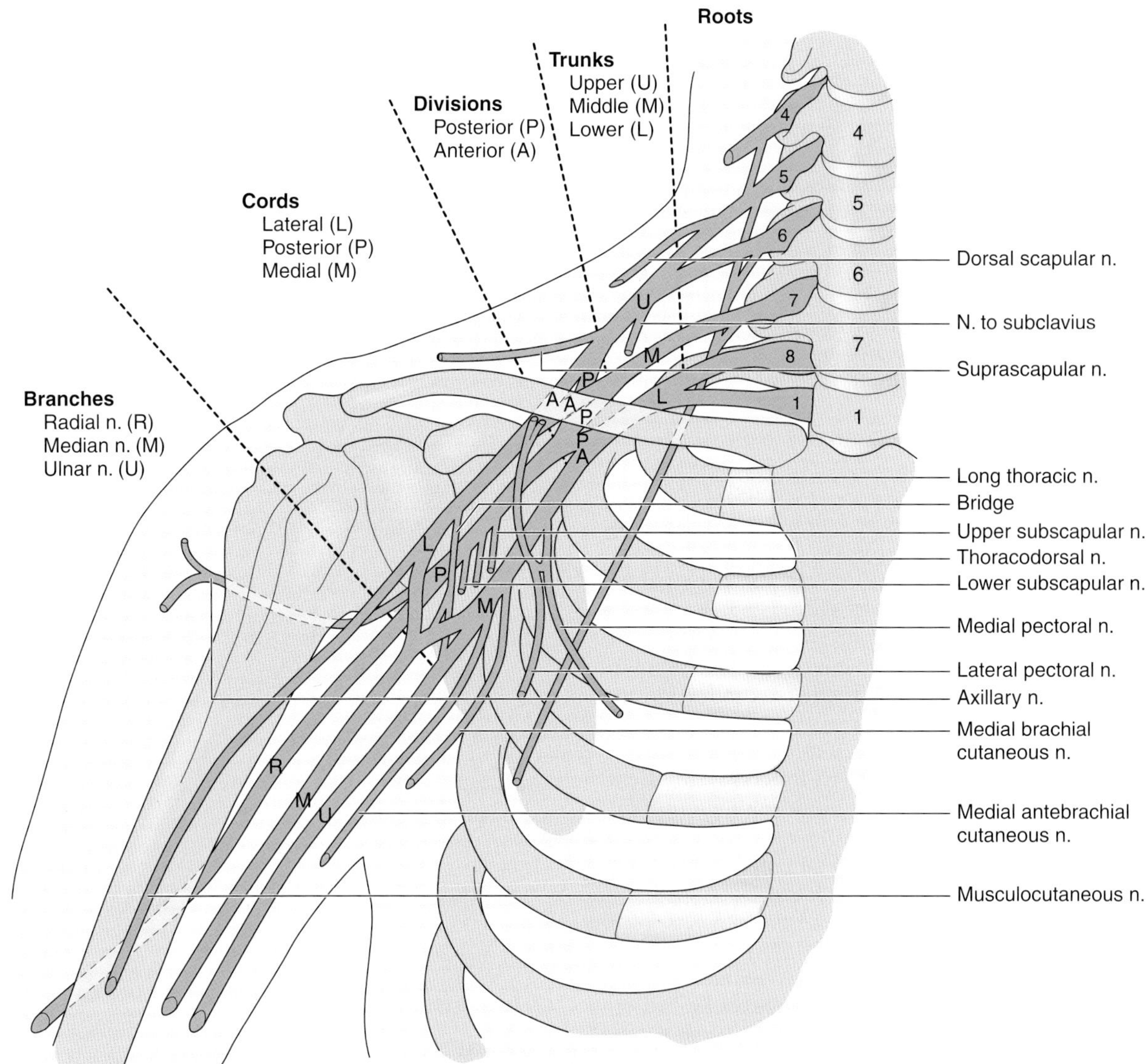

FIGURE 143.1 The brachial plexus. The clinician must be able to visualize this structure in performing electrodiagnostic examination so that an appropriate number of muscles and nerves are sampled to localize a lesion. *(From Dumitru D, Amato A, Zwarts M. Electrodiagnostic Medicine, 2nd ed. Philadelphia, Hanley & Belfus, 2002.)*

entire extremity need to be exposed during examination to allow close inspection of muscle bulk and fasciculations. Assessment of atrophy of muscles is often assisted by side-to-side comparisons. Muscle strength examination needs to be thorough and to include proximal muscles not commonly tested, such as infraspinatus, supraspinatus, rhomboids, and serratus anterior. Sensory testing also must be thorough, with both dermatomal and peripheral nerve sensory distributions examined. A musculoskeletal examination of the shoulder joint is helpful; joint disease can be both a possible primary cause of pain and a secondary effect of plexopathy. Shoulder range of motion and signs of tendinosis as well as reflexes and any muscle atrophy need to be assessed. The lack of pain exacerbation with neck movement and multi-root distribution of sensory or motor deficits can help distinguish brachial plexopathy from cervical radiculopathy, which more commonly affects a single root [3]. It is often not possible to determine the exact location of a brachial plexus lesion from physical examination, but the examination is usually helpful in focusing electrodiagnostic and radiologic testing.

Functional Limitations

Depending on whether the brachial plexopathy involves the upper plexus, lower plexus, or entire plexus, the proximal shoulder muscles, the distal muscles involved in fine finger movements, or the entire extremity can be weak or numb. Activities of daily living, such as dressing, feeding, and grooming, can be significantly affected. These impairments can result in disabilities in many activities, including computer use, writing, and driving. Brachial plexopathy secondary to birth trauma may subsequently cause difficulty for children and teens with sports and other recreational activity.

Diagnostic Studies

Electromyography (EMG) can be helpful in localizing the pathologic area in brachial plexopathy as well as in determining the severity of axonal injury and the potential for recovery. However, many brachial plexopathies cannot be definitely localized by EMG because of subtle findings encountered with incomplete nerve injury and the complexity of plexus-related innervation. The nerve conduction and needle EMG assessment is best directed by both symptoms and physical examination findings. Both nerve conduction studies and needle EMG are required for complete assessment. Sensory nerve conduction studies can help in localization by the pattern of abnormalities seen and in judging injury severity based on reductions of amplitudes or absence of potentials. The nerve conduction study may not detect abnormality if the lesion is mild in severity or too recent to allow axonal degeneration.

The following five basic sensory nerve conduction studies are suggested as a screen for brachial plexus evaluation: lateral antebrachial cutaneous, median recording from the thumb, median recording from the index finger, superficial radial, and ulnar recording from the little finger [2]. The presence of fibrillation potentials in EMG is particularly sensitive for motor axon loss and helps localize the site of lesions. The choice of muscles sampled on EMG is usually focused on the area of interest, but other areas are also included for the exclusion of wider disease. It is important to include paraspinal muscles of the relevant areas to investigate the possibility of radiculopathy (paraspinals are supplied by the posterior primary rami of the nerve roots, which do not supply the brachial plexus). EMG evaluation of the brachial plexus is complex and best performed by experienced electromyographers.

Radiologic studies of the plexus are helpful to evaluate the severity of trauma, presence of mass lesions, and inflammation of the brachial plexus nerve elements [4]. Magnetic resonance imaging (MRI) has become the study of choice in evaluation of traumatic brachial plexus injuries [5]. More than 80% of traumatic nerve root avulsions will show pseudomeningoceles, which are tears in the meningeal sheath surrounding the nerve roots that allow extravasation of cerebrospinal fluid into nearby tissues. They appear bright on T2-weighted images. MRI is also the most useful study for evaluation of other causes of brachial plexopathy, such as tumors, both secondary and primary [6]. An early MRI sign in Pancoast tumor is obliteration of the interscalene fat pad, which is best visualized on coronal T1-weighted MRI [7]. Inflammatory changes in the brachial plexus may be visualized with MRI, including brachial neuralgic amyotrophy [8].

Computed tomography myelography is increasingly becoming the study of choice in the preoperative evaluation of infants with obstetric brachial plexopathy, given its usefulness in identifying nerve root avulsion, which affects operative interventions [9,10].

Musculoskeletal ultrasonography has been used in the evaluation of suspected neoplastic brachial plexopathy. Sonography may identify the neoplastic lesion as a hypoechoic mass or present evidence consistent with a compressive lesion, such as segmental neuronal swelling of the involved portion of the brachial plexus [11].

Chest radiographs are valuable for the evaluation of diaphragmatic paralysis in traumatic brachial plexopathy, which usually indicates an irreparable lesion of the brachial plexus [12].

Differential Diagnosis

Generalized peripheral neuropathy
Focal peripheral neuropathy
Cervical radiculopathy
Motor neuron disorder
Neuromuscular junction disorder
Myopathy
Spinal cord injury
Stroke
Complex regional pain syndrome

Differential Diagnosis

Etiology of Brachial Plexopathy

It is helpful to approach the differential diagnosis of brachial plexopathy by the common causes in the different anatomic regions where the brachial plexus is affected. The anatomic areas of interest are the supraclavicular, retroclavicular, and infraclavicular. There are also causes of brachial plexopathy that tend to produce more diffuse plexus injury.

Supraclavicular

Birth Trauma

Lateral deviation of the head and neck to free the infant's shoulder, during both vaginal delivery and cesarean section, can lead to stretch injury of the upper brachial plexus. Such injuries can also occur from in utero causes, including compression of the fetal shoulder by the maternal symphysis pubis or sacral promontory, as well as by uterine anomalies that result in abnormally elevated intrauterine pressures [13]. The incidence of brachial plexopathy from birth trauma is 0.4 to 4 per 1000 live births [14]. It is called Erb palsy when the C5-C6 nerve roots are affected, resulting primarily in proximal arm weakness. When the C8-T1 roots are affected, the results are hand weakness, called Klumpke paralysis.

Trauma

Most commonly, trauma involves the upper plexus and is especially seen with closed traction, as in "burner" or "stinger" sports injuries (sudden separation of the shoulder and head due to contact) and pressure from backpack straps ("rucksack palsy"). The roots can be stretched but remain continuous, tear, or avulse from the spinal cord as possibilities. More direct trauma, such as from a stab wound or gunshot wound, can affect any portion of the plexus, but the supraclavicular portion is the most susceptible.

Intraoperative Arm Malpositioning

Postoperative brachial plexopathy may result from malpositioning of the arm during surgery [15].

Pancoast Syndrome

An apical lung tumor (usually small cell carcinoma) can extend into the supraclavicular brachial plexus, often being manifested with shoulder pain [16].

Neurogenic Thoracic Outlet

This syndrome is a rare condition in which a fibrous band extends from the lower cervical spine (cervical rib or transverse process) to the first rib. The T1 fibers are deflected and injured further by this fibrous band more than the C8 fibers are.

Infraclavicular

Postirradiation

Radiation therapy directed at the axillary lymph nodes can result in brachial plexopathy, which can occur months to years after radiation therapy. EMG studies may reveal evidence of conduction block and classic myokymia.

Metastatic Lymphadenopathy

A secondary neoplastic injury is usually due to compression from enlargement of involved axillary lymph nodes.

Regional Blocks

Infraclavicular brachial plexus injury has been identified as a complication of axillary regional blocks [17].

Heterotopic Ossification

The growing mass of heterotopic ossification about the shoulder can envelop and compromise the brachial plexus [18]. In midclavicular fractures, brachial plexopathy can be secondary to the initial trauma and also result from the development of heterotopic ossification [18].

Retroclavicular

Midclavicular Fractures

In midclavicular fractures, brachial plexopathy can be secondary to the initial trauma but also can result late from exuberant callus compression of the brachial plexus [18]. Retroclavicular brachial plexopathy, however, is rare and most often occurs in the context of wider spread plexopathy.

Diffuse Localization

Neuralgic Amyotrophy

Also called Parsonage-Turner syndrome, brachial amyotrophy, idiopathic shoulder girdle neuropathy [19], and brachial plexitis, neuralgic amyotrophy is a well-described syndrome of idiopathic monophasic brachial plexopathy that was well characterized by a large case series [20]. The initial symptom is onset during a few hours of severe continuous proximal upper extremity pain, which occurred in 90% of patients in this case series. After the onset of pain, weakness of the extremity usually develops within 2 weeks. Whereas sensory symptoms in the affected extremity are usually less pronounced than pain and weakness, they occur in 70% of patients. Pain decreases first, with an average pain duration of 28 days. Motor recovery begins within 6 months in most patients and with significant functional improvement; but in this case series, more than 70% of patients still had at least mild weakness detected on thorough strength examination at 3 years after weakness onset. Neuralgic amyotrophy can involve any part of the brachial plexus but tends to affect the upper plexus; 49% of patients have shoulder–proximal arm involvement.

Hereditary Neuralgic Amyotrophy

This is a similar condition but with a known genetic etiology, which is often autosomal dominant but is genetically heterogeneous.

Diabetic Cervical Radiculoplexus Neuropathy

Distinct from neuralgic amyotrophy is the recently described diabetic cervical radiculoplexus neuropathy [21]. This condition is associated with type 2 diabetes mellitus. Patients initially develop pain in the upper limb, often acutely, followed later by weakness and sensory changes, such as paresthesias, dysesthesias, or numbness. Associated autonomic symptoms (orthostasis, sudomotor changes) are common, as is weight loss. Electrodiagnosis reveals predominantly axonal neuropathy, whereas biopsy findings of involved nerves show axonal degeneration, ischemic injury, and perivascular inflammation. The condition is typically monophasic with improvement, but 21% of patients demonstrated recurrence [21].

Primary Neoplastic Peripheral Nerve Tumors

Local primary peripheral nerve tumors can cause brachial plexopathies that occur anywhere in the brachial plexus but are rare and usually benign. Benign tumors are typically nerve sheath tumors, either schwannomas or neurofibromas (associated with neurofibromatosis type 1), and cause painless sensory loss and weakness [2]. In contrast, malignant peripheral nerve tumors in the brachial plexus tend to be painful [22,23].

Treatment

Initial

The treatment of brachial plexopathy needs to be customized to the individual patient and the cause of the brachial plexopathy. Pain can be the most disabling symptom but is usually effectively treated with neuropathic pain medications, such as gabapentin and tricyclic antidepressants, and analgesics, such as tramadol and opiates in cases of severe pain. Dosing is usually at the higher end of accepted ranges (such as gabapentin at 600 mg three times daily or more) secondary to the pain severity of acute plexopathy, although duration of therapy may be brief. Levetiracetam has been used successfully to reduce refractory brachial plexopathy pain and to decrease opioid need [24].

Rehabilitation

When the muscles of the shoulder girdle are involved, therapy focused on positioning and shoulder range of motion can prevent secondary complications, such as adhesive capsulitis [25]. Directed exercise can be beneficial, with the caveat that exercise of muscles with neurogenic weakness from brachial plexus lesions to full exhaustion may be counterproductive on the basis of findings in exercise in patients with peripheral neuropathy [26]. Occupational therapy is often indicated when weakness from brachial plexopathy results in loss of function. Adaptive aids can be helpful when they are indicated, such as a shoulder sling to help reduce imbalance from proximal arm weakness from brachial plexopathy. Vocational rehabilitation may be indicated when the resultant disability from weakness affects the patient's ability to perform in the job setting.

Procedures

Brachial plexus blocks are rarely used but are possible for the treatment of severe pain from metastatic brachial plexopathy or severe acute brachial plexopathy. Increasingly, botulinum toxin injections, combined with surgery, serial casting, and physical and occupational therapy, are used to treat and to prevent shoulder and forearm pronation contractures as well as to optimize elbow range of motion in infants with obstetric brachial plexus injury [27]. However, botulinum use in this scenario has yet to be tested by randomized controlled trials.

Surgery

Surgery is an option in cases of traumatic plexopathy but has variable results. Surgical techniques such as nerve grafting, free muscle transfer, neurolysis, and neurotization are used. Surgeons who use these techniques frequently differ considerably in their approach to them, making conclusions about their efficacy difficult. Surgery is an option in brachial plexus birth injuries, usually when persistent severe motor deficits are present after 3 to 8 months of age. A case series found improvement in surgically treated patients on a shoulder motion scale [28]. The location of injury affects selection of patients for surgery and surgical outcome. For example, postganglionic nerve root avulsion injuries may do better with earlier surgery [29]. Preganglionic avulsions are difficult to repair, but direct implantation into the spinal cord may help some patients [30].

Potential Disease Complications

Weakness from brachial plexopathy can result in joint instability or in joint and musculotendinous contractures of upper extremity joints. Complex regional pain syndrome may follow brachial plexopathy [31]. Secondary depression can be due to pain and loss of function. Insensate limbs are at risk for trauma neglect, infection, and amputation.

Potential Treatment Complications

Stretching and range of motion exercises for avoidance or treatment of contractures can acutely exacerbate neuropathic pain. Care to avoid shoulder impingement during range of motion exercises is important because of weak rotator cuff muscles. Insensate limbs become more susceptible to heat injuries, such as by hot packs or therapeutic ultrasound. Medicines used for brachial plexopathy pain can have side effects, which are specific to the particular medicine used. Surgery for brachial plexopathy may result in nerve or vascular injury.

References

[1] Slinghuff Jr CL, Terzis CK, Edgerton MT. The quantitative microanatomy of the brachial plexus in man: reconstructive relevance. In: Terzis JK, editor. Microreconstruction of nerve injuries. Philadelphia: WB Saunders; 1987. p. 285–324.

[2] Ferrante MA. Brachial plexopathies: classification, causes, and consequences. Muscle Nerve 2004;30:547–68.

[3] Mamula CJ, Erhard RE, Piva SR. Cervical radiculopathy or Parsonage-Turner syndrome: differential diagnosis of a patient with neck and upper extremity symptoms. J Orthop Sports Phys Ther 2005;35:659–64.

[4] Castillo M. Imaging the anatomy of the brachial plexus: review and self-assessment module. AJR Am J Roentgenol 2005;185:S196–204.

[5] Doi K, Otsuka K, Okamomo Y, et al. Cervical nerve root avulsion in brachial plexus injuries: magnetic resonance imaging classification and comparison with myelography and computerized tomography myelography. J Neurosurg Spine 2002;96:277–84.

[6] Saifuddin A. Imaging tumors of the brachial plexus. Skeletal Radiol 2003;32:375–87.

[7] Huang JH, Zagoul K, Zager EL. Surgical management of brachial plexus tumors. Surg Neurol 2004;61:372–8.

[8] Sarikaya S, Sumer M, Ozdolap S, Erdem CZ. Magnetic resonance neurography diagnosed brachial plexitis: a case report. Arch Phys Med Rehabil 2006;86:1058–9.

[9] Steens SCA, Pondaag W, Malessy MJA, Verbist BM. Obstetric brachial plexus lesions: CT myelography. Neuroradiology 2011;259: 508–15.

[10] VanderHave KL, Bovid K, Alpert H, et al. Utility of electrodiagnostic testing and computed tomography myelography in the preoperative evaluation of neonatal brachial plexus injury. J Neurosurg Pediatr 2012;9:283–9.

[11] Kesikurun S, Omac OK, Taskaynatan MA, et al. Neoplastic brachial plexopathy detected by ultrasonography in a patient with chronic cervicobrachialgia. J Rehabil Med 2012;44:181–3.

[12] Belzberg AJ, Dorsi MJ, Strom PB, Moriarty JL. Surgical repair of brachial plexus injury: a multinational survey of experienced peripheral nerve surgeons. J Neurosurg 2004;101:365–76.
[13] Doumouchtsis SK, Arulkumaran S. Are all brachial plexus injuries caused by shoulder dystocia? Obstet Gynecol Surv 2009;64:615–23.
[14] Hale HB, Bae DS, Waters PM. Current concepts in the management of brachial plexus birth palsy. J Hand Surg [Am] 2010;35:322–31.
[15] Wilbourn AJ. Iatrogenic nerve injuries. Neurol Clin 1998;16:55–82.
[16] Huehnergarth KV, Lipsky BA. Superior pulmonary sulcus tumor with Pancoast syndrome. Mayo Clin Proc 2004;79:1268.
[17] Tsao BE, Wilbourn AJ. Infraclavicular brachial plexus injury following axillary regional block. Muscle Nerve 2004;30:44–8.
[18] England JD, Tiel RL. AAEM case report 33: costoclavicular mass syndrome. American Association of Electrodiagnostic Medicine. Muscle Nerve 1999;22:412–8.
[19] Weaver K, Kraft GH. Idiopathic shoulder girdle neuropathy. Phys Med Rehabil Clin N Am 2001;12:353–64.
[20] van Alfen N, van Engelen BG. The clinical spectrum of neuralgic amyotrophy in 246 cases. Brain 2006;129(Pt 2):438–50.
[21] Massie R, Mauermann M, Staff N, et al. Diabetic cervical radiculoplexus neuropathy: a distinct syndrome expanding the spectrum of diabetic radiculoplexus neuropathies. Brain 2012;135:3074–88.
[22] Park JK. Peripheral nerve tumors. In: Samuels MA, Feske SK, editors. Office practice of neurology. 2nd ed. Philadelphia: Churchill Livingstone; 2003. p. 1118–21.
[23] Pacelli J, Whitaker C. Brachial plexopathy due to malignant peripheral nerve sheath tumor in neurofibromatosis type 1: case report and subject review. Muscle Nerve 2006;33:697–700.
[24] Dunteman ED. Levetiracetam as an adjunctive analgesic in neoplastic plexopathies: case series and commentary. J Pain Palliat Care Pharmacother 2005;19:35–43.
[25] Langer JS, Sueoka SS, Wang AA. The importance of shoulder external rotation in activities of daily living: improving outcomes in traumatic brachial plexus palsy. J Hand Surg Am 2012;37:1430–6.
[26] Carter GT. Rehabilitation management of peripheral neuropathy. Semin Neurol 2005;25:229–37.
[27] Gobets D, Beckerman H, de Groot V, et al. Indications and effects of botulinum toxin A for obstetric brachial plexus injury: a systematic literature review. Dev Med Child Neurol 2010;52:517–28.
[28] Grossman JA, DiTaranto P, Yaylali I, et al. Shoulder function following late neurolysis and bypass grafting for upper brachial plexus birth injuries. J Hand Surg [Br] 2004;29:356–8.
[29] Waters PM. Update on management of pediatric brachial plexus palsy. J Pediatr Orthop B 2005;14:233–44.
[30] Bertelli JA, Ghizoni MF. Brachial plexus avulsion injury repairs with nerve transfers and nerve grafts directly implanted into the spinal cord yield partial recovery of shoulder and elbow movements. Neurosurgery 2003;52:1385–9.
[31] de Carvalho M. Reflex sympathetic dystrophy precipitated by brachial plexitis. Electromyogr Clin Neurophysiol 1998;38:459–61.

CHAPTER 144

Plexopathy—Lumbosacral

Hope S. Hacker, MD
John C. King, MD
John D. Alfonso, MD

Synonyms

Lumbosacral plexitis
Neuralgic amyotrophy of the lumbosacral plexus
Lumbosacral plexus neuropathy
Lumbosacral radiculoplexus neuropathy
Diabetic amyotrophy

ICD-9 Codes

353.1 Lumbosacral plexus lesions
353.8 Other nerve root and plexus disorders
353.9 Unspecified nerve root and plexus disorder
907.3 Late effects of injury to nerve root, spinal plexus, and other nerve of trunk
953.5 Injury to lumbosacral plexus
953.8 Injury to multiple sites of nerve roots and spinal plexus
953.9 Injury to nerve root and spinal plexus, unspecified site

ICD-10 Codes

G54.1 Lumbosacral plexus disorders
G54.8 Other nerve root and plexus disorders
G54.9 Nerve root and plexus disorder, unspecified
S34.21 Injury of nerve root of lumbar spine
S34.22 Injury of nerve root of sacral spine
S34.4 Injury of lumbosacral plexus
M54.15 Radiculopathy, thoracolumbar region
M54.16 Radiculopathy, lumbar region
M54.17 Radiculopathy, lumbosacral region
M54.18 Radiculopathy, sacral and sacrococcygeal region
Add seventh character for episode of care (S—late effects)

Definition

Lumbosacral plexopathy is an injury to or involvement of one or more nerves that combine to form or branch from the lumbosacral plexus. This involvement is distal to the root level.

The lumbar plexus originates from the first, second, third, and fourth lumbar nerves (Fig. 144.1). The fourth lumbar nerve makes a contribution to both the lumbar and the sacral plexus. There is typically a small communication from the twelfth thoracic nerve as well. As in the brachial plexus, these nerve roots divide into the dorsal rami and the ventral rami as they exit through the intervertebral foramina. The dorsal or posterior rami innervate the paraspinal muscles and supply nearby cutaneous sensation. The ventral or anterior rami of the lumbar plexus form the motor and sensory nerves to the anterior and medial sides of the thigh and the sensation on the medial aspect of the leg and foot. The undivided anterior primary rami of the lumbar and sacral nerves also carry postganglionic sympathetic fibers that are mainly responsible for vasoregulation of the lower extremities. The branches of the lumbar plexus include the iliohypogastric, ilioinguinal, genitofemoral, femoral, lateral femoral cutaneous, and obturator nerves [1]. The lumbar portion of the plexus lies just anterior to the psoas muscle [2].

The sacral plexus innervates the muscles of the buttocks, posterior thigh, and leg below the knee and the skin of the posterior thigh and leg, lateral leg, foot, and perineum. It is formed from the lumbosacral trunk to include L5 and a portion of L4 as well as the S1 to S3 (or S4) nerve roots (Fig. 144.2). The anterior primary rami of S2 and S3 nerve roots carry parasympathetic fibers that mainly control the urinary bladder and anal sphincters. The triangular sacral plexus lies on the anterior surface of the sacrum, in the immediate vicinity of the sacroiliac joint and lateral to the cervix or prostate [1]. The branches of the sacral plexus include the superior and inferior gluteal nerves, the posterior cutaneous nerves of the thigh, the

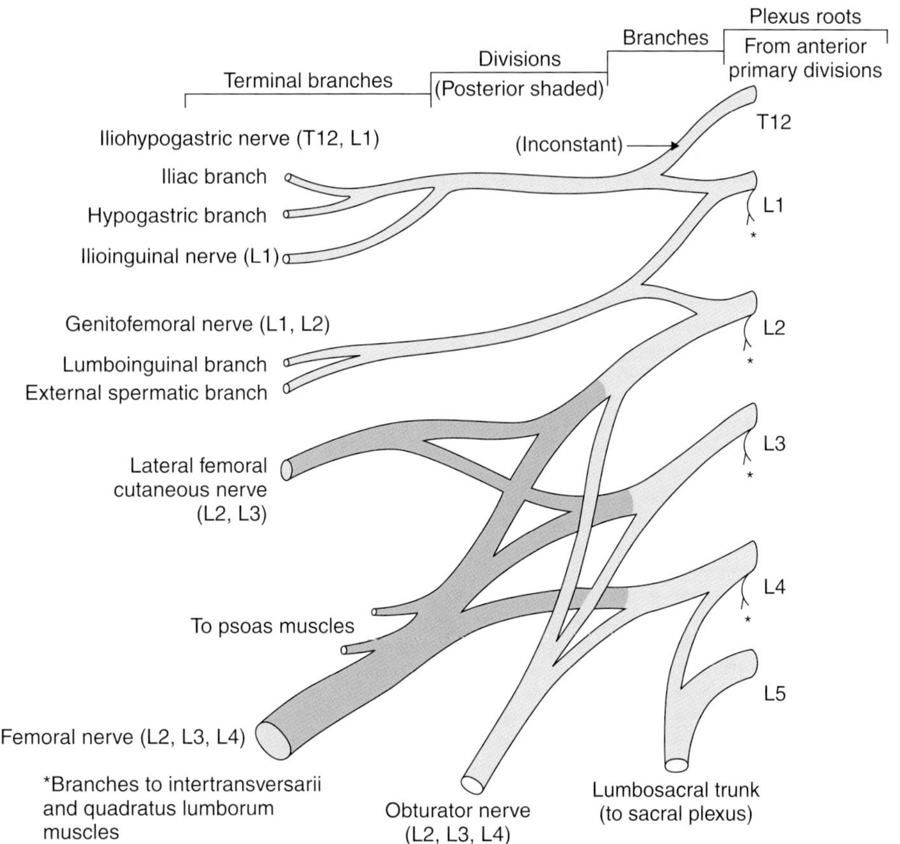

FIGURE 144.1 The lumbar plexus and its peripheral terminal branches. The shaded portions represent the posterior divisions of the ventral primary rami; those not shaded are either the ventral primary rami or their anterior branches. In this diagram, the nerve to the psoas major arises from the femoral nerve, as opposed to directly from the spinal nerve region. *(From de Groot J, Chusid JG. Correlative Neuroanatomy, 21st ed. Norwalk, Conn, Appleton & Lange, 1991.)*

lumbosacral trunk that becomes the sciatic nerve with both tibial and peroneal divisions, and the pudendal nerve.

Etiology

Lumbosacral plexopathy has been recognized as a clinical entity or complication in a variety of surgical procedures, trauma, and obstetric surgery or delivery and as a clinical finding or sequela in treatment of pelvic tumors.

Trauma

Traumatic pelvic fractures have a 30.8% incidence of lumbosacral plexus injury [3,4]. The incidence and severity of traumatic lumbosacral plexopathy increase with the number of pelvic fracture sites and fracture instability [4]. Sacral fractures have typically been considered of secondary importance in conjunction with pelvic trauma [5]. However, sacral fractures have become recognized as an essential consideration in pelvic trauma because of their high association with lumbosacral nerve deficits. This can have a profound influence on prognosis and level of functional recovery [3,6]. The more common sacral fractures are typically the compression or avulsion fractures of the sacral ala, which can occur in lateral compression and anterior-posterior compression pelvic fractures [7]. Fractures of the sacral neuroforamina or midline sacral fractures may also occur. Fractures of the sacrum can increase the incidence of neurologic injury in pelvic trauma to between 34% and 50% because of its proximity to the sacral nerve roots [7].

Gunshot wounds and motor vehicle accidents have long been recognized as potential causes of lumbosacral plexus injuries. In a retrospective comparison of patterns of lumbosacral plexus injury in motor vehicle crashes and gunshot wounds, individuals with gunshot wounds had a greater chance of involvement of the upper portion of the plexus in comparison to individuals who sustained a motor vehicle crash. Lower plexus injuries were more common in victims of motor vehicle accidents as opposed to gunshot wounds [8].

Finally, trauma is a common cause of retroperitoneal hemorrhage, which can injure the lumbosacral plexus.

Labor and Delivery

The lumbosacral plexus may be compressed as a complication of labor and delivery. The incidence of neurologic injury that is reported in the literature for postpartum sensory and motor dysfunction is relatively low at 0.008% to 0.5% [9,10]. Factors associated with nerve injury were nulliparity and a prolonged second stage of labor; assisted vacuum or forceps vaginal delivery also had some positive association. Women with nerve injury spent more time pushing in the semi-Fowler lithotomy position. During the second stage of labor, direct pressure of the fetal head may compress the lumbosacral plexus against the pelvic rim, which may result in nerve injury [11,12].

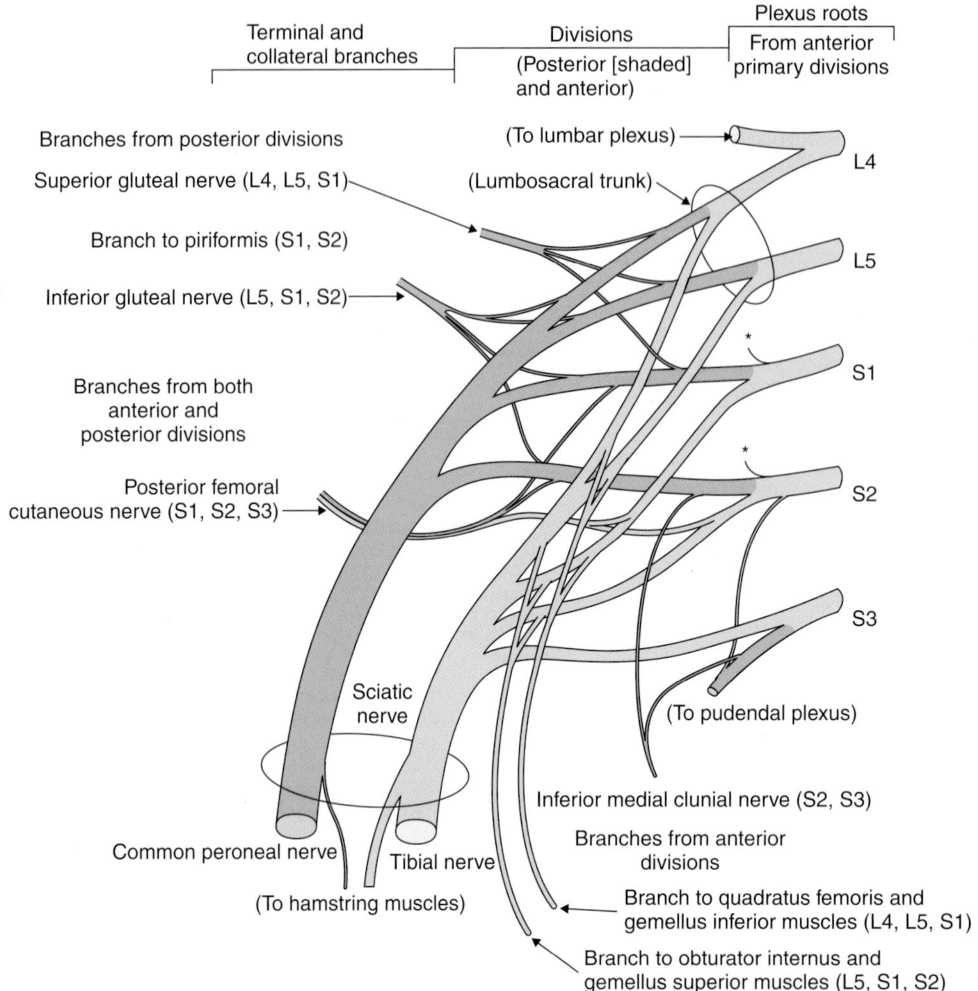

FIGURE 144.2 Schematic representation of the sacral plexus. The shaded portions signify the posterior divisions of the ventral primary rami; the unshaded aspects are the anterior branches of the ventral primary rami. *(From de Groot J, Chausid JG. Correlative Neuroanatomy, 21st ed. Norwalk, Conn, Appleton & Lange, 1991.)*

Iatrogenic

Gynecologic surgery is thought to be one of the most common causes of femoral nerve injury (see Chapter 54) and lumbosacral plexus nerve injuries. Abdominal hysterectomy is the surgical procedure that has been most frequently implicated [13,14]. The mechanisms of neurologic injury that have been established include improper placement or positioning of self-retaining or fixed retractors, incorrect positioning of the patient in lithotomy position preoperatively or prolonged lithotomy positioning without repositioning, and radical surgical dissection resulting in autonomic nerve disruption [15].

Lumbosacral injury has also been noted after appendectomy and inguinal herniorrhaphy. Patients who are thin, diabetic, or elderly are at increased risk for such an injury. Injury to the lumbosacral plexus with clinical findings occurs in up to 10% of hip replacement procedures, and injury that is subclinical but detected electromyographically occurred in up to 70% of patients [16].

In individuals receiving anticoagulant therapy or with acquired or congenital coagulopathies, retroperitoneal hemorrhage causing lumbosacral plexopathy may occur with no precipitating injury [17,18].

Retroperitoneal hematoma has also been documented as a rare but potentially serious complication after cardiac catheterization [19,20]. In a review of 9585 femoral artery catheterizations, a reported retroperitoneal hematoma rate of 0.5% occurred. In patients undergoing stent placement, there was evidence of lumbar plexopathy involving the femoral, obturator, and lateral femoral cutaneous nerves, and the condition was typically completely reversible [21,22]. Femoral vein catheterization for dialysis has also been documented as a cause of hemorrhagic complications and retroperitoneal hemorrhage [23].

Case reports have also identified patients sustaining lumbosacral plexopathy after undergoing aortoiliac bypass grafting for abdominal aortic aneurysm. The proposed mechanism for this rare complication, with fewer than 80 patients reported in the literature, is neural ischemia secondary to interruption of the blood supply to the lumbosacral plexus or caudal portion of the spinal cord [24,25].

Oncologic

Both pelvic malignant neoplasms and treatment of pelvic tumors can damage the lumbosacral plexus. Lumbosacral radiculopathy is most common with gynecologic tumors, sarcomas, and lymphomas. Neoplastic plexopathy is characterized by severe and unrelenting pain, typically followed by weakness and sensory disturbances [26]. Pelvic radiation therapy may cause a delayed lumbosacral plexopathy that can occur 3 months to 22 years after completion of treatment; the median amount of time from the completion of treatment to onset of symptoms is about 5 years [27–29]. Chemotherapeutic agents can also cause symptoms of lumbosacral radiculopathy. Cisplatin, 5-fluorouracil, mitomycin C, and bleomycin have been implicated in the majority of these plexopathies [2]. Metastatic or tumor extension into the lumbosacral plexus and malignant psoas syndrome have been described in the literature. Malignant psoas syndrome was first reported in 1990. It is characterized by proximal lumbosacral plexopathy, painful fixed flexion of the ipsilateral hip, and radiologic or pathologic evidence of ipsilateral psoas major muscle malignant involvement [2].

Diabetic Amyotrophy

Diabetic and nondiabetic lumbosacral radiculoplexus neuropathies have been documented in the literature. Diabetic lumbosacral radiculoplexus neuropathy is a subacute, painful asymmetric lower limb neuropathy that is associated with significant weight loss (at least 10 pounds), type 2 diabetes mellitus, and relatively recent diagnosis of diabetes with relatively good glucose control [30]. The underlying pathophysiologic mechanism is thought to be immune mediated with microvasculitis of the nerve rather than a metabolic issue caused by diabetes; nondiabetic lumbosacral radiculoplexus neuropathy has also been documented with similar clinical and pathophysiologic features [30–34]. The similar clinical symptoms, findings, and response to treatment suggest that the metabolic changes from diabetes may not be the cause of these symptoms, although impaired glucose tolerance has been noted in nondiabetic lumbosacral radiculoplexus neuropathy [32].

Vascular

Vascular causes of lumbosacral plexopathies may include diabetic amyotrophy and connective tissue diseases that may be associated with vasculitis, such as systemic lupus erythematosus, rheumatoid arthritis, and polyarteritis nodosa [35]. Further, a recently published case report described acute lumbosacral plexus injury secondary to direct compression by an internal iliac artery aneurysm [36]. If a vascular cause is suspected, the aorta and iliac vessels must be evaluated for disease or occlusion [37–39].

Symptoms

Plexopathies may vary considerably in their presentation, depending on the location and degree of involvement. Lumbosacral plexopathy often begins with leg pain radiating to the low back and buttocks and progressing posterolaterally down the leg, soon followed by symptoms of numbness and weakness. Lumbosacral plexus injuries are often associated with a footdrop and sensory changes to the top of the foot. A plexopathy involving the upper lumbar roots may primarily be manifested by femoral and obturator nerve symptoms. Femoral nerve injury typically is manifested with iliopsoas or quadriceps weakness, and there may be sensory deficits over the anterior and medial thigh as well as the anterior medial aspect of the leg [13]. Obturator injury has also been seen in upper plexus injuries with weakness of the hip adductors [10] and sensory changes in the upper medial thigh.

Diabetic plexopathy typically starts as an identifiable onset of asymmetric lower extremity symptoms that most typically involve the thigh and hip with pain that progresses to include weakness, which then becomes the main disabling symptom. In a few months, this usually evolves into bilateral symmetric weakness and pain with distal as well as proximal involvement. Although motor findings are prominent, sensory and autonomic nerves have also been shown to be involved [29].

Bowel and bladder injuries tend to occur in cases in which there is bilateral sacral root involvement. Sexual dysfunction has been documented in both bilateral and unilateral sacral injuries and pelvic trauma. Lumbosacral plexus injuries are much more common in pelvic and sacral fractures but have been documented in acetabular fractures and midshaft femoral fractures as well [3,6,26].

Physical Examination

Clinical examination to evaluate for a lumbosacral plexopathy involves neurologic assessment to include motor strength testing, sensory testing, muscle stretch reflexes, tone, and bowel and bladder function. The pattern of sensory loss, asymmetric reflexes, or weakness is suggestive of multiple nerve or root level involvement. It is important to differentiate a suspected plexus injury from single root level involvement, suggesting a radiculopathy, or more generalized nerve changes consistent with peripheral neuropathy. A detailed examination of the bilateral lower limbs, including skin sensory testing of all dermatomes, manual muscle testing of all myotomes, and examination of the patellar and Achilles deep tendon reflexes, can reveal neurologic deficits that can aid in this differentiation. In addition, it may be necessary to evaluate lower sacral involvement by physical examination of a patient's external anal sphincter tone, particularly if complaints include bowel and bladder incontinence. Edema or swelling in one lower extremity may be suggestive of a pelvic mass or lumbosacral plexus involvement rather than a more global peripheral neuropathy [38] or possible retroperitoneal hematoma or pelvic malignant neoplasm [2].

Functional Limitations

Functional limitations depend on which portions of the lumbar or lumbosacral plexus have been injured and the severity of the injury. Patients frequently present with some type of difficulty with mobility and ambulation. Activities such as transferring from one surface to another, rising from a chair, ambulation, grooming, bathing, dressing, and cooking may potentially be affected. These functional limitations may have far-reaching consequences on one's ability to live independently and to continue in one's chosen vocation.

Diagnostic Studies

Electrodiagnostic Testing

The electrodiagnostic evaluation of lumbosacral plexopathy is one of the most effective tools available for differentiation of a specific pattern and severity of nerve involvement. Guided by a focused history and physical examination, the skilled electromyographer can use testing of both proximal and distal sensory and motor nerves as well as muscle needle examination to determine whether there is radicular involvement, lumbar or lumbosacral plexus involvement with multiple nerves involved but no paraspinal involvement, or a more generalized picture consistent with a peripheral neuropathy.

Testing for upper lumbar plexopathy may include lateral femoral cutaneous nerve, saphenous nerve, posterior femoral cutaneous sensory nerve, and femoral motor nerve studies. Side-to-side comparison is recommended to assess for asymmetry in these technically challenging studies. Sensory involvement without motor involvement suggests a lesion distal to the dorsal root ganglion. Studies to evaluate the lumbosacral plexus and lumbosacral roots include sural and superficial peroneal sensory studies, H reflex, and peroneal and tibial motor conduction studies. Depending on the timing of the injury, nerve conduction studies can demonstrate a decrease in amplitude for the sensory nerve action potentials starting at 5 to 6 days and for compound muscle action potentials starting at 2 to 4 days [8].

The needle electromyographic examination is likely to be the most useful electrodiagnostic technique [8]. Careful examination of proximal and distal musculature demonstrates a pattern of muscle membrane instability in more than one peripheral nerve from different root levels without involvement of the paraspinal muscles. The pattern of muscle membrane instability indicates whether the injury appears to be a neurapraxia with conduction block, axonotmesis, or neurotmesis with wallerian degeneration and poor prognosis for reinnervation. Increased insertional activity may be seen in the involved musculature after 7 to 8 days, with positive waves and fibrillations starting at 10 to 30 days but being most prominent at 21 to 30 days after injury [8]. Decreased recruitment is noted immediately after injury, and this may be the only change on needle electromyographic examination in the first few days if the nerve is partially intact.

Imaging Studies

Computed tomography and positron emission tomography can be useful in determining the presence of a structural mass in the pelvic region. Computed tomographic scans, along with abdominal ultrasonography, may be used to diagnose a retroperitoneal hemorrhage. Both computed tomographic scanning and magnetic resonance imaging have been used to evaluate the lumbosacral plexus. Magnetic resonance imaging has been found to be more sensitive than computed tomography for diagnosis of cancer-related lumbosacral plexopathy [40]. High-resolution magnetic resonance neurography with T1-weighted fast spin echo and fat-saturated T2-weighted fast spin echo has been used to study the lumbosacral plexus and the sciatic nerve [41]. Plain radiographs are useful as a screening tool for suspected aneurysms or malignant disease.

Differential Diagnosis

Spinal cord injury
Cauda equina injury
Lumbosacral nerve root injury
Multiple peripheral nerve injuries
Anterior horn cell diseases
Myopathies
Occlusion of the aorta

Treatment

Initial

Initial treatment is based on both the presenting symptoms and the cause of the lumbosacral plexopathy. For example, many obstetric lumbosacral plexus symptoms are treated conservatively. Pelvic masses or a retroperitoneal hemorrhage may require surgical or medical intervention. Neoplastic or radiation-based plexopathy symptoms may need specific medical management, chemotherapy, or possibly surgery. If edema control is necessary, leg elevation and compressive stockings may be of some benefit. Medication for neuropathic pain might include gabapentin, duloxetine, or pregabalin. Tricyclic antidepressants may also be helpful. Opioids and nonsteroidal anti-inflammatory drugs may also provide pain relief. Use of nonsteroidal anti-inflammatory drugs is contraindicated, however, when hemorrhage is suspected. Various immunomodulation therapies for diabetic amyotrophy, including corticosteroids, cyclophosphamide, intravenous immune globulin, and plasmapheresis, have been described in a number of case series, most of which report positive outcomes with regard to resolution of pain and weakness [29,34]. To date, only one multicenter, double-blind controlled study of intravenous methylprednisolone in diabetic amyotrophy exists, but it is as yet unpublished [42]. Therefore, at this time, the literature still lacks strong evidence from randomized controlled trials to definitively recommend the use of immunotherapy for diabetic lumbosacral radiculoplexus neuropathies.

Rehabilitation

Rehabilitation aims to maximize mobility and functional independence. The goals of rehabilitation are preservation of joint range of motion and flexibility, joint protection, and pain management; these goals depend on a good physical examination to determine what neurologic and functional deficits are present.

One of the primary rehabilitation concerns in an individual with nerve involvement in the lumbar or lumbosacral plexus is safe mobility and ambulation. The patient should be evaluated for the need for an assistive device, such as a cane or a walker, with ambulation. Patients with significant footdrop impairing gait benefit from prescription of ankle-foot orthoses, with dorsiflexion assist as an option. Energy conservation techniques and care of insensate feet are key treatment tools. Symptoms of lumbosacral plexopathy may be subtle and may be difficult to appreciate in a clinical setting. Physicians need to address potentially sensitive issues such as work limitations, sexual functioning, and sensory changes in the pelvic and inguinal areas.

Procedures

Sympathetic nerve blocks and chemodenervation have both been used to ameliorate pain. This can be both diagnostic and treatment oriented in helping to confirm the suspected diagnosis. Sacral nerve stimulation has been evaluated for adjunctive treatment of lumbosacral plexopathy, but further research is required for its effectiveness to be determined [17].

Surgery

Lumbosacral plexus injuries associated with pelvic or sacral fractures or with gynecologic surgery are often treated conservatively [13], although it has been documented that long-term sequelae can occur. Nerve reconstruction including nerve grafting has been reported in an attempt to restore some lower extremity function [43]. Microsurgical treatment of lumbosacral plexopathies for neurolysis and nerve grafting has been used in the retroperitoneal space. In a series of 15 cases, the muscles that benefited the most from surgery were the gluteal and femoral innervated muscles. The more distal musculature did not seem to show much benefit [44]. Whereas motor improvement is an important consideration, pain is often extremely debilitating in patients with a lumbosacral plexopathy and may block or limit rehabilitation. Pain relief is one of the major goals for surgical intervention. Surgical resection of a tumor may also be indicated in certain cases with lumbosacral plexopathy [26].

Potential Disease Complications

Potential complications of lumbosacral plexopathy include joint contractures, limited mobility, weakness, falls secondary to weakness or sensory loss, bowel or bladder incontinence, diminished or absent sensation, skin breakdown, sexual dysfunction, and significant decrease in functional independence from these complications. The rare complication of complex regional pain syndrome type II has also been reported [45].

Potential Treatment Complications

Treatment complications may include skin breakdown under orthoses and increased weakness if the rehabilitation program is too aggressive. Medication side effects are dizziness, somnolence, gastrointestinal irritation, and ataxia due to anticonvulsants; dry mouth, urinary retention, and atrioventricular conduction block due to tricyclic antidepressants; and dependence, dizziness, somnolence, and constipation due to opioid pain medications. Nonsteroidal anti-inflammatory drugs and analgesics can also have significant side effects that affect the gastrointestinal and renal systems as well as the liver.

References

[1] Moore KL, Dalley AF, editors. Clinically oriented anatomy. 4th ed. Philadelphia: Lippincott Williams & Wilkins; 1999.

[2] Agar M, Broadbent A, Chye R. The management of malignant psoas syndrome: case reports and literature review. J Pain Symptom Manage 2004;28:282–93.

[3] Kutsy RL, Robinson LR, Routt ML. Lumbosacral plexopathy in pelvic trauma. Muscle Nerve 2000;23:1757–60.

[4] Jang D-H, Byun SH, Jeon SY, Lee SJ. The relationship between lumbosacral plexopathy and pelvic fractures. Am J Phys Med Rehabil 2011;90:707–12.

[5] Medelman JP. Fractures of the sacrum: their incidence in fractures of the pelvis. Am J Roentgenol Radium Ther Nucl Med 1939;42:100–3.

[6] Gibbons KJ, Soloniuk DS, Razack N. Neurological injury and patterns of sacral fractures. J Neurosurg 1990;72:889–93.

[7] Bellabarba C, Stewart JD, Ricci WM, et al. Midline sagittal sacral fractures in anterior-posterior compression pelvic ring injuries. J Orthop Trauma 2003;17:32–7.

[8] Chiou-Tan FY, Kemp K, Elfenbaum M, et al. Lumbosacral plexopathy in gunshot wounds and motor vehicle accidents: comparison of electrophysiologic findings. Am J Phys Med Rehabil 2001;80:280–5.

[9] Holdcroft A, Gibberd FB, Hargrove RL, et al. Neurological complications associated with pregnancy. Br J Anaesth 1995;75:522–6.

[10] Wong CA, Scavone BM, Dugan S, et al. Incidence of postpartum lumbosacral spine and lower extremity nerve injuries. Obstet Gynecol 2003;101:279–88.

[11] Dawson DM, Krarup C. Perioperative nerve lesions. Arch Neurol 1989;46:1355–60.

[12] Feasby TE, Burton SR, Hahn AF. Obstetrical lumbosacral plexus injury. Muscle Nerve 1992;15:937–40.

[13] Irvin W, Andersen W, Taylor P, et al. Minimizing the risk of neurologic injury in gynecologic surgery. Obstet Gynecol 2004;103:374–82.

[14] Fardin P, Benettello P, Negrin P. Iatrogenic femoral neuropathy. Considerations on its prognosis. Electromyogr Clin Neurophysiol 1980;20:153–5.

[15] Whiteside JL, Barber MD, Walters MD, et al. Anatomy of ilioinguinal and iliohypogastric nerves in relation to trocar placement and low transverse incisions. Am J Obstet Gynecol 2003;189:1574–8, discussion 1578.

[16] Solheim LF, Hagen R. Femoral and sciatic neuropathies after total hip arthroplasty. Acta Orthop Scand 1980;51:531–4.

[17] Chad DA, Bradley WG. Lumbosacral plexopathy. Semin Neurol 1987;7:97–107.

[18] Rajashekhar RP, Herbison GJ. Lumbosacral plexopathy caused by retroperitoneal hemorrhage: report of two cases. Arch Phys Med Rehabil 1974;55:91–3.

[19] Ozcakar L, Sivri A, Aydinli M, et al. Lumbosacral plexopathy as the harbinger of a silent retroperitoneal hematoma. South Med J 2003;96:109–10.

[20] Kent KC, Moscucci M, Mansour KA, et al. Retroperitoneal hematoma after cardiac catheterization: prevalence, risk factors, and optimal management. J Vasc Surg 1994;20:905–10, discussion 910–913.

[21] Lumsden AB, Miller JM, Kosinski AS, et al. A prospective evaluation of surgically treated groin complications following percutaneous cardiac procedures. Am Surg 1994;60:132–7.

[22] Kent KC, Moscucci M, Gallagher SG, et al. Neuropathy after cardiac catheterization: incidence, clinical patterns, and long-term outcome. J Vasc Surg 1994;19:1008–13, discussion 1013–1014.

[23] Kaymak B, Ozcakar L, Cetin A, et al. Bilateral lumbosacral plexopathy after femoral vein dialysis: synopsis of a case. Joint Bone Spine 2004;71:347–8.

[24] Adbelhamid MF, Sandler D, Awad RW. Ischaemic lumbosacral plexopathy following aorto-iliac bypass graft: case report and review of literature. Ann R Coll Surg Engl 2007;89:W12–3.

[25] Abdellaoui A, West NJ, Tomlinson MA, et al. Lower limb paralysis from ischaemic neuropathy of the lumbosacral plexus following aorto-iliac procedures. Interact Cardiovasc Thorac Surg 2007;6:501–2.

[26] Jaeckle KA. Neurological manifestations of neoplastic and radiation-induced plexopathies. Semin Neurol 2004;24:385–93.

[27] Georgiou A, Grigsby PW, Perez CA. Radiation induced lumbosacral plexopathy in gynecologic tumors: clinical findings and dosimetric analysis. Int J Radiat Oncol Biol Phys 1993;26:479–82.

[28] Taphoorn MJB, Bromberg JEC. Neurological effects of therapeutic irradiation. Continuum: lifelong learning in neurology. Neuro Oncol 2005;11:93–115.
[29] Thomas JE, Cascino TL, Earle JD. Differential diagnosis between radiation and tumor plexopathy of the pelvis. Neurology 1985;35:1–7.
[30] Fann A. Plexopathy—lumbosacral. In: Frontera WR, Silver JK, editors. Essentials of physical medicine and rehabilitation. Philadelphia: Hanley & Belfus; 2001. p. 671.
[31] Dyck PJB, Windebank AJ. Diabetic and nondiabetic lumbosacral radiculoplexus neuropathies: new insights into pathophysiology and treatment. Muscle Nerve 2002;25:477–91.
[32] Dyck PJB, Norell JE, Dyck PJ. Non-diabetic lumbosacral radiculoplexus neuropathy: natural history, outcome and comparison with the diabetic variety. Brain 2001;124:1197–207.
[33] Kelkar P, Hammer-White S. Impaired glucose tolerance in nondiabetic lumbosacral radiculoplexus neuropathy [letter]. Muscle Nerve 2005;31:273–4.
[34] Zochodne DW, Isaac D, Jones C. Failure of immunotherapy to prevent, arrest, or reverse diabetic lumbosacral plexopathy. Acta Neurol Scand 2003;107:299–301.
[35] Dumitru D, Zwarts MJ. Lumbosacral plexopathies and proximal mononeuropathies. In: Dumitru D, Amato A, Zwarts M, editors. Electrodiagnostic medicine. 2nd ed. Philadelphia: Hanley & Belfus; 2002. p. 777–836.
[36] Wong CJ, Kraus EE. An unusual case of acute foot drop caused by a pseudoaneurysm. Case Rep Med 2011;2011:515078.
[37] van Alfen N, van Engelen BG. Lumbosacral plexus neuropathy: a case report and review of the literature. Clin Neurol Neurosurg 1997;99:138–41.
[38] Frontera W, Silver JK, editors. Essentials of physical medicine and rehabilitation. Philadelphia: Hanley & Belfus; 2001. p. 671–7.
[39] Larson WL, Wald JJ. Foot drop as a harbinger of aortic occlusion. Muscle Nerve 1995;18:899–903.
[40] Taylor BV, Kimmel DW, Krecke KN, et al. Magnetic resonance imaging in cancer-related lumbosacral plexopathy. Mayo Clin Proc 1997;72:823–9.
[41] Moore KR, Tsuruda JS, Dailey AT. The value of MR neurography for evaluating extraspinal neuropathic leg pain: a pictorial essay. Am J Neuroradiol 2001;22:786–94.
[42] Chan YC, Lo YL, Chan ESY. Immunotherapy for diabetic amyotrophy. Cochrane Database Syst Rev 2012;6:1–15.
[43] Tung TH, Martin DZ, Novak CB, et al. Nerve reconstruction in lumbosacral plexopathy. Case report and review of the literature. J Neurosurg 2005;102(Suppl.):86–91.
[44] Alexandre A, Coro L, Azuelos A. Microsurgical treatment of lumbosacral plexus injuries [abstract]. Acta Neurochir Suppl 2005;92:53–9.
[45] Gallo AC, Codispoti VT. Complex regional pain syndrome type II associated with lumbosacral plexopathy: a case report. Pain Med 2010;11:1834–6.

CHAPTER 145

Polytrauma Rehabilitation

Marissa McCarthy, MD
Robert Kent, DO, MHA, MPH
Neil Kirschbaum, DO
Gail Latlief, DO
Rafael Mascarinas, MD
Bryan Merritt, MD
S. Jit Mookerjee, DO
Steven Scott, DO
Joseph Standley, DO
Jill Massengale, MS, ARNP

Synonyms

Blast injury
Multiple injuries
Multiple trauma

ICD-9 Codes

344.0 Quadriplegia and quadriparesis
344.1 Paraplegia
804 Multiple fractures involving skull or face with other bones
850 Concussion
854.0 Intracranial injury of other and unspecified nature without mention of open intracranial wound
854.1 Intracranial injury of other and unspecified nature with open intracranial wound
905.0 Late effect of traumatic amputation
906.8 Late effect of burn of unspecified site
907.0 Late effect of intracranial injury without mention of skull fracture
997.63 Infection (chronic)

ICD-10 Codes

G82.50 Quadriplegia, unspecified
G82.20 Paraplegia, unspecified
S02.91 Unspecified fracture of skill
S02.92 Unspecified fracture of facial bones
Add seventh character for S02 (A—initial encounter for closed fracture, B—initial encounter for open fracture, D—subsequent encounter for fracture with routine healing, G—subsequent encounter for fracture with delayed healing, K—subsequent encounter for fracture with nonunion, P—subsequent encounter for fracture with malunion, S—sequela)
S06.0 Concussion
S06.9X Unspecified intracranial injury; add seventh digit for duration of loss of consciousness
Add seventh character to S06 for episode of care
B99.9 Unspecified infectious disease

Definition

In 2005, the U.S. Department of Veterans Affairs officially adopted the term *polytrauma*, originally defined as an injury to the brain in addition to other body parts. The definition changed in 2009 to be more encompassing: "two or more injuries sustained in the same incident that affect multiple body parts or organ systems and result in physical, cognitive, psychological, or psychosocial impairments and functional disabilities [1,2]."

The sequelae of polytrauma may include physical, cognitive, and psychological impairments. If a brain injury is involved, the severity typically guides the course of rehabilitation [3]. Other common disabling conditions include limb extremity trauma or amputation, spinal cord injury, neurosensory impairments, mental health disorders, and extreme soft tissue injury.

Because of the nature of modern military combat and violence in society, there is an increased risk for polytrauma injuries. Current combat-related polytrauma injuries are frequently caused by exposure to high-energy blasts or explosions [4]. Other causes of polytrauma may include severe motor vehicle accidents, falls, suicide attempts, accidental drug overdoses, and assaults. Advanced trauma life support permits increased survival among those with even the most devastating injuries (Table 145.1).

Polytrauma war-related injuries as well as civilian-based injuries occur more frequently in the younger population and predominantly in males. In noncombat conditions, active-duty men are 2.5 times more likely to have a traumatic brain injury. Military reports indicate that more than 27,000 service members serving in the current conflicts were injured between December 2001 and April 2012; of those, 49% sustained injuries classified as polytrauma. Of those injured as a result of combat operations, 62% had polytrauma injuries (K. Gross, personal communication, February 1, 2013). In the military polytrauma population, 1581 amputees have been treated in the military treatment facilities [5]. Civilian polytrauma frequency statistics are not available at this time [6,7].

Symptoms

Whereas many symptoms of polytrauma are immediately recognized, others are more subtle. Symptoms related to traumatic brain injury include cognitive, emotional, and physical impairments (see Chapter 162).

Cognitive deficits in patients with moderate to severe brain injury may include difficulties with speech and language, executive function, memory, concentration, and judgment. Irritability, anxiety, depression, and emotional lability are commonly observed. Physical symptoms of polytrauma commonly include motor and sensory deficits as well as more subtle complaints, such as headache, dizziness, fatigue, and dyssomnias. Pain is common and arises from multiple causes, complicating pain management.

Physical Examination

A thorough physical examination is essential in the evaluation of a patient who has sustained polytrauma. A mechanism of injury–directed review of systems is suggested [5]. If the mechanism of injury is blast related, the examination emphasizes testing for barotrauma to air- or fluid-filled organs. A thorough neurologic examination with complete assessment of cranial nerves (including olfactory), motor strength, sensation, reflexes, and coordination and a neuropsychological evaluation are recommended when central nervous system involvement is suspected.

A multidisciplinary approach commonly requiring specialty consultants to participate in the assessment is necessary for comprehensive care of these complex patients. Special attention is paid to the assessment of skin and soft tissue. The ideal approach is a patient-centered interdisciplinary evaluation and treatment plan coordinated by physiatry.

Functional Limitations

Polytrauma patients have multiple functional limitations based on the severity and number of physical and cognitive impairments. Hearing and visual field deficits affect everyday life functions and can make educational and vocational goals difficult to achieve. Lower extremity muscle weakness often impairs ambulation and creates a safety risk from falls. Upper extremity weakness and spasticity impair the patient's ability to do everyday activities such as dressing, hygiene, and handwriting. Cognitive deficits affect the ability to work and to perform roles related to parenting and living independently. Particularly in the early phase of recovery, some patients may require continuous surveillance to prevent wandering or self-injurious behavior. Later in recovery, driving can be achieved in some patients after passing of a driving evaluation, which may identify necessary modifications to the current vehicle. Many polytrauma patients will experience psychosocial problems. Traumatic brain injury, stress, and mental health–related issues predispose patients to depression, anger, and mood swings. Those with brain injuries may experience significant personality changes affecting interpersonal relationships, vocational rehabilitation, and quality of life.

Diagnostic Studies

Imaging Studies

Because of the complex nature of injuries, several different imaging modalities are used to assess the central nervous

Table 145.1 Blast Injury

	Etiology of Injury	Organ Systems Affected	Examples
Primary	Barotrauma	Organs with gas-fluid interface	Ear, lung, and bowel perforations
Secondary	Fragment, shrapnel	Soft tissue, penetrating head injuries	Penetrating traumatic brain injury
Tertiary	Displacement of body from combined pressure loads	Soft tissue, orthopedic, head injury	Broken femur from forceful displacement
Quaternary	Miscellaneous (e.g., crush, burns, object displacement)	Any organ system can be affected	Falling building causing crush injury

system in the polytrauma patient. In general, central nervous system injury is assessed by a combination of computed tomography and magnetic resonance imaging. Magnetic resonance imaging may be challenging in both military and civilian populations because of the higher incidence of retained fragments or past medical history involving a metal implant. Post-traumatic encephalomalacia, hydrocephalus, intracranial hemorrhage, diffuse axonal injury, cerebral contusions, mass effect, degree of atrophy, and spinal cord injury can be assessed by magnetic resonance or computed tomographic imaging.

Routine radiographs are often sufficient to assess axial, musculoskeletal, and visceral injuries. Other imaging techniques, such as computed tomography, bone scan, magnetic resonance, and ultrasonography, can be used when more detailed examination is necessary or for assessment of secondary complications.

Electrodiagnostics

Patients with polytrauma often sustain damage to the peripheral nervous system. A review of 33 active-duty patients admitted to the Tampa Polytrauma Rehabilitation Center revealed multiple cases of plexopathy and peripheral nerve damage due to exposure to blasts, penetrating wounds, crush injuries, and motor vehicle collisions. In this study, upper extremity nerve damage was more common than lower extremity nerve damage; multiple nerve injuries were more common than mononeuropathy [7]. Electromyography and nerve conduction studies should be considered as part of the assessment of a polytrauma patient.

Electroencephalography is a useful tool in diagnosis of post-traumatic epilepsy or encephalopathy. Seizure control and treatment of post-traumatic epilepsy are important for maximizing goal attainment during the rehabilitation process. Long-term electroencephalographic monitoring can aid in diagnosis of post-traumatic epilepsy as well as in the identification of subclinical seizures or seizure activity in patients with severe brain injuries who have not regained consciousness.

Polysomnography and actigraphy can be helpful in assessing for dyssomnias that may result after a polytrauma injury. Both sleep efficiency and sleep duration are important components of recovery, which is especially true in patients with concomitant brain injury [8].

Vascular Studies

Thromboembolic disease is a consequence of polytrauma and subsequent immobility after injury. Venous Doppler ultrasonography is frequently used to detect deep venous thrombosis in the extremities. In addition, computed tomography angiography is the diagnostic study of choice to evaluate for pulmonary embolism. Arterial Doppler ultrasonography may also be useful in the assessment of traumatic amputations to determine adequate perfusion of the residual limb.

Arterial dissection has also been documented to occur secondary to polytrauma. Traditional angiography and magnetic resonance angiography are both useful to explore the extent of dissection and superimposed thrombus after traumatic dissection.

Functional Testing

Functional testing uses sets of tests to determine performance or limitations. This testing is routinely performed by speech-language pathologists, physical therapists, and occupational therapists. Whereas overt injuries may be manifested with obvious functional deficits, milder or subclinical injuries in the presence of massive traumatic injuries may be unrecognized initially but need to be identified throughout the rehabilitation process. The intradisciplinary assessment of a polytrauma patient should include all members of the rehabilitation team to develop the full functional picture of each individual patient.

Disturbances in balance, hearing, and vision are commonly reported by polytrauma patients. Examples may include tinnitus, dizziness, and blurry vision. These disturbances result in sensory processing difficulties that affect cognitive functioning, mobility, independent performance of activities of daily living, and successful integration into the community. Evaluation and rehabilitation of the multisensory disturbances should be therapeutically integrated among specialty providers. Physical therapists with specialized training in balance disorders may perform computerized dynamic posturography to help determine the etiology of the impairment. Speech-language pathologists may be employed to evaluate dysphagia by bedside examination or video swallow study.

Neuropsychological and Psychological Evaluations

A comprehensive battery of neuropsychological and psychological tests is necessary to determine the full spectrum of cognitive and psychological sequelae from polytrauma injuries. This is typically completed once the person is medically stable, is in an acute rehabilitation program, and has emerged from a postinjury confusional state such as post-traumatic amnesia or delirium. Evaluations may be repeated to address different clinical questions during the course of recovery. Initially, assessment helps identify cognitive and emotional impairments that should be a focus of treatment. Repeated evaluations may be useful in making decisions about additional treatment needs, residential placement independence capacity, and future vocational or educational endeavors.

Differential Diagnosis

Differential diagnosis for patients sustaining polytrauma injuries is complex for seemingly simple problems. Even the cause of the injury is frequently debated. For example, brain injury can be caused by primary, secondary, and tertiary blast injuries or a combination of the three and may be traumatic or anoxic. A broad differential should be included when any problem with a polytrauma patient is considered.

The clinician must maintain a high index of suspicion for possible central nervous system infection when patients with a history of penetrating head injury present with such vague complaints as confusion, fatigue, and functional decline. Likewise, patients with a history of penetrating abdominal wounds may present with vague abdominal complaints, and an aggressive evaluation may be required for retained shrapnel and possible abscess. Musculoskeletal complaints may also be challenging, and evaluation for retained shrapnel causing impingement or nerve injury should be explored. Any complaint that does not respond to treatment as expected should be explored and the differential diagnosis widened in an effort to treat this challenging population of patients. In this regard, the potential for development of chronic pain or somatoform disorders, posttraumatic stress disorder, depression, or other psychological conditions should be considered.

Differential Diagnosis

Conversion disorder
Somatoform disorder
Malingering

Some potential diagnoses are actually the traumas or injuries of polytrauma:

Dementia or cognitive disorder NOS
Normal-pressure hydrocephalus
Toxic exposure
Fibromyalgia
Mycobacterial infection
Mycoplasmal infection
Infectious disease
Drug and alcohol abuse
Medication side effects

Others are potential differential diagnoses:

Progressive dementias
Sleep apnea
Multiple sclerosis
Neoplasms
Autoimmune disease (e.g., rheumatoid, lupus, vasculitis)
Other infectious diseases (Lyme disease, syphilis, poliomyelitis, human immunodeficiency virus infection, Epstein-Barr virus infection)

Treatment

Initial

Dramatic improvement in survival is attributed to advanced trauma life support. The initial treatment is predominantly focused on maintaining medical stability and preventing further injury. With enhanced survival of catastrophic injuries, disability and impairments are increased, thus dictating the complexity of multidisciplinary rehabilitation.

Rehabilitation

Polytrauma rehabilitation is challenging in that multiple impairments must be rehabilitated concurrently. The rehabilitation process begins in the acute medical setting, such as a military treatment facility or level I trauma hospital, with the initiation of individual physical, occupational, and speech therapy. Treatment in the acute medical setting will lay the foundation for the rest of the rehabilitation process.

Successful rehabilitation of polytrauma patients requires both multidisciplinary medical care and interdisciplinary rehabilitation care. The interdisciplinary patient-centered rehabilitation team led by a physiatrist should consist of speech therapists, physical therapists, occupational therapists, nurses, blind rehabilitation specialists or certified low vision therapists, audiologists, recreational therapists, psychologists, social workers, rehabilitation counselors, family therapists, prosthetists, and others working together to minimize disability, to maximize independence, to offer psychosocial support, and to provide a rehabilitation regimen specific to each patient's individual needs [9]. The polytrauma patients should be observed with a rehabilitation model of care from initial consultation to long-term rehabilitation care or community reintegration.

Mobility issues should be discussed with the patient or caregiver, and the most appropriate source of mobility should be considered for each individual patient. With choice of mobility, a provider must identify which type of mobility assistance provides the highest degree of independent function with the lowest degree of long-term loss of function. Some polytrauma patients are able to use manual wheelchairs, offering them a higher level of independence, whereas other polytrauma patients and their caregivers benefit from power mobility. Pressure mapping of chair cushions should also be considered in developing chairs for this population. Prosthetists and orthotists are integral members of the rehabilitation team when mobility needs of the amputee are addressed.

During the past years of conflicts in the Middle East, there has been an increase in the number and severity of urinary tract, rectal, and external genital injuries in polytrauma patients. Surgeons are faced with testicular salvage, reconstruction, and colostomies. There is an increased need for incorporating urologic care into the care of these complex injuries. The rehabilitation team faces challenges of voiding dysfunction, erectile dysfunction, infertility, and long-term psychological effects [5].

Patients with polytrauma also have increased metabolic demands. These metabolic demands are driven by factors such as healing tissue, diffuse spasticity, and rigors of the rehabilitation process. Nutrition can be further complicated by the risk of aspiration, which may require dietary changes, use of percutaneous endoscopic gastrostomy or jejunostomy, and parenteral nutrition. Including a registered dietitian on the team can be extremely beneficial to these patients.

Telemedicine is an emerging technology that has proved to be an effective tool to address rehabilitation needs in this population. In the VA Polytrauma System of Care, a telehealth network was developed in 2006 to connect the interdisciplinary rehabilitation teams. This has enabled provider continuity and coordination of care from initial contact to community reintegration. Telehealth also provides enhanced options for patient access to care [10].

Multifaceted aspects of physical, psychosocial, financial, and reintegration challenges are vast. Resources for polytrauma patients are extremely individualized on the basis of the nature of the injuries. For example, patients may require special adapted housing, durable medical equipment, cognitive and physical prosthetics, vehicle modification, and mobility devices. The physiatrist has a critical role as a patient advocate. A strong working relationship with social services and caregivers is integral to the effective definition of needs and available resources. This can be a challenging but rewarding process.

Procedures

During the rehabilitation process, various interventions may be used to augment the efforts of the multidisciplinary team. Chemodenervation, intrathecal baclofen pumps, and serial casting can help reduce spasticity and improve overall mobility, hygiene, pain, caregiver burden, and function. Negative pressure wound therapy with vacuum-assisted closure may be used for large or slowly healing traumatic or postsurgical wounds, and débridement may be necessary [11]. Interventional pain procedures, trigger point and peripheral joint injections, and peripheral nerve blocks are often used to treat nociceptive pain when more conservative treatments fail. Spinal cord and peripheral nerve stimulator trials and subsequent placement are becoming more common for treatment of refractory pain [12].

Surgery

Because of the complexity of management necessary for the polytrauma patient, multiple surgical interventions may be required during the initial acute medical setting and acute rehabilitation period. Surgical examples include but are not limited to tracheostomies, percutaneous gastrostomy tubes, and external fixators. Patients may also require readmission to the hospital for subsequent surgeries, and an additional stay in the rehabilitation unit may allow the attainment of further independence goals. Patients with hydrocephalus may require placement of a ventriculoperitoneal shunt. Finally, reconstructive procedures for facial deformities, revision of skin grafts and scars, and resection of heterotopic ossification may be required in the late post-acute rehabilitation stage.

Patients who have sustained crush injuries may require fasciotomies as a result of compartment syndrome. Many patients who have sustained severe head trauma will require partial craniectomy both for removal of blood accumulation and for avoidance of further damage from cerebral edema. The removed portion of the skull is frequently unsalvageable because of fragmentation injuries. If the skull plate is salvageable, it may be either frozen or implanted into the abdominal wall for use at a later date.

The polytrauma patient frequently requires repeated surgical interventions during the acute hospitalization phase. Multiple revisions of amputated limbs as well as staged interventions for burned patients, such as repeated skin grafting, may be required.

Potential Disease Complications

Explosions have the potential to inflict multiple and severe trauma that few U.S. health care providers outside the military and the Veterans Administration have experience treating. The acute complications vary by the mechanism and pattern of trauma. Such complications can include air embolism, compartment syndrome, rhabdomyolysis, renal failure, seizures, hemorrhage, increased intracranial pressure, infections, meningitis, and encephalopathy. Early complications that follow major burns include bacterial infections, septicemia, deep venous thrombosis, pulmonary embolism, renal failure, hypovolemic shock, jaundice, glottic edema, and ileus.

Table 145.2 Common Infections in Polytrauma

Traumatic Brain Injury [13,14]	Spinal Cord Injury [15]	Amputation	General and Orthopedic [16]
Pneumonia Surgical site Urinary tract infection	Urinary tract infection Pneumonia Infected pressure wound	Skin Surgical site	Urinary tract infection Pneumonia Skin or soft tissue infection

During the acute rehabilitation stage of care, there is overlap of potential complications. However, some variable patterns emerge, depending on whether the major injury is traumatic brain injury, spinal cord injury, burn, or limb amputation.

The risk of heterotopic ossification exists for traumatic brain injuries, spinal cord injuries, burns, and amputations independently; thus, concern for increased risk exists when concomitant injuries are present. Heterotopic ossification is of great concern in this population as it can decrease function, lead to increased pain, and limit rehabilitation potential (see Chapter 130).

Mental health complications are common in the polytrauma patient. Diagnoses include depression, posttraumatic stress and anxiety disorders, adjustment disorders, body image issues, and behavioral or emotional dysregulation. Any or all of these can have an impact on medication or treatment compliance and general recovery.

It is important to include an infectious disease specialist in the care of the polytrauma patient, particularly for those patients who have a recent history of exposure to endemic infections. An example of this may be an infection related to *Acinetobacter baumannii* in a combat-related polytrauma patient returning from Afghanistan [13] (Table 145.2).

Cognitively impaired polytrauma patients are prone to falls because of compounding spasticity, visual impairment, impulsivity, or vestibulocochlear deficits. Along with fall issues, understanding the etiology and ramifications of the patient's other injuries is important to map out a safe rehabilitation process. Patients' families need to be educated on issues such as skin integrity, appropriate transfers, fall avoidance, proper wheelchair transfer and use, physical limitations, weight-bearing precautions, balance issues, and emotional stability in specific patients [17].

Potential Treatment Complications

Polypharmacy, side effects of medications, addiction to prescription pain medications, and surgical and procedural complications exist in the polytrauma patient. The use of rehabilitation equipment, orthotics, prosthetics, and other medical or adaptive devices can sometimes result in complications. Splints used in polytrauma patients to prevent joint contractures can result in pressure ulcers. Compartment syndrome, nerve injury, and infections can develop under casts that are sometimes used to treat contractures in the polytrauma population. An amputee may develop skin irritation, abrasions, ulcerations, or other skin changes from the prosthetic liner or socket.

References

[1] U.S. Department of Veterans Affairs. VHA Directive 2005-024. http://www.federalpt.org/pdfs/PolytraumaCenter.pdf; [accessed January 2013].

[2] U.S. Department of Veterans Affairs. VHA Directive 2009-028. http://www1.va.gov/vhapublications/ViewPublication.asp?pub_ID=2032; [accessed January 2013].

[3] Nolan S. Traumatic brain injury: a review. Crit Care Nurs Q 2005;28:188–94.

[4] DePalma RG, Burris DG, Champion HR, Hodgson MJ. Blast injuries. N Engl J Med 2005;1335–42.

[5] Ficke JR, Eastridge BJ, Butler FK, et al. Dismounted complex blast injury. Report of the army dismounted complex blast injury task force. J Trauma Acute Care Surg 2012;73:S520–34.

[6] Belanger HG, Scott S, Scholten S, et al. Utility of mechanism-of-injury-based assessment and treatment. Blast Injury Program case illustration. J Rehabil Res Dev 2005;42:403–12.

[7] Merritt B, Humayun F, Tran H. Patterns of peripheral nerve injuries sustained by polytrauma active duty service members. Poster presented at the annual assembly of the American Academy of Physical Medicine and Rehabilitation, September 2007.

[8] Collen J, Orr N, Lettieri CJ, et al. Sleep disturbances among soldiers with combat-related traumatic brain injury. Chest 2012;142:622–30.

[9] Sayer NA, Cifu DX, McNamee S, et al. Rehabilitation needs of combat-injured service members admitted to the VA Polytrauma Rehabilitation Centers: the role of PM&R in the care of wounded warriors. PM R 2009;1:23–8.

[10] Darkins A, Cruise C, Armstrong M, et al. Enhancing access of combat-wounded veterans to specialist rehabilitation services: the VA Polytrauma Telehealth Network. Arch Phys Med Rehabil 2008;89:182–7.

[11] United States Army Institute of Surgical Research. Joint theater trauma system clinical practice guideline: initial management of war wounds: wound débridement and irrigation. http://usaisr.amedd.army.mil/clinical_practice:guidelines.html; [accessed February 2013].

[12] Falco F, Berger J, Vrable A, et al. Cross talk: a new method for peripheral nerve stimulation. An observational report with cadaveric verification. Pain Physician 2009;12:965–83.

[13] Massengale J, Tran J, Schwartz T, et al. Prevalence of intracranial infection among a consecutive series of VHA patients with disorders of consciousness. Poster presented at the federal interagency conference on traumatic brain injury, Washington, DC, 2011.

[14] Korbetti IS, Vakis AF, Papadakis JA, et al. Infections in traumatic brain injury patients. Clin Microbiol Infect 2012;18:359–64.

[15] Montgomerie J. Infections in patients with spinal cord injuries. http://www.lesionadomedular.com/archivos/almacen/infecciones%20urinarias%20y%20lesionados%20medulares.pdf; [accessed January 2013].

[16] Tinneli M, Mannino S, Lucchi S, et al. Healthcare acquired infections in rehabilitation units of the Lombardy region of Italy. Infection 2011;39:353–8.

[17] Latlief F, Elnitsky C, Hart-Hughes S, et al. Patient safety in the rehabilitation of the adult with an amputation. Phys Med Rehabil Clin N Am 2012;23:377–92.

CHAPTER 146

Postpoliomyelitis Syndrome

Jan Lexell, MD, PhD

Synonyms

Late effects of poliomyelitis
Poliomyelitis sequelae
Post-polio

ICD-9 Code

138 Late effects of acute poliomyelitis

ICD-10 Codes

B91 Sequelae of poliomyelitis
G14 Postpolio syndrome

Definition

Poliomyelitis, also referred to as infantile paralysis, has a special history among infectious diseases. During the first half of the 20th century, there were major epidemics throughout the world. As a viral infection, caused by an RNA virus, it affected mainly children and countries in the Western world with good hygienic and sanitary standards. This occurred when other infectious diseases were being successfully prevented. At the end of the 1940s, several research discoveries led to a better understanding of poliovirus and opened up new opportunities for the manufacture of vaccine. The American organization the March of Dimes invested large sums of money, and the American researcher Jonas Salk started to develop a vaccine, which in 1954 was shown to be effective. General vaccination began in 1956 in the United States and shortly thereafter in other parts of the Western world. This rapidly led to a large reduction in the number of polio cases. In 1988, the World Health Organization decided to try to eradicate polio from the world. The campaign has been highly successful, and there are now only a few countries in Africa (Nigeria) and Asia (mainly Pakistan and Afghanistan) where the virus still exists. The original goal was that polio should be totally eliminated by 2000, but this deadline has been postponed repeatedly. Today, fewer than a thousand new cases are being reported annually.

It is well known that many polio survivors later in life develop new symptoms, referred to as poliomyelitis sequelae, late effects of polio, or just post-polio. Although sequelae of prior polio have been known since the end of the 19th century, it was not until the early1980s that researchers came to agree on the term *postpoliomyelitis syndrome* (PPS) to describe the various symptoms that polio survivors may perceive. As there are no accurate statistics describing the number of people being affected by polio, we have no clear account of the number living with PPS. The figures in the literature vary, mostly depending on the definitions used, but it is generally agreed that around 60% of those who initially had paralytic polio will develop PPS [1]. In the United States, it is estimated that more than 1 million survivors of polio live in the country; in the European Union (with a population of approximately 500 million inhabitants), the number is approximated to 600,000 polio survivors. With many young polio survivors in Africa and Asia, it is estimated that up to 10 million people around the world will need health care and rehabilitation during the next decades as a result of their poliomyelitis infection. This makes PPS one of the most common neuromuscular conditions and a challenge to rehabilitation professionals.

PPS is a neurologic disorder characterized by a collection of symptoms occurring decades after the initial paralytic polio. There are different definitions of PPS, but all are more or less based on the original description by Halstead and Rossi in 1985 and consist of five diagnostic criteria (Table 146.1) [2]. At the March of Dimes international conference on PPS in 2000, diagnostic criteria were recommended, including a criterion that symptoms should persist for at least 1 year [3]. Individuals with prior polio may perceive a number of new symptoms, but the three most common are new muscle weakness, fatigue (muscle as well as generalized), and pain from muscles and joints (at rest and during activities). Other, less frequently occurring but equally disabling symptoms are respiratory problems, swallowing problems, and cold intolerance [4,5].

The cause of PPS is not entirely clear, but it is generally agreed that the new symptoms (muscle weakness and fatigue) are due to a distal degeneration of axons in greatly

Table 146.1 Diagnostic Criteria for Postpoliomyelitis Syndrome

- The patient must have had polio.
- Full or incomplete neurologic and functional recovery must have taken place.
- A stable period of 15 years must have occurred.
- Thereafter, two or more of the following health problems must have arisen: lack of stamina/tiredness, muscle or joint pain, recent weakening of muscles in previously known or unknown polio-damaged muscles, recent muscle atrophy, loss of functioning, or intolerance to cold.
- Symptoms persist for at least a year, and other medical reasons for these increased problems must have been excluded.

In practice, requirements for typical findings during medical examination and neurophysiologic tests have been added in recent years.

enlarged motor units that develop during recovery after the acute paralytic polio [5]. After the initial paralysis, motor units are enlarged as a compensatory mechanism. These enlarged motor units undergo a continuous remodeling, and at the age of around 50 years, people start to suffer from the "normal" age-related loss of motor neurons [6]. This process of denervation and reinnervation could be accelerated in PPS owing to a premature dropout of motor neurons caused by neuronal damage from the initial infection, increased metabolic demand in the enlarged motor units, or overuse. The loss of whole, enlarged motor units without reinnervation would also contribute and lead to a progressive dropout of muscle fibers. Other reasons underlying PPS have been discussed during the past decades, such as persistent poliovirus infection; overuse weakness due to transition in contractile properties and firing frequency; weight gain; and combined effects of muscle overuse, disuse, and weight gain. On the basis of recent findings of raised concentrations of cytokines in the cerebrospinal fluid, an inflammatory process might also be present as part of PPS [7]. This has led to the development of new treatment strategies that potentially could be beneficial for people with PPS (see the section on treatment).

Regardless of the underlying pathophysiologic mechanisms of PPS, it is a condition that is highly suitable for physicians in physical medicine and rehabilitation. There is no treatment that can cure PPS or any medication that can clearly delay its progression. However, those who have PPS can benefit from taking part in an interdisciplinary comprehensive goal-oriented rehabilitation program to reduce the consequences of the symptoms and the disability that these symptoms impose on their lives [8–10].

Symptoms

Weakness

Muscle weakness typically occurs in muscles involved during the acute infection but may also be experienced in muscles that were not clinically paralyzed originally. There is an association between the initial weakness and weakness occurring later in life. The greater the initial paralysis, the greater is the PPS-related weakness. Most people start to perceive the new weakness around the age of 50 years; however, the progression of strength losses is usually slow, with an approximate annual loss of 2% to 4% [11]. A history of more rapid progression of muscle weakness during weeks or months could indicate an alternative diagnosis, such as myopathy (e.g., polymyositis, thyroid myopathy), peripheral nerve disorders, or motor neuron disorder (e.g., amyotrophic lateral sclerosis), and should require a thorough investigation.

Fatigue

Fatigue in PPS can be either of muscle origin or more generalized. Muscle fatigue is commonly reported by people with PPS and is characterized by the inability to maintain muscle force. Muscle fatigue is linked to muscle weakness and muscle atrophy, and those with more pronounced muscle weakness also experience more muscle fatigue. Fatigue can also be described as more generalized and of central origin. This type of fatigue can be perceived as severe and persist for several years. It has been found to be associated with reduced physical functioning, increased body pain, reduced sleep quality, and more psychological distress [12]. Typically, this generalized fatigue is described as an influenza-like exhaustion that is often related to the amount of activities performed. Polio survivors usually feel fairly refreshed in the morning and become more fatigued as the day goes on. Some may even complain that they "hit a wall," sometimes experiencing an almost paralyzing tiredness, and just have to lie down and rest, something that usually relieves the fatigue. It is not unusual for people who have had severe meningitis as part of their acute polio to experience this type of fatigue. In addition, polio survivors who describe a fairly prominent fatigue can also complain about cognitive problems, such as impaired concentration and memory difficulties. Sleep disturbance, which is also reported in polio survivors, can exacerbate general fatigue. As fatigue is an unspecific symptom, commonly occurring in other disorders, alternative diagnoses should be ruled out (e.g., depression, thyroid dysfunction, anemia, other inflammatory diseases, or vitamin B_{12} deficiency).

Pain

Pain is common among people with PPS and often the symptom that drives them to seek medical help. It has been shown that 50% to 90% of those with PPS experience pain. Pain is common in the shoulders, lower back, legs, and hips and is usually most pronounced in the legs. It is associated with depression and fatigue [13] and can also affect sleep. Not everyone experiences pain, however, and many suffer from mild or no pain. In general, though, increasing pain is related to a lower perceived life satisfaction [14]. Pain can emanate from a joint, a muscle, ligaments, tendons or tendon sheaths, muscle and tendon insertions, and bursae close to a joint. The reason for this is usually the weakness that occurs as a result of muscle atrophy in PPS, which leads to muscle imbalance, stress, and overload and incorrect posture. Pain in PPS can be aching, burning, or cramping in the muscles. Joint pain commonly occurs as a result of the gradual development of osteoarthritis. Osteoarthritis after polio can affect joints in parts of the body with muscle weakness resulting from polio but also affects parts of the body not affected by polio because of compensatory overload. Osteoarthritis usually occurs in hip, knee, and foot joints. Typical symptoms are pain under strain, but pain at rest is also common.

Respiratory Problems

During the initial polio infection, breathing could be affected as a result of paralyzed respiratory muscles. This was treated with a ventilator for a longer or shorter time, and some have used a ventilator ever since their polio infection, whereas most improved and managed without it. These people may later in life experience new weakness in their respiratory muscles that can lead to an inability to maintain normal carbon dioxide levels in the blood because of reduced breathing volumes. This so-called underventilation is exacerbated by obesity and worsened by other restrictive lung diseases. However, respiratory problems usually occur in less than 10% of those with PPS. People with PPS-related underventilation can complain of morning headache, daytime tiredness, problems with concentration, restless sleep, waking up several times, nightmares, difficulty getting up in the morning, and increased breathlessness during and after exertion.

Swallowing

Swallowing problems occur only in those who had "bulbar" poliomyelitis that affected the swallowing muscles during the initial infection. Usual complaints are feelings of choking, gagging or coughing, and irritation in the throat or a feeling of a lump in the throat. Some people will also complain of voice problems, especially dysphonia [15].

Cold Intolerance

Cold intolerance is a feeling of coldness in the arms and legs and a general inability to thermoregulate. Cold intolerance may be caused by damage to the part of the brain that regulates body temperature, effects on nerves to arms and legs, or reduced muscle mass. It may also be exacerbated by other medical conditions, such as peripheral vascular disease.

Physical Examination

The findings during a clinical, musculoskeletal, and neurologic examination should support the diagnosis of a lower motor neuron disease process. This includes absent or diminished reflexes, decreased muscle tone, and atrophy (symmetric or asymmetric) and weakness of the muscles in the limbs or trunk. Sensory deficits are not part of PPS, but median and ulnar nerve entrapments are common in polio survivors; therefore, it is important to search for symptoms and signs of sensory disturbances in the hands.

Biomechanical symptoms and signs may also occur from musculoskeletal abnormalities in the lower extremities. This, in turn, is a result of contractures due to muscle weakness (hip and ankle), weakness of the quadriceps causing genu recurvatum at the knee, and reduced joint range of motion without apparent contributing weakness (common in the cervical spine and shoulders). Leg length discrepancies are common and may lead to scoliosis and kyphosis and pain from the spinal column.

Manual muscle testing is a quick and useful assessment of function. However, the occurrence and distribution of muscle weakness, as a hallmark of PPS, can be anything from obvious to subtle. It is therefore not always possible to rule out PPS solely by a clinical examination of muscle strength.

Visual assessment of gait and gait disturbances is a starting point for more mechanistic evaluations. Also, specific areas of the body that are reported as painful should be examined. Seating posture, turning, rising from a chair, and stair climbing are specific movements that can be affected, leading to pain, and may require interventions and corrections.

Fatigue is a common symptom and may be associated with other disorders. Therefore it is important to detect possible signs and symptoms of, for example, depression and sleep disorders. Respiratory problems should also be ruled out by a general physical examination complemented by a basic spirometer examination. Assessment of peripheral pulses and edema is also important.

Functional Limitations

Symptoms occurring as part of PPS can affect a person's ability to perform daily tasks, such as dressing, feeding, and grooming, as well as domestic life activities, such as managing one's household, cooking, cleaning, shopping, and participating in leisure activities. This is partly due to a reduced walking ability, including stair climbing, walking shorter and longer distances, and getting in and out of a car. It is also known that these limitations in activities of daily living can affect people with PPS, who may face a variety of challenges related to their participation, which in turn may have an impact on their autonomy and, ultimately, their life satisfaction. Areas that can be affected are family life, social roles, autonomy indoors and outdoors, work, and education [16].

PPS-related muscle and generalized fatigue as well as muscle weakness, muscle and joint pain, and breathing problems could limit the ability to perform usual daily activities, particularly activities that require some physical endurance. This, in turn, can contribute to a general deconditioning, which can cause even greater breathing problems and decreased endurance. It is therefore important to observe signs of a general reduction in physical activity, taking into account all types of daily activities, and to implement a variety of rehabilitation interventions that break this obvious vicious circle.

Diagnostic Studies

Weakness

As part of the routine clinical examination and verification of prior polio, electrodiagnostic studies, including electromyography (EMG) and nerve conduction studies, are highly recommended. Concentric needle EMG is performed to assess the distribution of neuromuscular changes and the degree of changes and also to rule out other neuromuscular diseases. On concentric needle EMG, motor unit action potentials in the limbs previously affected with paralytic polio are abnormally enlarged and polyphasic in configuration, and there is a decreased recruitment secondary to a reduction in the number of motor units available for activation during voluntary muscle contraction [1]. In many cases, EMG may be the only way to determine that signs of PPS are present.

To assess muscle weakness, as part of the routine clinical examination and in planning of appropriate interventions and evaluation, strength testing can be performed. Muscle strength can be assessed manually, with a hand-held dynamometer or with more sophisticated equipment, such as an isokinetic dynamometer. For research purposes, isokinetic dynamometers have been commonly used and are found to be both valid and reliable [17].

If it is clinically needed to establish an alternative or additional diagnosis, imaging of the spine (e.g., magnetic resonance imaging) can help evaluate whether a myelopathy or radiculopathy is present. Useful laboratory studies may include thyroid function studies to rule out thyroid myopathy and muscle enzymes, which can be mildly elevated in PPS.

Fatigue

Persons who experience generalized fatigue should be examined for an alternative diagnosis, for example, anemia, thyroid dysfunction, depression, sleep disorders, and respiratory problems. Other chronic conditions, such as congestive heart failure, diabetes, and chronic infections, can also contribute to fatigue and should lead to appropriate workup. In addition, cancer and other serious malignant diagnoses should also be ruled out.

Pain

For the underlying causes of pain to be understood, various diagnostic procedures are commonly performed, such as blood tests and plain radiographs of the spine and painful joints. Upper extremity neuropathies, such as carpal tunnel syndrome, should be considered and ruled out with electrodiagnostic studies.

Pain in PPS is of nociceptive origin. When pain is of neurogenic origin, alternative diagnoses should be considered, and magnetic resonance imaging and computed tomography can be performed. In rare cases, pain can also occur in persons who have had polio without paralysis or muscle weakness. Last but not least, pain can be due to reasons that are not related to PPS, and it is important that this is also considered.

Respiratory Problems

Respiratory problems can be initially evaluated by a baseline pulmonary function test with a portable desktop spirometer. When a reduced pulmonary function is found, a more thorough investigation with chest radiography and laboratory studies (e.g., arterial blood gas analysis) may be needed, and referral to a pulmonary specialist is recommended.

Swallowing Problems

Swallowing disorders can be diagnosed by imaging studies. A functional endoscopic evaluation of swallowing is most commonly performed.

Cold Intolerance

Cold intolerance can result from several factors, but diagnostic studies are generally not performed unless an alternative diagnosis (e.g., peripheral vascular disease) is suspected.

Treatment

Initial

Weakness

There is yet no treatment that can cure PPS and restore muscle strength. In a series of investigations, different medications (pyridostigmine, amantadine, prednisone, Q10) have been tested, but none has proved beneficial with regard to muscle weakness [18]. On the basis of the notion of an inflammatory process in the central nervous system of patients with PPS, intravenous immune globulin has been tested. In two larger randomized controlled trials, variable effects on muscle strength, pain, physical activity, and quality of life have been described [19,20]. The effect on muscle strength is, however, generally small and within the limits of random variability that would be seen from just repeated measurements [17]. However, the effect on other variables is more prominent. One clinically uncontrolled study showed that two thirds of 45 patients with PPS and pain reported a decrease on the visual analog scale for pain after treatment and 40% reported a decrease of more than 20 points [21]. A follow-up study of 41 patients [22] from the previous treatment trial [19] showed that scores of the physical component of the Short Form 36 (bodily pain and vitality), the visual analog scale for pain, and the 6-minute walk test were significantly better at 1 year compared with baseline and control subjects. These findings encourage further controlled trials to more firmly establish whether this treatment should be used in PPS.

Fatigue

Fatigue is managed by a multimodal approach. Primarily, any medical condition that may be contributing to it should be treated. Sleep disorders, depression, and other causes should be appropriately treated. Proper sleep hygiene is important (e.g., regular bedtimes, avoidance of caffeine late in the day); depression can be treated with medication or counseling or both. It is also important to address a person's daily activities; various fatigue management interventions, including pacing and taking rest breaks during the day, can be taught. The use of medication to treat fatigue has not been highly successful. Intravenous immune globulin has shown some promising results on fatigue and vitality in subgroups of fatigued patients with PPS [23]. More recently, modafinil has been used to treat fatigue pharmacologically; in more controlled studies, the results have not been particularly encouraging [24], whereas in clinical practice and individual cases, the medication may have an effect. The dose usually starts at 100 mg orally every morning and may be increased to 200 mg daily, 100 mg in the morning and 100 mg at lunchtime.

Pain

Treatment of pain should always start with a thorough analysis of the underlying cause and thereafter selection of appropriate interventions. Treatment of joint pain consists mainly of movement training (e.g., pool exercise) in combination with mobility aids, other aids, or orthotic devices. Transcutaneous electrical nerve stimulation, acupuncture, nonsteroidal anti-inflammatory drugs, and cortisone injections are other alternatives. Other medications, such as paracetamol and tramadol, can also be prescribed. In severe cases of osteoarthritis, joint replacements are necessary, which may then eliminate the pain completely.

Pain near joints (in tendons and ligaments) is usually due to a continuous overload as a result of muscle weakness. Polio survivors often need mobility aids to relieve this pain when they walk, stand, or engage in other activities. It is also important that they be given information on the importance of reducing the load on their bodies. Activity-related muscle pain is often caused by overuse of the weakened musculature. The most important part is to focus on the reason for the muscle pain. As it is often due to overuse of muscles, the person with PPS needs to understand this so that he or she can make necessary lifestyle changes. This is combined with the prescription of mobility aids to reduce overload during various activities, the provision of information about changed activity patterns, the correction of a sitting position, and the prescription of orthotic devices. Normally, pain is reduced when the load is reduced, but if the overuse continues, the pain can become more lasting and spread to the whole body. Postpoliomyelitis myalgias can be treated and have been reported to respond to low-dose tricyclic antidepressants and also to gabapentin and pregabalin.

Respiratory Problems

Respiratory problems, particularly sleep apnea, are often treated with significant improvement in symptoms by continuous positive airway pressure or bilevel positive airway pressure at night.

Swallowing Problems

Swallowing problems are treated conservatively, with specific recommendations from a speech and language pathologist.

Cold Intolerance

Cold intolerance is treated symptomatically, and recommendations to wear layered clothing, thermal underwear, and wool socks are given. Electrically heated stockings and insoles can also be tried.

Rehabilitation

Interdisciplinary rehabilitation is the cornerstone of appropriate management in PPS [25]. Several aspects of life are often affected, so it is important that the rehabilitation team have a thorough understanding and experience of PPS. Rehabilitation in PPS can be described as a process of change. In a qualitative study, the experiences of 12 persons with PPS who had participated in an individualized, goal-oriented, comprehensive interdisciplinary rehabilitation program were presented [26]. The focus of the program was to reduce self-perceived disability by providing a variety of interventions and thereby to maximize each individual's physical, mental, and social potential. The rehabilitation program was experienced as a turning point in the participants' lives (Fig. 146.1). Before rehabilitation, they felt that they were on a downward slope without control. Rehabilitation was the start of a process of change whereby they acquired new skills that, over time, contributed to a different but good life. After approximately a year, they had a sense of control and had accepted life with late effects of polio. They had also established new habits, had taken on a changed valued self, and could look to the future with confidence. The participants experienced the benefits of the program developed by an ongoing and iterative process that took at least a year to complete. This emphasizes that the outcome of a PPS rehabilitation program should be assessed from a long-term perspective. The results also indicate that the effect of an interdisciplinary rehabilitation program goes beyond that of simply reducing impairments. This, in turn, emphasizes the need to select outcome measures that address the impact of rehabilitation programs in a broad sense. One newly developed rating scale that specifically assesses self-reported impairments has been presented [27]. This scale, Self-reported

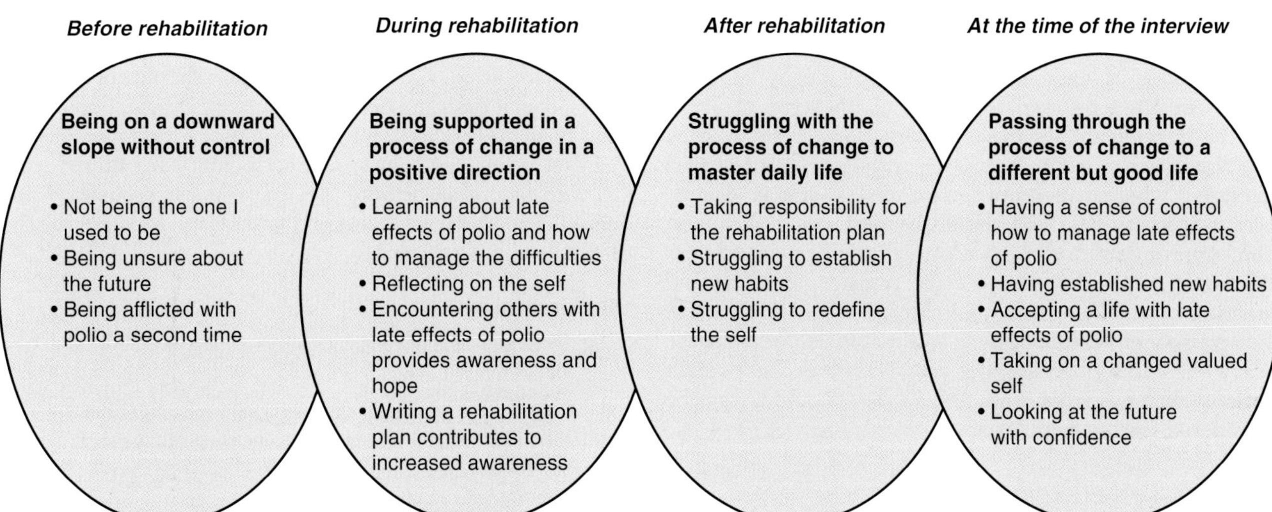

FIGURE 146.1 The core category, with the four categories and their subcategories, describing the experiences of persons with postpoliomyelitis syndrome and the influence of an individualized, goal-oriented, comprehensive interdisciplinary rehabilitation program. *(From Larsson Lund M, Lexell J. A positive turning point in life—how persons with late effects of polio experience the influence of an interdisciplinary rehabilitation program. J Rehabil Med 2010;42:559-565.)*

Impairments in Persons with late effects of Polio (SIPP), has been shown to have good psychometric properties and will facilitate the evaluation of impairments that people with PPS may experience.

Positive effects of rehabilitation were also reported in a pilot study of 27 participants with PPS. Significant improvements were noted for exercise endurance, depression, and fatigue but not for muscle strength and anxiety [28]. Another uncontrolled study found similar effects up to a year after multidisciplinary rehabilitation with emphasis on physiotherapy [29].

During a rehabilitation program, persons with PPS will be assessed by different team members and various interventions will be planned. Family members should also be encouraged to take part in the program. Many interventions cannot be evaluated until the person has actually tried them at home and later returns for follow-up. Examples of such interventions are prescription of mobility aids (scooter or power wheelchair), orthotic devices, and other adaptive equipment; teaching of compensatory techniques; medical and nonmedical interventions aimed at reducing pain, fatigue, and sleep disturbances; therapeutic home exercises, ergonomics, and vocational interventions to maintain workability; and home visits to assist in making appropriate environmental adaptation and driving adaptations [8–10]. It is therefore important that outcomes be assessed not only directly after a short rehabilitation period but also after the participants have been able to evaluate the different interventions in their preferred environment.

The exercise program should always be individualized and address flexibility, strength, and conditioning. The frequency, duration, and intensity depend very much on the distribution of PPS-related muscle weakness. For parts of the body and muscles that are not affected or only mildly affected, there are generally no restrictions. Exercise such as resistance training as well as an endurance type of training can be prescribed and may affect fatigue and quality of life positively [30]. On the other hand, whole-body vibration, a method that has gained popularity in the past decade, had no effect on muscle strength and gait performance [31]. When body parts and muscles are significantly affected by PPS, nonfatiguing protocols are preferred and the intensity of exercise must be individually tailored. EMG can often be used to decide on the type of activity, the frequency, and the duration. Non–weight-bearing exercises, such as pool exercise or cycling, are usually well tolerated, whereas high-impact exercises, such as jogging, may exacerbate pain and should be performed with caution. Appropriate prescription of orthotic devices will enable many polio survivors to walk, transfer, exercise, and function optimally within their limitations. Today, there are a variety of bracing options and materials, far from the heavy ones prescribed decades ago. Therefore, lightweight options, such as carbon fiber and Kevlar, should always be considered for this population.

Procedures

On occasion, therapeutic procedures are recommended on the basis of specific symptoms. Musculoskeletal symptoms may be treated with local steroid injections (e.g., tendinitis, osteoarthritis in the foot joints).

Surgery

Surgery should not be avoided when a disabling osteoarthritis is present. Joint replacements and carpal tunnel release can be successfully performed.

Potential Disease Complications

An important complication in PPS is falling, because of weakness and mobility problems, with subsequent injury (e.g., fracture or traumatic brain injury), and many persons with PPS complain about falls and a fear of falling [32]. Because of reduced bone mineral density, osteopenia, or osteoporosis in affected limbs, polio survivors may be more susceptible to fracture. Therefore bone mineral density studies should be considered in polio survivors with prominent weakness. Oral bisphosphonate treatment has led to significant increases in bone mineral density at the hip of PPS patients, which may have a protective effect on fracture risk [33]. Swallowing difficulties and respiratory problems can lead to pneumonia or aspiration. Also, polio survivors may be more prone to cardiovascular diseases [34], and therefore a general screening for cardiovascular risk factors in individuals diagnosed with PPS is recommended.

Potential Treatment Complications

Treatment complications may occur as a result of medication side effects and inappropriate interventions. Analgesics and nonsteroidal anti-inflammatory drugs have well-known side effects that most commonly affect the gastric, hepatic, and renal systems. Tricyclic antidepressants have cholinergic side effects, the most serious of which is the possibility of acute urinary retention in men (men with underlying prostate problems are generally at risk). Antihypertensive drugs such as beta blockers could potentially reduce muscle strength, and alternative medication for increased blood pressure should be considered. Statins can have a deleterious effect on muscle [35], which should be taken into account when they are prescribed. Polio survivors are reported to take longer to recover after general anesthesia and may require larger than the usual doses of postoperative pain medication. Careful consideration should therefore be given to the risks and benefits of surgery for this population.

During rehabilitation interventions, caution must always be used when someone's gait and mobility are altered, such as with use of an orthotic device. Too strenuous exercises could exacerbate weakness and fatigue and increase the risk for falls.

References

[1] Trojan DA, Cashman NR. Post-poliomyelitis syndrome. Muscle Nerve 2005;31:6–19.

[2] Halstead LS, Rossi CD. New problems in old polio patients: result of survey of 539 polio survivors. Orthopedics 1985;8:845–50.

[3] March of Dimes. Post-polio syndrome: identifying best practice in diagnosis and care. http://www.marchofdimes.com; [accessed 21.03.13].

[4] Farbu E, Gilhus NE, Barnes MP, et al. EFNS guideline on diagnosis and management of post-polio syndrome. Report of an EFNS task force. Eur J Neurol 2006;13:795–801.

[5] Boyer FC, Tiffreau V, Rapin A, et al. Post-polio syndrome: pathophysiological hypotheses, diagnosis criteria, medication therapeutics. Ann Phys Rehabil Med 2010;53:34–41.

[6] Laffont I, Julia M, Tiffreau V, et al. Aging and sequelae of poliomyelitis. Ann Phys Rehabil Med 2010;53:4–33.

[7] Gonzalez H, Olsson T, Borg K. Management of postpolio syndrome. Lancet Neurol 2010;9:634–42.

[8] Silver JK. Post-polio. A guide for polio survivors and their families. New Haven, Conn: Yale University Press; 2001.

[9] Halstead LS. Managing post-polio: a guide to living well with post-polio syndrome. Washington, DC: NRH Press; 1998.

[10] Lexell J, editor. Everything you need to know about post-polio syndrome (PPS). A guide for people who have had polio or who work in the health service. Stockholm, Sweden: Personskadeförbundet RTP; 2009.

[11] Stolwijk-Swuste JM, Beelen A, Lankhorst GJ, Nollet F. The course of functional status and muscle strength in patients with late-onset sequelae of poliomyelitis: a systematic review. Arch Phys Med Rehabil 2005;86:1693–701.

[12] Tersteeg IM, Koopmnan FS, Stolwijk-Swüste JM, et al. A 5-year longitudinal study of fatigue in patients with late-onset sequelae of poliomyelitis. Arch Phys Med Rehabil 2011;92:899–904.

[13] Jensen MP, Alschuler KN, Smith AE, et al. Pain and fatigue in persons with postpolio syndrome: independent effects of functioning. Arch Phys Med Rehabil 2011;92:1796–801.

[14] Lexell J, Brogårdh C. Life satisfaction and self-reported impairments in persons with late effects of polio. Ann Phys Rehabil Med 2012;55:577–89.

[15] Söderholm S, Lehtinen A, Valtonen K, Ylinen A. Dysphagia and dysphonia among persons with post-polio syndrome—a challenge in neurorehabilitation. Acta Neurol Scand 2010;122:343–9.

[16] Larsson Lund M, Lexell J. Perceived participation in the life situations in persons with late effects of polio. J Rehabil Med 2008;40:659–64.

[17] Flansbjer UB, Lexell J. Reliability of knee extensor and flexor muscle strength measurements in persons with late effects of polio. J Rehabil Med 2010;42:588–92.

[18] Koopman FS, Uegaki K, Gilhus NE, et al. Treatment for postpolio syndrome. Cochrane Database Syst Rev 2011;2, CD007818.

[19] Gonzalez H, Sunnerhagen KS, Sjöberg I, et al. Intravenous immunoglobulin for post-polio syndrome: a randomized controlled trial. Lancet Neurol 2006;5:493–500.

[20] Farbu E, Rekand T, Vik-Mo E, et al. Post-polio syndrome patients treated with intravenous immunoglobulin: a double-blinded randomized controlled pilot study. Eur J Neurol 2007;14:60–5.

[21] Werhagen L, Borg K. Effect of intravenous immunoglobulin on pain in patients with post-polio syndrome. J Rehabil Med 2011;43:1038–40.

[22] Gonzalez H, Khademi M, Borg K, Olsson T. Intravenous immunoglobulin treatment of the post-polio syndrome: sustained effects on quality of life variables and cytokine expression after a one year follow up. J Neuroinflammation 2012;9:167.

[23] Ostlund G, Broman L, Werhagen L, Borg K. IVIG treatment in post-polio patients: evaluation of responders. J Neurol 2012;259:2571–8.

[24] Vasconcelos OM, Prokhorenko OA, Salajegheh MK, et al. Modafinil for treatment of fatigue in post-polio syndrome: a randomized controlled trial. Neurology 2007;68:1680–6.

[25] Tiffreau V, Rapin A, Serafi R, et al. Post-polio syndrome and rehabilitation. Ann Phys Rehabil Med 2010;53:42–50.

[26] Larsson Lund M, Lexell J. A positive turning point in life—how persons with late effects of polio experience the influence of an interdisciplinary rehabilitation program. J Rehabil Med 2010;42:559–65.

[27] Brogårdh C, Lexell J, Lundgren-Nilsson A. Construct-validity of a new rating scale for self-reported impairments in persons with late effects of polio. PM R 2013;5:176–81.

[28] Davidson AC, Auyeung V, Luff R, et al. Prolonged benefit in post-polio syndrome from comprehensive rehabilitation: a pilot study. Disabil Rehabil 2009;31:309–17.

[29] Bertelsen M, Broberg S, Medsen E. Outcome of physiotherapy as part of a multidisciplinary rehabilitation in an unselected polio population with one-year follow-up: an uncontrolled study. J Rehabil Med 2009;41:85–7.

[30] Oncu J, Durmaz B, Karapolat H. Short-term effects of aerobic exercise on functional capacity, fatigue, and quality of life in patients with post-polio syndrome. Clin Rehabil 2009;23:155–63.

[31] Brogårdh C, Flansbjer UB, Lexell J. No specific effect of whole-body vibration training in chronic stroke: a double-blind randomized controlled study. Arch Phys Med Rehabil 2010;91:1474–7.

[32] Bickerstaffe A, Beelen A, Nollet F. Circumstances and consequences of falls in polio survivors. J Rehabil Med 2010;42:908–15.

[33] Alvarez A, Kremer R, Weiss DR, et al. Response of postpoliomyelitis patients to bisphosphonate treatment. PM R 2010;2:1094–1103.

[34] Gawne AC, Wells KR, Wilson KS. Cardiac risk factors in polio survivors. Arch Phys Med Rehabil 2003;84:694–6.

[35] Martikainen MH, Gardberg M, Kohonen I, Lähdesmäki J. Statin-induced myopathy in a patient with previous poliomyelitis. Am J Phys Med Rehabil 2013;92:1031–4.

CHAPTER 147

Postconcussion Symptoms

Mel B. Glenn, MD
Seth D. Herman, MD

Synonym

Postconcussive disorders

ICD-9 Code

310.2 Postconcussion syndrome

ICD-10 Code

F07.81 Postconcussional syndrome

Definition

Postconcussion symptoms are a set of symptoms commonly seen after concussion. The term *concussion* is generally used as a synonym for mild traumatic brain injury (mTBI). A number of definitions with varying lower and upper limits of severity for diagnosis have been proposed [1]. One commonly used definition of mTBI is a traumatically induced physiologic disruption of brain function, manifested by at least one of the following:

- any period of loss of consciousness;
- any loss of memory for events immediately before or after the accident;
- any alteration in mental state at the time of the accident (e.g., feeling dazed, disoriented, or confused); and
- focal neurologic deficits, which may or may not be transient;

but in which the severity of injury does not exceed the following:

- loss of consciousness of approximately 30 minutes or less;
- after 30 minutes, an initial Glasgow Coma Scale score of 13-15; and
- post-traumatic amnesia not longer than 24 hours [1].

"Complicated" mTBI is characterized by the addition of intracranial abnormalities on computed tomography (CT) scan on the day of injury [2].

There are also several classification systems [3]. Table 147.1 presents a classification established by the American Academy of Neurology [4].

Bazarian and colleagues [5] reported the incidence of emergency department visits for mTBI to be 503 per 100,000, which is about 1.4 million emergency department visits for mTBI in the United States per year. This is similar to the Centers for Disease Control and Prevention estimate of 1.375 million [6]. However, the true numbers are probably considerably higher, given that a large percentage of people do not seek hospital treatment.

Symptoms

The most common postconcussion symptoms are headache, dizziness (often vertiginous) or poor balance, forgetfulness, difficulty in learning or remembering, difficulty in concentrating, slowed thinking, hypersomnolence, fatigue, insomnia, depression, anxiety, irritability, sensitivity to noise and light, and visual problems [7,8]. The most commonly used instrument for assessing the number and severity of postconcussion symptoms is the Rivermead Post-Concussion Symptoms Questionnaire, which has been found to have adequate divergent validity and reliability [9–11]. Criteria for "postconcussion syndrome" have been established by the *International Classification of Diseases, Ninth Revision* [12], the *International Statistical Classification of Diseases and Related Health Problems, Tenth Revision* [13], and the fourth edition of the *Diagnostic and Statistical Manual of Mental Disorders* [14]. However, symptoms may be present in a wide variety of both limited and extensive constellations and as such do not constitute a true syndrome [7,8]. There may be a lag of days or weeks between the concussion and the patient's first complaints, and some related phenomena, such as depression, may not become manifest until months after the initial injury. Although these symptoms can be seen with any severity of injury, they are often most pronounced in the context of mTBI. Over time, most people make a complete clinical recovery [11]. Although some authors have estimated that less than 5% still have symptoms 1 year after injury [15], studies vary considerably in this regard [16–18]. The prevalence of postconcussion symptoms is relatively high in healthy populations [15]; in people with whiplash and other painful conditions, depression, post-traumatic stress disorder (PTSD), and acute stress; and in

Table 147.1 American Academy of Neurology Classification of Mild Traumatic Brain Injury

Grade of Concussion	Characteristics
Grade 1	Transient confusion All symptoms <15 minutes and Mental status changes <15 minutes
Grade 2	Transient confusion Any symptoms >15 minutes and/or Mental status changes >15 minutes
Grade 3a	Brief loss of consciousness (seconds)
Grade 3b	Prolonged loss of consciousness (minutes)

From Practice parameter: the management of concussion in sports (summary statement). Report of the Quality Standards Subcommittee. Neurology 1997;48:581-585.

people litigating non-head injuries [19]. Nevertheless, one study found a difference of 31% between those who had mTBI and a non–head-injured control group with orthopedic injuries with respect to the number who had three or more symptoms 1 year after injury. However, these differences were significant only among those who were married and those who had higher levels of education [17].

The etiology of postconcussion symptoms is often multifactorial, and much of it is still not well understood. The usual inciting factors are mTBI with residual impairment of cognition, whiplash or other soft tissue injury to the head and neck, and at times disruption of the vestibular apparatus or central vestibular insult. Problems with attention, forgetfulness, and fatigue coupled with the frequent development of headaches, insomnia, and vertigo often lead to considerable anxiety and depression and a "shaken sense of self" [20]. In those who have persistent problems, a complex of symptoms often feed one on the other [7], exacerbating the cognitive impairment, which may then take on a life of its own even as the underlying brain injury continues to recover [20,21]. A common scenario is one in which pain, anxiety (including, at times, PTSD), and depression contribute to insomnia, which in turn exacerbates headaches, and all of these symptoms contribute to cognitive impairment [11]. Early on, as the symptoms attributable to brain injury gradually improve, the patient may not experience any cognitive improvement because other factors are driving these symptoms. The lack of improvement often increases the patient's anxiety and can bring about depressive feelings. A vicious circle ensues (Fig. 147.1). Difficulty in concentrating can also result in headaches, which exacerbates the complex. PTSD should be suspected in individuals who have reexperiences of the original injury ("flashbacks"), avoidance of situations similar to that which caused the injury (e.g., riding in a car), a feeling of emotional "numbness," and hyperarousal. There are high prevalence rates of PTSD, mTBI, and their co-occurrence in recently deployed soldiers [5].

There is evidence to suggest that persistence of symptoms is associated with a high number of early symptoms: acute headache, multiple painful areas, nausea, dizziness, or balance problems; early impaired memory; intoxication at the time of injury; intracranial lesions on the day of injury

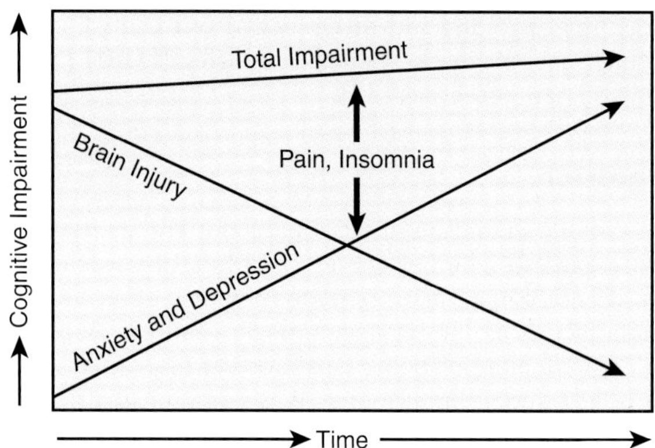

FIGURE 147.1 A possible postconcussion scenario: relationship between brain injury, emotions, pain, insomnia, and cognitive recovery.

CT scan; loss of white matter integrity on diffusion tensor imaging; preexisting social, psychological, and vocational difficulties; lack of social support; less education; lower socioeconomic status; age older than 40 years; being married; female gender; current student status; litigation or compensation; being out of work secondary to injury; motor vehicle crash as cause of injury; lack of fault for a collision; preexisting physical impairment; APOε4 genotype; and preexisting brain (including prior mTBI) and other neurologic problems. Studies vary with respect to some of these findings [8,11,15,22–26]. However, the total body of evidence regarding the causes of poor outcome after mTBI suggests a complex interaction among biologic, psychological, and social factors, with different factors varying in significance by the individual [27]. It is notable that people with mTBI have been found to underestimate the frequency of symptoms that they had *before* the injury, demonstrating a bias toward attributing current symptoms to the mTBI ("good old days bias") [17].

Most authors have not defined a particular time frame for the designation of "persistent" postconcussion symptoms; those who have done so have used 3 months as a cutoff [16,28]. The question of persistence of cognitive impairment after mTBI has been a subject of considerable controversy. Most controlled studies and meta-analyses indicate that cognitive deficits found on neuropsychological testing resolve within 3 months of mTBI, with the notable exception of complicated mTBI [2,29]. Most studies have been done with relatively young people, often athletes. Some studies have found subtle differences from controls [30,31] or differences on more demanding tests, such as dual-task performance, months or years after injury [32]. Subtle differences in balance have also been found among college football players who have had one or more concussions compared with those who have not [32]. Athletes who have had multiple concussions have been found to do worse on neuropsychological testing than controls [22,33]. There is a greater prevalence of mild cognitive impairment in later life [34] among professional football players who have had concussions than among those who have not had a concussion. These findings suggest that a single concussion may result in some loss of brain function, possibly subclinical in most people. In addition, individuals who have had one or more concussions months or years ago have been found to have evidence for loss of white matter integrity on diffusion tensor imaging [26] and differences from control subjects on functional magnetic resonance imaging (fMRI) [35] and event-related potentials [32].

Cognition

The patient should be questioned about the inciting event with regard to whether there was a loss of consciousness, loss of anterograde or retrograde memory, other alteration in mental status, or focal neurologic findings. A patient's subjective feeling of being dazed or confused may or may not reflect actual brain injury. It is common for people to feel dazed because of the emotional shock experienced after an accident. There is often limited or no documentation of the details of the patient's mental status immediately after the accident, and a clinician must do his or her best to reconstruct the situation largely on the basis of the history given by the patient. The observations of others may help clarify whether the patient was responding slowly or otherwise appeared confused. Emergency medical records should be obtained whenever possible but may or may not reflect the patient's mental status at the scene of the accident and may not pick up more subtle deficits if only orientation is evaluated.

Headaches

Tension, migraine, cervicogenic (musculoskeletal), and mixed headaches are the most frequent types seen after concussion. Pain from soft tissue injury at the site of impact, occipital neuralgic pain, and dysautonomic cephalgia can be seen as well. The patient should be questioned with respect to severity, quality, location and radiation, date of onset, duration, frequency, exacerbating or ameliorating factors, and frequency of medication use in addition to associated symptoms, such as nausea, vomiting, visual phenomenon, diaphoresis, rhinorrhea, and sensitivity to light and noise [36,37].

Vestibular/Balance Disorder

Vertigo and other illusory motion related to head movement or position as well as impaired balance can be caused by cupulolithiasis or canalithiasis (benign paroxysmal positional vertigo), brainstem injury, migraine-associated vertigo, labyrinthine concussion, or perilymph fistula or may be cervicogenic. Perilymph fistula and labyrinthine concussion are usually associated with hearing loss and tinnitus as well. Nonvertiginous dizziness is not usually directly related to concussion; medication-induced dizziness (e.g., by nonsteroidal anti-inflammatory drugs and antidepressants) and other causes should be considered, including psychogenic dizziness [38]. See also Chapter 8.

Sleep

A history of fatigue or daytime sleepiness should suggest the possibility of a sleep disorder. Delayed sleep phase syndrome and disrupted sleep-wake cycles can usually be diagnosed by history. Being overweight or obese or heavy snoring suggests obstructive sleep apnea. Difficulty in falling asleep and maintaining sleep can be determined by history [11].

Other

The physician's history of the events surrounding the initial accident should also include exploration of other associated injuries, seizure, vomiting, and drug or alcohol intoxication. A preinjury medical, social, psychological, vocational, and educational history should be obtained, including any history of attention deficit disorder or learning disability.

Physical Examination

Cognition

The examination of the individual with postconcussion symptoms will often elicit problems with attention, memory, and executive function on mental status evaluation. Memory problems are most often related to attention deficits or difficulty with retrieval [39]. The contribution of attention, encoding, and retrieval problems to verbal memory can be evaluated with the presentation of a word list followed by immediate recall, recall after 5 minutes, and then a multiple choice recognition task, which provides the structure needed to assist retrieval when information has been encoded. The Montreal Cognitive Assessment, which contains subtests that challenge executive function as well as memory and attention, is a useful tool to assess for cognitive impairment, although it has not been studied in traumatic brain injury [40]. However, findings on mental status testing may be normal; more extensive evaluation by neuropsychological testing, including reaction time [31] and continuous performance tasks, may be necessary to reveal the deficits. Findings inconsistent with daily functioning or more severe than would be expected for someone with mTBI indicate that there may be poor effort or other contributing factors [19,41]. See the section on differential diagnosis for potential contributing factors [20].

Psychological

Assessment of affect, demeanor, and behavior may reveal evidence of depression, anxiety, and other psychological characteristics. The Patient Health Questionnaire-9 is one approach to assessing depression. It is a brief questionnaire that mirrors the diagnostic criteria of the *Diagnostic and Statistical Manual of Mental Disorders* (fourth edition) for major depression. It has been found to be valid and reliable in people with traumatic brain injury [42]. The Primary Care PTSD Screen is another useful instrument. Those who screen in for PTSD should then receive a more thorough assessment [43].

Headaches

Examination of the head and neck often elicits restriction of motion, tender points, or trigger points radiating to the head. There may be tenderness at the site of the original head injury and occasionally pain elicited by compression of the occipital nerves [36,37]. See Chapters 102 and 105.

Vestibular/Balance Disorder

During acute vertigo, nystagmus will often be present, generally stronger with peripheral than with central vertigo.

As adaptation begins to occur, nystagmus may be seen only with certain maneuvers (e.g., after 20 horizontal head shakes) or may not be seen at all. When benign paroxysmal positional vertigo is the cause, the Hallpike-Dix maneuver is usually positive. This maneuver is performed from the sitting position on a flat surface with the head rotated 45 degrees to either side. The patient is quickly lowered from the sitting to the lying position, until the head, still rotated, is extended over the edge of the examining table. Vertigo is experienced and nystagmus seen after a lag of up to 30 seconds [38]. Neck range of motion and tender points or trigger points should be assessed for contributions from cervicogenic dizziness (see also Chapter 8). Patients with vertigo and other illusory movement may also have balance problems, but impaired balance with difficulty on tandem walk, standing on one leg, hopping, and other maneuvers may be seen without vertigo. The Balance Error Scoring System can provide a quantifiable assessment of balance [11].

Visual

Some patients complain of a feeling of visual disorientation or intermittent blurred vision. The symptoms can be related to a need for changes in refraction, accommodative dysfunction [44], or vascular, vestibular, attentional, or psychological problems. Frequently nothing will be found on routine examination.

Olfactory

The sense of smell may be affected by damage to branches of the olfactory nerve as they pass through the cribriform plate or by focal cortical contusion.

Other cranial nerve testing, muscle strength, cerebellar testing, deep tendon reflexes, plantar stimulation, and sensation are usually normal.

Functional Limitations

The extent to which postconcussion symptoms interfere with function varies with the extent of the associated pathologic process but depends also on the psychological reaction to the postconcussion impairments. The most common consequences of postconcussion symptoms are limitations in home and community living skills or social, academic, or vocational disability. Patients may be forgetful and inattentive, may have difficulty following conversations, and may find crowded, noisy environments difficult to tolerate. Headaches are often exacerbated by attentional demands and other stresses and may themselves contribute to inattentiveness. Vertigo or other illusory motion causes difficulty in tolerating motion, including, for some, moving vehicles, and may be associated with balance problems. Depression, anxiety, and irritability can contribute heavily to functional limitations.

Diagnostic Testing

The brain CT scan is the standard for the acute assessment of intracranial lesions after mTBI [45]. Indications for emergent CT scan include headache, vomiting, loss of consciousness or amnesia, alcohol intoxication, age older than 60 years, post-traumatic seizure, physical evidence of trauma above the clavicles, and current anticoagulant use [45,46]. Although definitive criteria have not been established for those who have had no loss of consciousness, it is probably wise to obtain a CT scan or MRI study for anyone who continues to have frequent headaches, severe lethargy, confusion, or anterograde memory loss or who has focal neurologic findings and has not had any neuroimaging acutely. MRI with susceptibility-weighted imaging is more likely to show microhemorrhage related to diffuse axonal injury [26]. Event-related potentials [32], serum biomarkers (such as S100B [47]), advanced magnetic resonance techniques (such as diffusion tensor imaging [26] and fMRI [35]), and metabolic imaging (such as positron emission tomography, single-photon emission computed tomography, and magnetic resonance spectroscopy [48]) have shown promise but have not yet been studied thoroughly enough to be used routinely to answer clinical questions after mTBI [49].

Cervical spine radiographs should be obtained for patients with significant neck pain shortly after the accident to assess for fracture or subluxation.

Neuropsychological evaluation should be performed if cognitive deficits persist, particularly when rehabilitation therapies are to be pursued. Testing can provide the patient and the treatment team with a more thorough understanding of the patient's neuropsychological strengths and weaknesses and in some instances can assist with understanding of the interplay between neurocognitive and other psychological contributions to cognitive disturbance. Tests for assessment of malingering and symptom magnification ("effort testing") can be incorporated when necessary. In one study, people with mTBI for whom financial compensation was available, and who were referred for neuropsychological testing an average of 19.4 months after injury, had a 26.7% failure rate for effort testing (Test of Memory Malingering). Those with better benefits had a higher rate than those with modest benefits [50]. However, symptom magnification does not eliminate the possibility that the person has real cognitive deficits as well. It is useful for sports teams to have their players undergo at least a brief baseline cognitive testing or, if the resources are available, formal neuropsychological testing so that any changes can be identified after the concussion [51]. A history of attention deficit/hyperactivity disorder or learning disability, certain medications or abused substances, depression, anxiety, pain, sleep disorders, malingering, symptom exaggeration, and even expectation of the cognitive effects of mTBI can lower test performance [52]. On the other hand, normal findings on testing do not preclude a more subtle but significant underlying cognitive impairment.

A sleep study (polysomnography) is indicated to rule out sleep apnea and other disorders when excessive daytime sleepiness does not improve despite the absence of sedating medications. The threshold for obtaining polysomnography should be lower for overweight or obese patients or those who snore prominently. When vestibular complaints are prominent or are not improving in the early months after the injury, a thorough vestibular evaluation, including electronystagmography, may be indicated. Audiologic evaluations should be done when hearing loss is suspected or when tinnitus persists [38]. Ophthalmology or optometry evaluation by someone with particular expertise in visual problems related to brain injury should be considered when visual symptoms are present. Although post-traumatic neuroendocrine dysfunction is more commonly found among those with more severe traumatic brain injury, even mTBI may be associated with pituitary dysfunction. Schneider and coworkers [53] found a prevalence of endocrine disorders of 16.8% among patients with mTBI and persistent postconcussion symptoms. Neuroendocrine testing should be considered in individuals with mTBI who have persistent fatigue, cognitive difficulties, behavioral changes, or depression as these can be symptoms of post-traumatic hypopituitarism. Other manifestations include decreased libido, amenorrhea, myopathy, and life-threatening complications such as sodium dysregulation and adrenal crisis [54]. Recommended screening includes serum free thyroxine, thyroid-stimulating hormone, morning cortisol, prolactin, and insulin-like growth factor 1 levels; testosterone concentration in men; and follicle-stimulating hormone concentration in postmenopausal women or premenopausal women with amenorrhea [55].

Differential Diagnosis [11,23]

Depressive disorders
Anxiety disorders, including post-traumatic stress disorder
Somatoform disorder
Whiplash injury with associated headache (myofascial pain syndrome)
Other chronic pain
Insomnia
Sleep apnea
Endocrine disorders
Other medical illness
Substance abuse
Prescription medications
Early progressive dementias
Malingering and symptom magnification

Treatment

Initial

Treatment will depend on the specific constellation of symptoms and their severity. In general, if the patient is seen in the first few weeks after the injury, the major emphasis should be placed on caring for acute problems with headache, neck pain, and insomnia as these symptoms tend to be more responsive to early treatment than cognitive impairment and dizziness. However, education of the patient and significant others is the most important early intervention. Explanations should integrate the physical, cognitive, and psychological dimensions of the symptoms in as clear and simple a manner as possible. This is no small task, given the diversity of symptoms and possible causes and our limited understanding of postconcussion disorders at this time. Some patients are very sensitive to discussions of psychological etiology and may not return if they believe that this has been overemphasized. The patient's experience, including the psychological reactions, should be validated and normalized [20]. The patient should be told that improvement is to be expected, and after concussions without high-risk factors (e.g., numerous previous concussions, complicated mTBI), reasonable reassurance should be given that a good recovery is likely without dismissing what the patient is experiencing. Establishing a reasonable expectation for recovery can be helpful in preventing postconcussion symptoms [56,57]. Anticipating the psychological reactions to postconcussion symptoms that occur in some patients allows the patients to recognize these reactions if they begin and leaves the door open for them to seek psychological help. Follow-up should be planned and more extensive counseling provided at the first signs of significant distress. Patients with significant symptoms should be instructed to take time off from work, school, or other taxing activities as the attentional demands and accompanying psychological stresses of attempting to perform under these circumstances can exacerbate the symptoms [23]. All patients should be instructed not to drive for at least the first 24 hours, longer when they have had post-traumatic seizures, slow processing speed, attention deficits, dizziness, and visual or other symptoms that are likely to interfere [11].

Athletes should not go back to competitive sports on the day of injury until they are free of symptoms and have gone through a program of graded exertion symptom free. Those with more severe concussions should move through this program more slowly [51]. Refer to Table 147.2 for guidelines for the stepwise return to sports activities.

Table 147.2 Template for Stepwise Return to Sports

Stage	Activity	Objective
No activity	Symptom-limited physical and cognitive	Rest and recovery
Light aerobic exercise	Walking, swimming, or stationary bicycle, keeping intensity less than 70% of maximum predicted heart rate; no resistance training	Modest increase in heart rate
Sport-specific exercise	Skating drills in ice hockey, running drills in soccer; no head impact activities	Further increase in heart rate in sport-specific context
Noncontact training drills	Progression to more complex training drills (e.g., passing drills in football and ice hockey); may start progressive resistance training	Challenge agility, coordination, and cognitive aspects of sport
Full-contact practice	Following medical clearance, participate in normal training activities	Full physical and cognitive challenge; restore confidence and allow coaching staff to assess functional skills
Return to play	Normal game play	

Modified from McCrory P, Meeuwisse W, Johnston K, et al. Consensus statement on concussion in sport—the 3rd International Conference on Concussion in Sport held in Zurich, November 2008. PM R 2009;1:406-420.

Severe acute vertigo may require a few days of bed rest [38], but only if it is absolutely necessary. The management of acute neck pain is described in Chapter 6.

Rehabilitation

Cognition

If symptoms persist, patients may benefit from speech or occupational therapy to learn strategies for compensating for problems with arousal, attention, memory, and executive function and, later, training for internal compensation and restoration of cognitive skills [58–61]. The timing of therapies depends on the severity of the disability and the pace of recovery, which can often be determined within the first 3 months after injury. There are no published data on the optimal timing of these interventions, and no specific guidelines are available. Therapies should address the specific functional tasks that the individual faces on a daily basis and may need to include community outings. Foam earplugs or sunglasses can be tried for those sensitive to noise and light, respectively. Paper or electronic memory aids may be helpful. Psychostimulants and dopaminergic drugs (e.g., methylphenidate, amphetamines, atomoxetine, donepezil, modafinil, armodafinil, amantadine) and cholinesterase inhibitors (e.g., donepezil, 5-23 mg daily) that treat attentional and arousal disorders may be useful for reducing the extent of attention deficits and underarousal [62,63]. When sleep apnea is contributing to cognitive problems, positive airway pressure therapy, sleep position changes, or custom dental devices are indicated. Both resistance and aerobic exercises can result in improved cognitive function [64,65]. Exercise may also benefit other postconcussion symptoms when heart rate is kept below the rate that provokes symptoms [66]. There is some evidence to suggest that acupressure may also result in improved cognitive function [67].

Psychological

If symptoms persist beyond a few months, psychological counseling is almost always indicated. Some individuals benefit from learning relaxation techniques and sleep hygiene. Cognitive-behavioral therapy focused on sleep issues can help insomnia [68]. Education of the patient and significant others should continue to emphasize the interaction between the cognitive, psychological, and physical sequelae. It is important that the rehabilitation team communicate on a regular basis for treatment planning and to ensure that all clinicians approach these issues from a common framework so that mixed messages are not delivered to the patient. Support groups are often useful as well and offer an opportunity for further education about the various contributing factors. Cognitive-behavioral therapy can be helpful in concert with other treatments [69] even when symptoms do not seem to be explained by the medical condition [70]. It can target depression, anxiety, insomnia, pain, and probably other postconcussion symptoms as well. Other psychotherapy approaches include acceptance and commitment therapy and self-management, both of which focus on improving daily function rather than on improving symptoms [52]. Family counseling should be offered when there is evidence of significant stress on family members or problem family dynamics.

Depression and anxiety can also be addressed pharmacologically when they are severe and prolonged, contributing to cognitive impairment, or interfering with progress in rehabilitation, usually after or simultaneously with counseling interventions. It is generally best to begin with nonsedating, nonanticholinergic agents, such as the selective serotonin reuptake inhibitors (e.g., sertraline), to avoid further exacerbation of neuropsychological problems [62]. Cognitive status has been found to improve after treatment with sertraline [71]. Sedating agents, such as trazodone, zolpidem, or eszopiclone, may be necessary for those with significant insomnia [62] if treatment of depression and anxiety and sleep hygiene approaches are not successful. Zolpidem (10 mg at bedtime) can cause cognitive impairment in the morning [72]. Melatonin (0.5-3 mg) can be helpful, especially with delayed sleep phase disorder.

Headaches

Post-traumatic headaches can have a number of different causes and may be multifactorial [21,23,24,36–38]. They are therefore best addressed on multiple levels, with the emphasis depending on the headache type [73]. Treating problems with attention, sleep disorders, and psychological stresses may reduce the tension component of headaches. Relaxation techniques, including electromyographic biofeedback, can be taught. When myofascial pain originating in the neck, upper back, or temporomandibular joints contributes, physical therapy including stretching and strengthening exercises, postural retraining, environmental modification, trigger point massage, modalities, electromyographic biofeedback, or massage should be tried. However, headaches often persist despite these interventions. Trigger point, facet joint, and other injections can be helpful, as can acupuncture and pharmacologic approaches. Patients with temporomandibular joint problems can be treated with myofascial techniques, mouthguards, and exercises.

Those headaches that fit the criteria for migraine headaches may respond to acetaminophen, nonsteroidal anti-inflammatory drugs, or vasoconstrictive agents commonly used to abort migraine headaches (e.g., sumatriptan). Overuse of these agents can cause rebound headaches. For prophylaxis, anticonvulsants (particularly gabapentin and valproic acid), beta blockers (e.g., propranolol), calcium channel blockers (e.g., verapamil), and antidepressants (e.g., amitriptyline, nortriptyline, fluoxetine, venlafaxine) can be helpful. Topiramate often provides some relief but causes too much cognitive decline to be used as a first-line drug [74]. However, if it relieves frequent headaches that themselves are causing cognitive impairment, the tradeoff may be favorable. Tension headaches may respond to some of these agents as well, although not to calcium channel blockers. Injection of local anesthetics or corticosteroids can be considered for greater or lesser occipital neuralgia that does not respond to more conservative approaches. Injection should be done at the site along the nerve that replicates the headache when it is palpated [36,73] (see Chapter 102).

Vestibular/Balance Disorder

When vestibular symptoms persist beyond 3 months, vestibular rehabilitation may both encourage central nervous system accommodation under controlled circumstances and assist the patient in learning compensatory strategies [75]. Canalith repositioning maneuvers may bring relief from benign paroxysmal positional vertigo by displacing and dispersing calcium stones [76]. Suppressive medications (e.g., clonazepam, scopolamine, meclizine) should be used judiciously, if at all, when other approaches have failed [38]. The evidence for their efficacy is not strong, and they can cause worsening of problems with attention and memory. Frequent vertigo or other illusory motion in people with migraine headaches (migraine-associated vertigo) is best treated preventively with tricyclic antidepressants, beta blockers, or calcium channel blockers and vestibular rehabilitation. Cervicogenic dizziness can be treated by addressing the underlying cervical musculoskeletal problems (see Chapter 8). Physical therapy can help improve balance.

Vocational

The extent to which an employer or academic institution is supportive after mTBI can be crucial to successful return to work for those with persistent postconcussion symptoms. Vocational counselors can facilitate communication between the patient and the workplace. Therapies should attempt to simulate workplace tasks. A gradual return to work can ease the transition [20].

Procedures

Procedures are discussed in the preceding sections.

Surgery

There is little that can be done surgically to manage postconcussion disorders.

Potential Disease Complications

Persistence of postconcussion symptoms beyond a few months is a possible outcome. Individuals who sustain a second concussion while still symptomatic from a recent concussion may be susceptible to cerebral edema and dangerous increases in intracranial pressure ("second impact syndrome") [77], although some have questioned the existence of such a syndrome [78]. Multiple concussions, even after apparent clinical recovery from earlier episodes, can result in cumulative brain injury with permanent cognitive impairment or even dementia, at times with parkinsonian motor features, depression, or aggression in later life. Unique patterns of pathologic findings consistent with chronic traumatic encephalopathy have been found on autopsy in 68 of 85 people who have had multiple concussions who donated their brains. Most were boxers, football and hockey players, or military veterans. Most had developed cognitive impairment, sometimes associated with depression and suicide [79,80]. The incidence of chronic traumatic encephalopathy is unknown. Athletes and their parents (in youth) may want to discontinue involvement in high-risk sports after one or more concussions or may want to avoid such sports altogether. Caution must be exercised by those responsible for returning athletes to play.

Potential Treatment Complications

Those treating the patient with postconcussion symptoms may contribute to the persistence of symptoms either by overemphasizing the role of brain injury in causing symptoms with another etiology or, conversely, by overemphasizing psychological factors when brain injury and other physiologic variables are prominent [20,23]. There is often a fine line to be walked, and each patient must be approached individually in this regard, although there are few data available to guide the clinician.

Some of the complications related to medications can appear paradoxical. The frequent use of analgesics (nonsteroidal anti-inflammatory drugs, acetaminophen, and narcotics) can cause rebound headaches, as can the too frequent use of ergotamine and the "triptans." Although they are generally well tolerated, psychostimulants and dopaminergic agents can lead to sedation, worsening attention, irritability, or psychosis. There are myriad other complications possible from the use of the medications mentioned.

References

[1] Carroll LJ, Cassidy JD, Holm L, et al. Methodological issues and research recommendations for mild traumatic brain injury: the WHO Collaborating Centre Task Force on Mild Traumatic Brain Injury. J Rehabil Med 2004;43(Suppl.):113–25.

[2] Williams DH, Levin HS, Eisenberg HM. Mild head injury classification. Neurosurgery 1990;27:422–8.

[3] McCrea M. Mild traumatic brain injury and post concussion syndrome: the new evidence base for diagnosis and treatment. New York: Oxford University Press; 2008, Oxford Workshop Series, American Academy of Clinical Neuropsychology.

[4] Practice parameter: the management of concussion in sports (summary statement). Report of the Quality Standards Subcommittee. Neurology 1997;48:581–5.

[5] Bazarian JJ, Donnelly K, Peterson DR, et al. The relation between posttraumatic stress disorder and mild traumatic brain injury acquired during Operations Enduring Freedom and Iraqi Freedom. J Head Trauma Rehabil 2013;28:1–12.

[6] Centers for Disease Control and Prevention. Traumatic brain injury. http://www.cdc.gov/traumaticbraininjury/statistics.html; [accessed 31.01.13].

[7] Cicerone KD, Kalmar K. Persistent postconcussion syndrome: the structure of subjective complaints after mild traumatic brain injury. J Head Trauma Rehabil 1995;10:1–17.

[8] Kraus J, Hsu P, Schaffer K, et al. Preinjury factors and 3-month outcomes following emergency department diagnosis of mild traumatic brain injury. J Head Trauma Rehabil 2009;24:344–54.

[9] King NS, Crawford S, Wenden FJ, et al. The Rivermead Post Concussion Symptoms Questionnaire: a measure of symptoms commonly experienced after head injury and its reliability. J Neurol 1995;242:587–92.

[10] Eyres S, Carey A, Gilworth G, et al. Construct validity and reliability of the Rivermead Post-Concussion Symptoms Questionnaire. Clin Rehabil 2005;19:878–87.

[11] Guidelines Development Team. Guidelines for mild traumatic brain injury and persistent symptoms. Ontario Neurotrauma Foundation; 2010.

[12] International classification of diseases, 9th revision, clinical modification (ICD-9-CM). Geneva: World Health Organization; 1975, updated 2012.

[13] International statistical classification of disease and related health problems. 10th ed. Geneva: World Health Organization; 1992, updated 2012.

[14] Diagnostic and statistical manual of mental disorders. 4th ed. Washington, DC: American Psychiatric Association; 1994.

[15] Iverson GL. Outcome from mild traumatic brain injury. Curr Opin Psychiatry 2005;18:301–17.

[16] Ingebrigtsen T, Waterloo K, Marup-Jensen S, et al. Quantification of post-concussion symptoms 3 months after minor head injury in 100 consecutive patients. J Neurol 1998;245:609–12.

[17] Mickeviciene D, Schrader H, Obelieniene D, et al. A controlled prospective inception cohort study on the post-concussion syndrome outside the medicolegal context. Eur J Neurol 2004;11:411–9.

[18] Masson F, Maurette P, Salmi LR, et al. Prevalence of impairments 5 years after a head injury, and their relationship with disabilities and outcome. Brain Inj 1996;10:487–97.

[19] Rohling ML, Demakis GJ. Bowden, Shores, & Mathias (2006): failure to replicate or just failure to notice. Does effort still account for more variance in neuropsychological test scores than TBI severity? Clin Neuropsychol 2010;24:119–36.

[20] Kay T. Neuropsychological treatment of mild traumatic brain injury. J Head Trauma Rehabil 1993;8:74–85.

[21] Martelli MF, Grayson RL, Zasler ND. Posttraumatic headache: neuropsychological and psychological effects and treatment implications. J Head Trauma Rehabil 1999;14:49–69.

[22] Collins MW, Grindel SH, Lovell MR, et al. Relationship between concussion and neuropsychological performance in college football players. JAMA 1999;282:964–70.

[23] Alexander MP. Minor traumatic brain injury: a review of physiogenesis and psychogenesis. Semin Clin Neuropsychiatry 1997;2:177–87.

[24] Fenton G, McClelland R, Montgomery A, et al. The postconcussional syndrome: social antecedents and psychological sequelae. Br J Psychiatry 1993;162:493–7.

[25] Muller K, Ingebrigtsen T, Wilsgaard T, et al. Prediction of time trends in recovery of cognitive function after mild head injury. Neurosurgery 2009;64:698–704, discussion 704.

[26] Shenton ME, Hamoda HM, Schneiderman JS, et al. A review of magnetic resonance imaging and diffusion tensor imaging findings in mild traumatic brain injury. Brain Imaging Behav 2012;6:137–92.

[27] Iverson GL. A biopsychosocial conceptualization of poor outcome from mild traumatic brain injury. In: Vateling J, Bryant R, Keane T, editors. PTSD and mild traumatic brain injury. New York: Guilford Press; 2012.

[28] McHugh T, Laforce Jr R, Gallagher P, et al. Natural history of the long-term cognitive, affective, and physical sequelae of mild traumatic brain injury. Brain Cogn 2006;60:209–11.

[29] Kashluba S, Hanks RA, Casey JE, Millis SR. Neuropsychologic and functional outcome after complicated mild traumatic brain injury. Arch Phys Med Rehabil 2008;89:904–11.

[30] Vanderploeg RD, Curtiss G, Belanger HG. Long-term neuropsychological outcomes following mild traumatic brain injury. J Int Neuropsychol Soc 2005;11:228–36.

[31] Bleiberg J, Halpern EL, Reeves D, Daniel JC. Future directions for the neuropsychological assessment of sports concussion. J Head Trauma Rehabil 1998;13:36–44.

[32] Broglio SP, Eckner JT, Paulson HL, Kutcher JS. Cognitive decline and aging: the role of concussive and subconcussive impacts. Exerc Sport Sci Rev 2012;40:138–44.

[33] Belanger HG, Spiegel E, Vanderploeg RD. Neuropsychological performance following a history of multiple self-reported concussions: a meta-analysis. J Int Neuropsychol Soc 2010;16:262–7.

[34] Guskiewicz KM, Marshall SW, Bailes J, et al. Association between recurrent concussion and late-life cognitive impairment in retired professional football players. Neurosurgery 2005;57:719–26, discussion 719–726.

[35] McDonald BC, Saykin AJ, McAllister TW. Functional MRI of mild traumatic brain injury (mTBI): progress and perspectives from the first decade of studies. Brain Imaging Behav 2012;6:193–207.

[36] Lew HL, Lin PH, Fuh JL, et al. Characteristics and treatment of headache after traumatic brain injury: a focused review. Am J Phys Med Rehabil 2006;85:619–27.

[37] Zafonte RD, Horn LJ. Clinical assessment of posttraumatic headaches. J Head Trauma Rehabil 1999;14:22–33.

[38] Tusa RJ, Brown SB. Neuro-otologic trauma and dizziness. In: Rizzo M, Tranel D, editors. Head Injury and postconcussive syndrome. New York: Churchill Livingstone; 1996. p. 177–200.

[39] Nolin P. Executive memory dysfunctions following mild traumatic brain injury. J Head Trauma Rehabil 2006;21:68–75.

[40] Nasreddine Z. The Montreal Cognitive Assessment. Available at http://mocatest.org/. Accessed December 11, 2012.

[41] Larson EB, Kondiles BR, Starr CR, Zollman FS. Postconcussive complaints, cognition, symptom attribution, and effort among veterans. J Int Neuropsychol Soc 2013;19:1–18.

[42] Fann JR, Bombardier CH, Dikmen S, et al. Validity of the Patient Health Questionnaire-9 in assessing depression following traumatic brain injury. J Head Trauma Rehabil 2005;20:501–11.

[43] Prins A, Ouimette PC, Kimerling R, et al. The primary care PTSD screen (PC-PTSD): development and operating characteristics. Prim Care Psychiatr 2004;9:9–14.

[44] Leslie S. Accommodation in acquired brain injury. In: Suchoff IB, Ciuffreda KJ, Kapoor N, editors. Visual and vestibular consequences of acquired brain injury. Santa Ana, Calif: Optometric Extension Program; 2001. p. 56–76.

[45] Sharif-Alhoseini M, Khodadadi H, Chardoli M, Rahimi-Movaghar V. Indications for brain computed tomography scan after minor head injury. J Emerg Trauma Shock 2011;4:472–6.

[46] Haydel MJ, Preston CA, Mills TJ, et al. Indications for computed tomography in patients with minor head injury. N Engl J Med 2000;343:100–5.

[47] Unden J, Romner B. Can low serum levels of S100B predict normal CT findings after minor head injury in adults? An evidence-based review and meta-analysis. J Head Trauma Rehabil 2010;25:228–40.

[48] Lin AP, Liao HJ, Merugumala SK, et al. Metabolic imaging of mild traumatic brain injury. Brain Imaging Behav 2012;6:208–23.

[49] Kou Z, Wu Z, Tong KA, et al. The role of advanced MR imaging findings as biomarkers of traumatic brain injury. J Head Trauma Rehabil 2010;25:267–82.

[50] Bianchini KJ, Curtis KL, Greve KW. Compensation and malingering in traumatic brain injury: a dose-response relationship? Clin Neuropsychol 2006;20:831–47.

[51] McCrory P, Meeuwisse W, Johnston K, et al. Consensus statement on concussion in sport: the 3rd international conference on concussion in sport held in Zurich, November 2008. Br J Sports Med 2009;43(Suppl. 1):i76–90.

[52] Iverson GL, Silverberg N, Lange RT, Zasler ND. Conceptualizing outcome from mild traumatic brain injury. In: Zasler ND, Katz DI, Zafonte RD, editors. Brain injury medicine: principles and practice. 2nd ed. New York: Demos Medical; 2013. p. 470–97.

[53] Schneider HJ, Kreitschmann-Andermahr I, Ghigo E, et al. Hypothalamopituitary dysfunction following traumatic brain injury and aneurysmal subarachnoid hemorrhage: a systematic review. JAMA 2007;298:1429–38.

[54] Zaben M, El Ghoul W, Belli A. Post-traumatic head injury pituitary dysfunction. Disabil Rehabil 2013;35:522–5.

[55] Ghigo E, Masel B, Aimaretti G, et al. Consensus guidelines on screening for hypopituitarism following traumatic brain injury. Brain Inj 2005;19:711–24.

[56] Mittenberg W, Tremont G, Zielinski RE, et al. Cognitive-behavioral prevention of postconcussion syndrome. Arch Clin Neuropsychol 1996;11:139–45.

[57] Ponsford J, Willmott C, Rothwell A, et al. Impact of early intervention on outcome following mild head injury in adults. J Neurol Neurosurg Psychiatry 2002;73:330–2.

[58] Cicerone KD, Dahlberg C, Kalmar K, et al. Evidence-based cognitive rehabilitation: recommendations for clinical practice. Arch Phys Med Rehabil 2000;81:1596–615.

[59] Cicerone KD, Dahlberg C, Malec JF, et al. Evidence-based cognitive rehabilitation: updated review of the literature from 1998 through 2002. Arch Phys Med Rehabil 2005;86:1681–92.

[60] Cicerone KD, Langenbahn DM, Braden C, et al. Evidence-based cognitive rehabilitation: updated review of the literature from 2003 through 2008. Arch Phys Med Rehabil 2011;92:519–30.

[61] O'Neil-Pirozzi TM, Strangman GE, Goldstein R, et al. A controlled treatment study of internal memory strategies (I-MEMS) following traumatic brain injury. J Head Trauma Rehabil 2010;25:43–51.

[62] Glenn MB, Wroblewski B. Twenty years of pharmacology. J Head Trauma Rehabil 2005;20:51–61.

[63] Chew E, Zafonte RD. Pharmacological management of neurobehavioral disorders following traumatic brain injury—a state-of-the-art review. J Rehabil Res Dev 2009;46:851–79.

[64] Angevaren M, Aufdemkampe G, Verhaar HJ, et al. Physical activity and enhanced fitness to improve cognitive function in older people without known cognitive impairment. Cochrane Database Syst Rev 2008;3, CD005381.

[65] Liu-Ambrose T, Eng JJ, Boyd LA, et al. Promotion of the mind through exercise (PROMoTE): a proof-of-concept randomized controlled trial of aerobic exercise training in older adults with vascular cognitive impairment. BMC Neurol 2013;10:14.

[66] Leddy JJ, Kozlowski K, Donnelly JP, et al. A preliminary study of subsymptom threshold exercise training for refractory post-concussion syndrome. Clin J Sport Med 2010;20:21–7.

[67] McFadden KL, Healy KM, Dettmann ML, et al. Acupressure as a non-pharmacological intervention for traumatic brain injury (TBI). J Neurotrauma 2011;28:21–34.

[68] Mitchell MD, Gehrman P, Perlis M, Umscheid CA. Comparative effectiveness of cognitive behavioral therapy for insomnia: a systematic review. BMC Fam Pract 2012;13:40.

[69] Andersson G, Asmundson GJ, Denev J, et al. A controlled trial of cognitive-behavior therapy combined with vestibular rehabilitation in the treatment of dizziness. Behav Res Ther 2006;44:1265–73.

[70] Smith RC, Lyles JS, Gardiner JC, et al. Primary care clinicians treat patients with medically unexplained symptoms: a randomized controlled trial. J Gen Intern Med 2006;21:671–7.

[71] Fann JR, Uomoto JM, Katon WJ. Cognitive improvement with treatment of depression following mild traumatic brain injury. Psychosomatics 2001;42:48–54.

[72] Larson EB, Zollman FS. The effect of sleep medications on cognitive recovery from traumatic brain injury. J Head Trauma Rehabil 2010;25:61–7.

[73] Watanabe TK, Bell KR, Walker WC, Schomer K. Systematic review of interventions for post-traumatic headache. PM R 2012;4:129–40.

[74] Gomer B, Wagner K, Frings L, et al. Cognitive effects of levetiracetam versus topiramate. Epilepsy Current 2008;8:64–5.

[75] Wrisley DM, Pavlou M. Physical therapy for balance disorders. Neurol Clin 2005;23:855–74, Vii–viii.

[76] White J, Savvides P, Cherian N, Oas J. Canalith repositioning for benign paroxysmal positional vertigo. Otol Neurotol 2005;26:704–10.

[77] Thomas M, Haas TS, Doerer JJ, et al. Epidemiology of sudden death in young, competitive athletes due to blunt trauma. Pediatrics 2011;128:e1–8.

[78] McCrory P, Davis G, Makdissi M. Second impact syndrome or cerebral swelling after sporting head injury. Curr Sports Med Rep 2012;11:21–3.

[79] McKee AC, Stein TD, Nowinski CJ, et al. The spectrum of disease in chronic traumatic encephalopathy. Brain 2012;136(Pt 1):43–64.

[80] Baugh CM, Stamm JM, Riley DO, et al. Chronic traumatic encephalopathy: neurodegeneration following repetitive concussive and subconcussive brain trauma. Brain Imaging Behav 2012;6:244–54.

CHAPTER 148

Pressure Ulcers

Chester H. Ho, MD
Kath Bogie, DPhil

Synonyms

Decubitus ulcers
Pressure sores
Bedsores

ICD-9 Codes

707.00 Decubitus ulcer, unspecified site
707.20 Decubitus ulcer, unspecified stage

ICD-10 Code

L89.90 Pressure ulcer of unspecified site, unspecified stage

Definition

A pressure ulcer is a localized injury to the skin or underlying tissue, usually over a bone prominence, as a result of pressure or pressure in combination with shear [1]. The development of pressure ulcers due to tissue breakdown and cell necrosis is a significant problem for many patients, including the elderly and those with impaired mobility or paralysis. Pressure ulcers are associated with significant morbidity and even mortality; they can cause pain as well as decreased activities of daily living and quality of life [2]. Therefore this is a pertinent issue for many patients in rehabilitation. Furthermore, they are extremely costly; the burden on the U.S. health care system has recently been estimated at $6 to $15 billion per year [3].

Tissue breakdown is referred to by many terms, including decubitus ulcers, pressure sores, ischemic sores, and bedsores. The term *pressure ulcer* is the most accurate nomenclature to describe both the cause and nature of chronic, nonhealing wounds due primarily to excessive applied pressure. This term is used throughout the chapter.

The incidence of pressure ulcers among patients in acute care hospitals ranges from 1% to 33%, with prevalence rates of 3% to 69% [4,5]. Higher rates have been associated with increasing age and duration of hospital stay in the elderly [6]. In those with spinal cord injury, individuals with paraplegia are more likely to be rehospitalized because of pressure ulcers [7]. The prevalence of pressure ulcers on admission to skilled nursing facilities ranges between 10% and 26% [8,9]. A multicenter study of pressure ulcer incidence in spinal cord injury conducted across the U.S. Model Spinal Cord Injury System [10] found a significant trend toward increasing pressure ulcer prevalence more recently; the most recent period covered by this study was 2002. A consideration of the risk factors in pressure ulcer development is of vital importance because they contribute to the formulation of treatment and rehabilitation strategies. There are many factors that can lead to the development of pressure ulcers. These can be generally classified as intrinsic factors, which are related to the clinical and physiologic profile of the individual, and extrinsic factors, which are primarily attributed to the external environment (Table 148.1). These intrinsic and extrinsic factors can overlap. They highlight the complex nature of the development of pressure ulcers and are indicative of the need for a holistic and systematic approach to prevent their formation.

Intrinsic Risk Factors

Intrinsic risk factors in pressure ulcer development are related to the conditions of the individual patient. Decreased muscle activity and paralysis lead to loss of muscle bulk, thus reducing soft tissue coverage over the bone prominences of the pelvic and other anatomic regions. As muscle bulk decreases, regional vascularity diminishes and the proportion of avascular fatty tissue increases. Loss of normal muscle tone leads to abnormal responses to environmental stimuli, such as applied pressure, thus increasing the risk for blood flow to become compromised.

Furthermore, motor paralysis will directly affect a person's ability to respond unconsciously to potential noxious stimuli (e.g., fidgeting while sitting or turning while asleep). Reduced mobility also profoundly alters the individual's ability to consciously perform postural maneuvers necessary to relieve prolonged applied pressure, from weight shifting while sitting to walking. The loss or reduction of mobility may be further complicated by sensory impairment, leading to the absence or alteration of normal perception of environmental stimuli, such as pain or temperature. Patients with impaired sensation or proprioception are at increased

Table 148.1 Risk Factors in Pressure Ulcer Development

Extrinsic Factors	Intrinsic Factors
Applied pressure Surface shear Local microenvironment	Reduced or absent sensation Impaired mobility Decreased blood flow Muscle atrophy Poor nutrition Systemic diseases (e.g., diabetes) Altered mental status

risk for pressure ulcer development because they cannot sense the warning signals that precede tissue damage.

The malnourished patient is at increased risk for pressure ulcer development and will also have an impaired response to healing. Normal tissue integrity depends on correct nitrogen balance and vitamin intake. Protein depletion will lead to decreased perfusion and impaired immune response. The presence of an exuding pressure ulcer will cause massive protein loss, and the patient will move into increasingly negative nitrogen balance. The severity of a pressure ulcer can be directly related to the degree of hypoalbuminemia [11]. Fluid balance must also be considered in conjunction with nutritional status because dehydration will decrease cellular nutrient delivery.

Patients with systemic diseases may be at higher risk of pressure ulcers. For instance, those with renal disease and diabetes may be more prone to pressure ulcer formation because of their peripheral vascular status. The cognitive and mental status of an individual may also affect the ability to perform pressure relief for at-risk body areas, hence potentially increasing the risk of pressure ulcer formation.

Bowel and bladder incontinence causing excessive local moisture may alter the microenvironment of the skin surface, making it more susceptible to maceration and skin breakdown.

Extrinsic Risk Factors

The primary extrinsic risk factor is external applied pressure. Body tissues can support high levels of hydrostatic pressure, such as in deep sea diving. When pressure is the same in all directions, there is no resulting tissue damage. However, nonuniform applied pressures cause tissue distortion, leading to localized tissue damage. This will occur when a patient is in contact with an external load-supporting device, such as a bed or wheelchair. The pressure at the interface between the patient and the support surface must be maintained at a level such that the local blood supply and lymphatic circulation are not impaired. This threshold varies between individuals, and a specialized support system is often required in high-risk individuals, such as acute spinal cord–injured patients.

Any external load that can cause tissue distortion is also likely to cause shear stresses. When only shear forces are present, slipping occurs, and tissue damage will be minimized. However, shear and normal applied loads generally tend to occur together. The normal applied load required to occlude blood flow can be halved when shear forces are also present [12]. Significant clinical problems can arise from propping patients up in bed at angles of less than 90 degrees. In contrast, in the side-lying position, it has been found that blood flow is severely impaired by fully lying on the trochanteric region; but at a partial, 30-degree side-lying position, blood flow is maintained [13].

Symptoms

The primary symptoms of a pressure ulcer are due to an area of persistent tissue breakdown involving the skin and underlying tissues. The patients may complain of an open area in the skin, drainage, bleeding, odor, fever, and pain. The severity of pressure ulcers has traditionally been characterized by the extent of breakdown, as described by a staging system.

Physical Examination

Physical examination for a pressure ulcer starts with an overall assessment of the risk factors of the individual and his or her environment. During general examination, evaluation of overall strength, muscle tone, spasticity, range of motion, and presence of contractures is important. Abnormalities in these areas can contribute to both the development and the persistence of pressure ulcers. In addition, it is important to note whether the individual is malnourished, anemic, incontinent of feces or urine, cognitively impaired, or immobile from medical conditions such as stroke or spinal cord injury as well as whether appropriate pressure-relieving surfaces for seating and sleeping have been used. The Braden Scale is a commonly used nursing risk assessment tool to determine whether an individual is at risk for pressure ulcer development [14]. An individual with a score of 18 or lower is found to be at risk. A systematic approach to the examination of the pressure ulcer is necessary to provide accurate assessment and monitoring of the pressure ulcer. The following parameters are to be noted:

- Location of the ulcer
- Size of the pressure ulcer (length to be measured as the maximum measurement craniocaudally; width as the maximum measurement from side to side; depth to be measured at the deepest part of the wound perpendicular to the skin surface)
- Staging of the ulcer
- Presence of undermining or tunneling
- Ulcer bed appearance
- Presence of necrotic materials, slough, eschar, fibrous tissues
- Presence of rolled wound edges
- Presence and amount of drainage (exudate versus transudate)
- Presence of foul odor
- Health of the periulcer tissues, including any surrounding erythema, maceration, edema, or associated fungal infection

Staging of pressure ulcers describes the extent of tissue breakdown at initial examination. There have been multiple staging systems for pressure ulcers. The National Pressure Ulcer Advisory Panel (NPUAP) and European Pressure Ulcer Advisory Panel (EPUAP) have agreed on the following staging system [1].

Category/Stage I: Non-Blanchable Erythema

Intact skin with non-blanchable redness of a localized area usually over a bony prominence. Darkly pigmented skin may not have visible blanching; its color may differ from the surrounding area. The area may be painful, firm, soft, warmer or cooler as compared to adjacent tissue. Category I may be difficult to detect in individuals with dark skin tones. May indicate "at risk" persons.

Category/Stage II: Partial Thickness

Partial thickness loss of dermis presenting as a shallow open ulcer with a red pink wound bed, without slough. May also present as an intact or open/ruptured serum-filled or serosanguinous filled blister. Presents as a shiny or dry shallow ulcer without slough or bruising (may indicate deep tissue injury). This category should not be used to describe skin tears, tape burns, incontinence associated dermatitis, maceration or excoriation.

Category/Stage III: Full Thickness Skin Loss

Full thickness tissue loss. Subcutaneous fat may be visible but bone, tendon or muscle is *not* exposed. Slough may be present but does not obscure the depth of tissue loss. *May* include undermining and tunneling. The depth of a Category/Stage III pressure ulcer varies by anatomical location. The bridge of the nose, ear, occiput and malleolus do not have (adipose) subcutaneous tissue and Category/Stage III ulcers can be shallow. In contrast, areas of significant adiposity can develop extremely deep Category/Stage III pressure ulcers. Bone/tendon is not visible or directly palpable.

Category/Stage IV: Full Thickness Tissue Loss

Full thickness tissue loss with exposed bone, tendon or muscle. Slough or eschar may be present. Often includes undermining and tunneling. The depth of a Category/Stage IV pressure ulcer varies by anatomical location. The bridge of the nose, ear, occiput and malleolus do not have (adipose) subcutaneous tissue and these ulcers can be shallow. Category/Stage IV ulcers can extend into muscle or supporting structures (e.g., fascia, tendon or joint capsule) making osteomyelitis or osteitis likely to occur. Exposed bone/muscle is visible or directly palpable.

In addition, the EPUAP/NPUAP recommends use of the following categories/stages.

Unstageable/Unclassified: Full Thickness Skin or Tissue Loss—Depth Unknown

Full thickness tissue loss in which actual depth of the ulcer is completely obscured by slough (yellow, tan, gray, green or brown) or eschar (tan, brown or black) in the wound bed. Until enough slough and/or eschar are removed to expose the base of the wound, the true depth cannot be determined; but it will be either a Category/Stage III or IV. Stable (dry, adherent, intact without erythema or fluctuance) eschar on the heels serves as "the body's natural (biological) cover" and should not be removed.

Suspected Deep Tissue Injury—Depth Unknown

Purple or maroon localized area of discolored intact skin or blood-filled blister due to damage of underlying soft tissue from pressure or ***shear***. The area may be preceded by tissue that is painful, firm, mushy, boggy, warmer or cooler as compared to adjacent tissue. Deep tissue injury may be difficult to detect in individuals with dark skin tones. Evolution may include a thin blister over a dark wound bed. The wound may further evolve and become covered by thin eschar. Evolution may be rapid, exposing additional layers of tissue even with optimal treatment.

This staging system can be used *only* for initial description of the wound. It cannot be used for repeated assessments or reverse staging, primarily because it is not a physiologic description and cannot characterize what is happening in a healing wound. Reepithelialization will occur before lost muscle, subcutaneous fat, or dermis is replaced, resulting in mistakes when healed wounds are staged again.

Care must also be taken in the evaluation of the skin of patients with darkly pigmented skin. Sprigle and colleagues [15] found that erythema in subjects with dark skin is more likely to be nonblanching and to have poor resilience. This indicates that clinicians should use persistence of erythema rather than blanching status to judge incipient pressure ulcers. The staging system defined here includes both visual and nonvisual indicators in the definition of a stage I ulcer, in part to address this issue.

All pressure ulcers are associated with some degree of bacterial colonization, which may or may not lead to local wound infection. The presence of bacterial biofilms in the wound bed may be both a cause and effect of delayed healing [16,17]. Biofilms are typically polymicrobial and are not detected by routine clinical microbiology. They may inhibit healing even in the absence of clinical signs of infection [18]. The possible clinical signs and symptoms of local infection include increasing pain in the wound; erythema, edema, and heat of the periwound area; foul odor; and purulent drainage [19]. Individuals with spinal cord injury may not have intact sensation; in such cases, infected wounds are painless but can cause systemic responses, such as autonomic dysreflexia.

Pressure ulcers also frequently exhibit wound drainage. However, this drainage is not necessarily due to wound infection, and unless it is clinically indicated, routine wound swab culture may not be warranted because this would give a false-positive result. On the other hand, in some cases, increased volumes of exudate may indicate wound infection. Systemic infection may develop if the initial local wound infection is not adequately treated. In such cases, patients may exhibit fever, malaise, and chills. Cellulitis, osteomyelitis, and bacteremia may also develop.

Manual measurement of the wounds by length, width, and depth is the conventional method, but there is poor interrater reliability and the actual surface area of the wound is not known. Electronic technologies allow more accurate documentation and measurements of the surface areas; for instance, the Visitrak device allows easy measurement of wound surface area by a tracing method (Fig. 148.1) [20]. Newer digital stereophotogrammetry systems, such as the LifeViz (Quantificare, San Mateo, Calif) (Fig. 148.2) and Silhouette (ARANZ Medical Ltd, New Zealand) systems, can also provide three-dimensional wound geometry (Fig. 148.3).

Once a pressure ulcer develops, it must be examined regularly for treatment progress to be monitored. At the minimum, weekly assessments should be performed to ensure that the treatment plan is having the desired effect. The NPUAP Pressure Ulcer Scale for Healing (PUSH Tool) has been developed as a clinical tool to monitor changes in pressure ulcer status over time [21]. It takes into account the length and width, exudate amount, and tissue type, forming a composite score that can be tracked

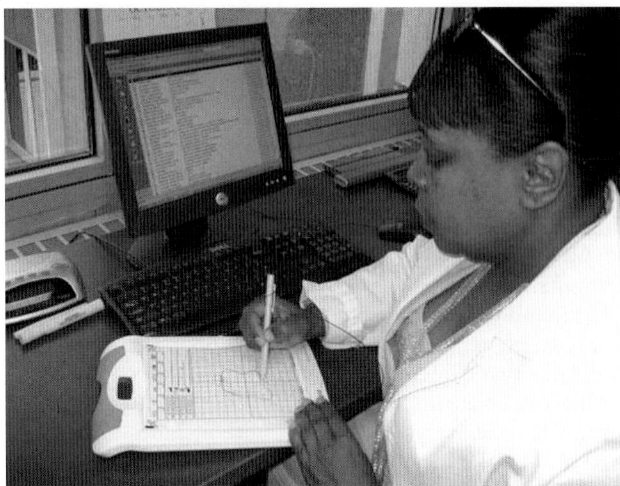

FIGURE 148.1 Visitrak wound measurement device. *(Courtesy Smith & Nephew, Largo, Fla.)*

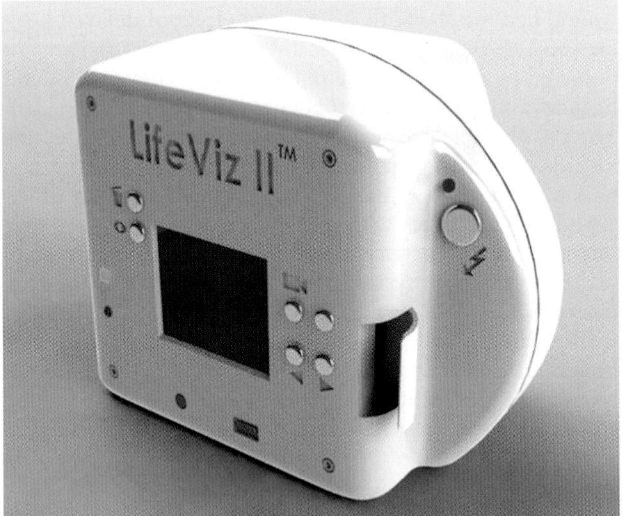

FIGURE 148.2 LifeViz system. *(Courtesy Quantificare, San Mateo, Calif.)*

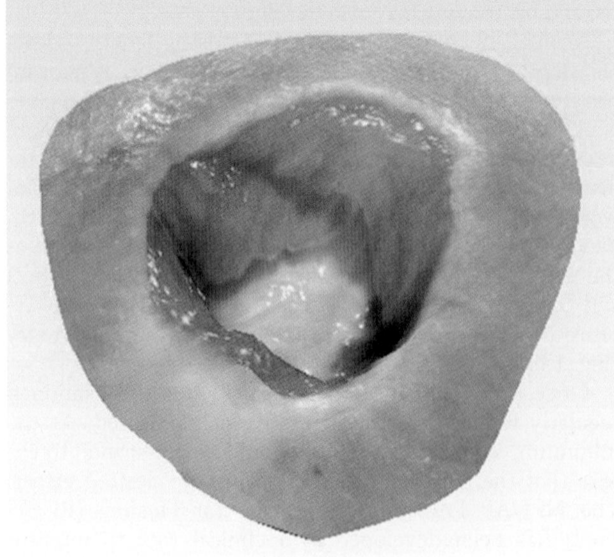

FIGURE 148.3 Pressure ulcer reconstructed as a three-dimensional object.

over time. The Bates-Jensen Wound Assessment Tool is a more comprehensive tool that takes into account 12 parameters, including periwound tissue and epithelialization status [22]. These tools have been validated and are used in clinical practice.

Once they are evaluated, it is critically important for pressure ulcers to be clearly documented in medical records. In the United States, accurate identification and documentation of pressure ulcers are required for reimbursement in addition to provision of appropriate patient care. Gunningberg and Ehrenberg [23] found that pressure ulcer prevalence determined by audit of clinical records is less than 50% of the rate found when the patient's skin is examined. Electronic point-of-care wound documentation has the potential to improve wound management with easy-to-use information technology [24]. Dahlstrom and colleagues [25] reported that education on pressure ulcer documentation improved the quality of pressure ulcer documentation by clinical staff. Unfortunately, the same study showed that the implementation of electronic medical records for nursing notes can have a detrimental impact on pressure ulcer documentation in the longer term. This highlights the importance of accurate wound documentation with well-designed templates in the electronic medical record together with ongoing quality improvement.

Functional Limitations

If a pressure ulcer develops, functional limitations are generally exacerbated. For example, the mobility status of a wheelchair user who develops an ischial region pressure ulcer may be affected because treatment can potentially require prolonged periods of total bed rest. Less obvious is a hemiplegic patient who always rolls and pivots to one side to get out of bed; if a greater trochanter pressure ulcer develops on the side that is aggravated by the pressure, shear, and friction of getting out of bed, either that individual will be limited in being able to get out of bed independently or a new technique must be explored.

The development and location of a pressure ulcer may sometimes give an indication of changes in the patient's activity level. For example, an active wheelchair user may develop an ischial region pressure ulcer from sitting for long periods without adequate pressure relief. However, if that same individual presented with a trochanteric pressure ulcer, most likely due to lying in bed for long periods, the clinician would question whether the patient is not getting up and about for physical or mental health reasons that may need further exploration. Changes in body mass should also be evaluated to determine whether the wheelchair and cushion are still appropriate; if a patient gains weight, the wheelchair and cushion can become too narrow, and increased pressures may develop at the greater trochanteric areas because of impingement.

The development of a pressure ulcer will affect many aspects of a patient's daily living activities. Patients in active rehabilitation programs may not be able to participate in therapy; independent mobility and transfers will be restricted, and it may not be possible for appropriate bracing or orthotics to be worn.

Diagnostic Studies

It is well accepted that malnutrition is linked to both the development of pressure ulcers and their ability to heal. A nutritional assessment that indicates malnutrition is a serum albumin level of less than 3.5 g/L, total protein level of less than 6.4 g/dL, or body weight decreased by more than 15% since the prior assessment. Prealbumin has a short half-life of only 2 or 3 days. Prealbumin concentration is an even more sensitive measure than serum albumin level and should be obtained in the determination of acute response to nutritional intervention. A nutritional assessment should be repeated every 12 weeks [10]. It has been proposed that the Mini Nutritional Assessment tool may be a reliable questionnaire-based approach to obtain repeated evaluations in the elderly [26].

Anemia is another important factor that may affect pressure ulcer healing. Therefore, appropriate management of anemia may positively influence the healing of pressure ulcers.

Once a patient has a pressure ulcer, the determination of whether bacterial infection, underlying osteomyelitis, related abscess, or sinus tracks are hindering the healing process becomes important. There are many studies that can help us determine the diagnosis of osteomyelitis. High serum erythrocyte sedimentation rate and C-reactive protein level, although nonspecific, may be an indication of osteomyelitis. Plain radiography of the underlying bone, computed tomography, bone scan, and magnetic resonance imaging can all be used to better assess the underlying and surrounding tissue and bones for possible associated complications. The proper imaging for each patient depends on the history and desired focus of the study. The most definitive and yet most invasive diagnostic study is bone biopsy. This can be done either bedside with a needle or in the interventional radiology suite or the operating room. Culture of the bone biopsy specimen will give the most accurate microbiologic diagnosis of the underlying osteomyelitis, allowing use of the most specific antimicrobial agent for treatment. Routine swab culture of the wounds is not recommended because all wounds are colonized with bacteria; such cultures will only bring about false-positive results, leading to unnecessary and inappropriate antimicrobial treatments.

Matrix metalloproteinases are produced by the wound and inflammatory cells during normal wound healing. However, when they are present in excessive quantities, they have a negative effect on wound healing [27]. Therefore, regulation of excessive matrix metalloproteinases through local treatments such as collagen-based dressings may facilitate healing [28]. Bedside diagnostic testing has been developed to determine protease activity in the wound to facilitate the [29].

Differential Diagnosis

Ischemic ulcer
Diabetic ulcer
Venous stasis ulcer
Dermatologic neoplasms
Surgical wound dehiscence
Abscess
Abrasion

Treatment

Initial

Unfortunately, pressure ulcers remain one of the most common reasons for readmission to the hospital for many patients with impaired mobility. The patient with a major pressure ulcer will require an average of 180 days of nursing time. Allman and colleagues [30] found that development of a nosocomial pressure ulcer was associated with significant and substantial increases in both hospital costs and length of stay in a group of patients admitted to the hospital with reduced mobility due to a primary diagnosis of hip fracture. Xakellis and Frantz [31] found that the cost of treating pressure ulcers was greatly increased when a patient required hospitalization. Therefore prevention is key to the management of pressure ulcers.

Both the NPUAP/EPUAP [32] and the Consortium for Spinal Cord Medicine [33] have issued comprehensive clinical guidelines for the prevention and treatment of pressure ulcers. Prevention of pressure ulcers aims to address the risk factors listed before. Once a pressure ulcer develops, therapy must focus on local management of the ulcer and systemic treatment of the factors that may affect the healing rate while concurrently addressing factors that led to ulcer formation. Local management of the pressure ulcer should follow the TIME framework for wound bed preparation: *t*issue (nonviable or deficient) management, *i*nflammation (and infection control), *m*oisture (imbalance), and *e*dge (nonadvancing or undermined) [34]. This framework systematically addresses wound bed preparation to optimize healing conditions. Following this framework, nonviable tissue will be débrided. Inflammation or infection will be addressed by appropriate methods, such as the use of an antimicrobial dressing (e.g., silver dressing). Moisture imbalance will be addressed by the retention or removal of fluid by appropriate dressings. Nonadvancing edges will be addressed by the use of débridement, skin grafts, biologic agents, or adjunctive therapies. Figure 148.4 demonstrates the paradigm modified from Sibbald and coworkers [35]; it provides a helpful guideline for chronic wound preparation for treatment.

Wound irrigation with normal saline must be done with adequate pressure to be effective for wound cleaning and mechanical débridement; the pressure of 4 to 15 psi has been found to be safe and nontraumatic to the wound bed. This can be achieved with an appropriate syringe or a pulsatile lavage [36] device that produces irrigation pressure within this recommended range.

With regard to systemic treatments, positioning should be evaluated in both the lying and seated positions. Patients should be positioned to avoid direct pressure and shearing force on the ulcer area (see the section on extrinsic factors). Immobile patients in bed should be turned on a scheduled basis, at least every 2 hours. If necessary, pillows or foam wedges should be used to help patients maintain a position that keeps the ulcer area pressure free. Multiple mattresses and overlays are available, depending on the patient, extent and location of the pressure ulcer, and goals of therapy. For the individuals who can tolerate lying prone, use of a prone cart allows the patient to be out of bed but avoids any pressure on the sacral area. Sitting should be avoided if pressure cannot be relieved from the ulcer area in the sitting position.

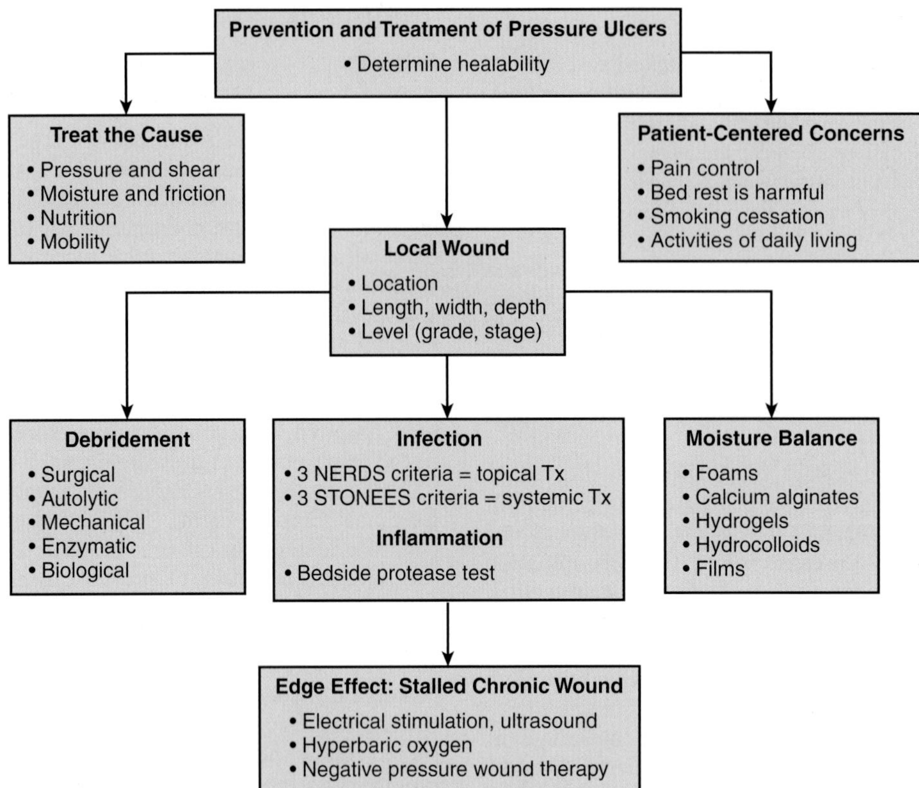

FIGURE 148.4 Wound bed preparation paradigm for holistic patient care. NERDS criteria: nonhealing, exudate increase, red friable or easily bleeding granulation tissue, new slough or debris on the wound surface, and smell. STONEES criteria: size increase, temperature of surrounding skin elevated, os probing or exposed bone, new satellite areas of breakdown, erythema or edema (cellulitis), exudate increase, and smell. *Tx*, treatment. *(From Sibbald RG, Goodman L, Norton L, et al. Prevention and treatment of pressure ulcers. Skin Therapy Lett 2012;17:4-7. © Sibbald RG, et al. 2000, 2003, 2006-2007, WHO 2010, 2011-2012.)*

The comorbid conditions shown to delay ulcer healing are peripheral vascular disease, diabetes mellitus, immune deficiencies, collagen vascular diseases, malignant neoplasms, psychosis, smoking, and depression. Identification and treatment of these conditions in patients with pressure ulcers are important.

If malnutrition is a factor, aggressive nutritional supplementation or support should be instituted to place the patient into a positive nitrogen balance. Nutritional support should occur if it is likely to change the patient's prognosis. Supplemental arginine, vitamin C, and zinc have been shown to enhance the rate of pressure ulcer healing in patients with low serum albumin and zinc levels and elevated C-reactive protein concentration [37].

Pain should also be addressed and treated appropriately. Some pain may be eliminated or controlled by covering the wound and appropriate positioning. If the pain persists, analgesia is provided as needed during manipulations of the wound and for chronic wound pain.

Within 1 to 2 weeks of the initiation of treatment, partial-thickness pressure ulcers should show signs of healing. Full-thickness ulcers should show reduction in size after 2 to 4 weeks of treatment. This should be determined with some caution; pressure ulcers often appear to be initially larger after treatment because of the effect of débridement and cleaning, exposing the real extent of ulceration. There also appears to be a proportion of pressure ulcers that develop as the result of deep tissue damage, at the interface between the soft tissues and the bone rather than at the skin surface. These ulcers will often progress to full-thickness ulcers even when appropriate intervention is provided and should be treated more aggressively.

With this in mind, if the ulcer is truly not healing, the different aspects of the treatment plan previously outlined should be reviewed. In addition, biophysical therapies, such as electrical stimulation, ultrasound, hyperbaric oxygenation [38], or negative pressure wound therapy, should be considered together with the possible need for surgical intervention for stage III and stage IV ulcers that are recalcitrant to standard therapy. Electrical stimulation has been shown in multiple studies to improve the rate and degree of healing when it is used in addition to standard interventions on recalcitrant ulcers [32]. Negative pressure wound therapy, such as vacuum-assisted closure, may also be useful for the appropriate wounds. The guidelines for the use of vacuum-assisted closure are as follows [39]:

- There is no untreated, underlying osteomyelitis.
- The wound is free of fistulas to internal organs or body cavities.
- The wound has not decreased in size for 2 to 4 weeks, despite the use of best practices.
- The wound has been sufficiently débrided.
- The wound has not decreased in size by more than 30% 4 weeks after major débridement.

Many different therapeutic modalities for the treatment of pressure ulcers are being investigated, such as growth factors and tissue-engineered skin substitutes. Basic science research continues to increase our understanding of the chronic wound pathogenesis and can guide the development of clinical interventions. Clinical research in the field of wound treatment is broadening the options for both the treatment and prevention of wounds through many different pathways.

Rehabilitation

Many of the major factors that increase susceptibility to pressure ulcer development are interrelated intrinsic changes in body characteristics and functional abilities. In many conditions, these changes are irreversible. Nutritional status can be altered by adequate diet, but a complete spinal cord injury is permanent. Clinical approaches to pressure ulcer prevention generally focus on extrinsic factors that can be changed. These include educational methods, device-oriented methods, and comprehensive systems of preventive care. These approaches to pressure ulcer prevention are complementary and should be reviewed periodically.

It is critically important during initial rehabilitation that every patient and caregiver be thoroughly educated in the causes of pressure ulcers and what they should do to prevent them. Skills to be learned include the ability to carry out a pressure relief regimen, both through postural changes, when possible, and through the provision of appropriate equipment (e.g., cushions, wheelchairs, mattresses). The need for routine skin inspection and care must also be emphasized, with particular regard to pressure areas such as the ischii, sacrum, greater trochanters, heels, and occiput. Increased care contact time is associated with reduced pressure ulcer incidence, although automated pressure relief systems can also provide an effective intervention during inpatient rehabilitation. Turning every 2 hours while in bed is a commonly accepted practice, but the evidence to support this turning frequency is still lacking. After initial rehabilitation, the at-risk patient must maintain a high level of skin care at all times to prevent the occurrence of pressure ulcers.

The provision of appropriate equipment for postural support and pressure relief, such as mattresses and wheelchair seating cushions, is an important component of rehabilitation. For a patient with impaired mobility who is being discharged to the community or to long-term care, this requires the selection of a wheelchair seating system, including both a wheelchair and a support cushion, to meet his or her individualized requirements. An inappropriate seating system can lead to poor posture, reduce functional abilities, and isolate the user from the environment. All these factors can in turn exacerbate the risk for pressure ulcer development in the rehabilitating patient.

Seating requirements of each patient must be thoroughly assessed during acute rehabilitation and when he or she presents with a pressure ulcer so that appropriate seating and other support surfaces can be recommended. Special seating and cushions are available to help distribute weight off of a pressure ulcer. Cushions can be divided into four categories: foam, viscoelastic foam, gel, and fluid flotation. Which cushion is best for a patient depends on pressure evaluation, lifestyle, postural stability, continence, and cost [40]. Pressure mapping can be a useful component in the objective determination of the interactions between the seating surface and the skin, helping the clinician to choose the most appropriate seating surface with the best pressure-relieving properties. Pressure relief maneuvers should be done every 15 minutes while the patient is sitting to prevent the development of ischial region pressure ulcers.

Tertiary prevention of pressure ulcers seeks to decrease the number of patients who exhibit chronic recurrence of tissue breakdown. Device-oriented prevention techniques continue to be developed and refined. Active pressure relief mattresses often incorporate temperature sensors to control the microenvironment, and this type of technology is now starting to be applied in wheelchair cushions. Wheelchair cushions that can dynamically alter pressure distribution at the seating interface may provide a method for pressure ulcer prevention in individuals with compromised mobility. Advances in system components have increased the reliability and robustness of these cushions, although they remain relatively expensive. Advanced technologies and new pharmacologic approaches are being explored that can affect the intrinsic clinical status of at-risk patients. The long-term application of implanted electrical stimulation devices offers a unique means to alter the intrinsic characteristics of paralyzed muscle, leading to sustained improvements in regional tissue health [41]. The use of anabolic steroids has also been investigated for both the treatment and prevention of pressure ulcers in the population with spinal cord injury [42].

In addition to altering the intrinsic susceptibility of at-risk patients, the incidence of pressure ulcers may be decreased by ensuring effective delivery of care and education by a multidisciplinary clinical team, at all stages of rehabilitation. A survey of the prevalence of pressure ulcers in 5000 hospitalized patients throughout Europe, carried out by the EPUAP [43], indicated that clinical expertise and standard treatment guidelines are not in themselves sufficient. They should be considered the starting point for effective prevention of pressure ulcers, rather than the endpoint. Personalized interactive programs have the potential to decrease readmission rates for high-risk individuals. An increase in the involvement of the patient in his or her care whenever possible may also decrease susceptibility to pressure ulcer development.

Outpatients at risk for pressure ulcers, such as residents of long-term care facilities, often have restricted ease of community mobility that limits both their desire and ability to access clinical expertise. Telemedicine represents a relatively new model for health care delivery that can eliminate or greatly reduce the need for transportation of the patient and improve standard of care.

Procedures

Débridement of necrotic tissue from the wound is essential for healing to occur. Débridement can be accomplished by several different approaches. Sharp débridement is performed by a qualified clinician who uses a scalpel either at the bedside or in surgery. Mechanical débridement is commonly done with wet to dry dressings changed two or three times a day. Autolytic débridement permits the enzymes in the wound to dissolve the necrotic tissue by covering of the wound with a moisture-retentive dressing. Last, enzymatic débridement uses exogenous enzymes in commercial preparations, such as papain, to dissolve the necrotic tissue. The determination of débridement method depends on the condition of the wound. Sharp débridement is often performed when there is a large amount of necrotic material; for instance, the presence of eschar tissue often leads to sharp débridement. This will allow efficient removal of necrotic materials from the wound. However, for chronic wounds that do not have easily removable necrotic tissues (e.g., adherent, yellow, necrotic tissues at the base of the wound), enzymatic débridement through the use of collagenase may be the method of choice, allowing nontraumatic débridement of the wound.

Surgery

A variety of surgical options are available to close stage III and stage IV pressure ulcers that do not heal by conservative means. Possible surgeries are as follows: direct closure, split- or full-thickness skin grafts, skin flaps, musculocutaneous flaps, and free flaps. The type of surgical repair depends on the location of the ulcer, the primary diagnosis of the patient, the comorbid conditions, and the goals of treatment. The long-term outcomes of surgical intervention are variable [44]. Predictors of surgical success correlate with the compliance of the patient with postoperative bed rest as well as preoperative risk factors for wound healing.

Potential Disease Complications

The following complications are associated with pressure ulcers: bacteremia, osteomyelitis, cellulitis, amyloidosis, endocarditis, heterotopic bone formation, perineal-urethral fistula, pseudoaneurysm, septic arthritis, sinus track or abscess, and squamous cell carcinoma in the ulcer.

Potential Treatment Complications

Failure to heal and recurrence of pressure ulcers are potential treatment complications. The need to maintain pressure relief over the area of the ulcer may lead to the formation of another pressure ulcer in a different location. Asymmetric sitting posture due to unilateral removal of necrotic bone may cause pressure ulcer development.

Prolonged bed rest and reduced activity levels will decondition the patient and may lead to or exacerbate other comorbidities. Increased pain may occur with dressing changes and sharp or mechanical débridement. Surgical complications of infection, bleeding, and wound dehiscence are possible.

References

[1] NPUAP Pressure Ulcer Stages/Categories. http://www.npuap.org/resources/educational-and-clinical-resources/npuap-pressure-ulcer-stagescategories. Accessed November 14, 2012.

[2] Gorecki C, Brown JM, Nelson EA, et al. European Quality of Life Pressure Ulcer Project group. Impact of pressure ulcers on quality of life in older patients: a systematic review. J Am Geriatr Soc 2009;57:1175–83.

[3] Markova A, Mostow EN. US skin disease assessment: ulcer and wound care. Dermatol Clin 2012;30:107–11, ix.

[4] Jenkins ML, O'Neal E. Pressure ulcer prevalence and incidence in acute care. Adv Skin Wound Care 2010;23:556–9.

[5] Suriadi, Sanada H, Sugama J, et al. A new instrument for predicting pressure ulcer risk in an intensive care unit. J Tissue Viability 2006;16:21–6.

[6] Chan EY, Tan SL, Lee CK, Lee JY. Prevalence, incidence and predictors of pressure ulcers in a tertiary hospital in Singapore. J Wound Care 2005;14:383–4, 386–388.

[7] Cardenas DD, Hoffman JM, Kirshblum S, McKinley W. Etiology and incidence of rehospitalization after traumatic spinal cord injury: a multicenter analysis. Arch Phys Med Rehabil 2004;85:1757–63.

[8] Siem CA, Wipke-Tevis DD, Rantz MJ, Popejoy LL. Skin assessment and pressure ulcer care in hospital-based skilled nursing facilities. Ostomy Wound Manage 2003;49:42–4, 46, 48 passim, contd.

[9] Baumgarten M, Margolis D, Gruber-Baldini AL, et al. Pressure ulcers and the transition to long-term care. Adv Skin Wound Care 2003;16:299–304.

[10] Chen Y, Devivo MJ, Jackson AB. Pressure ulcer prevalence in people with spinal cord injury: age-period-duration effects. Arch Phys Med Rehabil 2005;86:1208–13.

[11] Verbrugghe M, Beeckman D, Van Hecke A, et al. Malnutrition and associated factors in nursing home residents: a cross-sectional, multicentre study. Clin Nutr 2013;32:438–43.

[12] Zhang M, Roberts VC. The effect of shear forces externally applied to skin surface on underlying tissues. J Biomed Eng 1993;15:451–6.

[13] Colin D, Abraham P, Preault L, et al. Comparison of 90 degrees and 30 degrees laterally inclined positions in the prevention of pressure ulcers using transcutaneous oxygen and carbon dioxide pressures. Adv Wound Care 1996;9:35–8.

[14] Bergstrom N, Braden BJ, Laguzza A, Holman V. The Braden Scale for predicting pressure sore risk. Nurs Res 1987;36:205–10.

[15] Sprigle S, Linden M, Riordan B. Analysis of localized erythema using clinical indicators and spectroscopy. Ostomy Wound Manage 2003;49:42–52.

[16] Scales BS, Huffnagle GB. The microbiome in wound repair and tissue fibrosis. J Pathol 2013;229:323–31.

[17] Percival SL, Hill KE, Williams DW, et al. A review of the scientific evidence for biofilms in wounds. Wound Repair Regen 2012;20:647–57.

[18] Dowd SE, Wolcott RD, Sun Y, et al. Polymicrobial nature of chronic diabetic foot ulcer biofilm infections determined using bacterial tag encoded FLX amplicon pyrosequencing (bTEFAP). PLoS One 2008;3:e3326.

[19] National Pressure Ulcer Advisory Panel. Wound infection and infection control. http://www.npuap.org/woundinfection.html.

[20] Haghpanah S, Bogie KM, Wang XF, et al. Reliability of electronic versus manual wound measurement techniques. Arch Phys Med Rehabil 2006;87:1396–402.

[21] The Pressure Ulcer Scale for Healing (PUSH Tool). http://www.npuap.org/resources/educational-and-clinical-resources/push-tool/; [accessed 14.11.12].

[22] Bates-Jensen Wound Assessment Tool. http://www.geronet.med.ucla.edu/centers/borun/modules/Pressure_ulcer_prevention/puBWAT.pdf; [accessed 14.11.12].

[23] Gunningberg L, Ehrenberg A. Accuracy and quality in the nursing documentation of pressure ulcers: a comparison of record content and patient examination. J Wound Ostomy Continence Nurs 2004;31:328–35.

[24] Florczak B, Scheurich A, Croghan J, et al. An observational study to assess an electronic point-of-care wound documentation and reporting system regarding user satisfaction and potential for improved care. Ostomy Wound Manage 2012;58:46–51.

[25] Dahlstrom M, Best T, Baker C, et al. Improving identification and documentation of pressure ulcers at an urban academic hospital. Jt Comm J Qual Patient Saf 2011;37:123–30.

[26] Langkamp-Henken B, Hudgens J, Stechmiller JK, Herrlinger-Garcia KA. Mini nutritional assessment and screening scores are associated with nutritional indicators in elderly people with pressure ulcers. J Am Diet Assoc 2005;105:1590–6.

[27] McCarty SM, Cochrane CA, Clegg PD, Percival SL. The role of endogenous and exogenous enzymes in chronic wounds: a focus on the implications of aberrant levels of both host and bacterial proteases in wound healing. Wound Repair Regen 2012;20:125–36.

[28] Piatkowski A, Ulrich D, Seidel D, et al. Randomised, controlled pilot to compare collagen and foam in stagnating pressure ulcers. J Wound Care 2012;21:505–11.

[29] Sibbald RG, Snyder RJ, Botros M, et al. Role of a point-of-care protease activity diagnostic test in Canadian clinical practice: a Canadian expert consensus. Adv Skin Wound Care 2012;25:267–75.

[30] Allman RM, Goode PS, Burst N, et al. Pressure ulcers, hospital complications, and disease severity: impact on hospital costs and length of stay. Adv Wound Care 1999;12:22–30.

[31] Xakellis GC, Frantz R. The cost of healing pressure ulcers across multiple health care settings. Adv Wound Care 1996;9:18–22.
[32] National Pressure Ulcer Advisory Panel, European Pressure Ulcer Advisory Panel. Pressure ulcer prevention and treatment: clinical practice guideline. Washington, DC: National Pressure Ulcer Advisory Panel; 2009.
[33] Consortium for Spinal Cord Medicine. Pressure ulcer prevention and treatment following spinal cord injury: a clinical practice guideline for health care professionals. Washington, DC: Paralyzed Veterans of America; 2000.
[34] Schultz G, Mozingo D, Romanelli M, Claxton K. Wound healing and TIME; new concepts and scientific applications. Wound Repair Regen 2005;13(Suppl.):S1–S11.
[35] Sibbald RG, Goodman L, Norton L, et al. Prevention and treatment of pressure ulcers. Skin Therapy Lett 2012;17:4–7.
[36] Ho CH, Bensitel T, Wang X, Bogie KM. Pulsatile lavage for the enhancement of pressure ulcer healing: a randomized controlled trial. Phys Ther 2012;92:38–48.
[37] Desneves KJ, Todorovic BE, Cassar A, Crowe TC. Treatment with supplementary arginine, vitamin C and zinc in patients with pressure ulcers: a randomised controlled trial. Clin Nutr 2005;24:979–87.
[38] Warriner 3rd RA, Hopf HW. The effect of hyperbaric oxygen in the enhancement of healing in selected problem wounds. Undersea Hyperb Med 2012;39:923–35.
[39] Sibbald RG, Mahoney J, V.A.C. Therapy Canadian Consensus Group. A consensus report on the use of vacuum-assisted closure in chronic, difficult-to-heal wounds. Ostomy Wound Manage 2003;49:52–66.
[40] Ferguson-Pell MW. Seat cushion selection. J Rehabil Res Dev Clin Suppl 1990;2:49–73.
[41] Bogie KM, Wang X, Triolo RJ. Long-term prevention of pressure ulcers in high-risk patients: a single case study of the use of gluteal neuromuscular electric stimulation. Arch Phys Med Rehabil 2006;87:585–91.
[42] Spungen AM, Koehler KM, Modeste-Duncan R, et al. Nine clinical cases of nonhealing pressure ulcers in patients with spinal cord injury treated with an anabolic agent: a therapeutic trial. Adv Skin Wound Care 2001;14:139–44.
[43] European Pressure Ulcer Advisory Panel. The prevalence of pressure ulcers in European hospitals. EPUAP Review 2001;3. http://www.epuap.org/review3_3/index.html.
[44] Sameem M, Au M, Wood T, et al. A systematic review of complication and recurrence rates of musculocutaneous, fasciocutaneous, and perforator-based flaps for treatment of pressure sores. Plast Reconstr Surg 2012;130:67e–77e.

CHAPTER 149

Pulmonary Rehabilitation for Patients with Lung Disease

Andrew R. Berman, MD
Alpeshkumar Bavishi, MD
John R. Bach, MD

Synonyms

None

ICD-9 Codes

491.20	**Chronic obstructive bronchitis**
492.8	**Emphysema**
496	**Chronic obstructive pulmonary disease**
515	**Idiopathic pulmonary fibrosis**

ICD-10 Codes

J44.9	**Chronic obstructive pulmonary disease, unspecified, chronic obstructive bronchitis**
J43.9	**Emphysema, unspecified**
J84.112	**Idiopathic pulmonary fibrosis**

Definition

Pulmonary rehabilitation (PR) is a comprehensive intervention for patients who remain symptomatic with chronic respiratory disease despite standard medical treatment. Chronic diseases of the lung can be manifested in many forms. Chronic obstructive pulmonary disease (COPD) is among the most common, with an estimated prevalence of at least 8% in the United States. Idiopathic pulmonary fibrosis (IPF) is less common, although the incidence increases with older age, with patients typically presenting after the age of 60 years. PR programs are designed to optimize functional status and to reduce symptoms. A multidisciplinary health care team evaluates each patient's unique needs, with active collaboration among the patient, family members, and health care providers. Treatment programs are then devised and consist of education, physician-prescribed exercise training, nutritional and psychological counseling, and outcomes assessment. Each program includes a spectrum of intervention strategies that address both the primary condition and the secondary impairments and conditions associated with the respiratory disease, such as peripheral muscle dysfunction, anxiety, and depression. The American Thoracic Society and the European Respiratory Society, in a joint consensus statement, have endorsed the use of PR in the management of chronic respiratory disease regardless of cause [1]. Each prescription is individually specific for PR candidates with the conditions listed in Table 149.1 who have limited exercise tolerance despite standard medical treatment. This includes frequently hospitalized patients and patients undergoing lung volume reduction surgery or lung transplantation, who require PR both before and after surgery.

Symptoms

Symptoms of patients with chronic respiratory diseases such as COPD, due to persistent airflow limitation, and IPF, a condition associated with progressive scarring of the lungs (Fig. 149.1), include dyspnea, exercise intolerance, cough, and airway congestion. Initially, symptoms may be attributed to other conditions or age itself [2,3]. Whereas COPD patients are relieved by expectorating sputum, IPF patients typically are not. Both COPD and IPF patients may also have chest pain, orthopnea, sleep disordered breathing, poor endurance, anxiety, depression, and difficulty with concentration [3–5]. Inhalation of cigarette smoke is a risk factor for both conditions [3,6]. Disease progression is variable. Fatigue and any complicating conditions can further exacerbate restrictions in activities of daily living (ADLs) and quality of life [7,8]. Late-stage chronic lung disease patients tend to be home bound.

Table 149.1 Conditions Associated with Inadequate Oxygen Supply

Airway Disease	Interstitial Lung Disease*
COPD, emphysema	Idiopathic
COPD, chronic bronchitis	Environmental
Chronic asthma	Occupational
Cystic fibrosis	Granulomatous diseases
Bronchiectasis†	Collagen vascular diseases
Constrictive bronchiolitis	Drug-induced, radiation
Hypersensitivity pneumonitis†	Inherited

*Interstitial diseases are categorized by causes.
†Presents with mixed obstruction and restriction.
COPD, chronic obstructive pulmonary disease.

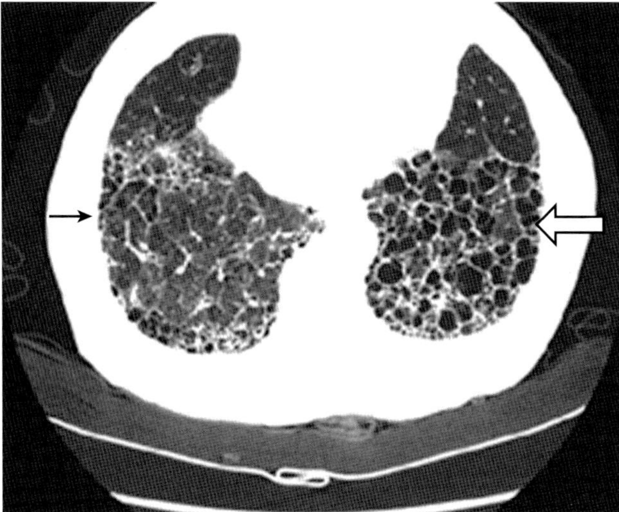

FIGURE 149.1 High-resolution computed tomography scan of the chest of an individual with idiopathic pulmonary fibrosis. Note subpleural fibrosis *(solid arrow)* and honeycombing *(open arrow)*.

Physical Examination

Abnormal physical findings are not usually detected early on. Auscultation in COPD may eventually reveal wheezing, hyperresonant lung sounds, prolonged expiratory phase, and rales. Chest percussion may reveal hyperresonance and hyperinflation. The chest may be barrel shaped, which is consistent with hyperinflation. Auxiliary respiratory muscle use and pursed-lip breathing are common with end-stage disease.

The most common finding in patients with IPF is inspiratory "Velcro-like" crackles heard on lung auscultation, mostly in the lower lung fields. Clubbing is found in up to 50% of patients. In advanced IPF, a loud pulmonic second heart sound and peripheral edema may be found, consistent with pulmonary hypertension or right-sided heart failure. Associated signs of arthritis and proximal muscle weakness are uncommon and may suggest interstitial lung disease occurring secondary to a collagen vascular disease.

Functional Limitations

Exercise tolerance and the ability to perform ADLs may be diminished by respiratory and skeletal muscle impairment including all limbs and the trunk [9–11]. Aerobic capacity is typically reduced with early lactate accumulation and muscle fatigue [9]. With diminished muscle strength, diminished mobility, and ADL restriction, patients become further deconditioned and dependent on others, leading to decreased social interaction, increased anxiety and depression, and being home bound [3,8]. In one study, 41% of COPD patients left the house less than once per month or never in their last year of life [12]. A cycle of diminished mobility leads to further deconditioning and, in turn, worsening exertional tolerance.

Diagnostic Studies

COPD and IPF are suspected for anyone with dyspnea, cough, or exercise intolerance. For IPF, a complete medical history with appropriate serologic tests is warranted to exclude secondary causes of pulmonary fibrosis.

Spirometry is most valuable for diagnosis of COPD and IPF. Spirometry provides quantifiable and reproducible parameters of airflow obstruction and lung restriction. The Global Initiative for Chronic Obstructive Lung Disease has established that a postbronchodilator forced expiratory volume in 1 second (FEV_1) to forced vital capacity (FVC) ratio (FEV_1/FVC) of less than 70% is required for the diagnosis of COPD to be made [3]. COPD severity is stratified by symptoms, postbronchodilator FEV_1 values, and frequency of exacerbations [3]. COPD patients demonstrate an increased total lung capacity, which is consistent with hyperinflation, and an increased residual volume/total lung capacity ratio, which suggests air trapping. IPF patients, in contrast, exhibit severe restrictive physiology with reduced FEV_1 and FVC but a normal or increased FEV_1/FVC ratio and reduced total lung capacity.

Patients with emphysema or IPF have decreased lung diffusion capacity for carbon monoxide consistent with loss of effective gas exchange. Oxyhemoglobin saturation and arterial blood gas values are usually normal at rest until the later disease stages. With exercise, hypoxemia and oxygen desaturation commonly occur.

Chest radiography in patients with advanced COPD commonly reveals evidence of hyperinflation. Other findings may include bullae and increased basilar lung markings. Computed tomography (CT) scan of the chest is not routinely used to diagnose COPD but may show evidence of emphysema and/or bullae.

Bilateral, symmetric reticular opacities, with lower lung field predominance, are usually seen in IPF. High-resolution CT (HRCT) scanning can demonstrate a reticular abnormality with a subpleural, basal predominance; honeycombing with or without bronchiectasis; and absence of findings suggestive of an alternative diagnosis, such as ground-glass opacities, nodules, or cysts [6]. When a patient presents with progressive dyspnea and dry cough without known cause and is found on HRCT to show these "typical" findings, surgical biopsy is not necessary to make the diagnosis. In most other cases, histopathologic correlation is warranted along with pulmonary function testing.

Other diagnostic studies can include testing for α_1-antitrypsin deficiency for COPD, especially if there is a family history of it. Pulse oximetry allows demonstration of worsening oxygenation with activity. Reduced oxyhemoglobin saturation is an indication for supplemental oxygen therapy. Last, echocardiography is performed when right-sided heart failure is suspected.

Differential Diagnosis

SHORTNESS OF BREATH
Lung disease
Heart disease
Neuromuscular disease
Anemia
Obesity
Deconditioning

Treatment

Management of COPD and IPF includes a comprehensive evaluation for contributing conditions as well as pharmacologic and nonpharmacologic approaches and rehabilitation as noted in Table 149.2. Pharmacologic treatment for COPD is considered in Table 149.3; it is used to reduce dyspnea and frequency of exacerbations and to improve health-related quality of life. For treatment of COPD, short-acting β-agonists and short-acting anticholinergics are equipotent in reducing dyspnea and improving exertional tolerance. In patients with more advanced disease, long-acting bronchodilators are indicated in addition to short-acting bronchodilators [3]. Inhaled corticosteroids are indicated for severe disease or repeated exacerbations despite use of long-acting bronchodilators [3]. Systemic steroids should not be prescribed for stable COPD patients because of an unfavorable risk-benefit ratio. There is insufficient evidence to support the use of any specific pharmacologic therapy for IPF [6].

Nonpharmacologic treatments include airway secretion mobilization, vaccinations (influenza and pneumococcal pneumonia), and education on smoking cessation interventions and the importance of medical regimen adherence and inhaler use techniques. Smoking cessation reduces chronic phlegm production and decreases the rate of loss of FEV_1 compared with continued smokers. Training for proper administration of nebulizers and inhalers promotes optimal medication deposition and efficacy. Thick respiratory secretions can augment dyspnea. *N*-Acetylcysteine is the only mucolytic readily available in clinical practice in the United States, but there is inconclusive evidence for its efficacy [13].

Patients with advanced COPD have a prevalence of osteoporosis of 36% to 60% and should be treated for osteoporosis [3]. Vertebral fractures have been found in 29% of patients [14]. Immobility as well as smoking, vitamin D deficiency, and the use of glucocorticoids can contribute to osteoporosis.

Long-term oxygen therapy is indicated for COPD patients with hypoxemia, demonstrated by arterial blood gas analysis ($Po_2 < 55$ mm Hg) or by pulse oximetry (oxygen saturation < 88%). Long-term oxygen therapy has been shown to increase endurance and to improve survival [15] as well as to improve sleep and cognitive performance [16]. Data for the use of long-term oxygen therapy in patients with IPF are lacking. Extrapolating from data of COPD patients, supplemental oxygen is recommended for clinically significant resting hypoxemia ($Spo_2 < 88\%$).

Table 149.2 Pulmonary Rehabilitation

Basic Outpatient Pulmonary Rehabilitation Program

Initial assessment of
- Respiratory disease process
- Underlying medical disorder
- General medical condition
- Functional status
- Patient's goals

Select treatment goals

Interdisciplinary Team Management

Medication optimization
Adjustment of supplemental oxygen therapy
Airway secretion elimination techniques and devices
Smoking cessation program
Exercise program
- Ventilatory muscle training
- Endurance and strength training

Breathing retraining
Alternative breathing techniques
Energy conservation techniques
Therapeutic modalities
Adaptive devices and mobility equipment
Psychosocial counseling
Nutritional counseling
Patient and caregiver education
Maintenance program

Rehabilitation

Goals and Objectives

The goals of a PR program are to reverse deconditioning and to optimize the individual's independence and functioning. A PR service aims to alleviate symptoms, to increase physical and social participation, to maximize independent functioning, and to enhance quality of life, all in the framework of reducing health care costs [1]. Specific objectives to improve exercise tolerance, strength, and flexibility as well as coping strategies and stress management require periodic reassessment. Patients, their families, and a multidisciplinary PR team work together to achieve the objectives.

Staffing

Specific PR team staffing varies and depends on resources and availability. All programs have a physician medical director who is responsible for initial patient assessment to determine candidacy for PR, to identify comorbidities, and to ensure an optimal medical regimen [17]. The physician must be accessible for emergencies when inpatient or outpatient services are being furnished.

A well-structured PR team also consists of therapists (physical, occupational, respiratory), a nutritionist, an exercise physiologist, and a social worker [18]. A psychiatrist or psychologist may also be part of the team. The main role of the physical or respiratory therapist is to carry out the prescribed exercise program (Table 149.4), whereas the occupational therapist evaluates the patient's environment and ADLs and makes recommendations for adaptive equipment to optimize ADLs. The respiratory therapist also teaches breathing exercises as well as proper use of aerosolized medications and oxygen. An exercise physiologist prescribes and monitors the therapeutic exercise program. The nutritionist formulates the nutritional goals and educates on proper diet. The social worker assesses any need for home services and counsels and instructs in coping strategies, especially if a psychiatrist or psychologist is not part of the team. All members' assessments are integrated into specific treatment plans.

Table 149.3 Commonly Prescribed Medications for Chronic Obstructive Pulmonary Disease

Drug Class	Commonly Prescribed Formulations	Modes of Delivery	Effect and Indication
Short-acting β_2-agonist	Albuterol	Inhaler, nebulizer solution, pill	Bronchodilator; used as needed for symptom relief
Short-acting anticholinergic	Ipratropium bromide	Inhaler, nebulizer solution	Bronchodilator; used as needed for symptom relief
Long-acting β_2-agonist	Salmeterol Formoterol	Inhaler, nebulizer solution	Bronchodilator; used daily for maintenance
Long-acting anticholinergic	Tiotropium bromide Aclidinium bromide	Inhaler	Bronchodilator; used daily for maintenance
Inhaled corticosteroid	Beclomethasone Budesonide Fluticasone	Inhaler, nebulizer solution	Anti-inflammatory; used daily for maintenance
Methylxanthine derivative	Theophylline	Pill	Bronchodilator (less effective than inhaled bronchodilators); used daily for maintenance
Phosphodiesterase type 4 inhibitors	Roflumilast	Pill	Anti-inflammatory (nonsteroid); used daily for maintenance (in patients with chronic bronchitis)

Combination inhalers are available in different formulations: short-acting β_2-agonist and short-acting anticholinergic; long acting β_2-agonist and inhaled corticosteroid.

Table 149.4 Types of Exercise [1,2,8,12,13,24,25]

Type of Exercise	Example
Ventilatory muscle training	Inspiratory resistive exercise: maximum sustained ventilation, inspiratory resistive loading, inspiratory threshold loading, sustained hyperpnea
Strength training	Upper extremity exercise: pulleys, elastic bands, supervised circuit training, weightlifting with low resistance Lower extremity exercise: supervised circuit training, weightlifting with low resistance
Endurance training	Upper extremity exercise: unsupported upper extremity activities ranging from activities of daily living to athletic activities, supervised arm cycling, low-impact aerobics, pool therapy Lower extremity exercise: incremental treadmill program, supervised walking, cycling and stair climbing program, low-impact aerobics, pool therapy

Setting

Most PR programs are carried out in the outpatient setting, although inpatient and home settings are also possibilities. Inpatient- and outpatient-based programs facilitate interaction with a more complete PR team in a safe environment. Inpatient PR is usually reserved for patients with severe impairments and multiple comorbidities or for difficult-to-transport severely disabled patients. Home-based rehabilitation is more convenient for the severely disabled, but team interaction is limited. PR is beneficial irrespective of setting [1,18–20]. Indeed, home-based PR can be of equivalent benefit to hospital-based programs [20]. Telemonitoring may now allow a hybrid of home- and hospital-based monitoring as well as enhanced clinical data collection and more prompt interventions from the PR team. Domiciliary telemonitoring and home-based PR may decrease hospitalizations for respiratory complications [21]. Whereas efficacy of PR for patients with IPF is limited, it seems that many would benefit. Swigris [22] reported an improved sense of well-being, a greater sense of control, more energy, and a better general outlook on life. Outpatient PR programs also resulted in improvements in 6-minute walk distance and health-related quality of life for IPF patients, although pulmonary function and oxygenation did not improve [23–25]. Home-based programs may be equally effective [26]. Larger controlled studies are needed.

Rehabilitation Treatment Modalities

Because there are insufficient resources to provide PR to all symptomatic patients, attention to the following increases the likelihood of success: the patient's respiratory condition should be stable on prescribed medical therapy including supplemental oxygen, with demonstrated adherence to the medical regimen before enrollment in PR; underlying medical conditions (e.g., cardiac disease or psychiatric illness) should be stable; and no medical conditions or physical impairments should be present that would interfere with the PR process [1]. The patient also needs to be able to understand the educational content of the program and be motivated and willing to devote the necessary time. PR dropout rates are highest among current smokers [27,28].

Although cigarette smoking is sometimes considered a contraindication to PR, clinical and physiologic gains can be similar in smokers and nonsmokers [27–29]. A trial of smoking cessation can be offered as an index of the patient's motivation for PR [29].

Morbidity due to trapping of airway secretions may be relieved by the many secretion mobilization systems now available, but there is no clear evidence that one system works better than any other. The least expensive and simplest methods to supplement airway secretion mobilization efforts, such as use of a flutter value, positive expiratory pressure mask, and chest vibrators, are probably as effective as the expensive chest vibrating and oscillating devices [30]. Supplemental respiratory therapeutic secretion mobilization methods that can be taught include chest percussion and postural drainage, huffing, and active cycle of breathing. The last is the most inexpensive technique of airway secretion mobilization because no assistive device is used. The patient simply breathes slowly and shallowly at lung volumes well below functional residual capacity. He or she gradually increases tidal volumes to approach functional residual capacity and, once reaching it, takes a deep breath and "huffs" out secretions. Other important strategies for these patients are to administer and to monitor compliance with medications.

Carefully prescribed maximally intense anaerobic exercise over 30- to 45-minute periods provides the greatest benefits for reducing dyspnea and respiratory rate and increasing exercise tolerance, maximum oxygen consumption, 6- and 12-minute walk distance, ADLs, work output, mechanical efficiency, and possibly gas exchange while decreasing anxiety and depression [31–35].

For advanced patients who cannot tolerate high-intensity training, low-intensity training can be prescribed on the basis of objective or subjective measures. Objective measures involve calculating or measuring the maximal oxygen consumption or maximum heart rate. If open-circuit spirometry and metabolic cart are available, specific target intensity may be 50% of peak rate of oxygen uptake. Heart rate parameters may be most useful for patients with cardiac conditions. Several formulas are used. One is the desired exercise intensity multiplied by the maximum predicted heart rate. Hence, if the desired exercise intensity is defined as 60% of maximum predicted heart rate (HR), then

$$\text{Target HR} = 0.60 \times [\text{HR}_{\text{max}} = 220 - \text{age}]$$

Another is the Karvonen formula. For the target HR range of 50% to 85%:

$$\begin{aligned}\text{HR reserve} &= [(\text{HR}_{\text{max}} - \text{HR}_{\text{rest}}) \times 0.50] + \text{HR}_{\text{rest}} \\ &= [(\text{HR}_{\text{max}} - \text{HR}_{\text{rest}}) \times 0.85] + \text{HR}_{\text{rest}}\end{aligned}$$

Initial targets can be 50% (range, 50% to 80%) of either objective measure or the level tolerated by the patient [36].

When objective measures are not applicable, as in the case of patients taking negative chronotropic medications (e.g., beta blockers or calcium channel blockers) and heart transplant patients, subjective measures may be more predictive of exercise tolerance. In addition, because patients are often limited by exertional dyspnea, subjective measures may be more desirable [36].

Subjective measures of exercise tolerance, such as the Borg Rating of Perceived Exertion Scale or dyspnea rating scale, provide patient feedback based on symptoms alone. The Borg Rating of Perceived Exertion Scale from 6 to 20 is linearly related to heart rate. This is illustrated by multiplying the chosen scale number by 10 to obtain the estimated predicted heart rate. For example, when the patient chooses the number 10 on the scale to describe exertion symptoms, heart rate is estimated by the following equation:

$$10 \times 10 = 100(\pm 10)$$

The original Borg scale uses this method [36,37].

Daily activities in mobility and exercise are tailored to the patient's form of mobility and baseline level of function. Mobility and endurance exercise programs can include walking, stair climbing, low-impact aerobics, stationary bicycling, and pool activities. For mobility, work, and recreational pursuits, assistive devices to improve ADLs can include wheelchair, walker, or cane. Strength training increases ADLs, mobility, and specific occupation-related tasks. Intermingled with endurance, strength, and task-specific training are energy conservation techniques that provide the patient with more energy efficient methods to perform daily activities. Increased endurance for exercise can occur independently of changes in ventilatory muscle endurance. The patient is made responsible for a progressive program to reinforce adherence and independence.

Breathing retraining goals modify the breathing pattern to decrease the work of breathing and to improve cough. Pursed-lip breathing and diaphragmatic breathing decrease the respiratory rate, coordinate the breathing pattern, and tend to prevent collapse of smaller bronchi. Air shifting is performed several times per hour. It involves a deep inspiration that is held with the glottis closed for 5 seconds. The air shifts to lesser ventilated areas of the lung and may help prevent microatelectasis. The subsequent expiration is through pursed lips. Pursed-lip breathing aids in relaxation as well. Other relaxation exercises, such as Jacobson exercises and biofeedback, can be used to decrease tension and anxiety [38,39].

For hypercapnic patients, interspersing periods of respiratory muscle rest with exercise of specific respiratory muscle groups is a principle of PR. Rest can be achieved by overnight use of nasal bilevel positive airway pressure, which improves daytime gas values, increases vital capacity, decreases fatigue, and increases well-being and quality of life [40,41].

After the acute rehabilitation period, continued surveillance and attention to abstinence from smoking, bronchial hygiene (Table 149.5), breathing retraining, physical reconditioning, oxygen therapy, and airway secretion mobilization have been shown to reduce hospital admissions, length of hospital stays, and cost [42,43]. The benefits of PR therapeutic exercise on exercise performance and quality of life are greatest during the first year and last up to 5 years [44–46].

Table 149.5 Pulmonary Hygiene Options [11,14,43]

Inhaled Treatments
Bronchodilators
Mucolytics
Methods of Airway Secretion Elimination
Oral, nasal, or transtracheal suctioning
Chest percussion and postural drainage
Positive expiratory pressure breathing
Flutter mucus clearance devices
Mechanical vibration devices to the chest wall
Intrapulmonary percussive ventilation with aerosolized medications
Mechanical insufflation-exsufflation applications
Autogenic drainage
Manual assisted cough
Abdominal binder

So far, there is not enough evidence to support improved survival with PR. As reported by Troosters and colleagues [47], in a pooled analysis of some small studies, 1-year to 18-month mortality risk was 7.8% in the PR group and 9.9% in the control group. The pooled odds of dying in the PR group was 0.69 compared with the control group. This suggests that PR reduces the short-term risk of dying by 31%, although this was not statistically significant. In 2011, a Cochrane review concluded that PR after an acute exacerbation of COPD was safe and associated with a reduction in mortality [48].

Surgery

Lung volume reduction surgery is an option for patients with predominantly upper lobe emphysema and low baseline exercise capacity. Results from the National Emphysema Treatment Trial demonstrated that lung volume reduction surgery in this subset of patients improved exercise capacity and quality of life and reduced mortality compared with a similar group of patients treated medically and that this benefit was maintained on a 5-year follow-up assessment [49]. Lung volume reduction surgery is contraindicated in patients with low FEV_1, homogeneous emphysema, or very low carbon monoxide diffusing capacity because of the increased risk of death after surgery [50]. More recently, lung volume reduction by bronchoscopic techniques has been introduced, and studies of the effectiveness of this approach are ongoing.

Lung transplantation is an option for selected patients with COPD or IPF. Appropriate patients for lung transplantation have severe disease as defined by a low FEV_1% predicted (<25%), resting hypoxemia, hypercapnia, and secondary pulmonary hypertension. Referral for lung transplantation should be considered for COPD patients with progressive deterioration despite optimal treatment. After lung transplantation, quality of life and functional capacity have been demonstrated to improve [51]. Appropriate IPF patients for transplantation have a lung diffusion capacity for carbon monoxide of less than 39% of predicted, a decrement in FVC of more than 10% during 6 months of follow-up, a decrease in oxygen saturation below 88% during a 6-minute walk test, and honeycombing on HRCT. Five-year survival rates after lung transplantation in IPF are about 50%, with improvement demonstrated in oxygenation and spirometry, lung volumes, and diffusing capacity [52].

Potential Treatment Complications

Treatment complications can result from oxygen toxicity, barotrauma from ventilator use, and patient comorbidities such as concomitant cardiac or atherosclerotic peripheral vascular disease and pharmacologic treatment. Routine evaluation of a patient's medication profile by the treating clinician is necessary. Immobility due to muscle weakness or acute illness can also exacerbate pulmonary secretion stasis and cause deep venous thromboses, cardiac deconditioning, skin ulceration, and bone decalcification. Each individual's progress with mobilization, exercise, and daily activity facilitation programs is monitored, and prescriptions are modified accordingly.

References

[1] Nici L, Donner C, Wouters E, et al. American Thoracic Society/European Respiratory Society statement on pulmonary rehabilitation. Am J Respir Crit Care Med 2006;173:1390–413.

[2] Kim DS, Collard HR, King Jr TE. Classification and natural history of the idiopathic interstitial pneumonias. Proc Am Thorac Soc 2006;3:285–92.

[3] Vestbo J, Hurd SS, Agusti AG, et al. Global strategy for the diagnosis, management and prevention of chronic obstructive pulmonary disease: GOLD executive summary. Am J Respir Crit Care Med 2013;187:347–65.

[4] De Vries J, Kessels BL, Drent M. Quality of life of idiopathic pulmonary fibrosis patients. Eur Respir J 2001;17:954–61.

[5] Mermigkis C, Stagaki E, Amfilochiou A, et al. Sleep quality and associated daytime consequences in patients with idiopathic pulmonary fibrosis. Med Princ Pract 2009;18:10–5.

[6] Raghu G, Collard HR, Egan JJ, et al. An official ATS/ERS/JRS/ALAT statement: idiopathic pulmonary fibrosis: evidence-based guidelines for diagnosis and management. Am J Respir Crit Care Med 2011;183:788–824.

[7] Rutten-van Mölken M, Oostenbrink J, Tashkin D, et al. Does quality of life of COPD patients as measured by the generic EuroQol five-dimension questionnaire differentiate between COPD severity stages? Chest 2006;130:1117–28.

[8] Swigris JJ, Anita L, Stewart AL, et al. Patients' perspectives on how idiopathic pulmonary fibrosis affects the quality of their lives. Health Qual Life Outcomes 2005;3:61.

[9] Casaburi R, Patessio A, Ioli F, et al. Reductions in exercise lactic acidosis and ventilation as a result of exercise training in patients with obstructive lung disease. Am Rev Respir Dis 1991;143:9–18.

[10] Eisner MD, Blanc PD, Yelin EH, et al. COPD as a systemic disease: impact on physical functional limitations. Am J Med 2008;121:789–96.

[11] Nishiyama O, Taniguchi H, Kondoh Y, et al. Quadriceps weakness is related to exercise capacity in idiopathic pulmonary fibrosis. Chest 2005;127:2028–33.

[12] Elkington H, White P, Addington-Hall J, et al. The healthcare needs of chronic obstructive pulmonary disease patients in the last year of life. Palliat Med 2005;19:485–91.

[13] Decramer M, Rutten-van Mölken M, Dekhuijzen P, et al. Effects of *N*-acetylcysteine on outcomes in chronic obstructive pulmonary disease (Bronchitis Randomized on NAC Cost-Utility Study, BRONCUS): a randomised placebo-controlled trial. Lancet 2005;365:1552–60.

[14] Shane E, Silverberg S, Donovan D, et al. Osteoporosis in lung transplantation candidates with end-stage pulmonary disease. Am J Med 1996;101:262–9.

[15] American Thoracic Society Consensus Statement. Dyspnea: mechanisms, assessment and management. Am J Respir Crit Care Med 1999;159:321–40.

[16] Celli B, MacNee W, Agusti A, et al. Standards for the diagnosis and treatment of patients with COPD: a summary of the ATS/ERS position paper. Eur Respir J 2004;23:932–46.

[17] Hill NS. Pulmonary rehabilitation. Proc Am Thorac Soc 2006;3:66–74.

[18] Ries AL, Bauldoff GS, Carlin BW, et al. Pulmonary rehabilitation: joint ACCP/AACVPR evidence-based clinical practice guidelines. Chest 2007;131:4S–42S.

[19] Lacasse Y, Goldstein R, Lasserson TJ, et al. Pulmonary rehabilitation for chronic obstructive pulmonary disease. Cochrane Database Syst Rev 2006;4, CD003793.

[20] Vieira DS, Maltais F, Bourbeau J. Home-based pulmonary rehabilitation in chronic obstructive pulmonary disease patients. Curr Opin Pulm Med 2010;16:134–43.

[21] Garuti G, Bagatti S, Verucchi E, et al. Pulmonary rehabilitation at home guided by telemonitoring and access to healthcare facilities for respiratory complications in patients with neuromuscular disease. Eur J Phys Rehabil Med 2013;49:51–7.

[22] Swigris JJ, Brown KK, Make BJ, Wamboldt FS. Pulmonary rehabilitation in idiopathic pulmonary fibrosis: a call for continued investigation. Respir Med 2008;102:1675–80.

[23] Nishiyama O, Kondoh Y, Kimura T, et al. Effects of pulmonary rehabilitation in patients with idiopathic pulmonary fibrosis. Respirology 2008;13:394–9.

[24] Holland AE, Hill CJ, Conron M, et al. Short term improvement in exercise capacity and symptoms following exercise training in interstitial lung disease. Thorax 2008;63:549–54.

[25] Holland AE, Hill CJ, Glaspole I, et al. Predictors of benefit following pulmonary rehabilitation for interstitial lung disease. Respir Med 2012;106:429–35.

[26] Ozalevli S, Karaali HK, Ilgin D, et al. Effect of home-based pulmonary rehabilitation in patients with idiopathic pulmonary fibrosis. Multidiscip Respir Med 2010;5:31–7.

[27] Selzler AM, Simmonds L, Rodgers WM, et al. Pulmonary rehabilitation in chronic obstructive pulmonary disease: predictors of program completion and success. COPD 2012;9:538–45.

[28] Giménez M, Saavedra P, Martin N, et al. A two-step stool aerobic training for smokers. Am J Phys Med Rehabil 2014;93:1–9.

[29] Lacasse Y, Maltais F, Goldstein RS. Smoking cessation in pulmonary rehabilitation: goal or prerequisite? J Cardiopulm Rehabil 2002;22:148–53.

[30] Hardy KA. A review of airway clearance: new techniques, indications, and recommendations. Respir Care 1994;39:440–55.

[31] Gozal D. Nocturnal ventilatory supports in patients with cystic fibrosis: comparison with supplemental oxygen. Eur Respir J 1997;10:1999–2003.

[32] Gimenez M, Servera E, Vergara P, et al. Endurance training in patients with chronic obstructive pulmonary disease: a comparison of high versus moderate intensity. Arch Phys Med Rehabil 2000;81: 102–9.

[33] Carter R, Nicotra B, Clark L, et al. Exercise conditioning in rehabilitation of patients with chronic obstructive pulmonary disease. Arch Phys Med Rehabil 1988;69:118–22.

[34] Troosters T, Gosselink R, Decramer M. Short and long-term effects of outpatient rehabilitation in patients with chronic obstructive pulmonary disease: a randomized trial. Am J Med 2000;109:207–12.

[35] Make B. Pulmonary rehabilitation and outcome measure. In: Baum GL, Crapo JD, Celli BR, Karlinsky JB, editors. Textbook of pulmonary diseases. 6th ed. Philadelphia: Lippincott-Raven; 1998. p. 987–1006.

[36] Jones NL, Campbell EJM. Clinical exercise testing. 2nd ed. Philadelphia: WB Saunders; 1982, 158.

[37] Noble BJ, Borg GAV. A category-ratio perceived exertion scale: relationship to blood and muscle lactates and heart rate. Med Sci Sports Exerc 1983;15:523–8.

[38] Reina-Rosenbaum R, Bach JR, Penek J. The cost/benefits of outpatient based pulmonary rehabilitation. Arch Phys Med Rehabil 1997;78:240–4.

[39] Kahn AU. Effectiveness of biofeedback and counter-conditioning in the treatment of bronchial asthma. J Psychosom Res 1977;21:97–104.

[40] Elliot MW, Mulvey D, Moxham J, et al. Domiciliary nocturnal nasal intermittent positive pressure ventilation in COPD: mechanisms underlying changes in arterial blood gas tensions. Eur Respir J 1991;4:1044–52.

[41] Gay P, Hubmayr RD, Stroetz RW. Efficacy of nocturnal nasal positive pressure ventilation combined with oxygen therapy and oxygen monotherapy in patients with severe COPD. Am J Respir Care Med 1996;154:353–8.

[42] Hudson LD, Tyler ML, Petty T. Hospitalization needs during an outpatient rehabilitation program for chronic airway obstruction. Chest 1976;70:606–10.

[43] Roselle S, D'Amico FJ. The effect of home respiratory therapy on hospital re-admission rates of patients with chronic obstructive pulmonary disease. Respir Care 1990;35:1208–13.

[44] Holle RHO, Williams DV, Vandree JC, et al. Increased muscle efficiency and sustained benefits in an outpatient community hospital-based pulmonary rehabilitation program. Chest 1988;94:1161–8.

[45] Ilowite J, Niederman M, Fein A, et al. Can benefits seen in pulmonary rehabilitation be sustained long term? Chest 1991;100:182.

[46] Mall RW, Medieros M. Objective evaluation of results of a pulmonary rehabilitation program in a community hospital. Chest 1988;94:1156–60.

[47] Troosters T, Casaburi R, Gosselink R, et al. Pulmonary rehabilitation in chronic obstructive pulmonary disease. Am J Respir Crit Care Med 2005;172:19–38.

[48] Puhan MA, Gimeno-Santos E, Scharplatz M, et al. Pulmonary rehabilitation following exacerbations of chronic obstructive pulmonary disease. Cochrane Database Syst Rev 2011;10, CD005305.

[49] Yusen R, Lefrak S, Gierda D, et al. A prospective evaluation of lung volume reduction surgery in 200 consecutive patients. Chest 2003;123:1026–37.

[50] National Emphysema Treatment Trial Research Group. Patients at high risk of death after lung volume reduction surgery. N Engl J Med 2001;345:1075–83.

[51] Smeritschnig B, Jaksch P, Kocher A, et al. Quality of life after lung transplantation: a cross-sectional study. J Heart Lung Transplant 2005;24:474–80.

[52] Keating D, Levey B, Kotsimbos T, et al. Lung transplantation in pulmonary fibrosis: challenging early outcomes counterbalanced by surprisingly good outcomes beyond 15 years. Transplant Proc 2009;41:289–91.

CHAPTER 150

Pulmonary Rehabilitation (Neuromuscular)

John R. Bach, MD

Synonyms

Neuromuscular respiratory dysfunction
Neuromuscular restrictive pulmonary syndrome

ICD-9 Codes

E0482 Mechanical insufflation-exsufflation
E0461 Noninvasive mechanical ventilation
E0450 Invasive mechanical ventilation
335.20 Amyotrophic lateral sclerosis
359.9 Myopathy disorders
V46.11 Dependence on ventilator

ICD-10 Codes

G12.21 Amyotrophic lateral sclerosis
G72.89 Myopathy

Definition

Neuromuscular disorders such as amyotrophic lateral sclerosis and myopathic disorders most often result in respiratory morbidity and mortality caused by weakness of the respiratory muscles. The three respiratory muscle groups are the inspiratory muscles, the expiratory (predominantly abdominal and upper chest wall) muscles for coughing, and the bulbar-innervated muscles. Whereas the inspiratory and expiratory muscles can be completely supported by physical aids such as continuous noninvasive ventilation (NIV), as presented here, and some patients have used this for more than 50 years without resort to tracheostomy (Fig. 150.1), there are no effective noninvasive measures to assist bulbar-innervated muscle function [1,2].

Symptoms

Patients with diminished ventilatory reserve who are able to walk complain of exertional dyspnea; but wheelchair users' symptoms may be minimal except during intercurrent respiratory infections, when they complain of anxiety, inability to fall asleep, and possibly dyspnea. Morning headaches, fatigue, sleep disturbances, and hypersomnolence result from nocturnal hypoventilation or the decreased ability to recruit accessory respiratory muscles during sleep [3].

Physical Examination

Signs of inspiratory muscle impairment and hypoventilation can include tachypnea, paradoxical breathing, hypophonia, nasal flaring, accessory respiratory muscle use, cyanosis, flushing or pallor, anxiety, and airway secretion congestion. Lethargy, obtundation, and confusion signal carbon dioxide (CO_2) narcosis. Often there are no signs at all despite symptoms of hypoventilation. The rest of the physical examination is usually typical for neuromuscular disorders (see, for example, Chapters 132 and 135).

Functional Limitations

With diminished respiratory reserve, walking becomes limited by dyspnea in going up stairs or walking long distances. Once a patient is wheelchair dependent and incapable of independently performing few activities of daily living, there are no additional functional limitations associated with chronic hypoventilation. However, symptoms of hypoventilation and CO_2 levels may increase until patients become obtunded or develop CO_2 narcosis.

Diagnostic Studies

Respiratory muscle dysfunction and hypoventilation are diagnosed by end-tidal CO_2 monitoring (capnography), oximetry, spirometry, and assessment of cough peak flows. The end-tidal CO_2 is 2 to 6 mm Hg less than arterial P_{CO_2}. The vital capacity (VC) is measured in sitting and supine positions and should not be significantly different in either position. Because hypoventilation is worse during sleep, the supine VC is more important. Orthopnea is common when the VC is less than 25% of normal or the VC in the supine position is at least 20% less than in the sitting position. The normal difference in VC between sitting and the supine position is less than 7%. Patients wearing thoracolumbar

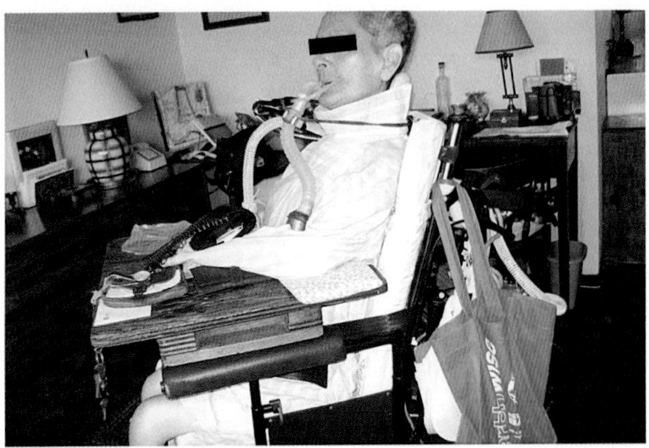

FIGURE 150.1 A 68-year-old woman who has depended on noninvasive mechanical ventilation around-the-clock since 1954 and used mouthpiece noninvasive intermittent positive pressure ventilation with the mouthpiece fixed adjacent to the sip and puff motorized wheelchair controls for daytime support since 1957.

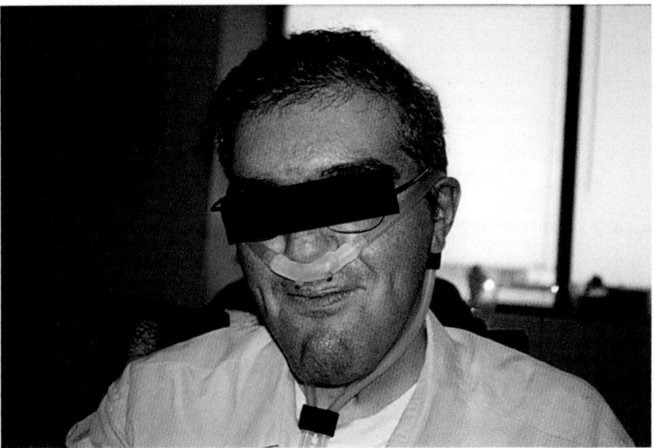

FIGURE 150.2 A 36-year-old man with Duchenne muscular dystrophy using nasal prongs interface for air stacking and for daytime ventilatory support.

bracing should have the VC measured both with the brace on and with it off because a brace that fits well can increase VC, whereas one that restricts respiratory muscle movement can decrease it.

Patients are taught glossopharyngeal breathing (GPB), and its progress is measured spirometrically, as is air stacking. Air stacking and GPB are used for lung volume recruitment. Patients air stack by receiving consecutively delivered volumes of air through a manual resuscitator or volume-cycled ventilator that are held by the glottis to the greatest volume possible. The maximum volume that can be held by the glottis, the maximum insufflation capacity (MIC), is determined spirometrically. Likewise, GPB can often provide volumes of air to or beyond those achieved by air stacking and is also measured spirometrically [4]. A nasal interface or oral-nasal interface can be used for air stacking when the lips are too weak for effective air stacking through the mouth (Fig. 150.2).

Cough peak flows are measured with a peak flow meter (Access Peak Flow Meter; Healthscan Products Inc, Cedar Grove, NJ). Cough peak flows of 160 L/min are minimal and often ineffective [4]. The attainment of (unassisted) cough peak flows above 160 L/min is the best indicator for successful tracheostomy tube removal irrespective of remaining pulmonary function [4]. Patients with VCs of less than 1500 mL have assisted cough peak flows measured from a maximally air stacked volume of air with an abdominal thrust delivered simultaneously with glottic opening [5]. A cough produced from a deep air stacked volume and with an abdominal thrust applied concomitantly with glottis opening is a "manually assisted cough"; its efficacy is also determined by peak flow meter.

For the stable patient without intrinsic pulmonary disease, arterial blood gas sampling is unnecessary. Besides the discomfort, 25% of patients hyperventilate as a result of anxiety or pain during the procedure [6].

For symptomatic patients with normal VC, an unclear pattern of oxyhemoglobin desaturation, and no apparent hypercapnia, polysomnography is warranted [7]. Polysomnography is unnecessary for symptomatic patients with decreased VC because it is programmed to interpret every apnea and hypopnea as resulting from central or obstructive events rather than from inspiratory muscle weakness.

Whereas all clearly symptomatic patients with diminished lung volumes require a trial of NIV to ease symptoms, if symptoms are questionable, nocturnal continuous capnography and oximetry are useful and most practically done in the home. A questionably symptomatic patient with decreased VC, multiple nocturnal oxyhemoglobin desaturations below 95%, and elevated nocturnal CO_2 should be encouraged to undergo a trial of nocturnal NIV.

Treatment

Initial and Habilitation

Lung Volume Recruitment

The initial intervention goals are to promote normal lung and chest wall growth for children; to maintain lung and chest wall compliance, lung growth, and chest wall mobility; and to increase cough peak flows to prevent intercurrent respiratory tract infections from developing into pneumonias and respiratory failure.

Pulmonary compliance is diminished and chest wall contractures and lung restriction occur when the lungs cannot be expanded to predicted inspiratory capacity. As the VC decreases, the largest breath one can take expands only a fraction of lung volume. Like limb articulations, regular mobilization is required. This can be achieved only by providing deep insufflations, air stacking, or nocturnal NIV [8]. The primary objectives of lung expansion therapy are to increase VC and voice volume, to maximize cough peak flows (Fig. 150.3), to maintain pulmonary compliance, to diminish atelectasis, and to master NIV because anyone who can air stack through a mouthpiece can use mouthpiece NIV and therefore be successfully extubated and decannulated even if not ventilator weaned (Table 150.1).

Bulbar muscle function and glottis function are objectively quantitated by the extent to which the MIC exceeds VC (MIC − VC). Thus, one who cannot air stack cannot close the glottis and must be passively insufflated by a pressure-cycled ventilator or CoughAssist (Respironics International Inc, Murrysville, Pa) at pressures of 40 to 70 cm H_2O or by a manual resuscitator with the exhalation

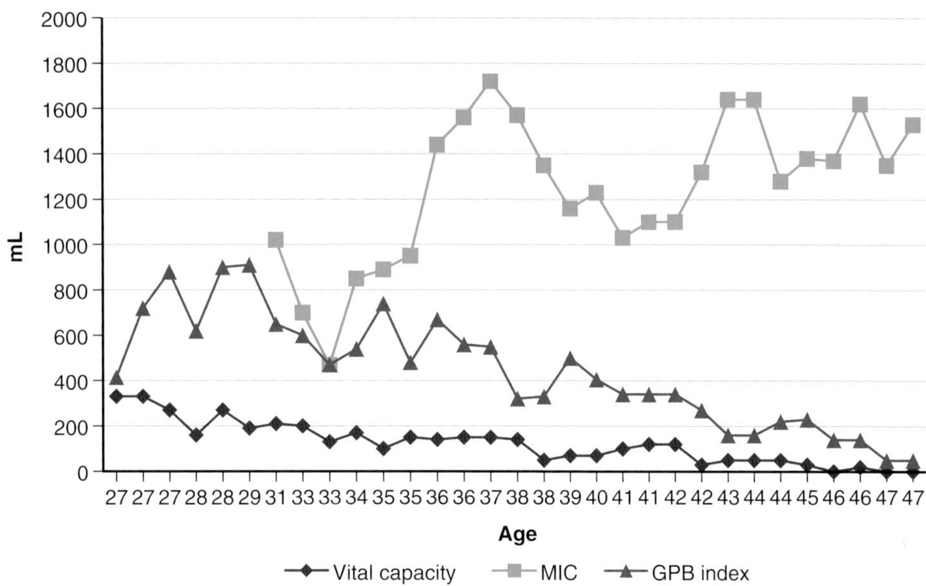

FIGURE 150.3 Graph over time of vital capacity, maximum insufflation capacity, and glossopharyngeal maximum single-breath capacity of a 47-year-old continuous mouthpiece/nasal intermittent positive pressure ventilation user with Duchenne muscular dystrophy. *GPB*, glossopharyngeal breathing; *MIC*, maximum insufflation capacity. *(From Bach JR, DeCicco A. Forty-eight years with Duchenne muscular dystrophy. Am J Phys Med Rehabil 2011;90:868-870.)*

Table 150.1 Extubation Criteria for "Unweanable" Ventilator Users

- Oxyhemoglobin saturation (Spo_2) ≥ 95% in ambient air
- $Paco_2$ ≤ 40 mm Hg at peak inspiratory pressures < 30 cm H_2O on ventilatory support up to full settings
- Afebrile and normal white blood cell count
- Any acute oxyhemoglobin desaturations below 95% reversed by mechanically assisted coughing
- Fully alert and cooperative, receiving no sedative medications
- Air leakage through upper airway sufficient for vocalization on cuff deflation
- Chest radiograph abnormalities cleared or clearing

valve blocked. The maximum passive insufflation volume has been termed the lung insufflation capacity [8]. In 282 evaluations of VC, MIC, and lung insufflation capacity, the mean values were 1131 ± 744 mL, 1712 ± 926 mL, and 2069 ± 867 mL, respectively [9].

Cough Flow Augmentation

Manually assisted coughing involves air stacking to a deep lung volume for any patient with less than 1500 mL of VC, then applying an abdominal thrust timed to glottic opening. For 364 patients able to air stack, whereas the mean VC was 997 mL, the mean MIC was 1648 mL, and although cough peak flows were 135 L/min, mean assisted cough peak flows were 235 L/min. This can be the difference between developing pneumonia and coughing effectively to prevent it [10]. The inability to generate 160 L/min of assisted cough peak flows despite having a VC or MIC greater than 1 L indicates upper airway obstruction, which can be due to severe bulbar muscle dysfunction or other lesion that should be identified by laryngoscopy so that reversible lesions can be corrected.

Mechanically assisted coughing (MAC) is the combination of the use of mechanical insufflation-exsufflation (CoughAssist) with an exsufflation-timed abdominal thrust. Deep insufflations followed immediately by deep exsufflations at pressures of 50 to −50 or greater cm H_2O are usually the most effective and preferred. MAC can be provided by an oral-nasal mask, a simple mouthpiece, or a translaryngeal or tracheostomy tube. When it is delivered by a translaryngeal or tracheostomy tube, the cuff, when present, should be inflated. The CoughAssist can be manually or automatically cycled. Manual cycling facilitates caregiver-patient coordination of inspiration and expiration with insufflation and exsufflation, but it requires hands to deliver an abdominal thrust, to hold the mask on the patient, and to operate machine cycling.

Procedures

Lung Volume Recruitment

Before patients' VCs decrease to 70% of predicted normal, they are instructed to air stack 10 to 15 times two or three times daily, usually with a manual resuscitator. Because of the importance of air stacking, NIV is provided through ventilators using volume rather than pressure cycling.

Infants cannot air stack or cooperate with passive insufflation therapy. All small children with paradoxical breathing require nocturnal NIV to prevent pectus excavatum and to promote lung growth as well as for inspiratory muscle assistance [11]. Deep insufflations can also be timed to the child's breathing and delivered through an oral-nasal interface. Children can become cooperative with deep insufflation therapy by 14 to 30 months of age.

Cough Flow Augmentation

Cough flows are augmented and sputum expulsed by delivery of about five cycles of MAC followed by a short period of normal breathing or ventilator use to avoid hyperventilation until offending sputum is expulsed and oxyhemoglobin saturation levels, if diminished, return to 95% or greater. Insufflation and exsufflation times are adjusted to provide maximum observable chest expansion and rapid full lung emptying. In general, 2 to 4 seconds are required. Treatment continues until no more secretions are expulsed and secretion-related oxyhemoglobin desaturations are reversed. Use can be required as often as every 30 minutes around-the-clock during chest infections.

The use of mechanical insufflation-exsufflation through the upper airway can be effective for children as young as 11 months, who can occasionally facilitate its efficacy by not crying or closing the glottis. Between 2.5 and 5 years of age, most children cooperate with it. Before that, the insufflations and exsufflations and exsufflation-timed abdominal thrusts are timed to the child's own breathing cycle.

Conventional airway suctioning misses the left main stem bronchus about 90% of the time [12]. However, MAC can provide effective flows in both left and right airways without the discomfort or airway trauma. Patients prefer MAC to suctioning [13]. Deep suctioning, whether by tube or upper airway, can be discontinued for most patients.

VC, pulmonary flow rates, and Spo_2, when abnormal, can improve immediately with clearing of airway secretions by MAC [14]. An increase in VC of 15% to 42% was noted immediately after treatment in 67 patients with "obstructive dyspnea," and a 55% increase in VC was noted after MAC for patients with neuromuscular disorders [15]. We have observed 15% to 400% (200 to 800 mL) improvements in VC and normalization of Spo_2 for patients during chest infections [16].

Of the three muscle groups required for effective coughing, MAC can take the place of only the inspiratory and expiratory muscles. Thus, ventilator users with intact bulbar muscles can usually air stack to volumes of 3 L or more and, unless very scoliotic or obese, can achieve effective assisted cough peak flows of 6 to 9 L/s and do not need MAC. The patients who need MAC the most have moderately impaired bulbar muscle function that limits assisted cough peak flows to less than 300 L/min. This is typical of Duchenne muscular dystrophy and other myopathies [10]. Patients with respiratory muscle weakness complicated by scoliosis and inability to capture the asymmetric diaphragm by abdominal thrusting can also greatly benefit from MAC (Table 150.2).

Surgery

No surgery is indicated in these patients.

Potential Disease Complications

The great majority of morbidity and mortality for patients with neuromuscular disease is due to complications of respiratory muscle weakness. In particular, these patients develop life-threatening chronic alveolar hypoventilation. Life can be prolonged by ventilatory assistance or support, which is usually administered invasively but can be administered noninvasively by use of physical medicine respiratory muscle aids. Respiratory orthopnea, symptoms of hypoventilation noted before, and paradoxical breathing in children indicate the need for nocturnal noninvasive intermittent positive pressure ventilation (NIV) [11]. Because, in general, only patients improperly treated with supplemental oxygen develop CO_2 narcosis and respiratory failure is generally caused by ineffective cough and airway secretion management, any patient finding that NIV use is more burdensome than his or her symptoms is told that it is all right to discontinue it for now but to return regularly for reevaluation.

Although the inspiratory muscles can be assisted by applying pressures to the body, negative pressure body ventilators cause obstructive apneas, are less effective than NIV, and become even less effective with age and decreasing pulmonary compliance [17]. A useful body ventilator, the intermittent abdominal pressure ventilator (IAPV) or Exsufflation Belt (Respironics International Inc, Murrysville, PA), involves the intermittent inflation of an elastic air sac that is contained in a corset or belt worn beneath the patient's outer clothing. The sac is cyclically inflated by a positive pressure ventilator. This moves the diaphragm upward to assist in expiration. With bladder deflation, gravity causes the abdominal contents and diaphragm to return to the resting position, and inspiration occurs. A trunk angle of 30 degrees or more from the horizontal is required for effectiveness. A patient can add to the IAPV-delivered volume by breathing or GPB along with it. The IAPV augments tidal volumes by 300 mL to as high as 1200 mL and is often preferred to mouthpiece NIV by patients with little autonomous breathing ability during daytime hours [18].

Noninvasive Intermittent Positive Pressure Ventilation

NIV can be delivered by lip seal, nasal, and oral-nasal interfaces during sleep or by a mouthpiece or nasal interface during daytime hours. Mouthpiece and nasal NIV are open systems that require the user to rely on central nervous system reflexes to prevent excessive insufflation leakage during

Table 150.2 Management of Patients with Spinal Cord Injury

Level*	Vital Capacity	Bulbar Function/Neck Function†	Daytime	Nocturnal
Above C1	0	Inadequate/inadequate	TIPPV	TIPPV
C2-C3	<200 mL	Adequate/inadequate	EPP/DP	NIPPV/MIPPV
Below C2	>200 mL	Adequate/adequate	MIPPV/IAPV	NIPPV/MIPPV

*Motor levels.

†Adequate neck function involves sufficient oral and neck muscle control to rotate, flex, and extend the neck to grab and use a mouthpiece for intermittent positive pressure ventilation. Adequate bulbar function prevents aspiration of saliva to the degree that the Spo_2 baseline decreases below 95%.

DP, diaphragm pacing; *EPP,* electrophrenic pacing; *IAPV,* intermittent abdominal pressure ventilation; *MIPPV,* mouthpiece intermittent positive pressure ventilation; *NIPPV,* nasal intermittent positive pressure ventilation; *TIPPV,* tracheostomy intermittent positive pressure ventilation.

sleep [3,19]; thus, supplemental oxygen and sedatives can render it ineffective. NIV can be introduced in the clinic or home setting.

There are numerous commercially available nasal interfaces (continuous positive airway pressure masks). Several should be tried and their use alternated to avoid prolonged skin pressure. Excessive insufflation leakage can be avoided, if necessary, by switching from an open to a closed system with use of a lip seal–nasal prongs system. Such interfaces deliver air through the mouth and nose during sleep and require minimal strap pressure. This optimizes skin comfort and minimizes air (insufflation) leakage.

The most useful method for daytime ventilatory support is NIV through a 15-mm angled mouthpiece. Some keep the mouthpiece in the mouth all day, but most have it fixed near the mouth by a metal clamp attached to a wheelchair for this purpose [20–22]. The mouthpiece can also be fixed onto motorized wheelchair controls (e.g., sip and puff, chin, and tongue controls). Large volumes of 800 to 1500 mL are delivered so that the patient can take as much air as desired for each breath to vary tidal volumes, speech volume, and cough flows as well as to air stack. Neck movement and lip function are needed to use mouthpiece NIV; otherwise, a nasal prongs system is used for daytime support [18]. Nasal NIV is also most practical for nocturnal and daytime use by infants. Other than perhaps for uncontrollable seizures and the inability to cooperate, there are no contraindications to the use of NIV long term.

Glossopharyngeal Breathing

Both inspiratory and, indirectly, expiratory muscle function can be assisted by GPB [23]. This is the glottis pistoning boluses of air into the lungs. One GPB breath usually consists of six to nine gulps of 40 to 200 mL each (Fig. 150.3). During the training period, its efficiency can be monitored by spirometrically measuring the milliliters of air per piston action, piston actions per breath, and breaths per minute. A training manual [24] and numerous videos are available [25], the most analytical of which was produced in 1999 [26]. GPB can provide an individual with no VC with ventilator-free breathing tolerance up to all day [23,27].

Severe oropharyngeal muscle weakness can limit or eliminate the usefulness of GPB. However, we have managed 13 Duchenne muscular dystrophy ventilator users who had no breathing tolerance other than by GPB [28]. Approximately 60% of ventilator users with no autonomous ability to breathe but with good bulbar muscle function can use GPB for ventilator-free breathing up to all day [23,27]. GPB is rarely useful in the presence of an indwelling tracheostomy tube. The safety and versatility afforded by GPB are key reasons for tube decannulation or avoidance of tracheostomy in favor of NIV and MAC. This frees patients from the fear of sudden ventilator failure or accidental ventilator disconnection [23,27,29].

Oximetry Monitoring and Feedback Protocol

For a hypercapnic patient with oxyhemoglobin desaturation due to chronic alveolar hypoventilation or for the patient being weaned from tracheostomy ventilation, introduction to and use of mouthpiece or nasal NIV are facilitated by oximetry feedback. An Spo_2 alarm set at 94% signals the patient to maintain normal Spo_2 by taking deeper breaths and to maintain Spo_2 above 94% all day [10]. When it is no longer possible to achieve this by unassisted breathing, it is done by mouthpiece or nasal NIV. With advancing disease and muscle weakness, the patient can require increasing periods of daytime NIV to maintain normal Spo_2 and intact central ventilatory drive.

Continuous Spo_2 feedback is especially important during respiratory tract infections. The cough of infants and small children who can never sit is inadequate to prevent chest cold–triggered pneumonia and acute respiratory failure. MAC is used for any dip in Spo_2 below 95%. When NIV is used continuously, such dips are usually due to bronchial mucous plugging rather than to hypoventilation, and if the mucus is not quickly cleared, atelectasis and pneumonia can quickly result. Thus, patients are instructed to use NIV and MAC to maintain normal Spo_2 to avert pneumonia and respiratory failure. For adults with infrequent chest colds, rapid access to MAC may be all that is necessary.

Potential Treatment Complications

Abdominal distention tends to occur sporadically in NIV users. The air usually passes as flatus once the patient is mobilized in the morning. When it is severe, however, it can increase ventilator dependence and necessitate burping the air out by opening a gastrostomy or nasogastric tube.

Despite aggressive lung mobilization and expansion three times daily, often to above 60 cm H_2O pressures and along with NIV support for more than 50 years in many cases, we have had one case of pneumothorax in more than 1000 NIV users [30]. Although it is often described as a complication of or limiting factor for NIV, secretion encumbrance most often results from failure to use MAC.

References

[1] Bach JR. Update and perspectives on noninvasive respiratory muscle aids: part 1—the inspiratory muscle aids. Chest 1994;105: 1230–40.
[2] Bach JR, Bianchi C, Aufiero E. Oximetry and indications for tracheotomy in amyotrophic lateral sclerosis. Chest 2004;126:1502–7.
[3] Bach JR, Alba AS. Management of chronic alveolar hypoventilation by nasal ventilation. Chest 1990;97:52–7.
[4] Bach JR, Saporito LR. Criteria for extubation and tracheostomy tube removal for patients with ventilatory failure. A different approach to weaning. Chest 1996;110:1566–71.
[5] Kang SW, Bach JR. Maximum insufflation capacity. Chest 2000;118:61–5.
[6] Currie DC, Munro C, Gaskell D, et al. Practice, problems and compliance with postural drainage: a survey of chronic sputum producers. Br J Dis Chest 1986;80:249–53.
[7] Williams AJ, Yu G, Santiago S, Stein M. Screening for sleep apnea using pulse oximetry and a clinical score. Chest 1991;100:631–5.
[8] Bach JR, Kang SW. Disorders of ventilation: weakness, stiffness, and mobilization. Chest 2000;117:301–3.
[9] Bach JR, Mahajan K, Lipa B, et al. Lung insufflation capacity in neuromuscular disease. Am J Phys Med Rehabil 2008;87:720–5.
[10] Gomez-Merino E, Bach JR. Duchenne muscular dystrophy: prolongation of life by noninvasive respiratory muscle aids. Am J Phys Med Rehabil 2002;81:411–5.
[11] Bach JR, Baird JS, Plosky D, et al. Spinal muscular atrophy type 1: management and outcomes. Pediatr Pulmonol 2002;34:16–22.
[12] Fishburn MJ, Marino RJ, Ditunno Jr JF. Atelectasis and pneumonia in acute spinal cord injury. Arch Phys Med Rehabil 1990;71: 197–200.

[13] Garstang SV, Kirshblum SC, Wood KE. Patient preference for in-exsufflation for secretion management with spinal cord injury. J Spinal Cord Med 2000;23:80–5.
[14] Bach JR, Smith WH, Michaels J, et al. Airway secretion clearance by mechanical exsufflation for post-poliomyelitis ventilator assisted individuals. Arch Phys Med Rehabil 1993;74:170–7.
[15] Barach AL, Beck GJ. Exsufflation with negative pressure: physiologic and clinical studies in poliomyelitis, bronchial asthma, pulmonary emphysema and bronchiectasis. Arch Intern Med 1954;93:825–41.
[16] Bach JR. Mechanical insufflation-exsufflation: comparison of peak expiratory flows with manually assisted and unassisted coughing techniques. Chest 1993;104:1553–62.
[17] Bach JR, Alba AS, Shin D. Management alternatives for post-polio respiratory insufficiency: assisted ventilation by nasal or oral-nasal interface. Am J Phys Med Rehabil 1989;68:264–71.
[18] Bach JR, Alba AS. Intermittent abdominal pressure ventilator in a regimen of noninvasive ventilatory support. Chest 1991;99:630–6.
[19] Bach JR, Robert D, Leger P, et al. Sleep fragmentation in kyphoscoliotic individuals with alveolar hypoventilation treated by nasal IPPV. Chest 1995;107:1552–8.
[20] Ishikawa Y, Miura T, Ishikawa Y, et al. Duchenne muscular dystrophy: survival by cardio-respiratory interventions. Neuromuscul Disord 2011;21:47–51.
[21] Bach JR, Alba AS, Saporito LR. Intermittent positive pressure ventilation via the mouth as an alternative to tracheostomy for 257 ventilator users. Chest 1993;103:174–82.
[22] Bach JR, Gonçalves MR, Hon AJ, et al. Changing trends in the management of end-stage respiratory muscle failure in neuromuscular disease: current recommendations of an international consensus. Am J Phys Med Rehabil 2013;92:267–77.
[23] Bach JR, Alba AS, Bodofsky E, et al. Glossopharyngeal breathing and noninvasive aids in the management of post-polio respiratory insufficiency. Birth Defects 1987;23:99–113.
[24] Dail C, Rodgers M, Guess V, et al. Glossopharyngeal breathing. Downey, Calif: Rancho Los Amigos Department of Physical Therapy; 1979.
[25] Dail CW, Affeldt JE. Glossopharyngeal breathing [video]. Los Angeles, Calif: Department of Visual Education, College of Medical Evangelists; 1954.
[26] Webber B, Higgens J. Glossopharyngeal breathing: what, when and how? [video]. Holbrook, Horsham, West Sussex, England: Aslan Studios Ltd; 1999.
[27] Bach JR. New approaches in the rehabilitation of the traumatic high level quadriplegic. Am J Phys Med Rehabil 1991;70:13–20.
[28] Bach JR, Bianchi C, Vidigal-Lopes M, et al. Lung inflation by glossopharyngeal breathing and "air stacking" in Duchenne muscular dystrophy. Am J Phys Med Rehabil 2007;86:295–300.
[29] Bach JR, Alba AS. Noninvasive options for ventilatory support of the traumatic high level quadriplegic. Chest 1990;98:613–9.
[30] Suri P, Burns SP, Bach JR. Pneumothorax associated with mechanical insufflation-exsufflation and related factors. Am J Phys Med Rehabil 2008;87:951–5.

CHAPTER 151

Rheumatoid Arthritis

Faren H. Williams, MD, MS

Synonyms

None

ICD-9 Code

714.0 Rheumatoid arthritis

ICD-10 Code

M06.9 Rheumatoid arthritis

Definition

Rheumatoid arthritis is a chronic inflammatory disorder that primarily affects joints but may also have prominent extra-articular features. The arthritis is classically symmetric and affects the peripheral joints. The prevalence of rheumatoid arthritis is approximately 1% in white individuals, and it affects women about 2 to 2.5 times more often than men, which may be related to the effect of sex hormones, such as estrogen, in regulating the immune response [1]. Peak incidence of rheumatoid arthritis is in the third and fourth decades, although the disease affects all ages and individuals from all racial and ethnic groups [2–4]. Classification criteria are available for rheumatoid arthritis and may be helpful in the evaluation of patients (Table 151.1). Many patients with early disease, however, may not fulfill these criteria [5].

Symptoms

Rheumatoid arthritis is a systemic disease, and symptoms vary according to the system involved [6–8].

General

Morning stiffness is a prominent feature of rheumatoid arthritis. Unlike the brief stiffness (5 to 10 minutes) that occurs in patients with osteoarthritis, the morning stiffness in rheumatoid arthritis may last for hours. Fatigue and generalized malaise are also common complaints.

Joint

Patients present with joint pain and swelling as well as loss of joint function, which may be due to joint inflammation or structural damage from cartilage destruction and bone erosion. A Baker cyst can develop and cause pain or swelling of the popliteal fossa. If the cyst ruptures, it may cause pain, swelling, and erythema of the calf. If the cricoarytenoid joint is involved, patients may complain of laryngeal pain, hoarseness, or difficulty in swallowing.

Eye

Up to one third of patients will complain of dry eyes (keratoconjunctivitis sicca). These patients may also complain of foreign body sensation, burning, or discharge. Patients with episcleritis will complain of red, painful eyes.

Skin

Patients may note small, painless subcutaneous nodules, mainly over the extensor surfaces. Rheumatoid vasculitis will cause a rash that may lead to ulceration. Patients with vasculitis may also complain of discoloration around the fingertips (digital infarcts).

Neurologic

Numbness and tingling are common symptoms of nerve involvement. Nerve entrapment may result from joint inflammation. The most common site is at the wrist, where median nerve involvement may cause carpal tunnel symptoms. Mononeuritis multiplex is the result of vasculitis and is manifested as weakness, numbness, or tingling in discrete nerve distributions (e.g., femoral, peroneal, or radial nerve, causing proximal leg weakness, footdrop, or wristdrop). Cervical spine instability may lead to myelopathy, causing sensory symptoms and weakness, most commonly in the upper extremities. This can occur in the absence of neck pain in patients with long-standing rheumatoid arthritis.

Cardiac

The incidence and prevalence of coronary artery disease are increased in any type of chronic inflammatory disorder, and this is especially evident in rheumatoid arthritis. Thus patients may present with complaints of chest pain,

Table 151.1 Classification Criteria for Rheumatoid Arthritis*

Criterion	Definition
Morning stiffness	Morning stiffness in or around the joints lasting at least 1 hour before maximal improvement
Arthritis of three or more joint areas	Soft tissue swelling or fluid in at least three joints observed by a clinician The 14 possible joints include right and left proximal interphalangeal, metacarpophalangeal, wrist, elbow, knee, ankle, and metatarsophalangeal joints.
Arthritis of the hand joints	At least one area swollen in a wrist, metacarpophalangeal, or proximal interphalangeal joint
Symmetric arthritis	Simultaneous involvement of the same joint areas on both sides of the body Involvement of the small joint groups (metacarpophalangeal joints, proximal interphalangeal joints, and metatarsophalangeal joints) is acceptable without absolute symmetry.
Rheumatoid nodules	Subcutaneous nodules occurring over bone prominences, extensor surfaces, or juxta-articular regions These must be observed by a clinician.
Serum rheumatoid factor	Abnormal amounts of serum rheumatoid factor by any method for which the result has been positive in <5% of normal control subjects
Radiographic changes	Posteroanterior hand and wrist films that demonstrate erosion or unequivocal bone decalcification localized in or most marked adjacent to the involved joints

*A patient is said to have rheumatoid arthritis if he or she satisfies at least four of the seven criteria. Criteria one through four must have been present for at least 6 weeks.

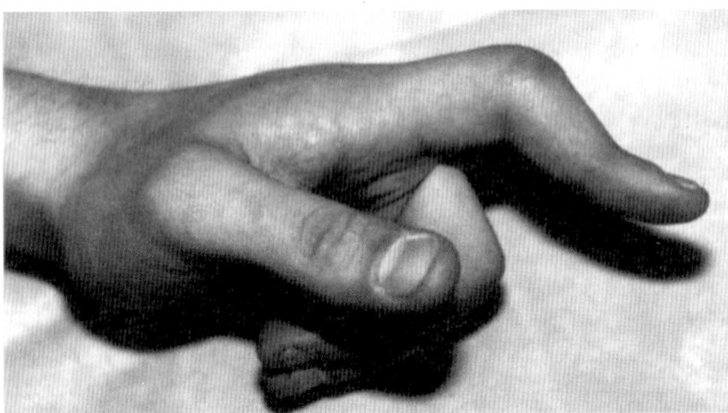

FIGURE 151.1 The boutonnière deformity, involving hyperextension of the distal interphalangeal joint with flexion of the proximal interphalangeal joint, is caused by a derangement of the extensor mechanism—typically a rupture of the central extensor tendon at its insertion in the middle phalanx. Early diagnosis and prolonged splinting of the proximal interphalangeal joint in extension are necessary for successful treatment of this difficult injury. *(From Concannon MJ. Common Hand Problems in Primary Care. Philadelphia, Hanley & Belfus, 1999.)*

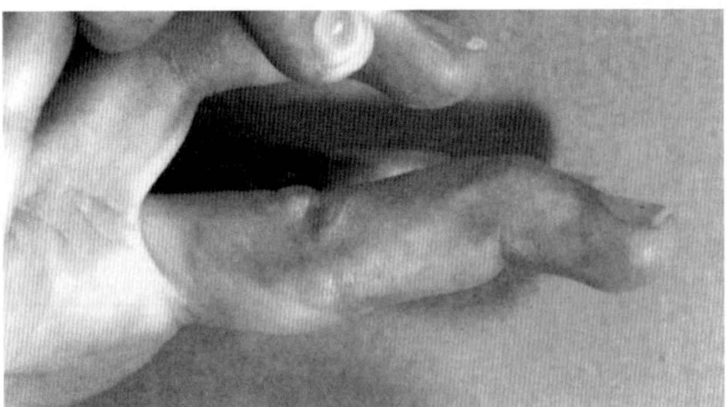

FIGURE 151.2 The swan-neck deformity (recurvatum) involves hyperextension of the proximal interphalangeal joint with flexion of the distal interphalangeal joint. This is caused by a derangement in the extensor mechanism, with a dorsal migration of the lateral bands. *(From Concannon MJ. Common Hand Problems in Primary Care. Philadelphia, Hanley & Belfus, 1999.)*

shortness of breath, diaphoresis, and other symptoms consistent with cardiac ischemia. Prevalence of angina in patients with rheumatoid arthritis may be less because of the relative inactivity. Other cardiac manifestations of rheumatoid arthritis include myocarditis, pericarditis, atrioventricular block, and cardiac rheumatoid nodules. Pericardial involvement is usually asymptomatic.

Pulmonary

Pleural inflammation or nodulosis may produce typical symptoms of pleurisy. Shortness of breath may occur secondary to pleural or interstitial disease.

Physical Examination

All joints are examined for swelling, warmth, effusion, range of motion, and deformity. Fingers, feet, wrists, and knees are most commonly involved. The distal interphalangeal joints are usually spared. In rare cases, patients will present with monarthritis (involvement of a single joint). Rheumatoid nodules are present in about 30% of patients and occur over bone prominences, over extensor surfaces, or in juxta-articular regions [6].

In the hands, early rheumatoid arthritis causes fusiform swelling at the proximal interphalangeal joint. Chronic inflammation may lead to subluxation of the metacarpophalangeal joints with ulnar deviation of the fingers. Damage to collateral ligaments at the proximal interphalangeal joints results in the classic boutonnière (proximal interphalangeal joint flexion and distal interphalangeal joint hyperextension) and swan-neck (proximal interphalangeal joint hyperextension and distal interphalangeal joint flexion) deformities (Figs. 151.1 and 151.2).

Symmetric wrist swelling is usually present. Subluxation results from synovitis and weakening of the ligaments and causes prominence of the ulnar styloid.

Inflammation of the synovial tendon sheath (tenosynovitis) may occur in the flexor or extensor tendons of the fingers. Examination reveals that passive motion is greater than active motion. Crepitus is often felt when the examiner's hands are placed over the tendon sheaths and the fingers are flexed and extended. If the patient has a trigger finger, placement of one finger over the flexor tendon while the affected finger is flexed and extended will allow palpation of a nodule.

Elbow involvement is common. In early disease, inflammation and effusion cause decreased extension. Effusions can be palpated in the para–olecranon groove. In some cases, there may be pressure on the ulnar nerve. With chronic inflammation and erosion of the cartilage between the radius and ulna, loss of elbow extension and flexion occurs. Rheumatoid nodules are often found over the extensor aspect of the proximal ulna. The olecranon bursa may be enlarged and filled with fluid or nodules.

The shoulder may be involved in rheumatoid arthritis. Effusions are best seen on the anterior aspect of the shoulder below the acromion. Evaluation of rotator cuff strength is important because inflammation of the rotator cuff may result in tendinous destruction. The biceps tendon may rupture, causing a bulge in the biceps when it is flexed against resistance.

The cervical spine may have decreased range of motion or pain with range of motion. Patients with suspected cervical instability should have a thorough neurologic examination, checking for upper motor neuron findings. Patients with cord involvement may demonstrate paresthesias, weakness, or pathologic reflexes. Tingling paresthesias descending the thoracolumbar spine on flexion of the cervical spine are called Lhermitte sign.

The hip joint is deep, limiting evaluation for synovitis and effusion. An inflamed hip will cause groin pain on active and passive range of motion. Patients may walk with an antalgic gait, rapidly taking weight off the affected leg, or shorten their stride length. Pain in the hip may also result from trochanteric bursitis. Application of pressure over the lateral hip region reproduces the pain from the trochanteric bursa. Lateral hip pain and lack of groin pain distinguish trochanteric bursitis from joint inflammation. Iliopsoas bursitis may result in an inguinal mass.

The knee is commonly involved in rheumatoid arthritis. Small effusions can be detected by looking for a "bulge" sign. For the performance of this maneuver, the patient should be lying down. With one hand, the clinician makes an upward stroke to depress the medial synovial pouch. A downward stroke on the lateral aspect of the knee will result in a bulge of the medial pouch if a small effusion is present. A ballottable patella (patellar tap) indicates a larger effusion. Baker cyst occurs as an extension of synovial fluid from the joint cavity. The cyst causes fullness in the popliteal fossa that can be seen when the patient is standing with his or her back facing the clinician. Erythema and swelling of the calf may be seen if the Baker cyst has ruptured. Evaluation for hemorrhage below the malleoli of the ankle (the "crescent" sign) can distinguish this from thrombophlebitis.

The ankle may have synovitis, effusion, or decreased range of motion in the patient with rheumatoid arthritis. Involvement of the hindfoot (subtalar and talonavicular joints) may result in valgus deformity and flatfoot. Metatarsophalangeal joint involvement is common. Synovitis causes pain and fullness with palpation. Hallux valgus deformity is also common. Progressive disease causes dorsal dislocation of the metatarsophalangeal joints and claw toes.

Table 151.2 Criteria for Classification of Functional Status in Rheumatoid Arthritis

Class I	Able to perform all activities of daily living (self-care, vocational, and avocational)
Class II	Able to perform self-care and vocational activities, but limited in avocational activities
Class III	Able to perform usual self-care activities, but limited in vocational and avocational activities
Class IV	Limited in all activities of daily living (self-care, vocational, and avocational)

Functional Limitations

Functional limitations depend on the location and severity of joint and extra-articular involvement. There may be limitations or pain with upper extremity movements or lower extremity motions, including gait. Criteria for the assessment of functional status have been established (Table 151.2) and are based on activities of daily living, including self-care (e.g., dressing, feeding, bathing, grooming, and toileting) and vocational (e.g., work, school, and homemaking) and avocational (e.g., recreational and leisure) activities [10].

Whereas radiologic changes have limited value in determining functional impairment and quality of life, disability from rheumatoid arthritis has been directly attributed to joint damage, disease activity, pain, and depressive symptoms [11]. Patients with rheumatoid arthritis may have less disability conviction than those with other problems, such as low back pain.

Diagnostic Studies

Laboratory histologic findings and radiographic findings may be suggestive of rheumatoid arthritis, but no test is diagnostic of the disease [6,12] (Figs. 151.3 and 151.4). Rheumatoid factor is present in the serum of 85% of patients [8]. However, because rheumatoid factor is often present in other inflammatory conditions, such as systemic lupus erythematosus, primary Sjögren syndrome, and chronic osteomyelitis, much debate exists about its utility in the diagnosis of rheumatoid arthritis as a result of low specificity [13]. Anti–cyclic citrullinated peptide antibodies have shown more promise as potential biologic markers because of sensitivities of 70% to 80% and specificities of 95% to 98% in patients with established rheumatoid arthritis [14]. Normochromic, normocytic anemia consistent with chronic disease is often found, and the degree of anemia often correlates with disease activity. Acute phase reactants, such as erythrocyte sedimentation rate, C-reactive protein concentration, and erythrocyte and platelet counts, are elevated. Eosinophilia may be found in patients with extra-articular manifestations. Patients with Felty syndrome (rheumatoid arthritis, splenomegaly, and leukopenia) exhibit low white blood cell counts and may have thrombocytopenia. A variant of Felty syndrome has been described in which patients have large granular lymphocytes in blood and bone marrow in addition to neutropenia. Liver enzymes including aspartate transaminase and alkaline phosphatase are often elevated in patients with active disease.

Evaluation of fluid taken from an affected joint will show an inflammatory cell count (more than 2000 white blood cells). Joint fluid should always be sent for culture to rule out infection and evaluated under a polarized microscope to

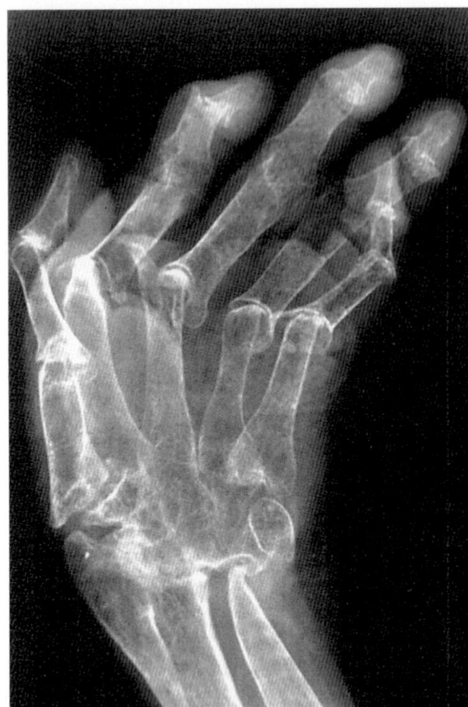

FIGURE 151.3 Advanced rheumatoid arthritis—hand and wrist. Bony ankylosis at the wrist, penciling of the distal ulna, and marked erosive changes at the metacarpophalangeal joints with ulnar deviation of the fingers are classic findings of rheumatoid arthritis. Also note the more severe involvement of the carpus and metacarpophalangeal joints; interphalangeal joints are typically less severely affected. *(From Katz DS, Math KR, Groskin SA. Radiology Secrets. Philadelphia, Hanley & Belfus, 1998.)*

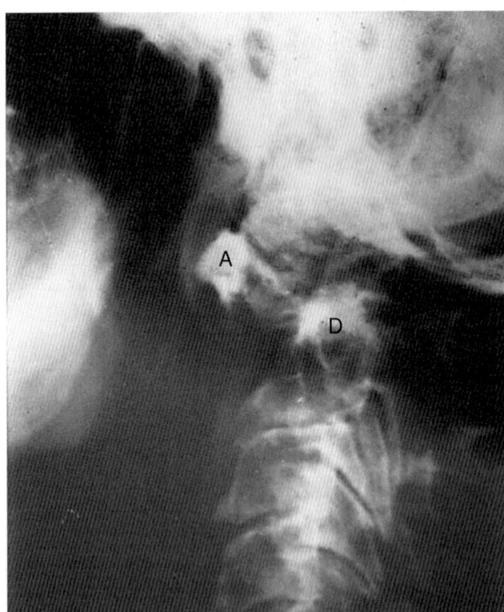

FIGURE 151.4 Atlantoaxial subluxation—rheumatoid arthritis. There is marked widening of the space between the anterior arch of the atlas (*A*) and the margin of the dens (*D*). *(From Katz DS, Math KR, Groskin SA. Radiology Secrets. Philadelphia, Hanley & Belfus, 1998.)*

exclude crystal disease. If pleurocentesis or pericardiocentesis is necessary, the fluid has a low complement concentration, a high protein concentration, and a predominance of lymphocytes. The glucose concentration is characteristically extremely low or may even be absent.

Characteristic changes on joint radiographs include periarticular osteopenia and marginal erosions. Early in the disease, joint films may be normal. Baseline hand and wrist films may aid in diagnosis and can be used to follow disease progression. Flexion and extension views of the cervical spine may demonstrate erosion of the odontoid and atlantoaxial subluxation. Pulmonary nodules or interstitial fibrosis can be seen on the chest radiograph. Echocardiography often reveals a small pericardial effusion, valvular thickening, or aortic root dilation, but these are most often asymptomatic. Electrocardiography may reveal conduction abnormalities due to involvement of the cardiac conduction system by rheumatoid nodules.

Differential Diagnosis

Crystal-induced arthritis
Gout
Pseudogout
Spondyloarthropathies
Psoriatic arthritis
Ankylosing spondylitis
Enteropathic arthritis

Treatment

Initial

Nonsteroidal anti-inflammatory drugs are effective in some patients.

For patients with inadequate response to nonsteroidal anti-inflammatory drugs or poor prognostic indicators, disease-modifying antirheumatic drugs (DMARDs) should be initiated. Poor prognostic factors include high-titer rheumatoid factor, early presence of bone erosion, many affected joints, extra-articular involvement, and considerable degree of physical disability at disease onset [9,15].

DMARDs that are prescribed include antimalarials, intramuscular administration of gold, sulfasalazine, azathioprine, methotrexate, leflunomide, cyclosporine, and cyclophosphamide [15,16]. Anticytokine therapies include the anti–tumor necrosis factor-α agents etanercept, infliximab, and adalimumab and the interleukin-1 receptor antagonist anakinra. Other biologic agents currently available include abatacept (CTLA4-Ig) and rituximab, which is a B cell–depleting monoclonal antibody. Several studies support the use of combination DMARD therapy [17]. Anti–tumor necrosis factor-α agents used in combination with small-molecule DMARDs such as methotrexate will often halt disease activity and radiologic progression of joint destruction [18]. Corticosteroids can be very useful and can be administered systemically as a bridge to therapy with DMARDs or intra-articularly for monarticular or oligoarticular involvement.

Patients who have persistent pain due to structural damage may need treatment specifically for the pain, with different medications. Depending on the patient, one may need to consider analgesics, anti-inflammatories, opioids, opioid-like drugs (tramadol), and neuromodulators to include antidepressants, anticonvulsants, and muscle relaxants [19].

Rehabilitation

Once the diagnosis is confirmed, it is important to work together with a rheumatologist to prescribe the most optimal rehabilitation treatment program. Static exercise regimens to maintain strength while protecting inflamed joints from adverse stress are recommended. Appropriate referrals to occupational or physical therapists for more specific treatment and splinting can be initiated by a physician, with close follow-up to determine whether the patient needs modifications or changes in the treatment program as the disease progresses. The physician can also address issues of pain, return to work, and maintenance of function important to the patient's lifestyle.

The role of occupational and physical therapy may be different in early or established disease and end-stage disease [20,21]. In early disease, occupational therapy is directed toward education of the patient about how to minimize joint stress in performing activities of daily living. Splints may be used to provide joint rest and to reduce inflammation during the acute inflammatory phase. Splints may also allow functional use of joints that would otherwise be limited by pain. However, not all clinicians advocate splints as they can facilitate more joint stiffness if they are used routinely. Paraffin baths can provide relief of pain and stiffness in the small joints of the hands. Contrast baths are used to increase superficial blood flow, although the benefit for patients with rheumatoid arthritis is not clear [22]. In end-stage disease, the occupational therapist plays an important role, providing aids and adaptive devices, such as raised toilet seats, special chairs and beds, and special grips that can assist in self-care. By maximizing one's functional ability, the occupational therapist can help prevent other physical or psychological problems [23]. Outcomes can include improvements in self-care, productivity at home and at work, and leisure time enjoyment [24].

Physical therapy can be helpful in reducing joint inflammation and pain. The therapist may employ a variety of techniques, including the application of heat in conjunction with passive stretch or cold for inflamed joints. Water exercise (hydrotherapy) is used to increase muscle strength without joint overload. In patients with foot involvement, small alterations to footwear or inserts may decrease pain and provide a more normal gait. In end-stage disease, the goals of therapy are to reduce joint inflammation, to enhance flexibility, to improve the function of damaged joints, and to improve strength in surrounding muscles and maintain a level of physical fitness.

Local immobilization may be used to reduce inflammation and pain. Nonfixed contractures may be prevented or improved with periods of splinting combined with goal-oriented exercise. Muscle strength and overall conditioning may be improved by static, range of motion, and relaxation exercises. In recent years, aerobic and weight-bearing exercises have been used without detrimental effect to the joints. These dynamic exercises are more effective in increasing muscle strength, range of motion, and physical capacity [25]. However, high-intensity weight-bearing exercises have been shown to accelerate joint destruction in individuals with preexisting extensive large-joint damage from rheumatoid arthritis [26]. Thus the exercise prescription must be appropriately tailored to the degree of disease present in each patient. The motivation and encouragement provided by the physician and therapist should not be underestimated. In one study, the communication skills and disease-specific knowledge exhibited by the therapists were most important in managing the patient's disease. The investigators also identified a need for therapists to have a good understanding of the disease process and to understand the role of a multidisciplinary team in treating the patient [27]. Some therapists may require more professional development to confidently educate and treat this patient population. In another study by O'Brien [28], there was significant improvement in arm function with patients who did home strengthening exercises versus stretching and education alone. Resistance exercise has been shown to be safe and efficacious as it improves isokinetic, static, and grip strength [29]. Community aquatic programs for arthritis help reduce stress on weight-bearing joints and provide some general conditioning [30,31].

Procedures

For monarticular or oligoarticular involvement, local steroid injection may be used when oral medications fail to control joint inflammation. If there is electrodiagnostically confirmed carpal tunnel syndrome, focal steroid injections may be helpful. If the neurophysiologic studies confirm more sensory axonal loss or motor involvement, surgical decompression may be recommended [32]. Ultrasonography is recognized as useful diagnostically, because a skilled examiner can differentiate tendinopathy from bursitis and determine whether there is any entrapment of these structures with movement. The goal of any diagnostic procedure is increase the specificity for the diagnosis. Sonography is dynamic and can be more specific than other diagnostic imaging in the hands of a skilled sonographer [33]. There is increasing use of ultrasonography for needle placement during procedures to ensure injection into the affected joints [34]. The goals of any procedure are to maintain the patient's functional level, to minimize pain, and to try to prevent more debility from the disease by slowing the progression or treating associated problems that impair function.

Surgery

Orthopedic intervention includes joint reconstruction (arthrodesis) or replacement (arthroplasty) (Fig. 151.5). For hand patients with low-demand activities, arthroplasty

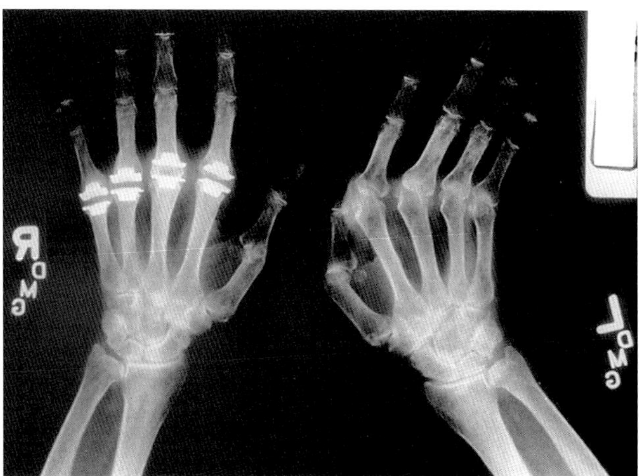

FIGURE 151.5 Hinged silicone prosthesis with grommets. Radiograph of implanted prostheses at the metacarpophalangeal joints of the index, middle, ring, and little fingers on the right hand. *(From Weinzweig J. Plastic Surgery Secrets. Philadelphia, Hanley & Belfus, 1999.)*

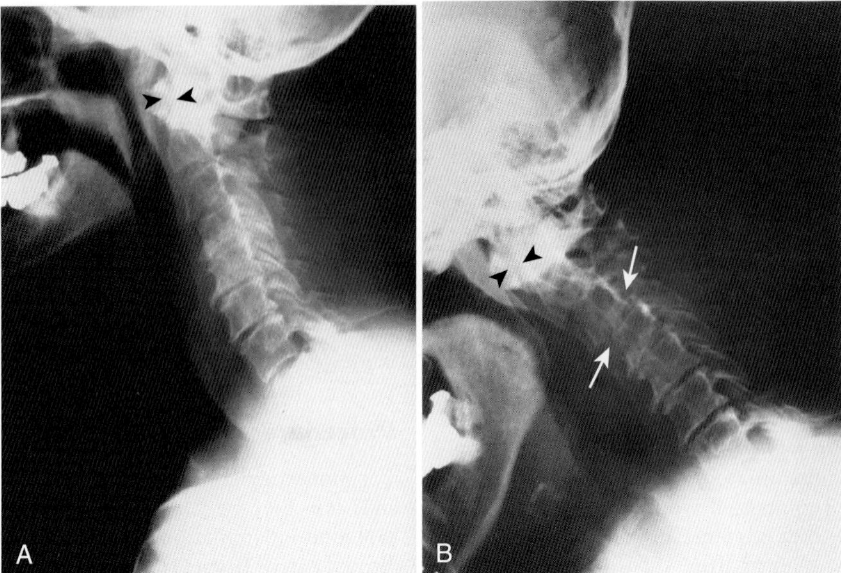

FIGURE 151.6 Subluxation of vertebrae in rheumatoid arthritis. The abnormal movement between vertebrae due to laxity of ligaments becomes more apparent in flexion of the cervical spine. Lateral flexion-extension views are requested if subluxation of cervical vertebrae is suspected. The radiograph in **A** is taken in the neutral position, and the one in **B** is taken in flexion. The arrowheads mark the distance between the anterior surface of the odontoid process and the posterior surface of the arch of the atlas. This space is increased in flexion because of subluxation of the arch of the atlas on the second vertebra. The arrows show anterior slippage of the third cervical vertebra on the fourth. In a normal cervical spine, the posterior surface of vertebral bodies forms a smooth curve that is convex anteriorly (lordosis). This curve is disturbed and a step-like deformity is seen *(arrows)* at the posteroinferior angle of the upper vertebra and the posterosuperior angle of the lower vertebra in subluxation. *(From Mehta AJ. Common Musculoskeletal Problems. Philadelphia, Hanley & Belfus, 1997.)*

may be helpful, whereas more active patients may do better with arthrodesis [35]. For patients with involvement of larger joints, arthroplasty can significantly improve one's activity level and lifestyle. Some patients may require tendon repair or synovectomy. Any surgical procedure should take into consideration the functionality of the entire upper or lower extremity [36]. Patients with suspected or confirmed cervical spine involvement will need special consideration and handling during intubation for anesthesia (Fig.151.6). Surgical cervical spine stabilization may be considered if the patient has neurologic symptoms.

Potential Disease Complications

The most common complication is joint destruction with subsequent decreased functional use of affected joints. Neuropathy may be due to entrapment, pressure, or deposition of amyloid. Cervical instability can lead to myelopathy. Irregular bone edges may result in tendon rupture. Nodules may break down and ulcerate. Skin ulcerations may also occur in pressure points in the immobilized patient. The kidneys and gastrointestinal tract may be sites of deposition in patients who develop secondary amyloidosis. Scleritis may result in scleromalacia. As previously mentioned, cardiovascular disease is almost always present in aggressive or untreated cases.

Potential Treatment Complications

Medication side effects vary according to the drug (Table 151.3) [16].

Overly aggressive physical or occupational therapy can cause increased joint inflammation, joint deformity, and pain.

Table 151.3 Side Effects of Medications Used to Treat Patients with Rheumatoid Arthritis

Medication	Side Effects
Nonsteroidal anti-inflammatory drugs	
Traditional	Dyspepsia, ulcer, or bleeding Renal insufficiency Hepatotoxicity Rash Inhibit platelet function
Cyclooxygenase-2 inhibitors	Same as traditional nonsteroidal anti-inflammatory drugs, but gastrointestinal side effects occur less often No platelet effect
Glucocorticoids	Increased appetite, weight gain Cushingoid habitus Acne Fluid retention Hypertension Diabetes Glaucoma, cataracts Atherosclerosis Avascular necrosis Osteoporosis Impaired wound healing Susceptibility to infection
Antimalarials	Dyspepsia Hemolysis (glucose-6-phosphate dehydrogenase–deficient patients) Macular damage Abnormal skin pigmentation Neuromyopathy Rash
Gold	Myelosuppression Proteinuria or hematuria Oral ulcers Rash Pruritus

Table 151.3 Side Effects of Medications Used to Treat Patients with Rheumatoid Arthritis—cont'd

Medication	Side Effects
Etanercept	Injection site reaction Exacerbation of infection
Cyclosporine	Renal insufficiency Hypertension Anemia
Sulfasalazine	Myelosuppression Hemolysis (glucose-6-phosphate dehydrogenase–deficient patients) Hepatotoxicity Photosensitivity, rash Dyspepsia, diarrhea Headaches Oligospermia
Azathioprine	Myelosuppression Hepatotoxicity Pancreatitis (rarely) Lymphoproliferative disorders (long-term risk)
Methotrexate	Hepatic fibrosis, cirrhosis Pneumonitis Myelosuppression Mucositis Dyspepsia Alopecia Increased rheumatoid nodules
Leflunomide	Hepatic fibrosis, cirrhosis Myelosuppression Dyspepsia Alopecia
Infliximab	Infusion reaction Exacerbation of infection
Cyclophosphamide	Dyspepsia, diarrhea Myelosuppression Alopecia Hemorrhagic cystitis Ovarian and testicular failure Teratogenicity Malignant neoplasia Opportunistic infection

References

[1] Gerosa M, DeAngelis V, Ribioldi P, Meroni PL. Rheumatoid arthritis: a female challenge. Womens Health (Lond Engl) 2008;4:195–201.

[2] MacGregor AJ, Silman AJ. Rheumatoid arthritis: classification and epidemiology. In: Klippel JH, Dieppe PA, editors. Rheumatology. 2nd ed. London: Mosby; 1998. p. 5.2.2–6.

[3] Del Rincon I, Williams K, Stern MP, et al. High incidence of cardiovascular events in rheumatoid arthritis cohort not explained by traditional cardiac risk factors. Arthritis Rheum 2001;44:2237–45.

[4] Maradit-Kremers H, Crowson CS, Nicola PJ, et al. Increased unrecognized coronary heart disease and sudden deaths in rheumatoid arthritis: a population-based cohort study. Arthritis Rheum 2005;52:402–11.

[5] Arnet FC, Edworthy SM, Bloch DA, et al. The American Rheumatism Association 1987 revised criteria for the classification of rheumatoid arthritis. Arthritis Rheum 1988;31:315–24.

[6] Fuchs HA, Sergent JS. Rheumatoid arthritis: the clinical picture. In: Koopman WJ, editor. Arthritis and allied conditions: a textbook of rheumatology. 13th ed. Baltimore: Williams & Wilkins; 1997. p. 1041–70.

[7] Gordon AG, Hastings DE. Rheumatoid arthritis: clinical features of early, progressive and late disease. In: Klippel JH, Dieppe PA, editors. Rheumatology. 2nd ed. London: Mosby; 1998. p. 5.3.1–14.

[8] Anderson RJ. Rheumatoid arthritis: clinical and laboratory features. In: Klippel JH, editor. Primer on the rheumatic diseases. 11th ed. Atlanta: Arthritis Foundation; 1997. p. 161–7.

[9] Mota LM, Laurindo IM, Santos Neto LL. General principles for the treatment of early rheumatoid arthritis. Rev Assoc Med Bras 2010;56:360–2.

[10] Hochberg MC, Chang RW, Dwosh I, et al. The American College of Rheumatology 1991 revised criteria for the classification of global functional status in rheumatoid arthritis. Arthritis Rheum 1992;35:493–502.

[11] Rupp I, Boshuizen HC, Dinant HJ, et al. Disability and health-related quality of life among patients with rheumatoid arthritis: association with radiographic joint damage, disease activity, pain, and depressive symptoms. Scand J Rheumatol 2006;35:175–81.

[12] Matteson EL, Cohen MD, Doyt DL. Rheumatoid arthritis: clinical features and systemic involvement. In: Klippel JH, Dieppe PA, editors. Rheumatology. 2nd ed. London: Mosby; 1998. p. 5.4.1–7.

[13] Symmons DP. Classification criteria for rheumatoid arthritis—time to abandon rheumatoid factor? Rheumatology (Oxford) 2007;46:725–6.

[14] Avouc J, Gossec L, Dougados M. Diagnostic and predictive value of anti-cyclic citrullinated protein antibodies in rheumatoid arthritis: a systematic review. Ann Rheum Dis 2006;65:845–51.

[15] Paget SA. Rheumatoid arthritis: treatment. In: Klippel JH, editor. Primer on the rheumatic diseases. 11th ed. Atlanta: Arthritis Foundation; 1997. p. 168–73.

[16] Cash JM, Klippel JH. Drug therapy: second-line drug therapy for rheumatoid arthritis. N Engl J Med 1994;330:1368–75.

[17] Perdriger A, Mariette X, Kuntz JL, et al. Safety of infliximab used in combination with leflunomide or azathioprine in daily clinical practice. J Rheumatol 2006;33:865–9.

[18] Hyrich KL, Symmons DP, Watson KD, Silman AJ. Comparison of the response to infliximab or etanercept monotherapy with the response to cotherapy with methotrexate or another disease modifying anti-rheumatic drug in patients with rheumatoid arthritis: results from the British Society for Rheumatology Biologics Register. Arthritis Rheum 2006;54:1786–94.

[19] Radner H, Ramiro S, Buchbinder R, et al. Pain management for inflammatory arthritis (rheumatoid arthritis, psoriatic arthritis, ankylosing spondylitis and other spondylarthritis) and gastrointestinal or liver comorbidity. Cochrane Database Syst Rev 2012;1, CD008951.

[20] van Riel PL, Wijnands MJH, van de Putte LBA. Rheumatoid arthritis: evaluation and management of active inflammatory disease. In: Klippel JH, Dieppe PA, editors. Rheumatology. 2nd ed. London: Mosby; 1998. p. 5.14.1–12.

[21] Hazes JMW, Cats A. Rheumatoid arthritis: management: end stage and complications. In: Klippel JH, Dieppe PA, editors. Rheumatology. 2nd ed. London: Mosby; 1998. p. 5.15.1–10.

[22] Breger Stanton DE, Lazaro R, Macdermid JC. A systematic review of the effectiveness of contrast baths. J Hand Ther 2009;22:57–69.

[23] Hammond A. What is the role of the occupational therapist? Best Pract Res Clin Rheumatol 2004;18:491–505.

[24] Hand C, Law M, McColl MA. Occupational therapy interventions for chronic diseases: a scoping review. Am J Occup Ther 2011;65:428–36.

[25] van den Ende CH, Breedveld FC, le Cessie S, et al. Effect of intensive exercise on patients with active rheumatoid arthritis: a randomised clinical trial. Ann Rheum Dis 2000;59:615–21.

[26] Munneke M, de Jong Z, Zwinderman AH, et al. Effect of a high-intensity weight-bearing exercise program on radiologic damage progression of the large joints in subgroups of patients with rheumatoid arthritis. Arthritis Rheum 2005;53:410–7.

[27] Briggs AM, Fary RE, Slater H, et al. Disease-specific knowledge and clinical skills required by community-based physiotherapists to co-manage patients with rheumatoid arthritis. Arthritis Care Res (Hoboken) 2012;64:1514–26.

[28] O'Brien AV, Jones P, Mullis R, et al. Conservative hand therapy treatments in rheumatoid arthritis—a randomized controlled trial. Rheumatology (Oxford) 2006;45:577–83.

[29] Baillet A, Vaillant M, Guinot M, et al. Efficacy of resistance exercises in rheumatoid arthritis: meta-analysis of randomized controlled trials. Rheumatology (Oxford) 2012;51:519–27.

[30] Skirven TM, Osterman AL, Fedorczyk JM, Amadio PC. Rehabilitation of the hand and upper extremity. 6th ed. Philadelphia: Elsevier; 2011.

[31] Stucki G, Liang MH. Efficacy of rehabilitation interventions in rheumatic conditions. Curr Opin Rheumatol 1994;6:153–8.

[32] Muramatsu K, Tanaka H, Taguchi T. Peripheral neuropathies of the forearm and hand in rheumatoid arthritis: diagnosis and options for treatment. Rheumatol Int 2008;28:951–7.

[33] Dinges H. Sonography of the rheumatoid hand. Orthopade 2005;34:36–8.

[34] Bruyn GA, Schmidt WA. How to perform ultrasound-guided injections. Best Pract Res Clin Rheumatol 2009;23:269–79.

[35] Chacko AT, Rozental TD. The rheumatoid thumb. Hand Clin 2008;24:307–14.

[36] Schill S, Thabe H. Differential therapy for the rheumatoid thumb. Orthopade 2005;34:21–8.

CHAPTER 152

Scoliosis and Kyphosis

Mark A. Thomas, MD
Maya Therattil, MD

Synonyms

Scoliosis
- **Curvature of the spine/back**
- **Curved spine/back**

Kyphosis
- **Hunchback**
- **Humpback**
- **Roundback**
- **Dorsum rotundum**
- **Dowager's hump**
- **Postural kyphosis**
- **Gibbus deformity**

ICD-9 Codes

737.30	**Scoliosis, idiopathic**
737.32	**Progressive scoliosis and progressive infantile scoliosis**
737.31	**Resolving infantile scoliosis**
737.34	**Thoracogenic scoliosis**
756.15	**Congenital spine fusion**
754.2	**Congenital musculoskeletal deformity of spine**
756.19	**Other congenital anomaly of spine**
737.33	**Scoliosis due to radiation**
737.39	**Other kyphoscoliosis and scoliosis**
737.43	**Scoliosis associated with other condition**
737.10	**Kyphosis, dorsal kyphosis, acquired postural kyphosis**
737.19	**Thoracic kyphosis**
737.0	**Adolescent postural kyphosis**
737.12	**Postlaminectomy kyphosis**
737.11	**Kyphosis due to radiation**
732.0	**Juvenile osteochondrosis of spine**
737.41	**Kyphosis associated with other conditions**

ICD-10 Codes

M41.20	**Other idiopathic scoliosis, site unspecified**
M41.30	**Thoracogenic scoliosis, site unspecified**
M41.00	**Infantile idiopathic scoliosis, site unspecified**
Q76.49	**Congenital fusion of spine, congenital malformation of spine**
Q67.5	**Congenital deformity of spine, congenital postural scoliosis**
M34.0	**Progressive systemic sclerosis**
M96.5	**Postradiation scoliosis**
M41.9	**Scoliosis, unspecified**
M40.00	**Postural kyphosis, site unspecified**
M40.204	**Unspecified kyphosis, thoracic region**
M41.119	**Juvenile idiopathic scoliosis, site unspecified**
M96.3	**Postlaminectomy kyphosis**
M96.2	**Postradiation kyphosis**
M42.00	**Juvenile osteochondrosis of spine, site unspecified**
M40.209	**Unspecified kyphosis, site unspecified**

Definition

Scoliosis

Scoliosis (Fig. 152.1) is a structural or postural deformity of the spine that results in a lateral (coronal) deviation or curve. Scoliosis is associated with rotation of the vertebral bodies located within the curve. It may also be associated with an arm or leg length difference, particularly in cases of idiopathic or congenital scoliosis.

Scoliosis is most commonly idiopathic, degenerative, or a result of vertebral anomalies. Less prevalent is scoliosis consequent to disease-related or iatrogenic causes. Growth asymmetry at the vertebral end plate, rib, and pelvic growth

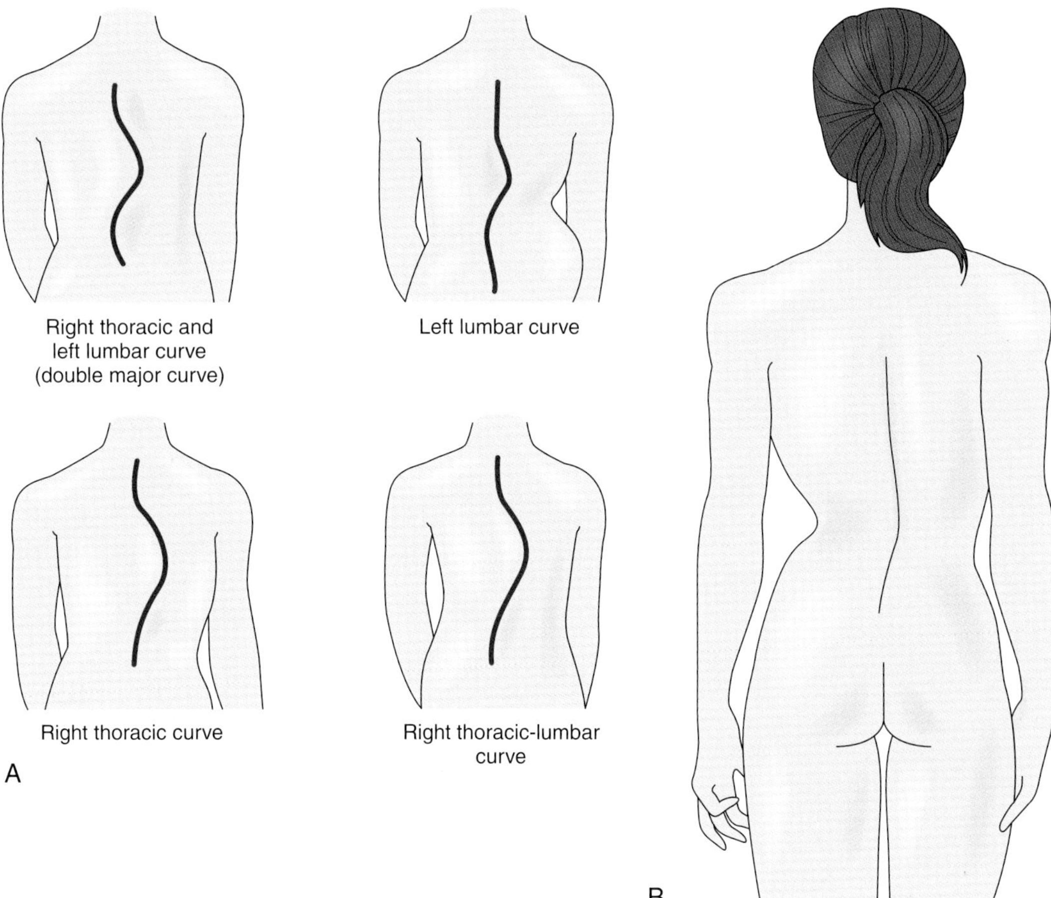

FIGURE 152.1 **A,** Examples of scoliosis curve patterns. **B,** Scoliosis.

centers can result in scoliosis and progression of a scoliotic curve [1,2].

Scoliosis affects between 3% and 30% of the population; about 0.25% require treatment [3]. The incidence of scoliosis increases with age [4] (Table 152.1). The scoliotic curve may be congenital; appear during infancy (infantile scoliosis); or develop in childhood (juvenile scoliosis), adolescence (adolescent scoliosis), or adulthood. When the diagnosis of scoliosis is made in an adult patient, the curve is identified as either adult onset (degenerative) or adult presenting (a previously undiagnosed idiopathic adolescent curve).

There is increasing evidence that idiopathic curves can result from genetic or epigenetic factors. Gene candidates have been identified in a genome-wide association study. Statistical associations with scoliosis exist for gene polymorphisms (interleukin receptor and vitamin D receptor genes; *ATRX* gene; and chromosomes 6, 9, 16, and 17) [5–8]. All are associated with idiopathic curves. Epigenetic factors that might contribute to the development of scoliosis relate to maternal age, spinal cord injury before the age of 5 years (96% prevalence of scoliosis), DNA methylation, and transient fetal hypoxia [9–12]. These are only associations, and at this time any causality or mechanism of action is unclear.

Other types of scoliotic curves can begin with degenerative changes in the spine, congenital malformation of the vertebrae (usually incomplete fusion—butterfly vertebrae or hemivertebrae), tumor, neuromuscular or connective tissue disease, trauma, surgery, or radiation therapy.

Kyphosis

Thoracic kyphosis is an excessive sagittal deviation in thoracic spine alignment, a dorsal apex curve exceeding 40 degrees. Possible causes include osteoporotic compression fractures (note that most of these fractures are asymptomatic and unidentified), direct trauma, chronic kyphotic posture, tumor, radiation therapy [13], and Scheuermann disease. A resulting wedge deformity of the vertebral bodies produces the malalignment. Animal studies suggest that gestational and neonatal hypovitaminosis D or alterations in calcium and phosphorus concentrations in neonatal feedings can play a role in the development of pathologic kyphosis. The incidence of kyphosis in animals studied with maternal vitamin D deficiency during gestation or with low calcium and phosphorus feed content was 32%. No similar humans studies have been published. Earlier presentation of the kyphotic deformity was seen in cases of maternal hypovitaminosis D [14].

Cervical kyphosis is pathologic. Infection (particularly tuberculosis), tumor, abnormal development of the cervical vertebrae, trauma, and advanced degenerative disease of the spine can produce cervical kyphosis. Kyphosis related to trauma (including laminectomy)

Table 152.1 Age at Presentation and Common Causes of Scoliosis

Time of Presentation	Most Common Causes	
Congenital	Abnormalities of development, vertebral body	Failure of fusion or development: hemivertebrae, butterfly vertebrae (types 1-4)
	Developmental, associated with abnormal development of other systems	Abnormal differentiation (especially weeks 1-6)
Infantile (0-3 years)	Postural	
	Idiopathic	Genetic or epigenetic (?)
	Related to disease or trauma	Trauma (especially spinal cord injury) Tumor (neurofibroma)
Juvenile (4-9 years)	Idiopathic	Genetic (?)
	Related to disease or trauma	Neuromuscular disease Connective tissue disease Tumor (neurofibroma) Metabolic disease Trauma (especially spinal cord injury)
Adolescent	Idiopathic	Genetic (?)
Adult	Adult presenting, idiopathic	Progression of idiopathic adolescent curve
	Adult, degenerative	Listhesis Spondylosis Facet arthropathy
	Adult, disease or treatment related	Laminectomy Radiation therapy Tumor (primary, metastatic)

or advanced degenerative changes in the cervical spine (due to disease such as rheumatoid arthritis or the mechanical changes that can occur over time) becomes more prevalent with advancing age. The most common tumors are manifested early in life as osseous or neural extramedullary masses. They include (in order of decreasing frequency) chordoma, bone cyst, Ewing sarcoma, meningioma, schwannoma, and neurofibroma [15]. As a feature of the congenital cervical vertebral dysmorphic syndromes, cervical kyphosis is noted in the following syndromes: Down, Morquio, Goldenhar, Klippel-Feil, Stickler, Williams, and Larsen [16].

Symptoms

Scoliosis

Scoliosis is usually asymptomatic. If symptoms are present, they generally are produced by scoliosis as it directly relates to the location and severity of the curve. Large or highly rotated curves can produce pain and have the potential to produce symptoms related to the cardiopulmonary or nervous systems. Curves that exceed 60 to 80 degrees begin to affect other organ systems. They can produce shortness of breath or poor endurance due to decreased lung capacity. If there is pressure on nerve roots or the spinal cord, the patient may experience paresthesia or hypesthesia, weakness, and bowel or bladder involvement.

There is some controversy as to whether cosmetic changes related to thoracic scoliosis contribute to low self-esteem, anxiety, and depression (particularly in adolescents). Quality of life indices do not differ for adults by the age of 30 years [17].

Musculoskeletal pain may occur in performing activities of daily living that require a full active range of shoulder motion, such as overhead or extended reach activities. There may be upper back and neck pain in lifting or carrying because of strain of the scapular or shoulder muscles.

Kyphosis

Thoracic kyphosis is usually asymptomatic. If symptoms do appear, they are commonly associated with intermittent aching back pain and stiffness that are most prominent at the apex of the curve. Compensatory lumbar lordosis can be associated with low back pain.

Kyphosis with a wide scapular spread and shoulder and head protraction restricts both shoulder range of motion and the ability to look upward. When the ability to compensate for this with cervical or lumbar motion is compromised, kyphosis results in difficulty in performing overhead activities. Patients with cervical kyphosis may also complain of neck pain and the inability to look upward.

Physical Examination

Scoliosis

Scoliosis is usually apparent on inspection, although small thoracic curves with minimal rotation or a small lumbar curve can be difficult to detect. Have the patient bend forward (Adam forward bend test). If pelvic and lower extremity asymmetries affect the appearance of the back, minimize these by examining the patient in a seated position. Vertebral body or rib rotation associated with scoliosis is most readily seen when the patient bends forward. The tilt of the back, reflective of the angle of rotation, can be quantified by the use of a type of level, the scoliometer. The level is placed on the forward bent back in the area of maximum tilt and measures that angle. In idiopathic thoracic scoliosis, an angle of 7 degrees roughly corresponds to a scoliotic curve between 10 and 20 degrees.

Scoliosis can produce apparent asymmetry of breast size, asymmetry of the waist fold contour, asymmetric appearance of arm or leg length, or unequal iliac crest and shoulder height. A true leg length discrepancy exceeding 2.2 cm is indicative of asymmetric growth and possible scoliosis [18].

Serial assessment of scoliosis is advisable. The frequency of evaluation varies with curve parameters and treatment but is generally between 6 and 12 months, more frequently with curves that are progressing or being treated. These assessments focus on the degree of curvature, location and extent of the curve, degree of rotation, degree of skeletal maturity, flexibility of the curve, height, vital capacity, and expiratory pulmonary function tests.

Patients with degenerative scoliosis should be examined for neurologic deficits. Lower extremity strength, sensation, and reflexes can be impaired if the curvature exceeds 40 degrees.

Congenital vertebral malformations arise during the first 6 weeks of gestation. Symptoms and signs may be identified that relate to other systems in early development at that same time, particularly cardiac and renal.

Kyphosis

Increased thoracic kyphosis displaces the head and neck forward, and this forward displacement can be measured as an occiput to wall distance. A compensatory increase in lumbar lordosis can occur. These are apparent on inspection. The rounding of the back will not fully correct with trunk extension in a prone position, but the degree to which the curve decreases with active extension of the neck and upper back should be used as a benchmark for subsequent evaluations. Severe cervical kyphosis can produce a chin on chest appearance, but smaller curves are also readily apparent. Thoracolumbar and lumbar kyphoses are less easily identified on inspection. Prominence of the spinous processes can indicate lower spine kyphosis [19]. Kyphosis-associated scoliosis will be present in about one third of patients [20]. Restrictions in active trunk and neck extension can result from either deformity or pain. Tightness of the pectoral muscles is common.

A neurologic examination should be performed if there are radicular or myelopathic symptoms.

Functional Limitations

The functional limitations related to scoliosis and kyphosis result from the loss of spinal motion. Restriction in upper back extension can reduce upward gaze and affect driving or cause discomfort in lying prone or swimming in a prone position. Loss of shoulder range of motion, particularly forward flexion and abduction, can result from a decreased range of scapular excursion over the scoliotic or kyphotic thorax. This impedes overhead activities of daily living. When present, pain and stiffness can limit sitting, standing, or walking tolerance.

Disruption of spinal balance displaces the center of gravity, particularly with large uncompensated curves. This increases the energy costs for standing and ambulation. It can also impair balance. With severe deformity and cardiopulmonary compromise, endurance is diminished. Cosmetic deformities that affect self-image or self-esteem can lead to social isolation. Age-related changes in anatomy and physiology can compound the impairments and restrict mobility or cause disability associated with the activities of daily living.

Diagnostic Studies

Standing anteroposterior and lateral radiographs are the standard diagnostic tests used to evaluate scoliosis and kyphosis. Radiographs can reveal congenital abnormalities of the vertebral body, Scheuermann disease, or lateral vertebral body wedging [21]. Bending or supine radiographs are not usually obtained but can help determine the flexibility of the curve. Non–weight-bearing radiographs and serial radiographs, both in the brace and out of the brace, may offer some advantage in estimating possible correction, actual correction, and the effectiveness of bracing [22].

Rib-vertebral angle and space available for lung (reported to be useful in cases of infantile scoliosis) are less common but available x-ray assessments. The difference in angle magnitude or ratio of angles between the convex and larger concave rib-vertebral angles in the thorax can be sensitive indicators of change [23,24].

X-ray measurement of the scoliotic curve is commonly done by the Cobb method. The Cobb angle is the angle at the intersection of lines drawn perpendicular to the vertebral end plates that frame the curve—those with the maximal tilt (Fig. 152.2).

Radiographs can demonstrate vertebral body rotation and the status of growth centers in the ilium, vertebrae, and humerus. The degree of vertebral body rotation is gauged by the deviation from midline of the spinous process or fullness of the pedicle silhouette. Rotation is graded 0 (no rotation) to 4 (rotation of 90 degrees or more). Closure of the growth plates proceeds in a cephalad manner. Because vertebral growth plates are usually not visualized, iliac and femur epiphyses are useful sites for assessing spine growth status. Growth status is graded 0 (no mineralization) to 5 (fusion of the growth plate). Radiographs can help assess the growth or degenerative status of the spine, useful information for determining a plan of care.

Magnetic resonance imaging can identify an unsuspected pathologic process, for example, a neurofibroma, diastematomyelia, or tethered cord. Magnetic resonance imaging is recommended before surgery as an otherwise undetectable spinal cord abnormality is present in about 10% of cases slated for surgery [25].

Bone scans can help exclude discitis or tumor as a cause of pain or spinal deformity. Bone densitometry demonstrates increased density on the convex side of the curve. This occurs even in osteoporotic patients [26]. Pulmonary function testing, particularly volume and expiratory studies, should be performed when curves exceed 50 degrees. Genetic testing for markers associated with scoliosis is available but not useful at this time.

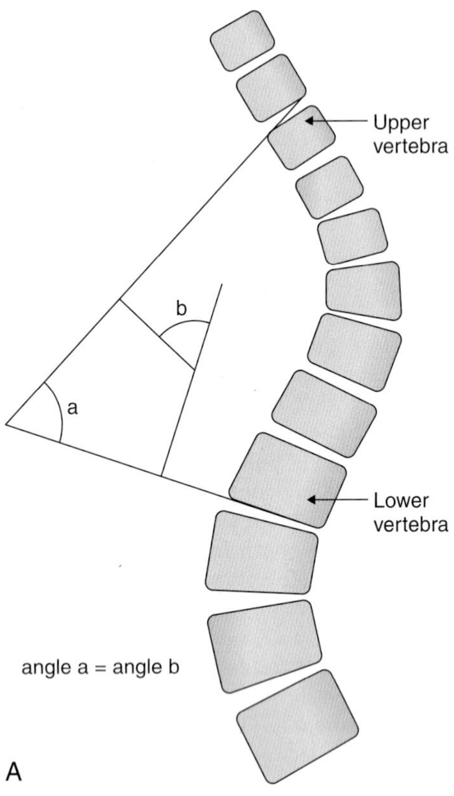

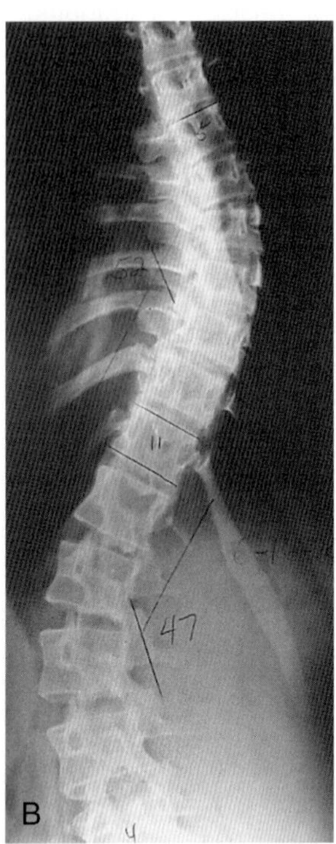

FIGURE 152.2 **A,** Measurement of idiopathic scoliosis by the Cobb angle. **B,** Idiopathic adolescent scoliosis. There is a primary thoracic dextroscoliosis (convexity to the right side) measuring 52 degrees and a compensatory lumbar levoscoliosis (convexity to the left side) measuring 47 degrees. *(From Katz DS, Math KR, Groskin SA. Radiology Secrets. Philadelphia, Hanley & Belfus, 1998.)*

Differential Diagnosis

Differential Diagnosis for Spine Deformity	Differential Diagnosis for Disease Underlying Spine Deformity
Scoliosis	Spina bifida
Congenital	Myelomeningocele
Infantile	Syringomyelia
Neuromuscular	Klippel-Feil syndrome
Juvenile idiopathic	Thoracic insufficiency syndrome
Adolescent idiopathic	Traumatic brain injury
Adult presenting	Cerebral palsy
Idiopathic	Myopathy
Degenerative (lumbar)	Muscular dystrophy
Kyphosis	Spinal cord injury
Lateral listhesis	Spinal muscular atrophy
Spondylolisthesis	Marfan syndrome
Postural scoliosis	Ehlers-Danlos syndrome
Spondyloepiphyseal dysplasia tarda	Friedreich ataxia
Congenital vertebral malformation	Osteogenesis imperfecta
Postural kyphosis	Rheumatoid arthritis
	Fracture
	Tumor
	Tuberculosis
	Scheuermann disease

Treatment

Initial

The broad categories of treatment for scoliosis and kyphosis include observation, bracing, and surgery. The problems needing treatment fall into the categories of pain, deformity, deficit, and disability.

In all patients, regardless of age, it is important to identify curves that are likely to progress. Curves that are large (degree of curvature), particularly if they are "unbalanced" (e.g., a single major curve without a compensatory curve), are likely to progress. Other curves that tend to progress are those with a closely packed configuration (a small number of spinal segments between the apex and ends of the curve), congenital vertebral body malformation, and neuromuscular or lumbar degenerative disease etiology [27].

Lumbar degenerative scoliosis (this includes adult-presenting idiopathic scoliosis with subsequent degenerative change) is most likely to progress when L5 is involved or there are asymmetric changes in the L2-3 or L3-4 disc space.

In general, scoliotic curves that measure less than 20 degrees or kyphotic curves measuring less than 40 degrees are observed rather than treated with bracing or surgery. Observation can be supplemented by an exercise program.

Pain can be treated with bracing or exercise. Anti-inflammatory medication, analgesics, acupuncture, and transcutaneous electrical nerve stimulation may be useful.

There is no clear role for electrical stimulation of paraspinal muscles in the treatment of scoliosis. Treatment of coincident disease, such as osteoporosis, complements the treatment of scoliosis and its attendant symptoms and disability.

Rehabilitation

Exercise is beneficial for general well-being, flexibility, and improvement of posture. There is no clear evidence that exercise is a disease-modifying intervention for idiopathic scoliosis [28]. There is, however, a specific exercise protocol for scoliosis, the Schroth method. These exercises attempt to correct growth imbalances in the back and to improve spinal alignment. There is anecdotal evidence that the

Schroth method is useful in the treatment of small curves, particularly the component exercises of spinal extension, abdominal strengthening, and hamstring stretch. These exercises may also be helpful in treating back pain. Kyphosis may improve with cervicothoracic extension exercise and pelvic tilt to reduce lumbar lordosis, along with stretching and strengthening exercise of the hamstrings, hip flexors, and pectoralis muscles.

Physical therapy and occupational therapy should be prescribed as an appropriate part of a pain management plan as well as to optimize independent mobility and function in activities of daily living.

Bracing is an important part of the rehabilitation intervention when scoliosis is symptomatic or progressive. Scoliotic curves exceeding 20 degrees are 20% to 40% more likely to progress if a brace is not used, as is kyphosis in excess of 40 degrees.

Bracing for scoliosis is most effective for lower thoracic and lumbar curves. In the case of idiopathic adolescent scoliosis, an orthosis has the potential to provide good control. Stabilization of the curve occurs in 42% to 92% of cases, depending on the accuracy of brace prescription and patient compliance. Actual correction (reduction of the coronal deviation and rotation) with bracing, including serial casting, is more likely to happen in cases of infantile or juvenile idiopathic curves than it is for scoliosis at other ages [29].

There are many different orthoses in use, with a plethora of names [30]. The mechanics of bracing varies with brace type. Braces can be static (constant pressure and rigid containment) (Fig. 152.3) or dynamic (movement opposing the spine deviations, facilitated by flexible bands). Braces can work by derotation, three-point pressure correction, or distraction. Braces may need to be worn full-time or at intervals throughout the day (usually at night or during episodes of pain). Selection of the brace with the best control effect and the least discomfort or inconvenience depends on several factors. These factors include curve parameters, such as etiology, location, and rotation of the curve, but also symptoms and likely compliance with prescribed use [31].

In adolescent idiopathic scoliosis, the goal of orthotic treatment is to limit progression of the curve. There is no clear consensus regarding daily brace wear-time. Recommendations range from 8 to 23 hours. Bracing for idiopathic curves in a growing child or adolescent is maintained until the spinal growth centers fuse.

When a brace is used to decrease pain and to improve posture for patients with degenerative scoliosis, the brace is worn when needed. The most commonly prescribed brace is the thoracolumbosacral orthosis, such as a body jacket with wedges or pads. High thoracic and cervical scoliosis and kyphotic curves require a Milwaukee cervicothoracolumbosacral orthosis.

In cases of scoliosis associated with neuromuscular diseases, bracing guidelines are less clear. Bracing may be withheld while the patient is ambulatory. Braces can be useful as a means to delay surgical intervention. If a body jacket is provided, an abdominal window is needed to allow respiratory excursion.

Contoured or custom-molded seating systems that align and support the trunk can be useful in patients with neuromuscular disease. These accommodate the scoliotic curve while allowing the patient to maintain an upright posture while seated, improving head control and upper extremity function.

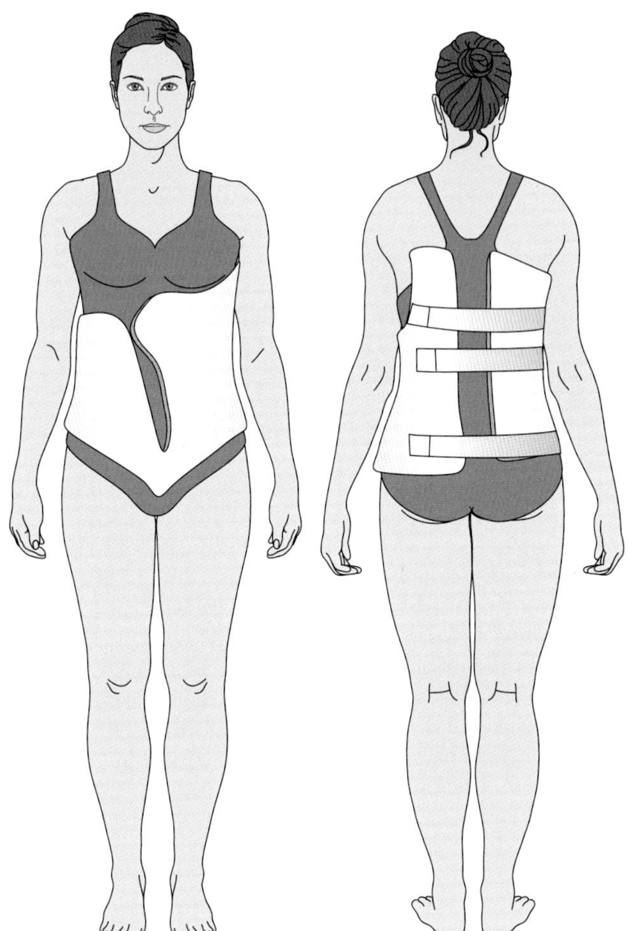

FIGURE 152.3 Body jacket thoracolumbosacral orthosis, posterior opening.

Procedures

There are no invasive physiatric procedures for the treatment of scoliosis or kyphosis.

Surgery

The goal of surgery is to stabilize the spine through correction or control of the deformity. Indications for surgical correction of scoliosis or kyphosis include progressive deformity, segmental instability, progressive or new neurologic deficit, and cardiopulmonary compromise. Pain, even when it is refractory to conservative management, is a controversial indication for surgery. Inability to use a brace or severe cosmetic deformity can be an indication for surgery in specific instances.

Scoliosis

A variety of surgical techniques and approaches address the coronal and rotational deformities. There are procedures that provide decompression to relieve scoliosis-related stenosis. There are surgical strategies to preserve or to promote growth of the spine in children and adolescents. Stabilization of the spine is the primary goal in any surgery, but there are multiple ways to achieve this stability.

Surgery for idiopathic (adolescent, adult presenting) scoliosis addresses the coronal and rotational deformities by derotation or distraction. The spine is stabilized with hardware with or without bone fusion.

Static stabilization of the spine is achieved through fusion. This eliminates any future growth at the fused segment and may not be the procedure of choice for a growing child, for whom dynamic stabilization may be the better option. For these patients, the goal of treatment is to foster balanced growth of the spine. In the youngest patients, a rib cage implant can do this. In cases of infantile or juvenile idiopathic scoliosis, some success with thoracoscopic stapling has been reported [32]. Semirigid rods or cords can be used to control spinal motion while promoting growth [33,34]. Growth rods are lengthened either surgically or magnetically about every 6 months [35]. A similar technique with dynamic stabilization (but without growth rods) that reduces or eliminates the adverse effects associated with static stabilization has also been reported in cases of degenerative scoliosis [36].

Lumbar degenerative scoliosis can be associated with radicular disease. Surgical options in such instances include various degrees of decompression and long (extending above and below the curve) or short fusion. The selection of the procedure is influenced by the location of the scoliosis, but when possible, long fusion is the better option [37,38].

Kyphosis

Various surgical approaches have been used to correct thoracic kyphosis. Combined anterior plus posterior instrumentation with fusion currently provides the highest success rate for lasting correction and pain relief [39].

Potential Disease Complications

Scoliosis and kyphosis can produce pain and reduce joint or segmental motion and result in disability. The deformity can progress and contribute to the development or worsening of spondylosis, facet arthropathy, spondylolysis, and spondylolisthesis. Such changes in spine structure and mechanics correlate well with large angles and angles of rotation at the curve apex [40]. Foraminal, lateral recess, or canal stenosis can occur with signs and symptoms of neurologic compromise. Root entrapment usually occurs on the concave side of the curve (rarely both convex and concave sides). Cauda equina compression has been reported, as has myelopathy [41].

Shortness of breath, poor endurance, and poor activity tolerance due to restrictive lung disease can occur as a complication of scoliotic curves exceeding 40 degrees or kyphosis in excess of 50 degrees.

Potential Treatment Complications

Most treatment complications follow surgery or bracing. Exercise-related complications are uncommon but include overuse conditions of the soft tissues (tendinitis, bursitis, sprain, strain).

Complications of bracing include skin breakdown, dermatitis due to an allergy to the orthotic material, hyperhidrosis, cutaneous infection, gastroesophageal reflux disease, esophagitis, and altered gastrointestinal motility. There can be shortness of breath, difficulty in sitting, low self-esteem, and altered body image.

Surgical complications include vascular or neurologic injury, pseudarthrosis, infection, graft donor site pain, progressive pelvic obliquity, painful degenerative changes in the segment adjacent to the level of fusion (especially low lumbar or at T11-T12), spine segment instability, hardware prominence or failure, and thromboembolism. Hardware complications include slippage of anchoring hooks, bending or fracture of a rod, wire pull-out, and hardware migration [42]. High complication rates are associated with the placement of growth rods. Progression of the curve is possible despite surgical fixation. The patient with degenerative scoliosis who has undergone otherwise successful surgery may continue to experience pain or restricted mobility and may need revision surgery at a later time.

References

[1] Burwell RG, Aujla RK, Grevitt MP, et al. Upper arm length model suggests transient bilateral asymmetry is associated with right thoracic adolescent idiopathic scoliosis with implications for pathogenesis and estimation of linear skeletal overgrowth. Stud Health Technol Inform 2012;176:188–94.

[2] D'Amico M, Roncoletta P, Di Felice F, et al. Leg length discrepancy in scoliotic patients. Stud Health Technol Inform 2012;176:146–50.

[3] Asher MA, Burton DC. Adolescent idiopathic scoliosis: natural history and long term treatment effects. Scoliosis 2006;1:2.

[4] Ogilvie JW. Adult scoliosis: evaluation and nonsurgical treatment. Instr Course Lect 1992;41:251–5.

[5] Gorman KF, Julien C, Moreau A. The genetic epidemiology of idiopathic scoliosis. Eur Spine J 2012;21:1905–19.

[6] Suh K, Eun IE, Lee J. Polymorphism in vitamin D receptor is associated with bone mineral density in patients with adolescent idiopathic scoliosis. Eur Spine J 2010;19:1545–50.

[7] Zhou S, Qiu XS, Zhu ZZ, et al. A single-nucleotide polymorphism rs708567 in the IL-17RC gene is associated with a susceptibility to and the curve severity of adolescent idiopathic scoliosis in a Chinese Han Population: a case-control study. BMC Musculoskelet Disord 2012;13:181.

[8] Miller NH, Justice CM, Marosy B, et al. Identification of candidate regions for familial idiopathic scoliosis. Spine (Phila Pa 1976) 2005;30:1181–7.

[9] Burwell RG, Dangerfield PH, Moulton A, Grivas TB. Adolescent idiopathic scoliosis (AIS) environment, exposome and epigenetics: a molecular perspective of postnatal normal spinal growth and the etiopathogenesis of AIS with consideration of a network approach and possible implications for medical therapy. Scoliosis 2011;6:26.

[10] Grivas TB, Mihas C, Mazioti C, et al. Maternal age at birth: does it dictate the epigenotypic expression of the trunkal asymmetry of a child? Stud Health Technol Inform 2012;176:36–42.

[11] Sparrow DB, Chapman G, Smith AJ, et al. A mechanism for gene-environment interaction in the etiology of congenital scoliosis. Cell 2012;149:295–306.

[12] Schottler J, Vogel LC, Sturm P. Spinal cord injuries in young children: a review of children injured at 5 years of age and younger. Dev Med Child Neurol 2012;54:1138–43.

[13] de Jonge T, Slullitel H, Dubousset J, et al. Late-onset spinal deformities in children treated by laminectomy and radiation therapy for malignant tumors. Eur Spine J 2005;14:765–71.

[14] Rortvedt LA, Crenshaw TD. Expression of kyphosis in young pigs is induced by a reduction of supplemental vitamin D in maternal diets and vitamin D, Ca and P concentrations in nursery diets. J Anim Sci 2012;90:4905–15.

[15] Menezes AH. Craniovertebral junction neoplasms in the pediatric population. Childs Nerv Syst 2008;24:1173–86.

[16] McKay SD, Al-Omari A, Tomlinson LA, Dormans JP. Review of cervical spine anomalies in genetic syndromes. Spine (Phila Pa 1976) 2012;37:E269–77.

[17] Danielsson AJ, Hasserius R, Ohlin A, Nachemson AL. Health-related quality of life in untreated versus brace-treated patients with adolescent idiopathic scoliosis: long term follow-up. Spine (Phila Pa 1976) 2010;35:199–205.
[18] Papaiaonnou T, Stokes I, Kenwright J. Scoliosis associated with limb-length inequality. J Bone Joint Surg Am 1982;64:59–62.
[19] Outland T. Juvenile dorsal kyphosis. Clin Orthop 1955;5:155.
[20] Ali RM, Green DW, Patel TC. Scheuermann's kyphosis. Curr Opin Pediatr 1999;11:70–5.
[21] Sorenson KH. Scheuermann's juvenile kyphosis: clinical appearance, radiography, aetiology and prognosis. Copenhagen: Munksgaard; 1964.
[22] Kuroki H, Inomata N, Hamanaka H, et al. Significance of hanging total spine x-ray to estimate the indicative correction angle by brace wearing in idiopathic scoliosis patients. Scoliosis 2012;7:8.
[23] Corona J, Sanders JO, Luhman SJ, et al. Reliability of radiographic measures for infantile idiopathic scoliosis. J Bone Joint Surg Am 2012;94:e86.
[24] Canavese F, Holveck J, De Coulon G, Kaelin A. Analysis of concave and convex rib-vertebral angle, angle difference, and angle ratio in patients with Lenke type 1 main thoracic adolescent idiopathic scoliosis treated by observation, bracing or posterior fusion and instrumentation. J Spinal Disord Tech 2011;24:506–13.
[25] Singhai R, Perry DC, Prasad S, et al. The use of routine preoperative magnetic resonance imaging in identifying intraspinal anomalies in patients with idiopathic scoliosis: a 10-year review. Eur Spine J 2013;22:355–9.
[26] Routh RH, Rumancik S, Pathak RD, et al. The relationship between bone mineral density and biomechanics in patients with osteoporosis and scoliosis. Osteoporos Int 2005;16:1857–63.
[27] Kobayashi T, Atsuta Y, Takemitsu M, et al. A prospective study of de novo scoliosis in a community based cohort. Spine (Phila Pa 1976) 2006;31:178–82.
[28] Romano M, Minozzi S, Bettany-Saltikov J, et al. Exercises for adolescent idiopathic scoliosis. Cochrane Database Syst Rev 2012;8, CD007637.
[29] Baulesh DM, Huj J, Judkins T, et al. The role of serial casting in early-onset scoliosis. J Pediatr Orthop 2012;32:658–63.
[30] Grivas TB, Kaspiris A. European braces widely used for conservative scoliosis treatment. Stud Health Technol Inform 2012;158:157–66.
[31] Canavese F, Kaelin A. Adolescent idiopathic scoliosis: indications and efficacy of nonoperative treatment. Indian J Orthop 2011;45:7–14.
[32] Laituri CA, Schwend RM, Holcomb 3rd GW. Thoracoscopic vertebral body stapling for treatment of scoliosis in young children. J Laparoendosc Adv Surg Tech A 2012;22:830–3.
[33] Olgun ZD, Ahmadiadli H, Alanay A, Yazici M. Vertebral body growth during growing rod instrumentation: growth preservation or stimulation? J Pediatr Orthop 2012;32:184–9.
[34] Miladi L, Journe A, Mousny M. H3S2 (3 hooks, 2 screws) construct: a simple growing rod technique for early onset scoliosis. Eur Spine J 2013;22(Suppl. 2):S96–105.
[35] Akbarnia BA, Cheung K, Noordeen H, et al. Next generation of growth-sparing technique: preliminary clinical results of a magnetically controlled growing rod in 14 patients with early-onset scoliosis. Spine (Phila Pa 1976) 2013;38:665–70.
[36] Coe JD, Kitchel SH, Meisel HJ, et al. NFlex dynamic stabilization system: two-year clinical outcomes of multicenter study. J Korean Neurosurg Soc 2012;51:343–9.
[37] Zhao D, Deng SC, Sun ZM, et al. Influences of clinical symptoms on the selection of surgical options for adult degenerative scoliosis [abstract]. Zhonghua Yi Xue Za Zhi 2012;92:1201–5.
[38] Che KJ, Suk SI, Park SR, et al. Selection of proximal fusion level for adult degenerative lumbar scoliosis. Eur Spine J 2013;22:394–401.
[39] Herndon WA, Emans JB, Micheli LJ, Hall JE. Combined anterior and posterior fusion for Scheuermann's kyphosis. Spine 1981;6:125–30.
[40] Richter DE, Nash Jr CL, Moskowitz RW, et al. Idiopathic adolescent scoliosis—a prototype of degenerative joint disease. The relation of biomechanic factors to osteophyte formation. Clin Orthop Relat Res 1985;193:221–9.
[41] Bennini A. Root compression in lumbar scoliosis—clinical picture and treatment based on 13 personal cases. Neurochirugia (Stuttg) 1982;25:195–201.
[42] Greggi T, Lolli F, DiSilvestre M, et al. Complications incidence in the treatment of early onset scoliosis with growing spinal implants. Stud Health Technol Inform 2012;176:334–7.

CHAPTER 153

Spasticity

Joel E. Frontera, MD
Monica Verduzco-Gutierrez, MD

Synonyms

Increased muscle tone
Spastic dystonia

ICD-9 Codes

728.85	**Spasm of muscle**
781.0	**Abnormal involuntary movements**
781.92	**Abnormal posture**
333.2	**Myoclonus**

ICD-10 Codes

M62.838	**Muscle spasm**
R25.9	**Abnormal involuntary movements**
R29.3	**Abnormal posture**
G25.3	**Myoclonus**

Definition

Spasticity is commonly defined as a velocity-dependent increase in muscle tone with exaggerated tendon jerks, resulting from hyperexcitability of the stretch reflex. This means that the faster the passive movement of the limb through its range, the greater the increase in muscle tone. This definition makes spasticity a component of an upper motor neuron syndrome, which is also associated with other findings that include hyperreflexia, clonus, muscle co-contraction, and muscle weakness.

Spasticity can be caused by a variety of upper motor neuron conditions. It is often noted to be a major problem in conditions like spinal cord injury, multiple sclerosis, and traumatic brain injury. It is estimated to affect between 40% and 80% of patients with a spinal cord injury or multiple sclerosis and as much as 80% of the traumatic brain injury population. It can also be present in other conditions like amyotrophic lateral sclerosis, brain and spinal cord tumors, and cerebral palsy.

Symptoms

Patients may complain of increased tightness, worsening spasms, and pain when they come to the clinic, but more important, the main complaint can be worsening of functional activities. The ability to move affected limbs actively or passively is reduced. Spasticity significantly interferes with routine tasks and even hygiene (e.g., increased elbow flexor spasticity in a stroke survivor while walking; adductor spasticity in a paraplegic individual during urinary catheterization) while at the same time causing pain and muscle co-contraction. These symptoms may be due to a secondary condition that may increase spasticity, such as an infectious process, skin problems, and cord tethering. Thus, when a patient comes to the clinic complaining of worsening spasticity, a thorough history and physical examination should be performed to identify the cause.

Physical Examination

Spasticity occurs in the presence of other signs and symptoms of upper motor neuron damage. Other positive signs include hyperreflexia, Babinski responses, and clonus. Negatives signs include muscle weakness, fatigue, reduced motor control, and loss of coordination. Increased muscle tone in the absence of these findings should lead to consideration of alternative causes of increased muscle tone, such as dystonia, Parkinson disease, or pain-associated muscle spasm. Strength testing may not be reliable as the spasticity may affect both range of motion because of contractures and co-contraction of antagonist muscles.

Muscle contracture as well as other soft tissue changes can be a part of this upper motor neuron syndrome, and it may be difficult in some cases to determine how much contracture is present in an individual with severe spasticity. A thorough physical examination can discover other issues associated with spasticity that could affect the individual, such as sensory disturbances (proprioception and spatial orientation), dysphagia, dysarthria, and skin issues. The skin should be inspected because abnormal positioning due to spasticity may directly cause skin injury (e.g., maceration of the palm due to a clenched fist) or contribute to pressure ulcer formation.

Sometimes it is important to differentiate spasticity from rigidity, commonly seen in conditions like Parkinson disease. One must look at some physical examination findings that occur with spasticity, such as the clasp-knife phenomenon.

There is also variability when antagonistic muscles are evaluated. In spasticity, for example, some muscle groups are more affected than their antagonist muscles. Rigidity is not velocity dependent; it is constant throughout the full range of motion.

Functional Limitations

Spasticity can cause significant functional limitations. In a patient with spinal cord injury, for example, spasticity can have a serious impact on positioning. It can affect wheelchair positioning as well as transfers. Hygiene and catheterization may be affected by significant hip adductor tone or spasticity. It will affect dexterity and fine motor coordination in the upper extremities. The use of bracing or other modalities to assist with ambulation may be limited if the spasticity is significant. Studies have found that a significant number of patients with both spinal cord injury and traumatic brain injury have noted that spasticity affects quality of life. In some cases, spasticity may serve as a partial substitute for voluntary muscle contraction. A common example of substitution for voluntary muscle function is the hip and knee extensor spasticity seen after stroke that may allow successful weight bearing through the weak leg and contribute to restoration of walking ability.

Diagnostic Studies

Spasticity is a clinical diagnosis, without any specific laboratory confirmation. Clinical measurement scales to quantify the severity of spasticity may be useful to monitor the efficacy of treatment. The most commonly used scales are the Ashworth scale (and a modified version of this scale) [1], which measures resistance of the muscle to passive stretch, and the Penn Spasm Frequency scale, which characterizes the frequency of muscle spasms [2] (Tables 153.1 and 153.2).

Table 153.1 Modified Ashworth Scale [1]

0	No increase in muscle tone
1	Slight increase in muscle tone, manifested by a catch and release or by minimal resistance at the end range of motion when the part is moved in flexion or extension/abduction or adduction
1+	Slight increase in muscle tone, manifested by a catch, followed by minimal resistance throughout the remainder (less than half) of the range of motion
2	More marked increase in muscle tone through most of the range of motion, but the affected part is easily moved
3	Considerable increase in muscle tone, passive movement is difficult
4	Affected part is rigid in flexion or extension (abduction or adduction)

Table 153.2 Penn Spasm Frequency Scale [2]

How often are muscle spasms occurring?

0	No spasms
1	Spasms induced only by stimulation
2	Spasms occurring less than once per hour
3	Spasms occurring between 1 and 10 times per hour
4	Spasms occurring more than 10 times per hour

Differential Diagnosis

Dystonia
Rigidity (e.g., Parkinson disease)
Paratonia
Pain-associated muscle spasm
Contracture

Treatment

Initial

Management of spasticity should always be decided in the setting of functional and clinical scenarios. As noted before, spasticity can be used to the patient's advantage, such as ambulation in the setting of spastic hemiparesis. Treatment should be started when spasticity becomes an obstacle to functional goals as well as to safety (spasms while transferring that could lead to a fall), hygiene, and skin integrity management. A change in previously well controlled spasticity should always lead to consideration of possible irritants or nociceptive stimuli that might be "triggering" the spasticity. Examples are urinary tract infections, skin breakdown, occult fractures, and an ingrown toenail in an insensate limb (e.g., in a paraplegic person).

There are several options for oral medications (Table 153.3) that have had mixed results in the different diseases that cause spasticity. Spasticity caused by injury to the spinal cord tends to respond better to oral medications such as baclofen and tizanidine than does spasticity caused by a traumatic brain injury or a stroke. Some of the centrally acting medications, such as baclofen, tizanidine [3], and the benzodiazepines, have significant side effects that may impair cognition and overall recovery after an acquired brain injury [4]. Another commonly used drug is dantrolene [5], which works directly at the muscle level, preventing calcium flux at the sarcoplasmic reticulum and thereby reducing muscle force.

Rehabilitation

A physical management program of therapeutic exercise, stretching, and passive range of motion initiated by trained physical and occupational therapists is imperative for the management of spasticity, regardless of cause. Goals of therapeutic exercise are to maintain range of motion, to prevent contractures, to reduce muscle overactivity, and to disrupt maladaptive spasticity patterns. Active exercise can also increase muscle strength [6].

Stretching and passive range of motion serve to prevent contracture formation and temporarily reduce increased muscle tone, especially in patients who are not capable of active movement. Therapists can instruct the patient and caregivers in appropriate stretching techniques. Standing has been shown to be helpful in tone management as well as to have many other benefits. Physical modalities including ultrasound treatment have been used to facilitate stretching, although ultrasound had no effect in minimizing the spasticity at the gastrocnemius compared with passive stretching exercises in one trial [7]. The results of a different study did show that neuromuscular electrical stimulation with

Table 153.3 Commonly Used Oral Antispasticity Medications

Medication	Mechanism of Action	Starting Dose	Common Side Effects	Relative Contraindications
Baclofen	$GABA_B$ agonist Increases presynaptic and postsynaptic inhibition	5-10 mg tid (maximum dose: 80 mg/day)	Sedation, rare hepatotoxicity, withdrawal symptoms	Cognitive impairment, seizures
Diazepam (benzodiazepines)	$GABA_A$ agonist	2 mg tid	Sedation, respiratory ataxia	History of benzodiazepine or other substance abuse
Tizanidine	α_2-Agonist Suppresses polysynaptic reflexes	2 mg tid (maximum dose: 32 mg/day)	Sedation, hypotension, hepatotoxicity	Cognitive impairment
Dantrolene	Prevents calcium influx at the sarcoplasmic reticulum in the muscle	25 mg daily	Weakness, hepatotoxicity, occasional sedation	Liver disease

Table 153.4 Characteristics of Different Botulinum Toxins

	OnabotulinumtoxinA*	AbobotulinumtoxinA†	IncobotulinumtoxinA‡	RimabotulinumtoxinB§
Serotype	A	A	A	B
Packaging, units/vial	100 or 200	300 or 500	50 or 100	2500, 5000, or 10,000
Preparation	Vacuum dried	Lyophilized	Lyophilized	Solution (5000 units/mL)
Storage for packaged product	Refrigerator	Refrigerator	Room temperature, refrigerator, or freezer	Refrigerator
Storage after reconstitution	2° C-8° C for 24 hours	2° C-8° C for 4 hours	2° C-8° C for 24 hours	2° C-8° C for 4 hours

*Botox medication guide. Allergan. www.allergan.com
†Dysport medication guide. Ipsen Biopharmaceuticals. www.dysport.com
‡Xeomin medication guide. Merz Pharma. www.xeomin.com
§Myobloc medication guide. Solstice Neurosciences. www.myobloc.com

stretching of the wrist extensor muscles was more effective than stretching alone in reducing spasticity [8]. External cooling of a spastic limb may provide a temporary reduction in spasticity, but this modality is generally impractical as a long-term therapy.

Splinting is another imperative treatment in a comprehensive spasticity rehabilitation program. This can include prefabricated splints, low-temperature thermoplastic custom orthotics, and plaster or fiberglass casts. Serial casting has been shown to be effective both on its own and after botulinum toxin treatment in improving both passive range of motion and the modified Ashworth scale score [9].

Procedures

Treatment with injections is an effective means of obtaining substantial reduction in spasticity in specific muscles while minimizing the risks of systemic or sedating side effects. Prior to botulinum toxin, two compounds have been used for local muscle relaxation: local anesthetics (lidocaine, etidocaine, and bupivacaine) and alcohols (ethyl alcohol and phenol). Local anesthetic injections have a fully reversible action and are of short duration; therefore, they can be useful in assessing the efficacy and benefits of more permanent injections. Chemical neurolysis with phenol in concentrations of 5% to 7% and alcohol in concentrations of 45% to 100% have an advantage of lower cost, rapid onset of action, and potency but have risks of dysesthesias and muscle fibrosis and require more skill and time to perform [10].

Chemodenervation with botulinum toxin has become a mainstay of practice in the treatment of spasticity for graded relief in selected muscles. Intramuscular injection of botulinum toxin provides local relief of spasticity for 2 to 6 months. There are currently four toxins available: onabotulinumtoxinA, rimabotulinumtoxinB, abobotulinumtoxinA, and incobotulinumtoxinA. There is ample literature on and Food and Drug Administration approval of all four agents for the treatment of cervical dystonia. There are now more publications on the type A products that document their utility in the management of spasticity [11–14]. The American Academy of Neurology published an evidence-based position paper on spasticity in 2008 supporting the use of botulinum toxin as a treatment to decrease tone and to improve passive function. In addition, it should be considered to improve active function [15]. Furthermore, with all injection procedures, adjunctive treatments such as physical and occupational therapy will improve the delivery of therapy and improve the outcome [16]. The dosing and administration of botulinum toxins are not standardized and must be managed with great care as they are not clinically equivalent. Some differences in the four botulinum toxins are shown in Table 153.4.

Surgery

Several surgical interventions are used for spasticity. An important neurosurgical intervention is placement of an intrathecal baclofen pump into the abdominal wall. In this system, there is an infusion of a prescribed rate of baclofen that is administered to the intrathecal space through a catheter system. This intervention has been found to reduce severe spasticity of cerebral and spinal origin, including in patients with cerebral palsy, spinal cord injury, brain injury, multiple sclerosis, and stroke. Evidence suggests that not only can intrathecal baclofen reduce spasticity, it can also improve function and quality of life [17] as well as improve gait in ambulatory patients [18,19].

Other neurosurgical techniques include stereotactic ablation or stimulation and cerebellar stimulation, which have been shown to have variable to uncertain results. Spinal cord surgeries such as selective posterior rhizotomy and myelotomy have been used as well in specially selected patients.

Neuro-orthopedic consultation can be obtained for further correction of limb deformities when conservative measures performed by a multidisciplinary team have been ineffective. Surgical procedures including tendon release or lengthening, tenotomy, and joint fusion can lead to improvement in functional outcome, pain, and subjective satisfaction [20,21].

Potential Disease Complications

Permanent loss of range of motion and contracture can result from inadequately controlled spasticity or insufficient stretching and splinting. Lost range of motion can also lead to difficulty with dressing, hygiene, and grooming activities. Skin issues can result, including accumulation of moisture, skin irritation, bacterial overgrowth, infection, and skin breakdown. Bone and joint issues, such as adhesive capsulitis, complex regional pain syndrome, and subluxation of joints, can occur.

Potential Treatment Complications

All of the centrally acting medications can cause significant sedation, which limits and therefore determines the dosage that can be tolerated. In individuals with preexisting cognitive impairments (e.g., stroke, traumatic brain injury), the sedative side effects can hinder rehabilitation goals, and the maximally tolerated dosage may be insufficient to control the symptoms of spasticity. Alternative treatments or use of the agents only before bedtime can be considered. Abrupt discontinuation of oral antispasticity medications is inadvisable. Seizures have been described after abrupt discontinuation of baclofen, and rebound spasticity is a concern with all of these medications.

In individuals with marginal motor function who may be relying in part on spasticity as a substitution for voluntary motor control, excessive reduction in spasticity may lead to reduced functional ability (e.g., loss of the ability to stand in a patient with paraparesis). Oral medication or intrathecal baclofen doses can generally be titrated to avoid this side effect; however, injected treatments (botulinum toxin, phenol) are more of a problem if overtreatment occurs.

Phenol carries some risk for painful dysesthesia, muscle fibrosis, scarring, and edema after injection. Botulinum toxin is generally well tolerated in therapeutic doses but does carry a Food and Drug Administration–mandated black box warning of a rare but potentially life-threatening complication when the effects of the toxin spread far beyond the injection site, causing systemic weakness, vision changes, dysarthria, dysphonia, dysphagia, and respiratory insufficiency. This can be avoided by careful selection of muscles, proper method of injection guidance (e.g., electromyography, ultrasonography, or motor point electrical stimulation), appropriate dilution of toxin, and restriction of dosage to the minimal dose needed to obtain a therapeutic effect. Antibodies to botulinum toxin can develop after repeated injection, which can render treatment ineffective.

Intrathecal baclofen pump treatment can result in post–dural puncture headache, iatrogenic meningitis, or infection of the external surface of the pump. Complications can also involve the medication (e.g., known adverse effects of baclofen are drowsiness and weakness) but are more frequently the result of malfunction of the intrathecal baclofen therapy system due to the pump, catheter, or human error. Interruption or underdosing of drug delivery can lead to a life-threatening withdrawal syndrome. Catheter failures can result in need for surgical intervention.

References

[1] Bohannon RW, Smith MB. Interrater reliability of a modified Ashworth scale of muscle spasticity. Phys Ther 1987;67:206–7.

[2] Penn RD, Savoy SM, Corcos D, et al. Intrathecal baclofen for severe spinal spasticity. N Engl J Med 1989;320:1517–54.

[3] Nance PW, Bugaresti J, Shellenberger K, et al. Efficacy and safety of tizanidine in the treatment of spasticity in patients with spinal cord injury. North American Tizanidine Study Group. Neurology 1994;44:S44–5.

[4] Goldstein LB, the Sygen in Acute Stroke Investigators. Common drugs may influence motor recovery after stroke. Neurology 1995;45:865–71.

[5] Kita M, Goodkin DE. Drugs used to treat spasticity. Drugs 2000;59:487–95.

[6] Stevenson VL. Rehabilitation in practice: spasticity management. Clin Rehabil 2010;24:293–304.

[7] Sahin N, Ugurlu H, Karahan AY. Efficacy of therapeutic ultrasound in the treatment of spasticity: a randomized controlled study. NeuroRehabilitation 2011;29:61–6.

[8] Sahin N, Ugurlu H, Albayrak I. The efficacy of electrical stimulation in reducing the post-stroke spasticity: a randomized controlled study. Disabil Rehabil 2012;34:151–6.

[9] Logan LR. Rehabilitation techniques to maximize spasticity management. Top Stroke Rehabil 2011;18:203–11.

[10] Elovic E, Esquenazi A, Alter K, et al. Chemodenervation and nerve blocks in the diagnosis and management of spasticity and overactivity. PM R 2009;1:842–51.

[11] Brashear A, Gordon MF, Elovic E, et al, Botox Post-Stroke Spasticity Study Group. Intramuscular injection of botulinum toxin for the treatment of wrist and finger spasticity after a stroke. N Engl J Med 2002;347:395–400.

[12] Elovic EP, Brashear A, Kaelin D, et al. Repeated treatments with botulinum toxin type A produce sustained decreases in the limitations associated with focal upper-limb poststroke spasticity for caregivers and patients. Arch Phys Med Rehabil 2008;89:799–806.

[13] Bakheit AM, Pittock S, Moore AP, et al. A randomized, double-blind, placebo-controlled, dose-ranging study to compare the efficacy and safety of three doses of botulinum toxin type A (Dysport) with placebo in upper limb spasticity after stroke. Stroke 2000;31:2402–6.

[14] Santamato A, Panza F, Ranieri M, Frisardi V, et al. Efficacy and safety of higher doses of botulinum toxin type A NT 201 free from complexing proteins in the upper and lower limb spasticity after stroke. J Neural Transm 2013;120:469–76.

[15] Simpson DM, Gracies JM, Graham HK, et al. Assessment: botulinum neurotoxin for the treatment of spasticity (an evidence-based review): report of the Therapeutics and Technology Assessment Subcommittee of the American Academy of Neurology. Neurology 2008;70:1691–8.

[16] Esquenazi A, Mayer N, Lee S, et al, PROS Study Group. Patient registry of outcomes in spasticity care. Am J Phys Med Rehabil 2012;91:729–46.

[17] Ivanhoe CB, Francisco GE, McGuire JR, et al. Intrathecal baclofen management of poststroke spastic hypertonia: implications for function and quality of life. Arch Phys Med Rehabil 2006;87:1509–15.

[18] Sadiq SA, Wang GC. Long-term intrathecal baclofen therapy in ambulatory stroke patients with spasticity. J Neurol 2006;253:563–9.

[19] Francisco GE, Boake C. Improvement in walking speed in poststroke spastic hemiplegia after intrathecal baclofen therapy: a preliminary study. Arch Phys Med Rehabil 2003;84:1194–9.

[20] Namdari S, Park MJ, Baldwin K, et al. Effect of age, sex, and timing on correction of spastic equinovarus following cerebrovascular accident. Foot Ankle Int 2009;30:923–7.

[21] Gong HS, Chung CY, Park MS, et al. Functional outcomes after upper extremity surgery for cerebral palsy: comparison of high and low manual ability classification system levels. J Hand Surg [Am] 2010;35:277–3.

CHAPTER 154

Speech and Language Disorders

Jason H. Kortte, MS, CCC-SLP

Jeffrey B. Palmer, MD

Synonyms

Aphasia
- **Dysphasia**

Dysarthria
- **Slurred speech**

Dysphonia
- **Voice disturbance**
- **Change in voice**
- **Hoarseness**
- **Hypernasality**
- **Hyponasality**

ICD-9 Codes

483.11 **Aphasia, late effect of stroke**
784.49 **Dysphonia**
784.5 **Dysarthria**

ICD-10 Codes

I69.320 **Aphasia following cerebral infarction**
R49.0 **Dysphonia**
R47.1 **Dysarthria and anarthria**

Definitions

A summary of the speech and language disorders described in this chapter is presented in Table 154.1.

Aphasia is an acquired, neurogenic language processing impairment that can disrupt the modalities of language, including speaking, listening, reading, and writing. Aphasia is commonly caused by stroke; it occurs in 21% to 38% of cases of acute stroke and is associated with high morbidity, mortality, and financial cost [1]. However, aphasia can result from brain injuries other than stroke, such as tumors and head trauma, and it must be differentiated from motor or sensory dysfunction, psychiatric illness, confusion, or general intellectual impairment [2]. In the United States, there are approximately 100,000 new cases of aphasia per year; the majority are women and 65 years of age or older [3]. Primary progressive aphasia is a term reserved for subtle, insidious progressive language impairments associated with frontal-temporal dementia. In primary progressive aphasia, there is relative preservation of other mental and cognitive functions for at least the first 2 years of the condition [4].

Aphasia is classified into subtypes according to the ability to produce, to understand, and to repeat language [5]. The ability to produce language is assessed in terms of fluency, defined as the rate of speech and the amount of effort in producing speech. Each subtype of aphasia is associated with a specific profile of language capabilities and disabilities (Table 154.2). For example, an individual with Wernicke aphasia produces fluent language, has impaired auditory comprehension, and has poor repetition skills. In contrast, Broca aphasia is characterized by nonfluent language, relatively intact auditory comprehension, and poor repetition skills.

Motor speech disorders, which include dysarthria and apraxia of speech, result from neurologic impairment affecting motor planning, neuromuscular control, or execution of speech [6]. Apraxia of speech results from a disruption in programming of the volitional movements for speech and is characterized by difficulty in orchestrating the movements of the lips, tongue, jaw, soft palate, vocal cords, and respiratory system for the production of speech. It can occur without muscle weakness or impairments in receptive and expressive language. Apraxia of speech is a distinct disorder, although some of its symptoms can co-occur in the presence of dysarthria and aphasia [7].

Dysarthria, a group of motor speech disorders resulting from damage to the central or the peripheral nervous system, affects 10% to 65% of individuals with acquired brain injury, depending on the type, extent, and duration of injury [8]. Dysarthria results from weakness, paralysis, or dyscoordination of the speech muscles that impairs articulation, respiration, resonance, and phonation (voice production). Dysarthria is divided into subtypes according to the speech characteristics and underlying pathophysiologic process. Neurogenic speech disorders should be differentiated from those resulting from structural problems (such as cleft palate or post-laryngectomy status) or psychogenic disorders [6].

Table 154.1 Speech and Language Disorders

Disorder	Definition
Aphasia	Language processing disturbance that can involve the expression of language, the comprehension of language, or both Word finding errors and difficulty in understanding language are classic indicators of aphasia.
Dysarthria	Group of motor speech disorders associated with muscle paralysis, weakness, or incoordination Dysarthria often is manifested as slurred speech and does *not* involve language (receptive or expressive) processes.
Apraxia of speech	Motor speech disorder disrupting the motor programming of the volitional movements for speech Individuals struggle to find correct position of articulators (i.e., lips, tongue). It can occur without muscle weakness or impairments in receptive and expressive language.
Dysphonia	Faulty or abnormal phonation (voice production) Vocal quality may sound hoarse, harsh, strained, or breathy.

The extreme form of dysarthria is anarthria, in which the individual is entirely incapable of producing articulated speech. Individuals with dysarthria often have dysphagia, or impaired swallowing, regardless of the etiology or duration [9]. This is readily understood, considering the overlap of structures and functions used in speaking and swallowing (see Chapter 129).

Dysphonia is faulty or abnormal phonation (voice production). Although prevalence rates are not well established, dysphonia is common in any condition causing abnormal motion of the vocal cords or dyscoordination of breathing and speaking. These include brainstem stroke, Parkinson disease, amyotrophic lateral sclerosis, Guillain-Barré syndrome, myasthenia gravis, spastic dysphonia, and multiple sclerosis, among others [6], as well as secondary processes that alter the structure or function of the vocal cords, including vocal abuse (such as excessive talking, screaming, or smoking), trauma (traumatic or prolonged intubation, arytenoid dislocation), status post–laryngeal surgery, and a variety of disorders (laryngeal cancer, reflux laryngitis) [10]. Dysphonia is distinguished from dysarthria in that dysphonia involves only the sound of the voice, whereas dysarthria involves the overall sound of speech, including resonance and articulation.

Symptoms

Individuals with aphasia often complain of difficulty in speaking, reading, writing, or understanding speech. They often report difficulty in finding the word they wish to say and can become frustrated; however, some are unaware of their deficits. Individuals who solely have a motor speech disorder (e.g., dysarthria, dysphonia, or apraxia of speech) have no difficulty in finding the words they wish to say and report no difficulties with reading, writing, or auditory comprehension but complain primarily of difficulty in producing intelligible speech. Aphasia develops most commonly after left hemisphere stroke even in people who are left handed, whereas neglect, visual-spatial impairments, and other cognitive syndromes are more common after right hemisphere strokes [11].

Physical Examination

During the initial history and physical, the physiatrist should attend to speech intelligibility, vocal quality, language content, fluency, and auditory comprehension. Deficits in these areas warrant referral to a certified speech-language pathologist for comprehensive evaluation including standardized testing. In the rehabilitation setting, the Functional Independence Measure is widely used to measure functional abilities including communication [12]. Typical findings are described here for the four main categories of speech and language disorders.

Aphasia

Findings indicative of aphasia vary according to the location and size of the brain lesion (see Table 154.2). One classic sign of aphasia is difficulty in comprehending language

Table 154.2 Aphasia Syndromes

Aphasia Type	Predicted Lesion Site	Comprehension	Fluency	Repetition
Broca	Inferior frontal gyrus; Brodmann area	Relatively intact	Nonfluent	Poor
Wernicke	Posterior superior temporal gyrus; Brodmann area	Impaired	Fluent	Poor
Conduction	Superior marginal gyrus and underlying white matter (arcuate fasciculus)	Relatively intact	Fluent	Poor
Transcortical motor	Anterior and superior to Broca area (watershed area)	Relatively intact	Nonfluent	Good or less impaired than spontaneous speech
Transcortical sensory	Posterior and inferior to Wernicke area (watershed area)	Impaired	Fluent	Good
Transcortical mixed (isolation)	Anterior and posterior association areas (watershed areas)	Impaired	Nonfluent	Less impaired than spontaneous speech
Anomic	Angular gyrus or anywhere in left hemisphere	Relatively intact	Fluent	Good
Global	Left frontal, parietal, and temporal lobes	Impaired	Nonfluent	Poor

Modified from Helm-Estabrooks N, Albert ML. Manual of Aphasia and Aphasia Therapy, 2nd ed. Austin, Texas, Pro-Ed, 2004.

(spoken, gestural, or written). Significant impairment can be characterized by difficulty in following simple commands, whereas milder impairments may be obvious only during lengthy or complicated messages. Individuals who have aphasia may also have deficits in verbal expression (producing meaningful verbal output), which may be manifested as a total loss of language, with the production of only jargon (multiple whole-word substitutions) or meaningless sounds. A person with less severe aphasia may be able to express basic wants and needs but have difficulty in expressing complex ideas in conversation. Paraphasias, or naming errors, are a classic symptom of aphasia. Phonemic paraphasias involve the substitution, addition, or omission of target sounds (phonemes). For example, an individual may say "bable" for "table." A semantic paraphasia occurs when an individual produces a word related in meaning to the target word (i.e., "fork" for "spoon"). The severity of impairment can vary for each modality of language (listening, reading, writing, recognition of numbers, and gesturing). Aphasia is *not* a result of decreased auditory or visual perceptual skills, disordered thought processes, impaired motor programming, or weakness or incoordination of speech musculature [1].

Table 154.3 Classification of Dysarthria

Type	Localization	Motor Deficit
Flaccid	Lower motor neuron	Weakness, hypotonia
Spastic	Bilateral upper motor neuron	Spasticity
Ataxia	Cerebellum	Incoordination; inaccurate range, timing, direction; slow rate
Hypokinetic	Extrapyramidal system (basal ganglia circuit)	Variable speed of repetitive movements, rigidity
Hyperkinetic	Extrapyramidal system	Involuntary movements
Mixed	Multiple motor systems (amyotrophic lateral sclerosis, multiple sclerosis)	Weakness, reduced rate and range of motion

Modified from Duffy JR. Motor Speech Disorders: Substrates, Differential Diagnosis, and Management, 2nd ed. St. Louis, Elsevier Mosby, 2005.

Apraxia of Speech

The most common sign of apraxia of speech is a struggle to speak. This struggle is a direct result of the difficulty in finding the correct position of the articulators (i.e., lips, tongue). Speech is often halting and may contain sound substitutions, distortions, omissions, additions, and repetitions [6]. The individual is aware of his or her speech errors and will attempt to correct them with varying degrees of success. Severe forms of apraxia of speech may result in the inability to produce simple words. Interestingly, most people with apraxia of speech can produce common everyday phrases or sayings (e.g., *How are you? Have a nice day. Thank you.*) without error. A symptom that commonly coincides with apraxia of speech is nonverbal oral apraxia, which is the inability to imitate or to follow commands to perform volitional movements with the mouth or tongue [6]. Apraxia of speech is not caused by muscle weakness, decreased tone, or incoordination, nor is it the result of linguistic disturbances as in aphasia. Sound-level errors in apraxia of speech are thought to result from difficulty with motor execution and not with the selection of phonemes found in aphasia [4]. Apraxia of speech differs from dysarthria in that apraxia of speech is not a result of paresis or paralysis or the uncoordinated movements of speech muscles. Rather, it is believed to reflect a disturbance in the programming of movements used for speech [7]. In contrast to dysarthric errors, which are typically consistent and predictable, errors in apraxia of speech are highly irregular.

Dysarthria

In dysarthria, speech is often characterized as being slurred; the predominant errors are distortions of speech sounds. Dysarthria may also be characterized by changes in a person's rate, volume, and rhythm of speech. The findings vary greatly, depending on the pathophysiologic mechanism. Table 154.3 presents an overview of dysarthria classification.

Dysphonia

Dysphonia is characterized by a reduction or alteration in voice quality. Vocal quality can vary by degrees of loudness, breathiness, hoarseness, or harshness. A common example of dysphonia is the hoarse vocal quality of individuals with laryngitis. In the extreme form, aphonia, the individual is incapable of producing any voice but may be able to produce voiceless speech (e.g., whispering).

Functional Limitations

Functional limitations depend on the nature and severity of the communication impairment. Severe deficits can impair the ability to express basic daily needs or to understand simple directions. The individual may not be able to effectively interact with family members or health care providers. Less severe deficits allow the individual to express and to understand basic information but impair high-level activities. These include the expression and understanding of complex and lengthy information to meet vocational or social needs. Speech and language impairments can affect an individual's ability to complete a range of daily life tasks, including the ability to read bills and newspapers or environmental signs, to communicate using the telephone, and to participate effectively in conversations or school or employment activities. Speech and language impairments may result in frustration and can cause disruptions in personal relationships, community and religious participation, and vocational functioning. Individuals with aphasia often participate in fewer activities and report worse quality of life even when physical limitations, well-being, and social support are comparable to those of other individuals [13].

Diagnostic Studies

The speech-language pathologist or neuropsychologist can administer a variety of standardized instruments to diagnose aphasia. The aim of these instruments is to identify the pattern of symptoms to classify the aphasic syndrome, which is critical for the development of individualized interventions. Similarly, there are structured assessments for the diagnosis of dysarthria, dysphonia, and apraxia of speech. Performed by a speech-language pathologist, these in-depth assessments involve an oral-motor examination to identify the structure and function of oral, pharyngeal, and laryngeal musculature as well as speech characteristics (i.e., rate, volume, and intelligibility). For determination of the etiology and pathophysiology of dysphonia, a referral to an otolaryngologist is warranted. Laryngoscopy is often necessary to evaluate both the structure and the function of the larynx. Biopsy is indicated when a mass lesion is noted. Stroboscopic examination of the larynx, electroglottography, and acoustic voice analysis may reveal subtle abnormalities of vocal fold motion and resulting acoustic parameters [14,15]. The voice spectrogram is sometimes useful for quantitative assessment of vocal features.

Differential Diagnosis

APHASIA
Confusion, delirium, or dementia
Psychosis
Apraxia of speech
Dysarthria
Neurogenic stuttering
Echolalia
Palilalia
Selective mutism
Depression

APRAXIA OF SPEECH
Dysarthria
Aphasia
Neurogenic stuttering

DYSARTHRIA
Apraxia of speech
Aphasia
Depression
Abulia

DYSPHONIA
Acute and chronic laryngitis
Laryngeal hyperfunction (abuse and misuse)
Neurogenic disorders
Psychogenic disorders (i.e., conversion dysphonia)
Spasmodic dysphonia
Structural disorders of the larynx (congenital, traumatic, arthritic, neoplastic)

Treatment

Initial

Treatment of speech and language disorders usually requires referral to a speech-language pathologist. Initial treatment depends on the nature and severity of the disorder. The treatment plans for aphasia, apraxia of speech, dysarthria, and dysphonia vary greatly and must be individualized to meet each patient's communication needs. Initial intervention may include education of the patient and family about the communication impairment and compensatory strategies to facilitate communication.

Rehabilitation

To maximize a patient's communication skills, a speech-language pathologist can offer specific strategies, exercises, and activities to regain functional communication abilities.

Aphasia

Aphasia rehabilitation is efficacious in the stroke population [16,17]. Intervention depends on the aphasia subtype and the individual's specific strengths and weaknesses. General models of aphasia therapy involve stimulating intact language processes, facilitating maximal language and speech processes through hierarchical cues and prompts, and compensating for refractory deficits through alternative communication systems and partner-facilitated communication strategies [18]. Common therapeutic activities may involve naming tasks that use hierarchical cueing techniques to improve language content and structure. Therapy may begin with the production of automatic speech tasks, such as stating numbers or the days of the week. More difficult tasks may involve individually naming objects and describing pictures using appropriate sentence and word forms. Errorless naming techniques and gestural training can promote recovery of word retrieval [19]. The training of scripts can allow the individual to produce rehearsed sentences to meet needs in specific situations [20]. Written expression can be targeted through functional activities such as writing and copying biographical information. Common activities to improve auditory comprehension include following simple or complex commands and answering spoken questions correctly. Therapy to improve reading comprehension may involve matching objects to written words, following written directions, or reading functional information (bills, medication labels, environmental signs). Activities that involve attention training, problem solving, and executive functioning skills were shown to have a positive effect on verbal expression and auditory comprehension [21,22]. Furthermore, collaboration between the speech-language pathologist and other skilled services, such as occupational therapy, can improve the patient's daily living skills.

Treatment for aphasia includes education. It is important to teach the individual with aphasia, family, and health care providers compensatory strategies to facilitate communication. Environmental modification and partner-facilitated approaches can dramatically improve communication success [23–25]. These can include turning off the television to reduce distractions, speaking slowly, using simple language, offering a pen and paper, checking that you are understood, and paraphrasing. Effective word-finding strategies include the use of circumlocutions, such as descriptions, definitions, or even sound effects during communication breakdowns. Training of volunteers to serve as conversation partners by the Supported Conversation for Adults with Aphasia intervention has been shown to be effective [26].

Advances in computer technology have provided therapists with new options in treating aphasia. Computer programs allow clinicians to easily design activities, to select stimulus items, to present cues, and to individualize reinforcements [27,28]. Software programs also can be used to turn a computer into a speech output communication device, allowing people with severe aphasia to produce phrases and sentences of varying degrees of complexity [29–31]. These programs often contain features such as word prediction and graphic cues to facilitate correct sentence structure. Video technology has allowed individuals with aphasia to follow pre-recorded mouth movements with auditory and written cues to aid word retrieval for full sentences and even longer narratives [32,33]. The growing popularity of user-friendly smart phones has allowed individuals with aphasia and other speech disorders easy access to tools for enhancing communication including photos, videos, maps, pre-recorded messages, and text support.

Recent changes in reimbursement for aphasia therapy encouraged development of the Life Participation Approach to Aphasia. This philosophy focuses on long-term life goals, incorporating "aphasia-friendly" environments, use of communication partners, and identification of barriers to life participation [34].

Dysarthria

Rehabilitation for dysarthria also depends on the specific subtype. Approaches to treatment include medical intervention, oral prosthetic devices, and behavioral management [6]. For example, people with dysarthria due to Parkinson disease may benefit from dopamine agonists. Palatal lifts and voice amplifiers are commonly used to improve intelligibility. A palatal lift and augmentation prosthesis have been used successfully in conjunction with behavioral management [35]. Behavioral management of dysarthria involves muscle strengthening (e.g., lip closure, tongue protrusion, tongue elevation), improvement of breath support, and modification of posture. The person with dysarthria learns to use compensatory techniques to decrease rate of speech, to increase loudness, and to "overarticulate." As with aphasia, the family is educated in strategies to maximize communication. Treatment of severe dysarthria or aphasia can include use of an augmentative communication system in which the individual uses pictures, written words, and alphabet or pictograph boards to enhance communication. Some individuals can use computer systems that produce synthesized speech. These offer a wide variety of communication topics and can be personalized to the individual's needs.

Apraxia of Speech

Treatment of apraxia of speech involves techniques to elicit accurate voluntary speech production. The speech-language pathologist incorporates multimodality cues, such as modeling mouth and lip movements, using verbal cues to describe accurate tongue and lip placement, and intoning words and sentences. Treatment approaches often incorporate the use of rate and rhythm control strategies [4]. For severe cases, alternative communication strategies, such as writing, drawing, and communication books, are used to augment or to replace speech.

Dysphonia

Management of dysphonia is based on the underlying disorder and the pathophysiologic process [36]. Vocal hygiene education and proper voicing techniques can improve vocal quality for individuals with vocal nodules due to laryngeal hyperfunction (vocal abuse). Techniques to enhance vocal fold approximation are useful in individuals with vocal cord motion impairments. Laryngitis due to gastroesophageal reflux disease is treated with a combination of voice therapy and vigorous antireflux regimen including proton pump inhibitors [37].

Procedures

Injection of a paralyzed vocal cord with Gelfoam or Teflon can increase its mass, bringing the medial edge of the cord closer to the midline. This facilitates contact with the mobile contralateral vocal cord, thereby improving phonation. This solution is usually only temporary; however, surgery is helpful in some cases. For cases of spasmodic dysphonia, an injection of botulinum toxin into the affected muscles can result in improved voice by correcting the abnormal motion of the vocal folds [38].

Surgery

Surgery is sometimes needed for treatment of voice disorders. Individuals with mass lesions of the larynx may need surgical excision. For individuals with unilateral vocal cord paralysis, a surgical procedure can bring the paralyzed cord closer to midline to achieve appropriate glottal closure. Implantation of a small device into the paralyzed hemilarynx, pushing the paralyzed cord toward the midline, can provide a lasting improvement in voice quality.

Structural lesions (e.g., cleft palate) or functional disorders (e.g., weakness of the palatal elevators) may cause inadequate seal of the velopharyngeal isthmus (the space between the soft palate and the pharyngeal walls). In either case, a surgical procedure to narrow the defect can sometimes provide improved speech quality.

Potential Disease Complications

Individuals with severe speech and language disorders may suffer extreme psychosocial consequences, including isolation, unemployment, depression [39], alienation, ostracism, and inability to fulfill essential family roles. Aphasia has been shown to be a risk factor for disability after stroke and plays a significant role in quality of life issues [40].

Potential Treatment Complications

Injection or surgical implant of the larynx may result in complications including infection, hemorrhage, and local tissue trauma. Injected material may gradually slip out of place and lose effectiveness, but this rarely leads to serious sequelae. Botulinum toxin injection rarely causes airway obstruction if the vocal folds become immobilized in the medial position. Leakage of the toxin into adjacent muscles may worsen the voice disorder or produce dysphagia.

References

[1] Berthier ML. Poststroke aphasia: epidemiology, pathophysiology and treatment. Drugs Aging 2005;22:163–82.
[2] Hallowell B, Chapey R. Introduction to language intervention strategies in adult aphasia. In: Chapey R, editor. Language intervention strategies in aphasia and related neurogenic communication disorders. 5th ed. Baltimore: Lippincott Williams & Wilkins; 2008. p. 3–19.

[3] Ellis C, Dismuke C, Edwards KK. Longitudinal trends in aphasia in the United States. NeuroRehabilitation 2010;27:327–33.

[4] Duffy J, McNeil MR. Primary progressive aphasia and apraxia of speech. In: Chapey R, editor. Language intervention strategies in aphasia and related neurogenic communication disorders. 5th ed. Baltimore: Lippincott Williams & Wilkins; 2008. p. 543–64.

[5] Helm-Estabrooks N, Albert ML. Manual of aphasia and aphasia therapy. 2nd ed. Austin, Texas: Pro-Ed; 2004.

[6] Duffy JR. Motor speech disorders: substrates, differential diagnosis, and management. 2nd ed. St. Louis: Elsevier Mosby; 2005.

[7] Ogar J, Slama H, Dronkers N, et al. Apraxia of speech: an overview. Neurocase 2005;11:427–32.

[8] Wang YT, Kent RD, Duffy JR, Thomas JE. Dysarthria associated with traumatic brain injury: speaking rate and emphatic stress. J Commun Dis 2005;38:231–60.

[9] Nishio M, Niimi S. Relationship between speech and swallowing disorders in patients with neuromuscular disease. Folia Phoniatr Logop 2004;56:291–304.

[10] Prater RJ, Swift RW. Manual of voice therapy. Austin, Texas: Pro-Ed; 1984.

[11] Jordan LC, Hillis AE. Aphasia and right hemisphere syndromes in stroke. Curr Neurol Neurosci Rep 2005;5:458–64.

[12] Linacre JM, Heinemann AW, Wright BD, et al. The structure and stability of the Functional Independence Measure. Arch Phys Med Rehabil 1994;75:127–32.

[13] Hilari K. The impact of stroke: are people with aphasia different to those without? Disabil Rehabil 2011;33:211–8.

[14] Akyildiz SM, Ogut F, Varis A, et al. Impact of laryngeal findings on acoustic parameters of patients with laryngopharyngeal reflux. ORL J Otorhinolaryngol Relat Spec 2012;74:215–9.

[15] Ayazi S, Pearson J, Hashemi M. Gastroesophageal reflux and voice changes: objective assessment of voice quality and impact of antireflux therapy. J Clin Gastroenterol 2012;46:119–23.

[16] Robey RR. The efficacy of treatment for aphasic persons: a meta-analysis. Brain Lang 1994;47:582–608.

[17] Nickels L. Therapy for naming disorders: revisiting, revising, and reviewing. Aphasiology 2002;16:935–79.

[18] Burns MS, Halper AS. Speech/language treatment of the aphasias: an integrated clinical approach. Rockville, Md: Aspen; 1988.

[19] Raymer AM, McHose B, Smith KG, et al. Contrasting effects of errorless naming treatment and gestural facilitation for word retrieval in aphasia. Neuropsychol Rehabil 2012;22:235–66.

[20] Cherney LR, Halper AS, Holland AL, Cole R. Computerized script training for aphasia: preliminary results. Am J Speech Lang Pathol 2008;17:19–34.

[21] Helm-Estabrooks N. Treating attention to improve auditory comprehension deficits associated with aphasia. Perspect Neurophysiol Neurogenic Speech Lang Disord 2011;21:64–71.

[22] Hatfield B, Millet D, Coles J, et al. Characterizing speech and language pathology outcomes in stroke rehabilitation. Arch Phys Med Rehabil 2005;86:S61–72.

[23] Lubinski R. Environmental considerations for elderly patients. In: Lubinski R, editor. Dementia and communication. Philadelphia: BC Decker; 1991.

[24] Lubinski R, Welland RJ. Normal aging and environmental effects on communication. Semin Speech Lang 1997;18:107–25.

[25] Hengst JA, Frame SR, Neuman-Stritzel T, et al. Using others' words: conversational use of reported speech by individuals with aphasia and their communication partners. J Speech Lang Hear Res 2005;48:137–56.

[26] Kagan A, Black SE, Duchan FJ, et al. Training volunteers as conversational partners using "Supported Conversation for Adults with Aphasia" (SCA): a controlled trial. J Speech Lang Hear Res 2001;44:624–38.

[27] Katz RC, Hallowell B. Technological applications in the treatment of acquired neurogenic communication and swallowing disorders in adults. Semin Speech Lang 1999;20:251–68.

[28] Fink RB, Brecher A, Schwartz MF, et al. A computer-implemented protocol for treatment for naming disorders: evaluation of clinician-guided and partially guided instruction. Aphasiology 2002;16:1061–86.

[29] Koul R, Corwin M, Hayes S. Production of graphic symbol sentences by individuals with aphasia: efficacy of a computer-based augmentative and alternative communication intervention. Brain Lang 2005;92:58–77.

[30] McCall D. Steps to success with technology for individuals with aphasia. Semin Speech Lang 2012;33:234–42.

[31] McCall D, Virata T, Linbarger M, et al. Integrating technology and targeted treatment to improve narrative production in aphasia: a case study. Aphasiology 2009;23:438–61.

[32] Williamson D. Speak-in-motion—VAST. http://www.speakinmotion.com. Accessed October 2012.

[33] Fridriksson J, Baker J, Whiteside J, et al. Treating visual speech perception to improve speech production in nonfluent aphasia. Stroke 2009;40:853–8.

[34] Silverman ME. Community: the key to building and extending engagement for individuals with aphasia. Semin Speech Lang 2011;32:256–67.

[35] Ono T, Hamamura M, Honda K, Nokubi T. Collaboration of a dentist and speech-language pathologist in the rehabilitation of a stroke patient with dysarthria: a case study. Gerodontology 2005;22:116–9.

[36] Chang JI, Bevans SE, Swartz SR. Evidence-based practice: management of hoarseness/dysphonia. Otolaryngol Clin North Am 2012;45:1109–26.

[37] Park J, Shim M, Hwang Y, et al. Combination of voice therapy and antireflux therapy rapidly recovers voice-related symptoms in laryngopharyngeal reflux patients. Otolaryngol Head Neck Surg 2012;146:92–7.

[38] Blitzer A, Brin MF, Fahn S, et al. Localized injections of botulinum toxin for the treatment of focal laryngeal dystonia (spastic dysphonia). Laryngoscope 1988;98:193–7.

[39] Kauhenen M, Korpelainen J, Hiltunen P, et al. Post stroke depression correlates with cognitive impairment and neurological deficits. Stroke 1999;30:1875–80.

[40] Flick CL. Stroke rehabilitation: stroke outcome and psychosocial consequences. Arch Phys Med Rehabil 1999;80:S21–6.

CHAPTER 155

Spinal Cord Injury (Cervical)

Sunil Sabharwal, MD

Synonyms

Tetraplegia
Quadriplegia

ICD-9 Codes

344.00 Quadriplegia, unspecified
344.01 Quadriplegia, C1-C4, complete
344.02 Quadriplegia, C1-C4, incomplete
344.03 Quadriplegia, C5-C7, complete
344.04 Quadriplegia, C5-C7, incomplete
344.09 Other quadriplegia

ICD-10 Codes

G82.50 Quadriplegia, unspecified
G82.51 Quadriplegia, C1-C4 complete
G82.52 Quadriplegia, C1-C4 incomplete
G82.53 Quadriplegia, C5-C7 complete
G82.54 Quadriplegia, C5-C7 incomplete

Definition

Cervical spinal cord injury (SCI) results in tetraplegia. The term *tetraplegia* (preferred to quadriplegia) refers to an impairment or loss of motor or sensory function in the cervical segments of the spinal cord due to damage of neural elements within the spinal canal [1]. The result is impairment of function in the arms as well as in the trunk, legs, and pelvic organs. Impairment of sensorimotor involvement outside the spinal canal, such as brachial plexus lesions or injury to peripheral nerves, should not be referred to as tetraplegia.

In a complete cervical SCI, sensory or motor function is absent in the lowest sacral segments S4-S5 (i.e., no anal sensation or voluntary anal contraction is present). If sensory or motor function is partially preserved below the neurologic level and includes the lowest sacral segments, the injury is defined as incomplete [1,2]. The American Spinal Injury Association Impairment Scale (AIS) is used in grading the degree of impairment (Table 155.1). Central cord syndrome is an incomplete SCI syndrome that applies almost exclusively to cervical SCI. It is characterized by greater weakness in the upper limbs than in the lower limbs and sacral sensory sparing [1].

SCI primarily affects young men. However, the average age at injury has increased from 28.7 years in the 1970s to 41.0 years since 2005, and the proportion of new SCI in adults older than 60 years has increased from 4.7% to 13.2% in the same time period in the national Spinal Cord Injury Model Systems database [3]. Males account for about 80% of injuries. The most common cause is motor vehicle accidents, followed by falls, violence (primarily gunshot wounds), and recreational sporting activities [2,3]. The proportion of injuries due to falls has increased over time. Cervical injuries occur more frequently than thoracic and lumbar injuries and accounted for 56.6% of the SCI database between 2005 and 2008. Since 2005, the most frequent neurologic category at discharge reported to the database is incomplete tetraplegia (40.8% of all SCI).

Symptoms

Primary symptoms of cervical SCI are related to muscle paralysis, sensory impairment, and autonomic impairment (including bladder, bowel, and sexual dysfunction). The patient can present in the outpatient setting with a multitude of secondary conditions [4] and associated problems. Symptoms may be vague and nonspecific. For example, urinary tract infections may be manifested not with classic symptoms of urgency and dysuria but with increased spasticity, increased frequency of spontaneous voiding, and lethargy [5]. The patient with pneumonia may present with fever, shortness of breath, or increasing anxiety. Headache may be indicative of autonomic dysreflexia and may be the primary or only presentation of a variety of pathologic processes ranging from bladder distention, urinary infection, constipation, or ingrown toenail to myocardial infarction or acute abdominal emergencies [6]. Table 155.2 lists common presenting symptoms of autonomic dysreflexia and underlying causes.

Because symptoms can reflect a variety of underlying conditions, these need to be evaluated carefully. For example, pain in cervical SCI may be multifactorial and needs to be further assessed by characteristics reported in the history, including quality, location, onset, timing, relieving and exacerbating factors, and associated

Table 155.1 American Spinal Injury Association Impairment Scale

Grade	Category	Description
A	Complete	No sensory or motor function is preserved in the sacral segments S4-S5.
B	Sensory incomplete	Sensory but no motor function is preserved below the neurologic level including the sacral segments S4-S5.
C	Motor incomplete*	Motor function is preserved below the neurologic level, and more than half of key muscles below the neurologic level have a muscle grade less than 3.
D	Motor incomplete*	Motor function is preserved below the neurologic level, and at least half of key muscles below the neurologic level have a muscle grade 3 or more.
E	Normal	Sensory function and motor function are normal; the patient may have abnormalities in reflex examination.

*There must be some sparing of sensory or motor function in S4-S5 segments to be classified as motor incomplete.

Table 155.2 Etiology of Common Symptoms in Spinal Cord Injury

Symptom	Possible Cause
Fever	Infectious Urinary tract infection Pneumonia Infected pressure ulcer, cellulitis, osteomyelitis Intra-abdominal or pelvic infection Hot environment (due to poikilothermia) Deep venous thrombosis Heterotopic ossification Pathologic limb fracture Drug fever (e.g., from antibiotics or anticonvulsant pain medications)
Fatigue	Nonspecific, but could be the only symptom of serious illness Infection Respiratory or cardiac failure Side effect of medications Depression (inquire about associated dysphoric symptoms)
Daytime drowsiness	Side effect of medications (e.g., narcotics, antispasticity agents) Nocturnal sleep apnea Ventilatory failure with carbon dioxide retention Depression
Shortness of breath	Pneumonia Abdominal distention (e.g., postprandial, obstipation) Pulmonary embolus Ventilatory impairment (can be postural with sitting up if borderline) Cardiac causes
Diarrhea	Altered bowel management schedule *Clostridium difficile* infection Spurious diarrhea with bowel impaction Side effect of medications (antibiotic, excess laxative or stool softener)
Rectal bleeding	Hemorrhoids Trauma from bowel care Colorectal cancer
Hematuria	Urinary tract infection Urinary stones Traumatic bladder catheterization Bladder cancer
Headache	Autonomic dysreflexia; may be associated with any noxious stimulus below injury level Consider other causes in absence of increased blood pressure
Increased spasticity	Urine infection Pressure ulcer Bowel impaction Any noxious stimulus Syringomyelia
Pain	Multiple nociceptive and neuropathic causes (see Table 155.3)
Unilateral leg swelling	Osteoporotic fracture of the lower extremity Deep venous thrombosis Heterotopic ossification Cellulitis Hematoma Invasive pelvic cancer
New weakness or numbness	Syringomyelia Entrapment neuropathy (median at wrist, ulnar at elbow)

Table 155.3 International Spinal Cord Injury Pain Classification

Tier 1: Pain Type	Tier 2: Pain Subtype	Tier 3: Primary Pain Source or Pathologic Process
Nociceptive pain	Musculoskeletal pain	Example: glenohumeral arthritis, lateral epicondylitis, femur fracture
	Visceral pain	Example: myocardial infarction, abdominal pain due to bowel impaction, cholecystitis
	Other nociceptive pain	Example: autonomic dysreflexia headache, migraine headache, surgical skin incision
Neuropathic pain	At-level SCI pain	Example: spinal cord compression, nerve root compression
	Below-level SCI pain	Example: spinal cord ischemia, spinal cord compression
	Other neuropathic pain	Example: carpal tunnel syndrome, trigeminal neuralgia, diabetic polyneuropathy
Other pain		Example: fibromyalgia, complex regional pain syndrome type I, irritable bowel syndrome
Unknown pain		

symptoms. Various SCI pain classification systems have been described. The International Spinal Cord Injury Pain classification (Table 155.3) organizes SCI pain into three tiers: tier 1 classifies pain type as nociceptive, neuropathic, other, and unknown; tier 2 includes various subtypes for neuropathic and nociceptive pain; and tier 3 is used to specify the primary pain source or pathologic process [7].

Physical Examination

The neurologic examination is conducted by systematic examination of the dermatomes and myotomes (Tables 155.4 and 155.5) in accordance with the *International Standards for Neurological and Functional Classification of Spinal Cord Injury*, published by the American Spinal Injury Association [1]. Depending on the presentation, specific elements of the physical examination of various body systems that are relevant in evaluation of SCI-related conditions may include the following.

Neurologic

- Determine the level and completeness of the injury (Fig. 155.1). Conduct the examination in the supine position.
    - Sensory examination for pinprick and light touch sensation in key points bilaterally (see Table 155.4)
    - Motor examination for strength in key muscle groups bilaterally (see Table 155.5)
    - Neurologic rectal examination (voluntary anal contraction, deep anal sensation)
- Determine completeness of injury and AIS grade (see Table 155.1). If the AIS grade is A, determine the zone of partial preservation.
- Additional elements of the neurologic examination include
    - Position and deep pressure sensation, testing of additional muscles
    - Muscle tone and spasticity
    - Muscle stretch reflexes, bulbocavernosus reflex, plantar reflex

Respiratory

- Assess respiratory effort, including effect of posture (e.g., sitting versus supine).
- Check for paradoxical respiration and chest expansion.
- Auscultate to assess for decreased breath sounds, rales, and wheeze.

Table 155.4 Key Sensory Points for Cervical Spinal Segments

Level	Key Sensory Point
C2	Occipital protuberance
C3	Supraclavicular fossa
C4	Top of the acromioclavicular joint
C5	Lateral side of the antecubital fossa
C6	Thumb, dorsal surface, proximal phalanx
C7	Middle finger, dorsal surface, proximal phalanx
C8	Little finger, dorsal surface, proximal phalanx
T1	Medial side of antecubital fossa

Table 155.5 Key Muscle Groups for Cervical Myotomes*

Level	Muscle Group	Positions for Testing Key Muscles for Grades 4 and 5
C5	Elbow flexors (biceps, brachialis)	Elbow flexed at 90°, arm at patient's side, forearm supinated
C6	Wrist extensors (extensor carpi radialis longus and brevis)	Wrist in full extension
C7	Elbow extensors (triceps)	Shoulder in neutral rotation, adducted, and in 90° of flexion, with elbow in 45° of flexion
C8	Finger flexors (flexor digitorum profundus) to the middle finger	Full-flexed position of the distal phalanx with the proximal finger joints stabilized in extended position
T1	Small finger abductors (abductor digiti minimi)	Full-abducted position of the fifth digit of the hand

*For those myotomes that are not clinically testable by manual muscle examination (e.g., C1 to C4), the motor level is presumed to be the same as the sensory level.

Cardiac

- Low baseline blood pressure is often a "normal" finding in SCI.
- Look for orthostatic symptoms or excess fall in blood pressure with sitting or upright position.

ASIA AMERICAN SPINAL INJURY ASSOCIATION
INTERNATIONAL STANDARDS FOR NEUROLOGICAL CLASSIFICATION OF SPINAL CORD INJURY (ISNCSCI)
ISCOS INTERNATIONAL SPINAL CORD SOCIETY

Patient Name ______ Date/Time of Exam ______
Examiner Name ______ Signature ______

RIGHT — MOTOR KEY MUSCLES — SENSORY KEY SENSORY POINTS Light Touch (LTR) Pin Prick (PPR)

C2 C3 C4

UER (Upper Extremity Right): Elbow flexors C5; Wrist extensors C6; Elbow extensors C7; Finger flexors C8; Finger abductors (little finger) T1

Comments (Non-key Muscle? Reason for NT? Pain?):

T2 T3 T4 T5 T6 T7 T8 T9 T10 T11 T12 L1

LER (Lower Extremity Right): Hip flexors L2; Knee extensors L3; Ankle dorsiflexors L4; Long toe extensors L5; Ankle plantar flexors S1

S2 S3 S4-5

(VAC) Voluntary anal contraction (Yes/No)

RIGHT TOTALS (MAXIMUM) (50) (56) (56)

SENSORY KEY SENSORY POINTS Light Touch (LTL) Pin Prick (PPL) — MOTOR KEY MUSCLES — LEFT

C2 C3 C4

UEL (Upper Extremity Left): C5 Elbow flexors; C6 Wrist extensors; C7 Elbow extensors; C8 Finger flexors; T1 Finger abductors (little finger)

T2 T3 T4 T5 T6 T7 T8 T9 T10 T11 T12 L1

MOTOR (SCORING ON REVERSE SIDE)
0 = total paralysis
1 = palpable or visible contraction
2 = active movement, gravity eliminated
3 = active movement, against gravity
4 = active movement, against some resistance
5 = active movement, against full resistance
5* = normal corrected for pain/disuse
NT = not testable

SENSORY (SCORING ON REVERSE SIDE)
0 = absent 2 = normal
1 = altered NT = not testable

LEL (Lower Extremity Left): L2 Hip flexors; L3 Knee extensors; L4 Ankle dorsiflexors; L5 Long toe extensors; S1 Ankle plantar flexors

S2 S3 S4-5

(DAP) Deep anal pressure (Yes/No)

LEFT TOTALS (MAXIMUM) (56) (56) (50)

• Key Sensory Points
Palm
Dorsum

MOTOR SUBSCORES
UER ___ + UEL ___ = UEMS TOTAL ___ MAX (25) (25) (50)
LER ___ + LEL ___ = LEMS TOTAL ___ MAX (25) (25) (50)

SENSORY SUBSCORES
LTR ___ + LTL ___ = LT TOTAL ___ MAX (56) (56) (112)
PPR ___ + PPL ___ = PP TOTAL ___ MAX (56) (56) (112)

NEUROLOGICAL LEVELS — Steps 1-5 for classification as on reverse
R L
1. SENSORY
2. MOTOR
3. NEUROLOGICAL LEVEL OF INJURY (NLI)
4. COMPLETE OR INCOMPLETE? Incomplete = Any sensory or motor function in S4-5
5. ASIA IMPAIRMENT SCALE (AIS)
ZONE OF PARTIAL PRESERVATION (In complete injuries only) Most caudal level with any innervation — R L SENSORY MOTOR

This form may be copied freely but should not be altered without permission from the American Spinal Injury Association. REV 02/13

FIGURE 155.1 Standard neurologic classification of spinal cord injury. *(From American Spinal Injury Association. International Standards for Neurologic Classification of Spinal Cord Injury. Chicago, American Spinal Injury Association, 1996.)*

- High blood pressure may indicate autonomic dysreflexia (Table 155.6).
- Examination of peripheral pulses may be especially important for identification of peripheral vascular disease in the absence of claudication and pain symptoms.

Table 155.6 Symptoms and Signs of Autonomic Dysreflexia

Sudden, significant increase in blood pressure
Pounding headache
Flushing of the skin above the level of the SCI, or possibly below
Blurred vision, appearance of spots in the patient's visual fields
Nasal congestion
Profuse sweating above the level of the SCI, or possibly below the level
Piloerection or goose bumps above the level of the SCI, or possibly below
Bradycardia (may be a relative slowing only and still within normal range)
Cardiac arrhythmias
Feelings of apprehension or anxiety
Minimal or no symptoms, despite a significantly elevated blood pressure

Abdomen

- Examine for abdominal distention; examine bowel sounds for evidence of ileus.
- Perform anorectal examination for hemorrhoids and fissures.

Spine

- Identify spinal deformity and tenderness.
- Observe spinal precautions if the examination is being conducted in the acute or postoperative state.

Extremities

- Examine for range of motion, contractures, and swelling.
- Identify nociceptive sources of pain; palpate for tenderness.
- Differentiate effects of SCI (pedal edema, cool extremities) from additional pathologic processes.

Skin

- Examine bone prominences for erythema or skin breakdown.

- Describe any pressure ulcers: location, appearance, size, stage, exudate, odor, necrosis, undermining, sinus tracks; evidence of healing in form of granulation and epithelialization; wound margins and surrounding tissues [8].

Functional Limitations

Tetraplegia is associated with several functional limitations based on the level and completeness of injury [9]. Additional factors, such as age, comorbid conditions, pain, spasticity, body habitus, and psychosocial and environmental factors, can affect function after cervical SCI. A survey of individuals with tetraplegia conducted to rank seven functions in order of importance to their quality of life revealed that the greatest percentage ranked recovery of arm and hand function as their highest priority [10] (Table 155.7).

The Consortium for Spinal Cord Medicine has developed clinical practice guidelines on outcomes after SCI with expected functional outcomes for each level of injury in a number of domains [9,11]. Expected functional outcomes and equipment needs for each level of complete cervical SCI are summarized in Tables 155.8 and 155.9.

Table 155.7 Functional Recovery Priorities of Persons with Cervical Spinal Cord Injury

Area of Functional Recovery	Percentage Surveyed Ranking as the Most Important Item
Arm and hand function	48.7
Sexual function	13.0
Trunk stability	11.5
Bladder and bowel	8.9
Walking movement	7.8
Normal sensation	6.1
Chronic pain	4.0

From Anderson KD. Targeting recovery: priorities of the spinal cord–injured population. J Neurotrauma 2004;21:1371-1383.

Table 155.8 Pattern of Weakness and Functional Outcomes after Cervical Spinal Cord Injury*

Domain	C1-C4	C5	C6	C7-C8
Pattern of upper extremity weakness	Total paralysis of extremities	Absent elbow extension and pronation, all wrist and hand movements	Absent wrist flexion, elbow extension, and hand movement	Limited grasp release and hand dexterity due to intrinsic muscle weakness
Respiratory	Ventilator dependent (some C3, many C4 may be able to be weaned off ventilator)	Low endurance and vital capacity; may require assistance to clear secretions	Low endurance and vital capacity; may require assistance to clear secretions	Low endurance and vital capacity; may require assistance to clear secretions
Bowel management	Total assist	Total assist	Some to total assist	Some to total assist
Bladder management	Total assist	Total assist	Some to total assist with equipment; may be independent with leg bag emptying	Independent to some assist
Bed mobility	Total assist	Some assist	Some assist	Independent to some assist
Bed and wheelchair transfers	Total assist	Total assist	Level transfer: some assist to independent Uneven transfer: some to total assist	Level transfer: independent Uneven transfer: independent to some assist
Pressure relief/ positioning	Total assist; may be independent with equipment	Independent with equipment	Independent with equipment or adapted techniques	Independent
Wheelchair propulsion	Manual: total assist Power: independent with equipment	Power: independent Manual: independent to some assist indoors on non-carpet surface; some to total assist outdoors	Power: independent with standard arm drive on all surfaces Manual: independent indoors; some assist outdoors	Manual: independent on all indoor surfaces and level outdoor terrain; may need some assist or power for uneven terrain or long distances
Eating	Total assist	Total assist for setup, then independent eating with equipment	Independent with or without equipment, except total assist for cutting	Independent
Dressing	Total assist	Some assist for upper extremities; total assist for lower extremities	Independent upper extremities; some to total assist for lower extremities	Independent upper extremities; independent to some assist for lower extremities
Homemaking	Total assist	Total assist	Some assist with light meal preparation; total assist for other homemaking	Independent for light meal preparation and homemaking; some assist with heavy household tasks
Driving	Total assist, attendant-operated van (with lift, tie-downs)	Independent with highly specialized modified van	Independent driving a modified van from wheelchair	Car with hand controls or adapted van from captain's seat

*These outcomes pertain to expected function after motor complete SCI; functional outcomes after incomplete SCI vary on the basis of the extent of motor preservation.

Table 155.9 Equipment Needs after Cervical Spinal Cord Injury

Equipment Category	C1-C4	C5	C6	C7-C8
Respiratory	Ventilator (if not ventilator free) and suction equipment			
Bed	Electric hospital bed, pressure relief mattress	Electric hospital bed, pressure relief mattress	Electric hospital bed or full to king size standard bed, pressure relief mattress or overlay	Electric hospital bed or full to king size standard bed, pressure relief mattress or overlay
Transfers	Power or mechanical lift, transfer board	Power or mechanical lift, transfer board	Mechanical lift, transfer board	Transfer board may be needed
Wheelchair	Power wheelchair with tilt or recline (with postural support and head control devices as needed), vent tray, pressure relief cushion	Power wheelchair with tilt or recline with arm drive control, manual lightweight chair with hand rim modifications, pressure relief cushion	Lightweight manual wheelchair with hand rim modifications, may require power recline or standard upright power wheelchair, pressure relief cushion	Lightweight manual wheelchair with hand rim modifications, pressure relief cushion
Bathing and toileting	Reclining padded shower-commode chair (if roll-in shower available), shampoo tray, hand-held shower	Padded shower-commode chair or padded transfer tub bench with commode cutout, hand-held shower	Padded transfer tub bench with commode cutout or padded shower-commode chair, hand-held shower	Padded transfer tub bench with commode cutout or padded shower-commode chair, hand-held shower
Eating, dressing, and grooming	Total assist; specialized equipment, such as a balanced forearm orthosis, may allow limited feeding ability in those with C4 SCI and minimal (<3/5) strength in deltoid and biceps	Long opponens splint (with pocket for inserting utensils), long-handled mirror, adaptive devices as needed	Short opponens splint, universal cuff, long-handled mirror, adaptive devices as needed	Adaptive devices as needed, long-handled mirror
Communication	Mouthstick, high-tech computer access, environmental control unit	Adaptive devices as needed (e.g., for page turning, writing, button pushing, computer access)	Adaptive devices as needed (e.g., tenodesis splint, writing splint)	Adaptive devices as needed
Transportation	Attendant-operated van (with lift, tie-downs)	Highly specialized modified van with lift	Modified van with lift, tie-downs, hand controls	Modified vehicle

Diagnostic Studies

Spinal Imaging

Radiologic studies are performed to identify and to characterize the site of the pathologic change. Magnetic resonance imaging is especially helpful because of its ability to visualize the soft tissues, including ligamentous structures, intravertebral discs, epidural or subdural hematomas, and hemorrhage or edema in the spinal cord. Magnetic resonance imaging with gadolinium is helpful in diagnosis of post-traumatic syringomyelia.

Electrodiagnostic Testing

Electromyography and nerve conduction studies may be helpful in distinguishing lesions of the peripheral nerves or brachial plexus from those of the spinal cord when patients present with neurologic worsening [12].

Urologic Studies

Urodynamic studies assess neurogenic bladder and sphincter dysfunction. Tests to evaluate upper urinary tracts may be indicated on a periodic basis, but there currently is no uniform consensus on the type or frequency of these tests [4]. Periodic cystoscopy may be indicated in those with chronic indwelling urinary catheters because of increased risk of bladder cancer [13].

Pulmonary Function

Patients who are at high risk for pulmonary complications, such as those with high tetraplegia or with concomitant chronic obstructive airway disease, may require yearly measurements of forced vital capacity and repeated evaluations when new symptoms arise [14]. Chest radiographs will show evidence of pneumonia or atelectasis. Sputum culture and Gram stain will identify the involved pathogens and help guide antibiotic therapy.

Musculoskeletal Imaging

Radiographic evaluation may be needed in case of suspected fracture or to evaluate pain. Heterotopic ossification may be assessed with a bone scan in addition to plain radiographs [12]. If a pressure ulcer appears to involve the bone, magnetic resonance imaging or bone scan may be helpful to evaluate for osteomyelitis [5].

Differential Diagnosis

Cervical spinal stenosis with myelopathy
Spinal infections, abscess
Primary or metastatic tumors
Brainstem disease
Motor neuron disease
Lesions of the brachial plexus
Disorders involving multiple nerves (e.g., polyneuropathy, Guillain-Barré syndrome)

Treatment

Initial

Initial management includes adequate spinal immobilization and prevention of secondary injury. Physiatric consultation and intervention in an acute setting should address range of motion, positioning, bowel and bladder management programs, clearance of respiratory secretions, ventilatory management, consideration of venous thromboembolic prophylaxis, prevention of pressure ulcers, input about functional implications of options for surgery and spinal orthosis, and education of the patient and family [15].

Rehabilitation

Information about potential for motor recovery can be used to set functional goals and to plan for equipment needs (as described in Tables 155.8 and 155.9), keeping in mind that individual factors and coexisting conditions may affect achievable goals [9]. Important elements of rehabilitation include an interdisciplinary approach, establishment of an individualized rehabilitation program with consideration of unique barriers and facilitators, and inclusion of the patient as an active participant in establishment of goals [11]. Specialized equipment needs, based on the level of injury, are summarized in Table 155.9.

In addition to the post-acute rehabilitation that follows the injury, lifelong rehabilitation interventions are often indicated to address changes in neurologic status, new goals, changes in living situation, functional decline associated with medical complications and comorbidities, and aging [16]. Home modifications should be instituted to ensure accessibility [11].

Ongoing Management and Health Maintenance

There is general consensus that comprehensive preventive health evaluations for individuals with SCI are important [4], although uniform agreement about optimal frequency and specific elements is lacking. Because all body systems are potentially affected by cervical SCI, long-term management needs to be comprehensive as summarized here.

Respiratory

Respiratory infections should be promptly identified and treated [17]. Measures such as smoking cessation and pneumonia and annual influenza vaccinations are important for reducing respiratory problems [4]. Manually assisted cough methods can be taught to patients and caregivers. It is important to recognize and to address worsening ventilatory function that may occur with aging or after other complications.

Cardiovascular

Autonomic dysreflexia is a life-threatening emergency, and persons with tetraplegia can be at lifelong risk. Prompt identification and management are critical. The Consortium for Spinal Cord Medicine has published clinical practice guidelines for the acute management of autonomic dysreflexia [6]. If the patient has signs and symptoms of dysreflexia (see Table 155.6), the blood pressure is elevated, and the individual is supine, immediately sit the person up. Loosen any clothing or constrictive devices. Monitor the blood pressure and pulse frequently. Quickly survey for instigating causes, beginning with the urinary system. If an indwelling urinary catheter is not in place, catheterize the individual. Before the catheter is inserted, instill lidocaine jelly (if it is readily available) into the urethra. If the individual has an indwelling urinary catheter, check the system along its entire length for kinks, folds, constrictions, or obstructions and for correct placement of the indwelling catheter. If a problem is found, correct it immediately. Avoid manual compression of or tapping on the bladder. If the catheter is not draining and the blood pressure remains elevated, remove and replace the catheter. If the catheter cannot be replaced, consult a urologist. If acute symptoms of autonomic dysreflexia persist, including a sustained elevated blood pressure, suspect fecal impaction. If the elevated blood pressure is at or above 150 mm Hg systolic, consider pharmacologic management to reduce the systolic blood pressure without causing hypotension before checking for fecal impaction. Use an antihypertensive agent with rapid onset and short duration (e.g., nifedipine bite and swallow, 2% nitroglycerin ointment, or prazosin) while the causes of autonomic dysreflexia are being investigated, and monitor the individual for symptomatic hypotension. If fecal impaction is suspected, check the rectum for stool. If the precipitating cause of autonomic dysreflexia is not yet determined, check for other less frequent causes. Monitor the individual's symptoms and blood pressure for at least 2 hours after resolution of the autonomic dysreflexia episode to make sure that it does not recur. If there is poor response to the treatment specified or if the cause of the dysreflexia has not been identified, strongly consider admitting the individual to the hospital to be monitored, to maintain pharmacologic control of the blood pressure, and to investigate other causes of the dysreflexia. Document the episode in the individual's medical record. Once the individual with SCI has been stabilized, review the precipitating causes with the individual and caregivers and provide education as necessary [6]. Individuals with tetraplegia and their caregivers should be able to recognize and to treat autonomic dysreflexia and be taught to seek emergency treatment if it is not promptly resolved.

Treatment of symptomatic orthostatic hypotension [11] addresses any exacerbating causes (e.g., medications, dehydration, or sepsis). Nonpharmacologic measures include postural challenges, abdominal binder, compression stockings, and increased salt intake. Pharmacologic treatment is administered if it is needed (e.g., with ephedrine, fludrocortisone, or midodrine).

Primary and secondary prevention of cardiovascular disease includes smoking cessation, diet and weight control, lipid management, screening for and treatment of hypertension and glucose intolerance or diabetes, and individualized exercise program [18]. For evaluation of coronary artery disease, a modified or pharmacologic stress test is often needed in these individuals, and if a cardiac rehabilitation program is required, it can be adapted for wheelchair users.

Genitourinary

The goals of bladder management (Table 155.10) are to ensure low pressure and complete voiding, to minimize urinary tract complications, to preserve upper urinary tracts, and to be compatible with the individual's lifestyle [13]. Anticholinergic medications (e.g., oxybutynin, tolterodine) may be indicated for detrusor hyperreflexia and α-adrenergic blockers (prazosin, terazosin, tamsulosin) for detrusor-sphincter dyssynergia. Urinary infections should be identified and treated promptly, but antibiotics are generally not recommended for asymptomatic bacteriuria [5]. There is little role for prophylactic antibiotics, except before urologic procedures.

Counseling and education are key elements of managing sexual dysfunction [19]. Phosphodiesterase type 5 inhibitors (sildenafil, tadalafil, vardenafil) may be used to treat erectile impairment, although care needs to be taken to avoid simultaneous use of nitrate-based medications to treat autonomic dysreflexia, which could result in severe hypotension [4]. Other options include intracavernosal injections, devices, and implants. Advances in electroejaculation and fertility care have increased the fertility success rate for men with SCI. Female fertility is not affected once menses return, which typically occurs within 1 year of injury. Pregnancy and delivery in women with SCI carries risks, including autonomic dysreflexia, and close follow-up is recommended [4,19].

Table 155.10 Nonsurgical Options for Management of the Neurogenic Bladder in Spinal Cord Injury

Bladder Management	Indications
Intermittent catheterization	Often the first choice, if feasible Need sufficient hand skills or willing caregiver Must be willing and able to follow catheterization time schedule
Indwelling catheterization (urethral or suprapubic)	Consider for poor hand skills and lack of caregiver assistance Not able or willing to follow intermittent catheterization schedule High fluid intake Lack of success with less invasive measures Temporary management of vesicoureteral reflux Choose suprapubic with epididymo-orchitis, prostatitis
Credé and Valsalva	Generally avoided in cervical SCI (unless the patient had sphincterotomy)
Reflex voiding	Hand skills or willing caregiver to put on condom catheter, empty leg bag Confirmed small postvoid residual volumes, low voiding pressure Able to maintain condom catheter in place Need to also decrease detrusor-sphincter dyssynergia, if present (e.g., with alpha blocker, botulinum toxin injection, stent, sphincterotomy) Not an option for female patients

Gastrointestinal

The goals of bowel management are to facilitate predictable and effective elimination and to minimize bowel incontinence [20]. A scheduled individualized bowel program should be established, which typically includes reflex stimulation maneuvers, laxatives (stool softeners, stimulants), dietary interventions, and adequate fiber intake. Laxatives and enemas should be kept to a minimum. One should beware of fecal impaction presenting as spurious diarrhea and pay due attention to new bowel symptoms.

Skin

Education of the patient, regular pressure relief practices, and prescription of pressure-reducing support surfaces are vital for prevention of pressure ulcers [8]. Daily comprehensive skin inspections should be carried out by the patient or caregiver, with particular attention to vulnerable insensate areas (e.g., sacrum-coccyx, ischii, trochanters, and heels). Adequate nutritional intake is important. Management of pressure ulcers is discussed further in Chapter 148.

Neurologic

If spasticity is painful or continues to interfere with function after institution of a stretching and positioning program and treatment of any exacerbating factors, medications are often indicated [21]. Table 155.11 lists commonly used medications. Chapter 153 provides additional discussion about spasticity. Selective tightening (e.g., wrist extensors for tenodesis or back extensors for sitting balance) may be important for function in tetraplegia. Neurologic worsening (e.g., due to focal neuropathy, syringomyelia) should be investigated and addressed appropriately [12].

Musculoskeletal

Measures for upper extremity preservation after SCI should be instituted early and followed lifelong. These include optimization of equipment and wheelchair to minimize upper extremity stresses, activity modification to minimize repetitive or excessive upper extremity forces during daily activities and transfers, and individualized exercise program incorporating appropriate flexibility and strengthening components [22].

It is important to recognize and to address contributing factors to pain, which is often multifactorial [7] (see Table 155.3). Pain medications (see Table 155.11) often do not provide complete or optimal relief [21].

Heterotopic ossification is treated with etidronate sodium, nonsteroidals, and occasionally surgical resection, especially if it is interfering with function or comfort [11]. Pathologic fractures should be recognized and treated with padded splints or bivalved circular casts, monitoring of skin integrity, and often only a limited role for surgical treatment [12]. The role for pharmacologic treatment of osteoporosis in SCI is still evolving. Fall prevention (education, wheelchair lap belts) is important to prevent injuries.

Table 155.11 Medications Commonly Used for Spasticity and Pain in Spinal Cord Injury*

Problem	Drug Class	Medication
Spasticity	GABA related	Baclofen Gabapentin
	α_2-Agonist	Tizanidine Clonidine
	Benzodiazepine	Diazepam Clonazepam
	Calcium release inhibitor	Dantrolene
	Local injection	Botulinum toxin Phenol, alcohol
	Intrathecal agents	Baclofen
Pain	Nonopioid analgesic	Acetaminophen Tramadol Nonsteroidal anti-inflammatory drugs, salicylates
	Opioid	Morphine sulfate Oxycodone Hydrocodone Fentanyl (transdermal)
	Anticonvulsant	Gabapentin, pregabalin Carbamazepine Other (phenytoin, valproic acid, lamotrigine)
	Tricyclic antidepressant	Amitriptyline Nortriptyline
	Local anesthetic	Lidocaine patch
	Neuroblocking cream	Capsaicin
	Intrathecal agents	Morphine, clonidine

*The list is not meant to be exhaustive but includes examples of commonly used medications.

Psychosocial

It is important to address environmental barriers (physical and attitudinal), to promote self- efficacy, and to optimize participation and community integration in response to changes in the living situation and social support, functional decline, and aging. Depression should be identified and treated adequately, and substance abuse prevention and treatment programs should be offered [23].

Procedures

Pressure Ulcers

Sharp débridement of pressure ulcers may be done at the bedside to remove necrotic tissue, although if it is extensive, débridement may need to be done in the operating room.

Spasticity

Motor point or nerve blocks with phenol or alcohol may be helpful in treating localized spasticity that interferes with positioning, mobility, or hygiene. Intramuscular injections of botulinum toxin are another option.

Pain

Shoulder pain due to subacromial bursitis may be temporarily responsive to local corticosteroid injections, as is the discomfort from carpal tunnel syndrome [22].

Surgery

Spine Surgery

When cervical spine injury is accompanied by mechanical instability, pain, deformity, or progressive neural impairment, surgical decompression and segmental instrumentation may be indicated for reconstruction of spinal alignment, stability, and early mobilization [12,15].

Pressure Ulcers

Plastic surgery may be indicated for deep pressure ulcers. This includes excision of the ulcer and surrounding scar and muscle and musculocutaneous flap closure [22].

Spasticity

If spasticity is not controlled with maximum dosages of oral medications, or if a patient is unable to tolerate the medications, the placement of an intrathecal baclofen pump may be considered.

Motor Function

Reconstructive surgery of the upper extremity with tendon transfers may improve motor function by one level, typically in those with a neurologic level at C5, C6, or C7. Depending on the level of injury, restoration of wrist extension, elbow extension, and key grip strength or improvement of active grasp and hand control may be an appropriate goal [24].

Functional electrical stimulation has been used in SCI to improve motor function, including upper limb control, standing, and walking, as well as for electrophrenic respiration for ventilator-free breathing [11].

Bladder Dysfunction

Surgical treatment of urolithiasis includes cystoscopic removal of bladder stones, lithotripsy, and percutaneous nephrolithotomy for larger renal stones. Endourethral stents or transurethral sphincterotomy may be considered in individuals with detrusor-sphincter dyssynergia [13]. Electrical stimulation and posterior sacral rhizotomy may be considered for individuals who have problems with catheterization, have good bladder contractions, have no extensive bladder fibrosis, and are willing to lose reflex erections [13]. Bladder augmentation may be indicated for intractable bladder contractions with incontinence and in those at high risk for upper tract deterioration. Urinary diversion may be an appropriate option for unsalvageable bladders secondary to urethral fistula and in individuals with bladder cancer requiring cystectomy [13].

Bowel Dysfunction

Patients with neurogenic bowel who have significant difficulty or complications with typical bowel care may have improved quality of life after colostomy. Careful selection of patients and individualization are required in consideration of this surgery [20].

Upper Extremity Pain

Surgery may occasionally be considered for chronic upper extremity overuse-related symptoms that are unresponsive to medical and rehabilitative treatment (e.g., for carpal tunnel syndrome or rotator cuff disease). Outcomes are often poor if upper extremity overuse continues [22].

Post-traumatic Syringomyelia

Surgical placement of shunts may be indicated for post-traumatic syringomyelia associated with intractable pain or progressive neurologic decline.

Potential Disease Complications

Cervical SCI is associated with multiple complications that can involve every body system.

Respiratory

Respiratory problems include atelectasis, mucous plugs, and pneumonia secondary to impaired cough and retention of secretions; ventilatory failure with high tetraplegia; and sleep disordered breathing [17].

Cardiovascular

Patients with cervical SCI are prone to multiple cardiovascular complications throughout life [18]. Autonomic dysreflexia may occur in SCI above the T6 neurologic level and can be precipitated in response to any noxious stimulus below the level of injury. Symptomatic orthostatic hypotension often resolves after the first few months but may be persistent in some cases. Although venous thromboembolism risk is reduced after the initial months, it can increase even in chronic SCI in the setting of prolonged immobilization associated with medical illness or in the postsurgical state. Cardiovascular fitness is reduced and cardiovascular risk factors can be adversely affected (e.g., reduced high-density lipoprotein cholesterol, increased body fat and insulin resistance, decreased physical activity). Diagnosis of cardiovascular disease may be delayed because of confusing or absent symptoms and signs [18].

Genitourinary

Neurogenic bladder is associated with loss of voluntary control, detrusor-sphincter dyssynergia, and incomplete bladder emptying. Complications include urinary tract infection, bladder and kidney stones, vesicoureteral reflux, and hydronephrosis with renal impairment. Bladder cancer risk is increased with chronic indwelling catheter, especially in smokers [13]. Erectile and ejaculatory dysfunction occurs, and sperm quality may be impaired [4,19].

Gastrointestinal

There is loss of voluntary bowel control, anorectal dyssynergia, and reduced rectal expulsive force [20]. Fecal impaction may occur. Anorectal problems include hemorrhoids, fissures, proctitis, and prolapse. Gallstone risk is increased. Gastroesophageal reflux is common. False-positive results of examination for fecal occult blood may complicate colorectal cancer screening.

Skin

Pressure ulcers are common and may increase with duration of injury. Previous occurrence of a pressure ulcer is an important predictor of future pressure ulcers [8].

Metabolic and Endocrine

Hyponatremia may be a persistent problem in some patients. Carbohydrate and lipid metabolism is affected, and there may be glucose intolerance associated with relative insulin resistance [16]. A reduction in bone mineral density with secondary osteoporosis is common in chronic SCI and affects both the upper and lower extremities in those with tetraplegia.

Neurologic

Neuropathic pain can be persistent and have a negative impact on quality of life. Entrapment neuropathies (median nerve at wrist, ulnar nerve at elbow) and post-traumatic syringomyelia can result in neurologic deterioration [12].

Musculoskeletal

Overuse syndromes include shoulder pain and rotator cuff problems [12,22]. Contractures may occur without due attention to range of motion and positioning. Individuals with C5 level of injury are especially prone to elbow flexion and forearm supination contractures because of unopposed biceps activity. Heterotopic ossification, which is the development of ectopic bone within the soft tissues surrounding peripheral joints, occurs in SCI most commonly around the hip, followed by the knees, elbows, and shoulders [12]. It is further discussed in Chapter 130. Pathologic fractures may occur even with trivial injury because of severe osteoporosis [12].

Psychosocial

SCI can increase the potential for stress, isolation, and depression [23]. Alcohol and substance abuse risk seems to be increased.

Potential Treatment Complications

Spinal pain at the surgical site may result from loosening, infection, or broken hardware. Instability or neurologic deterioration may be due to inadequate spinal immobilization. Surgical shunts can become blocked or infected, and intrathecal pumps or catheters may malfunction.

Complications of urethral catheterization include urethral trauma, erosions, strictures, urinary infections, and epididymitis [13]. Chronic indwelling catheters increase the risk of stones and squamous cell carcinoma of the bladder. Complications may occur with surgical procedures for SCI-related problems, such as neurogenic bladder. For example, transurethral sphincterectomy may be associated with significant intraoperative and perioperative bleeding and erectile and ejaculatory dysfunction. Posterior sacral rhizotomy done in conjunction with electrical stimulation of the bladder may result in loss of reflex erection and ejaculation and reduction of reflex defecation. Urinary diversion procedures may be followed by intestinal or urinary leak, infection, ureteroileal stricture, stomal stenosis, and intestinal obstruction due to adhesions [13].

Because people with SCI are often prescribed multiple medications, drug-related side effects and complications are common. Cervical SCI can result in altered pharmacokinetics [25] in multiple ways (Table 155.12), which further increases unpredictability of side effects.

Table 155.12 Pharmacokinetic Changes in Spinal Cord Injury

SCI-Related Change	Impact on Pharmacokinetics
Delayed gastric emptying	Rapid absorption of acidic drugs Delayed absorption of basic drugs
Reduced gastrointestinal motility	Increased absorption of drugs that undergo enterohepatic circulation Decreased bioavailability of drugs that are destroyed by gut bacteria
Reduced blood flow to skin and muscle	Less reliable transcutaneous, subcutaneous, and intramuscular drug absorption below injury level
Increased percentage of body fat	Effect on fat- and water-soluble drug distribution
Reduced plasma protein level	Increased free fraction of protein-bound drugs
Impaired kidney function	Reduced renal elimination of drugs

References

[1] International standards for neurological and functional classification of spinal cord injury. revised 2011, Atlanta, Ga: American Spinal Injury Association; 2011.

[2] Devivo MJ. Epidemiology of traumatic spinal cord injury: trends and future implications. Spinal Cord 2012;50:365–72.

[3] National Spinal Cord Injury Statistical Center. Spinal cord injury: facts and figures at a glance. J Spinal Cord Med 2012;35:197–8.

[4] Chiodo AE, Scelza WM, Kirshblum SC, et al. Spinal cord injury medicine. 5. Long-term medical issues and health maintenance. Arch Phys Med Rehabil 2007;88(Suppl. 1):S76–83.

[5] Till M, Pertel P. Infections. In: Green D, editor. Medical management of long-term disability. Boston: Butterworth-Heinemann; 1996. p. 233–62.

[6] Consortium for Spinal Cord Medicine. Acute management of autonomic dysreflexia: individuals with spinal cord injury presenting to health care facilities. In: 2nd ed. Washington, DC: Paralyzed Veterans of America; 2001. Available at: www.pva.org.

[7] Bryce TN, Biering-Sørensen F, Finnerup NB, et al. International spinal cord injury pain classification: part I. Background and description. March 6-7, 2009, Spinal Cord 2012;50:413–7.

[8] Consortium for Spinal Cord Medicine. Pressure ulcer prevention and treatment following spinal cord injury. Clinical practice guidelines for health care professionals. In: Washington, DC: Paralyzed Veterans of America; 2000. Available at: www.pva.org.

[9] Consortium for Spinal Cord Medicine. Outcomes following traumatic spinal cord injury. Clinical practice guidelines for health care professionals. Washington, DC: Paralyzed Veterans of America; 1999. Available at: www.pva.org.

[10] Anderson KD. Targeting recovery: priorities of the spinal cord–injured population. J Neurotrauma 2004;21:1371–83.

[11] Kirshblum SC, Priebe MM, Ho CH, et al. Spinal cord injury medicine. 3. Rehabilitation phase after acute spinal cord injury. Arch Phys Med Rehabil 2007;88(Suppl. 1):S62–9.

[12] Scelza WM, Dyson-Hudson TA. Neuromusculoskeletal complications of spinal cord injury. In: Kirshblum SC, Campagnolo D, editors. Spinal cord medicine. 2nd ed. Philadelphia: Lippincott Williams & Wilkins; 2011. p. 282–308.

[13] Consortium for Spinal Cord Medicine. Bladder management for adults with spinal cord injury. Clinical practice guidelines for health care professionals. Washington, DC: Paralyzed Veterans of America; 2006. Available at: www.pva.org.

[14] Consortium for Spinal Cord Medicine. Respiratory management following spinal cord injury. Clinical practice guidelines for health care professionals. Washington, DC: Paralyzed Veterans of America; 2005. Available at: www.pva.org.

[15] Wuermser LA, Ho CH, Chiodo AE, et al. Spinal cord injury medicine. 2. Acute care management of traumatic and nontraumatic injury. Arch Phys Med Rehabil 2007;88(Suppl. 1):S55–9.

[16] Bauman WA, Spungen AM, Adkins RH, Kemp BJ. Metabolic and endocrine changes in persons aging with spinal cord injury. Assist Technol 2001;11:88–96.

[17] Lanig IS, Peterson WP. The respiratory system in spinal cord injury. Phys Med Rehabil Clin N Am 2000;11:29–43.

[18] Sabharwal S. Cardiovascular dysfunction in spinal cord disorders. In: Lin VW, editor. Spinal cord medicine: principles and practice. 2nd ed. New York: Demos; 2010. p. 241–55.

[19] Consortium for Spinal Cord Medicine. Sexuality and reproductive health in adults with spinal cord injury. Clinical practice guidelines for health care professionals. Washington, DC: Paralyzed Veterans of America; 2010. Available at: www.pva.org.

[20] Consortium for Spinal Cord Medicine. Neurogenic bowel management in adults with spinal cord injury. Clinical practice guidelines for health care professionals. Washington, DC: Paralyzed Veterans of America; 1998. Available at: www.pva.org.

[21] Burchiel KJ, Hsu FP. Pain and spasticity after spinal cord injury: mechanism and treatment. Spine 2001;26(Suppl.):S146–60.

[22] Consortium for Spinal Cord Medicine. Preservation of upper limb function following spinal cord injury. Clinical practice guidelines for health care professionals. Washington, DC: Paralyzed Veterans of America; 2005. Available at: www.pva.org.

[23] Consortium for Spinal Cord Medicine. Depression following spinal cord injury. Clinical practice guidelines for health care professionals. Washington, DC: Paralyzed Veterans of America; 1998. Available at: www.pva.org.

[24] Kirshblum S. New rehabilitation interventions in spinal cord injury. J Spinal Cord Med 2004;27:342–50.

[25] Mestre H, Alkon T, Salazar S, Ibarra A. Spinal cord injury sequelae alter drug pharmacokinetics: an overview. Spinal Cord 2011;49:955–60.

CHAPTER 156

Spinal Cord Injury (Thoracic)

Jesse D. Ennis, MD, FRCP(C)
Jane Wierbicky, RN, BSN
Shanker Nesathurai, MD, MPH, FRCP(C)

Synonym

Paraplegia

ICD-9 Code

344.1 Paraplegia

ICD-10 Codes

G82.20 Paraplegia of both lower limbs, unspecified
G82.21 Paraplegia of both lower limbs, complete
G82.22 Paraplegia of both lower limbs, incomplete

Definition

Spinal cord injury (SCI) is a common cause of paralysis, particularly in young men (Table 156.1). Just more than one third of all injuries to the spinal cord occur at the thoracic level, most commonly at T12 [1]. With thoracic SCI, 68% of patients will have complete injury, 8% will have a sensory incomplete injury, and 23% will have a motor incomplete injury. Mean age at the time of injury has increased over time: from 2005 to 2011, the mean age was 41 years, compared with 28.7 years from 1973 to 1979. Overall, there is still higher representation of males with SCI, with 80.6% of patients being male and 19.6% being female [1]. Compromise to the thoracic spinal cord typically results in paraplegia. Unlike paraplegia that results from compromise of the cauda equina associated with lumbar spine injuries, the clinical findings are consistent with upper motor neuron injury. However, lower limb paralysis is not the only impairment. The thoracic spinal cord also segmentally innervates the intercostal muscles as well as the upper and lower abdominal muscles. The intercostal muscles are innervated by the T1 to T12 spinal segments. The upper abdominal muscles are innervated by the T8 to T10 spinal segments; the T11 to T12 spinal segments innervate the lower abdominal muscles [2].

A quantitative three-dimensional anatomy of the thoracic spine reveals three distinct zones: the cervical-thoracic transition zone, the middle region, and the thoracic-lumbar transition zone [3,4]. The T1-T4 region is characterized by a narrowing of the vertebral end plate and spinal canal widths [3]. The middle thoracic region (T4-T9) is notable for its relatively narrow end plate and small spinal canal. The rib articulations provide an increased degree of protection at this level. An enlargement of the spinal canal characterizes the lower thoracic region (T10-T12) [3]. There is also less rigidity of the spine at the T11 and T12 segments because of the lack of ventral attachment of the ribs [3]. Therefore there is an increased vulnerability to SCI at the lower thoracic levels. Compared with the cervical and lumbar spinal levels, the blood supply is more tenuous in the thoracic spinal cord, and therefore ischemia poses a greater threat to neurologic function in this area [4].

Symptoms

The presenting symptoms of thoracic SCI are consistent with the alteration to the motor, sensory, and autonomic pathways. The chief symptoms are weakness or paralysis of the abdominal and lower extremity musculature and loss of sensation in the lower limbs, thorax, and perineum. Patients may also experience altered bowel or bladder function in addition to spasticity and sexual dysfunction.

With lesions above the T6 level, patients may experience the symptoms of autonomic dysreflexia. Autonomic dysreflexia is characterized by pounding headaches, nasal congestion, anxiety, visual disturbances, pallor below the level of injury, and sweating and flushing above the level of injury. In patients with an old, stable injury who are experiencing new or progressive symptoms (e.g., increasing weakness, loss of sensation), the clinician should consider the possibility of a syrinx.

Patients with SCI are often insensate to the pain that accompanies deep venous thrombosis, and therefore both the

Table 156.1 Demographic Comparison of Gunshot Spinal Cord Injury with Nonviolent Spinal Cord Trauma

	Gunshot SCI (%)	Nonviolent Traumatic SCI (%)
Gender		
Male	95.1	79.7
Female	4.9	20.3
Ethnicity		
White	9.8	51.5
Nonwhite	91.2	48.5
Marital status		
Never married	70.7	38.9
Married	19.5	44.3
Not married	9.8	16.8
Employment status		
Employed	41.5	75.4
Unemployed	58.5	24.5
Mean age	27.1	42.2

Modified from McKinley WO, Johns JS, Musgrove JJ. Clinical presentations, medical complications, and functional outcomes of individuals with gunshot wound–induced spinal cord injury. Am J Phys Med Rehabil 1999;78:102-107.

clinician and the patient should be attentive to clinical signs such as edema, erythema, and increased tone. Heterotopic ossification may mimic deep venous thrombosis because the symptoms include swelling, decreased range of motion, erythema, increased spasticity, pain, and low-grade fever.

Pain originating from either musculoskeletal or neurologic sources is common. Neuropathic pain resulting from central or peripheral nervous disruption may be described as burning or shooting. An analysis of several studies addressing prevalence of pain after SCI showed a variable overall prevalence of pain ranging from as low as 26% to as high as 96% [5].

Physical Examination

The diagnosis of a thoracic-level SCI necessitates a thorough physical examination, including a comprehensive neurologic assessment. Findings on physical examination include a motor and sensory level. Depending on whether the injury is partial or complete, there may be sparing of sacral sensation or anal sphincter motor function below the neurologic level of injury. In the acute period, the motor examination is characterized by loss of muscle tone and deep tendon reflexes. During subsequent days and weeks, there is emergence of increased muscle tone, reflexes, and pathologic reflexes. Cutaneous reflexes including the plantar response, cremasteric reflex, and bulbocavernosus reflex are initially depressed and follow a variable course to gradual return. The initial evaluation of the patient also includes the assessment of vital signs and the cardiovascular, respiratory, musculoskeletal, gastrointestinal, and genitourinary systems. A thorough examination of the skin is necessary. In thoracic SCI, pressure ulcers are more common over bone prominences such as the sacrum, calcaneus, and greater trochanter. In addition, it is important to evaluate the patient for spasticity and contractures.

New neurologic abnormalities on physical examination should alert the clinician to consider imaging studies to exclude syringomyelia. In this case, typical physical examination findings include change in sensory level, change in motor level, and reflex abnormality as well as spasticity.

Functional Limitations

Persons who suffer from thoracic SCI can have significantly different levels of disability, depending on their degree of paralysis and associated potential complications (e.g., contractures, spasticity). A patient with high thoracic paraplegia (i.e., T2 level) typically has some component of truncal instability; as a result, the patient's wheelchair requires a high back. In contrast, a person with low thoracic paraplegia generally has preservation of most of the intercostal and abdominal muscles and could opt for a chair with a low back. Intercostal muscle impairment in patients with SCI in the upper thoracic region may cause an impaired cough and a decreased ability to mobilize secretions.

Functional goals for individuals with thoracic SCI include the ability to complete activities of daily living and instrumental activities of daily living with or without the use of assistive equipment. Tasiemski and colleagues [6] have described a positive association of involvement in sports and recreational activities with increased life satisfaction in a community sample of people with SCI. Numerous sports and recreational organizations offer adaptive sports programs for people with disabilities.

Bowel and bladder function may cause social embarrassment, leading to self-imposed social isolation. Sexual dysfunction may result in a loss of intimacy. The availability of partners is a concern for many patients because their disability as well as environmental and social barriers may preclude their involvement in some of the more typical dating activities.

Depression is common in patients with SCI; reported rates of depression in the newly injured range between 20% and 44% [7]. The most recent large-scale retrospective study of veterans with SCI showed a depression rate of 22% [8]. Depression has been associated with an increase in secondary complications and poor compliance with self-care activities [7]. Referral to mental health professionals is encouraged for patients at risk.

Diagnostic Studies

The diagnosis of thoracic SCI is often corroborated with magnetic resonance imaging. The stability of the injury is assessed by evaluation of the anterior, middle, and posterior columns of the spine. Magnetic resonance imaging is also the study of choice when syringomyelia is suspected.

Urodynamic testing is commonly used to evaluate bladder function in the individual with SCI. Urodynamic studies involve filling of the bladder with fluid or gas and use of electromyographic and fluoroscopic techniques to evaluate voiding function. Annual evaluations often include an ultrasound examination to further assess the integrity of the renal system.

Patients with grade IV pressure ulcers may require a bone scan or magnetic resonance imaging study to detect osteomyelitis. The triple-phase bone scan is also used in the diagnosis of heterotopic ossification (see Chapter 130). Doppler surveillance studies are sometimes performed to detect deep venous thrombosis in this highly susceptible population (see Chapter 127). Routine colonoscopy and fecal occult blood testing may be appropriate for patients 50 years and older [9]. In patients susceptible to autonomic dysreflexia, appropriate precautions must be used during colonoscopy.

Differential Diagnosis

Amyotrophic lateral sclerosis
Post-traumatic syringomyelia
Guillain-Barré syndrome
Spinal cord infarction
Ischemic injury to spinal cord (i.e., secondary to abdominal and thoracic aneurysms)
Multiple sclerosis
Transverse myelitis

Treatment

Initial

Skin Management

In an analysis of long-term medical complications among subjects enrolled in the National Spinal Cord Injury Statistical Center database, pressure ulcers were the most commonly reported postinjury complication. McKinley and colleagues [10] reported a 15.2% incidence of pressure ulcers in the first annual follow-up postinjury year. The rates increased steadily during all follow-up years in both complete and incomplete SCIs. Common sites for pressure ulcers are the sacrum, greater trochanter, and heels. Excessive pressure, shearing, friction, and maceration can increase the risk for pressure ulcers. Other risk factors include spasticity, impaired sensation, immobility, poor nutrition, weight gain, and incontinence [11].

The maintenance of skin integrity is an ever-present goal in patients with SCI. Pressure ulcer formation will lead to the development of scar tissue and an even greater likelihood of ulcer recurrence. Seating surfaces should be reevaluated on a regular basis, ensuring that they have not worn out and still fit the patient's weight and size. Patients are encouraged to perform daily skin examinations, and most paraplegic patients are able to independently perform pressure-relieving strategies, such as wheelchair pushups. These techniques should be performed every 15 minutes to minimize excessive pressure.

Patients who have a pressure ulcer must minimize pressure to that area until the wound is healed. A variety of débridement methods are available for removal of necrotic debris from pressure ulcers (see Chapter 148).

Pain

The presentation of pain among the SCI population can be varied in nature; both neuropathic pain and pain resulting from abnormal mechanical stresses (e.g., tendinitis) are common. Many times, patients with musculoskeletal pain have a well-defined disorder that is amenable to standard physiatric treatment (e.g., rotator cuff tendinitis, lateral epicondylitis). Non-narcotic analgesics and nonsteroidal anti-inflammatory drugs can be used to treat musculoskeletal causes of pain. Neuropathic pain generally is not responsive to these medications; however, tricyclic antidepressants, antiseizure medications, and pregabalin have been effective in its treatment but should be prescribed with caution [12].

Bladder Management

Most patients with thoracic-level SCI will have upper motor neuron bladder dysfunction, characterized by low urinary volumes, high bladder pressures, bladder trabeculation, and diminished bladder compliance. Detrusor-sphincter dyssynergia (co-contraction of the bladder and sphincter) is common. This can contribute to vesicoureteral reflux, which may result in hydronephrosis and subsequent chronic renal failure. Detrusor-sphincter dyssynergia can be treated with medical interventions that decrease bladder tone (e.g., oxybutynin) or, alternatively, decrease sphincter tone (e.g., terazosin, tamsulosin, or sphincter chemodenervation) [13,14] (see Chapter 137).

Bladder management strategies should be individualized, but intermittent catheterization is the preferred treatment option. A typical intermittent catheterization program requires bladder emptying four to six times per day, with volumes remaining less than 500 mL. Most paraplegic patients have the manual dexterity to perform self-catheterization; some individuals, because of biologic or sociomedical factors, must use indwelling catheters (with suprapubic preferred to urethral). Indwelling catheters are associated with a higher incidence of bladder stones and bladder carcinoma [15]. In addition, in men, urethral catheters are associated with prostatitis, epididymitis, and urethral strictures. Long-term use of urethral catheters in women may result in urethral dilation.

Bowel Management

The patient with thoracic-level injuries will most likely have constipation; therefore a bowel program is necessary. A reasonable goal for a bowel regimen is to achieve socially acceptable fecal continence, with bowel evacuations at least three times per week. A bowel regimen may include medications (Table 156.2). In addition, bowel evacuation is scheduled after a meal to capitalize on the intrinsic increase in peristalsis after meals (i.e., the gastrocolic reflex). Bowel care programs done on a raised toilet seat use the benefits of gravity. Digital stimulation (gentle insertion of the finger) of the rectum or insertion of a suppository can activate the rectocolic reflex by stimulating peristalsis and promoting regular bowel movements. Enemas (Fleet, soapsuds) should not be part of a regular bowel program. However, these agents are useful in emptying the colon before initiation of a bowel program or treatment of fecal obstipation [9]. The administration of an enema can precipitate autonomic dysreflexia in susceptible patients. If administration of an oral osmotic laxative is required, consideration should be given to polyethylene glycol 3350 (PEG 3350) over the traditional use of lactulose. This is supported by a recent Cochrane review that demonstrated greater efficacy and less abdominal pain compared with lactulose for all-cause chronic constipation [16] (see Chapter 138).

Mental Health

Psychosocial adaptation subsequent to SCI is a lifelong process. There is no single "classic" presentation of this

Table 156.2 Oral Adjunctive Bowel Medications [9,16]

Medication	Brand	Mechanism of Action	Strength	Dose
Docusate sodium	Colace	Stool softener	100 mg (capsules)	1 tablet bid
Senna	Senokot	Colonic stimulant	8.6 mg (tablets)	1-2 tablets qhs
Bisacodyl	Dulcolax	Colonic irritant	5 mg (tablets)	2 tablets qd
Polyethylene glycol (PEG 3350)	Lax-A-Day, MiraLax	Osmotic laxative	17 g (powder)	17 g daily (dissolved in liquid)
Psyllium powder	Smooth Texture Sugar-Free Unflavored Metamucil	Bulk-forming agent	5.4 g per tsp	1 tsp qd-tid
Metoclopramide	Reglan	Prokinetic agent	10 mg (tablets)	1 tablet qid

Modified from Bergman S. Bowel Management. In Nesathurai S, ed. The Rehabilitation of People with Spinal Cord Injury, 3rd ed. Arbuckle Academic Publishers, 2013.

phenomenon. Anger, hostility, anxiety, and depression often result from overwhelming losses confronting this population. Suicide is among the leading causes of death in these patients. In individuals with depression or other psychological sequelae, consultation with an appropriate mental health care professional is recommended. Continued follow-up is encouraged, when appropriate.

Sexual and Reproductive Function

Sexual desire is not necessarily affected by SCI. However, associated depression, fears of inadequacy, and poor body image may consequently alter sexual desire. Sexual function (e.g., erection and ejaculation in men and lubrication in women) in patients with thoracic-level injuries may be altered. In general, patients with more complete lesions have more impairment. Men with thoracic-level lesions (with intact sacral reflexes) generally can achieve reflex erections with direct genital stimulation. However, many times, these reflex erections are of insufficient rigidity and duration for satisfactory vaginal penetration [17].

Many patients with SCI have numerous questions and fears about sexuality and sexual function. Treatment should address concerns related to body image, dating, and initiation and maintenance of intimate relationships. Peer counselors can share their experiences, and their advice can be beneficial. Peer counselors may be located through local independent living centers or through advocacy organizations such as the National Spinal Cord Injury Association or Canadian Paraplegia Association. In addition, mental health professionals (e.g., psychologists, psychiatrists, social workers) can be a valuable resource to the patient and rehabilitation team.

Several options available to men with erectile dysfunction include oral medications (e.g., sildenafil [18–24], tadalafil [18,24–26], vardenafil [24]), vacuum devices, penile injection programs (papaverine) [27], and surgically implanted prostheses. Ejaculatory dysfunction is also common, including retrograde ejaculation into the bladder [28]. Chronic SCI is also associated with poor semen quality and decreased spermatogenesis [29]. Elevated scrotal temperatures (from chronic sitting) and frequent urinary tract infections may negatively affect semen quality. Although studies have indicated that approximately 12% to 15% of men with SCI report ejaculation, fatherhood has become a possibility with use of semen retrieval methods such as penile vibrostimulation and electroejaculation along with improved assisted reproductive technology [30]. The risk of autonomic dysreflexia exists among susceptible patients with an injury level of T6 and above; therefore, assisted semen retrieval should be initiated by medical teams well trained in semen retrieval methods and the treatment of autonomic dysreflexia [31].

Women with thoracic-level lesions may note changes in vaginal lubrication. However, at this level, women may achieve reflex lubrication [32]. Direct stimulation of the genital region may result in sufficient lubrication. A water-soluble lubricant is recommended for patients with complaints of decreased vaginal lubrication. One randomized placebo-controlled study on the use of sildenafil to enhance sexual arousal in women with SCI failed to show a statistically significant benefit [33], despite an earlier pilot study that appeared to show benefit [34].

Orgasm for both men and women after injury may be nonexistent or described as a primarily emotional event or a pleasurable sensation in the pelvic region or sensory level with generalized muscle relaxation [32].

Women with thoracic-level SCI remain fertile. Contraceptive options include barrier methods (condoms, diaphragm) and oral contraceptives. Intrauterine contraceptive devices are contraindicated because of the lack of sensation and the risk for development of pelvic inflammatory disease. Patients with SCI are at increased risk for the development of thromboembolism, and the administration of oral contraceptives further increases this risk and should be discussed.

The care of pregnant women with SCI has special challenges. Potential complications include premature labor, increased risk of urinary tract infection, increased spasticity, autonomic dysreflexia, and constipation. In pregnancy, autonomic dysreflexia is manifested most frequently during labor; therefore hemodynamic monitoring is considered for all at-risk patients [35].

Pregnant women with thoracic SCI levels above T10 may be unable to sense fetal movements and contractions. Therefore, uterine palpation, serial cervical examinations, and fetal monitoring may be recommended. Regional anesthesia is preferred [36].

Deep Venous Thrombosis

SCI predisposes individuals to both deep venous thrombosis and pulmonary embolism. A systematic literature review revealed the prevalence of deep venous thrombosis in SCI to vary from 9% to 100% [37]. Of these, it is estimated that only 20% will extend into proximal veins, with associated elevated risk of pulmonary embolism. The rate of pulmonary embolism has been found to be 8% to 14% in acute SCI, with rates of fatal pulmonary embolism as high as 5% [37]. Putative mechanisms include immobility as a result of paralysis and failure of the venous-muscle pump as well as the possible contribution of a generalized hypercoagulable state.

Patients are administered fractionated or unfractionated heparin during the initial weeks after injury and may use thigh-high compression stockings and pneumatic compression. Current literature suggests continuation for 8 to 12 weeks after injury. For more details on the prevention and treatment of deep venous thrombosis, see Chapter 127.

Spasticity Management

Spasticity should be treated when it results in significant pain, contributes to contractures, impairs hygiene, interferes with functional tasks, or impedes nursing care. In the first instance, clinically significant spasticity should be treated by removal of noxious stimuli that may be contributing to the condition, such as urinary tract infection, ingrown toenails, and tight clothing. Second, physical interventions such as daily stretching of muscles with terminal sustained stretch can be considered. If these are unsuccessful, medications such as tizanidine and baclofen as well as interventional procedures (e.g., chemodenervation) can be considered (see Chapter 153 for details).

Heterotopic Ossification

Heterotopic ossification is most often seen in the first 6 months after injury in the spinal cord–injured population, especially in the first 2 months [38,39]. The incidence of heterotopic ossification among individuals with SCI ranges from 10% to 53% [39]. It is estimated that 20% to 30% of those with heterotopic ossification will experience a significant loss of joint mobility [38]. Treatment may include the administration of etidronate, which limits ossification, and physical therapy to maintain range of motion (see Chapter 130).

Osteoporosis

Osteoporosis among patients with SCI is common. Immobilization and the lack of weight-loading activities are among the chief causes of osteoporosis. Other factors may include alterations in blood circulation, lack of muscle traction on bone, and hormonal changes [40]. The loss of bone density develops in the acute stage of injury, with demineralization occurring below the level of injury [41]. Patients with SCI are at significant risk for long bone fracture, and care must be taken to prevent fractures resulting from range of motion exercises and falls. There is evidence from several studies that bisphosphonates may slow or stop the loss of bone density after SCI, but guidelines as to their use have not yet been developed [40]. In the absence of clear guidelines, investigation, treatment, and monitoring for osteoporosis in SCI patients remains somewhat empirical. Supplementation with vitamin D is often recommended, although calcium supplementation remains controversial because of the associated risk of urinary calculi [12] (see Chapter 140 for further details).

Autonomic Dysreflexia

For the treatment of autonomic dysreflexia, it is necessary to remove the precipitating noxious stimulus. Patients should be placed in an upright position, if possible, to decrease blood pressure, and a search for a causative agent is initiated. Most cases of autonomic dysreflexia are related to bladder distention or bowel distention [42]. However, noxious stimuli such as ingrown toenails, pressure ulcer, and renal calculi are not uncommon. Vasodilating medications such as nitropaste may be required to decrease the blood pressure while the clinician seeks the causative factor [43]. Nitrates are contraindicated in individuals who have ingested cyclic guanosine monophosphate–specific phosphodiesterase type 5 inhibitors, such as sildenafil, as the nitrates can potentiate the hypotensive effects of sildenafil and cause severe hypotension [37].

Rehabilitation

A comprehensive rehabilitation program is essential to optimize functional independence. The program should address functional goals related to mobility, transfers, and self-care as well as issues related to health maintenance and self-advocacy. Depending on the outstanding treatment goals, the treatment team may include a physical therapist, occupational therapist, orthotist, nurse, and mental health provider.

Mobility is a major issue that needs to be addressed both initially and then periodically as the patient's condition changes (e.g., women who become pregnant may require assistance with functional activities as the pregnancy progresses). Typically, patients with thoracic SCI are able to achieve mobility with a manual wheelchair. Higher levels of thoracic SCI are associated with greater truncal instability. This may affect stability in a wheelchair and should be addressed with the seating prescription. Most patients with thoracic injuries, with training, are able to transfer independently.

For assistance with independence in self-care, adaptive equipment, such as long-handled shoehorns and reachers, can be recommended. Home environmental modifications may also be necessary (i.e., ramp to enter home). Patients with thoracic SCI should be able to drive a modified car or van.

Passive interventions, such as therapeutic heat and cold as well as transcutaneous electrical nerve stimulation, may be beneficial in the management of pain. However, particular caution must be used with therapeutic heat or cold modalities over insensate areas.

As well, with higher levels of injury, there is increasing loss of intercostal muscle innervation and increased level of respiratory impairment. Techniques including incentive spirometry, manual assisted cough, and insufflation-exsufflation can be used to reduce pulmonary complications of thoracic SCI.

Physical interventions, such as daily stretching of muscles with terminal sustained stretch, can be considered a first-line rehabilitative treatment for spasticity. Positioning as well as serial casting and splinting of the affected limbs can minimize spasticity.

Other rehabilitation treatments may also be considered. Functional electrical stimulation may improve muscle strength, decrease muscle atrophy, and improve lower limb endurance [44]. Body weight–supported treadmill training is prescribed in many centers. This intervention has been shown to be as effective as traditional gait training practices in the first year after injury with regard to functional outcomes [44]. The use of lower limb bracing may be an option in individuals with thoracic SCI, predominantly in those with lower thoracic level.

Procedures

A number of procedures can be used to address issues such as spasticity and pain. Interventional approaches for the treatment of spasticity include botulinum toxin injection, motor branch blocks, and peripheral nerve blocks (see Chapter 153). To decrease sphincter tone in men, botulinum toxin can be injected into the sphincter. This treatment in women is associated with an unacceptably high incidence of urinary incontinence. A patient with dysreflexia caused by a bladder stone may require a urologic procedure for stone removal. For men with ejaculatory dysfunction, retrieval of sperm for insemination has been successfully accomplished by electroejaculation and vibrostimulation methods. These procedures may result in dysreflexia and are performed under medical supervision.

Surgery

Pressure ulcers that do not heal with conservative methods may require surgical closure. Direct closure, skin grafts, musculocutaneous flaps, and skin flaps are among the surgical treatments available for wound closure. Mobilization after surgical closure must be done under close supervision, with careful monitoring of the surgical wound.

A variety of surgical procedures are used in patients who cannot be satisfactorily maintained with an intermittent catheterization program. Sphincter tone can be reduced with a sphincterotomy for men. Men must wear external collection devices after this procedure because it results in continuous incontinence. Sphincterotomies may occasionally require revision because of the development of fibrosis that obstructs outflow. Sphincterotomies may result in erectile dysfunction in some men. In contemporary practice, sphincterotomies are performed less frequently.

Bladder augmentation is occasionally performed to increase bladder capacity. A piece of small bowel is interposed with the bladder tissue to increase vesical volume. Patients with chronic dysreflexia resulting from persistent bowel management difficulties, such as frequent impaction, may be candidates for ileostomy or colostomy procedures. Patients with hemorrhoids aggravated by digital stimulation occasionally require surgical consultation if the hemorrhoids are not relieved by more conservative methods (e.g., medicated suppositories or topical steroid creams).

On occasion, men with erectile dysfunction that is not amenable to less invasive therapies may opt for an implantable penile prosthesis. Again, with the introduction of medications to treat erectile dysfunction, these surgeries are less frequently performed. Surgical placement of an intrathecal morphine or baclofen pump may be beneficial for patients with severe pain or spasticity that is not responsive to noninvasive treatments. Surgical interventions are indicated in some cases of heterotopic ossification. Patients with functionally limited joint mobility or severe and chronic spasticity may benefit from surgical resection of the lesion.

Potential Disease Complications

Individuals with thoracic-level SCI are more likely to have associated injuries that are serious than are those with cervical or lumbosacral spinal cord lesions. In one study, patients with traumatic thoracic spine fractures had an 86.2% occurrence of additional traumatic injury, such as rib fractures (42.1%), pulmonary contusions (37.5%), pneumothorax or hemothorax (34.9%), cervical spine injury (31%), lumbar spine injuries (28.4%), clavicular fractures (11.9%), sternal fractures (10.7%), and scapular fractures (10.3%) [45]. Thoracic SCI may be associated with a lower life expectancy. The leading causes of death among people with SCI in the national Spinal Cord Injury Model Systems database are respiratory, infectious, and cardiovascular diseases [1]. Complications arising from a thoracic-level injury result from immobility, changing sensory patterns, and alterations in autonomic nervous system function.

Potential Treatment Complications

The anticholinergic side effects of tricyclic antidepressants, including dry mouth, blurred vision, and urinary retention, can pose additional difficulties for the patient with SCI. Sphincterotomies, performed to alleviate detrusor-sphincter dyssynergia, may result in urinary incontinence and occasionally sexual dysfunction in men. Voiding by the Credé maneuver may lead to vesicoureteral reflux. The long-term use of indwelling catheters is associated with prostatitis, epididymitis, strictures, bladder stones, and bladder carcinoma.

Digital stimulation of the bowel can result in autonomic dysreflexia and hemorrhoids.

Medications used to treat autonomic dysreflexia can result in hypotension. The blood pressure must be closely monitored.

When the less invasive methods of treating spasticity are ineffective, more interventional approaches to spasticity, including chemodenervation with botulinum toxin or neurolysis with phenol injections, motor branch blocks, peripheral nerve blocks, and intrathecal baclofen pump insertion, may be considered. Injections may result in bleeding or infection. Nerve blocks may result in dysesthesias and weakness. Patients with intrathecal baclofen pumps may experience drowsiness, weakness, catheter breakage, or infection.

References

[1] 2011 Annual statistical report for the spinal cord injury model systems. Birmingham, Ala: National Spinal Cord Injury Statistical Center; 2011.

[2] Nesathurai S. Functional outcomes by level of injury. In: Nesathurai S, editor. The rehabilitation of people with spinal cord injury, 3rd ed. Arbuckle Academic Publishers; 2013. p. 37–9.

[3] Panjabi MM, Takata K, Goel V, et al. Thoracic human vertebrae. Quantitative three-dimensional anatomy. Spine 1991;16:888–901.

[4] Yashon D. Spinal injury. New York: Appleton-Century-Crofts; 1978, 98.

[5] Dijkers M, Bryce T, Zanca J. Prevalence of chronic pain after traumatic spinal cord injury: a systematic review. J Rehabil Res Dev 2009;46:13–29.

[6] Tasiemski T, Kennedy P, Gardner BP, Taylor N. The association of sports and physical recreation with life satisfaction in a community sample of people with spinal cord injuries. NeuroRehabilitation 2005;20:253–65.
[7] Dryden DM, Saunders LD, Rowe BH, et al. Depression following traumatic spinal cord injury. Neuroepidemiology 2005;25:55–61.
[8] Smith BM, Weaver FM, Ullrich PM. Prevalence of depression diagnoses and use of antidepressant medications by veterans with spinal cord injury. Am J Phys Med Rehabil 2007;86:662–71.
[9] Bergman S. Bowel management. In: Nesathurai S, editor. The rehabilitation of people with spinal cord injury, 3rd ed. Arbuckle Academic Publishers; 2013. p. 59–64.
[10] McKinley WO, Jackson AB, Cardenas DD, DeVivo MJ. Long-term medical complications after traumatic spinal cord injury: a regional model systems analysis. Arch Phys Med Rehabil 1999;80:1402–10.
[11] Glover M. Pressure ulcers. In: Nesathurai S, editor. The rehabilitation of people with spinal cord injury, 3rd ed. Arbuckle Academic Publishers; 2013. p. 65–72.
[12] Roaf E. Aging and spinal cord injury. In: Nesathurai S, editor. The rehabilitation of people with spinal cord injury, 3rd ed. Arbuckle Academic Publishers; 2013. p. 101–8.
[13] Ahmed HU, Shergill IS, Arya M, Shah PJR. Management of detrusor–external sphincter dyssynergia. Nat Clin Pract Urol 2006;3:368–80.
[14] Gulamhusein A, Mangera A. OnabotulinumtoxinA in the treatment of neurogenic bladder. Biologics 2012;6:299–306.
[15] Hess MJ, Zhan EH, Foo DK, Yalla SV. Bladder cancer in patients with spinal cord injury. J Spinal Cord Med 2003;26:335–8.
[16] Lee-Robichaud H, Thomas K, Morgan J, Nelson RL. Lactulose versus polyethylene glycol for chronic constipation. Cochrane Database Syst Rev 2010;7, CD007570.
[17] Ducharme S, Gill K. Sexuality after spinal cord injury. Baltimore: Brookes; 1997.
[18] Del Popolo G, Li Marzi V, Mondaini N, Lombardi G. Time/duration effectiveness of sildenafil versus tadalafil in the treatment of erectile dysfunction in male spinal cord–injured patients. Spinal Cord 2004;42:643–8.
[19] Ergin S, Gunduz B, Ugurlu H, et al. A placebo-controlled, multicenter, randomized, double-blind, flexible-dose, two-way crossover study to evaluate the efficacy and safety of sildenafil in men with traumatic spinal cord injury and erectile dysfunction. J Spinal Cord Med 2008;31:522–31.
[20] Gans WH, Zaslau S, Wheeler S, et al. Efficacy and safety of oral sildenafil in men with erectile dysfunction and spinal cord injury. J Spinal Cord Med 2001;24:35–40.
[21] Hultling C, Giuliano F, Quirk F, et al. Quality of life in patients with spinal cord injury receiving Viagra (sildenafil citrate) for the treatment of erectile dysfunction. Spinal Cord 2000;38:363–70.
[22] Moemen MN, Fahmy I, AbdelAal M, et al. Erectile dysfunction in spinal cord–injured men: different treatment options. Int J Impot Res 2008;20:181–7.
[23] Sánchez Ramos A, Vidal J, Jáuregui ML, et al. Efficacy, safety and predictive factors of therapeutic success with sildenafil for erectile dysfunction in patients with different spinal cord injuries. Spinal Cord 2001;39:637–43.
[24] Soler JM, Previnaire JG, Denys P, Chartier-Kastler E. Phosphodiesterase inhibitors in the treatment of erectile dysfunction in spinal cord–injured men. Spinal Cord 2007;45:169–73.
[25] Giuliano F, Sanchez-Ramos A, Löchner-Ernst D, et al. Efficacy and safety of tadalafil in men with erectile dysfunction following spinal cord injury. Arch Neurol 2007;64:1584–92.
[26] Lombardi G, Macchiarella A, Cecconi F, Del Popolo G. Efficacy and safety of medium and long-term tadalafil use in spinal cord patients with erectile dysfunction. J Sex Med 2009;6:535–43.
[27] Rizio N, Tran C, Sorenson M. Efficacy and satisfaction rates of oral PDE5is in the treatment of erectile dysfunction secondary to spinal cord injury: a review of literature. J Spinal Cord Med 2012;35:219–28.
[28] Soler JM, Previnaire JG. Ejaculatory dysfunction in spinal cord injury men is suggestive of dyssynergic ejaculation. Eur J Phys Rehabil Med 2011;47:677–81.
[29] Patki P, Woodhouse J, Hamid R, et al. Effects of spinal cord injury on semen parameters. J Spinal Cord Med 2008;31:27–32.
[30] Dimitriadis F, Karakitsios K, Tsounapi P, et al. Erectile function and male reproduction in men with spinal cord injury: a review. Andrologia 2010;42:139–65.
[31] Elliot S. Sexual dysfunction and infertility in men with spinal cord disorders. In: Lin V, editor. Spinal cord medicine: principles and practice. New York: Demos; 2003. p. 349–65.
[32] Ducharme S. Sexuality and spinal cord injury. In: Nesathurai S, editor. The rehabilitation of people with spinal cord injury, 3rd ed. Arbuckle Academic Publishers; 2013. p. 95–100.
[33] Alexander MS, Rosen RC, Steinberg S, et al. Sildenafil in women with sexual arousal disorder following spinal cord injury. Spinal Cord 2011;49:273–9.
[34] Sipski ML, Rosen RC, Alexander CJ, Hamer RM. Sildenafil effects on sexual and cardiovascular responses in women with spinal cord injury. Urology 2000;55:812–5.
[35] ACOG committee opinion: number 275, September 2002. Obstetric management of patients with spinal cord injuries. Obstet Gynecol 2002;100:625–7.
[36] Kang AH. Traumatic spinal cord injury. Clin Obstet Gynecol 2005;48:67–72.
[37] Teasell RW, Hsieh JT, Aubut JL, et al. Venous thromboembolism after spinal cord injury. Arch Phys Med Rehabil 2009;90:232–45.
[38] Teasell RW, Mehta S, Aubut JL, et al. A systematic review of the therapeutic interventions for heterotopic ossification after spinal cord injury. Spinal Cord 2010;48:512–21.
[39] van Kuijk AA, Geurts ACH, van Kuppevelt HJM. Neurogenic heterotopic ossification in spinal cord injury. Spinal Cord 2002;40:313–26.
[40] Battaglino RA, Lazzari AA, Garshick E, Morse LR. Spinal cord injury–induced osteoporosis: pathogenesis and emerging therapies. Curr Osteoporos Rep 2012;10:278–85.
[41] Maïmoun L, Fattal C, Micallef J-P, et al. Bone loss in spinal cord–injured patients: from physiopathology to therapy. Spinal Cord 2006;44:203–10.
[42] Consortium for Spinal Cord Medicine. Acute management of autonomic dysreflexia: individuals with spinal cord injury presenting to health care facilities. 2nd ed. Washington, DC: Paralyzed Veterans of America; 2001.
[43] DeSantis N. Autonomic dysfunction. In: Nesathurai S, editor. The rehabilitation of people with spinal cord injury, 3rd ed. Arbuckle Academic Publishers; 2013. p. 77–80.
[44] Domingo A, Lam T, Wolfe D, Eng J. Lower limb rehabilitation following spinal cord injury. In: Eng J, Teasell R, Miller W, et al., editors. Spinal cord injury rehabilitation evidence. Vancouver: SCIRE Project; 2012. p. 1–55, Version 4.0.
[45] Singh R, McD Taylor D, D'Souza D, et al. Injuries significantly associated with thoracic spine fractures: a case-control study. Emerg Med Australas 2009;21:419–23.

CHAPTER 157

Spinal Cord Injury (Lumbosacral)

Sunil Sabharwal, MD

Synonyms

Paraplegia
Conus medullaris syndrome
Cauda equina syndrome

ICD-9 Codes

344.1	**Paraplegia**
344.6	**Cauda equina syndrome**
344.9	**Paralysis, unspecified**
806.4	**Fracture of the vertebral column with spinal cord injury: lumbar**
806.6	**Fracture of the vertebral column with spinal cord injury: sacral**

ICD-10 Codes

G82.20	**Paraplegia, unspecified**
G82.21	**Paraplegia, complete**
G82.22	**Paraplegia, incomplete**
G83.4	**Cauda equina syndrome**
G83.9	**Paralytic syndrome, unspecified**
S32.009	**Unspecified fracture of unspecified lumbar vertebra**
S34.109	**Unspecified injury to unspecified level of lumbar spinal cord**
S32.10	**Unspecified fracture of sacrum**
S34.139	**Unspecified injury to sacral spinal cord**

Add seventh character for S32 (A—initial encounter for closed fracture, B—initial encounter for open fracture, D—subsequent encounter for fracture with routine healing, G—subsequent encounter for fracture with delayed healing, K—subsequent encounter for fracture with nonunion, P—subsequent encounter for fracture with malunion, S—sequela)

Add seventh character for episode of care for S34

Definition

Lumbosacral spinal cord injury (SCI) refers to impairment or loss of motor or sensory function in the lumbar or sacral segments of the spinal cord, secondary to damage of neural elements within the spinal canal [1]. With this level of injury, arm and trunk functions are spared, but the legs and pelvic organs are involved.

The terms *lumbosacral* SCI and *paraplegia* are also used in referring to conus medullaris and cauda equina injuries but not to impaired sensorimotor function due to neural involvement outside the spinal canal (as in lumbosacral plexus lesions or injury to peripheral nerves). Conus medullaris syndrome results from an injury to the sacral spinal cord (conus) and lumbar nerve roots within the spinal canal. Cauda equina syndrome refers to injury to the lumbosacral nerve roots within the neural canal.

Lumbosacral injuries account for about 11% of SCI cases in the national Spinal Cord Injury Model Systems database [2]. The most common causes of injury include motor vehicle crashes, falls, acts of violence, and recreational sporting activities [3,4]. There is an association between level of injury and cause of injury, and acts of violence are more often associated with paraplegia than with cervical injury and tetraplegia [2].

Neurologic versus Skeletal Level of Injury

Lumbosacral SCI refers to the neurologic level of injury, which is different from the skeletal level of injury. Because of the discrepancy between the lengths of the spinal cord and the vertebral column, the L1-L5 lumbar spinal cord segments are typically located at the T11-T12 vertebral level, and the S1-S5 sacral spinal cord segments are at the L1 vertebral level. The spinal cord ends between T12 and L2 (most often at L1 vertebra), and injury within the neural canal below that bone level involves the cauda equina. Lesions at the level of the lowermost thoracic and first lumbar vertebrae may result in mixed cauda equina and conus medullaris lesions (Fig. 157.1).

Symptoms

Lumbosacral SCI may be manifested with weakness in the lower extremities, numbness and tingling, bladder and bowel disturbances (urinary retention, constipation, bladder or bowel incontinence), impotence, back pain, and burning perianal or lower extremity pain.

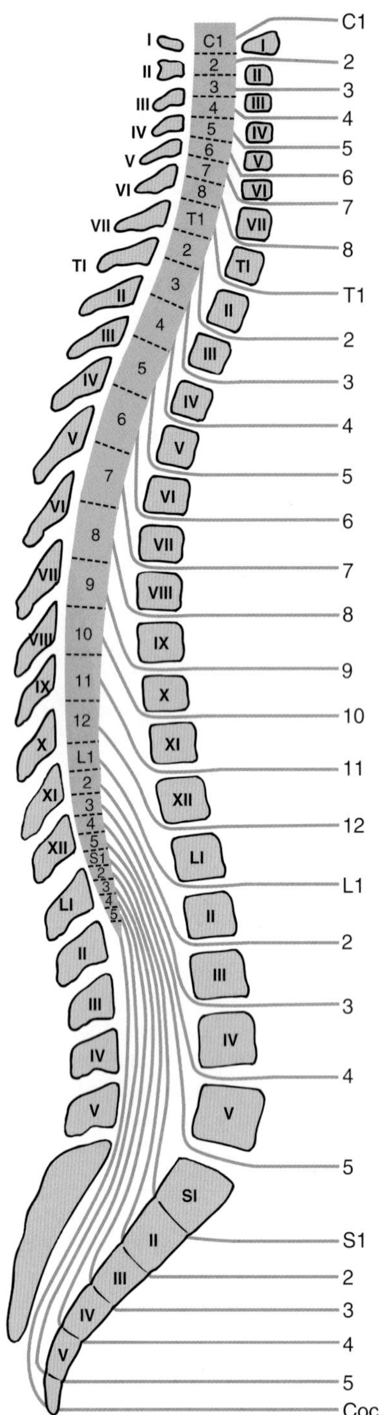

FIGURE 157.1 Discrepancy between spinal cord segments and vertebral levels due to difference in lengths of the vertebral column and spinal cord.

In the outpatient setting, patients may also present with secondary conditions and associated problems, such as urinary tract infections or pressure ulcers. Patients with SCI may have vague, atypical, or nonspecific symptoms. Classic symptoms of urinary tract infection, such as urinary frequency, urgency, and dysuria, may be absent, and patients may present instead with an increased frequency of spontaneous voiding or increased muscle spasms [5]. Fever and malaise may be indicative of a urinary tract infection but can also be due to other infections (such as osteomyelitis underlying a pressure ulcer) or noninfectious causes, such as osteoporotic long bone fracture, deep venous thrombosis, heterotopic ossification, or drug fever (e.g., due to antibiotics). Unilateral leg swelling may be the only presentation of osteoporotic lower limb fractures but could also be due to deep venous thrombosis, heterotopic ossification, hematoma, or cellulitis in the setting of SCI [6].

Pain is a common symptom in people with SCI, and some studies suggest that pain prevalence may be even higher with paraplegia than with cervical injury and tetraplegia [7,8]. A comprehensive history of pain characteristics is needed to accurately determine the underlying cause, which may be nociceptive, neuropathic, or a combination of both.

New weakness or sensory deficits in the upper extremities may indicate post-traumatic syringomyelia extending into the cervical spinal cord or a peripheral nerve entrapment, such as the median nerve at the carpal tunnel or ulnar nerve at the elbow [9]. Patients with chronic SCI who present with extension or worsening of lower extremity weakness or numbness may have post-traumatic syringomyelia or spinal cord or nerve root compression due to progressive spinal deformity or instability.

Rectal bleeding is often caused by hemorrhoids but may be a manifestation of more serious disease, such as colorectal cancer [10]. Similarly, hematuria may be due to urinary tract infection, stones, or catheter-induced trauma, but bladder cancer should be considered in the differential diagnosis, especially in smokers and those with chronic indwelling bladder catheters [5].

Mood disturbances are common in SCI [11]. Depression may be manifested with somatic symptoms such as appetite change and sleep disturbance, although symptoms like loss of energy may be difficult to interpret in the setting of SCI [11,12]. Because many medical diseases may produce similar somatic symptoms, it is helpful to inquire about specific symptoms typically associated with depression, such as suicidal thoughts, dysphoria, and feelings of hopelessness and worthlessness. Early morning awakening is suggestive of primary depression, and fatigue caused by depression is often worse in the morning.

Physical Examination

Spinal Inspection and Palpation

There may be reduced lumbar lordosis due to muscle spasm from pain. Spine fractures may result in deformity, and palpation may reveal areas of tenderness.

Evidence of Concurrent Injuries

Concurrent injuries, including head injury, extremity fractures, and abdominal visceral injury, may accompany lumbosacral SCI and should be considered during diagnostic examination.

Neurologic Examination

Neurologic examination is conducted in accordance with the *International Standards for Neurological and Functional*

Classification of Spinal Cord Injury published by the American Spinal Injury Association [1]. The neurologic findings may sometimes be subtle (e.g., limited to perineal anesthesia or urinary retention) and can be missed in the setting of acute trauma with routine placement of an indwelling catheter or drug-induced sedation, unless they are carefully considered [13]. The neurologic examination should be repeated at regular intervals to monitor for improvement or deterioration [14].

Sensory Examination

The required portion of the sensory examination is completed through testing of key points in each dermatome on the right and left sides of the body (Table 157.1) for pinprick (tested with a disposable safety pin) and light touch sensation (tested with cotton). Pinprick and light touch sensation are separately scored at each key point on a 3-point scale: 0, absent; 1, impaired; and 2, normal. In testing for pinprick sensation, inability to distinguish dull from sharp sensation is graded 0.

Motor Examination

Muscle strength is graded on a 6-point scale of 0 to 5; 0 is no contraction and 5 is normal strength. For the lumbosacral myotomes, five key muscle groups are tested bilaterally (Table 157.2).

Table 157.1 Key Sensory Points for Lumbosacral Spinal Segments

Level	Key Sensory Point
T12	Inguinal ligament at midpoint
L1	Half the distance between T12 and L2
L2	Mid anterior thigh
L3	Medial femoral condyle
L4	Medial malleolus
L5	Dorsum of the foot at the third metatarsophalangeal joint
S1	Lateral heel
S2	Popliteal fossa in the midline
S3	Ischial tuberosity
S4-S5	Perianal area (taken as one level)

Table 157.2 Key Muscle Groups for Lumbosacral Myotomes

Level	Muscle Group	Position for Testing Key Muscles for Grades 4 and 5
L2	Hip flexors (iliopsoas)	Hip flexed to 90°
L3	Knee extensors (quadriceps)	Knee flexed to 15°
L4	Ankle dorsiflexors (tibialis anterior)	Full-dorsiflexed position of the ankle
L5	Long toe extensors (extensor hallucis longus)	First toe fully extended
S1	Ankle plantar flexors (gastrocnemius, soleus)	Hip in neutral rotation, knee fully extended, and ankle in full plantar flexion

Neurologic Rectal Examination

Neurologic rectal examination includes determination of deep anal sensation and testing for voluntary contraction of the external anal sphincter around the examiner's finger (graded as present or absent). If there is voluntary contraction of the anal sphincter, the patient has a motor incomplete injury.

Additional Neurologic Examination

In addition to these required elements for neurologic classification of SCI, position and deep pressure sensation and muscle strength of additional lower extremity muscles, such as medial hamstrings and hip adductors, are also tested. Examination also includes assessment of muscle stretch reflexes, muscle tone, anal sphincter tone, bulbocavernosus reflex, and plantar reflexes.

Conus Medullaris and Cauda Equina Injuries

The examination will vary with the level of damage and the relative involvement of the conus and cauda equina and may include evidence of lower or upper motor neuron involvement. Patients with injury above the conus medullaris typically present with signs consistent with upper motor neuron or suprasacral SCI, whereas those with injury below this level present with a clinical picture consistent with lower motor neuron impairment. Lesions affecting the transition between the two regions (typically around L1 vertebral-level injury) can have a mixed picture. Conus medullaris lesions typically result in impaired sensation over the sacral dermatomes (saddle and perineal anesthesia), lax anal sphincter with loss of anal and bulbocavernosus reflexes, and sometimes weakness in the lower extremity muscles. Cauda equina involvement results in asymmetric atrophic, areflexic paralysis, radicular sensory loss, and sphincter impairment [1,13].

Skin Examination

Skin examination is conducted with particular attention to the areas most vulnerable to pressure ulcer development. These include the sacrum-coccyx, heels, trochanters, and ischial tuberosities [15].

Functional Limitations

Lumbosacral SCI can result in significant functional deficits. These include impaired mobility due to lower extremity paralysis and bladder, bowel, and sexual dysfunction due to autonomic dysregulation.

Expected Functional Outcomes

Predictions of function can be based on completeness and level of injury. The Consortium for Spinal Cord Medicine has developed clinical practice guidelines on outcomes after SCI with expected functional outcomes for each level of injury in a number of domains [14]. Expected outcomes for complete lumbosacral SCI are summarized in Table 157.3.

Ambulation

Persons with lumbosacral SCI should generally be independent at the wheelchair level and have the greatest

Table 157.3 Expected Functional Outcomes for Motor Complete Lumbosacral Spinal Cord Injury

Domain	Expected Functional Outcome	Equipment
Bowel	Independent	Padded toilet seat
Bladder	Independent	
Bed mobility	Independent	Full to king size standard bed
Bed and wheelchair transfers	Independent	
Pressure relief	Independent	Wheelchair pressure relief cushion
Wheelchair propulsion	Independent indoors and outdoors	Manual lightweight wheelchair
Standing and ambulation	Standing: independent	Standing frame
	Ambulation: functional, some assist to independent	Knee-ankle-foot orthosis or ankle-foot orthosis
	L1-L2: household ambulation	Forearm crutches or cane as indicated
	L3-S5: community ambulation	
Eating, grooming, dressing, and bathing	Independent	Padded tub bench Hand-held shower
Communication	Independent	
Transportation	Independent in car, including loading and unloading wheelchair	Hand controls
Homemaking	Independent complex cooking and light housekeeping, some assist with heavy housekeeping	

Modified from Consortium for Spinal Cord Medicine. Outcomes Following Traumatic Spinal Cord Injury. Clinical Practice Guidelines for Health Care Professionals. Washington, DC, Paralyzed Veterans of America, 1999.

potential for ambulation. If hip flexors and knee extensors demonstrate even minimal strength in the first few days after injury, functional recovery and community ambulation are likely. It has been reported that to ambulate independently after SCI, individuals need pelvic control, grade 3/5 (antigravity) hip flexor strength bilaterally to advance the lower extremities, and antigravity knee extensor strength on at least one side (so that no more than one knee-ankle-foot orthosis is needed) [16]. There is individual variation and additional factors than have an impact on ambulation outcome, but patients with motor complete lumbosacral SCI at the L1-L2 level can in general be expected to be household ambulators; community ambulation is an appropriate goal at L3-S5 levels. The lower extremity motor score can predict the likelihood of ambulation. In those with complete paraplegia, chance of walking at 1 year is less than 1% with a 30-day score of 0 and 45% with a score of 1 to 9. In those with incomplete paraplegia, chance of walking at 1 year is 33% with a score of 0, 70% with a score of 1 to 9, and 100% with a score above 10 [16].

Bowel, Bladder, and Sexual Dysfunction

Bowel, bladder, and sexual dysfunction may be significantly disabling in these patients. SCI above the sacral segments is typically associated with an upper motor neuron or reflexic bowel; lesions involving the S2-S4 anterior horn cells or cauda equina have areflexic or lower motor neuron bowel characterized by slow stool propulsion, dry and round stool referred to as scybalous, and risk of incontinence due to denervation of the external anal sphincter [10,17]. Depending on the location of injury and the extent of upper and lower motor neuron impairment, hyperreflexic, areflexic, or mixed type of neurogenic bladder may occur. Absent bulbocavernosus reflex and muscle stretch reflexes in the lower extremities suggest the likelihood of lower motor neuron impairment of the bladder and bowel. Sexual dysfunction is frequent [18]. Men with SCI at the sacral level often lose ability to have reflex erections, although psychogenic erections may be preserved in some. Ejaculation is often impaired, but it may be preserved in a higher proportion of those with incomplete lower motor neuron injuries.

Factors Affecting Functional Outcomes

Pain, whether nociceptive or neurogenic, may interfere with function [7,19]. Neuropathic pain is more common with cauda equina injuries than with injury limited to the conus medullaris. Age, concurrent injuries or comorbidities, body habitus, psychosocial and cultural factors, and personal goals and motivation can significantly affect functional outcomes.

Diagnostic Studies

Spinal Imaging

Radiologic and laboratory studies are used to localize the site of the pathologic change and the underlying cause [13]. Plain radiographs typically include anteroposterior, lateral, and oblique views. The entire spine should be visualized because multiple levels of injury are not unusual. Computed tomographic scanning allows optimal visualization of bone injury and canal occlusion due to bone fragments. Magnetic resonance imaging is especially helpful because of its ability to visualize the soft tissues, including ligamentous structures, intravertebral discs, epidural or subdural hematomas, and hemorrhage or edema in the spinal cord. Magnetic resonance imaging with gadolinium is helpful in diagnosis of post-traumatic syringomyelia.

Electrodiagnostic Testing

Electromyography and nerve conduction studies may be helpful in distinguishing lesions of the spinal cord or cauda equina from those of the lumbar plexus or peripheral nerves.

Urologic Studies

Urodynamic studies are useful to assess the type and extent of neurogenic bladder and sphincter dysfunction. Periodic cystoscopy may be indicated in those with chronic indwelling urinary catheters because of increased risk of bladder cancer [20]. Studies to evaluate upper urinary tracts in patients with neurogenic bladder include renal ultrasonography, renal scan, abdominal radiography, and abdominal computed tomography, but there is no current consensus on the type, indication, or frequency of these tests.

Differential Diagnosis

Lumbar spinal stenosis with spinal cord or cauda equina compression
Primary or metastatic spinal tumors
Spinal infections or abscess
Lesions of the lumbosacral plexus
Disorders involving multiple nerves (e.g., polyneuropathy, Guillain-Barré syndrome)

Treatment

Initial

Initial management [13] of anyone thought to have sustained spinal injury includes adequate spinal immobilization, with placement on a board in the neutral supine position. Stabilization of the airway and hemodynamic status takes precedence in the setting of acute trauma. Methylprednisolone has been advocated in patients presenting within 8 hours of SCI, although effectiveness of this pharmacologic intervention is not uniformly accepted.

Rehabilitation

Information about potential for motor recovery can be used to set functional goals and to plan for equipment needs (see Table 157.3), keeping in mind that individual factors and coexisting conditions may affect achievable goals [14]. Important elements of rehabilitation include an interdisciplinary approach, establishment of an individualized rehabilitation program with consideration of unique barriers and facilitators, and inclusion of the patient as an active participant in establishment of goals [16].

Bowel Management

An individualized bowel care program should be established [10,17]. For upper motor neuron (reflexic) bowel dysfunction, this includes digital rectal stimulation. For lower motor neuron (areflexic) bowel dysfunction, reflex stimulation will not be effective; digital manual evacuation by gloved lubricated fingers is needed, along with Valsalva maneuver or abdominal massage to increase pressure around the colon to push the stool out. Manual disimpaction is aided by use of bulking agents to keep stool consistency firm.

Bladder Management

Optimal bladder management minimizes urinary tract complications, preserves upper urinary tracts, and is compatible with the individual's lifestyle [20]. Because hand function is intact in individuals with lumbosacral injuries, they should be able to perform intermittent catheterization if it is needed for bladder management. If there is abnormal urethral anatomy, poor cognition or unwillingness to adhere to the catheterization schedule, or high fluid intake with consistently large bladder volumes, indwelling catheterization may be needed. Condom catheters can be an appropriate option for urinary drainage in men, provided low-pressure and complete voiding can be documented. For patients with lower motor neuron injuries with low outlet resistance, the use of Credé and Valsalva maneuvers may be considered.

In patients with suspected urinary tract infection, empirical antibiotic treatment may be started while waiting for urine culture results and modified as needed once results are available [5]. The presence of urinary tract obstruction, stones, reflux, abscess, or prostatitis should be considered if the patient fails to respond to antibiotic therapy or has a rapid recurrence with the same organism. Use of prophylactic antibiotics is usually not warranted but should be considered before urologic testing that involves instrumentation, especially in the presence of bacteriuria. Antibiotics to treat asymptomatic bacteriuria in patients with chronic indwelling bladder catheters are generally not indicated.

Pain and Spasticity

Nociceptive causes of pain should be identified and addressed [19]. Many medications, including anticonvulsants and tricyclic antidepressants, have been tried and may help in management of neuropathic pain after SCI, but none has been shown to be consistently effective. Nonpharmacologic interventions and education of the patient are important and should not be ignored. Transcutaneous nerve stimulation may help pain originating at the level of injury. Opioid prescription may be needed for pain unresponsive to other measures. Minimization of extreme or potentially injurious positions at all joints, reduction in the frequency of repetitive upper extremity tasks, proper instruction in transfer techniques to minimize upper extremity injury, optimal wheelchair selection and training, and incorporation of upper body flexibility and resistance exercises are important in preserving upper extremity function and reducing chronic pain due to upper extremity overuse [21].

Spasticity is less of a problem in lumbosacral SCI than in cervical or high thoracic injuries. Management of spasticity [22] includes elimination of the underlying noxious stimulus, use of physical interventions, systemic medications, chemical denervation, intrathecal agents, and rarely orthopedic or neurosurgical procedures. Nonpharmacologic interventions include positioning and stretching (e.g., prone lying to stretch hip flexors and stretching of hamstrings and heel cords to prevent tightness and contractures). Several medications are used for treatment of SCI-related spasticity, including baclofen, tizanidine, gabapentin, and benzodiazepines [23].

Pressure Ulcer Prevention

Education of the patient is critical in this area (see Chapter 148). Avoidance of prolonged positional immobilization, institution of pressure relief, and prescription of pressure-reducing seating systems and support surfaces are important in prevention of pressure ulcers. Daily comprehensive skin inspections should be carried out with particular attention to vulnerable insensate areas (e.g., sacrum-coccyx, ischii, trochanters, heels). Adequate nutritional intake and smoking cessation should be stressed [15].

Procedures

Spasticity

Motor point or nerve blocks with phenol or alcohol may be helpful in treatment of localized lower extremity spasticity (e.g., for hip adductors or ankle plantar flexors) that interferes with positioning, mobility, or hygiene. Intramuscular injections of botulinum toxin are another option.

Pain

Shoulder pain due to subacromial bursitis may be temporarily responsive to local corticosteroid injections, as is the discomfort from carpal tunnel syndrome.

Pressure Ulcers

Sharp débridement of pressure ulcers may be done at the bedside to remove necrotic tissue, although if it is extensive, débridement may need to be done in the operating room.

Surgery

Spine

When thoracolumbar fractures associated with lumbosacral SCI are accompanied by mechanical instability, pain, deformity, or progressive neural impairment, surgical decompression and segmental instrumentation may be indicated for reconstruction of spinal alignment, stability, and early mobilization [13,24]. The ideal timing of and indications for surgical intervention remain controversial.

Pressure Ulcers

Plastic surgery may be indicated for deep pressure ulcers. This includes excision of the ulcer and surrounding scar and muscle and musculocutaneous flap closure [4].

Upper Extremity Pain

Surgery may sometimes be considered for chronic upper extremity overuse-related symptoms that are unresponsive to medical and rehabilitative treatment (e.g., for carpal tunnel syndrome or rotator cuff disease). Outcomes are often poor, especially if upper extremity overuse continues [21].

Bladder and Bowel Dysfunction

Surgical treatment of urolithiasis includes cystoscopic removal of bladder stones, lithotripsy, and percutaneous nephrolithotomy for larger renal stones. Endourethral stents or transurethral sphincterotomy may be considered in individuals with detrusor-sphincter dyssynergia [20]. Patients with neurogenic bowel who have significant difficulty or complications with typical bowel care may be candidates for colostomy. This decision requires careful selection of the patient and individualization to make sure that it is appropriate [17].

Post-traumatic Syringomyelia

Surgical placement of shunts may be indicated for post-traumatic syringomyelia associated with intractable pain or progressive neurologic decline.

Potential Disease Complications

Patients with lumbosacral SCI are prone to multiple complications. Urinary tract infections and pressure ulcers are two of the most common causes of hospitalization in individuals with paraplegia and can result in systemic sepsis [25]. Delayed neurologic deterioration may be due to spinal instability, progressive spinal deformity, or post-traumatic syringomyelia. Upper extremity overuse can result in shoulder pain due to rotator cuff injury or entrapment neuropathies, such as carpal tunnel syndrome [21]. Lower extremity joint contractures (e.g., of the heel cords) can interfere with mobility and with wheelchair positioning. Untreated high bladder pressure in patients with detrusor-sphincter dyssynergia or low bladder compliance may result in upper urinary tract damage. Potential complications of neurogenic bowel include anorectal problems (hemorrhoids, fissures), toxic megacolon, and colonic perforation.

Potential Treatment Complications

Neurologic deterioration may occur from inadequate spinal immobilization or as a complication of surgical instrumentation. Other surgical complications include dural tears with cerebrospinal fluid leaks, infections at the surgical site, pseudarthrosis (which may cause progressive deformity), and chronic pain.

Because people with SCI are often prescribed multiple medications (e.g., to treat pain, spasticity, and bladder or bowel dysfunction), medication-related side effects and complications are common. Complications of urethral catheterization include urethral trauma, erosions, strictures, urinary infections, and epididymitis [20]. Chronic indwelling catheters increase the risk of stones and squamous cell carcinoma of the bladder.

References

[1] International standards for neurological and functional classification of spinal cord injury. revised 2011, Atlanta, Ga: American Spinal Injury Association; 2011.

[2] Devivo MJ. Epidemiology of traumatic spinal cord injury: trends and future implications. Spinal Cord 2012;50:365–72.

[3] National Spinal Cord Injury Statistical Center. Spinal cord injury: facts and figures at a glance. J Spinal Cord Med 2012;35:197–8.

[4] Jackson AB, Dijkers M, DeVivo MJ, et al. Demographic profile of new spinal cord injury: changes and stability over 30 years. Arch Phys Med Rehabil 2004;85:1740–8.

[5] Till M, Pertel P. Infections. In: Green D, editor. Medical management of long-term disability. Boston: Butterworth-Heinemann; 1996. p. 233–62.

[6] McKinley WO, Gittler MS, Kirshblum SC, et al. Spinal cord injury medicine. 2. Medical complications after spinal cord injury: identification and management. Arch Phys Med Rehabil 2002;83(Suppl. 1):S58–64.

[7] Cardenas DD, Bryce TN, Shem K, et al. Gender and minority differences in the pain experience of people with spinal cord injury. Arch Phys Med Rehabil 2004;85:1774–81.

[8] Rintala DH, Loubser PG, Castro J, et al. Chronic pain in a community-based sample of men with spinal cord injury: prevalence, severity, and relationship with impairment, disability, handicap, and subjective well-being. Arch Phys Med Rehabil 1998;79:604–14.

[9] Scelza WM, Dyson-Hudson TA. Neuromusculoskeletal complications of spinal cord injury. In: Kirshblum SC, Campagnolo D, editors. Spinal cord medicine. 2nd ed. Philadelphia: Lippincott Williams & Wilkins; 2011. p. 282–308.

[10] Stiens SA, Bergman SB, Goetz LL. Neurogenic bowel dysfunction after spinal cord injury: clinical evaluation and rehabilitative management. Arch Phys Med Rehabil 1997;78:S86–100.

[11] Consortium for Spinal Cord Medicine. Depression following spinal cord injury. Clinical practice guidelines for health care professionals.

Washington, DC: Paralyzed Veterans of America; 1998. Available at: www.pva.org.

[12] Bombardier CH, Richards S, Krause JS, et al. Symptoms of major depression in people with spinal cord injury: implications for screening. Arch Phys Med Rehabil 2004;85:1749–56.

[13] Harrop JS, Hunt Jr GE, Vaccaro AR. Conus medullaris and cauda equina syndrome as a result of traumatic injuries: management principles. Neurosurg Focus 2004;16:19–23.

[14] Consortium for Spinal Cord Medicine. Outcomes following traumatic spinal cord injury. Clinical practice guidelines for health care professionals. Washington, DC: Paralyzed Veterans of America; 1999. Available at: www.pva.org.

[15] Consortium for Spinal Cord Medicine. Pressure ulcer prevention and treatment following spinal cord injury. Clinical practice guidelines for health care professionals. Washington, DC: Paralyzed Veterans of America; 2000. Available at: www.pva.org.

[16] Kirshblum SC, Bloomgarden J, McClure I, et al. Rehabilitation after spinal cord injury. In: Kirshblum SC, Campagnolo D, editors. Spinal cord medicine. 2nd ed. Philadelphia: Lippincott Williams & Wilkins; 2011. p. 309–40.

[17] Consortium for Spinal Cord Medicine. Neurogenic bowel management in adults with spinal cord injury. Clinical practice guidelines for health care professionals. Washington, DC: Paralyzed Veterans of America; 1998. Available at: www.pva.org.

[18] Consortium for Spinal Cord Medicine. Sexuality and reproductive health in adults with spinal cord injury. Clinical practice guidelines for health care professionals. Washington, DC: Paralyzed Veterans of America; 2010. Available at: www.pva.org.

[19] Bryce TN, Biering-Sørensen F, Finnerup NB, et al. International spinal cord injury pain classification: part I. Background and description. March 6-7, 2009. Spinal Cord 2012;50:413–7.

[20] Consortium for Spinal Cord Medicine. Bladder management for adults with spinal cord injury. Clinical practice guidelines for health care professionals. Washington, DC: Paralyzed Veterans of America; 2006. Available at: www.pva.org.

[21] Consortium for Spinal Cord Medicine. Preservation of upper limb function following spinal cord injury. Clinical practice guidelines for health care professionals. Washington, DC: Paralyzed Veterans of America; 2005. Available at: www.pva.org.

[22] Kirshblum S. Treatment alternatives for spinal cord injury–related spasticity. J Spinal Cord Med 1999;22:199–217.

[23] Rekand T. Clinical assessment and management of spasticity: a review. Acta Neurol Scand Suppl 2010;190:62–6.

[24] McLain RF. Summary statement—thoracolumbar spine trauma. Spine 2006;31(Suppl.):S103.

[25] Cardenas DD, Hoffman JM, Kirshblum S, et al. Etiology and incidence of rehospitalization after traumatic spinal cord injury. Arch Phys Med Rehabil 2004;85:1757–63.

CHAPTER 158

Stroke

Joel Stein, MD

Synonyms

Cerebrovascular accident
Brain attack

ICD-9 Codes

430 Subarachnoid hemorrhage
431 Intracerebral hemorrhage
432 Other and unspecified intracranial hemorrhage
433 Occlusion and stenosis of precerebral arteries
434 Occlusion of cerebral arteries
435 Transient cerebral ischemia
436 Acute but ill-defined cerebrovascular disease
437 Other and ill-defined cerebrovascular disease
438 Late effects of cerebrovascular disease

ICD-10 Codes

I60.9 Nontraumatic subarachnoid hemorrhage
I61.9 Nontraumatic intracerebral hemorrhage
I62.9 Nontraumatic intracranial hemorrhage
I65.9 Occlusion and stenosis of precerebral artery
I66.9 Occlusion and stenosis of unspecified cerebral artery
G45.9 Transient cerebral ischemic attack, unspecified
I67.89 Other cerebrovascular disease
I67.9 Cerebrovascular disease, unspecified
I69.30 Unspecified sequelae of cerebral infarction

Definition

Stroke is an acquired injury of the brain caused by occlusion of a blood vessel or inadequate blood supply leading to infarction or a hemorrhage within the parenchyma of the brain. Ischemic stroke is most commonly due to atherosclerosis of large extracranial or intracranial blood vessels, hypertensive disease of small vessels (lipohyalinosis), or embolism from cardiac or other sources. Approximately 15% of strokes in the United States are hemorrhagic, resulting most commonly from hypertensive hemorrhages, aneurysms, vascular malformations, or cerebral amyloid angiopathy. Approximately 800,000 strokes occur annually in the United States, with a large population of survivors with permanent disability. Important modifiable risk factors for ischemic stroke include hypertension, smoking, diabetes, obesity, sedentary lifestyle, and hyperlipidemia; nonmodifiable risk factors include age, sex, and race/ethnicity. Risk factors for hemorrhage include hypertension and smoking as well as alcohol consumption.

Symptoms

The symptoms of stroke depend on the location of the injury in the brain. For example, a stroke in the distribution of the left middle cerebral artery will typically result in right hemiplegia, aphasia, and right homonymous hemianopia, whereas a lacunar infarct in the left internal capsule may result in a less severe degree of right-sided hemiparesis and few other symptoms. Left hemispatial neglect and impaired attention are common features of right hemispheric stroke. Ischemic strokes generally conform to the vascular territory of a specific artery within the brain and therefore result in characteristic combinations of neurologic impairments that constitute a particular stroke syndrome.

In general, difficulties in walking, performing activities of daily living, speaking, and swallowing are common manifestations of stroke. Cognitive impairments (memory, attention, visual-spatial perception) and impaired communication due to aphasia or dysarthria may be present. Impaired sexual function should be identified because patients may not volunteer functional impairments in this area unless the physician inquires. Loss of libido is common among both stroke survivors and their spouses or other partners and appears multifactorial in origin. Erectile dysfunction in men may result from comorbid conditions (such as diabetes or atherosclerosis), with frequent contributions from side effects of medications including antihypertensives, antidepressants, and anticonvulsant medications.

Weakness, difficulty in speaking or swallowing, aphasia, cognitive disturbance, sensory loss, and visual disturbance are the most common presenting symptoms of stroke, and deficits in these areas often persist even after initial rehabilitation. Weakness (typically hemiparesis) results from loss of motor control primarily, and some stroke survivors retain good strength despite limited ability to perform isolated precise movements of the affected side. Urinary urgency, increased muscle tone, fatigue, depression, and pain are symptoms that may be manifested after a stroke has already occurred. Reflex sympathetic dystrophy (also known as complex regional pain syndrome type I) may occur after stroke, although most post-stroke pain results from mechanical (e.g., joint subluxation) or central (e.g., thalamic pain syndromes) causes.

Depression is common after stroke, affecting as many as 40% of stroke survivors. Depression should be identified as a treatable complication of stroke rather than accepted as a consequence of functional loss.

Physical Examination

A full neurologic examination is appropriate. This includes evaluation of mental status, cranial nerves, sensation, deep tendon reflexes, abnormal reflexes (e.g., Babinski), motor strength and coordination, muscle tone, and functional mobility (sitting, transfers, and ambulation). The protean manifestations of stroke can cause many different combinations of abnormalities in these aspects of the neurologic examination. Common findings include hyperreflexia and hemiparesis on the affected side, with variable degrees of sensory loss. Dysarthria may be present, as can aphasia or hemineglect, depending on the areas affected. Hemiplegic gait is commonly seen, with reduced stride length, reduced knee flexion ("stiff-legged gait"), ankle plantar flexion and inversion, and circumduction to allow clearance of the affected leg. An assessment of mood and affect is important, given the high prevalence of post-stroke depression. Some degree of sadness is typically present as a normal grief reaction to a sudden disabling event and should be distinguished from true major depression on the basis of how pervasive the symptoms are and associated symptoms such as anhedonia. Emotional lability may also occur, with symptoms that tend to be fleeting and changeable. Range of motion in affected limbs should be measured; ankle plantar flexion contractures and upper limb contractures are common in patients with long-standing hemiplegic stroke and interfere with rehabilitation efforts. Shoulder subluxation may occur in hemiparetic patients and should be noted and quantified. Skin is examined for any areas of breakdown. Limb swelling is common and should be noted. The fit and function of leg braces, upper extremity splints, slings, wheelchairs, and ambulatory aids are assessed as part of the routine physical examination.

Functional Limitations

Depending on the impairments that patients have, they may be unable to drive or to use public transportation. Communication difficulties can lead to social isolation. Some individuals require ongoing supervision because of cognitive limitations. In severe cases, individuals with aphasia or cognitive impairments may not be able to live independently. Incontinence due to detrusor instability and urinary urgency can interfere with leaving the home and contribute to skin breakdown and social isolation.

Among stroke survivors older than 65 years who were evaluated 6 months after a stroke, 30% were unable to walk without some assistance, 26% were dependent for activities of daily living, and 26% were institutionalized in a nursing home [1].

Diagnostic Studies

In the acute setting, computed tomography is often the first diagnostic test performed because of the rapidity with which it can be obtained, its widespread availability, and its high sensitivity for cerebral hemorrhage. Magnetic resonance imaging provides greater anatomic resolution and avoids radiation exposure. With diffusion and perfusion-weighted sequences, magnetic resonance imaging abnormalities can be demonstrated at a very early stage, providing important information for acute treatments such as thrombolysis [2]. Magnetic resonance angiography, computed tomographic angiography, noninvasive flow studies, Holter monitoring, and echocardiography are important studies to help determine the cause of a stroke and to determine the best treatment for prevention of recurrent stroke. In selected patients (particularly young individuals or those without typical risk factors), an evaluation for a hypercoagulable state is indicated. In patients with prior stroke, diagnostic studies are typically directed to complications of stroke, such as persistent dysphagia or urinary incontinence. Videofluoroscopic swallowing studies can be useful in swallowing disorders, as can flexible endoscopic evaluation of swallowing. Urodynamic studies may be useful in the assessment of urinary symptoms, particularly if initial treatment with anticholinergic medications is unsuccessful.

Differential Diagnosis

Hemiplegic migraine
Post-seizure (Todd) paralysis
Brain neoplasm
Multiple sclerosis

Treatment

Initial

When ischemic stroke is diagnosed within the first 3 hours, thrombolytic therapy has been shown to reduce disability [3]. There is evidence that thrombolysis may be useful in selected individuals between 3 and 4.5 hours after stroke onset as well [4]. Mechanical clot retrieval and intra-arterial thrombolysis have been used successfully for patients who do not experience resumption of flow in the occluded artery with intravenous thrombolysis or who fall outside of the time window for this therapy [5]. Aspirin (between 80 and 325 mg) has been found to be effective when it is used in the acute setting. In younger patients with large ischemic strokes, increased intracranial pressure due to swelling may require hemicraniectomy to prevent herniation and death.

Secondary prevention depends on the cause of the stroke. Warfarin (Coumadin) is commonly used for the secondary prevention of embolic stroke, with the most extensive evidence for prevention of stroke in atrial fibrillation. Several new oral anticoagulants are increasingly used as alternatives to warfarin, including dabigatran (Pradaxa), apixaban (Eliquis), and rivaroxaban (Xarelto) [6,7]. Antiplatelet agents, including aspirin, clopidogrel (Plavix), or a combination of aspirin and dipyridamole (Aggrenox), are used for prevention of most non-cardioembolic strokes or when anticoagulation is desirable but contraindicated because of comorbid conditions. Risk factor modification, including treatment of hypertension, diabetes, hyperlipidemia, and obesity as well as smoking cessation and exercise, should be addressed for all stroke survivors.

Treatment of cerebral hemorrhage is based in part on the presumed cause. For hypertensive hemorrhages, control of blood pressure with antihypertensive medications is the mainstay of treatment. Large hemorrhages may require hematoma evacuation and removal of a portion of the skull to treat elevated intracranial pressure. For all causes of cerebral hemorrhage, avoidance of anticoagulants, antiplatelet medications, and alcohol is important.

Medications for the management of post-stroke symptoms on an outpatient basis are shown in Table 158.1. Anticholinergic medications are useful for bladder detrusor instability. Oral antispasticity medications are of limited efficacy in many cases (see Chapter 153). For sexual dysfunction in men, phosphodiesterase type 5 inhibitors may be effective. Treatment with selective serotonin reuptake inhibitors for post-stroke depression is widely employed, although a wide range of antidepressant medications can be effective. Psychostimulants (e.g., methylphenidate) and eugeroics (e.g., modafinil) may be useful for impaired attention. Anticonvulsants are used for central pain syndromes, but with variable benefit.

Rehabilitation

The rehabilitation program needs to be customized on the basis of the severity and nature of the impairments caused by the stroke. For individuals with moderate to severe stroke, a comprehensive multidisciplinary inpatient rehabilitation program in a rehabilitation hospital is often appropriate and may lead to improved outcomes [8]. Stroke patients with significant functional limitations in mobility, communication, cognition, or self-care who are capable of participating in and benefiting from an intensive rehabilitation program consisting of 3 hours or more of rehabilitation therapy per day commonly undergo an inpatient rehabilitation stay. For these individuals, rehabilitation commonly continues through home care or outpatient services after discharge from the rehabilitation hospital/unit. Patients with more circumscribed and less severe deficits may be discharged directly from the acute care hospital to home and participate in an outpatient rehabilitation program [9]. Patients who are unable to participate in an aggressive rehabilitation program because of poor motivation, severe cognitive deficits, or poor prognosis may receive inpatient rehabilitation at a subacute program (skilled nursing facility) instead, as may some patients with milder deficits who are unable to be discharged directly home. There is considerable practice variation regarding referral to an inpatient rehabilitation facility versus a skilled nursing facility and only limited observational data comparing outcomes in the two types of facilities [8,10]. Although not definitive, these studies suggest better outcomes for patients receiving inpatient care, and stroke patients who meet the admission criteria and have insurance coverage for this type of care should be preferentially referred to inpatient rehabilitation facilities when it is feasible.

Exercise

Therapeutic exercise programs are usually functionally oriented, with an emphasis on restoration of functional mobility and ability to perform activities of daily living (Fig. 158.1). Instruction in compensatory techniques and family teaching are important in assisting individuals to return home. There is growing evidence of the impact of therapeutic exercise on cortical reorganization after stroke, with associated improvements in motor control and functional use of the affected limbs [11]. Newer approaches being studied to enhance motor abilities include constraint-induced movement therapy, robot-assisted exercise training (Fig. 158.2), and virtual reality exercise training [11–14].

Table 158.1 Medications Commonly Used for Treatment of Post-Stroke Symptoms

Class of Medication	Examples	Indication
Anticholinergics	Oxybutynin (Ditropan) Tolterodine (Detrol)	Bladder detrusor instability
Antispasticity	Baclofen (Lioresal) Tizanidine (Zanaflex) Diazepam (Valium) Dantrolene (Dantrium)	Muscle spasticity
Phosphodiesterase type 5 inhibitors	Sildenafil (Viagra) Vardenafil (Levitra)	Erectile dysfunction
Selective serotonin reuptake inhibitors	Fluoxetine (Prozac) Paroxetine (Paxil) Sertraline (Zoloft)	Post-stroke depression
Stimulants	Methylphenidate (Ritalin) Dextroamphetamine (Dexedrine)	Impaired attention, arousal
Eugeroics	Modafinil (Provigil) Armodafinil (Nuvigil)	Impaired arousal, attention
Anticonvulsants	Gabapentin (Neurontin) Carbamazepine (Tegretol)	Central pain syndromes, seizure disorders

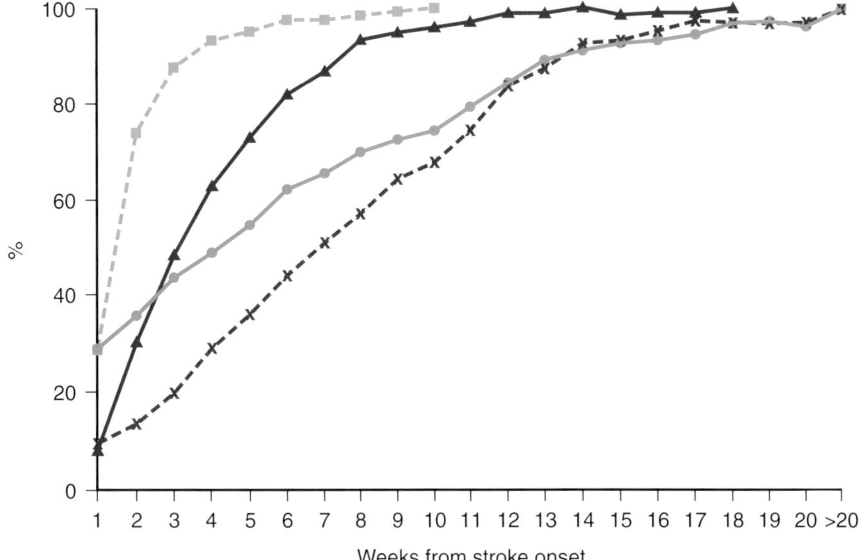

FIGURE 158.1 The time course of recovery after stroke is shown as the cumulative percentage of stroke survivors in each category who have reached their best function in activities of daily living relative to initial functional disability: ■, mild disability; ▲, moderate disability; ●, severe disability; and X, very severe disability. *(From Jorgensen HS, Nakayama H, Raaschou HO, et al. Outcome and time course of recovery in stroke. Part II. Time course of recovery. The Copenhagen Stroke Study. Arch Phys Med Rehabil 1995;76:406-412.)*

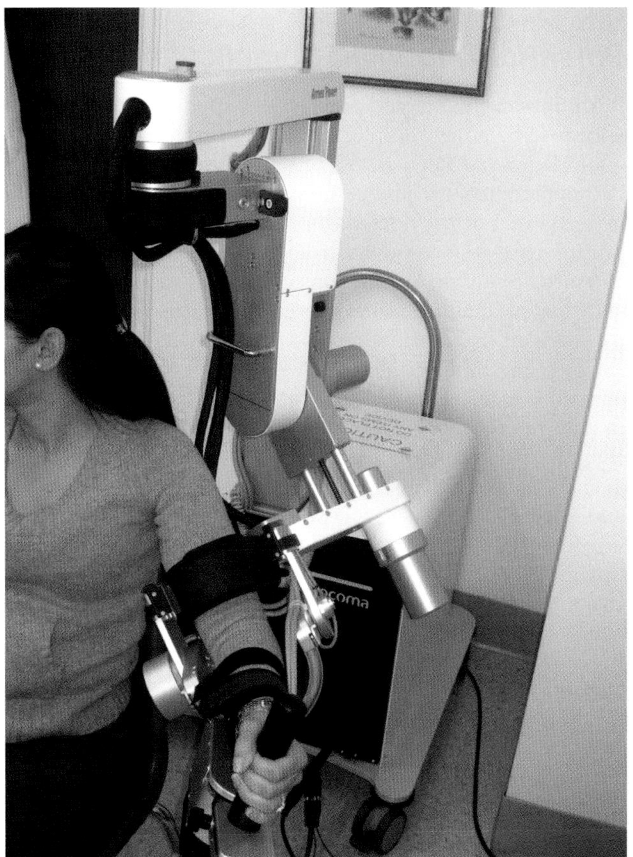

FIGURE 158.2 Robot-assisted upper limb exercise therapy using the ArmeoPower system (Hocoma, Zurich, Switzerland).

These novel techniques appear to improve motor function, but the optimal exercise program to facilitate recovery remains to be defined.

Electrical Stimulation

Noninvasive brain stimulation has been studied as a means of enhancing motor recovery and for treatment of aphasia after stroke. This can be delivered by transcranial magnetic stimulation or transcranial direct current stimulation. Preliminary studies suggest benefit of this therapy when it is combined with exercises, but definitive trials have not yet been performed [15].

Dysphagia

Management of dysphagia may include nasogastric or gastrostomy tube feedings, modified diets (e.g., thickened liquids, pureed foods), and swallowing therapy (e.g., the use of compensatory strategies, such as "tucking" the chin during swallowing).

Communication

The rehabilitation of aphasia relies on extensive speech therapy as its mainstay; selected patients benefit from communication aids, such as a picture board. Speech therapy may provide significant benefit for dysarthria as well, resulting in improved intelligibility. Severely dysarthric or anarthric patients may benefit from the use of computer-based communication aids, including those with speech synthesis, as well as "low-tech" solutions, such as spelling boards.

Cognition

Cognitive abilities are frequently affected by stroke; alterations in memory, attention, insight, and problem solving are common. Neuropsychological testing may be useful in defining the precise nature of these deficits and in helping to develop a remediation plan. Speech-language and occupational therapy approaches include attempts at remediation and teaching of compensatory techniques. Family education and training are important components of cognitive rehabilitation. Recognition and treatment of post-stroke depression are important because depression can contribute to reduced cognitive performance after stroke [16].

Bracing

Lower extremity bracing is frequently helpful in restoration of mobility in hemiparetic stroke survivors. Most commonly, a plastic or carbon-fiber ankle-foot orthosis is used, although other braces are appropriate in selected circumstances. Bracing is helpful as a compensation for impaired ankle dorsiflexion, controlling ankle inversion and plantar flexor spasticity as well as providing some stabilization at the knee. Electrical stimulation systems (e.g., Bioness L300, WalkAide) can be used to stimulate dorsiflexion as an alternative to a brace for selected patients.

Ambulatory Aids and Wheelchairs

Because of hemiparesis, many stroke survivors require ambulatory aids, which may include a straight cane, a four-pronged ("quad") cane, a hemi-walker, or, in some cases, a conventional walker. Wheelchairs are often needed for more severely impaired stroke survivors or for moderately impaired stroke survivors for longer distance travel. A hemi-wheelchair is lower to the ground and allows use of the nonparetic leg to assist with propulsion. On occasion, a one-arm drive wheelchair is useful; it allows control of both wheelchair wheels from one side. Active, nonambulatory individuals may benefit from a power wheelchair.

Shoulder Subluxation

Shoulder subluxation commonly occurs in the setting of hemiplegia after stroke, although the presence of pain is highly variable. Arm boards and the selective use of slings help in reducing subluxation. Electrical stimulation may have a beneficial effect as well [17].

Splints

Splints for proper positioning of the hemiplegic arm and ankle-foot are important to prevent contracture. These are particularly important when spasticity is present. Failure to properly splint and stretch the hand and wrist can result in progressive contracture leading to deformity, even with relatively mild spasticity.

Vocational Rehabilitation

Although stroke is predominantly a disease of older individuals, a significant portion of stroke survivors are of working age. Once activities of daily living have been mastered, vocational counseling may assist individuals seeking to return to work. Coordination with the rehabilitation team is important because retraining for certain job tasks may involve a multidisciplinary effort. Accommodations in the workplace may be necessary, and the Americans with Disabilities Act may require the employer to provide reasonable accommodation for individuals with disabilities.

Procedures

Botulinum toxin or phenol injections may be useful in the management of spasticity after stroke. These injections are described in greater detail in Chapter 153.

Surgery

Selected patients require craniotomy in the acute phase for evacuation of a large intracerebral hematoma or for severe swelling with increased intracranial pressure. Carotid endarterectomy or stenting in appropriately selected patients has been shown to reduce the risk of recurrent stroke [18]. Intrathecal baclofen pumps have been found to be effective in treatment of post-stroke spasticity [19,20] but are infrequently used for hemiplegic stroke at this time. In patients with chronic impairments from stroke, tendon lengthening procedures are occasionally needed for contractures.

Potential Disease Complications

Seizures can develop as an early or a late complication of stroke; strokes involving the cerebral cortex and hemorrhagic stroke carry greater risk. The risk of deep venous thrombosis is substantially elevated in hemiplegic stroke, and prophylactic treatment with subcutaneous heparin or low-molecular-weight heparin is advisable during the initial recovery phase [21]. The ideal duration of prophylaxis for deep venous thrombosis after stroke has not been established; in most cases, this is discontinued after a period of several weeks. Stroke recurrence is a feared complication of stroke, and individuals with a history of stroke remain at increased risk for recurrent stroke despite risk factor reduction. Aspiration pneumonia can occur as a complication of dysphagia, although this risk tends to abate over time except in the most severe cases.

Potential Treatment Complications

Both anticoagulants and antiplatelet medications can contribute to bleeding complications. Aspirin can cause gastritis. Clopidogrel has been associated with thrombotic thrombocytopenic purpura. The combined use of aspirin and clopidogrel does not provide additional protection against stroke but increases the risk of gastrointestinal hemorrhage [22].

Anticholinergic medications commonly cause dry mouth and may precipitate urinary retention. Antispasticity medications can cause sedation and may exacerbate cognitive impairments. Sildenafil is known to be hazardous when it is used concurrently with nitrates and should be avoided in patients receiving these medications. Selective serotonin reuptake inhibitors can cause gastrointestinal symptoms (especially nausea and anorexia) as well as interfere with libido and sexual function. Psychostimulants can cause anorexia, insomnia, anxiety, or agitation and should be slowly titrated upward. Gabapentin is usually well tolerated, although occasional sedation has been reported. Carbamazepine may cause leukopenia.

References

[1] Kelley-Hayes M, Beiser A, Kase CS, et al. The influence of gender and age on disability following ischemic stroke: the Framingham study. J Stroke Cerebrovasc Dis 2003;12:119–26.

[2] Lansberg MG, Albers GW, Beaulieu C, Marks MP. Comparison of diffusion-weighted MRI and CT in acute stroke. Neurology 2000;54:1557–61.

[3] Tissue plasminogen activator for acute ischemic stroke. The National Institute of Neurological Disorders and Stroke rt-PA Stroke Study Group. N Engl J Med 1995;333:1581–7.

[4] Hacke W, Kaste M, Bluhmki E, et al, ECASS Investigators. Thrombolysis with alteplase 3 to 4.5 hours after acute ischemic stroke. N Engl J Med 2008;359:1317–29.

[5] Smith WS, Sung G, Saver J, et al. Mechanical thrombectomy for acute ischemic stroke: final results of the Multi MERCI trial. Stroke 2008;39:1205–12.

[6] Connolly SJ, Ezekowitz MD, Yusuf S, et al. Dabigatran versus warfarin in patients with atrial fibrillation. N Engl J Med 2009;361:1139–51.

[7] Patel MR, Mahaffey KW, Garg J, et al. Rivaroxaban versus warfarin in nonvalvular atrial fibrillation. N Engl J Med 2011;365:883–91.

[8] Chan L, Sandel ME, Jette AM, et al. Does postacute care site matter? A longitudinal study assessing functional recovery after a stroke. Arch Phys Med Rehabil 2013;94:622–9.

[9] Mayo NE, Wood-Dauphinee S, Cote R, et al. There's no place like home: an evaluation of early supported discharge for stroke. Stroke 2000;31:1016–23.

[10] Terdiman J, Armstrong MA, Klatsky A, et al. Postacute care and ischemic stroke mortality: findings from an integrated health care system in northern California. PM R 2011;3:686–94.

[11] Liepert J, Bauder H, Miltner WH, et al. Treatment-induced cortical reorganization after stroke in humans. Stroke 2000;31:1210–6.

[12] Wolf SL, Winstein CJ, Miller JP, et al, EXCITE Investigators. Effect of constraint-induced movement therapy on upper extremity function 3 to 9 months after stroke: the EXCITE randomized clinical trial. JAMA 2006;296:2095–104.

[13] Lo AC, Guarino PD, Richards LG, et al. Robot-assisted therapy for long-term upper-limb impairment after stroke. N Engl J Med 2010;362:1772–83.

[14] You SH, Jang SH, Kim YH, et al. Virtual reality–induced cortical reorganization and associated locomotor recovery in chronic stroke: an experimenter-blind randomized study. Stroke 2005;36:1166–71.

[15] Lindenberg R, Renga V, Zhu LL, et al. Bihemispheric brain stimulation facilitates motor recovery in chronic stroke patients. Neurology 2010;75:2176–84.

[16] Kimura M, Robinson RG, Kosier JT. Treatment of cognitive impairment after poststroke depression: a double-blind treatment trial. Stroke 2000;31:1482–6.

[17] Chantraine A, Baribeault A, Uebelhart D, Gremion G. Shoulder pain and dysfunction in hemiplegia: effects of functional electrical stimulation. Arch Phys Med Rehabil 1999;80:328–31.

[18] Barnett HJ, Taylor DW, Eliasziw M, et al. Benefit of carotid endarterectomy in patients with symptomatic moderate or severe stenosis. North American Symptomatic Carotid Endarterectomy Trial Collaborators. N Engl J Med 1998;339:1415–25.

[19] Francisco GE, Boake C. Improvement in walking speed in poststroke spastic hemiplegia after intrathecal baclofen therapy: a preliminary study. Arch Phys Med Rehabil 2003;84:1194–9.

[20] Meythaler JM, Guin-Renfroe S, Brunner RC, Hadley MN. Intrathecal baclofen for spastic hypertonia from stroke. Stroke 2001;32:2099–109.

[21] Gresham G, Duncan PW, Stason WB, Post-Stroke Rehabilitation Guideline panel. Clinical practice guideline number 16. Post-stroke rehabilitation. Rockville, Md: U.S. Department of Health and Human Services, Agency for Health Care Policy and Research; 1995.

[22] Benavente OR, Hart RG, McClure LA, et al, SPS3 investigators. Effects of clopidogrel added to aspirin in patients with recent lacunar stroke. N Engl J Med 2012;367:817–24.

CHAPTER 159

Stroke in Young Adults

Antoinne C. Able, MD, MSCI

Synonyms

Cerebrovascular accident
Cerebral infarction
Intracerebral hemorrhage
Cerebral venous thrombosis
Subarachnoid hemorrhage

ICD-9 Codes

342.01	Flaccid hemiplegia, dominant side
342.02	Flaccid hemiplegia, nondominant side
342.11	Spastic hemiplegia, dominant side
342.12	Spastic hemiplegia, nondominant side
344.0	Quadriplegia, unspecified
438	Late effects of cerebrovascular disease
438.0	Cognitive deficits
438.10	Speech and language deficits, unspecified
438.11	Aphasia
438.12	Dysphasia
438.19	Other speech and language deficits
438.2	Hemiplegia/hemiparesis
438.20	Hemiplegia affecting unspecified side
438.21	Hemiplegia affecting dominant side
438.22	Hemiplegia affecting nondominant side

ICD-10 Codes

G81.00	Flaccid hemiplegia affecting unspecified side
G81.01	Flaccid hemiplegia affecting right dominant side
G81.02	Flaccid hemiplegia affecting left dominant side
G81.03	Flaccid hemiplegia affecting right nondominant side
G81.04	Flaccid hemiplegia affecting left nondominant side
G81.10	Spastic hemiplegia affecting unspecified side
G81.11	Spastic hemiplegia affecting right dominant side
G81.12	Spastic hemiplegia affecting left dominant side
G81.13	Spastic hemiplegia affecting right nondominant side
G81.14	Spastic hemiplegia affecting left nondominant side
G82.50	Quadriplegia, unspecified
G82.51	Quadriplegia, C1-C4 complete
G82.52	Quadriplegia, C1-C4 incomplete
G82.53	Quadriplegia, C5-C7 complete
G82.54	Quadriplegia, C5-C7 incomplete
I69.30	Unspecified sequelae of cerebral infarction
R41.89	Other symptoms and signs involving cognitive functions and awareness
R47.01	Aphasia
R47.02	Dysphasia
G81.90	Hemiplegia, unspecified affecting unspecified side
G81.91	Hemiplegia, unspecified affecting right dominant side
G81.92	Hemiplegia, unspecified affecting left dominant side
G81.93	Hemiplegia, unspecified affecting right nondominant side
G81.94	Hemiplegia, unspecified affecting left nondominant side

Definition

Four percent of strokes in the United States occur in adults younger than 45 years, and a collective review of reports provides estimates that range up to 21% or greater [1]. Although the 28,000 strokes in this age group are a small fraction of the 731,000 total events in the United States each year, stroke is an important cause of neurologic impairment in this group. Stroke occurs in those younger than 45 years more than twice as frequently as spinal cord injury (11,000 per year, all ages), and yet there has been limited awareness in American society of stroke as a disease affecting younger adults. *As overall stroke incidence declines, there is evidence that stroke is occurring at a younger age, with the incidence increasing in younger adults* [2]. Before the age of 30 years, more women than men have strokes because of the risks of pregnancy, childbirth, and oral contraceptive use [3,4]; this trend reverses with advancing age. In the United States, the incidence of stroke is two to five times higher in young urban blacks and twice as high in Hispanics than in whites [5]. Strokes in young adults are particularly devastating events because they often occur in otherwise healthy-seeming individuals who are in the prime of life and fully involved with family, community, and workplace responsibilities. Young adults also have high expectations of recovery and consequent difficulty in adjusting to residual disability.

Although more than 60 different disorders causing stroke in young adults have been identified, they can be grouped into several broad categories. Atherosclerotic disease accounts for approximately 20%; cardiac emboli, 20%; arteriopathies (particularly large-vessel dissection), 10%; coagulopathy, 10%; and peripartum cerebrovascular accidents, 5%. Another 20% may be related to mitral valve prolapse, migraine, and oral contraceptive use, and 15% remain unexplained after full evaluation [6]. In American studies, illicit drug use has been associated with stroke in 4% to 12% of cases [5,7]. The main clinical challenge in the management of young adults with acute stroke is the identification of its cause. Whereas cryptogenic stroke was the most common cause in the past, today specific causes are more readily identified resultant to improved capability in noninvasive imaging of brain vessels and heart arteries and valves, aortic electrophysiology, and genetic diagnostic instruments developed in recent decades [8,9]. The rate of thrombolysis use among young acute ischemic stroke patients has increased in the past decade, in part owing to stroke center certification and the availability of the stroke networks [10].

Approximately 75% of patients younger than 65 years will survive 5 years or more after their stroke [1]. Individual survival depends, of course, on the specific cause of the stroke and its treatment. In general, two thirds of young survivors achieve good functional recovery, although a history of diabetes mellitus, severe deficit at onset, or stroke involving the total anterior circulation may reduce that likelihood. Overall, the risk for recurrence in those who have suffered a first stroke averages 5% per year and varies with the survivor's burden of risk factors [11–13].

Symptoms

The presenting neurologic symptoms of stroke are the same in young as in elderly patients and are reviewed in Chapter 158. The clinician caring for young adult stroke survivors in the post-acute phase is likely to encounter, in addition to neurologic residua of the stroke, a number of secondary symptoms that will require ongoing management. The most common of these are emotional effects, pain, spasticity, bladder dysfunction, sexual dysfunction, and fatigue. These symptoms may also occur in older stroke patients; however, this chapter focuses on the impact they have on the young stroke survivor.

Emotional Effects

The common emotional consequences of stroke are depression, emotional lability, and anxiety. Clinical depression occurs in approximately 40% of patients after stroke; its incidence peaks 6 months to 2 years after the ictus. It is more likely in those with a prior history of alcoholism or depression and in patients who have suffered a severe stroke [14,15].

Depression can be difficult to identify in aphasic patients who cannot respond reliably to questions about mood and in patients with motor aprosodia (loss of emotional tone in facial expression and voice) due to right hemispheric stroke. Patients tend to become more socially isolated after stroke because of language, cognitive, and physical deficits. Loss of social interaction and support increases the likelihood of depression. Stress related to marital role reversal after a stroke in one member of a couple is common, as is depression in caregivers [15].

Neurologically mediated emotional lability, also known as pseudobulbar affect or emotional incontinence, in which the patient has abrupt episodes of crying or laughing in response to mention of an affectively charged topic, may be a source of distress to the patient and family. It may also complicate evaluation of the patient's true emotional state.

Patients may experience heightened anxiety chronically after stroke. In some cases, specific triggers of the anxiety, such as fear of falling while walking with a cane or fear of being left alone, can be identified in the history. The prevalence and severity of anxiety symptoms were comparable to those of depression symptoms, and the prevalence of both mood symptoms was similar during the acute period and 1 year after stroke. Both mood disturbances were also associated with a poorer health-related quality of life at 1 year, whereas only depression symptoms influenced functional recovery. More emphasis should be given to the role of anxiety in stroke rehabilitation interventions [16].

Pain

Pain is a common problem after stroke in young patients. It usually affects the hemiparetic extremities and may be centrally or peripherally mediated. Shoulder pain occurs in up to 85% of stroke patients, usually during the first 6 to 12 months after stroke [17]. The history should address its many potential causes [18] (Table 159.1). In addition, younger individuals with partially recovered motor function may have secondary sprains, tendinitis, skin breakdown, and nerve palsies in the paretic extremities as these are pushed beyond their physiologic limits in the effort to resume normal activities. The normal arm and leg may suffer similar overuse injuries in the course of compensating for the weak side. Heavy use of assistive devices, including canes, walkers, braces, and splints, may contribute to these injuries and consequent pain.

Muscle Stiffness due to Spasticity

Stiffness and heaviness of muscles and joints are common complaints of young stroke patients in the post-acute

Table 159.1 Post-Stroke Shoulder Pain [18]

Disorder	Inferior Subluxation	Rotator Cuff Tear	CRPS I (Shoulder-Hand)	Frozen Shoulder	Impingement Syndrome	Biceps Tendinitis
Examination	Acromiohumeral separation Flaccid	Positive abduction test result Positive drop arm test result Flaccid or spastic	Metacarpophalangeal joint compression test Skin color changes Flaccid or spastic	External rotation <15 degrees Early scapular motion Spastic	Pain with abduction of 70-90 degrees End-range pain with forward flexion Spastic	Positive Yergason test result Flaccid or spastic
Diagnostic test	Standing radiograph in scapular plane	Arthrography Subacromial injection of lidocaine Magnetic resonance imaging	Triple-phase bone scan Stellate ganglion block	Arthrography	Subacromial injection of lidocaine	Tendon sheath injection of lidocaine
Treatment						
Initial	Analgesics, nonsteroidals	Nonsteroidals, analgesics	Oral corticosteroids	Analgesics	Nonsteroidals, analgesics	Nonsteroidals, analgesics
Rehabilitation	Harris hemi-sling or wheelchair arm board	AAROM Electrical stimulation to supraspinatus	AAROM Heat modalities	PROM Manipulation	AAROM Scapular mobilization	AAROM
Procedures		Steroid injection Surgical repair	Stellate ganglion block	Subacromial, intra-articular steroids Débridement Reduction of internal rotator tone	Subacromial steroids Reduction of internal rotator tone	Tendon sheath injection of steroids

AAROM, active-assisted range of motion; *CRPS I,* chronic regional pain syndrome type I; *PROM,* passive range of motion.

setting. These symptoms are often due to the evolution of muscle tone from the flaccid to the spastic state that occurs during the first several months that follow a stroke. Although it is occasionally helpful in allowing weight bearing on a leg with little voluntary motor return, spasticity more often complicates the patient's efforts to resume normal motor function. The reader is referred to Chapter 153 for further discussion of spasticity symptoms. Joint stiffness may also be due to contracture, which is shortening of the muscles, ligaments, or tendons around a joint due to rheologic changes in the tissues. This is common in the finger joints of the affected hand. Frozen shoulder, with contracture of the glenohumeral joint capsule, also occurs.

Bladder Dysfunction

Chronically diminished bladder control with urge incontinence occurs commonly in younger stroke patients. The history should ascertain chronicity and frequency of the problem, diurnal pattern, and presence or absence of the sensation of needing to void; a relationship to coughing, laughing, or straining is noted. The patient is queried about abdominal pain and pain on urination.

Sexual Dysfunction

Whether the physiologic process of sexual function changes as a result of stroke, and if so, how it changes, has not been scientifically established. Nonetheless, most patients report diminished sexual function after stroke. This may involve diminished libido or decreased erectile or ejaculatory function. Decreased libido may correlate with the presence of depression and reduced physiologic sexual function with medical comorbidity. Neither clearly relates to size or location of stroke. There is evidence that patients' partners play a significant role in the decline of sexual activity, through fear of relapse, anguish, and lack of excitation. A small number of patients report increased libido after stroke, and rarely, troublesome hypersexuality appears [19,20]. The history should note change in interest and frequency of sexual activity, alteration in ability to achieve erection or ejaculation in men and lubrication or orgasm in women, and presence of depression or active medical comorbidities that may influence sexual activity level. Medications are reviewed for antihypertensives, antidepressants, and others that may hinder sexual function and possibly fertility, although there is little research on this topic.

Fatigue

Increased fatigue after stroke has been reported in 39% to 68% of patients in published series. It is frequently influenced by coexisting depression. Young adults who never before needed naps now do. Patients become fatigued, physically and mentally, with less effort than before the stroke. Return to active work and family life may be limited by fatigue [21,22]. The history should document a change in fatigue level after the stroke and probe the daily pattern of fatigue and sleep for symptoms of insomnia, sleep apnea, and the many medical conditions that produce fatigue. Medications are reviewed to identify sedative agents. Depression and loss of physical conditioning may affect energy levels, as may the increased energy cost of hemiplegic gait [23].

Physical Examination

In the post-acute setting, the examination of the younger patient after a stroke includes neurologic and functional status for evidence of improvement or deterioration. Improved motor control in the affected leg may allow trimming back of a brace and progression in gait training to a less supportive assistive device. Worsening motor or sensory function, on the other hand, may signal not only further cerebral events but also the presence of a systemic illness, medication intolerance, new peripheral nerve injuries related to positioning or assistive devices, or worsening neuropathy. Confrontation testing for visual fields and double sensory stimulation tests for visual and tactile neglect provide important information to the patient and physician about suitability for community mobility, particularly driving. Clock drawing, target cancellation, line bisection, and reading from a magazine can be quickly performed in the office and provide additional information about neglect and attention. The Mini-Mental State Examination is a rapid and helpful cognitive screen [24,25]. The affected arm and leg should be inspected for skin breakdown. Maceration of the palm in a tightly flexed hand and friction marks on the dorsum of the foot and calf of patients using ankle-foot orthoses are common. Ulnar palsy and olecranon bursitis related to a constantly flexed spastic elbow can occur. It is particularly important to identify and to treat these problems early in patients with diminished sensation.

Signs of unusual causative entities should be sought if the etiology of the stroke is unclear. These may include the skin laxity and hypermobility of Ehlers-Danlos syndrome, the ipsilateral ptosis and miosis (partial Horner syndrome) associated with carotid dissection, the multiple venipuncture marks of intravenous drug abuse, the livedo reticularis of Sneddon syndrome, the vasculitic rash of connective tissue diseases, and the arachnodactyly and tall habitus of Marfan syndrome.

Emotional Effects

Mood should be evaluated for signs of depression, lability, and anxiety. For patients with intact verbal function, the two questions *During the past 2 weeks, have you felt down, depressed, or hopeless?* and *During the past 2 weeks, have you felt little interest or pleasure in doing things?* may be as helpful as more extensive screening tools, such as the depression screening criteria of the *Diagnostic and Statistical Manual of Mental Disorders* [26,27]. In severely aphasic patients, the screen must, of necessity, consider facial expression, gestures, and posture and the reports of caretakers regarding appetite, sleep, and mood. If the caretaker shows signs of depression, it may be helpful to offer him or her referral for further evaluation. Lability can often be elicited by discussing affectively relevant topics, such as children or spouse. Physical examination signs of chronic anxiety may include hunched posture, fleeting eye contact, cold or moist hands, mild tachycardia, rapid and hypophonic speech, and ready startle reaction.

Pain

The examination addresses appearance, tenderness, pain pattern, and range of motion of the painful regions, looking for signs of specific medical and musculoskeletal disorders. See Table 159.1 for helpful physical examination signs in the diagnosis of post-stroke shoulder pain.

Muscle Stiffness due to Spasticity

Muscle tone at the shoulder adductors, elbow flexors and extensors, wrist and finger flexors, knee extensors, and ankle plantar flexors should be assessed and recorded at each visit with use of the Ashworth scale (Table 159.2). Pain encountered on range of motion is recorded. Reflexes are evaluated, assessing for sustained clonus, which at the ankle and knee can compromise gait and at the wrist and fingers may be mistaken for seizure activity.

Bladder Dysfunction

Palpatory examination of the abdomen may reveal suprapubic tenderness due to cystitis or an enlarged bladder indicative of retention with overflow incontinence.

Sexual Dysfunction

Full gynecologic and urologic examinations will screen for infectious, traumatic, neoplastic, and hormonal causes of sexual dysfunction in young stroke survivors. The neurologic examination may reveal a neuropathy (manifested by decreased sensation in the feet or hands, decreased ankle and knee reflexes, and occasionally distal weakness) that may be affecting sexual function.

Fatigue

Idiopathic post-stroke fatigue is a diagnosis of exclusion. The examination must screen the patient for the many illnesses that cause fatigue. Among the more prominent of these in this population are Epstein-Barr viral disease, sleep apnea, allergic rhinitis, anemia, dehydration, cerebral hypoperfusion, hypothyroidism, depression, malignant neoplasia, and medications.

Table 159.2 Modified Ashworth Scale for Measurement of Spasticity

0	No increase in muscle tone
1	Slight increase in muscle tone, manifested by a catch and release or by minimal resistance at the end range of motion
1+	Slight increase in muscle tone, manifested by a catch, followed by minimal resistance throughout the remainder (less than half) of the range of motion
2	More marked increase in muscle tone through most of the range of motion, but the affected part is easily moved
3	Considerable increase in muscle tone, passive movement difficult
4	Affected part is rigid in flexion or extension

Functional Limitations

Driving

Return to driving is a necessary step for return to a normal lifestyle and avoidance of social isolation in many communities. Once they have been discharged home, young adult stroke patients are generally eager to resume driving. Many rehabilitation clinics offer written tests of driving ability. Although these have not been shown to be adequate predictors of on-the-road performance, they serve a useful screening purpose. Recent work with a computerized driving simulator suggests that these may be helpful and safe tools for retraining of driving skills [28]. A number of factors have been shown to predict driving performance after stroke; right hemisphere location of stroke, visual-perceptual deficits, reduced sustained and selective attention, impulsivity, poor judgment, and lack of organizational skills all correlate with poor performance behind the wheel. Aphasia, although it may have a negative impact on performance on written and road tests because of compromised processing of verbal instructions, does not always interfere with self-directed driving.

Physicians are often consulted about a patient's readiness to resume driving; visual acuity and fields can be readily screened in an office setting, but evaluation for impulsivity, judgment, and selective and divided attention is more difficult. An on-the-road test performed either by a driving instructor or by the state licensing agency remains the "gold standard" for assessment of driving ability.

Return to Work

The ability to perform valued work is central to self-esteem and an important goal for most young stroke patients. Between 11% and 85% of patients achieve this goal; the wide range reported in this literature is due to differing age ranges, definitions of work, and disability compensation systems [29]. Of those who return to work after stroke, 70% do so at a reduced level. Factors predictive of success in return to work include pure motor or no hemiparesis, good self-care and mobility function at completion of rehabilitation, no aphasia or apraxia, advanced education, and a white-collar job. Barriers to successful vocational rehabilitation include, in addition to the reverse of these factors, cognitive impairment, visual-perceptual impairment, age older than 55 years, and economic disincentives related to disability and retirement benefits.

Patients who are able to resume work after a stroke on average do so within the first 6 months. The 1990 Americans with Disabilities Act has had a positive impact on employers' responsiveness to the requests of stroke survivors for job accommodations, not only regarding physical access and equipment but also for personal assistance, schedule flexibility, and task modification [29–31]. Most patients return to their previous employer, although young stroke survivors with minimal cognitive impairment may be able to take on new jobs.

Parenting

The young adult stroke survivor who needs to return to parenting faces particular challenges in the performance of child bathing, dressing, feeding, and transporting tasks. Problem solving of these tasks can be done with the assistance of other adult family members, home care occupational therapists, or hired child care assistants. Many helpful items of equipment are readily available (paper disposable diapers with easy to close tabs, microwaves for heating bottles, baby tub inserts). Even when frequent assistance is needed, the patient should be encouraged to assume the supervisory role in child care.

Diagnostic Studies

Because the use of illicit drugs has been linked to strokes in younger individuals, ongoing drug screening in the post-acute setting may occasionally be indicated. Despite the use of early and advanced neuroimaging techniques along with improved symptom recognition by patients, misdiagnosis of acute stroke in young adults in emerging reports occurs at 14%, with posterior circulation more likely to be misdiagnosed as peripheral vertigo. The initial misdiagnosis results in a potential lost opportunity for thrombolysis or admission to certified stroke centers in otherwise good candidates [32]. For other diagnostic testing, see Chapter 158.

Differential Diagnosis

Brain infection (abscess, encephalitis)
Brain neoplasm
Cranial nerve palsy
Peripheral nerve palsy
Hemiplegic migraine
Multiple sclerosis
Progressive multifocal leukoencephalopathy
Positional vertigo
Post-seizure (Todd) paralysis
Toxic metabolic encephalopathy
Conversion disorder

Treatment

The patient's motivation to comply with treatment for hypertension and diabetes, to develop a habit of compliance with newly prescribed anticoagulation therapy, to quit smoking, to avoid excessive alcohol intake, and to turn away from the use of street drugs will be maximal in the months that follow the stroke. Some available studies suggest that stroke rehabilitation should provide interventions designed especially for young adults, but more recent studies reflect that the young adult patient's needs are similar to those of the general stroke population [33].

Emotional Effects

Initial

Post-stroke depression responds to antidepressant medications of several classes. The lower cardiac risk profile of selective serotonin reuptake inhibitors makes them an attractive option for patients with arrhythmia. They should be used with caution in patients with sexual dysfunction. The sedative and urinary retentive properties of tricyclic antidepressants may be helpful for patients with concomitant neuropathic pain, excessive salivation, and sleep disturbance or urge incontinence. All of the major classes of antidepressants have the potential to lower seizure threshold. The family and community, including local and national stroke support and education groups, are important resources for the young patient who is struggling with emotional adjustment to residual disability and altered lifestyle. Referral to a psychiatrist, psychologist, home care social worker, or psychiatric nurse is often helpful. Emotional lability often responds to selective serotonin reuptake inhibitors and usually diminishes over time [34,35]. Management of anxiety in cognitively impaired young stroke patients should emphasize the less sedating anxiolytics, counseling, and environmental manipulation to reduce known triggers.

Rehabilitation

Neurologic and functional improvement is perhaps the best antidote to post-stroke depression. A multidisciplinary stroke rehabilitation program, by providing graded and progressive activities in many areas, gives the patient the opportunity to make and to appreciate numerous improvements in parameters of mobility, self-care, language, and cognition. Therapists are skilled at providing encouragement and positive reinforcement for successes, large and small, in the targeted activities. The rehabilitation therapy environment provides substantial psychological support to the patient, and it is common for depression first to become evident, or to worsen, at the time outpatient therapy finishes and this support system is withdrawn.

Procedures

Electroconvulsive therapy may be indicated for refractory depression.

Pain

Initial

Measures for soft tissue–based pain include non-narcotic analgesics and nonsteroidal anti-inflammatory drugs, with care taken to consider the cardiac, renal, hepatic, and gastrointestinal risks. When narcotic medication for pain relief is required, the fentanyl transdermal patch is a useful option. Neuropathic and central pain syndromes often respond to gabapentin. See Table 159.1 for treatment options for the several varieties of post-stroke shoulder pain.

Rehabilitation

Rehabilitation treatment of pain syndromes is useful both in itself and because it allows close monitoring by a qualified therapist of the patient's symptoms and response to treatments. Soft tissue injuries often respond to stretching and strengthening, positioning, electrical stimulation of the affected muscles, and heat modalities including hot packs and ultrasound when sensation is adequate to allow their use. Transcutaneous electrical nerve stimulation and functional electrical stimulation to the supraspinatus and upper trapezius are often helpful in poorly defined shoulder pain, as are arm slings, such as the Harris hemi-sling, that promote optimal glenohumeral alignment.

Procedures

Acupuncture can be beneficial for central pain syndromes, and subacromial bursa steroid injection will help approximately half of patients with post-stroke shoulder pain. Botulinum toxin and phenol injections provide relief when pain is due to spasticity in specific muscles.

Surgery

In post-stroke shoulder pain, surgical repair may be considered when rotator cuff tear can be established as the cause. Surgical débridement may be required for severe, unremitting frozen shoulder.

Muscle Stiffness due to Spasticity

Initial

The management of muscle stiffness due to spasticity is discussed in detail in Chapter 153. Intercurrent infections, localized sores, stress, and anxiety can worsen spasticity and should be treated before other interventions are added. Sedation in this cognitively fragile population is to be avoided and limits dosage titration of all the available antispasticity agents. Tizanidine and gabapentin, because of their analgesic as well as muscle relaxant actions, are logical choices for painful spasticity. Selective serotonin reuptake inhibitors occasionally exacerbate spasticity.

Rehabilitation

Mild post-stroke spasticity in the heel cord and finger and wrist flexors can often be adequately controlled with a stretching program performed two or three times per day by the patient. Range of motion in a spastic ankle or hand can be preserved with nighttime use of custom-fabricated resting splints.

Procedures

Injection of spastic muscles with botulinum toxin and of peripheral motor nerves with phenol can enhance gait pattern and hand function and reduce pain in young stroke survivors. Once a pattern of useful response to injection to specific muscles and nerves has been established, consideration should be given to surgical referral for more permanent intervention.

Surgery

Tendon lengthening, sectioning, and transfers infrequently performed in elderly stroke patients because of limited life expectancy and medical risks should be considered in younger patients when the pattern of hypertonicity has stabilized. Achilles tendon lengthening may allow improved heel strike in patients with chronic equinovarus posturing due to spastic triceps surae. Sectioning of short toe flexors can reduce painful toe clawing, and splitting and lateral reattachment of a portion of the anterior tibial tendon (SPLATT procedure) can rebalance a varus foot. Electrophysiologic evaluation of the extremity in a gait laboratory can provide useful information to supplement the physical examination and help ensure that the optimal muscles are targeted for surgical intervention.

Bladder Dysfunction

Initial

For the stroke survivor with urge incontinence due to spastic neurogenic bladder, helpful medications are available. The anticholinergics oxybutynin and tolterodine are first-line agents for management of detrusor instability. In addition, tricyclic antidepressants provide mild anticholinergic stimulation and can be used to increase bladder capacity.

Rehabilitation

Urinary incontinence can be successfully managed in the inpatient rehabilitation setting or at home with timed voiding (every 2 hours while awake), timed fluid intake (none after supper), use of padded clothing or condom catheter, and a commode or urinal by the bedside.

Pelvic floor strengthening exercises are helpful for stress incontinence. There are no specific rehabilitation treatments for detrusor instability, although the patient's therapists are often in a position to observe and to document the extent of the problem.

Surgery

Bladder suspension surgery may be indicated for stress incontinence.

Sexual Dysfunction

Treatment of depression with medications such as bupropion, mirtazapine, and nefazodone, which do not hinder sexual function [36], and of active concurrent medical illnesses can promote improved sexual function. Elimination of other medications that compromise ejaculatory or orgasmic function will obviously help as well. Treatment with testosterone to enhance libido and with sildenafil to improve erection or estrogen to improve lubrication may be considered.

Fatigue

Initial

Efforts to ensure a normal sleep-wake cycle should be made. These include maintenance of a consistent and appropriate bedtime, avoidance of stimulant beverages late in the day, and use of hypnotic agents at bedtime, if needed. For the patient who sleeps well at night but remains easily fatigued during the day, a trial of methylphenidate on arising and at noon may be considered. Loss of initiation due to frontal lobe disease may be perceived as fatigue and occasionally responds to amantadine. For the depressed patient with fatigue, a nonsedating antidepressant should be chosen. Short daytime naps in patients with normal nighttime sleep pattern should not be discouraged.

Rehabilitation

A tailored cardiovascular conditioning program is helpful to maximize the patient's aerobic capacity and physical stamina. Patients with significant physical impairment will benefit from a physical therapist's assistance in designing an adapted conditioning program, which may emphasize use of a stationary bicycle, arm ergometer, and therapeutic pool.

Patients with limiting cardiovascular comorbidities will require the physician's input for heart rate and blood pressure guidelines. Appropriate bracing and use of assistive devices and gait training by an experienced physical therapist can help reduce the energy cost of hemiplegic gait. For some patients, wheelchair propulsion is less fatiguing than walking.

Potential Disease Complications

The spectrum of neurologic and medical complications of stroke in young adults is similar to that in older stroke patients. See Chapter 158.

Potential Treatment Complications

Complications of stroke treatment are similar in young and older adults. They are discussed in Chapter 158.

References

[1] Weinfeld FD. National survey of stroke. Stroke 1981;12(Pt 2, Suppl. 1): I1–I90.
[2] Sultan S, Elkind MS. Stroke in young adults: on the rise? Neurology 2012;79:1752–3.
[3] Lidegaard O, Soe M, Andersen MV. Cerebral thromboembolism among young women and men in Denmark 1977-1982. Stroke 1986;17:670–5.
[4] Naess H, Nyland HI, Thomassen L, et al. Incidence and short-term outcome of cerebral infarction in young adults in western Norway. Stroke 2002;33:2105–8.
[5] Chong JY, Sacco RL. Epidemiology of stroke in young adults: race/ethnic differences. J Thromb Thrombolysis 2005;20:77–83.
[6] Hart RG, Miller VT. Cerebral infarction in young adults: a practical approach. Stroke 1983;14:110–4.
[7] Adams HP, Kappelle LJ, Biller J, et al. Ischemic stroke in young adults. Arch Neurol 1995;52:491–5.
[8] Ferro JM, Massaro AR, Mas J-L. Aetiological diagnosis of ischaemic stroke in young adults. Lancet Neurol 2010;9:1085–96.
[9] Varona JF, Guerra JM, Bermejo F, et al. Causes of ischemic stroke in young adults, and evolution of the etiological diagnosis over the long term. Eur Neurol 2007;57:212–8.
[10] Kansara A, Chaturvedi S, Bhattacharya P. Thrombolysis and outcome of young stroke patients over the last decade: insights from the Nationwide Inpatient Sample. J Stroke Cerebrovasc Dis 2013;22:799–804.
[11] Naess H, Nyland HI, Thomassen L, et al. Long-term outcome of cerebral infarction in young adults. Acta Neurol Scand 2004;110:107–12.
[12] Nedeltchev K, der Maur TA, Georgiadis D, et al. Ischaemic stroke in young adults: predictors of outcome and recurrence. J Neurol Neurosurg Psychiatry 2005;76:191–5.
[13] Sacco RL. Risk factors and outcomes for ischemic stroke. Neurology 1995;45(Suppl. 1):S10–4.
[14] Sobel RM, Lotkowski S, Mandel S. Update on depression in neurologic illness: stroke, epilepsy, and multiple sclerosis. Curr Psychiatry Rep 2005;7:396–403.
[15] Dennis M, O'Rourke S, Lewis S, et al. Emotional outcomes after stroke: factors associated with poor outcome. J Neurol Neurosurg Psychiatry 2000;68:47–52.
[16] Donnellan C, Hickey A, Hevey D, O'Neill D. Effect of mood symptoms on recovery one year after stroke. Int J Geriatr Psychiatry 2010;25:1288–95.
[17] Gresham G, Duncan PW, Stason WB, Post-Stroke Rehabilitation Guideline panel. Clinical practice guideline number 16. Post-stroke rehabilitation. Rockville, Md: U.S. Department of Health and Human Services, Agency for Health Care Policy and Research; 1995, 125.
[18] Black-Schaffer RM, Kirsteins AE, Harvey RL. Stroke rehabilitation. 2. Co-morbidities and complications. Arch Phys Med Rehabil 1999;80:S8–S16.
[19] Korpaelainen JT, Nieminen P, Myllyla VV. Sexual functioning among stroke patients and their spouses. Stroke 1999;30:715–9.
[20] Carod J, Egido J, Gonzalez JL, et al. Poststroke sexual dysfunction and quality of life. Stroke 1999;30:2238–9.
[21] Schepers VA, Visser-Meily AM, Ketelaar M, Lindeman E. Poststroke fatigue: course and its relation to personal and stroke-related factors. Arch Phys Med Rehabil 2006;87:184–8.
[22] Naess H, Nyland HL, Thomassen L, et al. Fatigue at long-term follow-up in young adults with cerebral infarction. Cerebrovasc Dis 2005;20:245–50.
[23] Waters RL, Mulroy S. The energy expenditure of normal and pathologic gait. Gait Posture 1999;9:207–23.
[24] Folstein MF, Folstein SE, McHugh PR. "Mini-mental state," a practical method for grading the cognitive state of patients for the clinician. J Psychiatr Res 1975;12:189–98.
[25] Azouvi P, Samuel C, Louis-Dreyfus A, et al. Sensitivity of clinical and behavioural tests of spatial neglect after right hemisphere stroke. J Neurol Neurosurg Psychiatry 2002;73:160–6.
[26] Whooley MA, Avins AL, Miranda J, Browner WS. Case-finding instruments for depression: two questions are as good as many. J Gen Intern Med 1997;12:439–45.
[27] American Psychiatric Association. Diagnostic and statistical manual of mental disorders. 4th ed. Washington, DC: American Psychiatric Association; 1994.
[28] Akinwuntan AE, DeWeerdt W, Feys H, et al. Effect of simulator training on driving after stroke: a randomized controlled trial. Neurology 2005;65:843–50.
[29] Wozniak MA, Kittner SJ. Return to work after ischemic stroke: a methodological review. Neuroepidemiology 2002;21:159–66.
[30] Gresham GF, Fitzpatrick TE, Wolf PA, et al. Residual disability in survivors of stroke. The Framingham study. N Engl J Med 1975;293:954–6.
[31] Black-Schaffer RM, Lemieux L. Vocational outcome after stroke. Top Stroke Rehabil 1994;1:74–86.
[32] Kuruvilla A, Bhattacharya P, Rajamani K, Chaturvedi S. Factors associated with misdiagnosis of acute stroke in young adults. Stroke 2011;20:523–7.
[33] Lawrence M, Kinn S. Needs, priorities, and desired rehabilitation outcomes of family members of young adults who have had a stroke: findings from a phenomenological study. Disabil Rehabil 2013;35:586–95.
[34] Robinson RG, Schultz SK, Castillo C, et al. Nortriptyline versus fluoxetine in the treatment of depression and in short-term recovery after stroke: a placebo-controlled, double-blind study. Am J Psychiatry 2000;157:351–9.
[35] Choi-Kwon S, Han SW, Kwon SU, et al. Fluoxetine treatment in poststroke depression, emotional incontinence, and anger proneness: a double-blind, placebo-controlled study. Stroke 2006;37:156–61.
[36] Hirschfield RM. Care of the sexually active depressed patient. J Clin Psychiatry 1999;60(Suppl. 17):32–5, discussion 46–48.

CHAPTER 160

Systemic Lupus Erythematosus

Sallaya Chinratanalab, MD
John Sergent, MD

Synonyms

Lupus
Lupus erythematosus

ICD-9 Code

710.0 Systemic lupus erythematosus

ICD-10 Code

M32.9 Systemic lupus erythematosus, unspecified

Definition

Systemic lupus erythematosus (SLE) is a multisystem autoimmune disease that is associated with autoantibody production and complement-fixing immune complex deposition. The immune system attack triggers an inflammatory process, resulting in tissue damage. SLE is the prototype of an autoimmune disease that can cause a wide spectrum of clinical presentations and is characterized by remissions and exacerbation. Periods of active illness are sometimes called flares. The course of the disease is unpredictable but can sometimes be triggered by environmental factors, such as ultraviolet light and certain drugs. Although the cause of SLE is not yet fully elucidated, there are known to be a variety of genes that make individuals susceptible to the disease and to its flares. SLE can affect skin, joints, kidneys, lungs, heart, blood vessels, liver, and the nervous system. The disease occurs nine times more often in women than in men, especially in the childbearing years between the ages of 15 and 45 years. The disease can also be found in pediatric and geriatric populations. The prevalence in the general population is approximately 1 in every 2000 persons, but it varies according to race, ethnicity, and socioeconomic background.

The American College of Rheumatology formulated a set of clinical and laboratory findings known as the classification criteria of SLE in 1985 and subsequently revised them in 1997 (Table 160.1). The classification criteria were designed for investigators recruiting SLE patients into clinical trials, but many clinicians also commonly use them in practice to establish a diagnosis in a given patient.

Symptoms

SLE can cause a variety of symptoms ranging from mild to severe. Patients can present with constitutional symptoms and organ-specific symptoms. Constitutional symptoms include fever, weight loss, and fatigue, which are typically present at some time during the course of the disease in most SLE patients. Mucocutaneous manifestations are important, as shown by the fact that they account for 4 of the 11 classification criteria (see Table 160.1). Skin lesions can be burning, tender, or itching. Rashes such as the classic malar (butterfly) rash and discoid lesions are characteristic. Patients may experience photosensitivity after a period of sun exposure. Photosensitivity is clinically defined as an abnormal response to ultraviolet light. These responses are manifested as exaggerated sunburn reactions and are often associated with systemic symptoms including fever, weakness, fatigue, and joint pain. Photosensitivity seems to correlate strongly with the presence of Ro/SSA antibodies [1]. Oral ulcerations are common and may be painless or asymptomatic. They are commonly on the hard palate and usually indicate active disease. The location and often asymptomatic nature of lupus-related oral ulcerations help differentiate them from non-lupus ulcerations, including aphthous stomatitis, lichen planus, herpes simplex, and drug-related lesions such as thrush due to corticosteroids and mucositis due to methotrexate. Nasal ulcers can also be found during disease activity and are often painful.

Patients may note thin hair, alopecia, or bald spots. Diffuse alopecia is nonspecific and can be caused by many systemic illnesses as well as by drugs such as cyclophosphamide and steroids. Focal bald spots, known as alopecia areata, are almost always due to autoimmune reactions and are characteristic of SLE. Painful red eyes from episcleritis, scleritis, or uveitis can be seen in SLE patients. Visual loss can occur in SLE patients with retinitis, vasculitis, optic neuritis, or thrombosis due to the antiphospholipid antibody syndrome. Some SLE patients experience sicca symptoms of dry eyes and dry mouth due to secondary Sjögren syndrome.

Table 160.1 The 1997 Revised Criteria for the Classification of Systemic Lupus Erythematosus

Criterion	Definition
1. Malar rash	Fixed malar erythema, flat or raised
2. Discoid rash	Erythematous raised patches with keratotic scaling and follicular plugging; atrophic scarring may occur in older lesions
3. Photosensitivity	Skin rash as an unusual reaction to sunlight, by patient history or physician observation
4. Oral ulcers	Oral or nasopharyngeal ulcers, usually painless, observed by physician
5. Arthritis	Nonerosive arthritis involving two or more peripheral joints, characterized by tenderness, swelling, or effusion
6. Serositis	a. Pleuritis (convincing history of pleuritic pain or rub heard by physician or evidence of pleural effusion) *or* b. Pericarditis (documented by electrocardiogram, rub, or evidence of pericardial effusion)
7. Renal disorder	a. Persistent proteinuria (>0.5 g/day or >3+) *or* b. Cellular casts of any type
8. Neurologic disorder	a. Seizures (in the absence of other causes) *or* b. Psychosis (in the absence of other causes)
9. Hematologic disorder	a. Hemolytic anemia *or* b. Leukopenia (<4000/μL on two or more occasions) *or* c. Lymphopenia (<1500/μL on two or more occasions) *or* d. Thrombocytopenia (<100,000/μL in the absence of offending drugs)
10. Immunologic disorder	a. Anti–double-stranded DNA *or* b. Anti-Sm *or* c. Positive finding of antiphospholipid antibodies based on (1) an abnormal serum level of immunoglobulin G or M anticardiolipin antibodies, (2) a positive test result for lupus anticoagulant using a standard method, or (3) a false-positive serologic test for syphilis known to be positive for at least 6 months and confirmed by *Treponema pallidum* immobilization or fluorescent treponemal antibody absorption test
11. Antinuclear antibody	An abnormal titer of antinuclear antibody by immunofluorescence or an equivalent assay at any time and in the absence of drugs known to be associated with "drug-induced lupus syndrome"

For identifying patients in clinical studies, a person shall be said to have SLE if any 4 or more of the 11 criteria are present, either serially or simultaneously, during any interval of observation.

From Hochberg MG. Updating the American College of Rheumatology revised criteria for the classification of systemic lupus erythematosus [letter]. Arthritis Rheum 1997;40:1725.

Patients may present with pleuritic chest pain related to serositis or pulmonary embolism. In addition, SLE patients have a very high incidence of premature atherosclerosis, and myocardial infarctions and strokes are not uncommon in young women with SLE. The authors have seen such events in a number of women in their late teens and 20s.

Epigastric pain in SLE patients can be due to nonsteroidal anti-inflammatory drugs, but the differential diagnosis must include pancreatitis, a life-threatening complication of SLE or of drugs used to treat it, such as azathioprine.

Patients presenting with dependent edema must be evaluated for lupus nephritis, which can cause the nephrotic syndrome. In the case of unilateral leg swelling, deep venous thrombosis needs to be ruled out. The hypercoagulable state in SLE patients is often associated with the antiphospholipid antibody syndrome. Antiphospholipid antibodies, including the lupus anticoagulant, are seen in approximately one fourth of SLE patients. Many remain asymptomatic, but the antibodies are associated with a number of clinical manifestations, including deep venous thrombosis and pulmonary embolism, arterial clots, recurrent spontaneous abortions, and strokes.

Articular symptoms are almost universal in SLE patients. Typical joint involvement in SLE affects the small joints of the hands as well as the wrists, feet, and knees. The joint symptoms are inflammatory in nature; therefore, they tend to be worse in the morning and are often accompanied by generalized stiffness. Patients generally experience significant joint pain out of proportion to objective physical findings. In patients who have received high doses of corticosteroids, avascular necrosis (osteonecrosis) needs to be in the differential diagnosis of severe joint pain, especially in the hips, knees, and shoulders. Raynaud phenomenon is an additional risk factor for this complication in SLE.

Raynaud phenomenon occurs in at least a third of SLE patients and may be the presenting manifestation. Raynaud phenomenon is caused by episodic vasospasm and ischemia of the extremities in response to cold or emotional stimuli. Typical color change is triphasic from white to blue to red, but many patients do not go through all three phases. Instead, they may just have periods of blanching followed by a return to normal color. In severe cases, digital ulcers may occur and can lead to shortening of the distal phalanx.

Neurologic symptoms, including headaches, numbness, tingling, and weakness, can vary from mild to severe. Strokes are found at an increased incidence in SLE because of both the accelerated atherosclerosis mentioned before and the hypercoagulable state due to associated antiphospholipid antibodies. SLE can also affect the spinal cord with rapidly progressive transverse myelitis, a consideration in any patient with lower extremity neurologic symptoms plus bladder or bowel incontinence.

Proximal muscle weakness involving the upper arms and thighs can be seen in SLE patients as a result of concomitant inflammatory muscle disease. SLE patients are also at risk for steroid myopathy, which is typically much worse in the proximal lower extremities. Patients with myopathy generally present with significant muscle weakness rather than with muscle pain. They have difficulty in using their arms for over-the-shoulder tasks and difficulty in getting up from a chair or a low position as well as using stairs.

Physical Examination

A thorough physical examination is important in evaluating SLE patients, given the nature of their multisystem involvement (Table 160.2). Articular manifestations can present as painful, nonerosive symmetric synovitis. Patients who have had repeated bouts of arthritis in their hands can also develop Jaccoud arthropathy, which is clinically characterized by reversible joint deformities including swan-neck changes, thumb subluxations, ulnar deviation, and boutonnière and hallux valgus deformities along with an absence of articular erosions on plain radiographs (Fig. 160.1). In general, its prevalence is around 5% to 10%.

Table 160.2 Organ Involvement in Systemic Lupus Erythematosus

Mucocutaneous	Facial rashes including malar or butterfly rash, discoid rash, alopecia, photosensitivity, oral ulcerations
Musculoskeletal	Joint pain with or without swelling, morning stiffness, Jaccoud arthropathy, muscle weakness, muscle aches and pain, osteonecrosis
Serosal	Pleuritis, pericarditis, peritonitis
Cardiovascular	Myocarditis, sterile endocarditis Premature atherosclerosis Raynaud phenomenon, digital ulcers
Pulmonary	Pulmonary hypertension, interstitial lung disease, diffuse alveolar hemorrhage, shrinking lung syndrome, pulmonary embolism
Hematologic	Leukopenia, anemia, thrombocytopenia
Renal	Nephritis, nephrotic syndrome
Neuropsychiatric	Headaches, seizures, stroke, peripheral neuropathy, cranial neuropathy, transverse myelitis, psychosis, cognitive dysfunction

The skin is second only to the joints as the most frequently affected organ system, and skin disease is the second most common way that SLE initially is manifested clinically [2]. There are three major types of lupus-specific skin disease.

1. The typical malar or butterfly rash involves the cheeks and bridge of the nose. Photosensitive lupus dermatitis is generalized throughout sun-exposed areas.
2. Subacute cutaneous lupus erythematosus. This is a distinct clinical subset of SLE. It is characterized by recurrent, erythematous, photosensitive, nonscarring skin lesions in a characteristic distribution involving the face, trunk, and arms and by mild systemic disease. Anti-Ro/SSA antibodies are found in 63% to 90% of patients with subacute cutaneous lupus erythematosus [3]. The major anti-Ro/SSA response in subacute cutaneous lupus erythematosus is directed against the native 60-kDa Ro protein [4]. Many drugs can induce SLE skin reactions, including photosensitizers such as spironolactone, angiotensin-converting enzyme inhibitors, calcium channel blockers, and hydrochlorothiazide. The skin lesions begin between 4 and 20 months after the initiation of drugs, and the lesions typically improve 6 to 12 weeks after the offending drug is withdrawn [5].
3. Chronic cutaneous lupus erythematosus. The most common form is classic discoid lupus erythematosus (DLE). Clinical features of DLE are induration, scarring, pigment changes, follicular plugging, and hyperkeratosis. Involvement of hair follicles is a prominent clinical feature of DLE lesions. Typical DLE lesions occur most often on the face, scalp, ears, V-neck area of the neck, and extensor aspects of the arms. Scarring alopecia is often observed in patients with scalp involvement. Other forms of chronic cutaneous lupus erythematosus include lupus profundus or panniculitis, mucosal DLE, and chilblain lupus or lupus pernio.

There are generally two common types of alopecia in SLE patients: irreversible scarring alopecia due to persistent DLE activity on the scalp; and the more widespread and often reversible nonscarring focal areas of alopecia that are often present during periods of disease activity. Hair in areas of alopecia is dry and coarse with increased fragility, making it break easily. This is often prominent over the frontal hairline.

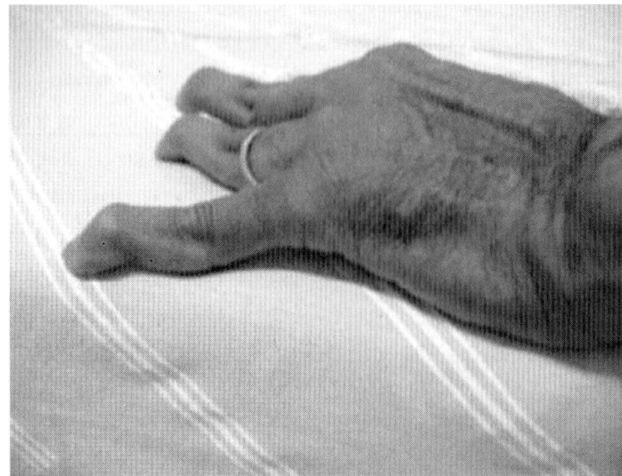

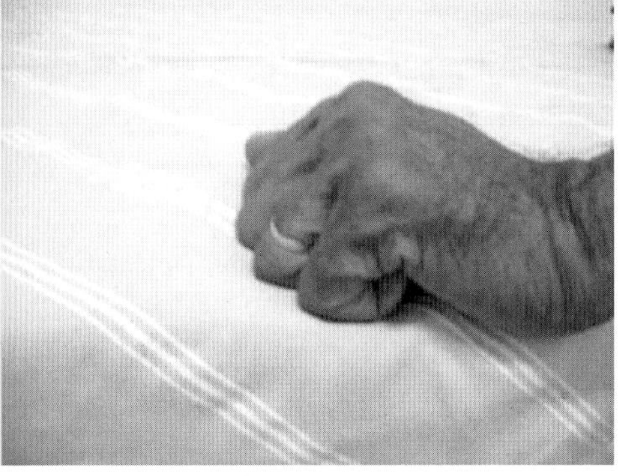

FIGURE 160.1 Reversible swan-neck deformities in a patient with SLE (Jaccoud arthropathy).

Because of the nature of painless oral ulceration in SLE, the lesions are often found by a physician on a thorough physical examination, and patients may not recognize them. In patients with inflammatory eye disease such as uveitis or retinitis, a careful examination by an ophthalmologist is needed.

Parotid gland enlargement, several dental cavities, very dry buccal mucosa, or oral thrush can be found in patients with secondary Sjögren syndrome. Oral thrush can also be found in patients who are treated with steroids.

Cardiac examination may reveal a pericardial rub or distant heart sounds in SLE patients with pericardial effusion from pericarditis. Heart murmurs due to noninfectious endocarditis can be detected in SLE patients. Split P_2, loud P_2, or right-sided heart heave may suggest pulmonary hypertension, a complication of SLE associated with a high mortality rate. Crackles can also be found in SLE patients from interstitial lung disease, which is treatable if it is detected early.

Splenomegaly is occasionally seen in SLE patients with or without overt hematologic complications of the disease. Focal neurologic deficits and altered mental status can be found in SLE patients with central nervous system involvement including central nervous system vasculitis or stroke from associated antiphospholipid antibody syndrome. The peripheral nervous system can also be involved in SLE patients, including peripheral stocking-glove neuropathies as well as mononeuritis due to vasculitis. In SLE patients with secondary Raynaud phenomenon, abnormal nail fold capillaries can be detected with the presentation of dilated, unorganized capillaries or dropout lesions. Digital ulcers may be evident, and they may be difficult to heal.

Functional Limitations

Because SLE can affect so many systems, disability is common, although it may be reversible once the disease is treated and in remission. However, there are many patients with a complicated course of illness resulting in joint deformity, muscle weakness, or deconditioning after prolonged illness. The functional limitations can be a major issue for these patients even if their acute disease is under control.

All forms of cutaneous lupus have a significant socioeconomic impact within the United States. It has been suggested that cutaneous lupus is the third most common cause of industrial disability from dermatologic disease, with 45% of cutaneous lupus patients experiencing some degree of vocational handicap [6].

Lupus is associated with the gradual development of cognitive dysfunction in a minority of patients. The presence of antiphospholipid antibody, hypertension, and stroke are key variables associated with cognitive impairment [7].

Fatigue is one of the most common complaints and can be debilitating. The cause of fatigue is most likely multifactorial. Many potential causes include cytokines associated with active inflammation, deconditioning from prolonged illness, sleep disturbances, sedentary lifestyle, anemia, hypothyroidism, depression, stress, and medications such as steroids and beta blockers. Fatigue symptoms from SLE may respond to steroids or antimalarial treatment in some cases. Fatigue does not always correlate with other evidence of disease activity. There is a strong association between fatigue and decreased exercise tolerance. In one study of women with SLE, the oxygen consumption kinetics was prolonged and the prolongation was accompanied by an increase in oxygen deficit. This may explain the performance fatigability in this group of patients [8].

Diagnostic Studies

The classification criteria (see Table 160.1) can be a useful guide in making the diagnosis. The diagnosis of SLE is made by the American College of Rheumatology criteria if four or more of the manifestations are present, either serially or simultaneously, during any interval of observation.

Specific laboratory findings include antinuclear antibodies (ANA), antiphospholipid antibodies, and complement levels (Table 160.3). The most characteristic laboratory finding in SLE is the presence of ANA, and a negative ANA titer makes a diagnosis of lupus extremely unlikely. Titers are typically 1:160 or higher. Whereas the ANA titer is very sensitive, it is not very specific; the false-positive rate in healthy controls varies from approximately 30% with ANA titers of 1:40 (high sensitivity, low specificity) to as little as 3% with ANA titers of 1:320 (low sensitivity, high specificity) [9]. On the other hand, anti–double-stranded DNA and anti-Smith antibodies are highly specific for SLE. Anti-Ro/SSA and anti-RNP antibodies can also be found in SLE patients. Complement levels, usually C3 and C4, tend to fall during periods of active disease, especially if there is renal involvement. If patients have venous or arterial thrombosis or recurrent second-trimester spontaneous abortions, tests for the lupus anticoagulant should be performed.

Nonspecific laboratory findings include leukopenia, anemia, and thrombocytopenia, which are present in many patients during periods of active disease. Anemia can often be due to chronic disease or iron deficiency. Less commonly, it can be Coombs-positive hemolytic anemia. Proteinuria and hematuria with an active urinary sediment including cellular or granular casts are typical in SLE patients with nephritis. Kidney function can be compromised, as evidenced by elevated creatinine concentration and abnormal electrolyte levels. Creatine kinase concentration can be elevated in SLE patients with muscle involvement. Inflammatory markers, including erythrocyte sedimentation rate and C-reactive protein level, are usually elevated in SLE patients with active disease.

Imaging testing is generally obtained in SLE patients with signs or symptoms concerning for organ-specific manifestations. Plain radiographs of involved joints may show evidence

Table 160.3 Laboratory Testing in Systemic Lupus Erythematosus

Autoantibody testing, including antinuclear antibody, antiphospholipid antibody, anti–double-stranded DNA antibody, and anti-Smith antibody
Complete blood count and differential counts
Complement C3 and C4
Urinalysis, spot urine protein and creatinine, or 24-hour urine collection for calculation of creatinine clearance and for quantitation of proteinuria
Erythrocyte sedimentation rate and C-reactive protein
Comprehensive metabolic profile
Creatine kinase

suggestive of inflammatory arthritis, such as periarticular osteopenia. Renal ultrasonography is useful to assess kidney size in patients with renal insufficiency, and magnetic resonance angiography is used to assess renal vein thrombosis in patients with the nephrotic syndrome. Chest radiography may be helpful in SLE patients with cough, chest pain, or shortness of breath as lupus can cause both interstitial and pleural disease. Echocardiography is obtained in cases of suspected pericardial involvement or cardiac disease as well as to assess pulmonary artery pressure. Computed tomography of the chest is useful in SLE patients with interstitial lung disease, and a computed tomography scan of the abdomen may be considered in the evaluation of abdominal pain, especially when pancreatitis is suspected. Magnetic resonance imaging of the brain or spinal cord can give evidence that suggests a cause of focal neurologic deficits or cognitive dysfunction in SLE patients. In vasculitis, angiography may be valuable. When osteonecrosis is suspected, magnetic resonance imaging of joints is helpful. Musculoskeletal ultrasonography has been reported as a useful tool for assessment and defining of complications of joint and tendon in SLE patients [10].

In some cases, in addition to clinical and laboratory findings, the diagnosis of SLE is made by surgical pathology, such as skin or kidney biopsy showing characteristics strongly suggestive of SLE. Interface dermatitis with immune complexes at the dermal-epidermal junction is characteristic of lupus skin biopsy specimens. Immunofluorescent staining of kidney biopsy specimens from SLE patients commonly reveals "full-house staining" of immunoglobulin G, immunoglobulin M, immunoglobulin A, C3, and C1q.

Treatment

Treatment of SLE must be personalized for each patient by the extent of organ involvement. The purpose of treatment focuses on inducing remission, maintaining normal function, and preventing damage. Corticosteroid therapy is used in SLE at various dosages according to the severity of the disease. With serious organ involvement, such as kidney, lung, or central nervous system disease, cyclophosphamide therapy is commonly given along with corticosteroids. Other agents, such as azathioprine, mycophenolate mofetil, leflunomide, rituximab, abatacept, intravenous immune globulin, and interferon alfa blockade, have been used in SLE.

Treatment of cutaneous lupus includes nonpharmacologic and pharmacologic approaches. Nonpharmacologic treatments are photoprotection from both ultraviolet A and B rays, smoking cessation, and avoidance of trauma to the skin (such as tattoos or tanning beds). Pharmacologic treatments include topical and systemic medications. Topical corticosteroids, intralesional corticosteroids, topical calcineurin inhibitors, and topical retinoids have been recommended in cutaneous lupus. The most common systemic medication used in cutaneous lupus is hydroxychloroquine. The combination of hydroxychloroquine and quinacrine or of chloroquine and quinacrine is an alternative when patients do not respond well to hydroxychloroquine alone. Other medications, such as methotrexate, oral retinoids, dapsone, mycophenolate mofetil, and thalidomide, have been used in cutaneous lupus.

The treatment of Jaccoud arthropathy is conservative. Medical treatment is recommended with nonsteroidal anti-inflammatory drugs, low-dose corticosteroids, antimalarials, or methotrexate.

Hydroxychloroquine is effective for the amelioration of joint symptoms and for the prevention of clinical lupus relapse [11]. The dose is weight based at less than 6.5 mg/kg/day, which is generally 200 to 400 mg/day. The recommendations on eye screening for hydroxychloroquine or chloroquine retinopathy have been revised by the American Academy of Ophthalmology [12]. It is strongly recommended that all patients beginning hydroxychloroquine or chloroquine therapy have a baseline examination within the first year of starting the drug to document any complicating ocular conditions and to establish a record of the fundus appearance and functional status. Annual screening should be performed after 5 years of drug use in all patients. In patients with maculopathy or risk factors such as liver or renal disease or advanced age, annual screening should be performed from the initiation of therapy.

Belimumab is the first biologic agent approved for the treatment of SLE by the U.S. Food and Drug Administration. It is the first drug approved in 55 years after hydroxychloroquine and corticosteroids were approved in 1955 and aspirin was approved in 1948. Belimumab is a fully humanized recombinant immunoglobulin G1λ monoclonal antibody that inhibits the binding of soluble B-lymphocyte stimulator to B cells and hence prevents the survival and differentiation of selected B-cell subsets. It is for the treatment of adult patients with active, autoantibody-positive SLE with a high degree of disease activity despite receiving standard therapy. It is well tolerated and appears to be efficacious in the treatment of SLE, although it is not approved for treatment of lupus nephritis or neuropsychiatric lupus [13,14].

Rehabilitation

In lupus patients with fatigue, supervised graded exercise programs show an improvement in aerobic capacity, quality of life, and depression [15,16]. The beneficial effects disappeared on stopping of exercise.

In some early cases of avascular necrosis, reduced weight bearing, limitation of activities, or use of crutches can occasionally slow the damage and permit natural healing [17]. Range of motion exercises are helpful for maintaining joint function.

In SLE patients with pulmonary hypertension, interstitial lung disease, or cardiac disease, cardiopulmonary rehabilitation is important once the patients are clinically stable.

Procedures

In lupus patients with active synovitis, tendinitis, or bursitis, local corticosteroid injections are helpful and can sometimes be used in lieu of systemic corticosteroids.

Osteonecrosis or avascular necrosis of the hip is a progressive disease. The prevention of femoral head collapse is highly desirable in the young lupus patient. In early-stage disease, before femoral head collapse (Ficat and Arlet stages I to III), core decompression of the femoral head is currently the most widely used procedure to try to relieve intraosseous pressure in the femoral head and to restore blood supply (Table 160.4).

Table 160.4 Avascular Necrosis of Femoral Head Classification: Ficat and Arlet

Stage 0: preclinical or preradiologic	Normal findings on a plain radiograph in an asymptomatic patient with a positive diagnosis in the contralateral hip The magnetic resonance image shows a double-line sign, consistent with a necrotic process.
Stage I: preradiologic	Normal findings on radiographs and abnormal findings on magnetic resonance imaging or bone scintigraphy
Stage II: reparative stage	
Stage IIA	Radiographic changes are demineralization, patchy sclerosis in the superolateral aspect of the femoral head, and small cysts within the femoral head
Stage IIB	A transition phase characterized by the presence of the crescent sign, seen as a linear subcortical lucency situated immediately beneath the subcortical bone, representing a fracture line
Stage III	Flattened or collapsed femoral head
Stage IV	Progressive degenerative joint disease with severe collapse and destruction of the femoral head, joint space narrowing, and osteophyte and subchondral cyst formation

Surgery

Lupus patients are prone to spontaneous tendon ruptures, including the Achilles tendon, the patellar tendon, and the long tendons of the hands. Early surgical repair is usually the treatment of choice.

In severe avascular necrosis of hips, knees, or shoulders, arthroplasty is required. Studies of the natural history of the disease suggest that femoral head collapse occurs within 2 to 3 years of the first symptoms, and at that stage arthroplasty is the most reliable treatment option. The outcome of hip arthroplasty showed an overall survival probability of 94.6% at 5 years and of 81.8% at 9 years with minimal perioperative morbidity [18]. Besides standard total hip arthroplasty, bipolar hemiarthroplasty, limited femoral resurfacing, and metal-on-metal resurfacing are alternatives. Because of the incidence of gluteal and groin pain and migration, total hip arthroplasty is a better procedure than bipolar hemiarthroplasty for patients with Ficat stage III osteonecrosis of the femoral head [19].

Potential Disease Complications

Jaccoud Arthropathy

This arthropathy may compromise hand function and is also a risk factor for tendon rupture [20].

Increased Risk of Infection

Although SLE patients are often leukopenic, they typically can mobilize white blood cells normally, so that SLE patients not receiving immunosuppressive therapy do not have a significantly increased risk of infection. However, patients receiving corticosteroids and other immunosuppressives are at increased risk of opportunistic infections. In anticipation of the need for immunosuppression, SLE patients should receive appropriate immunizations including pneumococcal and influenza vaccines. Live vaccines, such as the herpes zoster vaccine, should not be given to patients receiving immunosuppressive agents.

Hypertension

Hypertension can be seen in SLE patients with lupus nephritis and should be treated aggressively, preferably to 130/80 mm Hg or lower.

Premature Atherosclerosis

It has been recognized that premature coronary artery disease is a major cause of illness and death in SLE patients. Coronary atherosclerosis is much more prevalent among patients with lupus than in the general population and cannot be predicted by the measurement of traditional risk factors or markers of disease activity [21]. Many factors influence this process, including dysfunctional immune regulation, inflammation, traditional risk factors, defective endothelial cell function, and vascular repair as well the therapeutic used to treat the underlying autoimmune disease. SLE-specific factors including disease activity, disease duration, damage, and proinflammatory high-density lipoprotein could also contribute to increased atherosclerotic risk [22].

Potential Treatment Complications

The potential side effects and toxicities of hydroxychloroquine are retinal toxicity, hyperpigmented skin lesions, myopathy with vacuolization on muscle biopsy, and cardiomyopathy (Table 160.5).

Table 160.5 Potential Treatment Complications

Treatment	Complication
Nonsteroidal anti-inflammatory drugs	Dyspepsia, peptic ulcer, gastrointestinal bleeding, platelet dysfunction, renal insufficiency, hepatotoxicity, aseptic meningitis
Glucocorticoids	Cushingoid appearance, weight gain, fluid retention, acne, hypertension, diabetes, cataracts, glaucoma, avascular necrosis, osteoporosis, impaired wound healing, increased susceptibility to infection
Antimalarials	Retinopathy, abnormal skin pigmentation, neuromyopathy, cardiomyopathy
Cyclophosphamide	Myelosuppression, hemorrhagic cystitis, bladder cancer, infertility, alopecia
Azathioprine	Myelosuppression, hepatotoxicity, pancreatitis
Methotrexate	Myelosuppression, hepatotoxicity, mucositis, alopecia, pneumonitis
Mycophenolate mofetil	Myelosuppression, dyspepsia, diarrhea

References

[1] Chien JW, Lin CY, Yang LY. Correlation between anti-Ro/LA titers and clinical findings of patients with systemic lupus erythematosus. Zhonghua Yi Xue Za Zhi (Taipei) 2001;64:283–91.

[2] Cervera R, Khamashta MA, Font J, et al. Systemic lupus erythematosus: clinical and immunologic patterns of disease expression in a cohort of 1,000 patients. Medicine (Baltimore) 1993;72:113–24.

[3] Gilliam JN, Sontheimer RD. Distinctive cutaneous subsets in the spectrum of lupus erythematosus. J Am Acad Dermatol 1981;4:471–5.

[4] Lopez-Longo FJ, Monteagudo I, Gonzalez CM, et al. Systemic lupus erythematosus: clinical expression and anti-Ro/SSA. A response in patients with and without lesions of subacute cutaneous lupus. Lupus 1997;6:32–9.

[5] Srivastava M, Rencic A, Diglio G, et al. Drug-induced, Ro/SSA-positive cutaneous lupus erythematosus. Arch Dermatol 2003;139:45–9.

[6] O'Quinn S, Cole J, Many H. Problems of disability in patients with chronic skin diseases. Arch Dermatol 1972;105:35–40.

[7] Murray SG, Yazdany J, Kaiser R, et al. Cardiovascular disease and cognitive dysfunction in systemic lupus erythematosus. Arthritis Care Res (Hoboken) 2012;64:1328–33.

[8] Keyser RE, Rus V, Mikdashi JA, et al. Exploratory study on oxygen consumption on-kinetics during treadmill walking in women with systemic lupus erythematosus. Arch Phys Med Rehabil 2010;91:1402–9.

[9] Tan EM, Feltkamp TE, Smolen JS, et al. Range of antinuclear antibodies in "healthy" individuals. Arthritis Rheum 1997;40:1601.

[10] Gabba A, Piga M, Vacca A, et al. Joint and tendon involvement in systemic lupus erythematosus: an ultrasound study of hands and wrists in 108 patients. Rheumatology (Oxford) 2012;51:2278–85.

[11] Wallace DJ. Antimalarial agents and lupus. Rheum Dis Clin North Am 1994;20:243.

[12] Marmor F, Kellner U, Lai TY, et al. Revised recommendations on screening for chloroquine and hydroxychloroquine retinopathy. Ophthalmology 2011;118:415–22.

[13] Furie R, Petri M, Zamani O, et al. A phase III, randomized, placebo-controlled study of belimumab, a monoclonal antibody that inhibits B lymphocyte stimulator, in patients with systemic lupus erythematosus. Arthritis Rheum 2011;63:3918–30.

[14] Boyce EG, Fusco BE. Belimumab: review of use in systemic lupus erythematosus. Clin Ther 2012;34:1006–22.

[15] Tench CM, McCarthy J, McCurdie I, et al. Fatigue in systemic lupus erythematosus: a randomized controlled trial of exercise. Rheumatology (Oxford) 2003;42:1050–4.

[16] Carvalho MR, Sato EI, Tebexreni AS, et al. Effects of supervised cardiovascular training program on exercise tolerance, aerobic capacity, and quality of life in patients with systemic lupus erythematosus. Arthritis Care Res (Hoboken) 2005;53:838–44.

[17] Schoenstadt A. Avascular necrosis, http://bones.emedtv.com/avascular-necrosis.html

[18] Huo MH, Salvati EA, Browne MG, et al. Primary total hip arthroplasty in systemic lupus erythematosus. J Arthroplasty 1992;7:51–6.

[19] Lee SB, Sugano N, Nakata K, et al. Comparison between bipolar hemiarthroplasty and THA for osteonecrosis of the femoral head. Clin Orthop Relat Res 2004;424:161–5.

[20] Alves EM, Macieira JC, Borba E, et al. Spontaneous tendon rupture in systemic lupus erythematosus: association with Jaccoud's arthropathy. Lupus 2010;19:247–54.

[21] Asanuma Y, Oeser A, Shintani AK, et al. Premature coronary-artery atherosclerosis in systemic lupus erythematosus. N Engl J Med 2003;349:2407–15.

[22] Skaggs BJ, Hahn BH, McMahon M. Accelerated atherosclerosis in patients with SLE—mechanisms and management. Nat Rev Rheumatol 2012;8:214–23.

CHAPTER 161

Transverse Myelitis

Peter A.C. Lim, MD

Synonyms

Transverse myelitis
Acute transverse myelitis
Idiopathic transverse myelitis
Myelitis
Acute myelopathy

ICD-9 Codes

323.9	**Unspecified cause of encephalitis**
344.11	**Chronic paraplegia**
344.12	**Acute paraplegia**

ICD-10 Codes

G04.90	**Encephalitis, and encephalomyelitis, unspecified**
G04.91	**Myelitis, unspecified**
G82.20	**Paraplegia, unspecified**
G82.21	**Paraplegia, complete**
G82.22	**Paraplegia, incomplete**
G82.50	**Quadriplegia, unspecified**
G82.51	**Quadriplegia, C1-C4 complete**
G82.52	**Quadriplegia, C1-C4 incomplete**
G82.53	**Quadriplegia, C5-C7 complete**
G82.54	**Quadriplegia, C5-C7 incomplete**

Definition

Transverse myelitis is a focal inflammation across the spinal cord along one or more levels. This inflammation can cause damage to the ensheathing nerve cell fiber myelin, with resultant nervous system dysfunction [1]. The diagnosis may incorporate the terms *acute,* meaning arising suddenly and intensely, and *idiopathic,* in which no specific bacterial, viral, or other obvious inflammatory cause can be found. Other descriptors include *acute partial, acute complete,* and *longitudinally extensive.* Few population-based studies are available, and comparative or meta-analysis of the literature is difficult because of the different presentations of transverse myelitis being reported. It appears, however, that acute transverse myelitis is rare, with only 1400 new cases annually in the United States, or 1 to 4 cases per million population per year [1,2].

An older study from 1993 in the United States on acute or subacute noncompressive myelopathy showed these cases to be 45% parainfectious, 21% multiple sclerosis, 12% spinal cord ischemia, and 21% idiopathic [3]. With the availability of improved diagnostic tools, possible changes in disease patterns, and longer follow-up, the etiology of transverse myelitis may be clearer. A 2012 study from France on acute partial transverse myelitis with a median follow-up period of 104.8 months reported the etiology of cases as 62% multiple sclerosis, 1% postinfectious myelitis, 1% neuromyelitis optica, 1% Sjögren syndrome, and 34% undetermined (i.e., idiopathic) [4]. However, another French multicenter retrospective study applying the Transverse Myelitis Consortium Working Group criteria [2] for acute transverse myelitis to 288 subjects was more evenly spread. It reported the etiology as 20.5% systemic disease (systemic lupus erythematosus, Sjögren syndrome, antiphospholipid syndrome), 18.8% spinal cord infarct, 10.8% multiple sclerosis, 17.3% infectious or parainfectious, 17% neuromyelitis optica, and 15.6% idiopathic acute transverse myelitis [5].

There is a female predominance of 60% to 75% [4–9] and a bimodal age distribution. Patients having transverse myelitis related to multiple sclerosis, postinfectious transverse myelitis, or idiopathic transverse myelitis are younger, whereas those with transverse myelitis related to spinal cord infarcts or delayed radiation effects are older [4,6,8,10]. Transverse myelitis may recur, with reported rates ranging from 17.5% [9] to 61% [8], and relapse appears to be more common with acute partial transverse myelitis [11].

According to one magnetic resonance imaging (MRI) study, idiopathic acute transverse myelitis most commonly affects the cervical region (60%), followed by the thoracic region (33%) [5]. The onset of transverse myelitis can be acute (within hours or days) or subacute (between 1 and 4 weeks) [1,3]. The period from onset to complete weakness in idiopathic transverse myelitis has been reported to range from 10 hours to 28 days, with a mean of 5 days [10]. Subacute presentations, progressing over days to weeks and ascending, are associated with a good to fair prognosis. Acute and catastrophic presentations with back pain have a poorer outcome [12].

Symptoms

Patients with transverse myelitis may present in the ambulatory clinic or hospital setting with complaints of weakness of the arms and legs, pain, sensory impairments, or difficulties with the bowel and bladder. Weakness may affect the lower limbs or all four limbs with varying severity. Sensory complaints may include hypersensitivity, numbness, tingling, coldness, or burning. Pain is a common symptom in a third to one half of patients and may be localized or shooting in character. Bowel frequency or constipation may occur, and bladder symptoms include increased frequency, retention, and incontinence [1,10].

The history may reveal symptoms of recent infection, immunocompromised or autoimmune condition, space-occupying lesion, demyelinating disease, travel, vaccination, trauma, sexual exposure, animal bites, and insect or tick bites. A careful review may yield systemic symptoms, including the upper respiratory tract with cough and difficulty in breathing, chest pain, rashes, joint aches, muscle pain, vision changes, nausea, diarrhea, constipation, and problems with urinary function. Particular attention should be paid to details pointing toward potentially treatable or reversible conditions responsive to antimicrobials or surgical decompression.

Any history of invasive spinal intervention for pain management should be explored. Cases of acute paraplegia with sensory, bowel, and bladder dysfunction have been reported after epidural steroid injections and lumbosacral nerve root blocks. Inadvertent direct cord injury may occur, or a vascular injury resulting in cord infarction may be the cause [13–15]. Damage to an abnormally low artery of Adamkiewicz as it travels with the nerve root through the neural foramen has been postulated. This dominant radiculomedullary artery arises between T9 and L2 levels in 85% of people, but it may arise from the lower lumbar region to as low as S1 [15]. There has also been a report of transverse myelitis resulting from the infected catheter tip of an intrathecal morphine pump for chronic pain [12].

Physical Examination

The physical examination follows a thorough history taking and will focus on the manifestations and findings relating to myelopathy, such as motor weakness, changes in sensation (pinprick, light touch, vibration, position sense, or temperature), tone, muscle stretch reflexes, coordination, and bowel and bladder functioning. Changes affecting the brain, such as cognitive dysfunction and cranial nerve and visual abnormalities, are generally not seen with idiopathic transverse myelitis and suggest other diagnoses.

Temperature elevation, tachycardia, and tachypnea may indicate an infectious etiology. Infections and autoimmune conditions that cause acute inflammation of the spinal cord may also be manifested in the other body systems. The respiratory, cardiovascular, gastrointestinal, and genitourinary tracts as well as the musculoskeletal and integumentary systems should be assessed accordingly. The findings may assist in determining the level of spinal involvement, guide diagnostic testing for the myelitis, and help rule out other diagnoses.

Functional Limitations

The physiatrist is likely to encounter the patient as a consultation or referral for rehabilitation assessment and management or for specific problems, such as spasticity and pain intervention. As with other spinal cord injuries, the functional limitations in transverse myelitis usually depend on the level or levels of injury and the muscles that are affected or continue to be innervated normally. Debilitation and deconditioning from associated illnesses and prolonged recumbence will also affect function secondarily.

Recovery is often related to the clinical presentation and may or may not be complete. In general, one third of patients with acute transverse myelitis make a good recovery, another third have fair recovery, and the rest either fail to improve or die [5,7,10,16]. In idiopathic transverse myelitis treated with methylprednisolone, by use of the Medical Research Council (MRC) scale for muscle strength (5, normal; 0, no movement is observed), 37.5% were reported to have complete recovery or minimal residual deficit (MRC 5-4), 43% had partial recovery (MRC 3), and 19.4% had severe disability or absent recovery (MRC 0-2). Factors associated with poor outcomes include severe initial symptoms with spinal shock, delayed presentation to the hospital after maximum deficits have already occurred, development of syringomyelia, and extensive MRI lesions [5,10]. If no recovery has occurred by 1 to 3 months, complete recovery is less likely [3,12].

The following functional capability review according to spinal level may be influenced by whether the cord injury is unilateral or bilateral and the degree of completeness. A patient with only C4 innervation preserved and loss of function distally may or may not have respiratory difficulties but will be dependent for most self-care activities. Using appropriate technology and devices, whether they are customized or commercially available, the patient may be able to control the immediate home environment, summon assistance, and mobilize in an electric wheelchair with a chin control or a sip-and-puff interface. Devices that can be controlled by moving and positioning the head, cheek, or tongue and by infrared-sensitive or voice-activated mechanisms include door openers and various electronic devices such as the television and personal computer.

A patient with C5 level may be able to self-feed and groom with equipment such as a glove with universal cuff allowing attachment of tools (e.g., fork, spoon, or comb). The patient can independently use a powered wheelchair and propel a lightweight manual wheelchair with rim projections ("quad knobs") for limited distances over level ground. C6 innervation allows independence with upper extremity dressing, bathing with equipment, and functional use of a manual wheelchair indoors. The patient with superior balance and motor control could potentially perform independent or supervised transfers with a sliding board, self-catheterize with appropriate aids, and drive a specially adapted automatic transmission vehicle with powered steering, hand-controlled accelerator and brake. A C7 level allows independence in all self-care activities with equipment and independent transfers because of preserved ability to push off with the elbow extensors, and the patient may be able to live alone. A patient with C8 and T1 innervation will have improved manual dexterity and strength for self-care, is independent with a manual wheelchair, and should be able to self-catheterize.

The patient with preservation of upper thoracic innervation has a degree of trunk control that increases stability during use and propulsion of a manual wheelchair. It also adds to ease and independence with bladder and bowel self-management. With bracing of the hips, knees, and ankles (knee-ankle-foot orthoses), minimal ambulation can be attempted, although this would be more for encouragement and exercise purposes than truly functional. Independent ambulation even with bracing and bilateral axillary or forearm crutches is usually not realistic unless the patient has preservation of some upper lumbar innervation. Further preservation of lumbar and sacral innervation will increase ease of ambulation with better trunk and pelvic control. There have been developments in exoskeleton systems to assist standing and ambulation, such as the ReWalk (Argo Medical Technologies Inc., Marlborough, Mass) and Ekso (Ekso Bionics, Richmond, Calif), although these are currently still limited by the individual patient's abilities, terrain, and need for safety supervision. The patient with incomplete spinal injury is less predictable, and functional abilities will largely depend on the degree and nature of neurologic preservation.

Diagnostic Studies

With increasingly greater resolution, T1 versus T2 weighting, and other techniques to enhance and to suppress the appearance of tissues of different densities, the best tool when transverse myelitis is suspected is MRI. MRI not only allows visualization of the lesion but also helps rule out potentially treatable causes, such as tumor, abscess, and other lesions causing compressive myelopathy. Contrast material can be given to highlight lesions [17], and myelography may be considered if MRI is not available.

Although it is not definitive, there are MRI features that help differentiate transverse myelitis from other disorders, such as multiple sclerosis (Figs. 161.1 and 161.2). Transverse myelitis is more likely to have high signal intensity on T2-weighted images extending longitudinally over more segments [17,18]. The number of segments involved may be 1 or 2, to as many as 11. The entire cord or sometimes only the medulla may be affected [17–20]. In transverse myelitis, the lesion appears more likely to affect the central region of the cord and to involve more than two thirds of the cord diameter.

In multiple sclerosis, the lesion appears more peripheral and generally involves less than half of the diameter of the cord [17]. The lesion in transverse myelitis is more likely to resemble a spinal cord tumor, and biopsy may even be mistakenly performed [17,18]. MRI of the brain with contrast enhancement is often performed to help determine whether the patient's condition is a prelude to multiple sclerosis rather than "idiopathic" transverse myelitis. In idiopathic partial transverse myelitis, a study that does not show brain lesions translates to the likelihood of evolving multiple sclerosis at 15% to 44%. When brain lesions such as white matter plaques (especially periventricular) are seen, the chance for development of multiple sclerosis increases to 44% to 93% [21]. Asymmetric motor or sensory symptoms and absence of peripheral nervous system involvement at presentation suggest acute myelopathic multiple sclerosis, whereas symmetric symptoms and neurophysiologic evidence of peripheral nervous system involvement suggest acute transverse myelitis [22,23].

Immunoglobulin G antibodies may be useful for determining neuromyelitis optica as the etiology in patients with acute complete transverse myelitis. Longitudinally extensive transverse myelitis spanning three or more vertebral segments is an important feature of neuromyelitis optica, and detection of anti–aquaporin 4–specific antibodies (anti-AQP4) is useful to determine both increased risk for recurrence and conversion to neuromyelitis optica [11,24].

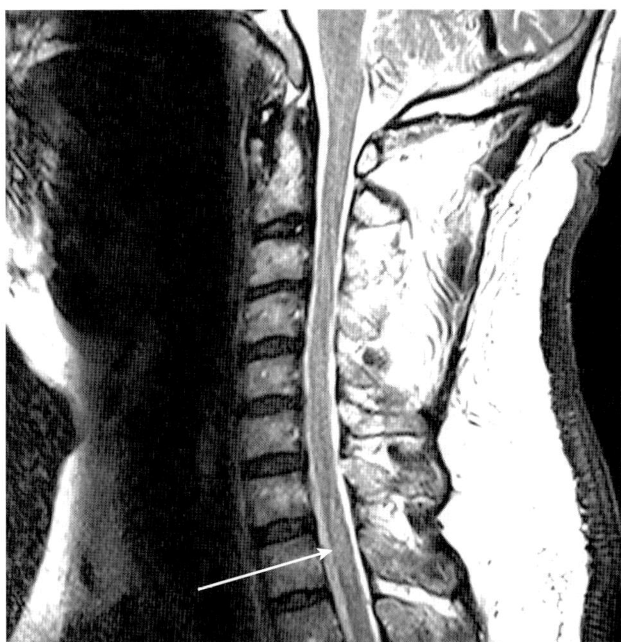

FIGURE 161.1 Myelitis: T2-weighted magnetic resonance image of the sagittal cervical spine with fusiform lesion at C7-T1 *(arrow)*.

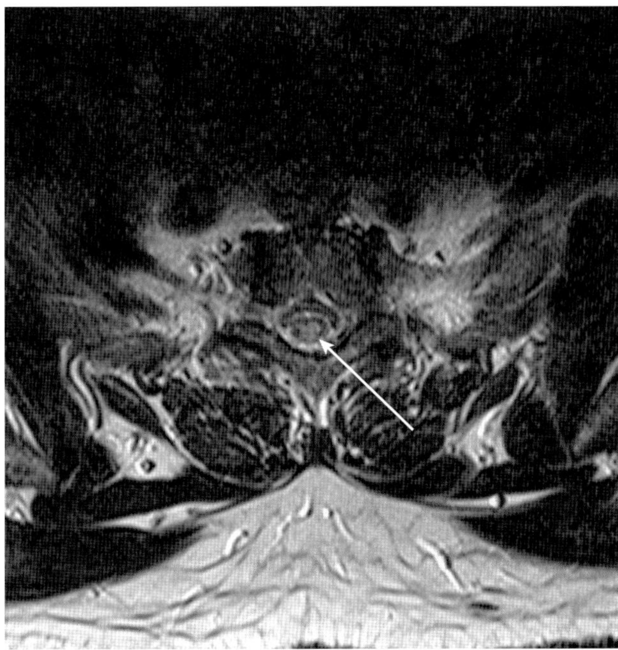

FIGURE 161.2 Myelitis: T2-weighted magnetic resonance image of the axial cervical spine showing lesion across most of the spinal cord *(arrow)*.

Other tests include blood counts and chemistry; tests for autoimmune conditions, such as antinuclear antibodies, anti–double-stranded DNA antibodies, anti-Sm antibodies, and erythrocyte sedimentation rate; SS-A antibody for Sjögren disease; immunoglobulin levels; and VDRL test.

Vitamin B_{12} levels may be tested, and *Mycoplasma pneumoniae* or *Mycobacterium* cultures may be performed. Lyme titers and titers for various viruses including human immunodeficiency virus, West Nile virus, poliovirus, hepatitis virus, Epstein-Barr virus, cytomegalovirus, and enteric cytopathic human orphan virus may be elevated.

A lumbar puncture allows the assessment of central nervous system pressure as well as obtains cerebrospinal fluid for cell count, determination of protein and glucose concentrations, measurement of immunoglobulins, and protein electrophoresis. Oligoclonal bands detected in the cerebrospinal fluid are useful in making a diagnosis. In one report, they were present in three of five patients with multiple sclerosis–associated transverse myelitis but in none of four patients with parainfectious transverse myelitis [3]. Vascular flow studies or clotting parameters may be needed if spinal hematoma, thrombosis, or vasculitis is suspected. Electrodiagnostic studies, including somatosensory and motor evoked potentials, may be useful for both diagnostic purposes and monitoring of treatment progress [25]. A urinary evaluation may include cystography, voiding cystourethrography, and cystoscopy. Baseline renal ultrasound and urodynamic evaluation have been recommended because of the very high rates of persistent long-term bladder dysfunction [26,27]. Bowel evaluation may require radiography, computed tomography, MRI, or colonoscopy to rule out obstruction.

In 2002, the Transverse Myelitis Consortium Working Group proposed the criteria in Table 161.1 for the diagnosis of idiopathic acute transverse myelitis [2].

A comparison by de Seze [6] of the clinical findings, MRI results, laboratory profiles, and outcomes of patients with acute myelopathy according to etiology is presented in Table 161.2.

Table 161.1 Criteria for the Diagnosis of Idiopathic Acute Transverse Myelitis

Inclusion Criteria	Exclusion Criteria
• Development of sensory, motor, or autonomic dysfunction attributable to the spinal cord • Bilateral signs or symptoms (although not necessarily symmetric) • Clearly defined sensory level • Exclusion of extra-axial compressive etiology by neuroimaging (MRI or myelography; CT of spine not adequate) • Inflammation within the spinal cord demonstrated by CSF pleocytosis or elevated IgG index or gadolinium enhancement. If no inflammatory criterion is met at symptom onset, repeated MRI and lumbar puncture evaluation between 2 and 7 days after symptom onset meet criteria. • Progression to nadir between 4 hours and 21 days after the onset of symptoms (if patient awakens with symptoms, symptoms must become more pronounced from point of awakening)	• History of previous radiation to the spine within the last 10 years • Clear arterial distribution clinical deficit consistent with thrombosis of the anterior spinal artery • Abnormal flow voids on the surface of the spinal cord consistent with AVM • Serologic or clinical evidence of connective tissue disease (e.g., sarcoidosis, Behçet disease, Sjögren syndrome, SLE, mixed connective tissue disorder)* • CNS manifestations of syphilis, Lyme disease, HIV, HTLV-1, mycoplasma, other viral infection (e.g., HSV-1, HSV-2, VZV, EBV, CMV, HHV-6, enteroviruses)* • Brain MRI abnormalities suggestive of multiple sclerosis* • History of clinically apparent optic neuritis*

*Do not exclude disease-associated acute transverse myelitis.

AVM, arteriovenous malformation; *CMV,* cytomegalovirus; *CNS,* central nervous system; *CSF,* cerebrospinal fluid; *CT,* computed tomography; *EBV,* Epstein-Barr virus; *HSV,* herpes simplex virus; *IgG,* immunoglobulin G; *HHV,* human herpes virus; *HIV,* human immunodeficiency virus; *HTLV-1,* human T-lymphotropic virus 1; *MRI,* magnetic resonance imaging; *SLE,* systemic lupus erythematosus; *VZV,* varicella-zoster virus.

Modified from Transverse Myelitis Consortium Working Group. Proposed diagnostic criteria and nosology of acute transverse myelitis. Neurology 2002;59:499-505.

Table 161.2 Comparison of Findings Based on Etiology [6]

Etiology	Findings	Prognosis
Multiple sclerosis	MRI: lesions small, localized in lateral or posterior cord, more cervical CSF: oligoclonal bands	Clinical outcome good but relapse in 47% at mean of 21 months
Systemic disease (SLE, Sjögren syndrome)	Severe motor and sphincter problems MRI in SLE: large and centromedullary lesions CSF: > 30 cells	Clinical outcome poor
Spinal cord infarct	No clear diagnostic criteria acutely; > 50 years old; severe motor and sphincter problems MRI: isolated centromedullary lesions CSF: absent or low cells, no oligoclonal bands	Outcome poor or fair in 91% of cases
Parainfectious myelopathy	Severe motor and sphincter problems MRI: large centromedullary lesions, cervicodorsal frequently CSF: > 30 cells, no oligoclonal bands Serologic confirmation rarely obtained	Clinical outcome good
Delayed radiation myelopathy	History of irradiation; delay can exceed 10 years MRI: high-intensity cord signals with focal swelling, follow-up cord atrophy CSF: normal	Clinical outcome good in early (10-16 weeks after) radiation myelopathy, poor in delayed
Unknown etiology	Long-term follow-up produces diagnosis in 50% of cases	

CSF, cerebrospinal fluid; *MRI,* magnetic resonance imaging; *SLE,* systemic lupus erythematosus.

Differential Diagnosis [1,3,8,13–17,19–21,28–30]

Demyelinating disease
Multiple sclerosis
Neuromyelitis optica (Devic disease)

POSTINFECTIOUS OR PARAINFECTIOUS
Viral: Epstein-Barr virus, herpes simplex, varicella-zoster, cytomegalovirus, human immunodeficiency virus, enteroviruses (poliovirus, coxsackievirus, enteric cytopathic human orphan virus, echovirus), mumps, adenovirus, rubella, measles, angiotropic large-cell lymphoma, leukemia virus, influenza, rabies, West Nile virus
Bacterial: Lyme borreliosis, syphilis, tuberculosis, pneumonia *(Mycoplasma pneumoniae),* cat-scratch disease *(Bartonella henselae),* histoplasmosis

AUTOIMMUNE
Systemic lupus erythematosus
Sjögren syndrome
Sarcoidosis
Behçet disease
Mixed connective tissue disease

SPINAL CORD ISCHEMIA OR INJURY
Space-occupying lesions: tumors, herniated nucleus pulposus, spinal abscess, hematoma, spinal stenosis
Vascular: atherosclerosis, thrombosis of spinal arteries, arteriovenous malformations, vasculitis in heroin abuse, iatrogenic

OTHERS
Idiopathic
Post-vaccination (measles, mumps, chickenpox, rabies)
Paraneoplastic syndrome

Treatment

Initial

Although the physiatrist may manage stable long-standing transverse myelitis on an outpatient basis, hospitalization may be necessary to monitor vital signs, to manage respiratory status and bowel or bladder complications, and to carry out diagnostic investigations, particularly during the acute presentation [26,31]. Abnormalities of the vital signs, such as tachypnea or tachycardia, may suggest impaired oxygenation or blood flow that may need to be managed urgently. The ability to provide antiviral agents, antibacterial agents, and surgical decompression may also be critical, depending on whether a specific cause has been identified.

Various medications have been tried for idiopathic transverse myelitis without clear success in changing the course. Intravenous methylprednisolone has been advocated to prevent further damage to the spinal cord as a result of swelling [19,20]. During the acute phase, it may lead to faster recovery and less disability, and it is well tolerated according to several small observational studies [21]. Cyclophosphamide exerts an immunosuppressive and immunomodulatory effect through suppression of cell-mediated and humoral immunity (i.e., on the T cells and B cells) [21]. Cyclophosphamide in combination with methylprednisolone has some success on lupus-related lesions [20,29]. However, there appears to be an absence of any beneficial effect of immunosuppressive drugs (cyclophosphamide, azathioprine, intravenous immune globulin) in patients with idiopathic acute transverse myelitis [5]. Plasma exchange to remove autoreactive antibodies and other toxic molecules from plasma can be effective, especially within 20 days of onset, to increase chances of a good clinical response [21].

Rehabilitation

Rehabilitation is a crucial component of the treatment for any spinal cord injury, and the more affected or severe cases of transverse myelitis will require a comprehensive multidisciplinary rehabilitation program led by a physiatrist. Physical and occupational therapists on the team can work with patients on strengthening, endurance, balance, coordination, joint range of motion, reconditioning, mobility, and independence with activities of daily living. If pain is present, appropriate medications and heat, cold, and electrical modalities including transcutaneous electrical stimulation may be helpful.

An orthotist can improve mobility with bracing devices such as an ankle-foot orthosis or knee-ankle-foot orthosis. An assessment for appropriate equipment, such as wheelchair, and other assistive and walking devices, is needed. Education of the patient and family about the disease, resultant impairments, potential complications, and plans and prognosis for rehabilitation is important. The psychological state of the patient should not be neglected, and there should be monitoring for depression. Discharge planning needs and issues potentially affecting the patient's community reintegration should be assessed.

Transverse myelitis may or may not be a transient condition. Recovery may occur, and it is important to minimize the effects of even temporary denervation. All muscles and joints should be kept as active as possible, and having the joints go through a full range of motion daily will help prevent contractures. Passive and active exercises at all times and electrical stimulation are methods to keep muscles as flexible and strong as possible. If respiration is compromised, exercises for muscles of inspiration may be started, glossopharyngeal breathing may need to be taught, and electrical stimulation of the diaphragm may need to be considered [31].

Spasticity is a possible complication as with other upper motor neuron lesions. Regular stretching and use of antispasticity medications, such as baclofen, diazepam, and tizanidine, can minimize and decrease development of joint contractures. An antiepileptic drug (e.g., gabapentin) can also have a degree of antispasticity effect. Checking the skin thoroughly on a daily basis can potentially avoid skin breakdown and associated infections. Insensate areas of high pressure should be relieved with special cushions and mattresses, such as egg crate foam and alternating pressure overlays, and pressure-relieving ankle-foot orthoses may be helpful.

Bladder and bowel programs should be started immediately because a neglected neurogenic bowel or bladder may lead to stool obstruction or kidney damage. An indwelling catheter can initially be used for bladder drainage, but intermittent catheterization, independently or otherwise, is commonly instituted whenever possible. Long-term follow-up of 2 to 10 years in pediatric patients with transverse myelitis has shown that residual bladder dysfunction is common even with improvement of paraparesis and lack of urologic symptoms. In one study, 86% had persistent bladder dysfunction and 77% had persistent bowel dysfunction [27].

A bowel program includes adequate fluids, proper diet, activity, and scheduled bowel movements. Upper motor neuron bowels may need a stool softener (e.g., docusate), osmotic laxative (lactulose), or stimulant laxative (senna or bisacodyl) for evacuation. Digital stimulation of the rectum is often effective and needs to be taught. With areflexic lower motor neuron bowels, use of bulk laxatives like psyllium or methylcellulose to obtain formed stools may help during digital manual evacuation. Bowel training is often started on a daily basis in the hospital, but the frequency can be extended to every 2 or 3 days once an individual returns home.

Individuals who require assistive devices for mobility must be trained in use of a wheelchair, walker, crutches, or cane, including maneuvering over steps and curbs. If transfers and ambulation require assistance, training of family members or assistants becomes crucial.

For patients with transverse myelitis at the cervical level, various types of equipment and temporary or permanent orthoses can be provided to help with self-care activities. Proper bathroom equipment and modifications, such as a tub bench, commode, hand-held shower, raised toilet seat, and grab bars, may make the difference between dependence and independence. Selection of appropriate aids is essential to maximize function, and many are expensive. Timing of these purchases may need to be carefully considered in this possibly transient condition. Despite a reasonable prognosis for eventual recovery, inaction may result in secondary complications, and it is important to keep an individual as functionally independent and active as possible throughout the entire recovery period.

Procedures

Procedures in transverse myelitis are determined by which systems are affected by the spinal cord injury. Renal ultrasound and urodynamic evaluations are relatively routine procedures for these patients to assess and monitor bladder dysfunction. Intramuscular botulinum toxin injections or alcohol or phenol nerve and motor point blocks may be needed for spastic limb muscles. An intrathecal baclofen pump may be effective in intractable cases and allows much smaller doses and concomitantly fewer side effects. Other procedures include implantation of diaphragmatic electrodes (phrenic nerve stimulation) when respiratory muscles have been affected. Some patients receive functional electrical stimulation systems to help maintain fitness or to increase hand and ambulatory function. Although not routinely done presently, anterior sacral root stimulation may be effective for bladder management.

Surgery

There is no specific curative surgical procedure for idiopathic transverse myelitis. However, when there are compressive abnormalities such as abscess, herniated nucleus pulposus, spinal stenosis, and tumor, surgery may be needed as soon as possible to relieve pressure on the spinal cord. Timely management of compressive lesions may reverse neurologic injury to the cord or at the least stop further injury.

Secondary complications from spinal cord dysfunction may require surgical intervention. These include skin breakdown, accidental injury including fractures from lack of sensation in muscles and joints, development of kidney stones, and infections. Tendon transfers may be considered at a later stage to increase an individual's functioning. Nerve transfer in patients with permanent upper limb deficits may be considered to restore or to improve ability to voluntarily activate a muscle. In a recent case report, a child who underwent multiple fascicle transfers from median and ulnar nerves to the musculocutaneous nerve, spinal accessory to suprascapular nerve, and medial cord to axillary nerve had excellent recovery of elbow flexion. However, shoulder abduction had improved only minimally after 22 months [32].

Potential Disease Complications

Potential disease complications resulting from spinal cord injury with its attendant sequelae are generally similar irrespective of the etiology. A common complication is pressure ulcer of the skin if pressure relief is not done regularly. Awareness of and monitoring for deep venous thrombosis and pulmonary embolism should be routine. There may be varying degrees of respiratory muscle weakness, and when it is severe, mechanical ventilation assistance may be required. Patients are at increased risk for pneumonia or sleep apnea from the illness, compounded by any sedating medications or respiration-depressing narcotics given.

Spasticity and joint contractures may result over time. Heterotopic ossification may surround a joint, further promoting contractures. Gastrointestinal complications may begin with an acute ileus followed by chronic constipation. Urinary tract infections are common because retained urine and instrumentation both increase the likelihood of infection. Autonomic dysreflexia may occur, especially for lesions above T6. Pain, a frequent complaint after spinal cord injury, is often attributed to either musculoskeletal sources or a "central" or neurogenic pain mechanism and in some studies affects more than 90% of individuals. Treatment initiated for this pain includes tricyclic antidepressants, anticonvulsants, analgesics, nonsteroidal anti-inflammatory drugs, or short courses of cyclooxygenase-2 inhibitors. Depression and anxiety may occur and usually respond to supportive counseling but may need antidepressants such as the selective serotonin reuptake inhibitor or the serotonin-norepinephrine reuptake inhibitor drugs.

Overuse syndromes can result because muscles and joints are commonly stressed in trying to maintain or to learn new functions. Shoulder pain is a prominent issue, and the problems of tendinitis, arthritis, rotator cuff tear, impingement, and contracture must be properly identified and managed or rehabilitated. Steroid and local anesthetic injections in the joint may sometimes be needed, but use of proper transfer techniques or specific adaptive equipment is often helpful. Pressure from prolonged resting on superficial nerves can also cause pain or weakness. There may be difficulty with reproduction and fertility problems in the younger patients, and sexuality issues and solutions should be addressed or referred to a specialist.

Potential Treatment Complications

Treatment complications may result from side effects of medications and equipment required to treat the disease manifestations. Skin complications may result from ill-fitting devices or poorly applied dressings. Strictures or tracheal inflammation can result from tracheostomy tubes; if mechanical ventilation is required, failure of equipment can result in hypoxia or worse. Respiratory infections occur frequently with prolonged mechanical ventilation in high tetraplegia. High-dose steroids used to treat initial inflammation may cause gastritis, ulceration, or hemorrhage in the gastrointestinal tract. Deep venous thrombosis prophylaxis and anticoagulant treatment may result in or exacerbate bleeding tendencies. Catheterization may cause urinary tract infections or false passages in the urethra, making further catheterization difficult, with possible development of strictures. If bowel programs are not well managed, anal irritation may go on to skin maceration and breakdown around the sacral region.

Acknowledgment

Deborah Reiss Schneider, MD, for the chapter in the first edition on which this is based.

References

[1] National Institute of Neurological Disorders and Stroke. Transverse myelitis fact sheet, http://www.ninds.nih.gov/disorders/transverse-myelitis/detail_transversemyelitis.htm; [accessed October 2012].

[2] Transverse Myelitis Consortium Working Group. Proposed diagnostic criteria and nosology of acute transverse myelitis. Neurology 2002;59:499–505.

[3] Jeffery DR, Mandler RN, Davis LE. Transverse myelitis: retrospective analysis of 33 cases, with differentiation of cases associated with multiple sclerosis and parainfectious events. Arch Neurol 1993;50:532–5.

[4] Bourre B, Zephir H, Ongagna JC, et al. Long-term follow-up of acute partial transverse myelitis. Arch Neurol 2012;69:357–62.

[5] de Seze J, Lanctin C, Lebrun C, et al. Idiopathic acute transverse myelitis: application of the recent diagnostic criteria. Neurology 2005;65:1950–3.

[6] de Seze, Stojkovic T, Breteau G, et al. Acute myelopathies: clinical, laboratory and outcome profiles in 79 cases. Brain 2001;124:1509–21.

[7] Sepulveda M, Blanco Y, Rovira A, et al. Analysis of prognostic factors associated with longitudinally extensive transverse myelitis [published online ahead of print October 4, 2012]. Mult Scler 2013;19:742–8. http://www.ncbi.nlm.nih.gov/pubmed/23037550, Accessed October 9, 2012.

[8] Alvarenga MP, Thuler LC, Neto SP, et al. The clinical course of idiopathic acute transverse myelitis in patients from Rio de Janeiro. J Neurol 2010;257:992–8.

[9] Chaves M, Rojas JI, Patrucco L, Crsitiano E. Acute transverse myelitis in Buenos Aires, Argentina. A retrospective cohort study of 8 years follow-up. Neurologia 2012;27:348–53.

[10] Shahbaz NN, Amanat S, Soomro S, et al. Idiopathic transverse myelitis: an experience in a tertiary care setup. J Dow University Health Sciences Karachi 2012;6:12–6.

[11] Scott TF, Frohman EM, de Seze J, et al. Evidence-based guideline: clinical evaluation and treatment of transverse myelitis: report of the Therapeutics and Technology Assessment Subcommittee of the American Academy of Neurology. Neurology 2011;77:2128–34.

[12] Ropper AH, Poskanzer DC. The prognosis of acute and subacute transverse myelopathy based on early signs and symptoms. Ann Neurol 1978;4:451–9.

[13] Glaser SE, Falco F. Paraplegia following a thoracolumbar transforaminal epidural steroid injection. Pain Physician 2005;8:309–14.

[14] Tripathi M, Nath SS, Gupta RK. Paraplegia after intracord injection during attempted epidural steroid injection in an awake patient. Anesth Analg 2005;101:1209–11.

[15] Houten JK, Errico TJ. Paraplegia after lumbosacral nerve root block: report of three cases. Spine J 2002;2:70–5.

[16] Berman M, Feldman S, Alter M, et al. Acute transverse myelitis: incidence and etiological considerations. Neurology 1981;31:966–71.

[17] Murthy JM, Reddy JJ, Meena AK, Kaul S. Acute transverse myelitis: MR characteristics. Neurol India 1999;47:290–3.

[18] Bakshi R, Kinkel PR, Mechtler LL, et al. Magnetic resonance imaging findings in 22 cases of myelitis: comparison between patients with and without multiple sclerosis. Eur J Neurol 1998;5:35–48.

[19] Manabe Y, Sasaki C, Warita H, et al. Sjögren's syndrome with acute transverse myelopathy as the initial manifestation. J Neurol Sci 2000;176:158–61.

[20] Kovacs B, Lafferty TL, Brent LH, et al. Transverse myelopathy in systemic lupus erythematosus: an analysis of 14 cases and review of the literature. Ann Rheum Dis 2000;59:120–4.

[21] Awad A, Stuve O. Idiopathic transverse myelitis and neuromyelitis optica: clinical profiles, pathophysiology and therapeutic choices. Curr Neuropharmacol 2011;9:417–28.

[22] Scott TF, Bhagavatula K, Snyder PJ, Chieffe C. Transverse myelitis. Comparison of spinal cord presentations of multiple sclerosis. Neurology 1998;50:429–33.

[23] Harzheim M, Schlegel U, Urbach H, et al. Discriminatory features of acute transverse myelitis: a retrospective analysis of 45 patients. J Neurol Sci 2004;217:217–23.

[24] Chang KH, Lyu RK, Chen CM, et al. Distinct features between longitudinally extensive transverse myelitis presenting with and without anti-aquaporin 4 antibodies [published online ahead of print July 24, 2012]. Mult Scler 2013;19:299–307. http://www.ncbi.nlm.nih.gov/pubmed/22829325 [accessed 09.10.12].

[25] Kalita J, Guptar PM, Misra UK. Clinical and evoked potential changes in acute transverse myelitis following methyl prednisolone. Spinal Cord 1999;37:658–62.

[26] Cheng W, Chiu R, Tam P. Residual bladder dysfunction 2 to 10 years after acute transverse myelitis. J Paediatr Child Health 1999;35:476–8.

[27] Tanaka ST, Stone AR, Kurzrock EA. Transverse myelitis in children: long-term urological outcomes. J Urol 2006;175:1865–8.

[28] Ubogu EE, Lindenberg JR, Werz MA. Transverse myelitis associated with *Acinetobacter baumanii* intrathecal pump catheter-related infection. Reg Anesth Pain Med 2003;28:470–4.

[29] Neumann-Andersen G, Lindgren S. Involvement of the entire spinal cord and medulla oblongata in acute catastrophic-onset transverse myelitis in SLE. Clin Rheumatol 2000;19:156–60.

[30] Muranjan MN, Deshmukh CT. Acute transverse myelitis due to spinal epidural hematoma—first manifestation of severe hemophilia. Indian Pediatr 1999;36:1151–3.

[31] Alba AS. Concepts in pulmonary rehabilitation. In: Braddom RL, editor. Physical medicine and rehabilitation. 2nd ed. Philadelphia: WB Saunders; 2000. p. 687–701.

[32] Dorsi MJ, Belzberg AJ. Nerve transfers for restoration of upper extremity motor function in a child with upper extremity deficits due to transverse myelitis: case report. Microsurgery 2012;32:64–7.

CHAPTER 162

Traumatic Brain Injury

David T. Burke, MD, MA

Di Cui, MD

Synonyms

Head injury
Acquired brain injury
Concussion
Diffuse axonal injury

ICD-9 Codes

854.0 Intracranial injury of other and unspecified nature without mention of open intracranial wound
854.1 Intracranial injury of other and unspecified nature with open intracranial wound
907.0 Late effect of intracranial injury without mention of skull fracture

ICD-10 Codes

S06.2X0-8 Diffuse traumatic brain injury (sixth digit will define the level of consciousness)
S06.2X9 Diffuse traumatic brain injury with loss of consciousness of unspecified duration
S06.300-389 Focal traumatic brain injury (fifth digit will define the location of injury, sixth digit will define the level of consciousness)
S06.309 Unspecified focal traumatic brain injury with loss of consciousness of unspecified duration
Add seventh character for episode of code; S—late effect

Definition

Traumatic brain injury (TBI) is an insult to the brain from an external physical force and resulting in temporary or permanent impairment, functional disability, or psychosocial maladjustment. TBI occurs twice as frequently in males as in females. The incidence of TBI peaks among those 15 to 24 years old and again among those 75 years and older [1]. TBI usually is a consequence of motor vehicle accidents, falls, violence, and sports. Motor vehicle accidents and violence are more common in a younger population, and falls are more common in aging populations [2,3]. Recent trends have shown that TBI due to motor vehicle accidents is decreasing because of better traffic safety enforcement, whereas the percentage of TBI due to violence has increased, reported to be 7% to 10% [3]. These trends have consequences for the type of brain damage seen; contusion injury tends to be associated with falls, and diffuse injuries are more often seen in high-velocity traffic accidents [2].

In the United States, an average of 1.4 million TBIs occur each year, including 1.1 million emergency department visits, 235,000 hospitalizations, and 50,000 deaths [1,2,4,5]. The financial burden of TBI has been estimated at more than U.S. $60 billion per year [2]. However, routinely reported U.S. national data underestimate the true burden of TBI for several reasons. First, they do not include persons treated for TBI in other settings, including outpatient settings and physicians' offices. Second, patients seen in military facilities both in the United States and abroad are not recorded. Finally, the number of those who receive medical care but for whom the TBI is not diagnosed or who sustain a TBI and do not seek care is not known [4,5].

The pathophysiologic process of brain injury is usually divided into primary injury, which is the injury to the brain that results at the time of the insult, and secondary injury, which can be thought of as the summation of the biochemical or physiologic damage that develops during a period of hours, days, weeks, and perhaps months after the primary injury. The primary injury is sustained from external forces as a result of direct impact, rapid velocity changes, penetrating injuries, or blast injuries. The resulting injuries include contusion, hematomas, and diffuse axonal injuries. These are often associated with superimposed hypoxic or ischemic injury, often as a result of systemic insult. In patients with mild TBI, there is often a disruption of the sodium channels on axons, which can result in a transient disruption in function and, with it, an increased state of vulnerability to additional trauma [6]. Secondary insults include intracranial hemorrhage, swelling, hypoxia, brain shift, herniation, and numerous neurochemical and cellular events [2]. Although many of the mechanisms of secondary TBI have yet to be elucidated, it is thought that the processes include neurotransmitter release, free radical generation, calcium-mediated damage, inflammatory responses, and mitochondrial dysfunction [2,7].

Symptoms

Symptoms may vary according to the severity of the injury and the stage of recovery. The patient's history should include a detailed summary of the mechanism of injury, comorbid conditions, initial Glasgow Coma Scale score (Table 162.1), length of the coma (if any), and length of post-traumatic amnesia. Glasgow Coma Scale scores, however, can be obscured by confounders such as concurrent spinal cord injury, sedation, intubation, or other related injuries. Extracranial injuries (such as extremity fractures, thoracic or abdominal traumas), which have been reported to occur in about 35% of the cases, are associated with a higher incidence of secondary brain injuries [2,8].

Patients with severe injury and dramatically altered levels of arousal often can offer no subjective symptoms. After the acute phase of recovery, the clinician can expect symptoms to include seizures, contractures, spasticity, altered vision, vertigo or dizziness, and altered sense of smell. These may be the result of cranial nerve injuries or of central processing dysfunction. Symptoms of dysautonomia may still be seen at outpatient follow-up and may be characterized by increased body temperatures, tachycardia, tachypnea, increased posturing or tone, and profuse sweating [9]. Common late symptoms may include memory deficits, higher level executive dysfunction, headaches, difficulty with sleep-wake cycles, labile mood, depression, apathy, difficulty with attention, social disinhibition, sexual dysfunction, anxiety, impulsivity, fatigue, and difficulties with fine and gross motor control [10].

Table 162.1 The Glasgow Coma Scale

Patient Response	Score
Eye Opening	
Eyes open spontaneously	4
Eyes open when spoken to	3
Eyes open to painful stimuli	2
Eyes do not open	1
Motor	
Follows commands	6
Makes localized movements to painful stimuli	5
Makes withdrawal movements to painful stimuli	4
Demonstrates flexor posturing to painful stimuli	3
Demonstrates extensor posturing to painful stimuli	2
No motor response to pain	1
Verbal	
Oriented to place and date	5
Converses but is disoriented	4
Utters inappropriate words, though not conversing	3
Makes incomprehensible nonverbal sounds	2
Not vocalizing	1

Physical Examination

A thorough neurologic examination, including a neuropsychological evaluation, is important to assess the consequences of a brain injury. The neurologic examination evaluates mental status, cranial nerve function, vision, hearing, deep tendon reflexes, and abnormal reflexes. The examination should also evaluate muscle strength, tone, and coordination and assess gait or mobility in a wheelchair. It is important to create a thorough neuropsychological profile with the assistance of a neuropsychologist. This should be done to determine both physical abilities and the cognitive and emotional issues that will affect the patient's function. Cervical injury can be associated with TBI, especially in patients with a Glasgow Coma Scale score below 8 [11,12]. This must be recognized early to accurately assess injury severity and to determine treatment course.

Functional Limitations

Motor

Patients may have difficulty with mobility and self-care as a result of isolated motor weakness or coordination of either the upper or the lower extremities. Safe mobility may also be impeded by poor cognition, including deficits with planning and poor impulse control.

Behavior

Individuals often experience subtle or dramatic personality changes that alter relationships with others. These may include problems with the initiation of responses, verbal or physical aggression, altered emotional control, social disinhibition, depression, apathy, decreased sense of self-worth, and altered sexual function.

Social

Patients often are unable to return to work at their previous level of function. As a consequence, they may suffer significant economic strain and may have difficulty with their relationships, including their marriage. Studies have failed, however, to consistently show a significantly higher rate of divorce among those married at the time of injury [13]. Family members may be helpful in identifying issues of social isolation, depression, and anger.

Diagnostic Studies

Initial diagnostic studies can provide clues to the severity of the injury and will have prognostic implications. The IMPACT study suggests that in moderate to severe TBI, age, Glasgow Coma Scale motor scores, pupillary response, computed tomography characteristics, and the presence of subarachnoid hemorrhages are the most powerful independent prognostic factors for patient outcome. Other prognostic factors include hypotension, hypoxia, eye and verbal components of the Glasgow Coma Scale, glucose level, platelet number, and hemoglobin concentration [14].

Imaging Studies

The initial computed tomography scan has been shown to be useful as an outcome predictor with use of the Traumatic Coma Data Bank classification or the Rotterdam computed tomography score [15]. Previous studies and guidelines have recommended computed tomography scans for all TBI patients with a Glasgow Coma Scale score of 14 and of 15 in the presence of risk factors, such as emesis, advanced age, duration of amnesia, injury mechanism, neurologic deficits, or anticoagulation (Table 162.2) [2,15–17]. More sophisticated testing has been introduced, including single-photon emission computed tomography, functional magnetic resonance imaging, and positron emission tomography, but for the most part, these are of little use in assessing the functional limitations caused by the injury. In patients with otherwise normal findings on neuroimaging, diffusion tensor imaging is emerging as a potential diagnostic tool for mild brain injury as it can detect white matter microstructure changes (Fig. 162.1) [18,19]. Despite the potential of new imaging techniques, TBI remains primarily a clinical diagnosis [20,21].

At the time of outpatient follow-up, it may be necessary to remind the patient and his or her caregivers of the extreme limitations of these studies and to focus on that patient's functional abilities as the more important measure of the extent of the injury. In general, follow-up radiologic examinations are useful tools if the patient has excessively slow progress or has demonstrated a decline in function. These may be helpful in determining new or expanding lesions. Otherwise, these are generally of limited utility.

Table 162.2 Risk Factors for Intracranial Complications
Vomiting
Severe headaches
Age > 60 years
Coagulation disorder or anticoagulation
Trauma above the clavicle with clinical signs of skull fracture
Continued post-traumatic amnesia or retrograde amnesia longer than 30 minutes
Unclear mechanism of injury or intoxication with drug or alcohol

Biomarkers

The use of biomarkers to assess the magnitude of total brain injury and to localize brain injury is still in the investigatory phase. These markers may prove to be useful in patients with mild TBI with otherwise normal imaging findings as well as in patients whose injury severity cannot be accurately assessed because of confounders mentioned previously.

Biochemical markers of neuronal, glial, and axonal damage, such as neuron-specific enolase, S100B, and myelin basic protein, respectively, are readily detectable in biologic samples such as serum and cerebrospinal fluid and are being studied in patients with ischemic brain injury and TBI. These and others may soon be of use as an adjunct to neuroimaging in the early assessment of primary and evolving damage in traumatic and ischemic brain injury [22].

Functional Assessment Tools

One of the best diagnostic tools is the Glasgow Coma Scale, which is used for the initial evaluation of the severity of the patient's injury (see Table 162.1). A review of this initial score will help in the determination of the extent of the injury and thus with prognostication. Later, as a review of function in the outpatient setting, progress can be measured by the Disability Rating Scale. Post-traumatic amnesia is important for prognostication as well and can be assessed by the Galveston Orientation and Amnesia Test. For the current level of functional recovery to be characterized, the Rancho Los Amigos Scale is helpful in the assessment of the patient's awareness and interaction with the environment.

Neuropsychological Testing

This battery of tests, performed by a neuropsychologist, is the best means of determining the full spectrum of cognitive, affective, and emotional function of the individual. This may be completed before discharge from inpatient rehabilitation and should be repeated when a change in function needs to be documented. This testing may provide the clinician with critical information needed to understand the ability of the patient to progress toward more independence or responsibility at home or at work. This also may be a critical assessment tool for the documentation of the injury for insurance purposes.

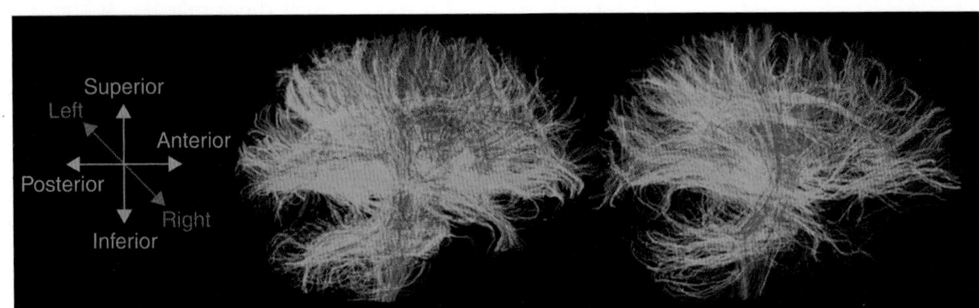

FIGURE 162.1 Diffusion tensor imaging in traumatic brain injury: loss of white matter tract fibers after traumatic brain injury (*right*) compared with an age-matched control (*left*). *(From Maas AI, Menon DK. Traumatic brain injury: rethinking ideas and approaches. Lancet Neurol 2012;11:12-13.)*

Differential Diagnosis

Anoxic brain injury
Metabolic encephalopathy
Affective disorder
Depression
Whiplash-associated disorder

Treatment

Initial

The initial focus of treating a patient with a TBI is to reduce the magnitude of the secondary injury. If the initial injury is of sufficient severity, computed tomography or magnetic resonance imaging is needed to determine the need for surgical intervention. The scans are reviewed for signs of excessive bleeding, edema, and shifting of the brain. If these signs are absent, medical intervention addresses the possible secondary injury that may result. Although it is still unclear as to how long a window of opportunity exists to affect the extent of secondary injury, it is generally accepted that this opportunity is likely to occur within the time of the initial acute hospitalization [4]. For this reason, there is little opportunity to affect this process in the outpatient setting.

Initially, metabolic issues such as blood pressure, electrolytes, hydration and nutrition, infectious processes, sleep disturbances including sleep apnea, and medications need to be addressed. Any imbalance in these may inhibit the function of the surviving brain tissue. Hydration and nutrition should be well maintained. An individual with a brain injury may be unable or unwilling to take nutrients by mouth, and this may necessitate either intravenous or direct gastrointestinal feedings. This may be a significant issue well into the post-acute phase of recovery. A survey for possible infectious processes includes, at a minimum, the pulmonary and genitourinary systems. Even infections that a clinician may otherwise label subclinical can disrupt the function of a damaged brain. For this reason, such infections should be treated as potentially symptomatic.

Medications can have undesired negative effects among those with a brain injury. These need to be reviewed carefully to eliminate any that may interfere with cognitive function. The list is long, but the most common offenders include antiseizure medications, antihypertensive medications, antispasticity medications, neuroleptics, sedatives, hypnotics, and gastrointestinal medications. Some of these may be unnecessary, whereas others may have less disruptive alternatives.

In addition to neuropsychological testing of the cognitive performance of the patient, psychological services are important in the assessment and treatment of affective disorders, which may include depression, apathy, and post-traumatic stress disorder. It is important to consider psychology services as being useful for the family and support system because the stress on these individuals may be tremendous. Psychologists and behavior specialists may be helpful for the intervention into behavior issues.

Arousal

Arousal will fluctuate throughout the day for a person with brain injury. Fatigue may become a long-standing problem. Frequent rests and naps may be needed, even at more than 1 year after injury. Pharmacologic interventions may be initiated for hypoarousal and excessive fatigue. These include amantadine, bromocriptine, carbidopa/levodopa, methylphenidate, modafinil, atomoxetine, amphetamine, nortriptyline, and protriptyline [23]. In a double-blind clinical trial, amantadine has been shown to accelerate the pace of functional recovery in patients with severe brain injury [24].

Attention

Neuropharmacologic agents for attention are similar to those used for arousal. These include neurostimulants, such as methylphenidate, modafinil, and atomoxetine, and dopaminergic agents, including amantadine, bromocriptine, and carbidopa/levodopa. Antidepressants include a long list of mixed as well as selective serotonin reuptake inhibitors; these will be especially useful if there is an element of depression interfering with cognition.

Agitation

Because agitation is a common and often troubling issue among those recovering from a TBI, a careful selection of pharmacologic agents is important to prevent injury, to allow focus on rehabilitation, and to reduce the stress on caregivers. In general, the agents that are preferred help control behavior while producing the least reduction in cognition. Because benzodiazepines are thought to have the potential of interfering with the recovery of the injured brain, these are often not recommended in the early stages of recovery. Other medications are therefore used as first-line agents. As an anxiolytic, buspirone seems preferable. A clinician may use antiseizure medications as a mood stabilizer (e.g., divalproex sodium, carbamazepine), newer antipsychotic medications (e.g., risperidone, quetiapine), beta blockers (e.g., propranolol), and antidepressants for anxious or agitated patients. Because poor attention to the environment may result in behavioral agitation, medications such as amantadine and methylphenidate should also be considered useful agents.

Memory

Because memory requires both arousal and attention, the medications previously discussed may produce improvements in the ability to learn. In addition, there have been limited reports of positive results through the use of donepezil, memantine, and other similar drugs. Memory can also be enhanced through the use of compensatory strategies and services. Speech pathologists can be useful for the introduction of and training in some of these strategies. There are portable electronic devices that can be preprogrammed with important information, and these memory aids can be frequently updated for individuals whose TBI may interfere with the ability to program the electronic memory aids.

Seizures

There is a reasonable body of literature to suggest that the use of antiseizure medications is not warranted if no seizure occurs within the first week after the brain injury. If the patient experiences a seizure after 1 week, the use of anticonvulsant agents may be needed for an extended time until the patient is seizure free for a period of 2 to 5 years; the patient is then to be reevaluated and managed per standard guidelines for patients with new-onset seizures [25,26]. Recommended agents depend on seizure type and usually include carbamazepine, valproic acid, and gabapentin.

Spasticity

Spasticity is a common problem among patients with brain injury (see Chapter 153). Patients may also have hyperactive muscle stretch reflexes and clonus. If these problems are not addressed, early contracture of joints may result. The modified Ashworth scale can be used to measure the degree of spasticity. As a first step of intervention, the clinician should look to reduce noxious stimuli, including anything that may produce pain. Infectious issues, positioning, and seating should be addressed as potential offenders. Stretching should be initiated and may necessitate serial casting and splinting. If medications are needed, these may include tizanidine, clonidine, dantrolene, diazepam, and baclofen. All of these agents have potential side effects and should be used judiciously. Dantrolene is unique in its lack of central effect but often results in acute liver dysfunction.

Rehabilitation

The rehabilitation of patients with brain injury begins during the acute stage of treatment when the risks of secondary brain injury are the greatest. After the acute phase, it is important that the clinician review the potential pharmacologic management and combine this with an interdisciplinary group of therapies, depending on the specific deficits of the patient. Studies have suggested that early admission to a dedicated inpatient brain rehabilitation unit is associated with reduced overall cost as well as improved outcome [27].

Physical Therapy

Physical therapy is important for the restoration of range of motion of the lower extremities and, if needed, through the use of serial casting. This may be aided by neurolysis or blocks at the neuromuscular junction. Later, issues of wheelchair preparation and propulsion may be important for those with sufficient impairment of mobility. Ambulation training with the appropriate assistive device should be frequently reviewed as the patient progresses with ambulation. Safety must always be considered because the patient with TBI may be endangered by impulsivity or poor planning and judgment.

Occupational Therapy

Occupational therapy addresses the preservation of joints when a lack of strength or an excess in tone or spasticity threatens a joint. As strength and ataxia are often issues in the first year, these should be addressed individually. The issues of self-care, including daily activities such as dressing, bathing, and grooming, must be addressed and emphasize the need for a planning strategy for the patient. Cooking and driving evaluations may be needed to advise the patient before his or her return to the home.

Speech Therapy

Early in the care of the patient, the ability to swallow safely needs to be evaluated. In addition, the speech pathologist, ideally working with the neuropsychologist, can identify focal cognitive needs of the patient and addresses these over a length of time. These often involve memory strategies, such as mnemonic training, and pragmatics, which focus on the contextual and social aspects of communication skills. Published cognitive rehabilitation studies have generally supported the efficacy of interventions that target memory [28–31]. These memory strategies, as a part of a comprehensive cognitive rehabilitation program, may enhance a partial restoration of focal activities in regions of the brain associated with memory, such as the hippocampus [32].

Vocational Rehabilitation

Many patients will have difficulty in returning to their previous level of employment. Vocational rehabilitation counselors can evaluate a patient's skills and determine the need for training.

Procedures

For spasticity, local injections may be preferable to oral medications. These may include nerve root blocks, nerve blocks, motor unit blocks (all with phenol), and neuromuscular junction blocks (with botulinum toxin). When spasticity is severe and not responsive to these interventions, an intrathecal pump may be considered for continuous infusion of baclofen into the cerebrospinal fluid (refer to Chapter 153).

Surgery

Patients with new-onset hydrocephalus may need a shunt placed to reduce the pressure load at the brain. If medications and other measures fail to control spasticity and contractures result, surgery may be an option. If joint contractures occur, a surgical release may be indicated.

Potential Disease Complications

Seizures can result from a TBI. The risk is highest early after the injury but persists for years. Soon after the injury, patients are at risk for aspiration pneumonia and, if their swallowing is impaired, for malnutrition and dehydration. Sleep apnea is a frequent early issue. If not treated, it may exacerbate the symptoms of the TBI. Continuous positive airway pressure may be an effective treatment. As with all trauma patients, there is a risk for deep venous thrombosis (see Chapter 127). This must be treated with prophylactic heparin or, if hemorrhage is a risk, with pneumatic compression devices or an inferior vena cava filter.

Potential Treatment Complications

Medications that are used to treat attention and arousal may lead to excess arousal and agitation. This may also be manifested as somatic complaints or delirium. Medications for agitation and seizures may slow the patient's recovery over time and may reduce the patient's function while the medications are taken. Refer to Table 162.3.

Table 162.3 Medications Frequently Used in Traumatic Brain Injury

Symptoms	Medication	Initial Dose	End Dose
Arousal	Amantadine	50 mg, 8 AM and 2 PM	100 mg, 8 AM and 2 PM
	Bromocriptine*	1.25 mg, 8 AM and 2 PM	5.0 mg, 8 AM and 2 PM
	Carbidopa/levodopa*	10 mg/100 mg tid	25 mg/100 mg tid
	Methylphenidate	2.5 mg, AM and 2 PM	20 mg, AM and 2 PM
	Modafinil	100 mg qd	100 mg, 8 AM and 2 PM
	Dextroamphetamine (Dexedrine)	5 mg qd	30 mg, AM and 2 PM
Attention	Methylphenidate	2.5 mg, AM and 2 PM	20 mg, AM and 2 PM
	Adderall	5 mg bid	20 mg bid
	Modafinil	100 mg, AM	100 mg, AM and PM
	Amantadine	100 mg, AM	150 mg, AM and 2 PM
	Bromocriptine*	1.25 mg, AM	50 mg, 8 AM and 2 PM
	Carbidopa/levodopa*	10 mg/100 mg tid	25 mg/100 mg tid
	Sertraline (Zoloft)	50 mg qd	200 mg qd
	Citalopram (Celexa)	20 mg qd	40 mg qd
	Donepezil (Aricept)	2.5 mg qd	5 mg bid
	Memantine (Namenda)	5 mg qd	10 mg qd
	Atomoxetine (Strattera)	20 mg qd	60 mg qd
Agitation	Buspirone	7.5 mg bid	30 mg bid
	Carbamazepine	200 mg bid	600 mg bid
	Risperidone	1 mg bid	6 mg/day
	Morphine	10 mg q4h	10 mg q4h
	Propranolol	10 mg qd	Limited by heart rate and blood pressure
	Quetiapine (Seroquel)	25 mg qd	800 mg qd

*Limited by hypotension.

References

[1] Langlois JA, Rutland-Brown W, Thomas KE. The incidence of traumatic brain injury among children in the United States: differences by race. J Head Trauma Rehabil 2005;20:229–38.

[2] Maas AI, Stocchetti N, Bullock R. Moderate and severe traumatic brain injury in adults. Lancet Neurol 2008;7:728–41.

[3] Redelmeier DA, Tibshirani RJ, Evans L. Traffic-law enforcement and risk of death from motor-vehicle crashes: case-crossover study. Lancet 2003;361:2177–82.

[4] Langlois JA, Rutland-Brown W, Wald MM. The epidemiology and impact of traumatic brain injury: a brief overview. J Head Trauma Rehabil 2006;21:375–8.

[5] Coronado VG, Xu L, Basavaraju SV, et al. Surveillance for traumatic brain injury–related deaths—United States, 1997–2007. MMWR Surveill Summ 2011;60:1–32.

[6] Yuen TJ, Browne KD, Iwata A, Smith DH. Sodium channelopathy induced by mild axonal trauma worsens outcome after a repeat injury. J Neurosci Res 2009;87:3620–5.

[7] Mondello S, Muller U, Jeromin A, et al. Blood-based diagnostics of traumatic brain injuries. Expert Rev Mol Diagn 2011;11:65–78.

[8] Gennarelli TA, Champion HR, Sacco WJ, et al. Mortality of patients with head injury and extracranial injury treated in trauma centers. J Trauma 1989;29:1193–201, discussion 1201–1202.

[9] Fernandez-Ortega JF, Prieto-Palomino MA, Garcia-Caballero M, et al. Paroxysmal sympathetic hyperactivity after traumatic brain injury: clinical and prognostic implications. J Neurotrauma 2012;29:1364–70.

[10] Englander J, Bushnik T, Oggins J, Katznelson L. Fatigue after traumatic brain injury: association with neuroendocrine, sleep, depression and other factors. Brain Inj 2010;24:1379–88.

[11] Holly LT, Kelly DF, Counelis GJ, et al. Cervical spine trauma associated with moderate and severe head injury: incidence, risk factors, and injury characteristics. J Neurosurg 2002;96(Suppl.):285–91.

[12] Paiva WS, Oliveira AM, Andrade AF, et al. Spinal cord injury and its association with blunt head trauma. Int J Gen Med 2011;4:613–5.

[13] Arango-Lasprilla JC, Ketchum JM, Dezfulian T, et al. Predictors of marital stability 2 years following traumatic brain injury. Brain Inj 2008;22:565–74.

[14] Murray GD, Butcher I, McHugh GS, et al. Multivariable prognostic analysis in traumatic brain injury: results from the IMPACT study. J Neurotrauma 2007;24:329–37.

[15] Smits M, Dippel DW, Steyerberg EW, et al. Predicting intracranial traumatic findings on computed tomography in patients with minor head injury: the CHIP prediction rule. Ann Intern Med 2007;146:397–405.

[16] Vos PE, Battistin L, Birbamer G, et al. EFNS guideline on mild traumatic brain injury: report of an EFNS task force. Eur J Neurol 2002;9:207–19.

[17] Ebell MH. Computed tomography after minor head injury. Am Fam Physician 2006;73:2205–7.

[18] Bigler ED, Bazarian JJ. Diffusion tensor imaging: a biomarker for mild traumatic brain injury? Neurology 2010;74:626–7.

[19] Maas AI, Menon DK. Traumatic brain injury: rethinking ideas and approaches. Lancet Neurol 2012;11:12–3.

[20] Mac Donald CL, Johnson AM, Cooper D, et al. Detection of blast-related traumatic brain injury in U.S. military personnel. N Engl J Med 2011;364:2091–100.

[21] Aoki Y, Inokuchi R, Gunshin M, et al. Diffusion tensor imaging studies of mild traumatic brain injury: a meta-analysis. J Neurol Neurosurg Psychiatry 2012;83:870–6.

[22] Kochanek PM, Berger RP, Bayir H, et al. Biomarkers of primary and evolving damage in traumatic and ischemic brain injury: diagnosis, prognosis, probing mechanisms, and therapeutic decision making. Curr Opin Crit Care 2008;14:135–41.

[23] Gordon WA, Zafonte R, Cicerone K, et al. Traumatic brain injury rehabilitation: state of the science. Am J Phys Med Rehabil 2006;85:343–82.

[24] Giacino JT, Whyte J, Bagiella E, et al. Placebo-controlled trial of amantadine for severe traumatic brain injury. N Engl J Med 2012;366:819–26.

[25] Bratton SL, Chestnut RM, Ghajar J, et al. Guidelines for the management of severe traumatic brain injury. XIII. Antiseizure prophylaxis. J Neurotrauma 2007;24(Suppl. 1):S83–6.

[26] Hixson JD. Stopping antiepileptic drugs: when and why? Curr Treat Options Neurol 2010;12:434–42.

[27] Cardenas DD, Haselkorn JK, McElligott JM, Gnatz SM. A bibliography of cost-effectiveness practices in physical medicine and rehabilitation: AAPM&R white paper. Arch Phys Med Rehabil 2001;82:711–9.

[28] Stringer AY. Ecologically-oriented neurorehabilitation of memory: robustness of outcome across diagnosis and severity. Brain Inj 2011;25:169–78.

[29] Chesnut RM, Carney N, Maynard H, et al. Summary report: evidence for the effectiveness of rehabilitation for persons with traumatic brain injury. J Head Trauma Rehabil 1999;14:176–88.

[30] Cicerone KD, Dahlberg C, Malec JF, et al. Evidence-based cognitive rehabilitation: updated review of the literature from 1998 through 2002. Arch Phys Med Rehabil 2005;86:1681–92.

[31] Cicerone KD, Dahlberg C, Kalmar K, et al. Evidence-based cognitive rehabilitation: recommendations for clinical practice. Arch Phys Med Rehabil 2000;81:1596–615.

[32] Hampstead BM, Stringer AY, Stilla RF, et al. Mnemonic strategy training partially restores hippocampal activity in patients with mild cognitive impairment. Hippocampus 2012;22:1652–8.

Index

Page numbers followed by *f* indicate figures; *t*, tables.

D

G

O

S

T